NURSE PRACTITIONER'S
DRUG HANDBOOK

FOURTH EDITION

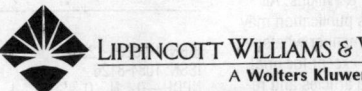

LIPPINCOTT WILLIAMS & WILKINS
A **Wolters Kluwer** Company

Philadelphia • Baltimore • New York • London
Buenos Aires • Hong Kong • Sydney • Tokyo

Staff

Publisher
Judith A. Schilling McCann, RN, MSN

Editorial Director
William J. Kelly

Clinical Director
Marguerite S. Ambrose, RN, MSN, CS

Art Director
Elaine Kasmer

Project Editor
Catherine E. Harold

Drug Information Editor
Melissa M. Devlin, PharmD

Senior Associate Editor
Elizabeth P. Lowe

Clinical Project Editor
Eileen Cassin Gallen, RN, BSN

Clinical Editors
Shari A. Regina Cammon, RN, MSN, CCRN;
Christine M. Damico, RN, MSN, CPNP;
Tracy A. Farnese, PharmD; Nancy Laplante,
RN, BSN; Kimberly A. Zalewski, RN, MSN

Copy Editors
Caryl Knutsen, Dolores Connors Matthews,
Beth Pitcher

Designers
Arlene Putterman (associate art director),
Joseph John Clark, Donald G. Knauss

Electronic Production Services
Diane Paluba (manager), Joyce Rossi Biletz
(technician)

Manufacturing
Patricia K. Dorshaw (manager), Beth Janae
Orr

Editorial Assistants
Danielle J. Barsky, Carol A. Caputo, Arlene
P. Claffee

Indexer
Barbara Hodgson

Visit our Web site at eDrugInfo.com

ISBN: 1-58255-129-4
ISSN: 1084-8126
NPDH—D N O S A J J M A M
03 02   10 9 8 7 6 5 4 3 2 1

Contents

Clinical consultants

Steven R. Abel, PharmD
Professor
Head, Department of Pharmacy Practice
Purdue University
West Lafayette, Ind.

Anita M. Bargardi, RN, MA, CS, CCRN, ACNP
Clinical Director, Advanced Practice Nursing
Cardiology Section
VA Ann Arbor Healthcare System
Ann Arbor, Mich.

Tricia M. Berry, PharmD, BCPS
Assistant Professor of Pharmacy Practice
St. Louis College of Pharmacy
St. Louis, Mo.

Susan C. Beylotte, PhD, ANP, CS
Nurse Practitioner
Ralph H. Johnson VA Medical Center
Charleston, S.C.

Lisa Morris Bonsall, RN, MSN, CRNP
Staff Nurse
University of Pennsylvania Medical Center
Philadelphia

Leanne C. Busby, DSN, RNC, FNP, FAANP
Professor & Chair, Division of Nursing
Cumberland University
Lebanon, Tenn.

James M. Camamo, PharmD
Clinical Pharmacist Supervisor
University Medical Center
Tucson, Ariz.

Lawrence Carey, PharmD
Clinical Pharmacist Supervisor
Jefferson Home Infusion Service
Philadelphia

Jennifer L. Defilippi, PharmD, BCPP
Clinical Pharmacy Specialist, Psychiatry
Central Texas Veteran's Health Care System
Waco, Tex.

Joseph Dufour, RN, MS, CS, FNP
Lecturer
State University of New York
New Paltz, N.Y.

Patricia L. Eltz, RN, MSN, CEN
Community Health Educator
Pottstown Memorial Medical Center
Pottstown, Pa.

Carmel A. Esposito, RN, MSN, EdD
Nurse Educator
Trinity Health System School of Nursing
Steubenville, Ohio

Ronald Greenberg, PharmD, BCPS
Clinical Pharmacy Coordinator
Fairview Ridges Hospital
Burnsville, Minn.

Tatyana Gurvich, PharmD
Clinical Pharmacologist
Glendale Adventist Family Practice Residency
    Program
Glendale, Calif.

Julia Anne Isen, BSN, MS, FNP-C
Assistant Clinical Professor
University of California San Francisco
Veterans Administration Medical Center
San Francisco

Michelle Kosich, PharmD
Clinical Pharmacist
Mercy Community Hospital
Havertown, Pa.

Thomas Lodise, PharmD
Infectious Diseases Pharmacotherapy and
    Outcomes Fellow
Wayne State University
Anti-Infective Research Laboratory
Detroit Receiving Hospital and University Health
    Center
Detroit, Mich.

Kristy Lucas, PharmD
Clinical Assistant Professor of Pharmacy and
    Internal Medicine
West Virginia University
Schools of Pharmacy and Medicine
Charleston, W.V.

Randall A. Lynch, PharmD
Assistant Director, Pharmacy Services
Presbyterian Medical Center
University of Pennsylvania Health System
Philadelphia

Marie Maloney, PharmD
Clinical Pharmacist
University Medical Center
Tucson, Ariz.

Erin M. McMenamin, MSN, CRNP, AOCN
Pain Medicine Nurse Practitioner
University of Pennsylvania
Philadelphia

George Melko, PharmD
Independent Consultant
West Chester, Pa.

Jolynne Myers, RNCS, MSN, MSEd, ANP
Coordinator, Hepatitis C Program
Consultants in Gastroenterology
Independence, Mo.

William O'Hara, BS, PharmD
Clinical Coordinator
Thomas Jefferson University Hospital
Philadelphia

Robert Lee Page II, PharmD, BCPS
Assistant Professor
School of Pharmacy
University of Colorado Health Sciences Center
Denver, Colo.

David Pipher, PharmD
Director of Pharmacy
Forbes Regional Hospital
Monroeville, Pa.

Christine Price, PharmD
Clinical Coordinator
Morton Plant Mease Health Care
Dunedin, Fla.

Ruthie Robinson, RN, MSN, CCRN, CEN
Nursing Instructor
Lamar University
Beaumont, Tex.

Gary Smith, PharmD, RPh
Manager, Clinical Pharmacy Services
Fairview Physician Associates
Edina, Minn.

Robert T. Smithing, MSN, FNP
President
Nurse Practitioner Support Systems
Kent, Wash.

Joseph F. Steiner, PharmD
Dean and Professor of Pharmacy Practice
College of Pharmacy, Idaho State University
Pocatello, Idaho

Leonora P. Thomas, APRN, MS
Acute Care Nurse Practitioner
Cardiology, PC
Hartford, Conn.

Barbara S. Wiggins, PharmD
Clinical Pharmacist
Cardiology Clinical Instructor
University of Washington Medical Center
Seattle, Wash.

Foreword

When I became a nurse practitioner more than 25 years ago, patients were vastly different than they are today. Today's patients ask more questions. They want more information. And they take a more active role in their care than ever before. What's more, the popularity of the Internet and direct-to-consumer advertising means that some patients come to their appointments already convinced that a certain drug is right for them—sometimes even before the health care provider has researched it.

The problem is that much of what consumers hear about drugs today either isn't accurate or isn't applicable. Direct-to-consumer ads commonly minimize important drug information. And although the Internet hosts a vast array of medical sites, consumers have no way of knowing which sites contain scientifically valid information and which contain junk science or blatant hoaxes designed simply to separate them from their money. Other public sources of information, such as books, magazines, and television shows, commonly are self-serving, or they emphasize drug information that has little to do with the average person's health.

At a time when patients are more hungry than ever for reliable teaching, it's more important than ever that you have the resources at hand to quickly zero in on accurate, pertinent drug information. That's why I recommend the *Nurse Practitioner's Drug Handbook*. It's a must-have reference for advanced practice nurses and other health care professionals who want to efficiently and effectively prescribe drugs and monitor their effects.

This updated and expanded edition of the *Nurse Practitioner's Drug Handbook* provides easy-to-understand information at your fingertips. You can quickly find the drug you need because the roughly 1,000 generic drugs are organized alphabetically. Or you can use the index, which lists both generic and trade names. Each drug entry includes indications, dosages, drug forms, contraindications, interactions, adverse reactions, treatment for overdose, nursing considerations, and patient education. To make finding the information you need even easier, drug interactions in each entry are broken down into four categories: drug-drug, drug-herb, drug-food, and drug-lifestyle. Interacting agents are italicized for quick-scan access. And dosage adjustment information is highlighted.

And there's more! In addition to the comprehensive drug entries, the *Nurse Practitioner's Drug Handbook* offers you a host of extra information hand-picked for its importance to advanced practice nurses. In the front of the book, you'll find an overview of all the major pharmacologic classes—more than 3 dozen in all. And in the back of the book, you'll find 15 practical and convenient appendices. They include an overview of each state's prescribing authority for advanced practice nurses; selected narcotic and nonnarcotic combination analgesics; a summary of topical drugs; selected local and topical anesthetics; guidelines for using selected antimicrobials and for therapeutic drug monitoring; a guide to dialyzable drugs; therapeutic management guidelines for asthma, cancer pain, dyslipidemia, hypertension, and status epilepticus; and a guide to the most popular herbal medicines.

As patients become more involved in their health care, you have an ever increasing need for handy access to dependable drug information. The *Nurse Practitioner's Drug Handbook* is an essential guide for advanced practice nurses and other health care professionals looking for the most comprehensive information available today.

Linda J. Pearson, RN, MSN, FNP
Editor-in-Chief, *The Nurse Practitioner:*
The American Journal of Primary
Health Care

How to use this book

The fourth edition of the *Nurse Practitioner's Drug Handbook* maintains the high standards that readers have come to expect from this valuable reference—exhaustively reviewed, completely updated drug information on virtually every drug in clinical use. This handy book covers the gamut of drug information, from fundamental pharmacology to specific management of toxicity and overdose. It also includes several unique features, including a review of major pharmacologic classes, a comprehensive listing of indications (including clinically approved but unlabeled uses), and more than a dozen helpful appendices specially selected for their usefulness to advanced practice nurses.

Pharmacologic classes

Listed alphabetically at the front of the book are synopses of 38 major pharmacologic classes. This section lets you compare the effects and uses of drugs within their classes. Each entry describes the pharmacology, clinical indications and actions, adverse reactions, and nursing considerations for drugs that belong to that pharmacologic group, along with tips for use in pregnant, breast-feeding, pediatric, and geriatric patients. In addition, you'll find tables throughout this section that allow you to compare drugs within and between pharmacologic classes.

Generic drugs

Individual drug entries provide detailed information on virtually all drugs in clinical use; they're arranged alphabetically by generic name for easy access. This new edition includes 56 new generic drug entries, most of which have been recently approved. Each generic entry is complete where it falls and doesn't require cross-referencing to other sections of the book.

In each drug entry, the generic name (with alternative generic names following in parentheses if needed) precedes an alphabetically arranged list of current trade names. (An asterisk signals products available only in Canada.) Several drugs available solely as combinations—such as acetaminophen and oxycodone hydrochloride (Percocet)—are listed in an appendix.

Just beneath each drug's trade names are its pharmacologic and therapeutic classifications. Considering both of these classifications helps you grasp the multiple, varying, and sometimes overlapping uses of drugs within a single pharmacologic class and among different classes. As appropriate, the next line identifies the controlled substance schedule (II, III, IV, or V) assigned to the drug by the Drug Enforcement Agency. Next, the entry lists the drug's pregnancy risk category as determined by the Food and Drug Administration (see *Pregnancy risk categories,* page viii).

Indications and dosages

The next section includes all approved and clinically accepted indications along with general dosage recommendations for adults and children. Dosage adjustments for specific patient groups, such as elderly patients and patients with renal or hepatic impairment, are included when appropriate. (Additional information may be found in the Special considerations section.) An open diamond signals a clinically accepted but unlabeled use. Dosage instructions reflect current clinical trends in therapeutics and should not be considered absolute and universal recommendations. For individual application, dosage must be considered according to the patient's condition.

How supplied

In this section, you'll find the preparations available for each drug (for example, tablets, capsules, solution, or injection), along with available dosage forms and strengths.

Pharmacodynamics

This section explains the mechanism and effects of the drug's physiologic action.

Pharmacokinetics

Here you'll find a description of the drug's absorption, distribution, metabolism, and excretion. The section also includes a table that specifies onset, peak, and duration for all routes and forms for which information is available.

Contraindications and precautions

This section lists disorders and other conditions that create special risks in patients who receive the drug.

Interactions

This section specifies the clinically significant additive, synergistic, or antagonistic effects that result from combined use of the drug with other agents. Interactions are broken down into four categories: drug-drug, drug-herb, drug-food, and drug-lifestyle. The interacting agent is italicized.

Adverse reactions

This section lists undesirable reactions that may follow use of the drug. They're arranged by body system (CNS, CV, EENT, GI, GU, Hematologic, Hepatic, Metabolic, Musculoskeletal, Respiratory, Skin, and Other). Adverse reactions not specific to a single body system (for example, the effects of hypersensitivity) are listed under Other.

Pregnancy risk categories

The Food and Drug Administration has assigned a pregnancy risk category to each systemically absorbed drug based on available clinical and preclinical information. The five categories (A, B, C, D, and X) reflect a drug's potential to cause birth defects or fetal death. Although drugs are best avoided during pregnancy, this rating system permits rapid assessment of the risk-benefit ratio if a pregnant woman needs drug therapy.

- A: Adequate studies in pregnant women have failed to show a risk to the fetus.
- B: Animal studies haven't shown a risk to the fetus, but there are no adequate clinical studies in pregnant women. Or, animal studies have a shown a risk to the fetus, but adequate clinical studies in pregnant women haven't shown a risk.
- C: Animal studies have shown an adverse effect on the fetus, but there are no adequate studies in humans. The drug may be useful in pregnant women despite its potential risks.
- D: There is evidence of risk to the human fetus, but the potential benefits of use in pregnant women may be acceptable despite the risks (such as a life-threatening situation or a serious disease for which safer drugs can't be used or are ineffective).
- X: Studies in animals or humans show fetal abnormalities, or adverse reaction reports indicate evidence of fetal risk. The risks clearly outweigh potential benefits.
- NR: Not rated.

Throughout, the most common adverse reactions (those experienced by a least 10% of people taking the drug in clinical trials) are in *italic* type; less common reactions are in roman type; life-threatening reactions are in ***bold italic*** type; and reactions that are both common and life-threatening are in BOLD SMALL CAPITAL letters.

Overdose and treatment

This section summarizes the signs and symptoms of drug overdose and recommends specific treatment as appropriate. Usually, it recommends emesis or gastric lavage, followed by activated charcoal to reduce the amount of drug absorbed and possibly a cathartic to eliminate the toxin. This section outlines antidotes, drug therapy, and other special care, if known. It also specifies the effects of hemodialysis or peritoneal dialysis for dialyzable drugs.

Special considerations

Here you'll find detailed recommendations for preparing and administering the drug, caring for the patient during drug therapy, preventing and treating adverse reactions, and storing the drug. The section also includes special tips for monitoring the effects of drug therapy and for administering the drug to pregnant, breast-feeding, pediatric, and geriatric patients. A special ☒ ALERT logo draws attention to particularly important information. Keep in mind that additional recommendations common to all members of the drug's pharmacologic class are listed in the relevant pharmacologic class entry at the front of the book.

Patient education

This section lists important teaching topics, including methods for preparing, taking, and storing the drug correctly. It also provides guidelines for patients to report adverse reactions to the prescriber.

Appendices

The appendices provide a wide range of helpful information, including an illustrated overview of prescribing authority by state for advanced practice nurses; summaries of combination analgesic products; guidelines for using selected antimicrobials; an overview of topical drugs; a review of local and topical anesthetics; a list of dialyzable drugs; guidelines for therapeutic drug monitoring; guidelines for therapeutic management of asthma, cancer pain, dyslipidemia, hypertension, and status epilepticus; and a guide to herbal medicines.

Index

The index makes the *Nurse Practitioner's Drug Handbook* even easier to use by listing generic drug names, trade names, and indications.

Guide to abbreviations

AIDS	acquired immunodeficiency syndrome
ALT	alanine transaminase
AST	aspartate transaminase
AV	atrioventricular
b.i.d.	twice daily
BPH	benign prostatic hypertrophy
BUN	blood urea nitrogen
cAMP	cyclic adenosine monophosphate
CBC	complete blood count
CK	creatine kinase
CNS	central nervous system
COPD	chronic obstructive pulmonary disease
CSF	cerebrospinal fluid
CV	cardiovascular
CVA	cerebrovascular accident
CVP	central venous pressure
D_5W	dextrose 5% in water
dl	deciliter
DNA	deoxyribonucleic acid
ECG	electrocardiogram
EEG	electroencephalogram
EENT	eyes, ears, nose, throat
g	gram
G	gauge
GGT	gamma-glutamyltransferase
GI	gastrointestinal
GU	genitourinary
G6PD	glucose-6-phosphate dehydrogenase
HIV	human immunodeficiency virus
h.s.	at bedtime
I.D.	intradermal
I.M.	intramuscular
INR	international normalized ratio
IU	international unit
I.V.	intravenous
kg	kilogram

L	liter
LD	lactate dehydrogenase
M	molar
m^2	square meter
MAO	monoamine oxidase
mcg	microgram
mEq	milliequivalent
mg	milligram
MI	myocardial infarction
ml	milliliter
mm^3	cubic millimeter
ng	nanogram
NSAID	nonsteroidal anti-inflammatory drug
OTC	over-the-counter
P.O.	by mouth
P.R.	by rectum
p.r.n.	as needed
PT	prothrombin time
PVC	premature ventricular contraction
q	every
q.i.d.	four times daily
RBC	red blood cell
RDA	recommended daily allowance
RNA	ribonucleic acid
SA	sinoatrial
S.C.	subcutaneous
SIADH	syndrome of inappropriate antidiuretic hormone
S.L.	sublingual
sp.	species
T_3	triiodothyronine
T_4	thyroxine
t.i.d.	three times daily
USP	United States Pharmacopeia
WBC	white blood cell

Pharmacologic Classes

adrenergics, direct- and indirect-acting

albuterol sulfate, arbutamine hydrochloride, bitolterol mesylate, brimonidine tartrate, dobutamine hydrochloride, dopamine hydrochloride, ephedrine, ephedrine hydrochloride, ephedrine sulfate, epinephrine, epinephrine bitartrate, epinephrine hydrochloride, epinephryl borate, isoproterenol, isoproterenol hydrochloride, isoproterenol sulfate, metaproterenol sulfate, metaraminol bitartrate, naphazoline hydrochloride, norepinephrine bitartrate, phenylephrine hydrochloride, pirbuterol acetate, pseudoephedrine hydrochloride, pseudoephedrine sulfate, ritodrine hydrochloride, salmeterol xinafoate, terbutaline sulfate, tetrahydrozoline hydrochloride, xylometazoline hydrochloride

Beta-receptor activation is associated with the activation of adenylate cyclase and the accumulation of cAMP; the cellular consequences of alpha-receptor activation are less well understood.

Alpha$_1$ receptors are located on smooth muscle and glands and are excitatory; alpha$_2$ receptors are prejunctional regulatory receptors in the CNS and postjunctional receptors in many peripheral tissues. Beta$_1$ receptors are located in cardiac tissues and are excitatory; beta$_2$ receptors are located primarily on smooth muscle and glands and are inhibitory.

Adrenergic drugs may mimic the naturally occurring catecholamines norepinephrine, epinephrine, and dopamine or may function by stimulating the release of norepinephrine.

Pharmacology

Most actions of clinically useful adrenergics involve peripheral excitatory actions on glands and vascular smooth muscle; cardiac and CNS excitatory actions; peripheral inhibitory actions on smooth muscle of the bronchial tree and blood vessels supplying skeletal muscles and gut; and metabolic and endocrine effects. Because different tissues respond in varying degrees to adrenergic agonists, differences in the actions of catecholamines are attributed to the presence of different receptor types within the tissues (alpha and beta).

Indications and actions

Most agents act on two or more receptor sites; the net effect is the sum of alpha and beta activity. Dopaminergic and serotonergic activity may occur, possibly stimulating receptors in the CNS to release histamine.

Temporary appetite suppression is another effect, often resulting in a reboundlike weight gain after tolerance to the anorexic effect develops or after withdrawal of the drug. Other uses include support of blood pressure, suppression of urinary incontinence and enuresis, and relief from pain of dysmenorrhea.

Hypotension

Alpha agonists, such as norepinephrine, metaraminol, phenylephrine, and pseudoephedrine, cause arteriolar and venous constriction, resulting in increased blood pressure. This action helps support blood pressure in hypotension and in management of serious allergic conditions. Topical formulations are used to induce local vasoconstriction (decongestion), arrest superficial hemorrhage (styptic), stimulate radial smooth muscle of the iris (mydriasis), and, with local anesthetics, localize anesthesia and prolong duration of action. Ophthalmic preparations reduce aqueous humor production and increase uveoscleral outflow.

Cardiac stimulation

Beta$_1$ agonists, such as dobutamine, act primarily in the heart, producing a positive inotropic effect. Because they increase heart rate, enhance AV conduction, and increase the strength of the heartbeat, beta$_1$ agonists may be used to restore heartbeat in cardiac arrest and for heart block in syncopal seizures, which isn't a treatment of choice, or to treat acute heart failure and cardiogenic or other types of shock. Their use in shock is somewhat controversial, because beta$_1$ agonists induce lipolysis (increase of free fatty acids in plasma), which promotes a metabolic acidosis, and because they favor arrhythmias, which pose a special threat in cardiogenic shock.

Bronchodilation

Beta$_2$ agonists, such as albuterol, bitolterol, isoetharine, metaproterenol, salmeterol, pirbuterol, and terbutaline, act primarily on smooth muscle of the bronchial tree, vasculature, intestines, and uterus. They also induce hepatic and muscle glycogenolysis, which results in hyperglycemia (sometimes useful in insulin overdose) and hyperlactic acidemia.

---

* Canada only   ◇ Unlabeled clinical use

Some are used as bronchodilators, some as vasodilators. They're also used to relax the uterus, to delay delivery in premature labor, and for dysmenorrhea. Some degree of cardiostimulation may occur, because all beta$_2$ agonists have some degree of beta$_1$ activity.

Renal vasodilation

Dopamine is currently the only commercially available sympathomimetic with significant dopaminergic activity, although some other sympathomimetics appear to act on dopamine receptors in the CNS. Dopamine receptors are prominent in the periphery (splanchnic and renal vasculature), where they mediate vasodilation, which is useful in inducing diuresis in patients with acute renal failure, heart failure, and shock.

Overview of adverse reactions

Geriatric patients, infants, and patients with thyrotoxicosis or CV disease are more sensitive to the effects of these drugs.

Alpha agonists commonly produce CV reactions. An excessive increase in blood pressure is a major adverse reaction of systemically administered alpha agonists. Exaggerated pressor response may occur in hypertensive or geriatric patients, which may evoke vagal reflex responses and result in bradycardia and AV block. Alpha agonists also interfere with lactation and may cause nausea, vomiting, sweating, piloerection, rebound congestion or miosis, difficult urination, and headache. Ophthalmic use may cause mydriasis, photophobia, burning, stinging, and blurring.

Beta agonists most frequently cause tachycardia, palpitations, and other arrhythmias. Their other effects include premature atrial and ventricular contractions; tachyarrhythmias; and myocardial necrosis. Reflex tachycardia and palpitations occur with beta$_2$ agonists because of decreased blood pressure.

Metabolic reactions to beta agonists include hyperglycemia, increased metabolic rate, hyperlactic acidosis, and local and systemic acidosis (decreased bronchodilator response).

Respiratory reactions include increased perfusion of nonfunctioning portions of lungs (COPD); mucous plugs may develop as a result of increased mucus secretion. Other reactions include tremors, vertigo, insomnia, sweating, headache, nausea, vomiting, and anxiety.

Centrally acting adrenergics have similar effects, which may also be associated with dry mouth, flushing, diarrhea, impotence, hyperthermia (excessive doses), agitation, anorexia, dizziness, dyskinesia, and changes in libido. Chronic use of adrenergics in children may cause endocrine disturbances that arrest growth; however, growth usually rebounds after withdrawal of drug.

Special considerations

Parenteral preparations

● If drug is used as a pressor agent, recommend correcting fluid volume depletion before administration. Adrenergics aren't a substitute for blood, plasma, fluid, or electrolytes.
● Carefully monitor blood pressure, pulse, and respiratory and urinary output during therapy.
● Tachyphylaxis or tolerance may develop after prolonged or excessive use.

Inhalation therapy

● The preservative sodium bisulfite is present in many adrenergic formulations. Patients with a history of allergy to sulfites should avoid drugs that contain this preservative.
● Administer drug when patient arises in morning and before meals, to reduce fatigue by improving ventilation.
● For unknown reasons, paradoxical airway resistance, evidenced by sudden increase in dyspnea, may result from repeated excessive use of isoetharine. If this occurs, tell patient to discontinue drug and use alternative therapy, such as epinephrine.
● Adrenergic inhalation may be alternated with other drug administration (steroids, other adrenergics), if necessary, but avoid giving simultaneously because of danger of excessive tachycardia.
● Don't use discolored or precipitated solutions.
● Protect solutions from light, freezing, and heat. Store at controlled room temperature.
● Systemic absorption, although infrequent, can follow applications to nasal and conjunctival membranes. Advise patient to stop drug if symptoms of systemic absorption occur.
● Prolonged or too-frequent use may cause tolerance to bronchodilating and cardiac stimulant effect. Rebound bronchospasm may follow end of drug effect.

Pregnant patients

● Pregnancy risk categories range from B to D in this group. Refer to specific package insert for manufacturer recommendations.

Breast-feeding patients

● The use of adrenergics during breast-feeding usually isn't recommended.

Pediatric patients

● Lower doses of adrenergics are recommended.

Geriatric patients

● May be more sensitive to therapeutic and adverse effects of some adrenergics and may require lower doses.

Patient education

Inhalation therapy

● Instruct patient in correct use of nebulizer and warn to use lowest effective dose.
● Explain that overuse of adrenergic bronchodilators may cause tachycardia, headache,

nausea and dizziness, loss of effectiveness, possible paradoxical reaction, and cardiac arrest.
● Tell patient to contact his health care provider if bronchodilator causes dizziness, chest pain, or lack of therapeutic response to usual dose.
● Advise patient to avoid other adrenergic medications unless they're prescribed.
● Inform patient that saliva and sputum may appear pink after inhalation treatment.
● Instruct patient to begin treatment with first symptoms of bronchospasm.
● Caution patient to keep spray away from eyes.
● Tell patient not to discard drug applicator. Refill units are available.

Nasal therapy
● Instruct patient to blow nose gently, with both nostrils open, to clear nasal passages before administration of medication.
● Instruct patient on proper method of instillation, as follows. *Drops:* Tilt head back while sitting or standing up, or lie on bed with head over side. Stay in position a few minutes to permit medication to spread through nose. *Spray:* With head upright, squeeze bottle quickly and firmly to produce 1 or 2 sprays into each nostril; wait 3 to 5 minutes, blow nose, and repeat dose. *Jelly:* Place in each nostril and sniff it well back into nose.
● Tell patient not to use nasal decongestant for longer than 3 to 5 days.

Ophthalmic therapy
● Tell patient to apply pressure to lacrimal sac during and for 1 to 2 minutes after instillation of drops to avoid excessive systemic absorption.
● Inform patient that after instillation of ophthalmic preparation, pupils of eyes will be very large and eyes may be more sensitive to light than usual. Advise patient to wear dark glasses until pupils return to normal.
● Warn patient to use drug only as directed.
● Instruct patient to contact his health care provider if no relief occurs or condition worsens.
● Tell patient to store drug away from heat and light and out of reach of children.
● Advise patient not to use drug for longer than 48 to 72 hours without consulting prescriber.

Representative combinations
Ephedrine sulfate with guaifenesin and theophylline: Bronkolixir; with guaifenesin, theophylline, and phenobarbital: Bronkotabs; with belladonna extract, boric acid, zinc oxide, beeswax, and cocoa butter: Wyanoids Relief Factor.
Epinephrine with benzalkonium chloride: Glaucon; with pilocarpine: E-Pilo.
Isoproterenol hydrochloride with phenylephrine bitartrate: Duo-Medihaler.
Naphazoline with antazoline phosphate, boric acid, phenylmercuric acetate, and carbonate anhydrous: Vasocon-A Solution; with pheniramine maleate: Naphcon-A; with phenylephrine hydrochloride, pyrilamine maleate, and phenylpropanolamine hydrochloride: 4-Way Long Lasting Spray; with polyvinyl alcohol: Albalon.

Pseudoephedrine with chlorpheniramine maleate: Chlor-Trimeton; with codeine phosphate and guaifenesin: Alamine Expectorant, Deproist Expectorant with Codeine, Guiatussin DAC, Isoclor Expectorant, Novahistine Expectorant, Robitussin-DAC; with dextromethorphan and acetaminophen: Contac Severe Cold and Flu Nighttime; with dextromethorphan, acetaminophen, and guaifenesin: Vicks 44M Cough, Cold, and Flu Relief; with dexbrompheniramine: Disophrol, Drixoral; with dexchlorpheniramine: Polaramine; with guaifenesin: Robitussin PE, Zephrex; with hydrocordone bitartrate: De-Tuss, Detussin Liquid, Entuss-D, Tussend; with triprolidine: Actagen, Actamin, Actifed, Allerfrim Tablets, Aprodine, Cenafed Plus, Triposed.
See also *antihistamines, barbiturates, and xanthine derivatives.*

---

adrenocorticoids (nasal and oral inhalation)

Nasal: beclomethasone dipropionate, budesonide, flunisolide, fluticasone propionate, triamcinolone acetonide

Oral: beclomethasone dipropionate, budesonide, flunisolide, fluticasone propionate, fluticasone propionate and salmeterol inhalation powder, triamcinolone acetonide

---

Topical administration through oral aerosol and nasal spray delivers adrenocorticoids (also known as corticosteroids) to sites of inflammation in the nasal passages or the tracheobronchial tree. Because smaller doses are administered, less drug is absorbed systemically, with fewer systemic adverse effects.

Pharmacology
Inhaled glucocorticoid (a type of adrenocorticoid) is absorbed through the nasal mucosa or through the trachea, bronchi, and alveoli. The anti-inflammatory effects of glucocorticoids depend on the direct local action of the steroid. Glucocorticoids stimulate transcription of messenger RNA in individual cell nuclei to synthesize enzymes that decrease inflammation. These enzymes stimulate biochemical pathways that decrease the inflammatory response by stabilizing leukocyte lysosomal membranes, which prevent the release of destructive acid hydrolases from leukocytes; inhibiting macrophage accumulation in inflamed areas; reducing leukocyte adhesion to the capillary endothelium; reducing capillary wall permeability and edema formation; decreasing complement components; antagonizing histamine activity and release of kinin from substrates; reducing fibroblast proliferation, collagen deposition, and scar tissue formation; and by other unknown mechanisms.

Nasal adrenocorticoids for inflammation caused by allergic rhinitis

Drug	Pediatric daily dose†	Adult daily dose†
beclomethasone dipropionate	**Nasal aerosol** *Under age 6:* not recommended *Ages 6-12:* 84 mcg b.i.d. to q.i.d. *Maximum dose:* 168-336 mcg/day **Nasal solution** *Under age 6:* not recommended *Ages 6-12:* 84 mcg t.i.d. *Maximum dose:* 252 mcg/day	**Nasal aerosol** 84 mcg b.i.d. to q.i.d. *Maximum dose:* 168-336 mcg/day **Nasal solution** 84-168 mcg b.i.d. *Maximum dose:* 336 mcg/day
budesonide	**Nasal powder** *Under age 6:* not recommended *Ages 6-12:* 200-400 mcg/day *Maximum dose:* 400 mcg/day **Nasal solution** *Under age 6:* not recommended *Ages 6-12:* 64-256 mcg/day *Maximum dose:* 256 mcg/day	**Nasal powder** 200-400 mcg/day *Maximum dose:* 800 mcg/day **Nasal solution** 64-256 mcg/day *Maximum dose:* 256 mcg/day
flunisolide	**Nasal solution** *Under age 6:* not recommended *Ages 6-14:* 50-100 mcg b.i.d. *Maximum dose:* 200 mcg/day	**Nasal solution** 50-100 mcg b.i.d. to t.i.d. *Maximum dose:* 400 mcg/day
fluticasone propionate	**Nasal solution** *Under age 4:* not recommended *Ages 4-12:* 100-200 mcg once daily *Maximum dose:* 200 mcg/day	**Nasal solution** 100-200 mcg once daily *Maximum dose:* 200 mcg daily
triamcinolone acetonide	**Nasal aerosol** *Under age 5:* not recommended *Ages 6-12:* 110-220 mcg once daily *Maximum dose:* 220 mcg/day **Nasal solution** *Under age 6:* not recommended *Ages 6-12:* 110-220 mcg/day *Maximum dose:* 220 mcg/day	**Nasal aerosol** 110-220 mcg once daily *Maximum dose:* 440 mcg/day **Nasal solution** 110-220 mcg/day *Maximum dose:* 220 mcg/day

† Total doses to both nostrils.

Indications and actions
Nasal inflammation
Nasal solutions are used to relieve symptoms of seasonal or perennial rhinitis when antihistamines and decongestants are ineffective, to treat inflammatory conditions of the nasal passages, and to prevent recurrence after surgical removal of nasal polyps. (See *Nasal adrenocorticoids for inflammation caused by allergic rhinitis.*)

Chronic bronchial asthma
Aerosols treat chronic bronchial asthma not controlled by bronchodilators and other nonsteroidal drugs. (See *Oral inhalation adrenocorticoids for chronic bronchial asthma.*)

Overview of adverse reactions
Nasal: Local sensations of nasal burning and irritation occur in about 10% of patients; sneezing attacks occur immediately after nasal application in about 10% of patients; transient mild nosebleeds occur in 10% to 15% of patients. It's unknown whether these are effects of the nasal solution or of the dryness it induces in the nasal

passages. Localized candidal infections of the nose or pharynx rarely occur.
Oral: Localized infections with *Candida albicans* or *Aspergillus niger* occur commonly in the mouth and pharynx and occasionally in the larynx.
Systemic: Systemic absorption may occur, potentially leading to hypothalamic-pituitary-adrenal (HPA) axis suppression. This is more likely to occur with large doses or with combined nasal and oral corticosteroid therapy.
Other: Hypersensitivity reactions are possible. Some patients may be intolerant of the fluorocarbon propellants in the preparations.

Special considerations
● Full therapeutic benefit requires regular use and is usually evident within a few days, although a few patients may require up to 3 weeks of therapy for maximum benefit. Discontinue therapy in the absence of significant symptomatic improvement within recommended time frame (varies with drug used).

Oral inhalation adrenocorticoids for chronic bronchial asthma

Drug	Pediatric daily dose	Adult daily dose
beclomethasone dipropionate	**Inhalation aerosol** *Under age 6:* not recommended *Ages 6-12:* 42-84 mcg t.i.d. to q.i.d. or 168 mcg b.i.d. *Maximum dose:* 420 mcg/day	**Inhalation aerosol** 84 mcg t.i.d. to q.i.d. or 168 mcg b.i.d. *Maximum dose:* 840 mcg/day
budesonide	**Inhalation powder** *Under age 6:* not recommended *Ages 6-12:* 200-400 mcg b.i.d. *Maximum dose:* 800 mcg/day	**Inhalation powder** 200-400 mcg b.i.d. *Maximum dose:* 1600 mcg/day
flunisolide	**Inhalation aerosol** *Under age 6:* not recommended *Over age 6:* 500 mcg b.i.d. *Maximum dose:* 1 mg/day	**Inhalation aerosol** 500 mcg b.i.d. *Maximum dose:* 2 mg/day
fluticasone propionate	**Inhalation aerosol** *Under age 12:* not recommended **Inhalation powder** *Under age 4:* not recommended *Ages 4-11:* 50 mcg b.i.d. *Maximum dose:* 200 mcg/day	**Inhalation aerosol** 88-440 mcg b.i.d. *Maximum dose:* 1,760 mcg/day **Inhalation powder** 100-500 mcg b.i.d. *Maximum dose:* 2 mg/day
triamcinolone acetonide	**Inhalation aerosol** *Under age 6:* not recommended *Ages 6-12:* 100-200 mcg t.i.d. or q.i.d., or 200-400 mcg b.i.d. *Maximum dose:* 1,200 mcg/day	**Inhalation aerosol** 200 mcg t.i.d. or q.i.d., or 400 mcg b.i.d. *Maximum dose:* 1,600 mcg/day

• Use of nasal or oral inhalation therapy may allow a patient to discontinue systemic adrenocorticoid therapy.

• After the desired clinical effect is obtained, reduce maintenance dosage to the smallest amount necessary to control symptoms.

• Discontinue drug if signs of systemic absorption (such as Cushing's syndrome, hyperglycemia, or glucosuria), mucosal irritation or ulceration, hypersensitivity, or infection develop. If antifungals or antibiotics are being used with adrenocorticoids and the infection doesn't respond immediately, discontinue adrenocortocoids until the infection is controlled.

Pregnant patients
• Adrenocorticoids shouldn't be used, especially in large doses or for long periods of time. They should only be used when the potential benefits outweigh the potential risks.

Breast-feeding patients
• Use cautiously. Adrenocorticoids may cause growth suppression in infants if drug is secreted in breast milk.

Pediatric patients
• Nasal or oral inhalant adrenocorticoid therapy may be successfully substituted for systemic adrenocorticoid therapy. However, the risk of HPA axis suppression and Cushing's syndrome still exists.

Geriatric patients
• Many elderly patients have conditions that could be aggravated by the excessive use of adrenocorticoid inhalant therapy. Geriatric patients have a reduced ability to metabolize and eliminate drugs; monitor patient closely for adverse effects.

Patient education
Nasal therapy
• Instruct patient to use only as directed. Inform him that full therapeutic effect isn't immediate but requires regular use of inhaler.

• Encourage patient with blocked nasal passages to use an oral decongestant 30 minutes before intranasal adrenocorticoid administration to ensure adequate penetration. Advise patient to clear nasal passages of secretions before using the inhaler.

• Instruct patient to clean inhaler according to manufacturer's instructions.

Oral therapy
• Instruct patient to use only as directed.

• Advise patient receiving bronchodilators by inhalation to use the bronchodilator before the adrenocorticoid to enhance penetration of the adrenocorticoid into the bronchial tree. He should wait several minutes to allow time for the bronchodilator to relax the smooth muscle.

• Instruct patient to hold his breath for a few seconds to enhance placement and action of the drug and to wait 1 minute before taking subsequent puffs of medication.

• Tell patient to rinse mouth with water after using the inhaler to decrease the chance of oral fungal infections. Tell him to check nasal and oral mucous membranes frequently for signs of fungal infection.

• Instruct patient to clean inhaler properly.

• Warn asthmatic patient not to increase use of adrenocorticoid inhaler during a severe asthma attack, but to call for adjustment of therapy, possibly by adding a systemic adrenocorticoid.

• Inform patient that medication is for preventative therapy, not to abort an acute attack.

Nasal or oral therapy

• Tell patient to report decreased response; dosage adjustment or discontinuation of drug may be needed.

• Instruct patient to observe for adverse effects and, if fever or local irritation develops, to discontinue use and report the effect promptly.

Representative combinations
None.

adrenocorticoids (systemic)

Glucocorticoids: betamethasone, betamethasone sodium phosphate, betamethasone sodium phosphate and betamethasone sodium acetate, cortisone acetate, dexamethasone, dexamethasone acetate, dexamethasone sodium phosphate, hydrocortisone, hydrocortisone acetate, hydrocortisone cypionate, hydrocortisone sodium phosphate, hydrocortisone sodium succinate, methylprednisolone, methylprednisolone acetate, methylprednisolone sodium succinate, prednisolone, prednisolone acetate, prednisolone sodium phosphate, prednisolone tebutate, prednisone, triamcinolone, triamcinolone acetonide, triamcinolone diacetate, triamcinolone hexacetonide

Mineralocorticoid: fludrocortisone acetate

Adrenocorticoids (also known as corticosteroids) are classified according to their activity into two groups: glucocorticoids and mineralocorticoids. Glucocorticoids regulate carbohydrate, lipid, and protein metabolism; inflammation; and the body's immune responses to diverse stimuli. Mineralocorticoids regulate electrolyte homeostasis. Many adrenocorticoids exert both kinds of activity. (See *Comparing systemic glucocorticoids.*)

Pharmacology
Adrenocorticoids dramatically affect almost all body systems. They control the rate of protein synthesis, reacting with receptor proteins in the cytoplasm of sensitive cells to form a steroid-receptor complex. Steroid receptors have been identified in many tissues. The steroid-receptor complex migrates into the nucleus of the cell, where it binds to chromatin. Information carried by the steroid of the receptor protein directs the genetic apparatus to transcribe RNA, resulting in the synthesis of specific proteins that serve as enzymes in various biochemical pathways. Because the maximum pharmacologic activity lags behind peak blood levels, the effects of adrenocorticoids may result from modification of enzyme activity rather than from direct action by the drugs.

Glucocorticoids stimulate transcription of messenger RNA in individual cell nuclei to synthesize enzymes that decrease inflammation. These enzymes stimulate biochemical pathways that decrease the inflammatory response by stabilizing leukocyte lysosomal membranes, which prevent the release of destructive acid hydrolases from leukocytes; inhibiting macrophage accumulation in inflamed areas; reducing leukocyte adhesion to the capillary endothelium; reducing capillary wall permeability and edema formation; decreasing complement components; antagonizing histamine activity and release of kinin from substrates; reducing fibroblast proliferation, collagen deposition, and scar tissue formation; and by other unknown mechanisms.

Mineralocorticoids act renally at the distal tubules to enhance the reabsorption of sodium ions, and thus water, from the tubular fluid into the plasma, and the urinary excretion of both potassium and hydrogen ions. The primary features of excess mineralocorticoid activity are positive sodium balance and expansion of the extracellular fluid volume, normal or slight increase in the level of sodium in the plasma, hypokalemia, and alkalosis. In contrast, deficiency of mineralocorticoids produces sodium loss, hyponatremia, hyperkalemia, contraction of the extracellular fluid volume, and cellular dehydration.

Indications and actions
Asthma
Treatment of status asthmaticus and acute asthma episodes. Therapy is combined with sympathomimetics and aminophylline.

Sarcoidosis
Therapy is aimed at the management of ocular, CNS, glandular, myocardial, or severe pulmonary involvement. Systemic glucocorticoids may also be used for hypercalcemia or severe skin lesions.

Advanced pulmonary or extrapulmonary tuberculosis
Systemic glucocorticoids have been used to help decrease inflammation caused by *Mycobacterium tuberculosis.*

Comparing systemic glucocorticoids

Drug	Approximate equivalent dose (mg)	Relative glucocorticoid (anti-inflammatory) potency	Relative mineralo-corticoid potency	Plasma half-life (hr)	Biological half-life (hr)
betamethasone, oral	0.6-0.75	20-30	0	> 5	36-54
betamethasone acetate	0.6-0.75	20-30	0	> 5	36-54
betamethasone sodium phosphate	0.6-0.75	20-30	0	> 5	36-54
cortisone acetate	25	0.8	2	½	8-12
dexamethasone, oral	0.5-0.75	20-30	0	2-3½	36-54
dexamethasone acetate	0.5-0.75	20-30	0	2-3½	36-54
dexamethasone sodium phosphate	0.5-0.75	20-30	0	2-3½	36-54
hydrocortisone, oral	20	1	2	1½-2	8-12
hydrocortisone acetate	20	1	2	1½-2	8-12
hydrocortisone cypionate	20	1	2	1½-2	8-12
hydrocortisone sodium phosphate	20	1	2	1½-2	8-12
hydrocortisone sodium succinate	20	1	2	1½-2	8-12
methylprednisolone, oral	4	5	0	1-3	18-36
methylprednisolone acetate	4	5	0	1-3	18-36
methylprednisolone sodium succinate	4	5	0	1-3	18-36
prednisolone, oral	5	4	1	2¼-3½	18-36
prednisolone acetate	5	4	1	2¼-3½	18-36
prednisolone sodium phosphate	5	4	1	2¼-3½	18-36
prednisolone tebutate	5	4	1	2¼-3½	18-36
prednisone	5	4	1	1	18-36
triamcinolone, oral	4	5	0	> 3⅓	18-36
triamcinolone acetonide	4	5	0	> 3⅓	18-36
triamcinolone diacetate	4	5	0	> 3⅓	18-36
triamcinolone hexacetonide	4	5	0	> 3⅓	18-36

Pericarditis
Unlabeled use for systemic glucocorticoids for the treatment of pain, fever, and inflammation of pericarditis.

Inflammation
A major pharmacologic use of glucocorticoids is treatment of inflammation. The anti-inflammatory effects depend on the direct local action of the steroids. Glucocorticoids decrease the inflam-

◇ Unlabeled clinical use

matory response by stabilizing leukocyte lysosomal membranes, which prevent the release of destructive acid hydrolases from leukocytes; inhibiting macrophage accumulation in inflamed areas; reducing leukocyte adhesion to the capillary endothelium; reducing capillary wall permeability and edema formation; decreasing complement components; antagonizing histamine activity and release of kinin from substrates; reducing fibroblast proliferation, collagen deposition, and subsequent scar tissue formation; and by other unknown mechanisms.

Immunosuppression

The full mechanisms of immunosuppressive actions are unknown. Glucocorticoids reduce activity and volume of the lymphatic system, producing lymphocytopenia, decreasing immunoglobulin and complement concentrations, decreasing passage of immune complexes through basement membranes, and possibly depressing reactivity of tissue to antigen-antibody interaction.

Adrenal insufficiency

Combined mineralocorticoid and glucocorticoid therapy is used in treating adrenal insufficiency and in salt-losing forms of congenital adrenogenital syndrome.

Rheumatic and collagen diseases and other severe diseases

Glucocorticoids are used to treat rheumatic and collagen diseases, such as arthritis, polyarteritis nodosa, and systemic lupus erythematosus; thyroiditis; severe dermatologic diseases, such as pemphigus, exfoliative dermatitis, lichen planus, and psoriasis; allergic reactions; ocular disorders, such as inflammations; respiratory diseases, such as asthma, sarcoidosis, and lipid pneumonitis; hematologic diseases, such as autoimmune hemolytic anemia and idiopathic thrombocytopenia; neoplastic diseases, such as leukemias and lymphomas; and GI diseases, such as ulcerative colitis, regional enteritis, and celiac disease. Other indications include myasthenia gravis, organ transplantation, nephrotic syndrome, and septic shock.

Antenatal use in preterm labor

Dexamethasone and betamethasone have been used as short-course I.M. therapy in women with preterm labor to hasten fetal maturation of lungs and cerebral blood vessels.

Hypercalcemia

Glucocorticoids are used to treat hypercalcemia secondary to sarcoidosis, vitamin D intoxication, multiple myeloma, and breast cancer in postmenopausal women.

Cerebral edema

High-dose parenteral glucocorticoid administration may decrease cerebral edema in brain tumors and during neurosurgery.

Acute spinal cord injury

Large I.V. doses of glucocorticoids, when given shortly after injury, may improve motor and sensory function in patients with acute spinal cord injury.

Overview of adverse reactions

Suppression of the hypothalamic-pituitary-adrenal (HPA) axis is the major effect of systemic therapy with adrenocorticoids. When administered in high doses or for prolonged therapy, glucocorticoids suppress release of corticotropin from the pituitary gland; subsequently, the adrenal cortex stops secreting endogenous corticosteroids. The degree and duration of HPA axis suppression produced by the drugs is highly variable among patients and depends on the dose, frequency and time of administration, and duration of therapy.

Patients with a suppressed HPA axis resulting from exogenous glucocorticoid administration who abruptly discontinue therapy may experience severe withdrawal symptoms, such as fever, myalgia, arthralgia, malaise, anorexia, nausea, desquamation of skin, orthostatic hypotension, dizziness, fainting, dyspnea, and hypoglycemia. Therefore, adrenocorticoid therapy should always be withdrawn gradually.

Adrenal suppression may persist for as long as 12 months in patients who have received large doses for prolonged periods. Until complete recovery occurs, patients subjected to stress may show signs and symptoms of adrenal insufficiency and may need glucocorticoid and mineralocorticoid replacement therapy.

Cushingoid symptoms, the effects of excessive glucocorticoid therapy, may develop in patients receiving large doses of glucocorticoids over several weeks or longer. These include moon face, central obesity, striae, hirsutism, acne, ecchymoses, hypertension, osteoporosis, muscle atrophy, sexual dysfunction, diabetes, cataracts, hyperlipidemia, peptic ulcer, increased susceptibility to infection, and fluid and electrolyte imbalances.

Other adverse reactions to normal or high doses of adrenocorticoids may include CNS effects (euphoria, insomnia, psychotic behavior, pseudotumor cerebri, mental changes, nervousness, restlessness); CV effects (heart failure, hypertension, edema); GI effects (peptic ulcer, irritation, increased appetite); metabolic effects (hypokalemia, sodium retention, fluid retention, weight gain, hyperglycemia, osteoporosis); musculoskeletal effects (acute tendon rupture, muscle wasting and pain, myopathy); skin effects (delayed wound healing, acne, skin eruptions, muscle atrophy, striae, Kaposi's sarcoma); and immunosuppression (increased susceptibility to infection, activation of latent infection, exacerbation of intercurrent infections).

Special considerations

• The patient may experience sudden weight gain, edema, change in blood pressure, or change in electrolyte status.

• During times of physiologic stress, such as trauma, surgery, and infection, the patient may require additional steroids and may experience signs of steroid withdrawal; patients who were previously steroid-dependent may need systemic adrenocorticoids to prevent adrenal insufficiency.

• Reduce drug gradually in long-term therapy; rapid reduction may cause withdrawal symptoms.

• Caregivers should be aware of patient's psychological history and watch for behavioral changes.

• Observe patient for infection or delayed wound healing.

Pregnant patients
• Glucocorticoids may cause fetal abnormalities; avoid use if possible.

Breast-feeding patients
• Women taking pharmacologic doses of adrenocorticoids shouldn't breast-feed.

Pediatric patients
• Long-term administration of pharmacologic doses of glucocorticoids may retard bone growth. Signs and symptoms of adrenal suppression include retardation of linear growth, delayed weight gain, low plasma cortisol levels, and lack of response to corticotropin stimulation. Alternate-day therapy is recommended to minimize growth suppression. Benefits of therapy should strongly outweigh adverse effects.

Geriatric patients
• Many elderly patients have conditions that could easily be aggravated by adrenocorticoid therapy.

• Elderly patients have a reduced ability to metabolize and eliminate drugs; monitor patient closely.

Patient education

• Explain the need to take the adrenocorticoid as prescribed. Give patient instructions on what to do if a dose is inadvertently missed.

• Warn patient not to stop drug abruptly.

• Inform patient of therapeutic and adverse effects of drug and tell him to report complications right away.

• Tell patient to carry a medical identification card noting the need for more adrenocorticoids during stress.

Representative combinations

Betamethasone sodium phosphate with betamethasone acetate: Celestone Soluspan.

Dexamethasone sodium phosphate with lidocaine hydrochloride: Decadron with Xylocaine.

adrenocorticoids (topical)

amcinonide, betamethasone benzoate, betamethasone dipropionate, betamethasone valerate, clobetasol propionate, clocortolone pivalate, desonide, dexamethasone, dexamethasone sodium phosphate, diflorasone diacetate, fluocinonide, flurandrenolide, fluticasone propionate, halcinonide, halobetasol propionate, hydrocortisone, hydrocortisone acetate, hydrocortisone butyrate, hydrocortisone valerate, methylprednisolone acetate, triamcinolone acetonide

Since topical hydrocortisone was introduced in the 1950s, numerous analogues have been developed to provide a wide range of potencies in creams, ointments, lotions, and gels.

Pharmacology

The anti-inflammatory effects of topical adrenocorticoids (also known as corticosteroids) depend on the direct local action of the steroid. Although the exact mechanism of action is unclear, many researchers believe that glucocorticoids (a type of adrenocorticoid) stimulate transcription of messenger RNA in individual cell nuclei to synthesize enzymes that decrease inflammation. These enzymes stimulate biochemical pathways that decrease the inflammatory response by stabilizing leukocyte lysosomal membranes, which prevents the release of destructive acid hydrolases from leukocytes, inhibiting macrophage accumulation in inflamed areas; reducing leukocyte adhesion to the capillary endothelium; reducing capillary wall permeability and edema formation; decreasing complement components; antagonizing histamine activity and release of kinin from substrates; and reducing fibroblast proliferation, collagen deposition, and subsequent scar tissue formation; and by other unknown mechanisms.

Topical adrenocorticoids are minimally absorbed systemically and cause fewer adverse effects than systemically administered adrenocorticoids. Fluorinated derivatives are absorbed to a greater extent than are other topical steroids. The degree of absorption depends on the site of application, the amount applied, the relative potency, the presence of an occlusive dressing (may increase penetration by 10%), the condition of the skin, and the vehicle carrying the drug. Topical adrenocorticoids are used to relieve pruritus, inflammation, and other signs of adrenocorticoid-responsive dermatoses.

Ointments are preferred for dry, scaly areas; solutions, gels, aerosols, and lotions for hairy areas. Creams can be used for most areas except those in which dampness may cause maceration. Gels and lotions can be used for moist lesions; however, gels may contain alcohol, which can dry

Potencies of topical adrenocorticoids

Topical adrenocorticoid preparations can be grouped according to relative anti-inflammatory activity. The following table arranges groups of topical adrenocorticoids in decreasing order of potency (based mainly on vasoconstrictor assay or clinical effectiveness in psoriasis). Preparations within each group are approximately equivalent.

Group	Drug	Concentration (%)
I	betamethasone dipropionate (Diprolene)	0.05
	betamethasone dipropionate (Diprolene AF)	0.05
	clobetasol propionate (Temovate)	0.05
	diflorasone diacetate (Psorcon)	0.05
II	amcinonide (Cyclocort)	0.1
	betamethasone dipropionate ointment (Diprosone)	0.05
	diflorasone diacetate (Florone, Maxiflor)	0.05
	fluocinonide (Lidex)	0.05
	fluocinonide gel	0.05
	halcinonide (Halog)	0.1
III	betamethasone benzoate gel	0.025
	betamethasone dipropionate cream (Diprosone)	0.05
	betamethasone valerate ointment (Valisone)	0.1
	diflorasone diacetate cream (Florone, Maxiflor)	0.05
	triamcinolone acetonide cream (Aristocort)	0.5
IV	flurandrenolide (Cordran)	0.05
	fluticasone propionate (Cutivate)	0.005, 0.05
	triamcinolone acetonide ointment (Aristocort, Kenalog)	0.1
V	betamethasone benzoate cream	0.025
	betamethasone dipropionate lotion (Diprosone)	0.05
	betamethasone valerate cream or lotion (Valisone)	0.1
	flurandrenolide (Cordran)	0.05
	hydrocortisone butyrate (Locoid)	0.1
	hydrocortisone valerate (Westcort)	0.2
	triamcinolone acetonide cream or lotion (Kenalog)	0.1
VI	desonide (Tridesilon)	0.05

and irritate the skin. The topical preparations are classified by potency into six groups: group I is the most potent and group VI the least potent. (See *Potencies of topical adrenocorticoids*.)

Indications and actions
Inflammatory disorders of skin and mucous membranes
Topical adrenocorticoids relieve inflammatory and pruritic skin disorders, including localized neurodermatitis, psoriasis, atopic or seborrheic dermatitis, the inflammatory phase of xerosis, anogenital pruritus, discoid lupus erythematosus, lichen planus, granuloma annulare, and lupus erythematosus.

These drugs may also relieve irritant or allergic contact dermatitis; however, relief of acute dermatosis may require systemic adrenocorticoids.

Rectal disorders responsive to this class of drugs include ulcerative colitis, cryptitis, inflamed hemorrhoids, postirradiation or factitial proctitis, and pruritus ani.

Oral lesions, such as nonherpetic oral inflammatory and ulcerative lesions and routine gingivitis, may respond to treatment with topical adrenocorticoids.

OTC formulations of topical adrenocorticoids are indicated for minor skin irritation such as itching; rash caused by eczema, dermatitis, insect bites, poison ivy, poison oak, or poison sumac; or dermatitis caused by exposure to soaps, detergents, cosmetics, and jewelry.

Overview of adverse reactions
Local effects include burning, itching, irritation, dryness, folliculitis, striae, miliaria, acne, perioral dermatitis, hypopigmentation, hypertrichosis, allergic contact dermatitis, secondary infection, and atrophy.

Systemic absorption may occur, leading to hypothalamic-pituitary-adrenal (HPA) axis suppression.

The risk of adverse reactions increases with the use of occlusive dressings or more potent steroids, in patients with liver disease, and in children (because of their greater ratio of skin surface to body weight).

Prolonged application around the eyes may lead to cataracts or glaucoma.

Special considerations
- Wash hands before and after applying the drug.
- Gently clean the area of application. Washing or soaking the area before application may increase drug penetration.
- Apply sparingly in a light film; rub in lightly. Avoid contact with eyes, unless using an ophthalmic product.
- Avoid prolonged application of drug in areas near the eyes, genitals, rectum, face, and skin folds. High-potency topical adrenocorticoids are more likely to cause striae and atrophy in these areas because of their higher rates of absorption.
- Monitor response. Observe area of inflammation.
- Don't apply occlusive dressings over topical steroids.
- Stop drug if signs of systemic absorption develop.

Pregnant patients
- Safe use of topical adrenocorticoids during pregnancy hasn't been established. It's unknown whether these drugs affect fertility.

Breast-feeding patients
- Use topical adrenocorticoids cautiously.

Pediatric patients
- Limit topical adrenocorticoid therapy to the minimum amount necessary for therapeutic efficacy. Advise parents not to use tight-fitting diapers or plastic pants on a child whose diaper area is being treated, because such garments may act as occlusive dressings. Children may be more susceptible to topical adrenocorticoid-induced HPA-axis suppression and Cushing's syndrome than adults because of a greater skin surface area-to-body weight ratio.

Geriatric patients
- Loss of collagen may lead to friable and transparent skin with increased epidermal permeability to water and certain chemicals. Topically applied drugs such as steroid creams may have a greater effect locally than in younger patients. Elderly patients also have a reduced ability to metabolize and eliminate drugs and may have higher plasma drug levels and more adverse reactions. Monitor them closely.

Patient education
- Instruct patient on use of drug.
- Advise patient to discontinue drug and report local or systemic adverse reactions, worsening condition, or persistent symptoms.
- Warn patient not to use OTC topical products other than those specifically recommended.
- Tell patient to apply a missed dose as soon as it's remembered and to continue with his regular schedule of application. However, if it's almost time for the next application, tell him to wait and continue his regular schedule. He shouldn't apply a double dose.

Representative combinations
Betamethasone dipropionate with clotrimazole: Lotrisone.

Dexamethasone with neomycin sulfate: NeoDecadron Cream; with neomycin sulfate and polymyxin B sulfate: Dexacidin Ointment.

Flurandrenolide with neomycin: Cordran.

Hydrocortisone with iodoquinol: Vytone Cream; with iodochlorhydroxyquin: Vioform-Hydrocortisone Cream, AP, Corque Cream, Hysone; with neomycin: Hydrocortisone-Neomycin; with pramoxine: Pramosone, Zone-A Forte; with neomycin and polymyxin B: Cortisporin Cream; with neomycin, bacitracin, and polymyxin B sulfate: Cortisporin Ointment; with neomycin sulfate and polymyxin B sulfate: Cortisporin; with dibucaine: Corticaine; with pyrilamine maleate and chlorpheniramine maleate: HC Derma-Pax; with benzoyl peroxide and mineral oil: Vanoxide-HC; with lidocaine and glycerin: Lida-Mantle-HC; with sulfur and salicylic acid: Therac Lotion.

Triamcinolone acetonide with nystatin: Myco II, Myco-Biotic II, Mycogen II, Mycolog-II, Myco-Triacet II, Mykacet, Mytrex, N.G.T., Nystatin-Triamcinolone Acetonide, with neomycin, gramicidin, and nystatin: Myco-Triacet II, Tri-Statin II.

alpha-adrenergic blockers

carvedilol, dihydroergotamine mesylate, doxazosin mesylate, ergotamine tartrate, phentolamine mesylate, prazosin hydrochloride, tamsulosin hydrochloride, terazosin hydrochloride

Drugs that block the effects of peripheral neurohormonal transmitters (such as norepinephrine, epinephrine, and related sympathomimetic amines) on adrenergic receptors in various effector systems are designated as adrenergic-blocking agents. Just as adrenoreceptors are classified into two subtypes—alpha and beta—so too are the blocking agents. Essentially, those agents that antagonize mydriasis, vasoconstriction, nonvascular smooth muscle excitation, and other adrenergic responses caused by alpha receptor stimulation are termed alpha blockers.

Pharmacology
Nonselective alpha blockers
Ergotamine, and phentolamine antagonize both alpha$_1$ and alpha$_2$ receptors. Generally, alpha blockade results in tachycardia, palpitations, and increased secretion of renin caused by the abnormally large amounts of norepinephrine (transmitter "overflow") released from adrenergic nerve endings as a result of the concurrent blockade of alpha$_1$ and alpha$_2$ receptors. The effects of norepinephrine are clinically counterproductive to the major uses of nonselective alpha blockers, which include treating peripheral vascular disorders such as Raynaud's disease, acrocyanosis,

frostbite, acute atrial occlusion, phlebitis, phlebothrombosis, diabetic gangrene, shock, and pheochromocytoma.

Selective alpha blockers
Alpha$_1$ blockers have readily observable effects and are currently the only alpha-adrenergic agents with known clinical uses. They decrease vascular resistance and increase venous capacitance, thereby lowering blood pressure and causing pink warm skin, nasal and scleroconjunctival congestion, ptosis, orthostatic and exercise hypotension, mild to moderate miosis, and interference with ejaculation. They also relax nonvascular smooth muscle, notably in the prostate capsule, reducing urinary symptoms in men with BPH. Because alpha$_1$ blockers don't block alpha$_2$ receptors, they don't cause transmitter overflow. In theory, alpha$_1$ blockers should be useful in the same conditions as nonselective alpha blockers; however, doxazosin, prazosin, and terazosin are approved for treating hypertension. Terazosin and doxazosin are approved in treatment of prostatic outflow obstruction secondary to BPH.

Alpha$_2$ blockers produce more subtle physiologic effects and currently have no therapeutic applications. Yohimbine is one such agent.

Indications and actions
Peripheral vascular disorders
Alpha-adrenergic blockers are indicated for treating peripheral vascular disorders, including Raynaud's disease, acrocyanosis, frostbite, acute atrial occlusion, phlebitis, and diabetic gangrene. Dihydroergotamine and ergotamine have been used to treat vascular headaches. Prazosin has been used to treat Raynaud's disease. Phentolamine is indicated to treat dermal necrosis caused by extravasation of norepinephrine, dopamine, or phenylephrine (alpha agonists).

Hypertension
Prazosin, carvedilol, doxazosin, and terazosin are used in managing essential hypertension. Phentolamine is used to control hypertension and is a useful adjunct in surgical treatment of pheochromocytoma.

BPH
Terazosin, tamsulosin, and doxazosin are used to control mild to moderate urinary obstructive symptoms in men with BPH.

Overview of adverse reactions
Nonselective alpha-adrenergic blockers typically cause orthostatic hypotension, tachycardia, palpitations, fluid retention (from excess renin secretion), nasal and ocular congestion, and aggravation of the signs and symptoms of respiratory infection. Use of these drugs is contraindicated in patients with severe cerebral and coronary atherosclerosis and in those with renal insufficiency.

Selective alpha blockers may cause severe orthostatic hypotension and syncope, especially with the first dose; the most common adverse effects of alpha blockade are dizziness, headache, and malaise.

Special considerations
● Monitor vital signs, especially blood pressure.
● Administer dose at bedtime to reduce potential of dizziness or light-headedness.
● To avoid first-dose syncope, begin with a small dose.

Pregnant patients
● Avoid use in pregnant women.

Breast-feeding patients
● Women taking these drugs shouldn't breast-feed their infants.

Pediatric patients
● Safety and efficacy of many of these medications haven't been established for use in children. Refer to specific drug monograph for more information.

Geriatric patients
● Hypotensive effects may be more pronounced.

Patient education
● Warn patient about orthostatic hypotension. Tell him to avoid suddenly moving to an upright position.
● Tell patient to promptly report dizziness or irregular heartbeat.
● Advise patient to take dose at bedtime to reduce potential for dizziness or light-headedness.
● Warn patient to avoid driving and other hazardous tasks that require mental alertness until effects of medication are established.
● Reassure patient that adverse effects, including dizziness, should lessen after several doses.
● Tell patient that alcohol use, excessive exercise, prolonged standing, and exposure to heat will intensify adverse effects.
● Advise patient of the reason for taking the medication.

Representative combinations
None.

aminoglycosides

amikacin sulfate, gentamicin sulfate, kanamycin sulfate, neomycin sulfate, paromycin, streptomycin sulfate, tobramycin sulfate

Aminoglycoside antibiotics were discovered during the search for drugs to treat serious penicillin-resistant, gram-negative infections. Streptomycin, derived from soil actinomycetes, was the first therapeutically useful aminoglycoside. Bacterial resistance to this prototype and adverse reactions soon led to the development of kanamycin, gentamicin, neomycin, netilmicin, tobramycin, and amikacin.

The basic structure of aminoglycosides is an aminocyclitol nucleus joined with one to two amino sugars by glycosidic linkage, hence the name aminoglycosides.

Aminoglycosides share certain pharmacokinetic properties, such as poor oral absorption, poor CNS penetration, and renal excretion, as well as serious adverse reactions and toxicity; their clinical use may require close monitoring of serum levels.

Pharmacology

Aminoglycosides are bactericidal. Although the exact mechanism of action isn't fully known, the drugs appear to bind directly and irreversibly to 30S ribosomal subunits, inhibiting bacterial protein synthesis. Bacterial resistance to aminoglycosides may be from decreased bacterial cell wall permeability, low affinity of the drug for ribosomal binding sites, or enzymatic degradation by microbial enzymes.

Aminoglycosides are active against many aerobic gram-negative organisms and some aerobic gram-positive organisms; they don't kill fungi, viruses, or anaerobic bacteria.

Gram-negative organisms susceptible to aminoglycosides include *Acinetobacter, Citrobacter, Enterobacter, Escherichia coli, Klebsiella*, indole-positive and indole-negative *Proteus, Providencia, Pseudomonas aeruginosa, Salmonella, Serratia*, and *Shigella*. Streptomycin is active against *Brucella, Calymmatobacterium granulomatis, Francisella tularensis, Haemophilus influenzae, Haemophilus ducreyi, Pasteurella multocida*, and *Yersinia pestis*.

Susceptible aerobic gram-positive organisms include *Staphylococcus aureus* and *S. epidermidis*. Streptomycin is active against *Nocardia, Erysipelothrix, Enterococcus faecalis*, and some mycobacteria, including *Mycobacterium tuberculosis, Mycobacterium marinum*, and certain strains of *Mycobacterium kansasii* and *Mycobacterium leprae*.

Paromycin is active against protozoa, especially *Entamoeba histolytica* and is somewhat effective against *Taenia saginata, Hymenolepsis nana, Diphyllobothrium latum*, and *Taenia solium*. Neomycin and paromycin have some activity against *Acanthamoeba*.

Aminoglycosides aren't systemically absorbed after oral administration in patients with intact GI mucosa and usually are used parenterally for systemic infections; intraventricular or intrathecal administration is necessary for CNS infections. Kanamycin and neomycin are given orally for bowel sterilization.

Aminoglycosides are distributed widely throughout the body after parenteral administration; CSF concentrations are minimal even in patients with inflamed meninges. Over time,

aminoglycosides accumulate in body tissue, especially the kidney and inner ear, causing drug saturation. The drug is released slowly from these tissues. Most aminoglycosides are minimally protein-bound and aren't metabolized. They don't penetrate abscesses well.

Aminoglycosides are excreted primarily in urine, chiefly by glomerular filtration; neomycin is chiefly excreted unchanged in feces when taken orally. Elimination half-life ranges between 2 and 4 hours and is prolonged in patients with decreased renal function. (See *Aminoglycosides: Renal function and half-life*, page 14.)

Indications and actions
Infection caused by susceptible organisms

Aminoglycosides are used as sole therapy for the following disorders:
- infections caused by susceptible aerobic gram-negative bacilli, including septicemia; postoperative, pulmonary, intra-abdominal, and serious, recurrent urinary tract infections; and infections of skin, soft tissue, bones, and joints
- infections from aerobic gram-negative bacillary meningitis (not susceptible to other antibiotics); because of poor CNS penetration, drugs are given intrathecally or intraventricularly (in ventriculitis)
- ammonia-forming bacteria in the GI tract of patients with hepatic encephalopathy (kanamycin or paromycin used orally and neomycin used orally or as a retention enema as an adjunct therapy)
- disseminated *Mycobacterium avium* complex infections. (Gentamicin encapsulated in liposomes is being evaluated for this use.)

Aminoglycosides are combined with other antibacterials in many other types of infection, including these:
- serious staphylococcal infections (with an antistaphylococcal penicillin)
- serious *P. aeruginosa* infections (with such drugs as an antipseudomonal penicillin or cephalosporin)
- enterococcal infections, including endocarditis (with such drugs as penicillin G, ampicillin, or vancomycin)
- febrile, leukopenic compromised host (as initial empiric therapy with an antipseudomonal penicillin or cephalosporin)
- serious *Klebsiella* infections (with a cephalosporin)
- nosocomial pneumonia (with a cephalosporin)
- anaerobic infections involving *Bacteroides fragilis* (with such drugs as clindamycin, metronidazole, cefoxitin, doxycycline, chloramphenicol, or ticarcillin)
- tuberculosis (use of parenteral amikacin, kanamycin or streptomycin with other antitubercular agents)
- pelvic inflammatory disease (gentamicin with clindamycin).

Aminoglycosides: Renal function and half-life

As the table shows, aminoglycosides, which are excreted by the kidneys, have significantly prolonged half-lives in patients with end-stage renal disease. Knowing this can help you assess the patient's potential for drug accumulation and toxicity. Nephrotoxicity, a major hazard of therapy with aminoglycosides, is linked to serum levels that exceed the therapeutic levels listed below. Therefore, monitoring peak and trough levels is essential for safe use of these drugs.

| | Half-life (hr) | | Therapeutic levels (mcg/ml) | |
| | Normal renal function | End-stage renal disease | | |
Drug and route			Peak	Trough
amikacin I.M., I.V.	2-3	24-60	16-32	< 10
gentamicin I.M., I.V., topical	2	24-60	4-8	< 2
kanamycin I.M., I.V., topical	2-3	24-60	15-40	< 10
neomycin oral, topical	2-3	12-24	Not applicable	Not applicable
netilmicin I.M., I.V.	2-2½	< 10	6-10	< 2
streptomycin I.M., I.V.	2½	100	20-30	Not applicable
tobramycin I.M., I.V., topical	2-2½	24-60	4-8	< 2

Overview of adverse reactions

Systemic: Ototoxicity and nephrotoxicity are the most serious complications of aminoglycoside therapy. Ototoxicity involves both vestibular and auditory functions and usually is related to persistently high serum drug levels. Damage is reversible only if detected early and if drug is discontinued promptly.

Any aminoglycoside may cause usually reversible nephrotoxicity. The damage results in tubular necrosis. Mild proteinuria and casts are early signs of declining renal function; elevated serum creatinine levels follow several days after the decline has begun. Nephrotoxicity usually begins on day 4 to 7 of therapy and appears to be dose-related.

Neuromuscular blockade results in skeletal weakness and respiratory distress similar to that seen with the use of neuromuscular-blocking agents, such as tubocurarine and succinylcholine.

Oral aminoglycoside therapy most often causes nausea, vomiting, and diarrhea. Less common adverse reactions include hypersensitivity reactions (ranging from mild rashes, fever, and eosinophilia to fatal anaphylaxis) and hematologic reactions (hemolytic anemia, transient neutropenia, leukopenia, and thrombocytopenia). Transient elevations of liver function values also occur.

Local: Parenterally administered forms of aminoglycosides may cause vein irritation, phlebitis, and sterile abscess.

Special considerations

● Don't give an aminoglycoside to a patient with history of hypersensitivity reactions to any aminoglycoside.
● Culture and sensitivity tests should be done before first dose.
● Monitor vital signs, electrolyte levels, and renal function studies before and during therapy; be sure patient is well hydrated to minimize chemical irritation of renal tubules; watch for signs of declining renal function.
● Keep peak serum levels and trough serum levels at recommended levels, especially in patients with decreased renal function. Blood is drawn for peak level 1 hour after I.M. injection (30 minutes to 1 hour after I.V. infusion); for trough level, sample is drawn just before the next dose. Time and date all blood samples. Don't use heparinized tube to collect blood samples; it interferes with results.
● Evaluate patient's hearing before and during therapy; monitor patient for complaints of tinnitus, vertigo, or hearing loss.
● Avoid use of aminoglycosides with other ototoxic or nephrotoxic drugs.

• Usual duration of therapy is 7 to 10 days; if no response occurs in 3 to 5 days, discontinue drug and repeat cultures for reevaluation of therapy.
• Patients on long-term therapy should be closely monitored—especially elderly patients, debilitated patients, and patients receiving immunosuppressant or radiation therapy—for possible bacterial or fungal superinfection; monitor especially for fever.
• Don't add or mix other drugs with I.V. infusions, particularly penicillins, which inactivate aminoglycosides; the two groups are chemically and physically incompatible. If other drugs must be given I.V., temporarily stop infusion of primary drug.
• Oral aminoglycosides may be absorbed systemically in patients with ulcerative GI lesions; significant absorption may endanger patients with decreased renal function.

Oral and parenteral administration
• Rapid I.V. administration may cause neuromuscular blockade. Infuse I.V. drug continuously or intermittently over 30 to 60 minutes for adults, 1 to 2 hours for infants; dilution volume for children is determined individually.
• Solutions should always be clear, colorless to pale yellow (in most cases, darkening indicates deterioration), and free of particles; don't give solutions containing precipitates or other foreign matter.
• Amikacin, gentamicin (without preservatives), kanamycin, and tobramycin have been administered intrathecally or intraventricularly. Some clinicians prefer intraventricular administration to ensure adequate CSF levels in the treatment of ventriculitis.

Pregnant patients
• Pregnancy risk category is D; drugs cross the placenta, creating the potential for fetal toxicity and possibly causing congenital deafness.

Breast-feeding patients
• Small amounts of drugs appear in breast milk; recommend an alternative feeding method during therapy.

Pediatric patients
• Half-life of aminoglycosides is prolonged in neonates and premature infants because of immaturity of their renal systems; dosage alterations may be necessary.

Geriatric patients
• Geriatric patients often have decreased renal function and are at greater risk for nephrotoxicity; they often require lower drug dose and longer dosing intervals. They're also susceptible to ototoxicity and superinfection.

Patient education
• Tell patient signs and symptoms of hypersensitivity and other adverse reactions to aminoglycosides.

• Teach signs and symptoms of bacterial or fungal superinfection to geriatric patients, debilitated patients, and patients with low resistance from immunosuppressants or irradiation; emphasize the need to report them promptly.

Representative combinations
Neomycin with polymyxin B sulfates and bacitracin: Neosporin, Mycitracin, Foille Plus; with polymyxin B sulfates and gramicidin: Neosporin; with polymyxin B sulfates and hydrocortisone: Cortisporin, Drotic, Octicair, Otocort; with dexamethasone sodium phosphate: Neo-Decadron; with flurandrenolide: Cordran SP.
See also *adrenocorticoids (topical)*.

androgens

danazol, fluoxymesterone, testosterone, testosterone cypionate, testosterone enanthate, testosterone propionate, testosterone transdermal system

Testosterone is the endogenous androgen, or male sex hormone. The testosterone esters (cypionate, enanthate, propionate), methyltestosterone, and fluoxymesterone are synthetic derivatives with greater potency or longer duration of action than testosterone.

Pharmacology
Testosterone promotes maturation of the male sexual organs and the development of secondary sexual characteristics (facial and body hair and vocal cord thickening). Testosterone also causes the growth spurt of adolescence and terminates growth of the long bones by closing the epiphyses (growth plates at the ends of bones). Testosterone promotes retention of calcium, nitrogen, phosphorus, sodium, and potassium and enhances anabolism (tissue building). Through negative feedback on the pituitary, exogenously administered testosterone (and other androgenic drugs) decreases endogenous testosterone production and to some degree inhibits spermatogenesis in men. Androgens repeatedly stimulate production of erythrocytes, apparently by enhancing the production of erythropoietic stimulating factor.

Indications and actions
Androgen deficiency
Androgens (testosterone, all testosterone esters, methyltestosterone, fluoxymesterone) are indicated to treat androgen deficiency resulting from testicular failure or castration, or gonadotropin or luteinizing hormone-releasing hormone deficiency of pituitary origin. Methyltestosterone and testosterone cypionate are also indicated to treat male climacteric symptoms and impotence when these are caused by androgen deficiency.

Delayed male puberty
All androgens may be used to stimulate the onset of puberty when it's significantly delayed and psychological support proves insufficient.

Breast cancer
Testosterone, all testosterone esters, and fluoxymesterone are indicated for palliative treatment of metastatic breast cancer in women during the first 5 postmenopausal years. Androgens also may be used in premenopausal women with metastatic disease if the tumor is hormone-responsive.

Postpartum breast engorgement
Fluoxymesterone, testosterone, methyltestosterone, and testosterone propionate are indicated to treat painful postpartum breast engorgement in non-breast-feeding women.

Hereditary angioedema
Danazol is indicated in the prophylaxis of angioedema attacks.

Endometriosis
Danazol is indicated for palliative treatment of endometriosis. Danazol relieves pain and helps resolve endometrial lesions in 30% to 80% of patients who receive it. Endometriosis usually recurs 8 to 12 months after danazol is discontinued.

Fibrocystic breast disease
Danazol is indicated for palliative treatment of fibrocystic breast disease that's unresponsive to simple therapy. It usually relieves pain before it reduces nodularity. Fibrocystic breast disease recurs in about half of patients who have undergone successful treatment with danazol, usually 1 year after discontinuing the drug.

Danazol has been used for palliative treatment of virginal breast hypertrophy, for gynecomastia, and excessive menstrual blood loss; for contraception in men (in combination with testosterone) and women; for treatment of alpha$_1$-antitrypsin deficiency, systemic lupus erythematosus, gynecomastia in men, and Melkersson-Rosenthal syndrome; and for management of patients with hemophilia A (factor VIII deficiency, classic hemophilia), hemophilia B (factor IX deficiency, Christmas disease), and idiopathic thrombocytopenic purpura.

Overview of adverse reactions
The most common adverse effects of androgen therapy are extensions of the hormonal action. In men, frequent and prolonged erections, bladder irritability (causing frequent urination), and gynecomastia (swelling or tenderness of breast tissue) may occur. In women, clitoral enlargement, deepening of the voice, growth of facial or body hair, unusual hair loss, and irregular or absent menses may occur. Note that virilization, including hirsutism, deepening of voice, or clitoral enlargement may be irreversible even with prompt

discontinuation of the drug. Oily skin or acne occurs commonly in both sexes.

Metabolic adverse effects include retention of fluid and electrolytes (occasionally resulting in edema), increased serum calcium levels (hypercalcemia may occur, especially in women receiving the drug for breast cancer metastatic to bone), decreased blood glucose levels, and increased serum cholesterol levels.

Long-term administration of androgens may cause loss of libido and suppression of spermatogenesis in men. Although rare, serious hepatic dysfunction, including hepatic necrosis and hepatocellular carcinoma, has been reported in prolonged androgen administration.

Special considerations
● Don't administer androgens to men with breast or prostatic cancer or with symptomatic prostatic hypertrophy; to patients with severe cardiac, renal, or hepatic disease; or to patients with undiagnosed abnormal genital bleeding.
● Hypercalcemia symptoms may be difficult to distinguish from symptoms of the condition being treated unless anticipated and thought of as a cluster. Hypercalcemia is most likely to occur in women with breast cancer, particularly when metastatic to bone.
● Priapism indicates that dose is excessive.
● Yellowing of the sclera of the eyes or of skin may indicate hepatic dysfunction resulting from administration of androgens.

Pregnant patients
● Don't administer androgens during pregnancy because they may cause masculinization of a female fetus or other fetal harm.

Breast-feeding patients
● The degree of androgen excretion in breast milk is unknown. Because androgens may induce premature sexual development in boys or virilization in girls, women receiving androgens shouldn't breast-feed.

Pediatric patients
● Observe children receiving androgens carefully for excessive virilization and precocious puberty. Androgen therapy may cause premature epiphyseal closure and short stature. Regular X-ray examinations of hand bones may be used to monitor skeletal maturation during therapy.

Geriatric patients
● Elderly men receiving androgens may be at increased risk for prostatic hypertrophy and prostatic carcinoma. Androgens can aggravate prostatic hypertrophy with obstruction and are contraindicated in these cases.

Patient education
● Warn patient against using androgens to improve athletic performance. Androgens are clas-

sified as Schedule III controlled substances and their distribution is regulated by the Drug Enforcement Agency.
● Advise patient to report GI upset.
● Tell patient that virilization, including hirsutism, deepening of voice, or clitoral enlargement, may not be reversible.
● Explain to women that medication may cause menstrual cycle irregularities in premenopausal women and withdrawal bleeding in postmenopausal women.

Representative combinations
Fluoxymesterone with ethinyl estradiol: Halodrin.

   Testosterone cypionate with estradiol cypionate: De-Comberol, depAndrogyn, Depo-Testadiol, Depotestogen, Duo-Cyp, Duratestin, Menoject-L.A., Test-Estro Cypionate.

   Testosterone enanthate with estradiol valerate: Andrest 90-4, Andro-Estro 90-4, Androgyn L.A., Duo-Gen L.A., Duogex L.A.*, Neo-Pause*, Teev, Valertest No. 1.

angiotensin-converting enzyme inhibitors

benazepril hydrochloride, captopril, enalapril maleate, fosinopril sodium, lisinopril, moexipril hydrochloride, perindopril erbumine, quinapril hydrochloride, ramipril, trandolapril

Angiotensin-converting enzyme (ACE) inhibitors are used to manage hypertension, and most are used to treat heart failure. Captopril is indicated for the prevention of diabetic nephropathy, and captopril and lisinopril are useful in improving survival rate in patients after an MI.

Pharmacology
ACE inhibitors prevent the conversion of angiotensin I to angiotensin II, a potent vasoconstrictor. Besides decreasing vasoconstriction, and thus reducing peripheral arterial resistance, inhibition of angiotensin II decreases adrenocortical secretion of aldosterone. This results in decreased sodium and water retention and extracellular fluid volume.

Indications and actions
Hypertension, heart failure
ACE inhibitors are used to treat hypertension; their antihypertensive effects are secondary to decreased peripheral resistance and decreased sodium and water retention.

   ACE inhibitors are used to manage heart failure; they decrease systemic vascular resistance (afterload) and pulmonary capillary wedge pressure (preload). They're also used after MI to decrease mortality rate and to prevent diabetic nephropathy. (See *Comparing doses of angiotensin-converting enzyme inhibitors,* page 18.)

Overview of adverse reactions
The most common adverse effects of therapeutic doses of ACE inhibitors are headache, fatigue, hypotension, tachycardia, dysgeusia, proteinuria, hyperkalemia, rash, cough, and angioedema of the face and limbs. Severe hypotension may occur at toxic drug levels. ACE inhibitors should be used cautiously in patients with impaired renal function or serious autoimmune disease, and in patients taking other drugs known to depress WBC count or immune response.

Special considerations
● Diuretic therapy should be discontinued 2 to 3 days before starting ACE inhibitor therapy to reduce risk of hypotension; if drug doesn't adequately control blood pressure, reinstate diuretics. If diuretics can't be discontinued, begin ACE inhibitor at lowest dose.
● Periodically monitor WBC counts.
● Lower doses are necessary in patients with impaired renal function.
● Use potassium supplements cautiously because ACE inhibitors may cause potassium retention.

Pregnant patients
● Discontinue ACE inhibitors if pregnancy is detected. Drug may harm or cause fetal death during the second or third trimesters.

Breast-feeding patients
● Captopril and enalapril are distributed into breast milk. An alternative feeding method is recommended during therapy.

Pediatric patients
● Safety and efficacy of ACE inhibitors in children haven't been established; use only if potential benefit outweighs risk.

Geriatric patients
● Elderly patients may need lower doses because of impaired drug clearance. These patients may be more sensitive to hypotensive effects.

Patient education
● Tell patient that the agents may cause a dry, persistent, tickling cough, which is reversible when therapy is discontinued.
● Tell patient to report feelings of lightheadedness, especially in the first few days, so dose can be adjusted; signs of infection such as sore throat and fever because drugs may decrease WBC count; facial swelling or difficulty breathing because drugs may cause angioedema; and loss of taste, which may necessitate discontinuation of drug.
● Advise patient to avoid sudden position changes to minimize orthostatic hypotension.
● Warn patient to seek medical approval before taking OTC cold preparations.

Comparing doses of angiotensin-converting enzyme inhibitors

Drug	Target adult daily dose	Dosage adjustments
benazepril	10-40 mg in single or divided doses	Creatinine clearance < 30 ml/min or patient on concurrent diuretic: initially, 5 mg per day
captopril	25-150 mg in single or divided doses	Renal impairment, hyponatremia, or hypovolemia: 6.25 to 12.5 mg b.i.d. or t.i.d.
enalapril	P.O.: 10-40 mg in single or divided doses I.V.: 1.25 mg (≥ 5 minutes) q 6 hours	Creatinine clearance ≤ 30 ml/min or patient on concurrent diuretic: initially, 2.5 mg per day
fosinopril	20-40 mg in single or divided doses	Use cautiously if patient on concurrent diuretic: initially, 10 mg per day
lisinopril	20-40 mg in a single dose	Creatinine clearance ≤ 10-30 ml/min or patient on concurrent diuretic: initially, 5 mg per day Creatinine clearance < 10 ml/min: initially, 2.5 mg per day
moexipril	7.5-30 mg in single or divided doses	Creatinine clearance < 40 ml/min: initially, 3.75 mg per day
perindopril	4-8 mg in single or divided doses	Creatinine clearance 30-60 ml/min: initially, 2 mg per day
quinapril	20-80 mg in single or divided doses	Creatinine clearance 30-60 ml/min or patient on concurrent diuretic: initially, 5 mg per day Creatinine clearance 10-30 ml/min: initially, 2.5 mg per day
ramipril	2.5-20 mg in single or divided doses	Creatinine clearance < 40 ml/min or serum creatinine > 2.5 mg/dl: initially, 1.25 mg per day
trandolapril	1-4 mg in a single dose	Creatinine clearance < 30 ml/min, concurrent diuretic therapy, or hepatic cirrhosis: initially, 0.5 mg per day

● Tell patient to call if troublesome cough develops.
● Instruct patient to promptly report pregnancy.
● Tell patient not to take potassium-containing salt substitutes without medical approval.

Representative combinations
Captopril with hydrochlorothiazide: Capozide.
Benazepril hydrochloride with amlodipine: Lotrel; with hydrochlorothiazide: Lotensin HCT.
Enalapril with felodipine: Lexxel.
Enalapril with hydrochlorothiazide: Vaseretic.
Lisinopril with hydrochlorothiazide: Prinzide, Zestoretic.
Moexipril with hydrochlorothiazide: Uniretic.
Quinapril with hydrochlorothiazide: Accuretic.
Trandolapril with verapamil: Tarka.

angiotensin II receptor antagonists

candesartan cilexetil, eprosartan mesylate, irbesartan, losartan potassium, telmisartan, valsartan

Angiotensin II receptor antagonists (AIIRAs) are a class of antihypertensive drugs that exert their therapeutic effects by selectively blocking the binding of angiotensin II to the angiotensin II type 1 (AT$_1$) receptor. They're indicated as monotherapy and in combination with other antihypertensives. In comparison to ACE inhibitors, AIIRAs are associated with fewer adverse effects, such as cough and angioedema.

Pharmacology
Angiotensin II is a potent vasoconstrictor that's formed from angiotensin I by the enzyme ACE. Angiotensin II causes vasoconstriction, increased

Comparing angiotensin II receptor antagonists

Drug	Oral bio-availability (%)	Effect of food	Prodrug	Metabolized by cytochrome P-450 isoenzymes	Protein binding (%)	Half-life (hr)
candesartan	15	No effect	Yes	Unknown	> 99	9
eprosartan	13	↓AUC ~25%	No	No	98	5-9
irbesartan	60-80	No effect	No	Yes CYP2C9	90	11-15
losartan	33	↓AUC ~10%	Yes	Yes CYP2C9 and CYP3A4	~ 99	2 (6-9 for active metabolite)
telmisartan	42-58	↓AUC 6%-20%	No	No	> 99.5	24
valsartan	25	↓AUC ~ 40%	No	Unknown	95	6

aldosterone secretion, cardiac stimulation, and reabsorption of sodium by the kidney. AIIRAs selectively block the binding of angiotensin II to the AT_1 receptor. AT_1 receptors are found in many tissues throughout the body including vascular smooth muscle and the adrenal gland. Blockade of AT_1 receptors by the AIIRAs results in vasodilation, decreased aldosterone secretion, a 2- to 3-fold increase in plasma renin activity, and an increase in angiotensin II. The increase in renin and angiotensin II is due to removal of the negative feedback of angiotensin II and isn't enough to overcome the antihypertensive effects of AIIRAs. Another type of receptor is called the AT_2 receptor. The role of the AT_2 receptor isn't known, but it doesn't appear to be involved in CV homeostasis. AIIRAs are 1,000- to 20,000-fold more selective for the AT_1 than the AT_2 receptor. (See *Comparing angiotensin II receptor antagonists.*)

Indications and actions
Hypertension
All AIIRAs are indicated for hypertension, either as monotherapy or in combination with other agents. AIIRAs act by selectively blocking the binding of angiotensin II to the AT_1 receptor, resulting in vasodilation.

Heart failure
Heart failure is associated with elevated levels of angiotensin II and aldosterone. ACE inhibitors have been shown to decrease mortality rates in patients with heart failure and to increase quality of life related to their inhibition of the renin-angiotensin-aldosterone-system (RAAS). Whether AIIRAs will have similar effects on mortality rates as ACE inhibitors in patients with heart failure is being studied. Until more information is available, reserve AIIRAs for patients unable to tolerate ACE inhibitors.

Overview of adverse reactions
AIIRAs are well tolerated, with adverse effects similar to those of placebos. Adverse effects include dizziness, insomnia, headache, fatigue, anxiety, nervousness, diarrhea, dyspepsia, heart burn, nausea, vomiting, arthralgia, back or leg pain, muscle cramps, myalgia, upper respiratory infection, cough, nasal congestion, sinusitis, pharyngitis, rhinitis, influenza, bronchitis, viral infection, edema, chest pain, rash, tachycardia, urinary tract infection, peripheral edema, and albuminuria.

Symptomatic hypotension may occur in patients who are volume- or salt-depleted (such as patients taking diuretics). AIIRAs can cause deterioration in renal function, including oliguria, acute renal failure, and progressive azotemia. Decreased hemoglobin and hematocrit; increased serum potassium levels, and occasional increases in liver function tests have occurred in patients receiving valsartan.

Special considerations
● Use AIIRAs extremely cautiously with potassium supplements or potassium-sparing diuretics.
● Use cautiously in volume-depleted patients (such as patients taking diuretics); correct volume depletion before administration and use a lower starting dose.
● Use cautiously in patients with hepatic dysfunction; losartan requires dosing adjustment.
● Use cautiously in patients whose renal function may be dependent on the RAAS; a worsening of renal function may occur (such as heart failure or renal artery stenosis).

• Telmisartan increases peak digoxin levels by 49% and troughs by 20%. Monitor digoxin levels more frequently.

Pregnant patients
• AIIRAs are pregnancy risk category C in the first trimester and category D in the second and third trimester. Drugs that act on the RAAS have been associated with fetal and neonatal injury, and death when intrauterine exposure occurred during the second and third trimester of pregnancy. Patients taking AIIRAs who become pregnant should discontinued drug unless use is considered life-saving.

Breast-feeding patients
• It isn't known whether AIIRAs appear in breast milk; because of potential risk to the nursing infant, a decision should be made regarding drug discontinuation.

Pediatric patients
• The safety and efficacy of AIIRAs haven't been established in patients under age 18.

Geriatric patients
• No dosing adjustments are required.

Patient education
• Inform women about the risks associated with exposure to AIIRAs during the second and third trimester of pregnancy; adverse effects on the fetus don't appear to occur when intrauterine exposure is limited to the first trimester.
• Tell patient to report pregnancy to prescriber as soon as possible.
• Advise patient to continue taking drugs unless prescriber instructs her to stop.
• Instruct patient to take missed doses as soon as they're remembered unless it's almost time for the next dose.
• Tell patient to call if signs of allergy or dizziness develop.

Representative combinations
Hydrochlorothiazide and losartan: Hyzaar.
    Hydrochlorothiazide and irbesartan: Avapro HCT.
    Hydrochlorothiazide and valsartan: Diovan HCT.
    Irbesartan and hydrochlorothiazide: Avalide.

anticholinergics

Belladonna alkaloids: atropine sulfate, hyoscyamine sulfate, scopolamine hydrobromide

Synthetic quaternary anticholinergics: clidinium bromide, glycopyrrolate, ipratropium bromide, mepenzolate bromide, methscopalamine bromide, propantheline bromide

Tertiary synthetic and semisynthetic (antispasmodic) derivatives: dicyclomine hydrochloride, homatropine, oxybutynin chloride, tolterodine tartrate

Antiparkinsonians: benztropine mesylate, biperiden hydrochloride, biperiden lactate, trihexyphenidyl hydrochloride

Anticholinergics are used to treat various spastic conditions, including acute dystonic reactions, muscle rigidity, parkinsonism, and extrapyramidal disorders. They're also used to reverse neuromuscular blockade, prevent nausea and vomiting resulting from motion sickness, as adjunctive treatment for peptic ulcer disease and other GI disorders, and preoperatively to decrease secretions and block cardiac reflexes. Belladonna alkaloids are naturally occurring anticholinergics that have been used for centuries. Many semisynthetic alkaloids and synthetic anticholinergic compounds are available; however, most offer few advantages over naturally occurring alkaloids. (See *Comparing systemic anticholinergics.*)

Pharmacology
Anticholinergics competitively antagonize the actions of acetylcholine and other cholinergic agonists at muscarinic and nicotinic receptors within the parasympathetic nervous system and smooth muscles that lack cholinergic innervation. Lack of specificity for site of action increases the hazard of adverse effects in association with therapeutic effects.

Antispasmodics are structurally similar to anticholinergics; however, their anticholinergic activity usually occurs only at high doses. Their mechanism of action is unknown, but they're believed to directly relax smooth muscle.

Indications and actions
Hypersecretory conditions
Many anticholinergics, such as atropine, belladonna leaf, glycopyrrolate, hyoscyamine, levorotatory alkaloids of belladonna, and mepenzolate, are used therapeutically for their antisecretory properties. These properties derive from competitive blockade of cholinergic receptor sites, causing decreased gastric acid secretion, salivation, bronchial secretions, and sweating.

GI tract disorders
Some anticholinergics, such as atropine, belladonna leaf, glycopyrrolate, hyoscyamine, levorotatory alkaloids of belladonna, mepenzolate, and propantheline, as well as the antispasmodics such as dicyclomine, are used to treat spasms and other GI tract disorders. These drugs competitively block the actions of acetylcholine at cholinergic receptor sites. Antispasmodics presumably act by a nonspecific, direct spasmolytic action on smooth muscle. These agents are useful in treat-

Comparing systemic anticholinergics

Drug	Plasma half-life (hr)	Onset of action	Duration of action
atropine, oral	2½	Inhibition of saliva occurs in 30-60 min	4-6 hr
atropine, parenteral	2½	Peak increase in heart rate occurs after 2-4 min	Brief
benztropine	Unknown	P.O.: 1-2 hr I.V., I.M.: 15 min	24 hr
clidinium	Biphasic with initial half-life of 2½ and terminal half-life of 20	1 hr	3 hr
dicyclomine	9-10	Unknown	Unknown
glycopyrrolate	½-4½ I.V. 15-30 min I.M.	1 min I.V.	2-7 hr
homatropine	Unknown	40-60 min	1-3 days
hyoscyamine, oral	3½	20-30 min	4-6 hr
hyoscyamine, parenteral	3½	2-3 min	4-6 hr
mepenzolate	Unknown	Unknown	Unknown
methoscopolamine	Unknown	1 hr	6-8 hr
oxybutynin	Unknown	30-60 min	6-10 hr
propantheline	1½	1½ hr	6 hr
scopolamine, oral	1 hr	1-2 hr	Unknown
scopolamine, parenteral	30 min	Varies	Varies
tolterodine	Unknown	1 hr	5 hr
trihexyphenidyl	Unknown	Within 1 hr	6-12 hr

ing pylorospasm, ileitis, and irritable bowel syndrome. Transderm ' scopolamine is used to prevent nausea and vomiting associated with recovery from anesthesia and surgery. Atropine may be useful in treating nausea and vomiting associated with morphine used in treatment of an MI.

Sinus bradycardia

Atropine is used to treat sinus bradycardia caused by drugs, poisons, or sinus node dysfunction. It blocks normal vagal inhibition of the SA node and causes an increase in heart rate. Atropine may be used for the treatment of sustained bradycardia and hypotension associated with nitroglycerin used in treatment of an MI.

Dystonia and parkinsonism

Biperiden, benztropine, and trihexyphenidyl hydrochloride are used to treat acute dystonic reactions and drug-induced extrapyramidal adverse effects. They act centrally by blocking cholinergic receptor sites, balancing cholinergic activity with dopamine.

Perioperative use

Atropine, glycopyrrolate, and hyoscyamine are used postoperatively with anticholinesterase agents to reverse nondepolarizing neuromuscular blockade. These agents block muscarinic effects of anticholinesterase agents by competitively blocking muscarinic receptor sites.

Atropine, glycopyrrolate, and scopolamine are used preoperatively to decrease secretions and block cardiac vagal reflexes. They diminish secretions by competitively inhibiting muscarinic receptor sites; they block cardiac vagal reflexes by preventing normal vagal inhibition of the SA node.

Bronchospasm

Atropine and ipratropium are potent bronchodilators and are used to treat antigen-, methacholine-, histamine-, or exercise-induced bronchospasm (oral inhalation and I.M. atropine); oral inhalation of atropine or ipratropium is effective in the treatment of chronic bronchitis and asthma; oral inhalation of atropine sulfate has been used for the short-term treatment and prevention of bronchospasm associated with chronic bronchial asthma, bronchitis, and chronic obstructive pulmonary disease.

Genitourinary tract disorders
Atropine, oxybutynin, tolterodine, and propantheline have been used to treat reflex neurogenic bladder.

Poisoning
Atropine is used to reverse the cholinergic effects of toxic exposure to organophosphate, carbamate anticholinesterase pesticides, and ingestion of cholinomimetic plants and fungi.

Motion sickness
Scopolamine is effective in preventing nausea and vomiting from motion sickness. Its exact mechanism of action is unknown, but it's thought to affect neural pathways originating in the labyrinth of the ear.

Overview of adverse reactions
Dry mouth, decreased sweating or anhidrosis, headache, mydriasis, blurred vision, cycloplegia, xerophthalmia, dry skin, urinary hesitancy and urine retention, constipation, palpitations, and tachycardia most commonly occur with therapeutic doses and usually disappear once the drug is discontinued. Signs of drug toxicity include CNS signs resembling psychosis (disorientation, confusion, hallucinations, delusions, anxiety, agitation, and restlessness) and such peripheral effects as dilated, nonreactive pupils; blurred vision; hot, dry, flushed skin; dry mucous membranes; dysphagia; stupor, seizures, decreased or absent bowel sounds; urine retention; hyperthermia; tachycardia; hypertension; and increased respiration.

Special considerations
● Monitor patient's vital signs, urine output, visual changes, and signs of impending toxicity.
● Constipation may be relieved by stool softeners or bulk laxatives.

Pregnant patients
● The safety of anticholinergic therapy during pregnancy hasn't been determined. Use by pregnant women is indicated only when the benefits of drug outweigh potential risks to the fetus.

Breast-feeding patients
● Some anticholinergics may be excreted in breast milk, possibly resulting in infant toxicity; breast-feeding women should avoid these drugs. Anticholinergics may decrease milk production.

Pediatric patients
● Safety and efficacy haven't been established.

Geriatric patients
● Administer cautiously. Lower doses are usually indicated. Patients over age 40 may be more sensitive to the effects of these drugs.

Patient education
● Teach patient how and when to take drug.
● Warn patient to avoid driving and other hazardous tasks if he experiences dizziness, drowsiness, or blurred vision.
● Advise patient to avoid alcoholic beverages, because they may cause additive CNS effects.
● Advise patient to consume plenty of fluids and dietary fiber to help avoid constipation.
● Tell patient to promptly report dry mouth, blurred vision, rash, eye pain, or significant changes in urine volume, or pain or difficulty on urination.
● Warn patient that drug may cause increased sensitivity or intolerance to high temperatures, resulting in dizziness.
● Instruct patient to report confusion and rapid or pounding heartbeat.
● Advise women to report pregnancy or intent to conceive.
● Warn patient to avoid OTC agents such as Benadryl or Nytol, which also have anticholinergic activity.

Representative combinations
Atropine with meperidine: Atropine/Demerol injection; with scopolamine hydrobromide (hyoscine hydrobromide), hyoscyamine sulfate, and phenobarbital: Antispasmodic Elixir, Donnatal No. 2, Phenobarbital with Belladonna Alkaloids Elixir, Bellalphen, Donnatal, Haponal, Kinesed, Spasmolin; with scopolamine hydrobromide (hyoscine hydrobromide), hyoscyamine sulfate, kaolin, pectin, sodium benzoate, alcohol, and powdered opium: Donnagel-PG; with phenazopyridine, hyoscyamine, and scopolamine: Urogesic; with hyoscyamine, methenamine, phenyl salicylate, methylene blue, and benzoic acid: Urised; with scopolamine hydrobromide, hyoscyamine hydrobromide, and phenobarbital: Barbidonna No. 2 Tablets, Barbidonna Tablets, Belladonna Alkaloids with Phenobarbital Tablets, Barophen, Donnamor, Donnapine, Donnatal Extentabs, Hyosophen Tablets, Malatal Tablets, Spasmophen, Spasquid, Susano.

Belladonna alkaloids with ergotamine tartrate, caffeine, and phenacetin: Wigraine; with phenobarbital: Chardonna-2, Butibel Elixir; with powdered opium: B&O Supprettes No. 15A, B&O Supprettes No. 16A.

Belladonna extract with butabarbital: Butibel.

Hyoscyamine sulfate with phenobarbital: Levsin with Phenobarbital Tablets, Levsin-PB, Bellacane Tablets.

antihistamines

azelastine hydrochloride, cetirizine hydrochloride, chlorpheniramine maleate, clemastine fumarate, cyclizine hydrochloride, cyclizine lactate, cyproheptadine hydrochloride, dimenhydrinate, diphenhydramine hydrochloride, fexofenadine hydrochloride, loratadine, meclizine hydrochloride, promethazine hydrochloride, tripelennamine hydrochloride

Antihistamines, synthetically produced H_1-receptor antagonists, were discovered in the late 1930s and proliferated rapidly during the next decade. They have many applications related specifically to chemical structure, their widespread use testifying to their versatility and relative safety. Some antihistamines are used primarily to treat rhinitis or pruritus, whereas others are used more often for their antiemetic and antivertigo effects; still others are used as sedative-hypnotics, local anesthetics, and antitussives.

Pharmacology

Antihistamines are structurally related chemicals that compete with histamine for H_1-receptor sites on the smooth muscle of the bronchi, GI tract, uterus, and large blood vessels, binding to the cellular receptors and preventing access and subsequent activity of histamine. They don't directly alter histamine or prevent its release. Also, antihistamines antagonize the action of histamine that causes increased capillary permeability and resultant edema and suppress flare and pruritus associated with the endogenous release of histamine.

Indications and actions
Allergy
Most antihistamines (azelastine, brompheniramine, chlorpheniramine, clemastine, cyproheptadine, diphenhydramine, promethazine, and triprolidine) are used to treat allergic symptoms, such as rhinitis and urticaria. By preventing access of histamine to H_1-receptor sites, they suppress histamine-induced allergic symptoms.

Pruritus
Cyproheptadine and hydroxyzine are used systemically. It's believed that these drugs counteract histamine-induced pruritus by a combination of peripheral effects on nerve endings and local anesthetic and sedative activity.

Tripelennamine and diphenhydramine are used topically to relieve itching associated with minor skin irritation. Structurally related to local anesthetics, these compounds prevent initiation and transmission of nerve impulses.

Vertigo, nausea, and vomiting
Cyclizine, dimenhydrinate, and meclizine are used only as antiemetic and antivertigo drugs; their antihistaminic activity hasn't been evaluated. Diphenhydramine and promethazine are used as antiallergic and antivertigo drugs and as antiemetics and antinauseants. Although the mechanisms aren't fully understood, antiemetic and antivertigo effects probably result from central antimuscarinic activity.

Sedation
Diphenhydramine and promethazine are used for their sedative action; the mechanism of antihistamine-induced CNS depression is unknown.

Suppression of cough
Diphenhydramine syrup is used as an antitussive. The cough reflex is suppressed by a direct effect on the medullary cough center.

Dyskinesia
The central antimuscarinic action of diphenhydramine reduces drug-induced dyskinesias and parkinsonism through inhibition of acetylcholine (anticholinergic effect).

Overview of adverse reactions
At therapeutic dosage levels, all antihistamines except astemizole and loratadine are likely to cause drowsiness and impaired motor function during initial therapy. Also, their anticholinergic action usually causes dry mouth and throat, blurred vision, and constipation. Antihistamines that are also phenothiazines, such as promethazine, may cause other adverse effects, including cholestatic jaundice (thought to be a hypersensitivity reaction), and may predispose patients to photosensitivity; patients taking such drugs should avoid prolonged exposure to sunlight.

Toxic doses elicit a combination of CNS depression and excitation as well as atropine-like symptoms, including sedation, reduced mental alertness, apnea, CV collapse, hallucinations, tremors, seizures, dry mouth, flushed skin, and fixed, dilated pupils. Toxic effects reverse when medication is discontinued. Used appropriately, in correct doses, antihistamines are safe for prolonged use.

Special considerations
● Don't use antihistamines during an acute asthma attack because they may not alleviate the symptoms, and antimuscarinic effects can cause thickening of secretions.
● Use antihistamines cautiously in geriatric patients and in those with increased intraocular pressure, hyperthyroidism, CV or renal disease, diabetes, hypertension, bronchial asthma, urine retention, prostatic hypertrophy, bladder neck obstruction, or stenosing peptic ulcers.
● Monitor blood counts during long-term therapy; watch for signs of blood dyscrasias.
● Give antihistamines with food to reduce GI distress; recommend sugarless gum, sour hard candy, or ice chips to relieve dry mouth; increase

fluid intake (if allowed) or humidify air to decrease adverse effect of thickened secretions.
- If tolerance develops to one antihistamine, another may be substituted.
- Some antihistamines may mask ototoxicity from high doses of aspirin and other salicylates.

Pregnant patients
- Safe use of antihistamines during pregnancy hasn't been established. Some manufacturers recommend that drugs not be used during the third trimester of pregnancy because of the risk of severe reactions, such as seizures, in neonates and premature infants.

Breast-feeding patients
- Antihistamines shouldn't be used during breast-feeding.

Pediatric patients
- Children, especially those under age 6, may experience paradoxical hyperexcitability with restlessness, insomnia, nervousness, euphoria, tremors, and seizures.

Geriatric patients
- These patients are usually more sensitive to adverse effects of antihistamines and are especially likely to experience a greater degree of dizziness, sedation, hypotension, and urine retention.

Patient education
- Advise patient to take drug with meals or snacks to prevent gastric upset and to use any of the following measures to relieve dry mouth: warm water rinses, artificial saliva, ice chips, or sugarless gum or candy. The patient should avoid overusing mouthwash, which may add to dryness (alcohol content) and destroy normal flora.
- Warn patient to avoid hazardous activities, such as driving a car or operating machinery, until extent of CNS effects are known and to seek medical approval before using alcoholic beverages, tranquilizers, sedatives, pain relievers, or sleeping medications.
- Warn patient to stop taking antihistamines 4 days before diagnostic skin tests to preserve accuracy of tests.

Representative combinations
Carbinoxamine maleate with pseudoephedrine and dextromethorphan: Carbodec DM, Pseudo-Car DM, Rondec-DM, Tussafed; with pseudoephedrine hydrochloride: Rondec, Rondec-TR; with pseudoephedrine and guaifenesin: Brexin L.A.

Chlorpheniramine with phenylephrine and phenylpropanolamine: Naldecon; with dextromethorphan: Vicks Formula 44 Cough Mixture; with codeine and guaifenesin: Tussar SF; with acetaminophen: Coricidin Tablets; with pseudoephedrine and dextromethorphan: Rhinosyn-DM; with pseudoephedrine, dextromethorphan, and acetaminophen: Co-Apap; with phenylpropanolamine: Contac 12-hour, Dura-Vent, Or-

nade, Resaid S.R., Triaminic-12; with pseudoephedrine hydrochloride: Chlordrine S.R., Chlorphendrine SR, Chlorpheniramine Maleate/Pseudoephedrine HCl, Colfed-A, Cophene No. 2, Duralex, Klerist-D, Kronofed-A, ND Clear, Pseudo-Clor, Rescon Capsules, Rescon-ED, Time-Hist.

Diphenhydramine with pseudoephedrine: Benadryl Decongestant, Benylin DM; with acetaminophen: Tylenol Severe Allergy.

Promethazine with codeine: Phenergan with codeine; with dextromethorphan: Phenergan with Dextromethorphan; with phenylephrine: Phenergan VC; with phenylephrine and codeine: Phenergan VC with codeine.

Pyrilamine maleate with codeine: Tricodene Cough and Cold; with phenylephrine and codeine: Codimal; with phenylephrine and dextromethorphan: Codimal DM; with phenylephrine, dextromethorphan, and acetaminophen: Robitussin Night Relief; with phenylephrine and hydrocodone: Codimal; with phenylpropanolamine, chlorpheniramine maleate, and dextromethorphan: Tricodene Forte, Tricodene NN, Triminol Cough.

barbiturates

amobarbital, amobarbital sodium, aprobarbital, mephobarbital, metharbital, pentobarbital sodium, phenobarbital, phenobarbital sodium, primidone, secobarbital sodium

Barbituric acid was compounded in 1864. The first hypnotic barbiturate, barbital, was introduced into medicine in 1903. Although barbiturates have been used extensively as sedative-hypnotics and antianxiety agents, benzodiazepines are the current drugs of choice for sedative-hypnotic effects. Phenobarbital, mephobarbital, and metharbital remain effective for anticonvulsant therapy. A few short-acting barbiturates are used as general anesthetics.

Pharmacology
Barbiturates are structurally related compounds that act throughout the CNS, particularly in the mesencephalic reticular activating system, which controls the CNS arousal mechanism. Barbiturates induce an imbalance in central inhibitory and facilitatory mechanisms, which, in turn, influence the cerebral cortex and the reticular formation. Barbiturates decrease both presynaptic and postsynaptic membrane excitability.

The exact mechanisms of action of barbiturates at these sites aren't known, nor is it clear which cellular and synaptic actions result in sedative-hypnotic effects. Barbiturates can produce all levels of CNS depression, from mild sedation to coma to death. Barbiturates exert their effects by facilitating the actions of gamma-aminobutyric acid (GABA). Barbiturates also exert a central effect, which depresses respiration and GI motility. Barbiturates have no analgesic action and may increase the reaction to painful stimuli at subanesthetic doses. The principal anticonvulsant mechanism of action is reduction of nerve transmission and decreased excitability of the nerve cell. Barbiturates also raise the seizure threshold.

Indications and actions
Seizure disorders
Phenobarbital is used in the prophylactic treatment and acute management of seizure disorders. It's used mainly in tonic-clonic (grand mal) and partial seizures. At anesthetic doses, all barbiturates have anticonvulsant activity. Phenobarbital is an effective parenteral agent for status epilepticus (with airway support). Mephobarbital and metharbital may also be used.

Barbiturates suppress the spread of seizure activity produced by epileptogenic foci in the cortex, thalamus, and limbic systems by enhancing the effects of GABA.

Sedation, hypnosis
Most currently available barbiturates are used as sedative-hypnotics for short-term (up to 2 weeks) treatment of insomnia because of their nonspecific CNS effects.

Barbiturates aren't used routinely as sedatives. Barbiturate-induced sleep differs from physiologic sleep in that rapid-eye-movement sleep cycles are reduced.

Preanesthesia sedation
Barbiturates are also used as preanesthetic sedatives and for relief of anxiety.

Psychiatric use
Barbiturates (especially amobarbital) have been used parenterally in narcoanalysis and narcotherapy and in identifying schizophrenia.

Overview of adverse reactions
Drowsiness, lethargy, vertigo, headache, and CNS depression are common with barbiturates. After hypnotic doses, a hangover effect, subtle distortion of mood, and impairment of judgment or motor skills may continue for many hours. After a decrease in dose or discontinuation of barbiturates used for hypnosis, rebound insomnia or increased dreaming or nightmares may occur. Barbiturates cause hyperalgesia in subhypnotic doses. Hypersensitivity reactions (rash, fever, serum sickness) aren't common and are more likely to occur in patients with a history of asthma or allergies to other drugs; reactions include urticaria, rash, angioedema, and Stevens-Johnson syndrome. Barbiturates can cause paradoxical excitement at low doses, confusion in geriatric patients, and hyperactivity in children. High fever, severe headache, stomatitis, conjunctivitis, or rhinitis may precede skin eruptions. Because of the potential for fatal consequences, discontinue barbiturates if dermatologic reactions occur.

Withdrawal symptoms may occur after as little as 2 weeks of uninterrupted therapy. Symptoms of abstinence usually occur within 8 to 12 hours after the last dose, but may be delayed up to 5 days. They include weakness, anxiety, nausea, vomiting, insomnia, hallucinations, and possibly seizures.

Special considerations
- Doses of barbiturates must be individualized.
- Don't use barbiturates in patients with porphyria, liver impairment, severe respiratory disease, or previous addiction to barbiturates or in nephritic patients.
- Use barbiturates cautiously, if at all, in patients who are mentally depressed or have suicidal tendencies or history of drug abuse.
- Avoid administering barbiturates to patients with status asthmaticus.
- Parenteral solutions are highly alkaline and contain organic solvents (propylene glycol); infuse at 100 mg/min or less; avoid extravasation, which may cause local tissue damage and tissue necrosis; inject I.V. or deep I.M. only. Don't exceed 5 ml per I.M. injection site to avoid tissue damage.
- Rapid I.V. administration of barbiturates may cause respiratory depression, apnea, laryngospasm, or hypotension. Have resuscitative measures available. I.V. site should be assessed for signs of infiltration or phlebitis.
- Drug may be given P.R. if oral or parenteral route is inappropriate; it shouldn't be given intraarterially or S.C.
- Assess level of consciousness before and frequently during therapy to evaluate effectiveness of drug. Monitor neurologic status for possible alteration or deterioration, and monitor seizure character, frequency, and duration for changes.
- Vital signs must be checked frequently, especially during I.V. administration.
- Assess patient's sleeping patterns before and during therapy to ensure effectiveness of drug.
- Institute safety measures—side rails, assistance when out of bed, call light within reach—to prevent falls and injury.
- Consider airway support during I.V. administration.
- Anticipate possible rebound confusion and excitatory reactions in patient.
- Monitor patient for complaints of constipation. Advise diet high in fiber, if indicated.
- Carefully monitor PT and INR in patients taking anticoagulants; dose of anticoagulant may require adjustment to counteract possible interaction.
- Abrupt discontinuation may cause withdrawal symptoms; discontinue slowly.
- Death is common with an overdose of 2 to 10 g; it may occur at much smaller doses if alcohol is also ingested.

Pregnant patients
- Barbiturates may cause fetal harm. Postpartum hemorrhage and hemorrhagic disease of the newborn has occurred. The latter can be reversed

with vitamin K therapy. If a woman is taking these medications in the last trimester of pregnancy, neonates may exhibit withdrawal symptoms.

Breast-feeding patients
● Barbiturates appear in breast milk and may cause infant CNS depression. Use cautiously.

Pediatric patients
● Premature infants are more susceptible to the depressant effects of barbiturates because of immature hepatic metabolism. Children receiving barbiturates may experience hyperactivity, excitement, or hyperalgia.

Geriatric patients
● Elderly patients and patients receiving subhypnotic doses may experience hyperactivity, excitement, confusion, depression, or hyperalgesia. Use cautiously.

Patient education
● Warn patient to avoid use of other drugs with CNS depressant effects, such as antihistamines, analgesics, and alcohol, because they have additive effects and result in increased drowsiness. Instruct patient to seek medical approval before taking OTC cold or allergy preparations.
● Caution patient not to change dose or frequency without medical approval; abrupt discontinuation of medication may trigger rebound insomnia, with increased dreaming, nightmares, or seizures.
● Warn patient against driving and other hazardous tasks that require alertness while taking barbiturates. Instruct him in safety measures to prevent injury.
● Be sure pregnant women understand that barbiturates are capable of causing physical or psychological dependence (addiction), and that these effects may be transmitted to a fetus; withdrawal symptoms can occur in neonates whose mothers took barbiturates in the third trimester.
● Instruct patient to report skin eruption or other marked adverse effect.
● Explain that a morning hangover is common after therapeutic use of barbiturates.

Representative combinations
Amobarbital with secobarbital: Tuinal 100 mg Pulvules, Tuinal 200 mg Pulvules.

Phenobarbital with CNS stimulants: Bronkolixir, Bronkotabs, Quadrinal; with ergotamine tartrate: Bellergal-S; with phenytoin: Dilantin Kapseals; with aminophylline and ephedrine hydrochloride: Mudrane; with belladonna: Butibel, Butibel Elixir, Chardonna-2; with atropine: Antrocol; with hyoscyamine: Bellacane, Levsin-PB, Levsin and Phenobarbital,; with ASA and codeine phosphate: Phenaphen with Codeine No. 3, Phenaphen with Codeine No. 4; with atropine, hyoscyamine, and scopolamine hydrobromide: Barbidonna, Barbidonna No. 2, Barophen, Belladonna Alkaloids with Phenobarbital Tablets, Donnamor, Donnapine, Donnatal, Donnatal No. 2, Donnatal Extentabs, Hyoscyamine Compound, Hyosophen, Kinesed, Malatal, Phenobarbital with Belladonna Alkaloids Elixir, Spasmophen, Spasquid, Susano.

Pentobarbital sodium with ephedrine: Ephedrine and Nembutal Sodium; with ergotamine tartrate and caffeine: Cafergot-PB.

See also *anticholinergics (belladonna alkaloids)*.

---

benzodiazepines

alprazolam, chlordiazepoxide hydrochloride, clonazepam, clorazepate dipotassium, diazepam, estazolam, flurazepam hydrochloride, lorazepam, midazolam hydrochloride, oxazepam, quazepam, temazepam, triazolam

---

Benzodiazepines, synthetically produced sedative-hypnotics, gained popularity in the early 1960s, replacing barbiturates as the treatment of choice for anxiety, convulsive disorders, and sedation. These drugs are preferred over barbiturates because therapeutic doses produce less drowsiness, respiratory depression, and impairment of motor function, and toxic doses are less likely to be fatal.

Pharmacology
Benzodiazepines are a group of structurally related chemicals that selectively act on polysynaptic neuronal pathways throughout the CNS. Their precise sites and mechanisms of action aren't completely known. However, the benzodiazepines enhance or facilitate the action of gamma-aminobutyric acid (GABA), an inhibitory neurotransmitter in the CNS. The drugs appear to act at the limbic, thalamic, and hypothalamic levels of the CNS. These drugs produce anxiolytic, sedative, hypnotic, skeletal muscle relaxant, and anticonvulsant effects. All of the benzodiazepines have CNS-depressant activities; however, individual derivatives act more selectively at specific sites, allowing them to be subclassified into five categories based on their predominant clinical use.

Indications and actions
Seizure disorders
Five of the benzodiazepines (diazepam, clonazepam, clorazepate, midazolam and parenteral lorazepam) are used as anticonvulsants. Their anticonvulsant properties are derived from an ability to suppress the spread of seizure activity produced by epileptogenic foci in the cortex, thalamus, and limbic systems by enhancing presynaptic inhibition. Clonazepam is useful in the adjunctive treatment of petit mal variant (Lennox-Gastaut syndrome), myoclonic, or akinetic seizures. Benzodiazepines are also useful adjuncts for the prophylactic management of par-

tial seizures with elementary symptoms (Jacksonian seizures), psychomotor seizures, and petit mal seizures. The parenteral form of diazepam, midazolam and lorazepam is indicated to treat status epilepticus.

Anxiety, tension, and insomnia

Most benzodiazepines (alprazolam, chlordiazepoxide, clorazepate, diazepam, estazolam, flurazepam, lorazepam, oxazepam, quazepam, temazepam, and triazolam) are useful as antianxiety agents or sedative-hypnotic agents. They have a similar mechanism of action; they're believed to facilitate the effects of GABA in the ascending reticular activating system, increasing inhibition and blocking both cortical and limbic arousal.

They're used to treat anxiety and tension that occur alone or as an adverse effect of a primary disorder. They aren't recommended for tension associated with everyday stress. The choice of a specific benzodiazepine depends on individual metabolic characteristics of the drug. For instance, in patients with depressed renal or hepatic function, alprazolam, lorazepam, or oxazepam may be selected because they have a relatively short duration of action and have no active metabolites.

The sedative-hypnotic properties of chlordiazepoxide, clorazepate, diazepam, lorazepam, and oxazepam make these the drugs of choice as preoperative medication and as an adjunct in the rehabilitation of alcoholics.

Surgical adjuncts for conscious sedation or amnesia

Diazepam, midazolam, and lorazepam have amnesic effects. The mechanism of such action isn't known. Parenteral administration before such procedures as endoscopy or elective cardioversion causes impairment of recent memory and interferes with the establishment of memory trace, producing anterograde amnesia.

Skeletal muscle spasm, tremor

Because oral forms of diazepam and chlordiazepoxide have skeletal muscle relaxant properties, they're often used to treat neurologic conditions involving muscle spasms and tetanus. The mechanism of such action is unknown, but they're believed to inhibit spinal polysynaptic and monosynaptic afferent pathways.

Delirium

Benzodiazepines may be beneficial alone or in combination with antipsychotic agents to treat delirium. However, caution should be used because benzodiazepines can also exacerbate delirium.

Schizophrenia◇

Benzodiazepines have been used as an adjunct to antipsychotic drugs in the management of schizophrenia.

Chemotherapy-induced nausea and vomiting◇

Benzodiazepines have been used as an adjunct to control nausea and vomiting associated with emetogenic cancer chemotherapy.

Neonatal opiate withdrawal◇

Parenteral diazepam has been used to relieve agitation associated with neonatal opiate withdrawal.

Overview of adverse reactions

Therapeutic dosage of the benzodiazepines usually causes drowsiness and impaired motor function, which should be monitored early in treatment. It may or may not be persistent. GI discomfort, such as constipation, diarrhea, vomiting, and changes in appetite, with urinary alterations, also have been reported. Visual disturbances and CV irregularities also are common. Continuing problems with short-term memory, confusion, severe depression, shakiness, vertigo, slurred speech, staggering, bradycardia, shortness of breath or difficulty breathing, and severe weakness usually indicate a toxic dose level. Prolonged or frequent use of benzodiazepines can cause physical dependency and withdrawal syndrome when use is discontinued.

Special considerations

● Benzodiazepines shouldn't be used in patients with chronic pulmonary insufficiency, sleep apnea, depressive neuroses or psychotic reactions without predominant anxiety, or acute alcohol intoxication.
● Assess level of consciousness and neurologic status before and frequently during therapy for changes. Monitor patient for paradoxical reactions, especially early in therapy.
● Observe sleep patterns and quality, and for changes in seizure character, frequency, or duration.
● Recommend assessing vital signs frequently during therapy. Significant changes in blood pressure and heart rate may indicate impending toxicity.
● Administer dose with milk or immediately after meals to prevent GI upset. Give antacid, if needed, at least 1 hour before or after dose to prevent interaction and ensure maximum drug absorption and effectiveness.
● Periodically monitor renal and hepatic function to ensure adequate drug removal and prevent cumulative effects.
● Institute safety measures—raised side rails and ambulatory assistance—to prevent injury. Anticipate possible rebound excitement reactions.
● After prolonged use, abrupt discontinuation may cause withdrawal symptoms; discontinue gradually.

Pregnant patients

● Benzodiazepines can cause fetal harm if administered during pregnancy. There's an increased risk of congenital malformation if given during

◇ Unlabeled clinical use

the first trimester. Use of benzodiazepines during labor may cause neonatal flaccidity. Use should be determined if benefits outweigh risks.

Breast-feeding patients
• The breast-fed infant of a mother who uses a benzodiazepine drug may show sedation, feeding difficulties, and weight loss. Safe use hasn't been established.

Pediatric patients
• Because children, particularly very young ones, are sensitive to the CNS depressant effects of benzodiazepines, exercise caution. A neonate whose mother took a benzodiazepine during pregnancy may exhibit withdrawal symptoms.

Geriatric patients
• Because they're sensitive to CNS effects, elderly patients receiving benzodiazepines require lower doses; use cautiously.
• Parenteral administration of these drugs is more likely to cause apnea, hypotension, bradycardia, and cardiac arrest.
• Elderly patients may show prolonged elimination of benzodiazepines, except possibly of oxazepam, lorazepam, temazepam, and triazolam.

Patient education
• Warn patient to avoid use of alcohol or other CNS depressants, such as antihistamines, analgesics, MAO inhibitors, antidepressants, and barbiturates, to prevent additive depressant effects.
• Caution patient to take drug as prescribed and not to give medication to others. Tell him not to change the dose or frequency and to call before taking OTC cold or allergy preparations that may potentiate CNS depressant effects.
• Warn patient to avoid activities requiring alertness and good psychomotor coordination until the CNS response to the drug is determined. Instruct him in safety measures to prevent injury.
• Tell patient to avoid using antacids, which may delay drug absorption, unless prescribed.
• Be sure patient understands that benzodiazepines are capable of causing physical and psychological dependence with prolonged use.
• Warn patient not to stop taking the drug abruptly to prevent withdrawal symptoms after prolonged therapy.
• Tell patient that smoking decreases the effectiveness of the drug. Encourage patient to stop smoking during therapy.
• Tell patient to report adverse effects. These are often dose-related and can be relieved by dosage adjustments.
• Inform a woman of childbearing age who is taking drug to report if she suspects pregnancy or intends to become pregnant during therapy.

Representative combinations
Chlordiazepoxide with amitriptyline hydrochloride: Limbitrol DS; with clidinium bromide: Librax.

beta blockers

beta₁ blockers: acebutolol, atenolol, betaxolol hydrochloride, bisoprolol, esmolol, metoprolol tartrate

beta₁ and beta₂ blockers: carteolol hydrochloride, carvedilol, labetalol, levobunolol hydrochloride, metipranolol hydrochloride, nadolol, penbutolol sulfate, pindolol, propranolol, sotalol, timolol maleate

Beta blockers are widely used to treat hypertension, angina pectoris, and arrhythmias. These agents are well tolerated by most patients.

Pharmacology
Beta blockers are chemicals that compete with beta agonists for available beta-receptor sites; individual agents differ in their ability to affect beta receptors. Some available agents are considered nonselective; that is, they block both beta₁ receptors in cardiac muscle and beta₂ receptors in bronchial and vascular smooth muscle. Several agents are cardioselective and in lower doses primarily inhibit beta₁ receptors. Some beta blockers have intrinsic sympathomimetic activity and simultaneously stimulate and block beta receptors, decreasing cardiac output; still others also have membrane-stabilizing activity, which affects cardiac action potential. (See *Comparing beta blockers*.)

Indications and actions
Hypertension
Most beta blockers are used to treat hypertension. Although the exact mechanism of their antihypertensive effect is unknown, the action is thought to result from decreased cardiac output, decreased sympathetic outflow from the CNS, and suppression of renin release.

Angina
Propranolol, atenolol, nadolol, and metoprolol are used to treat angina pectoris; they decrease myocardial oxygen requirements through the blockade of catecholamine-induced increases in heart rate, blood pressure, and the extent of myocardial contraction.

Arrhythmias
Propranolol, acebutolol, sotalol, and esmolol are used to treat arrhythmias; they prolong the refractory period of the AV node and slow AV conduction.

Glaucoma
The mechanism by which betaxolol, levobunolol, metipranolol, and timolol reduce intraocular pressure is unknown, but the drug effect is at least partially caused by decreased production of aqueous humor.

Comparing beta blockers

Drug	Half-life (hr)	Lipid solubility	Membrane-stabilizing activity	Intrinsic sympathomimetic activity
Nonselective				
carteolol	6	low	0	++
carvedilol	7-10	high	not known	0
labetalol	6-8	moderate	0	0
metipranolol	4	low to moderate	0	0
nadolol	20	low	0	0
penbutolol	5	high	0	+
pindolol	3-4	moderate	+	+++
propranolol	4	high	++	0
timolol	4	low to moderate	0	0
Beta₁-selective				
acebutolol	3-4	low	+	+
atenolol	6-7	low	0	0
betaxolol	14-22	low	+	0
bisoprolol	9-12	low	0	0
esmolol	0.15	low	0	0
metoprolol	3-7	moderate	♦	0

♦ Only in higher-than-usual doses.
+ Activity that drug possesses in comparison to other beta blockers.

Myocardial infarction
Timolol, propranolol, atenolol, and metoprolol are used to prevent MI in susceptible patients.

Migraine prophylaxis
Atenolol, metoprolol, nadolol, propranolol and timolol are used to prevent recurrent attacks of migraine and other vascular headaches. The exact mechanism by which these decrease migraine headache attacks is unknown, but it's thought to result from inhibition of vasodilation of cerebral vessels.

Other uses
Some beta blockers have been used as antianxiety agents, for managing subaortic stenosis, as adjunctive therapy of bleeding esophageal varices or pheochromocytomas, and to treat portal hypertension or essential tremors. Carvedilol is used to treat heart failure with cardiac glycosides, diuretics, or ACE inhibitors.

Overview of adverse reactions
Therapeutic doses may cause bradycardia, fatigue, and dizziness; some cause other CNS disturbances, such as nightmares, depression, memory loss, or hallucinations. Impotence, cold limbs, and elevated cholesterol levels may also occur. Severe hypotension, bradycardia, heart failure, or bronchospasm usually indicates toxic dose levels.

Special considerations
● Recommend monitoring of BP, ECG, and apical heart rate and rhythm frequently; be alert for progression of AV block or severe bradycardia.
● Patients with heart failure must be weighed regularly; watch for gains of more than 5 lb (2.2 kg) per week.
● Signs of hypoglycemic shock are masked; watch diabetic patients for sweating, fatigue, and hunger. Tachycardia in hyperthyroidism is also masked.
● Don't discontinue these drugs before surgery for pheochromocytoma; before any surgical procedure, notify anesthesiologist that patient is taking a beta blocker.

• Glucagon may be prescribed to reverse signs and symptoms of beta blocker overdose.
• Don't dispense to patients with asthma, sinus bradycardia, first-degree heart block, cardiogenic shock, or overt cardiac failure.

Pregnant patients
• Pregnancy risk category is C/D. Avoid beta blocker therapy in pregnant women. Atenolol may cause intrauterine growth retardation.

Breast-feeding patients
• Beta blockers appear in breast milk. Recommendations for breast-feeding vary with individual drugs.

Pediatric patients
• Safety and efficacy of beta blockers in children haven't been established; they should be used only if potential benefit outweighs risk.

Geriatric patients
• Elderly patients may need lower maintenance dosages of beta blockers; they also may experience enhanced adverse effects.

Patient education
• Explain rationale for therapy, and emphasize importance of taking drug as prescribed, even when feeling well.
• Warn patient that abrupt discontinuation can exacerbate angina or precipitate MI.
• Teach patient to minimize dizziness from orthostatic hypotension by taking dose at bedtime, and by rising slowly and avoiding sudden position changes.
• Advise patient to seek medical approval before taking OTC cold preparations.

Representative combinations
Atenolol with chlorthalidone: Tenoretic.
   Bisoprolol with hydrochlorothiazide: Ziac Tablets.
   Metoprolol with hydrochlorothiazide: Lopressor HCT.
   Pindolol with hydrochlorothiazide: Viskazide.
   Propranolol hydrochloride with hydrochlorothiazide: Inderide, Inderide LA.
   Timolol with hydrochlorothiazide: Timolide.

calcium channel blockers

amlodipine besylate, bepridil hydrochloride, diltiazem hydrochloride, felodipine, isradipine, nicardipine hydrochloride, nifedipine, nimodipine, nisoldipine, verapamil hydrochloride

Calcium channel blockers have become increasingly popular as a treatment for classic and variant angina and have come to be the preferred drugs for Prinzmetal's variant angina (vasospas-

tic angina). They have been used as antihypertensives. Verapamil has proved effective in the acute treatment of supraventricular tachycardias (SVTs). (See *Comparing oral calcium channel blockers.*)

Pharmacology
The main physiologic action of calcium channel blockers is to inhibit calcium influx across the slow channels of myocardial and vascular smooth muscle cells. By inhibiting calcium influx into these cells, calcium channel blockers reduce intracellular calcium concentrations. This, in turn, dilates coronary arteries, peripheral arteries, and arterioles, and slows cardiac conduction.

When used to treat Prinzmetal's variant angina, calcium channel blockers inhibit coronary spasm, increasing oxygen delivery to the heart. Peripheral artery dilation leads to a decrease in total peripheral resistance; this reduces afterload, which, in turn, decreases myocardial oxygen consumption. Inhibition of calcium influx into the specialized cardiac conduction cells (specifically, those in the SA and AV nodes) slows conduction through the heart. This effect is most pronounced with verapamil and diltiazem.

Indications and actions
Angina
Calcium channel blockers are useful in managing Prinzmetal's variant angina, chronic stable angina, and unstable angina. In Prinzmetal's variant angina, they inhibit spontaneous and ergonovine-induced coronary spasm, thereby increasing coronary blood flow and maintaining myocardial oxygen delivery. In unstable and chronic stable angina, their effectiveness presumably stems from their ability to reduce afterload.

Arrhythmias
Of the calcium channel blockers, verapamil and diltiazem have the greatest effect on the AV node, slowing the ventricular rate in atrial fibrillation or flutter and converting SVT to normal sinus rhythm.

Hypertension
Because they dilate systemic arteries, most of these agents are useful in mild to moderate hypertension.

Other uses
Calcium channel blockers (especially verapamil) may also prove to be effective as a hypertrophic cardiomyopathy therapy adjunct by improving left ventricular outflow as a result of negative inotropic effects and possibly improved diastolic function. They've been used to treat migraine headaches, peripheral vascular disorders, subarachnoid hemorrhage (nimodipine), and as adjunctive therapy in the treatment of esophageal spasm.

Comparing oral calcium channel blockers

Drug	Onset of action	Peak serum level (hr)	Half-life (hr)	Therapeutic serum level
bepridil	1 hr	2-3	24	1-2 ng/ml
diltiazem	15 min	½	3-4	50-200 ng/ml
felodipine	2-5 hr	2.5-5	11-16	unknown
nicardipine	20 min	1	8.6	28-50 ng/ml
nifedipine	5-30 min	½-2	2-5	25-100 ng/ml
nimodipine	unknown	< 1	1-2	unknown
nisoldipine	unknown	6-12	7-12	unknown
verapamil	30 min	1-2.2	6-12	80-300 ng/ml

Overview of adverse reactions

Verapamil may cause adverse effects on the conduction system, including bradycardia and various degrees of heart block, exacerbate heart failure, and cause hypotension after rapid I.V. administration. Prolonged oral verapamil therapy may cause constipation.

Adverse effects of nifedipine include hypotension, reflex tachycardia, peripheral edema, flushing, light-headedness, and headache.

Diltiazem most commonly causes anorexia, nausea, various degrees of heart block, bradycardia, heart failure, and peripheral edema.

Special considerations

• Monitor cardiac rate and rhythm and blood pressure carefully when starting therapy or increasing dose.
• Use of calcium supplements may decrease the effectiveness of calcium channel blockers.
• Use cautiously in patients with impaired left ventricular function.

Pregnant patients

• Pregnancy risk category is C. Avoid use in pregnant women.

Breast-feeding patients

• Calcium channel blocking agents (verapamil and diltiazem) may be excreted in breast milk. To avoid possible adverse effects in infants, discontinue breast-feeding during therapy with these drugs.

Pediatric patients

• Adverse hemodynamic effects of parenteral verapamil have been observed in neonates and infants. Safety and effectiveness of diltiazem and nifedipine haven't been established.

Geriatric patients

• Use cautiously because the half-life of calcium channel blockers may be increased as a result of decreased clearance.

Patient education

• Tell patient not to abruptly discontinue drug; gradual dose reduction may be necessary.
• Instruct patient to report irregular heartbeat, shortness of breath, swelling of hands and feet, pronounced dizziness, constipation, nausea, or hypotension.
• Warn patient not to double the dose.

Representative combinations

Amlodipine and benazepril hydrochloride: Lotrel.

cephalosporins

First-generation cephalosporins:
cefadroxil, cefazolin sodium, cephalexin monohydrate, cephradine

Second-generation cephalosporins:
cefaclor, cefamandole nafate, cefotetan disodium, cefoxitin sodium, cefprozil, ceftibuten, cefuroxime axetil, cefuroxime sodium

Third-generation cephalosporins:
cefdinir, cefixime, cefoperazone sodium, cefotaxime sodium, cefpodoxime proxetil, ceftazidime, ceftizoxime sodium, ceftriaxone sodium

Fourth-generation cephalosporin:
cefepime hydrochloride

Cephalosporins are beta-lactam antibiotics first isolated from the fungus *Cephalosporium acremonium*. Their mechanism of action is similar to that of penicillins, but their antibacterial spectra differ.

Pharmacology

Cephalosporins are chemically and pharmacologically similar to penicillin; their structure con-

◇ Unlabeled clinical use

tains a beta-lactam ring, a dihydrothiazine ring, and side chains, and they act by inhibiting bacterial cell wall synthesis, causing rapid cell lysis. (See *Comparing cephalosporins*.)

The sites of action for cephalosporins are enzymes known as penicillin-binding proteins (PBP). The affinity of certain cephalosporins for PBP in various microorganisms helps explain the differing spectra of activity in this class of antibiotics.

Bacterial resistance to beta-lactam antibiotics is conferred most significantly by production of beta-lactamase enzymes (by both gram-negative and gram-positive bacteria) that destroy the beta-lactam ring and thus inactivate cephalosporins; decreased cell wall permeability and alteration in binding affinity to PBP also contribute to bacterial resistance.

Cephalosporins are bactericidal; they act against many gram-positive and gram-negative bacteria, and some anaerobic bacteria; they don't kill fungi or viruses.

First-generation cephalosporins act against many gram-positive cocci, including penicillinase-producing *Stapylococcus aureus* and *Staphylococcus epidermidis; Streptococcus pneumoniae, Streptococcus agalactiae* (group B streptococci), and *Streptococcus pyogenes* (group A beta-hemolytic streptococci); susceptible gram-negative organisms include *Escherichia coli, Klebsiella pneumoniae, Proteus mirabilis,* and *Shigella.*

Second-generation cephalosporins are effective against all organisms attacked by first-generation drugs and have additional activity against *Acinetobacter, Branhamella catarrhalis, Citrobacter, Enterobacter, Haemophilus influenzae, Neisseria, Providencia,* and *Serratia; Bacteroides fragilis* is susceptible to cefotetan and cefoxitin.

Third-generation cephalosporins are less active than first- and second-generation drugs against gram-positive bacteria, but more active against gram-negative organisms, including those resistant to first- and second-generation drugs; they have the greatest stability against beta-lactamases produced by gram-negative bacteria. Susceptible gram-negative organisms include *Acinetobacter, Enterobacter, E. coli, Klebsiella, Morganella, Neisseria, Proteus, Providencia,* and *Serratia;* some third-generation drugs are active against *B. fragilis* and *Pseudomonas.*

The fourth-generation cephalosporin cefepime is active against a wide range of gram-positive and gram-negative bacteria. Susceptible gram-negative organisms include *Enterobacter* spp., *E. coli, K. pneumoniae, P. mirabilis,* and *Pseudomonas aeruginosa;* susceptible gram-positive organisms include *S. aureus* (methicillin-susceptible strains only), *S. pneumoniae,* and *S. pyogenes* (Lancefield's group A streptococci).

Oral absorption of cephalosporins varies widely; many must be given parenterally. Most are distributed widely into the body, the actual amount varying with individual drugs. CSF penetration by first- and second-generation drugs is minimal; third-generation drugs achieve much greater penetration, and although the fourth-generation drug cefepime is known to cross the blood-brain barrier, it isn't known to what degree. Cephalosporins cross the placenta. Degree of metabolism varies with individual drugs; some aren't metabolized at all, whereas others are extensively metabolized.

Cephalosporins are excreted primarily in urine, chiefly by renal tubular effects; elimination half-life ranges from 30 minutes to 10 hours in patients with normal renal function. Some drug is excreted in breast milk. Most cephalosporins can be removed by hemodialysis or peritoneal dialysis. Patients on dialysis may require dosage adjustment.

Indications and actions
Infection caused by susceptible organisms
Parenteral cephalosporins: Cephalosporins are used to treat serious infections of the lungs, skin, soft tissue, bones, joints, urinary tract, blood (septicemia), abdomen, and heart (endocarditis).

Third-generation cephalosporins (except cefoperazone) and the second-generation drug cefuroxime are used to treat CNS infections caused by susceptible strains of *H. influenzae, N. meningitidis,* and *S. pneumoniae;* meningitis caused by *E. coli* or *Klebsiella* can be treated with ceftriaxone, cefotaxime, or ceftizoxime.

First-generation and some second-generation cephalosporins also can be given prophylactically to reduce postoperative infection after surgical procedures classified as contaminated or potentially contaminated; third-generation drugs aren't usually indicated.

Penicillinase-producing *N. gonorrhoeae* can be treated with cefoxitin, cefotaxime, ceftriaxone, ceftizoxime, or cefuroxime.

Oral cephalosporins: Cephalosporins can be used to treat otitis media and infections of the respiratory tract, urinary tract, and skin and soft tissue.

Ceftriaxone, cefotaxime, or cefuroxime axetil has been used in the treatment of Lyme disease ◊.

Cefepime, ceftazidime, and ceftriaxone have been used parenterally for empiric anti-infective therapy of probable bacterial infections in febrile neutropenic patients.

Overview of adverse reactions
Hypersensitivity reactions range from mild rash, fever, and eosinophilia to fatal anaphylaxis, and are more common in patients with penicillin allergy. Hematologic reactions include positive direct and indirect antiglobulin (Coombs' test), thrombocytopenia or thrombocythemia, transient neutropenia, and reversible leukopenia. Adverse renal effects, nausea, vomiting, diarrhea, abdominal pain, glossitis, dyspepsia, tenesmus, and minimal elevation of liver function test results have occurred. Hemolytic anemia with extravas-

Comparing cephalosporins

Drug and route	Elimination half-life (hr)		Sodium (mEq/g)	CSF penetration
	Normal renal function	End-stage renal disease		
cefaclor oral	0.5-1	3-5.5	Unknown	No
cefadroxil oral	1-2	20-25	Unknown	No
cefamandole I.M., I.V.	0.5-2	12-18	3.3	No
cefazolin I.M., I.V.	1.2-2.2	3-7	2.0-2.1	No
cefdinir P.O.	1.5	16	Unknown	Unknown
cefepime I.M., I.V.	2	17-21	Unknown	Yes
cefixime oral	3-4	11.5	Unknown	Unknown
cefoperazone I.M., I.V.	1.5-2.5	1.3-2.9	1.5	Sometimes
cefotaxime I.M., I.V.	1-1.5	3-11	2.2	Yes
cefotetan I.M., I.V.	2.8-4.6	13-35	3.5	No
cefoxitin I.M., I.V.	0.5-1	6.5-21.5	2.3	No
cefpodoxime oral	2-3	9.8	Unknown	Unknown
cefprozil oral	1-1.5	5.2-5.9	Unknown	Unknown
ceftazidime I.M., I.V.	1.5-2	35	2.3	Yes
ceftibuten oral	2.4	13.4-22.3	Unknown	Unknown
ceftizoxime I.M., I.V.	1.5-2	30	2.6	Yes
ceftriaxone I.M., I.V.	5.5-11	15.7	3.6	Yes
cefuroxime I.M., I.V.	1-2	15-22	2.4	Yes
cephalexin oral	0.5-1	19-22	Unknown	No
cephapirin I.M., I.V.	0.5-1	1.0-1.5	2.4	No
cephradine oral, I.M., I.V.	0.5-2	8-15	6	No

◇ Unlabeled clinical use

cular hemolysis and some fatalities have occurred in patients receiving cefotaxime, ceftizoxime, ceftriaxone, and cefotetan.

Local venous pain and irritation are common after I.M. injection; such reactions occur more often with higher doses and long-term therapy.

Disulfiram-type reactions occur when cefamandole, cefoperazone, cefonicid, or cefotetan are administered within 48 to 72 hours of alcohol ingestion.

Bacterial and fungal superinfection results from suppression of normal flora.

Special considerations
• Review patient's history of allergies.
• Monitor patient continuously for possible hypersensitivity reactions or other untoward effects.
• Monitor renal function studies; doses of certain cephalosporins must be lowered in patients with severe renal impairment. In decreased renal function, monitor BUN levels, serum creatinine levels, and urine output for significant changes.
• Monitor PT and platelet counts and assess patient for signs of hypoprothrombinemia, which may occur, with or without bleeding, during therapy with cefamandole, cefepime, cefoperazone, cefonicid, or cefotetan, usually in elderly, debilitated, or malnourished patients.
• Monitor patients on long-term therapy for possible bacterial and fungal superinfection, especially elderly patients, debilitated patients, and those receiving immunosuppressants or radiation therapy.
• Monitor susceptible patients receiving sodium salts of cephalosporins for possible fluid retention; consult individual drug entry for sodium content.
• Cephalosporins cause false-positive results in urine glucose tests using cupric sulfate solutions (Benedict's reagent or Clinitest); glucose oxidase tests aren't affected. Consult individual drug entries for other possible test interactions.

Administration
• Give cephalosporins at least 1 hour before giving bacteriostatic antibiotics (tetracyclines, erythromycins, and chloramphenicol); these drugs inhibit bacterial cell growth, decreasing cephalosporin uptake by bacterial cell walls.
• Give oral cephalosporin at least 1 hour before or 2 hours after meals for maximum absorption.
• Refrigerate oral suspensions; shake well before administering to assure correct dose.
• Give I.M. dose deep into large muscle mass (gluteal or midlateral thigh); rotate injection sites.
• Don't add or mix other drugs with I.V. infusions, particularly aminoglycosides, which are inactivated if mixed with cephalosporins; if other drugs must be given I.V., temporarily stop infusion of primary drug.
• Adequate dilution of I.V. infusion and rotation of the site every 48 hours help minimize local vein irritation; use of small-gauge needle in larger available vein may be helpful.

Pregnant patients
• Safety in pregnancy hasn't been established. Use only when clearly needed.

Breast-feeding patients
• Cephalosporins appear in breast milk; use cautiously in breast-feeding women.

Pediatric patients
• Serum half-life is prolonged in neonates and in infants up to age 1.

Geriatric patients
• Use cautiously; elderly patients are susceptible to superinfection and to coagulopathies.
• They commonly have renal impairment and may need lower doses of cephalosporins.

Patient education
• Explain the disease process and rationale for therapy.
• Teach patient signs and symptoms of hypersensitivity and other adverse reactions, and emphasize need to report any unusual effects.
• Teach signs and symptoms of bacterial and fungal superinfection to geriatric and debilitated patients and others with low resistance from immunosuppressants or irradiation; emphasize need to report them promptly.
• Warn patient not to ingest alcohol in any form within 72 hours of treatment with cefamandole, cefoperazone, cefonicid, or cefotetan.
• Suggest patient add yogurt or buttermilk to diet to prevent intestinal superinfection resulting from suppression of normal intestinal flora.
• Advise diabetic patients to monitor urine glucose level with Diastix, Chemstrip uG, or glucose enzymatic test strip and not to use Clinitest.
• Tell patient to take oral drug with food if GI irritation occurs.
• Be sure patient understands how and when to take drug; urge patient to complete entire prescribed regimen, to comply with instructions for around-the-clock dosing, and to keep follow-up appointments.
• Counsel patient to check expiration date of drug, how to store drug, and to discard unused drug.

Representative combinations
None.

diuretics, loop

bumetanide, ethacrynate sodium, ethacrynic acid, furosemide, torsemide

Loop diuretics are sometimes referred to as high-ceiling diuretics because they produce a peak diuresis greater than that produced by other agents. Loop diuretics are particularly useful in edema associated with heart failure, hepatic cirrhosis, and renal disease. Ethacrynic acid was synthesized during the search for compounds that might

Comparing loop diuretics

Drug and route	Onset (min)	Peak (hr)	Duration (hr)	Usual dosage
bumetanide				
I.V.	≤ 5	¼-¾	4-6	0.5-1 mg ≤ t.i.d
P.O.	30-60	1-2	½-1	0.5 2 mg/day
ethacrynic acid				
I.V.	≤ 5	¼-½	2	50 mg/day
P.O.	≤ 30	2	6-8	50-100 mg/day
furosemide				
I.V.	≤ 5	⅓-1	2	20-40 mg q 2 hr, p.r.n.
P.O.	30-60	1-2	6-8	20-80 mg ≤ b.i.d.
torsemide				
I.V.	≤ 10	≤ 1	6-8	5-20 mg/day
P.O.	≤ 60	1-2	6-8	5-20 mg/day

interact with renal sulfhydryl groups like mercurial diuretics. However, ethacrynic acid is associated with ototoxicity and a higher risk of GI reactions and is therefore used less frequently. Structurally similar to furosemide, bumetanide is about 40 times more potent. Torsemide is the newest loop diuretic. (See *Comparing loop diuretics.*)

Pharmacology

Loop diuretics inhibit sodium and chloride reabsorption in the ascending loop of Henle, thus increasing renal excretion of sodium, chloride, and water; like thiazide diuretics, loop diuretics increase excretion of potassium. Loop diuretics produce greater maximum diuresis and electrolyte loss than thiazide diuretics.

Indications and actions
Edema

Loop diuretics effectively relieve edema associated with heart failure. They may be useful in patients refractory to other diuretics; because furosemide and bumetanide may increase glomerular filtration rate, they're useful in patients with renal impairment. I.V. loop diuretics are used adjunctively in acute pulmonary edema to decrease peripheral vascular resistance. Loop diuretics also are used to treat edema associated with hepatic cirrhosis and nephrotic syndrome.

Hypertension

Loop diuretics are used in patients with mild to moderate hypertension, although thiazides are the initial diuretics of choice in most patients. Loop diuretics are preferred in patients with heart failure or renal impairment; used I.V., they're a helpful adjunct in managing hypertensive crises.

Loop diuretics have been used to increase excretion of calcium in patients with hypercalcemia ◇.

Loop diuretics have been used to enhance the elimination of drugs and toxic substances following intoxication ◇.

Overview of adverse reactions

The most common adverse effects associated with therapeutic doses of loop diuretics are metabolic and electrolyte disturbances (particularly potassium depletion), hypochloremic alkalosis, hyperglycemia, hyperuricemia, and hypomagnesemia. Rapid parenteral administration of loop diuretics may cause hearing loss (including deafness) and tinnitus. High doses may produce profound diuresis, leading to hypovolemia and CV collapse.

Special considerations

● Institute safety measures for all ambulatory patients until response to the diuretic is known.
● Patients taking cardiac glycosides are at increased risk of digitalis toxicity from potassium depletion.
● Patients with hepatic disease are especially susceptible to diuretic-induced electrolyte imbalance; in extreme cases, stupor, coma, and death can result.
● Consider possible dosage adjustment in the following circumstances: reduced doses for patients with hepatic dysfunction; increased doses in patients with renal impairment, oliguria, or decreased diuresis (inadequate urine output may result in circulatory overload, causing water intoxication, pulmonary edema, and heart failure); increased doses of insulin or oral hypoglycemics in diabetic patients; and reduced doses of other antihypertensive agents.
● Monitor blood pressure and pulse rate (especially during rapid diuresis), establish baseline values before therapy, and watch for significant changes.
● Establish baseline and periodically review CBC, including WBC count; serum electrolytes; carbon

dioxide; magnesium; BUN and creatinine levels; and results of liver function tests.
- Administer diuretics in the morning so major diuresis occurs before bedtime. To prevent nocturia, don't prescribe diuretics for use after 6 p.m.
- Watch for signs of excessive diuresis: hypotension, tachycardia, poor skin turgor, and excessive thirst.
- Monitor patient for edema and ascites.

Pregnant patients
- There are no adequately controlled studies for use of loop diuretics in pregnant women. Avoid use if possible.

Breast-feeding patients
- Don't use loop diuretics in breast-feeding women.

Pediatric patients
- Use loop diuretics cautiously in neonates; don't use ethacrynic acid and ethacrynate sodium in infants. The usual pediatric dose can be used, but extend dose intervals.

Geriatric patients
- Elderly and debilitated patients need close observation because they're more susceptible to drug-induced diuresis. Excessive diuresis can quickly lead to dehydration, hypovolemia, hypokalemia, and hyponatremia and may cause circulatory collapse. Reduced doses may be indicated.

Patient education
- Explain to patient the rationale for therapy and diuretic effect of these drugs (increased volume and frequency of urination).
- Teach patient signs of adverse effects, especially hypokalemia (weakness, fatigue, muscle cramps, paresthesias, confusion, nausea, vomiting, diarrhea, headache, dizziness, or palpitations), and importance of reporting such symptoms promptly.
- Advise patient to eat potassium-rich foods.
- Tell patient to report increased edema or weight or excess diuresis (more than 2-lb. [0.9-kg] weight loss per day).
- With initial doses, caution patient to change position slowly, especially when rising to upright position, to prevent dizziness from orthostatic hypotension.
- Instruct patient to call at once if he experiences chest, back, or leg pain; shortness of breath; or dyspnea.
- Inform patient that photosensitivity may occur in some patients. Caution patient to take protective measures, such as using sunscreens and protective clothing, against exposure to ultraviolet light or sunlight.

Representative combinations
None.

diuretics, potassium-sparing

amiloride hydrochloride, spironolactone, triamterene

Potassium-sparing diuretics are less potent than many others; in particular, amiloride and triamterene have little clinical effect when used alone. However, they protect against potassium loss and are used with more potent diuretics. Spironolactone, an aldosterone antagonist, is particularly useful in patients with edema and hypertension associated with hyperaldosteronism.

Pharmacology
Amiloride and triamterene act directly on the distal renal tubules, inhibiting sodium reabsorption and potassium excretion, thereby reducing potassium loss. Spironolactone competitively inhibits aldosterone at the distal renal tubules, also promoting sodium excretion and potassium retention.

Indications and actions
Edema
All potassium-sparing diuretics are used to manage edema associated with hepatic cirrhosis, nephrotic syndrome, and heart failure.

Hypertension
Amiloride and spironolactone are used to treat mild and moderate hypertension; the exact mechanism is unknown. Spironolactone may block the effect of aldosterone on arteriolar smooth muscle.

Diagnosis of primary hyperaldosteronism
Because spironolactone inhibits aldosterone, correction of hypokalemia and hypertension is presumptive evidence of primary hyperaldosteronism.

Other uses
Amiloride has been used to correct metabolic alkalosis produced by thiazide and other kaliuretic diuretics, and in combination with hydrochlorothiazide in patients with recurrent calcium nephrolithiasis. It has also been used to manage lithium-induced polyuria secondary to lithium-induced nephrogenic diabetes insipidus.

Spironolactone has been used to aid in the treatment of hypokalemia and for prophylaxis of hypokalemia in patients taking cardiac glycosides. It has also been used in the treatment of precocious puberty, female hirsutism, and as an adjunct to treatment in myasthenia gravis and familial periodic paralysis.

Overview of adverse reactions
Hyperkalemia is the most important adverse reaction; it may occur with all drugs in this class and could lead to arrhythmias. Other adverse reactions include nausea, vomiting, headache, weak-

ness, fatigue, bowel disturbances, cough, and dyspnea.

Potassium-sparing diuretics are contraindicated in patients with serum potassium levels above 5.5 mEq/L, in those receiving other potassium-sparing diuretics or potassium supplements, and in patients with anuria, acute or chronic renal insufficiency, diabetic nephropathy, or known hypersensitivity to the drug. They should be used cautiously in patients with severe hepatic insufficiency because electrolyte imbalance may precipitate hepatic encephalopathy, and in patients with diabetes, who are at increased risk of hyperkalemia.

Special considerations
● Administer diuretics in the morning to ensure that major diuresis occurs before bedtime. To prevent nocturia, don't prescribe diuretics for use after 6 p.m.
● Establish safety measures for ambulatory patients until response is known; diuretics may cause orthostatic hypotension, weakness, ataxia, and confusion.
● Consider possible dosage adjustments in the following circumstances: reduced doses for patients with hepatic dysfunction and for those taking other antihypertensive agents; increased doses in patients with renal impairment; and changes in insulin requirements in diabetic patients.
● Monitor patient for hyperkalemia and arrhythmias; measure serum potassium and other electrolyte levels frequently, and check for significant changes. Monitor the following at baseline and periodic intervals: CBC including WBC count; carbon dioxide, BUN, and creatinine levels; and especially, liver function studies.
● Monitor vital signs, intake and output, weight, and blood pressure daily; also, check patient for edema, oliguria, or lack of diuresis, which may indicate drug tolerance.
● Monitor patient with hepatic disease in whom mild drug-induced acidosis may be hazardous; watch for mental confusion, lethargy, or stupor. Patients with hepatic disease are especially susceptible to diuretic-induced electrolyte imbalance; in extreme cases, coma and death can result.
● Watch for other signs of toxicity.

Pregnant patients
● There are no adequately controlled studies for use in pregnant women.

Breast-feeding patients
● Safety hasn't been established; drug may appear in breast milk.

Pediatric patients
● If indicated, use drugs cautiously; children are more susceptible to hyperkalemia.

Geriatric patients
● Elderly and debilitated patients need close observation because they're more susceptible to drug-induced diuresis and hyperkalemia. Reduced doses may be indicated.

Patient education
● Explain to patient the signs and symptoms of possible adverse effects and the importance of reporting unusual effects.
● Tell patient to report increased edema or weight loss (more than 2 lb [0.9 kg] per day) or excess diuresis and to record weight each morning after voiding and before dressing and breakfast, using the same scale.
● Teach patient how to minimize dizziness from orthostatic hypotension by avoiding sudden postural changes.
● Advise patient to avoid potassium-rich food and potassium-containing salt substitutes or supplements, which increase the hazard of hyperkalemia.
● Tell patient to take drug at same time each morning to avoid interrupted sleep from nighttime diuresis.
● Advise patient to take drug with or after meals to minimize GI distress.
● Caution patient to avoid hazardous activities, such as driving or operating machinery, until response to drug is known.
● Tell patient to seek medical approval before taking OTC drugs; many contain sodium and potassium and can cause electrolyte imbalance.

Representative combinations
Amiloride with hydrochlorothiazide: Moduretic.
    Spironolactone with hydrochlorothiazide: Aldactazide.
    Triamterene with hydrochlorothiazide: Dyazide, Maxzide.

diuretics, thiazide

bendroflumethiazide, chlorothiazide, chlorothiazide sodium, hydrochlorothiazide, hydroflumethiazide, methyclothiazide, polythiazide, trichlormethiazide

diuretics, thiazide-like

chlorthalidone, indapamide, metolazone

Thiazide diuretics were discovered and synthesized as an outgrowth of studies on carbonic anhydrase inhibitors. Until the 1950s, organic mercurials were the only effective diuretics available; though potent, they were also toxic. Introduction of thiazides in 1957 proved a major advance because these were the first potent, and safe, diuretics.

Pharmacology
Thiazide diuretics interfere with sodium transport across tubules of the cortical diluting segment of the nephron, thereby increasing renal

Comparing thiazides

Drug	Equivalent dose (mg)	Onset (hr)	Peak (hr)	Duration (hr)
bendroflumethiazide	5	within 2	4	6-12
chlorothiazide	500	within 2	4	6-12
hydrochlorothiazide	50	within 2	4-6	6-12
methyclothiazide	5	within 2	4-6	24

excretion of sodium, chloride, water, potassium, and calcium. Bicarbonate, magnesium, phosphate, bromide, and iodide excretion are also increased. These drugs may also decrease excretion of ammonia, causing increased serum ammonia levels. Long-term thiazide therapy can cause mild metabolic alkalosis associated with hypokalemia and hypochloremia.

The exact mechanism of thiazides' antihypertensive effect is unknown; however, it's thought to be partially caused by direct arteriolar dilatation. Thiazides initially decrease extracellular fluid volume, plasma volume, and cardiac output; extracellular fluid volume and plasma volume revert to near baseline levels in several weeks but remain slightly below normal. Cardiac output returns to normal or slightly above. Total body sodium level remains slightly below pretreatment levels. Peripheral vascular resistance is initially elevated but falls below pretreatment levels with chronic diuretic therapy. (See *Comparing thiazides*.)

In patients with diabetes insipidus, thiazides cause a paradoxical decrease in urine volume and increase in renal concentration of urine, possibly because of sodium depletion and decreased plasma volume, which leads to an increase in renal water and sodium reabsorption. In addition, thiazides can cause hyperglycemia, exacerbation of diabetes mellitus, or precipitation of diabetes mellitus.

Indications and actions
Edema
Thiazide diuretics are used to treat edema caused by heart failure and nephrotic syndrome and, with spironolactone, to treat edema and ascites secondary to hepatic cirrhosis. Thiazides may also be used to control edema during pregnancy except if caused by renal disease. This treatment isn't indicated for mild edema.

Efficacy and toxicity profiles of thiazide and thiazide-like diuretics are equivalent at comparable doses; the single exception is metolazone, which may be more effective in patients with impaired renal function. Usually, thiazide diuretics are less effective than loop diuretics in patients with renal insufficiency.

Hypertension
Thiazide diuretics are commonly used for initial management of all degrees of hypertension. Used alone, they reduce mean blood pressure by only 10 to 15 mm Hg; in mild hypertension, thiazide diuresis alone will usually reduce blood pressure to desired levels. However, in moderate to severe hypertension that doesn't respond to thiazides alone, combination therapy with another antihypertensive is necessary.

Diabetes insipidus ◇
In diabetes insipidus, thiazides cause a paradoxical decrease in urine volume; urine becomes more concentrated, possibly because of sodium depletion and decreased plasma volume. Thiazides are particularly effective in nephrogenic diabetes insipidus.

Other uses
Prophylaxis of renal calculi formation associated with hypercalciuria and in the treatment of electrolyte disturbances associated with renal tubular necrosis.

Overview of adverse reactions
Therapeutic doses of thiazide diuretics cause electrolyte and metabolic disturbances, the most common being potassium depletion; patients may require dietary supplementation.

Other abnormalities include hypochloremic alkalosis, hypomagnesemia, hyponatremia, hypercalcemia, hyperuricemia, elevated cholesterol levels, and hyperglycemia. Overdose of thiazides may produce lethargy that can progress to coma within a few hours.

Special considerations
● Thiazides and thiazide-like diuretics (except metolazone) are ineffective in patients with a glomerular filtration rate below 25 ml per minute.
● Because thiazides may cause adverse lipid effects, consider an alternative agent in patients with significant hyperlipidemia.
● Monitor intake and output, weight, and serum electrolyte levels regularly.
● Monitor serum potassium levels and consult a dietitian to provide high-potassium diet. Foods rich in potassium include citrus fruits, tomatoes, bananas, dates, and apricots. Watch for signs of

hypokalemia, such as muscle weakness or cramps. Patients also taking a cardiac glycoside have an increased risk of digitalis toxicity from the potassium-depleting effect of these diuretics.
● Thiazides may be used with potassium-sparing diuretics or potassium supplements to prevent potassium loss.
● Monitor blood glucose values in diabetic patients. Thiazides may cause hyperglycemia and a need to adjust insulin or oral hypoglycemic doses.
● Monitor serum creatinine and BUN levels regularly. Drug isn't as effective if these levels are more than twice normal.
● Monitor blood uric acid levels, especially in patients with history of gout; these agents may cause an increase in uric acid levels.
● Antihypertensive effects persist for about 1 week after discontinuation of drug.

Pregnant patients
● Thiazides cross the placenta and appear in cord blood. Risks and benefits must be evaluated. There are some reports of teratogenic effects, but results are inconclusive. Some clinicians recommend avoiding use in the first trimester. Routine use isn't recommended with mild edema.

Breast-feeding patients
● Thiazides appear in breast milk; safety and effectiveness in breast-feeding women haven't been established.

Pediatric patients
● Safety and effectiveness in children haven't been established for all thiazide diuretics. Indapamide and metolazone aren't recommended for use in children.

Geriatric patients
● Elderly and debilitated patients require close observation and may require reduced doses. They're more sensitive to excess diuresis because of age-related changes in CV and renal function. In elderly patients, excess diuresis can quickly lead to dehydration, hypovolemia, hyponatremia, hypomagnesemia, and hypokalemia.

Patient education
● Explain rationale of therapy and diuretic effects of these drugs (increased volume and frequency of urination).
● Instruct patient to report joint swelling, pain, or redness; these signs may indicate hyperuricemia.
● Warn patient to call immediately if signs of electrolyte imbalance occur; these include weakness, fatigue, muscle cramps, paresthesia, confusion, nausea, vomiting, diarrhea, headache, dizziness, and palpitations.
● Tell patient to report increased edema, excess diuresis, or weight loss (more than a 2 lb [0.9 kg] per day); advise him to record weight each morning after voiding and before dressing and breakfast, using the same scale.

● Advise patient to take drug in the morning to prevent nocturia.
● Instruct patient to take drug with food to minimize gastric irritation; to eat potassium-rich foods; and not to add salt to other foods. Recommend use of salt substitutes.
● Counsel patient to avoid smoking because nicotine increases blood pressure.
● Tell patient to seek medical approval before taking OTC drugs.
● Warn patient about photosensitivity reactions.
Initial doses
● Caution patient to change position slowly, especially when rising to upright position, to prevent dizziness from orthostatic hypotension.
● Instruct patient to call immediately if he experiences chest, back, or leg pain; shortness of breath; or dyspnea.
● Tell patient to take drug only as prescribed and at the same time each day, to prevent nighttime diuresis and interrupted sleep.

Representative combinations
Chlorthalidone with atenolol: Atenolol/Chlorthalidone Tablets, Tenoretic; with reserpine: Regroton. *Hydrochlorothiazide* with bisoprolol: Ziac Tablets; with deserpidine: Orcticyl; with guanethidine monosulfate: Esimil; with hydralazine: Apresazide, Hydrochlorothiazide/Hydralazine Caps; with hydralazine hydrochloride and reserpine: Hydrap-ES Tablets, Marpres Tablets, Tri-Hydroserpine Tablets; with methyldopa: Aldoril, Methyldopa and Hydrochlorothiazide Tablets; with propranolol: Inderide, Propranolol/Hydrochlorothiazide Tablets; with reserpine: Hydrochlorothiazide/Reserpine Tablets, Hydropine, Hydropres, Hydro-Serp, Hydroserpine, Hydrotensin, Mallopres; with hydralazine and reserpine: Ser-Ap-Es, Unipres; with spironolactone: Aldactazide; with timolol maleate: Timolide; with triamterene: Dyazide, Maxzide; with amiloride hydrochloride: Moduretic.
 Hydroflumethiazide with reserpine: Salutensin Tablets.

---

estrogens

dienestrol, esterified estrogens, estradiol, estradiol cypionate, estradiol valerate, estrogen and progestin, estrogenic substances (conjugated), estropipate, ethinyl estradiol

---

Estrogens were first discovered in the urine of humans and animals in 1930. Since that time, numerous synthetic modifications of naturally occurring estrogen molecules and completely synthetic estrogenic compounds have been developed.
 Estrogens have several uses: in treating the symptoms of menopause, atrophic vaginitis, breast cancer, and other diseases; in the prophylaxis of

osteoporosis; and as contraceptives when used in combination with progestins.

Pharmacology

Estrogens are hormones secreted by ovarian follicles and also by the adrenals, corpeus luteum, placenta, and testes. Conjugated estrogens and estrogenic substances are normally obtained from the urine of pregnant mares. Other estrogens are manufactured synthetically. Of the six naturally occurring estrogens, three (estradiol, estrone, and estriol) are present in significant quantities.

Estrogens promote the development and maintenance of the female reproductive system and secondary sexual characteristics. Estrogens inhibit the release of pituitary gonadotropins and also have various metabolic effects, including retention of fluid and electrolytes, retention and deposition in bone of calcium and phosphorus, and mild anabolic activity. They also increase high-density lipoproteins and decrease low-density lipoproteins.

Estrogens and estrogenic substances administered as drugs have effects related to endogenous estrogen's mechanism of action. They can mimic the action of endogenous estrogen when used as replacement therapy or produce such useful effects as inhibiting ovulation or inhibiting growth of certain hormone-sensitive cancers.

Use of estrogens isn't without risk. Long-term use is linked to an increased risk of endometrial cancer, gallbladder disease, and thromboembolic disease. Elevations in blood pressure often occur as well.

Indications and actions
Moderate to severe vasomotor symptoms of menopause

Endogenous estrogens are markedly reduced in concentration after menopause. This commonly results in vasomotor symptoms, such as hot flashes and dizziness. Estradiol cypionate and ethinyl estradiol serve to mimic the action of endogenous estrogens in preventing these symptoms.

Carcinoma of the breast

Conjugated estrogens, diethylstilbestrol, esterified estrogens, estradiol, and ethinyl estradiol inhibit the growth of hormone-sensitive cancers in certain carefully selected men and postmenopausal women.

Carcinoma of the prostate

Conjugated estrogens, esterified estrogens, estradiol, estradiol valerate, and ethinyl estradiol inhibit growth of hormone-sensitive cancer tissue in men with advanced disease.

Cardiovascular risk prevention

Although somewhat controversial, estrogen and estrogen/progestin has shown to reduce the risk of ischemic heart disease by 50%. Therapy initiation should be highly individualized.

Prophylaxis of postmenopausal osteoporosis

Conjugated estrogens replace or augment activity of endogenous estrogen in causing calcium and phosphate retention and preventing bone decalcification.

Contraception

Estrogens are also used with progestins for ovulation control to prevent conception.

Overview of adverse reactions

Acute reactions include changes in menstrual bleeding patterns (spotting, prolongation or absence of bleeding), abdominal cramps, swollen feet or ankles, bloated sensation (fluid and electrolyte retention), breast swelling and tenderness, weight gain, nausea, loss of appetite, headache, photosensitivity, loss of libido.

With long-term administration, adverse reactions include increased blood pressure (sometimes into the hypertensive range), thromboembolic disease, cholestatic jaundice, benign hepatomas, endometrial carcinoma (rare). Risk of thromboembolic disease increases markedly with cigarette smoking, especially in women over age 35. Increased risk of thromboembolic events also seen in postmenopausal women, women undergoing surgery, and those with fractures or who are immobilized.

Special considerations

● Some clinicians recommend that women discontinue estrogen replacement therapy during immobilization caused by fracture, CVA, or severe illness; estrogen replacement therapy can be restarted when normal activity is resumed.
● Don't use estrogens in patients with thrombophlebitis or thromboembolic disorders; cancer of the breast, reproductive organs, or genitals; or undiagnosed abnormal genital bleeding.
● Use cautiously in patients with hypertension, asthma, mental depression, bone disease, blood dyscrasias, gallbladder disease, migraine, seizures, diabetes mellitus, amenorrhea, heart failure, hepatic or renal dysfunction, or a family history of breast or genital tract cancer. Development or worsening of these conditions may require discontinuation of the drug.
● Give patient package insert describing estrogen adverse reactions, and also provide verbal explanation.
● Closely monitor patients with diabetes mellitus for loss of diabetes control.
● If patient is receiving a warfarin-type anticoagulant, monitor PT and INR for anticoagulant dosage adjustment.
● Estrogen therapy is usually administered cyclically. The drugs are usually given once daily for 3 weeks, followed by 1 week without the drugs; this regimen is repeated as necessary.

Pregnant patients
● Estrogens are contraindicated for use in pregnancy.

Breast-feeding patients
● Estrogens are contraindicated in breast-feeding women.

Pediatric patients
● Because of the effects of estrogen on epiphyseal closure, use estrogens cautiously in adolescents whose bone growth isn't complete.
● Estrogens aren't used in children.

Geriatric patients
● Postmenopausal women with long-term estrogen use have an increased risk of endometrial cancer if they have a uterus. This risk can be reduced by adding a progestin to the regimen.

Patient education
● Warn patient to report adverse reactions immediately.
● Tell men on long-term therapy about possible gynecomastia and impotence.
● Explain to patient on cyclic therapy for postmenopausal symptoms that, although withdrawal bleeding may occur in week off drug, fertility hasn't been restored; ovulation doesn't occur.
● Diabetic patients should report symptoms of hyperglycemia or glycosuria.
● Tell women who are planning to breast-feed not to take estrogens.

Representative combinations
Estradiol cypionate with testosterone cypionate and chlorobutanol: Depo-Testadiol, Duo-Cyp, Menoject, testosterone cypionate and estradiol cypionate, depAndrogyn, Depotestogen, Test-Estro Cypionate.

Estradiol valerate with testosterone enanthate: Deladumone, Delatestadiol, Teev, Testosterone Enanthate and Estradiol Valerate Injection, Valertest.

Estrogen with methyltestosterone: Estratest, Estratest H.S.

Estrogenic substances (conjugated) with methyltestosterone: Premarin with methyltestosterone; with medroxyprogesterone: Premphase, Prempro.

Ethinyl estradiol with norethindrone: Brevicon, Estrostep, Genora 1/35, Jenest, Loestrin Fe 1.5/30, ModiCon, Nelova 1/35E, Ortho-Novum 1/35, Ortho-Novum 7/7/7, Ortho-Novum 10/11, Ovcon, Tri-Norinyl; with norgestimate: Cyclen, Ortho-Cyclen, Ortho Tri-Cyclen; with ethynodiol diacetate: Demulen 1/35, Demulen 1/50; with desogestrel: Desogen, Marvelon, Mircette, Ortho-Cept; with norgestrel: Lo/Ovral, Ovral; with levonorgestrel: Alesse, Levlen, Min-Ovral, Nordette, Tri-Levlen, Triphasil, Triquilar, Trivora.

Ethynodiol diacetate with ethinyl estradiol: Demulen 1/35, Demulen 1/50.

fluoroquinolones

ciprofloxacin, enoxacin, gatifloxacin, levofloxacin, lomefloxacin hydrochloride, moxifloxacin, norfloxacin, ofloxacin, sparfloxacin, trovafloxacin esylate/alatrofloxacin mesylate

Fluoroquinolones are broad-spectrum, systemic antibacterial agents active against a wide range of aerobic gram-positive and gram-negative organisms. Gram-positive aerobic bacteria include *Staphlococcus aureus, S. epidermis, S. hemolyticus, S. saprophyticus,* penicillinase- and nonpenicillinase-producing staphlococci as well as some methicillin-resistant strains, *Streptococcus pneumoniae,* group A (beta) hemolytic streptococci *(S. pyogenes),* group B streptococci *(S. agalactiae), viridans streptococci,* groups C, F, and G streptococci and nonenterococcal group D streptococci, *Enterococcus faecalis.* These drugs are active against gram-positive aerobic bacilli including *Corynebacterium, Listeria monocytogenes,* and *Nocardia asteroides*

Fluoroquinolones are effective against gram-negative aerobic bacteria including, but not limited to, *Neisseria meningitidis* and most strains of penicillinase- and non-penicillinase-producing *Haemophilus ducreyi, H. influenzae, H. parainfluenzae, Moraxella catarrhalis, Neisseria gonorrhoeae,* and most clinically important Enterobacteriaceae, *P. aeruginosa, Vibrio cholerae,* and *V. parahaemolyticus.* Certain fluoroquinolones are active against *Chlamydia trachomatis, Legionella pneumophila, Mycobacterium avium-intracellulare, Mycoplasma homini,* and *M. pneumoniae.*

Pharmacology
Fluoroquinolones produce a bactericidal effect by inhibiting intracellular DNA topoisomerase II (DNA gyrase) or topoisomerase IV. These enzymes are essential catalysts in the duplication, transcription, and repair of bacterial DNA. (See *Comparing fluoroquinolones,* see pages 42 and 43.)

Indications and actions
Fluoroquinolones are indicated for the treatment of the following infections when caused by susceptible organisms: bone and joint infections, bacterial bronchitis, endocervical and urethral chlamydial infections, bacterial gastroenteritis, endocervical and urethral gonorrhea, intraabdominal infections, empiric therapy for febrile neutropenia, pelvic inflammatory disease, bacterial pneumonia, bacterial prostatitis, acute sinusitis, skin and soft tissue infections, typhoid fever, bacterial urinary tract infections, chancroid, meningococcal carriers, and bacterial septicemia. Fluoroquinolones may be used for the prevention of bacterial urinary tract infections.

Comparing fluoroquinolones

Drug	Oral bioavailability (%)	Plasma protein binding (%)	Half-life (hr)
ciprofloxacin	70-80 (with food)	20-40	Normal renal function: 4-6 Severe renal failure: 6-8
enoxacin	90	40	Normal renal function: 3-6 Severe renal failure: 9-10
gatifloxacin	96 (without regard to food)	20	Normal renal function: 7-14 Severe renal failure: 36
levofloxacin	100 (without regard to food)	50	Normal renal function: 6 Severe renal failure: 76
lomefloxacin	78-86 (without regard to food)	10	Normal renal function: not stated Severe renal failure: 21-45
moxifloxacin	90 (without regard to food)	50	Normal renal function: 10-14
norfloxacin	30-40 (without regard to food)	10-15	Normal renal function: 3-4 Severe renal failure: 9-10
ofloxacin	98 (without regard to food)	20-25	Normal renal function: 4½-7 Severe renal failure: 28-37
sparfloxacin	92 (without regard to food)	45	Normal renal function: 16-30 Severe renal failure: 38.5
trovafloxacin/ alatrofloxacin	88 (with food)	76	Normal renal function: 9-11¼

Overview of adverse reactions

The following adverse effects are observed rarely with fluoroquinolones, but require medical attention: CNS stimulation (acute psychosis, agitation, hallucinations, tremors); hepatotoxicity; hypersensitivity reactions; interstitial nephritis; phlebitis; pseudomembranous colitis; and tendinitis or tendon rupture. The following adverse effects require no medical attention unless they persist or become intolerable: CNS effects (dizziness, headache, nervousness, drowsiness, insomnia); GI reactions; and photosensitivity.

Special considerations

● Consider the risk-benefit ratio of therapy with fluoroquinolones on an individual basis when any of the following conditions is present: seizure disorders, cerebral ischemia, severe hepatic dysfunction, or renal insufficiency.
● Monitor renal and liver function tests in patients with impaired renal or hepatic function.
● Achilles and other tendon ruptures have been reported. Discontinue drug if patient experiences pain, inflammation, or rupture of a tendon.

Pregnant patients

● Pregnancy risk category is C. Adequate, well-controlled trials haven't been completed, but these drugs cross the placenta and may cause arthropathies.

Breast-feeding patients

● Whether fluoroquinolones are readily distributed into breast milk is unknown. Therefore, their use in nursing mothers isn't recommended because these drugs may cause arthropathies in newborns and infants.

Pediatric patients

● Fluoroquinolones aren't recommended because they can cause joint problems.

Geriatric patients

● Because renal function deteriorates over time, geriatric patients may require a reduction in their daily dose.

Patient education

● Instruct patient to take this medication as prescribed and to finish the full course of therapy.
● Tell patient to take the medication with an 8-oz glass of water.
● Enoxacin and norfloxacin should be taken on an empty stomach
● Instruct patient that if a dose is missed, the next dose should be taken as soon as possible; don't double the dose.

Peak concentration (hr)	Elimination	Dosage adjustment	Dialyzability
1-2	40-70% of drug is cleared unchanged by the kidneys in 24 hr	Renal impairment	< 10% removed by hemodialysis
1-3	40-60% of drug is cleared unchanged by the kidneys in 48 hr	Renal impairment	< 5% removed by hemodialysis
1-2	70% unchanged by the kidneys	Renal impairment	Not defiined
1	Almost entirely eliminated unchanged in the urine	Renal impairment	Not defiined
1½	60-80% of drug is cleared unchanged by the kidneys in 48 hr	Renal impairment	< 3% removed by hemodialysis
1-3	45% unchanged (20% in urine, 25% in feces)	None	Not defiined
1-2	26% of drug is cleared unchanged by the kidneys in 24 hr	Renal impairment	< 10% removed by hemodialysis
1-2	70-90% of drug is cleared unchanged by the kidneys in 36 hr	Renal impairment	< 10-30% removed by hemodialysis
3-6	10% is excreted unchanged in the urine	Renal Impairment	Not defiined
1-2	50% of oral dose (43% in feces and 6% in urine) excreted as unchanged drug	Cirrhosis	Not efficiently r-moved by dialysis

- Avoid concurrent use of antacids or sucralfate and orally administered fluoroquinolones.
- Don't take other medications without first checking with a pharmacist or prescriber.

Representative combinations
None.

histamine$_2$-receptor antagonists

cimetidine, famotidine, nizatidine, ranitidine, ranitidine bismuth citrate

The introduction of H$_2$-receptor antagonists has revolutionized the treatment of peptic ulcer disease. These drugs structurally resemble histamine and competitively inhibit the action of histamine on gastric H$_2$-receptor. Cimetidine, approved for clinical use in 1977, is the prototype of this class. (See *Adult dosages of histamine$_2$-receptor antagonists,* page 44.)

Pharmacology
All H$_2$-receptor antagonists inhibit the action of histamine at H$_2$-receptors in gastric parietal cells, reducing gastric acid output and concentration regardless of the stimulatory agent (histamine, food, insulin, caffeine, betazole, pentagastrin) or basal conditions.

Indications and actions
Duodenal ulcer
Cimetidine, famotidine, nizatidine, and ranitidine are used to treat acute duodenal ulcer and to prevent ulcer recurrence. Ranitidine bismuth citrate is used in combination with clarithromycin to treat active duodenal ulcer associated with *Helicobacter pylori* infection.

Gastric ulcer
Cimetidine famotidine, nizatidine, and ranitidine are indicated for acute gastric ulcer. However, the benefits of long-term therapy (over 8 weeks) with these drugs remain unproven.

Hypersecretory states
Cimetidine, famotidine, nizatidine, and ranitidine are used to treat hypersecretory states such as Zollinger-Ellison syndrome. Because patients with these conditions require much higher doses than patients with peptic ulcer disease, they may experience more pronounced adverse effects.

Reflux esophagitis
Cimetidine, famotidine, nizatidine, and ranitidine are used to provide short-term relief from gas-

◇ Unlabeled clinical use

Adult dosages of histamine$_2$-receptor antagonists

Indication	cimetidine	famotidine	nizatidine	ranitidine
Duodenal ulcer	P.O. 800 mg h.s. or 300 mg q.i.d. with meals and h.s. or 400 mg b.i.d.	P.O. 40 mg h.s. or 20 mg b.i.d..	P.O. 300 mg h.s. or 150 mg b.i.d..	P.O. 150 mg b.i.d. or 300 mg once per day after evening meal or h.s.
Duodenal ulcer maintenance	P.O. 400 mg h.s.	P.O. 20 mg h.s.	P.O. 150 mg h.s.	P.O. 150 mg h.s.
Gastric ulcer	P.O. 800 mg h.s. or 300 mg q.i.d. with meals and h.s.	P.O. 4 0 mg h.s.	P.O. 300 mg h.s. or 150 mg b.i.d.	P.O. 150 mg b.i.d.
Gastric ulcer maintenance	NA	NA	NA	P.O. 150 mg h.s.
Gastroesophageal reflux disease	P.O. 400 mg q.i.d. or 800 mg b.i.d.	P.O. 20 mg b.i.d.	P.O. 150 mg b.i.d.	P.O. 150 mg b.i.d.
Erosive esophagitis	P.O. 400 mg q.i.d. or 800 mg b.i.d.	P.O. 20-40 mg b.i.d.	P.O. 150 mg b.i.d.	P.O. 150 mg q.i.d.
Erosive esophagitis healing maintenance	NA	NA	NA	P.O. 150 mg b.i.d.
Pathological hypersecretory conditions	P.O. 300 mg q.i.d. with meals and h.s.	P.O. 20 mg Q 6 hours	NA	P.O. 150 mg b.i.d.
Prevention of upper GI bleeding	I.V.: 50 mg/hr continuous infusion	NA	NA	NA
Heartburn, acid indigestion,sour stomach	P.O. 200 mg, p.r.n., up to 200 mg b.i.d.	P.O. 10 mg, p.r.n., up to 10 mg b.i.d.	P.O. 75 mg, p.r.n., up to 75 mg b.i.d.	P.O. 75 mg p.r.n., up to 75 mg b.i.d.

NA: Not FDA-approved.

troesophageal reflux in patients who don't respond to conventional therapy (lifestyle changes, antacids, diet modification). They act by raising the stomach pH. Some clinicians prefer to combine the H$_2$-receptor antagonist with metoclopramide, but further study is necessary to confirm effectiveness of the combination.

Stress ulcer prophylaxis ◇
Cimetidine, famotidine, nizatidine, and ranitidine are used to prevent stress ulcers in critically ill patients, particularly those in intensive care units. However, this remains an unlabeled (FDA-unapproved) indication; some health care providers prefer intensive antacid therapy for such patients.

Other uses ◇
H$_2$-receptor antagonists have been used for a number of other unlabeled indications, including short-bowel syndrome, prophylaxis for allergic reactions to I.V. contrast medium, and to eradicate H. pylori in treatment of peptic ulcers. Ranitidine

bismuth citrate in combination with clarithromycin is used to treat H. pylori infection.

Other uses include relief of occasional heartburn, acid indigestion, or sour stomach.

Overview of adverse reactions
H$_2$-receptor antagonists rarely cause adverse reactions. However, mild transient diarrhea, neutropenia, dizziness, fatigue, arrhythmias, and gynecomastia have been reported.

Cimetidine may inhibit hepatic enzymes, thereby impairing the metabolism of certain drugs. Ranitidine may also produce this effect, but to a lesser extent. Famotidine and nizatidine haven't been shown to inhibit hepatic enzymes or drug clearance.

Special considerations
• Give a single daily dose at bedtime, twice-daily doses morning and evening, and multiple doses with meals and at bedtime. Most clinicians prefer the once-daily dose at bedtime regimen for improved compliance.

Histamine₂-receptor antagonists: Dosage adjustments for renal impairment

Drug	Estimated creatinine clearance (ml/min)	Recommended dosage adjustment
cimetidine	20-40	q 8 hr or 75% of normal dose
famotidine	< 10	q 24 hr or 50% of normal dose
nizatidine	20-50	150 mg/day (active treatment) or 150 mg every other day (maintenance)
ranitidine	< 50	150 mg q 24 hr; increase to q 12 hr as tolerated

● When administering drugs I.V., don't exceed recommended infusion rates because this may increase the risk of adverse CV effects. Continuous I.V. infusion may yield better suppression of acid secretion.

● Because antacids may decrease drug absorption, give them at least 1 hour apart from H₂-receptor antagonists.

● Patients with renal disease may need a modified schedule. (See *Histamine₂-receptor antagonists: Dosage adjustments for renal impairment.*)

● Avoid discontinuing these drugs abruptly.

● Many investigational uses for these drugs (particularly cimetidine) are being evaluated. Ranitidine bismuth citrate shouldn't be prescribed alone for the treatment of active duodenal ulcers.

● Symptomatic response to therapy doesn't rule out gastric malignancy.

Pregnant patients
● There are no adequate controlled studies in pregnant women. Cimetidine may potentially result in reversible decreased sperm concentrations in men.

Breast-feeding patients
● H₂-receptor antagonists may be secreted in breast milk. Ratio of risk to benefit must be considered.

Pediatric patients
● Safety and efficacy in children haven't been established.

Geriatric patients
● Use cautiously when administering these drugs to geriatric patients because of the increased risk of adverse reactions, particularly those affecting the CNS. Dosage adjustment is required in patients with impaired renal function.

Patient education
● Instruct patient to avoid smoking during drug therapy because smoking stimulates gastric acid secretion and worsens the disease.

Representative combinations
None.

HMG-CoA reductase inhibitors

atorvastatin, fluvastatin sodium, lovastatin, pravastatin sodium, simvastatin

HMG-CoA reductase inhibitors, also known as statins, are a highly effective class of medications that have become first line pharmacologic therapy for the management of hypercholesterolemia.

Pharmacology
Statins lower cholesterol by competitively inhibiting the enzyme 3-hydroxy-3-methyl-glutaryl-coenzyme A (HMG-CoA) reductase. This enzyme catalyzes the conversion of HMG-CoA to mevalonate, which is an early rate-limiting step in cholesterol biosynthesis. Statins decrease low-density lipoprotein cholesterol (LDL-C), total cholesterol (total-C), apoprotein B (apo-B), very low-density lipoprotein (VLDL) cholesterol, and plasma triglyceride levels, and they increase high-density lipoprotein cholesterol (HDL-C) levels. Coronary artery disease may be caused by increased levels of total cholesterol, apo-B, and LDL-C, as well as by decreased levels of HDL-C. In addition, CV morbidity and mortality rates vary directly with the level of total-C and LDL-C, and inversely with the level of HDL-C. The mechanism by which statins lower LDL-C may be related to both a reduction of VLDL cholesterol and an induction of the LDL receptor, which results in reduced synthesis or increased breakdown of LDL-C.

Statins are highly effective at lowering total and LDL-C in patients with heterozygous familial and nonfamilial forms of hypercholesterolemia. Initial cholesterol-lowering effects are seen within 1 to 2 weeks, with maximum lowering effects observed within 4 to 6 weeks. Because cholesterol synthesis occurs mainly at night, single daily doses of all the agents except atorvastatin should be given in the evening or at bedtime. Lovastatin should be taken with the evening meal because

Comparing HMG-CoA reductase inhibitors

Drug	Usual dose	Absolute bioavailability (%)	Metabolism enzymes	Active metabolite	Excretion (%)
atorvastatin	10-80 mg/day	14	CYP3A4	Yes	< 2 (urine)
fluvastatin	20-80 mg/day at bedtime	24	CYP2C9	Yes	< 6 (urine) ~ 90 (feces)
lovastatin	20-80 mg/day with evening meal	< 5	CYP3A4	No	10 (urine) 83 (feces)
pravastatin	10-40 mg/day at bedtime	17	not reported	No	~ 20 (urine) 70 (feces)
simvastatin	10-80 mg/day in evening	< 5	CYP3A4	No	13 (urine) 60 (feces)

food increases its absorption. (See *Comparing HMG-CoA reductase inhibitors.*)

Indications and actions
Cardiovascular events
All statins are indicated for the treatment of primary hypercholesterolemia and mixed dyslipidemia. Atorvastatin is indicated for hypertriglyceridemia and primary dysbetalipoproteinemia. Atorvastatin and simvastatin are indicated for homozygous familial hyperlipidemia. Pravastatin is indicated for the primary prevention of coronary events. All statins except atorvastatin are indicated for the secondary prevention of CV events.

Unlabeled uses ◊
Lovastatin: diabetic dyslipidemia; nephrotic hyperlipidemia; neck artery disease; familial beta dysbetalipoproteinemia; and familial combined hyperlipidemia
Pravastatin: heterozygous familial hypercholesterolemia; diabetic dyslipidemia in non-insulin-dependent diabetes; hypercholesterolemia secondary to the nephrotic syndrome; homozygous hypercholesterolemia in patients with reduced LDL receptor activity.
Simvastatin: heterozygous familial hypercholesterolemia, familial combined hyperlipidemia, diabetic dyslipidemia in type II diabetes, hyperlipidemia secondary to the nephrotic syndrome, and homozygous familial hypercholesterolemia in patients with defective LDL receptors.

Overview of adverse reactions
Statins are well tolerated and have very few adverse effects. Adverse reactions include photosensitivity, hepatotoxicity, defined as an increase in transaminase levels to greater than 3 times normal; mild, nonspecific GI complaints; transient and mild increase in creatine phosphokinase (CPK) levels; myopathy, characterized by myalgia; and muscle weakness associated with CPK values greater than 10 times the upper lim-

it of normal. Lovastatin and simvastatin may cause insomnia.

A rare hypersensitivity syndrome has been reported. It's characterized by at least one of the following features: anaphylaxis, angioedema, lupus erythematosus-like syndrome, polymyalgia rheumatica, vasculitis, purpura, thrombocytopenia, leukopenia, hemolytic anemia, positive antinuclear antibodies, increased erythrocyte sedimentation rate, eosinophilia, arthritis, asthenia, photosensitivity, fever, chills, flushing, malaise, dyspnea, toxic epidermal necrolysis, erythema multiforme, and dermatomyositis.

Special considerations
● Statins are contraindicated in pregnancy and lactation, as well as in patients with active liver disease or unexplained persistent elevations of liver function tests.
● Use statins cautiously in patients who consume large quantities of alcohol.
● Monitor LFTs before the initiation of statins and at 6 and 12 weeks following initiation of treatment or increasing the dose, and periodically (such as semiannually) thereafter. Discontinue drug if AST increases more than 3 times upper limits of normal.
● Closely monitor patients taking pravastatin with renal insufficiency.
● The absorption of lovastatin is increased when taken with food, and it should be taken with the evening meal. All other statins, except atorvastatin, may be taken without regard to meals, but should be taken in the evening or at bedtime, because most cholesterol synthesis occurs at night.
● The risk of myopathy is increased when statins are taken with cyclosporine, erythromycin, gemfibrozil, fibric acid derivatives, azole antifungals, or lipid-lowering doses of niacin.
● Because of increased risk of myopathy, avoid concurrent use of statins with fibrates.
● Consider myopathy in any patient with diffuse myalgias, muscle tenderness, weakness, or CPK

Protein binding (%)	Half-life (hr)	% LDL-C lowering
≥ 98	~ 14	26.5-60
98	< 1	18.9-35
> 95	3-4	21-40
~ 50	13/4	22-34
~ 95	3	14-47

increases greater than 10 times the upper limit of normal. Discontinue drug if markedly elevated CPK levels occur or if myopathy is suspected. Don't exceed 20 mg/day of lovastatin or 10 mg/day of simvastatin in patients taking cyclosporine or itraconazole.
● Withhold or discontinue statins in patients with risk factors for renal failure secondary to rhabdomyolysis including: severe acute infection; sepsis; hypotension; major surgery; trauma; severe metabolic, endocrine, or electrolyte disorders; and uncontrolled seizures.

Pregnant patients
● Statin drugs are pregnancy category X and are contraindicated during pregnancy.
● Cholesterol is essential for fetal development and drugs that inhibit cholesterol synthesis may have adverse effects on the developing fetus.
● If a patient becomes pregnant while taking a statin, discontinue the drug immediately.

Breast-feeding patients
● Some statins appear in breast milk. Because of the potential adverse effects, women shouldn't take statins while breast-feeding.

Pediatric patients
● Safety and efficacy in patients under age 18 haven't been established; use isn't recommended.

Geriatric patients
● Plasma levels don't vary with age for fluvastatin and atorvastatin. In patients over age 70, the area under the curve is increased with lovastatin and simvastatin. For pravastatin, patients over age 65 show a greater effect on LDL-C, total-C, and LDL:HDL ratio compared to patients under age 65.

Patient education
● Tell patient that statin drugs may cause photosensitivity and to avoid prolonged exposure to sun and other sources of ultraviolet light. Recommend wearing protective clothing and sunscreens.
● Instruct a woman of child-bearing age on the potential hazards of statin drugs in pregnancy. Tell her to discontinue drug immediately if she becomes pregnant and to notify prescriber.
● Instruct patient to promptly report any unexplained muscle pain, tenderness, or weakness, especially if accompanied by malaise or fever.
● Instruct patient on the importance of adhering to dietary recommendations.
● Tell patient to take lovastatin with the evening meal; fluvastatin, pravastatin, and simvastatin may be taken without regard to meals but should be taken in the evening or at bedtime for best results; atorvastatin may be taken without regard to meals and at any time of the day.

Representative combinations
None.

nitrates

amyl nitrite, isosorbide dinitrate, isosorbide mononitrate, nitroglycerin, pentaerythritol tetranitrate

Nitrates have been recognized as effective vasodilators for more than 100 years. The best-known drug of this group, nitroglycerin, remains the therapeutic mainstay for classic and variant angina. With the availability of a commercial I.V. nitroglycerin form, use of the drug in reducing afterload and preload in various cardiac disorders has generated renewed enthusiasm. Various other dosage forms of nitroglycerin and of other nitrates also are available, thereby improving and extending their clinical usefulness.

Pharmacology
The major pharmacologic property of nitrates is vascular smooth muscle relaxation, resulting in generalized vasodilation. Venous effects predominate; however, nitroglycerin produces dose-dependent dilatation of both arterial and venous beds. Nitrates are metabolized to a free radical nitric oxide, which is thought to be an endothelium-derived relaxing factor, which is usually impaired in patients with coronary artery disease. Decreased peripheral venous resistance results in venous pooling of blood and decreased venous return to the heart (preload); decreased arteriolar resistance reduces systemic vascular resistance and arterial pressure (afterload). These vascular effects lead to reduction of myocardial oxygen consumption, promoting a more favorable oxygen supply:demand ratio. Although nitrates reflexively increase heart rate and myocardial contractility, reduced ventricular wall tension results in a net decrease in myocardial oxygen consumption. In the coronary circulation, nitrates redistribute circulating blood flow

along collateral channels and preferentially increase subendocardial blood flow, improving perfusion to the ischemic myocardium.

Nitrates relax all smooth muscle—not just vascular smooth muscle—regardless of autonomic innervation, including bronchial, biliary, GI, ureteral, and uterine smooth muscle.

Indications and actions
Angina pectoris
By relaxing vascular smooth muscle in both the venous and arterial beds, nitrates cause a net decrease in myocardial oxygen consumption; by dilating coronary vessels, they lead to redistribution of blood flow to ischemic tissue. Although systemic and coronary vascular effects may vary slightly, depending on which nitrate is used, both smooth muscle relaxation and vasodilation probably account for the value of nitrates in treating angina. Because individual nitrates have similar pharmacologic and therapeutic properties, the best nitrate to use in a specific situation depends mainly on the onset of action and duration of effect required.

S.L. nitroglycerin is considered the drug of choice to treat acute angina pectoris because of its rapid onset of action, relatively low cost, and well-established effectiveness. Lingual or buccal nitroglycerin and other rapidly acting nitrates, such as amyl nitrite and S.L. or chewable isosorbide dinitrate, also may be useful for this indication. Amyl nitrite is rarely used because it's expensive, inconvenient, and carries a high risk of adverse effects. S.L., lingual, or buccal nitroglycerin or S.L. or chewable isosorbide dinitrate or mononitrate typically are effective in circumstances likely to provoke an angina attack.

Beta blockers usually are considered the drug of choice in the prophylactic management of angina pectoris. Nitrates with a relatively long duration of effect include oral preparations of isosorbide mononitrate and isosorbide dinitrate, and oral or topical nitroglycerin. Combination treatment of beta blockers and nitrates appears to be the therapy of choice.

The effectiveness of oral nitrates is debatable, although isosorbide dinitrate, isosorbide mononitrate, and nitroglycerin generally are considered effective. However, the effectiveness of topical nitroglycerin preparations haven't been fully determined. Some experts believe oral nitrates are ineffective or less effective than rapidly acting I.V. nitrates in reducing frequency of angina and increasing exercise tolerance. Also, prolonged use of oral nitrates may cause cross-tolerance to S.L. nitrates.

I.V. nitroglycerin may be used to treat unstable angina pectoris, Prinzmetal's angina, and angina pectoris in patients who haven't responded to recommended doses of nitrates or a beta blocker.

Sedatives may be useful in the adjunctive management of angina pectoris associated with psychogenic factors. However, if combination therapy is required, each drug should be adjusted individually; fixed combinations of oral nitrates and sedatives should be avoided.

Acute myocardial infarction
The hemodynamic effects of I.V., S.L., or topical nitroglycerin may prove beneficial in treating left ventricular failure and pulmonary congestion associated with acute MI. However, the effects of the drug on morbidity and mortality in patients with these conditions is controversial.

I.V., S.L., and topical nitroglycerin and isosorbide dinitrate are effective adjunctive agents in managing acute and chronic heart failure. S.L. administration can quickly reverse the signs and symptoms of pulmonary congestion in acute pulmonary edema; however, the I.V. form may control hemodynamic status more accurately.

Other uses
I.V. nitroglycerin is used to control perioperative hypertension, hypertensive emergencies, heart failure, and pulmonary edema associated with MI.

I.V. nitroglycerin has been used to treat severe hypertension and hypertensive crises ◇; other forms have been used to treat refractory heart failure ◇. Nitroglycerin also has been used for relief of pain, dysphagia, and spasm in patients with diffuse esophageal spasm without gastroesophageal reflux ◇.

Overview of adverse reactions
Headache is most common early in therapy; it may be severe, but usually diminishes rapidly. Orthostatic hypotension, dizziness, weakness, and transient flushing may occur. In patients sensitive to hypotensive effects, nausea, vomiting, weakness, restlessness, pallor, cold sweats, tachycardia, syncope, or CV collapse may occur. Dose reduction may control GI upset; discontinue therapy if blurred vision, dry mouth, or rash develops. Tolerance and dependence can occur with repeated, prolonged use.

Tolerance to both the vascular and antianginal effects of the drugs can develop, and cross-tolerance between the nitrates and nitrites has been demonstrated. Tolerance is associated with a high or sustained plasma drug level and occurs with oral, I.V., and topical therapy. It rarely occurs with intermittent S.L. use. However, patients taking oral isosorbide dinitrate or topical nitroglycerin haven't exhibited cross-tolerance to S.L. nitroglycerin.

To prevent tolerance, the lowest effective dose and an intermittent dosing schedule should be used. A nitrate-free interval of 10 to 12 hours daily may also be helpful.

Special considerations
Oral dosage form
● Provide a dosage regimen that incorporates a 10- to 12-hour nitrate-free interval.

• Best absorption occurs when taken on an empty stomach (1 hour before or 2 hours after meals) and with a full glass of water.

• Adjust dosage to patient response. Patient should avoid switching brands after they are stabilized on a particular formulation.

Buccal dosage form

• Place the tablet between the patient's upper lip or cheek and gum.

• Dissolution rate varies, but usually ranges from 3 to 5 hours. Hot liquids increase dissolution rate and should be avoided.

• Patient shouldn't use buccal form at bedtime because of risk of aspiration.

Sublingual dosage form

• Only the S.L. and translingual forms should be used to relieve acute anginal attack. Although a burning sensation was formerly an indication of the potency of a drug, many current preparations don't produce this sensation.

Translingual spray

• Only the S.L. and translingual forms should be used to relieve acute angina attack. Spray the translingual form onto or under the tongue. Patient shouldn't inhale the spray.

Topical dosage form

• To apply ointment, spread in uniform thin layer to any hairless part of the skin except distal parts of arms and legs, because absorption isn't maximal at these sites. Don't rub in. Cover with plastic film to aid absorption and to protect clothing. If using Tape-Surrounded Appli-Ruler (TSAR) system, keep TSAR on skin to protect clothing and ensure that ointment remains in place. If serious adverse reactions develop in patients using ointment or transdermal system, remove product at once or wipe ointment from skin. Be sure to avoid contact with ointment.

• Be sure to remove transdermal patch before defibrillation. Because of the aluminum backing of the patch, electric current may cause patch to explode.

• Don't administer with sildenafil (Viagra).

Pregnant patients

• Pregnancy risk category is C. There are no adequate controlled studies in pregnant women. Use only if clearly indicated.

Breast-feeding patients

• Excretion into breast milk is unknown. Use cautiously.

Pediatric patients

• Safety and effectiveness of nitrates in children haven't been established.

Patient education

• Advise patient to avoid alcohol while taking nitrates, because severe hypotension and CV collapse may occur.

• Instruct patient to sit or lie down when taking nitrates, to prevent injury from transient episodes

of dizziness, syncope, or other signs of cerebral ischemia that the drug may cause.

• Advise patient to treat headache with aspirin or acetaminophen.

• Tell patient to report blurred vision, dry mouth, or persistent headache.

• Warn patient not to stop taking drug abruptly because this may cause withdrawal symptoms.

• Advise patient that nitrates and sildenafil can't be taken together because the combination can produce life-threatening hypotension.

Representative combinations
None.

nonsteroidal anti-inflammatory drugs

celecoxib, choline magnesium trisalicylate, diclofenac potassium, diclofenac sodium, diflunisal, etodolac, fenoprofen calcium, flurbiprofen sodium, ibuprofen, indomethacin, indomethacin sodium trihydrate, ketoprofen, ketorolac tromethamine, mefenamic acid, meloxicam, tromethamine, nabumetone, naproxen, naproxen sodium, oxaprozin, piroxicam, rofecoxib, salsalate, sulindac, tolmetin sodium

NSAIDs are a growing class of drugs prescribed widely for their analgesic and anti-inflammatory effects; some members of this class have an antipyretic effect.

Pharmacology

The analgesic effect of NSAIDs may result from interference with the prostaglandins involved in pain. Prostaglandins appear to sensitize pain receptors to mechanical stimulation or to other chemical mediators (such as bradykinin and histamine). NSAIDs inhibit synthesis of prostaglandins peripherally and possibly centrally. Their anti-inflammatory action may also contribute indirectly to their analgesic effect.

Like the salicylates, the anti-inflammatory effects of NSAIDs may result in part from inhibition of prostaglandin synthesis and release during inflammation. The exact mechanism hasn't been established, but the anti-inflammatory effect of NSAIDs correlates with their ability to inhibit prostaglandin synthesis. Selective inhibition of the cyclo-oxygenase 2 (COX-2) enzyme by the COX-2 inhibitors results in the anti-inflammatory efficacy and pain relief equivalent to other NSAIDs but with improved safety in that these newer NSAIDs don't result in gastric and renal adverse effects resulting from the lack of inhibition of the COX-1 enzyme.

The antipyretic effect may be due to suppression of prostaglandin synthesis in the CNS (probably the hypothalamus).

Indications and actions
Pain, inflammation, and fever
NSAIDs are used principally for symptomatic relief of mild to moderate pain and inflammation. These agents usually provide temporary relief of mild to moderate pain, especially that associated with inflammation. NSAIDs are used to treat low-intensity pain of headache, arthralgia, myalgia, neuralgia, and mild to moderate pain from dental or surgical procedures or dysmenorrhea.

Oral NSAIDs are also used for long-term treatment of rheumatoid arthritis, juvenile arthritis, and osteoarthritis. In osteoarthritis, NSAIDs are used primarily for analgesia. NSAIDs offer only symptomatic treatment for rheumatoid conditions, and don't reverse or arrest the disease process. NSAIDs reduce pain, stiffness, swelling, and tenderness. COX-2 inhibitors such as celecoxib and rofecoxib are new NSAIDs which also exhibit anti-inflammatory and analgesic actions.

Overview of adverse reactions
Adverse reactions to oral NSAIDs chiefly involve the GI tract, particularly erosion of the gastric mucosa. Most common symptoms are dyspepsia, heartburn, epigastric distress, nausea, and abdominal pain. GI symptoms usually occur in the first few days of therapy, and often subside with continuous treatment. They can be minimized by administering NSAIDs with meals or food, antacids, or large quantities of water or milk.

CNS adverse effects (headache, dizziness, drowsiness) may also occur. Flank pain with other signs and symptoms of nephrotoxicity has occasionally been reported. Fluid retention may aggravate hypertension or heart failure. NSAIDs shouldn't be used in patients with renal insufficiency.

Special considerations
• Use NSAIDs cautiously in patients with history of GI disease, increased risk of GI bleeding, or decreased renal function.
• Patients with known "triad" symptoms (aspirin hypersensitivity, rhinitis or nasal polyps, and asthma) are at high risk of bronchospasm.
• NSAIDs may mask the signs and symptoms of acute infection.
• Administer oral NSAIDs with a full 8-oz (240-ml) glass of water to ensure adequate passage into stomach.
• Tablets may be crushed and mixed with food or fluids to aid swallowing, and with antacids to minimize gastric upset.
• Monitor patient for signs and symptoms of bleeding. Assess bleeding time if surgery is required.
• Monitor ophthalmic and auditory function before and periodically during therapy to prevent toxicity.

• Monitor CBC, platelets, PT, and hepatic and renal function studies periodically to detect abnormalities.
• Use of an NSAID with an opioid analgesic has an additive effect. Use of lower doses of the opioid analgesic may be possible.

Pregnant patients
• Pregnant women should avoid using all NSAIDs, especially during the third trimester, when prostaglandin inhibition may cause prolonged gestation, dystocia, and delayed parturition.

Breast-feeding patients
• Most NSAIDs are distributed into breast milk; NSAID therapy isn't recommended during breast-feeding.

Pediatric patients
• Don't use long-term NSAID therapy in children under age 14; safety hasn't been established.

Geriatric patients
• Patients over age 60 may be more susceptible to the toxic effects of NSAIDs because of decreased renal function, resulting in NSAID accumulation.
• The effects of NSAIDs on renal prostaglandins may cause fluid retention and edema, a significant drawback for geriatric patients, especially those with heart failure.

Patient education
• Tell patient to take medication with 8 oz (240 ml) of water or with food or milk if gastric irritation occurs.
• Explain to patient that taking drug as directed is necessary to achieve the desired effect; 2 to 4 weeks of treatment may be needed before benefit is seen.
• Advise patient on chronic NSAID therapy to arrange for monitoring of laboratory parameters, especially BUN, serum creatinine, liver function tests, and CBC.
• Warn patient with current rectal bleeding or history of rectal bleeding to avoid using rectal NSAID suppositories. Because they must be retained in the rectum for at least 1 hour, they may cause irritation and bleeding.
• Warn patient that use of alcoholic beverages while on NSAID therapy may cause increased GI irritation and, possibly, GI bleeding.

Representative combinations
Diclofenac sodium and misoprostil: Arthrotec.

nucleoside reverse transcriptase inhibitors

abacavir sulfate, didanosine, lamivudine, stavudine, zalcitidine, zidovudine

These antiviral agents act specifically against human immunodeficiency virus (HIV) through inhibition of HIV DNA polymerase (reverse transcriptase).

Pharmacology
Nucleoside reverse transcriptase inhibitors suppress HIV replication by inhibition of HIV DNA polymerase. Competitive inhibition of nucleoside reverse transcriptase inhibits DNA viral replication by chain termination, competitive inhibition of reverse transcriptase, or both. (See *Comparing nucleoside reverse transcriptase inhibitors*, pages 52 and 53.)

Indications and actions
Nucleoside reverse transcriptase inhibitors are indicated for the treatment of HIV infection and acquired immunodeficiency syndrome (AIDS). Note that two drug regimens containing only nucleoside reverse transcriptase inhibitors are now considered suboptimal. Combination therapy including protease inhibitors or nonnucleoside reverse transcriptase inhibitors are recommended. These agents may also be used for the prevention of maternal-fetal HIV transmission and in the prevention of HIV infection after occupational exposure (such as needlesticks or other parenteral exposures).

Overview of adverse reactions
Because of the complexity of HIV infection, it's often difficult to distinguish between disease-related symptoms and adverse drug reactions. The most frequently reported adverse effects of nucleoside reverse transcriptase inhibitors include anemia, leukopenia, and neutropenia. Less frequent adverse effects include thrombocytopenia. Rare adverse effects of nucleoside reverse transcriptase inhibitors include hepatotoxicity, myopathy, and neurotoxicity. The occurrence of any of the aforementioned adverse effects requires prompt medical attention. The following adverse effects don't require medical attention unless they persist or are bothersome: headache, severe insomnia, myalgias, nausea, or hyperpigmentation of nails.

Special considerations
● Consider the risk-benefit ratio of therapy with nucleoside reverse transcriptase inhibitors on an individual basis when any of the following conditions is present: alcoholism, cardiac disease, hypertriglyceridemia, pancreatitis, bone marrow suppression, fluid overload, folic acid or vitamin B_{12} deficiency, liver dysfunction, peripheral neuropathy, or renal or hepatic dysfunction. These conditions may predispose the patient to adverse drug reactions during treatment with nucleoside reverse transcriptase inhibitors.
● The bone marrow suppressant action of the nucleoside reverse transcriptase inhibitors may cause increased susceptibility to certain microbial infections; this effect may be accentuated by other medications that also cause bone marrow suppression.

Pregnant patients
● Pregnancy risk category is C (didanosine is category B). Adequate, well-controlled trials haven't been completed, but the risk of HIV transmission to the fetus is decreased with the use of nucleoside reverse transcriptase inhibitors during pregnancy. Teratogenicity or ill effects haven't been seen in neonates. This drug crosses the placenta and decreases the perinatal transmission of HIV. Prescribers are encouraged to contact the registry at 1-800-258-4263 to report pregnant women on therapy.

Breast-feeding patients
● The rate and extent of excretion of nucleoside reverse transcriptase inhibitors into breast milk is unknown. Therefore, their use in breast-feeding women isn't recommended. However, the risks and benefits to both the woman and infant must be considered in each case.

Pediatric patients
● Nucleoside reverse transcriptase inhibitors may be used in children age 3 months or older. The half-life of these agents may be prolonged in neonates, but otherwise the pharmacokinetic and safety profile of nucleoside reverse transcriptase inhibitors is similar in children and adults.

Geriatric patients
● Safety and efficacy of nucleoside reverse transcriptase inhibitors in elderly patients are unknown. Anecdotal evidence suggests that elderly patients respond well to this therapy, but that they may experience a more prolonged half-life of elimination.

Patient education
● Tell the patient to take the medication as prescribed, that it's important not to take more or less medication than instructed, and to finish the full course of therapy.
● Instruct patient not to miss a dose but, if a dose is missed, to take the next dose as soon as possible; don't double the dose.
● Advise patient to adhere to scheduled appointments because important blood tests are needed to evaluate the response to this drug.
● Tell patient not to take other medications without first checking with the pharmacist or prescriber.
● Instruct patient to floss and brush teeth carefully to prevent unnecessary bleeding from the gums.
● Tell patient to avoid sexual intercourse or to use a condom to decrease the risk of HIV transmission.

Representative combinations
Lamivudine and *zidovudine:* Combivir.

Comparing nucleoside reverse transcriptase inhibitors

Drug	Oral bioavailability	Plasma protein–binding (%)	Half-life (hr)	Elimination
abacavir sulfate	83% May be taken with or without food	About 50	1½	Renal clearance accounts for 82.2%; fecal elimination is 16%.
didanosine	Acid labile Variable absorption Taken on an empty stomach	< 5	Adults: ¾-2¾ Children: ½-1¼ Severe renal impairment: 4½	Renal clearance by glomerular filtration and active tubular secretion accounts for 50% of total body clearance.
lamivudine	60%-88% Food reduces the rate but not the extent of absorption	36	Adults: 2-11 Children: 1¾-2 Creatinine clearance (CrCl) 10-40 ml/min: 13½ CrCl < 10 ml/min: 19½	Renal clearance by glomerular filtration and active tubular secretion accounts for 68%-71% of total body clearance.
stavudine	78%-86% May take with or without food	Negligible	Adults: 1-1½ Children: 1-1¼ CrCl < 25 ml/min: 4¾	Renal clearance by glomerular filtration and active tubular secretion; 40% is excreted unchanged in 6-24 hr.
zalcitidine	80% in adults 54% in children Food decreases bioavailability by 14%.	< 4	Adults: 1-3 Children: ¾ CrCl < 55 ml/min: 8½	70% excreted unchanged in urine.
zidovudine	65% Effect of food on bioavailability is unknown.	34-38	Adults: 1 CrCl < 20 ml/min: 1½	90% excreted in urine.

opioids

alfentanil hydrochloride, codeine phosphate, codeine sulfate, difenoxin hydrochloride, diphenoxylate hydrochloride, fentanyl citrate, hydromorphone hydrochloride, levomethadyl acetate hydrochloride, meperidine hydrochloride, methadone hydrochloride, morphine sulfate, oxycodone hydrochloride, oxymorphone hydrochloride, propoxyphene hydrochloride, propoxyphene napsylate, remifentanil hydrochloride, sufentanil citrate

Opioids, previously called narcotic agonists, are usually understood to include natural and semisynthetic alkaloid derivatives from opium and their synthetic surrogates, whose actions mimic those of morphine. Most of these drugs are classified as Schedule II by the Federal Drug Enforcement Agency because they have a high potential for addiction and abuse. In the past, opioids were used indiscriminately for analgesia and sedation and to control diarrhea and cough. (See *Comparing opioids*, page 54.)

Pharmacology

Opioids act as agonists at specific opiate receptor binding sites in the CNS and other tissues; these are the same receptors occupied by endogenous opioid peptides (enkephalins and endorphins) to alter CNS response to painful stimuli. Opiate agonists don't alter the cause of pain, but only the patient's perception of the pain; they relieve pain without affecting other sensory functions. Opiate receptors are present in highest concentrations in the limbic system, thalamus, striatum, hypothalamus, midbrain, and spinal cord.

Opioids produce respiratory depression by a direct effect on the respiratory centers in the brain stem, resulting in decreased sensitivity and responsiveness to increases in carbon dioxide tension. The antitussive effects of these drugs are mediated by a direct suppression of the cough reflex center. They cause nausea, probably by

Dialyzability	Dosage	Dosage adjustment
Not known	Adults: 300 mg b.i.d. Children: 8 mg/kg b.i.d. up to a maximum of 300 mg b.i.d.	Not known
20% loss following a 4-hr dialysis	Adults > 132 lb (60 kg): 200 mg (tablets) q 12 hr, or 250 mg (buffered powder) q 12 hr Adults < 132 lb (60 kg): 125 mg (tablets) q 12 hr, or 167 mg (buffered powder) q 12 hr Children: 31 to 125 mg q 8-12 hr based on body surface area	No adjustment for renal or hepatic failure.
Not known	Adults > 110 lb (50 kg): 150 mg b.i.d. Adults < 110 lb (50 kg): 2 mg/kg b.i.d. Children: 4 mg/kg b.i.d. to maximum of 150 mg q 12 hr	Patients 16 or older with renal impairment require dosage adjustment.
Not known	Adults < 132 lb (60 kg): 30 mg q 12 hr Adults > 132 lb (60 kg): 40 mg q 12 hr Children 66-132 lb (30-60 kg): 30 mg q 12 hr Children < 66 lb (30 kg): 1 mg/kg q 12 hr	Patients with CrCl < 50 ml/min may require dosage adjustment.
Not known	Adults > 66 lb (30 kg): 0.75 mg q 8 hr	Patients with CrCl < 50 ml/min may require dosage adjustment.
Negligible effect	Adults: 600 mg/day in divided doses Children: 3 months to 12 years: 180 mg/m2 q 6 hr (720 mg/m²/day), not to exceed 200 mg q 6 hr	Patients with anemia, neutropenia, renal disease may require adjustment.

stimulation of the chemoreceptor trigger zone in the medulla oblongata; through orthostatic hypotension, which causes dizziness; and possibly by increasing vestibular sensitivity.

Opioids also cause drowsiness, sedation, euphoria, dysphoria, mental clouding, and EEG changes; higher than usual analgesic doses cause anesthesia. Most opioids cause miosis, although meperidine and its derivatives may also cause mydriasis or no pupillary change.

Because opioids decrease gastric, biliary, and pancreatic secretions and delay digestion, constipation is a common adverse reaction. At the same time, these drugs increase tone in the biliary tract and may cause biliary spasms. Some patients may have no biliary effects, whereas others may have biliary spasms that increase plasma amylase and lipase levels up to 15 times normal values.

Opioids increase smooth muscle tone in the urinary tract and induce spasms, causing urinary urgency. These drugs have little CV effect in a supine patient, but may cause orthostatic hypotension when the patient assumes upright pos-

ture. These drugs are also associated with manifestations of histamine release or peripheral vasodilation, including pruritus, flushing, red eyes, and sweating. These effects are often mistakenly attributed to allergy and should be evaluated carefully.

Opiates can be divided chemically into three groups: phenanthrenes (codeine, hydrocodone, hydromorphone, morphine, oxycodone, and oxymorphone); diphenylheptanes (levomethadyl, methadone, and propoxyphene); and phenylpiperidines (alfentanil, diphenoxylate, fentanyl, meperidine, and remifentanil, sufentanil). If a patient is hypersensitive to an opioid, agonist-antagonist, or antagonist of a given chemical group, use extreme caution when considering the use of another agent from the same chemical group; however, a drug from the other groups might be well tolerated.

Some opioids are well absorbed after oral or rectal administration; others must be administered parenterally. I.V. dosing is the most rapidly effective and reliable; absorption after I.M. or S.C. dosing may be erratic. Opioids vary in onset

Comparing opioids

Drug	Route	Onset (min)	Peak	Duration (hr)
alfentanil	I.V.	Immediate	Not available	Not available
codeine	I.M., P.O., S.C.	15-30	30-60 min	4-6
fentanyl	I.M., I.V.	7-8	Not available	1-2
hydrocodone	P.O.	30	60 min	4-6
hydromorphone	I.M., I.V., S.C.	15	30 min	4-5
	P.O., rectal	30	60 min	4-5
meperidine	I.M.	10-15	30-50 min	2-4
	P.O.	15-30	60 min	2-4
	S.C.	10-15	40-60 min	2-4
methadone	I.M., P.O., S.C.	30-60	30-60 min	4-6†
morphine	I.M.	≤ 20	30-60 min	3-7
	P.O., rectal	≤ 20	≤ 60 min	3-7
	S.C.	≤ 20	50-90 min	3-7
oxycodone	P.O.	15-30	30-60 min	4-6
oxymorphone	I.M., S.C.	10-15	30-60 min	3-6
	I.V.	5-10	30-60 min	3-6
	rectal	15-30	30-60 min	3-6
propoxyphene	P.O.	20-60	2-2½ hr	4-6
remifentanil	I.V.	Immediate	Not available	Not available
sufentanil	I.V.	1.3-3	Not available	Not available

† Because of cumulative effects, duration of action increases with repeated doses.

and duration of action; they are removed rapidly from the bloodstream and distributed, in decreasing order of concentration, into skeletal muscle, kidneys, liver, intestinal tract, lungs, spleen, and brain; they readily cross the placenta.

Opioids are metabolized mainly in the microsomes in the endoplasmic reticulum of the liver (first-pass effect) and also in the CNS, kidneys, lungs, and placenta. They undergo conjugation with glucuronic acid, hydrolysis, oxidation, or N-dealkylation. They are excreted primarily in the urine; small amounts are excreted in the feces.

Indications and actions

The opioids produce varying degrees of analgesia and have antitussive, antidiarrheal, and sedative effects. Clinical response is dose-related and varies with each patient.

Analgesia

Opioids may be used in the symptomatic management of moderate to severe pain associated with acute and some chronic disorders, including renal or biliary colic, MI, acute trauma, postoperative pain, or terminal cancer. They also may be used to provide analgesia during diagnostic

and orthopedic procedures and during labor. Drug selection, route of administration, and dose depend on a variety of factors. For example, in mild pain, oral therapy with codeine or oxycodone usually suffices. In acute pain of known short duration, such as that associated with diagnostic procedures or orthopedic manipulation, a short-acting drug such as meperidine or fentanyl is effective. These drugs are often given to alleviate postoperative pain, but because they influence CNS function, special care should be taken to monitor the course of recovery and to detect early signs of complications. Opioids are commonly used to manage severe, chronic pain associated with terminal cancer; this requires careful evaluation and titration of drug used, dose, and route of administration.

Pulmonary edema

Morphine, meperidine, oxymorphone, hydromorphone, and other similar drugs have been used to relieve anxiety in patients with dyspnea associated with acute pulmonary edema and acute left ventricular failure. These drugs shouldn't be used to treat pulmonary edema resulting from a chemical respiratory stimulant. Opioids decrease peripheral resistance, causing pooling of blood in the limbs and decreased venous return, cardiac workload, and pulmonary venous pressure; blood is shifted from the central to the peripheral circulation.

Preoperative sedation

Routine use of opioids for preoperative sedation in patients without pain isn't recommended because it may cause complications during and after surgery. To allay preoperative anxiety, a barbiturate or benzodiazepine is equally effective, with a lower risk of postoperative vomiting.

Anesthesia

Certain opioids, including alfentanil, fentanyl, remifentanil, and sufentanil, may be used for induction of anesthesia, as an adjunct in the maintenance of general and regional anesthesia, or as a primary anesthetic agent in surgery.

Cough suppression

Some opioids, most commonly codeine and its derivative, hydrocodone, are used as antitussives to relieve dry, nonproductive cough.

Diarrhea

Diphenoxylate and other opioids are used as antidiarrheal agents. All opioids cause constipation to some degree; however, only a few are indicated for this use. Usually, opiate antidiarrheals are empirically combined with antacids, absorbing agents, and belladonna alkaloids in commercial preparations.

Overview of adverse reactions

Respiratory depression and, to a lesser extent, circulatory depression (including orthostatic hypotension) are the major hazards of treatment with opioids. Rapid I.V. administration increases the risk of these serious adverse effects. Respiratory arrest, shock, and cardiac arrest have occurred. It's likely that equianalgesic doses of individual opiates produce a comparable degree of respiratory depression, but its duration may vary. Other adverse CNS effects include dizziness, visual disturbances, mental clouding or depression, sedation, coma, euphoria, dysphoria, weakness, faintness, agitation, restlessness, nervousness, seizures, and, rarely, delirium and insomnia. Adverse effects seem to be more common in ambulatory patients and those not experiencing severe pain. Adverse GI effects include nausea, vomiting, and constipation, as well as increased biliary tract pressure that may result in biliary spasm or colic. Tolerance, psychological dependence, and physical dependence (addiction) may follow prolonged, high-dose therapy (more than 100 mg of morphine daily for more than 1 month).

Use opiate agonists extremely cautiously during pregnancy and labor, because they readily cross the placenta. Premature infants appear especially sensitive to their respiratory and CNS depressant effects when used during delivery.

Opiate agonists have a high potential for addiction and should always be administered cautiously in patients susceptible to physical or psychological dependence. The agonist-antagonists have a lower potential for addiction and abuse, but the liability still exists.

Special considerations

● Administer extremely cautiously to patients with head injury, increased intracranial pressure, seizures, asthma, COPD, alcoholism, prostatic hypertrophy, severe hepatic or renal disease, acute abdominal conditions, arrhythmias, hypovolemia, or psychiatric disorders, and to geriatric or debilitated patients. Reduced doses may be necessary.

● Keep resuscitative equipment and a narcotic antagonist (naloxone) available. Prepare to provide support of ventilation and gastric lavage.

● Parenteral administration of opiates provides better analgesia than oral administration. Give I.V. administration by slow injection, preferably in diluted solution. Rapid I.V. injection increases the risk of adverse effects.

● Give parenteral injections by I.M. or S.C. route cautiously to patients who are chilled, hypovolemic, or in shock, because decreased perfusion may lead to accumulation of the drug and toxic effects. Rotate I.M. or S.C. injection sites to avoid induration.

● A regular dosing schedule (rather than "as needed for pain") is preferred to alleviate the symptoms and anxiety that accompany pain.

● Duration of respiratory depression may be longer than the analgesic effect. Monitor patient closely with repeated dosing.

● With long-term administration, evaluate patient's respiratory status before each dose. Because severe respiratory depression may occur (especially with accumulation from chronic dosing), watch for respiratory rate below the patient's baseline level. Evaluate patient for restlessness, which may be a sign of compensatory response for hypoxia.

● Opiates or agonist-antagonists may cause orthostatic hypotension in ambulatory patients. The patient should sit or lie down to relieve dizziness or fainting.

● Because opiates depress respiration when used postoperatively, encourage patient turning, coughing, and deep breathing to avoid atelectasis.

● If gastric irritation occurs, give oral products with food; food delays absorption and onset of analgesia.

● Opiates may obscure the signs and symptoms of an acute abdominal condition or worsen gallbladder pain.

● The antitussive activity of opiates is used to control persistent, exhausting cough or dry, nonproductive cough.

● The first sign of tolerance to the therapeutic effect of opioid agonists or agonist-antagonists is usually a shortened duration of effect.

• Preservative-free morphine (Astramorph, Duramorph) is available for epidural or intrathecal use.

Pregnant patients
• Meperidine and oxymorphone hydrochloride are classified as pregnancy risk category B, but D if used for a prolonged time or for high doses used at term. Most opioids are listed as pregnancy risk category C.
• Administration of an opiate to a woman shortly before delivery may cause respiratory depression in the neonate. Watch closely and be prepared to resuscitate.

Breast-feeding patients
• Codeine, meperidine, methadone, morphine, and propoxyphene appear in breast milk and should be used cautiously in breast-feeding women.
• Methadone may cause physical dependence in breast-feeding infants of women on maintenance therapy.

Pediatric patients
• Safety and efficacy in children haven't been established. Use care when administering to children.

Geriatric patients
• Lower doses are usually indicated for elderly patients, who may be more sensitive to the therapeutic and adverse effects of drug.

Patient education
• Instruct patient to use drug cautiously and to avoid hazardous activities that require full alertness and coordination.
• Tell patient to avoid drinking alcohol when taking opioid agonists, because alcohol causes additive CNS depression.
• Explain that constipation may result from taking an opiate. Suggest measures to increase dietary fiber content, or recommend a stool softener.
• If patient's condition allows, instruct patient to breathe deeply, cough, and change position every 2 hours to avoid respiratory complications.
• Encourage patient to void at least every 4 hours to avoid urine retention.
• Tell the patient to take drug as prescribed and to call if significant adverse effects occur.
• Tell patient not to increase dose if he isn't experiencing the desired effect, but to call for prescribed dosage adjustment.
• Instruct the patient not to double the dose. Tell him to take a missed dose as soon as he remembers unless it's almost time for the next dose. If this is the case, he should skip the missed dose and go back to the regular dosing schedule.
• Tell patient to call immediately for emergency help if he thinks he or someone else has taken an overdose.
• Explain signs of overdose to patient and his family.

Representative combinations
Codeine with acetaminophen: Aceta with codeine, Acetaminophen with Codeine Oral Solution, Acetaminophen with Codeine Tablets, Capital with codeine, Margesic No. 3, Phenaphen with codeine, Tylenol with codeine, Tylenol with Codeine No. 4, Phenaphen with Codeine No. 4; with caffeine: Fioricet with codeine; with calcium iodide and alcohol: Calcidrine.

Codeine phosphate with guaifenesin: Cheracol, Guiatuss AC, Guiatussin with Codeine Liquid, Mytussin AC, Robitussin A-C, Tolu-Sed Cough; with iodinated glycerol: Tussi-Organidin NR; with triprolidine hydrochloride and pseudoephedrine hydrochloride: Actifed with Codeine.

Codeine with aspirin: Aspirin with Codeine No. 3, Aspirin with Codeine No. 4, Empirin with codeine.

Codeine and aspirin with caffeine and butalbital: Fiorinal with Codeine; with carisoprodol: Soma Compound with Codeine.

Dihydrocodeine with acetaminophen and caffeine: Synalgos-DC.

Fentanyl with droperidol: Droperidol, Fentanyl Citrate, and Innovar.

Hydrocodone bitartrate with acetaminophen: Anexsia 5/500 Tablets, Anexsia 7.5/650 Tablets, Anexsia 10/660 Tablets, Bancap HC, Co-Gesic, Damason-P, Dolacet, Duocet, Hydrocet, Hydrocodone Bitartrate and Acetaminophen Tablets, Hydrogesic, Hy-phen, Lorcet-HD, Lorcet Plus, Lortab, Lortab Elixir, Vicodin, Vicodin ES, Zydone; with aspirin: Lortab ASA, Panasal 5/500; with aspirin and caffeine: Damason-P; with aspirin, acetaminophen, and caffeine: Hyco-Pap; with guaifenesin: Hycotuss Expectorant Syrup (with alcohol); with guaifenesin and pseudoephedrine hydrochloride: Detussin Expectorant, Entuss-D; with guaifenesin and phenindamine tartrate: P-V-Tussin tablets; with guaifenesin and phenylephrine: Donatussin DC; with potassium guaiacosulfonate: Codiclear DH, Entuss-D Liquid; with pseudoephedrine hydrochloride: Detussin Liquid; with homatropine methylbromide: Hycodan; with phenylephrine hydrochloride and pyrilamine maleate: Codimal DH; with phenylpropanolamine hydrochloride: Hycomine; with phenylephrine hydrochloride, pyrilamine maleate, chlorpheniramine maleate salicylamide, citric acid, and caffeine: Citra Forte; with pheniramine maleate, pyrilamine maleate, potassium citrate, and ascorbic acid: Citra forte; with phenylephrine hydrochloride, phenylpropanolamine hydrochloride, pheniramine maleate, pyrilamine maleate, and alcohol: Ru-Tuss with hydrocodone; with guaifenesin and alcohol: S-T Forte; with phenyltoloxamine: Tussionex.

Hydromorphone with guaifenesin: Dilaudid Cough.

Meperidine with promethazine: Mepergan, Mepergan Fortis; with atropine sulfate: Atropine and Demerol Injection.

Oxycodone hydrochloride with acetaminophen: Oxycocet*, Oxycodone with Acetaminophen

Capsules, Percocet, Percocet-Demi, Roxicet, Roxicet 5/500 Caplets, Roxicet Oral Solution, Roxilox Capsules, Tylox; with aspirin: Oxycodone with Aspirin Tablets, Roxiprin Tablets; with oxycodone terephthalate and aspirin: Percodan, Percodan-Demi.

Propoxyphene with acetaminophen: Darvocet-N, E-Lor Tablets, Genagesic, Lorcet, Propacet 100, Pro-poxyphene Napsylate and Acetaminophen, Wygesic.

Propoxyphene napsylate with acetaminophen: Darvocet-N 50, Darvocet-N 100, Propocet 100; with aspirin: Propoxyphene HCl Compound Capsules; with aspirin and caffeine: Darvon Compound, Propoxyphene Compound, PC-Cap.

opioid agonist-antagonists

buprenorphine hydrochloride, butorphanol tartate, nalbuphine hydrochloride, pentazocine hydrochloride

The term opioid (or narcotic) agonist-antagonist is somewhat imprecise. Drugs in this class have varying degrees of agonist and antagonist activity. These drugs are potent analgesics, with somewhat less addiction potential than the pure narcotic agonists.

Pharmacology

The detailed pharmacology of these drugs is poorly understood. Each agent is believed to act on different opiate receptors in the CNS to a greater or lesser degree, thus yielding slightly different effects. Like the opioid agonists, these drugs can be divided into related chemical groups. Buprenorphine, butorphanol, and nalbuphine are phenanthrenes, like morphine, whereas pentazocine falls into a unique class, the benzmorphans.

Indications and actions
Pain
Opioid agonist-antagonists are primarily used as analgesics, particularly in patients at high risk for drug dependence or abuse. Some are used as preoperative or preanesthetic medication, to supplement balanced anesthesia, or to relieve prepartum pain.

Other uses
Buprenorphine has been used to reverse fentanyl-induced anesthesia ◊. Buprenorphine and naloxone have been used to reduce opiate consumption in patients who are physically dependent on opiates.

Overview of adverse reactions
Major hazards of agonist-antagonists are respiratory depression, apnea, shock, and cardiopulmonary arrest, possibly causing death. All opioid agonist-antagonists can cause respiratory depression, but the severity of such depression

each drug can cause has a "ceiling"; for example, each drug depresses respiration to a certain point, but increased doses don't depress it further. All opioid agonist-antagonists have been reported to cause withdrawal symptoms after abrupt discontinuation of long-term use; they appear to have some addiction potential, but less than that of the pure opioid agonists.

CNS effects are the most common adverse reactions and may include drowsiness, sedation, light-headedness, dizziness, hallucinations, disorientation, agitation, euphoria, dysphoria, insomnia, confusion, headache, tremor, miosis, seizures, and psychological dependence. CV reactions may include tachycardia, bradycardia, palpitations, chest wall rigidity, hypertension, hypotension, syncope, and edema. GI reactions may include nausea, vomiting, and constipation (most common), dry mouth, anorexia, and biliary spasms (colic). Other effects include urine retention or hesitancy, decreased libido, flushing, rash, pruritus, and pain at the injection site.

Opioid agonist-antagonists can produce morphine-like dependence and thus have abuse potential. Psychological and physiologic dependence with drug tolerance can develop upon chronic repeated administration. Patients with dependence or tolerance to narcotic agonist-antagonists usually present with an acute abstinence syndrome or withdrawal signs and symptoms, of which the severity is related to the degree of dependence, abruptness of withdrawal, and the drug used.

Common signs and symptoms of withdrawal are yawning, lacrimation, and sweating (early); mydriasis, piloerection, flushing of face, tachycardia, tremor, irritability, and anorexia (intermediate); and muscle spasms, fever, nausea, vomiting, and diarrhea (late).

Special considerations
● Opioid agonist-antagonists are contraindicated in patients with known hypersensitivity to any drug of the same chemical group. Use these drugs with extreme caution in patients with supraventricular arrhythmias; avoid or administer drug extremely cautiously in patients with head injury or increased intracranial pressure, because neurologic parameters are obscured; during pregnancy and labor, because drug crosses placenta readily (premature infants are especially sensitive to respiratory and CNS depressant effects of opioid agonist-antagonists).

● Use opioid agonist-antagonists cautiously in patients with renal or hepatic dysfunction, because drug accumulation or prolonged duration of action may occur; in patients with pulmonary disease (asthma, COPD) because drug depresses respiration and suppresses cough reflex; in patients undergoing biliary tract surgery because drug may cause biliary spasm; in patients with convulsive disorders because drug may precipitate seizures; in geriatric and debilitated patients, who are more sensitive to both therapeutic and adverse drug effects; and in patients susceptible to physical or psychological addiction because of the high risk of addiction to this drug.

● Opioid agonist-antagonists have a lower potential for abuse than do opioid agonists, but the risk still exists.

● Before administration, visually inspect all parenteral products for particles and discoloration and note the strength of the solution.

● Parenteral administration of opioid agonist-antagonists provides better analgesia than does oral dosing. Give I.V. dosing by very slow injections, preferably in diluted solution. Rapid I.V. injection increases the risk of adverse effects.

● Give I.M. or S.C. injections cautiously to patients who are chilled, hypovolemic, or in shock, because decreased perfusion may lead to accumulation.

● Opioid agonist-antagonists, as well as opioid antagonists, can reverse the desired effects of opioids; thus, members of different pharmacologic groups (such as meperidine and buprenorphine) shouldn't be prescribed at the same time.

● Keep resuscitative equipment on hand and an opioid antagonist (naloxone) available. Be prepared to provide ventilation and gastric lavage.

● Patient tolerance may develop to the opiate agonist activity but doesn't develop to opiate antagonist activity.

● A regular dosing schedule (rather than an "as needed for pain" regimen) is preferable to alleviate the symptoms and anxiety that accompany pain.

● The duration of respiratory depression may be longer than the analgesic effect. Monitor patient closely with repeated dosing.

● During prolonged administration, regularly evaluate the patient's respiratory status. Because severe respiratory depression may occur (especially with accumulation on chronic dosing), watch for a respiratory rate that's less than the patient's baseline respiratory rate. Also evaluate patient for restlessness, which may be a compensatory response to hypoxia.

● Opioid agonist-antagonists may cause orthostatic hypotension in ambulatory patients. Advise patient to sit or lie down to relieve dizziness or fainting.

● Because opioid agonist-antagonists can depress respiration when used postoperatively, strongly encourage patient turning, coughing, and deep breathing to avoid atelectasis. Monitor respiratory status.

● Oral opioid agonist-antagonists may be taken with food to prevent gastric irritation. Food delays absorption and the onset of analgesia.

● Opioid agonist-antagonists may obscure the signs and symptoms of an acute abdominal condition or worsen gallbladder pain.

● The first sign of tolerance to the therapeutic effect of opioid agonist-antagonists is usually a reduced duration of effect.

Pregnant patients

● Most drugs in this class are pregnancy risk category C.

● Administering an opiate agonist-antagonist to a woman shortly before delivery may cause respiratory depression in the neonate. The infant must be closely monitored. Be prepared to resuscitate.

Breast-feeding patients

● These drugs aren't recommended for breast-feeding women.

Pediatric patients

● Neonates may be more susceptible to the respiratory depressant effects of opiate agonist-antagonists.

Geriatric patients

● Lower doses are usually indicated for elderly patients, who may be more sensitive to the therapeutic and adverse effects of these drugs.

Patient education

● Advise ambulatory patients to be cautious when performing tasks that require alertness, such as driving, if they're taking an opioid agonist-antagonist.

● Warn patient not to stop taking an opioid agonist-antagonist abruptly if he has been taking it for a prolonged period or at a high dose.

● Tell patient not to increase dose if it isn't producing the desired effect, but to call for prescribed dosage adjustment.

● Advise patient to avoid drinking alcohol when taking opioid agonist-antagonists because additive CNS depression will occur.

● Tell patient that constipation may result. Suggest measures to increase dietary fiber content or recommend a stool softener.

● Instruct patient not to double the dose. Tell him to take a missed dose as soon as he remembers unless it's almost time for the next dose. If this is the case, tell him to skip the missed dose and go back to regular dosing schedule.

● Tell patient to call for emergency help if he thinks he or someone else has taken an overdose.

● Explain signs of overdose to patient and to his family.

● Instruct patient to breathe deeply, cough, and change position every 2 hours to avoid respiratory complications.

● Encourage patient to void at least every 4 hours to avoid urine retention.

● Tell patient to take the drug as prescribed and to promptly report any significant adverse effects.

● Inform a woman taking an opioid agonist-antagonist to call promptly if she is planning or suspects pregnancy; warn her that her fetus may become addicted to drug.

Representative combinations

Pentazocine with acetaminophen: Talacen; with aspirin: Talwin Compound; with naloxone: Talwin NX.

Buprenorphine and naloxone.

penicillins

Natural penicillins: penicillin G benzathine, penicillin G potassium, penicillin G procaine, penicillin G sodium, penicillin V potassium

Aminopenicillins: amoxicillin trihydrate with clavulanate potassium, ampicillin, ampicillin sodium with sulbactam sodium, ampicillin trihydrate

Penicillinase-resistant penicillins: cloxacillin sodium, dicloxacillin sodium, nafcillin sodium, oxacillin sodium

Extended spectrum penicillins: mezlocillin sodium, piperacillin sodium, piperacillin sodium with tazobactam sodium, ticarcillin disodium, ticarcillin with clavulanate potassium

Penicillins are very effective antibiotics with low toxicity. Their activity was first discovered by Sir Alexander Fleming in 1928, but they weren't developed for use against systemic infections until 1940. Penicillin is naturally derived from a mold, *Penicillium chrysogenum.* New synthetic derivatives are created by chemical reactions that modify their structure, resulting in increased GI absorption, resistance to destruction by beta-lactamase (penicillinase), and a broader spectrum of susceptible organisms.

Pharmacology

The basic structure of penicillin is a thiazolidine ring connected to a beta-lactam ring that contains a side chain. This nucleus is the main structural requirement for antibacterial activity; modifications of the side chain alter the antibacterial and pharmacologic effects of penicillin.

Penicillins are generally bactericidal. They inhibit synthesis of the bacterial cell wall, causing rapid cell lysis, and are most effective against fast-growing susceptible bacteria.

The sites of action for penicillins are enzymes known as penicillin-binding proteins (PBPs). The affinity of certain penicillins for PBPs in various microorganisms helps explain differing spectra of activity in this class of antibiotics.

Bacterial resistance to beta-lactam antibiotics is conferred most significantly by bacterial production of beta-lactamase enzymes, which destroy the beta-lactam ring and thus inactivate peni-

cillin; decreased cell wall permeability and alteration in binding affinity to PBP also contribute to such resistance.

Oral absorption of penicillin varies widely; the most acid labile is penicillin G. Side-chain modifications in penicillin V, ampicillin, amoxicillin, and other orally administered penicillins are more stable in gastric acid and permit better absorption from the GI tract. (See *Comparing penicillins,* page 60.)

Penicillins are distributed widely throughout the body; CSF penetration is minimal but is enhanced in patients with inflamed meninges. Most penicillins are only partially metabolized. With the exception of nafcillin, penicillins are excreted primarily in urine, chiefly through renal tubular effects; nafcillin undergoes enterohepatic circulation and is excreted chiefly through the biliary tract.

Indications and actions
Infection caused by susceptible organisms

Natural penicillins. Penicillin G is the prototype of this group; derivatives such as penicillin V are more acid stable and thus better absorbed by the oral route. All natural penicillins are vulnerable to inactivation by beta-lactamase-producing bacteria. Natural penicillins act primarily against gram-positive organisms.

Clinical indications for natural penicillins include streptococcal pneumonia, enterococcal and nonenterococcal group D endocarditis, diphtheria, anthrax, meningitis, tetanus, botulism, actinomycosis, syphilis, relapsing fever, Lyme disease, rat-bite fever, Whipple's disease, and others. Natural penicillins are used prophylactically against pneumococcal infections, rheumatic fever, bacterial endocarditis, and neonatal group B streptococcal disease.

Susceptible aerobic gram-positive cocci include nonpenicillinase-producing *Staphylococcus aureus, S. epidermis*; nonenterococcal group D streptococci, groups A, B, C, D, G, H, K, L, and M streptococci, *Streptococcus viridans*; and enterococcus (usually in combination with an aminoglycoside). Susceptible aerobic gram-negative cocci include *Neisseria meningitidis* and non–penicillinase-producing *N. gonorrhoeae.*

Susceptible aerobic gram-positive bacilli include *Bacillus anthracis, Corynebacterium* (both diphtheria and opportunistic species), and *Listeria.* Susceptible anaerobes include *Actinomyces, Clostridium, Fusobacterium, Peptococcus, Peptostreptococcus, Veillonella,* and non-beta-lactamase-producing strains of *Streptococcus pneumoniae.* The drugs are also active against some gram-negative aerobic bacilli, including some strains of *Haemophilus influenzae, Pasturella multocida, Streptobacillus moniliformis,* and *Spirillum minus.*

Susceptible spirochetes include *Borrelia recurrentis, Leptospira, Treponema pallidum,* and *T. pertenue,* and possibly *B. burgdorferi.*

Comparing penicillins

Drug	Route	Adult dosage	Penicillinase-resistant
amoxicillin	P.O.	250 to 500 mg q 8 hr 3 g with 1 g probenecid for gonorrhea as single dose	No
amoxicillin/clavulanate potassium	P.O.	250 mg q 8 hr 500 mg q 12 hr	Yes
ampicillin	I.M., I.V. P.O.	2 to 14 g daily in divided doses given q 4 to 6 hr 250 to 500 mg q 6 hr 2.5 g with 1 g probenecid (for gonorrhea) as single dose	No
ampicillin sodium/ sulbactam sodium	I.M., I.V.	1.5 to 3 g q 6 to 8 hr	Yes
cloxacillin	P.O.	250 mg to 1 g q 6 hr	Yes
dicloxacillin	P.O.	125 to 500 mg q 6 hr	Yes
mezlocillin	I.M., I.V.	3 to 4 g q 4 to 6 hr	No
nafcillin	I.M., I.V. P.O.	250 mg to 2 g q 4 to 6 hr 500 mg to 1 g q 6 hr	Yes
oxacillin	I.M., I.V. P.O.	250 mg to 2 g q 4 to 6 hr 500 mg to 1 g q 6 hr	Yes
penicillin G benzathine	I.M.	1.2 to 2.4 million units as single dose	No
penicillin G potassium	I.M., I.V.	200,000 to 4 million units q 4 hr	No
penicillin G procaine	I.M.	600,000 to 1.2 million units q 1 to 3 days 4.8 million units with 1 g probenecid as single dose for primary, secondary, and early latent syphilis; weekly for 3 weeks for late latent syphilis	No
penicillin G sodium	I.M., I.V.	200,000 to 4 million units q 4 hr	No
penicillin V potassium	P.O.	250 to 500 mg q 6 to 8 hr	No
piperacillin	I.M., I.V.	100 to 300 mg/kg daily as divided doses given q 4 to 6 hr	No
piperacillin sodium/ tazobactam sodium	I.V.	3.375 g q 6 hr	Yes
ticarcillin	I.M., I.V.	150 to 300 mg/kg daily as divided doses given q 3 to 6 hr	No
ticarcillin/clavulanate potassium	I.V.	3.1 g q 4 to 6 hr	Yes

Aminopenicillins (amoxicillin and ampicillin) offer a broader spectrum of activity including many gram-negative organisms. Like natural penicillins, aminopenicillins are vulnerable to inactivation by penicillinase. They are primarily used to treat septicemia, gynecologic infections, and infections of the urinary, respiratory, and GI tracts, and skin, soft tissue, bones, and joints. Their activity spectrum includes *Escherichia coli, H.* *influenzae, Listeria monocytogenes, N. gonorrhoeae, Proteus mirabilis, Salmonella, Shigella, S. aureus, S. epidermidis* (non–penicillinase-producing *Staphylococcus*), and *S. pneumoniae.*

Penicillinase-resistant penicillins (cloxacillin, dicloxacillin, nafcillin, and oxacillin) are semisynthetic penicillins designed to remain stable against hydrolysis by most staphylococcal penicillinases and thus are the drugs of choice against susceptible penicillinase-producing staphylococci. They also retain activity against most organisms susceptible to natural penicillins. Clinical indications are much the same as for aminopenicillins.

Extended-spectrum penicillins (carbenicillin, mezlocillin, piperacillin, and ticarcillin), as their name implies, offer a wider range of bactericidal action than the other three classes, are used in hard-to-treat gram-negative infections, and are usually given in combination with aminoglycosides. They are used most often against susceptible strains of *Bacteroides fragilis, Citrobacter, Enterobacter, Klebsiella, Pseudomonas aeruginosa,* and *Serratia;* their gram-negative spectrum also includes *Morganella morganii, Proteus mirabilis, P. vulgaris, Providencia rettgeri, Salmonella,* and *Shigella.* These penicillins are also vulnerable to destruction by beta-lactamase or penicillinases.

Overview of adverse reactions

Systemic: Hypersensitivity reactions range from mild rash, fever, and eosinophilia to fatal anaphylaxis. Hematologic reactions include hemolytic anemia, transient neutropenia, leukopenia, and thrombocytopenia.

Certain adverse reactions are more common with specific classes of penicillin: bleeding episodes are usually seen at high-dose levels of extended-spectrum penicillins; acute interstitial nephritis is reported most often with methicillin; GI adverse effects are most common with but not limited to ampicillin. High doses, especially of penicillin G, irritate the CNS in patients with renal disease, causing confusion, twitching, lethargy, dysphagia, seizures, and coma. Hepatotoxicity is most common with penicillinase resistant penicillins; hyperkalemia, and hypernatremia with extended-spectrum penicillins.

Jarisch-Herxheimer reaction can occur when penicillin G is used in secondary syphilis; signs and symptoms are chills, fever, headache, myalgia, tachycardia, malaise, sweating, hypotension, and sore throat—attributed to release of endotoxin following spirochete death.

Local: Local irritation from parenteral therapy may be severe enough to require discontinuation of the drug or administration by subclavian catheter if drug therapy is to continue.

Special considerations

● Assess patient's history of allergies.
● Keep in mind that a negative history for penicillin hypersensitivity doesn't preclude future allergic reactions; monitor patient continuously for possible allergic reactions or other untoward effects.
● Reduce dose in patients with renal impairment based on creatinine clearance and manufacturer's guidelines.
● Assess level of consciousness, neurologic status, and renal function when large doses are used,

because excessive blood levels can cause CNS toxicity.
● Monitor vital signs, electrolytes, and renal function studies; monitor body weight for fluid retention with extended-spectrum penicillins for possible hypokalemia or hypernatremia.
● Coagulation abnormalities, even frank bleeding, can follow high doses, especially of extended-spectrum penicillins. Monitor PT and platelet counts, and assess patient for signs of occult or frank bleeding.
● Monitor patients on long-term therapy for possible superinfection, especially geriatric and debilitated patients and others receiving immunosuppressants or radiation therapy; watch closely, especially for fever.

Oral and parenteral administration
● Give penicillins at least 1 hour before giving bacteriostatic antibiotics (tetracyclines, erythromycins, and chloramphenicol); these drugs inhibit bacterial cell growth, decreasing rate of penicillin uptake by bacterial cell walls.
● Refrigerate oral suspensions; shake well before administering to ensure correct dose.
● Give oral penicillin at least 1 hour before or 2 hours after meals to enhance gastric absorption; food may or may not decrease absorption.
● Administer I.M. dose deep into large muscle mass (gluteal or midlateral thigh); rotate injection sites to minimize tissue injury; don't inject more than 2 g of drug per injection site. Apply ice to injection site for pain.
● Don't add or mix other drugs with I.V. infusions, particularly aminoglycosides, which are inactivated if mixed with penicillins; they're chemically and physically incompatible. If other drugs must be given I.V., temporarily stop infusion of primary drug.
● Infuse I.V. drug continuously or intermittently (over 30 minutes) and assess I.V. site frequently to prevent infiltration or phlebitis; rotate infusion site every 48 hours; intermittent I.V. infusion may be diluted in 50 to 100 ml sterile water, normal saline solution, D_5W, D_5W with 0.45% saline solution, or lactated Ringer's solution.

Pregnant patients

● Safe use of penicillins in pregnancy hasn't been definitely established. However, penicillin G has been used for the treatment of syphilis without adverse effects, and amoxicillin and ampicillin have been used for the treatment of urinary tract infections without adverse effects.

Breast-feeding patients

● Consult individual drug recommendations.

Pediatric patients

● Specific dosage recommendations have been established for most penicillins.

Geriatric patients

● Use cautiously; elderly patients are susceptible to superinfection.

● Many elderly patients have renal impairment, which decreases penicillin excretion; lower the dose in elderly patients with diminished creatinine clearance.

Patient education

● Teach patient signs and symptoms of hypersensitivity and other adverse reactions; emphasize need to report unusual reactions.

● Teach patient signs and symptoms of bacterial and fungal superinfection, especially geriatric and debilitated patients and others with low resistance from immunosuppressants or irradiation; emphasize need to report signs of infection.

● Be sure patient understands how and when to take drugs; urge him to complete entire prescribed regimen, to comply with instructions for around-the-clock dosing, and to keep follow-up appointments.

● Counsel patient to check expiration date of drug and to discard unused drug and not give it to family members or friends.

Representative combinations

Amoxicillin with clavulanate potassium: Augmentin.

Ampicillin with probenecid: Polycillin-PRB.

Ampicillin sodium with sulbactam sodium: Unasyn.

Ampicillin trihydrate with probenecid: Polycillin-PRB, Principen with Probenecid.

Penicillin G benzathine with penicillin G procaine: Bicillin C-R, Bicillin C-R 900/300.

Piperacillin sodium with tazobactam sodium: Zosyn.

Ticarcillin disodium with clavulanate potassium: Timentin.

---

phenothiazines

Aliphatic derivatives: chlorpromazine hydrochloride, promethazine hydrochloride, triflupromazine, trimeprazine

Piperazine derivatives: fluphenazine hydrochloride, perphenazine, prochlorperazine, trifluoperazine hydrochloride

Piperidine derivatives: mesoridazine besylate, thioridazine

Thioxanthene: thiothixene

Phenothiazines were originally synthesized by European scientists seeking aniline-like dyes in the late 1800s. Several decades later, in the 1930s, promethazine was identified and found to have sedative, antihistaminic, and narcotic-potentiating

effects. Chlorpromazine was synthesized in the 1950s; this drug has many effects, among them strong antipsychotic activity.

Pharmacology

Phenothiazines are classified in terms of chemical structure: the aliphatic agent (chlorpromazine) has a greater sedative, hypotensive, and allergic activity. Piperazines (perphenazine, prochlorperazine, fluphenazine, and trifluoperazine) are more likely to produce extrapyramidal symptoms. Piperidines (thioridazine and mesoridazine) have intermediate effects. Thioxanthenes are chemically similar to phenothiazines and are pharmacologically similar to piperazine phenothiazines. Promethazine is a derivative that has antihistamine qualities.

All antipsychotics have fundamentally similar mechanisms of action; they're believed to function as dopamine antagonists, blocking postsynaptic dopamine receptors in various parts of the CNS; their antiemetic effects result from blockage of the chemoreceptor trigger zone. They also produce varying degrees of anticholinergic and alpha-adrenergic receptor blocking actions. The drugs are structurally similar to tricyclic antidepressants (TCAs) and share many adverse reactions.

All antipsychotics have equal clinical efficacy when given in equivalent doses; choice of specific therapy is determined primarily by the individual patient's response and adverse reaction profile. A patient who doesn't respond to one drug may respond to another.

Onset of full therapeutic effects requires 6 weeks to 6 months; therefore, dosage adjustment is recommended at not less than weekly intervals.

Indications and actions
Psychoses

Phenothiazines (except promethazine) and thiothixene are indicated to treat agitated psychotic states. They're especially effective in controlling hallucinations in schizophrenic patients, the manic phase of manic-depressive illness, and excessive motor and autonomic activity.

Nausea and vomiting

Chlorpromazine, perphenazine, promethazine, and prochlorperazine are effective in controlling severe nausea and vomiting induced by CNS disturbances. They don't prevent motion sickness or vertigo.

Anxiety ◇

Chlorpromazine, mesoridazine, promethazine, prochlorperazine, and trifluoperazine also may be used for short-term treatment of moderate anxiety in selected nonpsychotic patients, for example, to control anxiety before surgery.

Severe behavior problems
Chlorpromazine and thioridazine are indicated to control combativeness and hyperexcitability in children with severe behavior problems. They're also used in hyperactive children for short-term treatment of excessive motor activity with labile moods, impulsive behavior, aggressiveness, attention deficit, and poor tolerance of frustration. Mesoridazine is used to manage hypersensitivity and to promote cooperative behavior in patients with mental deficiency and chronic brain syndrome.

Tetanus
Chlorpromazine is an effective adjunct in treating tetanus.

Porphyria
Because of its effects on the autonomic nervous system, chlorpromazine is effective in controlling abdominal pain in patients with acute intermittent porphyria.

Delirium
Phenothiazines have been used in the treatment of delirium. Antipsychotics remain first-line therapy.

Intractable hiccups
Chlorpromazine has been used to treat patients with intractable hiccups. The mechanism is unknown.

Neurogenic pain
Fluphenazine is a useful adjunct, managing selected chronic pain states.

Allergies and pruritus
Because of their potent antihistaminic effects, many of these drugs (including promethazine and trimeprazine) are used to relieve itching or symptomatic rhinitis.

Overview of adverse reactions
Phenothiazines may produce extrapyramidal symptoms (dystonic movements, torticollis, oculogyric crises, parkinsonian symptoms) from akathisia during early treatment, to tardive dyskinesia after long-term use.

In rare cases, a neuroleptic malignant syndrome resembling severe parkinsonism may occur; it consists of rapid onset of hyperthermia, muscular hyperreflexia, marked extrapyramidal and autonomic dysfunction, arrhythmias, and sweating.

Other adverse reactions are similar to those seen with TCAs, including sedative and anticholinergic effects, orthostatic hypotension, reflex tachycardia, fainting, dizziness, arrhythmias, anorexia, nausea, vomiting, abdominal pain, local gastric irritation, seizures, endocrine effects, hematologic disorders, ocular changes, skin eruptions, and photosensitivity. Allergic manifestations

are usually marked by elevation of liver enzymes progressing to obstructive jaundice.

Piperidine derivatives have the most pronounced CV effects; piperazine derivatives have the least. Parenteral administration is often associated with CV effects because of more rapid absorption. Seizures are common with aliphatic derivatives.

Special considerations
• Phenothiazines are contraindicated in patients with known hypersensitivity to phenothiazines and related compounds.
• Use cautiously in patients with cardiac disease (arrhythmias, heart failure, angina pectoris, valvular disease, or heart block).
• Use cautiously in patients with encephalitis, Reye's syndrome, head injury, epilepsy, or other seizure disorders.
• Use phenothiazines cautiously in patients with glaucoma, prostatic hypertrophy, paralytic ileus, urine retention, hepatic or renal dysfunction, Parkinson's disease, pheochromocytoma, and hypocalcemia.
• Check vital signs regularly for decreased blood pressure (especially before and after parenteral therapy) or tachycardia; observe patient carefully for other adverse reactions.
• Monitor intake and output for urine retention or constipation, which may require dose reduction.
• Monitor bilirubin levels weekly for first 4 weeks; monitor CBC, ECG (for quinidine-like effects), liver and renal function studies, electrolyte levels (especially potassium), and eye examinations at baseline and periodically thereafter, especially in patients on long-term therapy.
• Observe patient for mood changes to monitor progress; benefits may not be apparent for several weeks.
• Monitor patient for involuntary movements. Check patient receiving prolonged treatment at least once every 6 months.
• Don't withdraw drug abruptly; although physical dependence doesn't occur with antipsychotic drugs, rebound exacerbation of psychotic symptoms may occur, and many drug effects persist.
• Carefully follow manufacturer's instructions regarding drug color for reconstitution, dilution, administration, and storage of drugs; slightly discolored liquids may or may not be usable.

Pregnant patients
• Safety of phenothiazine use during pregnancy hasn't been established.

Breast-feeding patients
• If possible, patient shouldn't breast-feed while taking antipsychotics; most phenothiazines appear in breast milk and have a direct effect on prolactin levels. Benefit to mother must outweigh hazard to infant.

Pediatric patients
● Unless otherwise specified, antipsychotics aren't recommended for children under age 12; be careful when using phenothiazines for nausea and vomiting because acutely ill children (suffering from chickenpox, measles, CNS infections, dehydration) are at greatly increased risk of dystonic reactions.

Geriatric patients
● Lower doses are indicated in elderly patients, who are more sensitive to therapeutic and adverse effects, especially cardiac toxicity, tardive dyskinesia, and other extrapyramidal effects. Adjust dose to patient response.

Patient education
● Explain to patient rationale and anticipated risks and benefits of therapy, and that full therapeutic effect may not occur for several weeks.
● Teach patient signs and symptoms of adverse reactions and importance of reporting unusual effects, especially involuntary movements.
● Tell patient to avoid beverages and drugs containing alcohol, and not to take other drugs (especially CNS depressants) including OTC products without medical approval.
● Instruct diabetic patient to monitor blood glucose because drug may alter insulin needs.
● Teach patient how and when to take drug, not to increase dose without medical approval, and never to discontinue drug abruptly; suggest taking full dose at bedtime if daytime sedation is troublesome.
● Advise patient to lie down for 30 minutes after first dose (1 hour if I.M.) and to rise slowly from sitting or supine position to prevent orthostatic hypotension.
● Warn patient to avoid tasks requiring mental alertness and psychomotor coordination such as driving until full effects of drug are established; emphasize that sedative effects will lessen after several weeks.
● Advise patient to take drug with milk or food to minimize GI distress because drugs are locally irritating. Warn that oral concentrates and solutions will irritate skin, and tell patient not to crush or open sustained-release products, but to swallow them whole.
● Warn patient that photosensitivity reactions, such as burns and abnormal hyperpigmentation, may occur.
● Tell patient to avoid exposure to extremes of heat or cold, because of risk of hypothermia or hyperthermia induced by alteration in thermoregulatory function.
● Explain to patient that phenothiazines may cause pink to brown discoloration of urine.

Representative combinations
None.

progestins
hydroxyprogesterone caproate, medroxyprogesterone acetate, megestrol acetate, norethindrone, norethindrone acetate, norgestrel, progesterone

Progesterone is the endogenous progestin, secreted by the corpus luteum within the female ovary. Several synthetic progesterone derivatives with greater potency or duration of action have been synthesized. Some of these derivatives also possess weak androgenic or estrogenic activity. Progestins are used to treat dysfunctional uterine bleeding and certain cancers. They're also used as contraceptives, either alone or in combination with estrogens.

Pharmacology
Progesterone is formed from steroid precursors in the ovary, testis, adrenal cortex, and placenta. Luteinizing hormone stimulates the synthesis and secretion of progesterone from the corpus luteum. Progesterone causes secretory changes in the endometrium, changes in the vaginal epithelium, increases in body temperature, relaxation of uterine smooth muscle, stimulation of growth of breast alveolar tissue, inhibition of gonadotropin release from the pituitary, and withdrawal bleeding (in the presence of estrogens). Synthetic progesterone derivatives have these properties as well.

Indications and actions
Hormonal imbalance in women
Hydroxyprogesterone, medroxyprogesterone, norethindrone, and progesterone are indicated to treat amenorrhea and dysfunctional uterine bleeding resulting from hormonal imbalance. Hydroxyprogesterone also is indicated to produce desquamation and a secretory endometrium.

Endometriosis
Norethindrone and norethindrone acetate are used to treat endometriosis.

Carcinoma
Hydroxyprogesterone, medroxyprogesterone, and megestrol are used in the adjunctive and palliative treatment of certain types of metastatic tumors. They're not considered primary therapy. See individual agents for specific indications.

Contraception
Norethindrone, medroxyprogesterone acetate, and norgestrel are approved for use with estrogens or alone as oral contraceptives.
    Progestins are no longer indicated to detect pregnancy (because of teratogenicity) or to treat threatened or habitual abortion, for which they're not effective.

Overview of adverse reactions

The most common adverse effect is a change in menstrual bleeding pattern, ranging from spotting or breakthrough bleeding to complete amenorrhea. Other reactions include breast tenderness and secretion, weight changes, increases in body temperature, edema, nausea, acne, somnolence, insomnia, hirsutism, hair loss, depression, cholestatic jaundice, and allergic reactions (rare). Some patients taking parenteral progestins have also suffered localized reactions at the injection site.

Special considerations

• Progestins are contraindicated during pregnancy and in patients with thromboembolic disorders, breast cancer, undiagnosed abnormal vaginal bleeding, or severe hepatic disease.
• Use cautiously in patients with diabetes mellitus, cardiac or renal disease, seizure disorder, migraine, or mental depression.
• Give oil injections I.M., deep into gluteal muscles. I.M. injections may be painful; observe injection site for sterile abscess formation.
• Glucose tolerance may be altered in diabetic patients. Monitor patient closely because antidiabetic may need to be adjusted.
• When used as an oral contraceptive, progestins are administered daily without interruption, regardless of menstrual cycle.
• Use of progestins may lead to gingival bleeding and hyperplasia.
• Because oral contraceptive combinations contain progestins, consider the precautions associated with oral contraceptives in patients receiving progestins.

Pregnant patients

• Progestins are listed as pregnancy category X. Potential adverse effects include masculinization of the female fetus, hypospadias in males, and potential CV and limb defects.
• A patient exposed to progestins during the first 4 months of pregnancy or who becomes pregnant while receiving the drug should be informed of the potential risks to the fetus.

Breast-feeding patients

• Don't use progestins in breast-feeding women, except for Depo-Provera, which may be used in breast-feeding women after 6 weeks.

Patient education

• Tell patient that GI distress may subside with use, after a few cycles.
• Instruct patient receiving progestins to have a full physical examination, including a gynecologic examination and a Papanicolaou test, every 6 to 12 months.
• Advise patient to discontinue therapy and call immediately if migraine or visual disturbances occur, or if sudden severe headache or vomiting develops.

• Teach patient how to perform breast self-examination.
• Tell patient to call promptly if period is missed or unusual bleeding occurs; and to call and discontinue drug immediately if pregnancy is suspected.
• Advise patient who misses a dose to take the missed dose as soon as possible or omit it.
• Advise patient who misses consecutive doses when used as a contraceptive to discontinue the drug and use an alternative contraception method until period begins or pregnancy is ruled out.
• Inform patient that drug may cause possible dental problems (tenderness, swelling, or bleeding of gums). Advise patient to brush and floss teeth, massage gums, and have dentist clean teeth regularly. She should check with dentist if there are questions about care of teeth or gums or if tenderness, swelling, or bleeding of gums is noticed.
• Advise patient to use extra care to avoid pregnancy when starting use of drug as an oral contraceptive and for at least 3 months after discontinuing it.
• Advise patient to keep an extra 1-month supply available.
• Tell patient to keep tablets in original container.
• Emphasize to patient the importance of not giving medication to anyone else.

Representative combinations

Hydroxyprogesterone caproate with estradiol valerate: Hylutin.

Norethindrone acetate with ethinyl estradiol: Brevicon, Loestrin 1.5/30, Loestrin Fe 1.5/30, Loestrin 21 1/20, Loestrin Fe 1/20, Modicon, Norinyl 1 + 35, Ortho 1/35*, Ortho 7/7/7*, Ortho 10/11*, Ortho-Novum 7/7/7, Ovcon-35, Ovcon-50, Tri-Norinyl; with mestranol: Norinyl 1/50, Ortho-Novum 0.5/35*, Ortho-Novum 1/50, Ortho-Novum 1/35.

Norgestrel with ethinyl estradiol: Lo/Ovral, Ovral.

---

protease inhibitors

amprenavir, indinavir sulfate, lopinavir, nelfinavir mesylate, ritonavir, saquinavir, saquinavir mesylate

These antiviral agents act specifically against human immunodeficiency virus (HIV) through inhibition of HIV protease.

Pharmacology

Protease inhibitors bind to the protease active site and inhibit the activity of HIV protease. This enzyme is required for the proteolysis of viral polyprotein precursors into individual functional proteins found in infectious HIV. The net effect is formation of noninfectious, immature viral particles. Note that two drug regimens containing only nucleoside reverse transcriptase inhibitors

Comparing protease inhibitors

Drug	Oral bioavailability	Plasma protein–binding (%)	Half-life (hr)	Peak concentration (hr)
amprenavir	May be taken without food, but shouldn't be taken with a high-fat meal, which reduces absorption. Absolute bioavailability hasn't been established.	90	Adults: 7-10½	1-2
indinavir	Meals rich in fats, proteins, or calories reduce bioavailability by 77%.	60	Adults: 1¾	Fasting: ¾
nelfinavir	Food produces 2- to 3-fold increase in bioavailability.	>98	Adults: 3½-5	Fed: 2-4
ritonavir	Food produces 15% increase in bioavailability.	98-99	Adults: 3-5	Fasted: 2 Fed: 4
saquinavir	High fat meals produce a 4% increase in bioavailability of Invirase. Soft gelatin capsule formulation (Fortovase) has a 33% increase in bioavailability.	98	Not defined	Not defined

are now considered suboptimal. Combination therapy including protease inhibitors or nonnucleoside reverse transcriptase inhibitors are recommended. (See *Comparing protease inhibitors.*)

Indications and actions

Protease inhibitors are used as monotherapy or in combination with nucleoside analogues for the treatment of HIV infection and acquired immunodeficiency syndrome (AIDS).

◇ Protease inhibitors may be used in conjunction with zidovudine and lamivudine for postexposure prophylaxis of HIV infection.

Overview of adverse reactions

The most frequently reported adverse effects of protease inhibitors, for which immediate medical attention should be sought, include kidney stones, pancreatitis, diabetes or hyperglycemia, ketoacidosis, or paresthesias. Frequently reported adverse effects that don't require medical attention unless they persist or are bothersome include generalized weakness, GI disturbances, headache, insomnia, and taste perversion. Less frequent adverse effects include dizziness and somnolence.

Special considerations

● Consider the risk-benefit ratio of therapy with protease inhibitors on an individual basis when either hemophilia or liver dysfunction is present.
● Indinavir may cause nephrolithiasis. Advise increasing fluid intake.

Pregnant patients

● Pregnancy risk categories are B and C. Adequate, well-controlled trials haven't been completed, because the drug can produce hyperbilirubinemia; exercise caution in pregnant women to prevent ill effects in neonates. Prescribers are encouraged to contact the registry at 1-800-258-4263 to report pregnant women on therapy.

Breast-feeding patients

● The rate and extent of excretion of protease inhibitors into breast milk is unknown. Therefore, their use in breast-feeding women isn't recommended. However, the risks and benefits to both the woman and infant must be considered in each case.

Pediatric patients

● Refer to specific drug monographs for dosing information.

Geriatric patients

● Safety and efficacy haven't been evaluated systemically.

Patient education

● Instruct patient to take drug as prescribed and to finish the full course of therapy.
● Tell patient to take the next dose as soon as possible after a missed dose, but not to double the dose.
● Tell patient that drug should be taken with plenty of water, 1 or 2 hours before meals, and he should drink about 48 oz of water daily.

Elimination	Dosage	Dosage adjustment
14% renal, 75% fecal	Adults: 1,200 mg b.i.d. Children: 20-22.5 mg/kg b.i.d.	Reduce dose with impaired hepatic function
83% hepatic; 19% renal	Adults: 800 mg q 8 hr Adults with cirrhosis: 600 mg q 8 hr	Reduce dose in cirrhosis
87% fecal; 78% as metabolites; 1%-2% recovered unchanged in urine	Adults: 750 mg t.i.d. with food Children: 20-30 mg/kg t.i.d. with food	None
88% fecal; 34% as unchanged drug; 11% excreted in urine; 4% as unchanged drug	Adults: 600 mg b.i.d. with food Children: > 2: 250 mg/m^2-400 mg/m^2 b.i.d. with food	None
88% fecal as unchanged drug and metabolites; 1% recovered unchanged in urine	Fortovase: 1,200 mg t.i.d. with food or within 2 hr of a meal Invirase: 600 mg t.i.d. with food or within 2 hr of a meal	None

• Instruct patient not to take other medications without first checking with the pharmacist or prescriber.

Representative combinations
Ritonavir with lopinavir: Kaletra.

selective serotonin reuptake inhibitors

citalopram hydrobromide, fluoxetine, fluvoxamine maleate, sertraline hydrochloride, paroxetine

These drugs are antidepressant, antiobsessional, antipanic agents that selectively inhibit the reuptake of serotonin with little or no effects on other neurotransmitters such as norepinephrine or dopamine. (See *Comparing selective serotonin reuptake inhibitors,* pages 68 and 69.)

Pharmacology
The antidepressant, antiobsessional, antipanic actions of fluoxetine, fluvoxamine maleate, sertraline, and paroxetine are thought to be related to the potent and selective inhibition of serotonin uptake, but not of norepinephrine or dopamine uptake, in the CNS. These agents lack affinity for alpha-adrenergic receptors and muscarinic receptors.

Indications and actions
Selective serotonin reuptake inhibitors are used in the treatment of major depression, obsessive-compulsive disorder (OCD), bulimia nervosa, premenstrual dysphoric disorders, and panic disorders. Sertraline is the first drug approved for the treatment of posttraumatic stress disorder.

Fluoxetine has been used for the treatment of bipolar disorder ◊, symptomatic management of cataplexy ◊, and management of alcohol dependence ◊.

Paroxetine and sertraline have been used for the treatment of premature ejaculation and chronic headache ◊; paroxetine for the symptoms of diabetic neuropathy ◊.

Overview of adverse reactions
Frequent adverse effects include headache, tremor, dizziness, sleep disturbances, GI disturbances, and sexual dysfunction. Less frequent adverse effects include bleeding (red spots on skin, nose bleeds), akathisia (restlessness), breast tenderness or enlargement, extrapyramidal effects, dystonia, fever, hyponatremia, mania or hypomania, palpitations, serotonin syndrome, weight gain or loss, skin rash, hives, or itching.

Special considerations
• Hyponatremia usually results from inappropriate secretion of antidiuretic hormone. This problem is most often seen in elderly patients and those treated with diuretics.
• Diarrhea, fever, palpitations, mood swings, behavioral changes, restlessness, shaking, and shivering characterize serotonin syndrome. Hypertension and seizures may accompany the serotonin syndrome. This syndrome is most commonly seen within days following dosage increases or concurrent administration of a serotonergic agent.

Comparing selective serotonin reuptake inhibitors

Drug	Oral bioavailability	Plasma protein–binding (%)	Half-life (hr)	Onset of action (wk)
citalopram	No food effect	80	35	1-4
fluoxetine	Well absorbed; no food effect	94½	2-3 days for fluoxetine and 7-9 days for nor-fluoxetine	1-3; may be 5 for obsessive-compulsive disorder
fluvoxamine	No food effect	80	13½-15½	4-5
paroxetine	50%-100%; no food effect	95	Average of 21-24	1-3
sertraline	Food increases rate and extent of absorption	98	Sertraline: 24-26 N-desmethyl-sertraline: 62-104	2-4

Pregnant patients
● Pregnancy risk category is C. Data haven't shown evidence of teratogenicity or ill effects in neonates of women given SSRIs during the first trimester of pregnancy or throughout gestation. The effects of SSRIs on labor and delivery aren't known.

Breast-feeding patients
● SSRIs appear in breast milk and may cause diarrhea and sleep disturbance in neonates. Use of SSRIs in breast-feeding women isn't recommended. However, the risks and benefits to both the woman and infant must be considered in each case.

Pediatric patients
● There's insufficient information to establish the safety and efficacy of SSRIs in children, but there's evidence of beneficial response following SSRI treatment for depression or OCD in this population. Children appear to be more susceptible than adults to the behavioral adverse reactions of SSRIs (mania, social inhibition, irritability, restlessness, and insomnia).

Geriatric patients
● The use of SSRIs is safe and effective in elderly patients.
● Elderly patients are more sensitive to the insomniac effects of SSRIs.
● Plasma sertraline level may be decreased in these patients.

Patient education
● Tell patient that drug may take 4 to 5 weeks to produce its full-intended benefit. Drug should be

taken as prescribed. If a dose is missed, dose shouldn't be doubled.
● Instruct patient to stop taking medication and call as soon as possible if a rash or hives develops.
● Avoid alcoholic beverages and use of medications or substances that have serotonergic activity.
● Tell patient to use caution when driving or doing jobs requiring alertness since this medication may cause drowsiness or impairment of judgment or motor skills.

Representative combinations
None.

sulfonamides

co-trimoxazole (sulfamethoxazole-trimethoprim), sulfadiazine, sulfamethoxazole, sulfasalazine, sulfisoxazole

Sulfonamides were the first effective drugs used to treat systemic bacterial infections. The prototype, sulfanilamide, was discovered in 1908 and first used clinically in 1933. Since then, many derivatives have been synthesized, and many therapeutic milestones have been reached, including improved solubility of sulfonamides in urine (which reduces renal toxicity) and discovery of the advantages of combinations such as triple sulfa and, especially, of combined trimethoprim and sulfamethoxazole (co-trimoxazole). Development of other major antibiotics has reduced the clinical impact of sulfonamides; however, introduction of the combination agent co-trimoxazole has increased their usefulness in certain infections.

Peak concentration (hr)	Elimination	Adult dosage	Dosage adjustment
4 (after a single dose)	35% excreted in urine; 65% in feces	20-40 mg/day	Lower dosing recommended in the elderly
6-8 (after a single dose)	80% excreted in urine; 15% in feces	20-60 mg/day in single or divided doses	No adjustment for renal or hepatic impairment
3-8	94% renal excretion	50-300 mg/day h.s. Total daily dose >100 mg should be divided and given in two doses	Reduction of initial dosage and modification of subsequent doses in renal and hepatic impairment
2-8	64% excreted in urine; 36% in feces	20-60 mg/day in single or divided doses	Maximum dose of 40 mg/day in severe renal or hepatic impairment
4½-8½	45% renal; 45% in feces	25-50 mg once daily	Reduce dose or increase interval in severe hepatic impairment

Pharmacology

Sulfonamides are bacteriostatic. Their mechanism of action correlates directly with the structural similarities they share with para aminobenzoic acid. They inhibit biosynthesis of folic acid, which is needed for cell growth; susceptible bacteria are those that synthesize folic acid.

Sulfonamides are well absorbed from the GI tract after oral administration, except for sulfasalazine, which is absorbed minimally by the oral route. Sulfonamides are distributed widely into tissues and fluids, including pleural, peritoneal, synovial, and ocular fluids; some, including sulfisoxazole, penetrate CSF. Sulfonamides readily cross the placenta and are found in low concentrations in breast milk. Sulfonamides are metabolized by the liver and the parent drug and metabolites are excreted in urine by glomerular filtration. Hemodialysis removes both sulfamethoxazole and sulfisoxazole, but peritoneal dialysis removes only sulfisoxazole.

Indications and actions
Bacterial infections

When first introduced, sulfonamides were active against many gram-positive and gram-negative organisms; over time, many bacteria have become resistant. Currently, sulfonamides are active against some strains of staphylococci, streptococci, *Bacillus anthracis, Clostridium perfringens, C. tetani, Escherichia coli, Neisseria gonorrhoeae, N.meningitides, Nocardia asteroides,* and *N. brasiliensis.* Resistance to sulfonamides is common if therapy continues beyond 2 weeks; resistance to one sulfonamide usually means cross-resistance to others.

Sulfonamides are used to treat urinary tract infections caused by *Enterobacter, E. coli, Klebsiella, Proteus mirabilis, P. vulgaris,* and *Staphylococcus aureus,* and genital lesions caused by *Haemophilus ducreyi* (chancroid). They're the drugs of choice in nocardiosis, usually with surgical drainage or combined with other antibiotics, including ampicillin, erythromycin, cycloserine, or minocycline. Sulfonamides also are used to treat otitis media. Sulfadiazine is used to eradicate meningococci from the nasopharynx of asymptomatic carriers of *N. meningitidis.*

Co-trimoxazole is used to treat infections of the urinary tract, respiratory tract, and ear; to treat chronic bacterial prostatitis; and to prevent recurrent urinary tract infection in women and "traveler's diarrhea."

Co-trimoxazole is also used to treat *Pneumocystis carinii* pneumonia.

Parasitic infections

Sulfonamides combined with pyrimethamine are used to treat toxoplasmosis; certain sulfonamides are combined with quinine and pyrimethamine to treat chloroquine-resistant *Plasmodium falciparum* malaria.

Inflammation

Sulfasalazine, used to treat inflammatory bowel disease, is cleaved in the intestine to sulfapyridine and 5-aminosalicylic acid.

Plague

Co-trimazole is recommended by the CDC for anti-infective prophylaxis in adults 18 and over and children 2 months or over who are at high risk for exposure to pneumonic plague.

Overview of adverse reactions

Sulfonamides cause adverse reactions affecting many organs and systems. Many are considered to be caused by hypersensitivity, including the following: rash, fever, pruritus, erythema multiforme, erythema nodosum, Stevens-Johnson syndrome, Lyell's syndrome, exfoliative dermatitis, photosensitivity, joint pain, conjunctivitis, leukopenia, and bronchospasm. Hematologic reactions include granulocytopenia, thrombocytopenia, agranulocytosis, hypoprothrombinemia, and, in G6PD deficiency, hemolytic anemia. Renal effects usually result from crystalluria (precipitation of the sulfonamide in the renal system). GI reactions include anorexia, stomatitis, pancreatitis, diarrhea, and folic acid malabsorption. Oral therapy commonly causes nausea and vomiting. Hepatotoxicity and CNS reactions (dizziness, confusion, headache, ataxia, drowsiness, and insomnia) are rare.

Special considerations

● Assess patient's history of allergies; don't give a sulfonamide to patient with history of hypersensitivity reactions to sulfonamides or to other drugs containing sulfur.
● Sulfonamides are also contraindicated in patients with severe renal or hepatic dysfunction, or porphyria; during pregnancy at term, and during breast-feeding. Sulfonamides may cause kernicterus in infants, because they displace bilirubin at the binding site, cross the placenta, and are excreted in breast milk. Don't use in infants under age 2 months (except in the treatment of congenital toxoplasmosis as adjunctive therapy with pyrimethamine).
● Administer sulfonamides cautiously in patients with the following conditions: mild to moderate renal or hepatic impairment; urinary obstruction, because of the risk of drug accumulation; severe allergies; asthma; blood dyscrasia; or G6PD deficiency.
● Continuously monitor patient for possible hypersensitivity reactions or other untoward effects; patients with AIDS have a much higher risk of adverse reactions.
● Obtain cultures and sensitivity tests before giving first dose, but therapy may begin before laboratory tests are complete; check test results periodically to assess drug efficacy. Recommend monitoring urine cultures, CBCs, and urinalysis before and during therapy.
● Monitor patients on prolonged therapy for superinfection, especially elderly patients, debilitated patients, and patients receiving immunosuppressants or radiation therapy.
● Sulfonamides may interact with other drugs (oral anticoagulants, cyclosporine, digoxin, folic acid, hydantoins, methotrexate, and sulfonylureas) and may alter test results; consult individual drug entries for possible test interactions.
● Give oral dose with full 8-oz (240-ml) glass of water, and force fluids to 12 to 16 glasses per day, depending on the agent; patient's urine output should be at least 1,500 ml/day.
● Follow manufacturer's directions for reconstitution, dilution, and storage of drugs; check expiration dates.
● Give oral sulfonamide at least 1 hour before or 2 hours after meals for maximum absorption.
● Shake oral suspensions well before administering to ensure correct dose.

Pregnant patients

● Safe use during pregnancy hasn't been established. There's potential for cleft palate, other bony abnormalities, and kernicterus in the infant.

Breast-feeding patients

● Because sulfonamides appear in breast milk, a decision should be made to discontinue breast-feeding or to discontinue the drug, taking into account the importance of the drug to the woman. Premature infants, infants with hyperbilirubinemia, and those with G6PD deficiency are at risk for kernicterus.

Pediatric patients

● Sulfonamides are contraindicated in infants under age 2 months, unless there's no therapeutic alternative.
● Give sulfonamides cautiously to children with fragile X chromosome and mental retardation because they are vulnerable to psychomotor depression from folate depletion.

Geriatric patients

● Use cautiously; elderly patients are susceptible to bacterial and fungal superinfection, are at greater risk of folate deficiency anemia after sulfonamide therapy, and commonly are at greater risk of renal and hematologic effects because of diminished renal function.

Patient education

● Teach patient the signs and symptoms of hypersensitivity and other adverse reactions, and emphasize the need to report these; specifically, urge patient to report bloody urine, difficulty breathing, rash, fever, chills, or severe fatigue.
● Teach patient the signs and symptoms of bacterial and fungal superinfection to geriatric and debilitated patients and others with low resistance from immunosuppressants or irradiation; emphasize the need to report them.
● Advise diabetic patient that sulfonamides may increase effects of oral hypoglycemic and not to monitor urine glucose levels with Clinitest; sulfonamides alter results of tests using cupric sulfate.)
● Advise patient to avoid exposure to direct sunlight because of risk of photosensitivity reaction.
● Tell patient to take oral drug with a full glass of water and to drink at least 12 to 16 8-oz (240-ml) glasses of water daily depending on the agent;

explain that tablet may be crushed and swallowed with water to ensure maximal absorption.

• Be sure patient understands how and when to take drugs; urge him to complete entire prescribed regimen, to comply with instructions for around-the-clock dosing, and to keep follow-up appointments.

• Teach patient to check expiration date of drug and how to store drug, and to discard unused drug.

• For sulfasalazine, inform patient to take with food if GI irritation occurs and tell him that it may cause an orange-yellow discoloration of the urine or skin and may permanently stain soft contact lenses yellow.

• Photosensitization may occur; therefore, caution patient to take protective measures (such as wearing sunscreen and protective clothing) against exposure to ultraviolet light or sunlight until tolerance is determined.

Representative combinations

Sulfadiazine with sulfamerazine and sulfamethazine: Triple Sulfa.

Sulfamethizole with oxytetracycline hydrochloride and phenazopyridine: Urobiotic-250; with sulfathiazole, sulfacetamide, sulfabenzamide, and urea: Gyne-Sulf, Sultrin, Triple Sulfa, Trysul, V.V.S.

Sulfamethoxazole with phenazopyridine hydrochloride: Azo Gantanol, Azo-Sulfamethoxazole; with trimethoprim: Bactrim, Cotrim, Co-Trimoxazole, Septra, SMZ-TMP.

Sulfisoxazole with erythromycin ethylsuccinate: Pediazole; with phenazopyridine hydrochloride: Azo Gantrisin.

Sulfadoxine with pyrimethamine: Fansidar.

sulfonylureas

acetohexamide, chlorpropamide, glimepiride, glipizide, glyburide, tolazamide, tolbutamide

In 1942, sulfonamide, an antibacterial agent, was discovered to have hypoglycemic effects. Subsequent experiments showed that this drug didn't exert similar effects in pancreatectomized animals. Later, tolbutamide was introduced and became popular for managing certain diabetic patients. Sulfonylureas are useful only in patients with mild to moderately severe type 2, or non-insulin-dependent diabetes mellitus (NIDDM). These drugs can be used only in patients with functioning beta cells of the pancreas.

Pharmacology

Sulfonylurea antidiabetic agents are sulfonamide derivatives that exert no antibacterial activity.

Sulfonylureas lower blood glucose levels by stimulating insulin release from the pancreas. These agents work only in the presence of functioning beta cells in the islet tissue of the pan-

creas. After prolonged administration, they produce hypoglycemia through significant extrapancreatic effects, including reduction of hepatic glucose production and enhanced peripheral sensitivity to insulin. The latter may result from an increase in the number of insulin receptors or from changes in events after insulin binding. (See *Comparing sulfonylureas,* page 72.)

Sulfonylureas are divided into first-generation agents (chlorpropamide) and second-generation agents (glyburide, glipizide, and glimepiride). Although their mechanisms of action are similar, the second-generation agents carry a more lipophilic side chain, are more potent, and cause fewer adverse reactions. Their most important differences are their durations of action.

Indications and actions
Diabetes mellitus, non-insulin-dependent

Sulfonylureas are used to manage mild to moderately severe, stable, nonketotic NIDDM that can't be controlled by diet alone. Sulfonylureas stimulate insulin release from the pancreas. After long-term therapy, extrapancreatic hypoglycemic effects include reduced hepatic glucose production, an increased number of insulin receptors, and changes in insulin binding.

Neurogenic diabetes insipidus

Chlorpropamide has been used in selected patients to treat neurogenic diabetes insipidus. The drug appears to potentiate the effect of minimal levels of antidiuretic hormone.

Overview of adverse reactions

Dose-related adverse effects, which usually aren't serious and respond to decreased doses, include headache, nausea, vomiting, anorexia, heartburn, weakness, and paresthesia. Hypoglycemia may follow excessive doses, increased exercise, decreased food intake, or consumption of alcohol. Signs and symptoms of overdose include anxiety, chills, cold sweats, confusion, cool pale skin, difficulty concentrating, drowsiness, excessive hunger, headache, nausea, nervousness, rapid heartbeat, shakiness, unsteady gait, weakness, and unusual fatigue.

Special considerations

• Administer sulfonylureas 30 minutes before the morning meal for once-daily dosing, or 30 minutes before the morning and evening meals for twice-daily dosing.

• Contraindicated in patients with juvenile-onset, brittle, or severe diabetes; diabetes mellitus adequately controlled by diet; and maturity-onset diabetes complicated by ketosis, acidosis, diabetic coma, Raynaud's gangrene, renal or hepatic impairment, or thyroid or other endocrine dysfunction.

• Use cautiously in patients with sulfonamide hypersensitivity.

Comparing sulfonylureas

Typically, sulfonylureas have similar actions and produce similar effects. They differ mainly in duration of action and dosage.

Drug	Usual dosage	Onset (hr)	Peak (hr)	Duration (hr)
First generation				
acetohexamide	500 mg once daily or b.i.d.	1	2	12-24
chlorpropamide	250 mg once daily	1	3-6	24-60
tolazamide	250 mg once daily or b.i.d.	4-6	6-10	12-24
tolbutamide	1,000 mg b.i.d. or t.i.d.	½-1	4-8	6-12
Second generation				
glimepiride	1 to 4 mg once daily	1	2-3	24
glipizide	5 mg once daily	1-3	2-3	10-24
glyburide	5 mg once daily	2	3-4	12-24

● Closely monitor patients transferring from insulin therapy to a sulfonylurea for urine glucose and ketones at least three times daily, before meals; emphasize the need for testing a double-voided specimen. Patients may require hospitalization during such changes in therapy.

● Patients transferring from another sulfonylurea (except chlorpropamide) usually need no transition period.

● NIDDM patients may require insulin therapy during periods of increased stress, such as infection, fever, surgery, or trauma. Monitor patients closely for hyperglycemia in these situations.

Pregnant patients

● Don't use a sulfonylurea in pregnant women because of prolonged, severe hypoglycemia lasting from 4 to 10 days in neonates born to women taking these drugs. Also, use of insulin permits more rigid control of blood glucose levels, which should reduce the risk of congenital abnormalities, illness, and death from abnormal glucose levels.

Breast-feeding patients

● Oral antidiabetics appear in breast milk in minimal amounts and may cause hypoglycemia in the breast-feeding infant.

Pediatric patients

● Oral antidiabetics aren't effective in insulin-dependent (type 1, juvenile-onset) diabetes mellitus.

Geriatric patients

● Elderly patients and those with renal insufficiency may be more sensitive to these drugs because of decreased metabolism and excretion. They usually need lower doses and should be closely monitored.

● Hypoglycemia may be more difficult to recognize in elderly patients, although it usually causes neurologic symptoms. Avoid drugs with prolonged duration of action in elderly patients.

Patient education

● Teach patient about the nature of his disease.

● Instruct patient on how to measure his own blood glucose levels.

● Emphasize the importance of following therapeutic regimen and adhering to specific diet, weight reduction, exercise, and personal hygiene recommendations. Teach patient how to avoid infections, test for glycosuria and ketonuria, and know signs and symptoms of hypoglycemia (fatigue, excessive hunger, profuse sweating, numbness of limbs) and hyperglycemia (excessive thirst or urination, excessive urine glucose or ketones).

● Be sure patient knows that therapy relieves symptoms but doesn't cure the disease.

● Discourage patient from consuming moderate to large amounts of alcohol while taking sulfonylureas; disulfiram-type reactions are possible.

Representative combinations

None.

tetracyclines

demeclocycline hydrochloride,
doxycycline hyclate, minocycline
hydrochloride, oxytetracycline
hydrochloride, tetracycline hydrochloride

Tetracycline antibiotics were discovered during
the random screening of soil samples for
antibiotic-producing microorganisms. The prototype, chlortetracycline, was discovered in 1948;
tetracycline was developed in 1952. Structural
modifications that enhanced both antibacterial
activity and pharmacokinetic parameters led to
development of doxycycline in 1966 and minocycline in 1972.

Usually well tolerated with few serious adverse
effects, tetracyclines have an unusually broad
spectrum of antibacterial activity, including gram-
negative and gram-positive anaerobic and aerobic bacteria, *Chlamydia*, and protozoa; longer-
acting tetracyclines have enhanced activity against
Chlamydia and *Legionella*.

Demeclocycline has a higher risk of severe
photosensitivity reactions; also, because of its renal effects, it's rarely prescribed for clinical use,
although it's used investigationally to treat SIADH
secretion.

Pharmacology

Tetracyclines are bacteriostatic but may be bactericidal against certain organisms. They bind reversibly to 30S and 50S ribosomal subunits, inhibiting bacterial protein synthesis. Bacterial
resistance to tetracyclines is usually mediated by
plasmids (R-factor resistance), which decrease
bacterial cell wall permeability; this is the most
important cause of resistance by staphylococci,
streptococci, most aerobic gram-negative organisms, and *Pseudomonas aeruginosa*. With
two exceptions, cross-resistance occurs with all
tetracyclines; doxycycline is active against *Bacteroides fragilis*, and minocycline is active against
Acinetobacter, Enterobacteriaceae, and *Staphylococcus aureus*.

Tetracyclines attack many pathogens; they
aren't antifungal or antiviral.

Susceptible gram-positive organisms include
*Actinomyces israelii, Bacillus anthracis,
Clostridium perfringens, Clostridium tetani,
Listeria monocytogenes*, and *Nocardia*. Initial
but transient activity exists against staphylococci and streptococci; infections caused by these
organisms are usually treated with other drugs.

Susceptible gram-negative organisms include
*Bartonella bacilliformis, Bordetella pertussis,
Brucella, Calymmatobacterium granulomatis,
Campylobacter fetus, Francisella tularensis,
Haemophilus ducreyi, H. influenzae, Legionella
pneumophila, Leptotrichia buccalis, Neisseria
gonorrhoeae, N. meningitidis, Pasteurella multocida, Shigella, Spirillum minus, Strepto-*
*bacillus moniliformis, Vibrio cholerae, V. para-
haemolyticus, Yersinia enterocolitica, Y. pestis*,
and many other common pathogens.

Other susceptible organisms include *Borrelia recurrentis, Chlamydia psittaci, C. trachomatis, Coxiella burnetii, Leptospira, Mycoplasma hominis, M. pneumoniae, Rickettsia
akari, R. prowazekii, R. tsutsugamushi, R. typhi, Treponema pallidum*, and *T. pertenue*.

Tetracyclines are absorbed systemically after
oral administration, chiefly from the duodenum;
with the exception of doxycycline and minocycline, absorption is decreased by food, milk, and
divalent and trivalent cations. Oral absorption of
tetracyclines is affected by chelation with certain
minerals such as calcium (doxycycline is least
involved); chelation causes tetracyclines to localize in bones and teeth. Because of hepatotoxicity and thrombophlebitis, only doxycycline and,
to a lesser extent, minocycline, are used I.V.

Tetracyclines occur widely into body tissues
and fluid, but CSF penetration is minimal; lipid-
soluble minocycline and doxycycline penetrate
fluids and tissues better; all tetracyclines cross
the placenta.

Tetracyclines are excreted primarily in urine,
chiefly by glomerular filtration; some drug is excreted in breast milk, and some inactivated drug
is excreted in feces. Unlike other tetracyclines,
minocycline undergoes enterohepatic circulation and is excreted in feces.

Oxytetracycline is moderately hemodialyzable;
other tetracyclines are removed only minimally
by hemodialysis or peritoneal dialysis.

Indications and actions
Bacterial, antiprotozoal, rickettsial,
and fungal infections

Tetracyclines are used as first-line therapy for
chlamydial infections and are the drugs of choice
for lymphogranuloma venereum, nonlympho-
granuloma venereum strains of *C. trachomatis*
in sexually transmitted diseases, psittacosis, and
nongonococcal urethritis if the primary pathogen
is probably *M. hominis* or *C. trachomatis*.
They're also the drugs of choice for rickettsial
infections (Rocky Mountain spotted fever, scrub
and endemic typhus, rickettsial pox, and Q fever)
and brucellosis. Tetracyclines also are used to
treat infections caused by *Campylobacter*, mycoplasma pneumonia (after Legionnaire's disease is ruled out), pertussis, cholera (in United
States only), leprosy, and gonorrhea.

Tetracyclines are second-line drugs in therapy of syphilis, actinomycosis, listeriosis, chancroid, and infections caused by *P. multocida* and
Y. pestis. They also provide economic prophylaxis in chronic pulmonary disease.

Tetracyclines are used orally to treat inflammatory acne vulgaris, topically for mild to moderate inflammatory acne, and as eyedrops for superficial eye infections, inclusion conjunctivitis,
and prophylaxis of ophthalmia neonatorum.

◊ Unlabeled clinical use

Individual tetracyclines are more effective against certain species or strains of a particular organism.

Diuretic agent in SIADH ◇
Demeclocycline causes diuresis by blocking antidiuretic hormone-induced reabsorption of water in the distal convoluted tubules and collecting ducts of the kidney.

Sclerosing agent
Parenteral tetracycline hydrochloride has been administered by intracavitary injection as a sclerosing agent in pleural or pericardial effusion. Parenteral doxycycline hyclate has been used as a sclerosing agent to control pleural effusions associated with metastatic tumors.

Other uses
Tetracyline is used as an adjunct to therapy for *H. pylori* infection.

Doxycycline is used for the suppression or prophylactic treatment of malaria caused by *Plasmodium falciparum* (chloroquine-resistant or sulfadoxine- and pyrimethamine-resistant) in individuals traveling for less than 4 months.

Oral doxycycline and oral tetracycline have been used to treat Lyme disease.

Tetracyline is used to treat various GI infections including balantidiasis caused by *Balantidium coli* ◇, Whipple's disease ◇, blind-loop syndrome ◇, and tropical sprue ◇.

Overview of adverse reactions
The most common adverse effects of tetracyclines involve the GI tract and are dose-related. Among them are anorexia, flatulence, nausea, vomiting, bulky and loose stools, epigastric burning, and abdominal discomfort.

Hypersensitivity reactions are infrequent; they manifest as urticaria, rash, pruritus, eosinophilia, and exfoliative dermatitis.

Photosensitivity reactions may be severe; they commonly occur with demeclocycline, rarely with minocycline.

Renal effects are minor and include occasional elevations in BUN levels (without increase in serum creatinine level) and a reversible diabetes insipidus syndrome (reported only with demeclocycline); renal failure has been attributed to Fanconi's syndrome after use of outdated tetracycline.

Rare adverse effects include hepatotoxicity (often in pregnant women receiving more than 2 g I.V. daily), leukocytosis, thrombocytopenia, hemolytic anemia, leukopenia, neutropenia, and atypical lymphocytes. There have also been reports of vaginal candidiasis, microscopic thyroid discoloration (after long-term use), dizziness, light-headedness, drowsiness, vein irritation (after I.V. use), and permanent discoloration of teeth in children under age 8.

Drug use with oral contraceptives can decrease the effectiveness of the contraceptive and increase risk of pregnancy.

Special considerations
● Assess patient's allergic history; don't give tetracycline antibiotics to patient with history of hypersensitivity reactions to other tetracyclines; monitor patient continuously for this and other adverse reactions.
● Obtain results of cultures and sensitivity tests before giving first dose, but don't delay therapy; check cultures periodically to assess drug efficacy.
● Monitor vital signs, electrolytes, and renal function studies before and during therapy.
● Check expiration dates. Outdated tetracyclines may cause nephrotoxicity.
● Monitor patient for bacterial and fungal superinfection, especially elderly patients, debilitated patients, and patients receiving immunosuppressants or radiation therapy. Watch especially for oral candidiasis. If symptoms occur, discontinue drug.
● Tetracyclines may interfere with certain laboratory tests; consult individual drug entry.
● Give oral drugs 1 hour before or 2 hours after meals for maximum absorption; don't give with food, milk or other dairy products, sodium bicarbonate, iron compounds, or antacids, which may impair absorption.
● Give water with and after oral drug to facilitate passage to stomach because incomplete swallowing can cause severe esophageal irritation; don't administer within 1 hour of bedtime, to prevent esophageal reflux.
● Follow manufacturer's directions for reconstitution and storage; keep product refrigerated and out of light.
● Avoid I.V. use of drug in patients with decreased renal function.
● I.V. use of tetracyclines in pregnancy or in patients with renal impairment, especially when dose exceeds 2 g daily, can cause hepatic failure.
● Monitor I.V. injection sites and rotate routinely to reduce local irritation. I.V. use may cause severe phlebitis.

Pregnant patients
● Tetracyclines may cause fetal toxicity in pregnant women.

Breast-feeding patients
● Avoid use of tetracyclines by breast-feeding women.

Pediatric patients
● Don't use in children under age 8 unless there's no alternative. Tetracyclines can cause permanent discoloration of teeth, enamel hypoplasia, and a reversible decrease in bone calcification.

Geriatric patients
● Some elderly patients have decreased esophageal motility; use tetracyclines cautiously, and watch for local irritation from slowly passing oral dosage forms. Elderly patients are more susceptible to superinfection.

Patient education
● Explain to patient the disease process and rationale for therapy.
● Teach patient signs and symptoms of adverse reactions, and emphasize need to report these promptly; urge patient to report unusual effects.
● Teach patient signs and symptoms of bacterial and fungal superinfection to geriatric and debilitated patients and others with low resistance from immunosuppressants or irradiation.
● Advise patient using oral contraceptives to use a backup method of contraception during drug therapy.
● Advise patient to avoid direct sunlight and to use a sunscreen to prevent photosensitivity reactions.
● Tell patient to take oral tetracyclines with a full 8-oz (240-ml) glass of water (to facilitate passage to the stomach) 1 hour before or 2 hours after meals for maximum absorption, and not less than 1 hour before bedtime (to prevent irritation from esophageal reflux).
● Emphasize that taking drug with food, milk or other dairy products, sodium bicarbonate, or iron compounds may interfere with absorption. Tell patient to take antacids 3 hours after tetracycline.
● Stress importance of completing prescribed regimen exactly as ordered and keeping follow-up appointments.
● Tell patient that doxycycline and monocycline may be taken with food.
● Instruct patient to check expiration date before use.

Representative combinations
Oxytetracycline with polymyxin B sulfate: Terramycin with polymyxin B, Terramycin topical ointment.

Oxytetracycline hydrochloride with phenazopyridine hydrochloride and sulfamethizole: Urobiotic-250.

Tetracycline hydrochloride with citric acid: Achromycin V.

thrombolytic enzymes

alteplase, anistreplase, reteplase (recombinant), streptokinase, tenecteplase, urokinase

When a thrombus obstructs a blood vessel, permanent damage to the ischemic area may occur before the body can dissolve the clot. Thrombolytic agents were developed in the hope that speeding lysis of the clot would prevent permanent ischemic damage. Thrombolytic activity attributable to streptokinase was described in 1933; the effects of this compound have since been studied on various kinds of clots. It isn't clear whether such agents significantly reduce thrombosis-induced ischemic damage in all situations for which the drugs are currently used. (See *Comparing thrombolytic enzymes,* page 76.)

Pharmacology
Streptokinase is a protein-like substance produced by group C beta-hemolytic streptococci; urokinase is an enzyme isolated from human kidney tissue cultures. Alteplase and tenecteplase are tissue-type plasminogen activator synthesized by recombinant DNA technology. Anistreplase is anisoylated streptokinase-plasminogen activated complex; it's a fibrinolytic enzyme (plasminogen) plus activator complex (streptokinase) with the activator temporarily blocked by an anisoyl group. Reteplase is a recombinant-plasminogen activator. Thrombolytic enzymes act to lyse clots chiefly by converting plasminogen to plasmin; in contrast, anticoagulants act by preventing thrombi from developing. Thrombolytics are more likely to produce bleeding than are oral anticoagulants.

Indications and actions
Thrombosis, thromboembolism
Alteplase, streptokinase, and urokinase are used to treat acute pulmonary thromboembolism; streptokinase and urokinase are used to treat deep vein thrombosis, acute arterial thromboembolism, or acute coronary arterial thrombosis and to clear arteriovenous cannula occlusion and venous catheter obstruction. Anistreplase, alteplase, reteplase, streptokinase, tenecteplase and urokinase are indicated in acute MI. These agents are administered in an attempt to lyse coronary artery thrombi, which may result in improved ventricular function and decreased risk of heart failure. Alteplase is used in the management of acute ischemic CVA.

Overview of adverse reactions
Adverse reactions to these agents are essentially an extension of their actions; hemorrhage is the most common adverse effect. These agents cause bleeding twice as often as does heparin. Streptokinase is more likely to cause an allergic reaction than urokinase. Information regarding hypersensitivity to alteplase is limited.

Special considerations
● Thrombolytic therapy requires medical supervision with continuous clinical and laboratory monitoring.
● Thrombolytics act only on fibrin clots, not those formed by a precipitated drug.
● Follow instructions for reconstitution precisely and pass solution through a filter 0.45 microns or smaller to remove filaments in the solution; don't use with dextran because it can interfere

Comparing thrombolytic enzymes

Thrombolytic enzymes dissolve clots by accelerating the formation of plasmin by activated plasminogen. Plasminogen activators, found in most tissues and body fluids, help plasminogen (an inactive enzyme) convert to plasmin (an active enzyme), which dissolves the clot. Doses of the enzymes listed below may vary according to the patient's condition.

Drug	Action	Initial dose	Maintenance therapy
alteplase	Directly converts plasminogen to plasmin	I.V. bolus: 6 to 10 mg over 1 to 2 min	I.V. infusion: 60 mg/hr in the 1st hr; then 20 mg/hr for the next 2 hr for a total of 100 mg
anistreplase	Directly converts plasminogen to plasmin	I.V. push: 30 units over 2 to 5 min	Not necessary
reteplase	Enhances the cleavage of plasminogen to generate plasmin	Double I.V. bolus injection of 10 + 10 units	Not necessary
streptokinase	Indirectly activates plasminogen, which converts to plasmin	Intracoronary bolus: 15,000 to 20,000 IU I.V. bolus: none needed	Intracoronary infusion: 2,000 to 4,000 IU/min over 1 hr; total dose 140,000 IU I.V. infusion: 1,500,000 units over 1 hr
tenecteplace	Directly converts plasminogen to plasmin	I.V. bolus over 5 seconds. If patient weighs less than 60 kg, give 30 mg; if 60 to 69 kg, give 35 mg; if 70 to 79 kg, give 40 mg; if 80 to 89 kg, give 45 mg; if 90 kg or more, give 50 mg.	Not necessary
urokinase	Directly converts plasminogen to plasmin	Intracoronary bolus: none needed	Intracoronary infusion: 2,000 units/lb/hr (4,400 units/kg/hr); rate of 15 ml of solution/hr for total of 12 hr (total volume shouldn't exceed 200 ml)

with coagulation as well as blood typing and cross-matching.

• Obtain pretherapy baseline determinations of thrombin time, activated partial thromboplastin time, PT, INR, hematocrit, and platelet count for subsequent blood monitoring. During systemic thrombolytic therapy, as in pulmonary embolism or venous thrombosis, PT, INR, or thrombin time after 4 hours of therapy should be about twice the pretreatment value.

• Administer drugs by infusion pump to ensure accuracy; I.M. injections are contraindicated during therapy because of increased risk of bleeding at the injection site.

• Check vital signs frequently, monitoring for blood pressure alterations in excess of 25 mm Hg and any change in cardiac rhythm; checking pulses, color, and sensitivity of limbs every hour. Monitor patient for excessive bleeding every 15 minutes for first hour, every 30 minutes for second through eighth hours; then at least once every 8 hours. Stop therapy if bleeding is evident; pre-

treatment with heparin or drugs affecting platelets increases risk.

• Monitor patient for hypersensitivity as well as hemorrhage; keep available typed and cross-matched packed RBCs and whole blood, aminocaproic acid to treat bleeding, and corticosteroids to treat allergic reactions.

• Keep involved limb in straight alignment to prevent bleeding from infusion site. Establish precautions to prevent injury and avoid unnecessary handling of patient because bruising is likely.

• At end of infusion, flush remaining dose from pump tubing with I.V. 5% dextrose or normal saline solution.

• Continuous heparin infusion usually is started with the prescribed thrombolytic.

• Before using thrombolytic to clear an occluded catheter, try to gently aspirate or flush with heparinized saline solution. Avoid forcible flushing or vigorous suction, which could rupture the catheter or expel the clot into the circulation.

• When treating MI or CVA, the sooner treatment is administered, the greater the benefit.

Pregnant patients
• Thrombolytics should only be used in pregnancy if clearly indicated.

Breast-feeding patients
• Safety in breast-feeding women hasn't been established.

Pediatric patients
• Safety in children hasn't been established.

Geriatric patients
• Patients age 75 or over are at greater risk of cerebral hemorrhage, because they're more apt to have cerebrovascular disease.

Patient education
• Explain to patient the rationale for treatment and procedure, and necessity for bed rest.
• Ask patient to be alert for signs of bleeding.
• When using these drugs to clear catheter, tell patient to exhale and hold breath at any time catheter isn't connected, to prevent air entering the open catheter.

Representative combinations
None.

---

tricyclic antidepressants

amitriptyline hydrochloride,
amoxapine, clomipramine hydrochloride, desipramine hydrochloride,
doxepin hydrochloride, imipramine
hydrochloride, imipramine pamoate,
nortriptyline hydrochloride,
protriptyline, trimipramine maleate

The inherent mood-elevating activity of tricyclic antidepressants (TCAs) was discovered during research with iminodibenzyl, a compound originally investigated for sedative, analgesic, antihistaminic, and antiparkinsonian effects. Clinical trials in 1958 with the class prototype, imipramine, found no antipsychotic activity, but showed marked mood-elevating effects.

Pharmacology
Although the precise mechanism of their CNS effects isn't established, TCAs may exert their effects by inhibiting reuptake of the neurotransmitters norepinephrine and serotonin in CNS nerve terminals (presynaptic neurons), resulting in increased concentration and enhanced activity of neurotransmitters in the synaptic cleft. TCAs also have antihistaminic, sedative, anticholinergic, vasodilatory, and quinidine-like effects; the drugs are structurally similar to phenothiazines and share similar adverse reactions.

Individual TCAs differ somewhat in their degree of CNS inhibitory effect. The tertiary amines (amitriptyline, doxepin, imipramine, and trimipramine) exert greater sedative effects; tertiary amines and protriptyline have more profound effects on cardiac conduction, whereas desipramine has the least anticholinergic activity. All of the currently available TCAs have equal clinical efficacy when given in equivalent therapeutic doses; choice of specific therapy is determined primarily by pharmacokinetic properties and the patient's adverse reaction profile. Patients may respond to some TCAs and not others; if patient doesn't respond to one drug, another should be tried.

Indications and actions
Depression
TCAs are used to treat major depression and dysthymic disorder. Depressed patients who are also anxious are helped most by the more sedating agents: doxepin, imipramine, and trimipramine. Protriptyline has a stimulant effect that evokes a favorable response in withdrawn depressed patients; only maprotiline has FDA approval for use in depression mixed with anxiety.

Obsessive-compulsive disorder
Clomipramine is used in the treatment of obsessive-compulsive disorder.

Enuresis
Imipramine is used for enuresis in children over age 6.

Severe, chronic pain
TCAs, especially amitriptyline, desipramine, doxepin, imipramine, and nortriptyline, are useful in the management of severe chronic pain.

Other psychiatric disorders ◇
TCAs have been used to treat phobic disorders with panic attacks, and eating disorders (bulimia nervosa), and in the short-term treatment of duodenal or gastric ulcer.

Overview of adverse reactions
Adverse reactions to TCAs are similar to those seen with phenothiazine antipsychotic agents, including varying degrees of sedation, anticholinergic effects, and orthostatic hypotension. The tertiary amines have the strongest sedative effects; tolerance to these effects usually develops in a few weeks. Protriptyline has the least sedative effect (and may be stimulatory), but shares with the tertiary amines the most pronounced effects on blood pressure and cardiac tissue. Maprotiline and amoxapine are most likely to cause seizures, especially in overdose situations. Desipramine has a greater margin of safety in patients with prostatic hypertrophy, paralytic ileus, glaucoma, and urine retention because of its relatively low level of anticholinergic activity.

Special considerations

- TCAs impair ability to perform tasks requiring mental alertness, such as driving a car.
- Check vital signs regularly for decreased blood pressure or tachycardia; observe patient carefully for adverse reactions and report changes. Obtain ECG in patients over age 40 before starting therapy.
- Have patient take the first dose in the office to allow close observation for adverse reactions.
- Check for anticholinergic adverse reactions, which may require dose reduction.
- Caregiver should be sure patient swallows each dose of drug when given; as depressed patients begin to improve, they may hoard pills for suicide attempt.
- Observe patient for mood changes to monitor progress; benefits may not occur for several (3 to 6) weeks.
- Don't withdraw full dose of drug abruptly; gradually reduce dose over a period of weeks to avoid rebound effect or other adverse reactions.
- Carefully follow manufacturer's instructions for reconstitution, dilution, and storage of drugs.
- Investigational uses include treating peptic ulcer, migraine prophylaxis, and allergy. Potential toxicity has, to date, outweighed most advantages.
- Because suicidal overdose with TCAs is usually fatal, prescribe only small amounts. If possible, entrust a reliable family member with the drug and warn him to store drug safely away from children.

Pregnant patients

- Safe use of TCAs in pregnancy hasn't been established. Fetal malformations, urine retention, CNS effects (lethargy), developmental delay, and withdrawal symptoms have occurred in neonates born to women taking TCAs during pregnancy.

Breast-feeding patients

- Safety in breast-feeding women hasn't been established.

Pediatric patients

- TCAs aren't advised for children under age 12.

Geriatric patients

- Use lower doses because these patients are more sensitive to both therapeutic and adverse effects of TCAs.

Patient education

- Explain to patient the rationale for therapy and anticipated risks and benefits; also explain that full therapeutic effect may not occur for several weeks.
- Teach patient the signs and symptoms of adverse reactions and the importance of reporting them.
- Tell patient to avoid beverages and drugs containing alcohol and not to take other drugs (including OTC products) without medical approval.

- Teach patient how and when to take drug, not to increase dose without medical approval, and never to discontinue drug abruptly.
- Tell patient to lie down for 30 minutes after first dose and to rise slowly to avoid orthostatic hypotension.
- Advise taking drug with milk or food to minimize GI distress; suggest taking full dose at bedtime if daytime sedation is troublesome.
- Urge diabetic patients to monitor blood glucose, as drug may alter insulin needs.
- Advise patient to avoid tasks that require mental alertness until full effect of drug is determined.
- Warn patient that excessive exposure to sunlight, heat lamps, or tanning beds may cause burns and abnormal hyperpigmentation.
- Recommend sugarless gum or hard candy, artificial saliva, or ice chips to relieve dry mouth.
- Advise patient that unpleasant adverse effects (except dry mouth) generally diminish over time.

Representative combinations

Amitriptyline hydrochloride with perphenazine: Etrafon, Triavil; with chlordiazepoxide: Limbitrol.

vitamins

Fat-soluble: vitamin A (retinol), vitamin A acid (retinoic acid), vitamin D, vitamin D_2 (ergocalciferol), vitamin D_3 (calcipotriene), vitamin E, vitamin K (phytonadione)

Water-soluble: vitamin B_1 (thiamine), vitamin B_2 (riboflavin), vitamin B_3 (niacin), vitamin B_6 (pyridoxine), vitamin B_9 (folic acid, folacin), vitamin B_{12} (cyanocobalamin), vitamin C (ascorbic acid)

Vitamins are chemically unrelated organic compounds that are required for normal growth and maintenance of metabolic functions. Because the body is unable to synthesize many vitamins, it must obtain them from exogenous sources. Vitamins don't furnish energy and aren't essential building blocks for the body; however, they're essential for the transformation of energy and for the regulation of metabolic processes.

Vitamins are classified as fat-soluble or water-soluble, and the Food and Nutrition Board of the National Research Council determines the RDAs for each. These allowances represent amounts that will provide adequate nutrition in most healthy persons; they're not minimum requirements. Note that a diet that includes ample intake of the major food groups provides sufficient amounts of vitamins. If needed, vitamins should be used as an adjunct to a regular diet and not as a food substitute.

Controversy has existed for years over the vitamin issue. Some argue that vitamin supple-

Vitamins: Recommended daily allowances for adults ages 23 to 50

Vitamin	Men	Women	Pregnant woment	Lactating woment
A	1,000 mcg	800 mcg	800 mcg	1,300 mcg
B_1	1.5 mg	1.1 mg	1.5 mg	1.6 mg
B_2	1.7 mg	1.3 mg	1.6 mg	1.8 mg
B_6	2 mg	1.6 mg	2.2 mg	2.1 mg
B_{12}	2 mcg	2 mcg	2.2 mcg	2.6 mcg
C	60 mg	60 mg	70 mg	95 mg
D	200 IU	200 IU	400 IU	400 IU
E	15 IU	12 IU	15 IU	18 IU
K	80 mcg	65 mcg	65 mcg	65 mcg
folic acid	200 mcg	180 mcg	400 mcg	280 mcg
niacin	19 mg	15 mg	17 mg	20 mg

† First 6 months.

mentation is unnecessary; some advise moderate supplementation, still others advocate the use of megavitamins.

Pharmacology

Vitamins are available as single drugs or in combination with several other vitamins with or without minerals, trace elements, iron, fluoride, or other nutritional supplements. Often, diets deficient in one vitamin are also deficient in other vitamins of similar dietary source. Malabsorption syndromes also affect the usage of several vitamins as do certain disease states that increase metabolic rates. Therefore, multiple vitamin therapy may be useful in these situations.

Fat-soluble vitamins are absorbed with dietary fats and stored in the body in moderate amounts; they aren't normally excreted in urine. Chronic ingestion leads to excessive build-up of these agents and toxicity.

Water-soluble vitamins aren't stored in the body in any appreciable amounts and are excreted in urine. These agents seldom cause toxicity in patients with normal renal function.

Both types of vitamins are needed for the maintenance of normal structure and metabolic functions of the body. (See *Vitamins: Recommended daily allowances for adults ages 23 to 50.*)

Indications and actions
Vitamin deficiency or malabsorption, conditions of metabolic stress
Vitamin supplementation is required when deficiencies exist, in malabsorption syndrome, in hypermetabolic disease states, during pregnancy and lactation, and in the elderly, alcoholics, or dieters. Multiple vitamins may be indicated for patients taking oral contraceptives, estrogens, prolonged antibiotic therapy, isoniazid, or for patients receiving prolonged total parenteral nutrition.

Persons with increased metabolic requirements such as infants and those suffering severe injury, trauma, major surgery, or severe infection also require supplementation. Prolonged diarrhea, severe GI disorders, malignancy, surgical removal of sections of GI tract, obstructive jaundice, cystic fibrosis, and other conditions leading to reduced or poor absorption are indications for multiple vitamin therapy. Refer to individual agents for specific indications.

Overview of adverse reactions
Common adverse reactions seen with both fat-soluble and water-soluble vitamins include nausea, vomiting, diarrhea, tiredness, weakness, headache, loss of appetite, rash, and itching.

Special considerations
• Monitoring may be required. See specific vitamin entries for details.
• Vitamins containing iron may cause constipation and black, tarry stools.
• Excessive fluoride supplements can result in hypocalcemia and tetany.
• Give with food or after meals to reduce GI distress.

Pregnant patients
• Vitamin supplementation in pregnancy should be regulated by a health care provider.

Breast-feeding patients
● RDAs may be increased in breast-feeding women.

Pediatric patients
● RDAs vary with age. Excessive amounts of vitamins, particularly in neonates, may be toxic.

Patient education
● Stress to patient the importance of adequate dietary intake. Vitamins aren't food substitutes.
● Tell patient to take vitamins only as directed, not to exceed RDA, and to take with food, milk, or after meals to reduce chance of stomach upset.
● Store vitamins away from heat and light, and out of the reach of small children.
● Warn patient that vitamins with iron may cause constipation and black, tarry stools.
● Tell patient to read all label directions. Warn him not to take large doses unless prescribed.
● Inform patient that liquid vitamins may be mixed with food or juice.
● Advise patient not to refer to vitamins or other drugs as candy and to avoid taking them indiscriminately.

Representative combinations
The following list includes selected combinations that are available only by prescription.
B vitamins (oral) niacin (B_3), pantothenic acid (B_5), pyridoxine (B_6), and cyanocobalamin (B_{12}), with folic acid (B_9), iron, manganese, zinc, and 13% alcohol: Megaton Elixir; with thiamine (B_1), riboflavin (B_2), ferric pyrophosphate, and 15% alcohol: Senilezol Liquid; with thiamine (B_1), riboflavin (B_2), ascorbic acid, and folic acid: Berocca, B-Plex, Strovite, B C with folic acid; with thiamine (B_1), riboflavin (B_2), ascorbic acid, folic acid, and biotin: Nephrocaps.

Multivitamins (oral) vitamins E, thiamine (B_1), riboflavin (B_2), niacin (B_3), pantothenic acid (B_5), pyridoxine (B_6), cyanocobalamin (B_{12}), ascorbic acid, and folic acid: Cefol Filmtabs; with vitamins A, D, E, thiamine (B_1), riboflavin (B_2), niacin (B_3), pantothenic acid (B_5), pyridoxine (B_6), cyanocobalamin (B_{12}), ascorbic acid, iron, and folic acid: Centrum Jr. with Iron, Cerovite Jr., Hi-Po-Vites, Monocaps, Quintabs-M, Unicap Sr., Unicomplex-T&M Tablets.

Multivitamins (parenteral) vitamins A, D, E, thiamine (B_1), riboflavin (B_2), niacin (B_3), pantothenic acid (B_5), pyridoxine (B_6), cyanocobalamin (B_{12}), ascorbic acid, biotin, and folic acid: Berocca Parenteral Nutrition, M.V.I.-12.

Multivitamins with fluoride (oral) vitamins A, D, thiamine (B_1), riboflavin (B_2), niacin (B_3), pantothenic acid (B_5), pyridoxine (B_6), cyanocobalamin (B_{12}), ascorbic acid, folic acid, and fluoride: Polyvitamin Fluoride, Mulvidren-F Softab Tablets, Polytabs-F; vitamins A, D, E, thiamine (B_1), riboflavin (B_2), niacin (B_3), pyridoxine (B_6), cyanocobalamin (B_{12}), ascorbic acid, folic acid, and fluoride: Poly-Vi-Flor, Florvite, Vi-Daylin/F.

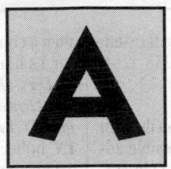

abacavir sulfate
Ziagen

Pharmacologic classification: nucleoside
analogue reverse transcriptase inhibitor
Therapeutic classification: antiviral
Pregnancy risk category: C

Indications and dosages
➤ *HIV-1 infection. Adults:* 300 mg P.O. twice
daily with other antiretrovirals.
Children ages 3 months to 16 years: 8 mg/kg
P.O. twice daily (up to maximum of 300 mg P.O.
twice daily) with other antiretrovirals.

How supplied
Available by prescription only
Oral solution: 20 mg/ml
Tablets: 300 mg

Pharmacodynamics
Antiviral action: Converted intracellularly to
the active metabolite carbovir triphosphate, which
inhibits the activity of HIV-1 reverse transcriptase by competing with the natural substrate
deoxyguanosine-5'-triphosphate and by incorporation into viral DNA.

Pharmacokinetics
Absorption: Rapidly and extensively absorbed
after oral administration; mean absolute bioavailability of the tablet is 83%.
Distribution: Distributed in the extravascular
space. About 50% of drug binds to plasma proteins.
Metabolism: Primarily metabolized by alcohol
dehydrogenase and glucuronyl transferase to form
two metabolites that lack antiviral activity.
Excretion: Primarily excreted in urine; about
16% in feces. Elimination half-life in single-dose
studies is 1 to 2 hours.

Route	Onset	Peak	Duration
P.O.	Unknown	Unknown	Unknown

Contraindications and precautions
Contraindicated in patients hypersensitive to drug
or its components. Use cautiously in patients with
risk factors for liver disease.

Interactions
Drug-lifestyle. *Alcohol use:* Reduces abacavir
elimination, increasing overall exposure to drug.
Monitor patient's alcohol consumption, and advise caution with concurrent use.

Adverse reactions
CNS: insomnia, sleep disorders, headache.
GI: *nausea, vomiting,* diarrhea, loss of appetite.
Skin: rash.
Other: *hypersensitivity reaction,* fever.

Overdose and treatment
There's no known antidote, and it isn't known
whether the drug is removed by peritoneal dialysis or hemodialysis.

Special considerations
● Abacavir should always be used with other antiretrovirals and shouldn't be added as a single
drug when an antiretroviral regimen is changed
because of loss of virologic response.
● Because the drug is absorbed equally well from
both dosage forms, solution and tablets can be
used interchangeably.
● The drug has caused fatal hypersensitivity reactions. If evidence of hypersensitivity (fever, skin
rash, fatigue, GI symptoms such as nausea, vomiting, diarrhea, or abdominal pain) develops, discontinue drug as soon as a reaction is suspected and provide immediate medical attention.
⚠ ALERT Don't start drug after a hypersensitivity reaction because more severe symptoms
will recur within hours and may include life-
threatening hypotension and death. Symptoms
usually appear within the first 6 weeks of treatment, but may occur at any time.
● To facilitate reporting of hypersensitivity reactions and collection of information on each case,
an abacavir hypersensitivity registry has been established at 1-800-270-0425.

Patient monitoring
● Lactic acidosis and severe (even fatal) hepatomegaly with steatosis have been reported with
use of nucleoside analogues alone or in combination, including abacavir and other antiretrovirals. Stop treatment if a patient develops clinical
or laboratory findings suggestive of lactic acidosis or pronounced hepatotoxicity (which may include hepatomegaly and steatosis even in the absence of marked transaminase elevations).
● Monitor patient for hypersensitivity reactions;
they may be fatal.

Pregnant patients
● There are no adequate controlled studies in
pregnant women. Report maternal-fetal outcomes

---

of pregnant women exposed to drug to the Anti-retroviral Pregnancy Registry at 1-800-258-4263.

Breast-feeding patients
• Because of the risk of HIV transmission through breast-feeding and because of the possible adverse effects of abacavir, women shouldn't breast-feed if receiving this drug.

Pediatric patients
• Safety and efficacy haven't been established in children ages 3 months to 13 years.

Geriatric patients
• Dose selection for geriatric patients should be cautious, taking into account the increased likelihood of decreased hepatic, renal, or cardiac function and of concomitant disease or other drug therapy.

Patient education
• Advise patient to take drug exactly as prescribed.
• Urge patient to read the medication guide that comes with each new prescription and refill.
• Tell patient that the drug may be taken without regard to meals.
• Advise patient about the risk of a life-threatening hypersensitivity reaction with this drug.
• Tell patient to immediately contact prescriber if signs or symptoms of hypersensitivity develop, including fever, skin rash, severe tiredness, GI symptoms (such as nausea, vomiting, diarrhea, or stomach pain), achiness, or a generally ill feeling.
• Instruct patient to carry a medical identification card that summarizes the symptoms of the hypersensitivity reaction.
• Explain that this drug doesn't cure HIV infection or reduce the risk of transmitting HIV to others through sexual contact or blood contamination. Advise patient to remain under medical care throughout drug therapy and to practice safe sex.
• Inform patient that long-term effects of this drug are unknown.

---

abciximab
ReoPro

Pharmacologic classification: antiplatelet aggregator
Therapeutic classification: platelet aggregation inhibitor
Pregnancy risk category: C

Indications and dosages
➤ *Adjunct to percutaneous transluminal coronary angioplasty (PTCA) or atherectomy for prevention of acute cardiac ischemic complications in patients at high risk for abrupt closure of treated coronary vessel.* Adults: 0.25 mg/kg as an I.V. bolus given 10 to 60 minutes before start of PTCA;

then a continuous I.V. infusion of 10 mcg/minute for 12 hours.
➤ *Unstable angina not responding to conventional therapy with plans to undergo PTCA within 24 hours.* Adults: 0.25 mg/kg I.V. bolus; then 18- or 24-hour I.V. infusion of 10 mcg/minute ending 1 hour after PTCA.

How supplied
Available by prescription only
Injection: 2 mg/ml

Pharmacodynamics
Platelet aggregation–inhibiting action: As the Fab fragment of the chimeric human-murine monoclonal immunoglobulin antibody 7E3, abciximab binds selectively to platelet glycoprotein (GP IIb/IIIa) receptors and inhibits platelet aggregation.

Pharmacokinetics
Absorption: Administered I.V.
Distribution: No information available.
Metabolism: No information available.
Excretion: Initial half-life is less than 10 minutes; second phase lasts about 30 minutes.

Route	Onset	Peak	Duration
I.V.	Unknown	Unknown	Unknown

Contraindications and precautions
Contraindicated in patients hypersensitive to any component of drug or to murine proteins and in those with active internal bleeding, significant GI or GU bleeding within 6 weeks, history of CVA within 2 years or CVA with significant residual neurologic deficit, bleeding diathesis, thrombocytopenia (less than 100,000/mm³), major surgery or trauma within 6 weeks, intracranial neoplasm, intracranial arteriovenous malformation, intracranial aneurysm, severe uncontrolled hypertension, or history of vasculitis. Also contraindicated when oral anticoagulants have been administered within past 7 days unless PT is 1.2 times control or less, or when I.V. dextran is being used before or is intended to be used during PTCA.

Use cautiously in patients who are at increased risk for bleeding, including those who weigh less than 165 lb (75 kg), those who are over age 65, those with history of GI disease, and those receiving thrombolytics. Conditions that also increase the risk of bleeding include PTCA within 12 hours of onset of symptoms for acute MI, PTCA lasting over 70 minutes, and failed PTCA. Heparin anticoagulation used with abciximab also may increase the risk of bleeding.

Interactions
Drug-drug. *Antiplatelet drugs, heparin, NSAIDs, thrombolytics, other anticoagulants:* Increased risk of bleeding. Monitor patient closely.

Adverse reactions
CNS: confusion, hypoesthesia.
CV: *bradycardia, hypotension,* peripheral edema.
EENT: abnormal vision.
GI: *nausea, vomiting.*
Hematologic: anemia, *bleeding,* leukocytosis, *thrombocytopenia.*
Respiratory: pleural effusion, pleurisy, pneumonia.
Other: pain.

Overdose and treatment
There are no reports of overdose. However, infusion should be discontinued after 12 hours to avoid effects of prolonged platelet receptor blockade.

Special considerations
● Patients at risk for abrupt closure (thus candidates for drug therapy) include those undergoing PTCA with at least one of the following conditions: unstable angina; non-Q-wave MI; acute Q-wave MI within 12 hours of symptom onset; or the presence of two type B lesions in the artery to be dilated, one type B lesion in the artery to be dilated in a woman age 65 or older or a diabetic patient, one type C lesion in the artery to be dilated, or angioplasty of an infarct-related lesion within 7 days of MI.
● Give drug with aspirin and heparin.
● Keep epinephrine, dopamine, theophylline, antihistamines, and corticosteroids readily available in case of anaphylaxis.
● Inspect solution for particulate matter before administration. If opaque particles are present, discard solution and obtain new vial.
● For bolus injection, withdraw needed amount of drug into a syringe through a sterile, nonpyrogenic, low-protein-binding, 0.2- or 0.22-millipore filter. Administer bolus 10 to 60 minutes before procedure.
● For continuous infusion, withdraw 4.5 ml of drug for continuous infusion through a sterile, nonpyrogenic, low-protein-binding, 0.2- or 0.22-micron filter into a syringe. Inject into 250 ml of sterile normal saline solution or D_5W and infuse at 17 ml/hour for 12 hours through a continuous infusion pump equipped with an in-line filter. Discard unused portion at end of 12-hour infusion.
● Administer drug in a separate I.V. line; don't add other drugs to infusion solution.

Patient monitoring
● Before infusion, platelet count, PT, activated clotting time, and APTT should be measured to identify hemostatic abnormalities.
● Monitor patient closely for bleeding. Bleeding may be at the arterial access site for cardiac catheterization, or it may be internal bleeding involving the GI or GU tracts or retroperitoneal sites.
● Institute bleeding precautions. Maintain patient on bed rest for 6 to 8 hours after sheath removal or drug discontinuation, whichever is later. Discontinue heparin at least 4 hours before sheath removal. Minimize or avoid, if possible, arterial and venous punctures, I.M. injections, nasotracheal intubation, and use of urinary catheters, nasogastric tubes, and automatic blood pressure cuffs.
● Monitor platelet counts before treatment, 2 to 4 hours after treatment, and at 24 hours after treatment or before discharge.
● Platelet function recovers in about 48 hours but drug remains in circulation for up to 10 days in a platelet-bound state.

Breast-feeding patients
● It's unknown if drug appears in breast milk or is absorbed systemically after ingestion. Use cautiously.

Pediatric patients
● Safety and effectiveness in children haven't been established.

Geriatric patients
● Use drug cautiously in patients over age 65.

Patient education
● Instruct patient to report bleeding promptly.

---

acarbose
Precose

Pharmacologic classification: alpha-glucosidase inhibitor
Therapeutic classification: antidiabetic
Pregnancy risk category: B

Indications and dosages
➤ *Dietary adjunct to lower blood glucose levels in patients with type 2 (non-insulin-dependent) diabetes mellitus whose hyperglycemia can't be managed by diet alone or by diet and a sulfonyl-urea, or adjunct to insulin or metformin; adjunct to insulin or metformin therapy in patients with type 2 (non-insulin-dependent) diabetes mellitus whose hyperglycemia can't be managed by diet, exercise, and insulin or metformin alone.*
Adults: Initially, 25 mg P.O. t.i.d. with the first bite of each main meal. Subsequent dosage adjustment made at 4- to 8-week intervals based on 1-hour postprandial glucose levels and tolerance. Maintenance dosage is 50 to 100 mg P.O. t.i.d. depending on patient's weight. Maximum dose for patients weighing 60 kg (132 lb) or less is 50 mg P.O. t.i.d.; for patients weighing over 60 kg, maximum dose is 100 mg P.O. t.i.d.

How supplied
Available by prescription only
Tablets: 25 mg, 50 mg, 100 mg

Pharmacodynamics
Antidiabetic action: The ability of acarbose to lower blood glucose results from a competitive, reversible inhibition of pancreatic alpha-amylase and membrane-bound intestinal alpha-glucoside hydrolase enzymes. In diabetic patients, this enzyme inhibition results in delayed glucose absorption and a lowering of postprandial hyperglycemia. The drug doesn't enhance insulin secretion.

Pharmacokinetics
Absorption: Minimally absorbed.
Distribution: Acts locally in the GI tract.
Metabolism: Metabolized exclusively within the GI tract, principally by intestinal bacteria with some metabolized action caused by digestive enzymes.
Excretion: Within 96 hours, 51% of dose is excreted in feces as unabsorbed drug. The fraction of drug absorbed is almost completely excreted by the kidneys. Plasma elimination half-life of acarbose is about 2 hours. Drug accumulation doesn't occur with t.i.d. oral dosing.

Route	Onset	Peak	Duration
P.O.	Unknown	1 hr	2-4 hr

Contraindications and precautions
Contraindicated in patients hypersensitive to drug and in those with diabetic ketoacidosis, cirrhosis, inflammatory bowel disease, colonic ulceration, partial intestinal obstruction, or predisposition to intestinal obstruction. Also contraindicated in patients with chronic intestinal diseases that cause marked disorders of digestion or absorption and in those with conditions that may deteriorate because of increased gas formation in the intestine. Avoid using drug in patients with serum creatinine levels above 2 mg/dl and in breast-feeding or pregnant women.

Use cautiously in patients with mild to moderate renal impairment.

Interactions
Drug-drug. *Calcium channel blockers, corticosteroids, estrogens, isoniazid, nicotinic acid, oral contraceptives, phenothiazines, phenytoin, sympathomimetics, thiazides and other diuretics, and thyroid products:* May cause hyperglycemia or hypoglycemia when withdrawn. Monitor patient's blood glucose levels.
Insulin, sulfonylureas: When used with acarbose, the hypoglycemic potential of these agents may be increased. Monitor patient's blood glucose level closely.
Intestinal adsorbents (activated charcoal), digestive enzyme preparations containing carbohydrate-splitting enzymes (amylase, pancreatin): May reduce the effect of acarbose. Don't administer together.

Adverse reactions
GI: *abdominal pain, diarrhea, flatulence.*

Hepatic: elevated serum transaminase levels.

Overdose and treatment
Unlike sulfonylureas or insulin, acarbose overdose doesn't result in hypoglycemia. An overdose may result in transient increases in flatulence, diarrhea, and abdominal discomfort, which quickly subside.

Special considerations
● Acarbose isn't effective as sole therapy in patients with diabetes mellitus complicated by acidosis, ketosis, or coma; management of these conditions requires the use of insulin.
● Because of its mechanism of action, acarbose shouldn't cause hypoglycemia when administered alone in the fasted or postprandial state.

Patient monitoring
● Acarbose alone doesn't cause hypoglycemia. However, when given with a sulfonylurea or insulin, it may increase the hypoglycemic potential of the sulfonylurea. Closely monitor patient receiving both drugs. If hypoglycemia occurs, treat with oral glucose (dextrose), whose absorption isn't inhibited by acarbose, rather than sucrose (cane sugar). Severe hypoglycemia may require I.V. glucose infusion or glucagon administration. Dosage adjustment in acarbose and sulfonylurea may be required to prevent further episodes of hypoglycemia.
● During periods of increased stress, such as infection, fever, surgery, or trauma, patient may require insulin therapy. Monitor patient closely for hyperglycemia in these situations.
● Monitor patient's 1-hour postprandial plasma glucose levels to determine effectiveness of acarbose and to identify appropriate dose. Thereafter, measure glycosylated hemoglobin every 3 months. Treatment goals include decreasing both postprandial plasma glucose and glycosylated hemoglobin levels to normal or near normal by using the lowest effective dose of acarbose either as monotherapy or with sulfonylureas.
● Monitor serum transaminase levels every 3 months during first year of therapy and then periodically thereafter in patients receiving doses exceeding 50 mg t.i.d. Abnormalities may require dosage adjustment or withdrawal of drug.

Breast-feeding patients
● It isn't known if drug appears in breast milk. Acarbose shouldn't be given to breast-feeding women.

Pediatric patients
● Safety and efficacy in patients under age 18 haven't been established.

Patient education
● Tell patient to take drug with the first bite of each of three main meals daily.
● Make sure patient understands that therapy relieves symptoms but doesn't cure disease.

Reactions may be *common,* uncommon, *life-threatening,* or COMMON AND LIFE-THREATENING.

• Stress the importance of adhering to specific diet, weight reduction, exercise, and personal hygiene programs. Explain how and when to monitor blood glucose level, and teach recognition of and intervention for hyperglycemia.

• Teach patient to recognize and intervene for hypoglycemia if a sulfonylurea drug is also taken. Tell patient to treat symptoms of hypoglycemia with a form of dextrose instead of products containing table sugar.

• Advise patient to wear or carry medical identification regarding diabetic status.

---

acebutolol
Sectral

Pharmacologic classification: beta blocker
Therapeutic classification: antihypertensive, antiarrhythmic
Pregnancy risk category: B

Indications and dosages
➤ *Hypertension. Adults:* 400 mg P.O. either as a single daily dose or 200 mg b.i.d. Patients may receive as much as 1,200 mg divided b.i.d.
➤ *Ventricular arrhythmias. Adults:* 200 mg P.O. b.i.d., increased to produce an adequate clinical response. Usual daily dose is 600 to 1,200 mg.
➤ *Angina ◇. Adults:* Initially, 200 mg b.i.d., increased to 800 mg daily until angina is controlled. Patients with severe angina may need higher doses.
✦ *Dosage adjustment.* Reduce dosage in geriatric patients and in those with impaired renal function. If creatinine clearance is 25 to 49 ml/minute, decrease dose by 50%. If creatinine clearance is less than 25 ml/minute, decrease dose by 75%. Avoid doses over 800 mg daily in geriatric patients.

How supplied
Available by prescription only
Capsules: 200 mg, 400 mg

Pharmacodynamics
Antihypertensive action: Exact mechanism of antihypertensive beta-adrenergic blocker effect is unknown. Drug has cardioselective beta blocking properties and mild intrinsic sympathomimetic activity.
Antiarrhythmic action: Drug decreases heart rate and prevents exercise-induced increases in heart rate; it also decreases myocardial contractility, cardiac output, and SA and AV nodal conduction velocity.

Pharmacokinetics
Absorption: Well absorbed after oral administration.
Distribution: About 26% protein-bound; minimal quantities are detected in CSF.
Metabolism: Undergoes extensive first-pass metabolism in the liver; peak levels of its major active metabolite, diacetolol, occur at about 3¼ hours.
Excretion: From 30% to 40% of a given dose is excreted in urine; remainder occurs in feces and bile. Half-life of acebutolol is 3 to 4 hours; half-life of diacetolol is 8 to 13 hours.

Route	Onset	Peak	Duration
P.O.	1½ hr	2½ hr	24 hr

Contraindications and precautions
Contraindicated in patients with persistent severe bradycardia, second- and third-degree heart block, overt cardiac failure, and cardiogenic shock. Use cautiously in patients at risk for heart failure, patients with impaired hepatic function, and patients with bronchospastic disease, diabetes, hyperthyroidism, and peripheral vascular disease.

Interactions
Drug-drug. *Alpha-adrenergic stimulants (such as those in OTC cold remedies), indomethacin, NSAIDs:* Hypotensive effects of acebutolol may be antagonized by these drugs. Use together cautiously.
Antihypertensives: Acebutolol may potentiate hypotensive effects. Monitor blood pressure.
Insulin, oral antidiabetics: Dosage requirements in stable diabetic patients may be altered. Monitor blood glucose levels.

Adverse reactions
CNS: depression, dizziness, fatigue, headache, hyperesthesia, hypoesthesia, insomnia.
CV: *bradycardia,* chest pain, edema, *heart failure,* hypotension.
GI: abdominal pain, constipation, diarrhea, dyspepsia, flatulence, nausea, vomiting.
GU: impotence.
Musculoskeletal: arthralgia, myalgia.
Respiratory: *bronchospasm,* cough, dyspnea.
Skin: rash.

Overdose and treatment
Signs of overdose include severe hypotension, bradycardia, heart failure, and bronchospasm.
After acute ingestion, empty stomach by emesis or gastric lavage; follow with activated charcoal to reduce absorption. Then provide symptomatic and supportive treatment.

Special considerations
Consider the recommendations relevant to all beta blockers as well as the following.
• Store capsules in well-closed containers, protected from light at room temperature.
• Adjust drug dose every 1 to 2 months if blood pressure control is inadequate.
• Don't discontinue drug abruptly because this may exacerbate angina symptoms or precipitate MI in patients with coronary artery disease. Discontinue gradually over 2 weeks.

Patient monitoring
• Carefully monitor blood pressure during dosage adjustment.

Pregnant patients
• There are no adequate and controlled studies in pregnant women. Infants born to women receiving acebutolol during pregnancy had lower birth weights and decreased systolic blood pressures and heart rates during the first 72 hours after delivery.

Breast-feeding patients
• Both acebutolol and its metabolite, diacetolol, appear in breast milk; breast-feeding isn't recommended.

Pediatric patients
• Safety and efficacy in children under age 12 haven't been established.

Geriatric patients
• Avoid doses over 800 mg.

Patient education
• Advise patient to promptly report wheezing.
• Warn patient not to discontinue drug suddenly, and to notify prescriber of adverse effects.
• Teach patient how to take his pulse and instruct him to withhold the dose and notify prescriber if pulse rate is below 60 beats/minute.

acetaminophen
Acephen, Anacin Aspirin Free, Feverall, Panadol, Tempra, Tylenol

Pharmacologic classification: para-aminophenol derivative
Therapeutic classification: nonnarcotic analgesic, antipyretic
Pregnancy risk category: B

Indications and dosages
➤ *Mild pain, fever. Adults and children over age 12:* 325 to 650 mg P.O. or P.R. q 4 to 6 hours p.r.n. Maximum dose shouldn't exceed 4 g daily. Maximum dose for long-term therapy is 2.6 g daily; alternatively, two 650-mg extended-release tablets every 8 hours p.r.n., not to exceed 4 g per day.
Children ages 11 to 12: 480 mg P.O. or P.R. q 4 to 6 hours p.r.n.
Children ages 9 to 10: 400 mg P.O. or P.R. q 4 to 6 hours p.r.n.
Children ages 6 to 8: 320 mg P.O. or P.R. q 4 to 6 hours p.r.n.
Children ages 4 to 5: 240 mg P.O. or P.R. q 4 to 6 hours p.r.n.
Children ages 2 to 3: 160 mg P.O. or P.R. q 4 to 6 hours p.r.n.
Children ages 12 to 23 months: 120 mg P.O. or P.R. q 4 to 6 hours p.r.n.

Children ages 4 to 11 months: 80 mg P.O. or P.R. q 4 to 6 hours p.r.n.
Children age 3 months or less: 40 mg P.O or P.R. q 4 to 6 hours p.r.n.
➤ *Osteoarthritis. Adults:* Up to 1 g P.O. q.i.d.; doses of 3 to 4 g per day common in these patients.

How supplied
Available without a prescription
Caplets: 160 mg, 500 mg, 650 mg
Capsules: 325 mg, 500 mg
Gelcaps: 500 mg
Solution: 48 mg/ml, 80 mg/0.8 ml, 80 mg/ml*, 80 mg/1.66 ml, 80 mg/2.5 ml, 80 mg/5 ml, 100 mg/ml, 120 mg/5 ml, 160 mg/5 ml, 500 mg/15 ml
Sprinkle capsules: 80 mg, 160 mg
Suppositories: 80 mg, 120 mg, 125 mg, 300 mg, 325 mg, 650 mg
Suspension: 80 mg/ml*, 100 mg/ml, 80 mg/5 ml*, 160 mg/5 ml
Syrup: 16 mg/ml
Tablets: 160 mg, 325 mg, 500 mg, 650 mg
Tablets (chewable): 80 mg
Tablets (extended-release): 650 mg

Pharmacodynamics
Mechanism and site of action may be related to inhibition of prostaglandin synthesis in CNS.
Analgesic action: Analgesic effect may be related to an elevation of the pain threshold.
Antipyretic action: Drug may exert antipyretic effect by direct action on hypothalamic heat-regulating center to block effects of endogenous pyrogen. This results in increased heat dissipation through sweating and vasodilation.

Pharmacokinetics
Absorption: Absorbed rapidly and completely via the GI tract.
Distribution: 25% protein-bound. Plasma levels don't correlate well with analgesic effect, but they do correlate with toxicity.
Metabolism: About 90% to 95% is metabolized in the liver.
Excretion: Excreted in urine. Average elimination half-life ranges from 1 to 4 hours. In acute overdose, prolongation of elimination half-life is correlated with toxic effects. Half-life over 4 hours is linked to hepatic necrosis; over 12 hours is linked to coma.

Route	Onset	Peak	Duration
P.O., P.R.	Unknown	1-3 hr	3-4 hr

Contraindications and precautions
No known contraindications. Use cautiously in patients with history of chronic alcohol abuse because hepatotoxicity has occurred after therapeutic doses. Also use cautiously in patients with hepatic or CV disease, renal function impairment, or viral infection.

Reactions may be *common*, uncommon, **life-threatening**, or COMMON AND LIFE-THREATENING.

Interactions

Drug-drug. *Antacids:* Delayed and decreased absorption of acetaminophen. Separate administration times.

Anticoagulants, thrombolytics: May potentiate effects of these drugs, but this appears to be clinically insignificant.

Anticonvulsants, isoniazid: Increased risk of hepatotoxicity. Use together cautiously.

Phenothiazines: If used with acetaminophen in large doses, hypothermia may result. Use together cautiously.

Drug-herb. *Feverfew, ginkgo biloba:* Possible increased risk of bleeding. Discourage concurrent use.

Red clover: Coumarin effects may enhance anticoagulation. Discourage use together. If concurrent therapy is unavoidable, monitor PT and INR closely.

Watercress: May inhibit oxidative metabolism of acetaminophen. Discourage use together.

Drug-food. *Caffeine:* May enhance therapeutic effect of acetaminophen. Discourage use together.

Foods: Delayed and decreased absorption of acetaminophen. Advise taking drug on an empty stomach.

Drug-lifestyle. *Alcohol use:* Increased risk of liver toxicity. Discourage alcohol use.

Adverse reactions

Hematologic: hemolytic anemia, *neutropenia, leukopenia, pancytopenia, thrombocytopenia.*
Hepatic: jaundice, *severe liver damage.*
Metabolic: hypoglycemia.
Skin: rash, urticaria.

Overdose and treatment

In all cases of suspected acetaminophen overdose, a regional poison center or the Rocky Mountain Poison Center (1-800-525-6115) may be called for assistance. In acute overdose, plasma levels of 300 mcg/ml 4 hours after ingestion or 50 mcg/ml 12 hours after ingestion are linked to hepatotoxicity. Signs and symptoms of overdose include cyanosis, anemia, jaundice, skin eruptions, fever, emesis, CNS stimulation, delirium, methemoglobinemia progressing to depression, coma, vascular collapse, seizures, and death. Acetaminophen poisoning develops in stages:

Stage 1 (12 to 24 hours after ingestion): nausea, vomiting, diaphoresis, anorexia

Stage 2 (24 to 48 hours after ingestion): clinically improved but elevated liver function test results

Stage 3 (72 to 96 hours after ingestion): peak hepatotoxicity

Stage 4 (7 to 8 days after ingestion): recovery.

To treat toxic overdose of acetaminophen, empty stomach immediately by inducing emesis with ipecac syrup (if patient is conscious) or by performing gastric lavage. Administer activated charcoal by way of nasogastric tube. Oral acetyl-cysteine (Mucomyst) is a specific antidote for acetaminophen poisoning and is most effective if started within 10 to 12 hours after ingestion, but it can help if started within 24 hours after ingestion. Administer a Mucomyst loading dose of 140 mg/kg P.O., followed by maintenance dosages of 70 mg/kg P.O. every 4 hours for an additional 17 doses. Doses vomited within 1 hour of administration must be repeated. Remove charcoal before giving acetylcysteine because it may interfere with absorption of this antidote.

Hemodialysis may be helpful to remove acetaminophen from the body. Monitor laboratory parameters and vital signs closely. Provide symptomatic and supportive measures (respiratory support, correction of fluid and electrolyte imbalances). Determine plasma acetaminophen levels at least 4 hours after overdose. If plasma acetaminophen levels indicate hepatotoxicity, perform liver function tests every 24 hours for at least 96 hours.

Special considerations

● Acetaminophen may cause a false-positive test result for urinary 5-hydroxyindoleacetic acid.

● Acetaminophen doesn't have a significant anti-inflammatory effect. Even so, studies have shown substantial benefit in patients with osteoarthritis of the knee. Therapeutic benefits may stem from the analgesic effects of the drug.

● Many OTC products contain acetaminophen. Be aware of this when recommending this drug.

⚠ ALERT Be aware of patient's total daily intake of acetaminophen, especially if he is also taking other prescribed drugs containing this component, such as Percocet. Toxicity can occur.

● Patients unable to tolerate aspirin may be able to tolerate acetaminophen.

● When buffered acetaminophen effervescent granules are prescribed, consider sodium content for sodium-restricted patients.

● Advise patients with phenylketonuria that many preparations contain aspartame.

● Many acetaminophen preparations contain sulfites.

● The extended-release tablet shouldn't be crushed, chewed, or dissolved in liquid.

● Store rectal acetaminophen suppositories in refrigerator.

Patient monitoring

● Address patient's level of pain and response before and after drug administration.

● Monitor vital signs, especially temperature, to evaluate effectiveness of drug.

● Monitor PT and INR values in patients receiving oral anticoagulants and sustained acetaminophen therapy.

Breast-feeding patients

● Drug appears in breast milk in low concentrations. No adverse effects have been reported.

Pediatric patients
● Children shouldn't take more than five doses per day or take drug for more than 5 days unless prescribed. Instruct caregivers on weight-based acetaminophen dosing, to use the provided calibrated measuring device with the preparation, and not to give more than the recommended dose. Also, caution caregivers not to use other OTC preparations that contain acetaminophen.

Geriatric patients
● Geriatric patients are more sensitive to drug. Use with caution.

Patient education
● Instruct patient in proper administration of prescribed form of drug.
● Advise patient on long-term high-dose drug therapy to arrange for monitoring of laboratory parameters, especially BUN, serum creatinine, liver function tests, and CBC.
● Warn patient with current or past rectal bleeding to avoid using rectal acetaminophen suppositories. If they're used, they must be retained in the rectum for at least 1 hour.
● Warn patient that high doses or unsupervised long-term use of acetaminophen can cause liver damage. Use of alcoholic beverages increases the risk of liver toxicity.
● Tell patient to avoid use if body temperature is above 103° F (39° C), if fever persists longer than 3 days, or if fever recurs.
● Tell patient not to take NSAIDs with acetaminophen on a regular basis.
● Warn patient to avoid taking tetracycline antibiotics within 1 hour after taking buffered acetaminophen effervescent granules.
● Tell patient not to use drug for arthritic or rheumatic conditions without medical approval. Drug may relieve pain but not other symptoms.
● Advise adult patient not to take drug for more than 10 days without medical approval.
● Tell patient on high-dose or long-term therapy that regular follow-up visits are essential.

---

acetazolamide
acetazolamide sodium
Dazamide, Diamox, Diamox Sequels

Pharmacologic classification: carbonic anhydrase inhibitor
Therapeutic classification: antiglaucoma agent, anticonvulsant, diuretic, altitude sickness agent (prevention and treatment)
Pregnancy risk category: C

Indications and dosages
➤ *Secondary glaucoma and preoperative management of acute angle-closure glaucoma.* *Adults:* 250 mg P.O. q 4 hours, or 250 mg P.O. b.i.d. for short-term therapy. In acute cases, 500 mg P.O. followed by 125 to 250 mg P.O. q 4

hours. To rapidly lower intraocular pressure, 500 mg I.V., which may be repeated in 2 to 4 hours, if necessary, followed by 125 to 250 mg P.O. q 4 hours.
Children: 5 to 10 mg/kg I.V. q 6 hours.
➤ *Edema in heart failure.* *Adults:* 250 to 375 mg P.O. daily in morning.
Children: 5 mg/kg or 150 mg/m² P.O. or I.V. daily in morning.
➤ *Drug-induced edema.* *Adults:* 250 to 375 mg (5 mg/kg) P.O. as single daily dose for 1 to 2 days alternating with 1 drug-free day.
➤ *Chronic open-angle glaucoma.* *Adults:* 250 mg to 1 g P.O. daily in divided doses, or 500 mg (extended-release) P.O. once daily or b.i.d. Doses over 1 g daily don't produce an increased effect.
Children: 8 to 30 mg/kg P.O. or 300 to 900 mg/m² daily in three divided doses.
➤ *Prevention or amelioration of acute mountain sickness.* *Adults:* 500 mg to 1 g P.O. daily in divided doses (such as 250 mg q 8 to 12 hours) or 500 mg (extended-release) P.O. q 12 to 24 hours, taken preferably 48 hours before ascent and continued for at least 48 hours after arrival at high altitude.
➤ *Myoclonic seizures, refractory generalized tonic-clonic (grand mal) or absence (petit mal) seizures, mixed seizures.* *Adults and children:* 8 to 30 mg/kg P.O. daily, divided into one to four doses. The optimum dose range is 375 mg to 1 g P.O. daily. When given with other anticonvulsants, the initial dose is 250 mg daily.
➤ *Periodic paralysis* ◊. *Adults:* 250 mg P.O. b.i.d. or t.i.d. Maximum dose is 1.5 g daily.

How supplied
Available by prescription only
Capsules (extended-release): 500 mg
Injection: 500 mg
Tablets: 125 mg, 250 mg

Pharmacodynamics
Antiglaucoma action: In open-angle glaucoma and perioperatively for acute angle-closure glaucoma, acetazolamide and acetazolamide sodium decrease the formation of aqueous humor, lowering intraocular pressure.
Anticonvulsant action: Inhibition of carbonic anhydrase in the CNS appears to slow abnormal paroxysmal discharge from the neurons.
Diuretic action: Acetazolamide and acetazolamide sodium act by noncompetitive reversible inhibition of the enzyme carbonic anhydrase, which is responsible for formation of hydrogen and bicarbonate ions from carbon dioxide and water. This inhibition results in decreased hydrogen concentration in the renal tubules, promoting excretion of bicarbonate, sodium, potassium, and water; systemic acidosis may occur because carbon dioxide isn't eliminated as rapidly.
Anti–altitude-sickness action: Acetazolamide shortens the period of high-altitude acclimatiza-

---

tion; by inhibiting conversion of carbon dioxide to bicarbonate, it may increase carbon dioxide tension in tissues and decrease it in the lungs. The resultant metabolic acidosis may also increase oxygenation during hypoxia.

Pharmacokinetics
Absorption: Well absorbed from the GI tract after oral administration.
Distribution: Distributed throughout body tissues.
Metabolism: None.
Excretion: Excreted primarily in urine via tubular secretion and passive reabsorption.

Route	Onset	Peak	Duration
P.O.			
Regular	1-1½ hr	1-3 hr	8-12 hr
Extended	2 hr	3-6 hr	18-24 hr
I.V.	2 min	15 min	1-5 hr

Contraindications and precautions
Contraindicated in patients hypersensitive to drug; in those receiving long-term therapy for chronic noncongestive angle-closure glaucoma; and in those with hyponatremia or hypokalemia, renal or hepatic disease or dysfunction, adrenal gland failure, and hyperchloremic acidosis. Use cautiously in patients with respiratory acidosis, emphysema, diabetes, or COPD and in those receiving other diuretics.

Interactions
Drug-drug. *Amphetamines, flecainide, procainamide, quinidine:* Acetazolamide alkalinizes urine and thus may decrease excretion of these drugs. Monitor patient closely.
Lithium, phenobarbital, salicylates: Increased excretion of these drugs causes low plasma levels, possibly necessitating dosage adjustments.

Adverse reactions
CNS: confusion, drowsiness, paresthesia.
EENT: hearing dysfunction, transient myopia, tinnitus.
GI: anorexia, altered taste, diarrhea, nausea, vomiting.
GU: hematuria, polyuria.
Hematologic: *aplastic anemia,* hemolytic anemia, *leukopenia.*
Metabolic: asymptomatic hyperuricemia, hyperchloremic acidosis, hypokalemia, decreased thyroid iodine uptake.
Skin: rash.

Overdose and treatment
Acetazolamide increases bicarbonate excretion and may cause hypokalemia and hyperchloremic acidosis.

Treatment is supportive and symptomatic. Induce emesis or perform gastric lavage. Don't induce catharsis because this may exacerbate electrolyte disturbances. Monitor fluid and electrolyte levels.

Special considerations
● Suspensions containing 250 mg/5 ml of syrup are the most palatable and can be made by the pharmacist. These remain stable for about 1 week. Tablets don't dissolve in fruit juice.
● Reconstitute powder by adding at least 5 ml sterile water for injection.
● Direct I.V. administration is preferred if drug must be given parenterally.

Patient monitoring
● Monitor electrolyte and serum glucose levels.
● Watch for hepatic coma or precoma in patients with hepatic cirrhosis, hypokalemia, or elevations in blood ammonia levels caused by drug therapy.
● Monitor patient's fluid intake and output.

Pregnant patients
● Acetazolamide may cause fetal toxicity when administered to pregnant women.

Breast-feeding patients
● Safety of drug in breast-feeding women hasn't been established.

Geriatric patients
● Observe geriatric and debilitated patients closely because they're more susceptible to drug-induced diuresis. Excessive diuresis promotes rapid dehydration, leading to hypovolemia, hypokalemia, and hyponatremia and may cause circulatory collapse. Reduced dosages may be indicated.

Patient education
● Warn patient to use caution while driving or performing tasks that require alertness, coordination, or physical dexterity because drug may cause drowsiness.
● Tell patient to take oral form with food if GI upset occurs.
● If drug is being used for diuretic therapy, have patient consult healthcare provider or dietitian regarding high-potassium diet.

acetylcholine chloride
Miochol

Pharmacologic classification: cholinergic agonist
Therapeutic classification: miotic
Pregnancy risk category: NR

Indications and dosages
➤ *To produce miosis during surgery.*
Adults and children: 0.5 to 2 ml of 1% solution instilled gently in anterior chamber of eye. Drug is used during ophthalmic surgery to cause rapid, complete miosis.

How supplied
Available by prescription only
Ophthalmic solution: 1%

Pharmacodynamics
Miotic action: The cholinergic activity of acetylcholine causes contraction of the sphincter muscles of the iris, resulting in miosis and contraction of the ciliary muscle, leading to accommodation. It also acts to deepen the anterior chamber and vasodilates conjunctival vessels of the outflow tract.

Pharmacokinetics
Absorption: Action begins in seconds.
Distribution: Unknown.
Metabolism: Probably locally metabolized by cholinesterases.
Excretion: Duration of activity is 10 minutes.

Route	Onset	Peak	Duration
Ophthalmic	Within sec	Unknown	10 min

Contraindications and precautions
Contraindicated in patients hypersensitive to drug or its components.

Interactions
None reported.

Adverse reactions
CV: *bradycardia,* hypotension, flushing.
EENT: corneal edema, clouding, decompensation.
Respiratory: breathing difficulties.
Skin: diaphoresis.

Overdose and treatment
Overdose is extremely rare after ophthalmic use but may cause miosis, flushing, vomiting, bradycardia, bronchospasm, increased bronchial secretion, sweating, tearing, involuntary urination, hypotension, and seizures. Flush eyes with normal saline solution or sterile water. If drug is accidentally swallowed, vomiting is usually spontaneous; if not, induce emesis with activated charcoal or a cathartic.

Treat accidental dermal exposure by washing the area twice with water. Epinephrine may be used to treat adverse CV reactions.

Special considerations
• Solutions of acetylcholine chloride are unstable; prepare solution immediately before use. Discard unused solution and one that is not clear and colorless.
• Don't use the vial if the center rubber plug seal doesn't go down or is already down when reconstituting.
• Don't gas-sterilize vial. Ethylene oxide may produce formic acid.

Patient monitoring
• Monitor patient for adverse effects.

Patient education
• Instruct patient to report breathing difficulties immediately.

---

acetylcysteine
Mucomyst, Mucosil, Parvolex*

Pharmacologic classification: amino acid (l-cysteine) derivative
Therapeutic classification: mucolytic, antidote for acetaminophen overdose
Pregnancy risk category: B

Indications and dosages
➤ *Acute and chronic bronchopulmonary disease, tracheostomy care, pulmonary complications of surgery, diagnostic bronchial studies.* Administer by nebulization, direct application, or intratracheal instillation. *Adults and children:* 1 to 2 ml of 10% or 20% solution by direct instillation into trachea as often as hourly; or 3 to 5 ml of 20% solution or 6 to 10 ml of 10% solution administered by nebulizer q 2 to 3 hours. For instillation via percutaneous intratracheal catheter, administer 1 to 2 ml of 20% solution or 2 to 4 ml of 10% solution q 1 to 4 hours; via tracheal catheter to treat a specific bronchopulmonary tree segment, administer 2 to 5 ml of 20% solution. For diagnostic bronchial studies (administered before procedure), administer 1 to 2 ml of 20% solution or 2 to 4 ml of 10% solution for two or three doses.
➤ *Acetaminophen toxicity. Adults and children:* Initially, 140 mg/kg P.O., followed by 70 mg/kg q 4 hours for 17 doses (a total of 1,330 mg/kg) or until acetaminophen assay reveals nontoxic level. Or, drug may be given I.V.: loading dose 150 mg/kg I.V. in 200 ml D_5W over 15 minutes, followed by 50 mg/kg I.V. in 500 ml D_5W over 4 hours, followed by 100 mg/kg I.V. in 1,000 ml D_5W over 16 hours.

How supplied
Available by prescription only
Injection*: 200 mg/ml
Solution: 10%, 20%

Pharmacodynamics
Mucolytic action: Drug produces its mucolytic effect by splitting the disulfide bonds of mucoprotein, the substance responsible for increased viscosity of mucus secretions in the lungs; thus, pulmonary secretions become less viscous and more liquid.
Acetaminophen antidote: Mechanism by which acetylcysteine reduces acetaminophen toxicity isn't fully understood; it's thought that acetylcysteine restores hepatic stores of glutathione or inactivates the toxic metabolite of acetaminophen

---

Reactions may be *common*, uncommon, *life-threatening*, or COMMON AND LIFE-THREATENING.

via a chemical interaction, thereby preventing hepatic damage.

Pharmacokinetics
Absorption: Most inhaled acetylcysteine acts directly on mucus in the lungs; the remainder is absorbed by pulmonary epithelium. After oral administration, drug is absorbed from the GI tract.
Distribution: Unknown.
Metabolism: Metabolized in the liver.
Excretion: Unknown.

Route	Onset	Peak	Duration
P.O., I.V., inhalation	Unknown	Unknown	Unknown

Contraindications and precautions
Contraindicated in patients hypersensitive to drug. Use cautiously in geriatric or debilitated patients with severe respiratory insufficiency.

Interactions
Drug-drug. *Activated charcoal:* Absorbs orally administered acetylcysteine, preventing its absorption. Remove charcoal before acetylcysteine administration.
Amphotericin B, ampicillin, chlortetracycline, chymotrypsin, erythromycin lactobionate, hydrogen peroxide, iodized oil, oxytetracycline, tetracycline, trypsin: Incompatible with these drugs. Administer drugs separately.

Adverse reactions
CV: chest tightness, hypotension, hypertension, tachycardia.
EENT: *rhinorrhea.*
GI: *nausea, stomatitis, vomiting.*
Respiratory: **bronchospasm** (especially in asthmatic patients).
Other: clamminess, fever.

Overdose and treatment
No information available.

Special considerations
● Acetylcysteine solutions release hydrogen sulfide and discolor on contact with rubber and some metals (especially iron, nickel, and copper); drug tarnishes silver (this doesn't affect drug potency).
● Solution may turn light purple; this doesn't affect safety or efficacy of the drug. Use plastic, stainless steel, or other inert metal when administering drug by nebulization. Don't use handheld bulb nebulizers; output is too small and particle size too large.
● After opening, store in refrigerator or use within 96 hours.
● When used orally for acetaminophen overdose, dilute with cola, fruit juice, or water to a 5% concentration and administer within 1 hour.
● Don't place directly in the chamber of a heated (hot pot) nebulizer.

● Optimal results occur when acetylcysteine is administered within 16 hours of acetaminophen ingestion, but preferably 8 hours; however, drug may be administered up to 24 hours after acetaminophen ingestion. A regional poison center or the Rocky Mountain Poison Center (1-800-525-6115) may be contacted for assistance when using acetylcysteine as an antidote.

Patient monitoring
● Monitor cough type and frequency; for maximum effect, instruct patient to clear airway by coughing before aerosol administration. Many clinicians pretreat with bronchodilators before administration of acetylcysteine. Keep suction equipment available; if patient has insufficient cough to clear increased secretions, suction will be needed to maintain open airway.
● If encephalopathy develops as a result of hepatic failure, stop acetylcysteine therapy to prevent further accumulation of nitrogenous substances.
● Obtain a 4-hour postingestion acetaminophen level (for peak concentration); the results are used with a nomogram to estimate the potential for hepatotoxicity. This guides the administration of acetylcysteine.

Pregnant patients
● There are no adequate studies in pregnant women. Use only if clearly indicated.

Breast-feeding patients
● It's unknown if drug appears in breast milk.

Pediatric patients
● Drug may be given by tent or croupette. Use a sufficient volume (up to 300 ml) of a 10% or 20% solution to maintain a heavy mist in the tent for the time prescribed. Administration may be continuous or intermittent.

Geriatric patients
● Geriatric patients may have inadequate cough and be unable to clear airway completely of mucus. Keep suction equipment available and monitor patient closely.

Patient education
● Warn patient about unpleasant odor (rotten egg odor of hydrogen sulfide), and explain that increased amounts of liquefied bronchial secretion plus unpleasant odor may cause nausea and vomiting; have patient rinse mouth with water after nebulizer treatment.
● For maximum effect, instruct patient to clear airway by coughing before aerosol administration.

activated charcoal

Actidose-Aqua, CharcoAid,
CharcoCaps, Liqui-Char

Pharmacologic classification: adsorbent
Therapeutic classification: antidote, antidiarrheal, antiflatulent
Pregnancy risk category: NR

Indications and dosages

➤**Poisoning.** *Adults and children:* Five to ten times the estimated weight of drug or chemical ingested. Dose is 30 to 100 g in 250 ml water to make a slurry.

Give orally, preferably within 30 minutes of toxin ingestion. Larger doses are necessary if food is in the stomach. Drug is used adjunctively in treating poisoning or overdose with acetaminophen, amphetamines, antimony, arsenic, aspirin, atropine, barbiturates, camphor, cardiac glycosides, cocaine, glutethimide, ipecac, malathion, morphine, opium, oxalic acid, parathion, phenol, phenothiazines, phenytoin, poisonous mushrooms, potassium permanganate, propoxyphene, quinine, strychnine, sulfonamides, or tricyclic antidepressants.

Activated charcoal may be given 20 to 60 g q 4 to 12 hours (gastric dialysis) to enhance removal of some drugs from the bloodstream. Monitor serum drug level.

➤**Flatulence or dyspepsia.** *Adults:* 600 mg to 5 g P.O. as a single dose, or 975 mg to 3.9 g t.i.d. after meals.

➤**To relieve GI disturbances (halitosis, anorexia, nausea, vomiting) in uremic patients**◇**.** *Adults:* 20 to 50 g P.O. daily.

How supplied

Available without a prescription
Capsules: 260 mg
Granules: 15 g in 120 ml
Hemoperfusion system: 300 g
Powder: 15-g, 30-g, 40-g, 120-g, 240-g unit dose
Suspension: 0.625 g/5 ml, 0.7 g/5 ml (50 g), 1 g/5 ml, 1.25 g/5 ml
Tablets: 250 mg
Tablets (delayed-release) with 80 mg simethicone: 250 mg

Pharmacodynamics

Antidote action: Drug adsorbs ingested toxins, thereby inhibiting GI absorption.
Antidiarrheal action: Activated charcoal adsorbs toxic and nontoxic irritants that cause diarrhea or GI discomfort.
Antiflatulent action: Activated charcoal adsorbs intestinal gas to relieve discomfort.

Pharmacokinetics

Absorption: Not absorbed from the GI tract.
Distribution: None.
Metabolism: None.

Excretion: Excreted in feces.

Route	Onset	Peak	Duration
P.O.	Immediate	Unknown	Unknown

Contraindications and precautions

No known contraindications.

Interactions

Drug-drug. *Oral acetylcysteine, syrup of ipecac:* Activated charcoal inactivates these medications and many other orally administered medications. Charcoal should be removed by gastric lavage before acetylcysteine is administered.
Drug-food. *Milk products:* Decreased effectiveness of activated charcoal. Don't dilute drug with dairy products.

Adverse reactions

GI: black stools, constipation, nausea.

Overdose and treatment

No information available.

Special considerations

● Don't use activated charcoal if poisoning involves corrosive agents, cyanide, iron, mineral acids, or organic solvents.
● Don't give activated charcoal by mouth to a semiconscious or unconscious patient; instead, administer the drug through a nasogastric tube.
● Because activated charcoal adsorbs and inactivates syrup of ipecac, give only after emesis is complete.
● Dose may need to be repeated if patient vomits shortly after administration.
● Activated charcoal is most effective when used within 30 minutes of toxin ingestion; a cathartic is commonly administered with or after activated charcoal to speed removal of the toxin/charcoal complex.
● Powder form is most effective. Mix with tap water to form consistency of thick syrup. A small amount of fruit juice or flavoring may be added to make mixture more palatable.
● If administering drug for indications other than poisoning, be sure to give other medications 1 hour before or 2 hours after activated charcoal.
● Activated charcoal may be used orally to decrease colostomy odor.

Patient monitoring

● Monitor patient's nutritional status; prolonged use (over 72 hours) may impair patient's nutritional status.
● Monitor serum electrolytes if repeated dosing of charcoal with sorbitol or in children who may be more sensitive to sorbitol.

Pediatric patients

● Don't use charcoal with sorbitol in children under 1 year old.

Reactions may be *common,* uncommon, *life-threatening,* or COMMON AND LIFE-THREATENING.

Patient education

• Tell patient to call poison information center or hospital emergency department before taking activated charcoal as an antidote.

• If patient is using activated charcoal as an antidiarrheal or antiflatulent, instruct him to take medications 1 hour before or 2 hours after activated charcoal. For antidiarrheal use, advise patient to report fever, diarrhea that persists after 2 days of therapy, or flatulence that persists after 7 days.

• Warn patient that activated charcoal turns stools black.

• Advise patient not to mix drug with milk products, which may lessen its effectiveness.

---

acyclovir (acycloguanosine)
acyclovir sodium
Zovirax

Pharmacologic classification: synthetic purine nucleoside
Therapeutic classification: antiviral
Pregnancy risk category: C

Indications and dosages

➤*Initial and recurrent mucocutaneous herpes simplex virus (HSV type 1 and HSV type 2) or severe initial genital herpes or herpes simplex in immunocompromised patients. Adults and children over age 12:* 5 mg/kg, given at a constant rate over 1 hour by I.V. infusion q 8 hours for 7 days (5 days for genital herpes).
Children under age 12: 10 mg/kg infused at a constant rate over 1 hour by I.V. infusion q 8 hours for 7 days (5 days for genital herpes).

➤*Mucocutaneous herpes simplex virus (HSV type 1 and HSV type 2) in immunocompromised patients. Adults:* 400 mg P.O. q 4 hours while awake (five times daily).
Children: 1 g P.O. daily divided into three to five doses for 7 to 14 days; dose shouldn't exceed 80 mg/kg daily.

➤*Disseminated herpes zoster◇. Adults:* 5 to 10 mg/kg I.V. q 8 hours for 7 to 10 days. Infuse over at least 1 hour.

➤*Initial genital herpes. Adults:* 200 mg P.O. q 4 hours while awake (a total of five capsules daily). Treatment should continue for 10 days. Or, 400 mg P.O. t.i.d. for 5 days.

➤*Genital herpes in immunocompromised patients◇. Adults:* 400 mg P.O. three to five times daily.

➤*Rectal herpes infection◇. Adults:* 400 mg P.O. five times daily for 10 days or until resolution; or, 800 mg P.O. q 8 hours for 7 to 10 days for initial infections.

➤*Acute herpes zoster infection. Adults:* 800 mg P.O. five times daily for 7 to 10 days. Start therapy within 48 hours of rash onset.

➤*Intermittent therapy for recurrent genital herpes. Adults:* 200 mg P.O. q 4 hours while awake (a total of five capsules daily). Continue treatment for 5 days. Start therapy at first sign of recurrence.

➤*Long-term suppressive therapy for recurrent genital herpes. Adults:* 400 mg P.O. b.i.d. for up to 1 year, followed by reevaluation.

➤*Genital herpes; non–life-threatening herpes simplex infection in immunocompromised patients. Adults and children:* Apply sufficient quantity of ointment to adequately cover all lesions q 3 hours, six times daily for 7 days.

➤*Neonatal herpes simplex virus infection. Neonates and infants up to 3 months:* 10 mg/kg I.V. q 8 hours for 10 days.
Preterm neonates: 10 mg/kg I.V. q 12 hours.

➤*Primary or recurrent HSV infections in patients with HIV. Adults:* 200 to 800 mg P.O. five times daily.

➤*Long-term suppressive or maintenance prophylaxis therapy for recurrent HSV infections in patients with HIV◇. Adults and adolescents:* 200 mg P.O. t.i.d. or 400 mg P.O. b.i.d.
Infants and children: 600 to 1,000 mg P.O. daily in three to five divided doses; alternatively, 80 mg/kg in three to four divided doses.

➤*Acute varicella (chickenpox) infections. Adults and children age 2 and older who weigh more than 88 lb (40 kg):* 800 mg P.O. q.i.d. for 5 days.
Children age 2 or over who weigh less than 88 lb: 20 mg/kg P.O. q.i.d. for 5 days.

➤*Acute herpes zoster ophthalmicus◇. Adults:* 600 mg P.O. q 4 hours five times daily for 10 days; within 7 days of rash onset, but preferably within 72 hours.

➤*Varicella in immunocompromised patients. Adults and children over age 12:* 10 mg/kg I.V. over 1 hour q 8 hours for 7 days.
Children under age 12: 20 mg/kg I.V. over 1 hour q 8 hours for 7 days.

➤*Herpes simplex encephalitis. Adults and children over age 12:* 10 mg/kg I.V. over 1 hour q 8 hours for 10 days.
Children ages 3 months to 12 years: 20 mg/kg I.V. over at least 1 hour for 10 days.

✦*Dosage adjustment.* In patients with renal failure, adjust normal oral dose (200 to 400 mg) to 200 mg q 12 hours if creatinine clearance drops below 10 ml/minute. If patient is on a regimen of 800 mg q 4 hours five times daily, give 800 mg P.O. q 8 hours if creatinine clearance is 10 to 25 ml/minute, or 800 mg P.O. q 12 hours if creatinine clearance is less than 10 ml/minute.

In patients with renal failure, give 100% of the I.V. dose q 8 hours if creatinine clearance exceeds 50 ml/minute. Give 100% of the dose q 12 hours if it's 25 to 50 ml/minute. Give 100% of the dose q 24 hours if it's 10 to 25 ml/minute. Give 50% of the dose q 24 hours if it falls below 10 ml/minute.

How supplied
Available by prescription only
Capsules: 200 mg
Injection: 500 mg/vial, 1 g/vial
Injection concentrate for I.V. infusion: 50 mg/ml
Ointment: 5%
Oral suspension: 200 mg/5 ml
Tablets: 400 mg, 800 mg

Pharmacodynamics
Antiviral action: Acyclovir is converted by the viral cell into its active form (triphosphate) and inhibits viral DNA polymerase. In vitro, acyclovir is active against herpes simplex virus type 1, herpes simplex virus type 2, varicella-zoster virus, Epstein-Barr virus, and cytomegalovirus. In vivo, acyclovir may reduce the duration of acute infection and speed lesion healing in initial genital herpes episodes. Patients with frequent herpes recurrences (more than six episodes a year) may receive oral acyclovir prophylactically to prevent recurrences or reduce their frequency.

Pharmacokinetics
Absorption: Oral form absorbed slowly and incompletely (15% to 30%). Absorption isn't affected by food. With topical administration, absorption is minimal.
Distribution: Distributed widely to organ tissues and body fluids. CSF levels equal about 50% of serum levels. About 9% to 33% of a dose binds to plasma proteins.
Metabolism: Metabolized inside the viral cell to its active form. About 10% of dose is metabolized extracellularly.
Excretion: Up to 92% of systemically absorbed acyclovir is excreted as unchanged drug by the kidneys by glomerular filtration and tubular secretion. In patients with normal renal function, half-life is 2 to 3½ hours. Renal failure may extend half-life to 19 hours.

Route	Onset	Peak	Duration
P.O.	Unknown	2-5 hr	Unknown
I.V.	Immediate	Immediate	Unknown
Topical	Unknown	Unknown	Unknown

Contraindications and precautions
Contraindicated in patients hypersensitive to drug. Use cautiously in patients with underlying neurologic problems, renal disease, or dehydration and in those receiving nephrotoxic drugs.

Interactions
Drug-drug. *Methotrexate:* Possible reaction in patients who have had a previous neurologic reaction to intrathecal methotrexate administration. Use I.V. acyclovir cautiously in these patients.
Probenecid: May reduce renal tubular secretion of acyclovir, leading to increased drug half-life, reduced elimination rate, and decreased urine excretion. This reduced clearance causes more sustained serum drug levels. Avoid use together.

Zidovudine: May result in increased levels of acyclovir, causing toxicity. Monitor acyclovir levels closely.

Adverse reactions
CNS: *encephalopathic changes (lethargy, obtundation, tremor, confusion, hallucinations, agitation, **seizures, coma**),* headache, malaise.
GI: diarrhea, *nausea, vomiting.*
GU: hematuria, *transient elevations of serum creatinine and BUN levels.*
Hematologic: ***bone marrow hypoplasia, leukopenia,*** megaloblastic hematopoiesis, thrombocytosis, ***thrombocytopenia.***
Skin: itching, rash, transient burning and stinging, pruritus, urticaria, vulvitis.
Other: *inflammation, phlebitis* (at injection site).

Overdose and treatment
Evidence of overdose includes signs of nephrotoxicity, including elevated serum creatinine and BUN levels, progressing to renal failure. Overdose has followed I.V. bolus administration in patients with unmonitored fluid status or in patients receiving inappropriately high parenteral dosages. Acute toxicity hasn't been reported after high oral dosage. Hemodialysis results in 60% decrease in plasma drug level.

Special considerations
• Drug shouldn't be given by S.C., I.M., or ophthalmic route or by I.V. bolus.
• Reconstitute drug by adding 10 to 20 ml of sterile water for injection to a 500 mg or 1 g acyclovir vial, respectively, to provide a solution containing 50 mg/ml. Don't use bacteriostatic water for injection. Use reconstituted solution within 12 hours. Further dilute in 50 to 125 ml of a compatible I.V. solution to no more than 7 mg/ml.
• Infuse I.V. dose over at least 1 hour to prevent renal tubular damage.
• Solubility of acyclovir in urine is low. Make sure patient taking the systemic form of drug is well hydrated to prevent nephrotoxicity.
• Don't apply topical preparation to vagina or cervix.

Patient monitoring
• Monitor serum creatinine level. If level doesn't return to normal within a few days after therapy begins, increase hydration, adjust dose, or discontinue drug.
• Monitor patient for encephalopathic signs; they're more likely in patients who have experienced neurologic reactions to cytotoxic drugs.

Pregnant patients
• Use only if benefits outweigh the risks.

Pediatric patients
• Safety and effectiveness of oral and topical acyclovir in children haven't been established.

Reactions may be *common,* uncommon, ***life-threatening,*** or COMMON AND LIFE-THREATENING.

• I.V. acyclovir has been used in only a few children.
• To reconstitute acyclovir for children, don't use bacteriostatic water for injection that contains benzyl alcohol.

Geriatric patients
• Administer drug cautiously to geriatric patients because they have an increased risk of renal dysfunction or dehydration.

Patient education
• Warn patient that although drug helps manage the disease, it doesn't cure it or prevent its spread to others.
• Tell patient to begin taking drug when early infection symptoms occur, such as tingling, itching, or pain.
• Instruct patient taking ointment to use a finger cot or rubber glove and to apply about a ¼" ribbon of ointment for every 4 square inches of area to be covered. Ointment should thoroughly cover each lesion. Warn patient to avoid getting ointment in eyes.
• Instruct patient to avoid sexual intercourse during active genital infection.

---

adenosine
Adenocard

Pharmacologic classification: nucleoside
Therapeutic classification: antiarrhythmic
Pregnancy risk category: C

Indications and dosages
➤ *Conversion of paroxysmal supraventricular tachycardia (PSVT) to sinus rhythm. Adults:* 6 mg I.V. by rapid bolus injection (over 1 to 2 seconds). If PSVT isn't eliminated in 1 to 2 minutes, give 12 mg by rapid I.V. push. Repeat 12-mg dose if necessary. Single doses over 12 mg aren't recommended.

How supplied
Available by prescription only
Injection: 3 mg/ml in 2-ml and 5-ml vials

Pharmacodynamics
Antiarrhythmic action: Adenosine is a naturally occurring nucleoside. In the heart, it acts on the AV node to slow conduction and inhibit reentry pathways. Adenosine is also useful for the treatment of PSVT linked to accessory bypass tracts (Wolff-Parkinson-White syndrome).

Pharmacokinetics
Absorption: Administered by rapid I.V. injection.
Distribution: Rapidly taken up by erythrocytes and vascular endothelial cells.
Metabolism: Metabolized within tissues to inosine and adenosine monophosphate.

Excretion: Unknown; circulating plasma half-life is less than 10 seconds.

Route	Onset	Peak	Duration
I.V.	Immediate	Immediate	Unknown

Contraindications and precautions
Contraindicated in patients hypersensitive to drug and in those with second- or third-degree heart block or sick sinus syndrome, unless an artificial pacemaker is present, because adenosine decreases conduction through the AV node and may produce first-, second-, or third-degree heart block. These effects are usually transient; however, patients in whom significant heart block develops after a dose of adenosine shouldn't receive additional doses.
Don't use in atrial fibrillation or atrial flutter. Use cautiously in patients with asthma because bronchoconstriction may occur.

Interactions
Drug-drug. *Carbamazepine:* Higher degrees of heart block occur in patients receiving concurrent therapy. Avoid use together.
Dipyridamole: May potentiate adenosine effects; smaller adenosine doses may be necessary.
Methylxanthines: Antagonized effects of adenosine. Therefore, patients receiving theophylline may require higher doses or may not respond to adenosine therapy.
Drug-herb. *Guarana:* May decrease response to adenosine. Monitor patient closely.
Drug-food. *Caffeine:* May antagonize the effects of adenosine. Patient may need higher doses or may not respond to adenosine therapy.

Adverse reactions
CNS: apprehension, burning sensation, dizziness, heaviness in arms, light-headedness, numbness, headache, tingling in arms.
CV: chest pain, *facial flushing,* hypotension, palpitations.
EENT: blurred vision.
GI: metallic taste, nausea.
Musculoskeletal: back pain, neck pain.
Respiratory: *chest pressure, dyspnea, shortness of breath,* hyperventilation.
Skin: diaphoresis.
Other: *throat tightness, groin pressure.*

Overdose and treatment
Because the half-life of adenosine is less than 10 seconds, the adverse effects of overdose usually dissipate rapidly and are self-limiting. Treat lingering adverse effects symptomatically.

Special considerations
• Check solution for crystals, which may form if solution is cold. If crystals are visible, gently warm solution to room temperature. Don't use solutions that aren't clear.

• Use Adenocard cautiously in patients with previous history of ventricular fibrillation or those taking digoxin and verapamil.
• Rapid I.V. injection is necessary for drug action. Administer directly into a vein if possible; if an I.V. line is used, use the most proximal port and follow with a rapid saline solution flush to ensure that drug reaches the systemic circulation rapidly.
• Discard unused drug because it contains no preservatives.
⚠ **ALERT** Don't confuse adenosine phosphate with adenosine (Adenocard).

Patient monitoring
• Monitor ECG rhythm during administration; drug may cause short-lasting first-, second-, or third-degree heart block or asystole.

Pediatric patients
• There have been no controlled studies.

Patient education
• Warn patient of adverse reactions and advise patient to notify prescriber if they occur.
• Tell patient to report discomfort at I.V. site.

---

albumin, human (normal serum albumin, human)
Albuminar-5, Albuminar-25, Albutein 5%, Albutein 25%, Buminate 5%, Buminate 25%, Plasbumin-5, Plasbumin-25

Pharmacologic classification: blood derivative
Therapeutic classification: plasma protein
Pregnancy risk category: C

Indications and dosages
➤ **Shock.** *Adults:* Initially, 500 ml (5% solution) by I.V. infusion, may repeat after 30 minutes. Dosage varies with patient's condition and response. Don't exceed 250 g in 48 hours.
Children: 10 to 20 ml/kg (5% solution) by I.V. infusion, at a rate up to 5 to 10 ml/minute.
➤ **Hypoproteinemia.** *Adults:* 1,000 to 1,500 ml 5% solution by I.V. infusion daily, maximum rate 5 to 10 ml/minute. Or, 200 to 300 ml of 25% solution by I.V. infusion daily, maximum rate 3 ml/minute. Dosage varies with patient's condition and response.
➤ **Burns.** *Adults and children:* Dosage varies based on extent of burn and patient's condition. Usually maintain plasma albumin level at 2 to 3 g/dl.
➤ **Hyperbilirubinemia**◇. *Infants:* 1 g/kg albumin (4 ml/kg of 25% solution) by I.V. infusion 1 to 2 hours before transfusion.
High-risk neonates with low serum protein levels: 1.4 to 1.8 ml/kg by I.V. infusion of 25% solution.

How supplied
Available by prescription only
Injection: 5% (50 mg/ml) in 50-ml, 250-ml, 500-ml, 1,000-ml vials; 25% (250 mg/ml) in 20-ml, 50-ml, 100-ml vials

Pharmacodynamics
Plasma volume–expanding action: Albumin 5% supplies colloid to the blood and expands plasma volume. Albumin 25% provides intravascular oncotic pressure at 5:1, causing fluid to shift from interstitial space to circulation and slightly increasing plasma protein level.

Pharmacokinetics
Absorption: Not adequately absorbed from the GI tract.
Distribution: Accounts for about 50% of plasma proteins; distributed into the intravascular space and extravascular sites, including skin, muscle, and lungs. In patients with reduced circulating blood volume, hemodilution secondary to albumin administration persists for many hours; in patients with normal blood volume, excess fluid and protein are lost.
Metabolism: Although synthesized in the liver, liver isn't involved in clearance of albumin from plasma in healthy individuals.
Excretion: Little is known about excretion in healthy people. Administration of albumin decreases hepatic albumin synthesis and increases albumin clearance if plasma oncotic pressure is high. In certain pathologic states, the liver, kidneys, or intestines may provide elimination mechanisms for albumin.

Route	Onset	Peak	Duration
I.V.	< 15 min	< 15 min	Several hr

Contraindications and precautions
Contraindicated in patients hypersensitive to drug. Use with extreme caution in patients with hypertension, cardiac disease, severe pulmonary infection, severe chronic anemia, or hypoalbuminemia with peripheral edema.

Interactions
Drug-drug. *ACE inhibitors:* Atypical reactions when used with plasma exchange of large volumes of albumin. Withhold ACE inhibitors for 24 hours before plasma exchange.

Adverse reactions
CNS: headache.
CV: hypotension, tachycardia, *vascular overload after rapid infusion.*
GI: increased salivation, nausea, vomiting.
Metabolic: increased serum alkaline phosphatase level, increased plasma albumin level.
Musculoskeletal: back pain.
Respiratory: altered respiration, dyspnea, *pulmonary edema.*
Skin: urticaria, rash.
Other: chills, fever.

Reactions may be *common*, uncommon, **life-threatening**, or COMMON AND LIFE-THREATENING.

Overdose and treatment

Overdose may cause signs of circulatory overload (such as increased venous pressure and distended neck veins) or pulmonary edema.

Slow flow to a keep-vein-open rate and reevaluate therapy.

Special considerations

• Be certain patient is properly hydrated before starting infusion; product may be administered without regard to blood typing and crossmatching.

• Solution should be a clear amber color; don't use if cloudy or contains sediment. Store at room temperature; freezing may break bottle.

• Use opened solution promptly, discarding unused portion after 4 hours; solution contains no preservatives and becomes unstable.

• One volume of 25% albumin produces the same hemodilution and relative anemia as five volumes of 5% albumin; reference to "1 unit" albumin usually indicates 50 ml of the 25% concentration containing 12.5 g of albumin.

• Dilute if necessary with normal saline solution or D_5W. Use 5-micron or larger filter; don't give through 0.22-micron I.V. filter.

• Avoid rapid I.V. infusion; rate is individualized based on patient's age, condition, and diagnosis. In patients with hypovolemic shock, infuse 5% solution at no more than 2 to 4 ml/minute, and 25% solution (diluted or undiluted) at no more than 1 ml/minute. In patients with normal blood volume, infuse 5% solution at no more than 5 to 10 ml/minute, and 25% solution (diluted or undiluted) at no more than 2 to 3 ml/minute. Don't give more than 250 g in 48 hours.

• Each liter contains 130 to 160 mEq of sodium before dilution with any additional I.V. fluids; a 50-ml bottle of solution contains 7 to 8 mEq sodium. This preparation was once known as salt-poor albumin.

Patient monitoring

• Vital signs must be monitored carefully and the patient observed for adverse reactions.

• Monitor intake and output, hematocrit, serum protein, hemoglobin, and electrolyte levels to help determine continuing dosage.

• The goal is to maintain plasma albumin levels at 2 to 3 g/dl or an oncotic pressure of 20 (total serum protein level of 5.2 g/dl).

Pediatric patients

• Premature infants with low serum protein levels may receive 1.4 to 1.8 ml/kg of a 25% albumin solution/kg by I.V. infusion (350 to 450 mg albumin).

Patient education

• Explain use and administration of albumin to patient and family.

• Tell patient to report adverse effects promptly.

albuterol sulfate
Airet, Proventil, Proventil HFA, Proventil Repetabs, Proventil Syrup, Ventolin, Ventolin Syrup, Volmax

Pharmacologic classification: adrenergic
Therapeutic classification: bronchodilator
Pregnancy risk category: C

Indications and dosages

➤ *Bronchospasm in patients with reversible obstructive airway disease.* Adults and children age 12 and older: 2 to 4 mg (immediate-release tablets) P.O. t.i.d. or q.i.d.; maximum dose, 8 mg q.i.d. Or, use sustained-release tablets. Usual starting dose is 4 mg q 12 hours. Increase to 8 mg q 12 hours if patient fails to respond. Cautiously increase in stepwise manner as needed and tolerated to 16 mg q 12 hours. Don't exceed 32 mg daily.

Oral solution

Children ages 6 to 14: 2 mg P.O. t.i.d. to q.i.d.; may increase to 24 mg daily in divided doses.

Aerosol solution

Adults and children age 4 and older: One to two inhalations q 4 to 6 hours. More frequent administration or a greater number of inhalations isn't usually recommended. However, because deposition of inhaled medications is variable, higher doses are occasionally used, especially in patients with acute bronchospasm.

Solution for inhalation

Adults: 2.5 mg t.i.d. or q.i.d. by nebulizer.

Children ages 2 to 12: 0.1 mg/kg to 0.15 mg/kg to maximum of 2.5 mg t.i.d. to q.i.d.

Capsules for inhalation

Adults and children age 4 and older: 200 mcg inhaled q 4 to 6 hours using a Rotahaler inhalation device.

Children ages 6 to 11: Administer 2 mg P.O. t.i.d. or q.i.d. or 4 mg extended-release preparation q 12 hours

Children ages 2 to 5: Administer 0.1 mg/kg P.O. t.i.d., not to exceed 2 mg t.i.d.

✦ *Dosage adjustment.* In adults over age 65, give 2 mg P.O. t.i.d. or q.i.d.

➤ *To prevent exercise-induced bronchospasm.* Adults and children age 4 and older: Two inhalations 15 minutes before exercise or 200 mcg (1 capsule) inhaled via the Rotahaler delivery device 15 minutes before exercise.

How supplied

Available by prescription only
Aerosol inhaler: 90 mcg/metered spray
Capsules for inhalation: 200 mcg microfine
Solution for nebulization: 0.083%, 0.5%
Syrup: 2 mg/5 ml
Tablets: 2 mg, 4 mg
Tablets (sustained-release): 4 mg, 8 mg

Pharmacodynamics

Bronchodilator action: Selectively stimulates beta-adrenergic receptors of the lungs, uterus, and vascular smooth muscle. Bronchodilation results from relaxation of bronchial smooth muscles, which relieves bronchospasm and reduces airway resistance.

Pharmacokinetics

Absorption: After oral inhalation, appears to be absorbed gradually, over several hours, from the respiratory tract; however, dose is mostly swallowed and absorbed through the GI tract.

Distribution: Doesn't cross the blood-brain barrier.

Metabolism: Extensively metabolized in the liver to inactive compounds.

Excretion: Rapidly excreted in urine and feces. After oral inhalation, 70% of dose is excreted in urine unchanged and as metabolites within 24 hours; 10% in feces. Elimination half-life is about 4 hours. After oral administration, 75% of dose is excreted in urine within 72 hours as metabolites; 4% in feces.

Route	Onset	Peak	Duration
P.O.	15-30 min	2-3 hr	6-12 hr
Inhalation	5-15 min	½-2 hr	2-6 hr

Contraindications and precautions

Contraindicated in patients hypersensitive to drug or any component of its formulation. Use cautiously in patients with CV disorders, including coronary insufficiency and hypertension; in patients with hyperthyroidism or diabetes mellitus; and in those who are unusually responsive to adrenergics.

Interactions

Drug-drug. *Epinephrine and other orally inhaled sympathomimetic amines:* May increase sympathomimetic effects and risk of toxicity. Avoid use together.

MAO inhibitors, tricyclic antidepressants: Serious CV effects may follow use. Avoid use together.

Propranolol and other beta blockers: May antagonize the effects of albuterol. Exercise caution when using together.

Adverse reactions

CNS: *tremor, nervousness,* dizziness, insomnia, *headache, hyperactivity,* weakness, CNS stimulation, malaise, hypesthesia, migraine, hypertonia.

CV: *tachycardia, palpitations,* hypertension.

EENT: dry and irritated nose and throat (with inhaled form), nasal congestion, epistaxis, hoarseness.

GI: increased appetite, heartburn, *nausea, vomiting,* anorexia, taste perversion.

Metabolic: hypokalemia with large doses.

Musculoskeletal: muscle cramps.

Respiratory: *bronchospasm,* cough, wheezing, dyspnea, bronchitis, increased sputum.

Other: *hypersensitivity reactions.*

Overdose and treatment

Signs and symptoms of overdose include exaggeration of common adverse reactions, particularly angina, hypertension, hypokalemia, and seizures. Cardiac arrest may occur.

To treat, use selective beta blockers (such as metoprolol) with extreme caution; they may induce asthmatic attack. Dialysis isn't appropriate. Monitor vital signs and electrolyte levels closely.

Special considerations

● Orally inhaled albuterol has been used investigationally to prevent or alleviate episodes of muscle paralysis in the treatment of some patients with hyperkalemic familial periodic paralysis.

⚡ **ALERT** Don't confuse Flomax (tamsulosin) 0.4 mg with Volmax (albuterol) 4 mg. These drugs sound and look alike.

Patient monitoring

● Small, transient increases in blood glucose levels may occur after oral inhalation.

● Serum potassium levels may decrease after I.V. and inhalation therapy administration, but potassium supplementation is usually unnecessary.

● Effectiveness of treatment is measured by periodic monitoring of patient's pulmonary function. Monitor patient for worsening symptoms or loss of control.

Pregnant patients

● The potential exists for cleft palate and limb defects; however, there's no consistent pattern of congenital abnormalities.

Breast-feeding patients

● Because it's unknown if albuterol appears in breast milk, alternative feeding methods are recommended.

Pediatric patients

● Safety and efficacy of extended-release tablets or immediate-release tablets in children under age 6 haven't been established.

Geriatric patients

● Lower doses may be required because geriatric patients are more sensitive to sympathomimetic amines.

Patient education

● Instruct patient in proper use of inhaler. Tell him to read directions before use, that dryness of mouth and throat may occur, and that rinsing with water after each dose may help.

● To administer by metered-dose nebulizer, give patient these instructions: Shake canister thoroughly to activate it, and place the mouthpiece well into mouth, aimed at back of throat. Close lips and teeth around mouthpiece, exhale through

---

Reactions may be *common*, uncommon, *life-threatening*, or COMMON AND LIFE-THREATENING.

nose as completely as possible, and then inhale through mouth slowly and deeply while actuating the nebulizer to release a dose. Hold breath 10 seconds (count "1-100, 2-100, 3-100," until reaching "10-100"). Remove the mouthpiece and exhale slowly.
• To administer by metered powder inhaler, caution patient not to take forced deep breath, but to breathe with normal force and depth. Observe patient closely for exaggerated systemic drug action.
• To administer by oxygen aerosolization, give over 15 to 20 minutes with oxygen flow rate adjusted to 4 L/minute. Turn on oxygen supply before patient places nebulizer in mouth. Lips don't have to be closed tightly around nebulizer opening. Placement of Y tube in rubber tubing permits patient to control administration. Advise patient to rinse mouth immediately after inhalation therapy to help prevent dryness and throat irritation. Rinse mouthpiece thoroughly with warm running water at least once daily to prevent clogging (it isn't dishwasher-safe.) After cleaning, wait until mouthpiece is completely dry before storing. Don't place near artificial heat, such as a dishwasher or oven. Replace reservoir bag every 2 to 3 weeks or as needed; replace mouthpiece every 6 to 9 months or as needed.
  Note: Replacement of bags or mouthpieces may require a prescription.
• Advise patient that repeated use may result in paradoxical bronchospasm. In such a case, patient should discontinue drug and contact prescriber immediately.
• Tell patient to contact prescriber if troubled breathing persists 1 hour after using medication, if symptoms return within 4 hours, if condition worsens, or if new (refill) canister is needed within 2 weeks.
• Advise patient to wait 15 minutes after using inhaled albuterol before using adrenocorticoids (beclomethasone, dexamethasone, flunisolide, or triamcinolone).
• Warn patient to use only as directed and not to use more than prescribed amount or more often than prescribed.

alclometasone dipropionate
Aclovate

Pharmacologic classification: topical corticosteroid
Therapeutic classification: anti-inflammatory
Pregnancy risk category: C

Indications and dosages
➤*Inflammation of corticosteroid-responsive dermatoses. Adults:* Apply a thin film to affected areas b.i.d. or t.i.d. Gently massage until medication disappears. Or apply a thick layer and cover with an occlusive dressing and tape and leave in place overnight or at least 6 hours. Course of treatment may last 2 to 6 weeks.

Use occlusive dressing for severe or resistant dermatoses.

How supplied
Available by prescription only
Cream, ointment: 0.05%

Pharmacodynamics
Anti-inflammatory action: Drug stimulates the synthesis of enzymes needed to decrease the inflammatory response. Alclometasone is a group VI nonfluorinated topical corticosteroid with less anti-inflammatory activity than hydrocortisone 0.2% or greater. It's similar in potency to desonide 0.05% and fluocinolone acetonide 0.01%. Applied topically, alclometasone may be used for refractory lesions of psoriasis and other deep-seated dermatoses such as localized neurodermatitis.

Pharmacokinetics
Absorption: Amount absorbed depends on amount of drug applied and on nature of the skin at the application site. It ranges from about 1% in areas with thick stratum corneum (such as the palms, soles, elbows, and knees) to as high as 36% in areas of the thinnest stratum corneum (face, eyelids, and genitals). Absorption increases in areas of skin damage, inflammation, or occlusion. Some systemic absorption of topical corticosteroids may occur, especially through the oral mucosa.
Distribution: After topical application, distributed throughout the local skin. If absorbed into the circulation, is rapidly removed from the blood and distributed into muscle, liver, skin, intestines, and kidneys.
Metabolism: After topical administration, metabolized primarily in the skin. The small amount absorbed into systemic circulation is metabolized primarily in the liver to inactive compounds.
Excretion: Inactive metabolites are excreted by the kidneys, primarily as glucuronides and sulfates, but also as unconjugated products. Small amounts of the metabolites are also excreted in feces.

Route	Onset	Peak	Duration
Topical	Unknown	Unknown	Unknown

Contraindications and precautions
Contraindicated in patients hypersensitive to corticosteroids.

Interactions
None reported.

Adverse reactions
EENT: cataracts, glaucoma (if used around eyes for a prolonged period).
Metabolic: hyperglycemia, glycosuria.
Skin: burning, pruritus, irritation, dryness, erythema, folliculitis, acneiform eruptions, perioral dermatitis, hypopigmentation, hypertrichosis, al-

lergic contact dermatitis, *secondary infection,* maceration, atrophy, striae, miliaria (with occlusive dressings).
Other: *hypothalamic-pituitary-adrenal axis suppression, Cushing's syndrome.*

Overdose and treatment
No information available.

Special considerations
● Recommendations for use of alclometasone and care and teaching of patient during therapy are the same as those for all topical corticosteroids.
● Alclometasone isn't for treatment of acne, rosacea, or perioral dermatitis.

Patient monitoring
● Monitor patient for worsened or improved condition.

Pregnant patients
● As with other corticosteroids, the potential exists for maternal toxicity.

Breast-feeding patients
● Recommendations for use of alclometasone in breast-feeding women are the same as those for all topical corticosteroids.

Pediatric patients
● Alclometasone has been used safely and effectively in children; observe usual precautions involving topical corticosteroid therapy in children.

Geriatric patients
● Recommendations for use of alclometasone in geriatric patients are the same as those for all topical corticosteroids.

Patient education
● Tell patient to use drug as directed.
● Advise patient to contact prescriber if condition worsens.

aldesleukin (interleukin-2, IL-2)
Proleukin

Pharmacologic classification: lymphokine
Therapeutic classification: immunoregulatory
Pregnancy risk category: C

Indications and dosages
➤ **Metastatic renal cell carcinoma, metastatic melanoma.** *Adults:* 600,000 IU/kg (0.037 mg/kg) I.V. q 8 hours for 5 days (a total of 14 doses). After a 9-day rest, repeat sequence for another 14 doses. Repeat courses may be administered after a rest period of at least 7 weeks from hospital discharge.

Continuous I.V. infusion of 18 million IU/m² for two 5-day cycles with a 5- to 8-day rest between cycles ◇.
18 million IU S.C. daily for 5 days, followed by 2-day rest period ◇.

How supplied
Available by prescription only
Injection: 22 million IU/vial

Pharmacodynamics
Immunoregulatory action: Aldesleukin is a lymphokine, a highly purified immunoregulatory protein synthesized using genetically engineered *Escherichia coli.* The drug produced is similar to human IL-2: it enhances lymphocyte mitogenesis, stimulates long-term growth of IL-2-dependent cell lines, enhances lymphocyte cytotoxicity, induces both lymphokine-activated and natural killer cell activity, and induces the production of interferon gamma.

Pharmacokinetics
Absorption: Onset is rapid after I.V. administration.
Distribution: Peak serum levels are proportional to dose. About 30% is rapidly distributed in plasma; the rest is rapidly distributed to the liver, kidneys, and lungs. Initial studies indicate that the distribution half-life is 13 minutes after a 5-minute I.V. infusion.
Metabolism: Metabolized by the kidneys to amino acids within the cells lining the proximal convoluted tubules.
Excretion: Excreted through the kidneys by peritubular extraction and glomerular filtration. Peritubular extraction ensures drug clearance as renal function diminishes and serum creatinine increases. Elimination half-life is 85 minutes.

Route	Onset	Peak	Duration
I.V.	4 wk	Unknown	< 12 mo

Contraindications and precautions
Contraindicated in patients hypersensitive to drug or any component of the formulation and in those with abnormal cardiac (thallium) stress test or pulmonary function tests or organ allografts. Retreatment is contraindicated in patients who experience the following adverse effects: pericardial tamponade; respiratory dysfunction requiring intubation; disturbances in cardiac rhythm that were uncontrolled or unresponsive to intervention; sustained ventricular tachycardia (five beats or more); chest pain accompanied by ECG changes, indicating MI or angina pectoris; renal dysfunction requiring dialysis for 72 hours or more; coma or toxic psychosis lasting 48 hours or more; seizures that are repetitive or difficult to control; ischemia or perforation of the bowel; GI bleeding requiring surgery.
Use with extreme caution in patients with cardiac or pulmonary disease or seizure disorders.

Interactions

Drug-drug. *Antihypertensives:* May increase risk of hypotension. Use together cautiously.
Cardiotoxic, hepatotoxic, myelotoxic, or nephrotoxic drugs: May enhance the toxicity of these drugs. Use together cautiously.
Corticosteroids: May decrease antitumor effectiveness of aldesleukin. Monitor drug effect.
Psychotropic drugs: Altered CNS function. Use together cautiously.

Adverse reactions

CNS: *malaise, headache, CVA, mental status changes, dizziness, sensory dysfunction, syncope, motor dysfunction, coma,* weakness, fatigue, *seizures.*
CV: *hypotension, sinus tachycardia, arrhythmias, bradycardia,* PVCs, *premature atrial contractions,* chest pain, *MI, heart failure, cardiac arrest,* myocarditis, endocarditis, pericardial effusion, thrombosis, edema, *capillary leak syndrome.*
EENT: conjunctivitis, *special senses disorders.*
GI: *nausea, vomiting, diarrhea,* abdominal pain, *stomatitis, anorexia, bleeding, dyspepsia, constipation, bowel perforation or infarction.*
GU: *elevated BUN and serum creatinine levels, oliguria, anuria, proteinuria, hematuria, dysuria,* urine retention, urinary frequency, urinary tract infection.
Hematologic: *anemia,* THROMBOCYTOPENIA, LEUKOPENIA, *coagulation disorders,* leukocytosis, eosinophilia.
Hepatic: *jaundice;* ascites; hepatomegaly; *elevated bilirubin, serum transaminase, and alkaline phosphatase levels.*
Metabolic: *hypomagnesemia, acidosis, hypocalcemia, hypophosphatemia, hypokalemia, hyperuricemia, hypoalbuminemia,* hypoproteinemia, hyponatremia, hyperkalemia, weight change.
Musculoskeletal: arthralgia, myalgia, back pain.
Respiratory: pulmonary congestion, dyspnea, *pulmonary edema, respiratory failure, pleural effusion, apnea,* pneumothorax, tachypnea.
Skin: pruritus, erythema, rash, dryness, exfoliative dermatitis, purpura, alopecia, petechiae.
Other: fever, chills, infections of catheter tip or injection site, phlebitis, SEPSIS, *gangrene.*

Overdose and treatment

Large doses produce rapid onset of expected adverse reactions, including dose-related cardiac, renal, and hepatic toxicity.
Treatment is supportive. Because of short serum half life, discontinuation of drug may ameliorate many adverse effects. Dexamethasone may decrease the toxicity of drug but also may impair effectiveness.

Special considerations

● Patients should be neurologically stable with a negative computed tomography scan for CNS metastases. Drug may worsen symptoms in patients with unrecognized or undiagnosed CNS metastases.
● Treat previous infections before starting therapy.
● Renal and hepatic impairment occur during treatment. Avoid administering other hepatotoxic or nephrotoxic drugs because toxicity may be additive. Be prepared to adjust dosage of other drugs to compensate for this impairment. Dosage modification because of toxicity is usually accomplished by holding a dose or interrupting therapy rather than by reducing the dose to be administered.
● Severe anemia or thrombocytopenia may occur. Packed RBCs or platelets may be necessary.
● Treat capillary leak syndrome with careful monitoring of fluid status, pulse, mental status, urine output, and organ perfusion. Central venous pressure monitoring is necessary.
● Because fluid management or administration of pressor agents may be essential to treat capillary leak syndrome, use cautiously in patients who require large volumes of fluid (such as patients with hypercalcemia).
● Reconstitute and dilute carefully to avoid altering the pharmacologic properties of drug; follow manufacturer's recommendations. Don't mix with other drugs.
● Reconstitute vial containing 22 million IU (1.3 mg) with 1.2 ml sterile water for injection. Don't use bacteriostatic water or normal saline solution for injection because these diluents cause increased aggregation of drug. Direct the stream at the sides of the vial and gently swirl to reconstitute. Don't shake.
● Reconstituted solution will contain 18 million IU (1.1 mg)/ml. Reconstituted drug should be particle-free and colorless to slightly yellow.
● Add the correct dose of reconstituted drug to 50 ml D_5W and infuse over 15 minutes. Don't use an in-line filter. Plastic infusion bags are preferred because they provide consistent drug delivery.
● Vials are for single use only and contain no preservatives. Discard unused drug.
● Powder for injection or reconstituted solutions must be stored in the refrigerator. After reconstitution and dilution, drug must be administered within 48 hours. Be sure that solutions are returned to room temperature before administering drug to patient.
● Preliminary studies indicate that over 75% of patients develop nonneutralizing antibodies to aldesleukin when treated with the every-8-hour dosing regimen. Neutralizing antibodies develop in less than 1%. The clinical significance of this finding isn't yet known.
● Aldesleukin has been investigated for various cancers, including Kaposi's sarcoma, metastatic melanoma, colorectal cancer, and malignant lymphoma.

Patient monitoring

• Perform standard hematologic tests, including CBC, differential, and platelet counts; serum electrolytes; and renal and hepatic function tests before therapy. Also obtain a chest X-ray daily during drug administration.

• Monitor CNS effects of drug, and discontinue drug if moderate to severe lethargy or somnolence develops because continued administration can result in coma.

• Take vital signs q 4 hours, and weigh patient daily.

Pregnant patients

• It's unknown if drug causes fetal harm. Don't use during pregnancy if possible.

Breast-feeding patients

• It's unknown if drug appears in breast milk. Consider risk and benefit and decide whether to discontinue drug or breast-feeding because of risk of serious adverse effects to the infant.

Pediatric patients

• Safety and efficacy haven't been established in children under age 18.

Patient education

• Make sure patient understands the serious toxicity related to drug. Adverse effects are expected with normal doses, and serious toxicity may occur despite close clinical monitoring.

• Explain administration schedule to patient and caregiver, and stress importance of compliance.

---

alendronate sodium

Fosamax

Pharmacologic classification: osteoclast-mediated bone resorption inhibitor
Therapeutic classification: antiosteoporotic
Pregnancy risk category: C

Indications and dosages

➤ *Osteoporosis in postmenopausal women; to increase bone mass in men with osteoporosis. Adults:* 10 mg P.O. daily or 70 mg P.O. once weekly taken with water at least 30 minutes before first food, beverage, or medication of the day.

➤ *Prevention of osteoporosis in postmenopausal women. Adults:* 5 mg P.O. daily taken with water at least 30 minutes before first food, beverage, or medication of the day.

➤ *In conjunction with calcium and vitamin D supplementation in the treatment of corticosteroid-induced osteoporosis. Adults:* 5 mg P.O. daily, taken with water at least 30 minutes before first food, beverage, or meal of day. In postmenopausal women not receiving estrogen replacement therapy, dose is 10 mg P.O. daily.

➤ *Paget's disease of bone. Adults:* 40 mg P.O. daily for 6 months taken with water at least 30 minutes before first food, beverage, or medication of the day.

How supplied

Available by prescription only
Tablets: 5 mg, 10 mg, 40 mg, 70 mg

Pharmacodynamics

Antiosteoporotic action: At the cellular level, alendronate suppresses osteoclast activity on newly formed resorption surfaces, which reduces bone turnover. Bone formation exceeds bone resorption at bone remodeling sites and thus leads to progressive gains in bone mass.

Pharmacokinetics

Absorption: Absorbed from the GI tract. Food or beverages can decrease bioavailability significantly.
Distribution: Distributed to soft tissues and then rapidly redistributed to bone or excreted in urine. Protein-binding is about 78%.
Metabolism: Doesn't appear to be metabolized.
Excretion: Excreted in urine.

Route	Onset	Peak	Duration
P.O.	Unknown	Unknown	Unknown

Contraindications and precautions

Contraindicated in patients hypersensitive to any component of drug and in patients with hypocalcemia or severe renal insufficiency (creatinine clearance below 35 ml/minute). Use cautiously in patients with active upper GI problems, such as dysphagia, symptomatic esophageal diseases, gastritis, duodenitis, or ulcers, and in patients with mild to moderate renal insufficiency (creatinine clearance between 35 and 60 ml/minute).

Interactions

Drug-drug. *Antacids, calcium supplements:* Interfere with absorption of alendronate. Instruct patient to wait at least 30 minutes after taking alendronate before taking these drugs.
Aspirin, NSAIDs: Increased risk of upper GI adverse reactions with alendronate doses above 10 mg daily. Monitor patient closely.
Hormone replacement therapy: Not recommended when used in treatment of osteoporosis with alendronate because of lack of clinical evidence regarding effectiveness.

Adverse reactions

CNS: headache.
GI: altered taste, abdominal pain, nausea, dyspepsia, constipation, diarrhea, flatulence, acid regurgitation, esophageal ulcer, vomiting, dysphagia, abdominal distention, gastritis.
Musculoskeletal: pain.

Reactions may be *common*, uncommon, *life-threatening*, or COMMON AND LIFE-THREATENING.

Overdose and treatment

Oral overdose may cause hypocalcemia, hypophosphatemia, and upper GI adverse effects, such as upset stomach, heartburn, esophagitis, gastritis, or ulcer.

Specific treatment information isn't available, but consider administration of milk or antacids (to bind alendronate). Dialysis isn't beneficial.

Special considerations

- Hypocalcemia must be corrected before drug therapy begins. Other disturbances of mineral metabolism (such as vitamin D deficiency) should also be corrected before starting therapy.
- When drug is used to treat osteoporosis in postmenopausal women, disease is confirmed by low bone mass findings on diagnostic studies or history of an osteoporotic fracture.
- Drug is indicated for patients with Paget's disease who have alkaline phosphatase levels at least twice the upper limit for normal, in those who are symptomatic, or in those at risk for future complications from the disease.

Patient monitoring

- Monitor patient's serum calcium and phosphate levels throughout therapy.
- Assess patient for dysphagia, odynophagia, or retrosternal pain.
- Monitor patient's renal function tests. Manufacturer recommends not using medication in patients with creatinine clearance less than 35 ml/minute.

Breast-feeding patients

- Drug may appear in breast milk; don't give it to breast-feeding women.

Pediatric patients

- Safety and efficacy in children haven't been established.

Geriatric patients

- Although no overall differences in efficacy or safety were observed in clinical trials between geriatric and younger patients, greater sensitivity of some older people can't be ruled out. Use cautiously in this age-group.

Patient education

◘ ALERT Advise patient to take drug with a full glass of water and sit upright for 30 minutes to avoid esophageal ulcer formation.
- Stress importance of taking each tablet with a glass of plain water (not mineral water or other beverage) first thing in the morning at least 30 minutes before ingesting food, beverages, or other drugs. Tell patient that waiting longer than 30 minutes improves absorption of drug.
- Tell patient to take supplemental calcium and vitamin D if daily dietary intake is inadequate.
- Inform patient about the benefit of weight-bearing exercises in increasing bone mass and the importance of modifying excessive cigarette smoking and alcohol consumption, if these factors are part of patient's lifestyle.

allopurinol
Purinol*, Zyloprim

allopurinol sodium
Aloprim

Pharmacologic classification: xanthine oxidase inhibitor
Therapeutic classification: antigout
Pregnancy risk category: C

Indications and dosages

➤ **Gout, primary or secondary hyperuricemia.** Dosage varies with severity of disease; drug can be given as single dose or divided, but should be divided if dose is larger than 300 mg.
Adults: Mild gout, 200 to 300 mg P.O. daily; severe gout with large tophi, 400 to 600 mg P.O. daily. Same dose for maintenance in secondary hyperuricemia.
➤ **Hyperuricemia secondary to malignancies.** *Children ages 6 to 10:* 300 mg P.O. daily (100 mg t.i.d.).
Children under age 6: 150 mg P.O. daily (50 mg t.i.d.).
➤ **Prevention of acute gouty attacks.** *Adults:* 100 mg P.O. daily; increase at weekly intervals by 100 mg without exceeding maximum dose (800 mg) until serum uric acid level decreases to 6 mg/dl or less.
➤ **Prevention of uric acid nephropathy during cancer chemotherapy.** *Adults:* 600 to 800 mg P.O. daily for 2 to 3 days in conjunction with high fluid intake. In those who can't tolerate oral therapy, 200 to 400 mg/m² I.V. daily as a single infusion or in divided infusions at 6-, 8-, or 12-hour intervals. Maximum daily I.V. dose is 600 mg.
Children: 200 mg/m² I.V. daily as a single infusion or in divided infusions at 6-, 8-, or 12-hour intervals.
✦ **Dosage adjustment.** For I.V. allopurinol sodium in patients with a creatinine clearance of less than 3 ml/minute, give 100 mg daily at extended intervals. For creatinine clearance of 3 to 10 ml/minute, give 100 mg daily. For 10 to 20 ml/minute, give 200 mg daily.
➤ **Recurrent calcium oxalate calculi.** *Adults:* 200 to 300 mg P.O. daily in single dose or divided doses.
✦ **Dosage adjustment.** In adults with creatinine clearance up to 9 ml/minute, give 100 mg P.O. q 3 days. For creatinine clearance of 10 to 19 ml/minute, give 100 mg P.O. every other day. For 20 to 39 ml/minute, give 100 mg P.O. daily. For 40 to 59 ml/minute, give 150 mg P.O. daily. For 60 to 79 ml/minute, give 200 mg P.O. daily. For 80 ml/minute, give 250 mg P.O. daily.

How supplied
Available by prescription only
Injection: 500 mg/30-ml vials
Tablets (scored): 100 mg, 200 mg*, 300 mg

Pharmacodynamics
Antigout action: Allopurinol inhibits xanthine oxidase, the enzyme catalyzing the conversion of hypoxanthine to xanthine, and the conversion of xanthine to uric acid. By blocking this enzyme, allopurinol and its metabolite, oxypurinol, prevent the conversion of oxypurines (xanthine and hypoxanthine) to uric acid, thus decreasing serum and urine levels of uric acid. Drug has no analgesic, anti-inflammatory, or uricosuric action.

Pharmacokinetics
Absorption: After oral administration, about 80% to 90% of dose is absorbed.
Distribution: Distributed widely throughout the body except in the brain, where drug levels are 50% of those found in the rest of the body. Allopurinol and oxypurinol aren't bound to plasma proteins.
Metabolism: Metabolized to oxypurinol by xanthine oxidase. Half-life of allopurinol is 1 to 2 hours; half-life of oxypurinol, about 15 hours.
Excretion: 5% to 7% of allopurinol dose is excreted in the urine unchanged within 6 hours of ingestion. Afterward, it's excreted by the kidneys as oxypurinol, allopurinol, and oxypurinol ribonucleosides. About 70% of the administered daily dose is excreted in the urine as oxypurinol and an additional 2% appears in the feces as unchanged drug within 48 to 72 hours.

Route	Onset	Peak	Duration
P.O.	Unknown	½-2 hr	1-2 wk
I.V.	Unknown	½ hr	Unknown

Contraindications and precautions
Contraindicated in patients hypersensitive to drug and in those with idiopathic hemochromatosis.

Interactions
Drug-drug. *Amoxicillin, ampicillin:* May increase the risk of rash. Monitor patient for this effect.
Azathioprine, mercaptopurine: May increase the toxic effects of these drugs, particularly bone marrow depression. Combined use of these drugs requires reduction of initial doses of azathioprine or mercaptopurine to 25% to 33% of the usual dose, with subsequent doses adjusted according to patient response and toxic effects.
Chlorpropamide: Because allopurinol or its metabolites may compete with chlorpropamide for renal tubular secretion, observe patients who receive these drugs together for signs of excessive hypoglycemia.
Co-trimoxazole: Use with allopurinol has been linked to thrombocytopenia. Monitor CBC with platelets.

Cyclophosphamide: May increase the risk of bone marrow depression through an unknown mechanism. Monitor patient for this effect.
Dicumarol: Allopurinol inhibits hepatic microsomal metabolism of this drug, thus increasing the half-life of dicumarol; observe patients receiving both drugs for increased anticoagulant effects.
Theophylline: Theophylline clearance can decrease with large doses (600 mg daily), leading to increased plasma theophylline levels. Monitor drug levels.
Thiazide diuretics: In patients with decreased renal function, the use of allopurinol with a thiazide diuretic may increase the risk of allopurinol-induced hypersensitivity reactions. Use together cautiously.

Adverse reactions
CNS: drowsiness, headache, paresthesia, peripheral neuropathy, neuritis.
CV: hypersensitivity vasculitis, necrotizing angiitis.
EENT: epistaxis.
GI: nausea, vomiting, diarrhea, abdominal pain, gastritis, dyspepsia, taste loss or perversion.
GU: *renal failure*, uremia.
Hematologic: *agranulocytosis*, anemia, *aplastic anemia, thrombocytopenia, leukopenia*, leukocytosis, eosinophilia, ecchymoses.
Hepatic: altered liver function studies, *hepatitis, hepatic necrosis*, hepatomegaly, cholestatic jaundice.
Musculoskeletal: arthralgia, myopathy.
Skin: alopecia; *rash* (usually maculopapular); *exfoliative, urticarial, and purpuric lesions; Stevens-Johnson syndrome; erythema multiforme;* severe furunculosis of nose; ichthyosis; *toxic epidermal necrolysis.*
Other: fever, chills.

Overdose and treatment
No information available.

Special considerations
• Gout may be secondary to diseases such as acute or chronic leukemia, polycythemia vera, multiple myeloma, or psoriasis or to administration of chemotherapeutic drug.
• Rash occurs mostly in patients taking diuretics and in those with renal disorders.
• If renal insufficiency occurs during treatment, reduce allopurinol dose.
• Acute gouty attacks may occur in first 6 weeks of therapy; concurrent use of colchicine or another anti-inflammatory agent may be prescribed prophylactically.
• Minimize GI adverse reactions by administering drug with meals or immediately after. Tablets may be crushed and administered with fluid or food.
• Allopurinol may predispose patient to ampicillin-induced rash if taken together.

Reactions may be *common*, uncommon, *life-threatening*, or COMMON AND LIFE-THREATENING.

- Allopurinol-induced rash may occur weeks after discontinuation of drug.
- When allopurinol is added to a therapeutic regimen of colchicine, uricosuric agents, or antiinflammatory agents, it may take months to discontinue the latter drugs.
- Allopurinol has been used to reduce hyperuricemia resulting from G6PD deficiency, Lesch-Nyhan syndrome, polycythemia vera, sarcoidosis, and administration of thiazides or ethambutol.
- Preparation of allopurinol sodium includes reconstitution and dilution. Dissolve each 30-ml vial with 25 ml of sterile water for injection. Dilute this solution to a desired concentration (no greater than 6 mg/ml) with normal saline solution or D5W. Solutions containing sodium bicarbonate shouldn't be used. Store at 68° to 77° F (20° to 25° C) and use within 10 hours. Don't use if particulate matter or discoloration is present. Refer to package insert for a full list of drugs with which Aloprim is incompatible in solution.

Patient monitoring
- Monitor patient's intake and output. Daily urine output of at least 2 L and maintenance of neutral or slightly alkaline urine is desirable.
- Monitor CBC, serum uric acid levels, and hepatic and renal function at start of therapy and periodically thereafter.

Breast-feeding patients
- Because oxypurinol and allopurinol appear in breast milk, use allopurinol with extreme caution in breast-feeding women.

Pediatric patients
- Don't use drug in children except to treat hyperuricemia resulting from malignancies.

Geriatric patients
- Follow dosage recommendations for adults. Watch for renal disorders or impaired renal function and treat according to dosage recommendations for patients with impaired renal function.

Patient education
- Encourage patient to drink 10 to 12 8-oz (240-ml) glasses of water daily while taking drug unless otherwise contraindicated.
- When using drug to treat recurrent calcium oxalate stones, advise patient to reduce dietary intake of animal protein, sodium, refined sugars, vitamin C, oxalate-rich foods, and calcium.
- Advise patient to avoid hazardous activities requiring alertness until CNS response to drug is known, because drowsiness may occur.
- Tell patient to report all adverse reactions immediately.
- Advise patient to take a missed dose when it's remembered unless it's time for next scheduled dose; he shouldn't double the dose.
- Tell patient to discontinue drug and contact prescriber at first sign of rash or other allergic reaction.

alprazolam
Alprazolam Intensol, Apo-Alpraz*, Novo-Alprazol*, Xanax

Pharmacologic classification: benzodiazepine
Therapeutic classification: antianxiety
Controlled substance schedule: IV
Pregnancy risk category: D

Indications and dosages
➤ *Anxiety. Adults:* Usual starting dose is 0.25 to 0.5 mg P.O. t.i.d. Increase dose p.r.n. q 3 to 4 days. Maximum total daily dose is 4 mg in divided doses.
✦ *Dosage adjustment.* In geriatric or debilitated patients or those with hepatic impairment, initial dose is 0.25 mg P.O. b.i.d. or t.i.d.
➤ *Panic disorder. Adults:* Initially, 0.5 mg P.O. t.i.d. Increase as needed and tolerated at intervals of 3 to 4 days in increments of 1 mg daily. Most patients require more than 4 mg daily; however, doses from 1 to 10 mg daily have been reported.

How supplied
Available by prescription only
Oral solution: 0.1 mg/1 ml
Oral solution (concentrated): 1 mg/1 ml
Tablets: 0.25 mg, 0.5 mg, 1 mg, 2 mg

Pharmacodynamics
Anxiolytic action: Alprazolam depresses the CNS at the limbic and subcortical levels of the brain. It produces an antianxiety effect by enhancing the effect of the neurotransmitter gamma-aminobutyric acid on its receptor in the ascending reticular activating system, which increases inhibition and blocks both cortical and limbic arousal.

Pharmacokinetics
Absorption: Well absorbed after oral administration.
Distribution: Distributed widely throughout the body. About 80% to 90% bound to plasma protein.
Metabolism: Metabolized in the liver equally to alpha-hydroxyalprazolam and inactive metabolites.
Excretion: Excreted in urine. Half-life of alprazolam is 12 to 15 hours.

Route	Onset	Peak	Duration
P.O.	15-30 min	1-2 hr	Unknown

Contraindications and precautions
Contraindicated in patients hypersensitive to drug or other benzodiazepines and in patients with acute angle-closure glaucoma. Use cautiously in patients with hepatic, renal, or pulmonary disease.

Interactions

Drug-drug. *Antidepressants, antihistamines, barbiturates, general anesthetics, MAO inhibitors, narcotics, phenothiazines:* Alprazolam potentiates the CNS depressant effects of these drugs. Avoid use together.

Cimetidine, possibly disulfiram: Diminished hepatic metabolism of alprazolam, increasing its plasma level. Monitor patient carefully.

Digoxin: Plasma levels of digoxin may increase. Monitor serum digoxin levels.

Haloperidol: Benzodiazepines may decrease serum levels of haloperidol.

Rifampin: The effects of alprazolam may decrease with use of rifampin. Monitor patient for clinical effect.

Theophylline: May increase the sedative effects of alprazolam. Use together cautiously.

Drug-herb. *Kava:* May induce lethargy, increased CNS effects, or coma if taken with alprazolam. Discourage use together.

Drug-lifestyle. *Alcohol use:* Alprazolam potentiates the CNS depressant effects of alcohol. Discourage use together.

Heavy smoking: Accelerates alprazolam metabolism, thus lowering clinical effectiveness. Advise patient to avoid smoking.

Adverse reactions

CNS: *drowsiness, light-headedness,* minor changes in EEG patterns, headache, confusion, tremor, dizziness, syncope, *depression,* insomnia, nervousness.
CV: hypotension, tachycardia.
EENT: blurred vision, nasal congestion.
GI: *dry mouth,* nausea, vomiting, *diarrhea, constipation.*
Hepatic: elevated liver function test results.
Metabolic: weight gain or loss.
Musculoskeletal: muscle rigidity.
Skin: dermatitis.

Overdose and treatment

Signs and symptoms of overdose include somnolence, confusion, coma, hypoactive reflexes, dyspnea, labored breathing, hypotension, bradycardia, slurred speech, unsteady gait, and impaired coordination.

Support blood pressure and respiration until drug effects subside; monitor vital signs. Flumazenil, a specific benzodiazepine antagonist, may be useful. Mechanical ventilatory assistance via endotracheal tube may be required to maintain a patent airway and support adequate oxygenation. As needed, use I.V. fluids and vasopressors, such as dopamine and phenylephrine, to treat hypotension. If the patient is conscious, induce emesis. Use gastric lavage if ingestion was recent, but only if an endotracheal tube is in place to prevent aspiration. After emesis or lavage, administer activated charcoal with a cathartic as a single dose. Dialysis is of limited value. Don't use barbiturates if excitation occurs because of possible exacerbation of excitation or CNS depression.

Special considerations

Consider the recommendations relevant to all benzodiazepines as well as the following.
● Lower doses are effective in geriatric patients and patients with renal or hepatic dysfunction.
● Anxiety with depression also responds to alprazolam, but patient may need more frequent dosing.
● Store drug in a cool, dry place away from direct light.

Patient monitoring

● Monitor patients during prolonged therapy with high doses because they should be weaned from the drug gradually to prevent withdrawal symptoms. A 2- to 3-month withdrawal may be necessary, decreasing at no more than 0.5 mg q 3 days.

Breast-feeding patients

● The breast-fed infant of a woman taking alprazolam may become sedated, have feeding difficulties, or lose weight. Avoid use in breast-feeding women.

Pediatric patients

● Closely observe neonate for withdrawal symptoms if mother took alprazolam during pregnancy. Use of alprazolam during labor may cause neonatal flaccidity. Safety hasn't been established in children or adolescents under age 18.

Geriatric patients

● Lower doses are usually effective in geriatric patients because of decreased elimination. During start of therapy or after an increase in dose, geriatric patients who receive drug need assistance with walking and activities of daily living.

Patient education

● Make sure patient understands potential for physical and psychological dependence with long-term use of alprazolam.
● Instruct patient not to alter drug regimen.
● Warn patient that sudden changes in position can cause dizziness. Advise him to dangle legs for a few minutes before getting out of bed to prevent falls and injury.

alprostadil
Prostin VR Pediatric

Pharmacologic classification: prostaglandin
Therapeutic classification: prostaglandin derivative
Pregnancy risk category: NR

Indications and dosages

➤ *Temporary maintenance of patency of ductus arteriosus until surgery can be performed.* *Infants:* Initial I.V. infusion of 0.05 to 0.1 mcg/kg/minute via infusion pump. After satisfactory response is achieved, reduce infusion rate to the lowest dose that will maintain response. Maintenance dosages vary. Infusion rate should be the lowest possible dose and is usually achieved by progressively halving the initial dose. Rates as low as 0.002 to 0.005 mcg/kg/minute have been effective.

How supplied
Available by prescription only
Injection: 500 mcg/ml

Pharmacodynamics
Ductus arteriosus patency adjunct action: Alprostadil, also known as prostaglandin E_1 or PGE_1 is a prostaglandin that relaxes or dilates the rings of smooth muscle of the ductus arteriosus and maintains patency in neonates when infused before natural closure.

Pharmacokinetics
Absorption: Administered I.V.
Distribution: Distributed rapidly throughout the body.
Metabolism: 68% of dose is metabolized in one pass through the lung, primarily by oxidation; 100% is metabolized within 24 hours.
Excretion: Excreted in urine within 24 hours.

Route	Onset	Peak	Duration
I.V.	20 min	1-2 hr	Length of infusion

Contraindications and precautions
Contraindicated in neonates with respiratory distress syndrome. Use cautiously in neonates with bleeding disorders.

Interactions
None reported.

Adverse reactions
CNS: *seizures.*
CV: *flushing,* ***bradycardia,*** hypotension, tachycardia, ***cardiac arrest,*** edema.
GI: diarrhea.
Hematologic: ***disseminated intravascular coagulation.***
Metabolic: *hypokalemia.*
Respiratory: APNEA.
Other: *fever,* ***sepsis.***

Overdose and treatment
Signs and symptoms are similar to adverse reactions and include apnea, bradycardia, pyrexia, hypotension, and flushing. Apnea most commonly occurs in neonates weighing under 2 kg (4.4 lb) at birth and usually develops during the first hour of drug therapy.

Treatment of apnea or bradycardia requires discontinuance of the infusion and appropriate supportive therapy, including mechanical ventilation as needed. Pyrexia or hypotension may be treated by reducing the infusion rate. Correct flushing by repositioning the intra-arterial catheter.

Special considerations
• Drug should be administered only by personnel trained in pediatric intensive care.
◾ **ALERT** Dilute drug before administration. Discard prepared solution after 24 hours.
• Adding a 500-mcg solution to 50 ml of D_5W or normal saline solution provides 10 mcg/ml. At this concentration, a 0.01-ml/kg/minute infusion rate delivers 0.1 mcg/kg/minute of alprostadil. During dilution, take care to avoid direct contact of the concentrate with the wall of the plastic volumetric infusion chamber; if a hazy solution develops, discard the chamber and solution.
• Apnea and bradycardia may indicate drug overdose. Stop the infusion immediately if they occur.
• Peripheral arterial vasodilation (flushing) may respond to repositioning of the catheter.
• Store ampules in refrigerator.

Patient monitoring
• Assess all vital functions closely and frequently to prevent adverse effects.
• Monitor arterial pressure by umbilical artery catheter, auscultation, or Doppler transducer. Slow the infusion if arterial pressure decreases significantly.
• Monitor respiratory status closely during treatment, and have ventilatory assistance immediately available.
• In infants with restricted pulmonary blood flow, measure effectiveness of drug by monitoring blood oxygenation. In infants with restricted systemic blood flow, measure effectiveness of drug by monitoring systemic blood pressure and blood pH.

Pregnant patients
• This drug isn't for use in pregnant patients.

Breast-feeding patients
• This drug isn't for use in breast-feeding patients.

Geriatric patients
• This drug isn't for use in geriatric patients.

Patient education
• Inform parents about child's need for drug, and explain its use.
• Encourage parents to ask questions.

alprostadil
Caverject, Edex, Muse

Pharmacologic classification: prostaglandin
Therapeutic classification: corrective agent for impotence
Pregnancy risk category: NR

Indications and dosages
➤ ***Erectile dysfunction of vasculogenic, psychogenic, or mixed etiology.*** *Adults:* Dosages are highly individualized. For injection:

Initial dose is 2.5 mcg intracavernously. If partial response occurs, increase second dose by 2.5 to 5 mcg, and then increase dose further in increments of 5 to 10 mcg until patient achieves an erection (suitable for intercourse but not lasting over 1 hour). If initial dose isn't effective, increase second dose to 7.5 mcg within 1 hour; then increase dose further in 5- to 10-mcg increments until patient achieves an erection. Patient must remain in prescriber's office until complete detumescence occurs. If patient responds, don't repeat procedure for 24 hours. For pellet, start initially with lower doses (125 or 250 mcg). Increases or decreases should be made on separate occasions in a stepwise manner until patient achieves an erection that's sufficient for sexual intercourse.

➤ *Erectile dysfunction of pure neurologic etiology (spinal cord injury).* Adults: Dosages are highly individualized. Initial dose is 1.25 mcg intracavernously. If partial response occurs, give second dose of 1.25 mcg and then a third dose of 2.5 mcg; increase dose further in 5-mcg increments until patient achieves an erection (suitable for intercourse but not lasting over 1 hour). If initial dose isn't effective, increase second dose to 2.5 mcg within 1 hour; then increase further in 5-mcg increments until patient achieves an erection. Patient must remain in prescriber's office until complete detumescence occurs. No more than two doses administered 1 hour apart should be given in 1 day. If patient responds, don't repeat procedure for 24 hours.

How supplied
Available by prescription only
Injection (frozen) intracavitary: 10.2 mcg/ml, 20.2 mcg/ml, 40.4 mcg/ml
Sterile powder for intracavernosal injection: 6.15-mcg, 6.225-mcg, 10.75-mcg, 11.9-mcg, 12.45-mcg, 21.5-mcg, 23.2-mcg, 24.9-mcg, 43-mcg, 49.8-mcg vials
Urethral suppository pellet: 125 mcg, 250 mcg, 500 mcg, 1,000 mcg

Pharmacodynamics
Corrective action in impotence: A prostaglandin derivative that induces erection by relaxation of trabecular smooth muscle and by dilation of cavernosal arteries. This leads to expansion of lacunar spaces and entrapment of blood by compressing the venules against the tunica albuginea, a process referred to as the corporal veno-occlusive mechanism.

Pharmacokinetics
Absorption: Absolute bioavailability hasn't been determined.
Distribution: Bound in plasma protein primarily to albumin (81%).
Metabolism: Rapidly converted to compounds that are further metabolized before excretion.

Excretion: Excreted primarily in urine, the remainder in feces.

Route	Onset	Peak	Duration
Intra-cavernous	Unknown	2-5 min	2 hr
Intra-urethral	5-10 min	Unknown	30-60 min

Contraindications and precautions
Contraindicated in patients hypersensitive to drug, in patients with disposition to priapism (those who have sickle cell anemia or trait, multiple myeloma, or leukemia), and in patients with penile deformation (angulation, cavernosal fibrosis, or Peyronie's disease). Don't administer to men with penile implants or in whom sexual activity is contraindicated. Also avoid use in women, children, and neonates. Muse shouldn't be used for sexual intercourse with a pregnant woman unless the couple uses a condom barrier.

Interactions
Drug-drug. *Anticoagulants:* Increased risk of bleeding from intracavernosal injection site. Monitor patient closely.
Cyclosporine: Decreased cyclosporine level. Use together cautiously.
Vasoactive agents: Safety and efficacy of use with other agents haven't been studied and, therefore, such use isn't recommended.

Adverse reactions
CNS: headache, dizziness, fainting.
CV: hypertension, hypotension, swelling of leg veins.
EENT: sinusitis, nasal congestion.
GU: *penile pain,* prolonged erection, penile fibrosis, penis disorder, penile rash, penile edema, prostatic disorder, testicular and perineal aching, urethral burning.
Musculoskeletal: back pain.
Respiratory: upper respiratory tract infection, cough.
Other: injection site hematoma, injection site ecchymosis, localized trauma, localized pain, flu syndrome.

Overdose and treatment
If intracavernous overdose of drug occurs, patient should be under medical supervision until systemic effects have resolved or penile detumescence has occurred. Symptomatic treatment of systemic symptoms is appropriate.

Special considerations
● Patient must have underlying treatable medical causes of erectile dysfunction diagnosed and treated before therapy starts.
● Regular follow-up of patient with careful examination of the penis is strongly recommended to detect signs of penile fibrosis. Discontinue drug in patient in whom penile angulation, cavernosal fibrosis, or Peyronie's disease develops.

• Female partners of Muse users may experience vaginal itching and burning.
• Intercavernosal alprostadil has been used as an adjunct to different diagnoses of erectile dysfunction and evaluation of the hemodynamic status of erectile tissue.

Patient monitoring
• Monitor patient for hypotension, and adjust drug to lowest effective dose.
• Monitor patient for adverse effects, and discontinue drug immediately if patient develops penile angulation, cavernosal fibrosis, or Peyronie's disease.

Breast-feeding patients
• Drug isn't indicated for use in women.

Pediatric patients
• Drug isn't indicated for use in neonates or children.

Patient education
• To ensure safe and effective use, thoroughly instruct patient how to prepare and administer alprostadil before beginning intracavernosal treatment at home. Stress importance of following instructions carefully.
• Tell patient to discard precipitated or discolored vials. Reconstituted vial is designed for only one use and should be discarded after withdrawal of proper volume of the solution.
• Instruct patient not to shake the contents of reconstituted vial.
• Stress importance of not reusing or sharing needles or syringes as well as not sharing medication.
• Make sure patient has the manufacturer's instructions for administration included in each package of alprostadil.
• Tell patient not to change the dose without medical approval.
• Inform patient that he can expect an erection to occur 5 to 20 minutes after drug administration and that standard treatment goal is to produce an erection not lasting more than 1 hour.
• Warn patient that an erection lasting over 6 hours has been known to occur after alprostadil injection. If this occurs, instruct patient to seek medical attention immediately.
• Tell patient that drug shouldn't be used more than three times weekly, with at least 24 hours between each use. The maximum frequency of using Muse is two administrations per 24-hour period.
• Review possible adverse reactions with patient. Tell him to immediately report priapism, penile pain that wasn't present before or that's increased in intensity, and the occurrence of nodules or hard tissue in the penis.
• Instruct patient to inspect penis daily for redness, swelling, tenderness, or curvature of the erect penis, which might suggest an infection.

The patient should contact prescriber if he suspects infection.
• Remind patient that regular follow-up visits are necessary to evaluate effectiveness and safety of therapy.
• Inform patient that drug doesn't offer protection from transmission of sexually transmitted diseases and that protective measures continue to be necessary.
• Warn patient that a small amount of bleeding can occur at the injection site. This can increase the risk of transmitting blood-borne diseases, if present, to his sexual partner.
• Caution patient using Muse to use a condom when having sexual intercourse with a pregnant partner; this will also prevent potential vaginal burning and itching in female partner.

alteplase (recombinant alteplase, tissue plasminogen activator)
Activase

Pharmacologic classification: enzyme
Therapeutic classification: thrombolytic enzyme
Pregnancy risk category: C

Indications and dosages
➤ *Lysis of thrombi obstructing coronary arteries in management of acute MI.* **Three-hour infusion.** *Adults who weigh more than 65 kg (143 lb):* 60 mg in first hour, with 6 to 10 mg I.V. bolus over first 1 to 2 minutes; then 20 mg/hour for an additional 2 hours. Total dose, 100 mg.
Adults who weigh 65 kg or less: 1.25 mg/kg given over 3 hours. Infuse 0.75 mg/kg during the first hour with an initial bolus of 0.045 to 0.075 mg/kg rapidly over 1 to 2 minutes. After the first hour, begin a maintenance infusion of 0.25 mg/kg for the remaining 2 hours.
Accelerated infusion
Adults who weigh more than 67 kg (148 lb): 15 mg I.V. push, 50 mg over 30 minutes, then 35 mg over 60 minutes.
Adults who weigh 67 kg or less: 15 mg I.V. push, 0.75 mg/kg over 30 minutes (not to exceed 50 mg), then 0.5 mg/kg over 60 minutes (not to exceed 35 mg).
➤ *Prevention of reocclusion after thrombolysis for acute MI. Adults:* 3.3 mcg/kg/min by I.V. infusion for 4 hours together with heparin therapy immediately after initial thrombolytic infusion.
➤ *Pulmonary embolism. Adults:* 100 mg by I.V. infusion over 2 hours. Start heparin therapy at the end of infusion. Or, 30 to 50 mg infused via the intrapulmonary artery over 1½ or 2 hours, respectively, in conjunction with heparin therapy.

➤ *Lysis of arterial occlusion in a peripheral vessel or bypass graft* ◇. *Adults:* 0.5 to 0.1 mg/kg/hour infused via the intrapulmonary artery for 1 to 8 hours.

➤ *Acute ischemic stroke. Adults:* 0.9 mg/kg (maximum dose, 90 mg). Administer 10% of dose as an I.V. bolus over 1 minute; remaining 90% over 1 hour.

How supplied
Available by prescription only
Injection: 50-mg (29 million IU), 100-mg (58 million IU) vials

Pharmacodynamics
Thrombolytic action: Alteplase is an enzyme that catalyzes the conversion of tissue plasminogen to plasmin in the presence of fibrin. This fibrin specificity produces local fibrinolysis in the area of recent clot formation, with limited systemic proteolysis. In patients with acute MI, this allows for reperfusion of ischemic cardiac muscle and improved left ventricular function with a decreased risk of heart failure after an MI.

Pharmacokinetics
Absorption: Must be given I.V.
Distribution: Rapidly cleared from the plasma by the liver; 80% of dose is cleared within 10 minutes after infusion is discontinued.
Metabolism: Primarily hepatic.
Excretion: Over 85% of drug is excreted in urine; 5% in feces. Plasma half-life is under 10 minutes.

Route	Onset	Peak	Duration
I.V.	Immediate	45 min	4 hr

Contraindications and precautions
Contraindicated in patients with history or evidence of intracranial hemorrhage, suspected subarachnoid hemorrhage, seizure at the onset of CVA, active internal bleeding, intracranial neoplasm, arteriovenous malformation, aneurysm, and severe uncontrolled hypertension (more than 185 mm Hg systolic or 110 mm Hg diastolic). Also contraindicated in patients with a history of CVA, recent (within 2 months) intraspinal or intracranial trauma or surgery, or bleeding diathesis (see package insert).

Use cautiously in patients with recent (within 10 days) major surgery; pregnant patients; patients within the first 10 days postpartum; and patients with recent organ biopsy, trauma (including cardiopulmonary resuscitation), GI or GU bleeding, cerebrovascular disease, hypertension, a likelihood of left-sided heart thrombus, hemostatic defects (including those secondary to severe hepatic or renal disease), hepatic dysfunction, occluded AV cannula, severe neurologic deficit (NIH Stroke Scale over 22), signs of major early infarct on a computed tomography scan, mitral stenosis, atrial fibrillation, acute pericarditis or subacute bacterial endocarditis, septic thrombophlebitis, or diabetic hemorrhagic retinopathy or other hemorrhagic ophthalmic conditions. Also use cautiously in those receiving anticoagulants and in patients age 75 and older.

Interactions
Drug-drug. *Drugs that antagonize platelet function (abciximab, aspirin, dipyridamole):* May increase risk of bleeding if given before, during, or after alteplase therapy. Use together cautiously.

Adverse reactions
CNS: *cerebral hemorrhage.*
CV: hypotension, *arrhythmias,* edema.
GI: nausea, vomiting.
Hematologic: *severe, spontaneous bleeding (cerebral, retroperitoneal, GU, GI).*
Other: fever, bleeding at puncture sites, *hypersensitivity reactions (anaphylaxis).*

Overdose and treatment
No information is available regarding accidental ingestion. Excessive I.V. dosage can lead to bleeding problems. Doses of 150 mg have been linked to a higher risk of intracranial bleeding. Discontinue infusion immediately if signs or symptoms of bleeding are observed.

Special considerations
● Altered results may be expected in coagulation and fibrinolytic tests. The use of aprotinin (150 to 200 units/ml) in the blood sample may attenuate this interference.
● Expect to begin alteplase infusions as soon as possible after onset of MI symptoms, such as angina or equivalent greater than 30 minutes' duration; angina that's unresponsive to nitroglycerin; or ECG evidence of MI.
● Administer drug within 3 hours after onset of CVA symptoms after exclusion of intracranial hemorrhage by CT scan or other diagnostic imaging methods capable of detecting presence of hemorrhage. Treatment should be performed only in facilities that can provide appropriate evaluation and management of intracranial hemorrhage.
● Heparin is usually administered during or after alteplase as part of the treatment regimen for acute MI or pulmonary embolism. The use of anticoagulant or antiplatelet therapy for 24 hours is contraindicated when alteplase is used for acute ischemic stroke.
● Discontinue drug therapy for acute ischemic stroke in patients who haven't recently used oral anticoagulants or heparin if pretreatment PT exceeds 15 seconds or if an elevated activated partial PT is identified.
● Staff should avoid I.M. injections, venipuncture, and arterial puncture during therapy. Use pressure dressings or ice packs on recent puncture sites to prevent bleeding. If arterial puncture is necessary, select a site on the arm and apply pressure for 30 minutes afterward.

Reactions may be *common*, uncommon, *life-threatening*, or COMMON AND LIFE-THREATENING.

• Prepare solution using supplied sterile water for injection. Don't use bacteriostatic water for injection.
• Don't mix other drugs with alteplase. Use 18G needle for preparing solution—aim water stream at lyophilized cake. Expect a slight foaming to occur. Don't use if vacuum isn't present.
• Drug may be further diluted with normal saline solution injection or D_5W to yield 0.5 mg/ml. Reconstituted or diluted solutions are stable for up to 8 hours at room temperature.

Patient monitoring
• Monitor patient for bleeding or hemorrhage.
• Monitor ECG for transient arrhythmias (sinus bradycardia, ventricular tachycardia, accelerated idioventricular rhythm, ventricular premature depolarizations) related to reperfusion after coronary thrombolysis. Antiarrhythmics should be available.

Pediatric patients
• Safety and efficacy of use in children haven't been established, but the drug has been used investigationally in children with some success.

Geriatric patients
• Use cautiously in patients over age 75 because they have an increased risk of adverse CV effects.

Patient education
• Teach patient signs and symptoms of internal bleeding and tell him to report these immediately.
• Advise patient to report adverse effects promptly.
• Advise patient about proper dental care to avoid excessive gum trauma resulting from vigorous brushing; drug increases chances of bleeding.

aluminum carbonate
Basaljel

Pharmacologic classification: inorganic aluminum salt
Therapeutic classification: antacid, hypophosphatemic agent
Pregnancy risk category: NR

Indications and dosages
➤ *Antacid.* Adults: 1 to 2 tablets or capsules q 2 hours p.r.n.
➤ *Hyperphosphatemia and prevention of urinary phosphate stone formation (with low-phosphate diet).* Adults: 1 g P.O. t.i.d. or q.i.d.; adjust to lowest possible dose after therapy is started, monitoring diet and serum levels.

How supplied
Available without a prescription
Tablets or capsules: aluminum hydroxide equivalent 500 mg

Pharmacodynamics
Antacid action: Exerts its antacid effect by neutralizing gastric acid; this increases pH, thereby decreasing pepsin activity.
Hypophosphatemic action: Aluminum carbonate reduces serum phosphate levels by complexing with phosphate in the gut. This results in formation of insoluble, nonabsorbable aluminum phosphate, which is then excreted in feces. Calcium absorption increases secondary to reduced phosphate absorption.

Pharmacokinetics
Absorption: Largely unabsorbed; small amounts may be absorbed systemically.
Distribution: None.
Metabolism: None.
Excretion: Excreted in feces; some may appear in breast milk.

Route	Onset	Peak	Duration
P.O.	20 min	Unknown	20-180 min

Contraindications and precautions
No known contraindications. Use cautiously in patients with chronic renal disease.

Interactions
Drug-drug. *Antimuscarinics, chenodiol, chlordiazepoxide, coumarin anticoagulants, diazepam, digoxin, indomethacin, iron salts, isoniazid, phenothiazines (especially chlorpromazine), potassium phosphate, quinolones, sodium phosphate, tetracycline, vitamin A:* Aluminum carbonate may decrease absorption of many drugs, thereby lessening their effectiveness. Separate administration by at least 2 hours.
Enteric-coated drugs: Premature drug release; these drugs shouldn't be taken together.

Adverse reactions
CNS: encephalopathy.
GI: *constipation,* intestinal obstruction, increased serum gastrin levels.
Metabolic: hypophosphatemia.
Musculoskeletal: osteomalacia.

Overdose and treatment
No information available. Patients with impaired renal function are at a higher risk of aluminum toxicity to brain, bone, and parathyroid glands.

Special considerations
• Aluminum carbonate may interfere with imaging techniques using sodium pertechnetate Tc99m and thus impair evaluation of Meckel's diverticulum. It also may interfere with reticuloendothelial imaging of liver, spleen, or bone marrow using technetium Tc99m sulfur colloid. It may antagonize the effect of pentagastrin during gastric acid secretion tests.
• When administering suspension, shake well and give with small amounts of water or fruit juice.

• After administration through a nasogastric tube, flush tube with water to prevent obstruction.
• When administering drug as an antiurolithic, encourage increased fluid intake to enhance drug effectiveness.
• Constipation may be managed with stool softeners or bulk laxatives, or administer alternately with magnesium-containing antacids (unless patient has renal disease).
• Long-term aluminum carbonate use can lead to calcium resorption and subsequent bone demineralization.

Patient monitoring
• Monitor serum calcium and phosphate levels periodically; reduced serum phosphate levels may lead to increased serum calcium levels.

Pediatric patients
• Use cautiously in children under age 6. Safety and efficacy haven't been established in children, but drug has been used in a few cases.

Geriatric patients
• Because geriatric patients commonly have decreased GI motility, they may become constipated from this drug.

Patient education
• Advise patient to take drug only as directed and not to take more than 24 capsules in a 24-hour period. Instruct patient to shake suspension well.
• As needed, advise patient to restrict sodium intake, to drink plenty of fluids, and to follow a low-phosphate diet.
• Advise patient not to switch antacids without medical approval.

aluminum hydroxide
AlternaGEL, Alu-Cap, Alu-Tab, Amphojel, Dialume

Pharmacologic classification: aluminum salt
Therapeutic classification: antacid, hypophosphatemic agent
Pregnancy risk category: C

Indications and dosages
➤ *To provide antacid effects, to treat hyperphosphatemia.* *Adults:* 500 to 1,500 mg P.O. (tablet or capsule) 1 hour after meals and h.s.; or 5 to 30 ml of suspension p.r.n. 1 hour after meals and h.s.

How supplied
Available without a prescription
Capsules: 475 mg, 500 mg
Liquid: 600 mg/5 ml
Suspension: 320 mg/5 ml, 450 mg/5 ml, 675 mg/5 ml
Tablets: 300 mg, 500 mg, 600 mg

Pharmacodynamics
Antacid action: Aluminum hydroxide neutralizes gastric acid, reducing the direct acid irritant effect. This increases pH, thereby decreasing pepsin activity.
Hypophosphatemic action: Aluminum hydroxide reduces serum phosphate levels by complexing with phosphate in the gut, resulting in insoluble, nonabsorbable aluminum phosphate, which is then excreted in feces. Calcium absorption increases as a result of decreased phosphate absorption.

Pharmacokinetics
Absorption: Absorbed minimally; small amounts may be absorbed systemically.
Distribution: None.
Metabolism: None.
Excretion: Excreted in feces; some may appear in breast milk.

Route	Onset	Peak	Duration
P.O.	Variable	Unknown	20-180 min

Contraindications and precautions
No known contraindications. Use cautiously in patients with renal disease.

Interactions
Drug-drug. *Antimuscarinics, chenodiol, chlordiazepoxide, coumarin anticoagulants, diazepam, digoxin, iron salts, isoniazid, phenothiazines (especially chlorpromazine), potassium phosphate, quinolones, sodium phosphate, tetracycline, vitamin A:* Aluminum hydroxide may decrease absorption of many drugs, thereby decreasing their effectiveness; separate administration by at least 2 hours.
Enteric-coated drugs: Aluminum hydroxide causes premature release of these drugs. Advise separation of doses by 1 hour.

Adverse reactions
CNS: encephalopathy.
GI: *constipation,* intestinal obstruction, elevated serum gastrin levels.
Metabolic: hypophosphatemia.
Musculoskeletal: osteomalacia.

Overdose and treatment
No information available. Patients with impaired renal function are at a higher risk of aluminum toxicity to brain, bone, and parathyroid glands.

Special considerations
• Drug therapy may interfere with imaging techniques using sodium pertechnetate Tc99m and thus impair evaluation of Meckel's diverticulum. It may also interfere with reticuloendothelial imaging of liver, spleen, and bone marrow using technetium Tc99m sulfur colloid. It may antagonize the effect of pentagastrin during gastric acid secretion tests.

Reactions may be *common*, uncommon, *life-threatening*, or COMMON AND LIFE-THREATENING.

• Shake suspension well (especially extra-strength suspension) and give with small amounts of water or fruit juice.
• After administering through nasogastric tube, flush tube with water to prevent obstruction.
• When drug is used as an antiurolithic, encourage increased fluid intake to enhance drug effectiveness.
• Constipation may be managed with stool softeners or bulk laxatives. Suggest alternating aluminum hydroxide with magnesium-containing antacids (unless patient has renal disease).

Patient monitoring
• Periodically monitor serum calcium and phosphate levels; decreased serum phosphate levels may lead to increased serum calcium levels.
• Observe patient for signs and symptoms of hypophosphatemia (anorexia, muscle weakness, and malaise).

Breast-feeding patients
• Although drug may appear in breast milk, no problems have been linked with its use in breast-feeding women.

Pediatric patients
• Use cautiously in children under age 6.

Geriatric patients
• Because geriatric patients commonly have decreased GI motility, they may become constipated from this drug.

Patient education
• Caution patient to take drug only as directed, to shake suspension well or chew tablets thoroughly, and to follow with sips of water or juice.
• As indicated, instruct patient to restrict sodium intake, drink plenty of fluids, or follow a low-phosphate diet.
• Advise patient not to switch to another antacid without medical approval.

---

amantadine hydrochloride
Symmetrel

Pharmacologic classification: synthetic cyclic primary amine
Therapeutic classification: antiviral, antiparkinsonian
Pregnancy risk category: C

Indications and dosages
➤ *Prophylaxis or symptomatic treatment of influenza type A virus, respiratory tract illnesses in geriatric or debilitated patients.* Adults up to age 64 and children age 10 and older who weigh more than 88 lb (40 kg): 200 mg P.O. daily in a single dose or divided b.i.d.
Children ages 1 to 9: 4.4 to 8.8 mg/kg P.O. daily up to a maximum of 150 mg daily. To reduce tox-

icity, 5 mg/kg daily given in one or two divided doses (up to a maximum of 150 mg daily) is recommended.
Adults over age 64: 100 mg P.O. once daily. Continue treatment for 24 to 48 hours after symptoms disappear. Prophylaxis should start as soon as possible after initial exposure and continue for at least 10 days after exposure. Prophylactic treatment may be continued up to 90 days for repeated or suspected exposures if influenza virus vaccine is unavailable. If used with influenza virus vaccine, continue dose for 2 to 4 weeks until protection from vaccine develops.
➤ *Drug-induced extrapyramidal reactions. Adults:* 100 to 300 mg P.O. daily in divided doses.
➤ *Idiopathic parkinsonism, parkinsonian syndrome. Adults:* 100 mg P.O. b.i.d.; in patients who are seriously ill or receiving other antiparkinsonian drugs, 100 mg daily for at least 1 week; then 100 mg b.i.d., p.r.n. Patient may benefit from as much as 400 mg daily, but doses over 200 mg must be closely supervised.
✦ *Dosage adjustment.* In patients with renal dysfunction, base maintenance dosage on creatinine clearance value, as follows. For syrup, give 200 mg P.O. on the first day. For capsules, give 200 mg P.O the first day, and then 100 mg daily if creatinine clearance is between 30 and 50 ml/minute. Give 200 mg on the first day and 100 mg q alternating day if it's 15 to 29 ml/minute. Give 200 mg q 7 days if it's below 15 ml/minute. Patients undergoing long-term hemodialysis should receive 200 mg P.O. q 7 days.

How supplied
Available by prescription only
Capsules: 100 mg
Syrup: 50 mg/5 ml
Tablets: 100 mg

Pharmacodynamics
Antiviral action: Amantadine interferes with viral uncoating of the RNA in lysosomes. In vitro, amantadine is active only against influenza type A virus. (However, spontaneous resistance commonly occurs.) In vivo, amantadine may protect against influenza type A virus in 70% to 90% of patients; when administered within 24 to 48 hours of onset of illness, it reduces duration of fever and other systemic symptoms.
Antiparkinsonian action: Amantadine is thought to cause the release of dopamine in the substantia nigra.

Pharmacokinetics
Absorption: Well absorbed from the GI tract with oral administration. Usual serum level is 0.2 to 0.9 mcg/ml. (Neurotoxicity may occur at levels exceeding 1.5 mcg/ml.)
Distribution: Distributed widely throughout body; crosses the blood-brain barrier.
Metabolism: About 10% of dose is metabolized.

Excretion: About 90% of dose is excreted unchanged in urine, primarily by tubular secretion. Portion of drug may appear in breast milk. Excretion rate depends on urine pH (acidic pH enhances excretion). Elimination half-life in patients with normal renal function is about 24 hours; in those with renal dysfunction, it may be prolonged to 10 days.

Route	Onset	Peak	Duration
P.O.	Unknown	1-4 hr	Unknown

Contraindications and precautions

Contraindicated in patients hypersensitive to drug. Don't use in patients with untreated angle-closure glaucoma. Use cautiously in elderly patients and in patients with seizure disorders, heart failure, peripheral edema, hepatic disease, mental illness, eczematoid rash, renal impairment, orthostatic hypotension, and CV disease.

Interactions

Drug-drug. *Benztropine and trihexyphenidyl in large doses:* Amantadine may potentiate anticholinergic adverse effects, possibly causing confusion and hallucinations.
CNS stimulants: May cause additive stimulation. Avoid use together.
Co-trimoxazole: Decreased renal clearance of amantadine with the potential for toxic delirium. Avoid use together.
Hydrochlorothiazide, triamterene: A combination of these drugs may decrease urinary amantadine excretion, resulting in increased serum amantadine levels and possible toxicity. Avoid use together.
Drug-herb. *Jimsonweed:* May adversely affect CV system function. Discourage use together.
Drug-lifestyle. *Alcohol use:* May result in lightheadedness, confusion, fainting, and hypotension. Discourage use together.

Adverse reactions

CNS: depression, fatigue, confusion, *dizziness,* hallucinations, anxiety, *irritability,* ataxia, *insomnia,* headache, *light-headedness.*
CV: peripheral edema, orthostatic hypotension, ***heart failure.***
GI: anorexia, *nausea,* constipation, vomiting, dry mouth.
Skin: livedo reticularis with prolonged use.

Overdose and treatment

Overdose may cause nausea, vomiting, anorexia, hyperexcitability, tremors, slurred speech, blurred vision, lethargy, anticholinergic symptoms, seizures, and possible ventricular arrhythmias, including torsades de pointes and ventricular fibrillation. CNS effects result from increased levels of dopamine in the brain.

Treatment includes immediate gastric lavage or emesis induction along with supportive measures, forced fluids, and, if necessary, I.V. administration of fluids. Urine acidification may be

used to increase drug excretion. Physostigmine may be given (1 to 2 mg by slow I.V. infusion at 1- to 2-hour intervals) to counteract CNS toxicity. Seizures or arrhythmias may be treated with conventional therapy. Monitor patient closely.

Special considerations

● To prevent orthostatic hypotension, advise patient to move slowly when changing positions (especially when standing up).
● If patient experiences insomnia, administer dose several hours before bedtime.
● Prophylactic drug use is recommended for selected high-risk patients who can't receive influenza virus vaccine. Manufacturer recommends prophylactic therapy lasting up to 90 days with possible repeated or unknown exposure.

Patient monitoring

● Monitor patient's blood pressure if dizziness or light-headedness occurs.

Pregnant patients

● There are no adequate controlled studies in pregnant women. Use drug only when benefits outweigh the risks.

Breast-feeding patients

● Drug appears in breast milk. Avoid breast-feeding during therapy with amantadine.

Pediatric patients

● Safety and effectiveness of drug in children under age 1 haven't been established.

Geriatric patients

● Geriatric patients are more susceptible to adverse neurologic effects; dividing daily dosage into two doses may reduce risk.

Patient education

● Warn patient that drug may impair mental alertness.
● Advise patient to take drug after meals to ensure best absorption.
● Caution patient to avoid abrupt position changes because these may cause light-headedness or dizziness.
● If drug is being taken to treat parkinsonism, warn patient not to discontinue it abruptly because doing so could precipitate a parkinsonian crisis.
● Warn patient to avoid alcohol while taking drug.
● Instruct patient to report adverse effects promptly, especially dizziness, depression, anxiety, nausea, and urine retention.

Reactions may be *common,* uncommon, ***life-threatening,*** or COMMON AND LIFE-THREATENING.

amifostine
Ethyol

Pharmacologic classification: organic thiophosphate
Therapeutic classification: cytoprotective drug
Pregnancy risk category: C

Indications and dosages
➤ *Reduction of cumulative renal toxicity caused by repeated administration of cisplatin in patients with advanced ovarian cancer. Adults:* 910 mg/m² daily as a 15-minute I.V. infusion, starting within 30 minutes before chemotherapy. If hypotension occurs and blood pressure doesn't return to normal within 5 minutes of treatment, subsequent cycles should use 740 mg/m².

How supplied
Available by prescription only
Injection: 500 mg anhydrous basis and 500 mg mannitol/10-ml vial

Pharmacodynamics
Cytoprotective action: Dephosphorylated by alkaline phosphatase in tissues to a pharmacologically active free thiol metabolite. The higher level of free thiol in normal tissues is available to bind to, and thereby detoxify, reactive metabolites of cisplatin, which can reduce the toxic effects of cisplatin on renal tissue. Free thiol can also act as a scavenger of free radicals that may be generated in tissues exposed to cisplatin.

Pharmacokinetics
Absorption: Administered I.V.
Distribution: Rapidly cleared from plasma with a distribution half-life of less than 1 minute. Found in bone marrow cells 5 to 8 minutes after administration.
Metabolism: Rapidly metabolized to an active free thiol metabolite. A disulfide metabolite is produced subsequently and is less active than the free thiol.
Excretion: Drug and its two metabolites are minimally excreted in urine.

Route	Onset	Peak	Duration
I.V.	Rapid	Unknown	6 min

Contraindications and precautions
Contraindicated in patients hypersensitive to aminothiol compounds or mannitol. Shouldn't be used in patients receiving chemotherapy for malignancies that are potentially curable (certain malignancies of germ-cell origin). Also contraindicated in hypotensive or dehydrated patients and in those receiving antihypertensives that can't be stopped for 24 hours before amifostine administration.

Use cautiously in elderly patients and in patients with ischemic heart disease, arrhythmias, heart failure, or history of CVA or transient ischemic attacks. Use cautiously in patients in whom the common adverse effects of nausea, vomiting, and hypotension are likely to have serious consequences.

Interactions
Drug-drug. *Antihypertensives, other drugs that could cause hypotension:* Enhanced hypotensive effects. Special consideration should be given regarding concomitant use.

Adverse reactions
CNS: loss of consciousness, dizziness, somnolence.
CV: *hypotension.*
EENT: sneezing.
GI: hiccups, *nausea, vomiting.*
Metabolic: hypocalcemia.
Other: flushing or feeling warm, chills or feeling cold, allergic reactions ranging from rash to rigors.

Overdose and treatment
The most likely symptom of overdose is hypotension, which should be managed by infusion of normal saline solution and other supportive measures, as indicated.

Special considerations
● Reconstitute each single-dose vial with 9.5 ml of sterile normal saline solution. Use of other solutions to reconstitute drug isn't recommended. Reconstituted solution (500 mg amifostine/10 ml) is chemically stable for up to 5 hours at room temperature (about 77° F [25° C]) or up to 24 hours under refrigeration (35° to 46° F [2° to 8° C]).
● Drug can be prepared in polyvinyl chloride bags at concentrations of 5 to 40 mg/ml and has the same stability as when reconstituted in the single-use vial.
● Inspect vial for particulate matter and discoloration before administration whenever solution and container permit. Don't use if cloudiness or precipitate is seen.
● If possible, stop antihypertensive therapy 24 hours before amifostine administration. If antihypertensive therapy can't be stopped, don't use drug because of severe hypotension risk.
● Patients receiving amifostine should be adequately hydrated before drug administration and be kept in a supine position during the infusion.
● Don't infuse for more than 15 minutes; longer infusion time has caused adverse reactions.
● Administer antiemetics, including dexamethasone 20 mg I.V. and a serotonin 5HT receptor antagonist, before and with amifostine. Additional antiemetics may be required based on the chemotherapy drugs administered.

Patient monitoring
• Monitor serum calcium level in patients at risk for hypocalcemia, such as those with nephrotic syndrome. If necessary, administer calcium supplements.
• Monitor blood pressure every 5 minutes during infusion. If hypotension occurs, requiring interruption of therapy, place patient in Trendelenburg's position and give an infusion of normal saline solution using a separate I.V. line. If blood pressure returns to normal within 5 minutes and patient is asymptomatic, infusion may be restarted so that full dose of drug can be given. If full dose of amifostine can't be administered, drug dose for later cycles should be 740 mg/m².
• When amifostine is used with highly emetogenic chemotherapy, monitor patient's fluid balance.

Breast-feeding patients
• It's unknown if drug or its metabolites appear in breast milk. Patient shouldn't breast-feed if taking drug.

Pediatric patients
• Safety and effectiveness in children haven't been established.

Geriatric patients
• Use drug with caution in elderly patients; safety hasn't been established in this age-group.

Patient education
• Instruct patient to remain in a supine position during infusion.

---

amikacin sulfate
Amikin

Pharmacologic classification: aminoglycoside
Therapeutic classification: antibiotic
Pregnancy risk category: D

Indications and dosages
➤ **Serious infections caused by susceptible organisms.** *Adults and children with normal renal function:* 15 mg/kg daily divided q 8 to 12 hours I.M. or I.V. (in 100 to 200 ml D₅W or normal saline solution administered over 30 to 60 minutes). Don't exceed 1.5 g daily or 15 mg/kg.
Adults◇: 4 to 20 mg given intrathecally or intraventricularly as a single dose in conjunction with I.M. or I.V. administration.
Neonates with normal renal function: Initially, 10 mg/kg I.M. or I.V. (in D₅W or normal saline solution administered over 1 to 2 hours), then 7.5 mg/kg q 12 hours.
➤ **Uncomplicated urinary tract infections.** *Adults:* 250 mg I.M. or I.V. b.i.d.
➤ **Clinical tuberculosis** ◇. *Adults, children, and older infants:* 15 mg/kg I.M. daily, 5 times weekly as an adjunct to other antitubercular drugs.

✦ **Dosage adjustment.** In renal failure, 7.5 mg/kg initially. Subsequent doses and frequency determined by blood amikacin levels and renal function studies. One method is to administer additional 7.5-mg/kg doses and alter dosing interval based on steady-state serum creatinine. To determine intervals (in hours) multiply patient's steady-state serum creatinine (in mg/dl) by 9. Keep peak serum levels between 15 and 35 mcg/ml; trough serum levels shouldn't exceed 5 to 10 mcg/ml.

How supplied
Available by prescription only
Injection: 50 mg/ml, 250 mg/ml

Pharmacodynamics
Antibiotic action: Amikacin is bactericidal; it binds directly to the 30S ribosomal subunit, thus inhibiting bacterial protein synthesis. Its spectrum of activity includes many aerobic gram-negative organisms (including most strains of *Pseudomonas aeruginosa*) and some aerobic gram-positive organisms. Amikacin may act against some organisms resistant to other aminoglycosides, such as *Proteus, Pseudomonas,* and *Serratia;* some strains of these may be resistant to amikacin. Drug is ineffective against anaerobes.

Pharmacokinetics
Absorption: Poorly absorbed after oral administration and is given parenterally.
Distribution: Distributed widely after parenteral administration; intraocular penetration is poor. Factors that increase volume of distribution (burns, peritonitis) may increase dosage requirements. CSF penetration is low, even in patients with inflamed meninges. Intraventricular administration produces high concentrations throughout the CNS. Protein binding is minimal. Amikacin crosses the placenta.
Metabolism: Not metabolized.
Excretion: Excreted primarily in urine by glomerular filtration; small amounts may be excreted in bile and breast milk. Elimination half-life in adults is 2 to 3 hours. In patients with severe renal damage, half-life may extend to 30 to 86 hours. Over time, amikacin accumulates in inner ear and kidneys; urine concentrations approach 800 mcg/ml 6 hours after a 500-mg I.M. dose.

Route	Onset	Peak	Duration
I.V.	Immediate	Immediate	8-12 hr
I.M.	Unknown	1 hr	8-12 hr

Contraindications and precautions
Contraindicated in patients hypersensitive to drug or other aminoglycosides. Use cautiously in patients with impaired renal function or neuromuscular disorders, in neonates and infants, and in elderly patients.

Reactions may be *common*, uncommon, **life-threatening**, or COMMON AND LIFE-THREATENING.

Interactions

Drug-drug. *Amphotericin B, capreomycin, cephalosporins, cisplatin, loop diuretics, methoxyflurane, polymyxin B, vancomycin, and other aminoglycosides:* Concurrent use may increase the hazard of nephrotoxicity, ototoxicity, and neurotoxicity. Use together cautiously.

Antiemetics, antivertigo drugs, dimenhydrinate: May mask amikacin-induced ototoxicity. Monitor patient closely.

Bumetanide, ethacrynic acid, furosemide, mannitol, urea: Increased risk of ototoxicity. Use together cautiously.

General anesthetics, neuromuscular blockers (such as succinylcholine, tubocurarine): Amikacin may potentiate neuromuscular blockade. Monitor patient closely.

Penicillins: Synergistic bactericidal effect against *P. aeruginosa, Escherichia coli, Klebsiella, Citrobacter, Enterobacter, Serratia,* and *Proteus mirabilis.* However, the drugs are physically and chemically incompatible and are inactivated when mixed or given together. Avoid use together.

Adverse reactions

CNS: *neuromuscular blockade.*
EENT: *ototoxicity.*
GU: *nephrotoxicity, azotemia.*
Musculoskeletal: arthralgia, acute muscular paralysis.

Overdose and treatment

Signs of overdose include ototoxicity, nephrotoxicity, and neuromuscular toxicity. Drug can be removed by hemodialysis or peritoneal dialysis. Treatment with calcium salts or anticholinesterases reverses neuromuscular blockade.

Special considerations

Consider the recommendations relevant to all aminoglycosides as well as the following.

• Because drug is dialyzable, patients undergoing hemodialysis need dosage adjustments.

• Recommendations for care and teaching of patients during therapy and use in geriatric patients and breast-feeding women are the same as for all aminoglycosides.

⚠ **ALERT** Don't confuse Amikin with Amicar.

• Prepare I.V. infusion by adding 500 mg of amikacin to 100 to 200 ml of I.V. infusion fluid. Or, prepare ADD-Vantage vials per manufacturer instructions. Infuse over 30 to 60 minutes. For infants, dilute enough to allow an infusion period of 1 to 2 hours.

Patient monitoring

• Monitor peak and trough levels. Peak serum levels should be no more than 35 mcg/ml and trough serum levels no more than 10 mcg/ml.

Pediatric patients

• Because risk of ototoxicity is unknown, use amikacin in infants only when other drugs are ineffective or contraindicated. Monitor patient closely during therapy.

Patient education

• Instruct patient to report adverse reactions promptly.
• Encourage adequate fluid intake.

---

amiloride hydrochloride
Midamor

Pharmacologic classification: potassium-sparing diuretic
Therapeutic classification: diuretic, antihypertensive
Pregnancy risk category: B

Indications and dosages

➤ *Hypertension; edema related to heart failure, usually in patients who are also taking thiazide or other potassium-wasting diuretics. Adults:* Usually 5 mg P.O. daily. Dose may be increased to 10 mg daily, if necessary. Don't exceed 20 mg daily.

➤ *Lithium-induced polyuria ◊. Adults:* 5 to 10 mg P.O. b.i.d.

How supplied

Available by prescription only
Tablets: 5 mg

Pharmacodynamics

Diuretic action: Amiloride acts directly on the distal renal tubule to inhibit sodium reabsorption and potassium excretion, thereby reducing potassium loss.

Antihypertensive action: Amiloride is commonly used with more effective diuretics to manage edema from heart failure, hepatic cirrhosis, and hyperaldosteronism. Mechanism of amiloride's hypotensive effect is unknown.

Pharmacokinetics

Absorption: About 50% is absorbed from GI tract. Food decreases absorption to 30%.
Distribution: Wide extravascular distribution.
Metabolism: Insignificant.
Excretion: Most is excreted in urine; half-life is 6 to 9 hours in patients with normal renal function.

Route	Onset	Peak	Duration
P.O.	2 hr	6-10 hr	24 hr

Contraindications and precautions

Contraindicated in patients with elevated serum potassium level (over 5.5 mEq/L). Don't administer to patients hypersensitive to drug or to those receiving other potassium-sparing diuretics, such as spironolactone and triamterene. Also contraindicated in patients with anuria, acute or chronic renal insufficiency, or diabetic nephropathy.

Use with extreme caution in patients who have diabetes mellitus.

Interactions
Drug-drug. *ACE inhibitors, potassium-containing drugs (parenteral penicillin G), potassium-sparing diuretics:* Amiloride increases the risk of hyperkalemia when administered with other drugs. Use together cautiously.
Antihypertensives: Amiloride may potentiate hypotensive effects. This may be used to therapeutic advantage.
Digoxin: Renal clearance of digoxin may be decreased, along with the inotropic effect. Use together cautiously.
Lithium: Amiloride may reduce renal clearance of lithium and increase lithium blood levels. Use together cautiously.
NSAIDs, such as ibuprofen or indomethacin: May alter renal function and thus affect potassium excretion. Use together cautiously.
Drug-herb. *Licorice:* Increased risk of hypokalemia. Discourage concomitant use.
Drug-food. *Potassium-containing salt substitutes:* Increased risk of hyperkalemia. Avoid use together.

Adverse reactions
CNS: *headache*, weakness, dizziness, encephalopathy, fatigue.
CV: orthostatic hypotension.
GI: *nausea, anorexia, diarrhea, vomiting,* abdominal pain, constipation, appetite changes.
GU: impotence, abnormal renal function test results.
Hematologic: *aplastic anemia, neutropenia.*
Hepatic: abnormal hepatic function test results.
Metabolic: hyperkalemia.
Musculoskeletal: muscle cramps.
Respiratory: dyspnea.

Overdose and treatment
Signs and symptoms of overdose are consistent with dehydration and electrolyte disturbance.

Treatment is supportive and symptomatic. In acute ingestion, empty stomach by emesis or lavage. In severe hyperkalemia (6.5 mEq/L or more), reduce serum potassium levels with I.V. sodium bicarbonate or glucose with insulin. A cation exchange resin, sodium polystyrene sulfonate (Kayexalate), given orally or as a retention enema, may also reduce serum potassium levels.

Special considerations
• Amiloride therapy causes severe hyperkalemia in diabetic patients following I.V. glucose tolerance testing; discontinue drug at least 3 days before testing.
• Recommendations for use of amiloride and for care and teaching of the patient during therapy are the same as those for all potassium-sparing diuretics.

Patient monitoring
• Monitor patient for signs of hyperkalemia, including paresthesia, muscular weakness, fatigue, flaccid paralysis of the limbs, bradycardia, shock, and ECG abnormalities.

Pregnant patients
• There are no adequate studies involving pregnant women.

Breast-feeding patients
• Amiloride appears in the breast milk of animals; no human data are available.

Pediatric patients
• Safety and efficacy in children haven't been established, but a dose of 0.625 mg/kg daily has been used in children weighing 13 to 44 lb (6 to 20 kg).

Geriatric patients
• Geriatric and debilitated patients need close observation because they're more susceptible to drug-induced diuresis and hyperkalemia. Reduced dosages may be indicated.

Patient education
• Tell patient that tablets and single-dose packets for oral suspension can be taken with or without food.
• Remind patient that multidose suspension should always be taken on an empty stomach because food and antacids decrease absorption.
• Advise patient to avoid consumption of large quantities of foods that are high in potassium.
• Tell patient to notify prescriber if symptoms of dehydration occur.

amino acid infusions
Aminosyn, Aminosyn with Dextrose, Aminosyn with Electrolytes, Aminosyn-PF, Aminosyn pH6, Aminosyn II, Aminosyn II in Dextrose, Aminosyn II with Electrolytes, Aminosyn II with Electrolytes in Dextrose, FreAmine III, FreAmine III with Electrolytes, Novamine, ProcalAmine, Travasol, Travasol with Electrolytes, TrophAmine

amino acid infusions for renal failure
Aminess, Aminosyn-RF, NephrAmine, RenAmin

amino acid infusions for high metabolic stress
Aminosyn-HBC, BranchAmin, FreAmine HBC

Reactions may be *common*, uncommon, *life-threatening*, or COMMON AND LIFE-THREATENING.

amino acid infusions for hepatic failure or hepatic encephalopathy
HepatAmine

Pharmacologic classification: protein substrates
Therapeutic classification: parenteral nutritional therapy, caloric drug
Pregnancy risk category: C

Indications and dosages

➤ **Hepatic encephalopathy in patients with cirrhosis or hepatitis; nutritional support.** *Adults:* 80 to 120 g of amino acids (12 to 18 g of nitrogen) daily. Use formulation specifically for hepatic failure or encephalopathy (HepatAmine). Typically, 500 ml amino acid injection is mixed with 500 ml dextrose 50% in water and administered over 8 to 12 hours. Add electrolytes, vitamins, and trace elements.

➤ **Total supportive or supplemental and protein-sparing parenteral nutrition to maintain normal nutrition and metabolism (amino acid infusions).** Individualize dosage to metabolic and clinical response as determined by nitrogen balance and body weight corrected for fluid balance. Add electrolytes, vitamins, trace elements, and nonprotein caloric drugs, p.r.n.
Adults: 1 to 1.5 g/kg I.V. daily.
Children: 2 to 3 g/kg I.V. daily.

How supplied
Available by prescription only
Injection without electrolytes: 1,000 ml (3.5%, 5%, 8.5%, 10%; 10% with 60 mg potassium metabisulfite, 11.4%, 15%); 500 ml (5%, 5.5% with sodium bisulfite, 7%, 8.5%, 8.5% with sodium bisulfite, 10%, 10% with sodium bisulfite, 11.4%, 15%); 250 ml (5%, 10% with sodium bisulfite, 11.4%)
Injection with electrolytes: 1,000 ml (3% with 50 mg potassium metabisulfite and 3 mEq calcium/L, 3% with potassium metabisulfite, 3.5%, 3.5% with 60 mg sodium hydrosulfite); 500 ml (3.5%, 5.5%, with 3 mEq sodium bisulfite/L, 7% with potassium bisulfite, 8% in 1,000-ml container with potassium metabisulfite, 8.5% with potassium metabisulfite, 8.5% with 3 mEq sodium bisulfite/L)

Pharmacodynamics
Nutritional action: Provide a substrate for protein synthesis in the protein-depleted patient or enhance conservation of body protein.

Pharmacokinetics
Absorption: Administered I.V.
Distribution: No information available.
Metabolism: No information available.

Excretion: No information available.

Route	Onset	Peak	Duration
I.V.	Unknown	Unknown	Unknown

Contraindications and precautions
Contraindicated in patients with anuria and in those with inborn errors of amino acid metabolism, such as maple syrup urine disease and isovaleric acidemia. Also contraindicated in patients with severe uncorrected electrolyte or acid-base imbalances, hyperammonemia, and decreased circulating blood volume.

Use cautiously in neonates (especially those with low birth weight), in children, and in patients with impaired renal, hepatic, or cardiac function.

Interactions
Drug-drug. *Acidic I.V. solutions for total parenteral nutrition (TPN):* May release bicarbonate as gas. Avoid using together.
Amino acid solutions: Don't mix because of risk of incompatibility.
Blood: Simultaneous administration with blood may cause pseudoagglutination. Don't give with blood.
Electrolytes, heparin, insulin, supplementary vitamins, trace minerals: May be added cautiously when needed; other drugs shouldn't be administered via the central venous catheter.
Folic acid: Calcium salts precipitate as calcium folate. Avoid concurrent use.
Sodium bicarbonate: May precipitate calcium and magnesium and decrease the activity of insulin and vitamin B complex with vitamin C. Avoid concurrent use.
Tetracycline: May reduce the protein-sparing effects of infused amino acids. Use together cautiously.
Vitamin K: Potential for incompatibility. Administer separately.

Adverse reactions
CV: flushing, thrombophlebitis, edema, thrombosis.
GI: nausea.
GU: glycosuria, osmotic diuresis.
Hepatic: elevated liver enzyme levels.
Metabolic: *rebound hypoglycemia* (when long-term infusions are abruptly stopped), hyperglycemia, metabolic acidosis, alkalosis, hypophosphatemia, *hyperosmolar hyperglycemic nonketotic syndrome,* hyperammonemia, *electrolyte imbalances,* weight gain.
Musculoskeletal: osteoporosis.
Other: *hypersensitivity reactions,* tissue sloughing at infusion site caused by extravasation, *catheter sepsis,* fever.

Special considerations
● Consult pharmacist about compatibility before combining amino acid infusions with other substances.

● Begin I.V. infusion slowly and increase over 1 to 2 days as tolerated to prevent hyperglycemia. Taper off over 1 to 2 days to prevent rebound hypoglycemia.
● Replace all I.V. equipment (I.V. lines, filter, and bottle) every 24 hours.
● Use TPN line solely for providing nutrition, not for collecting blood samples, transfusing blood, or administering drugs.
● High blood glucose levels may need supplementary insulin to prevent dehydration and coma.
● Essential fatty acid deficiency may result from long-term fat-free I.V. feedings. Fat emulsion (500 ml) weekly may be needed.
● If TPN must be interrupted, administer D₅W or D₁₀W by peripheral vein to prevent rebound hypoglycemia.
● Frequent, meticulous mouth care is important to prevent parotitis.
● Administer 10 mg of phytonadione weekly to prevent vitamin K deficiency.

Patient monitoring
● Check vital signs at least every 4 hours.
● Observe infusion site for signs of infection, drainage, edema, and extravasation. Check for fever or other possible signs of infection or hypersensitivity.
● Monitor intake, output, weight, and pattern as well as caloric intake for significant changes.
● Test patient's blood glucose level by fingerstick every 6 hours until infusion rate is stabilized, then twice daily.
● Watch for signs of circulatory overload.
● Regularly monitor the following laboratory values throughout TPN therapy: CBC with differential and platelet count, serum electrolytes, blood glucose, urine glucose and ketones, PT, renal and hepatic function tests, trace elements, and plasma lipids.
● Carefully monitor BUN and creatinine ratios. A BUN-to-creatinine ratio exceeding 10:1 may indicate that patient is receiving too much protein per unit of glucose. Reportedly, 100 to 150 g carbohydrate calories per gram of nitrogen are required to use amino acids effectively.
● In patients receiving protein-sparing therapy, check BUN determinations daily. If BUN levels increase 10 to 15 mg/dl for more than 3 days, therapy adjustment is usually required.

Pediatric patients
● The effect of amino acid infusions without dextrose on the carbohydrate metabolism of children is unknown.
● Take special precautions in children with acute renal failure and especially in low-birth-weight infants. In these patients, laboratory and clinical monitoring must be extensive and frequent.
● Monitor serum calcium levels frequently to check for signs of bone demineralization.

Patient education
● Tell patient receiving TPN that he may imagine taste or smell of food. Explain that these sensations are common, and suggest some distracting activity during mealtimes.
● Encourage patient to take special care with oral hygiene. Advise patient to use a soft toothbrush and fluoride toothpaste and floss teeth daily.
● Inform patient that fewer bowel movements occur while receiving TPN.

aminocaproic acid
Amicar

Pharmacologic classification: carboxylic acid derivative
Therapeutic classification: fibrinolysis inhibitor
Pregnancy risk category: C

Indications and dosages
➤ *Excessive acute bleeding from hyperfibrinolysis.* *Adults:* 4 to 5 g I.V. or P.O. over first hour, followed with constant infusion of 1 g/hour for about 8 hours or until bleeding is controlled. Maximum dose is 30 g over 24 hours. *Children:* 100 mg/kg I.V., or 3 g/m² I.V. first hour, followed by constant infusion of 33.3 mg/kg/hour or 1 g/m²/hour. Maximum dose is 18 g/m² over 24 hours.
➤ *Chronic bleeding tendency.* *Adults:* 5 to 30 g P.O. daily in divided doses at 3- to 6-hour intervals.
➤ *Antidote for excessive thrombolysis due to administration of streptokinase or urokinase◇.* *Adults:* 4 to 5 g I.V. in first hour, followed by continuous infusion of 1 g/hour. Continue treatment for 8 hours or until hemorrhage is controlled.
➤ *Secondary ocular hemorrhage in nonperforating traumatic hyphema◇.* *Adults:* 100 mg/kg P.O. q 4 hours for 5 days; maximum dose is 5 g, and 30 g daily.
➤ *Hereditary hemorrhagic telangiectasia◇.* *Adults:* 1 to 1.5 g P.O. b.i.d. for 1 to 2 months followed by 1 to 2 g daily.

How supplied
Available by prescription only
Injection: 5 g/20 ml for dilution; 24 g/96 ml for infusion
Syrup: 250 mg/ml
Tablets: 500 mg

Pharmacodynamics
Hemostatic action: Aminocaproic acid inhibits plasminogen activators; to a lesser degree, it blocks antiplasmin activity by inhibiting fibrinolysis.

Pharmacokinetics
Absorption: Rapidly and completely absorbed from GI tract.

Reactions may be *common*, uncommon, ***life-threatening***, or COMMON AND LIFE-THREATENING.

Distribution: Readily permeates human blood cells and other body cells; not protein-bound.
Metabolism: Insignificant.
Excretion: 40% to 60% of a single oral dose is excreted unchanged in urine in 12 hours.

Route	Onset	Peak	Duration
P.O.	1 hr	2 hr	Unknown
I.V.	1 hr	Unknown	3 hr

Contraindications and precautions

Contraindicated in patients with active intravascular clotting or presence of disseminated intravascular coagulation unless heparin is used concomitantly. Injectable form is contraindicated in neonates. Use cautiously in patients with cardiac, renal, or hepatic disease.

Interactions

Drug-drug. *Estrogens, oral contraceptives that contain estrogen:* Increased risk of hypercoagulability. Use with caution.

Adverse reactions

CNS: dizziness, malaise, headache, delirium, *seizures,* hallucinations, weakness.
CV: hypotension, *bradycardia, arrhythmias* (with rapid I.V. infusion), generalized thrombosis.
EENT: tinnitus, nasal congestion, conjunctival suffusion.
GI: nausea, cramps, diarrhea.
GU: *acute renal failure.*
Hepatic: increased AST and ALT levels.
Metabolic: *hyperkalemia.*
Musculoskeletal: myopathy.
Skin: rash.

Overdose and treatment

Overdose may cause nausea, diarrhea, delirium, thrombotic episodes, and cardiac and hepatic necrosis.

Discontinue drug immediately. Subendocardial hemorrhagic lesions have appeared in animal studies after long-term high-dose administration.

Special considerations

● Aminocaproic acid has been used investigationally to treat missed abortion, allergic reaction, dermatitides, prophylaxis for blood transfusion reaction, connective tissue disease, and rheumatoid arthritis.
⚠ ALERT Bulk doses and bulk packages must be further diluted.
● To prepare an I.V. infusion, use normal saline solution, D_5W, or lactated Ringer's injection for dilution. Dilute doses up to 5 g with 250 ml of solution, doses of 5 g or greater with at least 500 ml.
● Avoid rapid I.V. infusion to minimize risk of CV adverse reactions, such as hypotension, bradycardia, and arrhythmias; use infusion pump to ensure constancy of infusion.

Patient monitoring

● Monitor coagulation studies, heart rhythm, and blood pressure. Long-term use of drug requires routine creatine kinase determinations.
● Be alert for signs of phlebitis. If skeletal myopathy occurs, consider cardiomyopathy.

Pediatric patients

● Safety and efficacy in children haven't been established.

Patient education

● Advise patient to change positions slowly to minimize dizziness.
● Tell patient that routine CK determinations will be necessary with long-term use.
● Teach patient signs and symptoms of thrombophlebitis, and advise him to report them promptly.

aminophylline
Phyllocontin

Pharmacologic classification: xanthine derivative
Therapeutic classification: bronchodilator
Pregnancy risk category: C

Indications and dosages

➤ **Symptomatic relief of acute bronchospasm.** *Patients not currently receiving theophylline who need rapid relief of symptoms:* Loading dose is 6 mg/kg (equivalent to 4.7 mg/kg anhydrous theophylline) I.V. slowly (25 mg/minute or less); then maintenance infusion.
➤ **Maintenance infusions.** *Adults (nonsmokers):* 0.7 mg/kg/hour I.V. for 12 hours; then 0.5 mg/kg/hour I.V. Or, 3 mg/kg P.O. q 6 hours for two doses; then 3 mg/kg P.O. q 8 hours.
Otherwise healthy adult smokers: 1 mg/kg/hour I.V. for 12 hours; then 0.8 mg/kg/hour I.V. Or, 3 mg/kg P.O. q 4 hours for three doses; then 3 mg/kg P.O. q 6 hours.
Older patients; adults with cor pulmonale: 0.6 mg/kg/hour I.V. for 12 hours; then 0.3 mg/kg/hour I.V. Or, 2 mg/kg P.O. q 6 hours for two doses; then 2 mg/kg P.O. q 8 hours.
Adults with heart failure or liver disease: 0.5 mg/kg/hour I.V. for 12 hours; then 0.1 to 0.2 mg/kg/hour I.V. Or, 2 mg/kg P.O. q 8 hours for two doses; then 1 to 2 mg/kg P.O. q 12 hours.
Children ages 9 to 16: 1 mg/kg/hour I.V. for 12 hours; then 0.8 mg/kg/hour I.V. Or, 3 mg/kg P.O. q 4 hours for three doses; then 3 mg/kg P.O. q 6 hours.
Children ages 6 months to 9 years: 1.2 mg/kg/hour I.V. for 12 hours; then 1 mg/kg/hour I.V. Or, 4 mg/kg P.O. q 4 hours for three doses; then 4 mg/kg P.O. q 6 hours.
Patients currently receiving theophylline: Aminophylline loading infusions of 0.63 mg/kg (0.5 mg/kg anhydrous theophylline) will increase

plasma levels of theophylline by 1 mcg/ml, after serum levels have been evaluated. Some clinicians recommend a loading dose of 3.1 mg/kg I.V. (2.5 mg/kg anhydrous theophylline) if no obvious signs of theophylline toxicity are present; then maintenance infusion.

► *Chronic bronchial asthma. Adults and children:* 16 mg/kg or 400 mg (whichever is less) P.O. daily in three or four divided doses q 6 to 8 hours if using rapidly absorbed dosage forms. Dosage may be increased, if tolerated, in increments of 25% q 2 to 3 days. Alternatively, if using extended-release preparations, 12 mg/kg or 400 mg (whichever is less) P.O. daily in two or three divided doses q 8 to 12 hours. Dosage may be increased, if tolerated, by 2 to 3 mg/kg daily q 3 days.

Regardless of dosage form, the following are recommended maximum doses. For adults and children age 16 and older, 13 mg/kg daily or 900 mg daily (whichever is less); for children ages 12 to 16, 18 mg/kg daily; for children ages 9 to 12, 20 mg/kg daily; and for children ages 1 to 9, 24 mg/kg daily.

When recommended maximum dose is reached, dosage adjustment is based on peak serum theophylline levels. Monitor serum levels to ensure that theophylline levels range from 10 to 20 mcg/ml.

Note: Rectal dose is the same as that recommended for oral bolus.

► *To treat paroxysmal nocturnal dyspnea or periodic apnea with Cheyne-Stokes respirations; to promote diuresis ◇. Adults:* 200 to 400 mg I.V. bolus.

► *Reduction of severe bronchospasm in infants with cystic fibrosis ◇. Infants:* 10 to 12 mg/kg I.V. daily.

How supplied
Available by prescription only
Injection: 25 mg/ml
Liquid: 105 mg/5 ml
Rectal suppositories: 250 mg, 500 mg
Tablets: 100 mg, 200 mg
Tablets (controlled-release): 225 mg

Pharmacodynamics
Bronchodilating action: Aminophylline acts at the cellular level after it's converted to theophylline. (Aminophylline [theophylline ethylenediamine] is 79% theophylline.) Theophylline acts by either inhibiting phosphodiesterase or blocking adenosine receptors in the bronchi, thereby relaxing smooth muscle. Drug also stimulates the respiratory center in the medulla and prevents diaphragmatic fatigue.

Pharmacokinetics
Absorption: Most dosage forms are absorbed well; absorption of the suppository, however, is unreliable and slow. Rate and onset of action also depend on the dosage form selected. Food may alter the rate, but not the extent of absorption, of oral doses.

Distribution: Distributed in all tissues and extracellular fluids except fatty tissue.

Metabolism: Converted to theophylline, then metabolized to inactive compounds.

Excretion: Excreted in urine as theophylline (10%).

Route	Onset	Peak	Duration
P.O.	15-60 min	1-7 hr	Variable
I.V.	Rapid	Rapid	Unknown
P.R.	Unknown	Unknown	Unknown

Contraindications and precautions
Contraindicated in patients hypersensitive to xanthine compounds (caffeine, theobromine) and ethylenediamine and in patients with active peptic ulcer disease and seizure disorders (unless adequate anticonvulsant therapy is given). Rectal suppositories are also contraindicated in patients who have an irritation or infection of the rectum or lower colon.

Use cautiously in neonates, infants, young children, elderly patients, and patients with heart failure, CV disorders, COPD, cor pulmonale, renal or hepatic disease, hyperthyroidism, diabetes mellitus, peptic ulcer, severe hypoxemia, or hypertension.

Interactions
Drug-drug. *Alkali-sensitive drugs:* Reduced aminophylline activity. Don't add these drugs to I.V. fluids containing aminophylline.

Allopurinol (high dose), cimetidine, erythromycin, propranolol, quinolones, troleandomycin: May increase serum aminophylline level by decreasing hepatic clearance. Use together cautiously.

Aminoglutethimide, carbamazepine, marijuana, phenobarbital, phenytoin, rifampin, tobacco: Decreased aminophylline effects. Use together cautiously.

Lithium: Increased lithium excretion. Monitor lithium levels.

Drug-lifestyle. *Tobacco and marijuana use:* Decreased aminophylline effects. Discourage use.

Adverse reactions
CNS: *nervousness, restlessness,* headache, *insomnia, **seizures,*** muscle twitching, irritability.
CV: *palpitations, sinus tachycardia,* extrasystoles, flushing, marked hypotension, ***arrhythmias.***
GI: *nausea, vomiting,* diarrhea, epigastric pain, hematemesis.
Metabolic: hyperglycemia, increased plasma-free fatty acids and urinary catecholamines.
Respiratory: tachypnea, ***respiratory arrest.***
Skin: urticaria.
Other: local irritation (with rectal suppositories), fever.

Reactions may be *common*, uncommon, *life-threatening*, or COMMON AND LIFE-THREATENING.

Overdose and treatment

Signs and symptoms of overdose include nausea, vomiting, insomnia, irritability, tachycardia, extrasystoles, tachypnea, and tonic-clonic seizures. Onset of toxicity may be sudden and severe; arrhythmias and seizures are the first signs.

Induce emesis, except in patients with seizures, then use activated charcoal and cathartics. Charcoal hemoperfusion may be beneficial. Treat arrhythmias with lidocaine and seizures with I.V. benzodiazepine; support respiratory and CV systems.

Special considerations

● Aminophylline may alter the assay for uric acid, depending on method used. Theophylline levels are falsely elevated in the presence of furosemide, phenylbutazone, probenecid, theobromine, caffeine, tea, chocolate, cola beverages, and acetaminophen, depending on type of assay used. These substances don't interfere with levels if measured using high-pressure liquid chromatography.
● Check that patient hasn't had recent theophylline therapy before giving loading dose.
● Don't combine in fluids for I.V. infusion with ascorbic acid, chlorpromazine, codeine phosphate, dimenhydrinate, dobutamine, epinephrine, erythromycin gluceptate, hydralazine, insulin, levorphanol tartrate, meperidine, methadone, methicillin, morphine sulfate, norepinephrine bitartrate, oxytetracycline, penicillin G potassium, phenobarbital, phenytoin, prochlorperazine, promazine, promethazine, tetracycline, vancomycin, or vitamin B complex with vitamin C.
● Don't crush controlled-release tablets.
● I.V. drug administration includes I.V. push at a very slow rate or an infusion with 100 to 200 ml of D_5W or normal saline solution.
● GI symptoms may be relieved by taking oral drug with full glass of water at meals, although food in stomach delays absorption. Enteric-coated tablets may also delay absorption. There's no evidence that antacids reduce GI adverse reactions.
● Suppositories are slowly and erratically absorbed; retention enemas may be absorbed more rapidly. Rectally administered preparations can be given when patient can't take drug orally. Schedule after evacuation, if possible; may be retained better if given before meal. Advise patient to remain recumbent 15 to 20 minutes after insertion.

Patient monitoring

● Patients metabolize xanthines at different rates. Adjust dose by monitoring response, tolerance, pulmonary function, and theophylline blood levels. Therapeutic level is 10 to 20 mcg/ml, but some patients may respond at lower levels; toxicity occurs at levels over 20 mcg/ml.
● Monitor serum theophylline levels. Plasma clearance may be decreased in patients with heart failure, hepatic dysfunction, or pulmonary edema. Smokers show accelerated clearance. Dosage adjustments are necessary.

Breast-feeding patients

● Drug appears in breast milk and may cause irritability, insomnia, or fretfulness in the breast-fed infant.

Pediatric patients

● Drug isn't recommended for infants under age 6 months.

Geriatric patients

● Use reduced doses and monitor patient closely. Warn geriatric patients of dizziness, a common adverse reaction at start of therapy.

Patient education

● Teach patient rationale for therapy and importance of compliance with prescribed regimen; if a dose is missed, patient should take it as soon as possible, but shouldn't double the dose.
● Advise patient of adverse effects and possible signs of toxicity.
● Tell patient not to eat or drink large quantities of xanthine-containing foods and beverages.
● Warn patient that OTC remedies may contain ephedrine with theophylline salts; excessive CNS stimulation may result. Tell patient to seek medical approval before taking any other medications.

amiodarone hydrochloride
Cordarone

Pharmacologic classification: benzofuran derivative
Therapeutic classification: ventricular and supraventricular antiarrhythmic
Pregnancy risk category: D

Indications and dosages

➤ *Recurrent ventricular fibrillation and unstable ventricular tachycardia; atrial fibrillation; angina ◊; hypertrophic cardiomyopathy ◊.* **Adults:** Loading dose of 800 to 1,600 mg P.O. daily for 1 to 3 weeks until initial therapeutic response occurs. Reduce to 600 to 800 mg per day for 1 month. Maintenance dosage is 200 to 600 mg P.O. daily. Or, for first 24 hours, 150 mg I.V. over 10 minutes (mixed in 100 ml D_5W); then 360 mg I.V. over 6 hours (mix 900 mg in 500 ml D_5W); then maintenance dosage of 540 mg I.V. over 18 hours at 0.5 mg/minute. After first 24 hours, continue a maintenance infusion of 0.5 mg/minute in a 1- to 6-mg/ml concentration. For infusions greater than 1 hour, concentrations shouldn't exceed 2 mg/ml unless a central venous catheter is used. Don't use for more than 3 weeks.
Children ◊: 10 to 15 mg/kg P.O. daily or 600 to 800 mg/1.73 m^2 P.O. daily for 4 to 14 days or until response is seen. Then 5 mg/kg or 200 to 400 mg/1.73 m^2; usual maintenance dosage is 2.5 mg/kg or 200 mg/1.73 m^2 daily.

➤ *Supraventricular arrhythmias* ◇. *Adults:* 600 to 800 mg P.O. for 1 to 4 weeks or until supraventricular tachycardia is controlled. Maintenance dosage is 100 to 400 mg daily.

Conversion from I.V. to P.O.
Adults: Daily dose of 720 mg (rate 0.5 mg/minute): for 1 week, 800 to 1,600 mg daily; 1 to 3 weeks, 600 to 800 mg daily; more than 3 weeks, 400 mg daily.

How supplied
Available by prescription only
Injection: 50 mg/ml
Tablets: 100 mg*, 200 mg

Pharmacodynamics
Ventricular antiarrhythmic action: Although generally considered a class III drug, amiodarone hydrochloride has activity in each of the four Vaughn-Williams antiarrhythmic classes. It increases the action potential duration (repolarization inhibition). With prolonged therapy, the effective refractory period increases in the atria, ventricles, AV node, His-Purkinje system, and bypass tracts, and conduction slows in the atria, AV node, His-Purkinje system, and ventricles; sinus node automaticity decreases. Amiodarone also noncompetitively blocks beta-adrenergic receptors. Clinically, it has little, if any, negative inotropic effect. Coronary and peripheral vasodilator effects may occur with long-term therapy. Amiodarone is among the most effective antiarrhythmics, but its therapeutic applications are somewhat limited by its severe adverse reactions.

Pharmacokinetics
Absorption: Slow, variable absorption. Bioavailability is about 22% to 86%. Onset of action may be delayed from 2 to 3 days to 2 to 3 months—even with loading doses.
Distribution: Distributed widely because it accumulates in adipose tissue and in organs with marked perfusion, such as the lungs, liver, and spleen. It is also highly protein-bound (96%). The therapeutic serum level isn't well defined but may range from 1 to 2.5 mcg/ml.
Metabolism: Metabolized extensively in the liver to a pharmacologically active metabolite, desethyl amiodarone.
Excretion: Main excretory route is hepatic through the biliary tree (with enterohepatic recirculation). Because no renal excretion occurs, patients with impaired renal function don't require dosage reduction. Terminal elimination half-life is 25 to 110 days, the longest of any antiarrhythmic; in most patients, half-life ranges from 40 to 50 days.

Route	Onset	Peak	Duration
P.O.	Unknown	3-7 hr	Unknown
I.V.	Unknown	Unknown	Variable

Contraindications and precautions
Contraindicated in patients hypersensitive to drug and in those with severe SA node disease resulting in bradycardia. Unless an artificial pacemaker is present, drug is contraindicated in patients with second- or third-degree AV block and in those in whom bradycardia has caused syncope. Use with caution in patients already receiving antiarrhythmics, beta blockers, and calcium channel blockers. Use of amidoraone and ritonavir is contraindicated. Use cautiously with amprenavir.

Interactions
Drug-drug. *Beta blockers, calcium channel blockers:* Using amiodarone with these drugs may cause sinus bradycardia, sinus arrest, and AV block. Avoid use together.
Cholestyramine: Increased elimination of amiodarone. Avoid use together.
Cimetidine: Increased amiodarone levels. Avoid use together.
Cyclosporine, digoxin, flecainide, lidocaine, phenytoin, procainamide, quinidine, theophylline: May lead to increased serum levels of these drugs, resulting in enhanced effects. Monitor drug levels.
Disopyramide, phenothiazines, pimozide, quinidine, sparfloxacin, tricyclic antidepressants: May cause additive effects that lead to a prolonged QT interval, possibly resulting in torsades de pointes ventricular tachycardia. Use together very cautiously.
General anesthetics: Serious cardiac and CV effects may occur. Close perioperative monitoring of patient is needed.
Phenytoin: Decreased amiodarone levels. Monitor patient for drug effect.
Warfarin: May cause prolonged PT as a result of enhanced drug displacement from protein-binding sites. Monitor patient closely and decrease warfarin dosage.
Drug-herb. *Pennyroyal:* Amiodarone may alter the formation of toxic metabolites of pennyroyal. Discourage use together.
Drug-lifestyle. *Sunlight exposure:* Photosensitivity reactions may result. Encourage precautions.

Adverse reactions
CNS: peripheral neuropathy, ataxia, paresthesia, tremor, insomnia, sleep disturbances, headache, *malaise, fatigue.*
CV: *bradycardia,* edema, hypotension, *arrhythmias, heart failure, heart block, sinus arrest, asystole.*
EENT: *corneal microdeposits,* visual disturbances.
GI: *nausea, vomiting,* constipation, abdominal pain.
Hematologic: coagulation abnormalities, *pancytopenia, neutropenia.*
Hepatic: *altered liver enzyme levels,* hepatic dysfunction, *hepatic failure.*
Metabolic: hypothyroidism, hyperthyroidism.

Reactions may be *common,* uncommon, *life-threatening,* or COMMON AND LIFE-THREATENING.

Respiratory: SEVERE PULMONARY TOXICITY (PNEUMONITIS, ALVEOLITIS), hemoptysis, bronchiolitis obliterans, *organizing pneumonia*, pleuritis.
Skin: *photosensitivity*, blue-gray skin pigmentation, solar dermatitis.

Overdose and treatment
Overdose may cause bradyarrhythmias. Treatment may involve beta-adrenergic agonists, such as isoproterenol, or artificial pacing to help restore an acceptable heart rate. To treat hypotension, positive inotropic agents, such as dopamine or dobutamine, or vasopressors, such as epinephrine or norepinephrine, may be administered. General supportive measures should be used, as necessary. Drug can't be removed by dialysis.

Special considerations
• Drug is effective in treating arrhythmias resistant to other drug therapy. However, the high risk of adverse effects limits its use.
• Divide loading dose into three equal doses, and give with meals to minimize GI intolerance. Maintenance dosage may be given once daily but may be divided into two doses taken with meals if GI intolerance occurs.
• Decrease digoxin, quinidine, phenytoin, and procainamide doses during amiodarone therapy to avoid toxicity.
• Adverse effects are more prevalent with high doses but usually resolve within about 4 months after drug therapy stops.
• When mixed in D₅W, amiodarone is incompatible with aminophylline, cefamandole nafate, cefazolin sodium, mezlocillin, heparin sodium, and sodium bicarbonate.
• To produce the solution required for the first loading infusion or for supplemental infusions, add 3 ml of amiodarone concentrate to 100 ml of D₅W, resulting in 1.5 mg/ml. To produce the solution for slow infusion or maintenance infusion, add 18 ml of amiodarone concentrate to 500 ml of D₅W, resulting in 1.8 mg/ml. Subsequent maintenance infusions may contain 1 to 6 mg/ml of amiodarone. Administer solutions containing 2 mg/ml or more via a central venous catheter. Use an in-line filter. Infusions are administered in a three-step process: a rapid loading dose, a slow loading dose, and a maintenance infusion.
• Administer amiodarone I.V. infusions exceeding 2 hours in glass or polyolefin bottles containing D₅W.
• Store tablets and injection at room temperature and protected from light and excessive heat. Protect diluted solutions from light during administration.

Patient monitoring
• Monitor blood pressure and heart rate and rhythm frequently for significant change.

• Periodically monitor hepatic and thyroid function tests. Perform periodic eye exams to assess for corneal microdeposits.
• Patient needs monitoring for signs and symptoms of pneumonitis, such as exertional dyspnea, nonproductive cough, pleuritic chest pain, pulmonary function tests, and chest X-ray. (Pulmonary toxicity is more common when daily doses exceed 600 mg.) Pulmonary complications require discontinuation of amiodarone and possibly treatment with corticosteroids.
• Patient needs close monitoring during general anesthesia.

Pregnant patients
• Embryotoxic effects are possible in pregnant women. Avoid use.

Breast-feeding patients
• Drug appears in breast milk and shouldn't be given to breast-feeding women.

Pediatric patients
• Drug has been used in children for refractory SVT and ventricular tachycardia. Children receiving amiodarone with digoxin may experience more acute effects of interaction. Children may experience faster onset of action and shorter duration of effect than adults.

Geriatric patients
• Use cautiously in geriatric patients because ataxia may occur.

Patient education
• Advise patient to use sunscreen to prevent photosensitivity reactions to sunlight and UV light, which may cause sunburn and blistering.
• Although corneal microdeposits typically appear 1 to 4 months after therapy begins, only 2% to 3% of patients have visual disturbances. To minimize this complication, recommend frequent instillation of methylcellulose ophthalmic solution.

amitriptyline hydrochloride
Amitriptyline, Elavil, Levate*, Novotriptyn*

Pharmacologic classification: tricyclic antidepressant
Therapeutic classification: antidepressant
Pregnancy risk category: D

Indications and dosages
➤ *Depression, anorexia or bulimia related to depression◇, adjunctive treatment of neurogenic pain◇.* **Adults:** Initial outpatient, 75 to 100 mg P.O. daily in divided doses or 50 to 150 mg h.s. Inpatient, 100 to 300 mg daily. I.M. dosage is 20 to 30 mg q.i.d., which should be changed to oral route as soon as possible. Maintenance dosage is 50 to 100 mg daily.

✦ *Dosage adjustment.* In geriatric or adolescent patients, 10 mg P.O. t.i.d. and 20 mg h.s.

How supplied
Available by prescription only
Injection: 10 mg/ml
Tablets: 10 mg, 25 mg, 50 mg, 75 mg, 100 mg, 150 mg

Pharmacodynamics
Antidepressant action: Amitriptyline is thought to exert its antidepressant effects by inhibiting reuptake of norepinephrine and serotonin in CNS nerve terminals (presynaptic neurons), resulting in increased concentrations and enhanced activity of these neurotransmitters in the synaptic cleft. Amitriptyline more actively inhibits reuptake of serotonin than norepinephrine; it carries a high risk of undesirable sedation, but tolerance to this effect usually develops within a few weeks.

Pharmacokinetics
Absorption: Absorbed rapidly from the GI tract after oral administration and from muscle tissue after I.M. administration.
Distribution: Distributed widely into the body, including the CNS and breast milk; 96% protein-bound.
Metabolism: Metabolized by the liver to the active metabolite nortriptyline; a significant first-pass effect may account for variability of serum concentrations in different patients taking the same dosage.
Excretion: Excreted mostly in urine.

Route	Onset	Peak	Duration
P.O., I.M.	Unknown	2-12 hr	Unknown

Contraindications and precautions
Contraindicated in patients in acute recovery phase of MI, in patients hypersensitive to drug, and in patients who have taken an MAO inhibitor within the past 14 days.

Use cautiously in patients with recent history of MI and in those with unstable heart disease or renal or hepatic impairment.

Interactions
Drug-drug. *Antiarrhythmics (disopyramide, procainamide, quinidine), pimozide, thyroid hormones:* May increase risk of arrhythmias and conduction defects. Avoid use together.
Anticholinergics (including antihistamines, antiparkinsonians, atropine, meperidine, phenothiazines): May cause oversedation, paralytic ileus, visual changes, and severe constipation. Monitor clinical effects closely.
Barbiturates: Induce metabolism and decrease therapeutic efficacy of amitriptyline. Monitor drug effects closely.
Beta blockers, cimetidine, methylphenidate, oral contraceptives, propoxyphene, selective serotonin reuptake inhibitors: May inhibit amitriptyline metabolism, increasing plasma levels and toxicity. Use together cautiously.
Centrally acting antihypertensives (such as clonidine, guanabenz, guanadrel, guanethidine, methyldopa, reserpine): May decrease hypotensive effects of these drugs. Monitor blood pressure.
CNS depressants (including analgesics, anesthetics, barbiturates, narcotics, tranquilizers): Increased sedation. Monitor drug effects closely.
Disulfiram, ethchlorvynol: May cause delirium and tachycardia. Avoid use together.
Haloperidol, phenothiazines: Decreased amitriptyline metabolism and efficacy. Avoid use together.
Metrizamide: Increased risk of seizures. Avoid use together.
Sympathomimetics, including epinephrine, phenylephrine, phenylpropanolamine, and ephedrine (commonly found in nasal sprays): May increase blood pressure. Monitor patient's blood pressure.
Warfarin: May increase PT and cause bleeding. Monitor PT and INR, and decrease warfarin dosage.
Drug-herb. *Evening primrose oil:* Possible additive or synergistic effect resulting in lower seizure threshold and increasing the risk of seizures. Discourage concurrent use.
Drug-lifestyle. *Alcohol use:* Additive effects are likely. Discourage use together.
Heavy smoking: Induced amitriptyline metabolism and decreased therapeutic efficacy. Discourage use together.
Sun exposure: Photosensitivity reactions may result. Advise patient to take precautions.

Adverse reactions
CNS: ***coma, seizures,*** hallucinations, delusions, disorientation, ataxia, tremor, peripheral neuropathy, anxiety, insomnia, restlessness, drowsiness, dizziness, weakness, fatigue, headache, extrapyramidal reactions.
CV: edema, ***MI, CVA, arrhythmias,*** heart block, *orthostatic hypotension, tachycardia, ECG changes,* hypertension.
EENT: *blurred vision,* tinnitus, mydriasis, increased intraocular pressure.
GI: *dry mouth,* nausea, vomiting, anorexia, epigastric distress, diarrhea, constipation, paralytic ileus.
GU: urine retention.
Hematologic: ***agranulocytosis, thrombocytopenia, leukopenia,*** eosinophilia.
Hepatic: elevated liver function test results.
Metabolic: altered serum glucose levels.
Skin: *diaphoresis,* rash, urticaria, photosensitivity.
Other: ***hypersensitivity reaction.***

Overdose and treatment
The first 12 hours after acute ingestion are a stimulatory phase characterized by excessive anticholinergic activity (agitation, irritation, confu-

sion, hallucinations, hyperthermia, parkinsonian symptoms, seizure, urine retention, dry mucous membranes, pupillary dilation, constipation, and ileus). This is followed by CNS depressant effects, including hypothermia, decreased or absent reflexes, sedation, hypotension, cyanosis, and cardiac irregularities, including tachycardia, conduction disturbances, and quinidine-like effects on the ECG.

Severity of overdose is best indicated by widening of the QRS complex and usually represents a serum level in excess of 1,000 mg/ml; metabolic acidosis may follow hypotension, hypoventilation, and seizures. Delayed cardiac anomalies and death may occur.

Treatment is symptomatic and supportive, including maintaining airway, stable body temperature, and fluid and electrolyte balance. Induce emesis with ipecac if gag reflex is intact; follow with gastric lavage and activated charcoal to prevent further absorption. Dialysis is of little use. Physostigmine may be cautiously used to reverse the symptoms of tricyclic antidepressant poisoning in life-threatening situations. Treatment of seizures may include parenteral diazepam or phenytoin; treatment of arrhythmias, parenteral phenytoin or lidocaine; and treatment of acidosis, sodium bicarbonate. Don't give barbiturates; these may enhance CNS and respiratory depressant effects.

Special considerations
Consider the recommendations relevant to all tricyclic antidepressants as well as the following.
● Drug may be used to prevent migraine and cluster headaches, intractable hiccups, and posttherapeutic neuralgia.
● Amitriptyline causes a high risk of sedative effects. Tolerance to sedative effects may develop over several weeks.
● The full dose may be given at bedtime to help offset daytime sedation.
● Substitute oral administration route for parenteral route as soon as possible.
● **⚠ ALERT** Parenteral form of drug is for I.M. administration only. Drug shouldn't be given I.V.
● I.M. administration may result in a more rapid onset of action than oral administration.
● Don't withdraw drug abruptly.
● Discontinue drug at least 48 hours before surgical procedures.
● Sugarless chewing gum, hard candy, or ice may alleviate dry mouth. Stress the importance of regular dental hygiene because dry mouth can increase the risk of dental caries.
● Depressed patients, particularly those with known manic depressive illness, may experience a shift to mania or hypomania.

Patient monitoring
● Check vital signs regularly for decreased blood pressure or tachycardia; observe patient carefully for adverse reactions and report changes. Obtain ECG in patients over age 40 before starting therapy. Advise patient to take the first dose in the office to allow close observation for adverse reactions.
● Check for anticholinergic adverse reactions, which may require dose reduction.
● Observe patient for mood changes to monitor progress; benefits may not occur for several (3 to 6) weeks.
● After abrupt withdrawal of long-term therapy, patient may experience nausea, headache, or malaise. This doesn't indicate addiction.

Breast-feeding patients
● Drug appears in breast milk at levels equal to or greater than those in maternal serum. About 1% of ingested dose appears in the breast-fed infant's serum. The potential benefit to the woman should outweigh the possible adverse reactions in the infant.

Pediatric patients
● Drug isn't recommended for children under age 12.

Geriatric patients
● Geriatric patients may be at greater risk for adverse cardiac effects.

Patient education
● Tell patient to take drug exactly as prescribed and not to double missed doses.
● Advise patient that full dose may be taken at bedtime to alleviate daytime sedation. Alternatively, it may be taken in the early evening to avoid morning hangover.
● Explain that full effects of drug may not become apparent for up to 4 weeks.
● Warn patient that drug may cause drowsiness or dizziness. Tell him to avoid hazardous activities that require alertness until full effects of drug are known.
● Warn patient not to drink alcoholic beverages while taking drug.
● Suggest taking drug with food or milk if it causes stomach upset and using sugarless gum or candy to relieve dry mouth.
● After initial doses, advise patient to lie down for about 30 minutes and to rise slowly to prevent dizziness or fainting.
● Warn patient not to stop taking drug suddenly.
● Encourage patient to report troublesome or unusual effects, especially confusion, movement disorders, rapid heartbeat, dizziness, fainting, or difficulty urinating.

amlodipine besylate
Norvasc

Pharmacologic classification: dihydropyridine calcium channel blocker
Therapeutic classification: antianginal, antihypertensive
Pregnancy risk category: C

Indications and dosages
➤ *Chronic stable angina, vasospastic angina (Prinzmetal's or variant angina).*
Adults: Initially, 5 to 10 mg P.O. daily.
➤ *Hypertension. Adults:* Initially, 2.5 to 5 mg P.O. daily. Adjust dosage based on patient response and tolerance every 7 to 14 days. Maximum daily dose is 10 mg.
✦ *Dosage adjustment.* In small, frail, or geriatric patients, those receiving other antihypertensives, or those with hepatic insufficiency, give 2.5 mg daily.

How supplied
Available by prescription only
Tablets: 2.5 mg, 5 mg, 10 mg

Pharmacodynamics
Antianginal and antihypertensive actions: Contractility of cardiac muscle and vascular smooth muscle depends on movement of extracellular calcium ions into cardiac and smooth-muscle cells through specific ion channels. Amlodipine inhibits the transmembrane influx of calcium ions into vascular smooth muscle and cardiac muscle, thus decreasing myocardial contractility and oxygen demand. As a peripheral arterial vasodilator, the drug acts directly on vascular smooth muscle to reduce peripheral vascular resistance and blood pressure. It also dilates coronary arteries and arterioles.

Pharmacokinetics
Absorption: Absolute bioavailability has been estimated at 64% to 90%.
Distribution: About 93% of the circulating drug is bound to plasma proteins in hypertensive patients.
Metabolism: Extensively metabolized in the liver, with about 90% converted to inactive metabolites.
Excretion: Excreted primarily in urine.

Route	Onset	Peak	Duration
P.O.	Unknown	6-12 hr	24 hr

Contraindications and precautions
Contraindicated in patients hypersensitive to drug. Use cautiously in patients receiving other peripheral dilators and in those with aortic stenosis, heart failure, or severe hepatic disease.

Interactions
Drug-food. *Grapefruit juice:* Elevated amlodipine levels, increasing its pharmacologic and adverse effects. Tell patient to avoid concurrent use.

Adverse reactions
CNS: *headache,* somnolence, fatigue, dizziness, light-headedness, paresthesia.
CV: *edema,* flushing, palpitations.
GI: nausea, abdominal pain.
Musculoskeletal: muscle pain.
Respiratory: dyspnea.
Skin: rash, pruritus.

Overdose and treatment
Symptoms of overdose include nausea, weakness, dizziness, drowsiness, confusion, and slurred speech. Overdose also can cause excessive peripheral vasodilation with marked hypotension and bradycardia, both of which may reduce cardiac output. Junctional rhythms and second- or third-degree AV block also can occur.

Massive overdose warrants active cardiac and respiratory monitoring and frequent blood pressure measurements. Treatment of hypotension consists of CV support, including elevation of the limbs and judicious administration of fluids. If hypotension remains unresponsive to these conservative measures, consider administration of vasopressors (such as phenylephrine), with attention to circulating volume and urine output. I.V. calcium gluconate may help reverse the effects of calcium entry blockade. Because amlodipine is highly protein-bound, hemodialysis isn't likely to benefit the patient.

Special considerations
• Because the vasodilation induced by amlodipine is gradual in onset, acute hypotension has rarely been reported after oral administration. However, use caution when administering drug, particularly if patient has severe aortic stenosis.

Patient monitoring
• Some patients, especially those with severe obstructive coronary artery disease, have developed increased frequency, duration, or severity of angina or even acute MI after calcium channel blocker therapy starts or dosage increases.
• Blood pressure must be monitored closely, especially at the start of therapy.

Breast-feeding patients
• Because it isn't known if amlodipine appears in breast milk, breast-feeding isn't recommended during amlodipine therapy.

Pediatric patients
• Safety and efficacy in children haven't been established.

Geriatric patients
• Geriatric patients may require a smaller dosage of amlodipine.

Reactions may be *common*, uncommon, *life-threatening*, or COMMON AND LIFE-THREATENING.

Patient education

• Tell patient to take nitroglycerin S.L. as needed for acute anginal symptoms. If patient continues nitrate therapy during titration of amlodipine dosage, urge continued compliance.
• Caution patient to continue taking amlodipine even when feeling better.
• Tell patient to notify prescriber about signs of heart failure, such as swelling of hands and feet or shortness of breath.
• Tell patient to take drug with a liquid other than grapefruit juice.

amobarbital
amobarbital sodium
Amytal

Pharmacologic classification: barbiturate
Therapeutic classification: sedative-hypnotic, anticonvulsant
Controlled substance schedule: II
Pregnancy risk category: D

Indications and dosages

➤ *To produce sedation. Adults:* Usually 30 to 50 mg P.O. b.i.d. or t.i.d. but may range from 15 to 120 mg b.i.d. to q.i.d.
Children: 2 mg/kg P.O. daily divided into four equal doses.
➤ *To treat insomnia. Adults:* 65 to 200 mg P.O. or deep I.M. h.s.; I.M. injection not to exceed 5 ml in any one site. Maximum dose is 500 mg.
Children over age 6: 2 to 3 mg/kg deep I.M. h.s.
➤ *To produce preanesthetic sedation. Adults:* 200 mg P.O. 1 to 2 hours before surgery.
➤ *To produce sedation during labor. Adults:* 200 to 400 mg P.O.; may repeat at 1- to 3-hour intervals. Maximum dose is 1 g.
➤ *To produce anticonvulsant effects. Adults:* 65 to 500 mg by slow I.V. injection (rate not exceeding 100 mg/minute). Maximum dose is 1 g.

How supplied
Available by prescription only
Capsules: 200 mg
Powder for injection: 250-mg, 500-mg vials
Tablets: 30 mg

Pharmacodynamics
Anticonvulsant action: Exact cellular site and mechanism of action unknown. Parenteral amobarbital suppresses the spread of seizure activity produced by epileptogenic foci in the cortex, thalamus, and limbic systems by enhancing the effect of gamma-aminobutyric acid (GABA). Both presynaptic and postsynaptic excitability are decreased.
Sedative-hypnotic action: Acts throughout the CNS as a nonselective depressant with an intermediate onset and duration of action. Particularly sensitive to this drug is the mesencephalic

reticular activating system, which controls CNS arousal. Drug decreases both presynaptic and postsynaptic membrane excitability by facilitating the action of GABA.

Pharmacokinetics
Absorption: Absorbed well after oral administration. Absorption after I.M. administration is 100%. Onset of action is 10 to 30 minutes.
Distribution: Distributed well throughout body tissues and fluids.
Metabolism: Metabolized in the liver by oxidation to a tertiary alcohol.
Excretion: Less than 1% of dose is excreted unchanged in the urine; rest is excreted as metabolites. The half-life is biphasic, with a first phase half-life of about 40 minutes and a second phase of about 20 hours. Duration of action is 6 to 8 hours.

Route	Onset	Peak	Duration
P.O.	10-30 min	Unknown	6-8 hr
I.V.	Within 5 min	Within 30 min	3-6 hr
I.M.	Unknown	Unknown	Unknown

Contraindications and precautions
Contraindicated in patients hypersensitive to barbiturates and in those with bronchopneumonia, other severe pulmonary insufficiency, or porphyria.
Use cautiously in patients with suicidal tendencies, acute or chronic pain, history of drug abuse, hepatic or renal impairment, or pulmonary or CV disease.

Interactions
Drug-drug. *Antidepressants, antihistamines, MAO inhibitors, narcotics, sedative-hypnotics, tranquilizers:* May add to or potentiate CNS and respiratory depressant effects of these drugs. Use together cautiously.
Corticosteroids, digitoxin, doxycycline, oral contraceptives and other estrogens, theophylline and other xanthines: Enhanced hepatic metabolism of these drugs. Monitor patient carefully.
Disulfiram, MAO inhibitors, valproic acid: Decreased metabolism of amobarbital and increased toxicity. Monitor patient carefully.
Griseofulvin: Impaired effectiveness of griseofulvin. Use together cautiously.
Phenytoin: May cause unpredictable fluctuations in serum phenytoin levels. Monitor phenytoin levels.
Rifampin: May decrease amobarbital levels by increasing metabolism. Monitor patient for drug effect.
Warfarin, other oral anticoagulants: Enhanced enzymatic degradation of anticoagulants. Patient may need increased doses of anticoagulants.
Drug-food. *Food:* Decreased absorption of drug. Give on an empty stomach to enhance absorption.

◇ Unlabeled clinical use

Drug-lifestyle. *Alcohol use:* May add to or potentiate CNS and respiratory depressant effects. Discourage concurrent use.

Adverse reactions

CNS: *drowsiness, lethargy, hangover,* paradoxical excitement, somnolence, syncope.
CV: *bradycardia,* hypotension.
GI: nausea, vomiting.
Hematologic: exacerbation of porphyria.
Respiratory: *respiratory depression, apnea.*
Skin: rash; urticaria; *Stevens-Johnson syndrome;* pain, irritation, and sterile abscess at injection site.
Other: *angioedema,* physical and psychological dependence.

Overdose and treatment

Signs and symptoms of overdose include unsteady gait, slurred speech, sustained nystagmus, somnolence, confusion, respiratory depression, pulmonary edema, areflexia, and coma. Oliguria, jaundice, hypothermia, fever, and shock with tachycardia and hypotension may occur.

Treatment of overdose aims to maintain and support ventilation and pulmonary function as needed; support cardiac function and circulation with vasopressors and I.V. fluids as needed. If patient is conscious with a functioning gag reflex and ingestion has been recent, induce emesis by administering ipecac syrup. Gastric lavage may be performed if a cuffed endotracheal tube is in place to prevent aspiration when emesis is inappropriate. Follow with activated charcoal. Measure fluid intake and output, vital signs, and laboratory parameters. Maintain body temperature. Assess cardiopulmonary status frequently for possible alterations. Monitor blood counts for potential adverse reactions.

Alkalinization of urine may be helpful in removing amobarbital from the body; hemodialysis may be useful in severe overdose. Assess renal and hepatic laboratory studies to ensure adequate drug removal.

Special considerations

• Not commonly used as a sedative or aid to sleeping; barbiturates have been replaced by safer benzodiazepines for such use.
• Administer drug orally on an empty stomach to enhance absorption.
• Reconstitute powder for injection with sterile water for injection. Roll vial in hands; don't shake. Use 2.5 or 5 ml (for 250 or 500 mg of amobarbital) to make 10% solution. For I.M. use, prepare 20% solution by using 1.25 or 2.5 ml of sterile water for injection.
• Administer reconstituted parenteral solution within 30 minutes after opening vial.
• Don't administer solution that's cloudy or forms a precipitate after 5 minutes of reconstitution.
• Administer I.V. dose at no more than 100 mg/ minute in adults or 60 mg/m²/minute in children to prevent possible hypotension and respiratory

depression. Have emergency resuscitative equipment available.
• Administer I.M. dose deep into large muscle mass, giving no more than 5 ml in any one injection site. Sterile abscess or tissue damage may result from inadvertent superficial I.M. or S.C. injection.
• Administering full loading doses over short periods of time to treat status epilepticus may require ventilatory support in adults.
• Amobarbital may cause a false-positive phentolamine test.
• Physiologic effects of amobarbital may impair absorption of cyanocobalamin.
• Amobarbital may decrease serum bilirubin levels in neonates, epileptic patients, and patients with congenital nonhemolytic unconjugated hyperbilirubinemia.
• EEG patterns are altered, with a change in low-voltage, fast-activity; changes persist for a time after therapy is discontinued.

Patient monitoring

• Monitor PT carefully when patient on amobarbital starts or ends anticoagulant therapy. Anticoagulant dosage may need to be adjusted.
• Monitor patient for adverse effects.

Breast-feeding patients

• Drug appears in breast milk and may cause drowsiness in infant. If so, dosage adjustment or discontinuation of drug or breast-feeding may be needed. Use with caution.

Pediatric patients

• Safe use in children under age 6 hasn't been established. Drug may cause paradoxical excitement in some children.

Geriatric patients

• Elderly patients usually need lower doses.
• Confusion, disorientation, and excitability may occur in elderly patients. Use cautiously.

Patient education

• Warn patient of possible physical or psychological dependence with prolonged use.
• Tell patient to avoid alcohol while taking drug.

amoxapine

Pharmacologic classification: dibenzoxazepine, tricyclic antidepressant
Therapeutic classification: antidepressant
Pregnancy risk category: C

Indications and dosages

➤ *Depression.* **Adults:** Initial dose is 50 mg P.O. b.i.d. or t.i.d; may increase to 100 mg b.i.d. or t.i.d. by end of first week. Increases above 300 mg daily should be made only if this dose has been ineffective during a trial period of at least 2 weeks. When effective dose is established,

---

Reactions may be *common*, uncommon, *life-threatening*, or COMMON AND LIFE-THREATENING.

entire dose (not exceeding 300 mg) may be given h.s. No more than 400 mg daily for outpatients. Maximum dose in hospitalized patients is 600 mg. Don't give more than 300 mg in a single dose.

✦ **Dosage adjustment.** In geriatric patients, recommended starting dose is 25 mg P.O. b.i.d. to t.i.d.

How supplied
Available by prescription only
Tablets: 25 mg, 50 mg, 100 mg, 150 mg

Pharmacodynamics
Antidepressant action: Drug is thought to exert its antidepressant effects by inhibiting reuptake of norepinephrine and serotonin in CNS nerve terminals (presynaptic neurons), which results in increased levels and enhanced activity of these neurotransmitters in the synaptic cleft. Amoxapine has a greater inhibitory effect on norepinephrine reuptake than on serotonin. Drug also blocks CNS dopamine receptors, which may account for the higher occurrence of movement disorders during therapy.

Pharmacokinetics
Absorption: Absorbed rapidly and completely from the GI tract after oral administration
Distribution: Distributed widely into the body, including the CNS and breast milk. Drug is 92% protein-bound. Steady state is reached within 2 to 7 days. Proposed therapeutic plasma levels (parent drug and metabolite) range from 200 to 500 ng/ml.
Metabolism: Metabolized by the liver to the active metabolite 8-hydroxyamoxapine; a significant first-pass effect may explain variability of serum levels in different patients taking the same dosage.
Excretion: Excreted in urine and feces (7% to 18%); about 60% of a given dose is excreted as the conjugated form within 6 days.

Route	Onset	Peak	Duration
P.O.	Unknown	1½ hr	Unknown

Contraindications and precautions
Contraindicated in patients hypersensitive to amoxapine, in those in the acute recovery phase of MI, and in those who have taken an MAO inhibitor within 14 days.

Use cautiously in patients with history of urine retention, CV disease, angle-closure glaucoma, or increased intraocular pressure. Use with extreme caution in patients with history of seizures.

Interactions
Drug-drug. Antiarrhythmics (including disopyramide, procainamide, and quinidine), pimozide, thyroid drugs: Increased risk of arrhythmias and conduction defects. Avoid use together.

Anticholinergics (including antihistamines, antiparkinsonians, atropine, meperidine, and phenothiazines): Increased risk of oversedation, paralytic ileus, visual changes, and severe constipation. Use together cautiously.
Barbiturates: Induce amoxapine metabolism and decrease therapeutic efficacy. Monitor patient for clinical effects.
Beta blockers, cimetidine, methylphenidate, oral contraceptives, propoxyphene: May inhibit amoxapine metabolism, increasing plasma levels. Monitor patient for toxicity.
Centrally acting antihypertensives (such as clonidine, guanabenz, guanadrel, guanethidine, methyldopa, and reserpine): Amoxapine decreases hypotensive effects. Monitor clinical response.
CNS depressants (including analgesics, anesthetics, barbiturates, narcotics, and tranquilizers): Increased sedation. Use together cautiously.
Disulfiram, ethchlorvynol: May cause delirium and tachycardia. Use together cautiously.
Haloperidol, phenothiazines: Decreased metabolism, decreasing therapeutic efficacy. Monitor patient for clinical effects.
Metrizamide: Increased risk of seizures. Avoid use together.
Sympathomimetics, including epinephrine, phenylephrine, phenylpropanolamine, and ephedrine (commonly found in nasal sprays): May increase blood pressure. Avoid use together.
Warfarin: Increased PT, INR, and risk of bleeding. Monitor laboratory values, and decrease warfarin dosage.
Drug-herb. Evening primrose oil: Possible additive or synergistic effect resulting in lower seizure threshold and increased risk of seizures. Discourage concurrent use.
Drug-lifestyle. Alcohol use: Increased sedation. Discourage use together.
Heavy smoking: Induces amoxapine metabolism and decreases therapeutic efficacy. Discourage use together.
Sun exposure: Photosensitivity reactions may result. Advise patient to take precautions.

Adverse reactions
CNS: drowsiness, dizziness, excitation, tremor, weakness, confusion, anxiety, insomnia, restlessness, nightmares, ataxia, fatigue, headache, nervousness, tardive dyskinesia, EEG changes, **seizures,** extrapyramidal reactions, **neuroleptic malignant syndrome (high fever, tachycardia, tachypnea, profuse diaphoresis).**
CV: edema, orthostatic hypotension, tachycardia, hypertension, palpitations, prolonged conduction time (elongation of QT and PR intervals, flattened T waves on ECG).
EENT: blurred vision.
GI: dry mouth, constipation, nausea, excessive appetite.

◇ Unlabeled clinical use

GU: *urine retention, acute renal failure* (with overdose).
Hematologic: decreased WBC counts.
Hepatic: elevated liver function test results.
Metabolic: altered serum glucose levels.
Skin: rash, *diaphoresis.*

Overdose and treatment

The first 12 hours after acute ingestion are a stimulatory phase characterized by excessive anticholinergic activity (agitation, irritation, confusion, hallucinations, hyperthermia, parkinsonian symptoms, seizures, urine retention, dry mucous membranes, pupillary dilation, constipation, and ileus). This is followed by CNS depressant effects, including hypothermia, decreased or absent reflexes, sedation, hypotension, cyanosis, and cardiac irregularities, including tachycardia, conduction disturbances, and quinidine-like effects on the ECG.

Overdose with amoxapine produces a much higher risk of CNS toxicity than do other antidepressants. Acute deterioration of renal function (evidenced by myoglobin in urine) occurs in 5% of overdosed patients; this is most likely to occur in patients with repeated seizures after the overdose. Seizures may progress to status epilepticus within 12 hours.

Severity of overdose is best indicated by widening of the QRS complex, which generally represents a serum level in excess of 1,000 ng/ml; serum levels aren't usually helpful. Metabolic acidosis may follow hypotension, hypoventilation, and seizures.

Treatment is symptomatic and supportive, including maintaining airway, stable body temperature, and fluid and electrolyte balance; monitor renal status because of the risk of renal failure. Induce emesis with ipecac if patient is conscious; follow with gastric lavage and activated charcoal to prevent further absorption. Dialysis is of little use. Treat seizures with parenteral diazepam or phenytoin (the value of physostigmine is less certain); arrhythmias, with parenteral phenytoin or lidocaine; and acidosis, with sodium bicarbonate. Don't give barbiturates; these may enhance CNS and respiratory depressant effects.

Special considerations

⚠ ALERT Don't confuse amoxapine with amoxicillin.
● Amoxapine causes a high risk of seizures.
● Antidepressants can cause manic episodes during the depressed phase in patients with bipolar disorder.
● The full dose may be given at bedtime to help reduce daytime sedation.
● The full dose shouldn't be withdrawn abruptly. After abrupt withdrawal of long-term therapy patient may experience nausea, headache, and malaise. This doesn't indicate addiction.
● Tolerance to sedative effects usually develops over the first few weeks of therapy.

● Discontinue drug at least 48 hours before surgical procedures.
● Sugarless chewing gum, hard candy, or ice may alleviate dry mouth.

Patient monitoring

● Monitor patient for tardive dyskinesia and other extrapyramidal effects, which may occur because of the dopamine-blocking activity of amoxapine.
● Watch for gynecomastia in men and women because amoxapine may increase cellular division in breast tissue.

Pregnant patients

● Safe use of tricyclic antidepressants in pregnancy hasn't been established. Fetal malformations, urinary retention, CNS effects (lethargy), developmental delay, and withdrawal symptoms have occurred in neonates born to mothers taking tricyclic antidepressants during pregnancy.

Breast-feeding patients

● Amoxapine appears in breast milk at levels that are 20% those of maternal serum as parent drug and 30% as metabolites. The potential benefits to the woman should outweigh the possible adverse reactions in the infant.

Pediatric patients

● Drug isn't recommended for patients under age 16.

Geriatric patients

● Lower doses are indicated for geriatric patients because they're more sensitive to the therapeutic and adverse effects of drug.
● Geriatric patients are much more susceptible to tardive dyskinesia and extrapyramidal symptoms.

Patient education

● Explain that full effects of drug may not become apparent for 2 weeks or more after therapy begins, perhaps not for 4 to 6 weeks.
● Tell patient to take drug exactly as prescribed; however, full dose may be taken at bedtime to alleviate daytime sedation. Patient shouldn't double the dose for missed ones.
● Warn patient to avoid hazardous activities that require alertness until full effects of the drug are known; it may cause drowsiness or dizziness.
● Tell patient not to drink alcoholic beverages while taking drug.
● Suggest that patient take drug with food or milk if it causes stomach upset; dry mouth can be relieved with sugarless gum or hard candy.
● After initial doses, tell patient to lie down for about 30 minutes and rise slowly to prevent dizziness.
● Warn patient not to discontinue drug suddenly.
● Encourage patient to report unusual or troublesome reactions immediately, especially con-

---

fusion, movement disorders, rapid heartbeat, dizziness, fainting, or difficulty urinating.
• Inform patient that exposure to sunlight, sunlamps, or tanning beds may cause burning of the skin or abnormal pigmentary changes.

amoxicillin/clavulanate potassium
Augmentin, Clavulin*

Pharmacologic classification: aminopenicillin and beta-lactamase inhibitor
Therapeutic classification: antibiotic
Pregnancy risk category: B

Indications and dosages
➤ *Lower respiratory tract infections, otitis media, sinusitis, skin and skin structure infections, and urinary tract infections caused by susceptible organisms.*
Adults and children who weigh more than 40 kg (88 lb): 250 mg (based on amoxicillin component) P.O. q 8 hours or one 500-mg tablet q 12 hours. For more severe infections, 500 mg q 8 hours or 875 mg q 12 hours.
Children who weigh less than 40 kg: 25 to 45 mg/kg P.O. daily (based on amoxicillin component) given in divided doses q 8 to 12 hours.
Neonates and infants under 12 weeks: 30 mg/kg daily in divided doses q 12 hours.
✦ *Dosage adjustment.* In patients with creatinine clearance of 15 to 30 ml/minute, give usual dose q 12 to 18 hours. If clearance is 5 to 15 ml/minute, give usual dose q 20 to 36 hours. If clearance is less than 5 ml/minute, give usual dose every 48 hours. Some clinicians recommend not using drug if creatinine clearance is less than 30 ml/minute. In hemodialysis patients, give 500 mg P.O. midway through treatment and then 500 mg P.O. at the end of treatment.

How supplied
Available by prescription only
Oral suspension: 125 mg amoxicillin trihydrate and 31.25 mg clavulanic acid/5 ml (after reconstitution); 200 mg amoxicillin trihydrate and 28.5 mg clavulanic acid/5 ml (after reconstitution); 250 mg amoxicillin trihydrate and 62.5 mg clavulanic acid/5 ml (after reconstitution); 400 mg amoxicillin trihydrate and 57 mg clavulanic acid/5 ml (after reconstitution)
Tablets: 250 mg amoxicillin trihydrate, 125 mg clavulanic acid; 500 mg amoxicillin trihydrate, 125 mg clavulanic acid; 875 mg amoxicillin trihydrate, 125 mg clavulanic acid
Tablets (chewable): 125 mg amoxicillin trihydrate, 31.25 mg clavulanic acid; 200 mg amoxicillin trihydrate, 28.5 mg clavulanic acid; 250 mg amoxicillin trihydrate, 62.5 mg clavulanic acid; 400 mg amoxicillin trihydrate, 57 mg clavulanic acid

Pharmacodynamics
Antibiotic action: Amoxicillin is bactericidal; it adheres to bacterial penicillin-binding proteins, thus inhibiting bacterial cell wall synthesis.

Clavulanate has only weak antibacterial activity and doesn't affect mechanism of action of amoxicillin. However, clavulanic acid has a beta-lactam ring and is structurally similar to penicillin and cephalosporins; it binds irreversibly with certain beta-lactamases and prevents them from inactivating amoxicillin, enhancing its bactericidal activity.

This combination acts against penicillinase- and non-penicillinase-producing gram-positive bacteria, *Neisseria gonorrhoeae, Neisseria meningitidis, Haemophilus influenzae, Moraxella catarrhalis, Escherichia coli, Proteus mirabilis, Citrobacter diversus, Klebsiella pneumoniae, Proteus vulgaris, Salmonella,* and *Shigella, Clostridium, Peptococcus,* and *Peptostreptococcus.*

Pharmacokinetics
Absorption: Well absorbed after oral administration.
Distribution: Distributed into pleural fluid, lungs, and peritoneal fluid; high urine concentrations are attained. Amoxicillin also is distributed into synovial fluid, liver, prostate, muscle, and gallbladder and penetrates into middle ear effusions, maxillary sinus secretions, tonsils, sputum, and bronchial secretions. Amoxicillin and clavulanate cross the placenta, and low concentrations appear in breast milk. Amoxicillin and clavulanate potassium have minimal protein-binding of 17% to 20% and 22% to 30%, respectively.
Metabolism: Amoxicillin is metabolized only partially. The metabolic fate of clavulanate potassium isn't completely identified, but it appears to undergo extensive metabolism.
Excretion: Amoxicillin is excreted principally in urine by renal tubular secretion and glomerular filtration; drug also appears in breast milk.

Clavulanate potassium is excreted by glomerular filtration. Elimination half-life of amoxicillin in adults is 1 to 1½ hours; it is prolonged to 7½ hours in patients with severe renal impairment. Half-life of clavulanate in adults is about 1 to 1½ hours, prolonged to 4½ hours in patients with severe renal impairment.

Both drugs are removed readily by hemodialysis and minimally removed by peritoneal dialysis.

Route	Onset	Peak	Duration
P.O.	Unknown	1-2½ hr	6-8 hr

Contraindications and precautions
Contraindicated in patients hypersensitive to drug or other penicillins and in those with a previous history of amoxicillin-related cholestatic jaundice or hepatic dysfunction. An oral penicillin shouldn't be used in patients with severe pneumonia, empyema, bacteremia, pericarditis, menin-

gitis, and purulent or septic arthritis. Use with caution in patients with mononucleosis.

Interactions
Drug-drug. *Allopurinol:* Appears to increase the likelihood of rash from both drugs. Avoid use together.

Methotrexate: Large doses of penicillins may interfere with renal tubular secretion of methotrexate, thus delaying elimination and prolonging elevated serum levels of methotrexate. Monitor patient for adverse effects.

Oral contraceptives: Effectiveness of oral contraceptives may be reduced. Advise using alternative barrier method.

Probenecid: Blocks tubular secretion of amoxicillin, raising its serum levels; it has no effect on clavulanate. Avoid use together.

Adverse reactions
CNS: agitation, anxiety, insomnia, confusion, behavioral changes, dizziness.
GI: *nausea,* vomiting, *diarrhea,* indigestion, gastritis, stomatitis, glossitis, black "hairy" tongue, enterocolitis, pseudomembranous colitis.
GU: vaginitis.
Hematologic: anemia, ***thrombocytopenia,*** thrombocytopenic purpura, eosinophilia, ***leukopenia, agranulocytosis.***
Other: ***hypersensitivity reactions*** (erythematous maculopapular rash, urticaria, ***anaphylaxis***), overgrowth of nonsusceptible organisms.

Overdose and treatment
Evidence of overdose includes neuromuscular sensitivity and seizures.

After recent ingestion (4 hours or less), empty the stomach by induced emesis or gastric lavage; follow with activated charcoal to reduce absorption. Amoxicillin/clavulanate potassium can be removed by hemodialysis.

Special considerations
Consider the recommendations relevant to all penicillins as well as the following.
● Amoxicillin/potassium clavulanate alters results of urine glucose tests that use cupric sulfate (Benedict's reagent or Clinitest). Make urine glucose determinations with glucose oxidase methods (Chemstrip uG or Diastix or glucose enzymatic test strip). Positive Coombs' tests have been reported with other clavulanate combinations. Amoxicillin/potassium clavulanate may produce a positive direct antiglobulin test.
● Amoxicillin/clavulanate potassium has been used to treat infections caused by *Eikenella corrodens* or *Pasteurella multocida* and infections caused by anaerobic and mixed aerobic-anaerobic bacterial infections.
⊠ ALERT Both 250-mg and 500-mg film-coated tablets contain the same amount of clavulanic acid (125 mg). Therefore, two 250-mg tablets aren't equivalent to one 500-mg tablet.

● Oral dosage is maximally absorbed from an empty stomach, but food doesn't cause significant impairment of absorption.
● For reconstitution, add specified water in 2 parts and agitate well after each addition.
● Suspension is stable for 10 days in refrigerator after reconstitution.
● Because amoxicillin/clavulanate potassium is dialyzable, patients undergoing hemodialysis may need dosage adjustments.

Patient monitoring
● Monitor renal, hepatic, and hematologic function periodically.
● Test for *Clostridium difficile* in patients with diarrhea.

Pregnant patients
● There are no adequate and controlled studies of use of this drug in pregnant women. Use in pregnant women only if clearly needed.

Breast-feeding patients
● Both amoxicillin and potassium clavulanate appear in breast milk; use cautiously in breast-feeding women.

Pediatric patients
● Commercial products that contain aspartame shouldn't be used in children with phenylketonuria.

Geriatric patients
● In geriatric patients, diminished renal tubular secretion may prolong half-life of amoxicillin.

Patient education
● Tell patient to chew chewable tablets thoroughly or crush before swallowing and wash down with liquid to ensure adequate absorption of drug; capsule may be emptied and contents swallowed with water.
● Instruct patient to report diarrhea promptly.
● Inform patient to complete full course of medication.

amoxicillin trihydrate
Amoxil, Polymox, Trimox, Wymox

Pharmacologic classification: aminopenicillin
Therapeutic classification: antibiotic
Pregnancy risk category: B

Indications and dosages
➤ *Systemic infections, acute and chronic urinary or respiratory tract infections caused by susceptible organisms, uncomplicated urinary tract infections caused by susceptible organisms. Adults:* 250 mg P.O. q 8 hours or 500 mg q 12 hours. In adults who have severe infections or those caused by susceptible organisms, 500 mg q 8 hours or 875 mg q 12 hours may be needed.

Children: 20 to 40 mg/kg P.O. daily, divided into doses given q 8 hours.

Neonates and infants up to 12 weeks: 30 mg/kg P.O. daily in divided doses q 12 hours.

Pediatric drops

Children who weigh less than 6 kg (13 lb): 0.75 ml q 8 hours.

Children who weigh 6 to 7 kg (13 to 15 lb): 1 ml q 8 hours.

Children who weigh 7 to 8 kg (16 to 18 lb): 1.25 ml q 8 hours.

Children with lower respiratory tract infection who weigh less than 6 kg: 1.25 ml q 8 hours.

Children with lower respiratory tract infection who weigh 6 to 7 kg: 1.75 ml q 8 hours.

Children with lower respiratory tract infection who weigh 7 to 8 kg: 2.25 ml q 8 hours.

➤ *Uncomplicated gonorrhea. Adults:* 3 g P.O. as a single dose.

Children over age 2: 50 mg/kg given with 25 mg/kg probenecid as a single dose.

➤ *Chlamydial and mycoplasmal infections during pregnancy. Adults:* 500 mg P.O. t.i.d. for 7 to 10 days.

➤ *Lyme disease* ◇. *Adults:* 250 to 500 mg P.O. t.i.d. to q.i.d. for 10 to 30 days.

Children: 25 to 50 mg/kg daily (maximum 1 to 2 g daily) P.O. in three divided doses for 10 to 30 days.

➤ *Acute uncomplicated urinary tract infection in nonpregnant women* ◇. 3 g P.O. as a single dose.

✦ *Dosage adjustment.* In renal failure, patients who require repeated doses may need adjustment of dosing interval. If creatinine clearance is 10 to 30 ml/minute, increase interval to q 12 hours; if creatinine clearance is less than 10 ml/minute, administer q 24 hours. Supplemental doses may be necessary after hemodialysis. Don't administer 875-mg tablet if creatinine clearance is below 30 ml/minute.

➤ *Oral prophylaxis of bacterial endocarditis.* Consult current American Heart Association recommendations before administering drug. *Adults:* 2 g 1 hour before procedure. *Children:* 50 mg/kg 1 hour before procedure.

How supplied

Available by prescription only

Capsules: 250 mg, 500 mg

Pediatric drops: 50 mg/ml (after reconstitution)

Suspension: 125 mg/5 ml, 200 mg/5 ml, 250 mg/5 ml, 400 mg/5 ml

Tablets (chewable): 125 mg, 200 mg, 250 mg, 400 mg

Tablets (film-coated): 500 mg, 875 mg

Pharmacodynamics

Antibacterial action: Amoxicillin is bactericidal; it adheres to bacterial penicillin-binding proteins, thus inhibiting bacterial cell wall synthesis. Spectrum of action of amoxicillin includes non-penicillinase-producing gram-positive bacteria, *Streptococcus* group B, *Neisseria gonor-*rhoeae, *Proteus mirabilis, Salmonella,* and *Haemophilus influenzae.* It's also effective against non-penicillinase-producing *Staphylococcus aureus, Streptococcus pyogenes, Streptococcus bovis, Streptococcus pneumoniae, Streptococcus viridans, N. meningitidis, Escherichia coli, Salmonella typhi, Bordetella pertussis, Peptococcus,* and *Peptostreptococcus.*

Pharmacokinetics

Absorption: About 80% absorbed after oral administration.

Distribution: Distributed into pleural peritoneal and synovial fluids and into the lungs, prostate, muscle, liver, and gallbladder; it also penetrates middle ear, maxillary sinus and bronchial secretions, tonsils, and sputum. Amoxicillin readily crosses the placenta; about 17% to 20% is protein-bound.

Metabolism: Metabolized only partially.

Excretion: Excreted mainly in urine by renal tubular secretion and glomerular filtration; also excreted in breast milk. Elimination half-life in adults is about 1 to 1¼ hours; severe renal impairment increases half-life to 7¼ hours.

Route	Onset	Peak	Duration
P.O.	Unknown	1-2 hr	6-8 hr

Contraindications and precautions

Contraindicated in patients hypersensitive to drug or other penicillins. Use cautiously in patients with mononucleosis.

Interactions

Drug-drug. *Allopurinol:* Increased risk of rash from both drugs. Monitor patient.

Methotrexate: Large doses of penicillins may interfere with renal tubular secretion of methotrexate, thus delaying elimination and prolonging elevated serum levels of methotrexate. Monitor patient for toxicity.

Oral contraceptives: Effectiveness of oral contraceptives may be decreased. Advise a barrier method of contraception.

Probenecid: Blocks renal tubular secretion of amoxicillin, raising its serum concentrations. Probenecid may be used for this purpose.

Drug-herb. *Khat:* Antimicrobial effect of certain penicillins may be decreased. Discourage khat chewing, or tell patient to take amoxicillin 2 hours after chewing khat.

Adverse reactions

CNS: lethargy, hallucinations, *seizures,* anxiety, confusion, agitation, depression, dizziness, fatigue.

GI: *nausea,* vomiting, *diarrhea,* glossitis, stomatitis, gastritis, abdominal pain, enterocolitis, pseudomembranous colitis, black "hairy" tongue.

GU: interstitial nephritis, nephropathy, vaginitis.

Hematologic: anemia, *thrombocytopenia,* thrombocytopenic purpura, eosinophilia, *leukopenia, hemolytic anemia, agranulocytosis.*

Other: *hypersensitivity reactions* (erythematous maculopapular rash, urticaria, *anaphylaxis*), overgrowth of nonsusceptible organisms.

Overdose and treatment
Overdose may cause neuromuscular sensitivity or seizures. After recent ingestion (4 hours or less), empty the stomach by induced emesis or gastric lavage; follow with activated charcoal to reduce absorption. Drug can be removed by hemodialysis.

Special considerations
Consider the recommendations relevant to all penicillins as well as the following.
• Amoxicillin may alter results of urine glucose tests that use cupric sulfate (Benedict's reagent or Clinitest). Make urine glucose determinations with glucose oxidase methods (Chemstrip uG, Diastix, or glucose enzymatic test strip).
• 200-mg and 400-mg chewable Amoxil tablets contain aspartame and shouldn't be given to patients with phenylketonuria.
• Oral dosage is maximally absorbed from an empty stomach, but food doesn't cause significant loss of potency.
• Suspension and drops are stable for 14 days in refrigerator after reconstitution.
• Amoxicillin may cause less diarrhea than ampicillin.

Patient monitoring
• Monitor renal, hepatic, and hematologic tests if patient receives prolonged therapy.

Pregnant patients
• There are no adequate controlled studies in pregnant women, but drug has been used effectively without evidence of adverse effects.

Breast-feeding patients
• Drug is distributed readily into breast milk; safe use in breast-feeding women hasn't been established. Recommend an alternative feeding method during therapy.

Pediatric patients
• Pediatric drops may be placed on child's tongue or added to formula, milk, fruit juice, or soft drink. Make sure child ingests all of prepared dose.

Geriatric patients
• Because of diminished renal tubular secretion, half-life may be prolonged in geriatric patients.

Patient education
• Tell patient to chew chewable tablets thoroughly or crush before swallowing and wash down with liquid to ensure adequate absorption of drug; capsule may be emptied and contents swallowed with water.
• Tell patient to report diarrhea promptly.

• Instruct patient to complete full course of medication.

amphetamine sulfate
Pharmacologic classification: amphetamine
Therapeutic classification: CNS stimulant, short-term adjunctive anorexigenic, sympathomimetic amine
Controlled substance schedule: II
Pregnancy risk category: C

Indications and dosages
➤ *Attention deficit disorder with hyperactivity.* *Children age 6 and older:* 5 mg P.O. daily. Increase at 5-mg increments weekly until desired response. Dosage rarely exceeds 40 mg daily. Give first dose upon awakening; give additional doses at 4- to 6-hour intervals.
Children ages 3 to 5: 2.5 mg P.O. daily. Increased at 2.5-mg increments weekly until desired response is achieved.
➤ *Narcolepsy.* *Adults:* 5 to 60 mg P.O. daily in divided doses or a single dose.
Children over age 12: 10 mg P.O. daily, increased by 10-mg increments weekly, p.r.n.
Children ages 6 to 12: 5 mg P.O. daily, increased by 5-mg increments weekly, p.r.n.
➤ *Short-term adjunct in exogenous obesity.* *Adults:* 5 to 30 mg daily in divided doses of 5 to 10 mg.

How supplied
Available by prescription only
Tablets: 5 mg, 10 mg

Pharmacodynamics
CNS stimulant action: Amphetamines are sympathomimetic amines with CNS stimulant activity; in hyperactive children, they have a paradoxical calming effect. Amphetamines are used to treat narcolepsy and as adjuncts to psychosocial measures in attention deficit disorder in children. The cerebral cortex and reticular activating system appear to be their primary sites of activity; amphetamines release nerve terminal stores of norepinephrine, promoting nerve impulse transmission. At high doses, effects are mediated by dopamine.
Anorexigenic action: Anorexigenic effects are thought to occur in the hypothalamus, where decreased smell and taste acuity decreases the appetite. Amphetamines may be tried for short-term control of refractory obesity, with caloric restriction and behavior modification.

Pharmacokinetics
Absorption: Absorbed completely within 3 hours after oral administration; therapeutic effects persist for 4 to 24 hours.
Distribution: Distributed widely throughout body, with high concentrations in the brain. Therapeutic plasma levels are 5 to 10 mcg/dl.
Metabolism: Metabolized by hydroxylation and deamination in the liver.

Reactions may be *common*, uncommon, *life-threatening*, or COMMON AND LIFE-THREATENING.

Excretion: Excreted in urine.

Route	Onset	Peak	Duration
P.O.	Unknown	Unknown	4–24 hr

Contraindications and precautions

Contraindicated in agitated patients, patients who have taken an MAO inhibitor within 14 days, patients hypersensitive to sympathomimetic amines, patients with idiosyncratic reactions to sympathomimetic amines, and patients with symptomatic CV disease, hyperthyroidism, moderate to severe hypertension, glaucoma, advanced arteriosclerosis, or a history of drug abuse.

Use cautiously in geriatric, debilitated, or hyperexcitable patients or in those with suicidal or homicidal tendencies.

Interactions

Drug-drug. *Acetazolamide, antacids, sodium bicarbonate:* May enhance reabsorption of amphetamine and prolong its duration of action. Monitor patient for clinical effect.

Ammonium chloride, ascorbic acid: Enhanced amphetamine excretion and shortened duration of action. Monitor patient for clinical effect.

Antihypertensives: May antagonize hypertensive effects. Avoid use together.

Barbiturates: Counteract amphetamine by CNS depression; other CNS stimulants produce additive effects. Avoid use together.

Guanethidine: Amphetamines may decrease the effectiveness of guanethidine. Monitor patient for clinical effect.

Haloperidol, phenothiazines: Decreased amphetamine effects. Monitor patient for clinical effect.

Insulin: Amphetamines may alter insulin requirements. Monitor blood glucose levels.

MAO inhibitors (or drugs with MAO-inhibiting effects, such as furazolidone) or within 14 days of such therapy: May cause hypertensive crisis. Avoid use together.

Drug-food. *Caffeine:* Produces additive effects. Tell patient to avoid use together.

Adverse reactions

CNS: *restlessness,* tremor, *hyperactivity, talkativeness, insomnia,* irritability, dizziness, headache, chills, dysphoria, euphoria.

CV: *tachycardia, palpitations,* hypertension, **arrhythmias.**

GI: dry mouth, metallic taste, diarrhea, constipation, anorexia, weight loss.

GU: impotence.

Metabolic: elevated plasma corticosteroid levels.

Skin: urticaria.

Other: altered libido.

Overdose and treatment

Signs and symptoms of acute overdose include increasing restlessness, irritability, insomnia, tremor, hyperreflexia, diaphoresis, mydriasis, flushing, confusion, hypertension, tachypnea, fever, delirium, self-injury, arrhythmias, seizures, coma, circulatory collapse, and death.

Treat overdose symptomatically and supportively: If ingestion is recent (within 4 hours) use gastric lavage or emesis; activated charcoal and urinary acidification may enhance excretion. Forced fluid diuresis may help. In massive ingestion, hemodialysis or peritoneal dialysis may be needed. Keep patient in a cool room, monitor temperature, and minimize external stimulation. Haloperidol may be used for psychotic symptoms; diazepam, for hyperactivity.

Special considerations

● Amphetamines may interfere with urinary steroid determinations.

● Avoid administration late in the day (after 4 p.m.) to prevent insomnia.

● Amphetamine capsules shouldn't be used for initial or subsequent titration of dosage; however, once dosage has been established, capsules can be substituted if once-daily dosing is required.

● If therapy is prolonged, don't withdraw suddenly.

Patient monitoring

● Watch for adverse cardiac effects in susceptible patients.

● Monitor the patient's diet and calorie count when drug is used as an adjunct to weight reduction.

Pregnant patients

● Drug shouldn't be used during pregnancy, especially during first trimester.

Pediatric patients

● Amphetamines aren't recommended for weight reduction in children under age 12.

● Use of amphetamines for hyperactivity is contraindicated in children under age 3.

Patient education

● Instruct patient about the potential for drowsiness; recommend avoiding activities such as driving that require alertness.

● Tell patient to report signs of excessive stimulation.

● Warn patient with seizure disorder that drug may decrease seizure threshold. Instruct patient to notify prescriber if seizure occurs.

amphotericin B
Amphocin, Fungizone

Pharmacologic classification: polyene antibiotic
Therapeutic classification: antifungal
Pregnancy risk category: B

Indications and dosages

➤ *Systemic (potentially fatal) fungal infections caused by susceptible organisms,*

---

fungal endocarditis, fungal septicemia.
Adults and children: Some clinicians recommend an initial dose of 1 mg I.V. in 20 ml D₅W infused over 20 minutes. If test dose is tolerated, then give daily doses of 0.25 to 0.30 mg/kg, gradually increasing by 5 to 10 mg daily until daily dose is 1 mg/kg or 1.5 mg/kg q alternate day. Duration of therapy depends on the severity and nature of infection.

For sporotrichosis, give 0.4 to 0.5 mg/kg amphotericin B daily I.V. for up to 9 months. Total I.V. dosage of 2.5 g over 9 months.

For aspergillosis, give 0.5 to 0.6 mg/kg daily initially and a total I.V. dosage of 1.5 to 4 g over 11 months.

➤ *Fungal meningitis* ◇. *Adults:* Intrathecal injection of 25 mcg/0.1 ml diluted with 10 to 20 ml of CSF and administered by barbotage two or three times weekly. Initial dose shouldn't exceed 50 mcg.

➤ *Candidal cystitis* ◇. *Adults:* Bladder irrigations in concentrations of 5 to 50 mcg/ml instilled periodically or continuously for 5 to 7 days.

➤ *Oropharyngeal candidiasis. Adults and children:* 100 mg/ml oral suspension q.i.d. swish and swallow.

➤ *Topical fungal infections (3% cream, lotion, ointment). Adults and children:* Apply liberally and rub well into affected area b.i.d. to q.i.d.

➤ *Cutaneous or mucocutaneous candidal infections. Adults and children:* Apply topical product b.i.d., t.i.d., or q.i.d. for 1 to 3 weeks; apply up to several months for interdigital or paronychial lesions.

➤ *Sinus irrigation. Adults:* 1 mg/ml

➤ *Histoplasmal pulmonary and intrapleural effusion* ◇. *Adults:* 15 to 20 mg with 25 mg hydrocortisone sodium succinate.

➤ *Pulmonary coccidioidomycosis* ◇. *Adults:* Via intermittent positive pressure breathing device, 5 to 10 mg q.i.d.

➤ *Ophthalmic candidal infection* ◇. *Adults:* 0.1 to 1 mg/ml drop suspension q 30 minutes.

➤ *Empiric therapy of presumed fungal infections in febrile, neutropenic patients including cancer patients and bone marrow transplant or solid organ transplant recipients. Adults:* 0.8 mg/kg daily for 8 days.

How supplied
Available by prescription only
Cream: 3%
Lotion: 3%
Ointment: 3%
Oral suspension: 100 mg/ml
Powder for injection: 50 mg

Pharmacodynamics
Antifungal action: Amphotericin B is fungistatic or fungicidal, depending on the concentrations available in body fluids and on the susceptibility of the fungus. It binds to sterols in the fungal cell membrane, increasing membrane permeability of fungal cells, causing subsequent leakage of intracellular components; it also may interfere with some human cell membranes that contain sterols.

Spectrum of activity includes *Histoplasma capsulatum, Coccidioides immitis, Blastomyces dermatitidis, Cryptococcus neoformans, Candida* species, *Aspergillus fumigatus, Mucor* species, *Rhizopus* species, *Absidia* species, *Entomophthora* species, *Basidiobolus* species, *Paracoccidioides brasiliensis, Sporothrix schenckii,* and *Rhodotorula* species.

Pharmacokinetics
Absorption: Absorbed poorly from the GI tract.
Distribution: Distributed well into inflamed pleural cavities and joints; in low levels into aqueous humor, bronchial secretions, pancreas, bone, muscle, and parotids. CSF levels reach about 3% of serum levels. Drug is 90% to 95% bound to plasma proteins; it reportedly crosses the placenta.
Metabolism: Not well defined.
Excretion: Elimination is biphasic: initial serum half-life of 24 hours, followed by a second phase half-life of about 15 days. About 2% to 5% of drug is excreted unchanged in urine. Amphotericin B isn't readily removed by hemodialysis.

Route	Onset	Peak	Duration
P.O.	Unknown	Unknown	Unknown
I.V.	Immediate	Unknown	Unknown
Topical	Unknown	Unknown	Unknown

Contraindications and precautions
Contraindicated in patients hypersensitive to drug. Use cautiously in patients with renal impairment.

Interactions
Drug-drug. *Aminoglycosides, cisplatin, pentamidine, and other nephrotoxic drugs:* Added nephrotoxic effects. Avoid use together.
Clotrimazole, fluconazole, itraconazole, ketoconazole, miconazole: May antagonize amphotericin B. Monitor patient closely.
Corticosteroids, corticotropin: Electrolyte imbalances. Requires careful monitoring of serum electrolyte levels and cardiac function.
Digoxin: Increased risk of digitalis toxicity. Monitor serum digoxin level if drugs are used together.
Flucytosine and other antibiotics: Potentiated effects. Use together cautiously.
Skeletal muscle relaxants: Amphotericin B–induced hypokalemia may enhance effects of skeletal muscle relaxants. Use together cautiously.
Zidovudine: Increased myelotoxicity and nephrotoxicity. Monitor renal and hematologic function.
Drug-herb. *Gossypol:* May increase risk of renal toxicity. Discourage use together.

Adverse reactions
CNS: *malaise, headache,* peripheral neuropathy, *seizures* (with systemic form).

Reactions may be *common*, uncommon, *life-threatening*, or COMMON AND LIFE-THREATENING.

CV: *phlebitis, thrombophlebitis,* flushing, hypotension, **arrhythmias, asystole,** hypertension (with systemic form).

EENT: hearing loss, tinnitus, transient vertigo, blurred vision, diplopia (with systemic form).

GI: *anorexia, weight loss, nausea, vomiting, dyspepsia, diarrhea, epigastric pain, cramping,* melena, **hemorrhagic gastroenteritis** (with systemic form).

GU: *abnormal renal function with hypokalemia, azotemia, hyposthenuria, renal tubular acidosis, nephrocalcinosis;* with large doses, **permanent renal impairment,** anuria, oliguria (with systemic form).

Hematologic: *normochromic, normocytic anemia,* **thrombocytopenia, leukopenia, agranulocytosis,** eosinophilia, leukocytosis (with systemic form).

Hepatic: increased alkaline phosphatase and bilirubin levels, **hepatitis,** jaundice, **acute liver failure** (with systemic form).

Metabolic: hypokalemia and hypomagnesemia.

Musculoskeletal: arthralgia, myalgia.

Respiratory: dyspnea, tachypnea, **bronchospasm,** wheezing (with systemic form).

Skin: maculopapular rash, pruritus without rash (with systemic form); dryness, contact sensitivity, erythema, burning, pruritus (with topical administration).

Other: tissue damage with extravasation, *pain at injection site, fever, chills, generalized pain,* **anaphylactoid reactions** (with topical administration).

Overdose and treatment

Overdose may affect CV and respiratory function. Treatment is largely supportive. Hemodialysis isn't effective. Correction of electrolyte imbalances is usually necessary.

Special considerations

🔰 **ALERT** Amphotericin B preparations aren't interchangeable and dosages will vary.

● Cultures and histologic and sensitivity testing must be completed and diagnosis confirmed before starting therapy in nonimmunocompromised patient.

● Prepare infusion as manufacturer directs, with strict aseptic technique, using only 10 ml of sterile water to reconstitute. To avoid precipitation, don't mix with solutions containing sodium chloride, other electrolytes, or bacteriostatic agents such as benzyl alcohol.

● Don't use if reconstituted solution contains a precipitate or other foreign particles. Store the dry form at 36° to 46° F (2° to 8° C). Protect drug from light, and check expiration date.

● For I.V. infusion, use an in-line membrane with a mean pore diameter larger than 1 micron.

● Infuse slowly; rapid infusion may cause CV collapse.

● Don't mix or piggyback antibiotics with amphotericin B infusion; the I.V. solution appears compatible with small amounts of heparin sodium, hydrocortisone sodium succinate, and methylprednisolone sodium succinate.

● Severity of some adverse reactions can be reduced by premedication with aspirin or acetaminophen, antihistamines, antiemetics, meperidine, or small doses of corticosteroids; by addition of phosphate buffer to the solution; and by alternate-day dosing. If reactions are severe, drug may have to be discontinued for varying periods.

● Use topical products for folds of groin, neck, or armpit; avoid occlusive dressing with ointment, and discontinue if signs of hypersensitivity develop.

● Store at room temperature. Solution is stable at room temperature and in indoor light for 24 hours or in the refrigerator for 1 week.

● Intrathecal and intra-articular uses are unapproved.

Patient monitoring

● Give drug in distal veins, and monitor site for discomfort or thrombosis; if thrombosis occurs, consider alternate-day therapy.

● Check vital signs every 30 minutes for at least 4 hours after start of I.V. infusion; fever may appear in 1 to 2 hours but should subside within 4 hours of discontinuing drug.

● Watch for first-dose acute infusion reactions, which include fever, chills, hypotension, nausea, vomiting, headache, dyspnea, and tachycardia. Reaction may occur in 1 to 3 hours.

● Monitor intake and output, and check for changes in urine appearance or volume; renal damage may be reversible if drug is stopped at earliest sign of dysfunction.

● Monitor potassium and magnesium levels closely. Monitor calcium and magnesium levels twice weekly. Perform liver and renal function studies and CBC regularly (usually twice weekly).

Pregnant patients

● Safety during pregnancy hasn't been established, but the drug has been used without obvious adverse effects to the fetus.

Breast-feeding patients

● Safety hasn't been established in breast-feeding women.

Patient education

● Teach patient signs and symptoms of hypersensitivity and other adverse reactions, especially those that occur with I.V. therapy. Warn that fever and chills are likely to occur and can be severe when therapy begins. These symptoms usually subside with repeated doses. Encourage patient feedback during infusion.

● Warn patient that therapy may take several months; recommend personal hygiene and other measures to prevent spread and recurrence of lesions.

● Urge patient to adhere to regimen and to return, as instructed, for follow-up.

• Tell patient that topical products may stain skin and clothing; cream or lotion may be removed from clothing with soap and water.

---

amphotericin B cholesteryl sulfate complex
Amphotec

Pharmacologic classification: polyene antibiotic
Therapeutic classification: antifungal
Pregnancy risk category: B

Indications and dosages
➤ *Invasive aspergillosis in patients in whom renal impairment or unacceptable toxicity precludes use of conventional amphotericin B in effective doses and in those with invasive aspergillosis in whom prior amphotericin B therapy has failed;* Candida *and* Cryptococcus *infections unresponsive or tolerable to conventional amphotericin B* ◊. *Adults and children:* 3 to 4 mg/kg I.V. daily; may increase to 6 mg/kg daily if no improvement occurs or if fungal infection has progressed. Administer by continuous infusion at 1 mg/kg/hour. Perform a test dose before commencing new courses of treatment; infuse a small amount of drug (10 ml of final preparation containing 1.6 to 8.3 mg of drug) over 15 to 30 minutes and monitor patient for next 30 minutes.
➤ *Empiric therapy of presumed fungal infections in febrile, neutropenic patients including cancer patients and bone marrow transplant (BMT) or solid organ transplant recipients* ◊. *Adults:* 4 mg/kg I.V. daily for 8 days. Dosages up to 7.5 mg/kg have been used to treat invasive fungal infections in BMT patients.

How supplied
Available by prescription only
Injection: 50 mg/20 ml, 100 mg/50 ml

Pharmacodynamics
Fungistatic and fungicidal actions: Depend on concentration of drug and susceptibility of fungal organism. Drug binds to sterols in cell membranes of sensitive fungi, resulting in leakage of intracellular contents and causing cell death due to changes in membrane permeability. Also binds to sterols in mammalian cell membranes, which is believed to account for human toxicity. Spectrum of activity includes *Aspergillus fumigatus, Candida albicans, Coccidioides immitis,* and *Cryptococcus neoformans.*

Pharmacokinetics
Absorption: For an infusion of 1 mg/kg/hour and dosage ranges from 3 to 6 mg/kg daily, maximum plasma level at the end of an infusion ranges from 2.6 to 3.4 mcg/ml.

Distribution: Multicompartmental; steady-state volume increases with higher doses, possibly from uptake by tissues.
Metabolism: Unknown.
Excretion: Unclear; elimination half-life, 27 to 29 hours; increasing doses increase the elimination half-life. Drug may not be removed by dialysis.

Route	Onset	Peak	Duration
I.V.	Unknown	3 hr	Unknown

Contraindications and precautions
Contraindicated in patients hypersensitive to any component of drug unless the benefits outweigh the risk of hypersensitivity.

Interactions
No formal drug interaction studies have been done. However, the following drugs are known to interact with amphotericin B.
Drug-drug. *Antineoplastics:* Enhanced renal toxicity, bronchospasm, hypotension. Avoid use together.
Cardiac glycosides: Enhanced potassium excretion, which increases risk of digitalis toxicity. Monitor serum digoxin levels.
Corticosteroids, corticotropin: Enhanced potassium depletion, which could predispose patient to cardiac dysfunction. Monitor patient closely.
Cyclosporine, tacrolimus: May increase serum creatinine levels. Monitor serum creatinine levels.
Flucytosine: May cause synergistic effect and cause increased toxicity of flucytosine. Avoid use together.
Imidazoles (clotrimazole, fluconazole, ketoconazole, miconazole): May cause antagonistic effects. Monitor patient for adverse effects.
Nephrotoxic drugs (such as aminoglycosides, pentamidine): May enhance renal toxicity. Monitor renal function closely.
Skeletal muscle relaxants (such as tubocurarine): Amphotericin B-induced hypokalemia may enhance curariform effects of skeletal muscle relaxants due to hypokalemia. Use together cautiously.
Zidovudine: Increased myelotoxicity and nephrotoxicity. Monitor renal and hematologic function.
Drug-herb. *Gossypol:* Increased risk of renal toxicity. Discourage use together.

Adverse reactions
CNS: abnormal thoughts, anxiety, agitation, confusion, depression, dizziness, hallucinations, headache, hypertonia, neuropathy, paresthesia, *seizures,* somnolence, stupor, syncope, asthenia.
CV: *arrhythmias, atrial fibrillation, bradycardia, cardiac arrest, heart failure, hemorrhage,* hypertension, *hypotension,* edema, phlebitis, orthostatic hypotension, *shock, supraventricular tachycardia,* tachycardia, *ventricular extrasystoles.*

Reactions may be *common*, uncommon, *life-threatening*, or COMMON AND LIFE-THREATENING.

EENT: epistaxis, eye hemorrhage, tinnitus, mucous membrane disorder.
GI: anorexia, GI disorder, *GI hemorrhage,* hematemesis, melena, *nausea,* stomatitis, *vomiting.*
GU: *increased creatinine level,* abnormal renal function, increased BUN levels, hematuria, *renal failure.*
Hematologic: anemia, *agranulocytosis,* coagulation disorders, hypochromic anemia, increased PT, leukocytosis, *leukopenia, thrombocytopenia.*
Hepatic: *bilirubinemia;* jaundice; abnormal liver function test results; *hepatic failure;* increased alkaline phosphatase, AST, ALT, and LD levels.
Metabolic: *hypokalemia,* hypocalcemia, hyperglycemia, hypervolemia, hypophosphatemia, hyponatremia, hyperkalemia, hypomagnesemia,.
Musculoskeletal: arthralgia, myalgia, pain in abdomen, chest, or back.
Respiratory: *apnea,* asthma, dyspnea, hemoptysis, hyperventilation, hypoxia, increased cough, lung or respiratory disorders, *pulmonary edema.*
Skin: pruritus, rash, sweating, skin disorder.
Other: *allergic reaction, anaphylaxis, chills, fever,* peripheral or facial edema, infection, pain or reaction at injection site, *sepsis.*

Overdose and treatment
Amphotec isn't dialyzable. Amphotericin B overdose has been reported to result in cardiorespiratory arrest. If overdose is suspected, discontinue therapy, monitor clinical status, and administer supportive therapy.

Special considerations
● Pretreatment with antihistamines and corticosteroids or slowing the infusion (or both) may reduce acute infusion-related reactions.
◼ ALERT Amphotericin B products aren't interchangeable.
● Dilute in D₅W and administer by continuous infusion at 1 mg/kg/hour. If drug is well tolerated, can shorten infusion time to 2 hours or lengthen infusion time based on patient tolerance.
● Drug is incompatible with saline solution, electrolyte solutions, and bacteriostatic agents.
● Infuse drug over at least 2 hours.
● Don't mix with other drugs. If administered through an existing I.V. line, flush line with D₅W before infusion or use a separate line.
● Store vials at room temperature. Reconstitute 50-mg vial with rapid addition of 10 ml of sterile water for injection, and 100-mg vial with rapid addition of 20 ml sterile water with a sterile syringe and 20G needle. Shake vial gently. Don't use diluent other than sterile water for injection.
● Reconstituted drug is clear or opalescent liquid and is stable for 24 hours refrigerated. Discard partially used vials.
● Don't filter or use an in-line filter and don't freeze.

Patient monitoring
● Monitor vital signs every 30 minutes during initial therapy. Acute infusion-related reactions (fever, chills, hypotension, nausea, tachycardia) usually occur 1 to 3 hours after starting I.V. infusion. These reactions are usually more severe after initial doses and usually diminish with subsequent doses. If severe respiratory distress occurs, stop infusion immediately and don't treat further with drug.
● Monitor intake and output, and note changes in urine appearance or volume.
● Monitor renal and hepatic function tests, serum electrolytes (especially potassium, magnesium, and calcium), CBCs, and PT and INR.

Pregnant patients
● Safe use during pregnancy hasn't been established, but the drug has been used without obvious adverse effects to the fetus.

Breast-feeding patients
● It's unknown if drug appears in breast milk. Because of the potential for serious adverse reactions in breast-fed infants, a decision should be made to discontinue breast-feeding or to stop treatment, taking into account the importance of drug to the woman.

Pediatric patients
● No unexpected adverse events have been reported.

Geriatric patients
● No unexpected adverse events have been reported.

Patient education
● Instruct patient to report symptoms of hypersensitivity immediately.
● Warn patient of possible discomfort at I.V. site.
● Advise patient of potential adverse effects, such as fever, chills, nausea, and vomiting. Tell him that these can be severe with initial treatment but usually subside with repeated doses.

amphotericin B lipid complex
Abelcet

Pharmacologic classification: polyene antibiotic
Therapeutic classification: antifungal
Pregnancy risk category: B

Indications and dosages
➤ *Invasive fungal infections, including* Aspergillus sp. *and* Candida sp., *in patients who are refractory to or intolerant of conventional amphotericin B therapy.* *Adults and children:* 5 mg/kg daily I.V. as a single infusion administered at 2.5 mg/kg/hour.

How supplied
Available by prescription only
Suspension for injection: 100 mg/20-ml vial

Pharmacodynamics
Antifungal activity: The active component of Abelcet, amphotericin B, binds to sterols in fungal cell membranes, resulting in enhanced cellular permeability and cell damage. Amphotericin B has fungistatic or fungicidal effects depending on fungal susceptibility.

Pharmacokinetics
Absorption: Administered I.V.
Distribution: Well distributed. The distribution volume increases with increasing dose. Abelcet yields measurable amphotericin B levels in spleen, lungs, liver, lymph nodes, kidneys, heart, and brain.
Metabolism: Unknown.
Excretion: Although rapidly cleared from blood, Abelcet has a long terminal half-life (173 hr), probably due to slow elimination from tissues.

Route	Onset	Peak	Duration
I.V.	Unknown	Unknown	Unknown

Contraindications and precautions
Contraindicated in patients hypersensitive to amphotericin B or its components. Use cautiously in patients with renal impairment.

Interactions
Drug-drug. *Antineoplastics:* Increased risk of renal toxicity, bronchospasm, and hypotension. Use cautiously.
Cardiac glycosides: Increased risk of digitalis toxicity from amphotericin B-induced hypokalemia. Monitor serum potassium levels closely.
Clotrimazole, fluconazole, itraconazole, ketoconazole, miconazole: May antagonize amphotericin B. Monitor patient closely.
Corticosteroids, corticotropin: Enhanced hypokalemia, which may lead to cardiac toxicity. Monitor serum electrolyte levels and cardiac function.
Cyclosporine: Increased renal toxicity. Monitor patient closely.
Flucytosine: Increased risk of flucytosine toxicity from increased cellular uptake or impaired renal excretion. Use cautiously.
Nephrotoxic drugs (such as aminoglycosides, pentamidine): Increased risk of renal toxicity. Use cautiously. Monitor renal function closely.
Skeletal muscle relaxants: Enhanced effects of skeletal muscle relaxants resulting from amphotericin B-induced hypokalemia. Monitor serum potassium levels closely.
Zidovudine: Increased myelotoxicity and nephrotoxicity. Monitor renal and hematologic function.

Adverse reactions
CNS: headache, pain.
CV: chest pain, *cardiac arrest*, hypertension, hypotension.
GI: abdominal pain, diarrhea, *GI hemorrhage*, nausea, vomiting.
GU: *increased serum creatinine level, kidney failure*.
Hematologic: anemia, *leukopenia, thrombocytopenia*.
Hepatic: bilirubinemia.
Metabolic: hypokalemia.
Respiratory: dyspnea, respiratory disorder, *respiratory failure*.
Skin: rash.
Other: *chills, fever*, infection, MULTIPLE ORGAN FAILURE, *sepsis*.

Overdose and treatment
Overdose may raise the risk of cardiorespiratory arrest. Doses as high as 7 to 13 mg/kg haven't produced serious acute toxicity. If overdose is suspected, discontinue therapy, monitor patient's condition, and provide supportive treatment as needed. Drug isn't removed by hemodialysis.

Special considerations
⚡ **ALERT** Amphotericin B preparations aren't interchangeable and dosages will vary.
• Premedication with acetaminophen, antihistamines, and corticosteroids can prevent or lessen severity of infusion-related reactions, such as fever, chills, nausea, and vomiting, which occur 1 to 2 hours after start of infusion.
• If severe respiratory distress occurs, discontinue infusion, provide supportive therapy for anaphylaxis, and notify prescriber. Drug shouldn't be reinstituted in this situation.
• Leukocyte transfusions shouldn't be given with drug because acute pulmonary toxicity has been reported with concurrent administration.
• To prepare, shake vial gently until there's no yellow sediment. Using aseptic technique, withdraw calculated dose into one or more 20-ml syringes, using an 18-gauge needle. More than one vial will be required. Attach a 5-micron filter needle to the syringe and inject the dose into an I.V. bag of D₅W. One filter needle can be used for up to four vials of amphotericin B lipid complex. The volume of D₅W should be sufficient to yield a final concentration of 1 mg/ml.
• Drug has an unlabeled use for empiric therapy in febrile neutropenic patients.
• For children and patients with CV disease, recommended final concentration is 2 mg/ml.
• Don't mix with saline solution or infuse in same I.V. line as other drugs. Don't use an in-line filter.
• Discard any unused drug; it doesn't contain a preservative.
• Use an infusion pump and administer by continuous infusion at 2.5 mg/kg/hour. If infusion time exceeds 2 hours, mix contents by shaking infusion bag every 2 hours.
• If infusing through an existing I.V. line, flush first with D₅W.

Reactions may be *common*, uncommon, *life-threatening*, or COMMON AND LIFE-THREATENING.

• Infusions are stable for up to 48 hours if refrigerated at 36° to 46° F (2° to 8° C) and up to 6 hours at room temperature.

Patient monitoring
• Take vital signs frequently. Fever, shaking chills, and hypotension may appear within 2 hours after starting infusion. Slowing infusion rate may decrease infusion-related reactions.
• Monitor serum creatinine and electrolyte levels (especially magnesium and potassium), liver function, and CBC during therapy.
• The need for dosage adjustment should be based on the overall clinical status of the patient. Renal toxicity is more common at higher doses.

Breast-feeding patients
• It's unknown if drug appears in breast milk. The decision to administer Abelcet to a nursing woman should be based on the risk of adverse reactions in the infant compared to the benefits of treatment.

Pediatric patients
• No unexpected adverse reactions have been reported in children age 16 or under when given 5 mg/kg daily.

Geriatric patients
• No unexpected adverse reactions have been reported when treated with 5 mg/kg daily.

Patient education
• Inform patient that fever, chills, nausea, and vomiting may occur during infusion and that these reactions usually subside with subsequent doses.
• Instruct patient to report any redness or pain at infusion site.
• Teach patient to recognize and report any symptoms of acute hypersensitivity such as respiratory distress.
• Warn patient that therapy may take several months.
• Tell patient to expect frequent laboratory testing to monitor kidney and liver function.

---

amphotericin B liposomal
AmBisome

Pharmacologic classification: polyene antibiotic
Therapeutic classification: antifungal
Pregnancy risk category: B

Indications and dosages
➤ *Empirical therapy for presumed fungal infection in febrile, neutropenic patients. Adults and children:* 3 mg/kg I.V. infusion daily.
➤ *Systemic fungal infections caused by* Aspergillus *sp.,* Candida *sp., or* Cryptococcus *sp. refractory to amphotericin B or in patients in whom renal impairment or unacceptable toxicity precludes use of amphotericin B. Adults and children:* 3 to 5 mg/kg I.V. infusion daily.
➤ *Visceral leishmaniasis in immunocompetent patients. Adults and children:* 3 mg/kg I.V. infusion daily on days 1 to 5, 14, and 21. A repeat course of therapy may be beneficial if initial treatment fails to achieve parasitic clearance.
➤ *Visceral leishmaniasis in immunocompromised patients. Adults and children:* 4 mg/kg I.V. infusion daily on days 1 to 5, 10, 17, 24, 31, and 38. Expert advice regarding further treatment is recommended if initial therapy fails or patient experiences relapse.
➤ *Cryptococcal menigitis in HIV-infected patients. Adults and children:* 6 mg/kg I.V. daily over 60 to 120 minutes; adjust rate as tolerated.

How supplied
Available by prescription only
Injection: 50-mg vial

Pharmacodynamics
Antifungal activity: Amphotericin B, the active component of AmBisome, binds to the sterol component of a fungal cell membrane leading to alterations in cell permeability and cell death.

Pharmacokinetics
Absorption: Administered I.V.
Distribution: Unknown.
Metabolism: Unknown.
Excretion: The initial half-life is 7 to 10 hours with 24-hour dosing; terminal elimination half life is 100 to 153 hours.

Route	Onset	Peak	Duration
I.V.	Unknown	Unknown	Unknown

Contraindications and precautions
Contraindicated in patients hypersensitive to drug or its components. Use cautiously in patients with impaired renal function, in geriatric patients, and in pregnant women.

Interactions
Drug-drug. *Antineoplastics:* May enhance potential for renal toxicity, bronchospasm, and hypotension. Use cautiously.
Cardiac glycosides: Increased risk of digitalis toxicity from amphotericin B-induced hypokalemia. Monitor serum potassium level closely.
Clotrimazole, fluconazole, ketoconazole, miconazole: May induce fungal resistance to amphotericin B. Use together cautiously.
Corticosteroids, corticotropin: May potentiate potassium depletion, which could result in cardiac dysfunction. Monitor serum electrolyte level and cardiac function.

Flucytosine: May increase flucytosine toxicity by increasing cellular reuptake or impairing renal excretion of flucytosine. Use cautiously.

Other nephrotoxic drugs, such as antibiotics, antineoplastics: May cause additive nephrotoxicity. Administer cautiously. Monitor renal function closely.

Skeletal muscle relaxants: Enhanced effects of skeletal muscle relaxants resulting from amphotericin B-induced hypokalemia. Monitor serum potassium levels.

Adverse reactions

CNS: *anxiety, confusion, headache, insomnia, asthenia.*

CV: *flushing, chest pain, hypotension, tachycardia,* hypertension, *edema.*

EENT: *epistaxis, rhinitis.*

GI: *nausea, vomiting, abdominal pain, diarrhea,* **GI hemorrhage.**

GU: *hematuria, elevated creatinine and BUN levels.*

Hepatic: *elevated ALT and AST levels, increased alkaline phosphatase level, bilirubinemia.*

Metabolic: *hyperglycemia,* hypernatremia, *hypocalcemia, hypokalemia, hypomagnesemia.*

Musculoskeletal: *back pain.*

Respiratory: *increased cough, dyspnea,* hypoxia, *pleural effusion, lung disorder,* hyperventilation.

Skin: *pruritus, rash, sweating.*

Other: *chills, infection,* **anaphylaxis,** *pain,* **sepsis,** *fever, blood product infusion reaction.*

Overdose and treatment

Repeated daily doses of up to 7.5 mg/kg have been given without toxicity. If overdose occurs, cease administration immediately. Symptomatic supportive measures should be instituted. Pay particular attention to monitoring renal function. The drug isn't hemodialyzable.

Special considerations

● Patients also receiving chemotherapy or bone marrow transplantation are at greater risk for additional adverse reactions, including seizures, arrhythmias, and thrombocytopenia.

● Leukocyte transfusions shouldn't be given with drug because acute pulmonary toxicity has been reported with concurrent administration.

● To lessen risk or severity of adverse reactions, premedication with antipyretics, antihistamines, antiemetics, or corticosteroids can be ordered.

⚡ ALERT Amphotericin B preparations aren't interchangeable and dosages will vary.

● Patients given amphotericin B liposomal had a lower occurrence of chills, elevated BUN, hypokalemia, hypertension, and vomiting than patients treated with conventional amphotericin B.

● Reconstitute each 50-mg vial of amphotericin B liposomal with 12 ml of sterile water for injection to yield a solution of 4 mg amphotericin B/ml.

⚡ ALERT Don't reconstitute with bacteriostatic water for injection, and don't allow bacteriostatic agent in solution. Don't reconstitute with saline solution, add saline solution to reconstituted concentration, or mix with other drugs.

● After reconstitution, shake vial vigorously for 30 seconds or until particulate matter is dispersed.

● Withdraw calculated amount of reconstituted solution into a sterile syringe and inject through a 5-micron filter into the appropriate amount of D_5W to further dilute to 1 to 2 mg/ml. Lower concentrations (0.2 to 0.5 mg/ml) may be appropriate for children to provide sufficient volume of infusion.

● An existing I.V. line must be flushed with D_5W before infusion of drug. If this isn't feasible, administer drug through a separate line.

● Use a controlled infusion device and an in-line filter with a mean pore diameter larger than 1 micron. Initially, infuse drug over at least 2 hours. Infusion time may be reduced to 1 hour if treatment is well tolerated. If patient experiences discomfort during infusion, duration of infusion may be increased.

● Unopened drug is stored under refrigeration at 36° to 46° F (2° to 8° C). Once reconstituted, vial of reconstituted concentrate may be stored for up to 24 hours at 36° to 46° F. Don't freeze.

Patient monitoring

● Observe patient closely for adverse reactions during infusion. If anaphylaxis occurs, stop infusion immediately, provide supportive therapy, and notify prescriber.

● Monitor BUN and serum creatinine and electrolyte levels (particularly magnesium and potassium), liver function, and CBC. Therapy may take several weeks to months.

● Observe patient closely for signs of hypokalemia (ECG changes, muscle weakness, cramping, drowsiness).

Breast-feeding patients

● It's unknown if drug appears in breast milk, but because of the potential for serious adverse reactions in breast-fed infants, a decision should be made to discontinue either nursing or the drug, taking into account the importance of the drug to the woman.

Pediatric patients

● Safety and efficacy in children under age 1 month haven't been established.

Geriatric patients

● No dosage alteration is necessary. Carefully monitor geriatric patients.

Patient education

● Teach patient signs and symptoms of hypersensitivity, and stress importance of reporting them immediately.

Reactions may be *common,* uncommon, *life-threatening,* or COMMON AND LIFE-THREATENING.

- Warn patient that therapy may take several months; teach personal hygiene and other measures to prevent spread and recurrence of lesions.
- Instruct patient to report any adverse reactions that occur while receiving drug.
- Instruct patient to watch for and report signs of hypokalemia (muscle weakness, cramping, drowsiness).
- Advise patient that frequent laboratory testing will be necessary.

ampicillin
Apo-Ampi*, Novo-Ampicillin*, Omnipen, Penbritin*

ampicillin sodium
Ampicin*, Omnipen-N, Penbritin*

ampicillin trihydrate
Principen, Totacillin

Pharmacologic classification: aminopenicillin
Therapeutic classification: antibiotic
Pregnancy risk category: B

Indications and dosages
➤ *Systemic infections, acute and chronic urinary tract infections caused by susceptible organisms. Adults:* 250 to 500 mg P.O. q 6 hours.
Children who weigh less than 40 kg (88 lb): 25 to 100 mg/kg P.O. daily, divided into doses given q 6 hours; or 100 to 200 mg/kg I.V. daily for 3 days and then I.M., divided into doses given q 6 to 8 hours.
➤ *Meningitis. Adults:* 8 to 14 g I.V. or 150 to 200 mg/kg daily divided q 3 to 4 hours for 3 days; then may give I.M. if desired.
Children ages 2 months to 12 years: 200 to 400 mg/kg I.V. daily in divided doses q 4 to 6 hours. May be given along with chloramphenicol, pending culture results.
Neonates under 1 week old: 50 to 75 mg/kg I.V. q 12 hours (weight under 2 kg [4.4 lb]) or q 8 hours (weight over 2 kg).
Neonates over 1 week old: 50 mg/kg I.V. q 8 hours (weight under 2 kg) or q 6 hours (weight over 2 kg).
➤ *Neonatal group B streptococcal meningitis. Neonates age 7 days or under:* 200 mg/kg daily I.V. given in three divided doses.
Neonates age 7 days or over: 300 mg/kg/daily I.V. given in 4 to 6 divided doses.
➤ *Uncomplicated gonorrhea. Adults:* 3.5 g P.O. with 1 g probenecid given as a single dose.
✦ *Dosage adjustment.* Increase dosing interval to q 12 hours in patients with severe renal impairment (creatinine clearance 10 ml/minute or less).
➤ *Prophylaxis for bacterial endocarditis before dental or minor respiratory*

procedures. Adults: 2 g (I.V. or I.M.) 30 minutes before procedure.
Children: 50 mg/kg I.V. or I.M. 30 minutes before procedure.
➤ *Treatment of enterococcal endocarditis. Adults:* 12 g daily by continuous I.V. infusion or in six equally divided doses with gentamicin for 4 to 6 weeks.
➤ *Prophylaxis of neonatal group B streptococcus infections* ◊. *Adults:* 2 g I.V. given to the mother at least 4 hours before delivery, and then 1 to 2 g I.V. q 4 to 6 hours until delivery.

How supplied
Available by prescription only
Capsules: 250 mg, 500 mg
Infusion: 500 mg, 1 g, 2 g
Parenteral: 125 mg, 250 mg, 500 mg, 1 g, 2 g
Suspension: 125 mg/5 ml, 250 mg/5 ml

Pharmacodynamics
Antibiotic action: Ampicillin is bactericidal; it adheres to bacterial penicillin-binding proteins, inhibiting bacterial cell wall synthesis. Spectrum of activity includes non-penicillinase-producing gram-positive bacteria. It's also effective against many gram-negative organisms, including *Neisseria gonorrhoeae, Neisseria meningitidis, Haemophilus influenzae, Escherichia coli, Proteus mirabilis, Salmonella,* and *Shigella.* Ampicillin should be used in gram-negative systemic infections only when organism sensitivity is known.

Pharmacokinetics
Absorption: About 42% of ampicillin is absorbed after an oral dose.
Distribution: Distributed into pleural, peritoneal, and synovial fluids, lungs, prostate, liver, and gallbladder; it also penetrates middle ear effusions, maxillary sinus and bronchial secretions, tonsils, and sputum. Readily crosses the placenta; minimally protein-bound (15% to 25%).
Metabolism: Only partially metabolized.
Excretion: Excreted in urine by renal tubular secretion and glomerular filtration. It's also excreted in breast milk. Elimination half-life is about 1 to 1½ hours; in patients with extensive renal impairment, half-life is extended to 10 to 24 hours.

Route	Onset	Peak	Duration
P.O.	Unknown	2 hr	6-8 hr
I.V.	Immediate	Immediate	Unknown
I.M.	Unknown	1 hr	Unknown

Contraindications and precautions
Contraindicated in patients hypersensitive to drug or other penicillins. Use cautiously in patients with mononucleosis.

Interactions
Drug-drug. *Allopurinol:* Appears to increase occurrence of rash from both drugs. Monitor patient closely.

Aminoglycoside antibiotics: A synergistic bactericidal effect against some strains of enterococci and group B streptococci. However, the drugs are physically and chemically incompatible and are inactivated if mixed or given together. Don't mix together.

Methotrexate: Large doses of penicillins may interfere with renal tubular secretion of methotrexate, delaying elimination and elevating serum levels of methotrexate. Monitor patient for methotrexate toxicity.

Oral contraceptives: Effects of oral contraceptives may be decreased. Advise using alternative barrier method.

Probenecid: Inhibits renal tubular secretion of ampicillin, raising its serum concentrations. Avoid use together.

Drug-herb. *Khat:* Antimicrobial effect of certain penicillins may be decreased. Discourage khat chewing, or tell patient to take amoxicillin 2 hours after chewing khat.

Adverse reactions
CNS: lethargy, hallucinations, *seizures*, anxiety, confusion, agitation, depression, dizziness, fatigue.
CV: thrombophlebitis.
GI: *nausea*, vomiting, *diarrhea*, glossitis, stomatitis, gastritis, abdominal pain, enterocolitis, pseudomembranous colitis, black "hairy" tongue.
GU: interstitial nephritis, nephropathy, vaginitis.
Hematologic: anemia, *thrombocytopenia*, thrombocytopenic purpura, eosinophilia, *leukopenia, hemolytic anemia, agranulocytosis*.
Other: *hypersensitivity reactions* (erythematous maculopapular rash, urticaria, *anaphylaxis*), overgrowth of nonsusceptible organisms, pain at injection site, vein irritation.

Overdose and treatment
Signs of overdose include neuromuscular sensitivity and seizures. After recent ingestion (within 4 hours), empty the stomach by induced emesis or gastric lavage; follow with activated charcoal to reduce absorption. Drug can be removed by hemodialysis.

Special considerations
● Ampicillin alters results of urine glucose tests that use cupric sulfate (Benedict's reagent or Clinitest). Urine glucose determinations should be done with glucose oxidase methods (Chemstrip uG, Diastix, or glucose enzymatic test strip).
● Consider the recommendations relevant to all penicillins.
● Obtain patient's allergy history before dispensing drug.

● Administer I.M. or I.V. only when patient is too ill to take oral drug.

Patient monitoring
● Monitor renal, hepatic, and hematologic systems during prolonged therapy.

Pregnant patients
● Safe use during pregnancy hasn't been established, but drug has been used to treat urinary tract infections in pregnant women without affecting the fetus.

Breast-feeding patients
● Use cautiously. Ampicillin is distributed readily into breast milk; safety in breast-feeding women hasn't been established.

Geriatric patients
● Because of diminished renal tubular secretion in geriatric patients, half-life of drug may be prolonged.

Patient education
● Advise patient to report diarrhea promptly.
● Instruct patient to complete all of the prescribed drug.

ampicillin sodium/sulbactam sodium
Unasyn

Pharmacologic classification: aminopenicillin/beta-lactamase inhibitor combination
Therapeutic classification: antibiotic
Pregnancy risk category: B

Indications and dosages
➤ *Skin and skin-structure infections, intra-abdominal and gynecologic infections caused by susceptible gram positive bacteria, gram negative bacteria, beta-lactamase-producing strains of* Staphylococcus aureus, Escherichia coli, Klebsiella *(including* K. pneumoniae*),* Proteus mirabilis, Bacteroides *(including* B. fragilis*),* Enterobacter, Neisseria meningitidis, Neisseria gonorrhoeae, Moraxella catarrhalis, *and* Acinetobacter calcoaceticus.
Adults: 1.5 to 3 g I.M. or I.V. q 6 hours. Don't exceed 4 g daily sulbactam sodium.
➤ *Skin and skin-structure infections caused by susceptible organisms. Children who weigh less than 88 lb (40 kg):* same as adult dose.
Children age 1 and older who weigh less than 40 kg: 300 mg/kg I.V. daily in divided doses q 6 hours not to exceed 14 days of therapy.
✦ *Dosage adjustment.* For patients with renal impairment, give the usually recommended doses, but less frequently, as shown at the top of the next page.

Creatinine clearance (ml/min)	Half-life (hours)	Recommended dosage
≥ 30	1	1.5 to 3 g q 6 to 8 hr
15-29	5	1.5 to 3 g q 12 hr
5-14	9	1.5 to 3 g q 24 hr

How supplied
Available by prescription only
Injection: vials and piggyback vials containing 1.5 g (1 g ampicillin sodium with 500 mg sulbactam sodium) and 3 g (2 g ampicillin sodium with 1 g sulbactam sodium)

Pharmacodynamics
Antibiotic action: Ampicillin is bactericidal; it adheres to bacterial penicillin-binding proteins, thus inhibiting bacterial cell wall synthesis. Sulbactam inhibits beta-lactamase, an enzyme produced by ampicillin-resistant bacteria that degrades ampicillin.

Pharmacokinetics
Absorption: Well absorbed after I.V. and I.M. administration.
Distribution: Both distributed into pleural, peritoneal, and synovial fluids, lungs, prostate, liver, and gallbladder; they also penetrate middle ear effusions, maxillary sinus and bronchial secretions, tonsils, and sputum. Ampicillin readily crosses the placenta; it's minimally protein-bound at 15% to 25%; sulbactam is about 38% bound.
Metabolism: Both are metabolized only partially; only 15% to 25% of both are metabolized.
Excretion: Both are excreted in the urine by renal tubular secretion and glomerular filtration. They're also excreted in breast milk. Elimination half-life is 1 to 1¼ hours; in patients with extensive renal impairment, half-life can be as long as 10 to 24 hours.

Route	Onset	Peak	Duration
I.V.	Immediate	Immediately after infusion	Unknown
I.M.	Unknown	Unknown	Unknown

Contraindications and precautions
Contraindicated in patients hypersensitive to drug or other penicillins. Use cautiously in patients with maculopapular rash.

Interactions
Drug-drug. *Allopurinol*: May increase the risk of rash. Monitor patient closely.
Aminoglycosides: The ampicillin component may cause in vitro inactivation of aminoglycosides if these antibiotics are mixed in the same infusion container. Don't mix together.

Anticoagulants: Large doses of I.V. penicillins can increase bleeding risks of anticoagulants because of a prolongation of bleeding times. Monitor PT and INR.
Probenecid: Decreased excretion of both ampicillin and sulbactam. Monitor patient for toxicity.

Adverse reactions
CV: thrombophlebitis.
GI: *nausea,* vomiting, *diarrhea,* glossitis, stomatitis, gastritis, black "hairy" tongue, enterocolitis, pseudomembranous colitis.
Hematologic: anemia, *thrombocytopenia,* thrombocytopenic purpura, eosinophilia, *leukopenia, agranulocytosis.*
Other: *hypersensitivity reactions* (erythematous maculopapular rash, urticaria, *anaphylaxis*), *overgrowth of nonsusceptible organisms,* pain at injection site, vein irritation.

Overdose and treatment
Neurologic adverse reactions, including seizures, are likely. Treatment is supportive. Ampicillin and sulbactam are likely to be removed by hemodialysis.

Special considerations
• Ampicillin alters results of urine glucose tests that use cupric sulfate (Benedict's reagent or Clinitest). Make urine glucose determinations with glucose oxidase methods (Chemstrip uG, Diastix, or glucose enzymatic test strip).
🔲 **ALERT** Give I.V. drug by slow injection over at least 10 to 15 minutes or infuse in greater dilutions with 50 to 100 ml of a compatible diluent over 15 to 30 minutes to avoid risk for seizures.
• Store powder below 86° F (30° C).
• For I.V. use, reconstitute powder in piggyback units to desired concentrations with sterile water for injection, normal saline solution, D₅W, lactated Ringer's injection, 1/6 M sodium lactate injection, D₅W in half-normal saline solution, or 10% invert sugar.
• For I.M. injection, reconstitute with sterile water for injection, or 0.5% or 2% lidocaine hydrochloride injection. To obtain 375 mg/ml solutions (250 mg ampicillin/125 mg sulbactam/ml), add contents of the 1.5-g vial to 3.2 ml of diluent to produce 4 ml withdrawal volume; add 3-g vial to 6.4 ml of diluent to produce 8 ml withdrawal volume.
• Reconstituted solutions are stable for varying periods (from 2 to 72 hours) depending on diluent used. Refer to package insert for specific information. For patients on sodium restriction, note that a 1.5-g dose of ampicillin sodium/sulbactam sodium yields 5 mEq of sodium.

Patient monitoring
• Test for *Clostridium difficile* in patients with persistent diarrhea.
• Monitor patient for overgrowth of nonsusceptible organisms.

Pregnant patients
- Safety in pregnant women hasn't been established.
- Transient decreases in serum estradiol, conjugated estrone, conjugated estriol, and estriol glucuronide may occur.

Breast-feeding patients
- Distributed readily into breast milk. Because safety in breast-feeding women hasn't been established, recommend a different feeding method during therapy.

Pediatric patients
- Safety in children under age 1 hasn't been established. Safety and efficacy for use in children for treatment of skin and skin structure infections have been established. Not for use to treat other infections or for I.M. use.

Geriatric patients
- Because of diminished renal tubular secretion in geriatric patients, half-life of drug may be prolonged.

Patient education
- Tell patient to report a rash, fever, or chills. A rash is the most frequent allergic reaction.
- Advise patient to report discomfort at insertion site.
- Warn patient that I.M. injection may cause pain at the injection site.

amprenavir
Agenerase

Pharmacologic classification: protease inhibitor
Therapeutic classification: antiretroviral
Pregnancy risk category: C

Indications and dosages
➤ *Treatment of HIV-1 infection with other antiretrovirals.* Adults and children ages 13 to 16 who weigh 50 kg (110 lb) or more: 1,200 mg P.O. (eight 150-mg capsules) b.i.d. with other antiretrovirals.
Children ages 4 to 12 or 13 to 16 who weigh less than 50 kg: For capsules, 20 mg/kg P.O. b.i.d. or 15 mg/kg P.O. t.i.d. (to a maximum daily dose of 2,400 mg) with other antiretrovirals. For oral solution, 22.5 mg/kg P.O. (1.5 ml/kg) b.i.d. or 17 mg/kg P.O. (1.1 ml/kg) t.i.d. (to a maximum daily dose of 2,800 mg) with other antiretrovirals.
✦ *Dosage adjustment.* Patients with moderate or severe hepatic impairment should receive reduced dosage. Those with a Child-Pugh score of 5 to 8 should receive 450 mg (capsules) P.O. b.i.d. Those with a Child-Pugh score of 9 to 12 should receive 300 mg (capsules) P.O. b.i.d.

How supplied
Available by prescription only
Capsules: 50 mg, 150 mg
Oral solution: 15 mg/ml

Pharmacodynamics
Antiretroviral action: Amprenavir binds to the active site of HIV-1 protease and thereby prevents the processing of viral *gag* and *gag-pol* polyprotein precursors, resulting in the formation of immature noninfectious viral particles.

Pharmacokinetics
Absorption: Rapidly absorbed.
Distribution: About 90% bound to plasma proteins.
Metabolism: Metabolized in the liver by the cytochrome P-450 CYP3A4 enzyme system.
Excretion: Excretion of unchanged amprenavir in urine and feces is minimal. The plasma elimination half-life ranges from 7.1 to 10.6 hours.

Route	Onset	Peak	Duration
P.O.	Unknown	1-2 hr	Unknown

Contraindications and precautions
Contraindicated in patients hypersensitive to drug or any of its components. Contraindicated in infants, children younger than 4 years of age, pregnant women, patients with liver or kidney failure, and patients treated with disulfuram (Antabuse) or metronidazole (Flagyl). Use cautiously in patients with sulfonamide allergy, those with hepatic impairment, and those with hemophilia A and B.

Interactions
Drug-drug. *Antacids:* Separate administration of antacids and drug by at least 1 hour to avoid possible interference with absorption.
Antiarrhythmics (such as amiodarone, quinidine, systemic lidocaine), anticoagulants (such as warfarin), tricyclic antidepressants: Amprenavir serum levels may be affected. Monitor patient closely.
Bepridil, dihydroergotamine, midazolam, rifampin, triazolam: Serious or life-threatening interactions may occur. Avoid use together.
Hormonal contraceptives: Decreased contraceptive effectiveness. Encourage use of barrier contraception.
Macrolides: Increased amprenavir plasma levels. Dosage adjustment may be required.
Psychotherapeutic drugs: May increase CNS effects. Monitor patient closely.
Rifabutin: Decreased amprenavir levels and substantially increased rifabutin levels. Consider reducing dosage.
Sildenafil: Substantially increased sildenafil levels, which may increase drug effects, including hypotension, visual changes, and priapism. Avoid use together.

Reactions may be *common*, uncommon, *life-threatening*, or COMMON AND LIFE-THREATENING.

Drug-food. *High-fat meals:* Reduced drug absorption. Advise against taking drug with a high-fat meal.

Adverse reactions

CNS: *paresthesia*, depressive or mood disorders, headache.
GI: *nausea, vomiting, diarrhea or loose stools,* taste disorders.
Metabolic: *hyperglycemia, hypertriglyceridemia,* hypercholesterolemia.
Skin: *rash,* **Stevens-Johnson syndrome.**

Overdose and treatment

No known antidote. It isn't known whether amprenavir can be removed by peritoneal lavage or hemodialysis. If overdose occurs, monitor patient for evidence of toxicity and give supportive treatment as needed.

Special considerations

● Drug is a sulfonamide. Patients with a known sulfonamide allergy should be treated with caution.
● Amprenavir oral solution should be used only when the capsules or other protease inhibitor formulations aren't therapeutic options.
● Capsules and oral solution aren't interchangeable on milligram per milligram basis.
● Store capsules and oral solution at room temperature.

Patient monitoring

● Monitor patient for adverse reactions. Drug may cause redistribution or accumulation of body fat including central obesity, dorsocervical fat enlargement (buffalo hump), peripheral wasting, breast enlargement, or cushingoid appearance. Severe and life-threatening reactions, including Stevens-Johnson syndrome, have occurred.
● Perform CBC weekly and as clinically indicated to detect neutropenia in patients also receiving rifabutin.

Pregnant patients

● To monitor maternal-fetal outcomes of pregnant women exposed to drug, an Antiretroviral Pregnancy Registry has been established. Prescribers may call 1-800-258-4263 to register patients who have been exposed to drug during pregnancy.

Breast-feeding patients

● It isn't known if drug appears in breast milk, so instruct breast-feeding women not to breast-feed if they're receiving drug. In addition, it's recommended that HIV-infected women not breast-feed to avoid the risk of transmitting HIV to their infants.

Pediatric patients

● An adverse event profile similar to that in adults is seen in children. Safety, efficacy, and pharma-cokinetics of drug haven't been evaluated in children under age 4.

Geriatric patients

● Dosing in elderly patients should be cautious because of the likelihood of decreased hepatic, renal, or cardiac function, and of concomitant disease or other drug therapy.

Patient education

● Inform patient that drug isn't a cure for HIV infection and opportunistic infections and that other complications of the disease may continue to develop. The drug doesn't reduce the risk of transmitting HIV to others through sexual contact.
● Tell patient he may take drug without regard to meals but that he should avoid taking it with high-fat meals because absorption may be decreased.
● Advise patient to take drug each day as prescribed. It must always be taken with other antiretroviral drugs. Dose must not be altered or discontinued without consulting prescriber.
● Tell patient to take a missed dose as soon as possible and then return to the normal schedule. However, if a dose is skipped, don't double the next dose.
● Instruct patients taking hormonal contraceptives to use alternate contraceptive measures during drug therapy.

amyl nitrite

Pharmacologic classification: nitrate
Therapeutic classification: vasodilator, cyanide poisoning adjunct
Pregnancy risk category: C

Indications and dosages

➤ **Angina pectoris.** Adults: 0.18 to 0.3 ml by inhalation (one glass ampule inhaler), p.r.n.
➤ **Adjunct treatment of cyanide poisoning.** Adults and children: 0.3 ml by inhalation for 15 to 30 seconds; repeat q 60 seconds until I.V. sodium nitrite infusion and I.V. sodium thiosulfate infusion are available.

How supplied

Available by prescription only
Nasal inhalant: 0.3 ml

Pharmacodynamics

Vasodilating action: Drug reduces myocardial oxygen demand by decreasing left ventricular end-diastolic pressure (preload) and systemic vascular resistance and arterial pressure (afterload). It also increases collateral coronary blood flow. By relaxing vascular smooth muscle, it produces generalized vasodilation. Amyl nitrite also relaxes all other smooth muscle, including bronchial and biliary smooth muscle. In cyanide poisoning, it converts hemoglobin to methemoglobin, which reacts with cyanide to form cyanmethemoglobin.

Pharmacokinetics

Absorption: Inhaled drug is absorbed readily through the respiratory tract; action begins in 30 seconds and lasts 3 to 5 minutes.

Distribution: No information available.

Metabolism: Amyl nitrite, an organic nitrite, is metabolized by the liver to form inorganic nitrites, which are much less potent vasodilators than the parent drug.

Excretion: One-third of the inhaled dose is excreted in urine.

Route	Onset	Peak	Duration
Nasal	Within 30 sec	Unknown	3-5 min

Contraindications and precautions

Contraindicated in pregnant patients, patients hypersensitive to nitrites, and patients with severe anemia, angle-closure glaucoma, orthostatic hypotension, or increased intracranial pressure.

Use cautiously in patients with glaucoma, volume depletion, and hypotension.

Interactions

Drug-drug. *Antihypertensives, beta blockers, phenothiazines, sildenafil:* May cause excessive hypotension. Monitor patient's blood pressure.

Drug-lifestyle. *Alcohol use:* May cause excessive hypotension. Discourage concurrent use.

Adverse reactions

CNS: *headache,* sometimes with throbbing; dizziness; weakness.

CV: *orthostatic hypotension, tachycardia,* flushing, palpitations, fainting.

GI: nausea, vomiting.

Hematologic: methemoglobinemia.

Skin: cutaneous vasodilation, rash.

Other: *hypersensitivity reactions.*

Overdose and treatment

Overdose may cause methemoglobinemia, characterized by blue skin and mucous membranes, hypotension, tachycardia, palpitations, skin changes, diaphoresis, dizziness, syncope, vertigo, headache, nausea, vomiting, anorexia, increased intracranial pressure, confusion, moderate fever, and paralysis. Hypoxia may lead to metabolic acidosis, cyanosis, seizures, coma, and cardiac collapse.

Treat with high flow oxygen and methylene blue. Usual dose of methylene blue for adults and children is 1 to 2 mg/kg I.V. given slowly over several minutes. In severe cases, this dose may be repeated only once; doses exceeding 4 mg/kg may produce methemoglobinemia.

Special considerations

• Amyl nitrite therapy alters the Zlatkis-Zak color reaction, causing a false decrease in serum cholesterol levels.

• Drug is rarely used as an antianginal.

• Keep patient sitting or lying down during and immediately after inhalation. Crush ampule (has a woven gauze covering) between fingers and hold to nose for inhalation.

• Drug is highly flammable; keep away from open flame and extinguish all cigarettes before use.

• Drug is used illegally to enhance sexual pleasure. Street names include Amy and poppers.

Patient monitoring

• Monitor patient for orthostatic hypotension; don't allow patient to make rapid postural changes while inhaling drug.

Breast-feeding patients

• It isn't known if amyl nitrite appears in breast milk; risk and benefit must be considered.

Pediatric patients

• Safety and efficacy haven't been established.

Geriatric patients

• Orthostatic hypotensive effects may be more likely to occur in elderly patients.

Patient education

• Explain that ampule must be crushed to release drug.

• Warn patient to use drug only when seated or lying down.

---

anagrelide hydrochloride
Agrylin

Pharmacologic classification: platelet-reducing agent
Therapeutic classification: platelet-reducing agent
Pregnancy risk category C

Indications and dosages

➤ *Essential thrombocythemia to reduce elevated platelet count and risk of thrombosis and to ameliorate related symptoms.* *Adults:* 0.5 mg P.O. q.i.d. or 1 mg b.i.d. for at least 1 week; then adjust dosage to lowest effective dose required to maintain platelet count below 600,000/mm³, and ideally to the normal range. Don't increase to more than 0.5 mg daily in any 1 week; don't exceed 10 mg daily or 2.5 mg in a single dose.

How supplied

Available by prescription only
Capsules: 0.5 mg, 1 mg

Pharmacodynamics

Platelet-reducing action: Mechanism of action still under investigation; reduction in platelet production is thought to result from a decrease in megakaryocyte hypermaturation. Drug inhibits cAMP phosphodiesterase, as well as adenosine

---

Reactions may be *common*, uncommon, *life-threatening*, or COMMON AND LIFE-THREATENING.

diphosphate- and collagen-induced platelet aggregation.

Pharmacokinetics
Absorption: Following oral administration of 1 mg in healthy people, plasma levels peak in about 1 hour. Plasma levels decline to less than 10% of peak levels in 24 hours.
Distribution: Plasma half-life at fasting and at 0.5 mg doses is 1.3 hours. Drug doesn't accumulate in plasma after repeated administration and bioavailability is modestly reduced by food.
Metabolism: Drug is extensively metabolized before elimination in urine.
Excretion: Drug is eliminated in urine; less than 1% is recovered unchanged in urine.

Route	Onset	Peak	Duration
P.O.	Unknown	1 hr	Unknown

Contraindications and precautions
Use cautiously in patients with CV disease because drug may cause vasodilation, tachycardia, palpitations, and heart failure. Use cautiously in patients with creatinine clearance over 2 mg/dl and in those with liver function tests exceeding 1.5 times the upper limit of normal. Interruption of drug use will cause platelet counts to rise within 4 days of discontinuation.

Interactions
Drug-drug. *Sucralfate:* May interfere with anagrelide absorption; no other drug interaction studies have been performed.

Adverse reactions
CNS: malaise, amnesia, *asthenia,* confusion, *CVA,* depression, *dizziness, headache,* insomnia, migraine, nervousness, pain, paresthesia, syncope, somnolence.
CV: *arrhythmias, angina pectoris, chest pain,* CV disease, *edema, heart failure, hemorrhage,* hypertension, *palpitations,* orthostatic hypotension, vasodilatation, *tachycardia.*
EENT: sinusitis, abnormal vision, amblyopia, diplopia, tinnitus, visual field abnormality.
GI: anorexia, *abdominal pain,* aphthous stomatitis, constipation, *diarrhea,* dyspepsia, eructation, *flatulence,* GI distress, *GI hemorrhage,* gastritis, melena, *nausea,* vomiting.
GU: dysuria, hematuria.
Hematologic: anemia, ecchymoses, lymphadenoma, *thrombocytopenia.*
Metabolic: dehydration.
Musculoskeletal: arthralgia, back pain, leg cramps, myalgia, neck pain.
Respiratory: *dyspnea,* rhinitis, epistaxis, respiratory disease, pneumonia, bronchitis, asthma.
Skin: alopecia, pruritus, rash, skin disorder, urticaria, photosensitivity.
Other: chills, fever, flulike symptoms.

Overdose and treatment
Monitor patient closely; monitor platelet counts.

Special considerations
● Food has no clinically significant effect on anagrelide.

Patient monitoring
● Perform platelet counts every 2 days during first week, then weekly until maintenance dose is reached.
● During the first 2 weeks of treatment, monitor blood counts and liver and renal function tests.

Breast-feeding patients
● It isn't known if drug appears in breast milk. Use cautiously in breast-feeding women.

Pediatric patients
● Safety and efficacy of drug haven't been established in patients under age 16.

Geriatric patients
● Evaluate use of drug carefully in elderly patients with renal, liver, or CV disease.

Patient education
● Tell patient to use drug only as prescribed.
● Inform patient that drug can be taken without regard to meals.
● Instruct patient to report increased bleeding, bruising, or cardiac symptoms.

anastrozole
Arimidex

Pharmacologic classification: nonsteroidal aromatase inhibitor
Therapeutic classification: antineoplastic
Pregnancy risk category: D

Indications and dosages
➤ *Treatment of advanced breast cancer in postmenopausal women with disease progression following tamoxifen therapy, or initial treatment of postmenopausal women diagnosed with advanced or locally advanced hormone-receptive breast cancer.* Adults: 1 mg P.O. daily.

How supplied
Available by prescription only
Tablets: 1 mg

Pharmacodynamics
Antineoplastic action: A potent and selective nonsteroidal aromatase inhibitor, anastrozole significantly lowers serum estradiol concentrations. Estradiol is the principal estrogen circulating in postmenopausal women that has the ability to stimulate breast cancer cell growth.

Pharmacokinetics
Absorption: Absorbed from the GI tract; food affects the extent of absorption.

Distribution: 40% bound to plasma proteins in the therapeutic range.
Metabolism: Metabolized in the liver.
Excretion: About 11% of anastrozole is excreted in urine as parent drug and about 60% is excreted in urine as metabolites. Half-life is about 50 hours.

Route	Onset	Peak	Duration
P.O.	< 24 hr	Unknown	< 6 days

Contraindications and precautions
Contraindicated in pregnant women.

Interactions
None reported.

Adverse reactions
CNS: *asthenia, headache,* dizziness, depression, paresthesia.
CV: chest pain, edema, thromboembolic disease.
EENT: pharyngitis.
GI: dry mouth, *nausea,* vomiting, diarrhea, constipation, abdominal pain, anorexia, increased appetite.
GU: vaginal hemorrhage, vaginal dryness.
Metabolic: weight gain.
Musculoskeletal: *back pain,* bone pain, pelvic pain.
Respiratory: dyspnea, increased cough.
Skin: *hot flashes,* rash, sweating.
Other: *pain,* peripheral edema.

Overdose and treatment
A single dose of anastrozole that results in life-threatening symptoms hasn't been established. Single oral doses that exceed 100 mg/kg cause severe irritation of the stomach (necrosis, gastritis, ulceration, and hemorrhage) in animals.

There's no specific antidote to overdose and treatment must be symptomatic. Vomiting may be induced if the patient is alert. Dialysis may be helpful. General supportive care, including frequent monitoring of vital signs and close observation of the patient, is indicated.

Special considerations
● Exclude pregnancy before anastrozole therapy starts.
● Administer drug under supervision of qualified staff experienced in the use of anticancer drugs.
● Patients treated with drug don't need glucocorticoid or mineralocorticoid therapy.

Patient monitoring
● For patients with mild to moderate hepatic impairment, watch for adverse effects.

Breast-feeding patients
● It isn't known if anastrozole appears in breast milk. Drug shouldn't be given to breast-feeding women.

Pediatric patients
● Safety and efficacy in children haven't been established.

Patient education
● Instruct patient to report adverse reactions.
● Stress importance of follow-up care.

anistreplase (anisoylated plasminogen-streptokinase activator complex, APSAC)
Eminase

Pharmacologic classification: thrombolytic enzyme
Therapeutic classification: thrombolytic enzyme
Pregnancy risk category: C

Indications and dosages
➤ *Treatment of acute coronary arterial thrombosis. Adults:* 30 units by direct I.V. injection over 2 to 5 minutes.

How supplied
Available by prescription only
Injection: 30 units/single-dose vial

Pharmacodynamics
Enzymatic action: Anistreplase is derived from Lys-plasminogen and streptokinase. It activates the endogenous fibrinolytic system to produce plasmin, which degrades fibrin clots, fibrinogen, and other plasma proteins, including procoagulant factors V and VIII.

Pharmacokinetics
Absorption: Administered I.V.
Distribution: Information not available.
Metabolism: Immediately after injection, anistreplase is deacylated by a nonenzymatic process to form the active streptokinase-plasminogen complex. The half-life of acylated and deacylated anistreplase is 88 to 112 minutes.
Excretion: Unknown. Duration of fibrinolytic activity is 4 to 6 hours and is limited by the deacylation of the anistreplase.

Route	Onset	Peak	Duration
I.V.	Unknown	Unknown	Unknown

Contraindications and precautions
Contraindicated in patients with history of severe allergic reaction to anistreplase or streptokinase and in those with active internal bleeding, CVA, recent (within the past 2 months) intraspinal or intracranial surgery or trauma, aneurysm, arteriovenous malformation, intracranial neoplasm, uncontrolled hypertension, or known bleeding diathesis.

Use cautiously in patients with recent (within 10 days) major surgery, trauma (including cardiopulmonary resuscitation), GI or GU bleeding, cerebrovascular disease, hypertension, mitral stenosis, atrial fibrillation, acute pericarditis, subacute bacterial endocarditis, septic thrombophlebitis, and diabetic hemorrhagic retinopathy. Also use cautiously in women who are pregnant or within the first 10 days postpartum; in patients receiving anticoagulants; and in those older than age 75.

Interactions

Drug-drug. *Adrenocorticoids, cefamandole, cefoperazone, cefotetan, corticotropin (long-term therapy), ethacrynic acid, glucocorticoids, plicamycin, valproic acid:* May increase risk of severe hemorrhage. Use with extreme caution and monitor patient closely.
Drugs that alter platelet function (including NSAIDs, aspirin and dipyridamole), heparin, oral anticoagulants: May increase risk of bleeding. Monitor patient closely.

Adverse reactions

CNS: *intracranial hemorrhage.*
CV: flushing, **ARRHYTHMIAS**, *conduction disorders, hypotension.*
GI: *hemorrhage,* gum or mouth hemorrhage.
GU: hematuria.
Hematologic: *bleeding tendency,* bleeding at puncture sites, eosinophilia.
Musculoskeletal: arthralgia.
Respiratory: hemoptysis.
Skin: hematoma, urticaria, pruritus, delayed purpuric rash (2 weeks after therapy).
Other: *anaphylaxis.*

Overdose and treatment

Indications of overdose include signs of potentially serious bleeding: bleeding gums, epistaxis, hematoma, spontaneous ecchymoses, oozing at catheter site, increased pulse, and pain from internal bleeding. Discontinue drug and restart when bleeding stops.

Special considerations

● Anistreplase remains active in vitro and can cause degradation of fibrinogen in blood samples drawn for analysis.
● Start therapy as soon as possible after onset of clinical symptoms of acute MI.
● Anistreplase is derived from human plasma. No cases of hepatitis or HIV infection have been reported to date.
● Reconstitute by slowly adding 5 ml sterile water for injection. Direct the stream against the side of the vial, not at the drug itself. Gently roll the vial to mix the dry powder and water. To avoid excessive foaming, don't shake vial. Solution should be colorless to pale yellow.
● Don't mix with other medications or further dilute after reconstitution.
● Store lyophilized powder in the refrigerator.
● Discard drug that isn't administered within 30 minutes of reconstituting.

● To decrease risk of rethrombosis, heparin therapy may be started after administration.
● Addition of fibrinolysis inhibitor (for example, aprotinin) or aminocaproic acid to blood samples drawn to obtain specific measurement of fibrinogen will attenuate the degradation of fibrinogen in thrombolytic-treated patients.
● Keep patient on strict bed rest and apply pressure dressings to recently invaded sites. To minimize risk of bleeding, avoid nonessential handling or moving of patient, invasive procedures such as biopsies, and I.M. injections.

Patient monitoring

● The following tests may be needed before and after drug administration: aPTT, PT, thrombin time, hemoglobin, hematocrit, fibrinogen determination, platelet count, and fibrin-fibrinogen degradation products.
● Coronary angiography may be useful to monitor effectiveness.
● ECG monitoring is recommended to detect arrhythmias linked to acute MI or reperfusion and may help determine effectiveness of treatment.
● Monitor vital signs, mental status, and neurologic status.

Breast-feeding patients

● It isn't known if drug appears in breast milk. Use cautiously in breast-feeding women.

Pediatric patients

● Safety and efficacy in children haven't been established.

Geriatric patients

● No age-specific problems have been reported to date. Risk-benefit must be assessed in patients age 75 and over because preexisting conditions increase the risk of hemorrhagic complications.

Patient education

● Instruct patient and caregiver to recognize and report signs and symptoms of internal bleeding.
● Inform patient about importance of strict bed rest.

antihemophilic factor
Alphanate, Bioclate, Helixate, Hemofil M, Humate-P, Koate-HP, Kogenate, Monoclate-P, Recombinate

Pharmacologic classification: blood derivative
Therapeutic classification: antihemophilic
Pregnancy risk category: C

Indications and dosages
➤ *Hemophilia A (factor VIII deficiency).*
Adults and children: Dosage is highly individualized and depends on patient weight, severity of

deficiency, severity of hemorrhage, presence of inhibitors, and level of factor VIII desired.

How supplied
Available by prescription only
Injection: Vials, with diluent. Number of units on label. A porcine product is available for patients with congenital hemophilia A who have antibodies to human factor VIII:C.

Pharmacodynamics
Antihemophilic action: Antihemophilic factor (AHF) replaces deficient clotting factor that converts prothrombin to thrombin.

Pharmacokinetics
Absorption: Administered I.V.
Distribution: AHF equilibrates intravascular and extravascular compartments; it doesn't readily cross placenta.
Metabolism: AHF is cleared rapidly from plasma.
Excretion: AHF is consumed during blood clotting. Half-life ranges from 4 to 24 hours (average 12 hours).

Route	Onset	Peak	Duration
I.V.	Unknown	Unknown	Unknown

Contraindications and precautions
Contraindicated in patients hypersensitive to murine (mouse) protein or drug. Use cautiously in neonates, infants, and patients with hepatic disease.

Interactions
None significant.

Adverse reactions
CV: tightness in chest.
GI: nausea.
Respiratory: wheezing.
Skin: *urticaria*.
Other: *chills, fever, hypersensitivity reactions* (stinging at injection site, fever, *anaphylaxis*), *risk of hepatitis B and HIV*.

Overdose and treatment
Large or frequently repeated doses of AHF in patients with blood group A, B, or AB may cause intravascular hemolysis; monitor CBC and direct Coombs' test, and if intravascular hemolysis occurs, give serologically compatible type O RBCs.

Special considerations
● One AHF unit equals the activity present in 1 ml of normal pooled human plasma less than 1 hour old. Don't confuse commercial product with blood bank–produced cryoprecipitated factor VIII from individual human donors. AHF is designed for I.V. use; use a plastic syringe because solution adheres to glass.
● Refrigerate concentrate until needed; before reconstituting, warm concentrate and diluent bottles to room temperature. To mix, gently roll vial

between hands; don't shake or mix with other I.V. solutions. Keep product away from heat (but don't refrigerate because that may cause precipitation of active ingredient), and use within 3 hours.
● Prophylactic oral diphenhydramine may be prescribed if patient has history of transient allergic reactions to AHF.
● All products are heat-treated by special method similar to pasteurization to decrease risk of transmitting hepatitis. Patient should be immunized with hepatitis B vaccine to decrease the risk of transmission of hepatitis.

Patient monitoring
● Take baseline pulse rate before I.V. administration. If pulse rate increases significantly during administration, flow rate should be reduced or drug discontinued. Adverse reactions are usually related to too-rapid infusion.
● Monitor coagulation studies before and during therapy; monitor vital signs regularly, and be alert for allergic reactions.

Pediatric patients
● Administer cautiously to neonates and older infants because of susceptibility to hepatitis.

Patient education
● Teach patient how to use, inject, and store prescribed product.
● Advise patient not to take salicylates or other drugs that inhibit platelet formation.

anti-inhibitor coagulant complex
Autoplex T, Feiba VH Immuno

Pharmacologic classification: activated prothrombin complex
Therapeutic classification: hemostatic
Pregnancy risk category: C

Indications and dosages
➤ *Prevention and control of hemorrhagic episodes in some patients with hemophilia A in whom inhibitor antibodies to antihemophilic factor have developed; management of bleeding in patients with acquired hemophilia who have spontaneously acquired inhibitors to factor VIII.* *Adults and children:* Dosage is highly individualized and varies among manufacturers. For Autoplex T, give 25 to 100 unit/kg I.V. depending on the severity of hemorrhage. If no hemostatic improvement occurs within 6 hours after initial administration, repeat dose. For Feiba VH Immuno, give 50 to 100 unit/kg I.V. q 6 or 12 hours until patient shows signs of improvement. Maximum daily dose of Feiba VH Immuno is 200 unit/kg.

How supplied
Available by prescription only
Injection: Number of units of factor VIII correctional activity indicated on label of vial

Pharmacodynamics
Hemostatic action: Unknown. It has been suggested that efficacy of anti-inhibitor coagulant complex may be related in part to the presence of the activated factors, which leads to more complete factor X activation in conjunction with tissue factor, phospholipid, and ionic calcium and allows the coagulation process to proceed beyond those stages where factor VIII is needed.

Pharmacokinetics
Absorption: Administered I.V.
Distribution: Unknown.
Metabolism: Unknown.
Excretion: Unknown.

Route	Onset	Peak	Duration
I.V.	10-30 min	Unknown	Unknown

Contraindications and precautions
Contraindicated in patients with signs of fibrinolysis or disseminated intravascular coagulation and in those with normal coagulation mechanism. Use cautiously in patients with liver disease.

Interactions
Drug-drug. *Antifibrinolytics:* may alter the effects of anti-inhibitor coagulant complex. Don't use together.

Adverse reactions
CNS: headache.
CV: flushing, changes in blood pressure, *acute MI, thromboembolic events.*
GI: nausea, vomiting.
Hematologic: *dissmeinated intravascular coagulation.*
Skin: rash, urticaria.
Other: fever; chills; *hypersensitivity reactions; risk of infection, including viral hepatitis B and HIV.*

Overdose and treatment
None reported, although high doses may predispose the patient to thromboembolic events. Monitor patient closely and treat symptomatically.

Special considerations
• Administer hepatitis B vaccine before giving drug.
• Keep epinephrine readily available to treat anaphylaxis.
• For I.V. use, warm the drug and diluent to room temperature before reconstitution. Reconstitute according to manufacturer's directions. Use the filter needle provided by the manufacturer to withdraw the reconstituted anti-inhibitor coagulant complex solution from the vial into the syringe; the filter needle should then be replaced

with a sterile injection needle for administration. Administer drug as soon as possible. Autoplex T infusions should be completed within 1 hour following reconstitution, Feiba VH Immuno infusions within 3 hours.
• The rate of administration should be individualized according to patient's response. Autoplex T infusions may begin at 2 ml/minute; if well tolerated, may increase infusion rate gradually to 10 ml/minute. Feiba VH Immuno infusion rate shouldn't exceed 2 units/kg/minute.
• If flushing, lethargy, headache, transient chest discomfort, or changes in blood pressure or pulse rate develops because of rapid infusion, stop drug. These symptoms usually disappear with cessation of infusion. Infusion may be resumed at a slower rate.

Patient monitoring
• Assess patient closely for hypersensitivity reactions.

Pediatric patients
• Use cautiously in neonates because of risk of thrombosis or hepatitis.

Patient education
• Reassure patient that because of the manufacturing process, risk of HIV transmission is extremely low.

---

antithrombin III (heparin cofactor I)
ATnativ, Thrombate III

Pharmacologic classification: glycoprotein
Therapeutic classification: anticoagulant, antithrombotic
Pregnancy risk category: B

Indications and dosages
➤ *Prophylaxis and adjunct treatment of thromboembolism related to hereditary antithrombin III deficiency.* **Adults, adolescents, and children:** Initial dose is individualized to quantity required to increase antithrombin III activity to 120% of normal activity as determined 30 minutes after administration. Usual infusion rate is 50 to 100 IU/minute I.V., not to exceed 100 IU/minute. Dose is calculated based on anticipated 1% increase in plasma antithrombin III activity produced by 1 IU/kg of body weight using the formula:

$$\text{Dose} = \frac{\left[\begin{array}{c}\text{desired} \\ \text{level}\end{array} - \begin{array}{c}\text{baseline} \\ \text{level}\end{array}\right] \times \begin{array}{c}\text{body} \\ \text{weight} \\ \text{(kg)}\end{array}}{1.4 \text{ kg}}$$

Maintenance dose is individualized to quantity required to increase antithrombin III activity to 80% to 120%. This usually can be achieved with maintenance doses of 60% of the initial loading dose. Adjustments in maintenance dose or dosing interval should be based on actual plasma antithrombin III levels achieved.

Treatment usually continues for 2 to 8 days except during pregnancy, surgery, or lengthy immobilization, when more prolonged administration may be needed.

How supplied
Available by prescription only
Injection: 500 IU, 1,000 IU

Pharmacodynamics
Antithrombotic action: Administration of exogenous antithrombin III corrects hereditary antithrombin III deficiency, normalizing coagulation-inhibiting capability and inhibiting formation of thromboemboli. It also inactivates plasmin, but to a lesser extent than the clotting factor.

Pharmacokinetics
Absorption: Administered I.V.
Distribution: Binding to epithelium and redistribution into the extravascular compartment removes antithrombin III from the blood. Special receptors on hepatocytes bind antithrombin III clotting factor complexes, rapidly removing them from circulation.
Metabolism: Unknown.
Excretion: Unknown.

Route	Onset	Peak	Duration
I.V.	Unknown	Unknown	Unknown

Contraindications and precautions
No known contraindications. Use with extreme caution in children and neonates because safety hasn't been established.

Interactions
Drug-drug. *Heparin:* Increased anticoagulant effect. Reduction of heparin dosage may be necessary.

Adverse reactions
CV: vasodilation, lowered blood pressure.
GU: diuresis.

Overdose and treatment
No information available. Patients with antithrombin III levels of 150% to 210% were asymptomatic.

Special considerations
• Plasma levels of antithrombin III may be measured with clotting assays or amidolytic assays using synthetic chromogenic substrates. Immunoassays may not detect all congenital antithrombin III deficiencies.
• Transmission of viral disease by drug hasn't been reported to date.
• 1 IU equals the amount of endogenous antithrombin III present in 1 ml of normal human plasma.

• Heparin binds to antithrombin III lysine-binding sites in a 1:1 molar ratio, which results in increased efficacy of heparin.
• Drug isn't recommended for long-term prophylaxis of thrombotic episodes.
• Reconstitute using 10 ml sterile water (provided), normal saline solution, or D₅W. Don't shake vial. Further dilution in same diluent solution is acceptable.
• Solutions should be at room temperature for administration and should be used within 3 hours of reconstitution.

Patient monitoring
• Monitor patient for dyspnea and increased blood pressure if drug is given too rapidly (1,500 IU in 5 minutes).
• Determinations of antithrombin III activity should be performed twice daily until the dosage requirement has stabilized, then performed daily, immediately before dose. Functional assays are preferable because quantitative immunologic test results may be normal despite decreased drug activity.

Breast-feeding patients
• Distribution into breast milk is unlikely because of drug's large molecular size. No problems have been reported in breast-fed infants.

Pediatric patients
• No specific problems have been reported.

Geriatric patients
• No specific problems have been reported.

Patient education
• Reassure patient that risk of HIV transmission is extremely low.

---

apraclonidine hydrochloride
Iopidine

Pharmacologic classification: alpha-adrenergic agonist
Therapeutic classification: ocular hypotensive
Pregnancy risk category: C

Indications and dosages
➤ *Prevention or control of intraocular pressure elevations after argon laser trabeculoplasty or iridotomy. Adults:* Instill 1 drop (1% solution) in the eye 1 hour before laser surgery on the anterior segment, followed by 1 drop immediately after surgery.
➤ *Short-term adjunctive therapy in patients on maximally tolerated medical therapy who require additional intraocular pressure reduction. Adults:* Instill 1 to 2 drops (0.5% solution) in the eye t.i.d.
➤ *Open-angle glaucoma ◇. Adults:* Instill 1 drop (0.5% solution) in the eye b.i.d. or t.i.d.

Reactions may be *common*, uncommon, **life-threatening**, or COMMON AND LIFE-THREATENING.

How supplied
Available by prescription only
Ophthalmic solution: 0.5%, 1%

Pharmacodynamics
Ocular hypotensive action: Apraclonidine is an alpha-adrenergic agonist that reduces intraocular pressure, possibly by decreasing aqueous humor production.

Pharmacokinetics
Absorption: No information available.
Distribution: Onset of action is within 1 hour after instillation, and maximum effect on intraocular pressure reduction occurs in 3 to 5 hours.
Metabolism: No information available.
Excretion: No information available.

Route	Onset	Peak	Duration
Ophthalmic	1 hr	3-5 hr	12 hr

Contraindications and precautions
Contraindicated in patients hypersensitive to apraclonidine or clonidine and in those receiving concurrent MAO inhibitor therapy. Use cautiously in patients with severe cardiac disease, including hypertension and vasovagal attacks.

Interactions
Drug drug: *Topical beta blockers or pilocarpine:* May produce additive lowering of intraocular pressure. Use together cautiously.

Adverse reactions
CNS: insomnia, irritability, dream disturbances, headache, irritability, paresthesia.
CV: *bradycardia,* vasovagal attack, palpitations, hypotension, orthostatic hypotension.
EENT: upper eyelid elevation, conjunctival blanching and microhemorrhage, mydriasis, eye burning or discomfort, foreign body sensation in eye, eye dryness and *itching, hyperemia,* conjunctivitis, blurred vision, nasal burning or dryness or increased pharyngeal secretions.
GI: abdominal pain, discomfort, diarrhea, vomiting, taste disturbances, dry mouth.
Skin: pruritus not related to rash, sweaty palms.
Other: body heat sensation, decreased libido, limb pain or numbness, allergic response.

Overdose and treatment
No information available.

Special considerations
● Closely observe patients who tend to develop exaggerated decreases in intraocular pressure after drug therapy.
Protect stored drug from light and freezing.

Patient monitoring
● Patients with severe systemic disease, including hypertension, need close monitoring of CV status.

● Remind staff to watch closely for vasovagal attack during laser surgery.

Breast-feeding patients
● It isn't known if apraclonidine appears in breast milk. Advise breast-feeding women to consider discontinuing breast-feeding on the day of surgery.

Pediatric patients
● Safety and efficacy in children haven't been established.

Patient education
● Warn patient about the potential for dizziness and drowsiness.

aprotinin
Trasylol

Pharmacologic classification: naturally occurring protease inhibitor
Therapeutic classification: systemic hemostatic
Pregnancy risk category: B

Indications and dosages
➤ *Prophylactic reduction of perioperative blood loss and the need for blood transfusion in patients undergoing cardiopulmonary bypass during repeat coronary artery bypass graft surgery or in selected patients undergoing initial coronary artery bypass graft surgery in whom the risk of bleeding is high because of impaired hemostasis or in whom transfusion is unavailable or unacceptable; surgery on aortic arch* ◇. **Adults:** Usual test dose is 10,000 kallikrein inactivator units (KIU) (1.4 mg) I.V. If no adverse reactions occur within 10 minutes, give loading dose of 2 million KIU (280 mg) I.V. over 20 to 30 minutes while the patient is supine, after induction of anesthesia but before sternotomy. Follow loading dose with continuous I.V. infusion of 500,000 KIU/hour (70 mg/hour). Before cardiopulmonary bypass starts, 2 million KIU (280 mg) of aprotinin should be added to the priming fluid of the cardiopulmonary bypass circuit by replacement of an aliquot of the priming fluid.

If an allergic reaction occurs during injection or infusion of aprotinin, drug administration should be discontinued immediately. Severe acute hypersensitivity reactions should be treated immediately with appropriate therapy (for example, epinephrine, corticosteroids, maintenance of adequate airway, oxygen, I.V. fluids, antihistamines, maintenance of blood pressure), as indicated.

How supplied
Available by prescription only
Injection: 10,000 KIU/ml (1.4 mg/ml)

Pharmacodynamics

Systemic hemostatic action: The precise mechanism by which aprotinin minimizes perioperative bleeding related to coronary artery bypass graft surgery is unclear but appears to involve effects on platelet function as well as on coagulation and fibrinolysis. Aprotinin may improve hemostasis during and after cardiopulmonary bypass by preserving platelet membrane glycoproteins that maintain the adhesive and aggregative capacity of platelets. In addition, aprotinin inhibits fibrinolysis through inhibition of plasmin, plasma, and tissue kallikreins. Because of its effects on kallikrein, aprotinin also inhibits activation of the intrinsic clotting system, a process that initiates coagulation and promotes fibrinolysis.

Pharmacokinetics

Absorption: Not reported.
Distribution: After I.V. injection, aprotinin is rapidly distributed into the total extracellular space, leading to a rapid initial decrease in plasma levels. After this phase, a plasma half-life of about 150 minutes is observed, followed by a terminal elimination phase with a half-life of about 10 hours.
Metabolism: No information available.
Excretion: After a single I.V. dose, from 25% to 40% is excreted in urine over 48 hours.

Route	Onset	Peak	Duration
I.V.	Unknown	Unknown	Unknown

Contraindications and precautions

Contraindicated in patients hypersensitive to beef because drug is prepared from bovine lung.

Interactions

Drug-drug. *Fibrinolytics:* Fibrinolytic effects may be inhibited. Monitor patient.
Heparin: May prolong whole blood–activated clotting time. However, aprotinin shouldn't be used as a heparin-sparing agent.

Adverse reactions

CNS: *cerebral embolism, CVA.*
CV: phlebitis, *cardiac arrest, heart failure, ventricular tachycardia, MI, heart block, atrial fibrillation,* atrial flutter, hypotension, supraventricular tachycardia.
GU: *nephrotoxicity, renal failure.*
Hematologic: *hemolysis.*
Respiratory: pneumonia, respiratory disorder, *apnea,* asthma, dyspnea, pulmonary edema.
Other: *hypersensitivity reactions, anaphylaxis,* fever, *shock, sepsis.*

Overdose and treatment

Maximum amount of drug that can be safely administered in single or multiple doses hasn't been determined. Doses up to 17.5 million KIU have been administered within 24 hours without apparent toxicity.

Special considerations

● Aprotinin is recommended only for selected patients undergoing initial coronary artery bypass graft surgery because of the risks of anaphylaxis (should a second procedure be needed) and renal dysfunction linked to aprotinin therapy.
● Aprotinin is administered by I.V. injection and I.V. infusion through a central venous line; drug also is added to the priming fluid of the cardiopulmonary bypass circuit. No other drug should be administered concomitantly with aprotinin in the same I.V. line. Rapid I.V. administration of large (loading) doses of aprotinin should be avoided because of the potential for hypotension or anaphylactoid reactions.
● Dosage and potency of aprotinin usually are expressed in KIU, but mg also has been used; 1 mg of drug has a potency of about 7,143 KIU.
⚑ ALERT Use caution when administering aprotinin (even in test doses) to patients with previous exposure to drug because of risk of anaphylaxis. In such patients, I.V. administration of an antihistamine shortly before administration of the loading dose of aprotinin is recommended. Patients who experience an allergic reaction to the test dose shouldn't receive additional doses.
● A dosage reduction may be necessary in patients with renal failure. Liver damage occurs as often as renal damage.

Patient monitoring

● Because aprotinin inhibits contact activation of the intrinsic clotting system, therapy prolongs the results of coagulation assays that depend on contact activation, including partial thromboplastin time and celite-activated clotting time assays.
● Even after uneventful administration of the test dose or in patients without previous exposure to aprotinin, the full therapeutic dose of aprotinin may cause anaphylaxis.

Pediatric patients

● Safety and efficacy in children under age 18 haven't been established.

Patient education

● Advise patient to report adverse reactions.

arbutamine hydrochloride
GenESA

Pharmacologic classification: adrenergic agonist
Therapeutic classification: sympathomimetic diagnostic aid
Pregnancy risk category: B

Indications and dosages

➤ *Single-dose diagnostic aid in patients with suspected coronary artery disease (CAD) who cannot exercise adequately*

(stress induction with arbutamine is indicated as an aid in diagnosing the presence or absence of CAD). Adults: Dose is calculated and delivered via the GenESA Device, a closed-loop, computer-controlled, I.V. infusion device. This device initially delivers 0.1 mcg/kg/minute for 1 minute and adjusts dose until maximal heart rate limit (target heart rate set by user) is achieved or to maximum infusion rate of 0.8 mcg/kg/minute (maximum total dose 10 mcg/kg).

How supplied
Available by prescription only
Injection: 20-ml prefilled syringe containing a total of 1 mg (0.05 mg/ml)

Pharmacodynamics
Sympathomimetic diagnostic aid action: By increasing cardiac work through positive chronotropic and inotropic actions, arbutamine acts as a cardiac stress agent to mimic exercise and provoke myocardial ischemia in patients with compromised coronary arteries. Beta-agonist activity provides cardiac stress by increasing heart rate, contractility and systolic blood pressure; alpha-receptor activity decreases the potential for hypotension.

Pharmacokinetics
Absorption: Onset of effect on heart rate is about 1 minute after start of infusion. Drug isn't orally bioavailable.
Distribution: Because of sensitivity limitations of drug assay, pharmacokinetics have been characterized for first 20 to 30 minutes after stopping infusion. Apparent volume of distribution is 0.74 L/kg and plasma half-life is about 8 minutes. Drug is 58% bound to plasma proteins.
Metabolism: Drug is metabolized hepatically to methoxyarbutamine.
Excretion: Drug is 75% eliminated by metabolism to methoxyarbutamine, which is then excreted in either a free or conjugated form in the urine. After I.V. infusion, 84% of total dose is excreted in the urine and 9% in the feces within 48 hours.

Route	Onset	Peak	Duration
I.V.	1 min	Unknown	Unknown

Contraindications and precautions
Contraindicated in patients hypersensitive to drug and in patients with idiopathic hypertrophic subaortic stenosis, a history of recurrent sustained ventricular tachycardia, or heart failure (New York Heart Association class III or IV). Also contraindicated in patients with an implanted cardiac pacemaker or automated cardioverter or defibrillator. Drug contains sodium metabisulfite, a sulfite that may produce an allergic response in susceptible patients.

Avoid use of drug in patients with unstable angina, mechanical left ventricular outflow obstruction (such as severe valvular aortic stenosis), uncontrolled systemic hypertension, cardiac transplant, history of cerebrovascular disease, angle-closure glaucoma, or uncontrolled hyperthyroidism or in those receiving class I agents such as quinidine, lidocaine, or flecainide.

Interactions
Drug-drug. *Beta blockers:* May attenuate arbutamine effects. Discontinue at least 48 hours before giving arbutamine.

Adverse reactions
CNS: anxiety, dizziness, fatigue, headache, hypoesthesia, pain, paresthesia, *tremor*.
CV: *angina pectoris*, **ARRHYTHMIAS**, chest pain, flushing, hypotension, hot flashes, palpitations, vasodilatation.
GI: nausea, dry mouth, taste perversion.
Respiratory: dyspnea.
Skin: increased sweating.

Overdose and treatment
Risk of drug overdose is low, given the rapid onset and short half-life of drug and controlled administration. Signs and symptoms of overdose are those of catecholamine excess, such as tremor, headache, flushing, hypotension, dizziness, paresthesia, nausea, hot flashes, angina, increased sweating and anxiety, tachyarrhythmias, hypertension, MI, and ventricular fibrillation.

Management of overdose should include cessation of infusion, establishment of an airway, and adequate oxygenation. Severe signs and symptoms may be treated with I.V. beta blocker such as metoprolol (7.5 to 50 mg), esmolol (10 to 80 mg), or propranolol (0.5 to 2 mg). Sublingual nitrates should be considered if clinically appropriate.

Special considerations
● Don't dilute drug, and administer only via the prefilled syringe using the GenESA Device.
● Before using the GenESA Device, it is essential to read and understand the manufacturer's directions for use.
● Transient prolongation of corrected QT interval, as measured from surface ECG, occurs with administration. However, this doesn't appear to be linked with an increased risk of arrhythmias.
● Transient reductions in serum potassium levels can occur but rarely to hypokalemic levels.
● Don't administer atropine to enhance drug-induced chronotropic response; coadministration may lead to tachyarrhythmias.
● Safety and efficacy of drug in patients with recent history (within 30 days) of an MI haven't been evaluated; don't use drug in these patients.

Patient monitoring
● Monitor blood pressure, heart rate and a diagnostic quality ECG continuously throughout

drug infusion with cardiac emergency supplies available.

Breast-feeding
• It's unknown whether drug appears in breast milk; avoid use in breast-feeding women.

Patient education
• Tell patient to discontinue use of beta blockers at least 48 hours before test.

argatroban
Acova

Pharmacologic classification: direct thrombin inhibitor
Therapeutic classification: anticoagulant
Pregnancy risk category: B

Indications and dosages
➤ *Prophylaxis or treatment of thrombosis in patients with heparin-induced thrombocytopenia.* *Adults:* 2 mcg/kg/minute, administered as a continuous I.V. infusion; adjust dose until the steady state aPTT is 1.5 to 3 times the initial baseline value, not to exceed 100 seconds; maximum dose is 10 mcg/kg/minute.
✦ *Dosage adjustment.* For patients with moderate hepatic impairment, the initial dose should be reduced to 0.5 mcg/kg/min, administered as a continuous infusion. The aPTT should be monitored closely and the dosage should be adjusted as clinically indicated.

How supplied
Available by prescription only
Injection: 100 mg/ml.

Pharmacodynamics
Antithrombin action: Reversibly binds to the thrombin active site and inhibits thrombin-catalyzed or induced reactions, including fibrin formation, activation of coagulation factors V, VIII, and XIII, protein C, and platelet aggregation. Argatroban is capable of inhibiting the action of both free and clot-related thrombin.

Pharmacokinetics
Absorption: No information available.
Distribution: Argatroban is distributed mainly in the extracellular fluid. Argatroban is 54% bound to human proteins, of which 34% is bound to α1-acid glycoprotein and 20% to albumin.
Metabolism: Metabolized mainly in the liver by hydroxylation. The formation of four metabolites is catalyzed in the liver by the cytochrome P-450 enzymes CYP3A/45. The primary metabolite (M1) is 20% weaker than that of the parent drug. The other metabolites are detected in low concentrations in the urine. The terminal elimination half-life ranges from 39 to 51 minutes.

Excretion: Primary excretion of argatroban is in the feces, presumably through the biliary tract.

Route	Onset	Peak	Duration
I.V.	Rapid	1-3 hr	Until infusion stops

Contraindications and precautions
Argatroban is contraindicated in patients hypersensitive to argatroban or any of its constituents and in patients with overt major bleeding.

Use cautiously in patients with hepatic disease; disease states that create an increased risk of hemorrhage, such as severe hypertension; very recent lumbar puncture, spinal anesthesia, or major surgery, especially involving the brain, spinal cord, or eye; and hematologic conditions linked to increased bleeding tendencies, such as congenital or acquired bleeding disorders and GI lesions and ulcerations.

Interactions
Drug-drug. *Oral anticoagulants:* May prolong PT and INR and increase the risk of bleeding. Monitor patient closely.
Thrombolytics: Increased risk of intracranial bleeding. Avoid concomitant use.

Adverse reactions
CV: *atrial fibrillation, cardiac arrest, cerebrovascular disorder,* hypotension, *ventricular tachycardia.*
GI: abdominal pain, diarrhea, GI bleeding, hemoptysis, nausea, vomiting.
GU: abnormal renal function, groin bleeding, *hematuria,* urinary tract infection.
Hematologic: *decreased hemoglobin and hematocrit.*
Respiratory: coughing, dyspnea, pneumonia.
Other: *allergic reactions,* brachial bleeding, fever, infection, pain, *sepsis.*

Overdose and treatment
Excessive anticoagulation, with or without bleeding, may occur in argatroban overdose.

No specific antidote to argatroban is available if life-threatening bleeding occurs. Discontinue argatroban therapy immediately and monitor aPTT and other coagulation tests. Provide symptomatic and supportive therapy.

Special considerations
• Argatroban is intended for I.V. administration.
• All parenteral anticoagulants should be discontinued before administering argatroban.
• Administration of argatroban with antiplatelet drugs, thrombolytics, and other anticoagulants may increase the risk of bleeding.
• Hemorrhage can occur at any site in the body in patients receiving argatroban. Any unexplained drop in hematocrit or blood pressure or any other unexplained symptoms should lead to consideration of a hemorrhagic event.

Reactions may be *common*, uncommon, *life-threatening*, or COMMON AND LIFE-THREATENING.

• To convert to oral anticoagulant therapy, give warfarin with argatroban at doses of up to 2 mcg/kg/minute until the INR is above 4 on combined therapy. After argatroban is discontinued, repeat the INR in 4 to 6 hours. If the repeat INR is below the desired therapeutic range, resume the argatroban infusion. Repeat the procedure daily until the desired therapeutic range on warfarin alone is reached.

• Dilute in normal saline solution, D₅W, or lactated Ringer's injection to a final concentration of 1 mg/ml.

• Each 2.5-ml vial should be diluted 100-fold by mixing it with 250 ml of diluent.

• Mix the constituted solution by repeated inversion of the diluent bag for 1 minute.

• Prepared solutions are stable for up to 24 hours at 25° C (77° F).

Patient monitoring

• Obtain baseline coagulation tests, platelets, hemoglobin, and hematocrit before therapy. Note any abnormalities.

• Argatroban is monitored by the aPTT. Check aPTT 2 hours after giving argatroban; dose adjustments may be required to get a targeted aPTT (1.5 to 3 times the baseline not to exceed 100 seconds). Steady-state is achieved within 1 to 3 hours after starting argatroban.

Breast-feeding patients

• It's not known whether argatroban appears in breast milk. A decision should be made to discontinue nursing or to discontinue the drug, taking into account the importance of the drug to the mother.

Pediatric patients

• The safety and efficacy of argatroban in patients below age 18 haven't been established.

Geriatric patients

• Effectiveness of drug isn't affected by age.

Patient education

• Advise patient that this medication can cause bleeding, and urge patient to report any unusual bruising or bleeding (nosebleeds, bleeding gums) or tarry stools to the prescriber immediately.

• Advise patient to avoid activities that carry a risk of injury, and instruct patient to use soft toothbrush and electric razor while taking argatroban.

• Instruct patient to notify prescriber if wheezing, trouble breathing, or skin rash occurs.

• Tell patient to notify prescriber if she is pregnant or breast-feeding or recently had a baby.

• Tell patients to nofity prescriber if they have stomach ulcers or liver disease or if they've had recent surgery, radiation treatments, falls, or other injury.

arsenic trioxide
Trisenox

Pharmacologic classification: arsenic trioxide
Therapeutic classification: antineoplastic
Pregnancy risk category: D

Indications and dosages

➤ *Acute promyelocytic leukemia (APL) in patients who have relapsed from or are refractory to retinoid and anthracycline chemotherapy.* Adults and children age 5 and older: (Induction phase) 0.15 mg/kg I.V. daily until bone marrow remission. Maximum 60 doses. (Consolidation phase) 0.15 mg/kg I.V. daily for 25 doses over a period of up to 5 weeks, beginning 3 to 6 weeks after completion of induction therapy.

How supplied

Available by prescription only
Injection: 1 mg/ml

Pharmacodynamics

Arsenic trioxide causes morphological changes and DNA fragmentation resulting in death of promyelocytic leukemic cells.

Pharmacokinetics

Absorption: Unknown.
Distribution: Arsenic is stored mainly in the liver, kidneys, heart, lungs, hair, and nails.
Metabolism: Metabolized in the liver.
Excretion: Excreted in urine in the methylated form.

Route	Onset	Peak	Duration
I.V.	Unknown	Unknown	Unknown

Contraindications and precautions

Contraindicated in patients hypersensitive to arsenic. Use cautiously in patients with heart failure, renal failure, a history of torsades de pointes, QT interval prolongation, or conditions that result in hypokalemia or hypomagnesemia.

Interactions

Drug-drug. *Drugs that can lead to electrolyte abnormalities (diuretics or amphotericin B):* Increased risk of electrolyte abnormalities. Use cautiously.
Drugs that can prolong the QT interval (antiarrhythmics or thioridazine): May further prolong QT interval. Use cautiously.

Adverse reactions

CNS: *headache, insomnia, paresthesia, dizziness,* tremor, **seizures,** somnolence, **coma,** anxiety, depression, agitation, confusion, fatigue, weakness.
CV: tachycardia, **PROLONGED QT INTERVAL,** palpitations, edema, chest pain, ECG abnormalities, hypotension, flushing, hypertension.

EENT: *eye irritation, epistaxis, blurred vision,* dry eye, earache, tinnitus, *sore throat, post nasal drip,* eyelid edema, *sinusitis,* nasopharyngitis, painful red eye.

GI: *nausea, vomiting, diarrhea, anorexia, abdominal pain, constipation, loose stools, dyspepsia,* oral blistering, fecal incontinence, *GI hemorrhage,* dry mouth, abdominal tenderness or distension, bloody diarrhea, oral candidiasis.

GU: *renal failure,* renal impairment, oliguria, incontinence, *vaginal hemorrhage,* intermenstrual bleeding.

Hematologic: *leukocytosis, anemia,* THROMBOCYTOPENIA, NEUTROPENIA, *disseminated intravascular coagulation, hemorrhage,* lymphadenopathy, ecchymoses.

Hepatic: *increased ALT and AST levels.*

Metabolic: *hypokalemia, hypomagnesemia, hyperglycemia, hypocalcemia,* hypoglycemia, acidosis, *weight gain,* weight loss, *hyperkalemia.*

Musculoskeletal: *arthralgia, myalgia, bone pain, back pain, neck pain, limb pain.*

Respiratory: *cough, dyspnea, hypoxia, pleural effusion, wheezing, decreased breath sounds, crepitations, rales,* hemoptysis, tachypnea, rhonci, *upper respiratory tract infection.*

Skin: *dermatitis, pruritus, dry skin, erythema, increased sweating,* night sweats, petechiae, hyperpigmentation, urticaria, skin lesions, local exfoliation, *pallor.*

Other: *fever;* drug hypersensitivity; *pain, erythema, or edema at injection site; rigors;* lymphadenopathy; facial edema; *herpes simplex infection;* bacterial infection; herpes zoster; *sepsis.*

Overdose and treatment

Symptoms of acute arsenic toxicity include confusion, muscle weakness, and seizures. If overdose occurs, immediately discontinue Trisenox. Consider treatment with dimercaprol 3 mg/kg I.M. q 4 hours until life-threatening toxicity has subsided, followed by penicillamine 250 mg P.O. up to q.i.d. (1 gram daily or less).

Special considerations

⚠ ALERT Arsenic trioxide can cause fatal arrhythmias and complete AV block.

⚠ ALERT Arsenic trioxide has been linked to APL differentiation syndrome, characterized by fever, dyspnea, weight gain, pulmonary infiltrates and pleural or pericardial effusions, with or without leukocytosis. This syndrome can be fatal and requires treatment with high-dose steroids.

• Follow facility policy regarding preparation and handling of antineoplastic drugs. The active ingredient is a human carcinogen.

• Dilute with 100 to 250 ml of D_5W or normal saline solution. After dilution, drug is stable for 24 hours at room temperature and for 48 hours if refrigerated.

• Administer I.V. over 1 to 2 hours. Infusion time may be extended up to 4 hours if vasomotor reactions occur.

Patient monitoring

• Perform ECG and obtain potassium, calcium, magnesium, and creatinine levels before starting therapy. Correct electrolyte abnormalities before beginning drug.

• Monitor electrolytes and hematologic and coagulation profiles at least twice weekly during treatment. Keep potassium levels above 4 mEq/dL and magnesium levels above 1.8 mg/dL.

• Monitor patient for syncope and rapid or irregular heartrate. If these occur, discontinue drug, hospitalize patient and monitor serum electrolytes and QTc interval. Drug may be restarted when electrolyte abnormalities are corrected and QTc interval falls below 460 msec.

• Monitor ECG at least weekly during therapy. Prolonged QTc interval commonly occurs between 1 and 5 weeks after infusion, and returns to baseline about 8 weeks after infusion. If QTc interval is greater than 500 msec at any time during therapy, assess patient carefully and consider discontinuing drug.

Pregnant patients

• Caution women of childbearing age to avoid becoming pregnant during therapy. Also recommend consulting with prescriber before becoming pregnant.

• Instruct patient to notify prescriber of all the medications they are currently taking and to check with prescriber before staring any new medication.

Breast-feeding patients

• Arsenic appears in breast milk. Because of the potential for serious adverse reactions in nursing infants, breast-feeding should be discontinued during therapy.

Pediatric patients

• Safety and efficacy haven't been established in children younger than age 5.

Patient education

• Tell patient to report fever, shortness of breath, or weight gain immediately.

• Instruct patient to tell prescriber about all drugs being taken and to check with prescriber before starting any new drug.

• Inform diabetic patient that drug may cause hyperglycemia or hypoglycemia, and instruct him to monitor blood glucose level closely.

---

ascorbic acid (vitamin C)
Cecon, Cevi-Bid, Dull-C, Vita-C

Pharmacologic classification: water-soluble vitamin
Therapeutic classification: vitamin
Pregnancy risk category: A (C if exceeds RDA)

Indications and dosages
➤ *Recommended daily amount of ascorbic acid. Adults:* 60 mg daily.

Reactions may be *common*, uncommon, *life-threatening*, or COMMON AND LIFE-THREATENING.

Smokers: 100 mg daily.
Pregnant women: 70 mg daily.
Lactating women: 90 to 95 mg daily.
Infants and children: 30 to 60 mg daily.
Patients receiving long-term hemodialysis: 100 to 200 mg daily.
➤ *Frank and subclinical scurvy. Adults:* 100 to 250 mg, depending on severity, P.O., S.C., I.M., or I.V. daily or b.i.d.; then at least 50 mg daily for maintenance.
Infants and children: 100 to 300 mg, depending on severity, P.O., S.C., I.M., or I.V. daily; then at least 35 mg daily for maintenance.
➤ *Prevention of ascorbic acid deficiency in those with poor nutritional habits or increased requirements. Adults:* 45 to 60 mg P.O., S.C., I.M., or I.V. daily.
Pregnant or breast-feeding women: At least 60 to 80 mg P.O., S.C., I.M., or I.V. daily.
Children and infants over age 2 weeks: At least 20 to 50 mg P.O., S.C., I.M., or I.V. daily.
➤ *Potentiation of methenamine in urine acidification. Adults:* 4 to 12 g daily in divided doses.
➤ *Adjunctive therapy in the treatment of idiopathic methemoglobinemia. Adults:* 300 to 600 mg P.O. daily in divided doses.
➤ *Reduction of tyrosinemia in premature infants on high-protein diets. Premature infants:* 100 mg P.O. or I.M. daily.
➤ *To increase iron excretion resulting from deferoxamine administration. Adults:* 100 to 200 mg P.O. daily.
➤ *Prevention and treatment of the common cold. Adults:* 1 to 3 g or more P.O. per day.

How supplied

Available by prescription only
Injection: 100 mg/ ml, 250 mg/ml in 2-ml ampules and 2-ml and 30-ml vials; 500 mg/ml in 2-ml and 5-ml ampules and 50-ml vials; 500 mg/ml (with monothioglycerol) in 1-ml ampules
Available without a prescription
Capsules (extended-release): 500 mg
Crystals: 100 g (4 g/tsp), 1,000 g (4 g/tsp, sugar-free)
Liquid: 50 ml (35 mg/0.6 ml)
Lozenges: 60 mg
Powder: 100 g (4 g/tsp), 500 g (4 g/tsp)
Solution: 100 mg/ml
Syrup: 20 mg/ml in 120 ml and 480 ml; 500 mg/ 5 ml in 5 ml, 10 ml, 120 ml, and 473 ml
Tablets: 100 mg, 250 mg, 500 mg, 1,000 mg
Tablets (chewable): 100 mg, 250 mg, 500 mg, 1,000 mg
Tablets (extended-release): 500 mg, 1,000 mg, 1,500 mg

Pharmacodynamics

Nutritional action: Ascorbic acid, an essential vitamin, is involved with the biologic oxidations and reductions used in cellular respiration. It's essential for the formation and maintenance of intracellular ground substance and collagen. In the body, ascorbic acid is reversibly oxidized to dehydroascorbic acid and influences tyrosine metabolism, conversion of folic acid to folinic acid, carbohydrate metabolism, resistance to infections, and cellular respiration. Ascorbic acid deficiency causes scurvy, a condition marked by degenerative changes in the capillaries, bone, and connective tissues. Restoring adequate ascorbic acid intake completely reverses symptoms of ascorbic acid deficiency. Data regarding use of ascorbic acid as a urinary acidifier are conflicting.

Pharmacokinetics

Absorption: After oral administration, ascorbic acid is absorbed readily. After very large doses, absorption may be limited because absorption is an active process. Absorption also may be reduced in patients with diarrhea or GI diseases. Normal plasma levels of ascorbic acid are about 10 to 20 mcg/ml. Plasma levels below 1.5 mcg/ml are linked to scurvy. However, leukocyte levels (although not usually measured) may better reflect ascorbic acid tissue saturation. About 1.5 g of ascorbic acid is stored in the body. Within 3 to 5 months of ascorbic acid deficiency, clinical signs of scurvy become evident.
Distribution: Distributed widely in the body, with large concentrations found in the liver, leukocytes, platelets, glandular tissues, and lens of the eye. Ascorbic acid crosses the placenta; cord blood levels are usually two to four times the maternal blood levels. Ascorbic acid is distributed into breast milk.
Metabolism: Metabolized in the liver.
Excretion: Reversibly oxidized to dehydroascorbic acid. Some is metabolized to inactive compounds that are excreted in urine. The renal threshold is about 14 mcg/ml. When the body is saturated and blood levels exceed the threshold, unchanged ascorbic acid is excreted in urine. Renal excretion is directly proportional to blood levels. Ascorbic acid is also removed by hemodialysis.

Route	Onset	Peak	Duration
P.O., I.V., I.M., S.C.	Unknown	Unknown	Unknown

Contraindications and precautions

No known contraindications. Use cautiously in patients with renal insufficiency.

Interactions

Drug-drug. *Acidic drugs in large doses (more than 2 g daily):* May lower urine pH, causing renal tubular reabsorption of acidic drugs. Monitor patient for expected and adverse effects.
Basic drugs (such as amphetamines or tricyclic antidepressants): May cause decreased reabsorption and therapeutic effect. Monitor patient for expected and adverse effects.
Dicumarol: Influences the intensity and duration of anticoagulant effect. Monitor PT and INR.

Ethinyl estradiol: May increase plasma levels of ethinyl estradiol. Monitor these levels.

Iron: May increase iron absorption in the GI tract, but this increase may not be significant. A combination of 30 mg of iron with 200 mg of ascorbic acid is sometimes recommended.

Salicylates: Inhibited ascorbic acid uptake by leukocytes and platelets. Watch for symptoms of ascorbic acid deficiency.

Sulfonamides: May cause crystallization. Avoid use together.

Warfarin: May inhibit the anticoagulant effect. Monitor PT and INR.

Drug-lifestyle. *Smoking:* May decrease serum ascorbic acid levels, thus increasing dosage requirements of this vitamin. Monitor patient closely.

Adverse reactions

CNS: faintness, dizziness (with too-rapid I.V. administration).
GI: diarrhea.
GU: acid urine, oxaluria, renal calculi.
Other: discomfort at injection site.

Overdose and treatment

Excessively high doses of parenteral ascorbic acid are excreted renally after tissue saturation and rarely accumulate. Serious adverse effects or toxicity are uncommon. Severe effects require discontinuation of therapy.

Special considerations

● Ascorbic acid is a strong reducing agent; it alters results of tests that are based on oxidation-reduction reactions. Large doses of ascorbic acid (over 500 mg) may cause false-negative glucose determinations using the glucose oxidase method, or false-positive results using the copper reduction method or Benedict's reagent.

● Ascorbic acid shouldn't be used for 48 to 72 hours before an amine-dependent test for occult blood in the stool is conducted. A false-negative result may occur.

● Depending on the reagents used, ascorbic acid also may cause interactions with other diagnostic tests.

● Administer large doses of ascorbic acid (1,000 mg daily) in divided amounts because the body uses only a limited amount and excretes the rest in urine. Large doses may increase small intestine pH and impair vitamin B_{12} absorption.

● Administer oral solutions of ascorbic acid directly into the mouth or mix with food.

● Administer I.V. solution slowly.

● Conditions that elevate the metabolic rate (hyperthyroidism, fever, infection, burns and other severe trauma, postoperative states, neoplastic disease, and chronic alcoholism) significantly increase ascorbic acid requirements.

● Prolonged use of large doses results in increased metabolism of ascorbic acid; scurvy may result when reduced to normal.

● Reportedly, patients taking oral contraceptives require ascorbic acid supplements.

● Smokers appear to have increased requirements for ascorbic acid because the vitamin is oxidized and excreted more rapidly than in nonsmokers.

● Use ascorbic acid cautiously in patients with renal insufficiency because the vitamin is normally excreted in urine.

● Patients whose diets are chemically deficient in fruits and vegetables can develop subclinical ascorbic acid deficiency. Observe for such deficiency in elderly and indigent patients, patients on restricted diets, those receiving long-term treatment with I.V. fluids or hemodialysis, and drug addicts or alcoholics.

● Protect ascorbic acid solutions from light. Solution darkens with exposure to light, but this doesn't impair the therapeutic activity of the drug. Ascorbic acid is incompatible with many drugs.

Patient monitoring

● Monitor patient for symptoms of ascorbic acid deficiency, including irritability; emotional disturbances; general debility; pallor; anorexia; sensitivity to touch; limb and joint pain; follicular hyperkeratosis (particularly on thighs and buttocks); easy bruising; petechiae; bloody diarrhea; delayed healing; loosening of teeth; sensitive, swollen, and bleeding gums; and anemia.

Pregnant patients

● Ingestion of large doses during pregnancy has resulted in scurvy in neonates.

Breast-feeding patients

● Administer cautiously to breast-feeding women because ascorbic acid appears in breast milk.

Pediatric patients

● Infants fed on cow's milk alone require supplemental ascorbic acid.

Patient education

● Suggest good dietary sources of ascorbic acid, such as citrus fruits, leafy vegetables, tomatoes, green peppers, and potatoes.

● Instruct patient to cover foods and fruit juices tightly and to use them promptly.

● Advise patients with ascorbic acid deficiency to decrease or stop smoking. Replacement ascorbic acid dosages are greater for the smoker.

● Tell patient to avoid high doses of ascorbic acid if he is prone to renal calculi, has diabetes, is undergoing tests for occult blood in stools, follows a sodium-restricted diet, or takes an anticoagulant.

asparaginase
Elspar

Pharmacologic classification: enzyme
(l-asparagine amidohydrolase) (specific to G1
phase of cell cycle)
Therapeutic classification: antineoplastic
Pregnancy risk category: C

Indications and dosages
Indications and dosages may vary. Check current
literature for recommended protocol.
➤ *Acute lymphocytic leukemia. Adults and
children:* When used alone, 200 units/kg daily
I.V. for 28 days. When used with other chemotherapeutic agents, dosage is highly individualized.

How supplied
Available by prescription only
Injection: 10,000-unit vials

Pharmacodynamics
Antineoplastic action: Asparaginase exerts its
cytotoxic activity by inactivating the amino acid
asparagine, which is required by tumor cells to
synthesize proteins. Because the tumor cells can't
synthesize their own asparagine, protein synthesis and eventually synthesis of DNA and RNA are
inhibited.

Pharmacokinetics
Absorption: Not absorbed across the GI tract
after oral administration; therefore, drug must
be given I.V. or I.M.
Distribution: Distributed primarily in the intravascular space, with detectable levels in the
thoracic and cervical lymph. Crosses the blood-
brain barrier to a minimal extent.
Metabolism: Metabolic fate of asparaginase is
unclear; hepatic sequestration by the reticuloendothelial system may occur.
Excretion: Plasma elimination half-life, which
isn't related to dose or patient's sex, age, or hepatic or renal function, ranges from 8 to 30 hours.

Route	Onset	Peak	Duration
I.V.	Immediate	Immediate	23-33 days
I.M.	Unknown	14-24 hr	23-33 days

Contraindications and precautions
Contraindicated in patients with pancreatitis or
a history of pancreatitis. Also contraindicated in
patients with previous hypersensitivity unless desensitized. Use cautiously in patients with hepatic dysfunction.

Interactions
Drug-drug. *Methotrexate:* Decreased methotrexate effectiveness because asparaginase destroys
the actively replicating cells that methotrexate
needs for cytotoxic action. Avoid use together.

Prednisone: Hyperglycemia may result from an
additive effect on the pancreas. Monitor serum
blood glucose.
Vincristine: Additive neuropathy and disturbances
of erythropoiesis. Avoid use together.

Adverse reactions
CNS: confusion, drowsiness, depression, hallucinations, *intracranial hemorrhage,* fatigue,
coma, agitation, headache, lethargy, somnolence.
CV: *MI.*
GI: HEMORRHAGIC PANCREATITIS, *vomiting,
anorexia, nausea,* cramps.
GU: *azotemia, renal failure,* glycosuria,
polyuria.
**Hematologic: *anemia, hypofibrinogene-
mia,*** depression of other clotting factors,
leukopenia.
Hepatic: elevated AST and ALT levels, *hepatotoxicity.*
Metabolic: *hyperglycemia,* altered thyroid function test results, weight loss.
Skin: *rash, urticaria, hypersensitivity reactions.*
Other: ANAPHYLAXIS, chills, *fatal hyperthermia,* fever.

Overdose and treatment
Signs and symptoms of overdose include nausea
and diarrhea. Treatment is generally supportive
and includes antiemetics and antidiarrheals.

Special considerations
● Reconstitute drug for I.M. administration with
2 ml unpreserved normal saline solution. Don't
administer if precipitate forms.
● I.M. injections shouldn't contain more than
2 ml per injection. Multiple injections may be
used for each dose.
● For I.V. administration, reconstitute with 5 ml
of sterile water for injection or saline solution.
Solution will be clear or slightly cloudy. May further dilute with saline solution or D_5W and administer I.V. over 30 minutes. Filtration through
a 5-micron in-line filter during administration
removes particulate matter that may develop on
standing; filtration through a 0.22-micron filter
results in a loss of potency. Don't use if precipitate forms.
● Shake vial gently when reconstituting. Vigorous
shaking results in a decrease of potency.
● Refrigerate unopened dry powder. Use reconstituted solution within 8 hours.
● Don't use as sole drug to induce remission unless combination therapy is inappropriate. Not
recommended for maintenance therapy.
● Administer drug only in hospital settings with
close supervision.
● I.V. administration of asparaginase with or immediately before vincristine or prednisone may
increase toxicity reactions.
● A skin test should be done before initial dose.
Withdraw 0.1 ml from reconstituted vial and inject into vial containing 9.9 ml of saline solution

or sterile water. Inject 0.1 ml (2 units) intradermally and observe site for at least 1 hour. Erythema and wheal formation indicate a positive reaction.

• Risk of hypersensitivity increases with repeated doses. Patient may be desensitized, but this doesn't rule out risk of allergic reactions. Routine administration of 2-unit intradermal test dose may identify high-risk patients.

• Asparaginase has an unlabeled use as post induction intestification therapy for childhood acute myeloid leukemia.

• Because of vomiting, patient may need parenteral fluids for 24 hours or until oral fluids are tolerated.

• Tumor lysis can result in uric acid nephropathy. This can be prevented by increasing fluid intake. Allopurinol should be started before therapy begins.

• Epinephrine, diphenhydramine, and I.V. corticosteroids must be available for treatment of anaphylaxis.

Patient monitoring
• Monitor CBC and bone marrow function. Bone marrow regeneration may take 5 to 6 weeks.

• Obtain frequent serum amylase determinations to check pancreatic status. If levels are elevated, discontinue asparaginase.

• Monitor hepatic, renal, and CNS function.

• Monitor blood glucose and urine tests for glucose before and during therapy. Monitor patient for signs of hyperglycemia, such as glycosuria and polyuria.

Pregnant patients
• There are no adequate studies indicating safe use in pregnancy.

Breast-feeding patients
• It isn't known if drug appears in breast milk. However, because of the potential for serious adverse reactions and carcinogenicity in the infant, breast-feeding isn't recommended.

Pediatric patients
• Drug toxicity appears to be less severe in children than adults.

Patient education
• Encourage patient to maintain adequate intake of fluids to increase urine output and facilitate excretion of uric acid.

• Tell patient that because drowsiness may occur during therapy or for several weeks after treatment has ended, he should avoid hazardous activities requiring mental alertness.

• Advise patient to watch for signs of bleeding.

aspirin
A.S.A., Ascriptin, Aspergum, Bufferin, Ecotrin, Empirin, Halfprin, Novasen*, ZORprin

Pharmacologic classification: salicylate
Therapeutic classification: nonnarcotic analgesic, antipyretic, anti-inflammatory, antiplatelet
Pregnancy risk category: D

Indications and dosages
➤**Arthritis.** *Adults:* Initially, 2.4 to 3.6 g P.O. daily in divided doses. Increase 325 mg to 1.2 g daily no more frequently than at weekly intervals. Maintenance dosage is 3.6 to 5.4 g P.O. daily in divided doses.
Children: 60 to 130 mg/kg P.O. daily in divided doses.
➤**Juvenile arthritis.** *Children who weigh more than 25 kg (55 lb):* 2.4 to 3.6 g P.O. daily in divided doses.
Children who weigh 25 kg or less: 60 to 130 mg/kg P.O. daily in divided doses. Increase 10 mg/kg daily no more than at weekly intervals. Maintenance dosages usually range from 80 to 100 mg/kg daily; up to 130 mg/kg daily.
➤**Mild pain or fever.** *Adults:* 650 mg to 1.3 g extended-release tablets P.O. q 8 hours, p.r.n.; not to exceed 3.9 g daily.
Adults and children over age 11: 325 to 650 mg P.O. or P.R. q 4 hours, p.r.n.; not to exceed 4 g daily. Or, 454 mg chewing gum chewed for 15 minutes and discarded, p.r.n.; not to exceed 3.63 g daily.
Children ages 6 to 11: 227 mg to 454 mg chewed for 15 minutes and discarded, p.r.n.; not to exceed 1.82 g daily.
Children ages 3 to 5: 227 mg chewed for 15 minutes and discarded, p.r.n.; not to exceed 681 mg per day.
➤**Mild pain.** *Children ages 2 to 11:* 65 mg/kg P.O. or P.R. daily divided q 4 to 6 hours, p.r.n.; not to exceed 2.5 g/m^2.
➤**Transient ischemic attacks and thromboembolic disorders.** *Adults:* 50 to 325 mg P.O. daily (prophylactic in men) and 160 mg to 325 mg (treatment) P.O. daily immediately or within 48 hours of CVA onset.
➤**Treatment or reduction of the risk of MI in patients with previous MI or unstable angina.** *Adults:* For primary prevention, 75 to 325 mg P.O. daily. For secondary prevention, 75 to 325 mg P.O. daily. For treatment, 160 to 325 mg P.O. once daily.
➤**Kawasaki (mucocutaneous lymph node) syndrome.** *Adults:* 80 to 100 mg/kg P.O. daily in four divided doses. Some patients may require up to 120 mg/kg daily to maintain acceptable serum salicylate levels of over 200 mcg/ml during the febrile phase. After the fever subsides, reduce dosage to 3 to 5 mg/kg

---

Reactions may be *common*, uncommon, *life-threatening*, or COMMON AND LIFE-THREATENING.

once daily. Therapy is usually continued for 6 to 8 weeks.

➤ *Rheumatic fever*◊. *Adults:* 4.9 to 7.8 g P.O. daily divided q 4 to 6 hours for 1 to 2 weeks. Then decrease to 60 to 70 mg/kg daily for 1 to 6 weeks. Then gradually withdraw over 1 to 2 weeks. *Children:* 90 to 130 mg/kg P.O. daily divided q 4 to 6 hours.

➤ *Pericarditis following acute MI* ◊. *Adults:* 160 to 325 mg P.O. daily.

➤ *Prevention of reocclusion in coronary revascularization procedures. Adults:* 325 mg P.O. 6 hours after surgery and continued daily for at least 1 year.

➤ *Stent implantation* ◊. *Adults:* 160 to 325 mg P.O. 2 hours before stent placement and continued daily indefinitely.

How supplied
Available by prescription only
Tablets (enteric-coated): 975 mg
Tablets (extended-release): 800 mg
Available without a prescription
Chewing gum: 227.5 mg
Suppositories: 60 mg, 120 mg, 200 mg, 300 mg, 600 mg, 650 mg
Tablets: 325 mg (5 grains), 500 mg, 650 mg
Tablets (chewable): 81 mg
Tablets (enteric-coated): 81 mg, 162 mg, 165 mg, 325 mg, 500 mg, 650 mg
Tablets (extended-release): 650 mg

Pharmacodynamics
Analgesic action: Aspirin produces analgesia by an ill-defined effect on the hypothalamus (central action) and by blocking generation of pain impulses (peripheral action). The peripheral action may involve blocking of prostaglandin synthesis via inhibition of cyclo-oxygenase enzyme.
Anti-inflammatory action: Although the exact mechanism is unknown, aspirin is believed to inhibit prostaglandin synthesis; it may also inhibit the synthesis or action of other mediators of inflammation.
Antipyretic action: Aspirin relieves fever by acting on the hypothalamic heat-regulating center to produce peripheral vasodilation. This increases peripheral blood supply and promotes sweating, which leads to loss of heat and to cooling by evaporation.
Anticoagulant action: At low doses, aspirin appears to impede clotting by blocking prostaglandin synthetase action, which prevents formation of the platelet-aggregating substance thromboxane A_2. This interference with platelet activity is irreversible and can prolong bleeding time. However, at high doses, aspirin interferes with prostacyclin production, a potent vasoconstrictor and inhibitor of platelet aggregation, possibly negating its anticlotting properties.

Pharmacokinetics
Absorption: Absorbed rapidly and completely from the GI tract. Therapeutic blood salicylate

concentrations for analgesia and anti-inflammatory effect are 150 to 300 mcg/ml; responses vary with the patient.
Distribution: Distributed widely into most body tissues and fluids. Protein-binding to albumin is concentration dependent, ranges from 75% to 90%, and decreases as serum level increases. Severe toxic effects may occur at serum levels greater than 400 mcg/ml.
Metabolism: Hydrolyzed partially in the GI tract to salicylic acid with almost complete metabolism in the liver.
Excretion: Excreted in urine as salicylate and its metabolites. Elimination half-life ranges from 15 to 20 minutes.

Route	Onset	Peak	Duration
P.O.			
Tablets	5-30 min	25-40 min	1-4 hr
Buffered	5-30 min	1-2 hr	1-4 hr
Extended	5-30 min	1-4 hr	1-4 hr
Enteric-coated	5-30 min	4-8 hr	Unknown
Solution	5-30 min	15-40 min	1-4 hr
P.R.	Unknown	3-4 hr	Unknown

Contraindications and precautions
Contraindicated in patients hypersensitive to drug and in those with G6PD deficiency or bleeding disorders such as hemophilia, von Willebrand's disease, or telangiectasia. Also contraindicated in patients with NSAID-induced sensitivity reactions and in children with chickenpox or flulike symptoms.

Use cautiously in patients with GI lesions, impaired renal function, hypoprothrombinemia, vitamin K deficiency, thrombotic thrombocytopenic purpura, or hepatic impairment.

Interactions
Drug-drug. *Aminoglycosides, bumetanide, capreomycin, cisplatin, erythromycin, ethacrynic acid, furosemide, vancomycin:* May potentiate ototoxic effects. Monitor patient for this effect.
Ammonium chloride and other urine acidifiers: Increased aspirin blood levels. Monitor patient for aspirin toxicity.
Antacids in high doses and other urine alkalizers: Decreased aspirin blood levels. Monitor patient for decreased salicylate effect.
Antibiotics, corticosteroids, NSAIDs: May potentiate the adverse GI effects of aspirin. Use together cautiously.
Anticoagulants, thrombolytics: May potentiate the platelet-inhibiting effects of aspirin. Monitor PT and INR.
Corticosteroids: Enhanced aspirin elimination. Monitor patient for decreased salicylate effect.
Lithium: Aspirin decreases renal clearance of lithium carbonate, thus increasing serum lithium levels and the risk of adverse effects. Monitor lithium levels.

Phenylbutazone, probenecid, sulfinpyrazone: Aspirin is antagonistic to the uricosuric effect of these drugs. Avoid use together.

Phenytoin, sulfonylureas, warfarin: May cause displacement of either drug and adverse effects. Monitor therapy closely.

Drug-herb. *Feverfew, horse chestnut, ginkgo, kelpware, prickly ash, red clover:* Possible increased risk of bleeding. Discourage concurrent use.

Red clover: Coumarin effects may enhance anticoagulation. Avoid use together. If concurrent therapy is unavoidable, monitor PT and INR closely.

Drug-food. *Food:* Delays and decreases absorption of aspirin. Watch for decreased salicylate effect.

Drug-lifestyle. *Alcohol use*: May potentiate adverse GI effects of aspirin. Discourage use.

Adverse reactions

EENT: *tinnitus, hearing loss.*

GI: *nausea, GI distress, occult bleeding, dyspepsia,* **GI bleeding.**

Hematologic: **leukopenia, thrombocytopenia,** *prolonged bleeding time.*

Hepatic: abnormal liver function test results, **hepatitis.**

Skin: *rash,* bruising, urticaria.

Other: **hypersensitivity reactions (anaphylaxis,** asthma), **Reye's syndrome, angioedema.**

Overdose and treatment

Signs and symptoms of overdose include GI discomfort, oliguria, acute renal failure, hyperthermia, EEG abnormalities, and restlessness as well as metabolic acidosis with respiratory alkalosis, hyperpnea, and tachypnea because of increased carbon dioxide production and direct stimulation of the respiratory center.

To treat aspirin overdose, empty the patient's stomach immediately by inducing emesis with ipecac syrup if patient is conscious, or by gastric lavage. Administer activated charcoal via nasogastric tube. Provide symptomatic and supportive measures (respiratory support and correction of fluid and electrolyte imbalances). Closely monitor laboratory parameters and vital signs. Enhance renal excretion by administering sodium bicarbonate to alkalinize urine. Use cooling blanket or sponging if patient's rectal temperature is more than 104° F (40° C). Hemodialysis is effective in removing aspirin, but is only used in severely poisoned individuals or those at risk for pulmonary edema.

Special considerations

● Aspirin interferes with urinary glucose analysis performed with Diastix, Chemstrip uG, glucose enzymatic test strip, Clinitest, and Benedict's solution, and with urinary 5-hydroxyindoleacetic acid and vanillylmandelic acid tests. Serum uric acid levels may be falsely increased. Aspirin may interfere with the Gerhardt test for urine acetoacetic acid.

● Salicylates must be used cautiously in patients with history of GI disease (especially peptic ulcer disease), increased risk of GI bleeding, or decreased renal function.

● Tablets may be chewed, broken, or crumbled and administered with food or fluids to aid swallowing. Uncoated plain aspirin tablets allowed to remain in contact with mucous membranes of the mouth and aspirin-containing chewing gum have produced mucosal erosions and mouth ulcerations.

● Enteric-coated products are absorbed slowly and aren't suitable for acute therapy. They're ideal for long-term therapy, such as that for arthritis.

● There's no evidence that aspirin reduces the risk of transient ischemic attacks in women.

● Stop aspirin therapy 1 week before elective surgery, if possible.

● Adults shouldn't use drug for self-medication for longer than 10 days.

● Moisture may cause aspirin to lose potency. Store in a cool, dry place, and avoid using if tablets smell like vinegar.

● Patient should take 8 oz (240 ml) of water or milk with salicylates to ensure passage into stomach. Advise patient to sit up for 15 to 30 minutes after taking salicylates to prevent lodging of salicylate in esophagus.

● Consider dose reduction if fever or illness causes fluid depletion.

Patient monitoring

● Monitor vital signs frequently, especially temperature.

● Salicylates may mask the signs and symptoms of acute infection (fever, myalgia, erythema); carefully evaluate patients at risk for infections, such as those with diabetes.

● Monitor CBC, platelets, PT, BUN, serum creatinine, and liver function studies periodically during salicylate therapy to detect abnormalities.

● Assess patient for signs and symptoms of hemorrhage, such as petechiae, bruising, coffee ground vomitus, and black tarry stools.

Pregnant patients

● Aspirin has been used for the prevention of complications in pregnancy including preeclampsia, pregnancy loss with history of antiphospholipid syndrome, and recurrent loss. Generally, avoid use in pregnancy.

Breast-feeding patients

● Salicylates are distributed into breast milk; avoid use during breast-feeding.

Pediatric patients

● Because of epidemiologic association with Reye's syndrome, the Centers for Disease Control and Prevention recommend that children with chickenpox or flulike symptoms not be given aspirin or other salicylates. Don't use long-

---

Reactions may be *common*, uncommon, **life-threatening**, or COMMON AND LIFE-THREATENING.

term salicylate therapy in children under age 14; safety hasn't been established. Don't use more than 5 times per day or for more than 5 days.

Geriatric patients
• Patients over age 60 may be more susceptible to the toxic effects of aspirin. Use cautiously. Effects of aspirin on renal prostaglandins may cause fluid retention and edema, a significant drawback for geriatric patients and those with heart failure.

Patient education
• Tell parents to keep aspirin out of children's reach; encourage use of child-resistant closures because aspirin is a leading cause of poisoning.
• Advise patients receiving high-dose, long-term aspirin therapy to watch for petechiae, bleeding gums, and signs of GI bleeding.
• Instruct patient to avoid use of aspirin if allergic to tartrazine dye.
• Tell patient to take drug with food or after meals to avoid GI upset.

atenolol
Tenormin

Pharmacologic classification: beta blocker
Therapeutic classification: antihypertensive, antianginal
Pregnancy risk category: C

Indications and dosages
➤ *Hypertension. Adults:* Initially, 25 to 50 mg P.O. as a single daily dose. May increase dose to 100 mg daily after 7 to 14 days. Higher doses are unlikely to produce further benefit.
➤ *Chronic stable angina pectoris. Adults:* 50 mg P.O. once daily; may be increased to 100 mg daily after 7 days for optimal effect. Maximum daily dose is 200 mg daily.
➤ *To reduce risk of CV mortality in patients with acute MI. Adults:* 5 mg I.V. over 5 minutes, followed by another 5 mg I.V. 10 minutes later. Start oral therapy (50 mg) 10 minutes after the final dose in patients who tolerate the full I.V. dose. Then, 50 mg P.O. 12 hours later. Thereafter, 100 mg P.O. daily or 50 mg P.O. b.i.d. for 6 to 9 days or until discharged from the hospital.
➤ *To slow rapid ventricular response to atrial tachyarrythmias following AMI without LVD and AV block◇. Adults:* 2.5 to 5 mg I.V. over 2 minutes, p.r.n., to control rate; no more than 10 mg over a 10- to 15-minute period.
✦ *Dosage adjustment.* In patients with renal failure, adjust dosage if creatinine clearance is below 35 ml/minute. If patient has creatinine clearance of 15 to 35 ml/minute, give 50 mg daily. If patient has creatinine clearance below 15 ml/minute, give 25 mg daily. If patient is undergo-

ing hemodialysis, dosage is 25 to 50 mg after each treatment under close supervision.

How supplied
Available by prescription only
Tablets: 25 mg, 50 mg, 100 mg
Injection: 5 mg/10 ml

Pharmacodynamics
Antihypertensive action: Atenolol may reduce blood pressure by adrenergic receptor blockade, thereby decreasing cardiac output by decreasing the sympathetic outflow from the CNS and by suppressing renin release. At low doses, atenolol, like metoprolol, selectively inhibits cardiac beta$_1$-receptors; it has little effect on beta$_2$-receptors in bronchial and vascular smooth muscle.
Antianginal action: Atenolol aids in treating chronic stable angina by decreasing myocardial contractility and heart rate (negative inotropic and chronotropic effect), thus reducing myocardial oxygen consumption.
Cardioprotective action: The mechanism whereby atenolol improves survival in patients with MI is unknown. However, it does reduce the frequency of PVCs, chest pain, and enzyme elevation.

Pharmacokinetics
Absorption: About 50% to 60% of an atenolol dose is absorbed.
Distribution: Distributed into most tissues and fluids except the brain and CSF; about 5% to 15% is protein-bound.
Metabolism: Metabolized minimally.
Excretion: About 40% to 50% of a given dose is excreted unchanged in urine; remainder is excreted as unchanged drug and metabolites in feces. In patients with normal renal function, plasma half-life is 6 to 7 hours; half-life increases as renal function decreases.

Route	Onset	Peak	Duration
P.O.	1 hr	2-4 hr	24 hr
I.V.	5 min	5 min	12 hr

Contraindications and precautions
Contraindicated in patients with sinus bradycardia, greater than first-degree heart block, overt cardiac failure, or cardiogenic shock. Use cautiously in patients at risk for heart failure and in those with bronchospastic disease, diabetes, and hyperthyroidism.

Interactions
Drug-drug. *Alpha adrenergic drugs (such as those found in OTC cold remedies), indomethacin, NSAIDs:* Antihypertensive effects of atenolol may be antagonized. Monitor patient for effect.
Antihypertensives: Atenolol may potentiate antihypertensive effects. Monitor blood pressure.

Insulin, oral hypoglycemics: Altered dosage requirements in stable diabetic patients. Monitor serum glucose levels.

Adverse reactions
CNS: *fatigue,* lethargy, vertigo, drowsiness, *dizziness,* mental depression.
CV: *bradycardia, hypotension, heart failure,* intermittent claudication, changes in exercise tolerance and ECG.
GI: nausea, diarrhea, dry mouth.
GU: elevated BUN and creatinine.
Hematologic: *agranulocytosis, nonthrombocytopenic or thrombocytopenic purpura.*
Hepatic: elevated transaminase, alkaline phosphatase, and bilirubin levels.
Metabolic: hyperkalemia, hyperglycemia, hypoglycemia.
Musculoskeletal: leg pain.
Respiratory: dyspnea, *bronchospasm.*
Skin: rash.
Other: fever.

Overdose and treatment
Signs and symptoms of overdose include severe hypotension, bradycardia, heart failure, and bronchospasm.

After acute ingestion, empty stomach by emesis or gastric lavage; follow with activated charcoal to reduce absorption. Thereafter, treat symptomatically and supportively.

Special considerations
Consider the recommendations relevant to all beta blockers as well as the following.
• Patient should take oral single daily dose at same time each day.
• Drug may be taken without food.
• Dosage may need to be reduced in patients with renal insufficiency.
• I.V. atenolol affords a rapid onset of the protective effects of beta blockade against reinfarction.
• Patients who can't tolerate I.V. atenolol after an MI may be candidates for oral atenolol therapy. Some evidence suggests that gastric absorption of atenolol may be delayed in the early phase of MI. This may result from the physiologic changes that accompany MI or from the effects of morphine, which is commonly administered to treat chest pain. However, oral therapy alone may still provide benefits.
• I.V. atenolol may be given undiluted or diluted no more than 1 mg/minute.
• Protect medication from heat, direct light, and moisture and store at room temperature.
• Caution against abrupt withdrawal of medication; it may precipitate MI and increased angina.

Patient monitoring
• Monitor blood pressure, heart rate, and ECG during I.V. administration.

Pregnant patients
• Atenolol can cause fetal harm (intrauterine growth retardation).

Breast-feeding patients
• Safety hasn't been established. Recommend an alternative feeding method during therapy.

Pediatric patients
• Safety and efficacy in children haven't been established; use only if potential benefit outweighs risk.

Geriatric patients
• Geriatric patients may require lower maintenance dosages of atenolol because of increased bioavailability or delayed metabolism; they also may have greater adverse effects.

Patient education
• Stress importance of not missing doses, but tell patient not to double a missed dose, especially if taking drug once daily.
• Advise patient to seek medical approval before taking OTC cold preparations.

atorvastatin calcium
Lipitor

Pharmacologic classification: 3-hydroxy-3-methylglutaryl-coenzyme A (HMG-CoA) reductase inhibitor
Therapeutic classification: antilipemic
Pregnancy risk category: X

Indications and dosages
➤ *Adjunct to diet to reduce elevated low-density lipoprotein (LDL), total cholesterol, apo B, and triglyceride levels in patients with primary hypercholesterolemia and mixed dyslipidemia.* Adults: Initially, 10 mg P.O. once daily. Increase dose, p.r.n., to maximum of 80 mg daily as single dose. Dosage based on blood lipid levels drawn within 2 to 4 weeks after starting therapy.
➤ *Alone or as an adjunct to lipid-lowering treatments such as LDL apheresis in patients with homozygous familial hypercholesterolemia.* Adults and children over age 9: 10 to 80 mg P.O. once daily.

How supplied
Available by prescription only
Tablets: 10 mg, 20 mg, 40 mg

Pharmacodynamics
Antilipemic action: Inhibits HMG-CoA reductase, an early (and rate-limiting) step in cholesterol biosynthesis.

Pharmacokinetics
Absorption: Rapidly absorbed.

Reactions may be *common,* uncommon, *life-threatening,* or COMMON AND LIFE-THREATENING.

Distribution: Mean volume of distribution is about 565 L. Drug is 98% or more bound to plasma proteins with poor drug penetration into RBCs. It's likely to appear in breast milk.

Metabolism: Extensively metabolized to ortho-hydroxylated and parahydroxylated derivatives and various beta-oxidation products. In vitro inhibition of HMG-CoA reductase by orthohydroxylated and parahydroxylated metabolites is equivalent to that of atorvastatin. About 70% of circulating inhibitory activity for HMG-CoA reductase is attributed to active metabolites. In vitro studies suggest the importance of atorvastatin metabolism by cytochrome P-450 CYP3A4.

Excretion: Eliminated primarily in bile following hepatic or extrahepatic metabolism; however, drug doesn't appear to undergo enterohepatic recirculation. Mean plasma elimination half-life of atorvastatin is about 14 hours, but the half-life of inhibitory activity for HMG-CoA reductase is 20 to 30 hours because of the contribution of active metabolites. Less than 2% of a dose of atorvastatin is recovered in urine following oral administration.

Route	Onset	Peak	Duration
P.O.	Unknown	1-2 hr	Unknown

Contraindications and precautions

Contraindicated in patients hypersensitive to drug and in patients with active hepatic disease or conditions linked to unexplained persistent elevations of serum transaminase levels. Also contraindicated in pregnant or breast-feeding women and in women of childbearing age (except those with no risk of becoming pregnant).

Use cautiously in patients with history of hepatic disease or heavy alcohol use.

Interactions

Drug-drug. *Antacids:* May decrease atorvastatin levels. LDL-cholesterol reduction not affected. Monitor patient.

Azole antifungals, cyclosporine, erythromycin, fibric acid derivatives, niacin: May increase risk of rhabdomyolysis. Avoid use together.

Digoxin: May increase plasma digoxin levels. Monitor serum digoxin levels.

Erythromycin: Increased plasma drug level. Monitor patient.

Oral contraceptives: May increase levels of hormones. Consider when selecting an oral contraceptive.

Drug-food. *Grapefruit juice:* Elevated drug levels and increased risk of adverse effects. Tell patient to take drug with liquid other than grapefruit juice.

Adverse reactions

CNS: asthenia, *headache.*
EENT: pharyngitis, sinusitis.
GI: abdominal pain, constipation, diarrhea, dyspepsia, flatulence.
Hepatic: increased liver function test results.
Musculoskeletal: arthralgia, back pain, myalgia.
Skin: rash.
Other: accidental injury, *allergic reaction,* flulike syndrome, *infection.*

Overdose and treatment

There's no specific treatment for atorvastatin overdose. Treat patient symptomatically, and provide supportive measures as required. Because of extensive drug binding to plasma proteins, hemodialysis isn't expected to significantly enhance drug clearance.

Special considerations

● Withhold or discontinue drug in patients with serious, acute conditions that suggest myopathy or those at risk for renal failure secondary to rhabdomyolysis as a result of trauma; major surgery; severe metabolic, endocrine, and electrolyte disorders; severe acute infection; hypotension; or uncontrolled seizures.
● Use drug only after diet and other nonpharmacologic treatments prove ineffective. Patient should follow a standard low-cholesterol diet before and during therapy.
● Drug may be given as a single dose at any time of day without regard for food.

Patient monitoring

● Before starting drug, exclude secondary causes of hypercholesterolemia and perform a baseline lipid profile. Obtain periodic liver function tests and lipid levels before starting treatment, at 6 and 12 weeks after treatment starts, or after an increase in dosage and periodically thereafter.
● Watch for signs of myositis.

Breast-feeding patients

● Because of the potential for adverse reactions in breast-fed infants, women taking atorvastatin shouldn't breast-feed.

Pediatric patients

● Experience in children is limited to drug doses up to 80 mg daily for 1 year in eight patients with homozygous familial hypercholesteremia. No clinical or biochemical abnormalities were reported in these patients. Safety and efficacy haven't been established in children under age 9.

Geriatric patients

● Safety and efficacy in patients age 70 and older with drug doses up to 80 mg daily were similar to those of patients under age 70.

Patient education

● Teach patient proper dietary management, weight control, and exercise. Explain the importance of controlling elevated serum lipid levels.
● Warn patient to avoid alcohol.
● Tell patient to report adverse reactions, such as muscle pain, malaise, and fever.

• Warn women that drug is contraindicated during pregnancy because of potential danger to the fetus. Advise her to call immediately if pregnancy occurs.

atovaquone and proguanil hydrochloride
Malarone

Pharmacologic classification: hydroxynapthalenedione/biguanide hydrochloride
Therapeutic classification: antimalarial
Pregnancy risk category: C

Indications and dosages
➤ *Prevention of Plasmodium falciparum malaria, including in areas where chloroquine resistance has been reported.* Adults and children who weigh more than 40 kg (88 lb): One adult-strength tablet (250 mg atovaquone and 100 mg proguanil) P.O. once daily with food or milk. Begin 1 or 2 days before patient enters a malaria-endemic area. Continue prophylactic treatment during the stay and for 7 days after return.
Children who weigh 31 to 40 kg (68 to 88 lb): Three pediatric-strength tablets P.O. once daily with food or milk, beginning 1 or 2 days before entering endemic area. Total daily dose is 187.5 mg atovaquone and 75 mg proguanil. Treatment should continue during stay and for 7 days after return.
Children who weigh 21 to 30 kg (46 to 68 lb): Two pediatric-strength tablets P.O. once daily with food or milk, beginning 1 or 2 days before entering endemic area. Total daily dose is 125 mg atovaquone and 50 mg proguanil. Treatment should continue during stay and for 7 days after return.
Children who weigh 11 to 20 kg (24 to 45 lb): One pediatric-strength tablet P.O. daily with food or milk, beginning 1 or 2 days before entering endemic area. Continue treatment during stay and for 7 days after return.
➤ *Treatment of acute, uncomplicated P. falciparum malaria.* Adults and children who weigh more than 40 kg: Four adult-strength tablets, with food or milk, P.O. once daily for 3 consecutive days. Total daily dose is 1 g atovaquone and 400 mg proguanil.
Children who weigh 31 to 40 kg: Three adult-strength tablets P.O. once daily, with food or milk, for 3 consecutive days. Total daily dose is 750 mg atovaquone and 300 mg proguanil.
Children who weigh 21 to 30 kg: Two adult-strength tablets P.O. once daily, with food or milk, for 3 consecutive days. Total daily dose is 500 mg atovaquone and 200 mg proguanil.
Children who weigh 11 to 20 kg: One adult-strength tablet P.O. once daily, with food or milk, for 3 consecutive days.

How supplied
Available by prescription only
Tablets: 250 mg atovaquone and 100 mg proguanil; 62.5 mg atovaquone and 25 mg proguanil

Pharmacodynamics
Antimalarial action: Thought to interfere with nucleic acid replication in the malarial parasite by inhibiting the biosynthesis of pyrimidine compounds. Atovaquone selectively inhibits mitochondrial electron transport in the parasite. Cycloguanil, an active metabolite of proguanil, disrupts deoxythymidilate synthesis by inhibiting dihydrofolate reductase. Atovaquone and cycloguanil are active against the erythrocytic and exoerythrocytic stages of *Plasmodium* sp.

Pharmacokinetics
Absorption: Bioavailability of atovaquone is 23% when the tablet formulation is taken with food. Atovaquone bioavailability varies considerably among people. Dietary fat increases the rate and extent of atovaquone absorption compared with fasting. Proguanil is well absorbed independent of food consumption.
Distribution: Atovaquone is more than 99% protein-bound. Proguanil exhibits moderate (75%) protein binding.
Metabolism: Atovaquone undergoes virtually no metabolism. Proguanil is metabolized to cycloguanil (primarily via cytochrome P-450 2C19) and 4-chlorophenylbiguanide.
Excretion: More than 94% of atovaquone is eliminated unchanged in the feces over 21 days. Proguanil (40% to 60%) and its metabolites are eliminated by the kidneys. The elimination half-life of atovaquone is 2 to 3 days in adults. In adults and children, proguanil has an elimination half-life of 12 to 21 hours.

Route	Onset	Peak	Duration
P.O.	Unknown	Unknown	Unknown

Contraindications and precautions
Contraindicated in patients hypersensitive to atovaquone, proguanil, or any component of the formulation. Use cautiously in patients with severe renal failure because proguanil is renally eliminated. Use cautiously in vomiting patients.

Interactions
Drug-drug. *Metoclopramide:* May decrease atovaquone bioavailability. Consider alternative antiemetics.
Rifampin: Reduces atovaquone plasma level by about 50%. Avoid concurrent use.
Tetracycline: Reduces atovaquone plasma levels by about 40%. Parasitemia should be closely monitored in patients receiving concurrent tetracycline.

Adverse reactions
CNS: asthenia, dizziness, *headache.*

Reactions may be *common,* uncommon, *life-threatening,* or COMMON AND LIFE-THREATENING.

GI: *abdominal pain*, diarrhea, anorexia, dyspepsia, gastritis, *nausea, vomiting*.
Hepatic: elevated transaminase levels.
Musculoskeletal: back pain, *myalgia*.
Respiratory: cough, upper respiratory tract infection.
Skin: pruritus.
Other: fever, flu syndrome.

Overdose and treatment

There have been no reports of overdose of atovaquone and proguanil hydrochloride. In the event of an overdose, provide supportive measures.

Special considerations

● Atovaquone absorption may be decreased by persistent diarrhea or vomiting. Alternative antimalarial therapy may be necessary in patients with persistent diarrhea or vomiting.
● Atovaquone and proguanil haven't been studied in the treatment of cerebral malaria or other forms of complicated malaria.
● In the event of a treatment or prophylaxis failure, an alternative antimalarial is indicated.
● Administer atovaquone and proguanil at the same time each day with food or milk.
● Store tablets at room temperature of 59° to 86° F (15° to 30° C).

Breast-feeding patients

● It isn't known if atovaquone appears in breast milk.
● Proguanil appears in breast milk in small amounts. Therefore, use caution when administering to breast-feeding women.

Pediatric patients

● Safety and efficacy haven't been established in children weighing less than 11 kg.

Geriatric patients

● It isn't known whether older patients respond differently than younger patients. Use cautiously in geriatric patients since they are more likely to have decreased renal, hepatic, and cardiac function.

Patient education

● Tell patient to take dose at the same time each day.
● Advise patient to take medication with food or milk.
● If patient vomits within 1 hour after taking a dose, tell him to repeat dose.
● Advise patient to contact prescriber if he is unable to complete course of therapy as prescribed.
● Instruct patient that, in addition to drug therapy, malaria prophylaxis should include the use of protective clothing, bednets, and insect repellents.

atracurium besylate
Tracrium

Pharmacologic classification: nondepolarizing neuromuscular blocker
Therapeutic classification: skeletal muscle relaxant
Pregnancy risk category: C

Indications and dosages

➤ *Adjunct to general anesthesia, to facilitate endotracheal intubation, and to provide skeletal muscle relaxation during surgery or mechanical ventilation.*
Dosage depends on anesthetic used, individual needs, and response. Doses are representative and must be adjusted. *Adults and children over age 2:* Initially, 0.4 to 0.5 mg/kg by I.V. bolus. Maintenance dosage of 0.08 to 0.1 mg/kg within 20 to 45 minutes of initial dose should be administered during prolonged surgical procedures. Maintenance doses may be administered q 15 to 25 minutes in patients receiving balanced anesthesia.
Children ages 1 month to 2 years: Initially, 0.3 to 0.4 mg/kg by I.V. bolus when under halothane anesthesia. Frequent maintenance doses may be needed.

How supplied

Available by prescription only
Injection: 10 mg/ml

Pharmacodynamics

Skeletal muscle relaxant action: Atracurium produces skeletal muscle paralysis by causing a decreased response to acetylcholine (ACh) at the neuromuscular junction. Because of its high affinity to ACh receptor sites, atracurium competitively blocks access of ACh to the motor end-plate, thus blocking depolarization. At usual doses (0.45 mg/kg), atracurium produces minimal CV effects and doesn't affect intraocular pressure, lower esophageal sphincter pressure, barrier pressure, heart rate or rhythm, mean arterial pressure, systemic vascular resistance, cardiac output, or central venous pressure. CV effects such as decreased peripheral vascular resistance, usually seen at doses greater than 0.5 mg/kg, are caused by histamine release.

Pharmacokinetics

Absorption: Maximum neuromuscular blockade increases with increasing dose. Repeated administration doesn't appear to be cumulative, nor is recovery time prolonged.
Distribution: Distributed into the extracellular space after I.V. administration; about 82% protein-bound.
Metabolism: In plasma, drug is rapidly metabolized by Hofmann elimination and by nonspecific enzymatic ester hydrolysis. The liver doesn't appear to play a major role.

Excretion: Excreted in urine and feces by biliary elimination.

Route	Onset	Peak	Duration
I.V.	2 min	3-5 min	35-70 min

Contraindications and precautions

Contraindicated in patients hypersensitive to drug. Use cautiously in elderly patients, debilitated patients, and patients with CV disease; severe electrolyte disorder; bronchogenic carcinoma; hepatic, renal, or pulmonary impairment; neuromuscular disease; and myasthenia gravis.

Interactions

Drug-drug. *Aminoglycoside antibiotics, beta blockers, clindamycin, depolarizing neuromuscular blockers, enflurane, furosemide, isoflurane, lincomycin, lithium, nondepolarizing neuromuscular blockers, parenteral magnesium salts, polymyxin antibiotics, potassium-depleting drugs, quinidine, quinine, procainamide, thiazide diuretics:* The neuromuscular blockade related to atracurium may be enhanced by many general anesthetics. Carefully monitor patient.

Opioid analgesics: May cause additive respiratory depression. Use drug with extreme caution during and immediately after surgery.

Adverse reactions

CV: *flushing, **bradycardia,** hypotension, tachycardia.*
Respiratory: ***prolonged dose-related apnea,*** wheezing, increased bronchial secretions, dyspnea, ***bronchospasm, laryngospasm.***
Skin: erythema, pruritus, urticaria, rash.
Other: *anaphylaxis.*

Overdose and treatment

Signs and symptoms of overdose include prolonged respiratory depression or apnea and CV collapse. A sudden release of histamine may also occur. A peripheral nerve stimulator is recommended to monitor response and to determine the nature and degree of neuromuscular block. Maintain an adequate airway and manual or mechanical ventilation until patient can maintain respiration unassisted.

For treatment, administer cholinesterase inhibitors, such as edrophonium, neostigmine, or pyridostigmine, to reverse neuromuscular blockade; and atropine or glycopyrrolate to counteract muscarinic adverse effects of cholinesterase inhibitors. Monitor vital signs at least every 15 minutes until patient is stable, then every 30 minutes for next 2 hours. Observe airway until patient has fully recovered from drug effects. Note rate, depth, and pattern of respirations.

Special considerations

• Deliver drug by I.V. injection because I.M. injection causes tissue irritation.

• Dilute to desired concentration, usually 0.2 to 0.5 mg/ml.

• Reduce dose and administration rate in patients in whom histamine release may be hazardous.

• Prior administration of succinylcholine doesn't prolong duration of action of atracurium, but it quickens onset and may deepen neuromuscular blockade.

• Atracurium has a longer duration of action than succinylcholine and a shorter duration than tubocurarine or pancuronium.

• Drug has little or no effect on heart rate and doesn't counteract or reverse the bradycardia caused by anesthetics or vagal stimulation. Thus, bradycardia is seen more frequently with atracurium than with other neuromuscular blocking agents. Pretreatment with anticholinergics (atropine or glycopyrrolate) is advised.

• Alkaline solutions such as barbiturates shouldn't be mixed in the same syringe or given through the same needle with atracurium.

• Use drug only if endotracheal intubation, administration of oxygen under positive pressure, artificial respiration, and assisted or controlled ventilation are immediately available.

• Until head and neck muscles recover from blockade effects, patient may find speech difficult.

• Store in refrigerator at 2° to 8° C. Use within 14 days after removing from refrigerator, even if returned for storage.

• Drug is stable for 24 hours when diluted in most solutions except lactated Ringer's (8 hours); spontaneous degradation occurs more rapidly.

Patient monitoring

• If indicated, assess patient's need for pain medication or sedation. Drug doesn't affect consciousness or relieve pain.

• Watch for bradycardia during drug administration; patient may need I.V. atropine.

• Use a peripheral nerve stimulator to monitor responses during ICU administration; it may be used to detect residual paralysis during recovery and to avoid atracurium overdose.

Pregnant patients

• There are no adequate and controlled studies for use in this population.

Breast-feeding patients

• It's unknown whether drug appears in breast milk; therefore, use cautiously in breast-feeding women.

Pediatric patients

• Safety and efficacy haven't been established for children under age 1 month.

Geriatric patients

• Geriatric patients may be more sensitive to effects of drug.

Reactions may be *common*, uncommon, ***life-threatening***, or COMMON AND LIFE-THREATENING.

Patient education
• Explain all events and procedures because patient can still hear.

atropine sulfate

Pharmacologic classification: anticholinergic, belladonna alkaloid
Therapeutic classification: antiarrhythmic, vagolytic
Pregnancy risk category: C

Indications and dosages
➤*Symptomatic bradycardia, bradyarrhythmia (junctional or escape rhythm).*
Adults: Usually 0.5 to 1 mg by I.V. push; repeat q 3 to 5 minutes, to maximum of 0.03 mg/kg in patients with mild bradycardia or 2.5 mg (0.4 mg/kg) in patients with severe bradycardia or ventricular asystole. Lower doses (less than 0.5 mg) may cause bradycardia.
Children: 0.02 mg/kg I.V. up to maximum 1 mg; or 0.3 mg/m^2; may repeat q 5 minutes.
Note: Dose may be administered at 2½ times the I.V. dose and diluted in 10 ml of normal saline solution (adults) or 1 to 2 ml of half-normal or normal saline solution (child) and administered via the endotracheal tube during CPR if I.V. access unavailable.
➤*Preoperatively for diminishing secretions and blocking cardiac vagal reflexes.* Adults and children who weigh more than 20 kg (44 lb): 0.4 mg I.M. or S.C. 30 to 60 minutes before anesthesia.
Children who weigh less than 20 kg: 0.1 mg I.M. for 3 kg (6.6 lb), 0.2 mg I.M. for 4 to 9 kg (8.8 to 20 lb), 0.3 mg I.M. for 10 to 20 kg (22 to 44 lb) 30 to 60 minutes before anesthesia.
➤*To block adverse muscarinic effects of anticholinesterase agents when these agents are used to reverse neuromuscular blockade produced by curariform agents. Adults:* 0.6 to 1.2 mg for each 0.5 to 2.5 mg of neostigmine or 10 to 20 mg of pyridostigmine administered; administer I.V. a few minutes before the anticholinesterase agent.
➤*Antidote for anticholinesterase insecticide poisoning. Adults:* 1 to 2 mg I.M. or I.V. repeated q 5 to 60 minutes until muscarinic symptoms disappear. In severe cases, 2 to 6 mg may be given initially, repeating doses every 5 to 60 minutes.
Children: 0.05 mg/kg I.V. or I.M. repeated every 10 to 30 minutes until muscarinic signs and symptoms disappear.
➤*Hypotonic radiograph of the GI tract. Adults:* 1 mg I.M.
➤*Short-term treatment or prevention of bronchospasm. Adults:* 0.025 mg/kg administered via nebulizer t.i.d. or q.i.d. to maximum dose of 2.5 mg.
Children: 0.05 mg/kg t.i.d. or q.i.d.

➤*Acute iritis, uveitis. Adults:* 1 to 2 drops (0.5% or 1% solution) into the eye t.i.d. (in children use 0.5% solution) or a small amount of ointment in the conjunctival sac t.i.d.
➤*Cycloplegic refraction. Adults:* 1 drop (1% solution) 1 hour before refraction.
Children: 1 to 2 drops (0.5% solution) into each eye b.i.d. for 1 to 3 days before eye examination and 1 hour before examination.

How supplied
Available by prescription only
Injection: 0.05 mg/ml, 0.1 mg/ml, 0.3 mg/ml, 0.4 mg/ml, 0.5 mg/ml, 0.8 mg/ml, and 1 mg/ml
Ophthalmic ointment: 1%
Ophthalmic solution: 0.5%, 1%, 2%
Tablets: 0.4 mg

Pharmacodynamics
Antiarrhythmic action: An anticholinergic (parasympatholytic) agent with many uses, atropine remains the mainstay of pharmacologic treatment for bradyarrhythmias. It blocks the effects of acetylcholine on the SA and AV nodes, thereby increasing SA and AV node conduction velocity. It also increases sinus node discharge rate and decreases the effective refractory period of the AV node. These changes result in an increased heart rate (both atrial and ventricular).
    Atropine has variable—and clinically negligible—effects on the His-Purkinje system. Small doses (below 0.5 mg) and occasionally larger doses may lead to a paradoxical slowing of the heart rate, which may be followed by a more rapid rate.
Anticholinergic action: As a cholinergic blocking agent, atropine decreases the action of the parasympathetic nervous system on certain glands (bronchial, salivary, and sweat), resulting in decreased secretions. It also decreases cholinergic effects on the iris, ciliary body, and intestinal and bronchial smooth muscle.
Antidote for cholinesterase poisoning: Atropine blocks the cholinomimetic effects of these pesticides.

Pharmacokinetics
Absorption: I.V. administration is the most common route for bradyarrhythmia treatment. With endotracheal administration, atropine is well absorbed from the bronchial tree; drug has been used in 1-mg doses in acute bradyarrhythmia when an I.V. line hasn't been established.
Distribution: Well distributed throughout the body, including the CNS. Only 18% of drug binds with plasma protein (clinically insignificant).
Metabolism: Metabolized in the liver to several metabolites. About 30% to 50% of a dose is excreted by the kidneys as unchanged drug.
Excretion: Excreted primarily through the kidneys; however, small amounts may be excreted in the feces and expired air. Elimination half-life

is biphasic, with an initial 2-hour phase followed by a terminal half-life of about 12¼ hours.

Route	Onset	Peak	Duration
P.O.	½-2 hr	1-2 hr	4 hr
I.V.	Immediate	2-4 min	4 hr
I.M.	5-40 min	20-60 min	4 hr
S.C.	Unknown	Unknown	Unknown
Oph-thalmic	Unknown	½-3 hr	7-10 days

Contraindications and precautions

Contraindicated in patients hypersensitive to drug or sodium metabisulfite and in those with acute angle-closure glaucoma, obstructive uropathy, obstructive disease of the GI tract, paralytic ileus, toxic megacolon, intestinal atony, unstable CV status in acute hemorrhage, asthma, or myasthenia gravis.

Ophthalmic form is contraindicated in patients with glaucoma or hypersensitivity to drug or belladonna alkaloids and in those who have adhesions between the iris and lens. Atropine shouldn't be used during the first 3 months after birth because of the possible association between cycloplegia produced and development of amblyopia.

Use cautiously in patients with Down syndrome. Ophthalmic form should be used cautiously in elderly patients and patients with increased intraocular pressure.

Interactions

Drug-drug. *Amantadine:* May increase anticholinergic adverse effects. Monitor patient carefully.

Anticholinergics, drugs with anticholinergic effects: Additive effects. Monitor patient carefully.

Drug-herb. *Betel palm:* May cause reduced temperature, increasing effects and enhancing CNS effects. Discourage use together.

Jaborandi tree products: Decreased atropine effects. Monitor patient closely.

Jimsonweed: Adverse effects on CV function. Discourage use together.

Pill-bearing spurge: Choline in herb may decrease atropine effects. Tell patient to use together cautiously.

Squaw vine: Tannic acid may decrease metabolic breakdown of atropine. Monitor patient.

Adverse reactions

CNS: *headache, restlessness,* ataxia, disorientation, hallucinations, delirium, *insomnia, dizziness,* excitement, agitation, confusion, especially in geriatric patients (with systemic or oral form); confusion, somnolence, headache (with ophthalmic form).

CV: palpitations and **bradycardia** following low-dose atropine, tachycardia after higher doses (with systemic or oral form), tachycardia (with ophthalmic form).

EENT: photophobia, increased intraocular pressure, *blurred vision, mydriasis,* cycloplegia (with systemic or oral form), ocular congestion with long-term use, conjunctivitis, contact dermatitis of eye, ocular edema, eye dryness, transient stinging and burning, eye irritation, hyperemia (with ophthalmic form).

GI: *dry mouth,* thirst, *constipation,* nausea, vomiting (with systemic or oral form); dry mouth, abdominal distention in infants (with ophthalmic form).

GU: urine retention, impotence (with systemic or oral form).

Hematologic: leukocytosis (with systemic or oral form).

Skin: dryness (with ophthalmic form).

Other: severe allergic reactions, including *anaphylaxis* and urticaria (systemic or oral form).

Overdose and treatment

Signs of overdose reflect excessive anticholinergic activity, especially CV and CNS stimulation.

Treatment includes physostigmine administration to reverse excessive anticholinergic activity and general supportive measures, as necessary.

Special considerations

● With I.V. administration, drug may cause paradoxical initial bradycardia, which usually disappears within 2 minutes.

● High doses may cause hyperpyrexia, urinary retention, and CNS effects, including hallucinations and confusion (anticholinergic delirium). Other anticholinergic drugs may increase vagal blockage.

● Atropine sulfate injection is physically incompatible with norepinephrine bitartrate, mataraminol bitartrate, and sodium bicarbonate injection. A haze or precipitate will form within 15 minutes of mixing with methohexital solutions.

● Store drug at 59° to 86° F (15° to 30° C) and protect from heat, light, and air.

Patient monitoring

● If patient has a cardiac disorder, watch for tachycardia.

● Monitor patient's fluid intake and output; drug causes urine retention and hesitancy. If possible, patient should void before taking drug.

Geriatric patients

● Watch closely for urine retention in elderly men with BPH.

Patient education

● Tell patient to report serious adverse reactions promptly.

● Teach patient how to instill eye medication.

● Warn patient to avoid hazardous activities until blurry vision subsides.

● Advise patient to ease photophobia by wearing dark glasses.

Reactions may be *common,* uncommon, *life-threatening,* or COMMON AND LIFE-THREATENING.

attapulgite
Children's Kaopectate, Diasorb,
Donnagel, Fowler's*, Kaopectate,
Kaopectate Advanced Formula,
Kaopectate Maximum Strength,
K-Pek, Parepectolin, Rheaban,
Rheaban Maximum Strength

Pharmacologic classification: hydrated magnesium aluminum silicate
Therapeutic classification: anti-diarrheal
Pregnancy risk category: NR

Indications and dosages
➤ *Acute, nonspecific diarrhea. Adults and adolescents:* 1.2 to 1.5 g (unless using Diasorb, in which case dose can be as high as 3 g) P.O. after each loose bowel movement; don't exceed 9 g within 24 hours.
Children ages 6 to 12: 600 mg (suspension) or 750 mg (tablet) P.O. after each loose bowel movement; don't exceed 4.2 g (suspension and chewable tablets) or 4.5 g (tablet) within 24 hours.
Children ages 3 to 6: 300 mg P.O. after each loose bowel movement; don't exceed 2.1 g within 24 hours.

How supplied
Available without a prescription
Oral suspension: 600 mg/15 ml, 750 mg/5 ml, 750 mg/15 ml*, 900 mg/15 ml*
Tablets: 300 mg, 600 mg*, 630 mg*, 750 mg
Tablets (chewable): 600 mg

Pharmacodynamics
Antidiarrheal action: Although its exact action is unknown, it's believed that attapulgite absorbs large numbers of bacteria and toxins and reduces water loss in the GI tract.

Pharmacokinetics
Absorption: Not absorbed.
Distribution: Not applicable.
Metabolism: Not applicable.
Excretion: Excreted unchanged in feces.

Route	Onset	Peak	Duration
P.O.	Unknown	Unknown	Unknown

Contraindications and precautions
Contraindicated in patients with dysentery or suspected bowel obstruction. Use cautiously in dehydrated patients.

Interactions
Drug-drug. *Oral drugs:* Impaired absorption. Give attapulgite at least 2 hours before or 3 to 4 hours after oral drugs. Monitor patient for decreased effectiveness.

Adverse reactions
GI: constipation.

Overdose and treatment
Because attapulgite isn't absorbed, an overdose is unlikely to pose a significant health problem.

Special considerations
● Make sure patient achieves adequate fluid intake to compensate for fluid loss from diarrhea.
● Drug shouldn't be used if diarrhea is accompanied by fever or blood or mucus in the stool. Discontinue drug if any of these signs occurs during treatment.

Patient monitoring
● Monitor patient for signs and symptoms of dehydration.

Pediatric patients
● Use only under medical supervision in children under age 3.

Geriatric patients
● Use cautiously and only under medical supervision.

Patient education
● Tell patient to take drug after each loose bowel movement until diarrhea is controlled.
● Instruct patient to call if diarrhea isn't controlled within 48 hours or if fever develops.

auranofin
Ridaura

Pharmacologic classification: gold salt
Therapeutic classification: antiarthritic
Pregnancy risk category: C

Indications and dosages
➤ *Rheumatoid arthritis, psoriatic arthritis◊, active systemic lupus erythematosus◊, Felty's syndrome◊. Adults:* 6 mg P.O. daily, administered either as 3 mg b.i.d. or 6 mg once daily. After 4 to 6 months, may be increased to 9 mg daily (3 mg t.i.d.). If response remains inadequate after 3 months at 9 mg daily, discontinue drug.

How supplied
Available by prescription only
Capsules: 3 mg

Pharmacodynamics
Antiarthritic action: Auranofin suppresses or prevents, but doesn't cure, adult or juvenile arthritis and synovitis. It is anti-inflammatory in active arthritis. This drug is thought to reduce inflammation by altering the immune system. Auranofin has been shown to decrease high serum levels of immunoglobulins and rheumatoid factors in patients with arthritis. However, the exact mechanism of action remains unknown.

Pharmacokinetics

Absorption: When administered P.O., 25% of the gold in auranofin is absorbed through the GI tract.

Distribution: 60% protein-bound and distributed widely in body tissues. Oral gold from auranofin is bound to a higher degree than gold from the injectable form. Synovial fluid levels are about 50% of blood levels. No correlation between blood-gold levels and safety or efficacy has been determined.

Metabolism: The metabolic fate of auranofin isn't known, but it's believed that drug isn't broken down into elemental gold.

Excretion: 60% of absorbed auranofin (15% of the administered dose) is excreted in urine and the remainder in feces. Average plasma half-life is 26 days, compared with about 6 days for gold sodium thiomalate.

Route	Onset	Peak	Duration
P.O.	Unknown	2 hr	Unknown

Contraindications and precautions

Contraindicated in patients with history of severe gold toxicity, necrotizing enterocolitis, pulmonary fibrosis, exfoliative dermatitis, bone marrow aplasia, severe hematologic disorders, or history of severe toxicity caused by previous exposure to other heavy metals.

Use cautiously with other drugs that cause blood dyscrasias or in patients with renal, hepatic, or inflammatory bowel disease; rash; or bone marrow depression. Drug isn't recommended for use in pregnant women.

Interactions

Drug-drug. *Drugs that may cause blood dyscrasias:* Additive hematologic toxicity. Monitor hematologic studies.

Adverse reactions

CNS: confusion, hallucinations, *seizures.*
EENT: conjunctivitis.
GI: *diarrhea, abdominal pain, nausea, stomatitis,* glossitis, anorexia, metallic taste, dyspepsia, flatulence, constipation, dysgeusia, *ulcerative colitis.*
GU: proteinuria, hematuria, *nephrotic syndrome,* glomerulonephritis, *acute renal failure.*
Hematologic: *thrombocytopenia* (with or without purpura), *aplastic anemia, agranulocytosis, leukopenia,* eosinophilia, anemia.
Hepatic: jaundice, elevated liver enzyme levels.
Respiratory: interstitial pneumonitis.
Skin: *rash, pruritus, dermatitis,* exfoliative dermatitis, urticaria, erythema, alopecia.

Overdose and treatment

In acute overdose, empty gastric contents by induced emesis or gastric lavage. When severe reactions to gold occur, corticosteroids, dimercaprol (a chelating agent), or penicillamine may be given to aid recovery. Prednisone 40 to 100 mg daily in divided doses is recommended to manage severe renal, hematologic, pulmonary, or enterocolitic reactions to gold. Dimercaprol may be used together with steroids to facilitate the removal of the gold when steroid treatment alone is ineffective. Use of chelating agents is controversial, and caution is recommended. Appropriate supportive therapy is indicated as necessary.

Special considerations

● Serum protein–bound iodine test, especially when done by the chloric acid digestion method, gives false readings after gold therapy. TB skin test may have an enhanced response. Consider this when interpreting results.

● When switching from injectable gold, initial dose is 6 mg P.O. daily.

● To encourage patient compliance with follow-up, initial prescription should be for 2 weeks and subsequent prescriptions for 1 month.

Patient monitoring

● Discontinue drug if platelet count decreases to below 100,000/mm³.

● Monitor CBC, platelet count, urinalysis, and kidney and liver function tests before therapy for baseline and then monthly.

● Monitor patient for signs of toxicity, which include leukocyte count less than 400/mm³, granulocyte count less than 1,500/mm³, decreased platelet count to 150,000/mm³, proteinuria, hematuria, pruritus, rash, stomatitis, and persistent diarrhea.

● Advise monitoring for uncontrolled diarrhea; dose reduction or temporary discontinuance of drug may relieve diarrhea.

Pregnant patients

● There are no adequate and controlled studies, but clinical experience doesn't indicate evidence of adverse effects on the fetus.

Breast-feeding patients

● Drug isn't recommended for use during breast-feeding.

Pediatric patients

● Controlled clinical trials for the treatment of juvenile rheumatoid arthritis in children ages 4 to 16 are ongoing. Safe dosage hasn't been established; use in children isn't recommended.

Geriatric patients

● Administer usual adult dose. Use cautiously in patients with decreased renal function.

Patient education

● Emphasize importance of monthly follow-up to monitor patient's platelet count.

● Reassure patient that beneficial drug effect may be delayed for 3 months. However, if response is

---

Reactions may be *common,* uncommon, *life-threatening,* or COMMON AND LIFE-THREATENING.

inadequate after 6 to 9 months, auranofin will probably be discontinued.

• Encourage patient to take drug as prescribed and not to alter the dosage schedule.

• Diarrhea is the most common adverse reaction. Tell patient to continue taking drug if he experiences mild diarrhea; however, tell him to call immediately if blood appears in stool.

• Tell patient to continue taking concomitant drug therapy, such as NSAIDs, if prescribed.

• Dermatitis is a common adverse reaction. Advise patient to report rash or other skin problems immediately.

• Stomatitis is another common adverse reaction. Tell patient that stomatitis is often preceded by a metallic taste and advise him to call his prescriber immediately.

---

azathioprine
Imuran

azathioprine sodium
Imuran

Pharmacologic classification: purine antagonist
Therapeutic classification: immunosuppressive
Pregnancy risk category: D

Indications and dosages
➤ **Prevention of the rejection of kidney transplants.** *Adults and children:* Initially, 3 to 5 mg/kg P.O. as a single daily dose on day of transplantation or (rarely) 1 to 3 days before. After transplantation, dosage may be administered I.V., until patient is able to tolerate oral dosage. Usual maintenance dosage is 1 to 3 mg/kg daily. Dosage varies with patient response.
➤ **Severe, refractory rheumatoid arthritis.** *Adults:* Initially, 1 mg/kg (about 50 to 100 mg) P.O. taken as a single dose or in divided doses. If patient response is unsatisfactory after 6 to 8 weeks, dose may be increased by 0.5 mg/kg daily (up to a maximum of 2.5 mg/kg daily) at 4-week intervals. If no response after 12 weeks, discontinue.

How supplied
Available by prescription only
Injection: 100 mg/vial
Tablets: 50 mg

Pharmacodynamics
Immunosuppressant action: The mechanism of immunosuppressive activity is unknown; however, drug may inhibit RNA and DNA synthesis, mitosis, or (in patients undergoing renal transplantation) coenzyme formation and functioning. Azathioprine suppresses cell-mediated hypersensitivity and alters antibody production.

Pharmacokinetics
Absorption: Well absorbed orally.
Distribution: Drug and its major metabolite, mercaptopurine, are distributed throughout the body; both are 30% protein-bound. Azathioprine and its metabolites cross the placenta.
Metabolism: Metabolized primarily to mercaptopurine.
Excretion: Small amounts of azathioprine and mercaptopurine are excreted in urine intact; most of a given dose is excreted in urine as secondary metabolites.

Route	Onset	Peak	Duration
P.O., I.V.	4-8 wk	1-2 hr	Several days

Contraindications and precautions
Contraindicated in patients hypersensitive to drug and during pregnancy. Use cautiously in patients with impaired renal or hepatic function.

Interactions
Drug-drug. *ACE inhibitors:* Increased risk of anemia and severe leukopenia. Use together cautiously.
Allopurinol: Major metabolic pathway of azathioprine is inhibited by allopurinol, which competes for the oxidative enzyme xanthine oxidase. Avoid concurrent use if possible. If use together is unavoidable, reduce azathioprine dose by one-third to one-fourth the usual amount.
Cyclosporine: Decreased cyclosporine levels. Monitor patient for this effect.
Methotrexate: Increased plasma levels of 6-MP, a metabolite. Monitor patient for toxicity.
Pancuronium, tubocurarine: May reverse neuromuscular blockade caused by nondepolarizing muscle relaxants. Monitor patient for this effect.

Adverse reactions
GI: *nausea, vomiting, pancreatitis,* steatorrhea, diarrhea, abdominal pain.
Hematologic: LEUKOPENIA, *bone marrow suppression,* anemia, *pancytopenia, thrombocytopenia, immunosuppression* (possibly profound).
Hepatic: *hepatotoxicity,* jaundice.
Musculoskeletal: arthralgia, myalgia.
Skin: rash, alopecia.
Other: *infections,* fever, *increased risk of neoplasia.*

Overdose and treatment
Signs and symptoms of overdose include nausea, vomiting, diarrhea, and extension of hematologic effects. Supportive treatment may include blood products if necessary.

Special considerations
• If NSAIDs are used to treat rheumatoid arthritis, continue them when azathioprine therapy starts.
• Chronic immunosuppression with azathioprine is linked to an increased risk of neoplasia.

• Reconstitute 100 mg vial with 10 ml of sterile water for injection. The resulting concentration is 10 mg/ml. Visually inspect for particles before use. Drug may be administered by direct I.V. injection or further diluted in normal saline solution for injection or D_5W and infused over 30 to 60 minutes. Use only in patients who are unable to tolerate oral medications.
• If infection occurs, reduce drug dosage.
• If nausea and vomiting occur, dose may be divided or given with or after meals.
• Drug may cause temporary depression of spermatogenesis.

Patient monitoring
• Monitor patient for signs of hepatic damage: clay-colored stools, dark urine, jaundice, pruritus, and elevated liver enzyme levels.
• Watch for unusual bleeding or bruising, fever, or sore throat.
• Monitor hematologic status while patient is receiving azathioprine. CBCs, including platelet counts, should be taken at least weekly during the first month, twice monthly for the second and third months, then monthly.

Pregnant patients
• Drug may cause fetal harm.

Patient education
• Explain possible adverse effects of medication and importance of reporting them, especially unusual bleeding or bruising, fever, sore throat, mouth sores, abdominal pain, pale stools, or dark urine.
• Encourage compliance with therapy and follow-up visits.
• Advise patient to avoid pregnancy during therapy and for 4 months after stopping therapy.
• Tell patient with rheumatoid arthritis that clinical response may not be apparent for up to 12 weeks.
• Suggest taking drug with or after meals or in divided doses to prevent nausea.

azelaic acid cream
Azelex

Pharmacologic classification: naturally occurring saturated dicarboxylic acid
Therapeutic classification: antiacne
Pregnancy risk category: B

Indications and dosages
➤ **Mild to moderate inflammatory acne vulgaris.** *Adults:* Apply a thin film and gently but thoroughly massage into affected areas b.i.d. (morning and evening).

How supplied
Available by prescription only
Cream: 20%

Pharmacodynamics
Antiacne action: Unknown. Antimicrobial action may be attributed to inhibition of microbial cellular protein synthesis.

Pharmacokinetics
Absorption: Azelaic acid cream minimally penetrates the stratum corneum and other viable skin layers. About 4% of the topically applied drug is systemically absorbed.
Distribution: Minimal.
Metabolism: Azelaic acid cream has negligible cutaneous metabolism.
Excretion: Drug is mainly excreted unchanged in urine. Half-life after topical dosing is 12 hours.

Route	Onset	Peak	Duration
Topical	Unknown	Unknown	Unknown

Contraindications and precautions
Contraindicated in patients hypersensitive to any of drug's components. Use cautiously in pregnant and breast-feeding women.

Interactions
None reported.

Adverse reactions
Skin: pruritus, burning, stinging, tingling.

Overdose and treatment
Discontinue therapy.

Special considerations
• Apply drug after thoroughly washing affected areas and patting them dry.
• Wash hands well after applying drug.

Patient monitoring
• If patient has dark complexion, watch for early signs of hypopigmentation after use.

Breast-feeding patients
• Azelaic acid may appear in breast milk. Use cautiously in breast-feeding women.

Pediatric patients
• Safety and effectiveness in patients under age 12 haven't been established.

Patient education
• Tell patient to use drug for full prescribed treatment period.
• Teach patient how to apply drug. Advise against applying occlusive dressings or wrappings to affected areas.
• Tell patient to keep drug away from mouth, eyes, and other mucous membranes. If drug accidentally comes into contact with the eyes, instruct patient to wash eyes with abundant water and call if eye irritation persists.
• Advise patient with dark complexion to report abnormal changes in skin color.

Reactions may be *common*, uncommon, *life-threatening*, or COMMON AND LIFE-THREATENING.

• Warn patient that temporary skin irritation may occur when drug is applied to broken or inflamed skin, usually at the start of therapy. However, tell patient to call if it persists.

azelastine hydrochloride, ophthalmic solution
Optivar

Pharmacologic classification: H$_1$-receptor antagonist
Therapeutic classification: ophthalmic antihistamine
Pregnancy risk category: C

Indications and dosages
➤ *Ocular itching caused by allergic conjunctivitis.* Adults and children age 3 years and older: One drop instilled into affected eye b.i.d.

How supplied
Available by prescription only
Ophthalmic solution: 0.05%

Pharmacodynamics
Thought to be a relatively selective H$_1$-histamine antagonist. It inhibits the release of histamine and other mediators from cells, such as mast cells, involved in the allergic response. Decreased chemotaxis and activation of eosinophils also have been demonstrated.

Pharmacokinetics
Absorption: Relatively low following ocular administration.
Distribution: Unknown.
Metabolism: Unknown.
Excretion: Unknown.

Route	Onset	Peak	Duration
Ophthalmic	Within 3 min	Unknown	About 8 hr

Contraindications and precautions
Drug is contraindicated in patients hypersensitive to any of its components.

Interactions
None reported.

Adverse reactions
CNS: fatigue, *headache.*
EENT: transient eye burning, stinging, conjunctivitis, eye pain, pharyngitis, rhinitis, temporary blurring.
GI: bitter taste.
Respiratory: asthma, dyspnea.
Skin: pruritus.
Other: flulike symptoms.

Overdose and treatment
No information available.

Special considerations
• Indicated only for ocular use.
• Don't use to treat contact lens-related irritation.
• The preservative, benzalkonium, may be absorbed by soft contact lenses.

Patient monitoring
• Monitor patient's eyes for redness.

Breast-feeding patients
• It isn't known whether azelastine appears in breast milk. Because many drugs do, caution should be exercised when giving drug to a breast-feeding woman.

Pediatric patients
• Safety and effectiveness in children younger than age 3 haven't been established.

Patient education
• Instruct patient to prevent contamination of the eye drops by making sure the dropper tip doesn't touch any surface, the eyelids, or surrounding areas.
• Instruct patient to keep bottle tightly closed when not in use.
• Advise patient not to wear a contact lens if his eye is red.
• Warn patient that the preservative, benzalkonium, may be absorbed by soft contact lenses.
• Tell patient who wears soft contact lenses, and whose eyes aren't red, to wait at least 10 minutes after instilling Optivar before inserting contact lenses.

azithromycin
Zithromax

Pharmacologic classification: azalide macrolide
Therapeutic classification: antibiotic
Pregnancy risk category: B

Indications and dosages
➤ *Acute bacterial exacerbations of COPD caused by* Haemophilus influenzae, Moraxella catarrhalis, *or* Streptococcus pneumoniae; *uncomplicated skin and skin structure infections caused by* Staphylococcus aureus, Streptococcus pyogenes, *or* Streptococcus agalactiae; *and second-line therapy of pharyngitis or tonsillitis caused by* S. pyogenes. Adults and adolescents age 16 and older: Initially, 500 mg P.O. as a single dose on day 1, followed by 250 mg daily on days 2 through 5. Total cumulative dose is 1.5 g.
➤ *Community-acquired pneumonia caused by* Chlamydia pneumoniae, H. influenzae, Mycoplasma pneumoniae, S. pneumoniae; *I.V. form can be used for above infections and those caused by* Legionel-

◇ Unlabeled clinical use

la pneumophila, M. catarrhalis, *and* S. aureus. *Adults and adolescents age 16 and older:* 500 mg P.O. as a single dose on day 1, followed by 250 mg P.O. daily on days 2 to 5. Total dose is 1.5 g. For those who require initial I.V. therapy, 500 mg I.V. as a single daily dose for 2 days, followed by 500 mg P.O. as a single daily dose to complete a 7- to 10-day course of therapy. The timing of the change from I.V. to P.O. therapy should be based on patient's clinical response.

➤ *Nongonococcal urethritis or cervicitis caused by* Chlamydia trachomatis. *Adults and adolescents age 16 and older:* 1 g P.O. as a single dose.

➤ *Pelvic inflammatory disease caused by* C. trachomatis, Neisseria gonorrhoeae, *or* Mycoplasma hominis *in patients requiring initial I.V. therapy. Adults:* 500 mg I.V. as a single daily dose for 1 to 2 days, followed by 250 mg P.O. daily to complete a 7-day course of therapy. The timing of the change from I.V. to P.O. therapy should be directed by the prescriber based on patient's clinical response.

➤ *Otitis media. Children over age 6 months:* 10 mg/kg P.O. on day 1; then 5 mg/kg once daily on days 2 to 5.

➤ *Tonsillitis. Children over age 2:* 12 mg/kg P.O. daily for 5 days.

➤ *Chancroid. Adults:* 1 g P.O. as a single dose. *Infants and children:* 20 mg/kg (maximum of 1 g) as a single oral dose.

➤ *Prevention of disseminated* Mycobacterium avium *complex (MAC) in patients with advanced infection with HIV. Adults:* 1.2 g P.O. once weekly alone or with rifabutin. *Children:* 20 mg/kg P.O. (maximum of 1.2 g) weekly or 5 mg/kg (maximum of 250 mg) can be given P.O. daily.

➤ *Prophylaxis of bacterial endocarditis in penicillin-allergic adults at moderate to high risk. Adults:* 500 mg 1 hour before procedure.

➤ *Chlamydial ophthalmia neonatorum. Infants:* 20 mg/kg once daily P.O. for 3 days.

How supplied

Available by prescription only
Injection: 500 mg
Powder for oral suspension: 100 mg/5 ml, 200 mg/5 ml; 300 mg*, 600 mg*, 900 mg*, 1,000 mg/packet
Tablets: 250 mg, 500 mg

Pharmacodynamics

Antibiotic action: Azithromycin, a derivative of erythromycin, binds to the 50S subunit of bacterial ribosomes, blocking protein synthesis. It is bacteriostatic or bactericidal, depending on concentration. Azithromycin is effective against many gram-positive and gram-negative aerobic and anaerobic bacteria in addition to *Borrelia burgdorferi, C. pneumoniae, C. trachomatis, M. pneumoniae,* and MAC.

Pharmacokinetics

Absorption: Rapidly absorbed from the GI tract; food decreases both maximum plasma levels and amount of drug absorbed.
Distribution: Rapidly distributed throughout the body and readily penetrates cells; it doesn't readily enter the CNS. It concentrates in fibroblasts and phagocytes. Significantly higher levels of drug are reached in the tissues as compared with the plasma. Uptake and release of drug from tissues contribute to the long half-life. With a loading dose, peak and trough blood levels are stable within 48 hours. Without a loading dose, 5 to 7 days are required before steady state is reached.
Metabolism: Not metabolized.
Excretion: Excreted mostly in the feces after excretion into the bile. Less than 10% is excreted in the urine. Terminal elimination half-life is 68 hours.

Route	Onset	Peak	Duration
P.O.	Unknown	2½-4½ hr	Unknown
I.V.	Unknown	Unknown	Unknown

Contraindications and precautions

Contraindicated in patients hypersensitive to erythromycin or other macrolides. Use cautiously in patients with impaired hepatic function.

Interactions

Drug-drug. *Aluminum- and magnesium-containing antacids:* May reduce peak plasma levels of azithromycin. Separate administration times by at least 2 hours.
Dihydroergotamine, ergotamine: Acute ergot toxicity has been reported when macrolides have been administered with ergotamine or dihydroergotamine. Use together cautiously.
Drugs metabolized by the hepatic cytochrome P-450 system (such as barbiturates, carbamazepine, cyclosporine, and phenytoin): May result in impaired metabolism of these agents and increased risk of toxicity. Monitor patient for signs of drug toxicity.
Theophylline: Macrolides may increase plasma theophylline levels by decreasing theophylline clearance. Monitor theophylline levels carefully.
Triazolam: Clearance of triazolam may be decreased, increasing the risk of triazolam toxicity. Monitor patient for signs of drug toxicity.
Warfarin: Other macrolides may increase PT and INR; effect of azithromycin is unknown. Monitor PT and INR carefully.

Adverse reactions

CNS: dizziness, vertigo, headache, fatigue, somnolence.
CV: palpitations, chest pain.
GI: *nausea, vomiting, diarrhea, abdominal pain,* dyspepsia, flatulence, melena, cholestatic jaundice, pseudomembranous colitis.
GU: candidiasis, vaginitis, nephritis.
Skin: rash, photosensitivity.
Other: *angioedema.*

Reactions may be *common,* uncommon, *life-threatening,* or COMMON AND LIFE-THREATENING.

Overdose and treatment
No information available. Treat symptomatically.

Special considerations
● Azithromycin has been used investigationally in *Helicobacter pylori* regimens, infections caused by *Bartonella*, Lyme disease caused by *Borrelia burgdorferi*, *Toxoplasma gondii* encephalitis, babesiosis, granuloma inguanale, and AIDS-related cryptosporidiosis.
● Obtain culture and sensitivity tests before giving first dose. Therapy can begin before results are obtained.
● Reconstitute 500-mg vial with 4.8 ml of sterile water for injection. Shake well until drug is dissolved (yields 100 mg/ml). Dilute solution further in at least 250 ml of normal saline solution, half-normal saline solution, D₅W, or lactated Ringer's solution to yield 1 to 2 mg/ml.
◼ ALERT Infuse 500-mg dose of azithromycin I.V. over 1 hour or more. Don't give as a bolus or I.M. injection.
● Oral form shouldn't be used for moderate to severe pneumonia or when complicating risk factors exist.

Patient monitoring
● Monitor liver enzyme levels, especially in patients with impaired renal function.
● Obtain serologic tests for syphilis and cultures for gonorrhea in patients diagnosed with sexually transmitted urethritis or cervicitis. Drug shouldn't be used to treat gonorrhea or syphilis.
● Drug may cause overgrowth of nonsusceptible bacteria or fungi. Watch for signs and symptoms of superinfection.

Pregnant patients
● Preliminary studies have shown drug to be safe for the treatment of chlamydial infection in pregnant women, but there are insufficient data for routine use.

Breast-feeding patients
● It's unknown if drug appears in breast milk. Use cautiously in breast-feeding women.

Pediatric patients
● Safety and efficacy haven't been established in children age 16 and under for I.V. administration and 6 months and under for P.O. administration.

Geriatric patients
● Clinical trials of patients ages 65 to 85 with normal hepatic and renal function, in using the 5-day dosage regimen, yielded no significant pharmacokinetic differences.

Patient education
● Tell patient to take all of drug prescribed, even if he's feeling better.
● Remind patient to take oral suspension on an empty stomach because food and antacids decrease absorption. Patient should take oral suspension 1 hour before or 2 hours after a meal and shouldn't take antacids. Tablets and single-dose products can be taken with or without food or milk; GI distress may be reduced by taking drug with food or milk.
● Instruct patient to promptly report adverse reactions.

---

aztreonam
Azactam

Pharmacologic classification: monobactam
Therapeutic classification: antibiotic
Pregnancy risk category: B

Indications and dosages
➤ *Urinary tract, respiratory tract, intraabdominal, gynecologic, or skin infections; septicemia caused by gramnegative bacteria; adjunct therapy in pelvic inflammatory disease* ◊ *; gonorrhea* ◊. *Adults:* 500 mg to 2 g I.V. or I.M. q 8 to 12 hours. For severe systemic or life-threatening infections, 2 g q 6 to 8 hours may be given. Maximum dose is 8 g daily. For gonorrhea, give 1 g I.M. single dose.
✦ *Dosage adjustment.* In patients with a creatinine clearance of 10 to 30 ml/minute, reduce dose by one-half after an initial dose of 1 to 2 g. If creatinine clearance is below 10 ml/minute, an initial dose of 500 mg to 2 g should be followed by one-fourth of the usual dose at the usual intervals; give one-eighth the initial dose after each hemodialysis session.

How supplied
Available by prescription only
Injection: 500-mg, 1-g, 2-g vials

Pharmacodynamics
Antibacterial action: Aztreonam is a monobactam that inhibits mucopeptide synthesis of the bacterial cell wall. It preferentially binds to penicillin-binding protein 3 (PBP3) of susceptible organisms and often causes cell lysis and cell death.
Aztreonam has a narrow spectrum of activity and is usually bactericidal in action. Aztreonam is effective against *Escherichia coli, Enterobacter, Klebsiella pneumoniae, Proteus mirabilis,* and *Pseudomonas aeruginosa.* It has limited activity against *Citrobacter, Haemophilus influenzae, Klebsiella oxytoca, Hafnia, Serratia marcescens, Enterobacter aerogenes, Morganella morganii, Providencia, Moraxella catarrhalis, Proteus vulgaris,* and *Neisseria gonorrhoeae.*

Pharmacokinetics
Absorption: Absorbed poorly from GI tract after oral administration but is absorbed rapidly and completely after I.M. or I.V. administration.

Distribution: Distributed rapidly and widely to all body fluids and tissues, including bile, breast milk, and CSF. It crosses the placental barrier and is found in fetal circulation.

Metabolism: From 6% to 16% is metabolized to inactive metabolites by nonspecific hydrolysis of the beta-lactam ring; 56% to 60% is protein-bound, less if renal impairment is present.

Excretion: Excreted principally in urine as unchanged drug by glomerular filtration and tubular secretion; 1.25% to 3.25% is excreted in feces as unchanged drug. Half-life averages 1¾ hours. Drug appears in breast milk. It may be removed by hemodialysis and peritoneal dialysis.

Route	Onset	Peak	Duration
I.V.	Unknown	Immediate	Unknown
I.M.	Unknown	< 1 hr	Unknown

Contraindications and precautions
Contraindicated in patients hypersensitive to drug. Use cautiously in patients with impaired renal function and in elderly patients.

Interactions
Drug-drug. *Aminoglycosides, beta-lactam antibiotics (including cefoperazone, cefotaxime, clindamycin, metronidazole, piperacillin):* Synergistic or additive effects occur. Avoid use together.

Chloramphenicol: Antagonistic reaction. Give several hours apart.

Potent inducers of beta-lactamase production (cefoxitin, imipenem): May inactivate aztreonam. Avoid use together.

Probenecid: May prolong the tubular secretion of aztreonam. Avoid use together.

Adverse reactions
CNS: *seizures*, headache, insomnia, confusion.
CV: hypotension.
GI: diarrhea, nausea, vomiting.
GU: transient elevation of creatinine.
Hematologic: *neutropenia*, anemia, *pancytopenia*, *thrombocytopenia*, leukocytosis, thrombocytosis.
Hepatic: transient elevation of LD, ALT, and AST levels.
Other: *hypersensitivity reactions* (rash, *anaphylaxis*), thrombophlebitis at I.V. site, discomfort and swelling at I.M. injection site.

Overdose and treatment
No information is available on the symptoms of overdose. Hemodialysis or peritoneal dialysis increases elimination of aztreonam.

Special considerations
• Aztreonam therapy alters urinary glucose determinations using cupric sulfate (Clinitest or Benedict's solution) and gives false-positive Coombs' test results.

• Drug also has been used to treat bone and joint infection caused by susceptible aerobic, gram-negative bacteria.

• To reconstitute for I.M. use, dilute with at least 3 ml of sterile water for injection, bacteriostatic water for injection, normal saline solution, or bacteriostatic normal saline solution for each gram of aztreonam (15-ml vial).

• To reconstitute for I.V. use, add 6 to 10 ml of sterile water for injection to each 15-ml vial; for I.V. infusion, prepare as for I.M. solution. May be further diluted by adding to normal saline solution, Ringer's solution, lactated Ringer's solution, D_5W, $D_{10}W$, or other electrolyte-containing solutions. For I.V. piggyback (100-ml bottles), add at least 50 ml of diluent for each gram of aztreonam. Final concentration shouldn't exceed 20 mg/ml.

• I.V. route is preferred for doses larger than 1 g or in patients with bacterial septicemia, localized parenchymal abscesses, peritonitis, or other life-threatening infections; administer by direct I.V. push over 3 to 5 minutes or by intermittent infusion over 20 to 60 minutes.

• Solutions may be colorless or light straw yellow. On standing, they may develop a slight pink tint; potency isn't affected.

• Drug may be stored at room temperature for 48 hours or in refrigerator for 7 days.

Patient monitoring
• Monitor renal and hepatic function tests. Reduced dose may be required in patients with impaired renal function, cirrhosis, or other hepatic impairment.

• Test for *Clostridium difficile* in patients with prolonged diarrhea.

Pregnant patients
• There are no adequate controlled studies regarding use in pregnant women.

Breast-feeding patients
• Although drug appears in breast milk, it isn't absorbed from infant's GI tract and is unlikely to cause any serious problems.

Pediatric patients
• Manufacturer doesn't recommend use of drug in infants under age 1 month.

Geriatric patients
• Studies have shown that the half-life of aztreonam may be prolonged in patients ages 65 to 75 because of their diminished renal function.

Patient education
• Tell patient to call immediately if rash, redness, or itching develops.

Reactions may be *common*, uncommon, *life-threatening*, or COMMON AND LIFE-THREATENING.

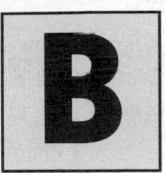

bacillus Calmette-Guérin (BCG), live intravesical
TheraCys, TICE BCG

Pharmacologic classification: biological response modifier
Therapeutic classification: antineoplastic
Pregnancy risk category: C

Indications and dosages
➤ **Treatment of in situ carcinoma of the urinary bladder (primary and relapsed).**
Adults: Consult published protocols, specialized references, and manufacturer's recommendations. Typical dose is 1 to 8×10^8 colony-forming units (CFUs). The Food and Drug Administration has reported errors in some treatment protocols that deliver 10 times the recommended dose.

How supplied
Available by prescription only
Suspension (powder form) for bladder instillation: 50 mg/vial, 81 mg/vial

Pharmacodynamics
Antitumor action: Exact mechanism unknown. Instillation of the live bacterial suspension causes a local inflammatory response. Local infiltration of histiocytes and leukocytes is followed by a decrease in the superficial tumors within the bladder.

Pharmacokinetics
No information available.

Route	Onset	Peak	Duration
Intravesical	Unknown	Unknown	Unknown

Contraindications and precautions
Contraindicated in immunocompromised patients, in those receiving immunosuppressive therapy, and in those with urinary tract infection or fever of unknown origin. If fever is caused by infection, withhold drug until patient recovers.

Interactions
Drug-drug. *Antimicrobial therapy for other infections:* May attenuate the response to BCG live. Avoid use together.
Drugs that depress bone marrow, immunosuppressants, radiation therapy: May impair the response to BCG intravesical because these treatments can decrease the patient's immune response. These treatments also may increase the

risk of osteomyelitis or disseminated BCG infection. Avoid use together.

Adverse reactions
CNS: *malaise.*
GI: *nausea, vomiting, anorexia,* diarrhea.
GU: *dysuria, urinary frequency, hematuria, cystitis, urinary urgency,* nocturia, urinary incontinence, *urinary tract infection,* cramps, pain, decreased bladder capacity, **nephrotoxicity,** genital pain.
Hematologic: *anemia,* **leukopenia.**
Hepatic: elevated liver enzyme levels.
Musculoskeletal: myalgia, arthralgia.
Other: **hypersensitivity reaction,** *fever,* chills, **disseminated mycobacterial infection.**

Overdose and treatment
Closely monitor the patient for signs of systemic BCG infection and treat with antituberculosis medication.

Special considerations
● Tuberculin sensitivity may be rendered positive by BCG intravesical treatment. Determine patient's reactivity to tuberculin before starting therapy.
● Reconstitute drug just before use, using only diluent provided. All persons handling drug should wear masks and gloves.
● Handle drug and all material used for instillation of the drug as infectious material because it contains live attenuated mycobacteria. Dispose of all materials (syringes, catheters, and containers) as biohazardous waste.
● The vial of TheraCys should be reconstituted with 3 ml of the supplied diluent. Don't remove the rubber stopper to prepare the solution. Further dilute in 50 ml of sterile, preservative-free saline solution (final volume, 53 ml). A urethral catheter is instilled into the bladder under aseptic conditions, the bladder is drained, and then the prepared solution is added by gravity feed. The catheter is then removed.
● Use strict aseptic technique to administer drug, thus minimizing trauma to the GU tract and preventing introduction of other contaminants to the area.
● If there's evidence of traumatic catheterization, don't administer drug and delay treatment for at least 1 week. Subsequent treatment may resume as if no interruption of the schedule has occurred.
● Bladder irritation can be treated symptomatically with phenazopyridine, acetaminophen, and propantheline bromide. Systemic adverse reac-

tions caused by hypersensitivity can be treated with diphenhydramine hydrochloride.
● Protect drug from light and store at less than 41° F (5° C). Drug expires 1 year after date of issue if stored at this temperature.

Patient monitoring
● Monitor patient for cystitis and hematuria.

Breast-feeding patients
● It isn't known if drug appears in breast milk. Use cautiously in breast-feeding women.

Pediatric patients
● Safety in children hasn't been established.

Patient education
● After instillation, patient should retain the fluid in bladder for 2 hours (if possible). For the first hour, tell patient to lie 15 minutes prone, 15 minutes supine, and 15 minutes on each side. Patient may be up for the second hour.
● For safety, patient should be seated when voiding. Instruct patient to disinfect urine for 6 hours after instillation of drug. Tell patient to add undiluted household bleach (5% sodium hypochlorite solution) in equal volume to voided urine to the toilet; let stand for 15 minutes before flushing.
● Tell patient to call if symptoms worsen or if the following occur: blood in the urine, fever and chills, frequent urge to urinate or painful urination, nausea, vomiting, joint pain, rash, or cough.

---

bacillus Calmette-Guérin (BCG), live
PACIS

Pharmacologic classification: live attenuated bacteria
Therapeutic classification: antineoplastic
Pregnancy risk category: C

Indications and dosages
➤ *Treatment of bladder carcinoma in situ (CIS) in the absence of an associated invasive cancer in the following situations: primary treatment of CIS with or without papillary tumors after transurethral resection; secondary treatment of CIS in patients failing to respond or relapsing after intravesical therapy with other drugs; primary or secondary treatment of CIS for patients with medical contraindications to radical surgery.* Adults: Instill 1 ampule (120 mg) intravesically into the bladder slowly by gravity flow, via catheter. The solution is retained in the bladder for 2 hours and then voided. The recommended induction course of therapy is a single dose of 120 mg instilled into the bladder once weekly for 6 weeks. Schedule may be repeated if tumor remission hasn't been achieved and if clinical circumstances warrant.

How supplied
Available by prescription only
Single-dose ampule of lyophilized BCG: 120 mg

Pharmacodynamics
Immunotherapeutic action: The mechanism of action in the treatment of CIS is unknown; however, evidence suggests that intravesical BCG is a form of immunotherapy. It induces tumor regression through specific and nonspecific actions. It promotes a local inflammatory reaction with histiocytic and leukocytic infiltration in the urinary bladder that apparently reduces or eliminates superficial cancerous lesions.

Pharmacokinetics
Absorption: None; not absorbed from the bladder.
Distribution: None.
Metabolism: None.
Excretion: Drug is excreted when the bladder is emptied.

Route	Onset	Peak	Duration
Intra-vesical	Not applicable	Not applicable	Not applicable

Contraindications and precautions
Contraindicated in immunosuppressed patients, patients with congenital or acquired immune deficiencies, patients receiving corticosteroids at immunosuppressive doses or other immunosuppressive therapies, patients with active tuberculosis, patients positive for HIV, and patients with a febrile illness, urinary tract infection, or gross hematuria. Also contraindicated within 7 to14 days of biopsy, transurethral resection of the prostate, or traumatic catheterization.

Use cautiously in patients at high risk for HIV infection and in those with small bladder capacity.

Interactions
Drug-drug. *Antimicrobials:* Therapy for other infections may interfere with the effectiveness of BCG. Avoid concomitant use.
Immunosuppressants, including bone marrow suppressants and radiation: Disrupted development of immune response, which decreases the efficacy of BCG. Avoid concomitant use.

Adverse reactions
GI: abdominal pain, diarrhea.
GU: bladder irritability, *dysuria, cystitis, urgency, frequency, hematuria, nocturia,* urinary incontinence, urine retention, urinary tract infection, foreign material in urine, local pain.
Other: *fever, flu syndrome,* chills, *BCG systemic infection.*

Overdose and treatment
Overdose occurs if more than 1 ampule is administered per instillation. If overdose occurs, monitor patient closely for active local or sys-

---

temic BCG infection (fever and acute localized inflammation such as epididymitis, prostatitis, or orchitis that persists longer than 2 to 3 days). If there are signs of active local or systemic infection, consult an infectious disease specialist experienced in BCG complications. BCG in this drug is sensitive to isoniazid, rifampin and ethambutol, clofazimine, cycloserine, ethionamide, para-aminosalicylic acid, rifabutin, and thiacetazone. It isn't sensitive to pyrazinamide. If infection is suspected, BCG treatment should be suspended and the patient should be treated with two or more antimycobacterials while diagnostic evaluation, including cultures, is conducted.

Special considerations

● May cause tuberculin sensitivity in patients previously negative to purified protein derivative (PPD).
● Intravesical treatment should begin 7 to 14 days after biopsy or transurethral resection.
● To avoid cross-contamination, parenteral drugs shouldn't be prepared in areas where BCG has been in use.
⚠ ALERT To prepare the suspension, use sterile technique and a biocontainment hood. If preparation can't be performed this way, wear gloves, mask, and gown to avoid inadvertent exposure to broken skin or inhalation of BCG organisms.
● Add 1 ml of sterile diluent (preservative-free saline injection USP) to 1 ampule of BCG to resuspend. Leave drug and diluent in contact for 1 minute. Then mix the suspension by withdrawing it into the syringe and expelling it gently back into the ampule two or three times. Avoid producing foam—don't shake. Dilute the reconstituted product in an additional 49 ml of saline solution, bringing the total volume to 50 ml.
● The suspension should be used immediately after preparation. Discard prepared suspension after 2 hours.
● After use, all equipment should be sterilized or disposed of properly as with other biohazardous waste.
● At no time should the reconstituted product be exposed to direct or indirect sunlight. Exposure to artificial light should be kept to a minimum.
● Don't allow patient to drink fluids for 4 hours before treatment, and have him empty his bladder before administration.
● The reconstituted suspension is instilled into the bladder slowly by gravity flow through the catheter. Don't force the flow of the suspension. Suspension is retained in the bladder for 2 hours and then voided.
● Patients unable to retain the suspension for 2 hours should be allowed to void sooner, if necessary.
● During the first hour after instillation, patient should lie for 15 minutes each in the prone and supine positions and on each side. He is then allowed to be up but should retain the suspension for another 60 minutes, for a total of 2 hours.

● Instruct patient to drink enough liquid after treatment to maintain adequate hydration.
● Instillation of BCG onto a bleeding mucosa may promote systemic BCG infection. Treatment should be postponed for at least 1 week after transurethral resection, biopsy, traumatic catheterization, or gross hematuria.
● Drug should be stored in a refrigerator at a temperature between 2° and 8° C (36° and 45° F).
● Flulike symptoms may be treated symptomatically with antihistamines.
● Drug may cause tuberculin sensitivity. If indicated, determine the tuberculin reactivity by PPD skin test before administration of BCG.

Patient monitoring
⚠ ALERT Monitor patient for symptoms and signs of toxicity after each intravesical treatment. Febrile episodes with flulike symptoms lasting more than 72 hours, fever higher than 39.4° C (103° F), systemic effects increasing in intensity with repeated instillations, or persistent abnormalities of liver function tests suggest BCG infection and may require antituberculosis therapy. Local symptoms (prostatitis, epididymitis, orchitis) lasting more than 2 to 3 days also may suggest active infection.
● Monitor patient for irritative bladder symptoms. These usually can be managed symptomatically with Pyridium, propantheline bromide, or oxybutynin chloride together with acetaminophen or ibuprofen.

Breast-feeding patients
● It's unknown if BCG appears in breast milk. Because many drugs do and because of the risk of serious adverse reactions from BCG in nursing infants, it's advisable to discontinue either nursing or drug, taking into consideration the importance of the drug to the mother.

Pediatric patients
● Safety and efficacy of BCG for treatment of CIS of the urinary bladder in children haven't been established.

Patient education
● Advise patient not to drink fluids for 4 hours before treatment and to empty his bladder before administration of the drug.
● Drug is retained in bladder for 2 hours, then voided.
● Advise patient to void in a seated position to avoid splashing of urine after treatment.
● Tell patient that urine voided during the 6 hours after instillation must be disinfected with an equal volume of 5% sodium hypochlorite solution (undiluted household bleach) and allowed to stand for 15 minutes before flushing.
● Instruct patient to increase fluid intake after BCG treatment to flush the bladder.
● Warn patient that he may experience burning with the first void after treatment.

bacitracin
AK-Tracin, Altracin, Baciguent,
Baci-IM

Pharmacologic classification: polypeptide
antibiotic
Therapeutic classification: antibiotic
Pregnancy risk category: C

Indications and dosages
➤ *Topical infections, impetigo, abrasions, cuts, minor wounds. Adults and children:* Apply thin film to cleansed area once daily
to t.i.d. for no more than 7 days.
➤ *Pneumonia and empyema caused by a
staphylococcal infection. Children who
weigh 2.5 kg (5.5 lb) or less:* 900 units/kg I.M.
daily in two or three divided doses.
Children who weigh more than 2.5 kg: 1,000
units/kg I.M. daily in two or three divided doses.
Adults ◇ : 10,000 to 25,000 units I.M. q 6 hours
not to exceed 100,000 units daily.
➤ *Treatment of antibiotic-related pseudomembranous colitis caused by* Clostridium difficile ◇ . *Adults:* 20,000 to 25,000 units
P.O. q 6 hours for 7 to 10 days.
➤ *Short-term topical treatment of superficial infections of the eye involving the
conjunctiva and cornea caused by baci-
tracin-susceptible organisms. Adults and
children:* Apply ophthalmic ointment to affected
area 1 or more times daily.

How supplied
Available by prescription only
Injection: 50,000-unit vials
Ophthalmic ointment: 500 units/g
Available without a prescription
Topical: ointment form (500 units/g) and in
combination products containing neomycin,
polymyxin B, and bacitracin

Pharmacodynamics
Antibacterial action: Bacitracin impairs bacterial cell wall synthesis, damaging the bacterial
plasma membrane and making the cell more vulnerable to osmotic pressure. Drug is effective
against many gram-positive organisms such as
staphylococci, streptococci, anaerobic cocci,
corynebacteria, and *C. difficile.* The drug is also
effective against gonococci, meningococci, fu-
sobacteria, *Actinomyces israelii, Treponema
pallidum,* and *Treponema vincenti.* Drug is only
minimally active against gram-negative organisms.

Pharmacokinetics
Absorption: Drug is absorbed rapidly and completely after I.M. use; serum levels range from
0.2 to 2 mcg/ml. Drug isn't absorbed from the
GI tract and isn't significantly absorbed from intact or denuded skin wounds or mucous membranes.

Distribution: Distributed widely throughout all
body organs and fluids except CSF (unless
meninges are inflamed). Binding to plasma protein is minimal.
Metabolism: Not significantly metabolized.
Excretion: When drug is given I.M., the kidneys
excrete 10% to 40% of dose.

Route	Onset	Peak	Duration
I.M.	Unknown	1-2 hr	Unknown
Ophthal-mic, topical	Unknown	Unknown	Unknown

Contraindications and precautions
Contraindicated in patients hypersensitive to drug
and in atopic patients. Use cautiously in patients
with myasthenia gravis and neuromuscular
disease.

Interactions
Drug-drug. *Anesthetics, neuromuscular blockers:* Prolonged or increased neuromuscular
blockade. Carefully monitor patient.
Other nephrotoxic drugs: Systemically administered bacitracin may induce additive damage
when given with bacitracin. Administer together
cautiously.

Adverse reactions
CV: tightness in chest, hypotension.
EENT: slowed corneal wound healing, temporary visual haze (with ophthalmic form), ototoxicity (when topical form is used over large areas for prolonged periods or with systemic use).
GU: *nephrotoxicity, renal failure.*
Skin: stinging, rash, other allergic reactions, pruritus, burning, swelling of lips or face (with topical form).
Other: *hypersensitivity reactions;* overgrowth of nonsusceptible organisms with ophthalmic form.

Overdose and treatment
With parenteral administration over several days,
bacitracin may cause nephrotoxicity. Acute oral
overdose may cause nausea, vomiting, and minor GI upset. Treatment is supportive.

Special considerations
• Bacitracin has been used orally as an intestinal antiseptic. Sterile solutions have been injected intrathecally for the treatment of meningitis,
intraperitoneally for peritoneal infections, in-
trapleurally for staphylococcal empyema, and intrasynovially after surgical treatment of chronic
osteomyelitis.
• Culture and sensitivity tests should be done before starting treatment.
• Patients allergic to neomycin also may be allergic to bacitracin.
• Injectable forms of drug may be used only for
I.M. administration. I.V. administration may cause
severe thrombophlebitis. Dilute injectable drug
in solution containing sodium chloride and 2%

procaine hydrochloride (if hospital policy permits). After reconstitution, bacitracin concentration should range from 5,000 to 10,000 units/ml. Inject deep into upper outer quadrant of buttocks (may be painful). Don't give if patient is sensitive to procaine or para-aminobenzoic acid derivatives.

• Drug may be used orally with neomycin as bowel preparation or in solution as wound irrigating agent.

Patient monitoring
• Obtain baseline renal function studies before starting therapy, and monitor results daily for signs of deterioration.
• Make sure patient has adequate fluid intake, and monitor output closely.
• Monitor patient's urine pH. It should be kept above 6 with good hydration, and alkalinizing agents (such as sodium bicarbonate) should be given, if necessary, to limit nephrotoxicity.

Pregnant patients
• Bacitracin shouldn't be used in pregnancy.

Patient education
• Advise patient to discontinue topical use of drug and to call promptly if condition worsens or doesn't respond to treatment.
• Warn patient with a skin infection to avoid sharing washcloths and towels with family members.
• Instruct patient to wash hands before and after applying ointment.
• Advise patient using ophthalmic ointment to clean eye area of excess exudate before applying ointment. Warn him not to touch tip of tube to eye or surrounding tissue.
• Warn patient that ophthalmic ointment may cause blurred vision. Tell him to stop drug immediately and report symptoms of sensitivity, such as itchy eyelids or constant burning.
• Instruct patient to store ophthalmic ointment in tightly closed, light-resistant container.
• Caution patient not to share eye medications with other people.

baclofen
Lioresal

Pharmacologic classification: chlorophenyl derivative
Therapeutic classification: skeletal muscle relaxant
Pregnancy risk category: C

Indications and dosages
➤ *Spasticity in multiple sclerosis and other spinal cord lesions.* *Adults:* Initially, 5 mg P.O. t.i.d. for 3 days. Dosage may be increased (based on response) at 3-day intervals by 15 mg (5 mg/dose) daily up to maximum of 80 mg daily. For geriatric patients, increase oral dose more gradually.

Intrathecal administration
Must be diluted with sterile preservative-free normal saline solution.
Adults: Initial intrathecal bolus of 50 mcg in 1 ml over not less than 1 minute. Observe patient for response over subsequent 4 to 8 hours. A positive response consists of a significant decrease in muscle tone or frequency or severity of spasm. If initial response is inadequate, repeat dose with 75 mcg in 1.5 ml 24 hours after last injection. Repeat observation of patient over 4 to 8 hours. If the response is still inadequate, repeat dosing at 100 mcg in 2 ml 24 hours later. If still no response, patient shouldn't be considered for an implantable pump for long-term baclofen administration. Ranges for long-term doses are 12 to 2,000 mcg daily.
Children under age 12: Test dose is the same as for adults (50 mcg); but for very small children, an initial dose of 25 mcg may be given. Maintenance dosage averages 274 mcg daily (range 24 to 1,200 mcg daily).

Postimplant dose adjustment
If the screening dose produces the desired effect for over 8 hours, the initial intrathecal dose is the same as the test dose; this dose is infused intrathecally for 24 hours. If the screening dose produces the desired effect for less than 8 hours, the initial intrathecal dose is twice the test dose, followed slowly by 10% to 30% increments at 24-hour intervals.

How supplied
Available by prescription only
Intrathecal kit: 500 mcg/ml, 2,000 mcg/ml
Tablets: 10 mg, 20 mg

Pharmacodynamics
Skeletal muscle relaxant action: Precise mechanism of action is unknown, but drug appears to act at the spinal cord level to inhibit transmission of monosynaptic and polysynaptic reflexes, possibly through hyperpolarization of afferent fiber terminals. It also may act at supraspinal sites because baclofen at high doses produces generalized CNS depression. Baclofen decreases the number and severity of spasms and relieves pain, clonus, and muscle rigidity and therefore improves mobility.

Pharmacokinetics
Absorption: Rapidly and extensively absorbed from the GI tract, but is subject to individual variation. As dose increases, rate and extent of absorption decreases. Onset of therapeutic effect may not be immediately evident; varying from hours to weeks. Peak effect is seen at 2 to 3 hours.
Distribution: Studies indicate that baclofen is widely distributed throughout the body, with small amounts crossing the blood-brain barrier. About 30% is plasma protein–bound.
Metabolism: About 15% is metabolized in the liver via deamination.

Excretion: 70% to 80% is excreted in urine unchanged or as its metabolites; remainder is excreted in feces.

Route	Onset	Peak	Duration
P.O.	Rapid	2-3 hr	Unknown
Intrathecal	½-1 hr	4 hr	4-8 hr

Contraindications and precautions
Contraindicated in patients hypersensitive to drug. Use cautiously in patients with renal impairment or seizure disorders or when spasticity is used to maintain motor function.

Interactions
Drug-drug. *Antidiabetics, insulin:* Baclofen may increase blood glucose levels and require dosage adjustments of antidiabetic drug or insulin. Monitor serum glucose levels.
CNS depressants, including antipsychotics, anxiolytics, general anesthetics, narcotics: May add to the CNS effects of drug. Use together cautiously.
MAO inhibitors, tricyclic antidepressants: May cause CNS depression, respiratory depression, and hypotension. Avoid use together.
Drug-lifestyle. *Alcohol use:* May add to the CNS effects of drug. Discourage use.

Adverse reactions
CNS: *CNS depression, drowsiness, dizziness,* headache, slurred speech, *weakness, fatigue, hypotonia, confusion,* insomnia, dysarthria, SEIZURES.
CV: *CV collapse,* hypotension, hypertension.
EENT: blurred vision, nasal congestion.
GI: *nausea,* constipation, *vomiting.*
GU: urinary frequency.
Hepatic: increased AST and alkaline phosphatase levels.
Metabolic: hyperglycemia, weight gain.
Respiratory: *respiratory failure,* dyspnea.
Skin: rash, pruritus.
Other: excessive perspiration.

Overdose and treatment
Signs and symptoms of overdose include absence of reflexes, vomiting, muscular hypotonia, marked salivation, drowsiness, visual disorders, seizures, respiratory depression, and coma.

Treatment involves supportive measures, including endotracheal intubation and positive-pressure ventilation. If patient is conscious, remove drug by inducing emesis followed by gastric lavage. If patient is comatose, don't induce emesis. Gastric lavage may be performed after endotracheal tube is in place with cuff inflated. Don't use respiratory stimulants. Monitor vital signs closely.

Special considerations
● Intrathecal administration should be performed only by qualified individuals familiar with administration techniques and patient management problems.

● Adverse reactions may be reduced by slowly decreasing the dosage. Abrupt withdrawal can result in hallucinations or seizures and acute exacerbation of spasticity.
● Baclofen is used investigationally to reduce choreiform movements in Huntington's chorea; to reduce rigidity in Parkinson's disease; to reduce spasticity in CVA, cerebral lesions, cerebral palsy, and rheumatic disorders; for analgesia in trigeminal neuralgia; and for treatment of unstable bladder.
● In some patients, smoother response may be obtained by giving daily dose in four divided doses.
● Patient may need supervision during walking. The initial loss of spasticity induced by baclofen may affect patient's ability to stand or walk. (In some patients, spasticity helps patient to maintain upright posture and balance.)
● Discontinue drug if signs of improvement don't occur within 1 to 2 months.
● Implantable pump or catheter failure can result in sudden loss of effectiveness of intrathecal baclofen.
● During prolonged intrathecal baclofen therapy for spasticity, about 10% of patients become refractory to baclofen therapy requiring a temporary suspension of treatment to regain sensitivity to its effects.
● Store tablets in a tight container.
● Store baclofen at temperatures below 86° F (30° C). Don't freeze. Each vial is for individual use. Use only sterile, preservative-free normal saline solution for dilution. Baclofen must be diluted to 50 mcg/ml before injecting into the subarachnoid space.

Patient monitoring
● Monitor blood glucose levels routinely in diabetic patients.
● Observe patient's response to drug. Signs of effective therapy may appear in a few hours to 1 week and may include diminished frequency of spasms and severity of foot and ankle clonus, increased ease and range of joint motion, and enhanced performance of daily activities.
⚠ ALERT Increased seizures may occur in patients with a seizure disorder. Closely monitor patients with seizure disorder using EEG and clinical observation. Assess patient for possible loss of seizure control.

Pregnant patients
● There are no adequate and controlled studies in pregnant women.

Pediatric patients
● Use of oral form isn't recommended for children under age 12. Safety of intrathecal administration in children under age 4 hasn't been established.

Geriatric patients
● Geriatric patients are especially sensitive to drug. Observe carefully for adverse reactions,

---

such as mental confusion, depression, and hallucinations. Lower doses are usually indicated.

Patient education
• Advise patient to report adverse reactions promptly. Most can be reduced by decreasing dosage. Drowsiness, dizziness, and ataxia are more common in patients over age 40.
• Warn patient of additive effects with use of other CNS depressants, including alcohol.
• Caution patient to avoid hazardous activities that require mental alertness.
• Tell diabetic patient that baclofen may elevate blood glucose levels and may require adjustment of insulin dosage during treatment with baclofen. Urge patient to promptly report changes in urine or blood glucose tests.
• Caution patient against taking OTC drugs without medical approval. Explain that hazardous drug interactions are possible.
• Inform patient that drug should be withdrawn gradually over 1 to 2 weeks. Abrupt withdrawal after prolonged use of drug may cause anxiety, agitated behavior, auditory and visual hallucinations, severe tachycardia, and acute spasticity.

---

balsalazide disodium
Colazal

Pharmacologic classification: GI agent
Therapeutic classification: anti-inflammatory agent
Pregnancy risk category: B

Indications and dosages
➤ *Ulcerative colitis. Adults:* 2.25 g P.O. (three 750-mg capsules) t.i.d for a total of 6.75 g daily for 8 weeks.

How supplied
Available by prescription only
Capsules: 750 mg

Pharmacodynamics
Balsalazide is converted in the colon to mesalamine, which is then converted to 5-aminosalicylic acid. The mechanism of action is unknown, but it appears to be topical. It may decrease inflammation by blocking production of arachidonic acid metabolites in the colon.

Pharmacokinetics
Absorption: Systemic absorption is very low and variable in healthy patients. Absorption is 60 times greater in patients with ulcerative colitis.
Distribution: Drug is 99% or more bound to plasma proteins.
Metabolism: Metabolized to mesalamine (5-aminosalicylic acid), the active component of the drug.

Excretion: Excreted by the kidneys. Less than 1% of dose recovered in urine.

Route	Onset	Peak	Duration
P.O.	Unknown	Unknown	Unknown

Contraindications and precautions
Contraindicated in patients hypersensitive to salicylates or to any component of Colazal capsules or balsalazide metabolites. Use cautiously in patients with history of renal disease or renal dysfunction.

Interactions
Drug-drug. *Oral antibiotics:* May interfere with release of mesalamine in the colon. Monitor patient for effect.

Adverse reactions
CNS: dizziness, fatigue, headache, insomnia.
EENT: pharyngitis, rhinitis, sinusitis.
GI: abdominal pain, anorexia, constipation, cramps, diarrhea, dyspepsia, flatulence, frequent stools, nausea, rectal bleeding, vomiting, dry mouth.
GU: urinary tract infection.
Musculoskeletal: arthralgia, back pain, myalgia.
Respiratory: cough, respiratory tract infection.
Other: fever, flu syndrome, pain.

Overdose and treatment
No case of overdose has been reported. If an overdose occurs, treatment should be supportive, with monitoring and correction of electrolyte abnormalities.

Special considerations
• Safety and effectiveness beyond 12 weeks haven't been established.
• Patients with pyloric stenosis may have prolonged retention of drug.

Patient monitoring
• Hepatotoxicity, including elevated liver function test results, jaundice, cirrhosis, liver necrosis, and liver failure, has occurred with other products containing or metabolized to mesalamine. Although no signs of hepatotoxicity have been reported with Colazal, patient should be monitored closely for evidence of hepatic dysfunction.

Breast-feeding patients
• It isn't known whether balsalazide appears in breast milk; use caution when administering drug to a nursing woman.

Pediatric patients
• Safety and effectiveness in children haven't been established.

Patient education
• Advise patient with allergy to aspirin not to take drug.
• Instruct patient to swallow capsules whole.

• Advise patient to report adverse reactions promptly.

basiliximab
Simulect

Pharmacologic classification: recombinant chimeric human monoclonal antibody IgG$_{1K}$
Therapeutic classification: immunosuppressive agent
Pregnancy risk category: B

Indications and dosages
➤ *Prophylaxis of acute organ rejection in patients receiving renal transplant when used as part of immunosuppressive regimen including cyclosporine and corticosteroids. Adults:* 20 mg I.V. given within 2 hours before transplant surgery and 20 mg I.V. given 4 days after transplantation.
Children ages 2 to 15: 12 mg/m^2 (up to a maximum of 20 mg) I.V. given within 2 hours of transplant surgery and 12 mg/m^2 (to a maximum of 20 mg) I.V. given 4 days after transplantation.

How supplied
Available by prescription only
Injection: 20-mg single-dose vials

Pharmacodynamics
Immunosuppressant action: Basiliximab binds specifically to and blocks the interleukin-2 receptor alpha-chain on the surface of activated T-lymphocytes. This inhibits interleukin-2–mediated activation of lymphocytes, a critical pathway in the cellular immune response involved in allograft rejection.

Pharmacokinetics
Absorption: Administered I.V.
Distribution: Unknown.
Metabolism: Unknown.
Excretion: Half-life is about 7.2 days in adults, 11.5 days in children.

Route	Onset	Peak	Duration
I.V.	Unknown	Unknown	Unknown

Contraindications and precautions
Contraindicated in patients hypersensitive to drug or its components. Anaphylactoid reactions may result after administration of proteins. Make sure that drugs used to treat severe hypersensitivity reactions are available for immediate use.

Interactions
None reported.

Adverse reactions
CNS: agitation, anxiety, *asthenia*, depression, *dizziness, headache,* hypoesthesia, *insomnia,* neuropathy, paresthesia, *tremor,* fatigue, malaise.

CV: angina pectoris, *arrhythmias,* atrial fibrillation, *cardiac failure,* chest pain, abnormal heart sounds, aggravated hypertension, *hypertension,* hypotension, tachycardia.
EENT: abnormal vision, cataract, conjunctivitis, *rhinitis, pharyngitis,* sinusitis.
GI: *abdominal pain, candidiasis, constipation, diarrhea, dyspepsia,* esophagitis, enlarged abdomen, flatulence, gastroenteritis, GI disorder, *GI hemorrhage,* gum hyperplasia, melena, *nausea,* ulcerative stomatitis, *vomiting.*
GU: abnormal renal function, albuminuria, bladder disorder, *dysuria,* frequent micturition, hematuria, *increased nonprotein nitrogen,* oliguria, renal tubular necrosis, ureteral disorder, *urinary tract infection,* urine retention.
Hematologic: *anemia,* hematoma, hemorrhage, polycythemia, purpura, *thrombocytopenia,* thrombosis.
Metabolic: *acidosis,* dehydration, diabetes mellitus, fluid overload, hypercalcemia, *hypercholesterolemia, hyperglycemia, hyperkalemia,* hyperlipemia, *hyperuricemia, hypocalcemia, hypokalemia,* hypomagnesemia, hypoglycemia, *hypophosphatemia,* hypoproteinemia, *weight increase.*
Musculoskeletal: arthralgia, arthropathy, *back pain,* bone fracture, cramps, hernia, *leg pain,* myalgia.
Respiratory: abnormal chest sounds, bronchitis, *bronchospasm, cough, dyspnea,* pneumonia, pulmonary disorder, pulmonary edema, *upper respiratory tract infection.*
Skin: *acne,* cyst, herpes simplex, herpes zoster, hypertrichosis, pruritus, rash, skin disorder or ulceration, *surgical wound complications.*
Other: accidental trauma, *viral infection, leg or peripheral edema, pain,* general edema, infection, rigors, *sepsis,* fever.

Overdose and treatment
No overdose reported. Single doses up to 60 mg have been given without significant adverse effects.

Special considerations
• Use cautiously and only under the supervision of a prescriber experienced in immunosuppression therapy and management of organ transplantation.
• Basiliximab should only be used with cyclosporine and corticosteroids; data are lacking regarding use with other immunosuppressants.
• It isn't known whether the response to vaccines will be altered with drug administration.
• Reconstitute with 5 ml sterile water for injection. Shake vial gently to dissolve powder. Dilute reconstituted solution to volume of 50 ml with normal saline solution or D$_5$W for infusion. When mixing solution, gently invert bag to avoid foaming. Don't shake.
• Infuse drug over 20 to 30 minutes via a central or peripheral vein. Don't add or infuse other drugs simultaneously through same I.V. line.

Reactions may be *common*, uncommon, *life-threatening*, or COMMON AND LIFE-THREATENING.

• Use reconstituted solution immediately; otherwise, refrigerate at 36° to 46° F (2° to 8° C) for up to 24 hours or at room temperature for 4 hours.

Patient monitoring
• Monitor patient for electrolyte imbalances and acidosis during drug therapy.
• Monitor patient's intake and output, vital signs, hemoglobin, and hematocrit during therapy.
• Monitor patient for signs of opportunistic infections during drug therapy.

Breast-feeding patients
• It isn't known if drug appears in breast milk. A decision should be made to discontinue the drug or to stop nursing depending upon the importance of the drug to the mother.

Pediatric patients
• Basiliximab may be administered to children as young as age 2.

Geriatric patients
• No significant difference has been seen between elderly and younger adults; however, caution should be used when prescribing immunosuppressive agents to this population.

Patient education
• Inform patient of potential benefits and risks of immunosuppressive therapy, including a decreased risk of graft loss or acute rejection.
• Advise patient that immunosuppressive therapy increases risk of developing lymphoproliferative disorders and opportunistic infections.
• Advise women of childbearing age to use effective contraception before beginning therapy and for 2 months after therapy stops.
• Instruct patient to report adverse effects or signs of infection immediately.

becaplermin
Regranex

Pharmacologic classification: recombinant human platelet-derived growth factor
Therapeutic classification: wound repair agent
Pregnancy risk category: C

Indications and dosages
➤ *Treatment of diabetic neuropathic leg ulcers that extend into the subcutaneous tissue and beyond and have an adequate blood supply. Adults:* Apply daily in ¼" layer of even thickness to entire surface of wound. Cover site with a saline solution–moistened dressing. Remove after 12 hours. Rinse gel from wound with saline solution or water and cover wound with moist dressing. Continue treatment until healing is complete. When squeezing gel from tube, length of gel to be applied varies with tube size and ulcer area.

Tube size (g)	Ulcer size (inches)	Ulcer size (centimeters)
2	length × width × 1.3	(length × width) ÷ 2
7.5, 15	length × width × 0.6	(length × width) ÷ 4

How supplied
Available by prescription only
Gel: 100 mcg/g in tubes of 2 g, 7.5 g, 15 g

Pharmacodynamics
Wound repair action: Recombinant of human platelet-derived growth factor that promotes the chemotactic recruitment and proliferation of cells involved in wound repair and enhances the formation of new granulation tissue.

Pharmacokinetics
Absorption: Minimal systemic absorption.
Distribution: Unknown.
Metabolism: Unknown.
Excretion: Unknown.

Route	Onset	Peak	Duration
Topical	Unknown	Unknown	Unknown

Contraindications and precautions
Contraindicated in patients hypersensitive to any component of product and in those with neoplasms at site of application. Gel is for external use only. If reaction occurs at application site, consider possibility of sensitization or irritation caused by parabens or m-cresol.

Interactions
None reported.

Adverse reactions
Skin: erythematous rash.

Overdose and treatment
No information available.

Special considerations
• When used as an adjunct to (not a substitute for) good ulcer care practices, including initial sharp debridement, pressure relief, and infection control, gel increases chance of complete healing of diabetic ulcers. Its efficacy in treating diabetic neuropathic ulcers that don't extend through the dermis into subcutaneous tissue or ischemic diabetic ulcers hasn't been evaluated.
• Don't use gel in wounds that close by primary intention.
• To apply gel, squeeze the calculated length onto a clean measuring surface, such as wax paper. Then transfer the measured gel from the measuring surface using an application aid.

• Use gel in addition to a good ulcer care program, including a strict non-weight-bearing program.

Patient monitoring

• Monitor patient for wound healing and application site reactions.
• Recalculate amount of gel to be applied weekly. If ulcer doesn't decrease in size by about one-third after 10 weeks or complete healing hasn't occurred by 20 weeks, reassess continued treatment.

Breast-feeding patients

• It isn't known if drug appears in breast milk. Use drug cautiously in breast-feeding women.

Pediatric patients

• Safety and efficacy in patients under age 16 haven't been established.

Patient education

• Instruct patient to wash hands thoroughly before applying gel.
• Advise patient not to touch tip of tube to ulcer or other surfaces.
• Tell patient to use a cotton swab, tongue blade, or other application aid to apply gel evenly over the surface of the ulcer, producing a thin (¼") continuous layer.
• Tell patient to apply drug once daily in a carefully measured quantity. Quantity will change on a weekly basis.
• Tell patient to refrigerate gel but never to freeze it.
• Urge patient not to use gel after expiration date on the crimped end of the tube.

beclomethasone dipropionate

beclomethasone dipropionate monohydrate

Nasal inhalants
Beconase, Vancenase

Nasal sprays
Beconase AQ, Vancenase AQ, Vancenase AQ 84 mcg, Vancenase Pockethaler

Oral inhalants
Becloforte*, Beclovent, Vanceril, Vanceril Double Strength

Pharmacologic classification: glucocorticoid
Therapeutic classification: anti-inflammatory, antiasthmatic
Pregnancy risk category: C

Indications and dosages

➤ *Corticosteroid-dependent asthma.* Oral inhalation. *Adults and children over age 12:*
For regular-strength form, two inhalations t.i.d. or q.i.d. or four inhalations b.i.d. For severe asthma, start with 12 to 16 sprays daily and then reduce the dosage to the lowest effective level. Maximum of 20 inhalations daily. For double-strength form, two inhalations b.i.d. For severe asthma, start with six to eight inhalations and adjust down. Don't exceed ten inhalations daily.
Children ages 6 to 12: For regular strength form, one to two inhalations t.i.d. or q.i.d. Maximum of ten inhalations daily. For double-strength form, two inhalations b.i.d. Don't exceed five inhalations daily.

➤ *Perennial or seasonal rhinitis; prevention of recurrence of nasal polyps after surgical removal.* Nasal inhalation. *Adults and children over age 12:* One spray (42 mcg) in each nostril b.i.d. to q.i.d. Usual total dose is 168 to 336 mcg daily.
Children ages 6 to 12: One spray in each nostril t.i.d. (252 mcg daily).

Nasal spray
Adults and children over age 6: One or two sprays of single-strength (42 to 84 mcg) in each nostril b.i.d. If the double-strength preparation is used, one or two sprays (84 to 168 mcg) into each nostril once daily (168 to 336 mcg). Maintenance dosage is one spray (42 mcg) into each nostril t.i.d.

How supplied

Available by prescription only
Nasal aerosol: 42 mcg/metered spray
Nasal spray: 42 mcg/metered spray, 84 mcg/metered spray
Oral inhalation aerosol: 42 mcg/metered spray, 84 mcg/metered spray

Pharmacodynamics

Anti-inflammatory action: Beclomethasone stimulates the synthesis of enzymes needed to decrease the inflammatory response. The anti-inflammatory and vasoconstrictor potency of topically applied beclomethasone is, on a weight basis, about 5,000 times greater than that of hydrocortisone, 500 times greater than that of betamethasone or dexamethasone, and about 5 times greater than fluocinolone or triamcinolone.
Antiasthmatic action: Beclomethasone is used as a nasal inhalant to treat symptoms of seasonal or perennial rhinitis and to prevent the recurrence of nasal polyps after surgical removal, and as an oral inhalant to treat bronchial asthma in patients who require long-term administration of corticosteroids to control symptoms.

Pharmacokinetics

Absorption: After nasal inhalation, drug is absorbed primarily through the nasal mucosa with minimal systemic absorption. After oral inhalation, drug is absorbed rapidly from the lungs and GI tract. Greater systemic absorption comes from oral inhalation, but systemic effects don't occur at usual doses because of rapid metabolism in

---

the liver and local metabolism of drug that reaches the lungs.

Distribution: Distribution after intranasal administration hasn't been described. There's no evidence of tissue storage of drug or its metabolites. About 10% to 25% of a nasal spray or orally inhaled dose is deposited in the respiratory tract. The remainder, deposited in the mouth and oropharynx, is swallowed. When absorbed, it's 87% bound to plasma proteins.

Metabolism: Swallowed drug undergoes rapid metabolism in the liver or GI tract to several metabolites, some of which have minor glucocorticoid activity. The portion inhaled into the respiratory tract is partially metabolized before absorption into systemic circulation. Mostly metabolized in the liver.

Excretion: Excretion of inhaled drug hasn't been described; however, when drug is administered systemically, its metabolites are excreted mainly in feces via biliary elimination and to a lesser extent in urine. Biological half-life of drug averages 15 hours.

Route	Onset	Peak	Duration
Nasal	Unknown	Unknown	Unknown
Inhalation	Unknown	Unknown	Unknown

Contraindications and precautions

Contraindicated in patients hypersensitive to drug and in those experiencing status asthmaticus or other acute episodes of asthma. Use cautiously in patients with tuberculosis, fungal or bacterial infection, herpes, or systemic viral infection.

Interactions

None reported.

Adverse reactions

CNS: headache.

EENT: *mild transient nasal burning and stinging,* nasal congestion, sneezing, dryness, epistaxis, nasopharyngeal fungal infections, hoarseness, fungal infection of throat, throat irritation.

GI: dry mouth, fungal infection of mouth.

Respiratory: *bronchospasm,* wheezing.

Other: *angioedema, hypersensitivity reactions* (urticaria, rash), *suppression of hypothalamic-pituitary-adrenal function, adrenal insufficiency,* facial edema.

Overdose and treatment

No information available.

Special considerations

● Don't use drug in patients with asthma controlled by bronchodilators or other noncorticosteroids alone or in patients with nonasthmatic bronchial diseases.

● Use drug cautiously in patients receiving systemic corticosteroid therapy.

● A spacer device may help ensure delivery of the proper dose and decrease local (oral) adverse effects.

● Therapy should last no longer than 3 weeks if symptoms don't improve substantially.

● Store Beconase inhalation at 36° to 86° F (2° to 30° C). Store Vancenase nasal inhaler at 59° to 86° F (15° to 30° C).

● During times of stress (trauma, surgery, or infection) systemic corticosteroids may be needed to prevent adrenal insufficiency in previously steroid-dependent patients.

⚠ ALERT Taper oral corticosteroid therapy slowly. Acute adrenal insufficiency and death have occurred in asthmatics who changed abruptly from oral corticosteroids to beclomethasone.

Patient monitoring

● Monitor patient for drug effectiveness.

● Periodic measurement of growth and development may be necessary during high-dose or prolonged therapy in children.

Pregnant patients

● Orally inhaled beclomethasone should be used in pregnant women only if the benefits outweigh the risks.

Pediatric patients

● Drug isn't recommended for children under age 6.

Patient education

● Inform patient that drug doesn't relieve acute asthma attacks.

● Tell patient who needs a bronchodilator to use it several minutes before using beclomethasone.

● Instruct patient to wear or carry medical identification that indicates his need for supplemental systemic corticosteroids during stress.

● If patient uses a metered-dose inhaler, instruct him to shake canister well before use.

● Advise patient to allow 1 minute to elapse before taking subsequent puffs of medication and to hold his breath for a few seconds to enhance action of drug.

● Instruct patient to contact prescriber if response to therapy decreases or if symptoms don't improve within 3 weeks; dosage may need to be adjusted. Tell him not to exceed recommended dosage on his own.

● Tell patient to keep inhaler clean and unobstructed. He should wash it with warm water and dry it thoroughly.

● Advise patient to prevent oral fungal infections by gargling or rinsing mouth with water after each use, but not to swallow the water.

● Tell patient to report symptoms of corticosteroid withdrawal, including fatigue, weakness, arthralgia, orthostatic hypotension, and dyspnea.

● Instruct patient to store drug between 59° and 86° F (15° and 30° C). Advise patient to ensure delivery of proper dose by gently warming canister to room temperature before using.

benazepril hydrochloride
Lotensin

Pharmacologic classification: ACE inhibitor
Therapeutic classification: antihypertensive
Pregnancy risk category: C (D in second and third trimesters)

Indications and dosages
➤**Hypertension.** *Adults:* Initially, 10 mg P.O. daily in patients not receiving diuretics. Adjust dosage as needed and tolerated; maintenance dosage range is 20 to 40 mg daily in one or two equally divided doses.
✦ *Dosage adjustment.* In patients with renal failure and creatinine clearance below 30 ml/ minute or serum creatinine levels above 3 mg/dl, initial dose is 5 mg P.O. daily. Don't exceed 40 mg daily.

How supplied
Available by prescription only
Tablets: 5 mg, 10 mg, 20 mg, 40 mg

Pharmacodynamics
Antihypertensive action: Benazepril and its active metabolite, benazeprilat, inhibit ACE, preventing conversion of angiotensin I to angiotensin II, a potent vasoconstrictor. Reduced formation of angiotensin II decreases peripheral arterial resistance and aldosterone secretion, which reduces sodium and water retention and lowers blood pressure.

Although the primary mechanism through which benazepril lowers blood pressure is believed to be suppression of the renin-angiotensin-aldosterone system, benazepril has an antihypertensive effect even in patients with low renin levels.

Pharmacokinetics
Absorption: At least 37% of drug is absorbed.
Distribution: Serum protein–binding of drug is about 97%; that of benazeprilat, 95%.
Metabolism: Almost completely metabolized in the liver to benazeprilat, which has much greater ACE inhibitory activity than benazepril, and to the glucuronide conjugates of benazepril and benazeprilat.
Excretion: Excreted primarily in the urine.

Route	Onset	Peak	Duration
P.O.	1 hr	2-4 hr	24 hr

Contraindications and precautions
Contraindicated in patients hypersensitive to ACE inhibitors. Use cautiously in patients with renal or hepatic impairment.

Interactions
Drug-drug. *Allopurinol:* Increased risk of hypersensitivity reaction. Monitor patient carefully.

Antihypertensives, including diuretics: Increased risk of excessive hypotension. The diuretic may need to be discontinued or benazepril dose lowered.
Digoxin: Increased plasma digoxin levels. Monitor digoxin levels.
Lithium: Increased serum lithium levels and lithium toxicity. Monitor blood levels closely.
Potassium-sparing diuretics, potassium supplements: Risk of hyperkalemia. Use together cautiously.
Drug-herb. *Capsaicin:* Increased risk of cough. Discourage concomitant use.
Drug-food. *Sodium substitutes containing potassium:* Risk of hyperkalemia. Discourage use together.

Adverse reactions
CNS: headache, dizziness, anxiety, fatigue, insomnia, nervousness, paresthesia.
CV: symptomatic hypotension, palpitations.
EENT: dysphagia, increased salivation.
GI: nausea, vomiting, abdominal pain, constipation.
GU: impotence.
Metabolic: hyperkalemia.
Musculoskeletal: arthralgia, arthritis, myalgia.
Respiratory: dry, persistent, tickling, nonproductive cough; dyspnea.
Skin: increased diaphoresis.
Other: *hypersensitivity reactions* (rash, pruritus), *angioedema.*

Overdose and treatment
Hypotension is the most common effect of overdose. No data suggest physiologic maneuvers that might accelerate elimination of benazepril and its metabolite if an overdose occurs. Drug is only slightly dialyzable, but dialysis might be considered in overdosed patients with severely impaired renal function. Angiotensin II could presumably serve as a specific antagonist-antidote, but angiotensin II is essentially unavailable outside of scattered research facilities. Because the hypotensive effect of the drug is achieved through vasodilation and effective hypovolemia, treatment of benazepril overdose by I.V. infusion of normal saline solution is reasonable.

Special considerations
⚠ **ALERT** Although rare, angioedema has been reported in patients receiving ACE inhibitors. Angioedema that causes laryngeal edema or shock may be fatal. If angioedema of the face, limbs, lips, tongue, glottis, or larynx occurs, discontinue treatment with benazepril and institute appropriate therapy immediately.
● Excessive hypotension can occur when drug is given with diuretics. If possible, discontinue diuretic therapy 2 to 3 days before starting benazepril to decrease the potential for excessive hypotensive response. If benazepril doesn't adequately control blood pressure, diuretic therapy may be reinstituted with care. If the diuretic

can't be discontinued, start benazepril therapy at 5 mg P.O. daily.

Patient monitoring
• Measure blood pressure when drug levels peak (2 to 6 hours after a dose) and trough (just before a dose) to verify adequate blood pressure control.
• Assess renal and hepatic function before and periodically throughout therapy. Also monitor serum potassium levels.
• Other ACE inhibitors have been linked to agranulocytosis and neutropenia. Monitor CBC with differential counts before therapy, every 2 weeks for first 3 months of therapy, and periodically thereafter.

Breast-feeding patients
• Minimal amounts of unchanged benazepril and benazeprilat appear in breast milk. Use cautiously when administering to breast-feeding women.

Pediatric patients
• Safety and efficacy in children haven't been established.

Patient education
• Advise patient to report signs or symptoms of infection (such as fever and sore throat); easy bruising or bleeding; swelling of tongue, lips, face, eyes, mucous membranes, or limbs; difficulty swallowing or breathing; and hoarseness.
• Because light-headedness can occur, especially during the first few days of therapy, tell patient to rise slowly to minimize this effect and to report symptoms. Patients who experience syncope should stop taking drug and call immediately.
• Tell patient to use caution in hot weather and during exercise. Inadequate fluid intake, vomiting, diarrhea, and excessive perspiration can lead to light-headedness and syncope.
• Tell patient to avoid sodium substitutes; these products may contain potassium, which can cause hyperkalemia in patients on drug therapy.
• Tell women of childbearing age about consequences of second- and third-trimester exposure to ACE inhibitors. Explain that these don't appear to result from exposure during the first trimester. Advise her to report suspected pregnancy as soon as possible.
• A persistent dry cough may occur and usually doesn't subside unless drug is stopped. Advise patient to call if this effect becomes bothersome.

benzocaine
Americaine, Dermoplast, Hurricaine, Lanacane, Maximum Strength Anbesol, Orabase Gel, Orajel Mouth Aid, Solarcaine

Pharmacologic classification: local anesthetic (ester)
Therapeutic classification: anesthetic
Pregnancy risk category: C

Indications and dosages
➤ *Local anesthetic for dental pain or dental procedures.* *Adults and children:* Apply topical gel (20%) or dental paste to area, p.r.n. or as directed by prescriber.
➤ *Local anesthetic for pruritic dermatoses, pruritus, or other irritations.* *Adults:* Apply topical preparation (1% to 20%) to affected area t.i.d. to q.i.d. or as directed by prescriber.
➤ *Relief of pain and pruritus in acute congestive and serous otitis media, acute swimmer's ear, and other forms of otitis externa.* *Adults:* 4 to 5 drops (otic) in external auditory canal; insert cotton into meatus; repeat q 1 to 2 hours.
➤ *Temporary relief of minor sore throat pain.* *Adults and children over age 3:* One lozenge dissolved slowly in the mouth and repeated, p.r.n. Don't use as self-medication for more than 2 days.
➤ *Male genital desensitization.* *Adults:* Apply a small amount of a topical preparation containing 3% to 7.5% of benzocaine in water-soluble base to head and shaft of penis before intercourse. Patient should wash off any remaining benzocaine after intercourse to reduce potential for allergic reaction.

How supplied
Available without a prescription
Gel: 20%
Lotion: 0.5% to 8%
Lozenges: 10 mg
Ointment, cream, and dental paste: 1% to 20%
Solution: 20%
Topical solution: 20%
Topical spray: 3%, 5%, 13.6%, 20%

Pharmacodynamics
Analgesic action: Acts at sensory neurons to produce a local anesthetic effect.

Pharmacokinetics
No information available.

Route	Onset	Peak	Duration
Topical	Unknown	Unknown	Unknown

Contraindications and precautions

Contraindicated in patients hypersensitive to any component of the preparation or related substances and in those with secondary infection in the area or serious burns. Don't use in eyes or in ears with a perforated tympanic membrane or discharge. Use cautiously in patients with severely traumatized mucosa or local sepsis.

Interactions

None significant.

Adverse reactions

CV: edema
Skin: urticaria, burning, stinging, tenderness, irritation, itching, erythema, rash.

Overdose and treatment

Maximum recommended daily dose is 5 g. Benzocaine overdose is unlikely; however, methemoglobinemia has been reported after topical application for teething pain.

Treat symptomatically; if necessary, administer methylene blue 1% 0.1 ml/kg I.V. over at least 10 minutes.

Special considerations

• Use drug with antibiotic to treat underlying cause of pain because using alone may mask more serious condition.
• Keep container tightly closed and dry.
• Drug is meant for temporary use, no more than 7 days.
🔃 ALERT Discontinue drug if symptoms of hypersensitivity occur.

Patient monitoring

• Monitor patient for worsening of condition.

Pediatric patients

• Excessive use may cause methemoglobinemia in infants. Don't use in children under age 2.

Patient education

• Tell patient to contact prescriber if pain lasts longer than 48 hours, if burning or itching occurs, or if condition persists.
• Instruct patient to keep container tightly closed and away from moisture.
• Advise patient not to eat or chew gum until effect of local anesthetic has worn off to avoid the risk of bite trauma.

---

benztropine mesylate
Cogentin

Pharmacologic classification: anticholinergic
Therapeutic classification: antiparkinsonian
Pregnancy risk category: C

Indications and dosages

➤ *Parkinsonism.* *Adults:* 0.5 to 6 mg P.O. daily. Initially, 0.5 to 1 mg I.M. or P.O. increased 0.5 mg

q 5 to 6 days. Adjust dosage to meet individual requirements. Maximum daily dose is 6 mg.
➤ *Drug-induced extrapyramidal reactions.* *Adults:* 1 to 4 mg P.O. or I.M. daily or b.i.d. Adjust dosage to meet individual requirements. Maximum daily dose is 6 mg.
➤ *Acute dystonic reaction.* *Adults:* 1 to 2 mg I.V. or I.M. followed by 1 to 2 mg P.O. b.i.d. to prevent recurrence.

How supplied

Available by prescription only
Injection: 1 mg/ml in 2-ml ampule
Tablets: 0.5 mg, 1 mg, 2 mg

Pharmacodynamics

Antiparkinsonian action: Benztropine blocks central cholinergic receptors, helping to balance cholinergic activity in the basal ganglia. It also may prolong effects of dopamine by blocking dopamine reuptake and storage at central receptor sites.

Pharmacokinetics

Absorption: Absorbed from the GI tract.
Distribution: Largely unknown; however, drug crosses the blood-brain barrier and may cross the placenta.
Metabolism: Unknown.
Excretion: Like other muscarinics, benztropine is excreted in urine as unchanged drug and metabolites. After oral therapy, small amounts are probably excreted in feces as unabsorbed drug.

Route	Onset	Peak	Duration
P.O.	1-2 hr	Unknown	24 hr
I.V., I.M.	15 min	Unknown	24 hr

Contraindications and precautions

Contraindicated in patients hypersensitive to drug or its components, in patients with acute angle-closure glaucoma, and in children under age 3. Use cautiously in hot weather, in patients with mental disorders, and in children over age 3.

Interactions

Drug-drug. *Amantadine:* May amplify such adverse anticholinergic effects as confusion and hallucinations. Decrease benztropine dosage before giving amantadine.
Antacids, antidiarrheals: May decrease benztropine absorption. Administer benztropine at least 1 hour before administering these agents.
CNS depressants: Increased sedative effects of benztropine. Use together cautiously.
Haloperidol, phenothiazines: Decreased effect of these drugs, possibly reflecting direct CNS antagonism. Monitor patient for clinical effect.
Phenothiazines: Increased risk of adverse anticholinergic effects. Use reduced phenothiazine dose.

Reactions may be *common*, uncommon, *life-threatening*, or COMMON AND LIFE-THREATENING.

Drug-lifestyle. *Alcohol use*: Increased sedative effects of benztropine. Discourage concurrent use.

Adverse reactions
CNS: disorientation, hallucinations, depression, toxic psychosis, confusion, memory impairment, nervousness.
CV: tachycardia.
EENT: dilated pupils, blurred vision.
GI: dry mouth, *constipation*, nausea, vomiting, paralytic ileus.
GU: urine retention, dysuria.

Overdose and treatment
Signs and symptoms of overdose include central stimulation followed by depression and psychotic symptoms such as disorientation, confusion, hallucinations, delusions, anxiety, agitation, and restlessness. Peripheral effects may include dilated, nonreactive pupils; blurred vision; hot, flushed, dry skin; dry mucous membranes; dysphagia; decreased or absent bowel sounds; urine retention; hyperthermia; tachycardia; hypertension; and increased respiration.

Treatment is primarily symptomatic and supportive, as necessary. Maintain a patent airway. If patient is alert, induce emesis (or use gastric lavage) and follow with a saline solution cathartic and activated charcoal to prevent further absorption. In severe cases, physostigmine may be administered to block the antimuscarinic effects of benztropine. Give fluids as needed to treat shock, diazepam to control psychotic symptoms, and pilocarpine (instilled into the eyes) to relieve mydriasis. If urine retention occurs, catheterization may be necessary.

Special considerations
Consider the recommendations relevant to all anticholinergics as well as the following.
• To help prevent gastric irritation, administer drug after meals.
• Never discontinue drug abruptly.
• Store in well-sealed containers between 59° and 86° F (15° and 30° C). Avoid freezing injectable preparation.
• Some adverse reactions may result from atropine-like toxicity and are dose related.

Patient monitoring
• Monitor patient for intermittent constipation and abdominal distention and pain, which may indicate paralytic ileus.
• Monitor patient periodically because effects are cumulative, especially if patient is prone to tachycardia and prostatic hypertrophy.
• Observe patients with mental disorders for worsening symptoms or toxic psychoses, especially at start of treatment and during dosage adjustment.

Pregnant patients
• Safe use during pregnancy hasn't been established.

Breast-feeding patients
• Drug may appear in breast milk, possibly causing infant toxicity. Avoid use in breast-feeding women.
• Benztropine may decrease milk production.

Pediatric patients
• Drug isn't recommended for children under age 3.

Patient education
• Explain to patient that the full effect of drug may not occur for 2 to 3 days.
• Caution patient not to stop drug suddenly; dosage should be reduced gradually.
• Tell patient that drug may increase sensitivity of eyes to light.

bepridil hydrochloride
Vascor

Pharmacologic classification: calcium channel blocker
Therapeutic classification: antianginal
Pregnancy risk category: C

Indications and dosages
➤ *Treatment of chronic stable angina (classic effort-related angina) in patients who are unresponsive or inadequately responsive to other antianginals. Adults:* Initially, 200 mg P.O. daily; after 10 days, adjust dosage based on patient tolerance and response. Most common maintenance dosage is 300 mg daily. Maximum daily dose is 400 mg.

How supplied
Available by prescription only
Tablets: 200 mg, 300 mg, 400 mg

Pharmacodynamics
Antianginal action: Precise mechanism of action is unknown. Drug inhibits calcium ion influx into cardiac and vascular smooth muscle and also inhibits the sodium inward influx, resulting in reductions in the maximal upstroke velocity and amplitude of the action potential. It's believed to reduce heart rate and arterial pressure by dilating peripheral arterioles and reducing total peripheral resistance (afterload). The effects are dose dependent. Bepridil has dose-related class I antiarrhythmic properties affecting electrophysiologic changes, such as prolongation of QT and QTc intervals.

Pharmacokinetics
Absorption: Rapidly and completely absorbed after oral administration.

Distribution: Over 99% of drug is bound to plasma proteins.
Metabolism: Metabolized in the liver.
Excretion: Elimination is biphasic. Bepridil has a distribution half-life of 2 hours. Over 10 days, 70% is excreted in urine, 22% in feces as metabolites. Terminal half-life after multiple dosing averages 42 hours (range, 26 to 64 hours).

Route	Onset	Peak	Duration
P.O.	1 hr	2-3 hr	24 hr

Contraindications and precautions

Contraindicated in patients hypersensitive to drug and in those with uncompensated cardiac insufficiency, sick sinus syndrome or second- or third-degree AV block (unless pacemaker is present); hypotension (below 90 mm Hg systolic); congenital QT interval prolongation; or history of serious ventricular arrhythmias. Also contraindicated in those receiving other drugs that prolong QT interval.

Use cautiously in patients with left bundle-branch block, sinus bradycardia, impaired renal or hepatic function, or heart failure. Drug isn't recommended for patients within 3 months of an MI.

Interactions

Drug-drug. *Beta blockers:* Excessive bradycardia and conduction abnormalities. Monitor patient closely.
Digoxin: Modest increases in steady-state serum digoxin levels. Monitor serum digoxin levels.
Potassium-wasting diuretics: Potential for hypokalemia, which increases risk of serious ventricular arrhythmias. Monitor serum potassium levels closely.
Procainamide, quinidine, tricyclic antidepressants: Additive prolongation of QT interval. Avoid use together.

Adverse reactions

CNS: *dizziness,* drowsiness, *nervousness, headache,* insomnia, paresthesia, *asthenia,* tremor.
CV: edema, flushing, palpitations, tachycardia, ***ventricular arrhythmias,*** including ***torsades de pointes, ventricular tachycardia, ventricular fibrillation.***
EENT: tinnitus.
GI: *nausea, diarrhea,* constipation, abdominal discomfort, dry mouth, anorexia.
Hematologic: ***agranulocytosis.***
Hepatic: increased ALT levels, abnormal liver function test results.
Respiratory: dyspnea, shortness of breath.
Skin: rash.
Other: flu syndrome.

Overdose and treatment

Exaggerated adverse reactions have been observed, especially clinically significant hypotension, high-degree AV block, and ventricular tachycardia.

Treat with appropriate supportive measures, including gastric lavage, beta-adrenergic stimulation, parenteral calcium solutions, vasopressor agents, and cardioversion, as necessary. Close observation in a cardiac care facility for a minimum of 48 hours is recommended.

Special considerations

⚑ ALERT Careful patient selection and monitoring are essential. Use the following selection criteria: Diagnosis of chronic stable angina with failure to respond or inadequate response to other therapies, QTc interval of less than 0.44 second, absence of hypokalemia, hypotension, severe left ventricular dysfunction, serious ventricular arrhythmias, unpacked sick sinus syndrome, second- or third-degree AV block, and no use of other drugs that prolong the QT interval.
● Beta blockers, nitrates, digoxin, insulin, and oral antidiabetic drugs may be used with bepridil.
● Food doesn't interfere with absorption of bepridil. Food may alleviate or prevent nausea.
● Use cautiously in patients with renal or hepatic disorders. No clinical data are available.

Patient monitoring
● Monitor serum potassium levels and correct hypokalemia before starting therapy. Use potassium-sparing diuretics for patients who need diuretic therapy.
● Monitor QTc interval before and during therapy. Reduced dosage is required if QTc prolongation is greater than 0.52 second or increases more than 25%. If prolongation of QTc interval persists, discontinue bepridil.
● Assess patient for development of cough or dyspnea; consider pulmonary infiltrates or fibroses as a potential cause.

Breast-feeding patients
● Drug appears in breast milk; risk-benefit must be assessed.

Pediatric patients
● Safety and efficacy in children under age 18 haven't been established.

Geriatric patients
● Recommended starting dose is same as in younger adult patients; however, more frequent monitoring may be required.

Patient education
● Instruct patient to recognize signs and symptoms of hypokalemia and the importance of compliance with prescribed potassium supplements.
● Tell patient to report signs or symptoms of infection, such as sore throat and fever.
● Instruct patient to take drug with food or at bedtime if nausea occurs.

Reactions may be *common*, uncommon, *life-threatening*, or COMMON AND LIFE-THREATENING.

beractant (natural lung surfactant)
Survanta

Pharmacologic classification: bovine lung extract
Therapeutic classification: lung surfactant
Pregnancy risk category: NR

Indications and dosages
➤ *Prevention and treatment (rescue) of respiratory distress syndrome (RDS, hyaline membrane disease) in premature infants. Infants:* 100 mg of phospholipids/kg of birth weight (4 ml/kg) administered by intratracheal instillation through a 5F end-hole catheter inserted into the infant's endotracheal tube with the tip of the catheter protruding just beyond the end of the tube above the carina. Shorten the length of the catheter before inserting it through the tube. Beractant shouldn't be instilled into a mainstem bronchus. Use the accompanying dosing table as a guide.

Guide to beractant doses

Weight (g)	Total dose (ml)
600-650	2.6
651-700	2.8
701-750	3
751-800	3.2
801-850	3.4
851-900	3.6
901-950	3.8
951-1,000	4
1,001-1,050	4.2
1,051-1,100	4.4
1,101-1,150	4.6
1,151-1,200	4.8
1,201-1,250	5
1,251-1,300	5.2
1,301-1,350	5.4
1,351-1,400	5.6
1,401-1,450	5.8
1,451-1,500	6
1,501-1,550	6.2
1,551-1,600	6.4
1,601-1,650	6.6
1,651-1,700	6.8
1,701-1,750	7
1,751-1,800	7.2
1,801-1,850	7.4
1,851-1,900	7.6
1,901-1,950	7.8
1,951-2,000	8

How supplied
Available by prescription only
Suspension: 25 mg of phospholipids/ml suspended in normal saline solution in 8-ml single-dose vials

Pharmacodynamics
Surfactant action: Beractant is a natural bovine lung extract containing phospholipids, neutral lipids, fatty acids, and surfactant-related proteins to which dipalmitoylphosphatidylcholine, palmitic acid, and tripalmitin are added to standardize and to mimic surface tension–lowering properties of natural lung surfactant. Endogenous lung surfactant lowers surface tension on alveolar surfaces during respiration and stabilizes the alveoli against collapse at resting transpulmonary pressures. Drug lowers minimum surface tension, restores pulmonary surfactant, and restores surface activity to the lungs of premature infants with RDS.

Pharmacokinetics
Absorption: Most of the administered dose becomes lung-associated within hours.
Distribution: Drug is distributed across the alveolar surface.
Metabolism: Lipids enter endogenous surfactant pathway of recycling and reutilization.
Excretion: Alveolar clearance of lipid components is rapid.

Route	Onset	Peak	Duration
Intratracheal	Unknown	Unknown	Unknown

Contraindications and precautions
No known contraindications.

Interactions
None significant.

Adverse reactions
CV: *transient bradycardia,* vasoconstriction, hypotension.
Hematologic: hypocapnia, hypercapnia.
Respiratory: decreased oxygen saturation, endotracheal tube reflux or blockage, *apnea.*
Skin: pallor.

Overdose and treatment
Overdose may result in acute airway obstruction. Treatment should be supportive and symptomatic.

Special considerations
● Transient crackles and moist breath sounds can occur after beractant administration. Endotracheal suctioning or other remedial action isn't needed unless clear signs of airway obstruction are present.
● There's an increased risk of post-treatment nosocomial sepsis.
● Ensure proper placement and patency of endotracheal tube before administration. Suction

endotracheal tube if needed and allow infant to stabilize before administration of beractant.
• Determine total dose and slowly withdraw entire contents of vial into syringe through at least a 20G needle. Don't filter. Avoid shaking. Attach premeasured French catheter to syringe and fill with beractant. Discard excess through the catheter so that syringe contains only the total dose to be given.
• To ensure homogeneous distribution of beractant, each dose is divided into quarter doses and administered with the infant in a different position: head and body inclined slightly down, head turned to the right; head and body inclined slightly down, head turned to the left; head and body inclined slightly up, head turned to the right; head and body inclined slightly up, head turned to the left. Four doses may be administered within the first 48 hours after birth at intervals not exceeding every 6 hours.
• Refrigerate stored beractant; warm to room temperature before administration (standing, at least 20 minutes; in hand, at least 8 minutes). Don't use artificial warming methods.
• Begin preparation before infant's birth if preventive dose is to be given.
• Prevention strategy: Weigh, intubate, and stabilize infant. Dose should be administered as soon as possible after birth, within 15 minutes. Position infant and gently instill first quarter dose through catheter over 2 to 3 seconds; remove catheter and manually ventilate with sufficient oxygen to prevent cyanosis, at 60 breaths/minute and with sufficient positive pressure to provide adequate air exchange and chest wall excursion.
• Rescue strategy: First dose should be given as soon as possible after the infant is placed on a ventilator for management of RDS, preferably by 8 hours of age. Position infant and gently instill first quarter dose through catheter over 2 to 3 seconds; remove catheter and return infant to mechanical ventilator.
• Both strategies: Ventilate infant for at least 30 seconds or until stable. Reposition infant and instill next quarter dose. Remaining doses should be instilled using same procedure. After final quarter dose is administered, remove catheter without flushing. Don't suction for 1 hour unless signs of significant airway obstruction occur. Resume usual ventilator management and clinical care once dosing procedure is completed.
• Repeat doses: Need for repeat doses is determined by evidence of continuing respiratory distress. Dose is 100 mg phospholipids/kg based on infant's birth weight. Infant shouldn't be reweighed.

Patient monitoring
• Frequently monitor infant. Transient bradycardia and decreased oxygen saturation have occurred during dosing. Take appropriate corrective measures.
• Marked improvements in oxygenation may occur within minutes of administration, and significant improvements may be sustained for 48 to 72 hours.

Patient education
• Inform parents of need for drug and explain drug action and administration.
• Encourage parents to ask questions and address any concerns raised by them.

17 beta-estradiol/ norgestimate
Ortho-Prefest

Pharmacologic classification: combined synthetic estrogen and progestin
Therapeutic classification: hormone replacement
Pregnancy risk category: X

Indications and dosages
➤ *Treatment of moderate to severe vasomotor symptoms related to menopause, symptoms of vulvar and vaginal atrophy, and the prevention of osteoporosis in women with an intact uterus. Adults:* 1 mg estradiol (pink tablet) P.O. daily for 3 days; then 1 mg estradiol/0.09 mg norgestimate (white tablet) P.O. daily for 3 days. Repeat until blister card is finished.

How supplied
Available by prescription only
Tablets: blister card of 15 pink and 15 white tablets, for a total of 30 tablets (pink tablets, 1 mg estradiol; white tablets, 1 mg estradiol and 0.09 mg norgestimate)

Pharmacodynamics
Hormonal replacement action: Estradiol mimics the action of endogenous estrogen in treating menopausal symptoms and atrophic vaginitis. Estradiol is more potent than its metabolites, estrone and estriol. After menopause, most endogenous estrogens are produced by conversion of androstenedione to estrone. Thus, estrone and the sulfate conjugated form, estrone sulfate, are the most abundant circulating estrogens in postmenopausal women.

Circulating estrogens modulate pituitary secretion of the gonadotropins, luteinizing hormone, and follicle stimulating hormone through a negative feedback mechanism. Estrogen replacement therapy reduces the elevated levels of these hormones in postmenopausal women. Estrogens contribute to the shaping of the skeleton.

Norgestimate mimics the natural hormone, progesterone. Progestins counter estrogenic effects by decreasing the number of nuclear estradiol receptors and suppressing epithelial DNA synthesis in endometrial tissue.

Pharmacokinetics

Absorption: Serum estradiol levels peak about 7 hours after a dose. The metabolite of norgestimate, 17-deacytlnorgestimate, reaches peak serum levels about 2 hours after a dose. When given with a high-fat meal, peak serum estrone and estrone sulfate levels increase by 14% and 24%, respectively. The peak serum level of 17-deacetylnorgestimate decreases by 16%.

Distribution: Estrogens are widely distributed throughout the body. Estradiol is bound mainly to sex hormone–binding globulin and to albumin; 17-deacetylnorgestimate, the primary active metabolite of norgestimate, is about 99% protein-bound.

Metabolism: Estrogens are mainly metabolized in the liver. Estradiol is converted reversibly to estrone, and both can be converted to estriol, which is the major urinary metabolite. Estrogens also undergo enterohepatic recirculation via sulfate and glucuronide conjugation in the liver; biliary secretion of conjugates in the intestine, and hydrolysis in the gut followed by reabsorption. Norgestimate is extensively metabolized by first-pass metabolism to 17-deacetylnorgestimate in the GI tract, liver, or both.

Excretion: Estradiol, estrone, and estriol are excreted in urine. Norgestimate metabolites are eliminated in urine or feces. The half-life of estradiol and 17-deacetylnorgestimate in postmenopausal women is about 16 and 37 hours, respectively.

Route	Onset	Peak	Duration
P.O.			
estradiol	Unknown	7 hr	Unknown
norgesti-mate	Unknown	2 hr	Unknown

Contraindications and precautions

Contraindicated in women with known or suspected pregnancy, patients hypersensitive to any component of Ortho-Prefest, and patients with cancer of the breast, estrogen-dependent neoplasia, undiagnosed abnormal genital bleeding, or active or previous thrombophlebitis or thromboembolic disorders.

Also use cautiously in women who have had a hysterectomy, are overweight, have abnormal lipid profiles, or have impaired liver function.

Interactions

None reported.

Adverse reactions

CNS: depression, dizziness, fatigue, pain, *headache*.

EENT: pharyngitis, sinusitis.

GI: flatulence, nausea, abdominal pain.

GU: dysmenorrhea, vaginal bleeding, vaginitis.

Musculoskeletal: arthralgia, myalgia, *back pain*.

Respiratory: cough, upper respiratory tract infection.

Other: flulike symptoms, viral infection, tooth disorder, *breast pain*.

Overdose and treatment

Overdose may cause nausea, vomiting, and withdrawal bleeding in women. No specific treatment is recommended.

Special considerations

● The following test results may be falsely elevated: thyroid-binding globulin; platelet count; factors II, VII antigen, VIII antigen, VIII coagulant activity, IX, X, XII, VII-X complex, and II-VII-X complex; beta-thromboglobulin; high-density lipoprotein levels; triglyceride levels; corticosteroid levels; sex steroid levels; angiotensinogen/renin substrate; alpha-1-antitrypsin; ceruloplasmin; fibrinogen; and plasminogen antigen. Also, PT, PTT, and platelet aggregation time may be accelerated.

● The following test results may be falsely decreased: T_3 resin uptake, serum folate, metyrapone, glucose tolerance, low-density lipoprotein levels, anti-factor Xa, and antithrombin III.

● Use of estrogens may induce malignant neoplasms. Using progestin therapy with estrogen therapy significantly reduces this risk.

● There's an increased risk of venous thromboembolism in users of estrogen replacement.

● Hormone replacement therapy has been reported to increase the risk of breast cancer in postmenopausal women.

Patient monitoring

● Reassess patient at 6-month intervals to determine whether treatment is still necessary.

● Estrogens can lead to severe hypercalcemia in patients with breast cancer and bone metastases. If this occurs, stop the drug and take the appropriate measures to reduce serum calcium level.

Breast-feeding patients

● Estrogens decrease the quantity and quality of breast milk. Avoid use in nursing mothers.

Pediatric patients

● Not indicated for use in children.

Patient education

● Inform patient about the risks of taking estrogen therapy, such as breast cancer, cancer of the uterus, abnormal blood clotting, and gallbladder disease.

● Tell patient to report immediately undiagnosed, persistent, or recurrent abnormal vaginal bleeding.

● Instruct women to perform monthly breast examinations, and advise them to receive mammograms if they are over age 50.

● Tell patient to report pain in calves or chest, sudden shortness of breath, coughing blood, severe headaches, vomiting, dizziness, faintness, changes in vision or speech, and weakness or numbness in arms or legs. These are warning signals of blood clots.

• Urge patient to report signs of liver problems, such as yellowing of skin or eyes and upper right quadrant pain.

• Instruct patient to report pain, swelling, or tenderness in abdomen, which may indicate gallbladder problems.

• Instruct patient to store Ortho-Prefest at room temperature away from excessive heat and moisture. Product will remain stable for 18 months.

betamethasone (systemic)
Betnelan*, Celestone

betamethasone sodium phosphate
Betnesol*, Celestone Phosphate, Cel-U-Jec

betamethasone sodium phosphate and betamethasone acetate
Celestone Soluspan

Pharmacologic classification: glucocorticoid
Therapeutic classification: anti-inflammatory
Pregnancy risk category: NR

Indications and dosages
Note: Betamethasone acetate suspension shouldn't be given I.V.

➤ *Severe inflammation or immunosuppression. Adults:* 0.6 to 7.2 mg P.O. daily; usually 2.4 to 4.8 mg daily divided into two to four doses.
Children: 0.0175 to 0.25 mg/kg P.O. daily or 0.5 to 7.5 mg/m² daily in three to four divided doses.
betamethasone sodium phosphate
Adults: 0.5 to 9 mg I.M., I.V., or into joint or soft tissue daily.
betamethasone sodium phosphate and betamethasone acetate suspension
Adults: 0.25 to 2 ml into joint or soft tissue q 1 to 2 weeks, p.r.n. Effects may last a few days or 1 to 2 weeks depending on the joint condition being treated.

➤ *Hyaline membrane disease◇. Adults:* Give 2 ml I.M. daily to expectant mothers for 2 to 3 days before delivery.

How supplied
Available by prescription only
betamethasone
Syrup: 0.6 mg/5 ml
Tablets: 0.6 mg
betamethasone sodium phosphate
Enema: 5 mg (base)*
Injection: 4 mg (3 mg base)/ml in 5-ml vials
Tablets (effervescent): 500 mcg*

betamethasone sodium phosphate and betamethasone acetate suspension
Injection: betamethasone acetate 3 mg and betamethasone sodium phosphate (equivalent to 3 mg base)/ml (not for I.V. use)

Pharmacodynamics
Anti-inflammatory action: Stimulates the synthesis of enzymes needed to decrease the inflammatory response. It's a long-acting corticosteroid with an anti-inflammatory potency 25 times that of an equal weight of hydrocortisone. It has essentially no mineralocorticoid activity. Betamethasone tablets and syrup are used as oral anti-inflammatory agents.

Betamethasone sodium phosphate is highly soluble, has a prompt onset of action, and may be given I.V. Betamethasone sodium phosphate and betamethasone acetate (Celestone Soluspan) combine the rapid-acting phosphate salt and the slightly soluble, slowly released acetate salt to provide rapid anti-inflammatory effects with a sustained duration of action. It's a suspension and isn't to be given I.V. It's particularly useful as an anti-inflammatory agent in intra-articular, intradermal, and intralesional injections.

Pharmacokinetics
Absorption: Absorbed readily after oral administration. Systemic absorption occurs slowly following intra-articular injections.
Distribution: Removed rapidly from the blood and distributed to muscle, liver, skin, intestines, and kidneys. Betamethasone is bound weakly to plasma proteins (transcortin and albumin). Only the unbound portion is active. Adrenocorticoids are distributed into breast milk and through the placenta.
Metabolism: Metabolized in the liver to inactive glucuronide and sulfate metabolites.
Excretion: Inactive metabolites and small amounts of unmetabolized drug are excreted by the kidneys. Insignificant quantities of drug also are excreted in feces. Biological half-life of drug is 36 to 54 hours.

Route	Onset	Peak	Duration
P.O.	Prompt	Unknown	3-25 days
I.M.	Unknown	Unknown	7-14 days

Contraindications and precautions
Contraindicated in patients hypersensitive to drug and in those with viral or bacterial infections (except in life-threatening situations) or systemic fungal infections.

Use cautiously in patients with renal disease, hypertension, osteoporosis, diabetes mellitus, hypothyroidism, cirrhosis, diverticulitis, nonspecific ulcerative colitis, recent intestinal anastomoses, thromboembolic disorders, seizures, myasthenia gravis, heart failure, tuberculosis, ocular herpes simplex, emotional instability, and psychotic tendencies.

Interactions
Drug-drug. *Amphotericin B, diuretics*: Betamethasone may enhance hypokalemia. Monitor serum potassium levels and observe patient carefully.

Antacids, cholestyramine, colestipol: Decreased effect of betamethasone by adsorbing the corticosteroid, decreasing the amount absorbed. Use together cautiously.

Antidiabetics, insulin: Hyperglycemia, requiring dosage adjustment in diabetic patients. Monitor serum glucose levels.

Barbiturates, phenytoin, rifampin: Decreased corticosteroid effects because of increased hepatic metabolism. Monitor patient for clinical effect.

Cardiac glycosides: Increased risk of toxicity in patients receiving cardiac glycosides. Use together cautiously.

Estrogens: Reduced corticosteroid metabolism by increasing transcortin level. Monitor patient for adverse effects.

Isoniazid, salicylates: Increased metabolism of these drugs. Monitor patient for clinical effect.

Oral anticoagulants: In rare cases, may decrease the effects of oral anticoagulants. Monitor PT and INR.

Ulcerogenic drugs, such as NSAIDs: May increase the risk of GI ulceration. Use together cautiously.

Adverse reactions
CNS: *euphoria, insomnia,* psychotic behavior, pseudotumor cerebri, vertigo, headache, paresthesia, *seizures.*

CV: *heart failure,* hypertension, edema, *arrhythmias,* thrombophlebitis, *thromboembolism.*

EENT: cataracts, glaucoma.

GI: *peptic ulceration,* GI irritation, increased appetite, *pancreatitis,* nausea, vomiting.

GU: menstrual irregularities.

Metabolic: hypokalemia, hyperglycemia, and carbohydrate intolerance; increased thyroxine, and triiodothyronine levels.

Musculoskeletal: muscle weakness, osteoporosis.

Skin: delayed wound healing, acne, various skin eruptions, hirsutism.

Other: cushingoid state (moonface, buffalo hump, central obesity); susceptibility to infections; growth suppression in children; *acute adrenal insufficiency,* which may follow increased stress (infection, surgery, or trauma) or abrupt withdrawal after long-term therapy.

Overdose and treatment
Acute ingestion, even in massive doses, rarely occurs. Toxic signs and symptoms rarely occur if drug is used for less than 3 weeks, even at large doses. However, long-term use causes adverse physiologic effects, including suppression of the hypothalamic-pituitary-adrenal axis, cushingoid appearance, muscle weakness, and osteoporosis.

Special considerations
● Adrenocorticoid therapy suppresses reactions to skin tests; causes false-negative results in the nitroblue tetrazolium tests for systemic bacterial infections.

● Most adverse reactions to corticosteroids are dose- or duration-dependent.

● Gradually reduce dose after long-term use.

◗ **ALERT** After abrupt withdrawal, patient may experience rebound inflammation, fatigue, weakness, arthralgia, fever, dizziness, lethargy, depression, fainting, orthostatic hypotension, dyspnea, anorexia, and hypoglycemia. After prolonged use, sudden withdrawal may be fatal.

● Store tablets in a well-closed container and protected from light at temperatures of 36° to 86° F (2° to 30° C).

● Protect betamethasone sodium phosphate injection from light and store at a temperature between 59° and 86° F (15° and 30° C). Avoid freezing.

● Protect betamethasone sodium phosphate and betamethasone acetate sterile solution from light and store at 36° to 77° F (2° to 25° C); avoid freezing. Don't mix the sterile solution with diluents or local anesthetics containing preservatives because flocculation of the suspension may occur.

Patient monitoring
● Monitor patient continuously for effect and dosage adjustment, remissions, exacerbations, and stress.

Breast-feeding patients
● Information is incomplete. Risk versus benefits must be determined and reviewed with patient.

Pediatric patients
● Long-term use of betamethasone in children and adolescents may delay growth and maturation.

Patient education
● Warn patient not to stop drug abruptly.

● Instruct patient to take drug with food or milk.

● Tell patient to report symptoms of corticosteroid withdrawal, including fatigue, weakness, arthralgia, orthostatic hypotension, and dyspnea.

● Instruct patient to wear or carry medical identification that indicates need for supplemental glucocorticoid therapy during stress.

betamethasone dipropionate, augmented

Diprolene, Diprolene AF

betamethasone dipropionate

Alphatrex, Diprosone, Maxivate, Teladar

betamethasone valerate

Betaderm*, Betatrex, Beta-Val, Betnovate*, Celestoderm-V*, Ectosone*, Luxiq, Metaderm*, Novobetamet*, Psorion, Valisone

Pharmacologic classification: topical gluco-corticoid
Therapeutic classification: anti-inflammatory
Pregnancy risk category: C

Indications and dosages

➤ *Inflammation of corticosteroid-responsive dermatoses.* betamethasone valerate. *Adults and children:* Apply cream, lotion, ointment, or gel in a thin layer once daily to q.i.d.
➤ *Relief of inflammatory and pruritic manifestations of corticosteroid-responsive dermatoses of scalp. Adults:* Gently massage small amounts of foam into affected scalp areas b.i.d. (once in the morning and once at night) until control is achieved. If no improvement is seen within 2 weeks, reassess diagnosis.
betamethasone dipropionate
Adults and children over age 12: Apply cream, lotion, or ointment sparingly daily or b.i.d. Dosage of augmented 0.05% gels or lotions shouldn't exceed 50 g or 50 ml per week. Dosage of Diprolene ointments or creams 0.05% shouldn't exceed 45 g per week. To apply aerosol, direct spray onto affected area from a distance of 6 in (15 cm) for only 3 seconds t.i.d. or q.i.d.

How supplied

Available by prescription only
betamethasone dipropionate, augmented
Cream, gel, lotion, ointment: 0.05%
betamethasone dipropionate
Aerosol: 0.1%
Lotion, ointment, cream: 0.05%
betamethasone valerate
Cream: 0.01%, 0.05%, 0.1%,
Foam: 0.12%
Lotion, ointment: 0.1%

Pharmacodynamics

Anti-inflammatory action: Stimulates the synthesis of enzymes needed to decrease the inflammatory response. Betamethasone, a fluorinated derivative, has the advantage of availability in various bases to vary the potency for individual conditions.

Pharmacokinetics

Absorption: Amount absorbed depends on the potency of the preparation, amount applied, and nature of the skin at the application site. It ranges from about 1% in areas with a thick stratum corneum to as high as 36% in areas with a thin stratum corneum. Absorption increases in areas of skin damage, inflammation, or occlusion. Some systemic absorption of topical steroids occurs.
Distribution: After topical application, drug is distributed throughout local skin. Drug absorbed into circulation is removed rapidly from the blood and distributed into muscle, liver, skin, intestines, and kidneys.
Metabolism: After topical administration, drug is metabolized primarily in skin. The small amount absorbed into systemic circulation is metabolized primarily in the liver to inactive compounds.
Excretion: Inactive metabolites are excreted by the kidneys, primarily as glucuronides and sulfates, but also as unconjugated products. Small amounts of metabolites also are excreted in feces.

Route	Onset	Peak	Duration
Topical	Unknown	Unknown	Unknown

Contraindications and precautions

Contraindicated in patients hypersensitive to corticosteroids.

Interactions

None significant.

Adverse reactions

GU: glycosuria (with betamethasone dipropionate).
Skin: burning, pruritus, irritation, dryness, erythema, folliculitis, acneiform eruptions, perioral dermatitis, hypopigmentation, hypertrichosis, allergic contact dermatitis; *secondary infection, maceration, atrophy, striae, miliaria* (with occlusive dressings).
Metabolic: hyperglycemia.
Other: *hypothalamic-pituitary-adrenal axis suppression,* Cushing's syndrome.

Overdose and treatment

No information available.

Special considerations

Consider the recommendations relevant to all topical adrenocorticoids as well as the following.
● Diprolene ointment may suppress the hypothalamic-pituitary-adrenal axis at doses as low as 7 g daily. Patient shouldn't use more than 45 g weekly and shouldn't use occlusive dressings.
● Gently wash skin before applying. To prevent skin damage, rub medication in gently, leaving a thin coat. When treating hairy sites, part hair and apply directly to lesions.
● For application to the scalp, invert the can of foam. Dispense a small amount of drug onto a cool surface (not directly onto the hand because

the drug will melt). Massage foam into scalp until foam disappears.

Patient monitoring
● Monitor patient for systemic adverse reactions during prolonged use or use on a large body surface area.

Pediatric patients
● Treatment with Diprolene ointment isn't recommended in children under age 12.

Patient education
● Teach patient how to apply drug.
● Tell patient to stop drug and report signs of systemic absorption, skin irritation or ulceration, hypersensitivity, or infection.

betaxolol hydrochloride
Betoptic, Betoptic S, Kerlone

Pharmacologic classification: beta blocker
Therapeutic classification: antiglaucoma, antihypertensive
Pregnancy risk category: C

Indications and dosages
➤ **Chronic open-angle glaucoma and ocular hypertension.** *Adults:* Instill one to two drops in eyes b.i.d.
➤ **Management of hypertension (alone or with other antihypertensives).** *Adults:* Initially, 10 mg P.O. once daily. After 7 to 14 days, full antihypertensive effect should be seen. If necessary, double the dose to 20 mg P.O. once daily. Doses up to 40 mg daily also have been used.
✦ **Dosage adjustment.** In elderly patients, those with renal impairment, and those receiving dialysis, initial dose is 5 mg P.O. daily. Increase by 5 mg daily q 2 weeks to maximum of 20 mg daily.

How supplied
Available by prescription only
Ophthalmic solution: 5 mg/ml (0.5%) in 2.5-ml, 5-ml, 10-ml, 15-ml dropper bottles
Ophthalmic suspension: 2.5 mg/ml (0.25%) in 2.5-ml, 5-ml, 10-ml, 15-ml dropper bottles
Tablets: 10 mg, 20 mg

Pharmacodynamics
Antihypertensive action: Cardioselective adrenergic blocking effects of betaxolol slow heart rate and decrease cardiac output.
Ocular hypotensive action: Betaxolol hydrochloride is a cardioselective beta$_1$-blocker that reduces intraocular pressure (IOP), possibly by reducing production of aqueous humor when administered as an ophthalmic solution.

Pharmacokinetics
Absorption: Essentially complete after oral administration; minimal after ophthalmic use. A small first-pass effect reduces bioavailability by about 10%. Absorption isn't affected by food or alcohol.
Distribution: About 50% bound to plasma proteins.
Metabolism: Hepatic; about 85% of drug is recovered in urine as metabolites. Elimination half-life is prolonged in patients with hepatic disease, but clearance isn't affected, so dosage adjustment is unnecessary.
Excretion: Primarily renal (about 80%). Plasma half-life is 14 to 22 hours.

Route	Onset	Peak	Duration
P.O.	Unknown	1½-6 hr	Unknown
Oph-thalmic	½-1 hr	2 hr	> 12 hr

Contraindications and precautions
Contraindicated in patients hypersensitive to drug and those with severe bradycardia, greater than first-degree heart block, cardiogenic shock, or uncontrolled heart failure.

Interactions
Drug-drug. *Beta blockers:* Betaxolol may increase the effects of these drugs. Monitor patient for clinical effect. Ophthalmic betaxolol may increase the systemic effect of oral beta blockers. Monitor patient closely.
Calcium channel blockers: Increased risk of hypotension, left-sided heart failure, and AV conduction disturbances. Use I.V. calcium antagonists cautiously.
Carbonic anhydrase inhibitors, epinephrine, pilocarpine: Ophthalmic betaxolol enhances the lowering of IOP with these drugs. Monitor patient for clinical effect.
Catecholamine-depleting drugs, reserpine: Ophthalmic betaxolol enhances the hypotensive and bradycardiac effect of these drugs. Use of oral betaxolol with these drugs may have an additive effect. Monitor patient closely.
General anesthetics: May increase hypotensive effects. Observe patient carefully for excessive hypotension, bradycardia, or orthostatic hypotension.

Adverse reactions
Ophthalmic form
CNS: insomnia, depressive neurosis.
EENT: *eye stinging and brief discomfort on instillation,* photophobia, erythema, itching, keratitis, occasional tearing.
Systemic form
CNS: dizziness, fatigue, headache, insomnia, lethargy, anxiety.
CV: *bradycardia,* chest pain, *heart failure,* edema.
EENT: pharyngitis.
GI: nausea, diarrhea, dyspepsia.
GU: impotence.
Metabolic: altered glucose tolerance test results.
Musculoskeletal: arthralgia.

Respiratory: dyspnea, *bronchospasm.*
Skin: rash.

Overdose and treatment

Signs and symptoms of overdose, which are extremely rare with ophthalmic use, may include diplopia, bradycardia, heart block, hypotension, shock, increased airway resistance, cyanosis, fatigue, sleepiness, headache, sedation, coma, respiratory depression, seizures, nausea, vomiting, diarrhea, hypoglycemia, hallucinations, and nightmares.

Discontinue drug and flush eye with normal saline solution or water. For treatment of accidental substantial ingestion, emesis is most effective if started within 30 minutes, providing the patient isn't obtunded, comatose, or having seizures. Activated charcoal may be used. Treat bradycardia, conduction defects, and hypotension with I.V. fluids, glucagon, atropine, or isoproterenol; refractory bradycardia may require a transvenous pacemaker. Treat bronchoconstriction with I.V. aminophylline; treat seizures with I.V. diazepam.

Special considerations
Ophthalmic use
• Betaxolol is a cardioselective beta blocker. Its pulmonary and systemic effects are considerably milder than those of timolol or levobunolol.
• Ophthalmic betaxolol is intended for twice-daily dosage. Encourage patient to comply with this regimen.
Systemic use
• Withdrawal of beta blocker therapy before surgery is controversial. Some clinicians advocate withdrawal to prevent impairment of cardiac responsiveness to reflex stimuli and to prevent decreased responsiveness to exogenous catecholamines.
• To withdraw drug, gradually reduce dosage over at least 2 weeks.

Patient monitoring
• In some patients, a few weeks' treatment may be needed to stabilize pressure-lowering response. Determine IOP during the first 4 weeks of drug therapy.
• Monitor blood pressure closely.
• Monitor serum glucose; signs of hypoglycemia may be masked in patients taking beta blockers.

Breast-feeding patients
• Use cautiously. After oral administration, betaxolol appears in breast milk in amounts sufficient to affect the breast-feeding infant.

Pediatric patients
• Ophthalmic preparation shouldn't be used in patients under age 18.

Geriatric patients
• Use cautiously in elderly patients with cardiac or pulmonary disease.

Patient education
Ophthalmic use
• Tell patient to shake suspension well before use.
• Instruct patient to tilt head back and, while looking up, instill drug into the lower lid.
• Warn patient not to touch dropper to eye or surrounding tissue.
• Instruct patient not to close eyes tightly or blink more than usual after instillation.
• Remind patient to wait at least 5 minutes before using other eyedrops.
• Advise patient to wear sunglasses or avoid exposure to bright lights.
Systemic use
• Instruct patient to take drug exactly as prescribed and warn against discontinuing it suddenly.
• Advise patient to report shortness of breath or difficulty breathing, unusually fast heartbeat, cough, or fatigue with exertion.

---

bethanechol chloride
Duvoid, Myotonachol, Urecholine

Pharmacologic classification: cholinergic agonist
Therapeutic classification: urinary tract and GI tract stimulant
Pregnancy risk category: C

Indications and dosages
➤ *Acute postoperative and postpartum nonobstructive (functional) urine retention, neurogenic atony of urinary bladder with retention.* Adults: 10 to 50 mg P.O. b.i.d., t.i.d, or q.i.d. Or 2.575 to 5.15 mg S.C. (use 10 mg S.C. with extreme caution). Never give drug I.M. or I.V. When used for urine retention, some patients may require 50 to 100 mg P.O. per dose. Use such doses with extreme caution. Test dose: 2.5 mg S.C. repeated at 15- to 30-minute intervals to a maximum of four doses to determine the minimal effective dose, then use minimal effective dose three or four times daily. Adjust dosage to meet individual requirements.
➤ *Restore bladder function in patients with chronic neurogenic bladder.* Adults: 7.5 to 10 mg S.C. q 4 hours around the clock. Dosage adjustments are made based on residual urine measurements.
➤ *Bladder dysfunction caused by phenothiazines* ◇. *Adults:* 50 to 100 mg P.O. q.i.d.
➤ *To lessen the adverse effects of tricyclic antidepressants* ◇. *Adults:* 25 mg P.O. t.i.d.
➤ *Chronic gastric reflux* ◇. *Adults:* 25 mg P.O. q.i.d.
➤ *Familial dysautonomia* ◇. *Children:* 0.2 to 0.4 mg/kg S.C. q.i.d. 30 minutes before meals with an oral antacid; then after 2 weeks, give 1 to 2 mg P.O. q.i.d.
➤ *To diagnose flaccid or atonic neurogenic bladder* ◇. *Adults:* 2.5 mg S.C.

Reactions may be *common*, uncommon, *life-threatening*, or COMMON AND LIFE-THREATENING.

► *To diagnose cystic fibrosis* ◇. Before administration, dilute 5 mg of drug in 3 ml of D₅W to yield 1.25 mg/ml. *Children over age 1:* 1 mg intradermally.
Children ages 2 months to 1 year: 0.5 mg intradermally.
Infants from birth to age 2 months: 0.25 mg intradermally.

How supplied
Available by prescription only
Injection: 5 mg/ml
Tablets: 5 mg, 10 mg, 25 mg, 50 mg

Pharmacodynamics
Urinary tract stimulant action: Bethanechol directly binds to and stimulates muscarinic receptors of the parasympathetic nervous system. This increases tone of the bladder detrusor muscle, usually resulting in contraction, decreased bladder capacity, and subsequent urination.
GI tract stimulant action: Bethanechol directly stimulates cholinergic receptors, leading to increased gastric tone and motility and peristalsis. Drug improves lower esophageal sphincter tone by directly stimulating cholinergic receptors, thereby alleviating gastric reflux.

Pharmacokinetics
Absorption: Poorly absorbed from the GI tract (absorption varies considerably among patients).
Distribution: Largely unknown; however, therapeutic doses don't penetrate the blood-brain barrier.
Metabolism: Unknown.
Excretion: Unknown.

Route	Onset	Peak	Duration
P.O.	30-90 min	Unknown	6 hr
S.C.	5-15 min	15-30 min	2 hr

Contraindications and precautions
Contraindicated for I.M. or I.V. use and in patients hypersensitive to drug or its components. Also contraindicated in patients with uncertain strength or integrity of the bladder wall, mechanical obstructions of the GI or urinary tract, hyperthyroidism, peptic ulceration, latent or active bronchial asthma, pronounced bradycardia or hypotension, vasomotor instability, cardiac or coronary artery disease, seizure disorder, Parkinson's disease, spastic GI disturbances, acute inflammatory lesions of the GI tract, peritonitis, or marked vagotonia. Also contraindicated when increased muscular activity of GI or urinary tract is harmful. Use cautiously in pregnant women.

Interactions
Drug-drug. *Cholinergic drugs, especially cholinesterase inhibitors:* Additive effects may occur. Avoid use together.
Ganglionic blockers such as mecamylamine: May cause a critical blood pressure decrease; this effect is usually preceded by abdominal symptoms. Avoid use together.
Procainamide, quinidine: May reverse the cholinergic effect of bethanechol on muscle. Monitor patient for clinical effect.

Adverse reactions
CNS: headache, malaise.
CV: flushing, hypotension, reflex tachycardia.
EENT: lacrimation, miosis.
GI: *abdominal cramps, diarrhea,* excessive salivation, nausea, belching, borborygmi.
GU: urinary urgency.
Hepatic: increased serum levels of amylase, lipase, bilirubin, and AST.
Respiratory: *bronchoconstriction,* increased bronchial secretions.
Skin: diaphoresis.

Overdose and treatment
Signs and symptoms of overdose include nausea, vomiting, abdominal cramps, diarrhea, involuntary defecation, urinary urgency, excessive salivation, miosis, excessive tearing, bronchospasm, increased bronchial secretions, hypotension, excessive sweating, bradycardia or reflex tachycardia, and substernal pain.

Treatment requires discontinuation of drug and administration of atropine by S.C., I.M., or I.V. route. (Atropine must be administered cautiously; an overdose could cause bronchial plug formation.) Contact local or regional poison control center for more information.

Special considerations
● Atropine sulfate should be readily available to counteract toxic reactions that may occur during treatment with bethanechol.
⚠ **ALERT** Never give bethanechol I.M. or I.V. because that could cause circulatory collapse, hypotension, severe abdominal cramps, bloody diarrhea, shock, or cardiac arrest. Give only by S.C. route when giving parenterally.
● For administration to treat urine retention, bedpan should be readily available.
● Give drug on an empty stomach; eating soon after drug administration may cause nausea and vomiting.
● Store drug in tight container between 59° and 86° F (15° and 30° C). Avoid freezing. The injection may be autoclaved at 248° F (120° C) for 20 minutes without discoloration or loss of potency.

Patient monitoring
● Monitor blood pressure; patients with hypertension receiving bethanechol may experience a precipitous decrease in blood pressure.

Pregnant patients
● Bethanechol shouldn't be used in pregnant women.

Pediatric patients

● Safety and efficacy haven't been established in children.

Patient education

● Instruct patient to take oral form on an empty stomach and at regular intervals.
● Inform patient that drug is usually effective within 30 to 90 minutes after oral administration and 5 to 15 minutes after S.C. administration.

bexarotene
Targretin

Pharmacologic classification: retinoid (selective retinoid X receptor activator)
Therapeutic classification: tumor cell growth inhibitor
Pregnancy risk category: X

Indications and dosages

➤ *Cutaneous effects of cutaneous T-cell lymphoma in patients refractory to at least one previous systemic therapy.*
Adults: 300 mg/m^2 P.O. daily as a single dose with a meal. If no response after 8 weeks, increase to 400 mg/m^2 daily if initial dose was tolerated.
✦ *Dosage adjustment.* For patients with hepatic insufficiency, lower doses may be needed. If toxicity occurs, dose may be adjusted to 200 mg/m^2 daily, then to 100 mg/m^2 daily; or drug may be temporarily suspended. When toxicity is controlled, doses may be carefully readjusted upward.

How supplied

Available by prescription only
Capsules: 75 mg

Pharmacodynamics

Antineoplastic action: Bexarotene selectively binds and activates retinoid X receptor subtypes. Once activated, these receptors function as transcription factors that regulate the expression of genes that control cellular differentiation and proliferation. Bexarotene inhibits the growth *in vitro* of some tumor cell lines of hematopoietic and squamous cell origin and it induces tumor cell regression *in vivo* in some animal models. The exact mechanism of action in the treatment of cutaneous T-cell lymphoma is unknown.

Pharmacokinetics

Absorption: Bexarotene is absorbed from the GI tract. Absorption is increased if given with a fat-containing meal.
Distribution: Bexarotene is more than 99% bound to plasma proteins.
Metabolism: Bexarotene is metabolized through oxidative pathways, primarily by the cytochrome P-450 3A4 system, to four metabolites. These metabolites may maintain retinoid receptor activity. The terminal half-life is 7 hours.
Excretion: Bexarotene is thought to be eliminated primarily through the hepatobiliary system.

Route	Onset	Peak	Duration
P.O.	Unknown	Unknown	Unknown

Contraindications and precautions

Contraindicated in pregnant women and in patients hypersensitive to drug or its components. Drug isn't recommended for patients who have risk factors for pancreatitis, such as previous pancreatitis, uncontrolled hyperlipidemia, excessive alcohol consumption, uncontrolled diabetes mellitus, or biliary tract disease. Also not recommended for patients taking drugs known to increase triglyceride levels or cause pancreatic toxicity.

Use cautiously in women of childbearing potential, patients with hepatic insufficiency, and patients hypersensitive to retinoids.

Interactions

Drug-drug. *Erythromycin, gemfibrozil, itraconazole, ketoconazole, other inhibitors of cytochrome P-450 3A4:* Increased plasma levels of bexarotene. Avoid concomitant use.
Insulin, sulfonylureas: May enhance hypoglycemic action of these drugs, resulting in hypoglycemia in patients with diabetes mellitus. Use together cautiously.
Phenobarbital, phenytoin, rifampin, other inducers of cytochrome P-450 3A4: Decreased plasma levels of bexarotene. Avoid concomitant use.
Vitamin A preparations: Increased risk of vitamin A toxicity. Avoid vitamin A supplements.
Drug-food. *Any food:* Increased drug absorption. Administer drug with food.
Grapefruit juice: May inhibit cytochrome P-450 3A4. Don't give concomitantly.
Drug-lifestyle. *Sun exposure:* Retinoids may cause photosensitivity. Tell patient to minimize exposure to sunlight and artificial ultraviolet light.

Adverse reactions

CNS: *headache,* insomnia, *asthenia,* fatigue, syncope, depression, agitation, ataxia, *CVA,* confusion, dizziness, hyperesthesia, hypoesthesia, neuropathy.
CV: *peripheral edema,* chest pain, *hemorrhage,* hypertension, angina, *heart failure,* tachycardia.
EENT: cataracts, pharyngitis, rhinitis, dry eyes, conjunctivitis, ear pain, blepharitis, corneal lesion, keratitis, otitis externa, visual field defect.
GI: *nausea,* diarrhea, vomiting, anorexia, *pancreatitis, abdominal pain,* elevated amylase level, constipation, dry mouth, flatulence, colitis, dyspepsia, cheilitis, gastroenteritis, gingivitis, melena.
GU: elevated creatinine level, albuminuria, hematuria, incontinence, urinary tract infection, uri-

nary urgency, dysuria, abnormal kidney function, breast pain.

Hematologic: *leukopenia,* anemia, eosinophilia, thrombocythemia, lymphocytosis, ***thrombocytopenia.***

Hepatic: increased LD, AST, and ALT levels; bilirubinemia; *liver failure.*

Metabolic: *hyperlipemia, hypercholesteremia, hypothyroidism,* hyperglycemia, hypoproteinemia, hypocalcemia, hyponatremia, weight change.

Musculoskeletal: arthralgia, myalgia, back pain, bone pain, myasthenia, arthrosis.

Respiratory: pneumonia, dyspnea, hemoptysis, pleural effusion, bronchitis, cough, lung edema, hypoxia.

Skin: *rash, dry skin, exfoliative dermatitis; alopecia, photosensitivity,* pruritus, cellulitis, acne, skin ulcer, skin nodule.

Other: *infection,* chills, fever, flu syndrome, *sepsis.*

Overdose and treatment

Overdose doesn't appear to produce acute toxic effects and should be treated with supportive care for the patient's signs and symptoms.

Special considerations

⚠ ALERT Women of childbearing potential should use effective contraception for at least one month before start of therapy, throughout therapy, and for at least one month after therapy stops. During therapy, two reliable forms of contraception should be used simultaneously unless abstinence is the chosen method. A negative pregnancy test should be obtained within one week before starting therapy and monthly during therapy.

• Therapy starts on the second or third day of a normal menstrual period.

• Men with sexual partners who are pregnant, could be pregnant, or could become pregnant must use condoms during sexual intercourse during and for at least one month after therapy.

• No more than a one-month supply of bexarotene should be given to a patient of childbearing potential so the results of pregnancy testing can be assessed and the patient can be counseled monthly to avoid pregnancy because of the risk of birth defects.

• CA 125 assay values in patients with ovarian cancer may be increased by bexarotene therapy.

Patient monitoring

• Obtain total cholesterol, high-density lipoprotin, and triglyceride levels at the start of drug therapy, weekly until the lipid response is established (2 to 4 weeks), and at 8-week intervals thereafter. Elevated triglycerides during treatment should be treated with antilipemic therapy and, if necessary, the dose of bexarotene should be reduced or suspended.

• Obtain baseline thyroid function tests and monitor them during treatment.

• Monitor WBC with differential at baseline and periodically during treatment.

• Monitor liver function tests at baseline and after 1, 2, and 4 weeks of treatment. If stable, monitor them every 8 weeks during treatment. Consider suspending treatment if results are three times the upper limit of normal.

• Obtain ophthalmologic evaluation for cataracts in patients who experience visual difficulties.

Breast-feeding patients

• Not recommended. A decision should be made to discontinue either nursing or the drug, taking into account the importance of the drug to the mother.

Pediatric patients

• Safety and effectiveness in children haven't been established.

Geriatric patients

• Bexarotene has been used in geriatric patients without any overall differences in safety or efficacy, but the greater sensitivity of some older people can't be ruled out.

Patient education

• Advise patient to minimize exposure to sunlight and artificial ultraviolet light and to take appropriate precautions.

• Teach patient that it may take several capsules to make the necessary dose and these capsules should all be taken at the same time and with a meal.

• Teach woman of childbearing potential the dangers of becoming pregnant while taking bexarotene, and emphasize the need for monthly pregnancy tests.

• Explain the need to obtain baseline laboratory tests and periodic tests throughout therapy.

• Tell patient to report vision changes.

bicalutamide
Casodex

Pharmacologic classification: nonsteroidal antiandrogen
Therapeutic classification: antineoplastic
Pregnancy risk category: X

Indications and dosages

➤ *Adjunct therapy for treatment of advanced prostate cancer. Adults:* 50 mg P.O. once daily in morning or evening.

How supplied

Available by prescription only
Tablets: 50 mg

Pharmacodynamics

Antineoplastic action: Drug competitively inhibits the action of androgens by binding to cytosol androgen receptors in the target tissue.

Prostatic carcinoma, known to be sensitive to androgens, responds to treatment that either counteracts the effect of androgen or removes its source.

Pharmacokinetics
Absorption: Well absorbed from GI tract.
Distribution: 96% protein-bound.
Metabolism: Undergoes stereospecific metabolism. The S (inactive) isomer is metabolized primarily by glucuronidation. The R (active) isomer also undergoes glucuronidation but is predominantly oxidized to an inactive metabolite followed by glucuronidation.
Excretion: Excreted in urine and feces.

Route	Onset	Peak	Duration
P.O.	Unknown	Unknown	Unknown

Contraindications and precautions
Contraindicated in pregnant women and in patients hypersensitive to drug or any component in the tablet. Use cautiously in patients with moderate to severe hepatic impairment because drug is extensively metabolized by the liver.

Interactions
Drug-drug. *Coumarin anticoagulants:* Bicalutamide displaces coumarin anticoagulants from their protein-binding sites. Monitor PT and INR closely. The anticoagulant dose may need adjustment.

Adverse reactions
CNS: *asthenia,* headache, dizziness, paresthesia, insomnia.
CV: *hot flashes,* hypertension, chest pain, peripheral edema.
GI: *constipation, nausea, diarrhea,* abdominal pain, flatulence, vomiting.
GU: nocturia, hematuria, urinary tract infection, impotence, urinary incontinence, increased BUN and creatinine levels.
Hematologic: hypochromic anemia, iron-deficiency anemia.
Hepatic: increased liver enzyme levels.
Metabolic: hyperglycemia, weight loss.
Musculoskeletal: *back or pelvic pain,* bone pain.
Respiratory: dyspnea.
Skin: rash, sweating.
Other: *general pain, infection,* flu syndrome, gynecomastia.

Overdose and treatment
A single dose of bicalutamide that results in symptoms of an overdose considered to be life-threatening hasn't been established. There's no specific antidote; treatment of an overdose should be symptomatic. Vomiting may be induced if patient is alert. Dialysis isn't likely to be helpful because bicalutamide is highly protein-bound and is extensively metabolized.

Special considerations
● Bicalutamide is used in combination therapy with a luteinizing hormone-releasing hormone (LHRH) analogue for the treatment of advanced prostate cancer. Treatment should begin at the same time as that with the prescribed LHRH analogue.
● Administer bicalutamide at the same time each day.
● Drug isn't indicated for use in women.

Patient monitoring
● Monitor serum prostate specific antigen (PSA) levels regularly. PSA levels help in assessing patient's response to therapy. Elevated levels require reevaluation of patient to determine disease progression.
● Monitor liver function studies. Discontinue drug when patient develops jaundice or has laboratory evidence of liver injury in the absence of liver metastases. Abnormalities are usually reversible with discontinuation of drug.

Pediatric patients
● Safety and efficacy in children haven't been established.

Patient education
● Inform patient that drug may be taken without regard to meals.
● Advise patient to take drug at the same time each day.
● Tell patient that bicalutamide is used with other drugs. Stress importance of not interrupting or stopping these drugs without medical consultation.

bimatoprost
LUMIGAN

Pharmacologic classification: prostaglandin analogue
Therapeutic classification: anti-glaucoma, ocular antihypertensive
Pregnancy risk category: C

Indications and dosages
➤ *Reduction of elevated intraocular pressure (IOP) in patients with open-angle glaucoma or ocular hypertension who are intolerant of or unresponsive to other IOP-lowering drugs.* **Adults:** Instill one drop in the conjunctival sac of the affected eye or eyes once daily in the evening.

How supplied
Available by prescription only
Ophthalmic solution: 0.03%

Pharmacodynamics
Ocular hypotensive activity: Bimatoprost is a prostamide, which is a synthetic analog of prostaglandin. It selectively mimics the effects of

naturally occurring prostaglandins. Bimatoprost is believed to lower IOP by increasing the outflow of aqueous humor through the trabecular meshwork and uveoscleral routes.

Pharmacokinetics
Absorption: Absorbed through the cornea.
Distribution: Moderately distributed into tissues. Bimatoprost resides mainly in plasma, and about 12% remains unbound in plasma.
Metabolism: Bimatoprost is mainly metabolized by oxidation.
Excretion: Metabolites are 67% eliminated in urine; 25% are eliminated in feces.

Route	Onset	Peak	Duration
Oph-thalmic	Unknown	10 min	1½ hr

Adverse reactions
CNS: headache, asthenia.
EENT: *conjunctival hyperemia, growth of eyelashes, ocular pruritus,* ocular dryness, visual disturbance, ocular burning, foreign body sensation, eye pain, pigmentation of the periocular skin, blepharitis, cataract, superficial punctate keratitis, eyelid erythema, ocular irritation, eyelash darkening, eye discharge, tearing, photophobia, allergic conjunctivitis, asthenopia, increased iris pigmentation, conjunctival edema.
Hepatic: abnormal liver function test results.
Respiratory: *upper respiratory tract infection.*
Skin: hirsutism.
Other: *infection.*

Interactions
None significant.

Overdose and treatment
No information available. Treatment should be symptomatic if overdose occurs.

Contraindications and precautions
Contraindicated in patients hypersensitive to bimatoprost, benzalkonium chloride, or other ingredients of this product. Use cautiously in patients with renal or hepatic impairment. Use cautiously in patients with active intraocular inflammation (iritis or uveitis), aphakic patients, pseudophakic patients with a torn posterior lens capsule, or patients at risk for macular edema.

Special considerations
• Don't use drug in patients with angle-closure glaucoma, inflammatory glaucoma, or neovascular glaucoma.
• Temporary or permanent increase in pigmentation of the iris, eyelid, and eyelashes may occur, as well as growth of the eyelashes.
• Contact lenses should be removed before instilling drug and may be reinserted 15 minutes afterward.
• If more than one ophthalmic drug is being used, they should be given at least 5 minutes apart.

• Store drug in original container between 59° and 77° F (15° to 25°C).

Patient monitoring
• Monitor patient for excessive ocular irritation, and evaluate the success of treatment.

Breast-feeding patients
• It isn't known if drug appears in breast milk. Use cautiously when administering drug to a nursing woman.

Pediatric patients
• Safety and efficacy in children haven't been established.

Geriatric patients
• No overall differences in safety or effectiveness have been observed between elderly and other adult patients.

Patient education
• Tell the patient receiving treatment in only one eye about the risk for increased brown pigmentation of the iris, darkening of the eyelid skin, and increased length, thickness, pigmentation, and number of lashes in the treated eye.
• Teach patient to instill drops. Tell him to wash his hands before and after doing so. Warn him not to touch the dropper tip to eye or surrounding tissue.
• Tell patient to remove contact lenses before instilling drops. Explain that they can be reinserted 15 minutes after administration.
• Advise patient to apply light pressure on lacrimal sac for 1 minute after instillation to minimize systemic absorption of the drug.
• Advise patient that if more than one ophthalmic drug is being used, they should be administered at least 5 minutes apart.
• Urge patient to immediately report conjunctivitis or lid reactions.
• Tell patient that if eye trauma or infection occurs or if eye surgery is needed, he should seek medical advice before continuing to use the multidose container.
• Stress the importance of compliance with the recommended therapy.

biperiden hydrochloride
biperiden lactate
Akineton

Pharmacologic classification: anticholinergic
Therapeutic classification: antiparkinsonian
Pregnancy risk category: C

Indications and dosages
➤ *Extrapyramidal disorders. Adults:* 2 mg P.O. daily, b.i.d., or t.i.d., depending on severity. Usual dose is 2 mg daily. For treatment of extrapyramidal symptoms induced by drugs, give

2 mg I.M. or slow I.V. q 30 minutes, not to exceed 8 mg in a 24-hour period.

➤ *Parkinsonism.* Adults: 2 mg P.O. t.i.d. or q.i.d. For prolonged therapy, adjust to maximum of 16 mg daily.

➤ *Treatment of unrelated spastic disorders (such as spinal cord injury)* ◇ . Adults: 2 mg P.O. b.i.d. to q.i.d.

How supplied
Available by prescription only
Injection: 5 mg/ml in 1-ml ampule
Tablets: 2 mg

Pharmacodynamics
Antiparkinsonian action: Drug blocks central cholinergic receptors, helping to balance cholinergic activity in the basal ganglia. It also may prolong the effects of dopamine by blocking dopamine reuptake and storage at central receptor sites.

Pharmacokinetics
Absorption: Well absorbed from the GI tract.
Distribution: Metabolized in the liver.
Metabolism: Unknown.
Excretion: Excreted in urine as unchanged drug and metabolites. After oral therapy, small amounts are probably excreted as unabsorbed drug.

Route	Onset	Peak	Duration
P.O.	1 hr	Unknown	6-12 hr
I.V.	Prompt	Unknown	1-8 hr
I.M.	10-30 min	Unknown	Unknown

Contraindications and precautions
Contraindicated in patients hypersensitive to drug and in those with angle-closure glaucoma, bowel obstruction, or megacolon. Use cautiously in patients with prostatic hyperplasia, arrhythmias, or seizure disorders.

Interactions
Drug-drug. *Amantadine:* Increased anticholinergic adverse effects of biperiden, such as confusion and hallucinations. Decrease biperiden dosage before amantadine administration.
Antacids, antidiarrheals: Decreased biperiden absorption. Administer biperiden at least 1 hour before these drugs.
CNS depressants: Increased sedative effects of biperiden. Use together cautiously.
Digoxin: Plasma digoxin levels may be elevated. Monitor digoxin level.
Haloperidol, phenothiazines: May decrease antipsychotic effectiveness of these drugs, possibly by direct CNS antagonism. Monitor patient for clinical effect.
Phenothiazines: Increased risk of anticholinergic adverse effects. Avoid use together.
Drug-lifestyle. *Alcohol use:* Increased sedative effects of biperiden. Discourage concurrent use.

Adverse reactions
CNS: disorientation, euphoria, drowsiness, agitation.
CV: transient orthostatic hypotension.
EENT: blurred vision.
GI: dry mouth, *constipation.*
GU: urine retention.

Overdose and treatment
Overdose may cause central stimulation followed by depression and psychotic symptoms, such as disorientation, confusion, hallucinations, delusions, anxiety, agitation, and restlessness. Peripheral effects may include dilated, nonreactive pupils; blurred vision; hot, dry, flushed skin; dry mucous membranes; dysphagia; decreased or absent bowel sounds; urine retention; hyperthermia; headache; tachycardia; hypertension; and increased respiration.

Treatment is primarily symptomatic and supportive, as necessary. Maintain patent airway. If the patient is alert, induce emesis (or use gastric lavage) and follow with a saline solution cathartic and activated charcoal to prevent further absorption of orally administered drug. In severe cases, physostigmine may be administered to block antimuscarinic effects of biperiden. Give fluids, as needed, to treat shock; diazepam to control psychotic symptoms; and pilocarpine (instilled into the eyes) to relieve mydriasis. If urine retention occurs, catheterization may be necessary.

Special considerations
● Adverse reactions are dose-related and may resemble atropine toxicity.
● When giving drug parenterally, keep patient supine; parenteral administration may cause transient orthostatic hypotension and disturbed coordination.
● When giving biperiden I.V., inject drug slowly.
● Because biperiden may cause dizziness, patient may need assistance when walking.
● If patient has severe parkinsonism, tremors may increase when drug is given to relieve spasticity.

Patient monitoring
● Monitor patient for adverse reactions related to anticholinergics.
● Monitor patient for tolerance to drug.

Breast-feeding patients
● Drug may appear in breast milk, possibly resulting in infant toxicity. Drug may also decrease milk production. Avoid use of drug in breast-feeding women.

Pediatric patients
● Drug isn't recommended for children.

Geriatric patients
● Use cautiously in geriatric patients. Lower doses are indicated.

Reactions may be *common*, uncommon, *life-threatening*, or COMMON AND LIFE-THREATENING.

Patient education
• Tell patient that tolerance to therapeutic and adverse effects can occur with long-term drug use.
• Advise patient that drug may increase sensitivity of the eyes to light.
• Instruct patient to take drug with food to avoid GI upset.

bisacodyl
Bisco-Lax, Correctol, Dulcolax, Fleet Laxative, Modane

Pharmacologic classification: diphenylmethane derivative
Therapeutic classification: stimulant laxative
Pregnancy risk category: B

Indications and dosages
➤ *Constipation, preparation for childbirth, surgery, or rectal or bowel examination.* *Adults and children over age 12:* 5 to 15 mg P.O. daily. In adults, up to 30 mg may be used for thorough evacuation needed for examinations or surgery. Or, give one suppository (10 mg) or 30 ml of rectal suspension P.R. daily.
Children ages 3 to 12: 5 to 10 mg P.O. daily or 0.3 mg/kg daily.
Children ages 2 to 11: ½ to 1 suppository (5 to 10 mg) or 15 ml of rectal suspension P.R. daily.
Children under age 2: ½ suppository (5 mg) P.R. daily.

How supplied
Available without a prescription
Rectal suspension: 10 mg/30 ml
Suppositories: 10 mg
Tablets: 5 mg

Pharmacodynamics
Laxative action: Bisacodyl has a direct stimulant effect on the colon, increasing peristalsis and enhancing bowel evacuation.

Pharmacokinetics
Absorption: Minimal.
Distribution: Distributed locally.
Metabolism: Metabolized in the liver.
Excretion: Excreted primarily in feces; some in urine.

Route	Onset	Peak	Duration
P.O.	6-12 hr	Variable	Variable
P.R.	15-60 min	Variable	Variable

Contraindications and precautions
Contraindicated in patients hypersensitive to drug; in patients with abdominal pain, nausea, vomiting, or other symptoms of appendicitis or acute surgical abdomen; and in patients with rectal bleeding, gastroenteritis, or intestinal obstruction.

Interactions
Drug-drug. *Antacids and drugs that increase gastric pH levels:* May cause premature dissolution of the enteric coating, resulting in intestinal or gastric irritation or cramping. Avoid use together.
Drug-food. *Milk:* May cause premature dissolution of the enteric coating, resulting in intestinal or gastric irritation or cramping. Discourage use together.

Adverse reactions
CNS: muscle weakness with excessive use, dizziness, faintness.
GI: nausea, vomiting, abdominal cramps, diarrhea (with high doses), *burning sensation in rectum* (with suppositories), laxative dependence with long-term or excessive use.
Metabolic: alkalosis, hypokalemia, tetany, protein-losing enteropathy with excessive use, fluid and electrolyte imbalance.

Overdose and treatment
No cases of overdose have been reported.

Special considerations
• To avoid GI irritation, patient should swallow tablets whole rather than crushing or chewing them.
• Administer tablets with 8 oz (240 ml) of fluid (but not milk).

Patient monitoring
• Monitor patient for diarrhea, electrolyte abnormalities (hypokalemia), and dehydration (with long-term use); drug is meant for short-term therapy.

Breast-feeding patients
• Drug may be used by breast-feeding women.

Patient education
• Instruct patient not to take drug within 1 hour of drinking milk or taking an antacid.
• Tell patient to take only as directed to avoid laxative dependence.

bismuth subsalicylate
Pepto-Bismol

Pharmacologic classification: adsorbent
Therapeutic classification: antidiarrheal
Pregnancy risk category: C (D in third trimester)

Indications and dosages
➤ *Mild, nonspecific diarrhea.* *Adults:* 30 ml or two tablets P.O. q 30 to 60 minutes up to a maximum of eight doses and for no more than 2 days.
Children ages 9 to 12: 15 ml or one tablet P.O.
Children ages 6 to 9: 10 ml or ⅔ tablet P.O.
Children ages 3 to 6: 5 ml or ⅓ tablet P.O.

Children's doses given q 30 to 60 minutes up to a maximum of eight doses in 24 hours and for no more than 2 days.

How supplied
Available without a prescription
Caplets: 262 mg
Suspension: 130 mg/15 ml, 262 mg/15 ml, 524 mg/15 ml
Tablets (chewable): 262 mg

Pharmacodynamics
Antidiarrheal action: Bismuth adsorbs extra water in the bowel during diarrhea. It also adsorbs toxins and forms a protective coating for the intestinal mucosa.

Pharmacokinetics
Absorption: Absorbed poorly; significant salicylate absorption may occur after using bismuth subsalicylate.
Distribution: Distributed locally in the gut.
Metabolism: Metabolized minimally.
Excretion: Excreted in urine.

Route	Onset	Peak	Duration
P.O.	1 hr	Unknown	Unknown

Contraindications and precautions
Contraindicated in patients hypersensitive to salicylates. Use cautiously in patients already taking aspirin or aspirin-containing medications.

Interactions
Drug-drug. *Salicylates:* Increased risk of aspirin toxicity. Monitor patient closely.
Sulfinpyrazone: Impaired uricosuric effect. Monitor patient for clinical effect.
Tetracycline: Bismuth subsalicylate may impair tetracycline absorption. Separate administration times.

Adverse reactions
GI: temporary darkening of tongue and stools.
Other: salicylism (with high doses).

Overdose and treatment
Overdose hasn't been reported. However, overdose is more likely with bismuth subsalicylate; probable clinical effects include CNS changes, such as tinnitus and fever.

Special considerations
● Because bismuth is radiopaque, it may interfere with radiologic examination of the GI tract.
● Bismuth subsalicylate has been used investigationally to treat peptic ulcer. Doses of 600 mg P.O. t.i.d. may be as effective as cimetidine 800 mg P.O. once daily.
● If giving drug by nasogastric tube, flush tube to clear it before giving drug to ensure delivery of drug to stomach; flush the tube afterward.
● If patient is also receiving tetracycline, administer drugs at least 1 hour apart; to avoid de-

creased drug absorption, dosages or schedules of other medications may need adjustment.
● Discontinue drug if patient develops tinnitus.
● Drug is useful for indigestion without causing constipation; for nausea; and for relief of flatulence and abdominal cramps.

Patient monitoring
● Monitor hydration status and serum electrolyte levels, and record number and consistency of stools.

Breast-feeding patients
● Small amounts of drug appear in breast milk. Patient should seek medical approval before use.

Pediatric patients
● Don't give drug to children or adolescents recovering from flu or chickenpox.

Patient education
● Advise patient taking anticoagulants or medication for diabetes or gout to seek medical approval before taking drug.
● As appropriate, instruct patient to chew tablets well or to shake suspension well before using.
● Tell patient to report persistent diarrhea.
● Warn patient that bismuth may temporarily darken stools and tongue.

bisoprolol fumarate
Zebeta

Pharmacologic classification: beta blocker
Therapeutic classification: antihypertensive
Pregnancy risk category: C

Indications and dosages
➤ **Hypertension (used alone or with other antihypertensives).** *Adults:* Initially, 2.5 to 5 mg P.O. once daily. If response is inadequate, increase to 10 mg once daily. Maximum recommended dose is 20 mg daily.
✦ *Dosage adjustment.* In adults with renal impairment (creatinine clearance less than 40 ml/minute), hepatic dysfunction, cirrhosis, or hepatitis, start at 2.5 mg P.O.; then increase cautiously.

How supplied
Available by prescription only
Tablets: 5 mg, 10 mg

Pharmacodynamics
Antihypertensive action: Mechanism of action isn't completely known. Possible antihypertensive effects include decreased cardiac output, inhibition of renin release by the kidneys, and diminution of tonic sympathetic outflow from the vasomotor centers in the brain.

Pharmacokinetics

Absorption: Bioavailability after a 10-mg oral dose is about 80%. Absorption isn't affected by the presence of food.
Distribution: About 30% bound to serum proteins.
Metabolism: First-pass metabolism is about 20%.
Excretion: Eliminated equally by renal and non-renal pathways, with about 50% of dose appearing unchanged in urine and the remainder appearing as inactive metabolites. Less than 2% of dose is excreted in feces. Plasma elimination half-life is 9 to 12 hours (slightly longer in elderly patients, in part because of their decreased renal function).

Route	Onset	Peak	Duration
P.O.	Unknown	1-4 hr	24 hr

Contraindications and precautions

Contraindicated in patients hypersensitive to drug and in those with cardiogenic shock, overt cardiac failure, marked sinus bradycardia, or second- or third-degree AV block. Use cautiously in patients with bronchospastic disease.

Interactions

Drug-drug. *Beta blockers:* Increased drug effects. Don't use bisoprolol with other beta blockers.
Catecholamine-depleting drugs, such as reserpine and guanethidine: Excessively reduced sympathetic activity. Monitor patient closely.
Clonidine: Additive effects. Discontinue bisoprolol for several days before clonidine withdrawal to avoid rebound hypertension.

Adverse reactions

CNS: asthenia, fatigue, dizziness, *headache,* hypesthesia, vivid dreams, depression, insomnia.
CV: *bradycardia,* peripheral edema, chest pain.
EENT: pharyngitis, rhinitis, sinusitis.
GI: nausea, vomiting, diarrhea, dry mouth.
Metabolic: hypoglycemia.
Musculoskeletal: arthralgia.
Respiratory: cough, dyspnea.

Overdose and treatment

The most common effects of overdose with a beta blocker such as bisoprolol are bradycardia, hypotension, heart failure, bronchospasm, and hypoglycemia. Discontinue drug and provide supportive and symptomatic treatment.

Special considerations

● Patients with renal or hepatic dysfunction or bronchospastic disease unresponsive to or intolerant of other antihypertensive therapies should start therapy at 2.5 mg P.O. daily. A beta$_2$-adrenergic agonist (bronchodilator) should be made available to patients with bronchospastic disease.

● Treatment with a beta blocker for heart failure (unlabeled use) should begin at a very low dose (1.25 mg P.O. daily for 2 to 4 weeks), although this low-dose strength isn't available in the U.S. If dose is tolerated, increase to 2.5 mg daily for 2 to 4 weeks. Subsequent doses can be doubled every 2 to 4 weeks if tolerated. May be adjusted up to 5 to 10 mg daily.
● Worsening of angina pectoris, MI, and ventricular arrhythmia has been observed in patients with coronary artery disease after abrupt cessation of therapy with beta blockers. It's advisable, even in patients without overt coronary artery disease, to taper bisoprolol therapy over 1 week while carefully observing the patient. If withdrawal symptoms occur, reinstitute bisoprolol therapy, at least temporarily.

Patient monitoring

● Monitor blood pressure closely.
● Monitor serum glucose levels; signs of hypoglycemia may be masked in patients taking beta blockers.
● Monitor patients with hyperthyroidism carefully; beta blockers mask symptoms (tachycardia).

Breast-feeding patients

● It isn't known if drug appears in breast milk. Use cautiously in breast-feeding women.

Pediatric patients

● Safety and efficacy in children haven't been established.

Patient education

● Inform diabetic patients subject to spontaneous hypoglycemia or those who need insulin or oral hypoglycemics that bisoprolol may mask some signs of hypoglycemia, particularly tachycardia.
● Warn patient not to drive, operate machinery, or perform tasks requiring alertness until reaction to bisoprolol has been established.
● Stress importance of taking drug as prescribed, even when feeling well. Advise patient not to discontinue drug abruptly because serious consequences can occur.
● Instruct patient to report adverse reactions.
● Tell patient to seek medical approval before taking OTC medications.

bitolterol mesylate
Tornalate

Pharmacologic classification: adrenergic, beta$_2$ agonist
Therapeutic classification: bronchodilator
Pregnancy risk category: C

Indications and dosages

➤ *To prevent and treat bronchial asthma and bronchospasm. Adults and children over age 12:* For symptomatic relief of bronchospasm, two inhalations at an interval of at least 1 to 3 minutes followed by a third inhalation, if needed; to prevent bronchospasm, two inhalations q 8 hours. Usually, dose shouldn't exceed three inhalations q 6 hours or two inhalations q 4 hours.

Nebulizer use: For intermittent flow, 1 mg t.i.d. For continuous flow, 2.5 mg t.i.d. However, because deposition of inhaled medications is variable, higher doses are occasionally used, especially in patients with acute bronchospasm. In some patients, higher doses (1.5 mg for intermittent flow and 3.5 mg for continuous flow nebulizer) or increased frequency may be required. The interval between treatments should be at least 4 hours. The maximum dose for intermittent flow is 8 mg and 14 mg for the continuous flow nebulizer system.

How supplied
Available by prescription only
Aerosol inhaler: 370 mcg/metered spray
Solution for nebulization: 0.2%

Pharmacodynamics
Bronchodilator action: Bitolterol selectively stimulates beta$_2$-adrenergic receptors of the lungs. Bronchodilation results from relaxation of bronchial smooth muscles, which relieves bronchospasm and reduces airway resistance. Some CV stimulation may occur as a result of beta$_2$-adrenergic stimulation, including mild tachycardia, palpitations, and changes in blood pressure or heart rate.

Pharmacokinetics
Absorption: After oral inhalation, bronchodilation results from local action on the bronchial tree, with most of the inhaled dose being swallowed.
Distribution: Widely distributed throughout body.
Metabolism: Hydrolyzed by esterases to active metabolites.
Excretion: After oral administration, excreted primarily in urine.

Route	Onset	Peak	Duration
Aerosol	3-5 min	½-2 hr	4-8 hr
Nebulizer	2-3 min	30-60 min	6-8 hr

Contraindications and precautions
Contraindicated in patients hypersensitive to drug. Use cautiously in patients with ischemic heart disease, hypertension, hyperthyroidism, diabetes mellitus, arrhythmias, seizure disorders, or a history of unusual responsiveness to beta-adrenergic agonists.

Interactions
Drug-drug. *Beta blockers, propranolol:* Antagonized effects of bitolterol. Use together cautiously.

Other orally inhaled beta-adrenergic agonists: Additive sympathomimetic effects. Use together cautiously.
Theophylline salt, such as aminophylline: Cardiotoxic effects may be increased. Monitor patient for these effects.

Adverse reactions
CNS: *tremor,* nervousness, headache, dizziness, light-headedness.
CV: palpitations, chest discomfort, tachycardia.
EENT: throat irritation.
GI: nausea, vomiting.
GU: proteinuria.
Hematologic: *leukopenia, thrombocytopenia.*
Hepatic: increased AST levels.
Respiratory: cough, dyspnea.
Other: *hypersensitivity reactions.*

Overdose and treatment
Signs and symptoms of overdose include exaggeration of common adverse reactions, especially arrhythmias, extreme tremor, nausea, and vomiting.

Treatment requires supportive measures. To reverse effects, use selective beta$_2$-adrenergic blockers (acebutolol, atenolol, metoprolol) with extreme caution (may induce asthmatic attack). Monitor vital signs and ECG closely.

Special considerations
Consider the recommendations relevant to all adrenergics as well as the following.
• Avoid excessive or prolonged use because it can lead to tolerance.
• Repeated use may result in paradoxical bronchospasm. Discontinue drug immediately if this occurs.
• May reduce the sensitivity of spirometry for diagnosing asthma.
• Store at 59° to 86° F (15° to 30° C). Nebulizer solution shouldn't be mixed with other medications (such as cromolyn sodium and acetylcysteine) in the nebulizer because of incompatibilities.

Patient monitoring
• Monitor patient for decreased effectiveness. Don't increase frequency or dose; fatal reactions have resulted from excessive oral inhalation of sympathomimetic amines.

Pregnant patients
• There are no adequate controlled studies of use in pregnant women.

Breast-feeding patients
• Administer cautiously to breast-feeding women. It's unknown if drug appears in breast milk.

Pediatric patients
• Drug isn't recommended for children under age 12.

Reactions may be *common*, uncommon, *life-threatening*, or COMMON AND LIFE-THREATENING.

Geriatric patients
● Lower doses are indicated in elderly patients, who may be more sensitive to the effects of the drug.

Patient education
● Tell patient to use drug only as directed and not to exceed the prescribed amount or shorten the time between doses.
● Teach patient to use drug correctly. Tell patient to ensure proper delivery of dose by cleaning plastic mouthpiece with warm tap water and drying thoroughly at least once daily. Tell him that dry mouth and throat may occur, but that rinsing with water after each dose may help.
● Tell patient to call promptly if troubled breathing persists 1 hour after using drug, if symptoms return within 4 hours, if condition worsens, or if new (refill) canister is needed within 2 weeks.
● Advise patient to wait 15 minutes after use of bitolterol before using adrenocorticoid inhaler.
● If patient uses a metered-dose nebulizer, give these instructions. Shake canister to activate. Place mouthpiece well into mouth, aimed at back of throat. Close lips and teeth around mouthpiece. Exhale through nose, and then inhale through mouth slowly and deeply while actuating the nebulizer to release a dose. Hold breath for 10 seconds (count "1-100, 2-100, 3-100" to "10-100"), remove mouthpiece, and then exhale slowly.
● If patient uses a metered powder inhaler, caution patient not to take forced deep breaths, but to breathe normally. Observe patient closely for exaggerated systemic drug action. Patients who need more than three aerosol treatments within 24 hours should be under close medical supervision.
● If drug is administered by oxygen aerosolization, give it over 15 to 20 minutes with the oxygen flow rate adjusted to 4 L/minute. Turn on oxygen supply before patient places nebulizer in mouth. Patient need not close lips tightly around nebulizer opening. Placement of Y tube in rubber tubing permits patient to control administration. Advise patient to rinse mouth immediately after inhalation therapy to help prevent dryness and throat irritation. Tell him to rinse mouthpiece with warm running water at least once daily to prevent clogging; it's not dishwasher-safe. Wait until mouthpiece is dry before storing. Don't place near artificial heat, such as a dishwasher or oven. Replace reservoir bag every 2 to 3 weeks or p.r.n.; replace mouthpiece every 6 to 9 months or p.r.n. Replacement of bags or mouthpieces may require a prescription.

bivalirudin
Angiomax

Pharmacologic classification: direct thrombin inhibitor
Therapeutic classification: anticoagulant
Pregnancy risk category: B

Indications and dosages
➤ *Unstable angina in patients undergoing percutaneous transluminal coronary angioplasty (PTCA).* Adults: 1 mg/kg I.V. bolus just before PTCA; then begin 4-hour I.V. infusion at 2.5mg/kg/hr. After the first 4-hour infusion, another I.V. infusion at 0.2 mg/kg/hr for up to 20 hours may be given as needed. Give with 300 to 325 mg of aspirin.
✦ *Dosage adjustment.* In patients with renal impairment, adjust dose according to glomerular filtration rate (GFR). For moderate renal impairment (GFR of 30 to 59 ml/minute), reduce dose by 20%. For severe renal impairment (GFR of 10 to 29 ml/minute), reduce dose by 60%. For dialysis-dependent patients (off dialysis), reduce dose by 90%.

How supplied
Available by prescription only
Injection: 250-mg vial

Pharmacodynamics
Thrombin-inhibiting action: Bivalirudin is highly specific for thrombin and directly inhibits both clot-bound and circulating thrombin. Therefore, bivalirudin prevents thrombin-induced generation of fibrin and further activation of the clotting cascade, and it inhibits thrombin-induced platelet activation, granule release, and aggregation. Bivalirudin doesn't require the presence of antithrombin to produce an anticoagulant effect.

Pharmacokinetics
Absorption: Administered I.V.
Distribution: Drug binds rapidly to thrombin and has a rapid onset of action. It doesn't bind to plasma proteins or RBCs.
Metabolism: Bivalirudin is rapidly cleared from plasma by a combination of renal mechanisms and proteolytic cleavage.
Excretion: Bivalirudin is eliminated renally. Total body clearance is similar in patients with normal and mild renal impairment. Clearance is reduced about 20% in patients with moderate and severe renal impairment and is reduced about 80% in dialysis-dependent patients. Bivalirudin is hemodialyzable. Half-life is 25 minutes in patients with normal renal function.

Route	Onset	Peak	Duration
I.V.	Rapid	Immediate	Duration of infusion

◇ Unlabeled clinical use

Adverse reactions

CNS: anxiety, *headache,* insomnia, nervousness.
CV: *bradycardia,* hypertension, *hypotension.*
GI: abdominal pain, dyspepsia, *nausea,* vomiting.
GU: urine retention.
Musculoskeletal: *back pain,* pelvic pain.
Hematologic: *severe, spontaneous bleeding* (cerebral, retroperitoneal, GU, GI)
Other: fever, *pain,* pain at injection site.

Interactions

Drug-drug. *Glycoprotein IIb/IIIa inhibitors:* Safety and effectiveness haven't been established. Avoid use together.
Heparin, warfarin, other oral anticoagulants: Increased risk of bleeding. Use together cautiously. Discontinue heparin at least 8 hours before giving bivalirudin.

Overdose and treatment

There has been no experience of overdose with bivalirudin. In case of overdose, stop drug and monitor patient for bleeding. There's no known antidote. The anticoagulant effects will gradually decline. Provide symptomatic and supportive therapy. Bivalirudin is hemodialyzable.

Contraindications and precautions

Bivalirudin is contraindicated in patients with active major bleeding and in patients hypersensitive to bivalirudin or its components. Don't use drug in patients with unstable angina who aren't undergoing PTCA or in patients with other acute coronary conditions.

Use cautiously in patients with heparin-induced thrombocytopenia or heparin-induced thrombocytopenia-thrombosis syndrome and in patients with diseases that increase the risk of bleeding.

Special considerations

● Don't give by I.M. route.
● Reconstitute with 5 ml of sterile water for injection, USP. Each reconstituted vial should be further diluted in 50 ml of D₅W or normal saline solution for injection to yield 5 mg/ml.
● To prepare the low-rate infusion, each reconstituted vial should be further diluted in 500 ml of D₅W or normal saline solution for injection to yield 0.5 mg/ml.
● Mix no other drugs with bivalirudin before or during administration.

Patient monitoring

● If the patient has an unexplained drop in hematocrit or blood pressure or other unexplained symptom, consider the possibility of hemorrhage.
● Monitor baseline coagulation tests, hemoglobin, and hematocrit before and periodically throughout therapy.
● Monitor venipuncture sites for bleeding, hematoma, or inflammation.

Breast-feeding patients

● It isn't known if bivalirudin appears in breast milk; therefore, use caution when giving bivalirudin to breast-feeding women.

Pediatric patients

● The safety and efficacy of bivalirudin in children haven't been established.

Geriatric patients

● Individual bleeding events seem to be no more likely with elderly patients than with other adults, although puncture site hemorrhage and catheterization site hematoma are more likely in patients over age 65.

Patient education

● Advise patient that drug can cause bleeding. Urge patient to report unusual bruising or bleeding (nosebleeds, bleeding gums) or tarry stools immediately.
● Counsel patient that bivalirudin is given with aspirin. Caution patient to avoid other aspirin-containing drugs and drugs used to treat swelling or pain (such as Motrin, Naprosyn, Aleve) while receiving bivalirudin.
● Advise patient to avoid activities that carry a risk of injury, and instruct patient to use a soft toothbrush and electric razor while taking bivalirudin.

bleomycin sulfate
Blenoxane

Pharmacologic classification: antibiotic, antineoplastic (specific to G2 and M phases of cell cycle)
Therapeutic classification: antineoplastic
Pregnancy risk category: D

Indications and dosages

Dosages and indications may vary. Check literature for current protocol.

➤ *Hodgkin's disease, squamous cell carcinoma, malignant lymphoma, testicular carcinoma.* Adults: 10 to 20 units/m² (0.25 to 0.5 units/kg) I.V., I.M., or S.C., one or two times weekly. After 50% response in regression of tumor size in Hodgkin's disease, maintenance dosage of 1 unit daily or 5 units weekly.
➤ *Malignant pleural effusion; to prevent recurrent pleural effusions or manage pneumothorax caused by AIDS and* Pneumocystis carinii *pneumonia* ◊. Adults: 50 to 60 units in 50 to 100 ml of normal saline solution by intracavitary administration not to exceed 1 unit/kg.
✦ *Dosage adjustment.* For geriatric patients receiving intracavitary administration in the pleural space, don't exceed 40 units/m².
➤ *Tumors of the head and neck* ◊. Adults: 10 to 20 units/m² daily by I.V. or regional arterial administration for 5 to 14 days.

▶ *AIDS-related Kaposi's sarcoma* ◇. *Adults:*
20 units/m² daily I.V. continuously over 72 hr
every 3 weeks.

How supplied
Available by prescription only
Injection: 15-unit, 30-unit vials

Pharmacodynamics
Antineoplastic action: The exact mechanism
of cytotoxicity is unknown. Drug's action may be
through scission of single- and double-stranded
DNA and inhibition of DNA, RNA, and protein synthesis. Bleomycin also appears to inhibit cell progression out of the G2 phase.

Pharmacokinetics
Absorption: Poorly absorbed across the GI tract.
I.M. administration results in lower serum levels
than those occurring after equivalent I.V. doses.
Distribution: Distributed widely into total body
water, mainly in the skin, lungs, kidneys, peri-
toneum, and lymphatic tissue.
Metabolism: Metabolic fate of drug is undetermined; however, extensive tissue inactivation occurs in the liver and kidneys and much less in
the skin and lungs.
Excretion: Excreted primarily in urine. The terminal plasma elimination phase half-life is 2
hours.

Route	Onset	Peak	Duration
I.V., S.C.	Unknown	Unknown	Unknown
I.M.	Unknown	½-1 hr	Unknown

Contraindications and precautions
Contraindicated in patients hypersensitive to drug.
Use cautiously in patients with renal or pulmonary
impairment.

Interactions
Drug-drug. *Digoxin, phenytoin:* Decreased
serum levels of these drugs. Monitor serum levels.

Adverse reactions
GI: stomatitis, anorexia, nausea, vomiting, diarrhea.
Metabolic: increased blood and urine levels of
uric acid, weight loss.
Respiratory: *pulmonary fibrosis,* pulmonary
toxicity such as PNEUMONITIS.
Skin: *erythema, hyperpigmentation, acne, rash,
reversible alopecia, striae, skin tenderness,
pruritus.*
Other: *chills;* fever; *severe idiosyncratic
reaction consisting of hypotension, mental confusion, fever, chills, and wheezing*
has occurred in about 1% of lymphoma patients.

Overdose and treatment
Signs and symptoms of bleomycin overdose include pulmonary fibrosis, fever, chills, vesiculation, and hyperpigmentation. Treatment is usually supportive and includes antipyretics for fever.

Special considerations
● To prepare solution for I.M. administration, reconstitute drug with 1 to 5 ml (15-unit vial) or
2 to 10 ml (30-unit vial) of normal saline solution, bacteriostatic water, or sterile water for injection. Don't use D₅W or dextrose-containing
diluents.
● For I.V. administration, dilute with at least 5 ml
(15-unit vial) or 10 ml (30-unit vial) of diluent
(don't exceed 3 units/ml) and administer over
10 minutes as I.V. push injection.
● For intrapleural administration, dissolve 60 units
of bleomycin in 50 to 100 ml of normal saline
solution and administer via thoracostomy tube.
● Use precautions in preparing and handling drug;
wear gloves and wash hands after preparing and
administering.
● Drug can be administered by intracavitary route
(see manufacturer's recommendation), intra-
arterially, or via intratumoral injection. It can also
be instilled into bladder for bladder tumors.
● Cumulative lifetime dosage shouldn't exceed
400 units.
● Response to bleomycin therapy may take 2 to
3 weeks.
● Administer a 1- to 2-unit test dose to lymphoma
patients for the first two doses to assess hypersensitivity to bleomycin. If no reaction occurs,
follow the dosing schedule. The test dose can be
incorporated as part of the total dose for the regimen.
● Keep epinephrine, diphenhydramine, I.V. corticosteroids, and oxygen available in case of anaphylaxis.
● Premedication with aspirin, corticosteroids,
and diphenhydramine may reduce drug fever and
risk of anaphylaxis.
● Reduce dosage in patients with renal or pulmonary impairment.
● Lung damage may occur at oxygen levels lower than normal. This is an important consideration for patients undergoing surgery.
● Drug concentrates in keratin of squamous epithelium. To prevent linear streaking, don't use
adhesive dressings on skin.
● Allergic reactions may be delayed, especially in
patients with lymphoma.
● Investigational uses for the drug include treatment of AIDS-related Kaposi's sarcoma, renal carcinomas, soft tissue sarcomas, otorhinolaryngeal
tumors, and mycosis fungoides.
● Bleomycin is stable for 24 hours at room temperature and 48 hours under refrigeration. Refrigerate unopened vials containing dry powder.

Patient monitoring
● Pulmonary function tests may be useful in
predicting fibrosis; they should be performed to
establish a baseline and then monitored periodically.
● Monitor chest X-rays and auscultate the lungs
to check for pulmonary toxicity.

Pregnant patients
● Drug may cause fetal toxicity in pregnant women. Don't give it to pregnant women.

Breast-feeding patients
● It isn't known if drug appears in breast milk. However, because of risk of serious adverse reactions, mutagenicity, and carcinogenicity in infants, breast-feeding isn't recommended.

Geriatric patients
● Use cautiously in patients over age 70 because they have an increased risk of pulmonary toxicity.

Patient education
● Explain that hair should grow back after treatment stops.

bretylium tosylate
Bretylate*, Bretylol

Pharmacologic classification: adrenergic blocker
Therapeutic classification: ventricular antiarrhythmic
Pregnancy risk category: C

Indications and dosages
➤ **Ventricular fibrillation and hemodynamically unstable ventricular tachycardia.** *Adults:* 5 mg/kg undiluted by rapid I.V. injection. If ventricular fibrillation persists, increase dosage to 10 mg/kg and repeat, p.r.n. (usually at 5- to 30-minute intervals) to total of 30 to 35 mg/kg. For continuous suppression, administer diluted solution by continuous I.V. infusion at 1 to 2 mg/minute, or infuse diluted solution at 5 to 10 mg/kg over more than 8 to 10 minutes q 6 hours.
➤ **Other ventricular arrhythmias.** *Adults:* Initially, 5 to 10 mg/kg I.M., undiluted, or I.V. diluted. Repeat in 1 to 2 hours if necessary. Maintenance dosage is 5 to 10 mg/kg q 6 to 8 hours I.M. or I.V. or 1 to 2 mg/minute I.V. infusion.
Children ◊ : For acute ventricular fibrillation, initially 5 mg/kg I.V., followed by 10 mg/kg q 15 to 30 minutes, with a maximum total dose of 30 mg/kg; maintenance dosage is 5 to 10 mg/kg q 6 hours. For other ventricular arrhythmias, 5 to 10 mg/kg q 6 hours or 2 to 5 mg/kg I.M. as a single dose.

How supplied
Available by prescription only
Injection: 50 mg/ml
Injection in dextrose: 500 mg in 250 mg D₅W, 1 g in 250 mg D₅W

Pharmacodynamics
Ventricular antiarrhythmic action: Bretylium is a class III antiarrhythmic used to treat ventricular fibrillation and tachycardia. Like other class III antiarrhythmics, it widens the action potential duration (repolarization inhibition) and increases the effective refractory period (ERP); it doesn't affect conduction velocity. These actions follow a transient increase in conduction velocity and shortening of the action potential duration and ERP.

Initial effects stem from norepinephrine release from sympathetic ganglia and postganglionic adrenergic neurons immediately after drug administration. Norepinephrine release also accounts for an increased threshold for successful defibrillation, increased blood pressure, and increased heart rate. This initial phase of drug's action is brief (up to 1 hour).

Bretylium also alters the disparity in action potential duration between ischemic and nonischemic myocardial tissue; its antiarrhythmic action may result from this activity.

Hemodynamic drug effects include increased blood pressure, heart rate, and possible cardiac irritability (all resulting from initial norepinephrine release). Drug-induced adrenergic blockade ultimately predominates, leading to vasodilation and a subsequent blood pressure drop (primarily orthostatic). This effect has been referred to as chemical sympathectomy.

Pharmacokinetics
Absorption: Incompletely and erratically absorbed from the GI tract; well absorbed after I.M. administration.
Distribution: Distributed widely throughout the body. Doesn't cross the blood-brain barrier. Only about 1% to 10% is plasma protein–bound.
Metabolism: No metabolites have been identified.
Excretion: Excreted in urine mostly as unchanged drug; half-life ranges from 5 to 10 hours (longer in patients with renal impairment).

Route	Onset	Peak	Duration
P.O.	Unknown	Unknown	Unknown
I.V.	Immediate	Immediate	6-24 hr
I.M.	5-40 min	1 hr	6-24 hr

Contraindications and precautions
Contraindicated in digitalized patients unless the arrhythmia is life-threatening, not caused by a cardiac glycoside, and unresponsive to other antiarrhythmics. Use cautiously in patients with aortic stenosis and pulmonary hypertension.

Interactions
Drug-drug. *Antiarrhythmics:* Additive toxic effects and additive or antagonistic cardiac effects. Avoid use if possible.
Cardiac glycosides: May worsen ventricular tachycardia from digitalis toxicity. Use together cautiously.
MAO inhibitors: May potentiate bretylium-induced release of catecholamines from nerve endings. Use together cautiously.

Reactions may be *common*, uncommon, *life-threatening*, or COMMON AND LIFE-THREATENING.

Pressor amines (sympathomimetics): Bretylium may potentiate the action of these drugs. Monitor patient for drug effects.

Adverse reactions
CNS: *vertigo, dizziness, light-headedness, syncope* (usually secondary to hypotension).
CV: SEVERE HYPOTENSION (especially orthostatic), **bradycardia,** angina, **transient arrhythmias,** transient hypertension, increased PVCs.
GI: severe nausea, vomiting.
Other: hyperthermia.

Overdose and treatment
The main effect of overdose is severe hypotension. Treatment includes administration of vasopressors to support blood pressure and general supportive measures. Volume expanders and positional changes also may be effective.

Special considerations
• Drug isn't a first-line agent according to American Heart Association advanced cardiac life-support guidelines.
• Administer I.V. infusion at appropriate rate to avoid or minimize adverse reactions.
• For I.M. injection, don't exceed 5-ml volume in any one site. Rotate sites.
• Avoid simultaneous start of therapy with a cardiac glycoside and bretylium.
• Because bretylium is excreted exclusively by the kidneys, patients with renal impairment require dosage modification. Increase dosage interval because the elimination half-life increases threefold to sixfold.
• Subtherapeutic doses (less than 5 mg/kg) may cause hypotension.
• Ventricular tachycardia and other ventricular arrhythmias respond less rapidly than ventricular fibrillation to drug.
• Drug is ineffective against atrial arrhythmias.
• Store bretylium between 59° and 86° F (15° and 30° C). Solutions in D_5W should be protected from freezing and stored at room temperature. Following dilution of bretylium injection to 10 mg/ml, the drug is stable for 48 hours at room temperature or 7 days at 40° F (4° C). Drug is compatible with most standard I.V. solutions.

Patient monitoring
• Monitor ECG and blood pressure throughout therapy.
• Monitor patient closely if he is receiving pressor amines (sympathomimetics) to correct hypotension; bretylium potentiates the effects of these drugs.
• Observe susceptible patients for increased angina.

Breast-feeding patients
• Safety in breast-feeding women hasn't been established.

Pediatric patients
• Safety and efficacy in children haven't been established.

Geriatric patients
• Start therapy at lower end of dosing range. Elderly patients are at greater risk for adverse effects and orthostatic hypotension.

Patient education
• Advise patient to remain supine and avoid sudden postural changes until tolerance to hypotension develops.
• Instruct patient to report adverse reactions immediately.

brimonidine tartrate
Alphagan

Pharmacologic classification: selective alpha$_2$-adrenergic agonist
Therapeutic classification: ophthalmic agent for glaucoma or ocular hypertension
Pregnancy risk category: B

Indications and dosages
➤ *Lowering of intraocular pressure in patients with open-angle glaucoma or ocular hypertension.* *Adults:* 1 drop in affected eye or eyes t.i.d., about 8 hours apart.

How supplied
Available by prescription only
Ophthalmic solution: 0.2%; 5 ml, 10 ml

Pharmacodynamics
Ocular antihypertensive action: Brimonidine is an alpha$_2$-adrenergic receptor agonist that reduces aqueous humor production and increases uveoscleral outflow.

Pharmacokinetics
Absorption: After ocular administration, plasma levels peak in 1 to 4 hours and decline, with a systemic half-life of about 3 hours.
Distribution: Not reported.
Metabolism: Systemically, drug is metabolized primarily by the liver.
Excretion: Systemically, urinary excretion is major route of elimination.

Route	Onset	Peak	Duration
Oph-thalmic	Unknown	1-4 hr	Unknown

Contraindications and precautions
Contraindicated in patients hypersensitive to brimonidine tartrate or benzalkonium chloride and in those taking an MAO inhibitor. Use cautiously in patients with cerebral or coronary insufficiency, CV disease, hepatic or renal impairment, depression, Raynaud's phenomenon, orthostatic hypotension, or thromboangiitis obliterans.

Interactions
Drug-drug. *Antihypertensives, beta blockers, cardiac glycosides:* May further decrease blood pressure. Monitor patient closely.
CNS depressants: May increase or potentiate the effects of these drugs. Use caution.
Tricyclic antidepressants: May interfere with intraocular pressure–lowering effects of brimonidine. Monitor patient closely.

Adverse reactions
CNS: anxiety, asthenia, depression, dizziness, syncope, *drowsiness, fatigue, headache,* insomnia.
CV: hypertension, palpitations.
EENT: abnormal vision or taste; blepharitis; *blurring, burning, or stinging;* conjunctival blanching, edema, hemorrhage, discharge, or *follicles;* corneal staining or erosion; eyelid erythema or eyelid edema; *foreign body sensation;* lid crusting; nasal dryness; *ocular hyperemia, allergic reactions, pruritus,* ache or pain, dryness, tearing, or irritation; photophobia.
GI: nausea, vomiting, diarrhea, dry mouth.
Musculoskeletal: muscle pain.
Respiratory: cough and cold symptoms.

Overdose and treatment
Supportive and symptomatic treatment. Maintain a patent airway.

Special considerations
● Monitor intraocular pressure because drug effects may decline after first month.

Breast-feeding patients
● It isn't known if drug appears in breast milk. Use cautiously in breast-feeding women.

Pediatric patients
● Safety and effectiveness in children haven't been established.

Patient education
● Tell patient to wait at least 15 minutes after instilling drug to insert soft contact lenses.
● Caution patient about risk of decreased mental alertness; drug may cause fatigue or drowsiness.

---

bromocriptine mesylate
Parlodel

Pharmacologic classification: dopamine receptor agonist
Therapeutic classification: semisynthetic ergot alkaloid, dopaminergic agonist, antiparkinsonian, inhibitor of prolactin release, inhibitor of growth hormone release
Pregnancy risk category: B

Indications and dosages
➤ *Amenorrhea and galactorrhea related to hyperprolactinemia; female infertil-*ity. *Adults:* 1.25 to 2.5 mg P.O. daily, increased by 2.5 mg daily at 3- to 7-day intervals as tolerated until optimal therapeutic effects are achieved. Maintenance dosage is usually 5 to 7.5 mg daily (range, 2.5 to 15 mg daily). Up to 40 mg daily have been used.
➤ *Acromegaly. Adults:* Initially, 1.25 to 2.5 mg P.O. daily h.s. for 3 days. Another 1.25 to 2.5 mg may be added q 3 to 7 days until patient receives therapeutic benefit. Therapeutic dose range varies from 20 to 30 mg daily in most patients. Maximum dose shouldn't exceed 100 mg daily. Dosages of 20 to 60 mg daily have been administered as divided doses.
➤ *Parkinson's disease. Adults:* Initially, 1.25 mg P.O. b.i.d. with meals. Dosage may be increased by 2.5 mg daily q 14 to 28 days, up to 100 mg daily or until a maximal therapeutic response is achieved. Safety in doses over 100 mg daily hasn't been established.
➤ *Premenstrual syndrome* ◇. *Adults:* 2.5 to 7.5 mg P.O. b.i.d. from day 10 of menstrual cycle until onset of menstruation.
➤ *Cushing's syndrome* ◇. *Adults:* 1.25 to 2.5 mg P.O. b.i.d. to q.i.d.
➤ *Hepatic encephalopathy* ◇. *Adults:* 1.25 mg P.O. daily, increased by 1.25 mg q 3 days until 15 mg is reached.
➤ *Neuroleptic malignant syndrome related to neuroleptic drug therapy* ◇. *Adults:* 2.5 to 5 mg P.O. 2 to 6 times per day.

How supplied
Available by prescription only
Capsules: 5 mg
Tablets: 2.5 mg

Pharmacodynamics
Prolactin-inhibiting action: Reduces prolactin levels by inhibiting release of prolactin from the anterior pituitary gland, a direct action on the pituitary. It also may stimulate postsynaptic dopamine receptors in the hypothalamus to release prolactin-inhibitory factor via a complicated catecholamine pathway. Drug reduces high serum prolactin levels and restores ovulation and ovarian function in amenorrheic women and suppresses puerperal or nonpuerperal lactation in women with adequate gonadotropin levels and ovarian function. The average time for reversing amenorrhea is 6 to 8 weeks, but it may take up to 24 weeks.
Antiparkinsonian action: Activates dopaminergic receptors in the neostriatum of the CNS, which may produce antiparkinsonism activity. Dysregulation of brain serotonin activity also may occur. The precise role of bromocriptine in long-term treatment of parkinsonism syndrome needs further study of safety and efficacy.

Pharmacokinetics
Absorption: 28% absorbed when given orally.
Distribution: About 90% to 96% is bound to serum albumin.

Metabolism: First-pass metabolism occurs with more than 90% of the absorbed dose. Metabolized completely in the liver, principally by hydrolysis, before excretion. The metabolites aren't active or toxic.

Excretion: Primarily excreted in bile. Only 2.5% to 5.5% of dose is excreted in urine. Almost all (85%) of dose is excreted in feces within 5 days.

Route	Onset	Peak	Duration
P.O.	2 hr	8 hr	24 hr

Contraindications and precautions

Contraindicated in patients hypersensitive to ergot derivatives and in those with uncontrolled hypertension or toxemia of pregnancy. Use cautiously in patients with renal or hepatic impairment and those with a history of MI and residual arrhythmias.

Interactions

Drug-drug. *Amitriptyline, butyrophenones, imipramine, methyldopa, phenothiazines, reserpine:* Increase prolactin levels. This may require increased dosage of bromocriptine.
Antihypertensives: Potentiation of effects. Reduced dosage prevents hypotension.

Drug-lifestyle. *Alcohol use:* Intolerance may result when high doses of bromocriptine are administered. Advise patient to limit alcohol consumption.

Adverse reactions

CNS: *dizziness, headache,* fatigue, mania, lightheadedness, drowsiness, delusions, nervousness, insomnia, depression, diarrhea, anorexia.
CV: *hypotension, CVA, acute MI.*
EENT: nasal congestion, blurred vision.
GI: *nausea,* vomiting, *abdominal cramps, constipation,* diarrhea, anorexia.
GU: urine retention, urinary frequency.
Skin: coolness and pallor of fingers and toes.

Overdose and treatment

Overdose may cause nausea, vomiting, and severe hypotension. Treatment includes emptying the stomach by aspiration and lavage, and administering I.V. fluids to treat hypotension.

Special considerations

• Patient must be examined carefully for pituitary tumor (Forbes-Albright syndrome). Use of bromocriptine doesn't affect tumor size, although it may alleviate amenorrhea or galactorrhea.
• First-dose phenomenon occurs in 1% of patients. Sensitive patients may experience syncope for 15 to 60 minutes but can usually tolerate subsequent treatment without ill effects. Patient should begin therapy with lowest dosage, taken at bedtime.
• Administer drug with meals, milk, or snacks to diminish GI distress.

• Alcohol intolerance may occur, especially with high doses of bromocriptine; advise patient to limit alcohol intake.
• As an antiparkinsonian, drug is usually given with levodopa or with levodopa-carbidopa. In treatment of Parkinson's disease, if levodopa dosage must be decreased because of adverse effects, daily bromocriptine doses may be increased gradually in 2.5-mg increments.
• Adverse reactions are more common when drug is given in large doses, as when treating parkinsonism.

Patient monitoring

• Monitor hepatic, hematopoietic, CV, and renal function in long-term use.
• Monitor blood pressure, especially during first few days of therapy.
• Monitor patient for pulmonary changes in long-term use.
• Monitor patient with acromegaly for cold-induced digital vasospasm and signs and symptoms of peptic ulcer.

Pregnant patients

• Discontinue drug if patient becomes pregnant. Recommend regular checks of the visual field if patient has underlying prolactin-secreting pituitary tumor.

Breast-feeding patients

• Because drug inhibits lactation, it shouldn't be used in women who intend to breast-feed.

Pediatric patients

• Drug isn't recommended for children under age 15.

Geriatric patients

• Use cautiously, particularly in patients receiving long-term, high-dose therapy. Perform regular physical assessment, paying particular attention to changes in pulmonary function and blood pressure.
• Safety hasn't been established for long-term use at the doses required to treat Parkinson's disease. Therapy should be started at the low end of the dosage range.

Patient education

• Advise patient that it may take 6 to 8 weeks or longer for menses to resume and for galactorrhea to be suppressed.
• Tell patient to take first dose where and when she can lie down because drowsiness commonly occurs after start of therapy.
• Instruct patient to report visual problems, severe nausea and vomiting, or acute headaches.
• Tell patient to take drug with meals to avoid GI upset.
• Warn patient that the CNS effects of drug may impair ability to perform tasks that require alertness and coordination.

- Instruct patient to use a nonhormonal contraceptive during treatment because of potential amenorrheic adverse effects.
- Advise patient to limit use of alcohol during treatment.

budesonide
Pulmicort Respules, Pulmicort Turbuhaler, Rhinocort

Pharmacologic classification: corticosteroid
Therapeutic classification: anti-inflammatory
Pregnancy risk category: C

Indications and dosages
➤ *Management of symptoms of seasonal or perennial allergic rhinitis or non-allergic perennial rhinitis. Adults and children over age 6:* Two sprays in each nostril in the morning and evening or four sprays in each nostril in the morning. Maintenance dosage is the fewest number of sprays needed to control symptoms. Doses exceeding 256 mcg daily (four sprays/nostril) aren't recommended.

Note: If improvement doesn't occur within 3 weeks, discontinue treatment.
➤ *Chronic asthma. Adults:* 200 to 400 mcg oral inhalation b.i.d. when patient previously used bronchodilators alone or inhaled corticosteroids; 400 to 800 mcg oral inhalation b.i.d. when patient previously used oral corticosteroids.
Children age 6 and over: Initially, 200 mcg oral inhalation b.i.d. Maximum dose is 400 mg b.i.d.
Children ages 1 to 8: (Respules) 0.25 mg via jet nebulizer with compressor once daily. Increase to 0.5 mg once daily or 0.25 mg b.i.d. in child not receiving systemic or inhaled corticosterids or 1 mg daily or 0.5 mg b.i.d. if child is receiving oral corticosteroids.

How supplied
Available by prescription only
Inhalation suspension: 0.25 mg/2 ml, 0.5 mg/2 ml
Nasal inhaler: 32 mcg/metered dose (200 doses per container)
Oral inhalation powder: 200 mcg/dose (200 doses per container)

Pharmacodynamics
Anti-inflammatory action: Precise mechanism by which corticosteroids such as budesonide act on allergic and nonallergic rhinitis isn't known. Corticosteroids show a wide range of inhibitory activities against multiple cell types (such as mast cells, eosinophils, neutrophils, macrophages, and lymphocytes) and mediators (such as histamine, eicosanoids, leukotrienes, and cytokines) involved in allergic and nonallergic, irritant-mediated inflammatory processes.

Pharmacokinetics
Absorption: The amount of an intranasal dose that reaches systemic circulation is usually low (about 20%).
Distribution: 88% protein-bound in the plasma; volume of distribution is 200 L.
Metabolism: Rapidly and extensively metabolized in the liver.
Excretion: Eliminated in urine (about 67%) and feces (about 33%).

Route	Onset	Peak	Duration
Inhalation	24 hr	1-2 wk	Unknown
Nasal	Unknown	Unknown	Unknown

Contraindications and precautions
Contraindicated in patients hypersensitive to drug or its components and in those who have had recent septal ulcers, nasal surgery, or nasal trauma until total healing has occurred.

Use cautiously in patients with tuberculosis infections; untreated fungal, bacterial, or systemic viral infections; or ocular herpes simplex.

Interactions
Drug-drug. *Alternate-day prednisone therapy, inhaled corticosteroids:* Increased risk of hypothalamic-pituitary-adrenal suppression. Monitor patient closely.
Ketoconazole: May increase plasma budesonide levels. Monitor patient.

Adverse reactions
CNS: *headache,* nervousness.
EENT: *nasal irritation, epistaxis, pharyngitis, sinusitis,* reduced sense of smell, nasal pain, hoarseness.
GI: taste perversion, dry mouth, dyspepsia, nausea, vomiting.
Respiratory: *cough,* candidiasis, wheezing, dyspnea.
Metabolic: weight gain.
Musculoskeletal: myalgia.
Skin: facial edema, rash, pruritus, contact dermatitis.
Other: *hypersensitivity reactions.*

Overdose and treatment
Acute overdose is unlikely as a result of the limited amount of product in each container. Chronic overdose may produce signs and symptoms of hyperadrenocorticism.

Special considerations
- Replacing a systemic corticosteroid with a topical corticosteroid can result in signs of adrenal insufficiency; in addition, some patients may experience withdrawal symptoms, such as joint or muscle pain, lassitude, and depression.
⚡ ALERT In patients with asthma or other conditions that require long-term systemic treatment, a too-rapid decrease in systemic corticosteroids may severely exacerbate symptoms.

• Excessive doses of budesonide or use of drug with other inhaled corticosteroids may lead to signs or symptoms of hyperadrenocorticism.

Patient monitoring

• Carefully monitor patient previously treated for prolonged period with systemic corticosteroids and subsequently given topical corticosteroids for acute adrenal insufficiency in response to stress.

• Because corticosteroids can affect growth, monitor children closely, weighing benefits of therapy against the possibility of growth suppression.

• Patients who take budesonide for several months or longer should be examined for evidence of *Candida* infection or other signs of adverse effects on the nasal mucosa.

Breast-feeding patients

• Use cautiously when giving drug to breast feeding women.

Pediatric patients

• Safety and efficacy of drug for treating seasonal or perennial allergic rhinitis in children under age 6 haven't been established.

• Drug isn't recommended for treating nonallergic rhinitis in children because adequate numbers of such children haven't been studied.

Patient education

• Warn patient not to exceed prescribed dosage or to use drug for long periods because of risk of hypothalamic-pituitary-adrenal axis suppression.

• Tell patient to follow these instructions for using a nasal inhaler: After opening aluminum pouch, use within 6 minutes. Shake canister well before using. Blow nose to clear nasal passages. Tilt head slightly forward and insert nozzle into nostril pointing away from septum. Hold the other nostril closed, inhale gently, and spray. Shake canister again and repeat in other nostril. Store with valve downward. Don't store in area of high humidity. Don't break, incinerate, or store canister in extreme heat; the contents are under pressure.

• Instruct patient to hold the inhaler upright when loading Pulmicort Turbuhaler, not to blow or exhale into the inhaler, not to shake it while loaded, and to hold inhaler upright while orally inhaling the dose. Tell patient to place the mouthpiece between the lips and inhale forcefully and deeply.

• Pulmicort Respules can be administered only via jet nebulizer connected to an air compressor with satisfactory airflow. System should be equipped with a mouthpiece or a facemask.

• Assure patient that drug rarely causes nasal irritation or burning; advise patient to call if such symptoms recur.

• Warn patient to avoid exposure to chickenpox or measles if at risk for contracting these diseases, and to consult prescriber immediately if exposed.

• Teach patient good nasal and oral hygiene.

• Tell patient to call if condition worsens or if symptoms don't improve within 3 weeks.

• Inform patient that effects aren't immediate; response requires regular use.

• Inform patient that with use of oral inhaler, improvement in asthma control can occur within 24 hours, with maximum benefit at 1 to 2 weeks or possibly longer.

⚠ ALERT Advise patient that Pulmicort Turbuhaler isn't indicated for relief of acute bronchospasm.

bumetanide
Bumex

Pharmacologic classification: loop diuretic
Therapeutic classification: diuretic
Pregnancy risk category: C

Indications and dosages

➤ *Edema (heart failure, hepatic and renal disease); postoperative edema◊; premenstrual syndrome◊; disseminated cancer◊.* *Adults:* 0.5 to 2 mg P.O. once daily. If diuretic response isn't adequate, give a second or third dose at 4- to 5-hour intervals. Maximum daily dose is 10 mg. Give parenterally when oral route isn't feasible. Usual initial dose is 0.5 to 1 mg I.V. over 1 to 2 minutes or I.M. If response isn't adequate, give a second or third dose at 2- to 3-hour intervals. Maximum daily dose is 10 mg.

➤ *Pediatric heart failure◊. Children:* 0.015 mg/kg every other day to 0.1 mg/kg daily. Use with extreme caution in neonates.

➤ *Hypertension◊. Adults:* 0.5 mg P.O. daily. Oral maintenance of 1 to 4 mg daily; a maximum of 5 mg has been used in patients with normal renal function.

✦ *Dosage adjustment.* In patients with impaired renal function, oral or I.V. doses up to 20 mg have been administered despite manufacturer recommendations for a maximum of 10 mg daily for the management of edema. In patients with severe chronic renal insufficiency, a continuous infusion of 12 mg over 12 hours may be less toxic and more effective than an intermittent dosing schedule.

How supplied
Available by prescription only
Injection: 0.25 mg/ml
Tablets: 0.5 mg, 1 mg, 2 mg

Pharmacodynamics
Diuretic action: Loop diuretics inhibit sodium and chloride reabsorption in the proximal part of the ascending loop of Henle, promoting the excretion of sodium, water, chloride, and potassium; bumetanide produces renal and peripheral vasodilation and may temporarily increase

---

glomerular filtration rate and decrease peripheral vascular resistance.

Pharmacokinetics
Absorption: After oral administration, 85% to 95% of dose is absorbed; food delays oral absorption. I.M. bumetanide is completely absorbed.
Distribution: About 92% to 96% protein-bound; it's unknown whether bumetanide enters CSF or breast milk or crosses the placenta.
Metabolism: Metabolized by the liver to at least five metabolites.
Excretion: Excreted in urine (80%) and feces (10% to 20%). Half-life ranges from 1 to 1½ hours.

Route	Onset	Peak	Duration
P.O.	½-1 hr	1-2 hr	4-6 hr
I.V.	Rapid	15-30 min	½-1 hr
I.M.	40 min	Unknown	5-6 hr

Contraindications and precautions
Contraindicated in patients hypersensitive to drug or sulfonamides (possible cross-sensitivity), patients with anuria or hepatic coma, and patients in states of severe electrolyte depletion.

Use cautiously in patients with hepatic cirrhosis and ascites and in those with depressed renal function.

Interactions
Drug-drug. *Antihypertensives, diuretics:* Potentiated hypotensive effects. These actions may be used to therapeutic advantage.
Indomethacin, probenecid: May reduce the diuretic effect of bumetanide. Combined use isn't recommended; however, if there's no therapeutic alternative, an increased dose of bumetanide may be needed.
Lithium: Reduced renal lithium clearance and increased lithium levels. Lithium dosage may need adjustment.
Ototoxic or nephrotoxic drugs: May result in increased toxicity. Use together cautiously.
Potassium-depleting drugs, such as amphotericin B and corticosteroids: May cause severe potassium loss. Use together cautiously.
Potassium-sparing diuretics (amiloride, spironolactone, triamterene): May decrease bumetanide-induced potassium loss. Monitor serum potassium levels.
Drug-herb. *Dandelion:* Possible interference with diuretic activity. Discourage concurrent use.

Adverse reactions
CNS: dizziness, weakness, headache, vertigo.
CV: volume depletion and dehydration, orthostatic hypotension, ECG changes, chest pain.
EENT: transient deafness, tinnitus.
GI: nausea, vomiting, upset stomach, dry mouth, diarrhea, pain.
GU: *renal failure*, premature ejaculation, difficulty maintaining erection, oliguria.
Hematologic: azotemia, *thrombocytopenia*.

Metabolic: hypokalemia; hypochloremic alkalosis; asymptomatic hyperuricemia; impaired glucose tolerance; fluid and electrolyte imbalances, including dilutional hyponatremia, hypocalcemia, and hyperglycemia.
Musculoskeletal: arthritic pain, muscle pain and tenderness.
Skin: rash, pruritus, diaphoresis.

Overdose and treatment
Signs and symptoms of overdose include profound electrolyte and volume depletion, which may cause circulatory collapse. Treatment is primarily supportive; replace fluid and electrolytes as needed.

Special considerations
Consider the recommendations relevant to all loop diuretics as well as the following.
● Give I.V. bumetanide slowly, over 1 to 2 minutes, for I.V. infusion.
● Dilute bumetanide in D$_5$W, normal saline solution, or lactated Ringer's solution and use within 24 hours.

Patient monitoring
● Monitor drug effect in patients with renal or hepatic impairment.
● With increased dosage, monitor patient for ototoxicity.
● Monitor patient for electrolyte imbalance, especially hypokalemia.

Breast-feeding patients
● Drug shouldn't be used in breast-feeding women.

Pediatric patients
● Safety and efficacy in children under age 18 haven't been established.

Geriatric patients
● Geriatric and debilitated patients need close observation because they're more susceptible to drug-induced diuresis. Excessive diuresis promotes rapid dehydration, hypovolemia, hypokalemia, and hyponatremia in these patients, and may cause circulatory collapse. Reduced dosages may be indicated.

Patient education
● Tell patient to take drug in the morning to prevent nocturia, and if second dose is prescribed, to take it in early afternoon.
● Instruct patient to take drug with food or milk.
● Advise patient to stand up slowly to prevent dizziness, and to limit alcohol intake and strenuous exercise in hot weather to avoid worsening orthostatic hypertension.
● Instruct patient to weigh himself daily to monitor fluid status.

Reactions may be *common*, uncommon, *life-threatening*, or COMMON AND LIFE-THREATENING.

bupivacaine hydrochloride
Marcaine, Sensorcaine, Sensorcaine MPF, Sensorcaine MPF Spinal

Pharmacologic classification: amide local anesthetic
Therapeutic classification: local anesthetic
Pregnancy risk category: C

Indications and dosages
Dosages given are for the drug without epinephrine. Dose will differ depending on anesthetic procedure, area to be anesthetized, vascularity of area, number of neuronal segments to be blocked, degree of block, duration of anesthesia desired, and individual patient conditions and tolerance. Always use incremental doses.
➤ *Epidural block. Adults:* 25 to 50 mg (10 to 20 ml) 0.25% solution, 50 to 100 mg (10 to 20 ml) 0.5% solution, 75 to 100 mg (15 to 30 ml) 0.75% solution, single-dose only.
➤ *Caudal block. Adults:* 37.5 to 75 mg (15 to 30 ml) 0.25% solution, 75 to 150 mg (15 to 30 ml) 0.5% solution.
➤ *Spinal block. Adults:* 7.5 to 12 mg (1 to 1.6 ml) 0.75% solution (in dextrose 8.25%).
➤ *Peripheral nerve block. Adults:* 12.5 mg (5 ml) 0.25% solution, 25 mg (5 ml) 0.5% solution.
➤ *Retrobulbar block. Adults:* 15 to 30 mg (2 to 4 ml) 0.75% solution.

How supplied
Available by prescription only
Injection: 0.25%, 0.5%, 0.75%

Pharmacodynamics
Local anesthetic action: Thought to block the generation and conduction of nerve impulses by increasing the threshold for electrical excitation in the nerve, slowing propagation of the nerve impulse, and reducing the action potential.

Pharmacokinetics
Absorption: Absorption from the site of administration is affected by vascularity of tissue and depends on dose, concentration, and route of administration. After injection for caudal, epidural, or peripheral nerve block, levels peak in 30 to 45 minutes.
Distribution: Bupivacaine is 95% protein-bound and is distributed to some extent to all tissues.
Metabolism: Drug is metabolized primarily in the liver.
Excretion: Bupivacaine is mostly excreted by the kidneys with only 5% of unchanged drug in urine.

Route	Onset	Peak	Duration
Epidural, caudal, peripheral	Unknown	30-45 min	Unknown

Adverse reactions
CNS: anxiety, nervousness, *seizures* followed by drowsiness, dizziness, tremors.
CV: *arrhythmias, bradycardia, cardiac arrest,* hypotension, myocardial depression, edema, *heart block.*
EENT: blurred vision, tinnitus.
GI: nausea, vomiting.
Respiratory: status asthmaticus, *respiratory arrest.*
Skin: urticaria, erythema, pruritus.
Other: *anaphylactoid reactions, anaphylaxis,* angioneurotic edema.

Interactions
Drug-drug. *Beta blockers:* Enhanced sympathomimetic effects when used with bupivacaine and epinephrine. Use cautiously.
Butyrophenones, phenothiazines: May reduce or reverse pressor effect of epinephrine. Monitor patient.
Chloroprocaine: May lessen action of bupivacaine. Don't use together.
CNS depressants: May cause additive CNS effects. Reduce dosage of CNS depressants.
Enflurane, halothane, isoflurane, related drugs: Arrhythmias when used with bupivacaine and epinephrine. Use with extreme caution.
MAO inhibitors, tricyclic antidepressants: Severe, sustained hypertension when used with bupivacaine and epinephrine. Avoid using together.

Overdose and treatment
Acute emergencies are usually from high plasma levels. Toxic reactions usually involve CNS and CV systems. To treat, immediately establish and maintain a patent airway or administer controlled ventilation with 100% oxygen. If necessary, use drugs to control convulsions. Supportive treatment of circulatory depression may require administration of I.V. fluids and appropriate vasopressors. If difficulty is encountered in maintaining a patent airway, or if prolonged ventilatory support is needed, endotracheal intubation may be indicated. If maternal hypotension or fetal bradycardia occur in a pregnant patient, keep patient in the left lateral decubitus position, if possible, or manually displace the uterus off the great vessels.

Contraindications and precautions
Contraindicated in patients hypersensitive to bupivacaine or any local anesthetic of the amide type. Avoid 0.75% bupivacaine in obstetric patients, and don't use bupivacaine solutions to produce obstetric paracervical block anesthesia. Also not recommended for I.V. regional anesthesia (Bier block). Preservative-containing solutions shouldn't be used for caudal or epidural anesthesia.
Use cautiously in patients with hypotension, heart block, hepatic disease, or impaired CV function.

Special considerations

⚠ ALERT Local anesthetics should be administered only by clinicians experienced in the diagnosis and management of drug-related toxicity and other acute emergencies that may occur.
• Resuscitative equipment, drugs, and oxygen should be immediately available.
• Check solution before administering. Don't use if it contains particulate matter or if solution is pinkish or slightly darker than yellow.
• Don't use disinfectants that contain heavy metals for skin or mucous membrane disinfection because they may cause swelling and edema.
• Use solution with epinephrine cautiously in patients with CV disorders and in body areas with limited blood supply (ears, nose, fingers, toes).
• A test dose of a local anesthetic with a fast onset, preferably a solution containing epinephrine, should be given before epidural anesthesia with bupivacaine and the patient monitored for CNS and CV toxicity. Monitor patient for increased heart rate.
• Aspiration for blood or CSF should be performed before injecting dose of bupivacaine to avoid intravascular or intrathecal injection.
⚠ ALERT An intravascular injection is still possible even if aspirations for blood are negative.
• Administer the smallest dose and concentration needed to produce the desired result. Dosages should be reduced for young, elderly, and debilitated patients and those with cardiac or liver disease.
• During epidural administration, use incremental volumes of 3 to 5 ml with sufficient time between doses to detect toxicity.
• Local anesthetics rapidly cross the placenta and can cause maternal, fetal, and neonatal toxicity. Adverse reactions may involve alterations in the CNS, peripheral vascular tone, and cardiac function.
• The 0.75% concentration is indicated for nonobstetrical surgery patients who need a long duration of profound muscle relaxation.
• Discard partially used bottles of unpreserved solution.

Patient monitoring
• Continuously monitor CV and respiratory status and patient's state of consciousness after each injection. Restlessness, anxiety, incoherent speech, light-headedness, numbness and tingling of mouth and lips, metallic taste, tinnitus, dizziness, blurred vision, tremors, twitching, depression, or drowsiness may be early signs of CNS toxicity.
• Small doses of local anesthetics injected into the head and neck area may produce adverse reactions similar to systemic toxicity seen with unintentional intravascular injections of larger doses. Monitor patient's circulatory and respiratory status.

Breast-feeding patients
• It isn't known if drug appears in breast milk. Use cautiously in nursing women.

Pediatric patients
• Administration to children younger than age 12 isn't recommended.

Geriatric patients
• Dosage reductions are recommended.

Patient education
• Advise patient that temporary loss of sensation and motor activity in the anesthetized part of the body may occur.

buprenorphine hydrochloride
Buprenex

Pharmacologic classification: narcotic agonist-antagonist, opioid partial agonist
Therapeutic classification: analgesic
Controlled substance schedule: V
Pregnancy risk category: C

Indications and dosages
➤ **Moderate to severe pain.** *Adults and children over age 13:* 0.3 mg I.M. or slow I.V. q 6 hours, p.r.n. May repeat 0.3 mg 30 to 60 minutes after initial dose or increase to 0.6 mg per dose if necessary. S.C. administration isn't recommended.
Adults ◇: 25 to 250 mcg/hour via I.V. infusion (over 48 hours for postoperative pain).
◇*Adults:* 60 to 180 mcg via epidural injection.
➤ **Reverse fentanyl-induced anesthesia ◇.** *Adults:* 0.3 to 0.8 mg, I.V. or I.M., 1 to 4 hours after the induction of anesthesia and about 30 minutes before the end of surgery.
➤ **Circumcision ◇.** *Children ages 9 months to 9 years:* 3 mcg/kg I.M. with surgical anesthesia.

How supplied
Available by prescription only
Injection: 0.3 mg/ml in 1-ml ampules

Pharmacodynamics
Analgesic action: Exact mechanisms of action are unknown. Drug may be a competitive antagonist at some opiate receptors and an agonist at others, thus relieving moderate to severe pain.

Pharmacokinetics
Absorption: Absorbed rapidly after I.M. administration.
Distribution: About 96% is protein-bound.
Metabolism: Metabolized in the liver.
Excretion: Excreted primarily in feces as unchanged drug with about 30% excreted in urine.

Route	Onset	Peak	Duration
I.V.	Immediate	2 min	6 hr
I.M.	15 min	1 hr	6 hr

Contraindications and precautions

Contraindicated in patients hypersensitive to drug. Use cautiously in elderly or debilitated patients and in patients with head injuries, increased intracranial pressure, intracranial lesions, CNS depression or coma, thyroid irregularities, adrenal insufficiency, prostatic hyperplasia, urethral stricture, acute alcoholism, delirium tremens, kyphoscoliosis, or respiratory, kidney, or hepatic impairment.

Interactions

Drug-drug. *Barbiturate anesthetics, such as thiopental:* Additive CNS and respiratory depressant effects and possibly apnea. Use together cautiously.

CNS depressants (antihistamines, barbiturates, benzodiazepines, narcotic analgesics, phenothiazines, sedative-hypnotics), muscle relaxants, tricyclic antidepressants: Potentiated respiratory and CNS depression, sedation, and hypotensive effects. Reduced doses of buprenorphine are usually necessary.

Diazepam: Potential for respiratory and CV collapse. Avoid use together.

General anesthetics: Severe CV depression. Use together cautiously.

MAO inhibitors: Additive effects. Use together cautiously.

Drug-lifestyle. *Alcohol use:* May potentiate respiratory and CNS depression, sedation, and hypotensive effects. Discourage concurrent use.

Adverse reactions

CNS: *dizziness, sedation, headache,* confusion, nervousness, euphoria, *vertigo,* **increased intracranial pressure.**

CV: *hypotension,* **bradycardia,** tachycardia, hypertension.

EENT: *miosis,* blurred vision.

GI: *nausea,* vomiting, constipation, dry mouth.

GU: urine retention.

Respiratory: *respiratory depression,* hypoventilation, dyspnea.

Skin: pruritus, *diaphoresis.*

Overdose and treatment

Safety of buprenorphine in acute overdose is expected to be better than that of other opioid analgesics because of its antagonist properties at high doses. Overdose may cause CNS depression, respiratory depression, and miosis (pinpoint pupils). Other acute toxic effects might include hypotension, bradycardia, hypothermia, shock, apnea, cardiopulmonary arrest, circulatory collapse, pulmonary edema, and seizures.

To treat acute overdose, first establish adequate respiratory exchange via a patent airway and ventilation as needed; administer a narcotic antagonist (naloxone) to reverse respiratory depression. Because the duration of buprenorphine is longer than that of naloxone, repeated naloxone dosing is necessary. Naloxone shouldn't be given unless the patient has clinically significant respiratory or CV depression. Monitor vital signs closely.

Naloxone doesn't completely reverse buprenorphine-induced respiratory depression; mechanical ventilation and higher-than-usual doses of naloxone and doxaprane may be indicated.

Provide symptomatic and supportive treatment (continued respiratory support, correction of fluid or electrolyte imbalance). Closely monitor laboratory parameters, vital signs, and neurologic status.

Special considerations

● Adverse effects of drug may not be as readily reversed by naloxone as those of pure agonists.
● Patients who become physically dependent on this drug may have acute withdrawal syndrome if given an antagonist. Use cautiously and monitor patient closely.
● Buprenorphine 0.3 mg is equal to 10 mg morphine or 75 to 100 mg meperidine in analgesic potency; duration of analgesia is longer than both.
● Use I.M. injection in adults not at risk for respiratory depression.
● Buprenorphine has been diluted to 15 mcg/ml in normal saline solution for continuous I.V. infusion. For epidural injection, drug has been diluted to 6 to 30 mcg/ml in normal saline solution.
● Store ampules at 59° to 86° F (15° to 30° C) and protect from light.

Patient monitoring

● Monitor patient for respiratory depression. Avoid use in patients with pulmonary impairment or compromised respiratory function.

Breast-feeding patients

● It's unknown if drug appears in breast milk. Use cautiously in breast-feeding women.

Pediatric patients

● Buprenorphine has an unlabeled use as a supplement to anesthesia for children. Safety and efficacy hasn't been established in children under age 2.

Geriatric patients

● Administer cautiously; lower doses are usually indicated for elderly patients, who may be more sensitive to the therapeutic and adverse effects of these drugs.

Patient education

● Teach patient to avoid activities that require full alertness.
● Instruct patient to avoid alcohol and other CNS depressants.

bupropion hydrochloride
Wellbutrin, Wellbutrin SR

Pharmacologic classification: aminoketone
Therapeutic classification: antidepressant
Pregnancy risk category: B

Indications and dosages
➤ **Depression.** *Adults:* Initially, 100 mg P.O.
b.i.d. or 75 mg P.O. t.i.d. If necessary, increase
after 3 days to usual dosage of 100 mg P.O. t.i.d.
If no response occurs after several weeks of therapy, consider increasing dosage to 150 mg t.i.d.
Maximum, 450 mg daily. For sustained-release
tablets, start with 150 mg P.O. q morning; increase to target dose of 150 mg P.O. b.i.d. as tolerated as early as day 4 of dosing. If no response
after several weeks of therapy, increase to 200 mg
b.i.d. Maximum, 400 mg daily.

How supplied
Available by prescription only
Tablets: 75 mg, 100 mg
Tablets (sustained-release): 100 mg, 150 mg

Pharmacodynamics
Antidepressant action: Mechanism of action
is unknown. Bupropion doesn't inhibit MAO; it's
a weak inhibitor of norepinephrine, dopamine,
and serotonin reuptake.

Pharmacokinetics
Absorption: Only 5% to 20% is bioavailable in
animal studies.
Distribution: At plasma levels up to 200 mcg/ml,
drug appears to be about 80% bound to plasma
proteins.
Metabolism: Metabolism is probably hepatic;
several active metabolites have been identified.
With prolonged use, the active metabolites probably accumulate in plasma, and their level may
exceed that of the parent compound. Appears to
induce its own metabolism.
Excretion: Excretion is primarily renal; elimination half-life of parent compound in single-
dose studies ranges from 8 to 24 hours.

Route	Onset	Peak	Duration
P.O.			
Regular	Unknown	2 hr	Unknown
Sustained	Unknown	3 hr	Unknown

Contraindications and precautions
Contraindicated in patients hypersensitive to drug,
in patients with seizure disorders, and in patients
who have taken an MAO inhibitor within previous 14 days. Also contraindicated in patients taking the smoking cessation drug Zyban (also
bupropion) and in those with a history of bulimia
or anorexia nervosa because of an increased risk
of seizures. Use cautiously in patients with recent
MI, unstable heart disease, and renal or hepatic
impairment.

Interactions
Drug-drug. *Levodopa, MAO inhibitors, phenothiazines, recent and rapid withdrawal of
benzodiazepines, tricyclic antidepressants:* Increased risk of adverse effects, including seizures.
Monitor patient closely.

Adverse reactions
CNS: *headache, seizures,* anxiety, *confusion,*
delusions, euphoria, hostility, impaired sleep
quality, insomnia, sedation, tremor, akinesia,
akathisia, agitation, dizziness, syncope, fatigue.
CV: *arrhythmias,* hypertension, hypotension,
palpitations, *tachycardia.*
EENT: *auditory disturbances,* blurred vision.
GI: *dry mouth,* taste disturbance, increased ap-
petite, *constipation,* dyspepsia, *nausea, vom-
iting, anorexia,* diarrhea.
GU: impotence, menstrual complaints, urinary
frequency, urine retention.
Metabolic: *weight changes,* hyperglycemia.
Musculoskeletal: arthritis.
Skin: pruritus, rash, cutaneous temperature dis-
turbance, *excessive diaphoresis.*
Other: fever, chills, decreased libido.

Overdose and treatment
Overdose may cause labored breathing, salivation, arched back, ptosis, ataxia, and seizures.

If ingestion was recent, empty the stomach
using gastric lavage or induce emesis with ipecac,
as appropriate; follow with activated charcoal.
Treatment should be supportive. Control seizures
with I.V. benzodiazepines; stuporous, comatose,
or convulsing patients may need intubation. There
are no data to evaluate the benefits of dialysis,
hemoperfusion, or diuresis.

Special considerations
● Consider the inherent risk of suicide until depression improves significantly. High-risk patients
should be supervised closely at start of therapy.
To reduce risk of intentional overdose, prescribe
the smallest quantity of tablets consistent with
good management.
● Gradual increase of drug (no more than 75 to
100 mg daily q 2 to 3 days) reduces the risk of
seizures, agitation, motor restlessness, and insomnia.
● Many patients experience a period of increased
restlessness, especially at start of therapy. This
may include agitation, insomnia, and anxiety. In
clinical studies, some patients needed sedative-
hypnotic drugs and about 2% discontinued bupropion.
● Patients with bipolar disorder have an increased
risk of manic episodes when taking an antidepressant.
● Investigational uses of drug include treatment
of bipolar depression and attention deficit hyperactivity disorder in children.

Reactions may be *common*, uncommon, *life-threatening*, or COMMON AND LIFE-THREATENING.

Patient monitoring
• Monitor renal and hepatic function during therapy.

Pregnant patients
• Safety hasn't been established in pregnant women. Use drug only when absolutely necessary, and use pregnancy registry for monitoring outcomes: 800-336-2176.

Breast-feeding patients
• Because of the risk of serious adverse reactions in the infant, breast-feeding during therapy isn't recommended.

Pediatric patients
• Safety in children under age 18 hasn't been established.

Patient education
• Advise patient to take drug regularly as scheduled and to take each day's amount in three divided doses, preferably at 6-hour intervals, to minimize risk of seizures.
• Warn patient to avoid alcohol, which may increase the risk of seizures.
• Advise patient to avoid activities that require alertness and coordination until CNS effects of drug are known.
• Tell patient not to chew, divide, or crush sustained-release tablets.
• Instruct patient not to take Zyban with Wellbutrin or other medications, including OTC medications, without medical approval.

bupropion hydrochloride
Zyban

Pharmacologic classification: aminoketone
Therapeutic classification: nonnicotine aid to smoking cessation
Pregnancy risk category: B

Indications and dosages
➤ *Aid to smoking cessation. Adults:* 150 mg daily P.O. for 3 days; increased to maximum of 300 mg daily P.O. given as two doses of 150 mg taken at least 8 hours apart.

How supplied
Available by prescription only
Tablets (sustained-release): 150 mg

Pharmacodynamics
Smoking cessation action: Bupropion is a relatively weak inhibitor of the neuronal uptake of norepinephrine, serotonin, and dopamine. It doesn't inhibit MAO. The mechanism by which drug enhances the ability to abstain from smoking is unknown.

Pharmacokinetics
Absorption: Well absorbed after oral administration.
Distribution: Volume of distribution from a single 150-mg dose is estimated to be 1,950 L. It's 84% bound to plasma proteins at concentrations of up to 200 mcg/ml.
Metabolism: Extensively metabolized in the liver mainly by the P-450 2B6 isoenzyme system to three active metabolites.
Excretion: Mean elimination half-life is about 21 hours. Following oral administration, 87% of a dose is recovered in urine and 10% in feces. About 0.5% of a dose is excreted unchanged.

Route	Onset	Peak	Duration
P.O.	Unknown	3 hr	Unknown

Contraindications and precautions
Contraindicated in patients with seizure disorders or with a current or previous diagnosis of bulimia or anorexia nervosa because of increased risk of seizures.

Concurrent administration of MAO inhibitors is contraindicated; at least 14 days must elapse between stopping an MAO inhibitor and starting bupropion. Concurrent administration of Wellbutrin, Wellbutrin SR, or other medications containing bupropion is contraindicated because of increased risk of seizures. Also contraindicated in patients allergic to drug or to its formulation.

Interactions
Drug-drug. *Abrupt withdrawal of benzodiazepines, antidepressants, antipsychotics, systemic corticosteroids, theophylline:* Lower seizure threshold. Use together cautiously.
Carbamazepine, phenobarbital, phenytoin: Induced bupropion metabolism. Closely monitor patient.
Cimetidine: Inhibited bupropion metabolism. Closely monitor patient.
Drugs that affect enzyme metabolism, such as cyclophosphamide and orphenadrine: May cause an interaction because bupropion is metabolized to hydroxybupropion by the CYP2B6 isoenzyme. Closely monitor patient.
Levodopa: Higher risk of adverse reactions. If concurrent use is necessary, give small initial doses of bupropion and gradually increase dose.
MAO inhibitors, phenelzine: Enhanced acute toxicity of bupropion. Avoid use together.

Adverse reactions
CNS: agitation, dizziness, hot flashes, *insomnia,* somnolence, tremor.
CV: *complete AV block,* edema, hypertension, hypotension, tachycardia.
EENT: *dry mouth,* taste perversion.
GI: anorexia, dyspepsia, increased appetite.
GU: impotence, polyuria, urinary frequency and urgency.
Metabolic: weight gain, hyperglycemia.

Musculoskeletal: arthralgia, leg cramps and twitching, myalgia, neck pain.
Respiratory: bronchitis, *bronchospasm*.
Skin: dry skin, pruritus, rash, urticaria.
Other: *allergic reactions.*

Overdose and treatment

Hospitalization is recommended for overdoses. If patient is conscious, induce vomiting with syrup of ipecac. Activated charcoal also may be administered every 6 hours for first 12 hours. Perform ECG and EEG monitoring for first 48 hours. Provide adequate fluid intake and obtain baseline tests.

If patient is stuporous, comatose, or experiencing seizures, intubation is recommended before undertaking gastric lavage. Gastric lavage may be beneficial within first 12 hours after ingestion because drug absorption may not be complete. Although diuresis, dialysis, or hemoperfusion is sometimes used to treat drug overdose, there's no experience with their use in managing bupropion overdose. Based on animal studies, seizures can be treated with an I.V. benzodiazepine and other supportive measures.

Special considerations

● Because drug causes a dose-dependent risk of seizures, don't exceed 300 mg daily for smoking cessation.
● Therapy starts while patient is still smoking; about 1 week is needed to achieve steady-state blood levels of drug. Patient should set target cessation date during second week of treatment. Course of treatment is usually 7 to 12 weeks. If patient hasn't made significant progress toward abstinence by week 7 of therapy, discontinue treatment.
● Dose doesn't have to be tapered when stopping treatment.

Patient monitoring
● Monitor patient for development of hypertension when bupropion is used with transdermal nicotine.
● Monitor renal and hepatic function.

Pregnant patients
● Drug isn't for use in pregnant women.

Breast-feeding patients
● Drug and its metabolites appear in breast milk. Because of the risk of serious adverse reactions in infant, a choice must be made between breast-feeding and drug therapy.

Pediatric patients
● Safety and efficacy in children haven't been established.

Geriatric patients
● Experience in patients age 60 and older has been similar to that in younger patients.

Patient education
● Stress importance of combining behavioral interventions, counseling, and support services with drug therapy.
● Explain that risk of seizures is increased if patient has a seizure or eating disorder (bulimia or anorexia nervosa), exceeds the recommended dose, or takes other bupropion-containing drugs.
● Instruct patient to take doses at least 8 hours apart.
● Inform patient that drug is usually taken for 7 to 12 weeks.
● Advise patient that, although he may keep smoking during drug therapy, doing so reduces his chance of breaking the smoking habit.
● Tell patient that drug and nicotine patch should be used together only under medical supervision because his blood pressure may increase.

---

buspirone hydrochloride
BuSpar

Pharmacologic classification: azaspirodecanedione derivative
Therapeutic classification: antianxiety
Pregnancy risk category: B

Indications and dosages
➤*Management of anxiety disorders.*
Adults: Initially, 5 mg P.O. t.i.d. Dosage may be increased at 3-day intervals. Usual maintenance dosage is 20 to 30 mg daily in divided doses. Don't exceed 60 mg daily.

How supplied
Available by prescription only
Tablets: 5 mg, 10 mg, 15 mg, 30 mg

Pharmacodynamics
Anxiolytic action: Buspirone is an azaspirodecanedione derivative with anxiolytic activity. It suppresses conflict and aggressive behavior and inhibits conditioned avoidance responses. Its precise mechanism of action hasn't been determined, but it appears to depend on simultaneous effects on several neurotransmitters and receptor sites: decreasing serotonin neuronal activity, increasing norepinephrine metabolism, and exerting a partial action as a presynaptic dopamine antagonist. Studies suggest an indirect effect on benzodiazepine gamma-aminobutyric acid (GABA)–chloride receptor complex or GABA receptors, or on other neurotransmitter systems.

Buspirone isn't pharmacologically related to benzodiazepines, barbiturates, or other sedative and anxiolytics. It has a nontraditional clinical profile and is uniquely anxiolytic. It has no anticonvulsant or muscle relaxant activity and doesn't appear to cause physical dependence or significant sedation.

Pharmacokinetics

Absorption: Absorbed rapidly and completely after oral administration, but extensive first-pass metabolism limits absolute bioavailability to 1% to 13% of the oral dose. Food slows absorption but increases the amount of unchanged drug in systemic circulation.

Distribution: 95% protein-bound; it doesn't displace other highly protein-bound drugs such as warfarin.

Metabolism: Metabolized in the liver by hydroxylation and oxidation, resulting in at least one pharmacologically active metabolite, 1, pyrimidinylpiperazine (1-PP).

Excretion: 29% to 63% is excreted in urine in 24 hours, primarily as metabolites; 18% to 38% is excreted in feces.

Route	Onset	Peak	Duration
P.O.	Unknown	40-90 min	Unknown

Contraindications and precautions

Contraindicated in patients hypersensitive to drug or within 14 days of taking an MAO inhibitor. Use cautiously in patients with renal or hepatic impairment.

Interactions

Drug-drug. *CNS depressants:* Increased sedation. Avoid use together.

Digoxin: Buspirone may displace digoxin from serum-binding sites. Monitor digoxin levels.

Haloperidol: Increased serum haloperidol levels. Decrease haloperidol dosage.

MAO inhibitors: Elevated blood pressure. Avoid use together.

Drug-food. *Grapefruit juice:* Elevated buspirone levels and increased pharmacologic and adverse effects. Tell patient to take drug with liquid other than grapefruit juice.

Drug-lifestyle. *Alcohol use:* Increased sedation. Discourage alcohol use.

Adverse reactions

CNS: *dizziness, drowsiness,* nervousness, insomnia, headache, light-headedness, fatigue, numbness.

EENT: blurred vision.

GI: dry mouth, nausea, diarrhea, abdominal distress.

Overdose and treatment

Signs and symptoms of overdose include severe dizziness, drowsiness, unusual constriction of pupils, and stomach upset, including nausea and vomiting.

Treatment of overdose is symptomatic and supportive; empty stomach with immediate gastric lavage. Monitor respiration, pulse, and blood pressure. No specific antidote is known. Effect of dialysis is unknown.

Special considerations

● Buspirone has been used investigationally to treat nonmelancholic depression and parkinsonian syndrome.

● Patients previously given benzodiazepines may not show good clinical response to this agent.

● Although buspirone doesn't appear to cause tolerance or physical or psychological dependence, the possibility exists that a patient prone to drug abuse may experience these effects.

● Buspirone doesn't block the withdrawal syndrome linked to benzodiazepines or other common sedative and hypnotic agents; therefore, these agents should be withdrawn gradually before replacement with buspirone therapy.

● Store tablets in tight, light-resistant containers at temperatures less than 86° F (30° C).

Patient monitoring

● Monitor hepatic and renal function. Hepatic and renal impairment impedes metabolism and excretion of drug and may lead to toxic accumulation; dosage reduction may be necessary.

Breast-feeding patients

● It's unknown whether buspirone and its metabolites appear in breast milk. Avoid using buspirone in breast-feeding women.

Patient education

● Advise patient to take drug exactly as prescribed; explain that therapeutic effect may not occur for 2 weeks or more. Warn patient not to double a missed dose; a missed dose should be taken as soon as possible unless it's almost time for next dose.

● Caution patient to avoid hazardous tasks that demand alertness until effects of drug are known. The effects of alcohol and other CNS depressants, such as antihistamines, sedatives, tranquilizers, sleeping aids, prescription pain medication, barbiturates, seizure medicine, muscle relaxants, anesthetics, and medicines for colds, coughs, hay fever, or allergies, may be enhanced by additive sedation and drowsiness caused by buspirone.

● Tell patient to store drug away from heat and light and out of the reach of children.

● Explain importance of regular follow-up visits to check progress. Urge patient to report adverse reactions immediately.

● Inform patient that results may not be seen in 3 to 4 weeks; however, an improvement may be noted within 7 to 10 days.

● Instruct patient not to take drug with grapefruit juice but to take it with another liquid.

busulfan
Busulfex, Myleran

Pharmacologic classification: alkylating agent
(not specific to phase of cell cycle)
Therapeutic classification: antineoplastic
Pregnancy risk category: D

Indications and dosages
Dosages and indications may vary. Check package insert for recommended protocol.
➤ *Chronic myelogenous leukemia. Adults:*
For remission induction, usual dosage is 4 to 8 mg P.O. daily; however dosage may range from 1 to 12 mg P.O. daily (0.06 mg/kg or 1.8 mg/m^2). For maintenance therapy, 1 to 3 mg P.O. daily.
Children: 0.06 to 0.12 mg/kg or 1.8 to 4.6 mg/m^2 P.O. daily. Dosage should be adjusted to maintain WBC count of about 20,000/mm^3.
➤ *Myelofibrosis ◇. Adults:* Initially, 2 to 4 mg P.O. daily, followed by the same dose two to three times weekly.
➤ *Allogenic hematopoietic stem cell transplantation ◇. Adults:* 0.8 mg/kg of ideal body weight or actual body weight (whichever is lower) I.V. q 6 hr for 4 consecutive days for a total of 16 doses. Give phenytoin for seizure prophylaxis.

How supplied
Available by prescription only
Injection for I.V. infusion: 6 mg/ml
Tablets (scored): 2 mg

Pharmacodynamics
Antineoplastic action: Busulfan is an alkylating agent that exerts its cytotoxic activity by interfering with DNA replication and RNA transcription, causing a disruption of nucleic acid function.

Pharmacokinetics
Absorption: Well absorbed from the GI tract.
Distribution: Distribution into the brain and CSF is unknown.
Metabolism: Metabolized in the liver.
Excretion: Cleared rapidly from plasma. Drug and its metabolites are excreted in urine.

Route	Onset	Peak	Duration
P.O.	1-2 wk	Unknown	Unknown

Contraindications and precautions
Contraindicated in patients whose chronic myelogenous leukemia has shown previous resistance to drug. Also contraindicated in patients with chronic lymphocytic leukemia or acute leukemia and in those in blastic crisis of chronic myelogenous leukemia.
Use cautiously in patients recently given other myelosuppressants or radiation treatment; in those with depressed neutrophil or platelet counts, head trauma, or seizures; and in patients taking other drugs that reduce the seizure threshold.

Interactions
Drug-drug. *Acetaminophen, cyclophosphamide, phenytoin, thioguanine:* Increased busulfan clearance. Use together cautiously.
Itraconazole: Decreased busulfan clearance. Avoid concurrent use if possible.

Adverse reactions
CNS: weakness, fatigue.
EENT: cataracts.
GI: cheilosis, dry mouth, anorexia.
Hematologic: *leukopenia* (WBC count decreasing after about 10 days and continuing to decrease for 2 weeks after stopping drug), *thrombocytopenia,* anemia, *severe pancytopenia.*
Metabolic: profound hyperuricemia caused by increased cell lysis.
Respiratory: *irreversible pulmonary fibrosis* (commonly called busulfan lung).
Skin: alopecia, *transient hyperpigmentation,* rash, urticaria, anhidrosis, jaundice.
Other: gynecomastia, Addison-like wasting syndrome.

Overdose and treatment
Signs and symptoms of overdose include hematologic problems, such as leukopenia and thrombocytopenia. Treatment is supportive and includes transfusion of blood components and antibiotics for infections that may develop.

Special considerations
● Drug-induced cellular dysplasia may interfere with interpretation of cytologic studies.
● Avoid all I.M. injections when platelet count is below 100,000/mm^3.
● Patient response (increased appetite, sense of well-being, decreased total leukocyte count, reduction in size of spleen) usually begins 1 to 2 weeks after starting drug.
⚡ ALERT Pulmonary fibrosis may be delayed for 4 to 6 months.
● Minimize hyperuricemia by adequate hydration, alkalinization of urine, and administration of allopurinol.

Patient monitoring
● Observe patient for signs or symptoms of infection, such as fever and sore throat.
● Monitor uric acid, CBC, and kidney function.
● Monitor serum alkaline phosphatase, bilirubin, and serum aminotransferase levels for possible hepatotoxicity.
● Monitor leukocyte count; manufacturer recommends stopping busulfan when leukocyte count is 15,000/mm^3 or less.

Reactions may be *common*, uncommon, *life-threatening*, or COMMON AND LIFE-THREATENING.

Pregnant patients
● Busulfan may cause fetal harm (malformations, bone marrow depression, growth retardation, and death). Also, drug may impair fertility. Avoid use in pregnant women.

Breast-feeding patients
● It isn't known if drug appears in breast milk. However, potential for mutagenicity, carcinogenicity, and serious adverse reactions in the infant should be taken into consideration when patient decides whether to breast-feed.

Patient education
● Advise patient to use caution when taking aspirin-containing products and to promptly report signs and symptoms of bleeding.
● Tell patient to take drug at the same time each day.
● Emphasize importance of continuing to take drug despite nausea and vomiting.
● Persistent cough and progressive dyspnea with alveolar exudate may result from drug toxicity, not pneumonia. Instruct patient to report symptoms so dosage adjustments can be made.
● Review the signs and symptoms of infection, and tell patient to report them promptly if they occur.
● Advise patient to use contraception during therapy.

---

butoconazole nitrate
Femstat

Pharmacologic classification: synthetic imidazole derivative
Therapeutic classification: topical fungistat
Pregnancy risk category: C

Indications and dosages
➤ *Vulvovaginal candidiasis. Nonpregnant women:* One applicatorful intravaginally h.s. for 3 days. May be extended to 6 days if necessary. *Pregnant women:* One applicatorful intravaginally h.s. for 6 days. Use only during second or third trimester.

How supplied
Available by prescription only
Vaginal cream: 2% supplied with applicators

Pharmacodynamics
Antifungal action: Although the exact mechanism is unknown, butoconazole probably controls or destroys fungi by disrupting the permeability of the cell membrane and reducing its osmotic pressure resistance. Drug is active against many fungi, including dermatophytes and yeasts. It's also active in vitro against some gram-positive bacteria.

Pharmacokinetics
Absorption: About 5.5% is absorbed through vaginal walls.
Distribution: Unknown.
Metabolism: Systemically absorbed drug appears to be metabolized, probably in the liver.
Excretion: Systemically absorbed drug appears to be excreted in urine and feces.

Route	Onset	Peak	Duration
Intra-vaginal	Unknown	Unknown	Unknown

Contraindications and precautions
Contraindicated in patients hypersensitive to drug.

Interactions
None reported.

Adverse reactions
GU: vulvovaginal burning and itching, soreness, and swelling.
Skin: finger itching.

Overdose and treatment
No information available.

Special considerations
● Make sure patient understands directions for use and length of therapy.
● Drug may be used with oral contraceptives and antibiotics.
● Store drug at room temperature.

Patient monitoring
● Monitor patient for recurrent infection. It may be caused by resistant strains (*Candida albicans, Candida glabrata*), underlying disease (HIV, diabetes mellitus), or pregnancy.

Pregnant patients
● Drug isn't for use during the first trimester.

Pediatric patients
● Drug isn't for self-medication in children under age 12.

Breast-feeding patients
● Use drug cautiously in breast-feeding women because it isn't known whether drug appears in breast milk.

Patient education
● Instruct patient to follow the package directions, to insert the applicator high into the vagina, and to wash hands after use.
● Tell patient to complete the full course of therapy, including during menstrual period. However, advise her not to use tampons during treatment.
● Advise patient to either refrain from sexual contact or to have partner use a condom to avoid reinfection during therapy.

• Tell patient to use a sanitary napkin to prevent staining clothing and to absorb discharge.
• Tell patient to report symptoms that persist after full course of therapy.

---

butorphanol tartrate
Stadol, Stadol NS

Pharmacologic classification: narcotic agonist-antagonist; opioid partial agonist
Therapeutic classification: analgesic, adjunct to anesthesia
Controlled substance schedule: IV
Pregnancy risk category: C

Indications and dosages
➤ *Moderate to severe pain.* *Adults:* 1 to 4 mg I.M. q 3 to 4 hours, p.r.n. Or, 0.5 to 2 mg I.V. q 3 to 4 hours, p.r.n., or around the clock. Or, give 1 mg by nasal spray (one spray in one nostril). Repeat if pain relief is inadequate after 60 to 90 minutes. Repeat q 3 to 4 hours, p.r.n. For severe pain, an initial 2 mg by nasal spray in patients able to remain recumbent (one spray in each nostril). Repeat no more than q 3 to 4 hours, p.r.n.
➤ *Pain during labor.* *Adults:* 1 to 2 mg I.M. or I.V. q 4 hours but not within 4 hours before delivery.
➤ *Preoperative anesthesia.* *Adults:* 2 mg I.M. 60 to 90 minutes before surgery or 2 mg I.V. shortly before induction.
✦ *Dosage adjustment.* Patients with hepatic or renal impairment and elderly patients should receive one-half of the usual parenteral adult dose at 6-hour intervals, p.r.n. For nasal spray, the initial dose (one spray in one nostril) is the same but repeated in 90 to 120 minutes, p.r.n. Repeat doses thereafter q 6 hours, p.r.n.

How supplied
Available by prescription only
Injection: 1-ml vials (1 mg/ml); 1-ml, 2-ml, and 10-ml vials (2 mg/ml)
Nasal spray: 10 mg/ml

Pharmacodynamics
Analgesic action: The exact mechanisms of action are unknown. Drug is believed to competitively antagonize some opiate receptors and agonize others, thus relieving moderate to severe pain. Like narcotic agonists, it causes respiratory depression, sedation, and miosis.

Pharmacokinetics
Absorption: Well absorbed after I.M. administration.
Distribution: Rapidly crosses the placenta, and neonatal serum levels are 0.4 to 1.4 times maternal levels.
Metabolism: Metabolized extensively in the liver, primarily by hydroxylation, to inactive metabolites.

Excretion: Excreted in inactive form, mainly by the kidneys. About 11% to 14% of a parenteral dose is excreted in feces.

Route	Onset	Peak	Duration
I.V.	2-3 min	30-60 min	3-4 hr
I.M.	10-15 min	30-60 min	3-4 hr
Nasal	15 min	1-2 hr	4-5 hr

Contraindications and precautions
Contraindicated in patients receiving repeated doses of narcotic drugs or with narcotic addiction; may precipitate withdrawal syndrome. Also contraindicated in patients hypersensitive to drug or to the preservative benzethonium chloride.

Use cautiously in emotionally unstable patients and in those with a history of drug abuse, head injury, increased intracranial pressure, acute MI, ventricular dysfunction, coronary insufficiency, respiratory disease or depression, and renal or hepatic dysfunction.

Interactions
Drug-drug. *Barbiturate anesthetics such as thiopental:* Additive CNS and respiratory depressant effects and possibly apnea. Monitor patient closely.
Cimetidine: May potentiate butorphanol toxicity, causing disorientation, respiratory depression, apnea, and seizures. Use cautiously and be prepared to administer a narcotic antagonist if toxicity occurs.
CNS depressants (antihistamines, barbiturates, benzodiazepines, muscle relaxants, narcotic analgesics, phenothiazines, sedative-hypnotics, tricyclic antidepressants): Potentiated respiratory and CNS depression, sedation, and hypotensive effects. Reduced butorphanol dosage is usually needed.
Digitoxin, phenytoin, rifampin: Drug accumulation and enhanced effects. Reduce butorphanol dosage.
General anesthetics: Severe CV depression. Avoid use together.
Narcotic antagonists: Patients who become physically dependent on opioids may experience acute withdrawal syndrome. Use cautiously and monitor patient closely.
Pancuronium: May increase conjunctival changes. Monitor patient.
Drug-lifestyle. *Alcohol use:* May potentiate respiratory and CNS depression, sedation, and hypotensive effects of drug. Discourage use together.

Adverse reactions
CNS: *confusion,* nervousness, lethargy, headache, *somnolence, dizziness, insomnia,* anxiety, paresthesia, euphoria, hallucinations, *increased intracranial pressure.*
CV: palpitations, flushing, vasodilation, hypotension.
EENT: blurred vision, *nasal congestion* (with nasal spray), tinnitus.

Reactions may be *common*, uncommon, *life-threatening*, or COMMON AND LIFE-THREATENING.

GI: taste perversion, *nausea, vomiting, constipation,* anorexia.
Respiratory: *respiratory depression.*
Skin: rash, hives, *clamminess, excessive diaphoresis.*
Other: sensation of heat.

Overdose and treatment
No information available.

Special considerations
● Patients using nasal form for severe pain may start with 2 mg (one spray in each nostril) provided they remain recumbent. Dose isn't repeated for 3 to 4 hours.
● Mild withdrawal symptoms have been reported with long-term use of the injectable form.

Patient monitoring
● Drug has the potential to be abused. Closely supervise emotionally unstable patients and those with a history of drug abuse when long-term therapy is necessary.
● Monitor patient for respiratory depression.

Pregnant patients
● Safe use during pregnancy (except during labor) hasn't been established.

Breast-feeding patients
● Use of drug in breast-feeding women isn't recommended.

Pediatric patients
● Safety and efficacy in children under age 18 haven't been established.

Geriatric patients
● Lower doses are usually indicated for elderly patients because they may be more sensitive to therapeutic and adverse effects of the drug. Plasma half-life is increased by 25% in patients over age 65.

Patient education
● Teach patient how to use nasal spray. Patient should use one spray in one nostril unless otherwise directed.

◇ Unlabeled clinical use

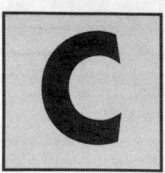

caffeine
Caffedrine, NoDoz, Quick Pep, Vivarin

Pharmacologic classification: methylxanthine
Therapeutic classification: CNS stimulant, analeptic, respiratory stimulant
Pregnancy risk category: C

Indications and dosages
➤**Neonatal apnea.** *Neonates:* 20 mg/kg I.V. infusion over 30 minutes as loading dose; 24 hours later, start 5 mg/kg P.O. or I.V. infusion q 24 hours. *Neonates◇:* 5 to 10 mg/kg (base) I.V., I.M., or P.O. as loading dose; then 2.5 to 5 mg/kg I.V., I.M., or P.O. daily. Adjust dosage according to patient tolerance and plasma caffeine levels.
➤**CNS depression.** (*Note:* This use is strongly discouraged by many clinicians.) *Adults:* 100 to 200 mg P.O. q 3 to 4 hours, p.r.n. For emergencies, 250 to 500 mg I.M. or I.V.
Infants and children◇: 4 mg/kg I.M., I.V., or S.C. q 4 hours, p.r.n.

How supplied
Available by prescription only
Injection: 250 mg/ml, caffeine (121.25 mg/ml) with sodium benzoate (128.75 mg/ml)
Available without a prescription
Chewable tablets: 100 mg
Tablets: 150 mg, 200 mg

Pharmacodynamics
CNS stimulant action: A xanthine derivative; increases levels of cAMP by inhibiting phosphodiesterase. Caffeine stimulates all levels of the CNS. It hastens and clarifies thinking and improves arousal and psychomotor coordination.
Respiratory stimulant action: In respiratory depression and neonatal apnea, larger doses of caffeine increase respiratory rate. Caffeine increases contractile force and decreases fatigue of skeletal muscle.

Pharmacokinetics
Absorption: Well absorbed from GI tract; absorption after I.M. injection may be slower.
Distribution: Distributed rapidly throughout body; crosses blood-brain barrier and placenta. About 17% protein-bound.
Metabolism: Metabolized by the liver; in neonates, liver metabolism is much less evident and half-life may approach 80 hours. Plasma half-life in adults is 3 to 4 hours.

Excretion: Excreted in urine.

Route	Onset	Peak	Duration
P.O.	Unknown	50-75 min	Unknown
I.M., I.V.	Unknown	Unknown	Unknown

Contraindications and precautions
Contraindicated in patients hypersensitive to drug. Use cautiously in patients with history of peptic ulcer, symptomatic arrhythmias, or palpitations, and after an acute MI.

Interactions
Drug-drug. *Beta agonists (albuterol, metaproterenol, terbutaline):* Increased cardiac effects and tremors. Monitor patient closely.
Fluoroquinolones such as cimetidine, ciprofloxacin, disulfiram, enoxacin; oral contraceptives: Inhibited caffeine metabolism and increased effects. Use together cautiously.
Xanthine derivatives (theophylline): May increase stimulant-induced adverse reactions, such as tremor, tachycardia, insomnia, and nervousness. Use together cautiously.
Drug-herb. *Ephedra:* Increased CNS effects. Discourage use together.
Drug-lifestyle. *Smoking:* May enhance elimination of caffeine. Discourage smoking.

Adverse reactions
CNS: *insomnia,* restlessness, nervousness, headache, excitement, agitation, muscle tremor, twitching.
CV: *tachycardia, palpitations,* extrasystoles.
EENT: tinnitus.
GI: nausea, vomiting, diarrhea, stomach pain.
GU: *diuresis.*
Other: abrupt withdrawal symptoms (headache, irritability).

Overdose and treatment
Signs and symptoms of overdose in adults may include insomnia, dyspnea, altered states of consciousness, muscle twitching, seizure, diuresis, arrhythmias, and fever. In infants, symptoms of overdose may include alternating hypotonicity and hypertonicity, opisthotonoid posture, tremors, bradycardia, hypotension, and severe acidosis.

Treat overdose symptomatically and supportively; lavage and charcoal may help. Carefully monitor vital signs, ECG, and fluid and electrolyte balance. Seizures may be treated with diazepam or phenobarbital; diazepam may exacerbate respiratory depression.

Special considerations

● Restrict caffeine-containing beverages in patients with arrhythmic symptoms and in those taking aminophylline or theophylline.

● Caffeine content in beverages (mg/cup) is the following: cola drinks, 24 to 64; brewed tea, 20 to 110; instant coffee, 30 to 120; brewed coffee, 40 to 180; decaffeinated coffee, 3 to 5.

● Many OTC pain relievers contain caffeine, but evidence concerning its analgesic effects is conflicting. Caffeine (30%) may be used in a hydrophilic base or hydrocortisone cream to treat atopic dermatitis.

● Caffeine has been used to relieve headache after lumbar puncture and, in topical creams, to treat atopic dermatitis.

● Caffeine may cause false-positive urate levels measured by the Bittner method. It also may cause false-positive test results for pheochromocytoma or neuroblastoma by increasing certain urinary catecholamines.

Patient monitoring

● Monitor patient for adverse effects.

Breast-feeding patients

● Caffeine appears in breast milk. Alternative feeding method is recommended during therapy with caffeine.

Pediatric patients

● For control of neonatal apnea, maintain plasma caffeine level at 5 to 20 mcg/ml.

● Adverse CNS effects are usually more severe in children.

● In neonates, avoid using caffeine products containing sodium benzoate; they may cause kernicterus.

Geriatric patients

● Elderly patients are more sensitive to caffeine and should take lower doses.

Patient education

● Advise patient to avoid excessive caffeine consumption, and therefore CNS stimulation, by learning caffeine content of beverages and foods.

● Warn patient not to exceed recommended dosage, not to substitute caffeine for needed sleep, and to stop drug if dizziness or tachycardia occurs.

---

calcifediol
Calderol

Pharmacologic classification: vitamin D analogue
Therapeutic classification: antihypocalcemic
Pregnancy risk category: C

Indications and dosages

➤ *Management of metabolic bone disease or hypocalcemia in patients on long-term renal dialysis. Adults:* Initially, 300 to 350 mcg/week P.O. given daily or every other day. May increase dosage at 4-week intervals based on serum levels. Most patients respond to 50 to 100 mcg daily or 100 to 200 mcg every other day.

How supplied

Available by prescription only
Capsules: 20 mcg, 50 mcg

Pharmacodynamics

Antihypocalcemic action: Vitamin D analogue (25-hydroxycholecalciferol) that works with parathyroid hormone to regulate serum calcium; drug must be activated for its full effect, but appears to have some intrinsic activity.

Pharmacokinetics

Absorption*: Absorbed readily from small intestine.

Distribution*: Distributed widely; highly protein-bound.

Metabolism: Metabolized in liver and kidney; half-life is 16 days. It's activated to 1,25 dihydroxycholecalciferol.

Excretion: Excreted in urine and bile.

Route	Onset	Peak	Duration
P.O.	Unknown	4 hr	15-20 days

Contraindications and precautions

Contraindicated in patients with hypercalcemia or vitamin D toxicity.

Interactions

Drug-drug. *Antacids, mineral oil:* May alter calcifediol absorption. Don't use concomitantly.
Barbiturates, phenytoin, primidone: May increase metabolism and reduce activity of calcifediol. Monitor patient closely.
Cardiac glycosides: Increased effect of cardiac glycosides. Monitor patient closely.
Cholestyramine, colestipol hydrochloride: May reduce intestinal absorption. Separate administration times.
Corticosteroids: Counteract effects of vitamin D analogues. Don't use together, if possible.
Thiazide diuretics: May result in hypercalcemia. Monitor serum calcium level.

Adverse reactions

Adverse reactions stem from vitamin D intoxication related to hypercalcemia.
CNS: headache, somnolence, weakness, irritability.
CV: hypertension, ***arrhythmias.***
EENT: conjunctivitis, rhinorrhea.
GI: constipation, nausea, vomiting, polydipsia, ***pancreatitis,*** metallic taste, dry mouth, anorexia, diarrhea.
GU: polyuria, nocturia, nephrocalcinosis.
Metabolic: weight loss.
Musculoskeletal: bone and muscle pain.
Skin: pruritus, photosensitivity.

◇ Unlabeled clinical use

Other: hyperthermia, decreased libido.

Overdose and treatment
Only sign of overdose is hypercalcemia. Treatment involves discontinuing therapy, instituting a low-calcium diet, and increasing fluid intake. Provide supportive measures. Severe overdose has led to death from cardiac and renal failure.

Special considerations
● Calcitonin administration may be useful in treating hypercalcemia.
● Calciferol may falsely elevate cholesterol determinations using the Zlatkis-Zak reaction.

Patient monitoring
● Before starting therapy, verify that serum phosphate levels are controlled. To avoid ectopic calcification, serum calcium (mg/dl) times phosphorus (mg/dl) shouldn't exceed 70.
● Monitor serum calcium levels several times weekly when starting therapy.
● There's some evidence that monitoring urine calcium and urine creatinine is very helpful in screening for hypercalciuria. Ratio of urine calcium to urine creatinine should be less than or equal to 0.18. A value above 0.2 suggests hypercalciuria; dose should be decreased regardless of serum calcium level.

Breast-feeding patients
● Very little drug appears in breast milk; however, the effect of vitamin D levels that exceed the RDA in infants is unknown. Use drug cautiously in breast-feeding women.

Pediatric patients
● Some infants may be hyperreactive to drug.

Patient education
● Explain importance of a calcium-rich diet.

calcipotriene
Dovonex

Pharmacologic classification: synthetic vitamin D₃ analogue
Therapeutic classification: topical antipsoriatic
Pregnancy risk category: C

Indications and dosages
➤ **Moderate plaque psoriasis.** *Adults:* Apply a thin layer to affected skin b.i.d. Rub in gently and completely.

How supplied
Available by prescription only
Cream, ointment, solution: 0.005%

Pharmacodynamics
Antipsoriatic action: Calcipotriene is a synthetic vitamin D₃ analogue that binds to vitamin D₃ receptors in skin cells (keratinocytes), regulating skin cell production and development.

Pharmacokinetics
Absorption: About 6% of the applied dose of calcipotriene is absorbed systemically when the ointment is applied topically to psoriasis plaques or 5% when applied to normal skin.
Distribution: Vitamin D and its metabolites are transported in the blood, bound to specific plasma proteins, to many parts of the body containing keratinocytes. (The scaly red patches of psoriasis are caused by the abnormal growth and production of keratinocytes.)
Metabolism: Drug metabolism after systemic uptake is rapid and occurs via a pathway similar to the natural hormone. The primary metabolites are much less potent than the parent compound.
Excretion: The active form of the vitamin, 1,25-dihydroxy vitamin D₃ (calcitriol), is recycled via the liver and excreted in bile.

Route	Onset	Peak	Duration
Topical	Unknown	Unknown	Unknown

Contraindications and precautions
Contraindicated in patients hypersensitive to drug or its components. Also contraindicated in patients with hypercalcemia or evidence of vitamin D toxicity. Use cautiously in breast-feeding patients and elderly patients. Drug shouldn't be used on the face.

Interactions
None reported.

Adverse reactions
Metabolic: hypercalcemia.
Skin: *burning, pruritus, irritation,* atrophy, dermatitis, dry skin, erythema, folliculitis, hyperpigmentation, peeling, rash, worsening of psoriasis.

Overdose and treatment
Topically applied calcipotriene can be absorbed in sufficient amounts to produce systemic effects. Serum calcium levels may increase with excessive use.

Special considerations
● Drug is for topical dermatologic use only. It isn't intended for ophthalmic, oral, or intravaginal use.
● Improvement usually begins after 2 weeks of therapy, and marked improvement occurs after 8 weeks; only about 10% of cases show complete clearing.
● Safety and effectiveness of topical calcipotriene in dermatoses other than psoriasis haven't been established.
● Use of calcipotriene may cause irritation of lesions and surrounding uninvolved skin. If irritation develops, discontinue drug.

Reactions may be *common*, uncommon, *life-threatening*, or COMMON AND LIFE-THREATENING.

Patient monitoring

• Transient, rapidly reversible elevation of serum calcium level may occur. If serum calcium level increases outside the normal range, discontinue treatment until normal calcium levels are restored.

Breast-feeding patients

• It isn't known if drug appears in breast milk. Use cautiously when administering calcipotriene ointment to breast-feeding women.

Pediatric patients

• Safety and effectiveness in children haven't been established.

Geriatric patients

• Adverse dermatologic effects of topical calcipotriene may be more severe in patients over age 65.

Patient education

• Tell patient that drug is for external use only, as directed, and that he should avoid contact with face or eyes.
• Instruct patient to wash hands thoroughly after application.
• Tell patient to report signs of local adverse reactions.

---

calcitonin (salmon)

Calcimar, Miacalcin, Osteocalcin, Salmonine

Pharmacologic classification: thyroid hormone
Therapeutic classification: hypocalcemic
Pregnancy risk category: C

Indications and dosages

➤ **Paget's bone disease (osteitis deformans).** *Adults:* Initially, 100 IU calcitonin S.C. or I.M. daily. Maintenance dosage is 50 to 100 IU calcitonin, three times weekly.
➤ **Hypercalcemia.** *Adults:* 4 IU/kg calcitonin (salmon) I.M. or S.C. q 12 hours; if no response in 1 to 2 days, increase to 8 IU/kg q 12 hours; if no response in 2 more days, increase to maximum of 8 IU/kg every 6 hours.
Or, 2 to 16 IU/kg I.V. infusion ◊ q 12 hours.
➤ **Postmenopausal osteoporosis.** *Adults:* 100 IU calcitonin S.C. or I.M. daily, or 200 IU (one spray) daily in alternating nostrils.
➤ **Osteogenesis imperfecta** ◊. *Adults:* 2 IU/kg calcitonin I.M. or S.C. three times weekly, with daily P.O. calcium supplementation.

How supplied

Available by prescription only
Injection: 200-IU/ml, 2-ml vials
Nasal spray: 200 IU/activation

Pharmacodynamics

Hypocalcemic action: Calcitonin directly inhibits the bone resorption of calcium. This effect is mediated by drug-induced increase of cAMP level in bone cells, which alters transport of calcium and phosphate across the plasma membrane of the osteoclast. A secondary effect occurs in the kidneys, where calcitonin directly inhibits tubular resorption of calcium, phosphate, and sodium, thereby increasing their excretion. A clinical effect may not be seen for several months in patients with Paget's disease.

Pharmacokinetics

Absorption: Drug can be administered parenterally or nasally. Plasma levels of 0.1 to 0.4 mg/ml are achieved within 15 minutes of a 200-IU S.C. dose. The maximum effect is seen in 2 to 4 hours; duration of action may be 8 to 24 hours for S.C. or I.M. doses, and ½ to 12 hours for I.V. doses. Plasma levels peak 31 to 39 minutes after using the nasal form.
Distribution: It isn't known if drug enters the CNS or crosses the placenta.
Metabolism: Rapid metabolism occurs in the kidneys, with additional activity in the blood and peripheral tissues.
Excretion: Excreted in urine as inactive metabolites.

Route	Onset	Peak	Duration
I.M., S.C.	15 min	4 hr	8-24 hr
Intranasal	Rapid	½ hr	1 hr
I.V.	Immediate	Unknown	½-12 hr

Contraindications and precautions

Contraindicated in patients hypersensitive to salmon calcitonin.

Interactions

None reported.

Adverse reactions

CNS: headache, weakness, dizziness, paresthesia.
CV: edema of feet, chest pressure, shortness of breath.
EENT: eye pain, nasal congestion.
GI: *transient nausea,* unusual taste, diarrhea, anorexia, *vomiting,* epigastric discomfort, abdominal pain.
GU: *increased urinary frequency,* nocturia.
Skin: *facial flushing,* rash, pruritus of ear lobes, *inflammation at injection site.*
Other: hypersensitivity reactions (*anaphylaxis*), tender palms and soles, chills.

Overdose and treatment

Signs and symptoms of overdose include hypocalcemia and hypocalcemic tetany. This usually occurs in patients at higher risk during the first few doses.
    Parenteral calcium will correct the symptoms and should be readily available.

Special considerations
- S.C. route is the preferred method of administration.
- Keep parenteral calcium available during the first doses in case of hypocalcemic tetany.
- Refrigerate solution. Once activated, nasal spray should be stored upright at room temperature.

Patient monitoring
- Consider a skin test using salmon calcitonin before starting therapy. If patient has allergic reactions to foreign proteins, test for hypersensitivity before therapy. Systemic allergic reactions are possible because hormone is a protein. Keep epinephrine readily available.
- Periodically monitor serum calcium levels during therapy.
- Observe patient for signs of hypocalcemic tetany during therapy (muscle twitching, tetanic spasms, and convulsions if hypocalcemia is severe).
- Watch for evidence of hypercalcemic relapse: Bone pain, renal calculi, polyuria, anorexia, nausea, vomiting, thirst, constipation, lethargy, bradycardia, muscle hypotonicity, pathologic fracture, psychosis, and coma. Patient with good initial clinical response to calcitonin who suffers relapse should be evaluated for antibody formation response to the hormone protein.
- Perform periodic nasal examination in patients using nasal spray.

Pregnant patients
- Use drug cautiously.

Breast-feeding patients
- Use drug cautiously.

Pediatric patients
- There are inadequate data to support the use of calcitonin in children.

Patient education
- Teach patient how to administer drug, and assist him until he learns proper technique.
- Tell patient to handle missed doses as follows: For daily dosing, take as soon as possible, and don't double the dose. For alternate day dosing, take as soon as possible, and then restart the alternate day schedule from this dose.
- Stress the importance of regular follow-up to assess progress.
- If given for postmenopausal osteoporosis, remind patient to take adequate calcium and vitamin D supplements.
- Instruct patient using the nasal spray to activate pump before using.
- Tell patient to report nasal irritation.

calcitriol
Calcijex, Rocaltrol

Pharmacologic classification: vitamin D analogue
Therapeutic classification: antihypocalcemic
Pregnancy risk category: C

Indications and dosages
➤*Management of hypocalcemia in patients undergoing long-term dialysis.*
Oral. *Adults:* Initially, 0.25 mcg P.O. daily. Dosage may be increased by 0.25 mcg daily at 4- to 8-week intervals. Maintenance dosage is 0.25 mcg every other day up to 0.5 to 1 mcg P.O. daily.
Parenteral
Adults: 1 to 2 mcg I.V. three times weekly, about every other day. Dosage may be increased by 0.25 to 0.5 mcg at 2- to 4-week intervals. Maintenance dosage is 0.5 to 4 mcg I.V. three times weekly.
➤*Management of hypoparathyroidism and pseudohypoparathyroidism. Adults and children age 6 and older:* Initially, 0.25 mcg P.O. daily in the morning. Dosage may be increased at 2- to 4-week intervals. Maintenance dosage is 0.5 to 2 mcg daily.
Children ages 1 to 5 (hypoparathyroidism only): Initially, 0.25 mcg P.O. daily. Dosage may be increased at 2- to 4-week intervals. Maintenance dosage is 0.25 to 0.75 mcg P.O. daily.
➤*Prevention or management of secondary hyperparathyroidism and resultant metabolic bone disease in predialysis patients (moderate to severe chronic renal failure with creatinine clearance of 15 to 55 ml/minute). Adults and children age 3 and older:* Initially, 0.25 mcg P.O. daily. Dosage may be increased to 0.5 mcg daily, if necessary.
Children under age 3: 0.01 to 0.015 mcg/kg P.O. daily.
➤*Psoriasis vulgaris* ◇. *Adults:* 0.25 mcg P.O. b.i.d. for 6 months and topically (0.1 to 0.5 mcg/g petroleum) daily for 8 weeks.

How supplied
Available by prescription only
Capsules: 0.25 mcg, 0.5 mcg
Injection: 1 mcg/ml, 2 mcg/ml
Oral solution: 1 mcg/ml

Pharmacodynamics
Antihypocalcemic action: Calcitriol is a vitamin D analogue (1,25-dihydroxycholecalciferol), or activated cholecalciferol. It promotes absorption of calcium from the intestine by forming a calcium-binding protein. It reverses the signs of rickets and osteomalacia in patients who can't activate or use ergocalciferol or cholecalciferol. In patients with renal failure, it reduces bone pain, muscle weakness, and parathyroid serum levels.

Reactions may be *common*, uncommon, *life-threatening*, or COMMON AND LIFE-THREATENING.

Pharmacokinetics

Absorption: Absorbed readily after oral administration.
Distribution: Distributed widely and is protein-bound.
Metabolism: Metabolized in the liver and kidneys, with a half-life of 3 to 8 hours. No activation step is required.
Excretion: Excreted primarily in feces.

Route	Onset	Peak	Duration
P.O.	2-6 hr	3-6 hr	3-5 days
I.V.	Immediate	Unknown	3-5 days

Contraindications and precautions

Contraindicated in patients with hypercalcemia or vitamin D toxicity. Withhold all preparations containing vitamin D.

Interactions

Drug-drug. *Cardiac glycosides:* Increased risk of arrhythmias. Avoid use together.
Cholestyramine, colestipol, mineral oil: May alter calcitriol absorption. Avoid use together.
Corticosteroids: May counteract the effects of vitamin D analogues. Don't use together.
Magnesium-containing antacids: May induce hypermagnesemia, especially in patients with chronic renal failure. Avoid use together.
Orlistat: Decreased absorption of vitamin D. Give at least 2 hours apart.

Adverse reactions

CNS: headache, somnolence, weakness, irritability.
CV: hypertension, *arrhythmias.*
EENT: conjunctivitis, photophobia, rhinorrhea.
GI: nausea, vomiting, constipation, polydipsia, *pancreatitis,* metallic taste, dry mouth, anorexia.
GU: nephrocalcinosis, polyuria, nocturia.
Metabolic: weight loss.
Musculoskeletal: bone and muscle pain.
Skin: pruritus.
Other: hyperthermia, decreased libido.

Overdose and treatment

Treatment of hypercalcemia (a sign of overdose) requires discontinuation of drug, a low-calcium diet, increased fluid intake, and supportive measures. Calcitonin administration may help reverse hypercalcemia. In severe cases, death has followed CV and renal failure.

Special considerations

● Drug may alter serum alkaline phosphatase levels and may alter electrolytes, such as magnesium, phosphate, and calcium in serum and urine.
● Vitamin D intoxication is linked to hypercalcemia.
● Protect drug from heat and light.
● Calcitriol therapy may falsely elevate cholesterol determinations made using the Zlatkis-Zak reaction

Patient monitoring

● Monitor serum calcium levels several times weekly after starting therapy.
● There's some evidence that monitoring urine calcium and urine creatinine is very helpful in screening for hypercalciuria. The ratio of urine calcium to urine creatinine should be less than or equal to 0.18. A value of more than 0.2 suggests hypercalciuria, and the dose should be decreased regardless of serum calcium level. The product of serum calcium times phosphate shouldn't exceed 70.

Breast-feeding patients

● Very little drug appears in breast milk; however, the effect of vitamin D levels exceeding the recommended daily allowance in infants isn't known. Therefore, large doses shouldn't be administered to breast-feeding women.

Pediatric patients

● Some infants may be hyperreactive to drug. Long-term treatment has been well-tolerated except for occasional episodes of electrolyte imbalance, which resolves with alteration of therapy.

Patient education

● Instruct patient on the importance of a calcium-rich diet.
● Tell patient that drug must not be taken by anyone for whom it wasn't prescribed. It's the most potent form of vitamin D.
● Advise patient to report adverse reactions immediately.
● Tell patient to avoid magnesium-containing antacids and other drugs without prescriber's approval.

calcium polycarbophil
Equalactin, Fiberall, FiberCon, Fiber-Lax, Mitrolan

Pharmacologic classification: hydrophilic
Therapeutic classification: bulk laxative, antidiarrheal
Pregnancy risk category: C

Indications and dosages

➤ *Constipation, acute nonspecific diarrhea related to irritable bowel syndrome.*
Adults: 1 g P.O. q.i.d. as required. Maximum dose is 6 g in 24-hour period.
Children ages 6 to 12: 500 mg P.O. once daily to t.i.d. as required. Maximum dose is 3 g in 24 hour period.
Children ages 3 to 6: 500 mg P.O. once daily to b.i.d. as required. Maximum dose is 1.5 g in 24-hour period.

How supplied

Available without a prescription
Tablets: 500 mg (FiberCon), 625 mg (Fiber-Lax)

Tablets (chewable): 500 mg (Equalactin, Fiber-Lax, Mitrolan), 1,000 mg (Fiberall)

Pharmacodynamics
Laxative action: Absorbs water and expands, thereby increasing stool bulk and moisture and promoting normal peristalsis and bowel motility.
Antidiarrheal action: Absorbs intestinal fluid, thereby restoring normal stool consistency and bulk.

Pharmacokinetics
Absorption: None.
Distribution: None.
Metabolism: None.
Excretion: Excreted in feces.

Route	Onset	Peak	Duration
P.O.	12-24 hr	3 days	Variable

Contraindications and precautions
Contraindicated in patients with GI obstruction; drug may worsen condition.

Interactions
Drug-drug. *Tetracycline:* Calcium polycarbophil may impair absorption. Use together cautiously.

Adverse reactions
GI: abdominal fullness and increased flatus, intestinal obstruction.
Other: laxative dependence (with long-term or excessive use).

Special considerations
• Patient must chew tablets (chewable) before swallowing; administer them with 8 oz (240 ml) of fluid. Administer less fluid for antidiarrheal effect.
• When using drug as an antidiarrheal, don't give if patient has high fever.

Patient monitoring
• Before starting drug, make sure patient has adequate fluid intake, diet, and exercise.
• Evaluate response to drug therapy.
• Monitor patient for signs of drug dependence.

Patient education
• For chewable tablets, instruct patient to chew tablets instead of swallowing them whole. If drug is being taken as a laxative, advise patient to drink a full glass (8 oz) of fluid after each tablet. Advise patient to take less fluid if drug is being used to treat diarrhea.
• Warn patient not to take more than 12 tablets in 24-hour period (six tablets for child age 6 to 12; three tablets for child age 3 to 6) and to take for length of time prescribed.
• If patient is taking drug as laxative, advise him to call promptly and stop drug if constipation persists after 1 week, or if fever, nausea, vomiting, or abdominal pain occurs.

• Instruct patient that dose may be taken every 30 minutes for acute diarrhea, but not to exceed maximum daily dosage.
• Tell patient that if abdominal discomfort or fullness occurs, smaller doses may be taken more frequently throughout the day, at regular intervals.

calcium salts

calcium acetate
Calphron, Phos-Lo

calcium carbonate
Calciday-667, Cal-Plus, Caltrate 600, Chooz, Os-Cal 500, Rolaids, Titralac, Tums, Tums E-X

calcium chloride

calcium citrate
Citracal

calcium glubionate
Neo-Calglucon

calcium gluceptate

calcium gluconate

calcium lactate

calcium phosphate, tribasic
Posture

Pharmacologic classification: calcium supplement
Therapeutic classification: therapeutic agent for electrolyte balance, cardiotonic
Pregnancy risk category: C

Indications and dosages
➤ *Emergency treatment of hypocalcemia.*
calcium chloride. *Adults:* 500 mg to 1 g I.V. slowly (not to exceed 1 ml/minute).
Children: 0.2 ml/kg I.V. slowly (not to exceed 1 ml/minute).
calcium gluconate
Adults: 7 to 14 mEq I.V. slowly (not to exceed 0.7 to 1.8 mEq/minute).
Children: 1 to 7 mEq I.V. slowly (not to exceed 0.7 to 1.8 mEq/minute).
Repeat above dosage based on laboratory value.
➤ *Cardiotonic use.* **calcium chloride.**
Adults: 500 mg to 1 g I.V. slowly (not to exceed 1 ml/minute); or 200 to 800 mg intraventricularly as a single dose.
➤ *Hyperkalemia.* **calcium gluconate.** *Adults:* 2.25 to 14 mEq I.V. slowly. Adjust administration based on ECG response.

➤ *Hypermagnesemia.* **calcium chloride.**
Adults: 500 mg I.V. initially, repeated based on clinical response.
calcium gluceptate
Adults: 2 to 5 ml I.M., or 5 to 20 ml I.V.
calcium gluconate
Adults: 4.5 to 9 mEq I.V. slowly.
➤ *During exchange transfusions. Adults:*
1.35 mEq I.V. with each 100-ml citrated blood exchange.
Neonates: 0.45 mEq I.V. after every 100 ml of citrated blood exchange.
➤ *Hypocalcemia.* **calcium acetate.** *Adults:*
2 to 4 tablets P.O. with meals.
calcium gluconate
Adults: For hypocalcemic tetany, 4.5 to 16 mEq I.V. until therapeutic response is obtained.
Children: For hypocalcemic tetany, 0.5 to 0.7 mEq/kg I.V. t.i.d. or q.i.d. or until tetany is controlled.
Neonates: 2.4 mEq/kg daily in divided doses until therapeutic response is obtained.
calcium lactate
Adults: 325 mg to 1.3 g P.O. t.i.d. with meals.
➤ *Osteoporosis prevention. Adults:* 1 to 1.5 g P.O. daily of elemental calcium.
➤ *Hyperphosphatemia in end-stage renal failure.* **calcium acetate.** *Adults:* 2 to 4 tablets P.O. with each meal.

How supplied
Available by prescription only
calcium chloride
Injection: 10% solution (1 g/10 ml; each ml of solution provides 27.2 mg or 1.36 mEq of calcium) in 10-ml ampules, vials, and syringes
calcium gluceptate
Injection: 1.1 g/5 ml ampules or 5-ml vials for preparation of I.V. admixtures (each ml of solution provides 18 mg or 0.9 mEq of calcium)
calcium gluconate
Injection: 10% solution (1 g/10 ml; each ml of solution provides 9.3 mg or 0.46 mEq of calcium) in 10-ml ampules and vials, or 20-ml vials
Available without a prescription
calcium acetate
Tablets: 668 mg (169 mg of calcium)
calcium carbonate
Capsules: 125 mg (50 mg of calcium), 1.25 g (500 mg of calcium)
Oral suspension: 1.25 g (500 mg of calcium) per 5 ml
Powder: 6.5 g
Tablets: 250 mg, 650 mg, 667 mg, 1.25 g, 1.5 g
Tablets (chewable): 750 mg, 1.25 g
calcium citrate
Tablets: 950 mg (contains 200 mg of elemental calcium/g)
Tablets (effervescent): 2,376 mg (500 mg of calcium)
calcium glubionate
Syrup: 1.8 g/5 ml (contains 115 mg of elemental calcium/g)

calcium gluconate
Tablets: 500 mg, 650 mg, 975 mg, 1 g (contains 90 mg of elemental calcium/g)
calcium lactate
Tablets: 325 mg, 650 mg (contains 130 mg of elemental calcium/g)
calcium phosphate, tribasic
Tablets: 600 mg elemental calcium

Pharmacodynamics
Calcium replacement: Calcium is essential for maintaining the functional integrity of the nervous, muscular, and skeletal systems and for cell membrane and capillary permeability. Calcium salts are used as a source of calcium cation to treat or prevent calcium depletion in patients in whom dietary measures are inadequate. Conditions linked to hypocalcemia are chronic diarrhea, vitamin D deficiency, steatorrhea, sprue, pregnancy and lactation, menopause, pancreatitis, renal failure, alkalosis, hyperphosphatemia, and hypoparathyroidism.

Pharmacokinetics
Absorption: I.M. and I.V. calcium salts are absorbed directly into the bloodstream. Oral dose is absorbed actively in the duodenum and proximal jejunum and, to a lesser extent, in the distal part of the small intestine. Calcium is absorbed only in the ionized form. Pregnancy and reduction of calcium intake may increase the efficiency of absorption. Vitamin D in its active form is required for calcium absorption.
Distribution: Enters the extracellular fluid and is incorporated rapidly into skeletal tissue. Bone contains 99% of the total calcium; 1% is distributed equally between the intracellular and extracellular fluids. CSF levels are about 50% of serum calcium levels.
Metabolism: None significant.
Excretion: Excreted mainly in the feces as unabsorbed calcium that was secreted through bile and pancreatic juice into the lumen of the GI tract. Most calcium entering the kidneys is reabsorbed in the loop of Henle and the proximal and distal convoluted tubules. Only small amounts of calcium are excreted in the urine.

Route	Onset	Peak	Duration
P.O.	Unknown	Unknown	Unknown
I.V.	Immediate	Immediate	½-2 hr

Contraindications and precautions
Contraindicated in patients with ventricular fibrillation, hypercalcemia, hypophosphatemia, or renal calculi. Use cautiously in digitalized patients and patients with sarcoidosis, renal or cardiac disease, cor pulmonale, respiratory acidosis, or respiratory failure.

Interactions
Drug-drug. *Atenolol, fluoroquinolones, tetracyclines:* Decreased bioavailability of these agents

and calcium when oral preparations are taken together. Separate administration times.

Calcium channel blockers (verapamil): Decreased calcium effectiveness. Avoid use together.

Cardiac glycosides: Increased digitalis toxicity. Administer calcium cautiously, if at all, to digitalized patients.

Phenytoin: Decreased absorption of both drugs. Avoid use together. Monitor levels closely if use together is required.

Sodium polystyrene sulfonate: Risk of metabolic acidosis in patients with renal disease. Avoid use together.

Thiazide diuretics: Risk of hypercalcemia. Avoid use together.

Drug-food. *Caffeine:* May affect calcium absorption. Advise patient to avoid caffeine-containing beverages.

Foods containing oxalic acid (rhubarb, spinach), phytic acid (bran, whole cereals), and phosphorus (milk, dairy products): May interfere with calcium absorption. Discourage use together.

Drug-lifestyle. *Alcohol use, tobacco use:* May affect calcium absorption. Discourage use together.

Adverse reactions

CNS: tingling sensations, sense of oppression or heat waves, headache, irritability, weakness (with I.V. use); syncope (with rapid I.V. injection).

CV: mild decrease in blood pressure; vasodilation, *bradycardia, arrhythmias, cardiac arrest* (with rapid I.V. injection).

GI: irritation, hemorrhage, *constipation* with oral use; chalky taste, rebound hyperacidity, nausea with I.V. use; hemorrhage, *nausea,* vomiting, thirst, abdominal pain with oral calcium chloride.

GU: hypercalcemia, polyuria, renal calculi.

Skin: local reactions, including burning, necrosis, tissue sloughing, cellulitis, soft tissue calcification (with I.M. use).

Other: pain and irritation with S.C. injection, *vein irritation* with I.V. use.

Overdose and treatment

Acute hypercalcemia syndrome is characterized by a markedly elevated plasma calcium level, lethargy, weakness, nausea and vomiting, and coma, and may lead to sudden death.

   In overdose, discontinue calcium immediately. After oral ingestion of calcium overdose, treatment includes removal by emesis or gastric lavage followed by supportive therapy, as needed.

Special considerations

• Give calcium chloride I.V. only.

• I.V. route is recommended in children, but not by scalp vein because calcium salts can cause tissue necrosis.

• Administer I.V. calcium slowly through a small-bore needle into a large vein to avoid extravasation and necrosis.

• Severe necrosis and tissue sloughing may occur after extravasation. Calcium gluconate is less irritating to veins and tissue than calcium chloride.

• After I.V. injection, patient should be recumbent for 15 minutes to prevent orthostasis.

• If perivascular infiltration occurs, discontinue I.V. immediately. Venospasm may be reduced by administering 1% procaine hydrochloride and hyaluronidase to the affected area.

• Use I.M. route only in emergencies when no I.V. route is available. Give I.M. injections in the gluteal region in adults, lateral thigh in infants.

• Hypercalcemia may result when large doses are given to patients with chronic renal failure.

• With oral product, patient may need laxatives or stool softeners to manage constipation.

• If GI upset occurs with oral calcium, give 2 to 3 hours after meals.

• I.V. calcium may produce transient elevation of plasma 11-hydroxycorticosteroid levels (Glen-Nelson technique) and false-negative values for serum and urine magnesium as measured by the Titan yellow method.

Patient monitoring

• Monitor ECG when giving calcium I.V. Give such injections slowly at a rate dependent on salt form used. Stop injection if patient complains of discomfort.

• Monitor serum calcium levels frequently, especially in patients with renal impairment.

• Assess Chvostek's and Trousseau's signs periodically to check for tetany.

• Monitor patient for symptoms of hypercalcemia (nausea, vomiting, headache, mental confusion, anorexia), and report them immediately. Calcium absorption of an oral dose is decreased in patients with certain disease states such as achlorhydria, renal osteodystrophy, steatorrhea, or uremia.

Breast-feeding patients

• Calcium passes into breast milk, but not in quantities large enough to affect the breast-feeding infant.

Pediatric patients

• Administer calcium cautiously to children by I.V. route (usually not administered I.M.).

Geriatric patients

• Calcium absorption (after oral administration) may be decreased in geriatric patients.

Patient education

• Tell patient not to exceed the manufacturer's recommended dosage of calcium.

• Warn patient not to use bone meal or dolomite as a source of calcium; they may contain lead.

• Advise patient to avoid tobacco and to limit intake of alcohol and caffeine-containing beverages.

---

candesartan cilexetil
Atacand

Pharmacologic classification: selective angiotensin II receptor antagonist
Therapeutic classification: antihypertensive
Pregnancy risk category: C (D in second and third trimesters)

Indications and dosages
➤ *Treatment of hypertension (alone or with other antihypertensives).* *Adults:* Initially, 16 mg P.O. once daily when used alone; usual dosage range is 8 to 32 mg P.O. daily as a single dose or divided b.i.d.

How supplied
Available by prescription only
Tablets: 4 mg, 8 mg, 16 mg, 32 mg

Pharmacodynamics
Antihypertensive action: Inhibits the vasoconstrictor and aldosterone-secreting effects of angiotensin II by selectively blocking the binding of angiotensin II to the AT_1 receptor in many tissues, such as vascular smooth muscle and the adrenal gland.

Pharmacokinetics
Absorption: Rapidly and completely bioactivated during absorption from the GI tract.
Distribution: Highly bound to plasma proteins (more than 99%).
Metabolism: Undergoes minor hepatic metabolism.
Excretion: Primarily recovered in the urine and feces. Elimination half life is about 9 hours.

Route	Onset	Peak	Duration
P.O.	Unknown	3-4 hr	24 hr

Contraindications and precautions
Contraindicated in patients hypersensitive to drug or its ingredients. Use cautiously in patients whose renal function depends on the renin-angiotensin-aldosterone system (such as patients with heart failure) because there's potential for oliguria and progressive azotemia with acute renal failure or death. Also use cautiously in patients who are volume- or salt-depleted because there's potential for symptomatic hypotension.

Interactions
None reported.

Adverse reactions
CNS: dizziness, fatigue, headache.
CV: chest pain, peripheral edema.
EENT: pharyngitis, rhinitis, sinusitis.
GI: abdominal pain, diarrhea, nausea, vomiting.
GU: albuminuria.
Musculoskeletal: arthralgia, back pain.

Respiratory: cough, bronchitis, upper respiratory tract infection.

Overdose and treatment
The most likely effects of overdose are hypotension, dizziness, and tachycardia; bradycardia could occur from parasympathetic (vagal) stimulation. Treatment should be supportive. Dialysis isn't effective.

Special considerations
● Drugs that act directly on the renin-angiotensin system (such as candesartan) can cause fetal and neonatal morbidity and death when administered to pregnant women. These problems haven't been detected when exposure was limited to first trimester. If pregnancy is suspected, discontinue drug immediately.
● In patients who are volume- or salt-depleted, start therapy with a lower dosage range, as ordered, and monitor blood pressure carefully.
● Most of the antihypertensive effect is present within 2 weeks. Maximal antihypertensive effect is obtained within 4 to 6 weeks. Diuretic may be added if blood pressure isn't controlled by drug alone.

Patient monitoring
● Monitor blood pressure. If hypotension occurs after a dose of candesartan, place patient in the supine position and, if necessary, give an I.V. infusion of normal saline solution.

Pregnant patients
● Inform woman of childbearing age of the consequences of second and third trimester exposure to drug. Advise her to notify prescriber immediately if pregnancy is suspected.

Breast-feeding patients
● It isn't known if drug appears in breast milk; therefore, breast-feeding during drug therapy isn't recommended.

Pediatric patients
● Safety and efficacy in children haven't been established.

Geriatric patients
● Serum levels of drug are higher in elderly persons than in younger adults; however, the drug and its inactive metabolite don't accumulate in the serum of elderly patients after repeated once-daily dosing.

Patient education
● Instruct patient to store medication at room temperature and to keep container tightly sealed.
● Inform patient to report adverse reactions promptly.
● Tell patient that drug may be taken without regard to meals.

candesartan cilexetil/ hydrochlorothiazide
Atacand HCT

Pharmacologic classification: angiotensin II (type 1) receptor antagonist/diuretic
Therapeutic classification: antihypertensive
Pregnancy risk category: C (first trimester), D (second and third trimesters)

Indications and dosages
➤ **Hypertension.** *Adults:* 16 mg candesartan and 12.5 mg hydrochlorothiazide, or 32 mg candesartan and 12.5 mg hydrochlorothiazide P.O. daily adjusted to effect.

How supplied
Tablets: 16 mg candesartan and 12.5 mg hydrochlorothiazide, or 32 mg candesartan and 12.5 mg hydrochlorothiazide

Pharmacodynamics
Antihypertensive action: Candesartan inhibits the vasoconstrictive action of angiotensin II by blocking the angiotensin II receptor on the surface of vascular smooth muscle and other tissue cells. Hydrochlorothiazide is a thiazide diuretic that acts by interfering with the reabsorption of sodium ions from renal tubules. As a result, the excretion of sodium, chloride, and water is enhanced.

Pharmacokinetics
Absorption: After oral administration, the bioavailability of candesartan is about 15%. The bioavailability of hydrochlorothiazide is between 65% and 75%. Candesartan levels peak 3 to 4 hours after oral administration, and hydrochlorothiazide peaks at 4 to 6 hours. The duration of action for candesartan is at least 24 hours; for hydrochlorothiazide, 6 to 12 hours.
Distribution: Candesartan is highly protein bound. Hydrochlorothiazide crosses the placenta and appears in breast milk.
Metabolism: Candesartan undergoes minor hepatic metabolism to an inactive metabolite. Hydrochlorothiazide isn't metabolized.
Excretion: About 30% of the candesartan dose is recovered in urine and 67% is recovered in feces via biliary excretion. Hydrochlorothiazide is eliminated by the kidneys. More than 60% of an oral dose of hydrochlorothiazide is eliminated via the kidneys. The half-life of candesartan is 9 hours. The half-life of hydrochlorothiazide ranges from 5 to 15 hours.

Route	Onset	Peak	Duration
P.O.			
candesartan	2-4 hr	3-4 hr	At least 24 hours
hydrochlorothiazide	2 hr	4 hr	6-12 hr

Contraindications and precautions
Drug is contraindicated in patients who are allergic to any of its components, in patients hypersensitive to sulfonamide-type drugs, and in patients with anuria.

Use cautiously in patients with impaired hepatic function, progressive liver disease, or severe renal disease. Use cautiously in patients with a history of allergy or bronchial asthma because hypersensitivity reactions are more common in these patients. Also use cautiously in patients with systemic lupus erythematosus because drug may worsen disease.

Interactions
hydrochlorothiazide
Drug-drug. *ACTH, corticosteroids:* May cause electrolyte abnormalities, including hypokalemia. Monitor patient closely.
Antidiabetics (insulin and oral drugs): Hydrochlorothiazide increases fasting blood glucose. Dose of the antidiabetic agent may need to be adjusted.
Antihypertensives: Potentiation of hypotensive effect. Monitor blood pressure.
Barbiturates, narcotics: Orthostatic hypotension may be potentiated. Monitor blood pressure.
Bile acid sequestrants (cholestyramine and colestipol resins): Reduced absorption of hydrochlorothiazide. Give thiazides at least 2 hours before resins.
candesartan cilexitil/hydrochlorothiazide
Drug-drug. *Lithium:* Thiazide diuretics decrease the excretion of lithium and increase the risk for lithium toxicity. Avoid use if possible.
Nondepolarizing muscle relaxants (tubocurarine): Neuromuscular blocking effects may be increased. Use cautiously.
NSAIDs: May decrease diuretic response of thiazides in some patients. Monitor patient for effectiveness.
Vasopressors (norepinephrine): Possible decreased pressor response. Dose may need to be adjusted.
Drug-lifestyle: *Alcohol use:* May potentiate orthostatic hypotension. Discourage concomitant use.

Adverse reactions
CNS: dizziness, headache.
Musculoskeletal: back pain.
Respiratory: upper respiratory tract infection.
Other: flulike symptoms.

Overdose and treatment
Overdose may cause hypotension, dizziness, tachycardia, bradycardia, hypokalemia, hypochloremia, and hyponatremia.

Hemodialysis won't remove candesartan, and the extent to which it removes hydrochlorothiazide is unknown. Therefore, supportive care measures should be utilized. Maintain the patient's airway, replace fluids intravenously, restore electrolytes, and use pressor agents, if need-

---

Reactions may be *common,* uncommon, *life-threatening,* or COMMON AND LIFE-THREATENING.

ed. Contact poison control center for up-to-date information on overdose.

Special considerations

• Drug isn't indicated for initial therapy of hypertension. The combination product should be used only after monotherapy has failed.

• Because symptomatic hypotension may occur in patients with intravascular volume depletion or sodium depletion, these conditions should be corrected before treatment, or treatment should start under close supervision.

• Patients at increased risk for hypokalemia include those with severe cirrhosis, those who have undergone brisk diuresis, and those on prolonged therapy.

• Dilutional hyponatremia may occur in edematous patients, especially in hot weather.

• Diabetic patients may need insulin or oral antidiabetics readjusted.

Patient monitoring

• Observe patient for signs and symptoms of fluid and electrolyte imbalance, such as a dry mouth, thirst, weakness, lethargy, drowsiness, restlessness, confusion, seizures, muscle pains or cramps, muscle fatigue, hypotension, oliguria, tachycardia, nausea, and vomiting.

• Periodically monitor electrolytes during therapy to check for imbalances, such as hypokalemia, hyponatremia, hypomagnesemia, and hyperchloremia

• Monitor patient for hyperuricemia and gout.

• Monitor patient's renal function. If progressive renal impairment occurs, consider withholding or discontinuing therapy.

Pregnant patients

• Intrauterine exposure to angiotensin II receptor antagonists during the second and third trimester has been linked to fetal and neonatal injury and death. Drug shouldn't be started in pregnant patients or patients considering pregnancy. If a patient becomes pregnant while receiving drug, drug should be discontinued as soon as possible.

Breast-feeding

• It isn't known whether candesartan appears in breast milk. Thiazide diuretics appear in breast milk.

Pediatric use

• Drug hasn't been studied in children.

Geriatric use

• Candesartan may have higher plasma levels in patients over age 65 than in younger patients. However, no initial dosage adjustment is needed in elderly patients.

Patient education

• Caution patient that light-headedness can occur, especially during the first few days of therapy.

• Advise patient to report light-headedness or syncope.

• Tell patient that inadequate fluid intake, excessive perspiration, diarrhea, or vomiting can lead to an excessive drop in blood pressure.

• Instruct patient to consult prescriber before taking potassium supplements, salt substitutes, or other OTC medications containing potassium.

• Advise woman of childbearing age to report pregnancy as soon as possible. Fetal abnormalities or death may occur if drug is taken during the second and third trimesters.

• Inform diabetic patients that blood glucose readings may become higher or lower than normal, and the dosage of diabetes medications may need adjustment.

capecitabine
Xeloda

Pharmacologic classification: fluoropyrimidine carbamate
Therapeutic classification: antineoplastic
Pregnancy risk category: D

Indications and dosages

➤ *Treatment of patients with metastatic breast cancer resistant to both paclitaxel and an anthracycline-containing chemotherapy regimen or resistant to paclitaxel and for whom further anthracycline therapy isn't indicated. Adults:* 2,500 mg/m² P.O. daily in two divided doses (about 12 hours apart) at end of a meal for 2 weeks, followed by a 1-week rest period and given as 3-week cycles.

✦ *Dosage adjustment.* Starting dose for patients with moderate renal impairment should be reduced to 75% of the recommended starting dose. Dosage also may need adjustment based on National Cancer Institute of Canada (NCIC) Common Toxicity Criteria:

NCIC grade 2: First appearance, interrupt treatment until resolved to grade 0 to 1, then restart at 100% of starting dose for next cycle; second appearance, interrupt treatment until resolved to grade 0 to 1 and use 75% of starting dose for next cycle; third appearance, interrupt treatment until resolved to grade 0 to 1 and use 50% of starting dose for next cycle; fourth appearance, discontinue treatment permanently.

NCIC grade 3: First appearance, interrupt treatment until resolved to grade 0 to 1 and use 75% of starting dose for next cycle; second appearance, interrupt treatment until resolved to grade 0 to 1 and use 50% of starting dose for next cycle; third appearance, discontinue treatment permanently.

NCIC grade 4: First appearance, discontinue treatment permanently or interrupt treatment until resolved to grade 0 to 1 and use 50% of starting dose for next cycle.

Toxicity criteria relate to degrees of severity of diarrhea, nausea, vomiting, stomatitis, and hand-and-foot syndrome. Refer to capecitabine package insert for specific toxicity definitions.

How supplied
Available by prescription only
Tablets: 150 mg, 500 mg

Pharmacodynamics
Antineoplastic action: Capecitabine is converted to the active drug 5-fluorouracil (5-FU). 5-FU is metabolized by both normal and tumor cells to metabolites that cause cellular injury by way of two different mechanisms: interference with DNA synthesis to inhibit cell division and interference with RNA processing and protein synthesis.

Pharmacokinetics
Absorption: Readily absorbed from the GI tract. The rate and extent of absorption are decreased with food.
Distribution: About 60% is bound to plasma proteins.
Metabolism: Extensively metabolized to 5-FU (an active metabolite).
Excretion: Elimination half-life of the parent drug and the active moiety is about 45 minutes with 70% excreted in the urine.

Route	Onset	Peak	Duration
P.O.	Unknown	1½-2 hr	Unknown

Contraindications and precautions
Contraindicated in patients hypersensitive to 5-FU. Severe diarrhea can occur; monitor electrolytes and ensure proper hydration. Also contraindicated in patients with severe renal impairment. Use cautiously in elderly patients and in patients with a history of coronary artery disease, mild-to-moderate hepatic dysfunction resulting from liver metastases, hyperbilirubinemia, and renal insufficiency.

Interactions
Drug-drug. *Antacids:* Increased rate of capecitabine absorption. Dosage change may be necessary.
Coumadin: Altered PT and bleeding. Monitor patient closely.
Leucovorin: Increased 5-FU level with enhanced toxicity. Patient needs close monitoring.

Adverse reactions
CNS: dizziness, *fatigue*, headache, insomnia, *paresthesia*.
CV: edema.
EENT: eye irritation.
GI: *diarrhea, nausea, vomiting, stomatitis, abdominal pain, constipation, anorexia*, intestinal obstruction, *dyspepsia*.

Hematologic: NEUTROPENIA, THROMBOCYTOPENIA, *anemia, lymphopenia*.
Hepatic: *hyperbilirubinemia*.
Musculoskeletal: myalgia, limb pain.
Skin: *hand-and-foot syndrome, dermatitis*, nail disorder.
Other: *pyrexia*, dehydration.

Overdose and treatment
Overdose should be managed by supportive care aimed at correcting the signs and symptoms. Dialysis may help in drug removal.

Special considerations
● Capecitabine therapy may need to be interrupted or decreased if hand-and-foot syndrome occurs (characterized by numbness, paresthesia, tingling, painless or painful swelling, erythema, desquamation, blistering, and severe pain of hands or feet, hyperbilirubinemia, and severe nausea).
● Altered coagulation parameters and bleeding may occur within several days up to several months after starting therapy and, rarely, within one month after stopping capecitabine therapy.
● Tablets should be taken within 30 minutes after a meal.
● Inform prescriber if patient is taking folic acid or warfarin.
● Store tablets at room temperature. Keep container tightly closed.

Patient monitoring
● Monitor liver function tests during therapy. Hyperbilirubinemia may require discontinuation of drug.
● Monitor patient for diarrhea. Drug may need to be immediately interrupted until diarrhea resolves or decreases in intensity. Fluid and electrolyte replacement may be needed for severe diarrhea.
● Monitor patient carefully for toxicity. Toxicity may be managed by symptomatic treatment, dose interruptions, and dosage adjustments.

Pregnant patients
● Because of teratogenic effects, women of childbearing age should avoid becoming pregnant while taking capecitabine.

Breast-feeding patients
● Patients should discontinue breast-feeding while on drug therapy.

Pediatric patients
● Safety and efficacy in patients under 18 years of age haven't been established.

Geriatric patients
● Patients over age 80 may experience greater GI adverse effects.

Patient education
● Inform patient and caregiver of expected adverse effects of drug, especially nausea, vomit-

---

Reactions may be *common*, uncommon, *life-threatening*, or COMMON AND LIFE-THREATENING.

ing, diarrhea, and hand-and-foot syndrome (pain, swelling or redness of hands or feet). Tell them that patient-specific dose adaptations during therapy are expected and necessary.

• Instruct patient to stop taking drug and contact prescriber immediately if the following adverse effects occur: diarrhea (more than four bowel movements daily or diarrhea at night), vomiting (two to five episodes in a 24-hour period), nausea, appetite loss or decrease in amount of food taken each day, stomatitis (pain, redness, swelling, or sores in mouth), hand-and-foot syndrome, temperature of 100.5° F (38° C) or greater, or other evidence of infection.

• Tell patient that most adverse effects improve within 2 to 3 days after stopping drug. If they don't improve, tell him to contact prescriber.

• Tell patient how to take the drug. Drug is usually taken for 14 days followed by a 7-day rest period (no drug) given as a 21-day cycle. The prescriber determines the number of treatment cycles.

• Instruct patient to take drug with water within 30 minutes after breakfast and dinner.

• If a combination of tablets is prescribed, teach patient importance of correctly identifying the tablets to avoid possible misdosing.

• For missed doses, instruct patient not to take the missed dose and not to double the next one. Instead, he should continue with regular dosing schedule and check with the prescriber.

• Tell patient to inform prescriber if he's taking the vitamin folic acid.

• Advise women of childbearing age to avoid becoming pregnant while receiving treatment.

capsaicin
Dolorac, Zostrix, Zostrix-HP

Pharmacologic classification: naturally occurring chemical derived from plants of the Solanaceae family
Therapeutic classification: topical analgesic
Pregnancy risk category: NR

Indications and dosages
➤ *Temporary pain relief from rheumatoid arthritis, osteoarthritis, and certain neuralgias, such as pain caused by shingles (herpes zoster) or diabetic neuropathy. Zostrix. Adults and children over age 2:* Apply to affected areas t.i.d. or q.i.d.
Dolorac
Adults and children over age 12: Apply thin film to affected areas b.i.d.

How supplied
Available without a prescription
Cream: 0.025% (Zostrix), 0.075% (Zostrix-HP), 0.25% (Dolorac)

Pharmacodynamics
Analgesic action: Exact mechanism unknown. Current evidence suggests that drug renders skin and joints insensitive to pain by depleting and preventing reaccumulation of substance P in peripheral sensory neurons. Substance P is thought to be the principal chemomediator of pain impulses from the periphery to the CNS. In addition, substance P is released into joint tissues and activates inflammatory mediators involved with the pathogenesis of rheumatoid arthritis.

Pharmacokinetics
No information available.

Route	Onset	Peak	Duration
Topical	Unknown	Unknown	Unknown

Contraindications and precautions
Contraindicated in patients hypersensitive to drug.

Interactions
None reported.

Adverse reactions
Respiratory: cough, irritation.
Skin: redness, *stinging or burning on application.*

Special considerations
• Transient burning or stinging with application is usually evident at start of therapy but will disappear in several days.
• Application schedules of less than t.i.d. or q.i.d. may not provide optimum pain relief, and the burning sensation may persist.
• Capsaicin is for external use only. Avoid contact with eyes and broken or irritated skin.

Patient monitoring
• Monitor patient for response to drug therapy.
• Monitor patient for signs of hypersensitivity.

Breast-feeding patients
• Safety and efficacy haven't been established. Use during breast-feeding isn't recommended.

Patient education
• Instruct patient how to apply cream, stressing importance of avoiding eyes and broken or irritated skin.
• Instruct patient to wash hands after applying cream, avoiding areas where drug was applied.
• Warn patient that transient burning or stinging with application may occur but will disappear with continued use after several days.
• Tell patient not to bandage areas tightly.
• Advise patient to stop drug and to call if condition worsens or doesn't improve after 28 days.

captopril
Capoten

Pharmacologic classification: ACE inhibitor
Therapeutic classification: antihypertensive,
adjunctive treatment of heart failure
Pregnancy risk category: C (D second and
third trimesters)

Indications and dosages
➤*Mild to severe hypertension; Idiopathic edema◇; Raynaud's phenome-
non◇.* *Adults:* Initially, 25 mg P.O. b.i.d. or
t.i.d.; if necessary, dosage may be increased to
50 mg b.i.d. or t.i.d. after 1 to 2 weeks. If control is still inadequate after 1 to 2 weeks more,
a diuretic may be added. Dosage may be increased to a maximum of 150 mg t.i.d. (450 mg
daily) while continuing the diuretic. Daily dose
may be given b.i.d.
➤*Heart failure.* *Adults:* 25 mg P.O. t.i.d. If
patient takes a diuretic or is hyponatremic or
hypovolemic, give an initial dose of 6.25 to
12.5 mg t.i.d. Maintenance dosage is 50 to
100 mg t.i.d.
➤*Prevention of diabetic nephropathy.*
Adults: 25 mg P.O. t.i.d.
➤*Left ventricular dysfunction after MI.*
Adults: 6.25 mg P.O. as a single dose 3 days after an MI; then 12.5 mg t.i.d., increasing dose to
25 mg t.i.d. Target dose is 50 mg t.i.d.
✦ *Dosage adjustment.* In elderly patients and
those with renal failure, use lower initial daily
doses and smaller increments for adjustment.
Adjust at 1- to 2-week intervals.

How supplied
Available by prescription only
Tablets: 12.5 mg, 25 mg, 50 mg, 100 mg

Pharmacodynamics
Antihypertensive action: Captopril inhibits
ACE, preventing conversion of angiotensin I to
angiotensin II, a potent vasoconstrictor. Reduced
formation of angiotensin II decreases peripheral arterial resistance, which results in decreased
aldosterone secretion, thus reducing sodium and
water retention and lowering blood pressure.
Cardiac load–reducing action: Captopril decreases systemic vascular resistance (afterload)
and pulmonary capillary wedge pressure (preload), thus increasing cardiac output in patients
with heart failure.

Pharmacokinetics
Absorption: 60% to 75% of an oral dose is absorbed through the GI tract; food may reduce absorption by up to 40%. Antihypertensive effect
begins in 15 minutes. Maximum therapeutic effect may take several weeks.
Distribution: Distributed into most body tissues
except CNS; drug is about 25% to 30% protein-
bound.

Metabolism: About 50% is metabolized in the
liver.
Excretion: Excreted primarily in urine; small
amounts are excreted in feces. Duration of effect
is usually 2 to 6 hours, increasing with higher
doses. Elimination half-life is less than 3 hours.
Duration of action may be increased in patients
with renal dysfunction.

Route	Onset	Peak	Duration
P.O.	½-1 hr	1-1½ hr	6-12 hr

Contraindications and precautions
Contraindicated in patients hypersensitive to drug
or other ACE inhibitors. Use cautiously in patients
with impaired renal function, renal artery stenosis, or serious autoimmune diseases (especially
lupus erythematosus) and in those taking drugs
that affect WBC counts or immune response.

Interactions
Drug-drug. *Antacids:* Decreased effects of captopril. Separate administration times.
Digoxin: May increase serum digoxin level by
15% to 30%. Patient needs close monitoring.
Diuretics, other antihypertensives: Risk of excessive hypotension. Diuretics may need to be
discontinued or captopril dosage lowered.
Insulin, oral antidiabetics: Risk of hypoglycemia
when captopril therapy starts. Monitor patient
closely.
Lithium: Increased lithium levels; toxicity may
occur. Monitor patient closely.
NSAIDs: May decrease antihypertensive effect of
captopril. Monitor patient closely.
*Potassium-sparing diuretics, potassium sup-
plements:* Increased risk of hyperkalemia. Avoid
these agents unless hypokalemic blood levels are
confirmed.
Drug-herb. *Black catechu:* May cause additional hypotensive effects. Discourage use together.
Capsaicin: Increased risk of cough. Discourage
use together.

Adverse reactions
CNS: dizziness, fainting, headache, malaise,
fatigue.
CV: tachycardia, hypotension, angina pectoris.
GI: anorexia, *dysgeusia,* nausea, vomiting, ab-
dominal pain, constipation, dry mouth.
Hematologic: *leukopenia, agranulocyto-
sis, pancytopenia,* anemia, *thrombocy-
topenia.*
Hepatic: transient increase in liver enzyme levels.
Metabolic: hyperkalemia.
Respiratory: *dry, persistent, tickling, non-
productive cough;* dyspnea.
Skin: *urticarial rash, maculopapular rash,* pru-
ritus, alopecia.
Other: fever, *angioedema of face and limbs.*

Reactions may be *common*, uncommon, *life-threatening*, or COMMON AND LIFE-THREATENING.

Overdose and treatment

Overdose may cause severe hypotension. After acute ingestion, stomach must be emptied by induced emesis or gastric lavage. Follow with activated charcoal to reduce absorption. Subsequent treatment is usually symptomatic and supportive. In severe cases, hemodialysis may be considered.

Special considerations

• Diuretic therapy is usually discontinued 2 to 3 days before starting ACE inhibitor therapy to reduce the risk of hypotension; if drug doesn't adequately control blood pressure, diuretics may be reinstated.
• Captopril may cause false-positive results for urinary acetone.
• Lower dosage or reduced dosing frequency is necessary in patients with impaired renal function. Adjust drug to effective levels over a 1- to 2-week interval, then reduce dosage to lowest effective level.
• Several weeks of therapy may be required before the beneficial effects of captopril are seen.
• Proteinuria and nephrotic syndrome may occur, especially in patients with renal disease or those treated with high doses of drug.

Patient monitoring
• Obtain WBC and differential counts before treatment, every 2 weeks for 3 months, and periodically thereafter; serum potassium levels must be checked because of potassium retention.

Pregnant patients
• Because ACE inhibitors can cause fetal harm or death, discontinue drug use as soon as pregnancy is detected.

Breast-feeding patients
• Captopril appears in breast milk, but its effect on breast-feeding infants is unknown; use drug with caution in breast-feeding women.

Pediatric patients
• Safety and efficacy in children haven't been established; use only if potential benefit outweighs risk.

Geriatric patients
• Elderly patients may need lower doses because of impaired drug clearance. They also may be more sensitive to the hypotensive effects of captopril.

Patient education
• Instruct patient to call prescriber immediately if she becomes pregnant.
• Tell patient to report light-headedness, especially in first few days, so dosage can be adjusted; signs of infection, such as sore throat or fever, because drug may decrease WBC count; facial swelling or difficulty breathing, because drug may

cause angioedema; and loss of taste, which may necessitate discontinuing drug.
• Instruct patient to take captopril 1 hour before meals to prevent decreased absorption.
• Advise patient to avoid sudden position changes to minimize orthostatic hypotension.
• Warn patient to seek medical approval before taking OTC cold preparations.
• Tell patient that a persistent, dry cough may occur and usually doesn't subside until medication is stopped. Call prescriber if this effect becomes bothersome.

carbachol
Carboptic, Isopto Carbachol, Miostat

Pharmacologic classification: cholinergic agonist
Therapeutic classification: miotic
Pregnancy risk category C

Indications and dosages
➤ *Ocular surgery (to produce pupillary miosis).* Adults: 0.5 ml of 0.01% (intraocular form) instilled gently into the anterior chamber for production of satisfactory miosis. May be instilled before or after securing sutures.
➤ *Open-angle or narrow-angle glaucoma.* Adults: 2 gtt of 0.75% to 3% solution up to t.i.d.

How supplied
Available by prescription only
Intraocular injection: 0.01%
Ophthalmic solution: 0.75%, 1.5%, 2.25%, 3%

Pharmacodynamics
Miotic action: Cholinergic activity causes contraction of the sphincter muscles of the iris, producing miosis, and contraction of the ciliary muscle, resulting in accommodation. Acts to deepen the anterior chamber and dilate conjunctival vessels of the outflow tract.

Pharmacokinetics
Absorption: Penetrates intact corneal epithelium very poorly.
Distribution: No information available.
Metabolism: No information available.
Excretion: No information available.

Route	Onset	Peak	Duration
Oph-thalmic	10-20 min	4 hr	8 hr
Intra-ocular	Unknown	2-5 min	24 hr

Contraindications and precautions
Contraindicated in patients hypersensitive to drug and in those in whom cholinergic effects, such as constriction, are undesirable (such as in those with acute iritis, some forms of secondary glaucoma, pupillary block glaucoma, or acute

◇ Unlabeled clinical use

inflammatory disease of the anterior ocular chamber).

Use cautiously in patients with acute heart failure, bronchial asthma, peptic ulcer, hyperthyroidism, GI spasm, Parkinson's disease, and urinary tract obstruction.

Interactions
Drug-drug. *Cyclopentolate, ophthalmic belladonna alkaloids (atropine, homatropine):* May interfere with antiglaucoma actions of carbachol. Use together cautiously.

Adverse reactions
CNS: headache, syncope.
CV: *arrhythmias,* hypotension, flushing.
EENT: spasm of eye accommodation, conjunctival vasodilation, eye and brow pain, transient stinging and burning, corneal clouding, bullous keratopathy.
GI: abdominal cramps, diarrhea, salivation.
GU: urinary urgency.
Respiratory: asthma.
Skin: diaphoresis.

Overdose and treatment
Signs and symptoms of overdose include miosis, flushing, vomiting, bradycardia, bronchospasm, increased bronchial secretion, sweating, tearing, involuntary urination, hypotension, and seizures.

With accidental oral ingestion, vomiting is usually spontaneous; if not, induce emesis and follow with activated charcoal or a cathartic. Treat dermal exposure by washing the area twice with water. Treat CV or blood pressure responses with epinephrine. Atropine has been suggested as a direct antagonist for toxicity.

Special considerations
• Drug is especially useful in glaucoma patients resistant or allergic to pilocarpine hydrochloride or nitrate.
• Premixed drugs should be used only for single-dose intraocular use.
• Discard unused portions of injectable drug.

Patient monitoring
• Obtain periodic tonometric readings.
• Monitor blood pressure and ECG as indicated.

Pregnant patients
• Safe use during pregnancy hasn't been established. Use during pregnancy only when the benefits justify possible risk to the fetus.

Breast feeding patients
• It isn't known whether carbachol appears in breast milk. Use cautiously in nursing women.

Pediatric patients
• Safety and efficacy haven't been established.

Patient education
• Tell patient with glaucoma that long-term use may be necessary. Stress compliance, and explain importance of medical supervision for tonometric readings before and during therapy.
• Instruct patient to apply finger pressure on the lacrimal sac for 1 to 2 minutes after topical instillation of drug.
• Reassure patient that blurred vision usually diminishes with continued use.
• Teach patient how to instill eyedrops correctly, and warn patient not to touch eye or surrounding area with dropper.
• Warn patient not to drive for 1 or 2 hours after administration until effect on vision is determined.

carbamazepine
Atretol, Carbatrol, Epitol, Tegretol, Tegretol-XR

Pharmacologic classification: iminostilbene derivative; chemically related to tricyclic antidepressants
Therapeutic classification: anticonvulsant, analgesic
Pregnancy risk category: D

Indications and dosages
➤ *Generalized tonic-clonic, complex-partial, mixed seizure patterns.* Adults and children over age 12: 200 mg P.O. b.i.d., or 100 mg P.O. q.i.d. of suspension, on day 1. May increase at weekly intervals by 200 mg P.O. daily, in divided doses at 6- to 8-hour intervals. Adjust to minimum effective level when control is achieved; don't exceed 1,000 mg daily in children ages 12 to 15, or 1,200 mg daily in those over age 15. In rare instances, doses up to 1,600 mg daily have been used in adults.

For extended-release capsules, initial dose is 200 mg P.O. b.i.d. Increase at weekly intervals by up to 200 mg daily until optimal response is obtained. Dose shouldn't exceed 1,000 mg daily in children ages 12 to 15 and 1,200 mg daily in patients over age 15. Some adult doses may be up to 1,600 mg daily. Maintenance dosage is usually 800 to 1,200 mg daily.
Children ages 6 to 12: Initially, 100 mg P.O. b.i.d., or 50 mg P.O. q.i.d. of suspension. Increase at weekly intervals by adding 100 mg P.O. daily, first using a t.i.d. schedule and then q.i.d. if necessary. Adjust dosage based on patient response. Generally, daily dose shouldn't exceed 1,000 mg. Children taking total daily dose of immediate-release form of 400 mg or more may be converted to same total daily dose of extended-release capsules using a b.i.d. regimen.
Children under age 6: Initially, 10 to 20 mg/kg daily P.O. b.i.d. or t.i.d. as tablets or q.i.d. as suspension. Increase weekly to achieve optimal clinical response administered t.i.d. or q.i.d. There's no recommendation for safe administration at

doses of more than 35 mg/kg daily. If optimal clinical response hasn't been achieved at a dose less than 35 mg/kg daily, check plasma levels to determine whether it's within the therapeutic range.

➤ *Oral loading dose for rapid seizure control. Adults and children age 12 and older:* 8 mg/kg P.O. of oral suspension.
Children younger than age 12: 10 mg/kg P.O. of oral suspension.

➤ *Bipolar affective disorder; intermittent explosive disorder* ◊. *Adults:* Initially, 200 mg P.O. b.i.d.; increase, p.r.n., q 3 to 4 days. Maintenance dosage may range from 600 to 1,600 mg daily.

➤ *Trigeminal neuralgia. Adults:* 100 mg P.O. b.i.d. or 50 mg P.O. q.i.d. of suspension with meals on day 1. Increase by 100 mg q 12 hours or 50 mg q.i.d. for suspension until pain is relieved. Don't exceed 1.2 g daily. Maintenance dosage is 200 to 1,200 mg P.O. daily. For extended-release capsules, 200 mg P.O. on day 1. Dosage may be increased by up to 200 mg daily q 12 hours, p.r.n., to achieve freedom from pain. Maintenance dosage is usually 400 to 800 mg daily.

➤ *Chorea* ◊. *Children:* 15 to 25 mg/kg P.O. daily.

➤ *Restless leg syndrome* ◊. *Adults:* 100 to 300 mg P.O. h.s.

How supplied

Available by prescription only
Capsules (extended-release): 200 mg, 300 mg
Oral suspension: 100 mg/5 ml
Tablets: 200 mg
Tablets (chewable): 100 mg
Tablets (extended-release): 100 mg, 200 mg, 400 mg

Pharmacodynamics

Anticonvulsant action: Carbamazepine is chemically unrelated to other anticonvulsants, and its mechanism of action is unknown. The anticonvulsant activity appears principally to involve limitations of seizure propagation by reduction of posttetanic potentiation of synaptic transmissions.
Analgesic action: In trigeminal neuralgia, carbamazepine is a specific analgesic through its reduction of synaptic neurotransmission.

Pharmacokinetics

Absorption: Absorbed slowly from the GI tract.
Distribution: Distributed widely throughout body; it crosses the placenta and accumulates in fetal tissue. About 75% is protein-bound. Therapeutic serum levels in adults are 4 to 12 mcg/ml; nystagmus may occur at serum levels of more than 4 mcg/ml, and ataxia, dizziness, and anorexia may occur at serum levels of 10 mcg/ml or more. Serum levels may be misleading because an unmeasured active metabolite also can cause toxicity. Carbamazepine levels in breast milk approach 60% of serum levels. There's poor cor-

relation between plasma levels and dose in children.
Metabolism: Metabolized by the liver to an active metabolite. It also may induce its own metabolism; over time, higher doses are needed to maintain plasma levels. Half-life is initially 25 to 65 hours and 12 to 17 hours with multiple dosing.
Excretion: Excreted in urine (70%) and feces (30%).

Route	Onset	Peak	Duration
P.O.	Unknown	1½-12 hr	Unknown

Contraindications and precautions

Contraindicated in patients hypersensitive to drug or tricyclic antidepressants, in those with history of previous bone marrow suppression, and in patients who have taken an MAO inhibitor within 14 days of therapy. Use cautiously in patients with mixed-type seizure disorders.

Interactions

Drug-drug. *Cimetidine, danazol, diltiazem, fluoxetine, fluvoxamine, isoniazid, macrolides (such as erythromycin), propoxyphene, valproic acid, verapamil:* May increase carbamazepine blood levels. Use cautiously.
Doxycycline, felbamate, haloperidol, oral contraceptives, phenytoin, theophylline, warfarin: May decrease blood levels of these drugs. Monitor patient for decreased effect.
Lithium: Increased CNS toxicity of lithium. Avoid use together.
MAO inhibitors: Increased depressant and anticholinergic effects. Don't use together.
Phenobarbital, phenytoin, primidone: May decrease carbamazepine levels. Monitor patient for decreased effect.
Drug-herb. *Plantain:* May decrease absorption, decreasing effect. Discourage use together.
Psyllium seed: May inhibit GI absorption. Discourage use together.

Adverse reactions

CNS: *dizziness, vertigo, drowsiness,* fatigue, *ataxia, worsening of seizures* (usually in patients with mixed-type seizure disorders, including atypical absence seizures), confusion, headache, syncope.
CV: *heart failure,* hypertension, hypotension, aggravation of coronary artery disease, *arrhythmias, AV block.*
EENT: conjunctivitis, dry mouth and pharynx, blurred vision, diplopia, nystagmus.
GI: *nausea, vomiting,* abdominal pain, diarrhea, anorexia, stomatitis, glossitis.
GU: urinary frequency, urine retention, impotence, albuminuria, glycosuria, elevated BUN.
Hematologic: *aplastic anemia, agranulocytosis,* eosinophilia, leukocytosis, *thrombocytopenia.*

Hepatic: abnormal liver function test results, *hepatitis.*
Metabolic: decreased values of thyroid function tests.
Respiratory: pulmonary hypersensitivity.
Skin: rash, urticaria, excessive diaphoresis, *erythema multiforme, Stevens-Johnson syndrome.*
Other: fever, chills, SIADH.

Overdose and treatment

Signs and symptoms of overdose may include irregular breathing, respiratory depression, tachycardia, blood pressure changes, shock, arrhythmias, impaired consciousness (ranging to deep coma), seizures, restlessness, drowsiness, psychomotor disturbances, nausea, vomiting, anuria, or oliguria.

Treat overdose with repeated gastric lavage, especially if patient ingested alcohol concurrently. Oral charcoal and laxatives may hasten excretion. Carefully monitor vital signs, ECG, and fluid and electrolyte balance. Diazepam may control seizures but can exacerbate respiratory depression.

Special considerations

● Adjust drug dosage based on individual response.
● Chewable tablets are available for children.
● Unlabeled uses of carbamazepine include hypophyseal diabetes insipidus, certain psychiatric disorders, and management of alcohol withdrawal.
● For administering through a nasogastric tube, mix with an equal volume of diluent (D_5W or normal saline solution) and administer; then flush with 100 ml of diluent.

Patient monitoring

● Hematologic toxicity is rare but serious. Hematologic and liver functions must be checked.
● Periodic eye examinations are recommended.

Breast-feeding patients

● Significant amounts of drug appear in breast milk; an alternative feeding method is recommended during therapy.

Pediatric patients

● Safety and efficacy haven't been established for children under age 6 in daily doses higher than 35 mg/kg.

Geriatric patients

● Drug may activate latent psychosis, confusion, or agitation in geriatric patients; use with caution.

Patient education

● Remind patient to store drug in a cool, dry place, and not in the medicine cabinet. Reduced bioavailability has been reported with use of improperly stored tablets.

● Tell patient that drug may cause GI distress. Patient should take drug with food at equally spaced intervals.
● Warn patient not to stop drug abruptly.
● Encourage patient to promptly report unusual bleeding, bruising, jaundice, dark urine, pale stools, abdominal pain, impotence, fever, chills, sore throat, mouth ulcers, edema, or disturbances in mood, alertness, or coordination.
● Warn patient that drug may cause drowsiness, dizziness, and blurred vision. Patient should avoid hazardous activities that require alertness, especially during first week of therapy and when dosage is increased.
● Remind patient to shake suspension well before using.
● Tell patient that the Carbatrol capsule can be opened and its contents sprinkled over food (such as a teaspoon of applesauce), but the capsule or its contents should never be crushed or chewed.
● Emphasize importance of follow-up laboratory tests and continued medical supervision.

carbamide peroxide
Auro Ear Drops, Debrox, Gly-Oxide Liquid, Murine Ear, Orajel, Orajel Perioseptic, Proxigel

Pharmacologic classification: urea hydrogen peroxide
Therapeutic classification: ceruminolytic, topical antiseptic
Pregnancy risk category: C

Indications and dosages

➤ *Impacted cerumen. Adults and children age 12 and older:* 5 to 10 drops otic solution into ear canal b.i.d. for 3 to 4 days.
➤ *Inflammation or irritation of lips, mouth, and gums. Adults and children over age 3:* Apply several drops of undiluted oral solution to affected area or place 10 drops on tongue (mix with saliva, swish for 1 to 3 minutes, and then expectorate) after meals and h.s.
Children: Apply undiluted gel to affected area (massage into area with finger or swab) q.i.d.

How supplied

Available without a prescription
Oral gel: 10% carbamide in water-free gel base
Oral solution: 10% carbamide with glycerin and propylene glycol; 15% with anhydrous glycerin, methylparaben, and propylene glycol
Otic solution: 6.5% carbamide in glycerin or glycerin and propylene glycol

Pharmacodynamics

Ceruminolytic action: Emulsifies and disperses accumulated cerumen.
Antiseptic action: Releases oxygen upon contact with oral mucosa, which results in a cleansing and mild anti-inflammatory action.

Reactions may be *common,* uncommon, *life-threatening,* or COMMON AND LIFE-THREATENING.

Pharmacokinetics
No information available.

Route	Onset	Peak	Duration
P.O.	Unknown	Unknown	Unknown
Otic	Unknown	Unknown	15-30 min

Contraindications and precautions
Contraindicated in patients with perforated eardrum.

Interactions
None reported.

Adverse reactions
GI: oral irritation or inflammation.

Overdose and treatment
Signs and symptoms of overdose include mild irritation to mucosal tissue or, if swallowed, irritation, inflammation, and burns in the mouth, throat, esophagus, or stomach. Gastric distention may result from liberation of oxygen. Accidental ocular exposure causes immediate pain and irritation, but severe injury is rare.

Irrigate eyes with large amounts of warm water for at least 15 minutes. Accidental dermal exposure bleaches the exposed area. Wash exposed skin twice with soap and water. Treat oral exposure by immediate dilution with water. Spontaneous vomiting may occur.

Special considerations
• Don't use drug to treat swimmer's ear or itching of the ear canal.
• Don't use drug if patient has a perforated eardrum.
• Irrigation of ear may be necessary to aid cerumen removal.
• Do not touch tip of dropper to ear or ear canal when using otic preparation.
• Remove cerumen remaining after instillation by using a soft rubber-bulb otic syringe to gently irrigate the ear canal with warm water.

Patient monitoring
• Patient should have regular checkup of mouth and throat by prescriber or dentist to check for signs of inflammation or irritation.

Pediatric patients
• Oral preparations shouldn't be used in children under age 2; otic forms shouldn't be used by children under age 12.

Patient education
• Teach patient correct way to use product.
• Tell patient to report inflammation or persistent irritation.
• Warn patient not to use otic form for more than 4 consecutive days and to avoid contact with eyes.
• Instruct patient to keep otic solution in ear for at least 15 minutes by tilting head sideways or putting cotton in ear.
• Tell patient not to rinse mouth or drink for 5 minutes after use of oral preparation.

---

carboplatin
Paraplatin

Pharmacologic classification: alkylating agent (not specific to phase of cell cycle)
Therapeutic classification: antineoplastic
Pregnancy risk category: D

Indications and dosages
►*Initial and secondary (palliative) treatment of ovarian carcinoma; retinoblastoma◇; advanced bladder cancer◇; lung cancer◇; head and neck cancer◇; Wilms' tumor◇; primary brain tumor◇; testicular neoplasm◇; cervical cancer◇.*
Adults: Initial recommended dose for single-agent therapy is 360 mg/m² I.V. on day 1. Dose is repeated q 4 weeks. In combination therapy (with cyclophosphamide), give 300 mg/m² I.V. on day 1 q 4 weeks for 6 cycles.
✦*Dosage adjustment.* Dosage adjustments are based on the lowest post-treatment platelet or neutrophil value obtained in weekly blood counts. In patients with impaired renal function, initial recommended dose is 250 mg/m² for creatinine clearance between 41 and 59 ml/minute; for creatinine clearance between 16 and 40 ml/minute, dose is 200 mg/m².

Lowest platelet count (per mm³)	Lowest neutrophil count (per mm³)	Adjusted dose
> 100,000	> 2,000	125%
50,000-100,000	500-2,000	No adjustment
< 50,000	< 500	75%

How supplied
Available by prescription only
Injection: 50-mg, 150-mg, 450-mg vials

Pharmacodynamics
Antitumor action: Carboplatin causes cross-linking of DNA strands.

Pharmacokinetics
Absorption: Administered I.V.
Distribution: Volume of distribution is about equal to total body water. Drug isn't protein-bound but degraded to platinum-containing products, which are 87% protein-bound at 24 hours.
Metabolism: Hydrolyzed to form hydroxylated and aquated species. Half-life of drug is 2 to 3 hours; terminal half-life for platinum is 4 to 6 days.

Excretion: 65% is excreted by the kidneys within 12 hours, 71% within 24 hours. Enterohepatic recirculation may occur.

Route	Onset	Peak	Duration
I.V.	Unknown	Unknown	Unknown

Contraindications and precautions
Contraindicated in patients with history of hypersensitivity to cisplatin, platinum-containing compounds, or mannitol or in patients with severe bone marrow suppression or bleeding.

Interactions
Drug-drug. *Aspirin:* Increased risk of bleeding. Avoid use together.
Bone marrow suppressants (including radiation therapy): Increased hematologic toxicity. Monitor patient closely.
Myelosuppressive drugs: Additive myelosuppression. Monitor patient.
Nephrotoxic drugs: Additive nephrotoxicity of carboplatin. Use cautiously.

Adverse reactions
CNS: dizziness, confusion, peripheral neuropathy, central neurotoxicity, paresthesia, asthenia, pain.
CV: *cardiac failure, embolism, CVA.*
EENT: visual disturbances, ototoxicity.
GI: constipation, diarrhea, *nausea, vomiting,* altered taste.
GU: increased BUN, creatinine.
Hematologic: THROMBOCYTOPENIA, *leukopenia,* NEUTROPENIA, *anemia,* BONE MARROW SUPPRESSION.
Hepatic: increased AST or alkaline phosphatase levels.
Metabolic: decreased serum electrolyte levels.
Skin: alopecia.
Other: *hypersensitivity reactions, anaphylaxis.*

Overdose and treatment
Signs and symptoms of overdose result from bone marrow suppression or hepatotoxicity. There's no known antidote for carboplatin overdose.

Special considerations
● Administration of carboplatin requires the supervision of a prescriber experienced in the use of chemotherapeutic agents.
● Needles or I.V. administration sets containing aluminum may precipitate drug and cause a loss of potency.
● Reconstitute with D₅W, normal saline solution, or sterile water for injection to make 10 mg/ml.
● Drug can be further diluted to as low as 0.5 mg/ml using normal saline solution or D₅W. Infuse over at least 15 minutes.
● Store unopened vials at room temperature. Once reconstituted and diluted as directed, solution is stable at room temperature for 8 hours. Because

drug doesn't contain antibacterial preservatives, discard unused drug after 8 hours.

Patient monitoring
● Although drug is promoted as causing less nausea and vomiting than cisplatin, it can cause severe emesis. Antiemetic therapy may be needed; monitor electrolyte levels regularly.

Pregnant patients
● May cause fetal harm. Carboplatin may be used during pregnancy if it's decided that the benefit outweighs the risk, or in life-threatening situations.
● Advise patient to avoid becoming pregnant while on carboplatin therapy.

Breast-feeding patients
● It isn't known if carboplatin appears in breast milk; however, because of the risk of toxicity in the infant, discontinue breast-feeding.

Pediatric patients
● Safety in children hasn't been established.

Geriatric patients
● Patients over age 65 have an increased risk of neurotoxicity.

Patient education
● Stress importance of adequate fluid intake and increase in urine output to facilitate uric acid excretion.
● Tell patient to report tinnitus immediately, to prevent permanent hearing loss. Patient should have audiometric testing before initial and subsequent course of drug therapy.
● Advise patient to avoid exposure to people with infections.
● Instruct patient to promptly report unusual bleeding or bruising.

carboprost tromethamine
Hemabate

Pharmacologic classification: prostaglandin
Therapeutic classification: oxytocic
Pregnancy risk category: C

Indications and dosages
➤ *To abort pregnancy between weeks 13 and 20 of gestation. Adults:* Initially, 250 mcg by deep I.M. injection. Subsequent 250-mcg doses at intervals of 1½ to 3½ hours depending on uterine response. Dose may be increased to 500 mcg if contractility is inadequate after several 250-mcg doses. Total dose shouldn't exceed 12 mg, and therapy shouldn't continue for more than 2 days.
➤ *Postpartum hemorrhage from uterine atony that hasn't responded to conventional management. Adults:* 250 mcg by deep I.M. injection. May repeat doses at 15- to 90-minute intervals. Maximum total dose is 2 mg.

Reactions may be *common*, uncommon, *life-threatening*, or COMMON AND LIFE-THREATENING.

How supplied
Available by prescription only
Injection: 250 mcg/ml carboprost and 83 mcg/ml tromethamine

Pharmacodynamics
Oxytocic action: Exact mechanism unknown. Stimulates myometrial contractions in the gravid uterus similar to the contractions of term labor. Effect may be due to one or more of the following: direct stimulation, regulation of cellular calcium transport, or regulation of intracellular levels of cAMP. Uterine response increases with the length of the pregnancy. Facilitates cervical dilation by softening the cervix. The mean abortion time is 16 hours.

Pharmacokinetics
Absorption: Following deep I.M. administration, levels peak in 15 minutes.
Distribution: No information available.
Metabolism: Primary site of oxidation appears to be liver.
Excretion: Excreted primarily as metabolites in urine.

Route	Onset	Peak	Duration
I.M.	Unknown	15-60 min	24 hr

Contraindications and precautions
Contraindicated in patients hypersensitive to drug and in those with acute pelvic inflammatory disease or active cardiac, pulmonary, renal, or hepatic disease. Use cautiously in patients with history of asthma; hypotension or hypertension; CV, renal, or hepatic disease; anemia; jaundice; diabetes; epilepsy; compromised uterus; or chorioamnionitis.

Interactions
Drug-drug. *Oxytocin, other oxytocics:* Enhanced effects of these drugs; however, cervical laceration and trauma have been reported with use of oxytocin. Use together cautiously.

Adverse reactions
CNS: headache, anxiety, hot flashes, paresthesia, syncope, weakness.
CV: chest pain, ***arrhythmias,*** flushing.
EENT: blurred vision, eye pain.
GI: *vomiting, diarrhea, nausea.*
GU: endometritis, uterine rupture, uterine or vaginal pain.
Musculoskeletal: backache.
Respiratory: cough, wheezing.
Skin: rash, diaphoresis.
Other: *fever,* chills, breast tenderness, leg cramps.

Overdose and treatment
Signs and symptoms of overdose are extensions of the adverse reactions. Because drug is metabolized rapidly, treatment of overdose involves stopping drug and providing supportive care.

Special considerations
● Administer only in hospitals in which intensive care and surgical facilities are available.
● Confirmation of fetal death is imperative before administration when used for missed abortion or intrauterine fetal death.
● Premedicate patient with antiemetics and antidiarrheals to minimize GI effects.
● Meperidine may be helpful to reduce abdominal cramps.
● Store drug in refrigerator. (Carboprost is stable at room temperature for 9 days.)
● If fever occurs, differentiate between drug-induced fever and endometritis pyrexia.
● If incomplete abortion occurs, use other measures to ensure complete abortion.

Patient monitoring
● Monitor patient for adverse effects.

Patient education
● Advise patient of expected adverse reactions.

carisoprodol
Soma

Pharmacologic classification: carbamate derivative
Therapeutic classification: skeletal muscle relaxant
Pregnancy risk category: NR

Indications and dosages
➤ *Adjunct for relief of discomfort in acute, painful musculoskeletal conditions. Adults and children over age 12:* Administer 350 mg P.O. t.i.d. and h.s.

How supplied
Available by prescription only
Tablets: 350 mg

Pharmacodynamics
Skeletal muscle relaxant action: Exact mechanism unknown. Doesn't relax skeletal muscle directly but apparently as a result of its sedative effects. Drug possibly modifies central perception of pain without eliminating peripheral pain reflexes and has slight antipyretic activity.

Pharmacokinetics
Absorption: With usual therapeutic doses, onset of action occurs within 30 minutes and persists 4 to 6 hours.
Distribution: Widely distributed throughout body.
Metabolism: Metabolized in liver. May induce microsomal enzymes in liver; half-life is 8 hours.
Excretion: Excreted in urine mainly as its metabolites; less than 1% of dose is excreted un-

changed. Drug may be removed by hemodialysis or peritoneal dialysis.

Route	Onset	Peak	Duration
P.O.	½ hr	4 hr	4-6 hr

Contraindications and precautions

Contraindicated in patients hypersensitive to related compounds (such as meprobamate or tybamate) and in those with intermittent porphyria. Use cautiously in patients with impaired renal or hepatic function.

Interactions

Drug-drug. *Other CNS depressants (antipsychotics, anxiolytics, general anesthetics, opioid analgesics, tricyclic antidepressants):* Produces additive CNS depression. Exercise care to avoid overdose; dosage adjustments may be needed.
Drug-lifestyle. *Alcohol use:* Produces additive CNS depression. Discourage use.

Adverse reactions

CNS: *drowsiness, dizziness,* vertigo, ataxia, tremor, agitation, irritability, headache, depressive reactions, insomnia.
CV: orthostatic hypotension, tachycardia, facial flushing.
GI: nausea, vomiting, hiccups, epigastric distress.
Hematologic: eosinophilia.
Respiratory: asthmatic episodes.
Skin: rash, *erythema multiforme,* pruritus.
Other: fever, *angioedema, anaphylaxis.*

Overdose and treatment

Signs and symptoms of overdose include exaggerated CNS depression, stupor, coma, shock, and respiratory depression.

Treatment of overdose in conscious patient requires emptying stomach by emesis or gastric lavage; activated charcoal may be used after gastric lavage to adsorb any remaining drug. If patient is comatose, secure endotracheal tube with cuff inflated before gastric lavage. Provide supportive therapy by maintaining adequate airway and assisted ventilation.

CNS stimulants and pressor drugs should be used cautiously. Monitor vital signs, fluid and electrolyte levels, and neurologic status closely. Monitor urine output, and avoid overhydration. Forced diuresis using mannitol, peritoneal dialysis, or hemodialysis may be beneficial. Continue to monitor patient for relapse from incomplete gastric emptying and delayed absorption.

Special considerations

• Use cautiously with other CNS depressants; effects may be cumulative.
• Initially, allergic or idiosyncratic reactions may occur (first to fourth dose). Symptoms usually subside after several hours; treat with supportive and symptomatic measures.
• Psychological dependence may follow longterm use.

• Withdrawal symptoms (abdominal cramps, insomnia, chills, headache, and nausea) may occur with abrupt termination of drug after prolonged use of higher-than-recommended doses.
• Commercially available formulations may contain sodium metabisulfite, which may cause an allergic reaction.

Patient monitoring

• Monitor patient's vital signs.
• Observe patient for adverse effects.

Breast-feeding patients

• Carisoprodol may appear in breast milk at two to four times maternal plasma levels.

Pediatric patients

• Safety and efficacy haven't been established in children under age 12. However, some clinicians suggest a dosage of 25 mg/kg or 750 mg/m² divided q.i.d. for children age 5 and older.

Geriatric patients

• Elderly patients may be more sensitive to drug's effects.

Patient education

• Inform patient that drug may cause dizziness and faintness. Symptoms may be controlled by making position changes slowly and in stages. Patient should report persistent symptoms.
• Tell patient to avoid alcoholic beverages and to use cough or cold preparations containing alcohol cautiously while taking this drug. Patient also should avoid other CNS depressants (effects may be additive) unless prescribed.
• Warn patient that drug may cause drowsiness. He should avoid hazardous activities that require alertness until CNS depressant effects can be determined.
• Advise patient to stop drug immediately and to call if rash, diplopia, dizziness, or other unusual signs or symptoms appear.
• Tell patient to store drug away from direct heat and light (not in bathroom medicine cabinet).
• Instruct patient to take missed dose only if remembered within 1 hour. If remembered later, patient should skip that dose and go back to regular schedule. Patient shouldn't double the dose.
• Tell patient that drug may be taken with food to avoid GI upset.

carmustine (BCNU)
BiCNU, Gliadel

Pharmacologic classification: alkylating agent, nitrosourea (not specific to cell cycle)
Therapeutic classification: antineoplastic
Pregnancy risk category: D

Indications and dosages

Dosage and indications may vary. Check current literature for recommended protocol.

Reactions may be *common,* uncommon, *life-threatening,* or COMMON AND LIFE-THREATENING.

➤*Hodgkin's disease; malignant lymphomas; multiple myeloma; brain, breast ◇, GI tract, lung, hepatic cancer; malignant melanomas ◇.* Adults: 150 to 200 mg/m^2 I.V. slow infusion as a single dose, repeated q 6 to 8 weeks. Or, 75 to 100 mg/m^2 I.V. by slow infusion daily for 2 consecutive days, repeated q 6 weeks if platelet count is above 100,000/mm^3 and WBC count is above 4,000/mm^3.

✦ *Dosage adjustment.* Reduce dosage, p.r.n., using the following guidelines.

Nadir after prior dose		Percentage of prior dose to be given
Leukocytes/ mm^3	Platelets/ mm^3	
≥ 3,000	≥ 75,000	100%
2,000-2,999	25,000-74,999	70%
< 2,000	< 25,000	50%

➤*Recurrent glioblastoma and metastatic brain tumors (adjunct to surgery to prolong survival)*
Adults: Eight wafers implanted in the resection cavity if allowed by size and shape of cavity.

How supplied
Available by prescription only
Injection: 100-mg vial (lyophilized), with a 3-ml vial of absolute alcohol supplied as a diluent
Implant: 7.7-mg wafer

Pharmacodynamics
Antineoplastic action: The cytotoxic action of carmustine is mediated through its metabolites, which inhibit several enzymes involved with DNA formation. This drug also can cause cross-linking of DNA. Cross-linking interferes with DNA, RNA, and protein synthesis. Cross-resistance between carmustine and lomustine has occurred.

Pharmacokinetics
Absorption: Not absorbed across the GI tract. Wafers are biodegradable in the human brain when implanted into the tumor resection cavity.
Distribution: Cleared rapidly from plasma. After I.V. administration, carmustine and its metabolites are distributed rapidly into CSF.
Metabolism: Metabolized extensively in the liver.
Excretion: About 60% to 70% of drug and its metabolites are excreted in urine within 96 hours, 6% to 10% is excreted as carbon dioxide by the lungs, and 1% is excreted in feces. Enterohepatic circulation and protein-binding can occur and may cause delayed hematologic toxicity.
Note: Absorption, distribution, metabolism, and excretion of the implant wafer copolymer are unknown.

Route	Onset	Peak	Duration
I.V.	Unknown	Unknown	Unknown

Contraindications and precautions
Contraindicated in patients hypersensitive to drug.

Interactions
Drug-drug. *Anticoagulants, aspirin:* Increased risk of bleeding. Avoid use together.
Cimetidine: Increases the bone marrow toxicity of carmustine. Avoid use together.
Myelosuppressive drugs: Concurrent use can cause additive myelosuppression. Monitor patient closely.

Adverse reactions
CNS: ataxia, drowsiness.
EENT: ocular toxicity.
GI: *severe nausea* beginning in 2 to 6 hours, *vomiting.*
GU: *nephrotoxicity,* azotemia, *renal failure.*
Hematologic: *cumulative bone marrow suppression* (delayed 4 to 6 weeks, lasting 1 to 2 weeks), *leukopenia, thrombocytopenia, acute leukemia, bone marrow dysplasia* (after long-term use), anemia.
Hepatic: *hepatotoxicity.*
Metabolic: possible hyperuricemia in lymphoma patients when rapid cell lysis occurs.
Respiratory: *pulmonary fibrosis.*
Skin: facial flushing, hyperpigmentation.
Other: *intense pain at infusion site from venous spasm.*

Overdose and treatment
Signs and symptoms of overdose include leukopenia, thrombocytopenia, nausea, and vomiting.

Treatment consists of supportive measures, including transfusion of blood components, antibiotics for infections that may develop, and antiemetics.

Special considerations
● Use double gloves and surgical instruments dedicated to handling implant wafers.
● Reconstitute 100-mg vial with the 3 ml of absolute alcohol provided by manufacturer; then dilute further with 27 ml sterile water for injection. Resulting solution contains 3.3 mg carmustine/ml in 10% ethanol. Dilute in normal saline solution or D$_5$W for I.V. infusion. Give at least 250 ml over 1 to 2 hours. Discard excess drug.
● Wear gloves to administer drug infusion and change I.V. tubing. Avoid contact with skin because carmustine causes a brown stain. If drug contacts skin, wash thoroughly.
● Solution is unstable in plastic I.V. bags. Administer only in glass containers.
● Carmustine may decompose at temperatures above 80° F (26.6° C).
● If powder liquefies or appears oily, discard it because it may have decomposed.
● Reconstituted solution may be stored in refrigerator for 24 hours (48 hours if reconstituted to 0.2 mg/ml in D$_5$W or normal saline solution).

- Don't mix with other drugs during administration.
- Avoid I.M. injections when platelet count is less than 100,000/mm³.
- To reduce pain of infusion, dilute further or slow infusion rate.
- Intense flushing of skin may occur during I.V. infusion but usually disappears in 2 to 4 hours.
- At first sign of extravasation, stop infusion and infiltrate area with liberal injections of 0.5 mEq/ml sodium bicarbonate solution.
- Drug has been applied topically in concentrations of 0.05% to 0.4% to treat mycosis fungoides.
- Because drug crosses the blood-brain barrier, it may be used to treat primary brain tumors.

Patient monitoring

- Monitor patient for nausea and vomiting, which may last up to 6 hours after administration. To reduce nausea, suggest giving antiemetic before administering.
- Monitor CBC weekly during therapy and for 6 weeks after treatment ends.
- Obtain pulmonary function tests before starting treatment and frequently throughout treatment. Pulmonary toxicity is more likely in people who smoke.
- Monitor liver and renal function tests periodically during therapy.

Pregnant patients

- Advise women to avoid becoming pregnant and to report suspected pregnancy.

Breast-feeding patients

- Active metabolites of drug have been found in breast milk. Therefore, it isn't advisable for women receiving drug to breast-feed their infants because of risk of serious adverse reactions, mutagenicity, and carcinogenicity in the infant.

Pediatric patients

- Safety and effectiveness of carmustine in children haven't been established.

Patient education

- Warn patient to watch for signs of infection and bone marrow toxicity (fever, sore throat, anemia, fatigue, easy bruising, nosebleeds, bleeding gums, melena). Patient should take temperature daily.
- Remind patient to return for follow-up blood work weekly, or as needed, and to watch for signs and symptoms of infection.
- Advise patient to avoid exposure to people with infections.
- Tell patient to avoid OTC products containing aspirin because they may precipitate bleeding. Advise patient to report signs of bleeding promptly.

carteolol hydrochloride
Cartrol, Ocupress

Pharmacologic classification: beta blocker
Therapeutic classification: antihypertensive
Pregnancy risk category: C

Indications and dosages

➤ *Hypertension. Adults:* Initially, 2.5 mg P.O. as a single daily dose. Gradually increase the dose as needed to 5 mg or 10 mg daily as a single dose.
➤ *Angina ◇. Adults:* 10 mg P.O. daily.
✦ *Dosage adjustment.* Patients with substantial renal impairment should receive the usual dose of carteolol scheduled at longer intervals. If creatinine clearance is 20 to 60 ml/minute, use a 48-hour interval. If creatinine clearance is less than 20 ml/minute, use a 72-hour interval.
➤ *Open-angle glaucoma. Adults:* 1 drop b.i.d. in affected eye or eyes.

How supplied

Available by prescription only
Ophthalmic solution: 1%
Tablets: 2.5 mg, 5 mg

Pharmacodynamics

Antihypertensive action: Drug is a nonselective beta blocker with intrinsic sympathomimetic activity. Its antihypertensive effects are probably caused by decreased sympathetic outflow from the brain and decreased cardiac output. Carteolol doesn't have a consistent effect on renin output.

Pharmacokinetics

Absorption: Absorbed rapidly. Bioavailability is about 85%.
Distribution: 20% to 30% bound to plasma proteins.
Metabolism: Only 30% to 50% is metabolized in the liver to 8-hydroxycarteolol, an active metabolite, and the inactive metabolite glucuronoside.
Excretion: Primarily renal. Plasma half-life is about 6 hours.

Route	Onset	Peak	Duration
P.O.	Unknown	1-3 hr	24 hr
Oph-thalmic	Unknown	Unknown	Unknown

Contraindications and precautions

Contraindicated in patients hypersensitive to any component of drug and in those with bronchial asthma, severe COPD, sinus bradycardia, second- or third-degree AV block, overt cardiac failure, or cardiogenic shock.

Use cautiously in breast-feeding women and in patients with nonallergic bronchospastic disease, diabetes mellitus, hyperthyroidism, or decreased pulmonary function.

Reactions may be *common*, uncommon, *life-threatening*, or COMMON AND LIFE-THREATENING.

Interactions
Drug-drug. *Calcium channel blockers:* Increased risk of hypotension, left ventricular failure, and AV conduction disturbances. Use I.V. calcium antagonists cautiously.
Cardiac glycosides: May produce additive effects on slowing AV node conduction. Avoid use together.
Catecholamine-depleting drugs, such as reserpine, oral adrenergic blockers: May have an additive effect and contribute to development of hypotension or bradycardia. Monitor patient closely.
General anesthetics: Increased hypotensive effects. Observe patient carefully for hypotension, bradycardia, and orthostatic hypotension.
Insulin, oral antidiabetics: May alter hypoglycemic response. Dose may need adjustment.
Drug-lifestyle. *Sun exposure:* Photophobia may occur with ophthalmic form. Advise patient to take precautions.

Adverse reactions
CNS: lassitude, fatigue, somnolence, *asthenia, paresthesia.*
CV: *conduction disturbances.*
EENT: transient irritation, conjunctival hyperemia, *edema.*
GI: diarrhea, nausea, abdominal pain.
Musculoskeletal: *muscle cramps,* arthralgia.
Skin: rash.

Overdose and treatment
No information available. The likely signs and symptoms are bradycardia, bronchospasm, heart failure, and hypotension.

Use atropine to treat symptomatic bradycardia. If no response occurs, cautiously use isoproterenol. Treat bronchospasm with a beta$_2$-agonist such as isoproterenol, or theophylline. Cardiac glycosides or diuretics may be useful in treating heart failure. Give vasopressors (epinephrine, dopamine, or norepinephrine) to combat hypotension.

Special considerations
Consider the recommendations relevant to all beta blockers as well as the following.
⚠ ALERT Discontinue drug at first sign of cardiac failure.
● Dosage of more than 10 mg daily doesn't produce a greater response and may decrease response.
● Food may slow the rate but not the extent of carteolol absorption.
● Steady-state levels occur rapidly (within 1 to 2 days) in patients with normal renal function.

Patient monitoring
● Monitor heart rate and blood pressure.

Breast-feeding patients
● Drug may appear in breast milk. Use cautiously in breast-feeding women.

Pediatric patients
● Safety in children hasn't been established.

Geriatric patients
● No specific age-related recommendations are available.

Patient education
● Advise patient to take drug exactly as prescribed and not to stop it suddenly.
● Tell patient to report shortness of breath, trouble breathing, an unusually fast heartbeat, cough, or fatigue with exertion.
● Inform patient that transient stinging or discomfort may occur with ophthalmic use; if reaction is severe, he should call prescriber immediately.
● If patient uses more than one topical ophthalmic drug, tell him to administer them at least 10 minutes apart.

carvedilol
Coreg

Pharmacologic classification: alpha-nonselective beta blocker
Therapeutic classification: antihypertensive, adjunct treatment for heart failure
Pregnancy risk category: C

Indications and dosages
➤**Hypertension.** *Adults:* Dosage individualized. Initially, 6.25 mg P.O. b.i.d. with food; obtain standing systolic pressure 1 hour after first dose. If tolerated, continue dosage for 7 to 14 days. Can increase to 12.5 mg P.O. b.i.d., repeating monitoring protocol as above. Maximum dose is 25 mg P.O. b.i.d. as tolerated.
➤**Heart failure.** *Adults:* Dosage individualized and adjusted carefully. Stabilize dosing of cardiac glycosides, diuretics, and ACE inhibitors before starting therapy. Initially, 3.125 mg P.O. b.i.d. with food for 2 weeks; if tolerated, possibly increased to 6.25 mg P.O. b.i.d. for 2 weeks. Dose can be doubled q 2 weeks to highest tolerated level. At start of new dose, observe patient for 1 hour for dizziness or light-headedness. If patient weighs less than 187 lb (85 kg), maximum dosage is 25 mg P.O. b.i.d.; if patient weighs more than 187 lb, maximum dosage is 50 mg P.O. b.i.d.

How supplied
Available by prescription only
Tablets: 3.125 mg, 6.25 mg, 12.5 mg, 25 mg

Pharmacodynamics
Antihypertensive action: Mechanism not established. Beta blockade reduces cardiac output and tachycardia. Alpha blockade is demonstrated by the attenuated pressor effects of phenylephrine, vasodilation, and decreased peripheral vascular resistance.

Heart failure: Not fully established. Drug decreases systemic blood pressure, pulmonary artery pressure, right atrial pressure, systemic vascular resistance, and heart rate while increasing stroke volume index.

Pharmacokinetics

Absorption: Rapidly and extensively metabolized after oral use, with absolute bioavailability of 25% to 35% because of significant first-pass metabolism.

Distribution: Plasma levels are proportional to oral dose. Absorption is slowed by food, as evidenced by a delay in reaching peak plasma levels, with no significant difference in extent of bioavailability.

Metabolism: Extensively metabolized, primarily by aromatic ring oxidation and glucuronidation. The oxidative metabolites are further metabolized by conjugation via glucuronidation and sulfation. Demethylation and hydroxylation at the phenol ring produce three active metabolites with beta-blocking activity.

Excretion: Metabolites are mainly excreted via bile into the feces. Less than 2% of dose is excreted unchanged in urine.

Route	Onset	Peak	Duration
P.O.	Unknown	1-2 hr	7-10 hr

Contraindications and precautions

Contraindicated in patients hypersensitive to drug and those with New York Heart Association (NYHA) class IV decompensated cardiac failure who need I.V. inotropic therapy, bronchial asthma or related bronchospastic conditions, second- or third-degree AV block, sick sinus syndrome (unless a permanent pacemaker is in place), cardiogenic shock, or severe bradycardia. Drug isn't recommended for patients with hepatic impairment.

Use cautiously in hypertensive patients with left ventricular failure, perioperative patients who receive anesthetics that depress myocardial function (such as ether, cyclopropane, trichloroethylene), diabetic patients receiving insulin or oral antidiabetics, or patients subject to spontaneous hypoglycemia. Also use cautiously in patients with thyroid disease (may mask hyperthyroidism and drug withdrawal may precipitate thyroid storm or an exacerbation of hyperthyroidism), pheochromocytoma, Prinzmetal's variant angina, or peripheral vascular disease (may precipitate or aggravate symptoms of arterial insufficiency).

Interactions

Drug-drug. *Calcium channel blockers:* May cause isolated conduction disturbances. Monitor ECG and blood pressure.

Catecholamine-depleting drugs, such as MAO inhibitors, reserpine: May cause severe bradycardia or hypotension. Monitor patient closely.

Cimetidine: Increased bioavailability of carvedilol. Monitor vital signs closely.

Clonidine: May potentiate blood pressure–lowering and heart rate–lowering effects. Monitor patient carefully.

Digoxin: Increased digoxin level (by about 15%). Evaluate digoxin levels.

Insulin, oral antidiabetics: May enhance hypoglycemic effects. Check blood glucose levels.

Rifampin: Decreased carvedilol levels (by 70%). Monitor vital signs.

Drug-food. *Any food:* Delays absorption but not extent of bioavailability. Tell patient to take drug with food to minimize orthostatic effects.

Adverse reactions

CNS: malaise, *dizziness, fatigue,* headache, hypesthesia, insomnia, pain, paresthesia, somnolence, vertigo.

CV: aggravated angina pectoris, **AV block**, **bradycardia**, chest pain, fluid overload, hypertension, hypotension, orthostatic hypertension, hypovolemia, syncope, peripheral edema, edema.

EENT: abnormal vision, pharyngitis, rhinitis, sinusitis.

GI: abdominal pain, *diarrhea,* melena, nausea, periodontitis, vomiting.

GU: abnormal renal function, albuminuria, glycosuria, hematuria, impotence, urinary tract infection, increased BUN.

Hematologic: decreased PT, purpura, **thrombocytopenia.**

Hepatic: increased ALT, AST, and alkaline phosphatase levels.

Metabolic: dehydration, gout, hypercholesterolemia, *hyperglycemia,* hypertriglyceridemia, hypervolemia, hyperuricemia, hypoglycemia, hyponatremia, weight gain, increased nonprotein nitrogen.

Musculoskeletal: arthralgia, back pain, myalgia.

Respiratory: bronchitis, dyspnea, *upper respiratory tract infection.*

Other: allergy, fever, **sudden death**, viral infection.

Overdose and treatment

Overdose may cause severe hypotension, bradycardia, cardiac insufficiency, cardiogenic shock, and cardiac arrest. Respiratory effects, bronchospasm, vomiting, lapses of consciousness, and generalized seizures also may occur.

Place patient in supine position. Gastric lavage or pharmacologically induced emesis may be effective shortly after ingestion. May use atropine 2 mg I.V. for bradycardia; glucagon 5 to 10 mg I.V. rapidly over 30 seconds, followed by continuous infusion at 5 mg/hour to support CV function; sympathomimetics (dobutamine, isoprenaline, adrenaline) at doses based on body weight and effect. If peripheral vasodilation dominates, administer epinephrine or norepinephrine, if necessary, and continuously monitor circulatory conditions. For therapy-resistant bradycardia,

---

Reactions may be *common*, uncommon, *life-threatening*, or COMMON AND LIFE-THREATENING.

perform pacemaker therapy. For bronchospasm, give beta-sympathomimetics by aerosol or I.V. or aminophylline I.V. If seizures occur, slow I.V. injection of diazepam or clonazepam may be effective. If severe toxicity and symptoms of shock occur, continue treatment with antidotes for a sufficient period of time consistent with the drug's 7- to 10-hour half-life.

Special considerations
● Discontinue drug gradually over 1 to 2 weeks. Decrease dosage if heart rate is less than 55 beats/minute.
● Patient taking beta blocker with a history of severe anaphylaxis to several allergens may be more reactive to repeated challenge, whether accidental, diagnostic, or therapeutic. Patient may be unresponsive to epinephrine doses usually used to treat allergic reactions.

Patient monitoring
● Mild hepatocellular injury may occur during therapy. At first sign of hepatic dysfunction, perform tests for hepatic injury or jaundice; if present, discontinue drug.
● Heart failure patients need monitoring for worsened condition, renal dysfunction, or fluid retention; diuretics may need to be increased. Monitor diabetic patient for worsening of hyperglycemia.

Breast-feeding patients
● It isn't known if drug appears in breast milk. Use cautiously.

Pediatric patients
● Safety of drug in patients under age 18 hasn't been established.

Geriatric patients
● Monitor plasma levels carefully; drug levels are about 50% higher in elderly patients than in younger patients.
● There seems to be no significant difference in adverse effects between older and younger patients, although dizziness may be more common in elderly patients.

Patient education
● Tell patient not to interrupt or stop drug without medical approval.
● Advise heart failure patient to report weight gain or shortness of breath.
● Inform patient that he may feel dizzy when he stands up. If he does, tell him to sit or lie down. Fainting is rare.
● Caution patient against performing hazardous tasks at the start of therapy. Tell him to report dizziness or fatigue; he may need a dosage adjustment.
● Advise diabetic patient to report changes in serum glucose level promptly.
● Inform patient who wears contact lenses that he may have decreased tearing.

cascara sagrada
cascara sagrada aromatic fluidextract

Pharmacologic classification: anthraquinone glycoside mixture
Therapeutic classification: laxative
Pregnancy risk category: C

Indications and dosages
➤ *Acute constipation, preparation for bowel or rectal examination.* Adults and children age 12 and older: 1 tablet P.O. h.s. or 2 to 6 ml of aromatic fluidextract P.O. once daily.
Children ages 2 to 11: ½ of adult dose.
Children under age 2: ¼ of adult dose.

How supplied
Available without a prescription
Aromatic fluidextract: 19% alcohol in 473 ml
Tablets: 325 mg

Pharmacodynamics
Laxative action: Cascara sagrada, obtained from dried bark of the buckthorn tree *(Rhamnus purshiana)*, contains cascarosides A and B (barbaloin glycosides) and cascarosides C and D (chrysaloin glycosides). Drug exerts a direct irritant action on the colon, which promotes peristalsis and bowel motility. It also enhances fluid accumulation in the colon.

Pharmacokinetics
Absorption: Minimal drug absorption occurs in the small intestine.
Distribution: Distributed in the bile, saliva, and colonic mucosa.
Metabolism: Metabolized in the liver.
Excretion: Excreted in feces via biliary elimination, in urine, or in both.

Route	Onset	Peak	Duration
P.O.	6-10 hr	Variable	Variable

Contraindications and precautions
Contraindicated in patients with abdominal pain, nausea, vomiting, or other symptoms of appendicitis or acute surgical abdomen; acute surgical delirium; fecal impaction; and intestinal obstruction or perforation. Use cautiously in patients with rectal bleeding.

Interactions
None reported.

Adverse reactions
GI: *nausea;* vomiting; diarrhea; loss of normal bowel function with excessive use; *abdominal cramps,* especially in severe constipation; malabsorption of nutrients; cathartic colon (syndrome resembling ulcerative colitis radiologi-

cally and pathologically) with long-term misuse; discoloration of rectal mucosa after long-term use.
Metabolic: hypokalemia, protein enteropathy, electrolyte imbalance (with excessive use).
Other: laxative dependence with long-term or excessive use.

Overdose and treatment
No information available.

Special considerations
● Prescribe doses carefully; fluidextract preparation is five times as potent as aromatic fluid extract.
● Aromatic fluidextract tastes better than fluidextract.
● Cascara is a common ingredient in many so-called natural laxatives available without a prescription.
● Cascara turns alkaline urine pink to red, red to violet, or red to brown and turns acidic urine yellow to brown in the phenolsulfonphthalein excretion test.

Patient monitoring
● Monitor patient's bowel patterns.

Pregnant patients
● Bulk-forming or surfactant laxatives are preferred during pregnancy.

Breast-feeding patients
● Cascara may appear in breast milk, which may result in increased risk of diarrhea in infant.

Pediatric patients
● Use cautiously in children.

Geriatric patients
● Because many elderly people use laxatives, they're at particularly high risk for development of laxative dependence. Encourage them to use laxatives only for short periods.

Patient education
● Warn patient that drug may turn urine reddish pink or brown.
● Tell patient to take each dose with a full glass of water.

caspofungin acetate
Cancidas

Pharmacologic classification: glucan synthesis inhibitor
Therapeutic classification: antifungal
Pregnancy risk category: C

Indications and dosages
➤ *Invasive aspergillosis in patients refractory to or intolerant of other therapies (such as amphotericin B, lipid forms of amphotericin B, itraconazole).* Adults:
A single 70-mg loading dose on day 1, followed by 50 mg daily thereafter. Administer by slow I.V. infusion over about 1 hour. Duration of treatment based on severity of patient's underlying disease, recovery from immunosuppression, and clinical response.
✦ *Dosage adjustment.* For patients with moderate hepatic insufficiency (Child-Pugh score 7 to 9), give 35 mg daily after the first 70-mg loading dose. There's no clinical experience in patients with severe hepatic insufficiency (Child-Pugh score above 9).

How supplied
Lyophilized powder for injection: 50-mg and 70-mg single-use vials

Pharmacodynamics
Caspofungin inhibits synthesis of $\beta(1,3)$-D-glucan, an integral component of the cell walls of susceptible filamentous fungi that isn't found in mammal cells. Caspofungin has in vitro activity against *Aspergillus fumigatus, Aspergillus flavus,* and *Aspergillus terreus.* Development of resistance to caspofungin by *Aspergillus* species in vitro hasn't been studied.

Pharmacokinetics
Absorption: Administered I.V.
Distribution: Distribution, rather than excretion or biotransformation, is the dominant mechanism influencing plasma clearance. Caspofungin is extensively bound to albumin (about 97%), and distribution into RBCs is minimal. There's little excretion or biotransformation of caspofungin during the first 30 hours after administration. There are three phases of decline in serum levels; the first is rapid, and the half-lives of the last two phases are 9 to 11 hours and 40 to 50 hours respectively.
Metabolism: Caspofungin is slowly metabolized by hydrolysis and N-acetylation. It also undergoes spontaneous chemical degradation to an open-ring peptide compound.
Excretion: After single-dose I.V. administration of caspofungin acetate, about 35% of drug and metabolites is excreted in feces and 41% in urine. Renal clearance of parent drug is very low.

Route	Onset	Peak	Duration
I.V.	Unknown	Unknown	Unknown

Contraindications and precautions
Caspofungin is contraindicated in patients hypersensitive to any of its components.

Interactions
Drug-drug. *Carbamazepine, dexamethasone, efavirenz, nelfinavir, nevirapine, phenytoin, rifampin:* Possible decreased caspofungin levels. Consider increasing caspofungin dosage if patient fails to respond.

Reactions may be *common,* uncommon, *life-threatening,* or COMMON AND LIFE-THREATENING.

Cyclosporine: Significantly increased caspofungin and ALT levels. Concurrent use isn't recommended unless potential benefit outweighs potential risk.

Tacrolimus: Decreased tacrolimus levels. Monitor tacrolimus levels and adjust tacrolimus dosage as needed.

Adverse reactions
CNS: headache, *paresthesia.*
CV: *tachycardia.*
GI: nausea, vomiting, diarrhea, abdominal pain, *anorexia.*
GU: proteinuria, hematuria.
Hematologic: eosinophilia, *anemia.*
Hepatic: increased alkaline phosphatase.
Metabolic: hypokalemia.
Musculoskeletal: *pain, myalgia.*
Respiratory: *tachypnea.*
Skin: histamine-mediated symptoms, including rash, facial swelling, pruritus, or sensation of warmth.
Other: fever, infused vein complications, phlebitis, *chills, sweating.*

Overdose and treatment
In clinical studies the highest dose was 100 mg, administered as a single dose to five patients; it was generally well tolerated. No overdoses have been reported. Caspofungin isn't dialyzable.

Special considerations
● The efficacy of a 70-mg dose regimen in patients who don't respond to 50-mg dose isn't known, although the increase seems to be well tolerated. The safety of treatment lasting longer than 2 weeks is unclear, but longer courses seem to be well tolerated.
● Monitor I.V. site carefully for phlebitis.
● Caspofungin should be administered by slow I.V. infusion over about 1 hour.
⚠ ALERT Caspofungin should never be mixed or diluted with dextrose solution. Don't mix or infuse it with other drugs.
● Reconstituted vials should be used within 1 hour or discarded.
● Caspofungin usually should be diluted in 250 ml of normal saline solution for all (70-mg, 50-mg, 35-mg) doses. In patients with fluid restrictions, the 50-mg and 35-mg doses may be diluted in 100 ml of normal saline solution.
● Refer to the manufacturer's instructions for specific reconstitution and I.V. dose preparation guidelines.
● Duration of treatment should be based on the severity of the patient's underlying disease, recovery from immunosuppression, and response.
● Patients with hepatic insufficiency may require dosage reduction.

Patient monitoring
● Observe patient for histamine-mediated reactions: rash, facial swelling, pruritis, sensation of warmth.

Breast-feeding patients
● It isn't known whether drug appears in breast milk. Because many drugs do, use cautiously when giving caspofungin to a nursing woman.

Pediatric patients
● Safety and effectiveness in patients under age 18 are unknown.

Geriatric patients
● No dosage adjustments are needed.

Patient education
● Instruct patient to report signs and symptoms of phlebitis.

castor oil
Emulsoil, Neoloid, Purge

Pharmacologic classification: glyceride, *Ricinus communis* derivative
Therapeutic classification: stimulant laxative
Pregnancy risk category: X

Indications and dosages
➤ *Preparation for rectal or bowel examination or surgery; acute constipation.* Liquid. *Adults:* 15 to 60 ml (or 30 to 60 ml, 95%) P.O.
Children ages 2 to 12: 5 to 15 ml P.O.
Liquid emulsion
Adults: 45 ml (36.4%) or 15 to 60 ml (95%) P.O. mixed with ½ to 1 glass liquid.
Children ages 2 to 12: 15 ml (36.4%) or 5 to 15 ml (95%) P.O. mixed with ½ to 1 glass liquid.

How supplied
Available without a prescription
Liquid: 60 ml, 120 ml, 480 ml
Liquid (95%): 30 ml, 60 ml
Liquid emulsion: 63 ml (95%), 118 ml (36.4%)

Pharmacodynamics
Laxative action: Castor oil acts primarily in the small intestine, where it's metabolized to ricinoleic acid, which stimulates the intestine, promoting peristalsis and bowel motility.

Pharmacokinetics
Absorption: Unknown.
Distribution: Distributed locally, primarily in the small intestine.
Metabolism: Like other fatty acids, castor oil is metabolized by intestinal enzymes into its active form, ricinoleic acid.
Excretion: Excreted in feces.

Route	Onset	Peak	Duration
P.O.	2-6 hr	Variable	Variable

Contraindications and precautions

Contraindicated in pregnant women; menstruating women; patients with ulcerative bowel lesions; and patients with abdominal pain, nausea, vomiting, or other symptoms of appendicitis or acute surgical abdomen. Also contraindicated in patients with anal or rectal fissures, fecal impaction, or intestinal obstruction or perforation. Use cautiously in patients with rectal bleeding.

Interactions

Drug-drug. *Intestinally absorbed drugs:* Decreased absorption of these drugs. Monitor patient closely.
Drug-herb. *Male fern:* Increased absorption and risk of toxicity. Discourage use together.

Adverse reactions

GI: *nausea;* vomiting; diarrhea; loss of normal bowel function with excessive use; *abdominal cramps,* especially in severe constipation; malabsorption of nutrients; cathartic colon (syndrome resembling ulcerative colitis radiologically and pathologically) with long-term misuse; laxative dependence with long-term or excessive use; constipation after catharsis.
Metabolic: hypokalemia, other electrolyte imbalances (with excessive use).
Other: protein-losing enteropathy.

Overdose and treatment

No information available.

Special considerations

● Failure to respond to drug may indicate an acute condition that needs surgery.
● Castor oil isn't recommended for routine use in constipation; it's commonly used to evacuate the bowel before diagnostic or surgical procedures.
● Because of rapid onset of action, drug shouldn't be given at bedtime.
● Drug is most effective when taken on an empty stomach; shake it well before giving it.
● Flavored preparations are available.

Patient monitoring

● Observe patient for signs and symptoms of dehydration.

Pregnant patients

● Drug shouldn't be used in pregnant women because of possible fetal abnormalities.

Breast-feeding patients

● Breast-feeding women should seek medical approval before using castor oil.

Geriatric patients

● With prolonged use, geriatric patients may experience electrolyte depletion, resulting in weakness, incoordination, and orthostatic hypotension.

Patient education

● Advise pregnant women not to use castor oil.
● Recommend that drug be chilled or taken with juice or carbonated beverage to improve palatability.
● Instruct patient to shake emulsion well before taking it.
● Reassure patient that after response to drug he may not need to move his bowels again for up to a few days.

cefaclor
Ceclor, Ceclor CD

Pharmacologic classification: second-generation cephalosporin
Therapeutic classification: antibiotic
Pregnancy risk category: B

Indications and dosages

➤ *Infections of respiratory tract, urinary tract, and skin; otitis media caused by susceptible organisms.* Adults: 250 to 500 mg P.O. q 8 hours. Total daily dose shouldn't exceed 4 g. For extended-release tablets, 375 to 500 mg P.O. q 12 hours for 7 to 10 days.
Children: 20 mg/kg P.O. daily (40 mg/kg for severe infections and otitis media) in divided doses q 8 to 12 hours, not to exceed 1 g daily.
➤ *Acute uncomplicated urinary tract infection.* Adults: 2 g P.O. as single dose.
✦ *Dosage adjustment.* Because cefaclor is dialyzable, patients receiving treatment with hemodialysis or peritoneal dialysis may require dosage adjustment.

How supplied

Available by prescription only
Capsules: 250 mg, 500 mg
Suspension: 125 mg/5 ml, 187 mg/5 ml, 250 mg/5 ml, 375 mg/5 ml
Tablets (extended-release): 375 mg, 500 mg

Pharmacodynamics

Antibacterial action: Drug is primarily bactericidal; it also may be bacteriostatic. Activity depends on the specific organism, extent of tissue penetration, dosage, and rate of organism multiplication. Drug acts by adhering to bacterial penicillin-binding proteins, thereby inhibiting cell wall synthesis.

Cefaclor has the same bactericidal spectrum as other second-generation cephalosporins, except that it has increased activity against ampicillin- or amoxicillin-resistant *Haemophilus influenzae* and *Branhamella catarrhalis.*

Pharmacokinetics

Absorption: Well absorbed from the GI tract. Food delays but doesn't prevent complete GI absorption.

Distribution: Distributed widely into most body tissues and fluids; CSF penetration is poor. Cefaclor crosses the placenta; it's 25% protein-bound.
Metabolism: Not metabolized.
Excretion: Excreted mainly in urine by renal tubular secretion and glomerular filtration; small amounts of drug appear in breast milk. Elimination half-life is ½ to 1 hour in patients with normal renal function; end-stage renal disease prolongs half-life to 3 to 5½ hours. Hemodialysis removes cefaclor.

Route	Onset	Peak	Duration
P.O.			
Regular	Unknown	½-1 hr	Unknown
Extended	Unknown	½-2½ hr	Unknown

Contraindications and precautions

Contraindicated in patients hypersensitive to other cephalosporins. Use cautiously in breast-feeding women and in patients with impaired renal function or penicillin allergy.

Interactions

Drug-drug. *Antacids:* Absorption of extended-release cefaclor is decreased if taken within 1 hour. Separate administration by 1 hour.
Chloramphenicol: Antagonistic effect. Don't use together.
Loop diuretics, nephrotoxic drugs (aminoglycosides, colistin, polymyxin B, vancomycin): May increase the risk of nephrotoxicity. Patient must be monitored.
Probenecid: Competitively inhibits renal tubular excretion of cephalosporins, resulting in higher, prolonged serum levels of these drugs. Patient must be monitored.

Adverse reactions

CNS: dizziness, headache, somnolence, malaise.
GI: *nausea,* vomiting, *diarrhea,* anorexia, dyspepsia, abdominal cramps, pseudomembranous colitis, oral candidiasis.
GU: vaginal candidiasis, vaginitis.
Hematologic: *transient leukopenia,* anemia, eosinophilia, *thrombocytopenia,* lymphocytosis.
Hepatic: transient increases in liver enzyme levels.
Skin: *maculopapular rash,* dermatitis, pruritus.
Other: *hypersensitivity reactions* (serum sickness, *anaphylaxis*), fever, *Stevens-Johnson syndrome.*

Overdose and treatment

Overdose may cause neuromuscular hypersensitivity; seizure may follow high CNS levels. Remove cefaclor by hemodialysis or peritoneal dialysis.

Special considerations

Consider the recommendations relevant to all cephalosporins as well as the following.

• Total daily dose may be given b.i.d. rather than t.i.d. with similar therapeutic effect.
• Stock oral suspension is stable for 14 days if refrigerated.
• Cefaclor may cause false-positive Coombs' test results. Cefaclor also causes false-positive results in urine glucose tests using cupric sulfate (Benedict's reagent or Clinitest); use glucose oxidase tests (Chemstrip uG, Diastix, or glucose enzymatic test strip) instead.
• Cefaclor causes false elevations in serum or urine creatinine levels in tests using Jaffé's reaction.

Patient monitoring

• Monitor patient with impaired renal function closely. Obtain relevant laboratory tests.
• Monitor patient for serum sickness or hypersensitivity reactions.

Breast-feeding patients

• Drug appears in breast milk; use cautiously in breast-feeding women.

Pediatric patients

• Drug can be used safely in children older than 1 month. Extended-release tablets should be used only in children age 16 and older.

Geriatric patients

• No dosage adjustments are needed.

Patient education

• Instruct patient to take extended-release tablets with food and not to cut, crush, or chew them.
• Tell patient to take the entire amount of drug exactly as prescribed, even if he feels better.

---

cefadroxil
Duricef

Pharmacologic classification: first-generation cephalosporin
Therapeutic classification: antibiotic
Pregnancy risk category: B

Indications and dosages

➤ *Urinary tract, skin, and soft-tissue infections caused by susceptible organisms; pharyngitis; tonsillitis. Adults:* 1 to 2 g P.O. daily, depending on the infection treated. Usually given once or twice daily.
Children: 30 mg/kg P.O. daily in two divided doses.
✦ *Dosage adjustment.* Adjust dosage, based on creatinine clearance, as shown at the top of the next page. Because drug is dializable, patients receiving treatment with hemodialysis may require dosage adjustment.

Creatinine clearance (ml/min)	Dosage interval (hr)
25-50	12
10-25	24
< 10	36

How supplied
Available by prescription only
Capsules: 500 mg
Suspension: 125 mg/5 ml, 250 mg/5 ml, 500 mg/5 ml
Tablets: 1 g

Pharmacodynamics
Antibacterial action: Cefadroxil is primarily bactericidal; it also may be bacteriostatic. Activity depends on the organism, tissue penetration, dosage, and rate of organism multiplication. It acts by adhering to bacterial penicillin-binding proteins, thereby inhibiting cell wall synthesis.

Cefadroxil is active against many gram-positive cocci, including penicillinase-producing *Staphylococcus aureus* and *Staphylococcus epidermidis; Streptococcus pneumoniae,* group B streptococci, and group A beta-hemolytic streptococci; and susceptible gram-negative organisms, including *Klebsiella pneumoniae, Escherichia coli,* and *Proteus mirabilis.*

Pharmacokinetics
Absorption: Absorbed rapidly and completely from the GI tract after oral administration.
Distribution: Distributed widely into most body tissues and fluids, including the gallbladder, liver, kidneys, bone, bile, sputum, and pleural and synovial fluids; CSF penetration is poor. Drug crosses the placenta; it's 20% protein-bound.
Metabolism: Not metabolized.
Excretion: Excreted primarily unchanged in urine by way of glomerular filtration and renal tubular secretion; small amounts may appear in breast milk. End-stage renal disease prolongs half-life to 25 hours. Drug can be removed by hemodialysis.

Route	Onset	Peak	Duration
P.O.	Unknown	1-2 hr	Unknown

Contraindications and precautions
Contraindicated in patients hypersensitive to drug or other cephalosporins. Use cautiously in breast-feeding women and patients with impaired renal function or penicillin allergy.

Interactions
Drug-drug. *Bacteriostatic drugs (chloramphenicol, erythromycin, tetracyclines):* May interfere with bactericidal activity. Use cautiously. *Loop diuretics, nephrotoxic drugs (aminoglycosides, colistin, polymyxin B, vancomycin):*
May increase the risk of nephrotoxicity. Patients need close monitoring.
Probenecid: Competitively inhibits renal tubular secretion of cephalosporins, resulting in higher, prolonged serum levels of these drugs. Use together cautiously.

Adverse reactions
CNS: *seizures.*
GI: pseudomembranous colitis, *nausea,* vomiting, *diarrhea,* glossitis, abdominal cramps, oral candidiasis.
GU: genital pruritus, candidiasis, vaginitis, renal dysfunction.
Hematologic: *transient neutropenia,* eosinophilia, *leukopenia,* anemia, *agranulocytosis, thrombocytopenia.*
Hepatic: transient increases in liver enzyme levels.
Respiratory: dyspnea.
Skin: *maculopapular and erythematous rashes,* urticaria.
Other: *hypersensitivity reactions* (serum sickness, *anaphylaxis, angioedema*), fever.

Overdose and treatment
Overdose may cause neuromuscular hypersensitivity; seizures may follow high CNS levels. Remove cefadroxil by hemodialysis. Other treatment is supportive.

Special considerations
Consider the recommendations relevant to all cephalosporins as well as the following.
• Longer half-life of this drug permits once- or twice-daily dosing.
• Cefadroxil causes false-positive results in urine glucose tests using cupric sulfate (Benedict's reagent or Clinitest); use glucose oxidase test (Chemstrip uG, Diastix, or glucose enzymatic test strip) instead. Cefadroxil causes false elevations in serum or urine creatinine levels in tests using Jaffé's reaction.
• Positive Coombs' test results occur in about 3% of patients taking cephalosporins.

Patient monitoring
• With large doses or prolonged therapy, monitor patient for superinfection, especially if high-risk.
• In patients with suspected renal impairment, monitor renal function tests before and during therapy.

Breast-feeding patients
• Drug appears in breast milk; use cautiously in breast-feeding women.

Pediatric patients
• Serum half-life is prolonged in neonates and infants under age 1.

Geriatric patients
• Reduce dosage in elderly patients with diminished renal function.

Reactions may be *common,* uncommon, *life-threatening,* or COMMON AND LIFE-THREATENING.

Patient education
• Inform patient of potential adverse reactions.
• Instruct patient to take medication with food to lessen GI discomfort.

cefamandole nafate
Mandol

Pharmacologic classification: second-generation cephalosporin
Therapeutic classification: antibiotic
Pregnancy risk category: B

Indications and dosages
➤ *Serious respiratory, GU, skin, soft-tissue, bone, and joint infections; septicemia; peritonitis from susceptible organisms.* Adults: 500 mg to 1 g I.M. or I.V. q 4 to 8 hours. In life-threatening infections, up to 2 g q 4 hours may be needed.
Infants and children: 50 to 100 mg/kg I.M. or I.V. daily in equally divided doses q 4 to 8 hours. May be increased to total daily dose of 150 mg/kg (not to exceed maximum adult dose) for severe infections.

Total daily dose is same for I.M. or I.V. administration and depends on susceptibility of organism and severity of infection. Inject drug deep I.M. into a large muscle mass, such as the gluteus or the lateral aspect of the thigh.
✦ *Dosage adjustment.* The following table gives appropriate doses for adults. In patients with impaired renal function, doses or frequency of administration must be modified according to degree of renal impairment, severity of infection, and susceptibility of organism.

Creatinine clearance (ml/min)	Severe infections	Life-threatening infections (maximum)
> 80	1 to 2 g q 6 hr	2 g q 4 hr
50-80	750 mg to 1.5 g q 6 hr	1.5 g q 4 hr or 2 g q 6 hr
25-50	750 mg to 1.5 g q 8 hr	1.5 g q 6 hr or 2 g q 8 hr
10-25	500 mg to 1 g q 8 hr	1 g q 6 hr or 1.25 g q 8 hr
2-10	500 to 750 mg q 12 hr	670 mg q 8 hr or 1 g q 12 hr
< 2	250 to 500 mg q 12 hr	500 mg q 8 hr or 750 mg q 12 hr

How supplied
Available by prescription only
For injection: 1 g, 2 g

Pharmacodynamics
Antibacterial action: Cefamandole is primarily bactericidal; it also may be bacteriostatic.

Activity depends on the organism, tissue penetration, dosage, and rate of organism multiplication. It acts by adhering to bacterial penicillin-binding proteins, thereby inhibiting cell wall synthesis.

Cefamandole is active against *Escherichia coli* and other coliform bacteria, *Staphylococcus aureus* (penicillinase- and nonpenicillinase-producing), *Staphylococcus epidermidis*, group A beta-hemolytic streptococci, *Klebsiella, Haemophilus influenzae, Proteus mirabilis,* and *Enterobacter. Bacteroides fragilis* and *Acinetobacter* are resistant.

Pharmacokinetics
Absorption: Not absorbed from the GI tract; must be given parenterally.
Distribution: Distributed widely into most body tissues and fluids, including the gallbladder, liver, kidneys, bone, sputum, bile, and pleural and synovial fluids; CSF penetration is poor. Cefamandole crosses the placenta; it's 65% to 75% protein-bound.
Metabolism: Not metabolized.
Excretion: Excreted mainly in urine by renal tubular secretion and glomerular filtration; small amounts of drug appear in breast milk. Elimination half-life is about ½ to 1 hour in patients with normal renal function; severe renal disease prolongs half-life to 12 to 18 hours.

Route	Onset	Peak	Duration
I.V., I.M.	Unknown	1½-2 hr	Unknown

Contraindications and precautions
Contraindicated in patients hypersensitive to drug or other cephalosporins. Use cautiously in breast-feeding women and in patients with impaired renal function or penicillin allergy.

Interactions
Drug-drug. *Anticoagulants:* May increase risk of bleeding. Avoid use together.
Bacteriostatic drugs (chloramphenicol, erythromycin, tetracyclines): May impair bactericidal activity. Use cautiously.
Loop diuretics, nephrotoxic drugs (aminoglycosides, colistin, polymyxin B, vancomycin): May increase the risk of nephrotoxicity. Monitor patient closely.
Probenecid: Competitively inhibits renal tubular secretion of cephalosporins, resulting in higher, prolonged serum levels of these drugs. Monitor patient closely.
Drug-lifestyle. *Alcohol use:* May cause severe disulfiram-like reactions. Advise patient not to consume alcohol during therapy.

Adverse reactions
GI: pseudomembranous colitis, nausea, vomiting, *diarrhea,* oral candidiasis.
Hematologic: eosinophilia, coagulation abnormalities.
Hepatic: transient increases in liver enzyme levels.

Skin: *maculopapular and erythematous rashes, urticaria.*
Other: *hypersensitivity reactions* (serum sickness, **anaphylaxis**); *pain, induration, sterile abscesses,* temperature elevation, tissue sloughing at injection site; *phlebitis, thrombophlebitis* with I.V. injection.

Overdose and treatment
Overdose may cause neuromuscular hypersensitivity. Seizures may follow high CNS levels. Hypoprothrombinemia and bleeding may occur; they may be treated with vitamin K or blood products. Some drug may be removed by hemodialysis.

Special considerations
● For most cephalosporin-sensitive organisms, cefamandole offers little advantage over other cephalosporins; it's less effective than cefoxitin against anaerobic infections. Some clinicians consider it inappropriate for pediatric use, especially for serious infections such as *Haemophilus influenzae.*
● For I.V. use, reconstitute 1 g with 10 ml of sterile water for injection, D₅W, or normal saline solution. Administer slowly, over 3 to 5 minutes, or by intermittent infusion or continuous infusion in compatible solutions. Check package insert.
● Don't mix with I.V. infusions containing magnesium or calcium ions, which are chemically incompatible and may cause irreversible effects.
● For I.M. use, dilute 1 g of cefamandole in 3 ml of sterile water for injection, bacteriostatic water for injection, normal saline solution for injection, or 0.9% bacteriostatic saline solution for injection.
● Administer cefamandole deeply into large muscle mass to ensure maximum absorption. Rotate injection sites.
● I.M. cefamandole is less painful than cefoxitin injection; it doesn't require addition of lidocaine.
● After reconstitution, solution remains stable for 24 hours at room temperature or 96 hours under refrigeration. Solution should be light yellow to amber. Don't use solution if it's discolored or contains a precipitate.
● Cefamandole causes false-positive results in urine glucose tests using cupric sulfate (Benedict's reagent or Clinitest); use glucose oxidase tests (Chemstrip uG, Diastix, or glucose enzymatic test strip) instead. Cefamandole also causes false elevations in serum or urine creatinine levels in tests using Jaffé's reaction. Drug may cause positive Coombs' test results and may elevate liver function test results or PT.

Patient monitoring
● Monitor patient for bleeding, and evaluate PT and platelet level. Patient may need prophylactic use of vitamin K to prevent bleeding.
● Bleeding can be reversed by giving vitamin K or blood products.

● In patient with suspected renal impairment, monitor renal function before and during therapy.

Breast-feeding patients
● Drug appears in breast milk; use cautiously in breast-feeding women. Safety hasn't been established.

Pediatric patients
● Safety in infants under age 1 month hasn't been established.

Geriatric patients
● Hypoprothrombinemia and bleeding have been reported most frequently in geriatric, malnourished, and debilitated patients.

Patient education
● Inform patient of potential adverse reactions.

cefazolin sodium
Ancef, Kefzol, Zolicef

Pharmacologic classification: first-generation cephalosporin
Therapeutic classification: antibiotic
Pregnancy risk category: B

Indications and dosages
➤ *Serious respiratory, GU, skin, soft-tissue, bone, and joint infections; biliary tract infections; septicemia; endocarditis from susceptible organisms; perioperative prophylaxis; contaminated surgery*◇. *Adults:* 250 mg I.M. or I.V. q 8 hours to 1 g q 8 hours. Maximum daily dose is 12 g in life-threatening situations.
Children over age 1 month: 25 to 100 mg/kg I.M. or I.V. daily in divided doses q 8 hours.

Total daily dose is same for I.M. or I.V. administration and depends on the susceptibility of organism and severity of infection. Inject cefazolin deep I.M. into a large muscle mass, such as the gluteus or the lateral aspect of the thigh.
✦ *Dosage adjustment.* Dose or frequency of administration must be modified according to the degree of renal impairment, severity of infection, susceptibility of organism, and serum levels of drug. Because drug can be removed by hemodialysis, patients undergoing hemodialysis may need a dosage adjustment.

Creatinine clearance (ml/min)	Adult dosage
35-54	Full dose q 8 hr or less frequently
11-34	½ usual dose q 12 hr
≤ 10	½ usual dose q 18 to 24 hr

Creatinine clearance (ml/min)	Pediatric dosage
40-70	60% of normal daily dose q 12 hr
20-40	25% of normal daily dose q 12 hr
5-20	10% of normal daily dose q 24 hr

How supplied
Available by prescription only
Injection (parenteral): 250 mg, 500 mg, 1 g, 5 g, 10 g, 20 g
Infusion: 500-mg or 1-g Redi Vials, Faspaks, or ADD-Vantage vials

Pharmacodynamics
Antibacterial action: Cefazolin is primarily bactericidal; it also may be bacteriostatic. Activity depends on the organism, tissue penetration, dosage, and rate of organism multiplication. It acts by adhering to bacterial penicillin-binding proteins, thereby inhibiting cell wall synthesis.

Cefazolin is active against *Escherichia coli*, Enterobacteriaceae, *Haemophilus influenzae*, *Klebsiella*, *Proteus mirabilis*, *Staphylococcus aureus*, *Streptococcus pneumoniae*, and group A beta-hemolytic streptococci.

Pharmacokinetics
Absorption: Not well absorbed from the GI tract; must be given parenterally.
Distribution: Distributed widely into most body tissues and fluids, including the gallbladder, liver, kidneys, bone, sputum, bile, and pleural and synovial fluids; CSF penetration is poor. It crosses the placenta; it's 74% to 86% protein-bound.
Metabolism: Not metabolized.
Excretion: Excreted primarily unchanged in urine by renal tubular secretion and glomerular filtration; small amounts of drug appear in breast milk. Elimination half-life is about 1 to 2 hours in patients with normal renal function; end-stage renal disease prolongs half-life to 12 to 50 hours. Hemodialysis or peritoneal dialysis removes cefazolin.

Route	Onset	Peak	Duration
I.V.	Immediate	Immediate	Unknown
I.M.	Unknown	1-2 hr	Unknown

Contraindications and precautions
Contraindicated in patients hypersensitive to other cephalosporins. Use cautiously in breast-feeding women and patients with impaired renal function or penicillin allergy.

Interactions
Drug-drug. *Bacteriostatic drugs (chloramphenicol, erythromycin, tetracyclines):* May interfere with bactericidal activity. Avoid use together.

Loop diuretics, nephrotoxic drugs (aminoglycosides, colistin, polymyxin B, vancomycin): May increase the risk of nephrotoxicity. Patient needs close monitoring.
Probenecid: Competitively inhibits renal tubular secretion of cephalosporins, resulting in higher, prolonged serum levels of these drugs. Patient needs close monitoring.

Adverse reactions
GI: pseudomembranous colitis, nausea, anorexia, vomiting, *diarrhea*, glossitis, dyspepsia, abdominal cramps, anal pruritus, oral candidiasis.
GU: genital pruritus, candidiasis, vaginitis.
Hematologic: *neutropenia*, *leukopenia*, eosinophilia, *thrombocytopenia*.
Hepatic: transient increases in liver enzyme levels.
Skin: *maculopapular and erythematous rashes, urticaria, pruritus, Stevens-Johnson syndrome*.
Other: *hypersensitivity reactions* (serum sickness, *anaphylaxis*); *pain, induration, sterile abscesses, tissue sloughing* (at injection site); *phlebitis, thrombophlebitis* (with I.V. injection).

Overdose and treatment
Overdose may cause neuromuscular hypersensitivity, seizures may follow high CNS levels. Cefazolin may be removed by hemodialysis.

Special considerations
Consider the recommendations relevant to all cephalosporins as well as the following.
● For I.M. use, reconstitute with sterile water, bacteriostatic water, or normal saline solution: 2 ml to a 500-mg vial and 2.5 ml to a 1-g vial produces 225 mg/ml, and 330 mg/ml, respectively.
● Reconstituted solution is stable for 24 hours at room temperature and for 10 days if refrigerated.
● I.M. cefazolin injection is less painful than that of other cephalosporins.
● Cephalosporins cause false-positive results in urine glucose tests utilizing cupric sulfate (Benedict's reagent or Clinitest); use glucose oxidase tests (Chemstrip uG, Diastix, or glucose enzymatic test strip) instead. Cefazolin causes false elevations in serum or urine creatinine levels in tests using Jaffé's reaction. Cefazolin also causes positive Coombs' test results.

Patient monitoring
● For patients on sodium restriction, note that cefazolin injection contains 2 mEq of sodium per gram of drug.
● Obtain electrolyte studies.
● If patient has suspected renal impairment, monitor renal function tests.

Breast-feeding patients
● Safety hasn't been established. Use drug cautiously in breast-feeding women.

Pediatric patients
• Drug has been used in children. However, safety in infants under age 1 month hasn't been established.

Patient education
• Inform patient of potential adverse reactions.

cefdinir
Omnicef

Pharmacologic classification: third-generation cephalosporin
Therapeutic classification: antibiotic
Pregnancy risk category: B

Indications and dosages
➤ *Mild to moderate infection caused by susceptible strains of microorganisms resulting in community-acquired pneumonia, acute exacerbations of chronic bronchitis, acute maxillary sinusitis, acute bacterial otitis media, and uncomplicated skin and skin-structure infections.* Adults and adolescents age 13 and older: 300 mg P.O. q 12 hours or 600 mg P.O. q 24 hours for 10 days. (Use q-12-hour doses for pneumonia and skin infections.)
Children ages 6 months to 12 years: 7 mg/kg P.O. q 12 hours or 14 mg/kg P.O. q 24 hours for 10 days, up to maximum dose of 600 mg daily. (Use q-12-hour dosages for skin infections.)
➤ *Pharyngitis, tonsillitis.* Adults and adolescents age 13 and older: 300 mg P.O. q 12 hours for 5 to 10 days or 600 mg P.O. q 24 hours for 10 days.
Children ages 6 months to 12 years: 7 mg/kg P.O. q 12 hours for 5 to 10 days or 14 mg/kg P.O. q 24 hours for 10 days.
✦ *Dosage adjustment.* If creatinine clearance is less than 30 ml/minute, reduce dosage to 300 mg P.O. once daily for adults and 7 mg/kg P.O. (up to 300 mg) once daily for children. If patient undergoes long-term hemodialysis, give 300 mg or 7 mg/kg P.O. at end of each dialysis session and subsequently every other day.

How supplied
Available by prescription only
Capsules: 300 mg
Suspension: 125 mg/5 ml

Pharmacodynamics
Antibiotic action: The bactericidal activity of cefdinir results from inhibition of cell wall synthesis. Drug is stable in the presence of some beta-lactamase enzymes, causing some microorganisms resistant to penicillins and cephalosporins to be susceptible to cefdinir. Excluding *Pseudomonas, Enterobacter, Enterococcus,* and methicillin-resistant *Staphylococcus* species, the spectrum of activity of cefdinir includes a broad range of gram-positive and gram-negative aerobic microorganisms.

Pharmacokinetics
Absorption: Estimated bioavailability of drug is 21% following a 300-mg capsule dose, 16% following a 600-mg capsule dose, and 25% for the suspension.
Distribution: Mean volume of distribution for adults and children is 0.35 and 0.67 L/kg, respectively, and distribution to tonsil, sinus, lung, and middle ear tissue and fluid ranges from 15% to 35% of corresponding plasma levels. About 60% to 70% is bound to plasma proteins; binding is independent of concentration.
Metabolism: Not appreciably metabolized; its activity is due mainly to parent drug.
Excretion: Excreted mainly by kidneys; mean plasma elimination half-life is 1.7 hours. Drug clearance is reduced in patients with renal dysfunction.

Route	Onset	Peak	Duration
P.O.	Unknown	2-4 hr	Unknown

Contraindications and precautions
Contraindicated in patients allergic to cephalosporin class of antibiotics. Use cautiously in patients hypersensitive to penicillin because of possible cross-sensitivity with other beta-lactam antibiotics. Also use cautiously in patients with a history of colitis.

Interactions
Drug-drug. *Antacids that contain aluminum or magnesium, iron supplements:* Decreased absorption and bioavailability of cefdinir. Give these drugs 2 hours before or after cefdinir dose. *Probenecid:* Inhibits renal secretion of cefdinir. Monitor patient.
Drug-food. *Foods fortified with iron, such as infant formula:* Decreased absorption and bioavailability of cefdinir. Monitor patient.

Adverse reactions
CNS: headache.
GI: abdominal pain, *diarrhea,* nausea, vomiting.
GU: vaginal candidiasis, vaginitis.
Skin: rash.

Overdose and treatment
Information isn't available. Evidence of overdose with other beta-lactam antibiotics includes nausea, vomiting, epigastric distress, diarrhea, and seizures. Drug is removed by hemodialysis.

Special considerations
• Pseudomembranous colitis has been reported with many antibiotics, including cefdinir, and should be considered in patients whose symptoms include diarrhea subsequent to antibiotic therapy or in those with history of colitis.
• False-positive reactions for ketones (tests using nitroprusside only) and glucose (Clinitest,

Benedict's solution, Fehling's solution) in the urine have been reported. Generally, cephalosporins can induce a positive direct Coombs' test.

Patient monitoring
● In patient with suspected renal impairment, monitor renal function before and during therapy.
● As with many antibiotics, prolonged drug treatment may result in possible emergence and overgrowth of resistant organisms. Monitor patient for superinfection and consider alternative therapy if it occurs.

Breast-feeding patients
● Drug isn't detectable in breast milk following 600-mg doses.

Pediatric patients
● Safety and efficacy in infants under age 6 months haven't been established. Pharmacokinetic data for children are comparable to data for adults.

Geriatric patients
● Cefdinir is well tolerated in all age-groups. Safety and efficacy are comparable in geriatric patients and younger patients. Dosage adjustment isn't necessary unless patient has renal impairment.

Patient education
● Instruct patient to take antacids, iron supplements, and iron-fortified foods 2 hours before or after a cefdinir dose.
● Inform diabetic patient that each teaspoon of suspension contains 2.86 g of sucrose.
● Advise patient to report severe diarrhea or diarrhea accompanied by abdominal pain.

---

cefepime hydrochloride
Maxipime

Pharmacologic classification: semisynthetic third- or fourth-generation cephalosporin
Therapeutic classification: antibiotic
Pregnancy risk category: B

Indications and dosages
➤ *Mild to moderate urinary tract infections caused by* Escherichia coli, Klebsiella pneumoniae, *or* Proteus mirabilis, *including cases related to concurrent bacteremia with these microorganisms.* Adults: 0.5 to 1 g I.M. (use I.M. route only for infections caused by *E. coli*) or I.V. infused over 30 minutes q 12 hours for 7 to 10 days.
➤ *Severe urinary tract infections including pyelonephritis caused by* E. coli *or* K. pneumoniae. Adults: 2 g I.V. infused over 30 minutes q 12 hours for 10 days.
➤ *Moderate to severe pneumonia caused by* Streptococcus pneumoniae, Pseudomonas aeruginosa, K. pneumoniae, *or* Enterobacter species. Adults: 1 to 2 g I.V. infused over 30 minutes q 12 hours for 10 days.

➤ *Moderate to severe uncomplicated skin and skin structure infections from* Staphylococcus aureus *(methicillin-susceptible strains) or* Streptococcus pyogenes. Adults: 2 g I.V. infused over 30 minutes q 12 hours for 10 days.
➤ *Empiric therapy in febrile neutropenia.* Adults: 2 g I.V. q 8 hours for 7 days or until neutropenia resolves.
Children who weigh less than 40 kg (88 lb): 50 mg/kg I.V. q 8 hours.
➤ *Uncomplicated and complicated urinary tract infections, uncomplicated skin and skin-structure infections, or pneumonia. Children who weigh less than 40 kg:* 50 mg/kg I.V. q 12 hours. Or, the American Academy of Pediatrics recommends for children older than 1 month a dosage of 1 to 2 g daily, divided b.i.d. for mild to moderate infections, or 2 to 4 g daily divided b.i.d. for severe infections.
    Pediatric dosages shouldn't exceed recommended adult dosages.
✦ *Dosage adjustment.* Adjust dosage in patients with impaired renal function. Consult manufacturer's recommendations. Patients receiving hemodialysis should receive a repeat dose at the end of dialysis. Patients undergoing continuous ambulatory peritoneal dialysis (CAPD) should receive the usual dose q 48 hours.

How supplied
Available by prescription only
Injection: 500 mg, 1 g, 2 g

Pharmacodynamics
Antibiotic action: Cefepime exerts bactericidal action by inhibiting cell wall synthesis. It's usually active against gram-positive microorganisms such as *S. pneumoniae, S. aureus,* and *S. pyogenes* and gram-negative microorganisms such as *Enterobacter* species, *E. coli, K. pneumoniae, P. mirabilis,* and *P. aeruginosa.*

Pharmacokinetics
Absorption: Completely absorbed after I.M. administration.
Distribution: Widely distributed; about 20% bound to serum protein.
Metabolism: Metabolized rapidly.
Excretion: About 85% is excreted in urine as unchanged drug; less than 1% as the metabolite, 6.8% as the metabolite oxide, and 2.5% as an epimer of cefepime.

Route	Onset	Peak	Duration
I.V., I.M.	½ hr	1-2 hr	Unknown

Contraindications and precautions
Contraindicated in patients hypersensitive to drug, other cephalosporins, penicillins, or other beta-lactam antibiotics. Use cautiously in patients with history of GI disease (especially colitis), impaired renal function, or poor nutritional status and in

those receiving a protracted course of antimicrobial therapy.

Interactions
Drug-drug. *Aminoglycosides:* May increase risk of nephrotoxicity and ototoxicity. Monitor patient's renal and hearing functions closely.
Potent diuretics such as furosemide: May increase risk of nephrotoxicity. Monitor patient's renal function.

Adverse reactions
CNS: headache.
GI: colitis, diarrhea, nausea, vomiting, oral candidiasis.
GU: vaginitis.
Skin: rash, pruritus, urticaria.
Other: phlebitis, pain, inflammation, fever.

Overdose and treatment
Overdose may cause seizures, encephalopathy, and neuromuscular excitability. Patients who receive an overdose should be carefully observed and given supportive treatment. If the patient has renal insufficiency, hemodialysis, not peritoneal dialysis, is recommended to help remove cefepime from the body.

Special considerations
Consider the recommendations relevant to all cephalosporins as well as the following.
⚠ ALERT Names of some cephalosporins are similar. Use caution when dispensing.
• Perform culture and sensitivity tests before giving first dose, if appropriate. Therapy may begin pending results.
• For I.V. administration, follow manufacturer guidelines closely when reconstituting drug. Variations occur in constituting drug for administration and depend on concentration of drug required and how drug is packaged (piggyback vial, ADD-Vantage vial, or regular vial). Type of diluent used for constitution varies, depending on product used. Use only solutions recommended by manufacturer. Administer the resulting solution over 30 minutes.
• Intermittent I.V. infusion with a Y-type administration set can be accomplished with compatible solutions. However, during infusion of a solution containing cefepime, discontinuing the other solution is recommended.
• For I.M. administration, constitute drug using sterile water for injection, normal saline solution, D₅W, 5% or 1% lidocaine hydrochloride, or bacteriostatic water for injection with parabens or benzyl alcohol. Follow manufacturer guidelines for quantity of diluent to use.
• Inspect solution visually for particulate matter before administration. The powder and its solutions tend to darken depending on storage conditions. However, product potency isn't adversely affected when stored as recommended.
• Cefepime may result in a false-positive reaction for glucose in the urine when using Clinitest

tablets. Use glucose tests based on enzymatic glucose oxidase reactions (such as Chemstrip uG, Diastix, or glucose enzymatic test strip) instead. A positive direct Coombs' test may occur during treatment.

Patient monitoring
• Many cephalosporins may cause a decrease in prothrombin activity; patients at risk include those with renal or hepatic impairment or poor nutritional status and those receiving prolonged cefepime therapy. PT must be checked. Exogenous vitamin K can be given if necessary.
• In patient with suspected renal impairment, monitor renal function before and during therapy.

Pregnant patients
• Use drug only when clearly needed during pregnancy.

Breast-feeding patients
• Drug appears in breast milk at very low levels; use cautiously.

Pediatric patients
• Safety and effectiveness in children under age 2 months haven't been established.

Geriatric patients
• Use caution when administering cefepime to geriatric patients. Dosage adjustment may be necessary in patients with impaired renal function.

Patient education
• Warn patient receiving drug I.M. that pain may occur at injection site.
• Instruct patient to report adverse reactions promptly.

---

cefixime
Suprax

Pharmacologic classification: third-generation cephalosporin
Therapeutic classification: antibiotic
Pregnancy risk category: B

Indications and dosages
➤ *Otitis media; acute bronchitis; acute exacerbations of chronic bronchitis, pharyngitis, tonsillitis; uncomplicated urinary tract infections caused by* Escherichia coli *and* Proteus mirabilis; *uncomplicated gonorrhea; disseminated gonococcal infections.* Adults and children who weigh more than 50 kg (110 lb) or are over age 12: 400 mg P.O. daily in one or two divided doses; for uncomplicated gonorrhea, 400 mg as a single dose.
Children over age 6 months or under age 12 who weigh less than 50 kg: 8 mg/kg P.O. daily in one or two divided doses.

Reactions may be *common,* uncommon, ***life-threatening,*** or COMMON AND LIFE-THREATENING.

✦ Dosage adjustment. In renally impaired patients, dosage must be adjusted based on degree of renal impairment, severity of infection, and susceptibility of organism. To prevent toxic accumulation in patients with creatinine clearance less than 60 ml/minute, reduced dosage may be needed.

Creatinine clearance (ml/min)	Adult dosage
20-60	75% of the usual dose
< 20 or patients receiving continuous ambulatory peritoneal dialysis	50% of the usual dose

How supplied
Available by prescription only
Powder for oral suspension: 100 mg/5 ml
Tablets: 200 mg, 400 mg

Pharmacodynamics
Antibacterial action: Cefixime is primarily bactericidal; it acts by binding to penicillin-binding proteins in the bacterial cell wall, thereby inhibiting cell wall synthesis.

It's used in the treatment of otitis media caused by *Haemophilus influenzae* (penicillinase- and nonpenicillinase-producing), *Moraxella (Branhamella) catarrhalis* (which is penicillinase-producing), and *Streptococcus pyogenes.* Substantial drug resistance has been noted. Cefixime is also active in the treatment of acute bronchitis and acute exacerbations of chronic bronchitis caused by *Streptococcus pneumoniae* and *H. influenzae* (penicillinase- and nonpenicillinase-producing), pharyngitis and tonsillitis caused by *S. pyogenes,* and uncomplicated urinary tract infections caused by *E. coli* and *P. mirabilis.*

Pharmacokinetics
Absorption: About 30% to 50% is absorbed following oral administration. The suspension form provides a higher serum level than the tablet form. Absorption is delayed by food, but the total amount absorbed isn't affected.
Distribution: Widely distributed; about 65% is bound to plasma proteins.
Metabolism: About 50% is metabolized.
Excretion: Excreted primarily in the urine. In patients with end-stage renal disease, half-life may be prolonged to 11½ hours.

Route	Onset	Peak	Duration
P.O.	Unknown	3-4½ hr	Unknown

Contraindications and precautions
Contraindicated in patients hypersensitive to drug or other cephalosporins. Use cautiously in patients with impaired renal function.

Interactions
Drug-drug. *Carbamazepine:* Elevated carbamazepine levels reported when administered together. Avoid use together.
Probenecid: May inhibit excretion and increase blood levels of cefixime. Use together cautiously.
Salicylates: May increase serum level of cefixime. Use together cautiously.

Adverse reactions
CNS: headache, dizziness.
GI: *diarrhea,* loose stools, abdominal pain, nausea, vomiting, dyspepsia, flatulence, pseudomembranous colitis.
GU: genital pruritus, vaginitis, genital candidiasis, transient increases in BUN and serum creatinine levels.
Hematologic: *thrombocytopenia, leukopenia,* eosinophilia.
Hepatic: transient increases in liver enzyme levels.
Skin: pruritus, rash, urticaria, erythema multiforme, *Stevens-Johnson syndrome.*
Other: drug fever, *hypersensitivity reactions* (serum sickness, *anaphylaxis*).

Overdose and treatment
No specific antidote available. Gastric lavage and supportive treatment are recommended. Peritoneal dialysis and hemodialysis will remove substantial quantities of drug.

Special considerations
Consider the recommendations relevant to all cephalosporins as well as the following.
⚠ ALERT Names of some cephalosporins are similar. Use caution when dispensing.
● Some cephalosporins may cause seizures, especially in patients with renal failure who receive full therapeutic dosages. If seizures occur, stop drug and start anticonvulsant therapy.
● Cefixime is the first orally active, third-generation cephalosporin that's effective with once-daily dosing.
● Manufacturer suggests that tablets shouldn't be substituted for suspension when treating otitis media.
● Cefixime may cause false-positive results in urine glucose tests utilizing cupric sulfate (Benedict's reagent or Clinitest); use glucose oxidase tests (Chemstrip uG, Diastix, or glucose enzymatic test strip) instead. Cefixime may cause false-positive results in tests for urine ketones that utilize nitroprusside (but not nitroferricyanide).
● False-positive direct Coombs' test results have occurred with other cephalosporins.

Patient monitoring
● Evaluate patients with antibiotic-induced diarrhea for overgrowth of pseudomembranous colitis caused by *Clostridium difficile.* Mild cases usually respond to discontinuation of the drug; moderate to severe cases may require fluid, electrolyte, and protein supplementation. Oral vancomycin is the drug of choice for the treatment

of antibiotic-associated *C. difficile* pseudomembranous colitis.

• Observe patient for hypersensitivity. Treat acute hypersensitivity reactions immediately. Emergency measures, such as airway management, pressor amines, epinephrine, oxygen, antihistamines, and corticosteroids, may be required.

• In patient with suspected renal impairment, monitor renal function before and during therapy.

Pregnant patients

• Use during pregnancy only when clearly needed.

Breast-feeding patients

• Distribution of drug in breast milk is unknown. The manufacturer recommends discontinuation of breast-feeding during cefixime therapy.

Pediatric patients

• The risk of adverse GI effects in children receiving oral suspension is similar to that in adults receiving tablets.

Patient education

• Instruct patient to report rash or symptoms of superinfection.

• Advise patient that oral suspension is stable for 14 days after reconstitution and doesn't require refrigeration.

• Tell patient to take all medication exactly as prescribed, even if he feels better.

cefoperazone sodium
Cefobid

Pharmacologic classification: third-generation cephalosporin
Therapeutic classification: antibiotic
Pregnancy risk category: B

Indications and dosages

➤*Serious respiratory tract, intra-abdominal, gynecologic, skin, skin-structure, urinary tract, and enterococcal infections; bacterial septicemia caused by susceptible organisms; perioperative prophylaxis* ◇. *Adults:* Usual dose is 1 to 2 g q 12 hours I.M. or I.V. In severe infections or infections caused by less sensitive organisms, the dosage may be increased up to 16 g daily in certain situations.

✦ *Dosage adjustment.* No dosage adjustment is usually necessary in patients with renal impairment. However, give doses of 4 g daily cautiously to patients with hepatic disease. Adults with impaired hepatic and renal function shouldn't receive more than 1 g (base) daily without serum determinations. In patients receiving hemodialysis, schedule a dose to follow treatment.

How supplied

Available by prescription only
Infusion: 1 g, 2 g piggyback

Parenteral: 1 g, 2 g, 10 g

Pharmacodynamics

Antibacterial action: Cefoperazone is primarily bactericidal; it also may be bacteriostatic. Activity depends on the organism, tissue penetration, dosage, and rate of organism multiplication. Drug acts by adhering to bacterial penicillin-binding proteins, thereby inhibiting cell wall synthesis. Third-generation cephalosporins appear to be more active against some beta-lactamase-producing gram-negative organisms.

Cefoperazone is active against some gram-positive organisms and many enteric gram-negative bacilli, including *Streptococcus pneumoniae* and *Streptococcus pyogenes, Staphylococcus aureus* (penicillinase- and nonpenicillinase-producing), *Staphylococcus epidermidis, Escherichia coli, Klebsiella, Haemophilus influenzae, Enterobacter, Citrobacter, Proteus,* some *Pseudomonas* species (including *Pseudomonas aeruginosa*), and *Bacteroides fragilis. Acinetobacter* and *Listeria* usually are resistant. Cefoperazone is less effective than cefotaxime or ceftizoxime against Enterobacteriaceae but is slightly more active than those drugs against *Pseudomonas aeruginosa.*

Pharmacokinetics

Absorption: Not absorbed from the GI tract; must be given parenterally.

Distribution: Distributed widely into most body tissues and fluids, including the gallbladder, liver, kidneys, bone, sputum, bile, and pleural and synovial fluids; CSF penetration occurs in patients with inflamed meninges. It crosses the placenta. Protein-binding is dose-dependent and decreases as serum levels rise; average is 82% to 93%.

Metabolism: Not substantially metabolized.

Excretion: Excreted primarily in bile; some drug is excreted in urine by renal tubular secretion and glomerular filtration; and small amounts in breast milk. Elimination half-life is about 1½ to 2½ hours in patients with normal hepatorenal function; biliary obstruction or cirrhosis prolongs half-life to about 3½ to 7 hours. Hemodialysis removes cefoperazone.

Route	Onset	Peak	Duration
I.V.	Immediate	Immediate	Unknown
I.M.	Unknown	1-2 hr	Unknown

Contraindications and precautions

Contraindicated in patients hypersensitive to drug or other cephalosporins. Use cautiously in breast-feeding women and patients with impaired renal or hepatic function or penicillin allergy.

Interactions

Drug-drug. *Aminoglycosides:* Synergistic activity against *P. aeruginosa* and *Serratia marcescens;* slightly increased risk of nephrotoxicity. Use together cautiously.

Reactions may be *common,* uncommon, *life-threatening,* or COMMON AND LIFE-THREATENING.

Anticoagulants: May increase risk of bleeding. Use together cautiously.

Probenecid: Competitively inhibits renal tubular secretion of cephalosporins, causing prolonged serum levels of these drugs. Use together cautiously.

Drug-lifestyle. *Alcohol use:* May cause disulfiram-like reaction. Discourage use.

Adverse reactions

GI: pseudomembranous colitis, nausea, vomiting, *diarrhea.*

Hematologic: *transient neutropenia, eosinophilia,* anemia, hypoprothrombinemia, bleeding.

Hepatic: mildly elevated liver enzyme levels.

Skin: *maculopapular and erythematous rashes, urticaria.*

Other: *hypersensitivity reactions* (serum sickness, *anaphylaxis*); *pain, induration, sterile abscesses, temperature elevation, tissue sloughing* (at injection site); *phlebitis, thrombophlebitis,* drug fever (with I.V. injection).

Overdose and treatment

Overdose may cause neuromuscular hypersensitivity. Seizures may follow high CNS levels. Hypoprothrombinemia and bleeding may occur and may require treatment with vitamin K or blood products. Hemodialysis removes cefoperazone.

Special considerations

Consider the recommendations relevant to all cephalosporins as well as the following.

• Diarrhea may be more common with drug than with other cephalosporins because of high degree of biliary excretion.

• Patients with biliary disease may need lower doses.

• For patients on sodium restriction, note that cefoperazone injection contains 1.5 mEq of sodium per gram of drug.

• To prepare I.M. injection, use the appropriate diluent, including sterile water for injection or bacteriostatic water for injection. Follow manufacturer's recommendations for mixing drug with sterile water for injection and lidocaine 2% injection. Final solution for I.M. injection will contain 0.5% lidocaine and will be less painful upon administration (recommended for concentrations of 250 mg/ml or greater). Inject cefoperazone deep into a large muscle mass, such as the gluteus or the lateral aspect of the thigh.

• Store drug in refrigerator and away from light before reconstituting.

• Allow solution to stand after reconstituting to allow foam to dissipate and solution to clear. Solution can be shaken vigorously to ensure complete drug dissolution.

• After reconstitution, solution is stable for 24 hours at a controlled room temperature or 3 days if refrigerated. Protecting drug from light is unnecessary.

• Because cefoperazone is dialyzable, patients undergoing treatment with hemodialysis may require dosage adjustment.

• Cephalosporins cause false-positive results in urine glucose tests using cupric sulfate (Benedict's reagent or Clinitest); use glucose oxidase (Chemstrip uG, Diastix, or glucose enzymatic test strip) instead. Cefoperazone may cause positive Coombs' test results.

Patient monitoring

• Monitor INR regularly. Vitamin K promptly reverses bleeding if it occurs.

• In patient with suspected renal impairment, monitor renal function before and during therapy.

Pregnant patients

• Use during pregnancy only when clearly needed.

Breast-feeding patients

• Drug appears in breast milk; use cautiously in breast-feeding women.

Pediatric patients

• Safety and effectiveness in children under age 12 haven't been established.

Geriatric patients

• Hypoprothrombinemia and bleeding have been reported more frequently in geriatric patients. Use cautiously, and monitor PT and INR and check for signs of abnormal bleeding.

Patient education

• Inform patient of potential adverse reactions.

• Tell patient to report discomfort at I.V. site.

cefotaxime sodium
Claforan

Pharmacologic classification: third-generation cephalosporin
Therapeutic classification: antibiotic
Pregnancy risk category: B

Indications and dosages

➤ *Serious lower respiratory, urinary, CNS, bone, joint, intra-abdominal, gynecologic, and skin infections; bacteremia; septicemia caused by susceptible organisms; pelvic inflammatory disease. Adults and children who weigh more than 50 kg (110 lb):* Usual dose is 1 g I.V. or I.M. q 6 to 12 hours. Up to 12 g daily can be given in life-threatening infections.

Children ages 1 month to 12 years who weigh less than 50 kg: 50 to 180 mg/kg I.V. daily in four or six equally divided doses. Higher doses are reserved for serious infections (such as meningitis).

Neonates ages 1 to 4 weeks: 50 mg/kg I.V. q 8 hours.

Neonates up to age 1 week: 50 mg/kg I.V. q 12 hours.

Total daily dose is same for I.M. or I.V. administration and depends on susceptibility of organism and severity of infection. Inject cefotaxime deep into a large muscle mass, such as the gluteus or the lateral aspect of the thigh.

➤ *Uncomplicated gonorrhea. Adults and adolescents:* 1 g I.M. as a single dose.

➤ *Perioperative prophylaxis. Adults:* 1 g I.V. or I.M. 30 to 90 minutes before surgery.

➤ *Disseminated gonococcal infection◊. Adults:* 1 g I.V. q 8 hours.

Neonates and infants: 25 to 50 mg/kg I.V. q 8 to 12 hours for 7 days or 50 to 100 mg/kg I.M. or I.V. q 12 hours for 7 days.

➤ *Gonococcal ophthalmia ◊. Adults:* 500 mg I.V. q.i.d.

Neonates: 100 mg I.V. or I.M. for one dose; may continue until ocular cultures are negative at 48 to 72 hours.

➤ *Gonorrheal meningitis or arthritis ◊. Neonates and infants:* 25 to 50 mg/kg I.V. q 8 to 12 hours for 10 to 14 days or 50 to 100 mg/kg I.M. or I.V. q 12 hours for 10 to 14 days.

✦ *Dosage adjustment.* In patients with impaired renal function, modify dose or frequency of administration based on degree of renal impairment, severity of infection, and susceptibility of organism. To prevent toxic accumulation, reduced dosage may be required in patients with creatinine clearance below 20 ml/minute.

How supplied
Available by prescription only
Infusion: 1 g, 2 g
Injection: 500 mg, 1 g, 2 g
Pharmacy bulk package: 10-g vial

Pharmacodynamics
Antibacterial action: Cefotaxime is primarily bactericidal; it also may be bacteriostatic. Activity depends on the organism, tissue penetration, dosage, and rate of organism multiplication. It acts by adhering to bacterial penicillin-binding proteins, thereby inhibiting cell wall synthesis.

Third-generation cephalosporins appear to be more active against some beta-lactamase–producing gram-negative organisms. Cefotaxime is active against some gram-positive organisms and many enteric gram-negative bacilli, including streptococci (*Streptococcus pneumoniae* and *pyogenes*), *Staphylococcus aureus* (penicillinase- and nonpenicillinase-producing), *Staphylococcus epidermidis, Escherichia coli, Klebsiella* species, *Haemophilus influenzae, Enterobacter* species, *Proteus* species, *Peptostreptococcus* species, and some strains of *Pseudomonas aeruginosa. Listeria* and *Acinetobacter* are often resistant. The active metabolite of cefotaxime, desacetylcefotaxime, may act synergistically with the parent drug against some bacterial strains.

Pharmacokinetics
Absorption: Not absorbed from the GI tract; must be given parenterally.

Distribution: Distributed widely into most body tissues and fluids, including the gallbladder, liver, kidneys, bone, sputum, bile, and pleural and synovial fluids. Unlike most other cephalosporins, drug has adequate CSF penetration when meninges are inflamed; it crosses the placenta; 13% to 38% is protein-bound.

Metabolism: Metabolized partially to an active metabolite, desacetylcefotaxime.

Excretion: Excreted primarily in urine by renal tubular secretion; some drug may appear in breast milk. About 25% of cefotaxime is excreted in urine as the active metabolite; elimination half-life in normal adults is about 1 to 1½ hours for cefotaxime and about 1½ to 2 hours for desacetylcefotaxime; severe renal impairment prolongs the half-life of cefotaxime to 11½ hours and that of the metabolite to as much as 56 hours. Hemodialysis removes both drug and its metabolites.

Route	Onset	Peak	Duration
I.V.	Immediate	Immediate	Unknown
I.M.	Unknown	½ hr	Unknown

Contraindications and precautions
Contraindicated in patients hypersensitive to drug or other cephalosporins. Use cautiously in breast-feeding patients and patients with impaired renal function or penicillin allergies.

Interactions
Drug-drug. *Aminoglycosides:* Apparent synergistic activity against Enterobacteriaceae and some strains of *P. aeruginosa* and *Serratia marcescens;* may increase risk of nephrotoxicity. Patient needs close monitoring.

Probenecid: May block renal tubular secretion of cefotaxime and prolong its half-life. Use together carefully.

Adverse reactions
CNS: headache.
GI: pseudomembranous colitis, nausea, vomiting, *diarrhea.*
GU: vaginitis, candidiasis, interstitial nephritis.
Hematologic: *transient neutropenia*, eosinophilia, hemolytic anemia, *thrombocytopenia, agranulocytosis.*
Hepatic: transient increases in liver enzyme levels.
Skin: *maculopapular and erythematous rashes*, urticaria.
Other: *hypersensitivity reactions* (serum sickness, *anaphylaxis*); elevated temperature; *pain, induration, sterile abscesses, temperature elevation, tissue sloughing* (at injection site); *phlebitis, thrombophlebitis* (with I.V. injection).

Reactions may be *common*, uncommon, *life-threatening*, or COMMON AND LIFE-THREATENING.

Overdose and treatment
Overdose may cause neuromuscular hypersensitivity. Seizures may follow high CNS levels. Cefotaxime may be removed by hemodialysis.

Special considerations
Consider the recommendations relevant to all cephalosporins as well as the following.
⚠ ALERT Names of some cephalosporins are similar. Use caution when dispensing.
• For patients on sodium restriction, note that cefotaxime contains 2.2 mEq of sodium per gram of drug.
• For I.M. injection, add 2 ml, 3 ml, or 5 ml of sterile or bacteriostatic water for injection to each 500-mg, 1-g, or 2-g vial. Shake well to dissolve drug completely. Check solution for particles and discoloration. Color ranges from light yellow to amber.
• Don't inject more than 1 g into a single I.M. site to prevent pain and tissue reaction.
• Don't mix with aminoglycosides or sodium bicarbonate or fluids with a pH above 7.5.
• For I.V. use, reconstitute all strengths of an I.V. dose with 10 ml of sterile water for injection. For infusion bottles, add 50 to 100 ml of normal saline solution injection or D₅W. May be further reconstituted to 50 to 1,000 ml with fluids recommended by manufacturer.
• Give drug by direct intermittent I.V. infusion over 3 to 5 minutes. Cefotaxime also may be given more slowly into a flowing I.V. line of compatible solution.
• Solution is stable for 24 hours at room temperature and at least 10 days under refrigeration in the original container. Cefotaxime may be stored in disposable glass or plastic syringes for 24 hours at room temperature or 5 days in the refrigerator.
• Cephalosporins cause false-positive results in urine glucose tests using cupric sulfate (Benedict's reagent or Clinitest); use glucose oxidase (Chemstrip uG, Diastix, or glucose enzymatic test strip) instead. Cefotaxime also causes false elevations in urine creatinine levels in tests using Jaffé's reaction. Cefotaxime may cause positive Coombs' tests results.

Patient monitoring
• With large doses or prolonged therapy, monitor patient for superinfection, especially if high-risk.
• If patient has suspected renal impairment, monitor renal function before and during therapy.

Breast-feeding patients
• Drug appears in breast milk and should be used cautiously in breast-feeding women.

Pediatric patients
• Cefotaxime may be used in neonates, infants, and children.

Geriatric patients
• Use cautiously in geriatric patients with diminished renal function.

Patient education
• Inform patient of potential adverse reactions.
• Instruct patient to report discomfort at I.V. site.

cefotetan disodium
Cefotan

Pharmacologic classification: second-generation cephalosporin, cephamycin
Therapeutic classification: antibiotic
Pregnancy risk category: B

Indications and dosages
➤ *Serious urinary, lower respiratory, gynecologic, skin, intra-abdominal, bone, and joint infections caused by susceptible organisms.* Adults: 500 mg to 3 g I.V. or I.M. q 12 hours for 5 to 10 days. Up to 6 g daily in life-threatening infections.
Children: 40 to 60 mg/kg I.V. daily divided in equal doses q 12 hours.
➤ *Perioperative prophylaxis; use in contaminated surgery* ◊. Adults: 1 to 2 g I.V. 30 to 60 minutes before surgery.
➤ *Postcesarean.* Adults: 1 to 2 g I.V. as soon as umbilical cord is clamped.

Total daily dose is same for I.M. and I.V. administration and depends on the susceptibility of the organism and severity of infection. Inject cefotetan deep into a large muscle mass, such as the gluteus or the lateral aspect of the thigh.
✦ *Dosage adjustment.* In patients with impaired renal function, doses or frequency of administration must be modified based on degree of renal impairment, severity of infection, and susceptibility of organism. To prevent toxic accumulation, reduced dosage may be necessary in patients with creatinine clearance less than 30 ml/minute, as shown. For patients receiving hemodialysis, give one-fourth the usual adult dose q 24 hours on the days between dialysis sessions and one-half the usual adult dose on the day of hemodialysis.

Creatinine clearance (ml/min)	Adult dosage
10-30	Usual adult dose q 24 hours; or one-half the usual adult dose q 12 hours
< 10	Usual adult dose q 48 hours; or one-fourth the usual adult dose q 12 hours

How supplied
Available by prescription only
Bulk package: 10 g
Infusion: 1-g, 2-g piggyback vials; frozen, premixed solutions of 1 g, 2 g in 50 ml

Injection: 1 g, 2 g

Pharmacodynamics

Antibacterial action: Cefotetan is primarily bactericidal; it also may be bacteriostatic. Activity depends on the organism, tissue penetration, dosage, and rate of organism multiplication. It acts by adhering to bacterial penicillin-binding proteins, thereby inhibiting cell wall synthesis.

Cefotetan is active against many gram-positive organisms and enteric gram-negative bacilli, including streptococci, *Staphylococcus aureus* (penicillinase- and nonpenicillinase-producing), *Staphylococcus epidermidis, Escherichia coli, Klebsiella* species, *Enterobacter* species, *Proteus* species, *Haemophilus influenzae, Neisseria gonorrhoeae,* and *Bacteroides* species (including some strains of *B. fragilis*); however, some *B. fragilis* strains, *Pseudomonas,* and *Acinetobacter* are resistant to cefotetan. Most Enterobacteriaceae are more susceptible to cefotetan than to other second-generation cephalosporins.

Pharmacokinetics

Absorption: Not absorbed from the GI tract; must be given parenterally.

Distribution: Distributed widely into most body tissues and fluids, including the gallbladder, liver, kidneys, bone, sputum, bile, and pleural and synovial fluids; CSF penetration is poor. Biliary levels of cefotetan can be up to 20 times higher than serum levels in patients with good gallbladder function. Cefotetan crosses the placenta and is 75% to 90% protein-bound.

Metabolism: Not metabolized.

Excretion: Excreted mainly in urine by glomerular filtration and some renal tubular secretion; 20% is excreted in the bile. Small amounts of drug appear in breast milk. Elimination half-life is about 3 to 4½ hours in patients with normal renal function.

Route	Onset	Peak	Duration
I.V.	Immediate	Immediate	Unknown
I.M.	Unknown	1½-3 hr	Unknown

Contraindications and precautions

Contraindicated in patients hypersensitive to drug or other cephalosporins. Use cautiously in breast-feeding women and in patients with impaired renal function or penicillin allergy.

Interactions

Drug-drug. *Anticoagulants:* May increase risk of bleeding. Monitor patient closely.

Loop diuretics, nephrotoxic drugs (aminoglycosides, colistin, polymyxin B, vancomycin): May increase the risk of nephrotoxicity. Monitor patient closely.

Probenecid: May inhibit excretion and increase blood levels of cefotetan. Sometimes used for this effect. Monitor patient closely.

Drug-lifestyle. *Alcohol use:* May cause disulfiram-like reaction (flushing, sweating, tachycardia, headache, abdominal cramping). Patient should avoid alcohol consumption while on therapy and shouldn't drink alcohol for several days after stopping cefotetan.

Adverse reactions

GI: pseudomembranous colitis, nausea, d*iarrhea.*

GU: *nephrotoxicity.*

Hematologic: *transient neutropenia,* eosinophilia, hemolytic anemia, hypoprothrombinemia, bleeding, thrombocytosis, *agranulocytosis, thrombocytopenia.*

Hepatic: transient increases in liver enzyme levels.

Skin: *maculopapular and erythematous rashes, urticaria pain, induration, sterile abscesses, tissue sloughing* at injection site; *phlebitis, thrombophlebitis* with I.V. injection.

Other: *hypersensitivity reactions* (serum sickness, *anaphylaxis*), elevated temperature.

Overdose and treatment

Overdose may cause neuromuscular hypersensitivity. Seizures may follow high CNS levels. Hypoprothrombinemia and bleeding may occur; they may be treated with vitamin K or blood products. Cefotetan may be removed by hemodialysis.

Special considerations

Consider the recommendations relevant to all cephalosporins as well as the following.

❗ ALERT Names of some cephalosporins are similar. Use caution when dispensing.

● For I.V. use, reconstitute drug with sterile water for injection. Then it may be mixed with 50 to 100 ml D₅W or normal saline solution. Infuse intermittently over 30 to 60 minutes.

● For I.M. injection, cefotetan may be reconstituted with sterile water or bacteriostatic water for injection or with normal saline solution or 0.5% or 1% lidocaine hydrochloride. Shake to dissolve and let solution stand until clear.

● Reconstituted solution remains stable for 24 hours at room temperature or for 96 hours when refrigerated.

● Cefotetan causes false-positive results in urine glucose tests using cupric sulfate (Benedict's reagent or Clinitest); use glucose oxidase tests (Chemstrip uG, Diastix, or glucose enzymatic test strip) instead. Cefotetan causes false elevations in serum or urine creatinine levels in tests using Jaffé's reaction. It may cause positive Coombs' test results.

Patient monitoring

● Assess patient for overt and occult bleeding. Monitor vital signs. Check CBC with differential, platelet levels, and PT for abnormalities.

● Bleeding can be reversed promptly by administering vitamin K.

Reactions may be *common*, uncommon, *life-threatening*, or COMMON AND LIFE-THREATENING.

• If patient has suspected renal impairment, monitor renal function before and during therapy.

Pregnant patients
• Use only when clearly needed.

Breast-feeding patients
• Cephalosporins appear in breast milk; use cautiously in breast-feeding women. Safety in breast-feeding women hasn't been established.

Pediatric patients
• Safety in children hasn't been established.

Geriatric patients
• Hypoprothrombinemia and bleeding have been reported more frequently in geriatric and debilitated patients.

Patient education
• Inform patient of potential adverse reactions.
• Tell patient to promptly report signs of bleeding and discomfort at I.V. site.

cefoxitin sodium
Mefoxin

Pharmacologic classification: second-generation cephalosporin, cephamycin
Therapeutic classification: antibiotic
Pregnancy risk category: B

Indications and dosages
➤ *Serious respiratory, GU, gynecologic, skin, soft-tissue, bone, joint, blood, and intra-abdominal infections caused by susceptible organisms.* Adults: 1 to 2 g I.V. q 6 to 8 hours for uncomplicated forms of infection. Up to 12 g daily in life-threatening infections.
Children over age 3 months: 80 to 160 mg/kg I.V. daily given in four to six equally divided doses. Don't exceed 12 g daily.

Total daily dose is same for I.M. and I.V. administration and depends on susceptibility of organism and severity of infection. Inject cefoxitin deep into a large muscle mass, such as the gluteus or lateral aspect of the thigh.
➤ *Perioperative prophylaxis; use in contaminated surgery* ◇. Adults: 2 g I.V. 30 to 60 minutes before surgery; then 2 g I.V. q 6 hours for 24 hours postoperatively.
Children over age 3 months: 30 to 40 mg/kg I.V. 30 to 60 minutes before surgery; then 30 mg/kg I.V. q 6 hours for 24 hours postoperatively. For contaminated surgery, 1 to 2 g I.V. q 6 hours with or without I.V. gentamicin (1.5 mg/kg q 8 hours) for 5 days.
➤ *Uncomplicated gonorrhea* ◇. Adults: Give 2 g I.M. as a single dose with 1 g probenecid P.O. at the same time or up to 30 minutes beforehand.
➤ *Pelvic inflammatory disease.* Adults: 2 g I.V. q 6 hours. (If *Chlamydia trachomatis* is suspected, give additional antichlamydial coverage.)
✦ *Dosage adjustment.* In patients with impaired renal function, doses or frequency of administration must be modified based on degree of renal impairment, severity of infection, and susceptibility of organism. To prevent toxic accumulation, reduced dosage may be required in patients with creatinine clearance less than 50 ml/minute.

Creatinine clearance (ml/min)	Adult dosage
30-50	1 to 2 g q 8 to 12 hours
10-29	1 to 2 g q 12 to 24 hours
5-9	500 mg to 1 g q 12 to 24 hours
< 5	500 mg to 1 g q 24 to 48 hours

How supplied
Available by prescription only
Injection: 1 g, 2 g
Infusion: 1 g, 2 g in 50-ml containers
Pharmacy bulk package: 10 g

Pharmacodynamics
Antibacterial action: Cefoxitin is primarily bactericidal; it also may be bacteriostatic. Activity depends on the organism, tissue penetration, dosage, and rate of organism multiplication. It acts by adhering to bacterial penicillin-binding proteins, thereby inhibiting cell wall synthesis.

Cefoxitin is active against many gram-positive organisms and enteric gram-negative bacilli, including *Escherichia coli* and other coliform bacteria, *Staphylococcus aureus* (penicillinase- and nonpenicillinase-producing), *Staphylococcus epidermidis,* streptococci, *Klebsiella, Haemophilus influenzae,* and *Bacteroides* species (including *B. fragilis*). *Enterobacter, Pseudomonas,* and *Acinetobacter* are resistant to cefoxitin.

Pharmacokinetics
Absorption: Not absorbed from the GI tract; must be given parenterally.
Distribution: Distributed widely into most body tissues and fluids, including the gallbladder, liver, kidneys, bone, sputum, bile, and pleural and synovial fluids; CSF penetration is poor. Cefoxitin crosses the placenta, and is 50% to 80% protein-bound.
Metabolism: About 2% of a cefoxitin dose is metabolized.
Excretion: Excreted primarily in urine by renal tubular secretion and glomerular filtration; small amounts of drug appear in breast milk. Elimination half-life is about 0.7 to 1.1 hours in patients with normal renal function; half-life is prolonged in patients with severe renal dysfunction to 6.3

to 21.5 hours. Cefoxitin can be removed by hemodialysis but not by peritoneal dialysis.

Route	Onset	Peak	Duration
I.V.	Immediate	Immediate	Unknown
I.M.	Unknown	20-30 min	Unknown

Contraindications and precautions
Contraindicated in patients hypersensitive to drug or other cephalosporins. Use cautiously in breast-feeding women and patients with impaired renal function or penicillin allergy.

Interactions
Drug-drug. *Bacteriostatic drugs (chloramphenicol, erythromycin, tetracyclines):* May impair the bactericidal activity of cefoxitin. Avoid use together.
Loop diuretics, nephrotoxic drugs (aminoglycosides, colistin, polymyxin B, vancomycin): May increase the risk of nephrotoxicity. Monitor patient closely.
Probenecid: Competitively inhibits renal tubular secretion of cephalosporins, resulting in higher, prolonged serum levels of these drugs. Monitor patient closely.

Adverse reactions
CV: hypotension, *thrombophlebitis.*
GI: pseudomembranous colitis, nausea, vomiting, *diarrhea.*
GU: *acute renal failure.*
Hematologic: *transient neutropenia,* eosinophilia, *hemolytic anemia,* anemia, *thrombocytopenia.*
Hepatic: transient increases in liver enzyme levels.
Respiratory: dyspnea with I.V. injection.
Skin: *maculopapular and erythematous rash,* urticaria, exfoliative dermatitis, *pain, induration, sterile abscesses, tissue sloughing* at injection site.
Other: *hypersensitivity reactions* (serum sickness, *anaphylaxis*), elevated temperature, *phlebitis.*

Overdose and treatment
Overdose may cause neuromuscular hypersensitivity. Seizures may follow high CNS levels. Cefoxitin may be removed by hemodialysis.

Special considerations
Consider the recommendations relevant to all cephalosporins as well as the following.
⚠ ALERT Names of some cephalosporins are similar. Use caution when dispensing.
● For I.V. use, reconstitute 1 g of cefoxitin with at least 10 ml of sterile water for injection, or 2 g of cefoxitin with 10 to 20 ml. Solutions of D$_5$W and normal saline solution for injection can also be used.
● For I.M. injection, reconstitute with 0.5% to 1% lidocaine hydrochloride (without epinephrine)

to minimize pain at injection site; or with sterile water for injection.
● Administer cefoxitin I.M. deep into a large muscle mass. Aspirate before injecting to prevent inadvertent injection into a blood vessel, and rotate sites to prevent tissue damage.
● After reconstituting, shake vial and then let stand until clear to ensure complete drug dissolution. Solution is stable for 24 hours at room temperature, for 1 week if refrigerated, or 26 weeks if frozen.
● Solution may range from colorless to light amber and may darken during storage. Slight color change doesn't indicate loss of potency.
● Cefoxitin injection contains 2.3 mEq of sodium per gram of drug.
● Cefoxitin causes false-positive results in urine glucose tests using cupric sulfate (Benedict's reagent or Clinitest); use glucose oxidase tests (Chemstrip uG, Diastix, or glucose enzymatic test strip) instead. Cefoxitin also causes false elevations in serum or urine creatinine levels in tests using Jaffé's reaction. May cause positive Coombs' test results.

Patient monitoring
● Cefoxitin has been linked to thrombophlebitis. Frequently assess I.V. site for signs of infiltration or phlebitis.
● If patient has suspected renal impairment, monitor renal function before and during therapy.

Pregnant patients
● Use only when clearly needed.

Breast-feeding patients
● Drug appears in breast milk; use cautiously in breast-feeding women.

Pediatric patients
● Dosage may need to be reduced in infants under age 3 months. Safety hasn't been established.

Geriatric patients
● Dosage reduction may be necessary in patients with diminished renal function.

Patient education
● Inform patient of potential adverse reactions.

cefpodoxime proxetil
Vantin

Pharmacologic classification: third-generation cephalosporin
Therapeutic classification: antibiotic
Pregnancy risk category: B

Indications and dosages
➤ **Acute, community-acquired pneumonia caused by** Haemophilus influenzae **or** Streptococcus pneumoniae. *Adults:* 200 mg P.O. q 12 hours for 14 days.

Reactions may be *common*, uncommon, *life-threatening*, or COMMON AND LIFE-THREATENING.

➤*Acute bacterial exacerbations of chronic bronchitis caused by non–beta-lactamase-producing strains of* H. influenzae, S. pneumoniae, *or* Moraxella catarrhalis. *Adults:* 200 mg P.O. q 12 hours for 10 days.

➤*Uncomplicated gonorrhea in men and women; rectal gonococcal infections in women. Adults:* 200 mg P.O. as a single dose. Follow with doxycycline 100 mg P.O. b.i.d. for 7 days.

➤*Uncomplicated skin and skin-structure infections caused by* Staphylococcus aureus *or* Streptococcus pyogenes. *Adults:* 400 mg P.O. q 12 hours for 7 to 14 days.

➤*Acute otitis media caused by* S. pneumoniae, H. influenzae, *or* M. catarrhalis. *Children ages 2 months to 12 years:* 5 mg/kg (not to exceed 200 mg) P.O. q 12 hours for 5 days.

➤*Pharyngitis or tonsillitis caused by* S. pyogenes. *Adults:* 100 mg P.O. q 12 hours for 7 to 10 days.

Children ages 2 months to 12 years: 5 mg/kg (not to exceed 100 mg) P.O. q 12 hours for 5 to 10 days.

➤*Uncomplicated urinary tract infections caused by* Escherichia coli, Klebsiella pneumoniae, Proteus mirabilis, *or* Staphylococcus saprophyticus. *Adults:* 100 mg P.O. q 12 hours for 7 days.

➤*Acute maxillary sinusitis. Children ages 2 months to 12 years:* 5 mg/kg (up to 200 mg) q 12 hours for 10 days.

✦ *Dosage adjustment.* In patients with renal impairment when creatinine clearance is less than 30 ml/minute, increase dosage interval to q 24 hours. Patients receiving hemodialysis should receive drug three times weekly, after dialysis.

How supplied
Available by prescription only
Oral suspension: 50 mg/5 ml, 100 mg/5 ml
Tablets (film-coated): 100 mg, 200 mg

Pharmacodynamics
Antibiotic action: A second-generation cephalosporin, cefpodoxime proxetil is a bactericidal agent that inhibits cell wall synthesis. It's usually active against gram-positive aerobes, such as *S. aureus* (including penicillinase-producing strains), *S. saprophyticus, S. pneumoniae,* and *S. pyogenes,* and gram-negative aerobes, such as *E. coli, H. influenzae* (including beta-lactamase–producing strains), *K. pneumoniae, M. catarrhalis, Neisseria gonorrhoeae* (including penicillinase-producing strains), and *P. mirabilis.*

Pharmacokinetics
Absorption: Absorbed via the GI tract. Absorption and mean peak plasma levels increase when drug is given with food.
Distribution: Widely distributed to most tissues and fluids. Second-generation cephalosporins don't enter CSF even when the meninges are in-

flamed. Protein-binding ranges from 22% to 33% in serum and from 21% to 29% in plasma.
Metabolism: De-esterified to its active metabolite, cefpodoxime.
Excretion: Excreted primarily in urine.

Route	Onset	Peak	Duration
P.O.	Unknown	2-3 hr	Unknown

Contraindications and precautions
Contraindicated in patients hypersensitive to drug or other cephalosporins. Use cautiously in breast-feeding women and in patients with impaired renal function or penicillin allergy.

Interactions
Drug-drug. *Antacids, H₂-receptor antagonists:* Decreased cefpodoxime proxetil absorption. Avoid concurrent administration.
Probenecid: Decreased cefpodoxime proxetil excretion. Monitor patient for cefpodoxime toxicity.
Drug-food. *Any food:* Increased absorption. Give drug with food.

Adverse reactions
CNS: headache.
GI: *diarrhea,* nausea, vomiting, abdominal pain.
GU: vaginal fungal infections.
Skin: rash.
Other: *hypersensitivity reactions (anaphylaxis).*

Overdose and treatment
No information available. Toxic signs and symptoms after an overdose of beta-lactam antibiotics may include nausea, vomiting, epigastric distress, and diarrhea. In the event of serious toxic reaction from overdose, hemodialysis or peritoneal dialysis may help remove drug from the body, particularly if renal function is compromised.

Special considerations
❚ ALERT Names of some cephalosporins are similar. Use caution when dispensing.
● Drug is highly stable in presence of beta-lactamase enzymes. As a result, many organisms resistant to penicillins and some cephalosporins, because of presence of beta-lactamases, may be susceptible to cefpodoxime proxetil.
● Cefpodoxime is inactive against most strains of *Pseudomonas, Enterobacter,* and *Enterococcus.*
● Obtain specimens for culture and sensitivity tests before first dose. Therapy may begin pending test results.
● Store suspension in refrigerator (36° to 46° F [2° to 8° C]). Shake well before using. Discard unused portion after 14 days.
● Cefpodoxime proxetil may induce a positive direct Coombs' test.

Patient monitoring
● As with other antibiotics, prolonged use of cefpodoxime proxetil may result in overgrowth of nonsusceptible organisms. Repeated evaluation

of the patient's condition is essential, and appropriate measures should be taken if superinfection occurs during therapy.
• If patient has suspected renal impairment, monitor renal function before and during therapy.

Pregnant patients
• Use only when clearly needed.

Breast-feeding patients
• Drug appears in breast milk. Because of the risk of serious reactions in breast-fed infants, a decision must be made to discontinue breast-feeding or drug, taking into account the importance of drug to the woman.

Pediatric patients
• Safety and efficacy in infants under age 6 months haven't been established.

Geriatric patients
• No dosage adjustment is necessary. Any patient on dialysis, especially an elderly patient, should receive the dose after dialysis treatment.

Patient education
• Tell patient to report rash or signs and symptoms of superinfection.
• Advise patient to continue taking drug for the prescribed course of therapy, even after feeling better.

cefprozil
Cefzil

Pharmacologic classification: second-generation cephalosporin
Therapeutic classification: antibiotic
Pregnancy risk category: B

Indications and dosages
➤ *Pharyngitis or tonsillitis caused by* Streptococcus pyogenes. *Adults and children age 13 and older:* 500 mg P.O. daily for at least 10 days.
Children ages 2 to 12: 7.5 mg/kg P.O. q 12 hours for 10 days.
➤ *Otitis media caused by* Streptococcus pneumoniae, Haemophilus influenzae, *or* Moraxella catarrhalis. *Infants and children ages 6 months to 12 years:* 15 mg/kg P.O. q 12 hours for 10 days.
➤ *Secondary bacterial infections of acute bronchitis and acute bacterial exacerbation of chronic bronchitis caused by* S. pneumoniae, H. influenzae, *or* M. catarrhalis. *Adults:* 500 mg P.O. q 12 hours for 10 days.
➤ *Uncomplicated skin and skin-structure infections caused by* Staphylococcus aureus *or* S. pyogenes. *Adults and children age 13 and older:* 250 mg P.O. b.i.d. or 500 mg daily to b.i.d. for 10 days.

Children ages 2 to 12: 20 mg/kg P.O. q 24 hours for 10 days.
✦ *Dosage adjustment.* No adjustments are necessary for patients with creatinine clearance above 30 ml/minute. For patients with creatinine clearance of 30 ml/minute or less, reduce dose by 50% but maintain dosing interval. Because drug is partially removed by hemodialysis, administer after the hemodialysis session.

How supplied
Available by prescription only
Oral suspension: 125 mg/5 ml, 250 mg/5 ml
Tablets: 250 mg, 500 mg

Pharmacodynamics
Antibiotic action: Cefprozil interferes with bacterial cell wall synthesis during cell replication, leading to osmotic instability and cell lysis. Action is bactericidal or bacteriostatic, depending on concentration.

Pharmacokinetics
Pharmacokinetic data are derived from investigational studies that used an oral capsule form that isn't commercially available.
Absorption: About 95% absorbed from the GI tract.
Distribution: About 36% protein-bound.
Metabolism: Probably metabolized by the liver; plasma half-life increases only slightly in patients with impaired hepatic function.
Excretion: About 60% of a dose is recovered unchanged in the urine. Plasma half-life is 1⅓ hours in patients with normal renal function; 2 hours with impaired hepatic function; and 5¼ to 6 hours with end-stage renal disease. Drug is removed by hemodialysis.

Route	Onset	Peak	Duration
P.O.	Unknown	1½ hr	Unknown

Contraindications and precautions
Contraindicated in patients hypersensitive to drug or other cephalosporins. Use cautiously in breast-feeding women and patients with impaired renal function or penicillin allergy.

Interactions
Drug-drug. *Aminoglycosides:* May increase the risk of nephrotoxicity of cephalosporins. Monitor patient closely.
Probenecid: May decrease excretion and increase blood cefprozil levels. Use together cautiously.

Adverse reactions
CNS: dizziness, hyperactivity, headache, nervousness, insomnia, confusion, somnolence.
GI: *diarrhea, nausea,* vomiting, abdominal pain.
GU: elevated BUN level, elevated serum creatinine level, genital pruritus, vaginitis.
Hematologic: decreased leukocyte count, eosinophilia.
Hepatic: elevated liver enzyme levels.

Reactions may be *common*, uncommon, *life-threatening*, or COMMON AND LIFE-THREATENING.

Skin: rash, urticaria, diaper rash.
Other: superinfection, *hypersensitivity reactions* (serum sickness, *anaphylaxis*).

Overdose and treatment
Because drug is eliminated primarily by the kidneys, hemodialysis may aid in removing drug in cases of extreme overdose, especially in patients with decreased renal function.

Special considerations
Consider the recommendations relevant to all cephalosporins as well as the following.
⚠ **ALERT** Names of some cephalosporins are similar. Use caution when dispensing.
● Obtain specimens for culture and sensitivity tests before first dose. Therapy may begin pending test results.
● Cephalosporins may produce a false-positive test for urine glucose with tests that use copper reduction method (Benedict's test, Fehling's solution, or Clinitest tablets). Instead, use enzymatic methods, such as glucose enzymatic test strip. A false-negative reaction may occur in the ferricyanide test for blood glucose.

Patient monitoring
● In patient with suspected renal impairment, monitor renal function before and during therapy.
● Drug may cause overgrowth of nonsusceptible bacteria or fungi. Observe patient for signs and symptoms of superinfection.
● Monitor patient for pseudomembranous colitis, which has been reported with nearly all antibacterial agents. It may occur in patients in whom diarrhea develops secondary to antibiotic therapy. Although most patients respond to withdrawal of drug therapy alone, it may be necessary to institute treatment with an antibacterial agent effective against *Clostridium difficile,* an organism linked to this disorder.

Pregnant patients
● Use during pregnancy or labor and delivery only when clearly needed.

Breast-feeding patients
● It isn't known if drug appears in breast milk. Use cautiously in breast-feeding women.

Pediatric patients
● Oral suspensions contain drug in a bubble gum–flavored vehicle to improve palatability and compliance in children. Store reconstituted suspension in the refrigerator, and discard unused drug after 14 days. Shake suspension well before measuring dose.

Geriatric patients
● Elderly patients (age 65 and older) had a higher area under the plasma-concentration-versus-time curve and lower renal clearance compared with younger subjects.

Patient education
● Tell patient to take all of drug as prescribed, even if he feels better.
● Advise patients with phenylketonuria that oral suspension contains 28 mg/5 ml phenylalanine.
● Instruct patient to notify prescriber if rash or symptoms of superinfection occur.

---

ceftazidime
Ceptaz, Fortaz, Tazicef, Tazidime

Pharmacologic classification: third-generation cephalosporin
Therapeutic classification: antibiotic
Pregnancy risk category: B

Indications and dosages
➤ *Bacteremia, septicemia, and serious respiratory tract, urinary tract, gynecologic, bone and joint, intra-abdominal, CNS, and skin infections from susceptible organisms. Adults:* 1 g I.V. or I.M. q 8 to 12 hours; up to 6 g daily in life-threatening infections.
Children ages 1 month to 12 years: 30 to 50 mg/kg I.V. q 8 hours to a maximum of 6 g daily (Fortaz, Tazicef, and Tazidime only).
Neonates up to age 4 weeks: 30 mg/kg I.V. q 12 hours (Fortaz, Tazicef, and Tazidime only).
Total daily dose is the same for I.M. or I.V. administration and depends on susceptibility of organism and severity of infection. Inject ceftazidime deep into a large muscle mass, such as the gluteus or lateral aspect of the thigh.
➤ *Empiric therapy in febrile neutropenic patients* ◇. *Adults:* 100 mg/kg I.V. daily in three divided doses; or 2 g I.V. q 8 hours either alone or with an aminoglycoside such as amikacin.
Children age 2 and older: 50 mg/kg (maximum 2 g) q 8 hours given I.V.
✦ *Dosage adjustment.* In patients with impaired renal function, doses or frequency of administration must be modified according to the degree of renal impairment, severity of infection, and susceptibility of organism. To prevent toxic accumulation, reduced dosage may be required in patients with creatinine clearance of 50 ml/minute or less; initially give 1 g loading dose and then follow maintenance recommendations

Creatinine clearance (ml/min)	Adult dosage
31-50	1 g q 12 hours
16-30	1 g q 24 hours
6-15	500 mg q 24 hours
≤5	500 mg q 48 hours

For hemodialysis patients, give 1 g after each hemodialysis period. For peritoneal dialysis patients, give 500 mg q 24 hours.

How supplied
Available by prescription only
Infusion: 1 g, 2 g in 50- and 100-ml vials and bags
Injection: 500 mg, 1 g, 2 g

Pharmacodynamics
Antibacterial action: Ceftazidime is primarily bactericidal; it also may be bacteriostatic. Activity depends on the organism, tissue penetration, dosage, and rate of organism multiplication. It acts by adhering to bacterial penicillin-binding proteins, thereby inhibiting cell wall synthesis. Third-generation cephalosporins appear to be more active against some beta-lactamase–producing gram-negative organisms.

Ceftazidime is active against some gram-positive organisms and many enteric gram-negative bacilli, as well as streptococci (*Streptococcus pneumoniae* and *S. pyogenes*); *Staphylococcus aureus* (penicillinase- and nonpenicillinase-producing); *Escherichia coli; Klebsiella* species; *Proteus* species; *Enterobacter* species; *Haemophilus influenzae; Pseudomonas* species; and some strains of *Bacteroides* species. It's more effective than any cephalosporin or penicillin derivative against *Pseudomonas.* Some other third-generation cephalosporins are more active against gram-positive organisms and anaerobes.

Pharmacokinetics
Absorption: Not absorbed from the GI tract; must be given parenterally.
Distribution: Distributed widely into most body tissues and fluids, including the gallbladder, liver, kidneys, bone, sputum, bile, and pleural and synovial fluids; unlike most other cephalosporins, ceftazidime has good CSF penetration; it crosses the placenta. Ceftazidime is 5% to 24% protein-bound.
Metabolism: Not metabolized.
Excretion: Excreted mainly in urine by glomerular filtration; small amounts of drug appear in breast milk. Elimination half-life is about 1½ to 2 hours in patients with normal renal function; up to 35 hours in patients with severe renal disease. Hemodialysis or peritoneal dialysis removes ceftazidime.

Route	Onset	Peak	Duration
I.V.	Immediate	Immediate	Unknown
I.M.	Unknown	1 hr	Unknown

Contraindications and precautions
Contraindicated in patients hypersensitive to drug or other cephalosporins. Use cautiously in breast-feeding women and in patients with poor renal function or penicillin allergy.

Interactions
Drug-drug. *Aminoglycosides:* Synergistic activity against some strains of *Pseudomonas aeruginosa* and Enterobacteriaceae. Monitor patient for effects.
Chloramphenicol: Antagonistic effect. Avoid use together.
Quinolones: In vitro studies show synergistic effect against *Burkholderia cepacia.* May be used as a therapeutic effect.

Adverse reactions
CNS: headache, dizziness, paresthesia, *seizures.*
CV: *thrombophlebitis* with I.V. injection.
GI: pseudomembranous colitis, nausea, vomiting, diarrhea, candidiasis, abdominal cramps.
GU: vaginitis.
Hematologic: eosinophilia, thrombocytosis, *leukopenia,* hemolytic anemia, *agranulocytosis, thrombocytopenia.*
Hepatic: transient elevation in liver enzyme levels.
Skin: *maculopapular and erythematous rash, urticaria, pain, induration, sterile abscesses, tissue sloughing* (at injection site).
Other: *hypersensitivity reactions* (serum sickness, *anaphylaxis*), *phlebitis.*

Overdose and treatment
Overdose may cause neuromuscular hypersensitivity. Seizures may follow high CNS levels. Drug may be removed by hemodialysis or peritoneal dialysis.

Special considerations
Consider the recommendations relevant to all cephalosporins as well as the following.
⚠ ALERT Names of some cephalosporins are similar. Use caution when dispensing.
● For patients on sodium restriction, note that ceftazidime contains 2.3 mEq of sodium per gram of drug.
● Ceftazidime powders (excluding Ceptaz) for injection contain 118 mg sodium carbonate per gram of drug; ceftazidime sodium is more water-soluble and is formed in situ upon reconstitution.
● Vials are supplied under reduced pressure. When antibiotic is dissolved, carbon dioxide is released and a positive pressure develops. Each brand of ceftazidime includes specific instructions for reconstitution. Read instructions carefully.
● Because drug is hemodialyzable, patients undergoing treatments with hemodialysis or peritoneal dialysis may require dosage adjustment.
● Separate I.V. sites should be used for aminoglycosides and ceftazidime.
● Ceftazidime causes false-positive results in urine glucose tests using cupric sulfate (Benedict's reagent or Clinitest); use glucose oxidase (Chemstrip uG, Diastix, or glucose enzymatic test strip) instead. Ceftazidime also causes false elevations in urine creatinine levels in tests using Jaffé's reaction. Ceftazidime may cause positive Coombs' test results.

Reactions may be *common*, uncommon, *life-threatening*, or COMMON AND LIFE-THREATENING.

Patient monitoring
With large doses or prolonged therapy, patients, especially high-risk patients, must be observed for superinfection.

Pregnant patients
• Use only when clearly needed.

Breast-feeding patients
• Drug appears in breast milk; use cautiously in breast-feeding women. Safety hasn't been established.

Pediatric patients
• Only Fortaz, Tazicef, and Tazidime may be used in infants and children. Ceptaz shouldn't be used in children under age 12 because it contains arginine.

Geriatric patients
• Reduced dosage may be necessary in geriatric patients with diminished renal function.

Patient education
• Advise patient to report discomfort at I.V. site.
• Tell patient to report rash or symptoms of superinfection.

ceftibuten
Cedax

Pharmacologic classification: third-generation cephalosporin
Therapeutic classification: antibiotic
Pregnancy risk category: B

Indications and dosages
➤ *Acute bacterial exacerbations of chronic bronchitis caused by* Haemophilus influenzae, Moraxella catarrhalis, *or* Streptococcus pneumoniae. *Adults and children age 12 and older:* 400 mg P.O. daily for 10 days.
➤ *Pharyngitis and tonsillitis caused by* Streptococcus pyogenes; *acute bacterial otitis media due to* H. influenzae, M. catarrhalis, *or* S. pyogenes. *Adults and children age 12 and older:* 400 mg P.O. daily for 10 days.
Children younger than age 12: 9 mg/kg P.O. daily for 10 days. Children who weigh more than 45 kg (99 lb) should receive the maximum daily dose of 400 mg.
✦ *Dosage adjustment.* No adjustments are necessary for patients with creatinine clearance of more than 50 ml/minute. Give 4.5 mg/kg (or 200 mg) daily to patients with creatinine clearance between 30 and 49 ml/minute and 2.25 mg/kg (or 100 mg) daily for those with creatinine clearance of 5 to 29 ml/minute. For patients undergoing hemodialysis two or three times weekly, give a single 400-mg dose (capsule form) or administer a single dose of 9 mg/kg (maximum dose, 400 mg) using oral suspension at the end of each hemodialysis session.

How supplied
Available by prescription only
Capsules: 400 mg
Oral suspension: 90 mg/5 ml, 180 mg/5 ml

Pharmacodynamics
Antibiotic action: Ceftibuten exerts its bactericidal action by binding to essential target proteins of the bacterial cell wall. This binding leads to inhibition of cell wall synthesis. Drug is usually active against gram-positive aerobes (*S. pneumoniae, S. pyogenes*) and gram-negative aerobes (*H. influenzae, M. catarrhalis*).

Pharmacokinetics
Absorption: Rapidly absorbed from GI tract. Food decreases the bioavailability of drug.
Distribution: 65% bound to plasma proteins.
Metabolism: Metabolized to its predominant component, cis-ceftibuten. About 10% of ceftibuten is converted to the transisomer.
Excretion: Excreted in urine and feces.

Route	Onset	Peak	Duration
P.O.	Unknown	2-4 hr	Unknown

Contraindications and precautions
Contraindicated in patients hypersensitive to the cephalosporin group of antibiotics. Use cautiously if administering to patients with history of hypersensitivity to penicillin because up to 10% of these patients will exhibit cross-sensitivity to a cephalosporin. Also use cautiously in patients with impaired renal function and GI disease (especially colitis).

Interactions
Drug-food. *Any food:* Decreased bioavailability of drug, which slows its absorption. Advise patient to take drug 2 hours before or 1 hour after a meal.

Adverse reactions
CNS: headache, dizziness, fatigue, paresthesia, somnolence, agitation, hyperkinesia, insomnia, irritability.
EENT: nasal congestion.
GI: nausea, dyspepsia, abdominal pain, vomiting, anorexia, constipation, dry mouth, eructation, flatulence, loose stools, melena, taste perversion.
GU: dysuria, hematuria, elevated BUN and serum creatinine level, vaginitis.
Hematologic: elevated amount of eosinophils, decreased hemoglobin level, altered platelet count, decreased leukocyte count.
Hepatic: elevated liver enzyme, bilirubin, and alkaline phosphatase levels.
Respiratory: dyspnea.
Skin: rash, pruritus, diaper dermatitis, urticaria.
Other: candidiasis, dehydration, fever, rigors.

Overdose and treatment
Overdose can cause cerebral irritation leading to seizures. Ceftibuten is readily dialyzable and significant quantities (65% of plasma levels) can be removed from the circulation by a single hemodialysis session. No information is available regarding the removal of ceftibuten by peritoneal dialysis.

Special considerations
Consider the recommendations relevant to all cephalosporins as well as the following.
• Pseudomembranous colitis has been reported with nearly all antibacterial agents; it may occur in patients in whom diarrhea develops secondary to antibiotic therapy. Although most patients respond to withdrawal of drug therapy alone, it may be necessary to institute treatment with an antibacterial agent effective against *Clostridium difficile*, an organism linked to this disorder.
• Obtain specimens for culture and sensitivity testing before first dose. Therapy may begin pending test results.
• When preparing oral suspension, first tap the bottle to loosen powder. Follow chart supplied by manufacturer for amount of water to add to powder when mixing oral suspension form. Add water in two portions, shaking well after each aliquot. After mixing, the suspension may be stored for 14 days in the refrigerator.
• Although ceftibuten hasn't been known to affect the direct Coombs' test to date, other cephalosporins have caused a false-positive direct Coombs' test. Therefore, it should be recognized that a positive Coombs' test could be due to drug.

Patient monitoring
• Drug may cause overgrowth of nonsusceptible bacteria or fungi. Patient requires observation for signs and symptoms of superinfection.
• In patient with suspected renal impairment, monitor renal function before and during therapy.

Breast-feeding patients
• It isn't known whether drug appears in breast milk. Use cautiously in breast-feeding women.

Pediatric patients
• Safety and effectiveness in infants under age 6 months haven't been established.

Geriatric patients
• Use cautiously in geriatric patients. Dosage adjustment may be needed if patient has impaired renal function.

Patient education
• Tell patient to take all of drug as prescribed, even if he's feeling better.
• Inform diabetic patient that oral suspension contains 1 g of sucrose per teaspoon of suspension.

• Instruct patient using oral suspension to shake bottle well before measuring dose.

ceftizoxime sodium
Cefizox

Pharmacologic classification: third-generation cephalosporin
Therapeutic classification: antibiotic
Pregnancy risk category: B

Indications and dosages
➤ *Bacteremia, septicemia, meningitis, pelvic inflammatory disease, and serious respiratory tract, urinary tract, gynecologic, intra-abdominal, bone and joint, and skin infections from susceptible organisms. Adults:* Usual dosage is 500 mg to 2 g I.V. or I.M. q 8 to 12 hours. In life-threatening infections, 3 to 4 g I.V. q 8 hours.
Children age 6 months and older: 50 mg/kg I.V. or I.M. q 6 to 8 hours.

Total daily dose is same for I.M. or I.V. administration and depends on susceptibility of organism and severity of infection. Inject ceftizoxime deep into a large muscle mass, such as the gluteus or lateral aspect of the thigh.
➤ *Uncomplicated gonorrhea. Adults:* 1 g I.M. given as a single dose.
✦ *Dosage adjustment.* In patients with impaired renal function, modify doses or frequency of administration according to degree of renal impairment, severity of infection, and susceptibility of organism. To prevent toxic accumulation, reduced dosage may be required in patients with creatinine clearance of less than 80 ml/minute. The following table gives appropriate doses for adults.

Creatinine clearance (ml/min)	Less severe infections	Life-threatening infections
50-79	500 mg q 8 hours	750 mg to 1.5 g q 8 hours
5-49	250 to 500 mg q 12 hours	500 mg to 1 g q 12 hours
0-4	500 mg q 48 hours or 250 mg q 24 hours	500 mg to 1 g q 48 hours or 500 mg q 24 hours

How supplied
Available by prescription only
Infusion: 1 g, 2 g in 100-ml vials
Injection: 500 mg, 1 g, 2 g, 10 g (bulk package)

Pharmacodynamics
Antibacterial action: Ceftizoxime is primarily bactericidal; it also may be bacteriostatic. Activity depends on the organism, tissue penetration,

dosage, and rate of organism multiplication. It acts by adhering to bacterial penicillin-binding proteins, thereby inhibiting cell wall synthesis. Third-generation cephalosporins appear to be more active against some beta-lactamase–producing gram-negative organisms.

Drug is active against some gram-positive organisms and many enteric gram-negative bacilli, as well as streptococci (*Streptococcus pneumoniae* and *pyogenes*); *Staphylococcus aureus* (penicillinase- and non-penicillinase-producing); *Staphylococcus epidermidis; Escherichia coli; Klebsiella* species; *Haemophilus influenzae; Enterobacter* species; *Proteus* species; *Bacteroides* species (including *Bacteroides fragilis*); *Peptostreptococcus* species; some strains of *Pseudomonas* and *Acinetobacter*. Cefotaxime and moxalactam are slightly more active than ceftizoxime against gram-positive organisms but are less active against gram-negative organisms.

Pharmacokinetics
Absorption: Not absorbed from the GI tract; must be given parenterally.
Distribution: Distributed widely into most body tissues and fluids, including the gallbladder, liver, kidneys, bone, sputum, bile, and pleural and synovial fluids. Unlike most other cephalosporins, ceftizoxime has good CSF penetration and achieves adequate levels in inflamed meninges; ceftizoxime crosses the placenta and is 30% protein-bound.
Metabolism: Not metabolized.
Excretion: Excreted primarily in urine by renal tubular secretion and glomerular filtration; small amounts of drug appear in breast milk. Elimination half-life is about 1½ to 2 hours in patients with normal renal function; severe renal disease prolongs half-life up to 30 hours. Hemodialysis or peritoneal dialysis removes minimal amounts of ceftizoxime.

Route	Onset	Peak	Duration
I.V.	Immediate	Immediate	Unknown
I.M.	Unknown	½-1½ hr	Unknown

Contraindications and precautions
Contraindicated in patients hypersensitive to ceftizoxime or other cephalosporins. Use cautiously in breast-feeding women and in patients with impaired renal function or penicillin allergy.

Interactions
Drug-drug. *Aminoglycosides:* May slightly increase the risk of nephrotoxicity. Avoid use.
Probenecid: Competitively inhibits renal tubular secretion of cephalosporins, causing higher, prolonged serum levels. May be used for this effect.

Adverse reactions
CV: *thrombophlebitis.*
GI: pseudomembranous colitis, nausea, anorexia, vomiting, *diarrhea.*
GU: vaginitis.

Hematologic: *transient neutropenia,* eosinophilia, hemolytic anemia, thrombocytosis, anemia, *thrombocytopenia.*
Hepatic: transient elevation in liver enzyme levels with I.V. injection.
Respiratory: dyspnea.
Skin: *maculopapular and erythematous rash, urticaria pain, induration, sterile abscesses, tissue sloughing (at injection site).*
Other: *hypersensitivity reactions* (serum sickness, *anaphylaxis*), elevated temperature, *phlebitis.*

Overdose and treatment
Overdose may cause neuromuscular hypersensitivity. Seizures may follow high CNS levels. Ceftizoxime may be removed by hemodialysis.

Special considerations
Consider the recommendations relevant to all cephalosporins as well as the following.
⚠ ALERT Names of some cephalosporins are similar. Use caution when dispensing.
● For patients on sodium restriction, note that ceftizoxime contains 2.6 mEq of sodium per gram of drug.
● Drug may be supplied as frozen, sterile solution in plastic containers. Thaw at room temperature. Thawed solution is stable for 24 hours at room temperature or for 21 days if refrigerated. Don't refreeze.
● For I.M. use, reconstitute with sterile water for injection. Shake vial well to ensure complete dissolution of drug. To administer a dose that exceeds 1 g, divide the dose and inject it into separate sites to prevent tissue injury.
● For I.V. use, reconstitute I.V. dose with sterile water for injection. Solution should clear after shaking well and range in color from yellow to amber. If particles are visible, discard solution. Reconstituted solution is stable for 24 hours at room temperature or for 96 hours if refrigerated.
● Administer ceftizoxime I.V. as a direct injection slowly over 3 to 5 minutes directly or through tubing of compatible infusion fluid. If given as intermittent infusion, the reconstituted drug is diluted in 50 to 100 ml of compatible fluid. Check package insert.
● Ceftizoxime causes false-positive results in urine glucose tests utilizing cupric sulfate (Benedict's reagent or Clinitest); use glucose oxidase (Chemstrip uG, Diastix, or glucose enzymatic test strip) instead. Ceftizoxime also causes false elevations in urine creatinine levels using Jaffé's reaction. Ceftizoxime may cause positive Coombs' test results.

Patient monitoring
● Monitor patient for hypersensitivity. If a severe hypersensitivity reaction occurs during therapy, stop drug and start appropriate therapy (such as epinephrine, I.V. fluids, oxygen).
● Monitor renal function when maximum dose is given to severely ill patients.

Breast-feeding patients
• Drug appears in breast milk; use cautiously in breast-feeding women. Safety hasn't been established.

Pediatric patients
• Safety and efficacy haven't been established in infants under age 6 months.

Geriatric patients
• Reduced dosage may be necessary in geriatric patients with diminished renal function.

Patient education
• Inform patient of potential adverse reactions.
• Tell patient to report discomfort at I.V. site.

---

ceftriaxone sodium
Rocephin

Pharmacologic classification: third-generation cephalosporin
Therapeutic classification: antibiotic
Pregnancy risk category: B

Indications and dosages
➤ *Bacteremia, septicemia, and serious respiratory tract, bone, joint, urinary tract, gynecologic, intra-abdominal, and skin infections caused by susceptible organisms.* Adults and children age 12 and older: 1 to 2 g I.M. or I.V. once daily or in equally divided doses b.i.d. Total daily dose shouldn't exceed 4 g.
Children younger than age 12: Total daily dose is 50 to 75 mg/kg I.M. or I.V., given in divided doses q 12 hours. Maximum daily dose is 2 g.
➤ *Gonococcal meningitis, endocarditis* ◇.
Adults: 1 to 2 g I.V. q 12 hours for 10 to 14 days for meningitis and 3 to 4 weeks for endocarditis.
Children: 50 to 100 mg/kg (maximum daily dose is 4 g) I.M. or I.V. daily or divided q 12 hours for 7 to 14 days for meningitis and 28 days for endocarditis.
    May give an initial dose of 100 mg/kg (not to exceed 4 g) I.M. or I.V. to start therapy. Total daily dose is same for I.M. or I.V. administration and depends on susceptibility of organism and severity of infection. Inject ceftriaxone deep I.M. into a large muscle mass, such as the gluteus or lateral aspect of the thigh.
➤ *Preoperative prophylaxis.* Adults: 1 g I.M. or I.V. 30 minutes to 2 hours before surgery.
➤ *Uncomplicated gonorrhea.* Adults: 125 to 250 mg I.M. given as a single dose.
➤ *Haemophilus ducreyi infection* ◇. Adults: 250 mg I.M. as a single dose.
➤ *Sexually transmitted epididymitis* ◇. Adults: 250 mg I.M. as a single dose; follow up with other antibiotics.
➤ *Pelvic inflammatory disease.* Adults: 250 mg I.M. as a single dose; follow up with other antibiotics.
➤ *Anti-infectives for sexual assault victims* ◇. Adults: 125 mg I.M. as a single dose with other antibiotics.
➤ *Lyme disease* ◇. Adults: 1 to 2 g I.M. or I.V. q 12 to 24 hours.
➤ *Persisting or relapsing otitis media in children* ◇. Children age 3 months and older: 50 mg/kg I.M. once daily for 3 days.
✦ *Dosage adjustment.* In patients with impaired hepatic and renal function, daily dose shouldn't exceed 2 g without monitoring serum drug levels.

How supplied
Available by prescription only
Infusion: 1 g, 2 g
Injection: 250 mg, 500 mg, 1 g, 2 g, 10-g bulk package

Pharmacodynamics
Antibacterial action: Ceftriaxone is primarily bactericidal; it also may be bacteriostatic. Activity depends on organism, tissue penetration, and dosage, and rate of organism multiplication. It acts by adhering to bacterial penicillin-binding proteins, thereby inhibiting cell wall synthesis. Third-generation cephalosporins appear to be more active against some beta-lactamase–producing gram-negative organisms.
    Ceftriaxone is active against some gram-positive organisms and many enteric gram-negative bacilli, as well as streptococci; *Streptococcus pneumoniae* and *pyogenes; Staphylococcus aureus* (penicillinase- and non-penicillinase-producing); *Staphylococcus epidermidis; Escherichia coli; Klebsiella* species; *Haemophilus influenzae, Enterobacter; Proteus;* some strains of *Pseudomonas* and *Peptostreptococcus* and spirochetes such as *Borrelia burgdorferi* (the causative organism of Lyme disease). Most strains of *Listeria, Pseudomonas,* and *Acinetobacter* are resistant. Generally, the activity of ceftriaxone is most like that of cefotaxime and ceftizoxime.

Pharmacokinetics
Absorption: Not absorbed from the GI tract and must be given parenterally.
Distribution: Distributed widely into most body tissues and fluids, including the gallbladder, liver, kidneys, bone, sputum, bile, and pleural and synovial fluids; unlike most other cephalosporins, ceftriaxone has good CSF penetration. Ceftriaxone crosses the placenta. Protein-binding is dose-dependent and decreases as serum levels rise; average is 84% to 96%.
Metabolism: Partially metabolized.
Excretion: Excreted principally in urine; some drug is excreted in bile by biliary mechanisms, and small amounts appear in breast milk. Elimination half-life is 5½ to 11 hours in adults with normal renal function; severe renal disease prolongs half-life only moderately. Neither he-

---

modialysis nor peritoneal dialysis will remove ceftriaxone.

Route	Onset	Peak	Duration
I.V.	Immediate	Immediate	Unknown
I.M.	Unknown	1½-4 hr	Unknown

Contraindications and precautions

Contraindicated in patients hypersensitive to ceftriaxone or other cephalosporins. Use cautiously in breast-feeding women and in patients with penicillin allergy.

Interactions

Drug-drug. *Aminoglycosides:* Produces synergistic antimicrobial activity against *Pseudomonas aeruginosa* and some strains of Enterobacteriaceae. Monitor patient closely.
Probenecid: May increase clearance by blocking biliary secretion and displacement of ceftriaxone from plasma proteins. Avoid use together.
Quinolones: In vitro synergism against *S. pneumoniae.* Clinical relevance unknown.

Adverse reactions

CNS: headache, dizziness.
GI: pseudomembranous colitis, nausea, vomiting, diarrhea, urolithiasis, jaundice.
GU: genital pruritus, candidiasis, elevated BUN levels.
Hematologic: eosinophilia, thrombocytosis, *leukopenia.*
Hepatic: increased liver function test results.
Skin: pain, induration, and tenderness at injection site; phlebitis; *rash;* pruritus.
Other: *hypersensitivity reactions* (serum sickness, **anaphylaxis**), elevated temperature, chills.

Overdose and treatment

Overdose may cause neuromuscular hypersensitivity. Seizures may follow high CNS levels. Treatment is supportive.

Special considerations

Consider the recommendations relevant to all cephalosporins as well as the following.
⚠ ALERT Names of some cephalosporins are similar. Use caution when dispensing.
• For patients on sodium restriction, note that ceftriaxone injection contains 3.6 mEq of sodium per gram of drug.
• Dosage adjustment usually isn't necessary in patients with renal insufficiency because of partial biliary excretion.
• Ceftriaxone causes false-positive results in urine glucose tests that use cupric sulfate (Benedict's reagent or Clinitest); use glucose oxidase (Chemstrip uG, Diastix, or glucose enzymatic test strip) instead. Ceftriaxone also causes false elevations in urine creatinine levels in tests using Jaffé's reaction. Ceftriaxone may cause positive Coombs' test results.

Patient monitoring

• With large doses or prolonged therapy, watch for superinfection in high-risk patients.
• Monitor serum drug levels in patients with severe renal impairment or in patients with both renal and hepatic impairment.

Breast-feeding patients

• Drug appears in breast milk. Use cautiously in breast-feeding women.

Pediatric patients

• Ceftriaxone may be used in neonates and children. Use cautiously in hyperbilirubinemic neonates because of ability of drug to displace bilirubin.

Patient education

• Inform patient of potential adverse reactions.
• Tell patient to report discomfort at I.V. site.

cefuroxime axetil
Ceftin

cefuroxime sodium
Kefurox, Zinacef

Pharmacologic classification: second-generation cephalosporin
Therapeutic classification: antibiotic
Pregnancy risk category: B

Indications and dosages

➤ *Serious lower respiratory, urinary tract, skin, and skin-structure infections; septicemia; meningitis caused by susceptible organisms. Adults:* Usual dosage is 750 mg to 1.5 g I.M. or I.V. q 8 hours for 5 to 10 days. For life-threatening infections and infections caused by less susceptible organisms, 1.5 g I.M. or I.V. q 6 hours; for bacterial meningitis, up to 3 g I.V. q 8 hours.
Children and infants over age 3 months: 50 to 100 mg/kg I.M. or I.V. daily in divided doses q 6 to 8 hours. Some clinicians give 100 to 150 mg/kg daily. For meningitis, the usual starting dosage is 200 to 240 mg/kg I.V. daily in divided doses q 6 to 8 hours, reduced to 100 mg/kg daily when clinical improvement occurs. However, some clinicians prefer other agents for meningitis.

Total daily dose is same for I.M. and I.V. administration and depends on susceptibility of organism and severity of infection. Inject cefuroxime deep I.M. into a large muscle mass, such as the gluteus or lateral aspect of the thigh.
➤ *Pharyngitis, tonsillitis, lower respiratory tract infection, urinary tract infection. Adults and children over age 12:* 125 to 500 mg P.O. b.i.d. for 10 days.
Children under age 12 who can swallow pills: 125 to 250 mg P.O. b.i.d. (tablets) for 10 days.

Children ages 3 months to 12 years: 20 mg/kg P.O. daily in divided doses b.i.d. (oral suspension) to maximum dose of 500 mg for 10 days.

➤ *Otitis media, impetigo. Children ages 3 months to 12 years:* 30 mg/kg P.O. oral suspension daily divided into two doses (maximum dose is 1 g) for 10 days.

Children who can swallow pills: 250 mg P.O. b.i.d. for 10 days.

Note: Compliance may be a problem when treating otitis media in children. Order suspension form if child is unable to swallow pills.

➤ *Perioperative prophylaxis. Adults:* 1.5 g I.V. 30 to 60 minutes before surgery; then 750 mg I.M. or I.V. q 8 hours intraoperatively for a prolonged procedure. Open-heart surgery patients can receive 1.5 g I.V. at induction, then q 12 hours for three doses.

➤ *Gonorrhea (urethral, endocervical, rectal). Adults:* 1.5 g I.M. given as a single dose, alone or with other antibiotics.

➤ *Lyme disease (erythema migrans) caused by* **Borrelia burgdorferi.** *Adults and children age 13 and older:* 500 mg P.O. b.i.d. for 20 days.

✦ *Dosage adjustment.* Safety of drug in renal patients hasn't been established. In patients with impaired renal function, dose or frequency of administration must be modified based on degree of renal impairment, severity of infection, and susceptibility of organism. To prevent toxic accumulation, reduced I.M. or I.V. dosage may be required. In patients with creatinine clearance of 10 to 20 ml/minute, give 750 mg q 12 hours. In those with creatinine clearance below 10 ml/minute, give 750 mg q 24 hours. For hemodialysis patients, give 750 mg at end of each dialysis period in addition to regular dose.

How supplied
Available by prescription only
cefuroxime axetil
Suspension: 125 mg/5 ml, 250 mg/5 ml
Tablets (film-coated): 125 mg, 250 mg, 500 mg
cefuroxime sodium
Infusion: 750 mg, 1.5-g infusion packets
Injection: 750 mg, 1.5 g, 7.5 g

Pharmacodynamics
Antibacterial action: Cefuroxime is primarily bactericidal; it also may be bacteriostatic. Activity depends on the organism, tissue penetration, dosage, and rate of organism multiplication. It acts by adhering to bacterial penicillin-binding proteins, thereby inhibiting cell wall synthesis.

Cefuroxime is active against many gram-positive organisms and enteric gram-negative bacilli, including *Streptococcus pneumoniae* and *S. pyogenes, Haemophilus influenzae, Klebsiella* species, *Staphylococcus aureus, Escherichia coli, Enterobacter,* and *Neisseria gonorrhoeae; Bacteroides fragilis, Pseudomonas,* and *Acinetobacter* are resistant to cefuroxime.

Pharmacokinetics
Absorption: Cefuroxime sodium isn't well absorbed from the GI tract and must be given parenterally. Cefuroxime axetil is better absorbed orally, with between 37% and 52% of an oral dose reaching systemic circulation. Food appears to enhance absorption. Tablets and suspension aren't bioequivalent.

Distribution: Distributed widely into most body tissues and fluids, including the gallbladder, liver, kidneys, bone, bile, and pleural and synovial fluids; CSF penetration is greater than that of most first- and second-generation cephalosporins and achieves adequate therapeutic levels in inflamed meninges. Cefuroxime crosses the placenta and is 33% to 50% protein-bound.

Metabolism: Not metabolized.

Excretion: Primarily excreted in urine by renal tubular secretion and glomerular filtration; elimination half-life is 1 to 2 hours in patients with normal renal function; end-stage renal disease prolongs half-life 15 to 22 hours. Some drug appears in breast milk. Hemodialysis removes cefuroxime.

Route	Onset	Peak	Duration
P.O.	Unknown	15-60 min	Unknown
I.V.	Immediate	Immediate	Unknown
I.M.	Unknown	2 hr	Unknown

Contraindications and precautions
Contraindicated in patients hypersensitive to cefuroxime or other cephalosporins. Use cautiously in breast-feeding women and in patients with impaired renal function or penicillin allergy.

Interactions
Drug-drug. *Aminoglycosides:* Synergistic activity against some organisms; risk of increased nephrotoxicity. Monitor patient closely.

Diuretics: Increased risk of adverse effects. Monitor patient closely.

Probenecid: Competitively inhibits renal tubular secretion of cephalosporins, resulting in higher, prolonged serum levels of these drugs. Sometimes used for this effect.

Drug-food. *Any food:* Increased absorption. Advise patient to take drug with food.

Adverse reactions
CV: *thrombophlebitis* (with I.V. injection).

GI: pseudomembranous colitis, nausea, anorexia, vomiting, *diarrhea.*

Hematologic: *transient neutropenia,* eosinophilia, *hemolytic anemia, thrombocytopenia,* decreased hemoglobin and hematocrit levels.

Hepatic: transient increases in liver enzyme levels.

Skin: *maculopapular and erythematous rash,* urticaria, pain, induration, sterile abscesses, *temperature elevation, tissue sloughing* (at injection site).

Other: *hypersensitivity reactions* (serum sickness, *anaphylaxis*), *phlebitis* (with I.V. injection).

Overdose and treatment
Overdose may cause neuromuscular hypersensitivity. Seizures may follow high CNS levels. Hemodialysis or peritoneal dialysis will remove cefuroxime.

Special considerations
Consider the recommendations relevant to all cephalosporins as well as the following.

🔰 **ALERT** Names of some cephalosporins are similar. Use caution when dispensing.
• Tablets and suspension aren't bioequivalent and can't be substituted on a milligram-per-milligram basis.
• For patients on sodium restriction, note that cefuroxime sodium contains 2.4 mEq of sodium per gram of drug.
• Check solutions for particulate matter and discoloration. Solution may range in color from light yellow to amber without affecting potency.
• Shake I.M. solution gently before administration to ensure complete drug dissolution. Give deep into a large muscle mass, preferably the gluteus area. Aspirate before injecting to prevent inadvertent injection into a blood vessel. Rotate injection sites to prevent tissue damage. Ice to injection site may relieve pain.
• For direct intermittent I.V., inject solution slowly into vein over 3 to 5 minutes or slowly through tubing of free-running, compatible I.V. solution.
• Reconstituted solution retains potency for 24 hours at room temperature or for 48 hours if refrigerated.
• Because drug is hemodialyzable, patients undergoing treatment with hemodialysis or peritoneal dialysis may require dosage adjustments.
• Reconstituted suspension can be stored at room temperature or in refrigerator. Discard unused portion after 10 days. Shake well before each dose.
• Drug causes false-positive results in urine glucose tests using cupric sulfate (Benedict's reagent or Clinitest); use glucose oxidase tests (Chemstrip uG, Diastix, or glucose enzymatic test strip) instead. Cefuroxime also causes false elevations in serum or urine creatinine levels in tests using Jaffé's reaction. Cefuroxime may cause positive Coombs' test results.

Patient monitoring
• With large doses or prolonged therapy, monitor patient for superinfection, especially if high-risk.
• Monitor renal function during therapy, especially when maximum dose is used in a severely ill patient.

Breast-feeding patients
• Drug appears in breast milk; use cautiously in breast-feeding women.

Pediatric patients
• Safety in infants under age 3 months hasn't been established.

Geriatric patients
• Use cautiously in geriatric patients.

Patient education
• Inform patient of potential adverse reactions.
• Patient should report discomfort at I.V. site.

celecoxib
Celebrex

Pharmacologic classification: cyclooxygenase-2 (COX-2) inhibitor
Therapeutic classification: anti-inflammatory
Pregnancy risk category: C

Indications and dosages
➤ *Relief of signs and symptoms of osteoarthritis.* *Adults:* 200 mg P.O. daily as a single dose or divided equally b.i.d.
➤ *Relief of signs and symptoms of rheumatoid arthritis.* *Adults:* 100 to 200 mg P.O. b.i.d.
✦ *Dosage adjustment.* In patients who weigh less than 50 kg (110 lb), start at lowest recommended dosage. In patients with moderate hepatic impairment (Child-Pugh Class II), start at 50% of normal dose.

How supplied
Available by prescription only
Capsules: 100 mg, 200 mg

Pharmacodynamics
Anti-inflammatory, analgesic, and antipyretic actions: Celecoxib is thought to act by selective inhibition of COX-2, resulting in decreased prostaglandin synthesis. Because celecoxib doesn't inhibit COX-1 at therapeutic levels, the reduction in symptoms of osteoarthritis and rheumatoid arthritis may have a lower risk of adverse peripheral effects.

Pharmacokinetics
Absorption: Steady-state plasma levels can be expected within 5 days if celecoxib is given in multiple dosages.
Distribution: Highly protein-bound, primarily to albumin.
Metabolism: Primarily metabolized by cytochrome P-450 2C9.
Excretion: Eliminated primarily by hepatic metabolism; 27% is excreted into the urine. Elimination half-life under fasting conditions is about 11 hours.

Route	Onset	Peak	Duration
P.O.	Unknown	3 hr	Unknown

Contraindications and precautions

Contraindicated during the third trimester of pregnancy, in patients with severe hepatic impairment, and in patients hypersensitive to celecoxib, sulfonamides, aspirin, or other NSAIDs.

Use cautiously in patients with a history of ulcers or GI bleeding, advanced renal disease, anemia, symptomatic liver disease, hypertension, edema, heart failure, or asthma. Also use cautiously in patients who smoke or use alcohol, in those taking oral corticosteroids or anticoagulants, and in elderly or debilitated patients.

Interactions

Drug-drug. *ACE inhibitors:* Diminished antihypertensive effects. Monitor blood pressure.

Aluminum and magnesium antacids: May decrease plasma levels of celecoxib. These drugs must be given at least 1 hour apart.

Aspirin: Increased risk of ulcers; low aspirin dosages can be used safely for prevention of CV events. Observe patient for evidence of GI bleeding.

Fluconazole: May increase celecoxib level. May need to adjust celecoxib to minimal effective dosage.

Furosemide: NSAIDs can reduce sodium excretion from diuretics, leading to sodium retention. Observe patient for swelling and increased blood pressure.

Lithium: Increased lithium levels. Monitor lithium levels closely.

Warfarin: A direct interaction hasn't been reported; however, observe patient for signs and symptoms of bleeding.

Drug-lifestyle. *Alcohol use:* May cause increased risk of GI irritation or bleeding with long-term use. Discourage alcohol consumption. Observe patient for signs of bleeding.

Adverse reactions

CNS: dizziness, *headache,* insomnia.
EENT: pharyngitis, rhinitis, sinusitis.
GI: abdominal pain, diarrhea, dyspepsia, flatulence, nausea.
GU: elevated BUN level.
Hepatic: elevated liver enzyme levels.
Metabolic: hyperchloremia, hypophosphatemia.
Musculoskeletal: *back pain.*
Respiratory: upper respiratory tract infection.
Skin: rash.
Other: *peripheral edema, accidental injury.*

Overdose and treatment

Common signs and symptoms of overdose include lethargy, drowsiness, nausea, vomiting, epigastric pain, and GI bleeding. Other possible effects include hypertension, acute renal failure, respiratory depression, and coma.

Although there's no antidote for overdose, symptomatic and supportive care is usually sufficient. If a patient is seen within 4 hours of the overdose, induced emesis, activated charcoal, an osmotic cathartic, or a combination of these can be used. Because of the high protein-binding, dialysis is unlikely to be effective.

Special considerations

● Patients may be allergic to celecoxib if they have an allergy to sulfonamides, aspirin, or other NSAIDs.
● Patients with a history of ulcers or GI bleeding are at higher risk for GI bleeding.

Patient monitoring

● Assess patient for signs and symptoms of hepatic and renal toxicity, especially if dehydrated. Consider correction of dehydration before starting therapy.
● Monitor renal function in patients with severe renal impairment.

Breast-feeding patients

● It isn't known if celecoxib appears in breast milk. Risks and benefits must be weighed before giving celecoxib to breast-feeding women.

Pediatric patients

● Drug hasn't been studied in patients under age 18.

Geriatric patients

● Dosage adjustment isn't necessary unless the patient weighs less than 50 kg; however, geriatric patients experience more adverse effects overall.

Patient education

● Inform the patient that it may take several days before pain is relieved consistently and that he should notify prescriber if no relief occurs.
● Advise patient to immediately report signs of swelling, excessive fatigue, yellowing of the skin, flu-like symptoms, signs of bleeding, or difficulty breathing.
● Instruct the patient to take drug with food if stomach upset occurs.

---

cephalexin hydrochloride
Keftab

cephalexin monohydrate
Biocef, Keflex, Novo-Lexin*

Pharmacologic classification: first-generation cephalosporin
Therapeutic classification: antibiotic
Pregnancy risk category: B

Indications and dosages

➤ *Respiratory tract, GU tract, skin, soft-tissue, bone, and joint infections caused by susceptible organisms. Adults:* 250 mg to 1 g P.O. q 6 hours.
Children: 25 to 50 mg/kg P.O. daily divided into four doses. In patients over age 1 with strepto-

---

coccal pharyngitis or skin and structure infections, dose may be administered q 12 hours.
➤ *Otitis media.* *Adults:* 250 mg to 1 g P.O. q 6 hours.
Children: 75 to 100 mg/kg P.O. daily divided into four doses.
✦ *Dosage adjustment.* To prevent toxic accumulation in patients with impaired renal function and creatinine clearance of less than 40 ml/minute, give reduced dosage.

Creatinine clearance (ml/min)	Adult dosage
11-40	500 mg q 8 to 12 hours
5-10	250 mg q 12 hours
< 5	250 mg q 12 to 24 hours

How supplied
Available by prescription only
cephalexin hydrochloride
Tablets: 500 mg
cephalexin monohydrate
Capsules: 250 mg, 500 mg
Suspension: 125 mg/5 ml, 250 mg/5 ml
Tablets (film-coated): 250 mg, 500 mg, 1g

Pharmacodynamics
Antibacterial action: Cephalexin is primarily bactericidal; it also may be bacteriostatic. Activity depends on the organism, tissue penetration, dosage, and rate of organism multiplication. It acts by adhering to bacterial penicillin-binding proteins, thereby inhibiting cell wall synthesis.

Drug is active against many gram-positive organisms, including penicillinase-producing *Staphylococcus aureus* and *S. epidermidis*, *Streptococcus pneumoniae*, group B streptococci, and group A beta-hemolytic streptococci; susceptible gram-negative organisms include *Klebsiella pneumoniae, Escherichia coli, Proteus mirabilis,* and *Shigella.*

Pharmacokinetics
Absorption: Absorbed rapidly and completely from the GI tract after oral administration. The base monohydrate is probably converted to the hydrochloride in the stomach before absorption. Food delays but doesn't prevent complete absorption.
Distribution: Distributed widely into most body tissues and fluids, including the gallbladder, liver, kidneys, bone, sputum, bile, and pleural and synovial fluids; CSF penetration is poor. Cephalexin crosses the placenta and is 6% to 15% protein-bound.
Metabolism: Not metabolized.
Excretion: Excreted primarily unchanged in urine by glomerular filtration and renal tubular secretion; small amounts of drug may appear in breast milk. Elimination half-life is about ½ to 1

hour in patients with normal renal function; 7½ to 14 hours in patients with severe renal impairment. Hemodialysis or peritoneal dialysis removes cephalexin.

Route	Onset	Peak	Duration
P.O.	Unknown	1 hr	Unknown

Contraindications and precautions
Contraindicated in patients hypersensitive to cephalosporins. Use cautiously in breast-feeding women and in patients with impaired renal function or penicillin allergy.

Interactions
Drug-drug. *Loop diuretics, nephrotoxic drugs (aminoglycosides, colistin, polymyxin B, vancomycin):* May increase the risk of nephrotoxicity. Patient requires close monitoring.
Probenecid: Competitively inhibits renal tubular secretion of cephalosporins, resulting in higher prolonged serum levels of these drugs. May be used for this effect.

Adverse reactions
CNS. dizziness, headache, fatigue, agitation, confusion, hallucinations.
GI: pseudomembranous colitis, *nausea, anorexia,* vomiting, *diarrhea,* gastritis, glossitis, dyspepsia, abdominal pain, anal pruritus, tenesmus, oral candidiasis.
GU: genital pruritus and candidiasis, vaginitis, interstitial nephritis.
Hematologic: *neutropenia,* eosinophilia, anemia, *thrombocytopenia.*
Hepatic: transient increases in liver enzyme levels.
Musculoskeletal: arthritis, arthralgia, joint pain.
Skin: *maculopapular and erythematous rash, urticaria.*
Other: *hypersensitivity reactions* (serum sickness, *anaphylaxis*).

Overdose and treatment
Overdose may cause neuromuscular hypersensitivity; seizures may follow high CNS levels. Remove cephalexin by hemodialysis or peritoneal dialysis. Other treatment is supportive.

Special considerations
Consider the recommendations relevant to all cephalosporins as well as the following.
● To prepare the oral suspension, add the required amount of water to the powder in two portions. Shake well after each addition. After mixing, store in refrigerator. Suspension is stable for 14 days without significant loss of potency. Store mixture in tightly closed container. Shake well before using.
● Because cephalexin is dialyzable, patients undergoing treatment with hemodialysis or peritoneal dialysis may require dosage adjustment.
● Drug causes false-positive results in urine glucose tests utilizing cupric sulfate (Benedict's reagent or Clinitest); use glucose oxidase test

(Chemstrip uG, Diastix, or glucose enzymatic test strip) instead. Cephalexin also causes false elevations in serum or urine creatinine levels in tests using Jaffé's reaction. Positive Coombs' test results occur in about 3% of patients.

Patient monitoring
• With large doses or prolonged therapy, monitor patient for superinfection, especially if high-risk.
• If patient has suspected renal impairment, monitor renal function tests before and during therapy.

Breast-feeding patients
• Drug appears in breast milk; use cautiously in breast-feeding women.

Pediatric patients
• Serum half-life is prolonged in neonates and infants under age 1. Safety and effectiveness in children haven't been established.

Geriatric patients
• Reduce dosage in geriatric patients who have diminished renal function.

Patient education
• Inform patient of potential adverse reactions.
• Instruct patient to take drug with food to avoid GI upset.

cephradine
Velosef

Pharmacologic classification: first-generation cephalosporin
Therapeutic classification: antibiotic
Pregnancy risk category: B

Indications and dosages
➤ *Serious respiratory tract, GU tract, skin, soft-tissue, bone, and joint infections; septicemia; endocarditis; otitis media.*
Adults: 250 to 500 mg P.O. q 6 hours. Severe or chronic infections may require larger or more frequent doses (up to 1 g P.O. q 6 hours).
Children over age 9 months: 25 to 100 mg/kg P.O. daily in equally divided doses q 6 to 12 hours.
   Larger doses (up to 1 g q.i.d.) may be given for severe or chronic infections in all patients regardless of age and weight.
✦ *Dosage adjustment.* To prevent toxic accumulation, reduced dosage may be required if patient has reduced creatinine clearance. In patients with creatinine clearance of 5 to 20 ml/minute, give 250 mg q 6 hours. In those with creatinine clearance below 5 ml/minute, give 250 mg q 12 hours.
   For patients receiving long-term intermittent dialysis, give 250 mg initially; repeat in 12 hours and after 36 to 48 hours. Children may need dose modifications proportional to weight and severity of infection.

How supplied
Available by prescription only
Capsules: 250 mg, 500 mg
Suspension: 125 mg/5 ml, 250 mg/5 ml

Pharmacodynamics
Antibacterial action*: Primarily bactericidal; it also may be bacteriostatic. Activity depends on the organism, tissue penetration, dosage, and rate of organism multiplication. It acts by adhering to bacterial penicillin-binding proteins, inhibiting cell wall synthesis.
   Like other first-generation cephalosporins, cephradine is active against many gram-positive organisms and some gram-negative organisms. Susceptible organisms include *Escherichia coli* and other coliform bacteria, group A beta-hemolytic streptococci, *Haemophilus influenzae, Klebsiella, Proteus mirabilis, Staphylococcus aureus, Streptococcus pneumoniae,* staphylococci, and *Streptococcus viridans.*

Pharmacokinetics
Absorption: Well absorbed from the GI tract.
Distribution: Distributed widely into most body tissues and fluids, including the gallbladder, liver, kidneys, bone, sputum, bile, and pleural and synovial fluids; CSF penetration is poor. Cephradine crosses the placenta and is 6% to 20% protein-bound.
Metabolism: Not metabolized.
Excretion: Excreted primarily in urine by renal tubular and glomerular filtration; small amounts of drug appear in breast milk. Elimination half-life is about ½ to 2 hours in normal renal function; end-stage renal disease prolongs half-life to 8 to 15 hours. Hemodialysis or peritoneal dialysis removes drug.

Route	Onset	Peak	Duration
P.O.	Unknown	1 hr	Unknown

Contraindications and precautions
Contraindicated in patients hypersensitive to drug and other cephalosporins. Use cautiously in breast-feeding women and patients with impaired renal function or penicillin allergy.

Interactions
Drug-drug. *Bacteriostatic drugs (chloramphenicol, erythromycin, tetracyclines):* May interfere with bactericidal activity. Avoid use together.
Loop diuretics, nephrotoxic drugs (aminoglycosides, colistin, polymyxin B, or vancomycin): May increase the risk of nephrotoxicity. Monitor patient closely.
Probenecid: Competitively inhibits renal tubular secretion of cephalosporins, resulting in higher, prolonged serum levels of these drugs. Sometimes used for this effect.

Reactions may be *common*, uncommon, ***life-threatening***, or COMMON AND LIFE-THREATENING.

Adverse reactions
CNS: dizziness, headache, malaise, paresthesia.
GI: pseudomembranous colitis, *nausea, anorexia,* vomiting, heartburn, abdominal cramps, *diarrhea,* oral candidiasis.
GU: genital pruritus and candidiasis, vaginitis.
Hematologic: *transient neutropenia,* eosinophilia, *thrombocytopenia.*
Hepatic: transient increases in liver enzyme levels.
Skin: *maculopapular and erythematous rash, urticaria.*
Other: *hypersensitivity reactions* (serum sickness, *anaphylaxis*).

Overdose and treatment
Overdose may cause neuromuscular hypersensitivity; seizures may follow high CNS levels. Remove cephradine by hemodialysis.

Special considerations
Consider the recommendations relevant to all cephalosporins as well as the following.
⚠ ALERT Names of some cephalosporins are similar. Use caution when dispensing.
• Reconstituted oral suspension may be stored for 7 days at room temperature or for 14 days in the refrigerator.
• Because drug is dialyzable, patients undergoing treatment with hemodialysis may require dosage adjustments.
• Drug causes false-positive results in urine glucose tests utilizing cupric sulfate (Benedict's reagent or Clinitest); use glucose oxidase tests (Chemstrip uG, Diastix, or glucose enzymatic test strip) instead. Cephradine also causes false elevations in serum or urine creatinine levels in tests using Jaffé's reaction. Cephradine may cause positive Coombs' test results.

Patient monitoring
• With large doses or prolonged therapy, watch for superinfection, especially in high-risk patients.
• If patient has suspected renal impairment, monitor renal function before and during therapy.

Breast-feeding patients
• Drug appears in breast milk; use cautiously in breast-feeding women. Safety hasn't been established.

Pediatric patients
• Serum half-life is prolonged in neonates and infants under age 12 months. Safety hasn't been established.

Geriatric patients
• Reduced dosage may be required in patients with reduced renal function. Use cautiously.

Patient education
• Inform patient of potential adverse reactions.
• Inform patient to take drug with food to lessen GI upset.
• Inform patient to take all medication as prescribed, even if he feels better.

---

cetirizine hydrochloride
Zyrtec

Pharmacologic classification: selective H₁-receptor antagonist
Therapeutic classification: antihistamine
Pregnancy risk category: B

Indications and dosages
➤ *Seasonal allergic rhinitis, perennial allergic rhinitis, chronic urticaria.* Adults and children age 6 and older: 5 or 10 mg P.O. daily.
✦ *Dosage adjustment.* In hemodialysis patients or those with hepatic impairment or creatinine clearance less than 31 ml/minute, give 5 mg P.O. daily.

How supplied
Available by prescription only
Syrup: 5 mg/ml
Tablets (film-coated): 5 mg, 10 mg

Pharmacodynamics
Antihistaminic action: Cetirizine's principal effects are mediated by selective inhibition of peripheral H₁ receptors.

Pharmacokinetics
Absorption: Rapidly absorbed.
Distribution: About 93% bound to plasma protein.
Metabolism: Metabolized to a very limited extent by oxidative O-dealkylation to a metabolite with negligible antihistaminic activity.
Excretion: Primarily excreted in urine, 50% as unchanged drug. A small amount is excreted in feces.

Route	Onset	Peak	Duration
P.O.	20-60 min	½-1½ hr	24 hr

Contraindications and precautions
Contraindicated in patients hypersensitive to drug or hydroxyzine. Use cautiously in patients with impaired renal function.

Interactions
Drug-drug. *Anticholinergics, CNS depressants:* May cause additive effect. Avoid use together.
Theophylline: Decreased cetirizine clearance. Monitor patient closely.
Drug-lifestyle. *Alcohol use:* May cause additive effect. Discourage use together.

Adverse reactions
CNS: somnolence, fatigue, dizziness.
EENT: pharyngitis.
GI: dry mouth.

◊ Unlabeled clinical use

Overdose and treatment

Overdose may result in somnolence. Treatment should be symptomatic or supportive. There's no known antidote for cetirizine and the drug isn't effectively removed by dialysis.

Special considerations

• There's no information to indicate that abuse or dependency occurs with cetirizine use.
• Discontinue drug 4 days before diagnostic skin tests; it can prevent, reduce, or mask positive skin test response.

Patient monitoring

• Monitor patient for excessive somnolence.
• Observe patient for adverse effects.

Breast-feeding patients

• Drug may appear in breast milk. Avoid use of drug in breast-feeding women.

Pediatric patients

• Safety and efficacy in children younger than age 6 haven't been established.

Geriatric patients

• Half-life of the drug may be prolonged, as may total body clearance. No dosage adjustments are necessary, however.

Patient education

• Caution patient not to perform hazardous activities if somnolence occurs with drug use.
• Tell patient that coffee or tea may help reduce drowsiness.

---

cetrorelix acetate
Cetrotide

Pharmacologic classification: gonadotropin-releasing hormone (GnRH) analog
Therapeutic classification: infertility agent
Pregnancy risk category: X

Indications and dosages

➤ **Inhibition of premature luteinizing hormone (LH) surges in women undergoing controlled ovarian stimulation.**
Adults: 3 mg S.C. once during early to middle follicular phase, given when serum estradiol level indicates an appropriate stimulation response, usually on stimulation day 7 (range, days 5 to 9). If human chorionic gonadotropin (hCG) hasn't been administered within four days after injection, cetrorelix 0.25 mg should be given S.C. once daily until the day of hCG administration. Or, 0.25-mg S.C. multiple dose regimen is given on either stimulation day 5 (morning or evening) or day 6 (morning) and continued once daily until the day of hCG administration.

How supplied

Available by prescription only
Powder for injection: 0.25 mg, 3 mg

Pharmacodynamics

GnRH antagonist action: Drug competes with natural GnRH for binding to membrane receptors on pituitary cells, which controls the release of LH and follicle-stimulating hormone.

Pharmacokinetics

Absorption: Drug is rapidly absorbed following S.C. injection. Levels peak 1 to 2 hours after administration.
Distribution: Drug is 86% bound to plasma.
Metabolism: After S.C. administration of 10 mg cetrorelix, small amounts were found in bile samples over 24 hours.
Excretion: Drug is excreted unchanged in urine and as metabolites in bile.

Route	Onset	Peak	Duration
S.C.	1-2 hr	1-2 hr	≥ 4 days

Contraindications and precautions

Contraindicated in patients hypersensitive to cetrorelix acetate, extrinsic peptide hormones, mannitol, GnRH, or any other GnRH analogs. Drug is also contraindicated in women with known or suspected pregnancy or who are breast-feeding.

Interactions

None reported.

Adverse reactions

CNS: headache.
GI: nausea.
GU: ovarian hyperstimulation syndrome.
Hepatic: elevated ALT, AST, GGT, and alkaline phosphatase levels.

Overdose and treatment

No overdoses have been reported. Single doses up to 120 mg have been well tolerated and have produced no evidence of overdose in patients treated for other indications.

Special considerations

• Drug should be prescribed by clinicians experienced in fertility treatment.
• Dose is adjusted according to patient response.
• When ultrasound shows a sufficient number or follicles of adequate size, hCG is given to induce ovulation and maturation of oocytes.
• To reduce the risk of ovarian hyperstimulation syndrome, don't give hCG if ovaries show an excessive response to treatment.
• Drug can be administered by the patient after proper instruction.

Patient monitoring

• Pregnancy must be ruled out before starting treatment.

Reactions may be *common*, uncommon, **life-threatening**, or COMMON AND LIFE-THREATENING.

Breast-feeding patients
• It isn't known if drug appears in breast milk. Drug shouldn't be used by nursing mothers.

Patient education
• Instruct patient to store 3-mg form at room temperature (77° F [25° C]). Instruct her to store 0.25-mg form in refrigerator at 36° to 46° F (2° to 8° C). Keep this product away from children.
• Instruct patient to report any adverse effect that becomes bothersome.
• Educate patient on the importance of following the regimen exactly as prescribed to achieve optimal results.
• Instruct patient on the proper administration technique, as follows. Wash hands thoroughly with soap and water. Flip off the plastic cover of the vial and wipe the top with an alcohol swab. Attach the needle with the yellow mark to the prefilled syringe. Push the needle through the rubber stopper of the vial and slowly inject the liquid into the vial. Leave the syringe in place and gently swirl the vial until the solution is clear and without residue. Don't shake. Draw liquid from the vial into the syringe. If necessary, invert the vial and pull the needle back as far as needed to withdraw the entire contents of the vial. Detach the needle with the yellow mark from the syringe and replace it with the needle with the gray mark. Invert the syringe and push the plunger until all air bubbles are gone.
• Tell patient to choose an injection site on the lower abdomen, around the navel. If she receives a multiple dose (0.25-mg) regimen, tell her to choose a different site each day to minimize local irritation. Instruct her to clean the site with an alcohol swab and gently pinch a skinfold surrounding the site of injection. Instruct her to insert the needle completely into the skin at about a 45-degree angle and, once the needle has been inserted completely, to release her grasp of the skin. Tell her to gently pull back the plunger of the syringe to check for correct positioning of the needle. If no blood appears, tell her to inject the entire solution by slowly pushing the plunger. She should then withdraw the needle and gently press an alcohol swab on the injection site.
• If blood appears when the patient pulls back on the plunger, tell her to withdraw the needle and gently press an alcohol swab on the injection site. Explain that she'll need to discard the syringe and the drug vial and to repeat the procedure using a new pack.
• Urge the patient to use a syringe and needle only once and then to dispose of them properly. If available, suggest that she use a medical waste container for disposal.

cevimeline hydrochloride
Evoxac

Pharmacologic classification: cholinergic agonist
Therapeutic classification: pro-secretory
Pregnancy risk category: C

Indications and dosages
➤ *Dry mouth in patients with Sjögren's syndrome.* Adults: 30 mg P.O. t.i.d.

How supplied
Available by prescription only
Tablets: 30 mg

Pharmacodynamics
Pro-secretory action: As a cholinergic agonist, cevimeline binds to and stimulates muscarinic receptors. This increases secretion of exocrine glands that cause salivation, sweating, and increased tone of smooth muscles in the GI and GU tracts.

Pharmacokinetics
Absorption: Cevimeline is rapidly absorbed, reaching peak plasma levels between 1½ and 2 hours. Food decreases the rate of absorption, and the peak concentration is reduced by 17.3%.
Distribution: Cevimeline is less than 20% protein-bound.
Metabolism: Liver enzymes CYP2D6, CYP3A3, and CYP3A4 are involved in the metabolism of cevimeline, and the drug is metabolized to a number of metabolites.
Excretion: Cevimeline is mostly excreted in urine and has a half-life of about 5 hours.

Route	Onset	Peak	Duration
P.O.	Unknown	1½ to 2 hr	Unknown

Contraindications and precautions
Contraindicated in patients hypersensitive to drug. Also contraindicated in patients with uncontrolled asthma and in patients for whom miosis is undesirable, as in those with acute iritis or angle-closure glaucoma.

Use cautiously in patients with significant CV disease, evidenced by angina pectoris or MI, because it can alter cardiac conduction and heart rate. Use cautiously in patients with controlled asthma, chronic bronchitis, or COPD, because it can cause bronchial constriction and increase bronchial secretions. Use cautiously in patients with a history of nephrolithiasis because an increase in ureteral smooth muscle tone could cause renal colic or ureteral reflux. Use cautiously in patients with cholelithiasis because contractions of the gallbladder or biliary smooth muscle could cause cholecystitis, cholangitis, and biliary obstruction.

Interactions
Drug-drug. *Beta blockers:* Possible conduction disturbances. Use cautiously.
Drugs with parasympathomimetic effects: Additive effects. Use cautiously.
Drugs that inhibit CYP2D6, CYP3A4, CYP3A3: Inhibited cevimeline metabolism. Monitor patient closely.

Adverse reactions
CNS: anxiety, depression, dizziness, fatigue, *headache,* hypoesthesia, insomnia, migraine, pain, tremor, vertigo.
CV: chest pain, palpitations, peripheral edema, edema.
EENT: abnormal vision, conjunctivitis, earache, epistaxis, eye infection, eye pain, otitis media, pharyngitis, *rhinitis, sinusitis,* tooth disorder, toothache, xerophthalmia, eye abnormality.
GI: abdominal pain, anorexia, constipation, *diarrhea,* dry mouth, eructation, excessive salivation, flatulence, gastroesophageal reflux, *nausea,* salivary gland enlargement and pain, sialoadenitis, ulcerative stomatitis, vomiting, dyspepsia.
GU: cystitis, candidiasis, urinary tract infection, vaginitis.
Hematologic: anemia.
Hepatic: increased amylase.
Musculoskeletal: arthralgia, back pain, hypertonia, hyporeflexia, leg cramps, myalgia, rigors, skeletal pain.
Respiratory: *upper respiratory tract infection,* bronchitis, pneumonia, cough, hiccups.
Skin: rash, pruritus, skin disorder, erythematous rash, *excessive sweating.*
Other: fever, fungal infections, flulike symptoms, injury, surgical intervention, hot flushes, postoperative pain, allergic reaction, infection, abscess.

Overdose and treatment
Toxicity is characterized by exaggeration of parasympathomimetic effects. These may include headache, visual disturbance, lacrimation, sweating, respiratory distress, GI spasm, nausea, vomiting, diarrhea, atrioventricular block, tachycardia, bradycardia, hypotension, shock, mental confusion, cardiac arrhythmias and tremors.

General supportive treatment should be instituted. If medically indicated, atropine may be of value as an antidote. Epinephrine may be useful in the presence of severe CV depression or bronchoconstriction. It's not known whether cevimeline is dialyzable.

Special considerations
● Patient with CYP2D6 activity may have a higher risk of adverse effects.
● Excessive sweating and dehydration may occur.
● Patient may develop impaired depth perception and decreased visual acuity with ophthalmic form.

Patient monitoring
● Monitor patients with a history of asthma, COPD, or chronic bronchitis for an increase in symptoms such as wheezing, increased sputum production, or cough.
● Monitor patients with a history of cardiac disease for increased frequency, severity, or duration of angina or changes in heart rate.

Breast-feeding patients
● It isn't known if cevimeline appears in breast milk. A decision should be made to either discontinue nursing or discontinue the drug based on its importance to the mother.

Pediatric patients
● Safety and efficacy haven't been established.

Geriatric patients
● Monitor elderly patients closely because they are more likely to have decreased renal, hepatic, and cardiac function and concurrent disease and drug therapy.

Patient education
● Tell patient not to interrupt or discontinue treatment without medical approval.
● Tell patient that sweating is a common effect of the drug. Fluid intake is important to prevent dehydration.
● Inform patient that cevimeline may cause visual disturbances, especially at night, that can impair the ability to drive.

chloral hydrate
Aquachloral Supprettes,
Novo-Chlorhydrate*

Pharmacologic classification: general CNS depressant
Therapeutic classification: sedative-hypnotic
Controlled substance schedule: IV
Pregnancy risk category: C

Indications and dosages
➤**Sedation.** *Adults:* 250 mg P.O. t.i.d. after meals.
Children: 8 mg/kg P.O. t.i.d. Maximum dose is 500 mg t.i.d.
➤**Management of alcohol withdrawal symptoms.** *Adults:* 500 to 1,000 mg; may repeat q 6 hours, p.r.n.
➤**Insomnia.** *Adults:* 500 mg to 1 g P.O. or P.R. 15 to 30 minutes before bedtime.
Children: 50 mg/kg P.O. or P.R. single dose. Maximum dose is 1 g.
➤**Premedication for EEG.** *Children:* 20 to 25 mg/kg P.O. single dose. Maximum dose is 1 g.
➤**Hypnosis.** *Children:* 50 mg/kg P.O. or 1.5 g/m^2 as single dose. Maximum dose is 1 g.
✦**Dosage adjustment.** Decrease dosage in elderly patients.

Reactions may be common, *uncommon,* **life-threatening**, *or* COMMON AND LIFE-THREATENING.

How supplied
Available by prescription only
Capsules: 250 mg, 500 mg
Suppositories: 325 mg, 500 mg, 650 mg
Syrup: 250 mg/5 ml, 500 mg/5 ml

Pharmacodynamics
Sedative-hypnotic action: CNS depressant activities similar to those of barbiturates. Nonspecific CNS depression occurs at hypnotic doses; however, respiratory drive is only slightly affected. Drug's primary site of action is the reticular activating system, which controls arousal. The cellular site of action isn't known.

Pharmacokinetics
Absorption: Well absorbed after oral and rectal administration. Sleep occurs 30 to 60 minutes after a 500-mg to 1-g dose.
Distribution: Drug and active metabolite, trichloroethanol, are distributed throughout body tissue and fluids. Trichloroethanol is 35% to 41% protein-bound.
Metabolism: Metabolized rapidly and nearly completely in liver and erythrocytes to active metabolite trichloroethanol. Further metabolized in liver and kidneys to trichloroacetic acid and other inactive metabolites.
Excretion: Inactive metabolites of drug hydrate excreted primarily in urine. Minor amounts excreted in bile. Trichloroethanol half-life is 8 to 10 hours.

Route	Onset	Peak	Duration
P.O.	0.5 hr	Unknown	4-8 hr
P.R.	Unknown	Unknown	4-8 hr

Contraindications and precautions
Contraindicated in patients hypersensitive to drug and in those with impaired hepatic or renal function or severe cardiac disease. Oral administration is contraindicated in patients with gastric disorders. Use with extreme caution in patients with mental depression, suicidal tendencies, or history of drug abuse.

Interactions
Drug-drug. *Antihistamines, narcotics, sedative-hypnotics, tranquilizers, tricyclic antidepressants, other CNS depressants:* Chloral hydrate will add to or potentiate their effects. Monitor patient closely.
I.V. furosemide: May cause a hypermetabolic state by displacing thyroid hormone from binding sites, resulting in sweating, hot flashes, tachycardia, and variable blood pressure. Use together cautiously.
Oral anticoagulants: Possible increased hypoprothrombinemic effects. Monitor PT.
Phenytoin: Possible increased elimination of phenytoin. Monitor serum phenytoin levels.
Drug-lifestyle. *Alcohol use:* May cause vasodilation, tachycardia, sweating, and flushing in some patients. Discourage use together.

Adverse reactions
CNS: drowsiness, nightmares, dizziness, ataxia, paradoxical excitement, hangover, somnolence, disorientation, delirium, light-headedness, hallucinations, confusion, vertigo, malaise.
GI: *nausea, vomiting, diarrhea,* flatulence.
Hematologic: eosinophilia, *leukopenia.*
Other: physical and psychological dependence, *hypersensitivity reactions* (rash, urticaria).

Overdose and treatment
Overdose may cause stupor, coma, respiratory depression, pinpoint pupils, hypotension, and hypothermia. Esophageal stricture may follow gastric necrosis and perforation. GI hemorrhage has been reported. Hepatic damage and jaundice may occur.

Treatment of overdose is supportive of respiration (including mechanical ventilation if needed), blood pressure, and body temperature. If patient is conscious, empty stomach by emesis or gastric lavage. Hemodialysis removes drug and its metabolite. Peritoneal dialysis may be effective.

Special considerations
- Chloral hydrate isn't a first-line drug because of the risk of adverse or toxic effects.
- Some brands contain tartrazine, which may cause allergic reactions in susceptible patients.
- Give drug capsules with 8 oz (240 ml) of water to lessen GI upset; dilute syrup in a half-glass of water or juice to improve taste.
- Store in dark container away from heat and moisture to prevent breakdown of drug. Store suppositories in refrigerator.
- Drug therapy may produce false-positive results for urine glucose with tests using cupric sulfate, such as Benedict's reagent and possibly Clinitest.
- Drug doesn't interfere with Chemstrip uG, Diastix, or glucose enzymatic test strip results.
- Drug will interfere with fluorometric tests for urine catecholamines; don't use drug for 48 hours before test.
- Drug may interfere with Reddy-Jenkins-Thorn test for urinary 17-hydroxycorticosteroids.
- Drug may cause a false-positive phentolamine test.

Patient monitoring
- Assess patient's level of consciousness before administering drug to ensure appropriate baseline level.
- Monitor vital signs frequently.

Breast-feeding patients
- Small amounts appear in breast milk and may cause drowsiness in breast-fed infants. Avoid use in breast-feeding women.

Pediatric patients
- Drug is safe and effective in children as a premedication for EEG and other procedures.

Geriatric patients
● Elderly patients may be more susceptible to CNS-depressant effects because of decreased elimination. Lower doses are indicated.

Patient education
● Advise patient to take drug with 8 oz of water and to dilute syrup with juice or water before use.
● Instruct patient in proper administration of form prescribed.
● Warn patient not to attempt tasks that require mental alertness or physical coordination until the CNS effects of drug are known.
● Tell patient to avoid alcohol and other CNS depressants.
● Instruct patient to call before using OTC allergy or cold preparations.
● Warn patient not to increase dose or stop drug except as prescribed.

chlorambucil
Leukeran

Pharmacologic classification: alkylating agent (not specific to phase of cell cycle)
Therapeutic classification: antineoplastic
Pregnancy risk category: D

Indications and dosages
Dosages and indications may vary. Check current literature for recommended protocol.
➤ *Chronic lymphocytic leukemia; malignant lymphomas including lymphosarcoma, giant follicular lymphomas, and Hodgkin's disease; autoimmune hemolytic anemias; ovarian neoplasms.*
Adults: 100 to 200 mcg/kg P.O. daily or 3 to 6 mg/m^2 P.O. daily as a single dose or in divided doses for 3 to 6 weeks. Usual dose is 4 to 10 mg daily. Reduce dose if full course of radiation therapy is planned within 4 weeks.
Children: 100 to 200 mcg/kg or 4.5 mg/m^2 P.O. as a single daily dose.
➤ *Minimal change nephrotic syndrome* ◇.
Children: 100 to 200 mcg/kg P.O. daily for 8 to 12 weeks with prednisone. Maximum 8.2 mg/kg to 14 mg/kg in one course of therapy.
➤ *Macroglobulinemia* ◇. *Adults:* 2 to 10 mg P.O. daily.
➤ *Metastatic trophoblastic neoplasia* ◇.
Adults: 6 to 10 mg P.O. daily for 5 days; repeat q 1 to 2 weeks.
➤ *Idiopathic uveitis, Behcet's syndrome* ◇.
Adults: 6 to 12 mg P.O. daily for 1 year.
➤ *Rheumatoid arthritis* ◇. *Adults:* 0.1 to 0.3 mg/kg P.O. daily.

How supplied
Available by prescription only
Tablets (sugar-coated): 2 mg

Pharmacodynamics
Antineoplastic action: Drug exerts its cytotoxic activity by cross-linking strands of cellular DNA and RNA, disrupting normal nucleic acid function.

Pharmacokinetics
Absorption: Well absorbed from the GI tract.
Distribution: Not well understood. However, drug and its metabolites have been shown to be highly bound to plasma and tissue proteins.
Metabolism: Metabolized in the liver. Its primary metabolite, phenylacetic acid mustard, also possesses cytotoxic activity.
Excretion: Metabolites are excreted in urine. Half-life of parent compound is 2 hours; the phenylacetic acid metabolite, 2½ hours.

Route	Onset	Peak	Duration
P.O.	Unknown	1 hr	Unknown

Contraindications and precautions
Contraindicated in patients hypersensitive to drug or resistant to previous therapy. Patients hypersensitive to other alkylating agents also may be hypersensitive to drug. Use cautiously in patients with history of head trauma or seizures and in those receiving other drugs that lower seizure threshold.

Interactions
Drug-drug. *Anticoagulants, aspirin:* Increased risk of bleeding. Avoid use together.
Myelosuppressive drugs: Concurrent use can cause additive myelosuppression. Monitor patient closely.

Adverse reactions
CNS: *seizures,* peripheral neuropathy, tremor, muscle twitching, confusion, agitation, ataxia, flaccid paresis.
GI: *nausea, vomiting, stomatitis,* diarrhea.
GU: *azoospermia, infertility.*
Hematologic: *neutropenia,* delayed up to 3 weeks, lasting up to 10 days after last dose; *bone marrow suppression; thrombocytopenia; anemia.*
Hepatic: *hepatotoxicity.*
Respiratory: interstitial pneumonitis.
Skin: rash.
Other: allergic febrile reaction, *hypersensitivity reaction.*

Overdose and treatment
Evidence of overdose includes reversible pancytopenia in adults, and vomiting, ataxia, abdominal pain, muscle twitching, and major motor seizures in children.
    Treatment is usually supportive with transfusion of blood components, if necessary, and appropriate anticonvulsant therapy if seizures occur. Induction of emesis, activated charcoal, and gastric lavage may be useful in removing unabsorbed drug. Drug probably isn't dialyzable.

Reactions may be *common*, uncommon, *life-threatening*, or COMMON AND LIFE-THREATENING.

Special considerations
● Oral suspension can be prepared in the pharmacy by crushing tablets and mixing powder with a suspending agent and simple syrup.
● I.M. injections shouldn't be given when platelets are below 100,000/mm³.
● To prevent hyperuricemia with resulting uric acid nephropathy, allopurinol may be used with adequate hydration.
● Store tablets in a tightly closed, light-resistant container.

Patient monitoring
● Monitor CBC at least weekly during treatment and leukocyte counts 3 to 4 days after each weekly CBC for the first 3 to 6 weeks of treatment.
● In patients receiving intermittent therapy, perform CBC once weekly for 3 months, then at least once every 4 weeks.
● Drug-induced pancytopenia generally lasts 1 to 2 weeks but may persist for 3 to 4 weeks. It's reversible up to a cumulative dose of 6.5 mg/kg in a single course.

Pregnant patients
● Drug should be used in life-threatening cases or when safer drugs can't be used or are ineffective. Inform patient of potential hazards to fetus.

Breast-feeding patients
● It isn't known whether drug appears in breast milk. Consider the risk of serious adverse reactions, mutagenicity, and carcinogenicity in nursing infants and the woman's need for the drug in deciding whether to discontinue drug or breastfeeding.

Pediatric patients
● Safety and efficacy in children haven't been established. The potential benefits versus risks must be evaluated.

Patient education
● Emphasize importance of continuing medication despite nausea and vomiting, and of keeping appointments for periodic blood work.
● Advise patient to report vomiting that occurs shortly after taking a dose or symptoms of infection or bleeding.
● Tell patient to immediately report skin reactions or rash.
● Tell patient to avoid exposure to people with infections.

chloramphenicol
Chloromycetin, Chloroptic, Econochlor, Fenicol*, Ophthochlor, Pentamycetin*

chloramphenicol sodium succinate
Chloromycetin Sodium Succinate, Pentamycetin*

Pharmacologic classification: dichloroacetic acid derivative
Therapeutic classification: antibiotic
Pregnancy risk category: C

Indications and dosages
➤ *Severe meningitis, brain abscesses, bacteremia, other serious infections.*
Adults and children: 50 to 100 mg/kg I.V. daily, divided q 6 hours. Maximum dose is 100 mg/kg daily.
Premature infants and neonates who weigh less than 2 kg (4.4 lb) or are under age 7 days: 25 mg/kg I.V. daily.
Neonates who weigh more than 2 kg and are age 7 days or over: 25 mg/kg I.V. q 12 hours. I.V. route must be used to treat meningitis.
➤ *Superficial infections of the skin caused by susceptible bacteria.* Adults and children: Rub into affected area b.i.d. or t.i.d.
➤ *Infection of external ear canal.* Adults and children: Instill 2 to 3 drops into ear canal t.i.d or q.i.d.
➤ *Surface bacterial infection involving conjunctiva or cornea.* Adults and children: Instill 2 drops of solution in eye q hour until condition improves, or instill q.i.d., depending on severity of infection. Apply small amount of ointment to lower conjunctival sac h.s. as supplement to drops. To use ointment alone, apply small amount to lower conjunctival sac q 3 to 6 hours or more frequently, if necessary. Continue with treatment up to 48 hours after condition improves.

How supplied
Available by prescription only
Injection: 1-g vial
Ophthalmic ointment: 1%
Ophthalmic solution: 0.5%
Otic solution: 0.5%
Powder for solution: 25 mg/vial

Pharmacodynamics
Antibacterial action: Chloramphenicol palmitate and chloramphenicol sodium succinate must be hydrolyzed to chloramphenicol before antimicrobial activity can take place. The active compound then inhibits bacterial protein synthesis by binding to the 50S subunit of the ribosome, thus inhibiting peptide bond formation.
  Drug usually produces bacteriostatic effects on susceptible bacteria, including *Rickettsia,*

Chlamydia, Mycoplasma, and certain *Salmonella* strains, as well as most gram-positive and gram-negative organisms. Chloramphenicol is used to treat *Haemophilus influenzae* infection, Rocky Mountain spotted fever, meningitis, lymphogranuloma, psittacosis, severe meningitis, and bacteremia.

Pharmacokinetics
Absorption: With I.V. administration, serum levels vary greatly, depending on patient's metabolism.
Distribution: Distributed widely to most body tissues and fluids, including CSF, liver, and kidneys; it readily crosses the placenta. About 50% to 60% of drug binds to plasma proteins.
Metabolism: Parent drug is metabolized primarily by hepatic glucuronyl transferase to inactive metabolites.
Excretion: About 8% to 12% of dose is excreted by the kidneys as unchanged drug; the remainder is excreted as inactive metabolites. (However, some drug may appear in breast milk.) Plasma half-life ranges from about 1½ to 4½ hours in adults with normal hepatic and renal function. Plasma half-life of parent drug is prolonged in patients with hepatic dysfunction. Peritoneal hemodialysis doesn't remove significant drug amounts. Plasma chloramphenicol levels may be elevated in patients with renal impairment after I.V. chloramphenicol administration.

Route	Onset	Peak	Duration
I.V.	Unknown	1-3 hr	Unknown
Ophthalmic	Unknown	Unknown	Unknown
Otic	Unknown	Unknown	Unknown

Contraindications and precautions
Contraindicated in patients hypersensitive to chloramphenicol. Use cautiously in patients taking drugs that suppress bone marrow function and those with impaired renal or hepatic function, acute intermittent porphyria, or G6PD deficiency.

Interactions
Drug-drug. *Acetaminophen:* Elevated serum chloramphenicol level, possibly increasing pharmacologic effect. This may be useful.
Chlorpropamide, cyclophosphamide, dicumarol, phenobarbital, phenytoin, tolbutamide: Chloramphenicol inhibits hepatic metabolism by inhibiting microsomal enzyme activity, thus prolonging plasma half-life of these drugs and increasing the risk of toxicity from increased serum drug levels. Avoid use together.
Folic acid, iron salts, vitamin B₂: Reduced hematologic response to these substances. Monitor patient closely.
Penicillin: Chloramphenicol may antagonize bactericidal activity. Give penicillin 1 hour or more before chloramphenicol to avoid reducing bactericidal activity of penicillin.

Adverse reactions
CNS: headache, mild depression, confusion, delirium, peripheral neuropathy with prolonged therapy.
EENT: optic neuritis (in patients with cystic fibrosis), glossitis, decreased visual acuity, optic atrophy in children, stinging of eye after instillation, blurred vision (with ointment).
GI: nausea, vomiting, stomatitis, diarrhea, enterocolitis.
GU: hemoglobinuria.
Hematologic: *aplastic anemia, hypoplastic anemia, agranulocytosis, thrombocytopenia.*
Metabolic: lactic acidosis, *gray syndrome in neonates (abdominal distention, gray cyanosis, vasomotor collapse, respiratory distress, death within a few hours of onset of symptoms.*
Skin: jaundice; possible contact sensitivity; burning, urticaria, pruritus in hypersensitive patients.
Other: *angioedema* in hypersensitive patients, *hypersensitivity reactions* (fever, rash, urticaria, *anaphylaxis*).

Overdose and treatment
Signs and symptoms of parenterally administered overdose include anemia and metabolic acidosis followed by hypotension, hypothermia, abdominal distention, and possible death. Treatment is symptomatic and supportive. Drug may be removed by charcoal hemoperfusion.

Special considerations
• Culture and sensitivity tests may be done with first dose and repeated as needed.
• Use drug only when clearly indicated for severe infection. Because of risk of severe toxicity, it should be reserved for life-threatening infections.
• Refrigerate ophthalmic solution.
• For I.V. administration, reconstitute 1-g vial of powder for injection with 10 ml of sterile water for injection; concentration will be 100 mg/ml. Solution remains stable for 30 days at room temperature; however, refrigeration is recommended. Don't use cloudy solutions. Administer I.V. infusion slowly, over at least 1 minute. Check injection site daily for phlebitis and irritation.
• Therapeutic range is 10 to 20 mcg/ml for peak levels and 5 to 10 mcg/ml for trough levels.
• False elevation of urinary para-aminobenzoic acid levels will result if chloramphenicol is administered during a bentiromide test for pancreatic function. Drug therapy will cause false-positive results on tests for urine glucose level using cupric sulfate (Clinitest).

Patient monitoring
• Obtain CBC, platelet count, reticulocyte count, and serum iron level before therapy begins and every 2 days during therapy. Stop drug immediately if results indicate anemia, reticulocytopenia, leukopenia, or thrombocytopenia.
• Assess patient for superinfection by nonsusceptible organisms.

Reactions may be *common,* uncommon, *life-threatening,* or COMMON AND LIFE-THREATENING.

Pregnant patients
• Safe use during pregnancy hasn't been established.

Breast-feeding patients
• Drug appears in breast milk at low levels, posing a risk of bone marrow depression and slight risk of gray syndrome. An alternative feeding method is recommended during treatment.

Pediatric patients
• Use drug cautiously in children under age 2 because of risk of gray syndrome (although most cases occur in first 48 hours after birth). Drug has prolonged half-life in neonates, necessitating special dose.

Geriatric patients
• Administer drug cautiously to geriatric patients with impaired liver function.

Patient education
• Instruct patient to report adverse reactions, especially nausea, vomiting, diarrhea, bleeding, fever, confusion, sore throat, or mouth sores.
• Tell patient to take drug for prescribed period and to take it exactly as directed, even after he feels better.
• Instruct patient to wash hands before and after applying topical ointment or solution.
• Warn patient using otic solution not to touch ear with dropper.
• Caution patient using topical cream to avoid sharing washcloths and towels with family members.
• Tell patient using ophthalmic drug to clean eye area of excess exudate before applying drug; show him how to instill drug in eye. Warn him not to touch applicator tip to eye or surrounding tissue
• Instruct patient to be alert for signs and symptoms of sensitivity, such as itchy eyelids or constant burning, and to discontinue drug and call immediately should any occur.

chlordiazepoxide
Libritabs

chlordiazepoxide hydrochloride
Librium, Mitran, Reposans-10

Pharmacologic classification: benzodiazepine
Therapeutic classification: antianxiety, anticonvulsant, sedative-hypnotic
Controlled substance schedule: IV
Pregnancy risk category: D

Indications and dosages
➤ *Mild to moderate anxiety and tension.*
Adults: 5 to 10 mg P.O. t.i.d. or q.i.d.

Children over age 6 and geriatric or debilitated patients: 5 mg P.O. b.i.d. to q.i.d. Maximum dose is 10 mg P.O. b.i.d. or t.i.d.
➤ *Severe anxiety and tension. Adults:* 20 to 25 mg P.O. t.i.d. or q.i.d.
➤ *Withdrawal symptoms of acute alcoholism. Adults:* 50 to 100 mg P.O., I.M., or I.V. Maximum dose is 300 mg daily.
➤ *Preoperative apprehension and anxiety. Adults:* 5 to 10 mg P.O. t.i.d. or q.i.d. on day before surgery. Or, 50 to 100 mg I.M. 1 hour before surgery.

How supplied
Available by prescription only
Capsules: 5 mg, 10 mg, 25 mg
Powder for injection: 100 mg/ampule
Tablets: 5 mg, 10 mg, 25 mg

Pharmacodynamics
Anxiolytic action: Chlordiazepoxide depresses the CNS at the limbic and subcortical levels of the brain. It produces an antianxiety effect by influencing the effect of the neurotransmitter gamma-aminobutyric acid on its receptor in the ascending reticular activating system, which increases inhibition and blocks cortical and limbic arousal after stimulation of the reticular formation.
Anticonvulsant action: Drug suppresses the spread of seizure activity produced by the epileptogenic foci in the cortex, thalamus, and limbic structures by enhancing presynaptic inhibition.

Pharmacokinetics
Absorption: When given orally, drug is absorbed well through the GI tract. I.M. administration results in erratic absorption.
Distribution: Distributed widely throughout the body; 90% to 98% is protein-bound.
Metabolism: Metabolized in the liver to several active metabolites.
Excretion: Most metabolites are excreted in urine as glucuronide conjugates. Half-life of drug is 5 to 30 hours.

Route	Onset	Peak	Duration
P.O.	Unknown	½-4 hr	Unknown
I.V.	1-5 min	Unknown	15-60 min
I.M.	15-30 min	Unknown	Unknown

Contraindications and precautions
Contraindicated in patients hypersensitive to drug. Use cautiously in patients with impaired renal or hepatic function, mental depression, or porphyria.

Interactions
Drug-drug. *Antacids:* May delay chlordiazepoxide absorption. Monitor patient closely.
Antidepressants, antihistamines, barbiturates, general anesthetics, MAO inhibitors, narcotics, phenothiazines: Potentiated CNS depressant effects. Avoid use together.
Cimetidine, possibly disulfiram: Reduced hepatic metabolism of chlordiazepoxide, which in-

◇ Unlabeled clinical use

creases its plasma levels. Monitor patient carefully.

Digoxin, phenytoin: Levels of these drugs may be increased. Monitor patient for toxicity.

Levodopa: May decrease levodopa effects. Avoid use together.

Oral contraceptives: May impair chlordiazepoxide absorption. Avoid use together.

Drug-lifestyle. *Alcohol use:* Potentiated CNS depressant effects. Discourage use together.

Heavy smoking: Accelerated chlordiazepoxide metabolism and reduced effectiveness. Discourage smoking.

Adverse reactions
CNS: *drowsiness, lethargy,* ataxia, confusion, extrapyramidal symptoms, EEG changes.
CV: edema.
GI: nausea, constipation.
GU: menstrual irregularities.
Hematologic: *agranulocytosis.*
Hepatic: jaundice.
Skin: *swelling, pain at injection site,* skin eruptions.
Other: altered libido.

Overdose and treatment
Overdose may cause somnolence, confusion, coma, hypoactive reflexes, dyspnea, labored breathing, hypotension, bradycardia, slurred speech, and unsteady gait or impaired coordination.

Support blood pressure and respiration until drug effects subside; monitor vital signs. Flumazenil, a specific benzodiazepine antagonist, may be useful. Mechanical ventilatory assistance via endotracheal tube may be required to maintain a patent airway and support adequate oxygenation. Use I.V. fluids and vasopressors, such as dopamine and phenylephrine, to treat hypotension as needed. Use gastric lavage if ingestion was recent, but only if an endotracheal tube is in place to prevent aspiration. Induce emesis if the patient is conscious. After emesis or lavage, administer activated charcoal with a cathartic as a single dose. Don't administer barbiturates if excitation occurs. Dialysis is of limited value.

Special considerations
Consider the recommendations relevant to all benzodiazepines as well as the following.
● Parenteral form isn't recommended in children under age 12.
● I.M. administration isn't recommended because of erratic and slow absorption. However, if I.M. route is used, reconstitute with special diluent only. Don't use diluent if hazy. Discard unused portion. Inject I.M. deep into large muscle mass.
● For I.V. administration, reconstitute drug with sterile water or normal saline solution and infuse slowly, directly into a large vein, at a rate not exceeding 50 mg/minute for adults. Don't infuse chlordiazepoxide into small veins. Avoid extravasation into subcutaneous tissue. Observe in-

fusion site for phlebitis. Keep resuscitation equipment nearby in case of an emergency.
● Prepare solutions for I.V. or I.M. use immediately before administration. Discard unused portions.
● Lower doses are effective in patients with renal or hepatic dysfunction.
● Minor changes in EEG patterns, usually low-voltage, fast activity, may occur during and after chlordiazepoxide therapy.
● Chlordiazepoxide may cause a false-positive pregnancy test, depending on method used. It may also alter urinary 17-ketosteroids (Zimmerman reaction), urine alkaloid determination (Frings thin layer chromatography method), and urinary glucose determinations (with Chemstrip uG and Diastix, but not glucose enzymatic test strip).

Patient monitoring
● Patient should remain in bed under observation for at least 3 hours after parenteral administration of chlordiazepoxide.
● Closely monitor renal and hepatic studies for signs of dysfunction.

Breast-feeding patients
● The breast-fed infant of a woman who receives chlordiazepoxide may become sedated, have feeding difficulties, or lose weight. Drug shouldn't be given to breast-feeding women.

Pediatric patients
● Safety of oral form hasn't been established in children under age 6. Safety of parenteral form hasn't been established in children under age 12.

Geriatric patients
● Geriatric patients demonstrate a greater sensitivity to the CNS depressant effects of drug. Some may require supervision with walking and activities of daily living at start of therapy or after an increase in dose.
● Lower doses are usually effective in geriatric patients because of decreased elimination.
● Parenteral administration of drug is more likely to cause apnea, hypotension, and bradycardia in geriatric patients.

Patient education
● Warn patient that sudden changes in position may cause dizziness. Advise patient to dangle legs a few minutes before getting out of bed to prevent falls and injury.
● Warn patient not to abruptly stop using drug because withdrawal symptoms may occur.
● Tell patient to avoid hazardous activities until the CNS effects of the drug are known.

Reactions may be *common*, uncommon, *life-threatening*, or COMMON AND LIFE-THREATENING.

chloroquine hydrochloride
Aralen Hydrochloride

chloroquine phosphate
Aralen Phosphate

Pharmacologic classification: 4-aminoquinoline
Therapeutic classification: antimalarial, amebicide, anti-inflammatory
Pregnancy risk category: C

Indications and dosages

➤ **Suppressive prophylaxis.** *Adults:* 500 mg (300-mg base) P.O. on same day once weekly beginning 2 weeks before exposure.
Children: 5 mg (base)/kg P.O. on same day once weekly (not to exceed adult dosage) beginning 2 weeks before exposure.

➤ **Treatment of acute attacks of malaria.** *Adults:* 1 g (600-mg base) P.O. followed by 500 mg (300-mg base) P.O. after 6 to 8 hours; then a single dose of 500 mg (300-mg base) P.O. for next 2 days or 4 to 5 ml (160- to 200-mg base) I.M. and repeated in 6 hours if needed; change to P.O. as soon as possible.
Children: 10 mg (base)/kg P.O. initially; then 5 mg (base)/kg after 6 hours. Third dose is 5 mg (base)/kg 18 hours after second dose; fourth dose is 5 mg (base)/kg 24 hours after third dose; or 5 mg (base)/kg I.M. May repeat in 6 hours and change to P.O. as soon as possible.

➤ **Extraintestinal amebiasis.** *Adults:* 1 g (600-mg base) daily for 2 days, then 500 mg (300-mg base) daily for 2 to 3 weeks or 4 to 5 ml (160- to 200-mg base) I.M. for 10 to 12 days; change to P.O. as soon as possible. Administer with an intestinal amebicide.

➤ **Rheumatoid arthritis** ◊. *Adults:* 250 mg P.O. daily (chloroquine phosphate) with evening meal.

➤ **Lupus erythematosus** ◊. *Adults:* 250 mg P.O. daily (chloroquine phosphate) with evening meal; reduce dosage gradually over several months when lesions regress.

How supplied

Available by prescription only
chloroquine hydrochloride
Injection: 50 mg/ml (40 mg/ml base)
chloroquine phosphate
Tablets: 500 mg (300-mg base)

Pharmacodynamics

Antimalarial action: Chloroquine binds to DNA, interfering with protein synthesis. It also inhibits DNA and RNA polymerases.
Amebicidal action: Unknown.
Anti-inflammatory action: Unknown. Drug may antagonize histamine and serotonin and inhibit prostaglandin effects by inhibiting conversion of arachidonic acid to prostaglandin F_2; it

also may inhibit chemotaxis of polymorphonuclear leukocytes, macrophages, and eosinophils.
Chloroquine's spectrum of activity includes the asexual erythrocytic forms of *Plasmodium malariae, P. ovale, P. vivax,* many strains of *P. falciparum,* and *Entamoeba histolytica.*

Pharmacokinetics

Absorption: Absorbed readily and almost completely.
Distribution: 55% bound to plasma proteins. Concentrated in erythrocytes, liver, spleen, kidneys, heart, and brain and is strongly bound in melanin-containing cells.
Metabolism: About 30% of an administered dose is metabolized by the liver to monodesethylchloroquine and bidesethylchloroquine.
Excretion: About 70% of dose is excreted unchanged in urine; unabsorbed drug is excreted in feces. Small amounts of the drug may be present in urine for months after the drug is discontinued. Renal excretion is enhanced by urinary acidification. Drug appears in breast milk.

Route	Onset	Peak	Duration
P.O.	Unknown	1-3 hr	Unknown
I.M.	Unknown	½ hr	Unknown

Contraindications and precautions

Contraindicated in patients hypersensitive to drug and in those with retinal or visual field changes or porphyria. Use cautiously in patients with GI, neurologic, or blood disorders.

Interactions

Drug-drug. *Aluminum salts, kaolin, magnesium salts:* May decrease chloroquine absorption. Separate administration times.
Cimetidine: May reduce oral clearance and metabolism. Monitor patient for toxicity.
Intradermal human diploid cell rabies vaccine: May interfere with antibody response. Use together cautiously.
Drug-lifestyle. *Sun exposure:* May worsen drug-induced dermatoses. Urge patient to avoid excessive sun exposure.

Adverse reactions

CNS: mild and transient headache, psychic stimulation, *seizures,* dizziness, neuropathy.
CV: hypotension, ECG changes, AV block, cardiomyopathy.
EENT: visual disturbances (blurred vision; difficulty in focusing; reversible corneal changes; typically irreversible, sometimes progressive or delayed retinal changes, such as narrowing of arterioles; macular lesions; pallor of optic disk; optic atrophy; patchy retinal pigmentation, typically leading to blindness), ototoxicity (nerve deafness, vertigo, tinnitus).
GI: anorexia, abdominal cramps, diarrhea, nausea, vomiting, stomatitis.
Hematologic: *agranulocytosis, aplastic anemia,* hemolytic anemia, *thrombocytopenia.*

Skin: pruritus, lichen planus eruptions, skin and mucosal pigmentary changes, pleomorphic skin eruptions.

Overdose and treatment
Symptoms of overdose may appear within 30 minutes after ingestion and may include headache, drowsiness, visual changes, CV collapse, and seizures followed by respiratory and cardiac arrest. Treatment is symptomatic. Empty stomach by emesis or lavage. After lavage, activated charcoal in an amount at least five times the estimated amount of drug ingested may be helpful if given within 30 minutes of ingestion.

Ultra-short-acting barbiturates may help control seizures. Intubation may become necessary. Peritoneal dialysis and exchange transfusions also may be useful. Forced fluids and acidification of the urine are helpful after the acute phase.

Special considerations
◪ ALERT Drug dosage may be discussed in milligrams or milligrams base. Be aware of the difference.
● Resistance of *P. falciparum* to chloroquine has spread to most areas with malaria except the Dominican Republic, Haiti, Central America west of the Panama Canal, and Egypt.
● It may also be advisable for traveler to take along sulfadoxine and pyrimethamine (Fansidar). Instruct patient to take drug if a febrile illness occurs and professional medical care isn't available. Emphasize that such self-treatment is a temporary measure and that he must seek medical care as soon as possible. He should continue prophylaxis after the treatment dose of Fansidar.

Patient monitoring
● Baseline and periodic ophthalmologic examinations are necessary in prolonged or high-dosage therapy.
● Assist patient in obtaining audiometric examinations before, during, and after therapy, especially if therapy is long-term.

Breast-feeding patients
● Safety hasn't been established. Use cautiously in breast-feeding women.

Pediatric patients
● Children are extremely susceptible to toxicity; monitor children closely for adverse effects.

Patient education
● Tell patient to promptly report blurred vision, increased sensitivity to light, hearing loss, pronounced GI disturbances, or muscle weakness.
● Advise patient to take drug immediately before or after meals on the same day each week to minimize gastric distress. Patients who can't tolerate drug because of GI distress may tolerate hydroxychloroquine.

chlorpheniramine maleate
Aller-Chlor, Chlo-Amine, Chlor-Trimeton, Chlor-Tripolon*, Novo-Pheniram*, Phenetron, Teldrin

Pharmacologic classification: propylamine-derivative antihistamine
Therapeutic classification: antihistamine (H_1-receptor antagonist)
Pregnancy risk category: B

Indications and dosages
➤ *Rhinitis, allergy symptoms. Adults and children age 12 and older:* 4 mg tablets or syrup P.O. q 4 to 6 hours; or 8 to 12 mg extended-release tablets b.i.d. or t.i.d. Maximum dose is 24 mg daily; 10 to 20 mg S.C., I.V., or I.M. also may be used.
Children ages 6 to 11: 2 mg tablets or syrup P.O. q 4 to 6 hours; or one 8-mg extended-release tablet in 24 hours. Maximum dose is 12 mg daily.
Children ages 2 to 5: 1 mg syrup P.O. q 4 to 6 hours. Maximum dose is 6 mg daily. Safety and efficacy of extended release preparations for children under age 6 haven't been established.

How supplied
Available by prescription only
Injection: 10 mg/ml
Available without a prescription
Capsules (extended-release): 8 mg, 12 mg
Syrup: 2 mg/5 ml
Tablets: 4 mg
Tablets (chewable): 2 mg
Tablets (extended-release): 8 mg, 12 mg

Pharmacodynamics
Antihistamine action: Antihistamines compete with histamine for H_1-receptor sites on smooth muscle of the bronchi, GI tract, uterus, and large blood vessels; they bind to cellular receptors, preventing access of histamine, thereby suppressing histamine-induced allergic symptoms. They don't directly alter histamine or its release.

Pharmacokinetics
Absorption: Well absorbed from the GI tract. Food in the stomach delays absorption but doesn't affect bioavailability.
Distribution: Distributed extensively into the body; drug is about 72% protein-bound.
Metabolism: Metabolized largely in GI mucosal cells and liver (first-pass effect).
Excretion: Half-life is 12 to 43 hours in adults and 10 to 13 hours in children; drug and metabolites are excreted in urine.

Route	Onset	Peak	Duration
P.O.	15-60 min	2-6 hr	24 hr
I.V.	Unknown	Unknown	24 hr
I.M., S.C.	15-60 min	Unknown	24 hr

Contraindications and precautions
Contraindicated in patients having acute asthmatic attacks. Antihistamines aren't recommended for breast-feeding women because small amounts of drug appear in breast milk.

Use cautiously in elderly patients and patients with increased intraocular pressure, hyperthyroidism, CV or renal disease, hypertension, bronchial asthma, urine retention, prostatic hyperplasia, bladder neck obstruction, or stenosing peptic ulcers.

Interactions
Drug-drug. *CNS depressants:* Increased sedation. Use together cautiously.
Epinephrine: Enhanced epinephrine effects. Monitor patient.
Heparin: Anticoagulant action may be partly counteracted. Avoid using together.
MAO inhibitors: Increased anticholinergic effects. Monitor patient.
Sulfonylureas: May diminish the effects of these drugs. Advise patient to report effectiveness of treatment.
Drug-lifestyle. *Alcohol use:* Additive sedation may occur. Discourage use together.

Adverse reactions
CNS: *stimulation,* sedation, *drowsiness,* excitability (in children).
CV: hypotension, palpitations, weak pulse.
GI: epigastric distress, *dry mouth,* constipation.
GU: urine retention.
Respiratory: thick bronchial secretions.
Skin: rash, urticaria, local stinging, burning sensation (after parenteral administration), pallor.

Overdose and treatment
Signs and symptoms of overdose may include either CNS depression (sedation, reduced mental alertness, apnea, and CV collapse) or CNS stimulation (insomnia, hallucinations, tremors, and seizures). Atropine-like symptoms, such as dry mouth, flushed skin, fixed and dilated pupils, and GI symptoms, are common, especially in children.

Treat overdose by inducing emesis with ipecac syrup (in conscious patient), followed by activated charcoal to prevent further drug absorption. Use gastric lavage if patient is unconscious or ipecac fails. Treat hypotension with vasopressors, and control seizures with diazepam or phenytoin. Don't give stimulants. Administering ammonium chloride or vitamin C to acidify urine promotes drug excretion.

Special considerations
Consider the recommendations relevant to all antihistamines as well as the following.
• Don't use parenteral solutions intradermally.
• Administer I.V. solution slowly, over 1 minute.
• If symptoms occur during or after parenteral dose, discontinue drug and inform prescriber.

• Antihistamines can prevent, reduce, or mask positive skin test response. Discontinue drug 4 days before diagnostic skin tests.

Patient monitoring
• Monitor patient for adverse reactions.

Breast-feeding patients
• Antihistamines such as chlorpheniramine shouldn't be used during breast-feeding. Many of these drugs appear in breast milk, exposing the infant to risks of unusual excitability; premature infants are at particular risk for seizures.

Pediatric patients
• Drug isn't indicated for use in premature or newborn infants. Children, especially those under age 6, may experience paradoxical hyperexcitability.

Geriatric patients
• Geriatric patients are usually more sensitive to adverse effects of antihistamines and are especially likely to experience a greater degree of dizziness, sedation, hyperexcitability, dry mouth, constipation, and urine retention than younger patients. Symptoms usually respond to a decrease in dosage.

Patient education
• Instruct patient to swallow extended-release tablets whole; they shouldn't be crushed or chewed.
• Inform patient to store syrup and parenteral solution away from light.

chlorpromazine hydrochloride
Chlorpromanyl-20*, Largactil*, Novo-Chlorpromazine*, Thorazine

Pharmacologic classification: aliphatic phenothiazine
Therapeutic classification: antipsychotic, antiemetic
Pregnancy risk category: C

Indications and dosages
➤ **Psychosis.** *Adults:* 30 to 75 mg P.O. daily in two to four divided doses. Dosage may be increased twice weekly by 20 to 50 mg until symptoms are controlled. Most patients respond to 200 mg daily, but doses up to 800 mg may be necessary. 25 to 50 mg may be given I.M., and may be repeated in 1 hour, if needed. Gradually increase subsequent I.M. doses over several days to a maximum of 400 mg q 4 to 6 hours. Switch to oral therapy as soon as possible.
Children age 6 months and older: 0.55 mg/kg P.O. q 4 to 6 hours; or I.M. q 6 to 8 hours; or 1.1 mg/kg P.R. q 6 to 8 hours. Maximum I.M. dose is 40 mg in children under age 5 or weigh-

ing less than 22.7 kg (50 lb), and 75 mg in children ages 5 to 12 or weighing 22.7 to 45.5 kg (50 to 100 lb).

➤ *Nausea, vomiting. Adults:* 10 to 25 mg P.O. q 4 to 6 hours, p.r.n.; or 50 to 100 mg P.R. q 6 to 8 hours, p.r.n.; or 25 mg I.M. initially. If no hypotension occurs, 25 to 50 mg I.M. q 3 to 4 hours may be given, p.r.n., until vomiting stops. *Children age 6 months and older:* 0.55 mg/kg P.O. q 4 to 6 hours, p.r.n.; or I.M. q 6 to 8 hours, p.r.n.; or 1.1 mg/kg P.R. q 6 to 8 hours, p.r.n. Maximum I.M. dose in children under age 5 or weighing less than 22.7 kg (50 lb) is 40 mg. Maximum I.M. dose in children ages 5 to 12 or weighing 22.7 to 45.5 kg (50 to 100 lb) is 75 mg.

➤ *Intractable hiccups; acute intermittent porphyria. Adults:* 25 to 50 mg P.O. or I.M. t.i.d. or q.i.d. For hiccups, if symptoms persist, 25 to 50 mg diluted in 500 to 1,000 ml of normal saline solution and infuse I.V. slowly with patient in supine position.

➤ *Tetanus. Adults:* 25 mg to 50 mg I.M. or I.V. t.i.d. or q.i.d.
Children age 6 months and older: 0.55 mg/kg I.M. or I.V. q 6 to 8 hours. Maximum parenteral dose in children weighing less than 22.7 kg (50 lb) is 40 mg daily; for children weighing 22.7 to 45.5 kg (50 to 100), maximum parenteral dose is 75 mg daily, except in severe cases.

➤ *Surgery. Adults:* Preoperatively, 25 to 50 mg P.O. 2 to 3 hours before surgery or 12.5 to 25 mg I.M. 1 to 2 hours before surgery; during surgery, 12.5 mg I.M., repeated in 30 minutes, if needed, or fractional 2-mg doses I.V. at 2-minute intervals up to maximum of 25 mg; postoperatively, 10 to 25 mg P.O. q 4 to 6 hours or 12.5 to 25 mg I.M., repeated in 1 hour, if needed.
Children age 6 months and older: Preoperatively, 0.55 mg/kg P.O. 2 to 3 hours before surgery or I.M. 1 to 2 hours before surgery; during surgery, 0.275 mg/kg I.M., repeated in 30 minutes, if needed, or fractional 1-mg doses I.V. at 2-minute intervals, up to maximum of 0.275 mg/kg; postoperatively, 0.55 mg/kg P.O. or I.M., oral dose repeated q 4 to 6 hours or I.M. dose repeated in 1 hour, if needed, and if hypotension doesn't occur.

How supplied
Available by prescription only
Capsules (sustained-release): 30 mg, 75 mg, 150 mg
Injection: 25 mg/ml
Oral concentrate: 30 mg/ml, 100 mg/ml
Suppositories: 25 mg, 100 mg
Syrup: 10 mg/5 ml
Tablets: 10 mg, 25 mg, 50 mg, 100 mg, 200 mg

Pharmacodynamics
Antipsychotic action: Drug is thought to exert its antipsychotic effects by postsynaptic blockade of CNS dopamine receptors, thereby inhibiting dopamine-mediated effects; antiemetic effects are attributed to dopamine receptor blockade in the medullary chemoreceptor trigger zone. Drug has many other central and peripheral effects; it produces both alpha and ganglionic blockade and counteracts histamine- and serotonin-mediated activity. Its most prominent adverse reactions are antimuscarinic and sedative.

Pharmacokinetics
Absorption: Rate and extent of absorption vary with route of administration. Oral tablet absorption is erratic; sustained-release preparations have similar absorption. Oral concentrates and syrups are much more predictable; I.M. drug is absorbed rapidly.
Distribution: Distributed widely into the body, including breast milk; level is usually higher in CNS than in plasma. Steady-state serum level is achieved within 4 to 7 days. Drug is 91% to 99% protein-bound.
Metabolism: Metabolized extensively by the liver and forms 10 to 12 metabolites; some are pharmacologically active.
Excretion: Mostly excreted as metabolites in urine; some is excreted in feces via the biliary tract. It may undergo enterohepatic circulation.

Route	Onset	Peak	Duration
P.O.			
Regular	½-1 hr	Unknown	4-6 hr
Extended	½-1 hr	Unknown	10-12 hr
I.V., I.M.	Unknown	Unknown	Unknown
P.R.	>1 hr	Unknown	3-4 hr

Contraindications and precautions
Contraindicated in patients hypersensitive to drug and in patients with CNS depression, bone marrow suppression, subcortical damage, or coma.

Use cautiously in acutely ill or dehydrated children; geriatric or debilitated patients; and in patients with impaired renal or hepatic function, severe CV disease, glaucoma, prostatic hyperplasia, respiratory or seizure disorders, hypocalcemia, reaction to insulin or electroconvulsive therapy, or exposure to heat, cold, or organophosphate insecticides.

Interactions
Drug-drug. *Antiarrhythmics, disopyramide, procainamide, quinidine:* Increased risk of arrhythmias and conduction defects. Avoid use together.
Anticholinergics: Increased anticholinergic activity and aggravated parkinsonian symptoms. Use cautiously.
Beta blockers: May inhibit chlorpromazine metabolism, increasing plasma levels and toxicity. Monitor patient closely.
Centrally acting antihypertensives: Chlorpromazine may decrease blood pressure. Monitor patient closely.
CNS depressants, parenteral magnesium sulfate: Additive effects are likely. Avoid use together.

Reactions may be *common*, uncommon, *life-threatening*, or COMMON AND LIFE-THREATENING.

Epinephrine: Chlorpromazine may cause epinephrine reversal. Avoid use together.
Lithium: May cause severe neurologic toxicity and a decreased response to chlorpromazine. Avoid use together.
Propylthiouracil: Increased risk of agranulocytosis. Avoid use together.
Sympathomimetics: May decrease stimulatory and pressor effects. Avoid use together.
Warfarin: Decreased anticoagulant effect. Monitor INR and PT.
Drug-food. *Caffeine:* Pharmacokinetic alterations and decreased therapeutic response. Tell patient to avoid caffeinated foods and beverages.
Drug-lifestyle. *Alcohol use:* Additive effects are likely. Discourage use.
Heavy smoking: May reduce response to chlorpromazine. Discourage use.
Sun exposure: Photosensitivity reactions may result. Urge patient to take precautions.

Adverse reactions

CNS: extrapyramidal reactions, drowsiness, sedation, *seizures,* tardive dyskinesia, pseudoparkinsonism, dizziness, *neuroleptic malignant syndrome.*
CV: *orthostatic hypotension,* tachycardia, ECG changes.
EENT: ocular changes, blurred vision, nasal congestion.
GI: *dry mouth, constipation,* nausea.
GU: *urine retention,* menstrual irregularities, inhibited ejaculation, priapism.
Hematologic: *leukopenia, agranulocytosis,* eosinophilia, hemolytic anemia, *aplastic anemia, thrombocytopenia.*
Hepatic: jaundice, abnormal liver function test results.
Skin: *mild photosensitivity,* allergic reactions, *pain at I.M. injection site,* sterile abscess, skin pigmentation.
Other: gynecomastia.
After abrupt withdrawal of long-term therapy: gastritis, nausea, vomiting, dizziness, tremor.

Overdose and treatment

CNS depression is characterized by deep, unarousable sleep and possible coma, hypotension, or hypertension, extrapyramidal symptoms, abnormal involuntary muscle movements, agitation, seizures, arrhythmias, ECG changes, hypothermia or hyperthermia, and autonomic nervous system dysfunction.

Treatment is symptomatic and supportive and includes maintaining vital signs, airway, stable body temperature, and fluid and electrolyte balance.

Don't induce vomiting: Drug inhibits cough reflex, and aspiration may occur. Use gastric lavage, then activated charcoal and saline solution cathartics; dialysis doesn't help. Regulate body temperature as needed. Treat hypotension with I.V. fluids: don't give epinephrine. Treat seizures with parenteral diazepam or barbitu-

rates; arrhythmias with parenteral phenytoin (1 mg/kg with rate adjusted to blood pressure); extrapyramidal reactions with benztropine 1 to 2 mg or parenteral diphenhydramine 10 to 50 mg.

Special considerations

Consider the recommendations relevant to all phenothiazines as well as the following.
🔋 **ALERT** I.V. form should be used only during surgery or for severe hiccups. Dilute injection to 1 mg/ml with normal saline solution and administer at 1 mg/2 minutes for children and 1 mg/minute for adults.
● Sustained-release preparations shouldn't be crushed or opened, but swallowed whole.
● Oral formulations may cause stomach upset and may be administered with food or fluid.
● Dilute concentrate in 2 to 4 oz of liquid, preferably water, carbonated drinks, fruit juice, tomato juice, milk, pudding, or applesauce.
● Store suppository form in a cool place.
● Give I.M. injection deep in the upper outer quadrant of the buttocks. Injection is usually painful; massaging the area after administration may prevent abscess formation.
● If tissue irritation occurs, chlorpromazine injection may be diluted with normal saline solution or 2% procaine.
● Liquid and injectable forms may cause a rash if skin contact occurs.
● Solution for injection may be slightly discolored. Don't use if drug is excessively discolored or if a precipitate is evident. Monitor patient's blood pressure before and after parenteral administration.
● Drug causes false-positive test results for urinary porphyrins, urobilinogen, amylase, and 5-hydroxyindoleacetic acid because of darkening of urine by metabolites; it also causes false-positive results in urine pregnancy tests using human chorionic gonadotropin.

Patient monitoring

● Evaluate patient for signs and symptoms of tardive dyskinesia.
● Monitor CBC in patients receiving prolonged therapy.
● Monitor patient for cholestatic jaundice (upper abdominal pain, nausea, yellow skin, flu-like symptoms, rash, fever, eosinophilia, bile in the urine, elevated serum bilirubin, alkaline phosphatase and transaminase levels). Weekly urine bilirubin tests during the first month of treatment may detect cholestatic jaundice.

Breast-feeding patients

● Drug appears in breast milk. Potential benefits to the woman should outweigh potential harm to the infant.

Pediatric patients

● Drug isn't recommended for patients under age 6 months. Sudden infant death syndrome has been reported in children younger than age 1 receiving drug. Extrapyramidal effects may be more common in children.

Geriatric patients
● Older patients tend to require lower doses, adjusted individually. Adverse reactions, especially tardive dyskinesia and other extrapyramidal effects, are more likely to develop in geriatric patients.

Patient education
● Explain risks of dystonic reactions and tardive dyskinesia, and tell patient to report abnormal involuntary body movements or painful muscle contractions.
● Warn patient to avoid extremely hot or cold baths or exposure to temperature extremes, sunlamps, or tanning beds. Drug may cause thermoregulatory changes.
● Tell patient not to spill the liquid preparation on the skin because rash and irritation may result.
● Instruct patient to take drug exactly as prescribed and not to double dose to compensate for missed ones.
● Explain that many drug interactions are possible. Patient should seek medical approval before taking other medications.
● Tell patient not to stop taking drug suddenly.
● Encourage patient to report difficulty urinating, sore throat, dizziness, fever, or fainting.
● Advise patient to avoid hazardous activities that require alertness until the effect of the drug is established. Excessive sedative effects tend to subside after several weeks.
● Explain what fluids are appropriate for diluting the concentrate and the dropper technique for measuring dose. Teach patient how to use suppository form.
● Inform patient that sugarless chewing gum or hard candy, ice chips, or artificial saliva may alleviate dry mouth.

chlorpropamide
Diabinese, Novo-Propamide*

Pharmacologic classification: sulfonylurea
Therapeutic classification: antidiabetic
Pregnancy risk category: C

Indications and dosages
➤ *Adjunct to diet to lower blood glucose levels in patients with non-insulin-dependent diabetes mellitus (type 2).*
Adults: 250 mg P.O. daily with breakfast or in divided doses if GI disturbances occur. First dosage increase may be made after 5 to 7 days because of extended duration of action, then dosage may be increased q 3 to 5 days by 50 to 125 mg, if needed, to a maximum of 750 mg daily.
✦ *Dosage adjustment.* In adults over age 65, initial dose should be 100 to 125 mg daily.

➤ *To change from insulin to oral therapy.* *Adults:* If insulin dosage is less than 40 units daily, insulin may be stopped and oral therapy started as above. If insulin dosage is 40 units or more daily, start oral therapy as above, with insulin dose reduced 50% the first few days. Further insulin reductions should be made based on patient response.

How supplied
Available by prescription only
Tablets: 100 mg, 250 mg

Pharmacodynamics
Antidiabetic action: Chlorpropamide lowers blood glucose levels by stimulating insulin release from beta cells in the pancreas. After prolonged administration, it produces hypoglycemic effects through extrapancreatic mechanisms, including reduced basal hepatic glucose production and enhanced peripheral sensitivity to insulin; the latter may result either from an increased number of insulin receptors or from changes in events that follow insulin binding.
Antidiuretic action: Drug appears to potentiate the effects of minimal levels of antidiuretic hormone.

Pharmacokinetics
Absorption: Absorbed readily from the GI tract. Maximum decrease in serum glucose levels at 3 to 6 hours.
Distribution: Distribution isn't fully understood, but is probably similar to that of the other sulfonylureas. It's highly protein-bound.
Metabolism: About 80% of drug is metabolized by the liver. Whether the metabolites have hypoglycemic activity is unknown.
Excretion: Excreted in urine. Rate of excretion depends on urinary pH; it increases in alkaline urine and decreases in acidic urine. Duration of action is up to 60 hours; half-life is 36 hours.

Route	Onset	Peak	Duration
P.O.	1 hr	2-4 hr	24 hr

Contraindications and precautions
Contraindicated for treating type 1 diabetes (insulin-dependent) or diabetes that can be adequately controlled by diet. Also contraindicated in pregnant women, breast-feeding women, patients hypersensitive to drug, and patients with type 2 diabetes complicated by ketosis, acidosis, diabetic coma, major surgery, severe infections, or severe trauma.
    Use cautiously in geriatric, debilitated, or malnourished patients and in those with porphyria or impaired renal or hepatic function.

Interactions
Drug-drug. *Anticoagulants:* May increase plasma levels of both drugs and, after continued therapy, may reduce plasma levels and anticoagulant effects. Monitor patient closely.

Reactions may be *common,* uncommon, *life-threatening,* or COMMON AND LIFE-THREATENING.

Beta blockers: May increase the risk of hypoglycemia. Monitor patient closely.

Chloramphenicol, guanethidine, insulin, MAO inhibitors, probenecid, salicylates, sulfonamides: May enhance hypoglycemic effects by displacing chlorpropamide from its protein-binding sites. Avoid use together.

Drug-herb. *Bitter melon (karela), ginkgo biloba.* Possible increased risk of hypoglycemia. Discourage use together.

Drug-lifestyle. *Alcohol use:* May produce a disulfiram-like reaction. Discourage use together.

Smoking: Increases corticosteroid release. May require higher dosages of chlorpropamide.

Adverse reactions

CNS: paresthesia, fatigue, dizziness, vertigo, malaise, headache.

EENT: tinnitus.

GI: nausea, heartburn, epigastric distress.

GU: tea-colored urine, altered urine phenyl ketone level.

Hematologic: *leukopenia, thrombocytopenia, aplastic anemia, agranulocytosis,* hemolytic anemia.

Hepatic: altered alkaline phosphatase and bilirubin levels.

Metabolic: *prolonged hypoglycemia; dilutional hyponatremia;* altered cholesterol, porphyrin, and protein levels; altered cephalin flocculation.

Skin: rash, pruritus, erythema, urticaria.

Other: *hypersensitivity reactions.*

Overdose and treatment

Signs and symptoms of overdose include low blood glucose levels, tingling of lips and tongue, hunger, nausea, decreased cerebral function (lethargy, yawning, confusion, agitation, and nervousness), increased sympathetic activity (tachycardia, sweating, and tremor), and ultimately seizures, stupor, and coma.

Mild hypoglycemia (without loss of consciousness or neurologic findings) can be treated with oral glucose and dosage adjustments. If patient loses consciousness or experiences neurologic symptoms, he should receive rapid injection of $D_{50}W$, followed by a continuous infusion of $D_{10}W$ at a rate to maintain blood glucose levels greater than 100 mg/dl. Because of chlorpropamide's long half-life, monitor patient for 3 to 5 days.

Special considerations

Consider the recommendations relevant to all sulfonylureas as well as the following.

• To avoid GI intolerance in patients who require daily dosages of 250 mg or more and to improve control of hyperglycemia, divided doses are recommended. These are given before the morning and evening meals.

• Geriatric, debilitated, or malnourished patients and those with impaired renal or hepatic function usually require a lower initial dosage.

• Because of the long duration of action of the drug, adverse reactions, especially hypoglycemia, may be more frequent or severe than with some other sulfonylureas.

• Patients with severe diabetes who don't respond to 500 mg usually won't respond to higher doses.

• Oral hypoglycemics have been linked to an increased risk of CV mortality compared with diet or diet and insulin.

Patient monitoring

• Drug may accumulate in patients with renal insufficiency. Observe patient for signs such as dysuria, anuria, and hematuria.

• Patients switching from chlorpropamide to another sulfonylurea should be monitored closely for 1 week because of chlorpropamide's prolonged retention in the body.

• Chlorpropamide may potentiate antidiuretic effects of vasopressin. Monitor patient for drowsiness, muscle cramps, seizures, unconsciousness, water retention, and weakness.

Breast-feeding patients

• Drug appears in breast milk and shouldn't be given to breast-feeding women.

Pediatric patients

• Drug is ineffective in type 1 diabetes mellitus (insulin-dependent or juvenile-onset).

Geriatric patients

• Geriatric patients may be more sensitive to the effects of drug because of reduced metabolism and elimination. They're more likely to develop neurologic symptoms of hypoglycemia.

• Avoid drug in geriatric patients because of its longer duration of action.

• Geriatric patients usually require a lower initial dosage.

Patient education

• Emphasize importance of following prescribed diet, as well as the exercise and medical regimen.

• Instruct patient to take medication at the same time each day. If a dose is missed, it should be taken immediately, unless it's almost time for the next dose. Patient should never double the dose.

• Encourage patient to wear a medical identification bracelet or necklace.

• Instruct patient to take drug with food if it causes GI upset.

• Teach patient how to monitor blood glucose, urine glucose, and ketone levels, as needed.

• Teach patient to recognize the signs and symptoms of hypoglycemia and hyperglycemia and what to do if they occur.

chlorthalidone
Apo-Chlorthalidone*, Hygroton,
Novo-Thalidone*, Thalitone, Uridon*

Pharmacologic classification: thiazide-like
diuretic
Therapeutic classification: diuretic, antihypertensive
Pregnancy risk category: B

Indications and dosages
➤ *Edema. Adults:* 50 to 100 mg (Thalitone, 30
to 60 mg) P.O. daily or 100 mg (Thalitone, 60 mg)
P.O. every other day.
Children: 2 mg/kg P.O. three times weekly.
➤ *Hypertension. Adults:* 25 to 100 mg (Thali-
tone, 15 to 50 mg) P.O. daily.
Children: 2 mg/kg P.O. three times weekly.

How supplied
Available by prescription only
Tablets: 15 mg, 25 mg, 50 mg, 100 mg

Pharmacodynamics
Diuretic action: Increases urinary excretion of
sodium and water by inhibiting sodium reabsorption in the cortical diluting tubule of the
nephron, thus relieving edema.
Antihypertensive action: Exact mechanism unknown. This effect may partially result from direct arteriolar vasodilation and a decrease in total peripheral resistance.

Pharmacokinetics
Absorption: Absorbed from GI tract; extent of
absorption unknown.
Distribution: 90% bound to erythrocytes.
Metabolism: Limited data.
Excretion: Between 30% and 60% of a dose is
excreted unchanged in urine; half-life is 54 hours.
Duration of action is 24 to 72 hours.

Route	Onset	Peak	Duration
P.O.	2-3 hr	2-6 hr	2-3 days

Contraindications and precautions
Contraindicated in patients hypersensitive to thiazides or other sulfonamide-derived drugs and
in those with anuria. Use cautiously in patients
with impaired renal or hepatic function.

Interactions
Drug-drug. *Amphetamine, quinidine:* Makes
urine slightly more alkaline and may decrease
urinary excretion of some amines. Monitor patient closely.
Antihypertensives: Enhanced hypotensive effects.
Monitor patient closely.
Cholestyramine, colestipol: May bind to chlorthalidone, preventing its absorption. Give 1 hour apart.
Diazoxide: Enhanced hyperglycemic, hypotensive, and hyperuricemic effects of diazoxide. Monitor patient closely.

Lithium: May reduce renal clearance of lithium,
elevating serum lithium levels. Lithium dose may
need to be reduced by 50%.
*Methenamine compounds such as methena-
mine mandelate:* May decrease therapeutic efficacy of these drugs. Use together cautiously.
NSAIDs: Drug may increase risk of NSAID-induced
renal failure. Use together cautiously.

Adverse reactions
CNS: dizziness, vertigo, headache, paresthesia,
weakness, restlessness.
CV: volume depletion and dehydration, vasculitis.
GI: anorexia, nausea, *pancreatitis*, vomiting,
abdominal pain, diarrhea, constipation.
GU: impotence.
Hematologic: *aplastic anemia, agranulocytosis, leukopenia, thrombocytopenia.*
Hepatic: jaundice.
Metabolic: hypokalemia; asymptomatic hyperuricemia; hyperglycemia and impairment of glucose tolerance; increased serum urate, glucose,
cholesterol, and triglyceride levels; fluid and electrolyte imbalances, including dilutional hyponatremia and hypochloremia; metabolic alkalosis;
hypercalcemia; gout.
Skin: dermatitis, photosensitivity, rash, purpura, urticaria.
Other: *hypersensitivity reactions.*

Overdose and treatment
Signs and symptoms of overdose include GI irritation and hypermotility, diuresis, and lethargy,
which may progress to coma.
   Treatment is mainly supportive; monitor and
assist respiratory, CV, and renal function as indicated. Monitor fluid and electrolyte balance. Induce vomiting with ipecac in conscious patient;
otherwise, use gastric lavage to avoid aspiration.
Don't give cathartics; they cause additional loss
of fluids and electrolytes.

Special considerations
• To prevent nocturia, give drug in the morning.
• In patients with hypertension, therapeutic re-
sponse may be delayed several weeks.
• Drug may interfere with tests for parathyroid
function; discontinue drug before such tests.

Patient monitoring
• Serum electrolyte levels should be determined
before starting therapy and at periodic intervals
during therapy.

Breast-feeding patients
• Drug appears in breast milk; safety and effectiveness in breast-feeding women haven't been
established.

Pediatric patients
• Safety and effectiveness in children haven't been
established.

Reactions may be *common*, uncommon, *life-threatening*, or COMMON AND LIFE-THREATENING.

Geriatric patients
● Elderly and debilitated patients need close observation and may need reduced doses. They're more sensitive to excess diuresis because of age-related changes in CV and renal function. Excess diuresis promotes orthostatic hypotension, dehydration, hypovolemia, hyponatremia, hypomagnesemia, and hypokalemia.

Patient education
● Instruct patient to take drug in morning to prevent nocturia.
● Tell patient to avoid sudden posture changes and to rise slowly to avoid orthostatic hypotension.

chlorzoxazone
Paraflex, Parafon Forte DSC,
Remular-S

Pharmacologic classification: benzoxazole derivative
Therapeutic classification: skeletal muscle relaxant
Pregnancy risk category: NR

Indications and dosages
➤ *Adjunct in acute, painful musculo-skeletal conditions.* Adults: 250, 500, or 750 mg P.O. t.i.d. or q.i.d. Reduce to lowest effective dose after response occurs.
Children: 20 mg/kg or 600 mg/m^2 P.O. daily divided t.i.d. or q.i.d. Or, 125 to 500 mg t.i.d. or q.i.d., depending on age and weight.

How supplied
Available by prescription only
Tablets: 250 mg, 500 mg
Tablets (film-coated): 250 mg

Pharmacodynamics
Skeletal muscle relaxant action: Chlorzoxazone doesn't relax skeletal muscle directly, but apparently does so through its sedative effects. Exact mechanism of action is unknown. Animal studies suggest that drug modifies central perception of pain without eliminating peripheral pain reflexes.

Pharmacokinetics
Absorption: Rapidly and completely absorbed from the GI tract.
Distribution: Widely distributed in the body.
Metabolism: Metabolized in the liver to inactive metabolites.
Excretion: Excreted in urine as glucuronide metabolite. The half-life of chlorzoxazone is 66 minutes.

Route	Onset	Peak	Duration
P.O.	1 hr	1-2 hr	3-4 hr

Contraindications and precautions
Contraindicated in patients hypersensitive to drug and those with impaired hepatic function.

Interactions
Drug-drug. *CNS depressants:* Increased CNS depression. Avoid use together.
MAO inhibitors, tricyclic antidepressants: May result in increased CNS depression, respiratory depression, and hypotensive effects. Reduce dosage of one or both drugs.
Drug-herb. *Watercress:* May elevate drug level, increasing therapeutic and adverse effects. Discourage use together.
Drug-lifestyle. *Alcohol use:* Increased CNS depression. Discourage alcohol use.

Adverse reactions
CNS: *drowsiness, dizziness, light-headedness,* malaise, headache, overstimulation, tremor.
GI: anorexia, nausea, vomiting, heartburn, abdominal distress, constipation, diarrhea.
GU: urine discoloration (orange or purple-red).
Hepatic: hepatic dysfunction.
Skin: urticaria, redness, pruritus, petechiae, bruising.
Other: *angioedema, anaphylaxis.*

Overdose and treatment
Signs and symptoms of overdose include nausea, vomiting, diarrhea, drowsiness, dizziness, light-headedness, headache, malaise, or sluggishness, followed by loss of muscle tone, decreased or absent deep tendon reflexes, respiratory depression, and hypotension.

To treat overdose, induce emesis or perform gastric lavage followed by activated charcoal. Closely monitor vital signs and neurologic status. Provide general supportive measures, including maintenance of adequate airway and assisted ventilation. Use caution if administering pressor agents.

Special considerations
● Drug may cause drowsiness.
● Urine may turn orange or reddish purple.

Patient monitoring
● Monitor liver function tests in patients receiving long-term therapy. Watch for early signs of hepatic dysfunction or abnormal liver enzyme levels.

Pregnant patients
● Use only when benefits outweigh the risks. Safety hasn't been established.

Breast-feeding patients
● It isn't known whether drug appears in breast milk. No clinical problems have been reported.

Pediatric patients
● Tablets may be crushed and mixed with food, milk, or fruit juice to aid dosing in children.

Geriatric patients
● Geriatric patients may be more sensitive to the effects of the drug. Use cautiously and at lower doses.

Patient education
● Caution patient to avoid hazardous activities that require alertness or physical coordination until CNS depressant effects are determined.
● Advise patient to store drug away from direct heat or light (not in bathroom medicine cabinet, where heat and humidity cause deterioration of drug).
● Tell patient to take missed dose only if remembered within 1 hour of scheduled time. If beyond 1 hour, patient should skip dose and go back to regular schedule. Patient shouldn't double the dose.
● Inform patient not to stop taking drug without calling for specific instructions.
● Warn athletic patient that skeletal muscle relaxants are banned in competition sponsored by the U.S. Olympics Committee and the National Collegiate Athletic Association. Use can lead to disqualification.

cholera vaccine

Pharmacologic classification: vaccine
Therapeutic classification: cholera prophylaxis
Pregnancy risk category: C

Indications and dosages
➤ **Primary immunization.** *Adults and children over age 10:* Two doses of 0.5 ml I.M. or S.C., 1 week to 1 month apart, before traveling in cholera area. Booster dosage is 0.5 ml q 6 months for as long as protection is needed.
Children ages 5 to 10: 0.3 ml I.M. or S.C. Boosters of same dose should be given q 6 months for as long as protection is needed.
Children ages 6 months to 4 years: 0.2 ml I.M. or S.C. Boosters of same dose should be given q 6 months for as long as protection is needed.

How supplied
Available by prescription only
Injection: Suspension of killed *Vibrio cholerae* (each ml contains 8 units of Inaba and Ogawa serotypes) in 1.5-ml and 20-ml vials

Pharmacodynamics
Cholera prophylaxis: Promotes active immunity to cholera in about 50% of those immunized.

Pharmacokinetics
Absorption: No information available.
Distribution: No information available. Virus-induced immunity begins to taper off within 3 to 6 months.
Metabolism: No information available.

Excretion: No information available.

Route	Onset	Peak	Duration
I.M., S.C.	After 2nd dose	Unknown	3-6 mo

Contraindications and precautions
Contraindicated in patients with acute illness or history of severe systemic reaction or allergic response to vaccine.

Interactions
Drug-drug. *Corticosteroids, immunosuppressants:* May impair immune response to cholera vaccine. Avoid use together.
Yellow fever vaccine: Simultaneous administration may decrease response to both. Avoid concurrent administration.

Adverse reactions
CNS: headache, malaise.
Skin: *erythema, swelling, pain, and induration at injection site.*
Other: fever.

Overdose and treatment
No information.

Special considerations
● Obtain a thorough history of allergies and reactions to immunizations.
● Epinephrine solution 1:1,000 should be available to treat allergic reactions.
● When possible, cholera and yellow fever vaccines should be administered at least 3 weeks apart; however, they may be administered simultaneously if time constraints make this necessary.
● Cholera vaccine may be given intradermally (0.2 ml) in persons over age 5, but higher levels of antibody may be achieved in children under age 5 by the S.C. or I.M. route.
● Shake vial well before removing a dose.
● Administer I.M. in deltoid muscle in adults and children over age 3 and in the anterolateral thigh in children under age 3.
● Don't use I.M. route in patients with thrombocytopenia or other coagulation disorders that would contraindicate I.M. injection. Cholera vaccine shouldn't be administered I.V. Aspirate before S.C. or I.M. injection.
● Store vaccine at 36° to 46° F (2° to 8° C). Don't freeze.

Patient monitoring
● Monitor patient for adverse effects.

Breast-feeding patients
● It's unknown whether cholera vaccine appears in breast milk or whether transmission of cholera vaccine to a breast-fed infant presents any unusual risk.

Reactions may be *common*, uncommon, *life-threatening*, or COMMON AND LIFE-THREATENING.

Pediatric patients
● Drug isn't recommended for infants under age 6 months.

Geriatric patients
● Elderly patients may be more sensitive to drug's effects.

Patient education
● Tell patient to report skin changes, difficulty breathing, fever, or joint pain.
● Inform patient that acetaminophen may be taken to relieve minor adverse effects, such as pain and tenderness at injection site.
● Tell patient that use of vaccine doesn't prevent infection.
● Advise patient to avoid consumption of contaminated food or water.

---

cholestyramine
Questran, Questran Light

Pharmacologic classification: anion exchange resin
Therapeutic classification: antilipemic, bile acid sequestrant
Pregnancy risk category: NR

Indications and dosages
➤ *Primary hyperlipidemia and hypercholesterolemia unresponsive to dietary measures alone; to reduce the risks of atherosclerotic coronary artery disease and MI; to relieve pruritus from partial biliary obstruction; cardiac glycoside toxicity* ◇ . *Adults:* 4 g P.O. before meals and h.s. not to exceed 32 g daily. Can be given in one to six divided doses.
Children ages 6 to 12: 80 mg/kg or 2.35 g/m² P.O. t.i.d.

How supplied
Available by prescription only
Powder: 378-g cans, 9-g single-dose packets (Questran), 5-g single dose packets (Questran Light). Each scoop of powder or single-dose packet contains 4 g of cholestyramine resin.

Pharmacodynamics
Antilipemic action: Bile is normally excreted into the intestine to facilitate absorption of fat and other lipid materials. Cholestyramine binds with bile acid, forming an insoluble compound that's excreted in feces. With less bile available in the digestive system, less fat and lipid materials in food are absorbed, more cholesterol is used by the liver to replace its supply of bile acids, and the serum cholesterol level decreases. In partial biliary obstruction, excess bile acids accumulate in dermal tissue, resulting in pruritus; by reducing levels of dermal bile acids, cholestyramine combats pruritus.

Drug can also act as an antidiarrheal in postoperative diarrhea caused by bile acids in the colon.

Pharmacokinetics
Absorption: Not absorbed. Cholesterol levels may start decreasing 24 to 48 hours after therapy starts and may continue falling for up to 12 months. In some patients, the initial decrease is followed by a return to baseline levels (or higher) as therapy continues. Relief of cholestasis-related pruritus occurs 1 to 3 weeks after therapy starts. Diarrhea related to bile acids may stop in 24 hours.
Distribution: None.
Metabolism: None.
Excretion: Insoluble cholestyramine with bile acid complex is excreted in feces.

Route	Onset	Peak	Duration
P.O.	Unknown	Unknown	2-4 wk

Contraindications and precautions
Contraindicated in patients hypersensitive to bile-acid sequestering resins and in those with complete biliary obstruction. Use cautiously in patients with coronary artery disease or a predisposition to constipation.

Interactions
Drug-drug. *Acetaminophen, cardiac glycosides, corticosteroids, thiazide diuretics, thyroid preparations:* Absorption of these drugs may be reduced. Give other drugs 1 hour before or 4 to 6 hours after cholestyramine. To prevent high-dose toxicity, readjust dosages of these drugs when cholestyramine is withdrawn.
Warfarin: May decrease anticoagulant effects. Avoid use together. Monitor PT and INR carefully.

Adverse reactions
CNS: headache, anxiety, vertigo, dizziness, insomnia, fatigue, syncope.
EENT: tinnitus.
GI: constipation, *fecal impaction*, hemorrhoids, *abdominal discomfort*, flatulence, *nausea*, vomiting, steatorrhea, GI bleeding, diarrhea, anorexia.
GU: hematuria, dysuria.
Hematologic: anemia, ecchymoses, bleeding tendencies.
Hepatic: altered serum ALT and AST levels.
Metabolic: altered serum chloride, phosphorus, potassium, calcium, and sodium levels; hyperchloremic acidosis with long-term use or very high doses.
Musculoskeletal: backache, muscle and joint pain, osteoporosis.
Skin: *rash;* irritation of skin, tongue, and perianal area.
Other: *vitamin A, D, E, and K deficiencies from decreased absorption.*

Overdose and treatment
Drug overdose hasn't been reported. Chief risk is intestinal obstruction; treatment would depend

on location and degree of obstruction and on intestinal motility.

Special considerations
● To mix, sprinkle powder on surface of preferred beverage or wet food, let stand a few minutes and stir to obtain uniform suspension; avoid excess foaming by using large glass and mixing slowly. Use at least 90 ml of water or other fluid, soup, milk, or pulpy fruit; rinse container and have patient drink this liquid to be sure he ingests entire dose.
● Drug has been used to treat cardiac glycoside overdose because it binds these agents and prevents enterohepatic recycling. When used as an adjunct to hyperlipidemia, monitor levels of cardiac glycosides and other drugs to ensure appropriate dosage during and after therapy with cholestyramine.
● Questran Light contains aspartame and provides 1.6 calories per packet or scoop.
● Cholecystography using iopanoic acid will yield abnormal results because iopanoic acid is also bound by cholestyramine.

Patient monitoring
● Monitor serum cholesterol level frequently during first few months of therapy and periodically thereafter.
● Monitor bowel function. Treat constipation promptly by decreasing dosage, adding a stool softener, or stopping drug.
● Observe patient for signs of vitamin A, D, or K deficiency.

Pregnant patients
● Although drug wouldn't be expected to harm fetus, its known interference with absorption of fat-soluble vitamins may cause fetal harm. Use dietary management.

Breast-feeding patients
● Safety in breast-feeding women hasn't been established.

Pediatric patients
● Children may be at greater risk of hyperchloremic acidosis during cholestyramine therapy. Safe dosage hasn't been established for children under age 6.

Geriatric patients
● Patients over age 60 are more likely to experience adverse GI effects as well as adverse nutritional effects.

Patient education
● Urge patient to comply with continued blood testing and special diet; although therapy isn't curative, it helps control serum cholesterol level.
● Urge patient to control weight and to stop smoking as part of attempt to increase awareness of other cardiac risk factors.

● Tell patient not to take the powder in dry form; teach him to mix drug with fluids or pulpy fruits.

choline magnesium trisalicylates
Tricosal, Trilisate

choline salicylate
Arthropan

Pharmacologic classification: salicylate
Therapeutic classification: nonnarcotic analgesic, antipyretic, anti-inflammatory
Pregnancy risk category: C

Indications and dosages
➤ *Rheumatoid arthritis, osteoarthritis.*
Adults: 1,500 mg P.O. b.i.d. or 3,000 mg h.s.
✦ *Dosage adjustment.* In geriatric patients, give 750 mg t.i.d.
➤ *Mild arthritis; antipyresis. Adults:* 2,000 to 3,000 mg P.O. daily in divided doses b.i.d.
➤ *Mild to moderate pain and fever. Children:* Based on weight, and the doses should be divided b.i.d.
Children who weigh 12 to 13 kg (26 to 28.5 lb): 500 mg P.O. daily.
Children who weigh 14 to 17 kg (30 to 37.5 lb): 750 mg P.O. daily.
Children who weigh 18 to 22 kg (39 to 48.5 lb): 1,000 mg P.O. daily.
Children who weigh 23 to 27 kg (50 to 59.5 lb): 1,250 mg P.O. daily.
Children who weigh 28 to 32 kg (61 to 70.5 lb): 1,500 mg P.O. daily.
Children who weigh 33 to 37 kg (73 to 81.5 lb): 1,750 mg P.O. daily.

How supplied
Available by prescription only
Solution: 500 mg of salicylate/5 ml (as choline and magnesium salicylate); 870 mg/5 ml (as choline salicylate)
Tablets: 500 mg, 750 mg, 1,000 mg of salicylate (as choline and magnesium salicylate)

Pharmacodynamics
Analgesic action: Choline salicylates produce analgesia by an ill-defined effect on the hypothalamus (central action) and by blocking generation of pain impulses (peripheral action). The peripheral action may involve inhibition of prostaglandin synthesis.
Anti-inflammatory action: These drugs exert anti-inflammatory effects by inhibiting prostaglandin synthesis; they also may inhibit the synthesis or action of other inflammation mediators.
Antipyretic action: Choline salicylates relieve fever by acting on the hypothalamic heat-regulating center to produce peripheral vasodilation. This increases peripheral blood supply and promotes sweating, which leads to loss of heat and to cool-

ing by evaporation. These drugs don't affect platelet aggregation and shouldn't be used to prevent thrombosis.

Pharmacokinetics
Absorption: Absorbed rapidly and completely from the GI tract.
Distribution: Protein-binding depends on concentration and ranges from 75% to 90%, decreasing as serum level increases. Severe toxic effects may occur at serum levels above 400 mcg/ml.
Metabolism: Hydrolyzed to salicylate in the liver.
Excretion: Metabolites are excreted in urine.

Route	Onset	Peak	Duration
P.O.	Unknown	1-2 hr	Unknown

Contraindications and precautions
Contraindicated in patients hypersensitive to drug and patients who consume three or more alcoholic beverages daily. Also contraindicated in patients with hemophilia, bleeding ulcers, and hemorrhagic states. Use cautiously in patients with impaired renal or hepatic function, peptic ulcer disease, or gastritis. Don't give to children or teenagers with chickenpox or influenza-like illnesses.

Interactions
Drug-drug. *Ammonium chloride, urine acidifiers:* Increased choline salicylate blood levels; monitor choline salicylate blood levels and toxicity.
Antacids: Delayed and decreaseed absorption of choline salicylates. Monitor patient closely.
Antibiotics, corticosteroids, NSAIDs: Increased risk of adverse GI effects. Use together cautiously.
Corticosteroids: Increased salicylate elimination. Watch for decreased effect.
Lithium carbonate: Choline salicylates decrease renal clearance, increasing serum lithium levels and the risk of adverse effects. Monitor patient closely.
Methotrexate: Possible displacement of bound methotrexate and inhibition of renal excretion. Avoid using together.
Phenytoin, sulfonylureas, warfarin: Possible displacement of either drug, with adverse effects. Monitor patient closely.
Warfarin: Increased hypoprothrombinemic effects. Avoid using together.
Drug-food. *Food:* Delayed and decreased absorption of choline salicylates. Give drug on an empty stomach.
Drug-lifestyle. *Alcohol use:* Enhanced risk of adverse GI effects. Discourage use together.

Adverse reactions
EENT: tinnitus, hearing loss.
GI: GI distress, nausea, vomiting, bleeding ulcer.
GU: *acute tubular necrosis with renal failure.*
Metabolic: elevated free T_4 levels.

Skin: rash.
Other: *hypersensitivity reactions (anaphylaxis), Reye's syndrome.*

Overdose and treatment
Overdose may cause metabolic acidosis with respiratory alkalosis, hypcrpnea, and tachypnea from increased carbon dioxide production and direct stimulation of the respiratory center.

To treat choline salicylate overdose, empty stomach immediately by inducing emesis with ipecac syrup, if patient is conscious, or by gastric lavage. Give activated charcoal via nasogastric tube. Provide symptomatic and supportive measures (respiratory support and correction of fluid and electrolyte imbalances). Monitor laboratory parameters and vital signs closely. Hemodialysis is effective in removing choline salicylates but is used only in severe poisoning. Forced diuresis with alkalinizing agent accelerates salicylate excretion.

Special considerations
Consider the recommendations relevant to all salicylates as well as the following.
● Choline salicylates shouldn't be mixed with antacids.
● Mix oral choline salicylate solution with fruit juice. Follow with a full 8-oz (240-ml) glass of water to ensure passage into stomach.
● Choline salicylates may interfcre with urinary glucose analysis performed via Chemstrip uG, Diastix, glucose enzymatic test strip, Clinitest, and Benedict's solution. These drugs also interfere with urinary 5-hydroxyindole acetic acid and vanillymandelic acid.

Patient monitoring
● Monitor serum magnesium levels to prevent possible magnesium toxicity.

Pregnant patients
● Avoid use of choline salicylates in the third trimester of pregnancy.

Breast-feeding patients
● Salicylates appear in breast milk. Avoid use in breast-feeding women.

Pediatric patients
● Safety of long-term drug use in children under age 14 hasn't been established. Because of epidemiologic link to Reye's syndrome, the Centers for Disease Control and Prevention recommend not giving salicylates to children with chickenpox or flulike symptoms.
● Toxicity can develop rapidly in febrile, dehydrated children. Usually, they shouldn't receive more than five doses in 24 hours.

Geriatric patients
● Patients over age 60 may be more susceptible to the toxic effects of these drugs.

Patient education
• Warn patient not to take drug longer than prescribed or to increase dosage without consulting prescriber.
• Advise patient to take drug with food.

---

chorionic gonadotropin, human
A.P.L., Chorex-5, Chorex-10, Gonic, Pregnyl, Profasi, Profasi HP*

Pharmacologic classification: gonadotropin
Therapeutic classification: ovulation stimulant, spermatogenesis stimulant
Pregnancy risk category: X

Indications and dosages
➤ *To induce ovulation and pregnancy.*
Adults: 5,000 to 10,000 USP units I.M. 1 day after last dose of menotropins.
➤ *Hypogonadotropic hypogonadism.*
Adults: 500 to 1,000 USP units I.M. three times weekly for 3 weeks, and then twice weekly for 3 weeks. Or, 4,000 USP units I.M. three times weekly for 6 to 9 months, and then 2,000 USP units three times weekly for 3 more months.
➤ *Nonobstructive prepubertal cryptorchidism.* *Children ages 4 to 9:* 5,000 USP units I.M. every other day for four doses. Or, 4,000 USP units I.M. three times weekly for 3 weeks. Or, 15 doses of 500 to 1,000 USP units I.M. given over 6 weeks. Or, 500 USP units three times weekly for 4 to 6 weeks, which may be repeated if unsuccessful in 1 month, giving 1,000 USP units per injection.

How supplied
Available by prescription only
Injection: 500 USP units/ml, 1,000 USP units/ml, 2,000 USP units/ml

Pharmacodynamics
Ovulation stimulant action: Mimics action of luteinizing hormone in stimulating ovulation of mature ovarian follicle.
Spermatogenesis stimulant action: Stimulates androgen production in Leydig's cells of testes and causes maturation of cells lining seminiferous tubules of testes.

Pharmacokinetics
Absorption: Must administer I.M. Blood levels peak within 6 hours.
Distribution: Distributed primarily into testes and ovaries.
Metabolism: Initial half-life is 11 hours, with a terminal phase of 23 hours.
Excretion: Excreted in urine.

Route	Onset	Peak	Duration
I.M.	2 hr	6 hr	36 hr

Contraindications and precautions
Contraindicated in patients hypersensitive to human chorionic gonadotropin (HCG) and in those with precocious puberty or androgen-responsive cancer (prostatic, testicular, male breast) because drug stimulates androgen production. Use cautiously in patients with asthma, seizure disorders, migraines, or cardiac or renal diseases because it may worsen these conditions.

Interactions
None reported.

Adverse reactions
CNS: headache, fatigue, irritability, restlessness, depression.
GU: early puberty (growth of testes, penis, pubic and axillary hair; voice change; down on upper lip; growth of body hair), hyperstimulation (ovarian enlargement), *rupture of ovarian cysts.*
Skin: pain at injection site.
Other: gynecomastia, edema.

Overdose and treatment
No information.

Special considerations
• Only clinicians experienced in treating infertility disorders should administer drug.
• Pregnancies that occur after stimulation of ovulation with gonadotropins show a relatively high risk of multiple births.
• HCG is usually used only after failure of clomiphene in anovulatory patients.
• In infertility, encourage daily intercourse from day before HCG is given until ovulation occurs.
• Be alert to symptoms of ectopic pregnancy, usually evident between 8 and 12 weeks' gestation.
• May interfere with radioimmunoassays for gonadotropins.

Patient monitoring
• Carefully observe young men receiving HCG for development of precocious puberty.
• Carefully monitor patients with disorders that may be aggravated by fluid retention.

Breast-feeding patients
• It isn't known whether chorionic gonadotropins appear in breast milk. Use caution when giving to breast-feeding women.

Pediatric patients
• Treating prepubertal cryptorchidism with HCG can help predict future need for orchidopexy. Induction of androgen secretion may induce precocious puberty in patients treated for cryptorchidism. Instruct parent to report the following: axillary, facial, or pubic hair; penile growth; acne; or deepening of voice.

Geriatric patients
• Drug isn't indicated for use in elderly patients.

Reactions may be *common*, uncommon, *life-threatening*, or COMMON AND LIFE-THREATENING.

Patient education
● Teach patient and family how to assess for edema, and urge them to report it promptly.
● Advise patient and family to report signs of precocious puberty promptly.
● Inform patient receiving HCG for infertility that multiple births are possible.

cidofovir
Vistide

Pharmacologic classification: nucleotide analogue
Therapeutic classification: antiviral
Pregnancy risk category: C

Indications and dosages
➤ *Cytomegalovirus (CMV) retinitis in patients with AIDS; acyclovir-resistant herpes simplex infections in immunocompromised patients* ◇. *Adults:* Give 5 mg/kg I.V. infused over 1 hour once weekly for 2 consecutive weeks followed by a maintenance dosage of 5 mg/kg I.V. infused over 1 hour once q 2 weeks. Probenecid must be administered concomitantly.

✦ *Dosage adjustment.* Dosage may need adjustment as follows based on patient's creatinine clearance.

Creatinine clearance (ml/min)	Induction and maintenance dosage
41-55	2 mg/kg
30-40	1.5 mg/kg
20-29	1 mg/kg
≤ 19	0.5 mg/kg

How supplied
Available by prescription only
Injection: 75 mg/ml

Pharmacodynamics
Antiviral action: Drug suppresses CMV replication by selective inhibition of viral DNA synthesis.

Pharmacokinetics
Absorption: Administered I.V.
Distribution: Unknown.
Metabolism: Not metabolized.
Excretion: 80% to 100% excreted unchanged in urine.

Route	Onset	Peak	Duration
I.V.	Unknown	Unknown	Unknown

Contraindications and precautions
Contraindicated in patients hypersensitive to drug and in those with a history of clinically severe hypersensitivity to probenecid or other sulfa drugs.

Don't administer as a direct intraocular injection, which may significantly decrease intraocular pressure and impair vision. Use cautiously in patients with impaired renal function.

Interactions
Drug-drug. *Ganciclovir ocular implants:* May cause profound hypotony. Don't give cidofovir within 1 month of placement of implant.
Nephrotoxic drugs (aminoglycosides, amphotericin B, foscarnet, I.V. pentamidine): May increase nephrotoxicity. Avoid use together.

Adverse reactions
CNS: malaise, *asthenia, headache,* amnesia, anxiety, confusion, *seizures,* abnormal gait, hallucinations, neuropathy, syncope, paresthesia, vasodilation.
CV: orthostatic hypotension, pallor, tachycardia.
EENT: amblyopia, conjunctivitis, ocular hypotony, iritis, retinal detachment, uveitis, abnormal vision, rhinitis, sinusitis.
GI: *nausea, vomiting, diarrhea, anorexia, abdominal pain,* dry mouth, colitis, constipation, tongue discoloration, dyspepsia, dysphagia, flatulence, gastritis, melena, oral candidiasis, rectal disorders, stomatitis, aphthous stomatitis, mouth ulceration, taste perversion.
GU: *elevated creatinine levels, nephrotoxicity, proteinuria,* decreased creatinine clearance levels, glycosuria, hematuria, urinary incontinence, urinary tract infection.
Hepatic: hepatomegaly, increased alkaline phosphatase levels.
Metabolic: fluid imbalances, hyperglycemia, hyperlipemia, hypocalcemia, hypokalemia, weight loss.
Musculoskeletal: myasthenia; pain in back, chest, or neck.
Respiratory: asthma, bronchitis, coughing, dyspnea, hiccups, increased sputum, lung disorders, pneumonia.
Skin: *rash, alopecia,* acne, skin discoloration, dry skin, herpes simplex, pruritus, sweating, urticaria.
Other: *fever, infections, chills,* allergic reactions, facial edema, *sarcoma, sepsis.*

Overdose and treatment
No information available. However, hemodialysis and hydration may reduce drug levels in patients who receive an overdose. Probenecid may reduce the risk of nephrotoxicity in patients who receive an overdose through reduction of active tubular secretion.

Special considerations
● Don't start drug if patient has baseline serum creatinine exceeding 1.5 mg/dl or calculated creatinine clearances of 55 ml/minute or less unless potential benefits exceed risks.
● Renal impairment is the major toxicity. To minimize the risk, use I.V. prehydration with normal

saline solution and give probenecid with each cidofovir infusion.
- Give 1 liter of normal saline solution over a 1- to 2-hour period immediately before each cidofovir infusion. Give a second liter if patient can tolerate the additional fluid load. If the second liter is given, administer it either at the start of the cidofovir infusion or immediately afterward; infuse it over a 1- to 3-hour period.
- Give 2 g of probenecid P.O. 3 hours before cidofovir and 1 g at 2 hours, and again at 8 hours after completing the 1-hour infusion (total 4 g).
- To prepare infusion, extract the appropriate amount of cidofovir from the vial with a syringe and transfer the dose to an infusion bag containing 100 ml normal saline solution. Infuse entire volume I.V. at a constant rate over 1 hour. Use a standard infusion pump.
- Because of drug's mutagenic properties, prepare it in a class II laminar flow biological safety cabinet. Wear surgical gloves and a closed front surgical-type gown with knit cuffs.
- If drug contacts the skin, wash and flush thoroughly with water. Place excess drug and all other materials used in admixture preparation and administration in a leak-proof, puncture-proof container. The recommended method of disposal is high temperature incineration.
- Give cidofovir infusion admixtures within 24 hours of preparation; don't refrigerate or freeze to extend this 24-hour period. If admixtures aren't to be used immediately, they may be refrigerated at 36 to 46° F (2 to 8° C) for no more than 24 hours. Allow refrigerated admixtures to reach room temperature before use.
- No other drugs and supplements should be added to the cidofovir admixture for concurrent administration. Compatibility with Ringer's solution, lactated Ringer's solution, and bacteriostatic infusion fluids hasn't been evaluated.
- Drug is indicated only for CMV retinitis in patients with AIDS. Safety and efficacy haven't been established for other CMV infections, congenital or neonatal CMV disease, and CMV disease in patients not infected with HIV.
- In animal studies, cidofovir was carcinogenic and teratogenic and caused hypospermia.
- Fanconi's syndrome and decreased serum bicarbonate levels with evidence of renal tubular damage have been reported in patients receiving cidofovir. Monitor patient closely.
- Discontinue zidovudine therapy or reduce dosage by 50% in patients receiving zidovudine on the days cidofovir is given because probenecid reduces metabolic clearance of zidovudine.

Patient monitoring
- Monitor WBC counts with differential before each dose.
- Monitor renal function (serum creatinine and urine protein) before each dose, and modify the dosage for changes in renal function.

- Granulocytopenia has been observed with cidofovir treatment; monitor neutrophil counts during therapy.
- Monitor intraocular pressure, visual acuity, and ocular symptoms periodically.

Pregnant patients
- Instruct women of childbearing potential to use contraception during and for 1 month after treatment with cidofovir.
- Tell men to practice barrier contraceptive methods during and for 3 months after drug treatment.

Breast-feeding patients
- It isn't known if drug appears in breast milk. Drug shouldn't be given to breast-feeding women.

Pediatric patients
- Safety and effectiveness in children haven't been established.

Geriatric patients
- Use cautiously when administering cidofovir to geriatric patients. Dosage adjustment will be necessary if patient is renally impaired.

Patient education
- Inform patient that drug isn't a cure for CMV retinitis and that regular ophthalmologic follow-up is necessary.
- Alert patients on zidovudine therapy that they'll need to obtain dosage guidelines on days that cidofovir is administered.
- Tell patient that close monitoring of renal function will be needed during cidofovir therapy and that an abnormality may require a change in cidofovir therapy.
- Stress importance of completing a full course of probenecid with each cidofovir dose. Tell patient to take probenecid after a meal to decrease nausea.
- Advise patient that cidofovir is a carcinogen.

cilostazol
Pletal

Pharmacologic classification: quinolinone phosphodiesterase inhibitor
Therapeutic classification: antiplatelet agent
Pregnancy risk category: C

Indications and dosages
➤ *Intermittent claudication. Adults:* 100 mg P.O. b.i.d., taken ½ hour before or 2 hours after breakfast and dinner.

How supplied
Available by prescription only
Tablets: 50 mg, 100 mg

Pharmacodynamics
Antiplatelet action: Mechanism of action not fully understood. Drug is believed to inhibit the

enzyme phosphodiesterase (type III), causing an increase of cAMP in platelets and blood vessels, inhibition of platelet aggregation, and vasodilation. Cilostazol reversibly inhibits platelet aggregation induced by various stimuli, such as thrombin, adenosine diphosphate, collagen, arachidonic acid, epinephrine, and stress.

Pharmacokinetics

Absorption: Absorbed following oral administration. A high-fat meal increases peak serum levels by about 90% and bioavailability by 25%. Absolute bioavailability isn't known.
Distribution: 95% to 98% protein-bound, primarily to albumin.
Metabolism: Extensively metabolized by hepatic cytochrome P-450 enzyme system, primarily CYP3A4.
Excretion: Excreted primarily in urine, mostly as metabolites (about 74%). Remaining drug is eliminated in feces (about 20%). Half life of cilostazol and active metabolites is about 11 to 13 hours.

Route	Onset	Peak	Duration
P.O.	Unknown	Unknown	Unknown

Contraindications and precautions

Contraindicated in patients with heart failure of any severity. Also contraindicated in patients with known or suspected hypersensitivity to any of drug's components. Use cautiously in patients with severe underlying heart disease and with other drugs that have antiplatelet activity.

Interactions

Drug-drug. *Diltiazem; erythromycin and other macrolides; omeprazole; strong inhibitors of CYP3A4, such as ketoconazole, itraconazole, fluconazole, miconazole, fluvoxamine, fluoxetine, nefazodone, and sertraline:* Increased peak serum levels of cilostazol or one of its metabolites. Avoid use together.
Drug-food. *Grapefruit juice:* May increase cilostazol levels. Discourage use together.
Drug-lifestyle. *Smoking:* Decreases drug exposure by about 20%. Discourage smoking.

Adverse reactions

CNS: *headache, dizziness,* vertigo.
CV: *palpitations,* tachycardia.
EENT: *pharyngitis, rhinitis.*
GI: *abnormal stools, diarrhea,* dyspepsia, abdominal pain, flatulence, nausea.
Musculoskeletal: back pain, myalgia.
Respiratory: cough aggravation.
Other: *infection,* peripheral edema.

Overdose and treatment

Signs and symptoms of overdose include severe headache, diarrhea, hypotension, tachycardia, and, possibly, cardiac arrhythmias. Observe patient carefully, and give supportive treatment. Be-

cause drug is highly protein-bound, it may not be efficiently removed by hemodialysis.

Special considerations

● There's uncertainty concerning CV risk in long-term use or in patients with severe underlying heart disease.
● Obtain a thorough drug history before starting therapy.
● Several drugs that inhibit the enzyme phosphodiesterase have decreased survival in patients with class III-IV heart failure. Therefore, cilostazol is contraindicated in patients with congestive heart failure.

Patient monitoring

● Assess patient for effectiveness of drug. Improved walking performance should be observed.

Breast-feeding patients

● Because drug appears in breast milk, a decision should be made to discontinue nursing or discontinue drug.

Pediatric patients

● Safety and effectiveness haven't been established in children.

Geriatric patients

● No overall differences in safety, efficacy, or pharmacokinetics have been observed between geriatric and younger patients.

Patient education

● Instruct patient to take cilostazol at least ½ hour before or 2 hours after breakfast and dinner.
● Tell patient that a beneficial effect won't occur for 2 to 4 weeks, and that it may take as long as 12 weeks.
● To chart effects of drug therapy, advise patient to keep a log of how far he can walk without pain.

cimetidine
Tagamet, Tagamet HB

Pharmacologic classification: H₂-receptor antagonist
Therapeutic classification: antiulcer
Pregnancy risk category: B

Indications and dosages

➤ **Duodenal ulcer (short-term treatment).**
Adults: 800 mg P.O. h.s. for maximum of 8 weeks. Or, 400 mg P.O. b.i.d. or 300 mg P.O. q i d. with meals and h.s. When healing occurs, stop treatment or give h.s. dose only to control nocturnal hypersecretion.
Parenteral: 300 mg diluted to 20 ml with normal saline solution or other compatible I.V. solution by I.V. push over 5 minutes q 6 hours. Or 300 mg diluted in 50 ml D₅W or other compatible I.V. solution by I.V. infusion over 15 to 20

minutes q 6 to 8 hours. Or 300 mg I.M. q 6 to 8 hours (no dilution necessary). To increase dose, give more frequently to maximum daily dose of 2,400 mg.

➤ **Duodenal ulcer prophylaxis.** *Adults:* 400 mg P.O. h.s.

➤ **Active benign gastric ulcer.** *Adults:* 800 mg P.O. h.s., or 300 mg P.O. q.i.d. with meals and h.s. for up to 8 weeks.

➤ **Pathologic hypersecretory conditions (such as Zollinger-Ellison syndrome, systemic mastocytosis, and multiple endocrine adenomas); short-bowel syndrome**◇. *Adults:* 300 mg P.O. q.i.d. with meals and h.s.; adjust to patient needs. Maximum daily dose is 2,400 mg.

Parenteral: 300 mg diluted to 20 ml with normal saline solution or other compatible I.V. solution by I.V. push over 5 minutes q 6 to 8 hours. Or 300 mg diluted in 50 ml D₅W or other compatible I.V. solution by I.V. infusion over 15 to 20 minutes q 6 to 8 hours. To increase dosage, give 300-mg doses more frequently to maximum daily dose of 2,400 mg.

➤ **Symptomatic relief of gastroesophageal reflux.** *Adults:* 800 mg P.O. b.i.d. or 400 mg q.i.d., before meals and h.s.

➤ **Active upper GI bleeding, peptic esophagitis, stress ulcer**◇. *Adults:* 1 to 2 g I.V. or P.O. daily, in four divided doses.

➤ **Continuous infusion for patients unable to tolerate oral medication.** *Adults:* 37.5 mg/hour (900 mg daily) by continuous I.V. infusion. Use an infusion pump if total volume is below 250 ml daily.

➤ **Heartburn, acid indigestion, sour stomach.** *Adults:* 200 mg P.O. up to a maximum of b.i.d. (400 mg).

✦ **Dosage adjustment.** In patients with renal failure, recommended dosage is 300 mg P.O. or I.V. q 8 to 12 hours at end of dialysis. Dosage may be decreased further if hepatic failure is also present.

How supplied
Available by prescription only
Injection: 300 mg/2 ml, 300 mg/50 ml normal saline solution (premixed)
Liquid: 300 mg/5 ml
Tablets: 200 mg, 300 mg, 400 mg, 800 mg
Available without a prescription
Tablets: 200 mg

Pharmacodynamics
Antiulcer action: Cimetidine competitively inhibits histamine's action at H₂ receptors in gastric parietal cells, inhibiting basal and nocturnal gastric acid secretion (such as from stimulation by food, caffeine, insulin, histamine, betazole, or pentagastrin). Cimetidine also may enhance gastromucosal defense and healing.

A 300-mg oral or parenteral dose inhibits about 80% of gastric acid secretion for 4 to 5 hours.

Pharmacokinetics
Absorption: About 60% to 75% of oral dose is absorbed. Absorption rate (but not extent) may be affected by food.
Distribution: Distributed to many body tissues. About 15% to 20% of drug is protein-bound. Cimetidine apparently crosses the placenta and appears in breast milk.
Metabolism: About 30% to 40% of dose is metabolized in the liver. Drug has a half-life of 2 hours in patients with normal renal function; half-life increases with decreasing renal function.
Excretion: Excreted primarily in urine (48% of oral dose, 75% of parenteral dose); 10% of oral dose is excreted in feces. Some drug appears in breast milk.

Route	Onset	Peak	Duration
P.O.	Unknown	45-90 min	4-5 hr
I.V.	Unknown	Immediate	Unknown
I.M.	Unknown	Unknown	Unknown

Contraindications and precautions
Contraindicated in patients hypersensitive to drug. Use cautiously in elderly or debilitated patients.

Interactions
Drug-drug. *Benzodiazepines, beta blockers (such as propranolol), carmustine, disulfiram, isoniazid, lidocaine, metronidazole, oral contraceptives, phenytoin, procainamide, quinidine, triamterene, tricyclic antidepressants, warfarin, xanthines:* Decreased metabolism of these drugs, increasing the risk of toxicity and possibly necessitating a dosage reduction. Monitor patient closely.
Digoxin: Serum digoxin levels may be reduced. Patient requires close monitoring.
Ferrous salts, indomethacin, ketoconazole, tetracyclines: May affect the absorption of these drugs by altering gastric pH. Avoid use together.
Flecainide: Serum flecainide levels may be increased. Avoid use together.
Drug-herb. *Guarana:* May increase serum caffeine levels or prolong half-life. Monitor patient closely.
Pennyroyal: May change the rate at which toxic metabolites of pennyroyal form. Discourage use together.
Yerba maté: May decrease yerba maté methylxanthine clearance and cause toxicity. Discourage use together.
Drug-lifestyle. *Alcohol use, smoking:* May increase gastric acid secretion and worsen disease. Discourage use together.

Adverse reactions
CNS: confusion, dizziness, headache, peripheral neuropathy, somnolence, hallucinations.
GI: *mild and transient diarrhea.*
GU: transient elevations in serum creatinine levels, impotence.
Hematologic: *neutropenia.*

Reactions may be *common*, uncommon, **life-threatening**, or COMMON AND LIFE-THREATENING.

Hepatic: increased prolactin and serum alkaline phosphatase levels.
Musculoskeletal: muscle pain, arthralgia.
Other: *hypersensitivity reactions,* mild gynecomastia if used for over 1 month.

Overdose and treatment
Effects of overdose include respiratory failure and tachycardia. Overdose is rare; intake of up to 10 g has caused no adverse effects. Support respiration and maintain a patent airway. Induce emesis or use gastric lavage; follow with activated charcoal to prevent further absorption. Treat tachycardia with propranolol if necessary. Hemodialysis removes drug.

Special considerations
Consider the recommendations relevant to all H_2-receptor antagonists as well as the following.
⚠ ALERT For I.V. use, cimetidine must be diluted before administration. Don't dilute drug with sterile water for injection; use normal saline solution or D_5W to a total volume of 20 ml. FD&C blue dye #2 used in Tagamet tablets may impair interpretation of Hemoccult and Gastroccult tests on gastric content aspirate. Be sure to wait at least 15 minutes after tablet administration before drawing the sample, and follow test manufacturer's instructions closely.
• For I.M. administration, drug may be given undiluted. Injection may be painful.
• After administration of the liquid via nasogastric tube, flush tube to clear it and ensure passage of drug to stomach.
• Since hemodialysis removes drug, schedule dose after dialysis session.
• Cimetidine may antagonize pentagastrin's effect during gastric acid secretion tests; it may cause false-negative results in skin tests using allergen extracts.

Patient monitoring
• Assess for abdominal pain. Note blood in emesis, stool, or gastric aspirate.

Breast-feeding patients
• Drug appears in breast milk. Avoid use in breast-feeding women.

Geriatric patients
• Use with caution in elderly patients because of the risk of adverse reactions affecting the CNS.

Patient education
• Instruct patient to take drug as directed and to continue taking it even after pain subsides, to allow for adequate healing.
• Urge patient to avoid smoking and alcohol use, because they may increase gastric acid secretion and worsen disease.
• Advise patient to notify prescriber about use of other medications before starting treatment with cimetidine.

ciprofloxacin (systemic)
Cipro

Pharmacologic classification: fluoroquinolone antibiotic
Therapeutic classification: antibiotic
Pregnancy risk category: C

Indications and dosages
➤ *Mild to moderate urinary tract infection caused by susceptible bacteria. Adults:* 250 mg P.O. or 200 mg I.V. q 12 hours.
➤ *Infectious diarrhea, mild to moderate respiratory tract infections, bone and joint infections, severe or complicated urinary tract infections. Adults:* 500 mg P.O. q 12 hours or 400 mg I.V. q 12 hours.
➤ *Severe or complicated infections of the respiratory tract, bones, joints, skin, or skin structures; mycobacterial infections. Adults:* 750 mg P.O. q 12 hours or 400 mg I.V. q 12 hours.
➤ *Typhoid fever. Adults:* 500 mg P.O. q 12 hours.
➤ *Intra-abdominal infections (with metronidazole). Adults:* 500 mg P.O. q 12 hours.
➤ *Treatment of mild to moderate acute sinusitis caused by* Haemophilus influenzae, Streptococcus pneumoniae, *or* Moraxella catarrhalis; *mild to moderate chronic bacterial prostatitis caused by* Escherichia coli *or* Proteus mirabilis. *Adults:* 400 mg I.V. infusion given over 60 minutes every 12 hours.
➤ *Uncomplicated gonorrhea. Adults:* 250 mg P.O. as a single dose.
➤ Neisseria meningitidis *in nasal passages* ◊. *Adults:* 500 to 750 mg P.O. as a single dose, or 250 mg P.O. b.i.d. for 2 days, or 500 mg P.O. b.i.d. for 5 days.
➤ *To reduce the occurrence or progression of disease after exposure to aerosolized* Bacillus anthracis *(anthrax). Adults:* 500 mg P.O. every 12 hours for 60 days, beginning as soon as possible after suspected or confirmed exposure.
Children: 15 mg/kg P.O. every 12 hours for 60 days, beginning as soon as possible after suspected or confirmed exposure. Maximum 500 mg per dose.
✦ *Dosage adjustment.* For patients with renal impairment, refer to the following table.

Creatinine clearance (ml/min)	Adult dosage
30 50	P.O.—250 to 500 mg q 12 hr
5-29	P.O.—250 to 500 mg q 18 hr I.V.—200 to 400 mg q 18 to 24 hr

For patients receiving hemodialysis or peritoneal dialysis, give 250 to 500 mg P.O. q 24 hours (after dialysis). Or, for patients receiving hemodialysis, give 200 to 400 mg I.V. q 24 hours (after dialysis).

How supplied
Available by prescription only
Injection for infusion: 200 mg/20-ml vial; 400 mg/40-ml vial; 200 mg in 100 ml D_5W; 400 mg in 200 ml D_5W
Oral suspension: 250 mg/5 ml, 500 mg/5 ml
Tablets (film-coated): 100 mg, 250 mg, 500 mg, 750 mg

Pharmacodynamics
Antibiotic action: Ciprofloxacin inhibits DNA gyrase, preventing bacterial DNA replication. The following organisms have been reported to be susceptible (*in vitro*) to ciprofloxacin: *Campylobacter jejuni, Citrobacter diversus, Citrobacter freundii, E. coli* (including enterotoxigenic strains), *Enterobacter cloacae, Haemophilus parainfluenzae, Klebsiella pneumoniae, Morganella morganii, P. mirabilis, Proteus vulgaris, Providencia rettgeri, Providencia stuartii, Pseudomonas aeruginosa, Serratia marcescens, Shigella flexneri, Shigella sonnei, Staphylococcus aureus* (penicillinase- and non-penicillinase-producing strains), *Staphylococcus epidermidis, Streptococcus faecalis,* and *Streptococcus pyogenes.*

Pharmacokinetics
Absorption: About 70% is absorbed after oral tablet administration. Food delays rate of absorption but not extent.
Distribution: Peak serum levels occur within 1 to 2 hours after oral tablet dosing. Drug is 20% to 40% protein-bound; CSF levels are only about 10% of plasma levels.
Metabolism: Metabolism is probably hepatic. Four metabolites have been identified; each has less antimicrobial activity than the parent compound.
Excretion: Excretion is primarily renal. Serum half-life is about 4 hours in adults with normal renal function.

Route	Onset	Peak	Duration
P.O.			
Tablet	Unknown	½-2⅓ hr	Unknown
Suspension	Unknown	Unknown	Unknown
I.V.	Unknown	Immediate	Unknown

Contraindications and precautions
Contraindicated in patients sensitive to fluoroquinolone antibiotics. Use cautiously in patients with CNS disorders or those at risk for seizures.

Interactions
Drug-drug. *Aminoglycosides, beta-lactams:* Synergistic effects have occurred with concurrent use. Avoid use together.
Antacid supplements that contain aluminum, calcium, or magnesium: May interfere with ciprofloxacin absorption. Ciprofloxacin may be safely administered 2 hours before or 6 hours after antacids.
Probenecid: Concurrent use interferes with renal tubular secretion and results in higher plasma levels of ciprofloxacin. Avoid use together.
Sucralfate: Reduces absorption of ciprofloxacin by 50%. Avoid use together.
Theophylline: Increased risk of theophylline toxicity. Closer monitoring of theophylline levels may be necessary.
Warfarin: Increased PT. Avoid use together.
Drug-herb. *Yerba maté methylxanthines:* May decrease yerba maté methylxanthine clearance and cause toxicity. Discourage use together.
Drug-food. *Caffeine:* Ciprofloxacin prolongs elimination half-life of caffeine. Discourage use together.
Iron, minerals, vitamins: May interfere with ciprofloxacin absorption. Discourage use together.
Drug-lifestyle. *Sun exposure:* Photosensitivity reaction may occur. Advise patient to take precautions.

Adverse reactions
CNS: headache, restlessness, tremor, dizziness, fatigue, drowsiness, insomnia, depression, lightheadedness, confusion, hallucinations, *seizures,* paresthesia.
GI: *nausea, diarrhea,* vomiting, abdominal pain or discomfort, oral candidiasis, pseudomembranous colitis, dyspepsia, flatulence, constipation.
GU: crystalluria, increased serum creatinine and BUN levels, interstitial nephritis.
Hepatic: elevated liver enzyme levels.
Musculoskeletal: arthralgia, joint or back pain, joint inflammation, joint stiffness, aching, neck or chest pain.
Skin: *rash,* photosensitivity, toxic epidermal necrolysis, exfoliative dermatitis.
Other: *Stevens-Johnson syndrome, hypersensitivity reactions;* thrombophlebitis, burning, pruritus, erythema, edema (with I.V. administration).

Overdose and treatment
To treat overdose, empty the stomach via induced vomiting or lavage. Provide supportive measures and maintain hydration. Peritoneal dialysis or hemodialysis may be helpful, particularly if patient's renal function is compromised.

Special considerations
● Duration of therapy depends on type and severity of infection. Therapy should continue for 2 days after symptoms have abated. Most infections

---

Reactions may be *common*, uncommon, *life-threatening*, or COMMON AND LIFE-THREATENING.

are well controlled in 1 to 2 weeks, but bone or joint infections may take 4 weeks or longer.

Patient monitoring
• Monitor patient's intake and output, and watch for signs of crystalluria.

Breast-feeding patients
• Drug may appear in breast milk. Consider discontinuing breast-feeding or drug therapy to avoid serious toxicity in the infant.

Pediatric patients
• Avoid use in children.

Patient education
• Tell patient that drug may be taken without regard to meals. The preferred time is 2 hours after a meal.
• Advise patient to avoid taking drug with antacids, iron, or calcium and to drink plenty of fluids during therapy.
• Inform patient that because dizziness, lightheadedness, or drowsiness may occur, he should avoid hazardous activities that require mental alertness until CNS effects of drug are determined.

---

ciprofloxacin hydrochloride (ophthalmic)
Ciloxan

Pharmacologic classification: fluoroquinolone
Therapeutic classification: antibacterial
Pregnancy risk category: C

Indications and dosages
➤ *Corneal ulcers caused by* Pseudomonas aeruginosa, Staphylococcus aureus, Staphylococcus epidermidis, Streptococcus pneumoniae, *and possibly* Serratia marcescens *and* Streptococcus viridans. *Adults and children over age 12:* Instill 2 drops in the affected eye q 15 minutes for first 6 hours, and then 2 drops q 30 minutes for remainder of first day. On day 2, instill 2 drops hourly. On days 3 to 14, instill 2 drops q 4 hours.
➤ *Bacterial conjunctivitis caused by* S. aureus, S. epidermidis *and possibly* S. pneumoniae. *Adults and children over age 12:* Instill 1 or 2 drops into the conjunctival sac of affected eye q 2 hours while awake, for first 2 days. Then 1 or 2 drops q 4 hours while awake, for next 5 days.

How supplied
Available by prescription only
Ophthalmic solution: 0.3% in 2.5- and 5-ml containers

Pharmacodynamics
Antibacterial action: Inhibits bacterial DNA gyrase, an enzyme necessary for bacterial replica-

tion. Bacteriostatic or bactericidal, depending on concentration.

Pharmacokinetics
Absorption: Systemic absorption is limited. The maximum plasma concentration is less than 5 ng/ml, and the mean plasma concentration is usually below 2.5 ng/ml.
Distribution: Unknown.
Metabolism: Unknown.
Excretion: Unknown.

Route	Onset	Peak	Duration
Oph-thalmic	Unknown	Unknown	Unknown

Contraindications and precautions
Contraindicated in patients hypersensitive to drug or other fluoroquinolone antibiotics. Use cautiously in breast-feeding women.

Interactions
None reported.

Adverse reactions
EENT: *local burning or discomfort, white crystalline precipitate* (in the superficial portion of the corneal defect in patients with corneal ulcers), *margin crusting, crystals or scales, foreign body sensation, itching, conjunctival hyperemia,* bad or bitter taste, corneal staining, allergic reactions, keratopathy, lid edema, tearing, photophobia, decreased vision.
GI: nausea.

Overdose and treatment
An overdose of topical drug may be flushed from the eye with warm tap water.

Special considerations
• If corneal epithelium is still compromised after 14 days of treatment, continue therapy.

Patient monitoring
• Discontinue drug at first sign of hypersensitivity reactions, such as rash, itching eyelids, redness or swelling.

Breast-feeding patients
• It isn't known if drug appears in breast milk after application to the eye; systemic absorption is limited. However, systemically administered ciprofloxacin has been detected in breast milk. Use cautiously.

Pediatric patients
• Safety and efficacy in children under age 12 haven't been established.

Patient education
• Teach patient how to instill drug correctly. Remind him not to touch the tip of the bottle with his hands and to avoid contact of the tip with the eye or surrounding tissue.

• Remind patient not to share washcloths or towels with other family members to avoid spreading infection.
• Advise patient to wash hands before and after instilling solution.

cisatracurium besylate
Nimbex

Pharmacologic classification: nondepolarizing neuromuscular blocker
Therapeutic classification: skeletal muscle relaxant
Pregnancy risk category: B

Indications and dosages
➤ *Adjunct to general anesthesia, to facilitate tracheal intubation, and to provide skeletal muscle relaxation during surgery or mechanical ventilation in the intensive care unit. Adults and children age 12 and older:* Initially, 0.15 or 0.2 mg/kg I.V.; then 0.03 mg/kg I.V. q 40 to 50 minutes after an initial dose of 0.15 mg/kg and q 50 to 60 minutes following an initial dose of 0.2 mg/kg for maintenance in prolonged surgical procedures. Or, 3 mcg/kg/minute maintenance infusion after initial dose; then decreaseed to 1 to 2 mcg/kg/minute, p.r.n.
Children ages 2 to 12: 0.1 mg/kg I.V. over 5 to 10 seconds. Administer 3 mcg/kg/minute maintenance I.V. infusion after initial dose and then decrease to 1 to 2 mcg/kg/minute, p.r.n., in prolonged surgical procedures.
➤ *Maintenance of neuromuscular blockade in intensive care unit. Adults:* 3 mcg/kg/minute I.V. infusion.
Note: Dosage requirements vary widely. Also, dosages may increase or decrease over time.

How supplied
Available by prescription only
Injection: 2 mg/ml, 10 mg/ml

Pharmacodynamics
Skeletal muscle relaxation action: Cisatracurium binds competitively to cholinergic receptors on the motor end-plate to antagonize the action of acetylcholine, resulting in blockage of neuromuscular transmission.

Pharmacokinetics
Absorption: Administered I.V.
Distribution: Volume of distribution is limited by its large molecular weight and high polarity. Drug binding to plasma proteins hasn't been successfully studied because of its rapid degradation at physiologic pH.
Metabolism: The degradation of cisatracurium is largely independent of liver metabolism. It's believed drug undergoes Hofmann elimination (a pH- and temperature-dependent chemical

process) to form laudanosine and the monoquaternary acrylate metabolite.
Excretion: The metabolites of cisatracurium are excreted primarily in urine and feces. Elimination half-life is between 22 and 29 minutes.

Route	Onset	Peak	Duration
I.V.	1-3 min	2-5 min	25-44 min

Contraindications and precautions
Contraindicated in patients hypersensitive to drug, other bis-benzylisoquinolinium agents, or benzyl alcohol. Use cautiously in pregnant women.

Interactions
Drug-drug. *Aminoglycosides, bacitracin, clindamycin, colistimethate sodium, colistin, lincomycin, lithium, local anesthetics, magnesium salts, polymyxins, procainamide, quinidine, tetracyclines:* May enhance the neuromuscular blocking action of cisatracurium. Use together cautiously.
Carbamazepine, phenytoin: May cause slightly shorter duration of neuromuscular blockage requiring higher infusion rate requirements. Monitor patient closely.
Enflurane administered with nitrous oxide or oxygen, isoflurane: May prolong the clinically effective duration of action of initial and maintenance dosages of cisatracurium. In long surgical procedures, less frequent maintenance dosing, lower maintenance dosages, or reduced infusion rates of cisatracurium may be needed.
Succinylcholine: Shorter time to onset of maximum neuromuscular block. Monitor patient closely.

Adverse reactions
CV: *bradycardia,* hypotension, flushing.
Respiratory: *bronchospasm.*
Skin: rash.

Overdose and treatment
Overdose may result in neuromuscular block beyond the time needed for surgery and anesthesia. The primary treatment is maintenance of a patent airway and controlled ventilation until recovery of normal neuromuscular function is assured. Once recovery from neuromuscular block begins, further recovery may be facilitated by administration of an anticholinesterase agent (neostigmine, edrophonium) and an appropriate anticholinergic agent.

Special considerations
⚠ **ALERT** The 20-ml vial is intended for use only in the intensive care unit. Drug isn't compatible with propofol injection or ketorolac injection for Y-site administration. Drug is acidic and also may not be compatible with an alkaline solution having a pH greater than 8.5, such as barbiturate solutions for Y-site administration. Drug shouldn't be diluted in lactated Ringer's injection USP because of chemical instability.

Reactions may be *common*, uncommon, *life-threatening*, or COMMON AND LIFE-THREATENING.

• Drug isn't recommended for rapid sequence endotracheal intubation because of its intermediate onset of action.

• Cisatracurium has no known effect on consciousness, pain threshold, or cerebration. To avoid patient distress, neuromuscular block shouldn't be induced before patient is unconscious.

• Drug is a colorless to slightly yellow or greenish-yellow solution. Inspect vial visually for particulate matter and discoloration before administration. Solutions that aren't clear or contain visible particulates shouldn't be used.

• To avoid inaccurate dosing, perform neuromuscular monitoring on a nonparetic limb in patients with hemiparesis or paraparesis.

• In patients with neuromuscular disease (myasthenia gravis and myasthenic syndrome), prolonged neuromuscular block may occur. The use of a peripheral nerve stimulator and a dose not exceeding 0.02 mg/kg is recommended to assess the level of neuromuscular block and to monitor dosage requirements.

• Because patients with burns have been shown to develop resistance to nondepolarizing neuromuscular blocking agents, these patients may require increased dosing requirements and exhibit shortened duration of action. Monitor these patients closely.

Patient monitoring
• Monitor neuromuscular function during drug administration with a nerve stimulator. Additional doses of drug shouldn't be given before there's a definite response to nerve stimulation. If no response occurs, discontinue infusion until a response returns.

• Monitor patient's acid-base balance and electrolyte levels. Acid-base or serum electrolyte abnormalities may potentiate or antagonize the action of cisatracurium.

• Monitor patient for malignant hyperthermia.

Breast-feeding patients
• Use caution when administering cisatracurium to breast-feeding women because it isn't known if drug appears in breast milk.

Pediatric patients
• Safety and effectiveness in children under age 2 haven't been established.

Geriatric patients
• Use cautiously when administering cisatracurium to geriatric patients. The time to maximum block is about 1 minute slower in geriatric patients.

Patient education
• Reassure patient and family that patient will be monitored continuously throughout drug use; explain reason for its use.

• All procedures and events must be explained to the patient since the drug doesn't interfere with patient's ability to hear.

cisplatin (cis-platinum)
Platinol, Platinol-AQ

Pharmacologic classification: platinum coordination complex
Therapeutic classification: antineoplastic
Pregnancy risk category: D

Indications and dosages
Indications and dosages may vary. Check current literature for recommended protocol.
➤ *Adjunctive therapy in metastatic testicular cancer. Adults:* 20 mg/m² I.V. daily for 5 days. Repeat q 3 weeks for three cycles or more. Usually used with bleomycin and vinblastine.
➤ *Adjunctive therapy in metastatic ovarian cancer. Adults:* 75 to 100 mg/m² I.V. Repeat q 4 weeks or 50 mg/m² I.V. q 3 weeks with concurrent doxorubicin hydrochloride therapy.
➤ *Treatment of advanced bladder cancer. Adults:* 50 to 70 mg/m² I.V. once q 3 to 4 weeks. Patients who have received other antineoplastics or radiation therapy should receive 50 mg/m² q 4 weeks.
➤ *Head and neck cancer. Adults:* 80 to 120 mg/m² I.V. once q 3 weeks.
➤ *Cervical cancer*◊. *Adults:* 50 mg/m² I.V. once q 3 weeks.
➤ *Non-small-cell lung cancer*◊. *Adults:* 70 to 120 mg/m² I.V. once q 3 to 6 weeks.
➤ *Brain tumor*◊. *Children:* 60 mg/m² I.V. for 2 days q 3 to 4 weeks.
➤ *Osteogenic sarcoma or neuroblastoma*◊. *Children:* 90 mg/m² I.V. q 3 weeks.

How supplied
Available by prescription only
Injection: 1 mg/ml (50-mg or 100-mg vials)

Pharmacodynamics
Antineoplastic action: Cisplatin exerts its cytotoxic effects by binding with DNA and inhibiting DNA synthesis and, to a lesser extent, by inhibiting protein and RNA synthesis. Cisplatin also acts as a bifunctional alkylating agent, causing intrastrand and interstrand cross-links of DNA. Interstrand cross-linking appears to correlate well with the cytotoxicity of drug.

Pharmacokinetics
Absorption: Not administered orally or I.M.
Distribution: Distributed widely into tissues, with highest levels found in the kidneys, liver, and prostate. Drug can accumulate in body tissues, with drug being detected up to 6 months after the last dose. Cisplatin doesn't readily cross the blood-brain barrier. Drug is extensively and irreversibly bound to plasma proteins and tissue proteins.

Metabolism: Metabolic fate is unclear.
Excretion: Excreted primarily unchanged in urine. In patients with normal renal function, the half-life of the initial elimination phase is 25 to 79 minutes and the terminal phase is 58 to 78 hours. The terminal half-life of total cisplatin is up to 10 days.

Route	Onset	Peak	Duration
I.V.	Unknown	Unknown	Several days

Contraindications and precautions

Contraindicated in patients hypersensitive to drug or to other platinum-containing compounds and in those with severe renal disease, hearing impairment, or myelosuppression.

Interactions

Drug-drug. *Aminoglycosides:* Potentiated cumulative nephrotoxicity. Don't use aminoglycosides within 2 weeks of cisplatin, and monitor renal function studies carefully.
Aspirin: Increased risk of bleeding. Avoid use together.
Loop diuretics: Increased risk of ototoxicity. Closely monitor patient's audiologic status.
Phenytoin: May decrease serum phenytoin level. Monitor phenytoin level.

Adverse reactions

CNS: *peripheral neuritis, seizures,* neuropathy.
EENT: *tinnitus, hearing loss, ototoxicity,* vestibular toxicity.
GI: *nausea, vomiting* (beginning 1 to 4 hours after dose and lasting 24 hours), loss of taste.
GU: prolonged and SEVERE RENAL TOXICITY with repeated courses of therapy.
Hematologic: MYELOSUPPRESSION (nadirs in circulating platelet and WBC counts on days 18 to 23, with recovery by day 39).
Metabolic: *hypomagnesemia,* hypokalemia, hypocalcemia, hyponatremia, hypophosphatemia, hyperuricemia.
Other: *anaphylactoid reaction.*

Overdose and treatment

Signs and symptoms of overdose include leukopenia, thrombocytopenia, nausea, and vomiting. Treatment is generally supportive and includes transfusion of blood components, antibiotics for possible infections, and antiemetics. Cisplatin can be removed by dialysis, but only within 3 hours after administration.

Special considerations

• Prehydration and mannitol diuresis may significantly reduce renal toxicity and ototoxicity.
• Review hematologic status and creatinine clearance before therapy.
• Reconstitute 10-mg vial with 10 ml and 50-mg vial with 50 ml of sterile water for injection to yield a concentration of 1 mg/ml. The drug may be diluted further in a saline solution for I.V. infusion.
• Don't use aluminum needles for reconstitution or administration of cisplatin; a black precipitate may form. Use stainless steel needles.
• Drug is stable for 24 hours in normal saline solution at room temperature. Don't refrigerate because precipitation may occur. Discard solution containing precipitate.
• Infusions are most stable in normal saline solution, half-normal saline solution, or 0.225% saline solution.
• Mannitol may be given as a 12.5-g I.V. bolus before starting cisplatin infusion. Follow by infusion of mannitol at up to 10 g/hour, as necessary, to maintain urine output during cisplatin infusion and for 6 to 24 hours after infusion.
• I.V. sodium thiosulfate may be administered with cisplatin infusion to decrease risk of nephrotoxicity.
• Hydrate patient, with P.O. fluids if possible, or with normal saline solution before giving drug. Maintain urine output of 100 ml/hour for 4 consecutive hours before and 24 hours after infusion.
• Nausea and vomiting may be severe and protracted (up to 24 hours). Antiemetics can be started 24 hours before therapy. Monitor fluid intake and output. Continue I.V. hydration until patient can tolerate adequate oral intake.
• High-dose metoclopramide (2 mg/kg I.V.) has been used to prevent and treat nausea and vomiting. Dexamethasone 10 to 20 mg has been administered I.V. with metoclopramide to alleviate nausea and vomiting. Many patients respond favorably to treatment with ondansetron (Zofran). Pretreatment with this 5-HT$_3$ antagonist should begin 30 minutes before cisplatin therapy is started.
• Treat extravasation with local injections of a 1/6 M sodium thiosulfate solution (prepared by mixing 4 ml of sodium thiosulfate 10% and 6 ml of sterile water for injection).
• Anaphylactoid reaction usually responds to immediate treatment with epinephrine, corticosteroids, or antihistamines.
• Avoid contact with skin. If contact occurs, wash drug off immediately with soap and water.

Patient monitoring

• Monitor CBC, platelet count, and renal function studies before first and subsequent doses. Don't repeat dose unless platelet count is more than 100,000/mm³, WBC count is more than 4,000/mm³, serum creatinine level is less than 1.5 mg/dl, or BUN level is less than 25 mg/dl.
• Renal toxicity becomes more severe with repeated doses. Renal function must return to normal before next dose can be given.
• Monitor electrolytes extensively; aggressive supplementation is often required after a course of therapy.

Reactions may be *common,* uncommon, *life-threatening,* or COMMON AND LIFE-THREATENING.

Pregnant patients
● Caution women of childbearing age not to become pregnant during therapy. Also recommend consulting with prescriber before becoming pregnant.

Breast-feeding patients
● It isn't known if cisplatin appears in breast milk. However, because of risk to infant of serious adverse reactions, mutagenicity, and carcinogenicity, breast-feeding isn't recommended during therapy.

Pediatric patients
● Pediatric dosages of cisplatin haven't been fully established.
● Unlabeled uses of cisplatin include osteogenic sarcoma and neuroblastoma.
● Ototoxicity appears to be more severe in children.

Patient education
● Stress importance of adequate fluid intake and increase in urine output, to facilitate uric acid excretion.
● Tell patient to report tinnitus immediately, to prevent permanent hearing loss. Patient should have audiometric tests before first and subsequent courses of drug therapy.
● Advise patient to avoid exposure to people with infections.
● Inform patient to promptly report unusual bleeding or bruising.

---

citalopram hydrobromide
Celexa

Pharmacologic classification: selective serotonin reuptake inhibitor (SSRI)
Therapeutic classification: antidepressant
Pregnancy risk category: C

Indications and dosages
➤ *Depression. Adults:* Initially, 20 mg P.O. once daily, increasing to 40 mg daily after no less than 1 week. Maximum recommended dose is 40 mg daily.
Geriatric patients: 20 mg P.O. daily adjusted to 40 mg daily for nonresponding patients.
✦ *Dosage adjustment.* For patients with hepatic impairment, give 20 mg P.O. daily and adjust to 40 mg daily only if patient fails to respond.

How supplied
Available by prescription only
Tablets: 20 mg, 40 mg

Pharmacodynamics
Antidepressant action: An SSRI whose action is presumed to be linked to potentiation of serotonergic activity in the CNS resulting from inhibition of neuronal reuptake of serotonin.

Pharmacokinetics
Absorption: Absolute bioavailability is 80% following oral administration.
Distribution: Highly bound to plasma proteins (80%).
Metabolism: Extensively metabolized primarily by cytochrome P-450 3A4 and cytochrome P-450 2C19 to inactive metabolites.
Excretion: About 20% of drug is excreted in urine. Elimination half-life is about 35 hours. In patients over age 60, the half-life is increased up to 30%.

Route	Onset	Peak	Duration
P.O.	Unknown	2-4 hr	Unknown

Contraindications and precautions
Contraindicated in patients also taking MAO inhibitors or within 14 days of MAO inhibitor therapy and in those hypersensitive to drug or its inactive ingredients.

Interactions
Drug-drug. *Carbamazepine:* May increase citalopram clearance. Monitor patient.
CNS drugs: Additive effects. Use together cautiously
Drugs that inhibit cytochrome P-450 isoenzymes 3A4 and 2C19: Decreased citalopram clearance. Monitor patient closely.
Imipramine, other tricyclic antidepressants: Level of imipramine metabolite desipramine increased by about 50%. Use together cautiously.
Lithium: May enhance serotonergic effect of citalopram. Use cautiously, and monitor lithium level.
MAO inhibitors: Serious, sometimes fatal, reactions may occur; don't use drug within 14 days of MAO inhibitor.
Warfarin: PT is increased by 5%. Monitor patient carefully.
Drug-lifestyle. *Alcohol use:* May increase CNS effects. Discourage use together.

Adverse reactions
CNS: tremor, *somnolence, insomnia,* anxiety, agitation, dizziness, paresthesia, migraine, impaired concentration, amnesia, depression, apathy, *suicide attempt,* confusion, fatigue.
CV: tachycardia, orthostatic hypotension, hypotension.
EENT: rhinitis, sinusitis, abnormal accommodation.
GI: *dry mouth, nausea,* diarrhea, anorexia, dyspepsia, vomiting, abdominal pain, taste perversion, increased saliva, flatulence, increased appetite.
GU: dysmenorrhea, amenorrhea, ejaculation disorder, impotence, polyuria.
Metabolic: hyponatremia, weight changes.
Musculoskeletal: arthralgia, myalgia.
Respiratory: upper respiratory tract infection, cough.

Skin: rash, pruritus.
Other: *increased sweating,* fever, yawning, decreased libido, SIADH.

Special considerations
● Use cautiously in patients with history of mania, seizures, suicidal ideation, or hepatic or renal impairment.
● Be aware that, although drug hasn't been shown to impair psychomotor performance, any psychoactive drug has the potential to impair judgment, thinking, or motor skills.

Patient monitoring
● The possibility of a suicide attempt is inherent in depression and may persist until significant remission occurs. Closely observe high-risk patients at the start of drug therapy. Reduce risk of overdose by limiting the amount of drug available per refill.

Breast-feeding patients
● Drug appears in breast milk with subsequent effects in the infant; therefore, a decision to discontinue drug or breast-feeding should be made during drug therapy.

Pediatric patients
● Safety and effectiveness haven't been established.

Geriatric patients
● Use cautiously in the elderly because they may experience greater sensitivity to drug.

Patient education
● Inform patient that, although improvement may occur within 1 to 4 weeks, he should continue therapy as prescribed.
● Instruct patient to exercise caution when driving and operating hazardous machinery because of the potential of psychoactive drugs to impair judgment, thinking, and motor skills.
● Advise patient to consult prescriber before taking other prescription or OTC medications.
● Tell patient that drug may be taken in the morning or evening without regard to meals.

cladribine
Leustatin

Pharmacologic classification: purine nucleoside analogue
Therapeutic classification: antineoplastic
Pregnancy risk category: D

Indications and dosages
➤ *Active hairy cell leukemia. Adults:* 0.09 mg/kg daily by continuous I.V. infusion for 7 days.
➤ *Advanced cutaneous T-cell lymphomas* ◇, *chronic lymphocytic leukemia* ◇, *malignant lymphomas* ◇, *acute myeloid leukemias* ◇, *autoimmune hemolytic anemia* ◇, *mycosis fungoides* ◇, *Sézary syndrome* ◇. *Adults:* Usually 0.1 mg/kg daily by continuous I.V. infusion for 7 days.

How supplied
Available by prescription only
Injection: 1 mg/ml

Pharmacodynamics
Antineoplastic action: Cladribine enters tumor cells, where it's phosphorylated by deoxycytidine kinase and subsequently converted into an active triphosphate deoxynucleotide. This metabolite impairs synthesis of new DNA, inhibits repair of existing DNA, and disrupts cellular metabolism.

Pharmacokinetics
Absorption: Not administered P.O. or I.M.
Distribution: About 20% of cladribine is bound to plasma proteins.
Metabolism: No information available.
Excretion: For patients with normal renal function, the mean terminal half-life of cladribine is 5½ hours.

Route	Onset	Peak	Duration
I.V.	Unknown	Unknown	Unknown

Contraindications and precautions
Contraindicated in patients hypersensitive to drug. Use cautiously in patients with impaired renal or hepatic function.

Interactions
Drug-drug. *Amphotericin B:* May increase the risk of nephrotoxicity, hypotension, and bronchospasm. Monitor patient closely.

Adverse reactions
CNS: *malaise, headache, fatigue,* dizziness, insomnia, asthenia.
CV: tachycardia, edema.
EENT: epistaxis.
GI: *nausea, decreased appetite, vomiting, diarrhea,* constipation, abdominal pain.
GU: acute renal insufficiency.
Hematologic: NEUTROPENIA, *anemia, thrombocytopenia.*
Metabolic: hyperuricemia.
Musculoskeletal: *trunk pain, myalgia, arthralgia.*
Respiratory: *abnormal breath or chest sounds, cough,* shortness of breath.
Skin: *rash, pruritus, erythema, purpura,* petechiae, *local reaction at the injection site, diaphoresis.*
Other: *fever,* INFECTION, *chills.*

Overdose and treatment
High doses of cladribine have been linked to irreversible neurologic toxicity (paraparesis/quadriparesis), acute nephrotoxicity, and severe bone marrow suppression that results in neutropenia,

anemia, and thrombocytopenia. No antidote specific to cladribine overdose is known. Besides discontinuation of cladribine, treatment consists of careful observation and appropriate supportive measures. It isn't known if drug can be removed by dialysis or hemofiltration.

Special considerations
● Fever is commonly observed during the first month of therapy and frequently requires antibiotic therapy.
● Because of risk of hyperuricemia from tumor lysis, administer allopurinol during therapy.
● For a 24-hour infusion, add the calculated dose to a 500-ml infusion bag of normal saline solution injection. Once diluted, administer promptly or store in the refrigerator for no more than 8 hours before administration. Don't use solutions that contain dextrose because studies have shown increased degradation of drug. Because the product doesn't contain bacteriostatic agents, use strict aseptic technique to prepare the admixture. Solutions containing cladribine shouldn't be mixed with other I.V. drugs or infused simultaneously via a common I.V. line.
● Or, prepare a 7-day infusion solution, using bacteriostatic saline solution for injection, which contains 0.9% benzyl alcohol. First, pass the calculated amount of drug through a disposable 0.22-micron hydrophilic syringe filter into a sterile infusion reservoir. Next, add sufficient bacteriostatic saline solution for injection to bring the total volume to 100 ml. Clamp off the line; then disconnect and discard the filter. If necessary, aseptically aspirate air bubbles from the reservoir, using a new filter or sterile vent filter assembly.
● Physical and chemical stability are acceptable using Pharmacia Deltec medication cassettes.
● Refrigerate unopened vials at 36° to 46° F (2° to 8° C), and protect from light. Although freezing doesn't adversely affect the drug, a precipitate may form; this will disappear if the drug is allowed to warm to room temperature gradually and the vial is vigorously shaken. Don't heat, microwave, or refreeze.

Patient monitoring
● Cladribine is a toxic drug, and some toxicity is expected during treatment. Monitor hematologic function closely, especially during the first 4 to 8 weeks of therapy. Severe bone marrow suppression, including neutropenia, anemia, and thrombocytopenia, has commonly been observed in patients treated with drug; many patients also have hematologic impairment from their disease.

Pregnant patients
● Women of childbearing age should avoid pregnancy during drug therapy because of risk of fetal malformations.

Breast-feeding patients
● It isn't known if drug appears in breast milk. A decision should be made to discontinue either breast-feeding or drug, taking into account the importance of drug to the woman.

Pediatric patients
● Safety and effectiveness in children haven't been established.

Patient education
● Teach patient to watch for signs of infection and bleeding (easy bruising, nosebleeds).
● Tell patient to take his temperature daily.

clarithromycin
Biaxin

Pharmacologic classification: macrolide
Therapeutic classification: antibiotic
Pregnancy risk category: C

Indications and dosages
➤ *Pharyngitis or tonsillitis caused by* Streptococcus pyogenes. *Adults:* 250 mg P.O. q 12 hours for 10 days.
Children: 15 mg/kg P.O. daily divided q 12 hours for 10 days.
➤ *Acute maxillary sinusitis caused by* Streptococcus pneumoniae, Haemophilus influenzae, *or* Moraxella catarrhalis. *Adults:* 500 mg P.O. q 12 hours for 14 days.
Children: 15 mg/kg P.O. daily divided q 12 hours for 10 days.
➤ *Acute exacerbations of chronic bronchitis caused by* M. catarrhalis *or* S. pneumoniae; *pneumonia caused by* S. pneumoniae, Mycoplasma pneumoniae, *or* H. influenzae. *Adults:* 250 mg P.O. q 12 hours for 7 to 14 days.
➤ *Acute exacerbations of chronic bronchitis caused by* H. influenzae. *Adults:* 500 mg P.O. q 12 hours for 7 to 14 days.
➤ *Uncomplicated skin and skin structure infections caused by* Staphylococcus aureus *or* S. pyogenes. *Adults:* 250 mg P.O. q 12 hours for 7 to 14 days.
➤ *Prophylaxis and treatment of disseminated infection from* Mycobacterium avium complex. *Adults:* 500 mg P.O. b.i.d.
Children: 7.5 mg/kg P.O. b.i.d. up to 500 mg b.i.d.
➤ *Acute otitis media caused by* H. influenzae, M. catarrhalis, *or* S. pneumoniae. *Children:* 7.5 mg/kg P.O. b.i.d. up to 500 mg b.i.d.
➤ Helicobacter pylori *eradication to reduce risk of duodenal ulcer recurrence.* *Adults:* 500 mg Biaxin with 30 mg lansoprazole and 1 g amoxicilin, all given q 12 hours for 10 to 14 days. Or, dual therapy with 500 mg Biaxin q 8 hours and 40 mg omeprazole once daily for 14 days.

✦ *Dosage adjustment.* In patients with creatinine clearance of less than 30 ml/minute, cut dose in half or double frequency interval.

How supplied
Available by prescription only
Suspension: 125 mg/5 ml, 250 mg/5 ml
Tablets: 250 mg, 500 mg

Pharmacodynamics
Antibiotic action: Clarithromycin, a macrolide antibiotic, binds to the 50S subunit of bacterial ribosomes, blocking protein synthesis. It's bacteriostatic or bactericidal, depending on the concentration.

Pharmacokinetics
Absorption: Rapidly absorbed from the GI tract; absolute bioavailability is about 50%. Although food slightly delays onset of absorption, clarithromycin may be taken without regard to meals because food doesn't alter the total amount of drug absorbed.
Distribution: Widely distributed; because it readily penetrates cells, tissue concentrations are higher than plasma levels. Plasma half-life is dose-dependent; half-life is 3 to 4 hours at doses of 250 mg q 12 hours and increases to 5 to 7 hours at doses of 500 mg q 12 hours.
Metabolism: Clarithromycin's major metabolite, 14-hydroxy clarithromycin, has significant antimicrobial activity. It's about twice as active against *H. influenzae* as the parent drug.
Excretion: In patients taking 250 mg q 12 hours, about 20% is eliminated in the urine unchanged; this increases to 30% in patients taking 500 mg q 12 hours. The major metabolite accounts for about 15% of drug in the urine. Elimination half-life of the active metabolite is dose-dependent: 5 to 6 hours with 250 mg q 12 hours; 7 hours with 500 mg q 12 hours.

Route	Onset	Peak	Duration
P.O.	Unknown	2-4 hr	Unknown

Contraindications and precautions
Contraindicated in patients hypersensitive to erythromycin or other macrolides who have cardiac abnormalities or electrolyte disturbances. Use cautiously in patients with impaired renal or hepatic function.

Interactions
Drug-drug. *Carbamazepine, theophylline:* May increase levels of these drugs. Monitor drug levels carefully.
Cyclosporine, phenytoin, triazolam: Decreased metabolism of these drugs. Monitor patient closely.
Digoxin: Increased digoxin levels. Monitor patient for signs of digoxin toxicity.
Dihydroergotamine, ergotamine: Acute ergot toxicity. Avoid use together.

Warfarin: Increased INR with other macrolides, and possibly with clarithromycin. Monitor patient closely.

Adverse reactions
CNS: headache.
GI: *diarrhea, nausea, abnormal taste,* dyspepsia, abdominal pain or discomfort.
GU: elevated BUN and creatinine levels.
Hematologic: increased PT, decreased WBCs.
Hepatic: elevated liver function test results.

Overdose and treatment
No information available.

Special considerations
● Obtain specimen for culture and sensitivity tests before giving first dose. Therapy may begin pending test results.
● Reconstituted suspension shouldn't be refrigerated; discard unused portion after 14 days.

Patient monitoring
● Drug may cause overgrowth of nonsusceptible bacteria or fungi. Monitor for signs and symptoms of superinfection.

Breast-feeding patients
● It isn't known if drug appears in breast milk; however, other macrolides have been found in breast milk. Use with caution.

Pediatric patients
● Safety and efficacy in children under age 12 haven't been established.

Patient education
● Tell patient to take all of drug as prescribed, even if he feels better.
● Inform patient that he may take drug without regard to meals.
● Instruct patient to shake suspension well before use and not to refrigerate. Tell patient to discard unused portion after 14 days.

clemastine fumarate
Tavist, Tavist Allergy

Pharmacologic classification: ethanolamine-derivative antihistamine
Therapeutic classification: antihistamine (H_1-receptor antagonist)
Pregnancy risk category: C

Indications and dosages
➤*Rhinitis, allergy symptoms. Adults and children age 12 or over:* 1.34 to 2.68 mg P.O. b.i.d. or t.i.d. Maximum recommended daily dose is 8.04 mg.
Children ages 6 to 11: 0.67 mg P.O. b.i.d.; not to exceed 4.02 mg daily.

Reactions may be *common,* uncommon, *life-threatening,* or COMMON AND LIFE-THREATENING.

➤ *Allergic skin reactions of urticaria and angioedema. Adults and children age 12 or over:* 2.68 mg P.O. up to t.i.d. maximum. *Children ages 6 to 11:* 1.34 mg P.O. b.i.d.; not to exceed 4.02 mg daily.

How supplied
Available without a prescription
Syrup: 0.5 mg /5 ml
Tablets: 1.34 mg (Tavist Allergy), 2.68 mg (Tavist)

Pharmacodynamics
Antihistamine action: Antihistamines compete with histamine for histamine H_1-receptor sites on the smooth muscle of the bronchi, GI tract, uterus, and large blood vessels; by binding to cellular receptors, they prevent access of histamine and suppress histamine-induced allergic symptoms, even though they don't prevent its release.

Pharmacokinetics
Absorption: Absorbed readily from the GI tract.
Distribution: Unknown.
Metabolism: Extensively metabolized.
Excretion: Excreted in urine.

Route	Onset	Peak	Duration
P.O.	15-60 min	5-7 hr	12 hr

Contraindications and precautions
Contraindicated in patients hypersensitive to drug or other antihistamines of similar chemical structure, in those with acute asthma, in neonates or premature infants, and in breast-feeding women.

Use cautiously in elderly patients and patients with increased intraocular pressure, glaucoma, hyperthyroidism, CV or renal disease, hypertension, bronchial asthma, pyloroduodenal obstruction, prostatic hyperplasia, bladder neck obstruction, and stenosing peptic ulcers.

Interactions
Drug-drug. *CNS depressants:* Increased sedation. Use together cautiously.
Heparin: May partially counteract the anticoagulant effect. Monitor patient closely.
MAO inhibitors: Prolonged and intensified central depressant and anticholinergic effects. Don't use together.
Sulfonylureas: May diminish effects of these drugs. Monitor patient closely.
Drug-lifestyle. *Alcohol use:* Additive CNS depression. Discourage use together.
Sun exposure: Photosensitivity reactions. Advise patient to take precautions.

Adverse reactions
CNS: *sedation, drowsiness, seizures,* nervousness, tremor, confusion, restlessness, vertigo, headache, *dizziness, incoordination,* fatigue.
CV: hypotension, palpitations, tachycardia.

GI: *epigastric distress,* anorexia, diarrhea, nausea, vomiting, constipation, *dry mouth.*
GU: urine retention, urinary frequency.
Hematologic: hemolytic anemia, *thrombocytopenia, agranulocytosis.*
Respiratory: *thick bronchial secretions.*
Skin: rash, urticaria, photosensitivity, diaphoresis.
Other: *anaphylaxis.*

Overdose and treatment
Signs and symptoms of overdose may include either CNS depression (sedation, reduced mental alertness, apnea, and CV collapse) or CNS stimulation (insomnia, hallucinations, tremors, or seizures). Anticholinergic symptoms, such as dry mouth, flushed skin, fixed and dilated pupils, and GI symptoms, are common, especially in children.

Treat overdose by inducing emesis with ipecac syrup (in conscious patient), followed by activated charcoal to reduce further drug absorption. Use gastric lavage if patient is unconscious or if ipecac fails. Treat hypotension with vasopressors, and control seizures with diazepam or phenytoin. Don't give stimulants.

Special considerations
Consider the recommendations relevant to all antihistamines as well as the following.
● Drug is indicated for treatment of urticaria only at dosages of 2.68 mg up to t.i.d.
● Discontinue clemastine 4 days before diagnostic skin tests; antihistamines can prevent, reduce, or mask positive skin test response.

Patient monitoring
● Monitor blood counts during long-term therapy; observe for signs of blood dyscrasias.

Breast-feeding patients
● Drug shouldn't be used during breast-feeding because it appears in breast milk, exposing infant to risks of unusual excitability; premature infants are at particular risk for seizures.

Pediatric patients
● Drug isn't indicated for use in premature infants or neonates.
● Children, especially those under age 6, may experience paradoxical hyperexcitability.

Geriatric patients
● Geriatric patients are more susceptible to the sedative effect of drug and may experience dizziness or hypotension more readily than younger people. Instruct older patients to change positions slowly and gradually.

Patient education
● Inform patient of potential adverse reactions.
● Tell patient to report if tolerance develops because a different antihistamine may need to be prescribed.

clindamycin hydrochloride
Cleocin

clindamycin palmitate hydrochloride
Cleocin Pediatric

clindamycin phosphate
Cleocin Phosphate, Cleocin T

Pharmacologic classification: lincomycin derivative
Therapeutic classification: antibiotic
Pregnancy risk category: B

Indications and dosages
➤ *Infections caused by sensitive organisms. Adults:* 150 to 450 mg P.O. q 6 hours. Or, 600 to 2,700 mg I.M. or I.V. daily divided into two to four equal doses.
Children over age 1 month: 8 to 20 mg/kg P.O. daily or 20 to 40 mg/kg I.V. daily divided into three or four equal doses.
Children under age 1 month: 15 to 20 mg/kg I.V. daily divided into three or four equal doses.
➤ *Bacterial vaginosis. Adults:* 100 mg (one applicatorful of clindamycin phosphate) intravaginally h.s. for 7 days.
➤ *Acne vulgaris. Adults:* Apply thin film of topical solution, gel, or lotion to affected areas b.i.d.
➤ *Toxoplasmosis (cerebral or ocular) in immunocompromised patients◇. Adults and adolescents:* 300 to 450 mg P.O. q 6 to 8 hours with pyrimethamine (25 to 75 mg once daily) and leucovorin (10 to 25 mg once daily). *Infants and children:* 20 to 30 mg/kg daily P.O. in four divided doses with oral pyrimethamine (1 mg/kg daily) and oral leucovorin (5 mg once every 3 days).
➤ *Pneumocystis carinii pneumonia◇. Adults:* 600 mg I.V. q 6 hours or 300 to 450 mg P.O. q.i.d. With primaquine, give 15 to 30 mg P.O. daily.

How supplied
Available by prescription only
Capsules: 75 mg, 150 mg, 300 mg
Gel, lotion, pledgets, topical solution: 1%
Infusion for I.V. use: 150 mg/ml (300 mg, 600 mg, 900 mg)
Injection: 150 mg/ml
Solution (granules): 75 mg/5 ml
Vaginal cream: 2%

Pharmacodynamics
Antibacterial action: Drug inhibits bacterial protein synthesis by binding to ribosome's 50S subunit. Clindamycin may produce bacteriostatic or bactericidal effects on susceptible bacteria, including most aerobic gram-positive cocci and anaerobic gram-negative and gram-positive organisms. It's considered a first-line drug in the treatment of *Bacteroides fragilis* and most other gram-positive and gram-negative anaerobes. It's also effective against *Mycoplasma pneumoniae, Leptotrichia buccalis,* and some gram-positive cocci and bacilli.

Pharmacokinetics
Absorption: When administered orally, drug is absorbed rapidly and almost completely from the GI tract, regardless of formulation. Drug also may be given I.M. with good absorption. With 300-mg dose, peak levels are about 6 mcg/ml; with 600-mg dose, about 10 mcg/ml.
Distribution: Distributed widely to most body tissues and fluids (except CSF) and crosses the placenta. About 93% of drug is bound to plasma proteins.
Metabolism: Metabolized partially to inactive metabolites.
Excretion: About 10% of dose is excreted unchanged in urine; rest is excreted as inactive metabolites (with some drug appearing in breast milk). Plasma half-life is 2½ to 3 hours in patients with normal renal function; 3½ to 5 hours in anephric patients; and 7 to 14 hours in patients with hepatic disease. Peritoneal dialysis and hemodialysis don't remove drug.

Route	Onset	Peak	Duration
P.O.	Unknown	45-60 min	Unknown
I.V.	Unknown	Immediate	Unknown
I.M.	Unknown	3 hr	Unknown
Topical, intra-vaginal	Unknown	Unknown	Unknown

Contraindications and precautions
Contraindicated in patients hypersensitive to the antibiotic congener lincomycin; in those with a history of ulcerative colitis, regional enteritis, or antibiotic-associated colitis; and in those with a history of atopic reactions.

Use cautiously in patients with asthma, impaired renal or hepatic function, or history of GI diseases or significant allergies.

Interactions
Drug-drug. *Acne preparations:* Topical clindamycin may cause a cumulative irritant or drying effect. Monitor patient carefully.
Diphenoxylate, opiates: May prolong or worsen clindamycin-induced diarrhea. Monitor patient closely.
Erythromycin: May block clindamycin from reaching its site of action. Avoid use together.
Kaolin: May reduce GI absorption of clindamycin. Separate administration times.
Neuromuscular blockers: May potentiate neuromuscular blockade. Monitor patient closely.
Drug-food. *Diet foods with sodium cyclamate:* Decreased serum drug levels. Discourage use together.

Reactions may be *common,* uncommon, *life-threatening,* or COMMON AND LIFE-THREATENING.

Adverse reactions

GI: *nausea,* vomiting, abdominal pain, *diarrhea,* pseudomembranous colitis.

GU: *cervicitis, vaginitis, Candida albicans* overgrowth, *vulvar irritation.*

Hematologic: *transient leukopenia,* eosinophilia, *thrombocytopenia.*

Hepatic: jaundice, abnormal liver function test results.

Skin: maculopapular rash, urticaria, dryness, *redness,* pruritus, swelling, irritation, contact dermatitis, burning.

Other: *anaphylaxis.*

Overdose and treatment

No information available.

Special considerations

● Take culture and sensitivity tests before treatment starts; repeat as needed.

● Don't refrigerate reconstituted oral solution because it will thicken. Drug remains stable for 2 weeks at room temperature.

● I.M. preparation should be given deep I.M. Rotate sites. Doses exceeding 600 mg aren't recommended.

● I.M. injection may increase creatine kinase levels because of muscle irritation.

● For I.V. infusion, dilute each 300 mg in 50 ml of D₅W, normal saline solution, or lactated Ringer's solution and give no more than 30 mg/minute. Don't administer more than 1.2 g/hour.

● Topical form may produce adverse systemic effects.

Patient monitoring

● Monitor renal, hepatic, and hematopoietic functions during prolonged therapy.

Breast-feeding patients

● Drug appears in breast milk. Advise breast-feeding women to use an alternative feeding method during clindamycin therapy.

Pediatric patients

● Administer drug cautiously, if at all, to neonates and infants. Monitor patient closely, especially for diarrhea.

Geriatric patients

● Geriatric patients may tolerate drug-induced diarrhea poorly. Monitor patient closely for change in bowel frequency and dehydration.

Patient education

● Warn patient that I.M. injection may be painful.

● Instruct patient to report adverse effects, especially diarrhea. Warn patient not to self-treat diarrhea.

● Advise patient to take capsules with 8 oz (240 ml) of water to prevent dysphagia.

● Instruct patient using topical solution to wash, rinse, and dry affected areas before application. Warn patient not to use topical solution near eyes, nose, mouth, or other mucous membranes, and advise patient not to share washcloths and towels with family members.

clobetasol propionate
Dermovate*, Temovate

Pharmacologic classification: topical adrenocorticoid
Therapeutic classification: anti-inflammatory
Pregnancy risk category: C

Indications and dosages

➤ *Inflammation of corticosteroid-responsive dermatoses.* *Adults:* Apply a thin layer to affected skin areas b.i.d., once in the morning and once at night. Limit treatment to 14 days, with no more than 50 g of the cream or ointment or 50 ml of lotion (25 mg total) weekly.

How supplied

Available by prescription only
Cream: 0.05%
Gel: 0.05%
Ointment: 0.05%
Solution: 0.05%

Pharmacodynamics

Anti-inflammatory action: Drug is effective because of anti-inflammatory, antipruritic, and vasoconstrictive actions; however, the exact mechanism of its actions is unknown. Clobetasol is a high-potency group I fluorinated corticosteroid that's usually reserved for the management of severe dermatoses that haven't responded satisfactorily to a less potent formulation.

Pharmacokinetics

Absorption: Amount absorbed depends on the potency of the preparation, the amount applied, and the nature of the skin at the application site. It ranges from about 1% in areas with a thick stratum corneum (such as the palms, soles, elbows, and knees) to as high as 36% in areas with a thin stratum corneum (face, eyelids, and genitals). Absorption increases in areas of skin damage, inflammation, or occlusion. Some systemic absorption of topical corticosteroids occurs, especially through the oral mucosa.

Distribution: After topical application, clobetasol is distributed throughout the local skin. Any drug absorbed into the circulation is rapidly removed from the blood and distributed into muscle, liver, skin, intestines, and kidneys.

Metabolism: After topical administration, drug is metabolized primarily in the skin. The small amount absorbed into systemic circulation is metabolized primarily in the liver to inactive compounds.

Excretion: Inactive metabolites are excreted by the kidneys, primarily as glucuronides and sulfates, but also as unconjugated products. Small

◊ Unlabeled clinical use

amounts of the metabolites also are excreted in feces.

Route	Onset	Peak	Duration
Topical	Unknown	Unknown	Unknown

Contraindications and precautions
Contraindicated in patients hypersensitive to corticosteroids.

Interactions
None reported.

Adverse reactions
GU: glucosuria.
Metabolic: hyperglycemia.
Skin: burning, pruritus, irritation, dryness, erythema, folliculitis, perioral dermatitis, allergic contact dermatitis, hypopigmentation, hypertrichosis, acneiform eruptions.
Other: *hypothalamic-pituitary-adrenal (HPA) axis suppression,* Cushing's syndrome.

Overdose and treatment
No information available.

Special considerations
Consider the recommendations relevant to all topical adrenocorticoids as well as the following.
• Don't use occlusive dressings or bandages. Don't cover or wrap treated area unless instructed by prescriber.
• Apply sparingly in light film.
• Pulse therapy is sometimes used with topical corticosteroids of this potency; that is, b.i.d. for 3 days, then none for 3 days. Intermittent use prevents cumulative effects. Drug suppresses HPA axis at doses as low as 2 g daily.

Patient monitoring
• Discontinue drug and notify prescriber if skin infection, striae, or atrophy occurs.

Pregnant patients
• Because of the possibility of teratogenic effects, avoid use in pregnancy.

Pediatric patients
• Drug treatment isn't recommended in patients under age 12.

Patient education
• Inform patient of potential adverse reactions.
• Advise patient to avoid contact with eyes.
• Warn patient not to use drug for longer than 14 days.

clofazimine
Lamprene

Pharmacologic classification: substituted iminophenazine dye
Therapeutic classification: leprostatic
Pregnancy risk category: C

Indications and dosages
➤ *Dapsone-sensitive multibacillary leprosy. Adults:* Combination therapy with two other drugs for at least 2 years until skin smears are negative; then monotherapy.
➤ *Dapsone-resistant leprosy. Adults:* 100 mg P.O. once daily, usually with one or more other antileprotics for at least 3 years; then monotherapy of 100 mg Lamprene daily.
➤ *Erythema nodosum leprosum. Adults:* 100 to 200 mg P.O. daily for up to 3 months. Taper dosage to 100 mg daily as soon as possible. Dosages above 200 mg daily aren't recommended.
➤ *Atypical mycobacterial infections◊. Adults:* 100 mg P.O. q 8 hours. Usually given with several other antituberculotics.

How supplied
Available by prescription only
Capsules: 50 mg, 100 mg

Pharmacodynamics
Leprostatic action: A bright red iminophenazine dye, a relative of aniline dyes. Exerts a slow bactericidal effect on *Mycobacterium leprae* (Hansen's bacillus). Clinical benefit is usually noted in 1 to 3 months, with clearing observed by 6 months. Administration with dapsone produces a more rapid effect on leprosy lesions. No cross-resistance with dapsone or rifampin has been reported. Clofazimine inhibits mycobacterial growth and preferentially binds to mycobacterial DNA. Although exact mechanism is unknown, drug also exhibits anti-inflammatory properties in controlling erythema nodosum leprosum reactions.

Clofazimine also appears to have an important role in treatment of atypical mycobacterial infections, such as *Mycobacterium avium* infections, which are prominent in patients with AIDS. Some efficacy has been demonstrated when used with ansamycin, ethionamide, or ethambutol. Further clinical information is required.

Pharmacokinetics
Absorption: Variable absorption (45% to 62%) after oral administration.
Distribution: Highly lipophilic; distributed widely into fatty tissues and taken up by macrophages into reticuloendothelial system. Little, if any, crosses blood-brain barrier or enters CNS.
Metabolism: Not completely defined; some evidence exists of enterohepatic cycling. Serum half-lives of up to 70 days have been noted.

Reactions may be *common,* uncommon, *life-threatening,* or COMMON AND LIFE-THREATENING.

Excretion: Mostly excreted in feces; some in sputum, sebum, and sweat; very little in urine. Drug appears in breast milk.

Route	Onset	Peak	Duration
P.O.	Unknown	1-6 hr	Unknown

Contraindications and precautions
No known contraindications. Use cautiously in patients with GI dysfunction, such as abdominal pain or diarrhea.

Interactions
Drug-drug. *Dapsone:* May inhibit the anti-inflammatory activity of clofazimine. Monitor patient closely.
Isoniazid: May increase plasma and urinary levels of clofazimine and decrease levels in skin. Monitor patient closely.

Adverse reactions
EENT: *conjunctival and corneal pigmentation, dryness, burning, itching, irritation.*
GI: *epigastric pain, diarrhea, nausea, vomiting, GI intolerance,* **bowel obstruction, GI bleeding.**
Hematologic: eosinophilia.
Hepatic: elevated albumin, serum bilirubin, and AST levels.
Metabolic: hypokalemia, elevated blood glucose levels.
Skin: *pink to brownish black pigmentation, ichthyosis, dryness,* rash, pruritus.
Other: **splenic infarction,** discolored body fluids and excrement.

Overdose and treatment
In case of overdose, empty stomach by inducing vomiting or by gastric lavage. Treatment includes usual supportive measures.

Special considerations
● Administer with meals. Use clofazimine with other antileprotics.
● Severe GI symptoms may necessitate withdrawal of drug if dosage reduction doesn't relieve symptoms.
● Pink to brownish-black pigmentation of skin occurs in 75% to 100% of patients.

Patient monitoring
● Observe patient for signs of depression.

Breast-feeding patients
● Drug appears in breast milk; don't use in breast-feeding women unless potential benefit to mother exceeds risk to infant.

Patient education
● Tell patient to take drug with meals to minimize GI problems.
● Advise patient to store drug away from heat and light and out of children's reach.

● Explain that pink to brownish black pigmentation of skin may occur. Although reversible, it may take several months or years to disappear after drug is stopped. Also explain that discoloration of eyes, urine, feces, sputum, sweat, and tears also may occur.
● Tell patient not to expect benefits for 1 to 3 months; observable benefits may take up to 6 months.
● Recommend use of skin oil or cream to help relieve dryness or ichthyosis.

clofibrate
Atromid-S

Pharmacologic classification: fibric acid derivative
Therapeutic classification: antilipemic
Pregnancy risk category: C

Indications and dosages
➤ **Hyperlipidemia and xanthoma tuberosum; type III hyperlipidemia that doesn't respond adequately to diet.** *Adults:* 2 g P.O. daily in two to four divided doses. Some patients may respond to lower doses as assessed by serum lipid monitoring.
➤ **Diabetes insipidus** ◇. *Adults:* 1.5 to 2 g P.O. daily in divided doses.
✦ **Dosage adjustment.** Decreased renal function may require reduced dosage frequency (q 12 to 18 hours).

How supplied
Available by prescription only
Capsules: 500 mg

Pharmacodynamics
Antilipemic action: Clofibrate may lower serum triglyceride levels by accelerating catabolism of very low-density lipoproteins; drug lowers serum cholesterol levels (to a lesser degree) by inhibiting cholesterol biosynthesis. Both mechanisms are unknown. Drug is closely related to gemfibrozil.

Pharmacokinetics
Absorption: Absorbed slowly but completely from GI tract. Serum triglyceride levels decrease in 2 to 5 days, with peak clinical effect at 21 days.
Distribution: Distributed into extracellular space as its active form, clofibric acid, which is up to 98% protein-bound. Animal studies suggest that fetal concentration levels may exceed maternal concentration levels.
Metabolism: Hydrolyzed by serum enzymes to clofibric acid, which is metabolized by the liver.
Excretion: 20% is excreted unchanged in urine; 70% is eliminated in urine as conjugated metabolite. Plasma half-life after a single dose ranges from 6 to 25 hours; in patients with renal im-

pairment and cirrhosis, half-life can be as long as 113 hours.

Route	Onset	Peak	Duration
P.O.	Unknown	2-6 hr	Unknown

Contraindications and precautions
Contraindicated in pregnant women, in breast-feeding women, in patients hypersensitive to drug, and in patients with primary biliary cirrhosis or significant hepatic or renal dysfunction. Use cautiously in patients with peptic ulcer or history of gallbladder disease.

Interactions
Drug-drug. *Cholestyramine:* Reduced rate of clofibrate absorption. Avoid use together.
Furosemide: Increased diuresis. Use together cautiously.
Oral anticoagulants: Potentiated anticoagulant effects. If combination is necessary, reduce oral anticoagulant dosage by 50% and evaluate PT and INR frequently.
Sulfonylureas: Enhanced sulfonylurea effects, causing hypoglycemia. Dosage adjustment may be needed.

Adverse reactions
CNS: fatigue, weakness, drowsiness, dizziness, headache.
CV: *arrhythmias,* angina, *thromboembolic events,* intermittent claudication.
GI: *nausea, diarrhea, vomiting,* stomatitis, *dyspepsia,* flatulence, *cholelithiasis, cholecystitis.*
GU: impotence, renal dysfunction (dysuria, hematuria, proteinuria, decreased urine output).
Hematologic: *leukopenia,* anemia, eosinophilia.
Hepatic: gallstones, *transient and reversible elevations of liver function test results,* hepatomegaly.
Metabolic: *weight gain, polyphagia.*
Musculoskeletal: myalgia and arthralgia.
Skin: rash, urticaria, pruritus, dry skin and hair.
Other: decreased libido.

Overdose and treatment
No information available.

Special considerations
● Clofibrate shouldn't be used indiscriminately; it may pose an increased risk of gallstones, heart disease, and cancer.
● Clofibrate may increase risk of death from cancer, postcholecystectomy complications, and pancreatitis.

Patient monitoring
● Monitor serum cholesterol and triglyceride levels regularly during clofibrate therapy.
● Observe patient for the following serious adverse reactions: thrombophlebitis, pulmonary embolism, angina, and dysrhythmias; monitor renal and hepatic function, blood counts, and serum electrolyte and blood glucose levels.

Breast-feeding patients
● Clofibrate may appear in breast milk; alternative feeding method is recommended during therapy.

Pediatric patients
● Safety and efficacy haven't been established in children under age 14.

Patient education
● Warn patient to report flulike symptoms immediately.
● Stress importance of close medical supervision and of reporting adverse reactions; encourage compliance with prescribed regimen and diet.
● Warn patient not to exceed prescribed dose.
● Advise patient to take drug with food to minimize GI discomfort.
● Emphasize that drug therapy won't replace diet, exercise, and weight reduction for the control of hyperlipidemia.

clomiphene citrate
Clomid, Milophene, Serophene

Pharmacologic classification: chlorotrianisene derivative
Therapeutic classification: ovulation stimulant
Pregnancy risk category: X

Indications and dosages
➤ **To induce ovulation.** *Adults:* 50 mg P.O. daily for 5 days, starting any time in women who have had no recent uterine bleeding; or 50 mg P.O. daily starting on day 5 of menstrual cycle (first day of menstrual flow is day 1). Dose may be increased to 100 mg if ovulation doesn't occur. Repeat the 5-day course each ovulatory cycle until conception occurs or until three courses of therapy are completed.
➤ **Male infertility◇.** *Adults:* 50 to 400 mg P.O. daily for 2 to 12 months.

How supplied
Available by prescription only
Tablets: 50 mg

Pharmacodynamics
Ovulation stimulant action: Mechanism of action for inducing ovulation in anovulatory women is unknown. Drug may stimulate release of pituitary gonadotropin, follicle-stimulating hormone (FSH), and luteinizing hormone (LH), which results in development and maturation of the ovarian follicle, ovulation, and subsequent development and function of corpus luteum.

Pharmacokinetics
Absorption: Absorbed readily from the GI tract.

Distribution: May undergo enterohepatic recirculation or may be stored in body fat.
Metabolism: Metabolized by the liver.
Excretion: Half-life is about 5 days. Drug is excreted principally in feces via biliary elimination.

Route	Onset	Peak	Duration
P.O.	Unknown	Unknown	Unknown

Contraindications and precautions

Contraindicated during pregnancy and in patients with undiagnosed abnormal genital bleeding, ovarian cyst not due to polycystic ovarian syndrome, hepatic disease or dysfunction, uncontrolled thyroid or adrenal dysfunction, or presence of organic intracranial lesion (such as a pituitary tumor).

Interactions
None reported.

Adverse reactions
CNS: headache, restlessness, insomnia, dizziness, light-headedness, depression, fatigue, aggression.
EENT: blurred vision, diplopia, scotoma, photophobia, epistaxis, pharyngitis, rhinitis, sinusitis.
GI: nausea, vomiting, bloating, distention.
GU: urinary frequency and polyuria; abnormal uterine bleeding; *ovarian enlargement* and cyst formation, which regress spontaneously when drug is stopped; ovarian hyperstimulation syndrome.
Hematologic: *thrombocytopenia, leukopenia,* anemia.
Metabolic: weight gain.
Respiratory: cough, dyspnea.
Skin: alopecia, urticaria, rash, dermatitis.
Other: *hot flashes; reversible breast discomfort;* increased levels of serum thyronine, thyroxine-binding globulin, sex hormone–binding globulin; *sulfobromophthalein retention;* FSH and LH secretion.

Overdose and treatment
No information available.

Special considerations
● Advise patient to stop drug and notify prescriber immediately if abdominal symptoms or pain occur; these may indicate ovarian enlargement or ovarian cyst. Also, immediately report visual disturbances.
● Human chorionic gonadotropin (5,000 to 10,000 units) may be administered 5 to 7 days after the last dose of drug to stimulate ovulation.

Patient monitoring
● Monitor patient closely because of risk of serious adverse effects.

Pregnant patients
● Contraindicated during pregnancy because of teratogenic possibilities. Advise patient to discontinue drug and contact prescriber if she suspects she's pregnant.

Patient education
● Advise patient of possibility of multiple births, which increases with higher doses.
● Patient should take basal body temperature every morning (starting on day 1 of menstrual period) and chart on a graph to detect ovulation.
● Inform patient of importance of properly timed coitus.
● Warn patient to avoid hazardous tasks until response to drug is known because dizziness or visual disturbances may occur.

---

clomipramine hydrochloride
Anafranil

Pharmacologic classification: tricyclic antidepressant (TCA)
Therapeutic classification: antidepressant
Pregnancy risk category: C

Indications and dosages
➤ *Obsessive compulsive disorder (OCD).*
Adults: Initially, 25 mg P.O. daily, gradually increasing to 100 mg P.O. daily (in divided doses, with meals) during the first 2 weeks. Maximum dosage is 250 mg daily. After adjustment, entire daily dose may be given h.s.
Children and adolescents: Initially, 25 mg P.O. daily, gradually increased to a maximum of 3 mg/kg or 100 mg P.O. daily, whichever is smaller (in divided doses, with meals) over the first 2 weeks. Maximum daily dose is 3 mg/kg or 200 mg, whichever is smaller. After adjustment, entire daily dose may be given h.s.

How supplied
Available by prescription only
Capsules: 25 mg, 50 mg, 75 mg

Pharmacodynamics
Antiobsessional action: A selective inhibitor of serotonin (5-HT) reuptake into neurons within the CNS. It also may have some blocking activity at postsynaptic dopamine receptors. The exact mechanism by which clomipramine treats OCD is unknown.

Pharmacokinetics
Absorption: Well absorbed from GI tract, but extensive first-pass metabolism limits bioavailablity to about 50%.
Distribution: Distributed well into lipophilic tissues; the volume of distribution is about 12 L/kg; 98% is bound to plasma proteins.
Metabolism: Metabolism is primarily hepatic. Several metabolites have been identified; desmethylclomipramine is the primary active metabolite.
Excretion: About 66% is excreted in the urine and the remainder in the feces. Mean elimina-

tion half-life of the parent compound is about 36 hours; the mean elimination half-life of desmethyl-clomipramine is 69 hours. After multiple dosing, the half-life may increase.

Route	Onset	Peak	Duration
P.O.	Unknown	2-6 hr	Unknown

Contraindications and precautions
Contraindicated in patients hypersensitive to drug or other TCAs, in those who have taken an MAO inhibitor within the previous 14 days, and in patients during acute recovery period after MI.

Use cautiously in patients with CV disease, urine retention, suicidal tendencies, glaucoma, increased intraocular pressure, brain damage, or seizure disorders and in those taking medications that may lower the seizure threshold. Also use cautiously in patients with impaired renal or hepatic function, hyperthyroidism, or tumors of the adrenal medulla and in those undergoing elective surgery or receiving thyroid medication or electroconvulsive treatment.

Interactions
Drug-drug. *Barbiturates*: Decreased TCA blood levels. Monitor patient for decreased effectiveness.
Barbiturates, CNS depressants: May cause an exaggerated depressant effect. Avoid use together.
Epinephrine, norepinephrine: May produce an increased hypertensive effect. Avoid use together.
MAO inhibitors: May cause hyperpyretic crisis, seizures, coma, and death. Don't use together.
Methylphenidate: May increase TCA blood levels. Patient needs close monitoring.
Drug-herb. *Evening primrose oil:* Possible additive or synergistic effect resulting in lower seizure threshold and increasing the risk of seizure. Discourage use together.
Drug-food. *Grapefruit juice:* Elevated levels of clomipramine and reduced levels of the metabolite, desmethylclomipramine. Discourage fluctuations in ingestion of grapefruit juice.
Drug-lifestyle. *Alcohol use:* Exaggerated depressant effect. Discourage use together.
Smoking: Lower levels of clomipramine have been noted. Advise patient to avoid smoking.
Sun exposure: Increased risk of photosensitivity. Advise patient to take precautions.

Adverse reactions
CNS: *somnolence, tremor, dizziness, headache, insomnia, nervousness, myoclonus, fatigue,* syncope, EEG changes, *seizures,* confusion.
CV: orthostatic hypotension, palpitations, tachycardia, chest pain, ECG changes.
EENT: *pharyngitis, rhinitis, visual changes.*
GI: *dry mouth, constipation, nausea, dyspepsia, increased appetite,* diarrhea, *anorexia, abdominal pain.*
GU: *urinary hesitancy,* urinary tract infection, *dysmenorrhea, ejaculation failure, impotence.*
Hematologic: purpura, anemia.

Metabolic: *weight gain.*
Musculoskeletal: *myalgia.*
Skin: *diaphoresis,* rash, pruritus, dry skin.
Other: *altered libido.*

Overdose and treatment
Signs and symptoms of clomipramine overdose are similar to those of other TCAs and include sinus tachycardia, intraventricular block, hypotension, fixed and dilated pupils, drowsiness, delirium, stupor, hyperreflexia, and hyperpyrexia.

Treatment should include gastric lavage with large quantities of fluid. Continue lavage for 12 hours because the anticholinergic effects of the drug slow gastric emptying. Hemodialysis, peritoneal dialysis, and forced diuresis are ineffective because of the high degree of plasma protein binding. Support respirations and monitor cardiac function. Treat shock with plasma expanders or corticosteroids; treat seizures with diazepam.

Special considerations
⚠ ALERT To minimize risk of overdose, dispense drug in small quantities.
● Don't withdraw drug abruptly.
● Mania or hypomania may occur with clomipramine therapy.

Patient monitoring
● Observe patient for urine retention and constipation. Suggest stool softener or high-fiber diet, as needed, and encourage adequate fluid intake.

Breast-feeding patients
● It isn't known if drug appears in breast milk. Use cautiously in breast-feeding women.

Patient education
● Warn patient to avoid hazardous activities that require alertness or good psychomotor coordination until adverse CNS effects are known. This is especially important during initial titration period when daytime sedation and dizziness may occur.
● Suggest that patient relieve dry mouth with saliva substitutes or sugarless candy or gum.
● Tell patient that adverse GI effects can be minimized by taking drug with meals during the titration period. Later, the entire daily dose may be taken at bedtime to limit daytime drowsiness.
● Inform patient to avoid using OTC medications, particularly antihistamines and decongestants.
● Encourage patient to continue therapy, even if adverse reactions are troublesome. Advise patient not to stop taking it without notifying prescriber.

Reactions may be *common*, uncommon, *life-threatening*, or COMMON AND LIFE-THREATENING.

clonazepam
Klonopin, Rivotril*

Pharmacologic classification: benzodiazepine
Therapeutic classification: anticonvulsant
Controlled substance schedule: IV
Pregnancy risk category: C

Indications and dosages
➤ *Absence and atypical absence seizures; akinetic and myoclonic seizures; generalized tonic-clonic seizures* ◇. *Adults:* Initial dosage shouldn't exceed 1.5 mg P.O. daily, divided into three doses. May be increased by 0.5 to 1 mg q 3 days until seizures are controlled. Maximum recommended daily dose is 20 mg. *Children up to age 10 or weighing 66 lb (30 kg) or less:* 0.01 to 0.03 mg/kg P.O. daily (not to exceed 0.05 mg/kg daily), divided q 8 hours. Increase dosage by 0.25 to 0.5 mg q third day to a maximum maintenance dosage of 0.1 to 0.2 mg/kg daily.
➤ *Leg movements during sleep, adjunct treatment in schizophrenia* ◇. *Adults:* 0.5 to 2 mg P.O. h.s.
➤ *Parkinsonian dysarthria* ◇. *Adults:* 0.25 to 0.5 mg P.O. daily.
➤ *Acute manic episodes* ◇. *Adults:* 0.75 to 16 mg P.O. daily.
➤ *Multifocal tic disorders* ◇. *Adults:* 1.5 to 12 mg P.O. daily.
➤ *Neuralgia* ◇. *Adults:* 2 to 4 mg P.O. daily.

How supplied
Available by prescription only
Tablets: 0.5 mg, 1 mg, 2 mg

Pharmacodynamics
Anticonvulsant action: Mechanism of anticonvulsant activity is unknown; drug appears to act in the limbic system, thalamus, and hypothalamus. Drug is used to treat myoclonic, atonic, and absence seizures resistant to other anticonvulsants and to suppress or eliminate attacks of sleep-related nocturnal myoclonus (restless legs syndrome).

Pharmacokinetics
Absorption: Well absorbed from the GI tract.
Distribution: Distributed widely throughout the body; about 85% protein-bound.
Metabolism: Metabolized by the liver to several metabolites. The half-life of drug is 18 to 39 hours.
Excretion: Excreted in urine.

Route	Onset	Peak	Duration
P.O.	20-60 min	1-2 hr	6-12 hr

Contraindications and precautions
Contraindicated in patients with significant hepatic disease; in those with sensitivity to benzodiazepines; and in patients with acute angle-closure glaucoma. Use cautiously in children and in patients with mixed-type seizures, respiratory disease, or glaucoma.

Interactions
Drug-drug. *Anticonvulsants, CNS depressants:* Additive CNS depressant effects. Avoid use together.
Ritonavir: May significantly increase clonazepam levels. Monitor patient closely.
Valproic acid: May induce absence seizures. Don't use together.
Drug-lifestyle. *Alcohol use:* Additive CNS depressant effects. Discourage use together.

Adverse reactions
CNS: *drowsiness, ataxia, behavioral disturbances* (especially in children), slurred speech, tremor, confusion, psychosis, agitation.
CV: palpitations.
EENT: nystagmus, abnormal eye movements, sore gums.
GI: constipation, gastritis, change in appetite, nausea, anorexia, diarrhea.
GU: dysuria, enuresis, nocturia, urine retention.
Hematologic: *leukopenia, thrombocytopenia,* eosinophilia.
Hepatic: increased liver function test results.
Respiratory: *respiratory depression,* chest congestion, shortness of breath.
Skin: rash.

Overdose and treatment
Signs and symptoms of overdose may include ataxia, confusion, coma, decreased reflexes, and hypotension.

Treat overdose with gastric lavage and supportive therapy. Flumazenil, a specific benzodiazepine antagonist, may be useful. Vasopressors should be used to treat hypotension. Carefully monitor vital signs, ECG, and fluid and electrolyte balance. Clonazepam isn't dialyzable.

Special considerations
● Abrupt withdrawal may precipitate status epilepticus; after long-term use, lower dosage gradually.

Patient monitoring
● Monitor CBC and liver function tests periodically.
● Monitor patient for oversedation, especially in geriatric patients.

Breast-feeding patients
● Alternative feeding method is recommended during clonazepam therapy.

Pediatric patients
● Long-term safety in children hasn't been established.

Geriatric patients
• Geriatric patients may require lower doses because of diminished renal function; such patients also are at greater risk for oversedation from CNS depressants.

Patient education
• Explain rationale for therapy and potential risks and benefits.
• Teach patient signs and symptoms of adverse reactions and need to report them promptly.
• Warn patient not to discontinue drug or change dosage unless prescribed.
• Advise patient to avoid tasks that require mental alertness until degree of sedative effect is determined.

clonidine hydrochloride
Catapres, Catapres-TTS, Dixarit*

Pharmacologic classification: centrally acting alpha-adrenergic agonist
Therapeutic classification: antihypertensive
Pregnancy risk category: C

Indications and dosages
➤**Hypertension.** *Adults:* Initially, 0.1 mg P.O. b.i.d.; then increased by 0.1 to 0.2 mg daily or every few days until desired response is achieved. Usual dose range is 0.2 to 0.6 mg daily in divided doses. Maximum effective dose is 2.4 mg daily. If transdermal patch is used, apply to area of hairless intact skin once q 7 days.
➤**Adjunctive therapy in nicotine withdrawal** ◇. *Adults:* Initially, 0.15 mg P.O. daily, gradually increased to 0.4 mg P.O. daily as tolerated. Or, apply transdermal patch (0.2 mg/24 hours) and replace weekly for the first 2 or 3 weeks after smoking cessation.
➤**Prophylaxis for vascular headache** ◇. *Adults:* 0.025 mg P.O. b.i.d. to q.i.d. up to 0.15 mg P.O. daily in divided doses.
➤**Adjunctive treatment of menopausal symptoms** ◇. *Adults:* 0.025 to 0.075 mg P.O. b.i.d.
➤**Adjunctive therapy in opiate withdrawal** ◇. *Adults:* 5 to 17 mcg/kg P.O. daily in divided doses for up to 10 days. Adjust dosage to avoid hypotension and excessive sedation, and slowly withdraw drug.
➤**Ulcerative colitis** ◇. *Adults:* 0.3 mg P.O. t.i.d.
➤**Neuralgia** ◇. *Adults:* 0.2 mg P.O. daily.
➤**Tourette syndrome** ◇. *Adults:* 0.15 to 0.2 mg P.O. daily.
➤**Diabetic diarrhea** ◇. *Adults:* 0.15 to 1.2 mg P.O. daily or one to two patches weekly (0.3 mg/24 hours).
➤**Growth delay in children** ◇. *Children:* 0.0375 to 0.15 mg/m² P.O. daily.
➤**To diagnose pheochromocytoma** ◇. *Adults:* 0.3 mg given once.

How supplied
Available by prescription only
Tablets: 0.1 mg, 0.2 mg, 0.3 mg
Transdermal: TTS-1 (releases 0.1 mg/24 hours); TTS-2 (releases 0.2 mg/24 hours); TTS-3 (releases 0.3 mg/24 hours)

Pharmacodynamics
Antihypertensive action: Clonidine decreases peripheral vascular resistance by stimulating central alpha-adrenergic receptors, thus decreasing cerebral sympathetic outflow; drug also may inhibit renin release. Initially, clonidine may stimulate peripheral alpha-adrenergic receptors, producing transient vasoconstriction.

Pharmacokinetics
Absorption: Absorbed well from the GI tract when administered orally; absorbed well percutaneously after transdermal topical administration.
Distribution: Distributed widely throughout the body.
Metabolism: Metabolized in the liver, where nearly 50% is transformed to inactive metabolites.
Excretion: About 65% of a given dose is excreted in urine; 20% is excreted in feces. Half-life of clonidine ranges from 6 to 20 hours in patients with normal renal function. After oral administration, the antihypertensive effect lasts up to 8 hours; after transdermal application, the antihypertensive effect persists for up to 7 days.

Route	Onset	Peak	Duration
P.O.	½-1 hr	2-4 hr	12-24 hr
Trans-dermal	2-3 days	2-3 days	7-8 days

Contraindications and precautions
Contraindicated in patients hypersensitive to drug. Transdermal form is contraindicated in patients hypersensitive to any component of the adhesive layer. Use cautiously in patients with severe coronary disease, recent MI, cerebrovascular disease, and impaired hepatic or renal function.

Interactions
Drug-drug. *Barbiturates:* Clonidine may increase CNS depressant effects. Avoid using together.
MAO inhibitors, tolazoline, tricyclic antidepressants: May inhibit antihypertensive effects. Avoid use together.
Propranolol and other beta blockers: May have an additive effect, producing bradycardia. Avoid use together.
Drug-herb. *Capsicum:* May reduce antihypertensive effectiveness. Discourage use together.
Drug-lifestyle. *Alcohol use:* Increases CNS depressant effects. Discourage alcohol use.

Adverse reactions

CNS: *drowsiness, dizziness,* fatigue, *sedation, weakness,* malaise, agitation, depression.
CV: orthostatic hypotension, ***bradycardia, severe rebound hypertension.***
GI: *constipation, dry mouth,* nausea, vomiting, anorexia.
GU: urine retention, impotence.
Metabolic: possible slight increase in serum glucose levels, weight gain.
Skin: *pruritus, dermatitis* (with transdermal patch), rash.
Other: loss of libido.

Overdose and treatment

Signs and symptoms of overdose include bradycardia, CNS depression, respiratory depression, hypothermia, apnea, seizures, lethargy, agitation, irritability, diarrhea, and hypotension; hypertension also has been reported.

Don't induce emesis because rapid onset of CNS depression can lead to aspiration. After adequate airway is assured, empty stomach by gastric lavage followed by administration of activated charcoal. If overdose occurs in patients receiving transdermal therapy, remove transdermal patch. Further treatment is usually symptomatic and supportive.

Special considerations

⚠ ALERT Remove transdermal systems when attempting defibrillation or synchronized cardioversion because of electrical conductivity.
● Clonidine may be used to lower blood pressure quickly in some hypertensive emergencies.
● Don't discontinue abruptly; reduce dosage gradually over 2 to 4 days to prevent severe rebound hypertension.
● Patients with renal impairment may respond to smaller doses of drug.
● Give drug 4 to 6 hours before scheduled surgery.
● Patient may need oral antihypertensive therapy at start of transdermal therapy.
● Clonidine may decrease urinary excretion of vanillylmandelic acid and catecholamines. It may cause a weakly positive Coombs' test.

Patient monitoring

● Monitor pulse and blood pressure frequently; dosage is usually adjusted to patient's response and tolerance.
● Daily weight must be recorded at start of therapy to monitor for fluid retention.

Breast-feeding patients

● Clonidine appears in breast milk. An alternate feeding method is recommended during treatment.

Pediatric patients

● Efficacy and safety in children haven't been established; use drug only if potential benefit outweighs risk.

Geriatric patients

● Geriatric patients may require lower doses because they may be more sensitive to the hypotensive effects of clonidine. Monitor renal function closely.

Patient education

● Explain disease and rationale for therapy; emphasize importance of follow-up visits in establishing therapeutic regimen.
● Teach patient signs and symptoms of adverse effects and need to report them; patient also should report excessive weight gain (more than 2.27 kg [5 lb] weekly).
● Warn patient to avoid hazardous activities that require mental alertness until tolerance develops to CNS effects.
● Advise patient to avoid sudden position changes to minimize orthostatic hypotension.
● Inform patient that ice chips, hard candy, or gum will relieve dry mouth.
● Warn patient to call for specific instructions before taking OTC cold preparations.
● Advise taking last dose at bedtime to ensure night-time blood pressure control.
● Tell patient not to discontinue drug suddenly; rebound hypertension may develop.
● Teach patient to rotate transdermal patch site weekly.

---

clopidogrel bisulfate
Plavix

Pharmacologic classification: inhibitor of adenosine diphosphate (ADP)-induced platelet aggregation
Therapeutic classification: antiplatelet agent
Pregnancy risk category: B

Indications and dosages

▶ ***To reduce atherosclerotic events (MI, CVA, vascular death) in patients with atherosclerosis documented by recent CVA, MI, or peripheral arterial disease.*** *Adults:* 75 mg P.O. once daily with or without food.

How supplied

Available by prescription only
Tablets: 75 mg

Pharmacodynamics

Antiplatelet action: Inhibits the binding of ADP to its platelet receptor and the subsequent ADP-mediated activation of glycoprotein IIb/IIIa complex, thereby inhibiting platelet aggregation. Because clopidogrel acts by irreversibly modifying the platelet ADP receptor, platelets exposed to the drug are affected for their life span.

Pharmacokinetics

Absorption: After repeated oral doses, plasma levels of parent compound, which has no platelet-inhibiting effect, are very low and generally below quantification limit. Pharmacokinetic evaluations are generally stated in terms of the main circulating metabolite. Rapidly absorbed after oral dosing. Following oral administration, about 50% of dose is absorbed.

Distribution: Clopidogrel and main circulating metabolite binds reversibly to human plasma proteins (98% and 94%, respectively).

Metabolism: Extensively metabolized by the liver. Main circulating metabolite is the carboxylic acid derivative that has no effect on platelet aggregation. It represents about 85% of circulating drug. Elimination half-life of main circulating metabolite is 8 hours.

Excretion: Following oral administration, about 50% is excreted in the urine and 46% in feces.

Route	Onset	Peak	Duration
P.O.	2 hr	Unknown	5 days

Contraindications and precautions

Contraindicated in patients with pathologic bleeding, such as peptic ulcer or intracranial hemorrhage, and in those hypersensitive to drug or its components.

Use with caution in patients at risk for increased bleeding from trauma, surgery, or other pathologic conditions and in those with hepatic impairment or severe hepatic disease.

Interactions

Drug-drug. *Aspirin, NSAIDs:* May increase risk for GI bleeding. Use together cautiously.
Heparin, warfarin: Safety hasn't been established. Use together cautiously.
Drug-herb. *Red clover:* May cause increased bleeding. Discourage use together.

Adverse reactions

CNS: asthenia, depression, dizziness, fatigue, headache, paresthesia, syncope, pain.
CV: chest pain, edema, hypertension, palpitations.
EENT: epistaxis, rhinitis.
GI: abdominal pain, constipation, diarrhea, dyspepsia, gastritis, hemorrhage, nausea, vomiting.
GU: urinary tract infection.
Hematologic: purpura.
Musculoskeletal: arthralgia.
Respiratory: bronchitis, cough, dyspnea, upper respiratory tract infection.
Skin: rash, pruritus.
Other: flu symptoms.

Overdose and treatment

No adverse effects were reported after single oral administration of 600 mg (equivalent to eight standard 75-mg tablets). The bleeding time was prolonged by a factor of 1.7, which is similar to that observed with the therapeutic dosage of 75 mg daily.

Based on biological plausibility, platelet transfusion may be appropriate to reverse the pharmacologic effects of clopidogrel if quick reversal is required.

Special considerations

● Drug is usually used in patients who are hypersensitive or intolerant to aspirin.
● If patient is to undergo surgery and an antiplatelet effect isn't desired, drug should be stopped 7 days before surgery.

Patient monitoring

● Monitor patient for unusual bleeding or bruising.

Breast-feeding patients

● It isn't known if drug or its metabolites appear in breast milk. Assess risks and benefits before continuing drug in breast-feeding women.

Pediatric patients

● Safety and efficacy in children haven't been established.

Patient education

● Inform patient that it may take longer than usual to stop bleeding; therefore, advise him to refrain from activities in which trauma and bleeding may occur. Encourage use of seat belts.
● Tell patient to inform prescriber of clopidogrel use before scheduling surgery or taking new drugs.
● Inform patient that drug may be taken without regard to meals.

clorazepate dipotassium
Novo-Clopate*, Tranxene*,
Tranxene-SD, Tranxene-SD Half
Strength

Pharmacologic classification: benzodiazepine
Therapeutic classification: antianxiety agent, anticonvulsant, sedative-hypnotic
Controlled substance schedule: IV
Pregnancy risk category: NR

Indications and dosages

➤ *Acute alcohol withdrawal.* **Adults:** Day 1—initially, 30 mg P.O., followed by 30 to 60 mg P.O. in divided doses; day 2—45 to 90 mg P.O. in divided doses; day 3—22.5 to 45 mg P.O. in divided doses; day 4—15 to 30 mg P.O. in divided doses; gradually reduce daily dose to 7.5 to 15 mg.
➤ *Anxiety.* **Adults:** 15 to 60 mg P.O. daily.
➤ *As an adjunct in treatment of partial seizures.* **Adults and children over age 12:** Maximum recommended initial dose is 7.5 mg P.O. t.i.d. Dosage increases shouldn't exceed 7.5 mg/week. Maximum daily dose shouldn't exceed 90 mg.
Children ages 9 to 12: Maximum recommended initial dose is 7.5 mg P.O. b.i.d. Dosage in-

creases shouldn't exceed 7.5 mg/week. Maximum daily dose shouldn't exceed 60 mg.

How supplied
Available by prescription only
Capsules: 3.75 mg, 7.5 mg, 15 mg
Tablets: 3.75 mg, 7.5 mg, 11.25 mg, 15 mg, 22.5 mg

Pharmacodynamics
Anxiolytic and sedative actions: Clorazepate depresses the CNS at the limbic and subcortical levels of the brain. It produces an antianxiety effect by enhancing the effect of the neurotransmitter gamma-aminobutyric acid (GABA) on its receptor in the ascending reticular activating system, which increases inhibition and blocks both cortical and limbic arousal.
Anticonvulsant action: Drug suppresses spread of seizure activity produced by epileptogenic foci in the cortex, thalamus, and limbic structures by enhancing presynaptic inhibition.

Pharmacokinetics
Absorption: After oral administration, clorazepate is hydrolyzed in the stomach to desmethyldiazepam, which is absorbed completely and rapidly.
Distribution: Distributed widely throughout the body. About 80% to 95% is bound to plasma protein.
Metabolism: Metabolized in the liver to conjugated oxazepam.
Excretion: Inactive glucuronide metabolites are excreted in urine. The half-life of desmethyldiazepam ranges from 30 to 100 hours.

Route	Onset	Peak	Duration
P.O.	Unknown	½-2 hr	Unknown

Contraindications and precautions
Contraindicated in patients hypersensitive to drug or other benzodiazepines and in patients with acute angle-closure glaucoma. Avoid use in pregnant women, especially during the first trimester.

Use cautiously in patients with impaired renal or hepatic function, suicidal tendencies, or history of drug abuse.

Interactions
Drug-drug. *Antidepressants, antihistamines, barbiturates, general anesthetics, MAO inhibitors, narcotics, phenothiazines:* Potentiated CNS depressant effects. Avoid use together.
Cimetidine, disulfiram: Increased clorazepate level. Watch for enhanced benzodiazepine effects, and reduce clorazepate dosage if needed.
Levodopa: Decreased levodopa effectiveness. Use together cautiously.
Drug-lifestyle. *Alcohol use:* Potentiates CNS depressant effects. Discourage alcohol use.
Heavy smoking: Accelerates clorazepate's metabolism, thus lowering clinical effectiveness. Discourage smoking.

Adverse reactions
CNS: *drowsiness,* dizziness, nervousness, confusion, headache, insomnia, depression, irritability, tremor, minor changes in EEG patterns.
CV: hypotension.
EENT: blurred vision, diplopia.
GI: nausea, vomiting, abdominal discomfort, dry mouth.
GU: urine retention, incontinence.
Hepatic: elevated liver function test results.
Skin: rash.

Overdose and treatment
Signs and symptoms of overdose include somnolence, confusion, coma, hypoactive reflexes, dyspnea, labored breathing, hypotension, bradycardia, slurred speech, and unsteady gait or impaired coordination.

Support blood pressure and respiration until drug effects subside; monitor vital signs. Flumazenil, a specific benzodiazepine antagonist, may be useful. Mechanical ventilatory assistance via endotracheal tube may be required to maintain a patent airway and support adequate oxygenation. Treat hypotension with I.V. fluids and vasopressors such as dopamine and phenylephrine, as needed. Induce emesis if patient is conscious. Use gastric lavage if ingestion was recent, but only if an endotracheal tube is present to prevent aspiration. After emesis or lavage, administer activated charcoal with a cathartic as a single dose. Dialysis is of limited value. Don't use barbiturates because they may worsen CNS adverse effects.

Special considerations
Consider the recommendations relevant to all benzodiazepines as well as the following.
• Lower doses are effective in geriatric patients and patients with renal or hepatic dysfunction.
• Store in a cool, dry place away from direct light.

Patient monitoring
• Monitor liver, renal, and hematopoietic function studies periodically in patients receiving repeated or prolonged therapy.

Breast-feeding patients
• The breast-fed infant of a woman who uses clorazepate may become sedated, have feeding difficulties, or lose weight. Avoid use in breast-feeding women.

Pediatric patients
• Safety hasn't been established in children under age 9.

Geriatric patients
• Lower doses are usually effective in geriatric patients because of decreased elimination. Use with caution. Geriatric patients who receive this drug require supervision with walking and activities of daily living at start of therapy or after a dosage increase.

Patient education
- Advise patient of potential for physical and psychological dependence with long-term use of clorazepate.
- Instruct patient not to alter drug regimen without medical approval.
- Warn patient that sudden position changes may cause dizziness. Advise patient to dangle legs for a few minutes before getting out of bed to prevent falls and injury.
- Advise patient to take antacids 1 hour before or after clorazepate.
- Inform patient not to suddenly stop taking drug.

clotrimazole
FemCare, Gyne-Lotrimin, Lotrimin, Lotrimin AF, Mycelex, Mycelex-G, Mycelex OTC, Mycelex-7

Pharmacologic classification: synthetic imidazole derivative
Therapeutic classification: topical antifungal
Pregnancy risk category: B (C, oral form)

Indications and dosages
➤ *Tinea pedis, tinea cruris, tinea versicolor, tinea corporis, cutaneous candidiasis.* *Adults and children:* Apply thin layer and massage into cleansed affected and surrounding area, morning and evening, for prescribed period (usually 1 to 4 weeks; however, therapy may take up to 8 weeks).
➤ *Vulvovaginal candidiasis.* *Adults:* Insert one tablet intravaginally h.s. for 7 consecutive days. If vaginal cream is used, insert one applicatorful intravaginally, h.s. for 7 to 14 consecutive days.
➤ *Treatment of oropharyngeal candidiasis.* *Adults and children:* Usual dosage is one lozenge P.O. five times daily for 14 consecutive days.
➤ *Prophylaxis of oropharyngeal candidiasis in immunocompromised patients.* *Adults:* One lozenge t.i.d. for duration of chemotherapy.
➤ *Keratitis ◇.* *Adults:* 1% ointment in sterile peanut oil q 2 to 4 hours for up to 6 weeks.

How supplied
Available by prescription only
Oral lozenges: 10 mg
Topical cream: 1%
Topical lotion: 1%
Topical solution: 1%
Vaginal tablets: 100 mg, 200 mg, 500 mg
Available without a prescription
Combination pack: Vaginal tablets 500 mg/topical cream 1% 7 g
Vaginal cream: 1%
Vaginal tablets: 100 mg

Pharmacodynamics
Antifungal action: Clotrimazole alters cell membrane permeability by binding with phospholipids in the fungal cell membrane. Clotrimazole inhibits or kills many fungi, including yeast and dermatophytes, and also is active against various species of gram-positive bacteria.

Pharmacokinetics
Absorption: Absorption is limited with topical administration. Absorption following dissolution of a lozenge in the mouth not determined.
Distribution: Distributed minimally with local application.
Metabolism: Unknown.
Excretion: Unknown.

Route	Onset	Peak	Duration
P.O.	Unknown	Unknown	3 hr
Topical, intra-vaginal	Unknown	Unknown	Unknown

Contraindications and precautions
Contraindicated in patients hypersensitive to drug. Also contraindicated for ophthalmic use.

Interactions
None reported.

Adverse reactions
GI: nausea, vomiting, unpleasant mouth sensation (with lozenges); lower abdominal cramps.
GU: *mild vaginal burning or irritation* (with vaginal use), cramping, urinary frequency.
Hepatic: abnormal liver function test results.
Skin: blistering, *erythema,* edema, pruritus, burning, stinging, peeling, urticaria, skin fissures, general irritation.

Overdose and treatment
No information available.

Special considerations
- Improvement usually occurs within 1 week; if no improvement occurs in 4 weeks, review diagnosis.

Patient monitoring
- Patients given clotrimazole oral lozenges, especially those who have liver dysfunction, should have periodic liver function tests.

Pregnant patients
- Use lozenges only when potential benefits outweigh the risks.

Breast-feeding patients
- It's unknown if drug appears in breast milk. Use cautiously in breast-feeding women.

Pediatric patients
- Drug isn't recommended for use in children under age 3.

Patient education
● Advise patient that lozenges must dissolve slowly (15 to 30 minutes) in the mouth to achieve maximum effect. Tell patient not to chew lozenges.
● Instruct patients using intravaginal application to insert drug high into the vagina and to refrain from sexual contact during treatment period to avoid reinfection. Also tell patient to use a sanitary napkin to prevent staining of clothing and to absorb discharge.
● Tell patient to complete the full course of therapy. Improvement usually will be noted within 1 week. Patient should call if no improvement occurs in 4 weeks or if condition worsens.
● Advise patient to watch for and report irritation or sensitivity and, if this occurs, to discontinue use.

cloxacillin sodium
Tegopen

Pharmacologic classification: penicillinase-resistant penicillin
Therapeutic classification: antibiotic
Pregnancy risk category: B

Indications and dosages
➤ *Systemic infections by penicillinase-producing staphylococci organisms. Adults:* 250 to 500 mg P.O. q 6 hours.
Children: 50 to 100 mg/kg P.O. daily, divided into doses given q 6 hours.

How supplied
Available by prescription only
Capsules: 250 mg, 500 mg
Oral solution: 125 mg/5 ml (after reconstitution)

Pharmacodynamics
Antibiotic action: Cloxacillin is bactericidal; it adheres to bacterial penicillin-binding proteins, thereby inhibiting bacterial cell wall synthesis. Cloxacillin resists the effects of penicillinases—enzymes that inactivate penicillin—and therefore is active against many strains of penicillinase-producing bacteria; this activity is most pronounced against penicillinase-producing staphylococci; some strains may remain resistant. Cloxacillin is also active against gram-positive aerobic and anaerobic bacilli but has no significant effect on gram-negative bacilli.

Pharmacokinetics
Absorption: Absorbed rapidly but incompletely (37% to 60%) from the GI tract; it's relatively acid stable. Food may decrease both rate and extent of absorption.
Distribution: Distributed widely. CSF penetration is poor but enhanced by meningeal inflammation. Cloxacillin crosses the placenta and is 90% to 96% protein-bound.
Metabolism: Only partially metabolized.

Excretion: Excreted in urine by renal tubular secretion and glomerular filtration; also excreted in breast milk. Elimination half-life in adults is ½ to 1 hour, extended to 2½ hours in patients with renal impairment.

Route	Onset	Peak	Duration
P.O.	Unknown	2 hr	6 hr

Contraindications and precautions
Contraindicated in patients hypersensitive to drug or other penicillins.

Interactions
Drug-drug. *Aminoglycosides:* Synergistic bactericidal effects against *Staphylococcus aureus.* However, the drugs are physically and chemically incompatible and are inactivated when mixed or given together. Avoid use together.
Probenecid: Increases serum cloxacillin levels. Probenecid may be used for this purpose.
Drug-food. *Foods:* Decreased drug absorption. Advise taking drug on an empty stomach.
Fruit juices and carbonated beverages: May inactivate drug. Discourage use together.

Adverse reactions
CNS: lethargy, hallucinations, *seizures,* anxiety, confusion, agitation, depression, dizziness, fatigue.
GI: *nausea,* vomiting, *epigastric distress, diarrhea,* enterocolitis, pseudomembranous colitis, black "hairy" tongue, abdominal pain.
GU: interstitial nephritis, nephropathy.
Hematologic: eosinophilia, anemia, *thrombocytopenia, leukopenia,* hemolytic anemia, *agranulocytosis.*
Hepatic: intrahepatic cholestasis, transient elevations in liver function test results.
Other: *hypersensitivity reactions* (rash, urticaria, chills, fever, sneezing, wheezing, *anaphylaxis*), overgrowth of nonsusceptible organisms.

Overdose and treatment
Overdose may cause neuromuscular irritability or seizures. No specific recommendation is available. Treatment is symptomatic. After recent ingestion (within 4 hours), empty the stomach by induced emesis or gastric lavage; follow with activated charcoal to reduce absorption. Cloxacillin isn't appreciably removed by hemodialysis or peritoneal dialysis.

Special considerations
Consider the recommendations relevant to all penicillins as well as the following.
● Give dose on empty stomach with water.
● Refrigerate oral suspension and discard unused medication after 14 days. Unrefrigerated suspension is stable for 3 days.
● Cloxacillin alters test results for urine and serum proteins; it produces false-positive or elevated results in turbidimetric urine and serum protein tests using sulfosalicylic acid or trichloroacetic

---

acid; it also may produce false results on the Bradshaw screening test for Bence Jones protein.
• Cloxacillin may falsely decrease serum aminoglycoside levels.

Patient monitoring
• Periodically assess renal, hepatic, and hematopoietic function in patients receiving long-term therapy.

Breast-feeding patients
• Drug appears in breast milk; use cautiously in breast-feeding women.

Pediatric patients
• Elimination of cloxacillin is reduced in neonates; safety of drug in neonates hasn't been established.

Patient education
• Inform patient of potential adverse reactions (such as fever, chills, or rash); advise him to report adverse reactions promptly.
• Instruct patient to take drug on an empty stomach and take with water only.
• Tell patient to refrigerate oral suspension and to discard unused suspension after the course of treatment.

clozapine
Clozaril

Pharmacologic classification: tricyclic dibenzodiazepine derivative
Therapeutic classification: antipsychotic
Pregnancy risk category: B

Indications and dosages
➤ *Treatment of schizophrenia in severely ill patients unresponsive to other therapies.* *Adults:* Initially, 12.5 mg P.O. once or twice daily, adjusted upward at 25 to 50 mg daily (if tolerated) to a daily dose of 300 to 450 mg by end of 2 weeks. Individual dosage is based on clinical response, patient tolerance, and adverse reactions. Subsequent dosage increases should occur no more than once or twice weekly and shouldn't exceed 100 mg. Many patients respond to doses of 300 to 600 mg daily, but some patients require as much as 900 mg daily. Don't exceed 900 mg daily.

How supplied
Available by prescription only
Tablets: 25 mg, 100 mg

Pharmacodynamics
Antipsychotic action: Clozapine binds to dopamine receptors (D-1, D-2, D-3, D-4, and D-5) within the limbic system of the CNS. It also may interfere with adrenergic, cholinergic, histaminergic, and serotoninergic receptors.

Pharmacokinetics
Absorption: Food doesn't appear to interfere with bioavailability. Only 27% to 50% of the dose reaches systemic circulation.
Distribution: About 95% bound to serum proteins.
Metabolism: Metabolism is nearly complete; very little unchanged drug appears in the urine.
Excretion: About 50% appears in the urine and 30% in the feces, mostly as metabolites. Elimination half-life appears to be proportional to dose and may range from 4 to 66 hours.

Route	Onset	Peak	Duration
P.O.	Unknown	2½ hr	4-12 hr

Contraindications and precautions
Contraindicated in patients with uncontrolled epilepsy or history of clozapine-induced agranulocytosis; in patients with a WBC count below 3,500/mm³; in patients with severe CNS depression or coma; in patients taking other drugs that suppress bone marrow function; and in those with myelosuppressive disorders.

Use cautiously in patients with renal, hepatic, or cardiac disease, prostatic hyperplasia, or angle-closure glaucoma and in those receiving general anesthesia.

Use cautiously with other drugs metabolized by cytochrome P-450 2D6, including antidepressants, phenothiazines, carbamazepine, and type IC antiarrhythmics (propafenone, flecainide, encainide) or drugs that inhibit this enzyme, such as quinidine.

Interactions
Drug-drug. *Anticholinergics:* May potentiate anticholinergic effects of clozapine. Avoid use together.
Antihypertensives: May potentiate hypotensive effects. Check blood pressure frequently.
Benzodiazepines: Risk of respiratory arrest and severe hypotension. Avoid use together.
Bone marrow suppressants: Increased bone marrow toxicity. Use together cautiously.
CNS-active drugs: Potential for additive effects. Use together cautiously.
Digoxin, highly protein-bound drugs, warfarin: Increased levels of these drugs. Monitor patient closely for adverse reactions.
Phenytoin: Decreased phenytoin levels. May lower the seizure threshold; avoid use together.
Drug-herb. *Nutmeg:* May reduce effectiveness of drug. Discourage use together.
Drug-food. *Caffeine-containing beverages:* May inhibit antipsychotic effects of clozapine. Monitor patient closely.
Drug-lifestyle. *Alcohol use:* Increased CNS depression. Advise patient to avoid alcohol.
Smoking: May reduce plasma clozapine levels. Discourage smoking.

Reactions may be *common*, uncommon, *life-threatening*, or COMMON AND LIFE-THREATENING.

Adverse reactions

CNS: *drowsiness, sedation, seizures,* dizziness, syncope, vertigo, headache, tremor, disturbed sleep or nightmares, restlessness, hypokinesia or akinesia, agitation, rigidity, akathisia, confusion, fatigue, insomnia, hyperkinesia, weakness, lethargy, ataxia, slurred speech, depression, myoclonus, anxiety, neuroleptic malignant syndrome.
CV: *tachycardia, hypotension,* hypertension, chest pain, ECG changes, orthostatic hypotension.
EENT: visual disturbances.
GI: *dry mouth,* nausea, vomiting, *excessive salivation,* heartburn, constipation, diarrhea.
GU: urinary abnormalities (urinary frequency or urgency, urine retention), incontinence, abnormal ejaculation.
Hematologic: *leukopenia, agranulocytosis,* eosinophilia, *neutropenia, thrombocytopenia.*
Metabolic: weight gain.
Musculoskeletal: muscle pain or spasm, muscle weakness.
Skin: rash, diaphoresis.
Other: fever.
After abrupt withdrawal of long-term therapy: Possible abrupt recurrence of psychotic symptoms. Monitor patient closely.

Overdose and treatment

Fatalities have occurred at doses exceeding 2.5 g. Symptoms include drowsiness, delirium, coma, hypotension, hypersalivation, tachycardia, respiratory depression, and, rarely, seizures.

Treat symptomatically. Establish an airway and ensure adequate ventilation. Gastric lavage with activated charcoal and sorbitol may be effective. Monitor vital signs. Avoid epinephrine (and derivatives), quinidine, and procainamide when treating hypotension and arrhythmias.

Special considerations

• When discontinuing clozapine therapy, drug must be withdrawn gradually (over a 1- to 2-week period). However, changes in the patient's clinical status (including the development of leukopenia) may require abrupt discontinuation of the drug. If so, monitor patient closely for recurrence of psychotic symptoms.
• To reinstate therapy in patients withdrawn from drug, follow usual guidelines for dosage buildup. However, re-exposure of the patient may increase the risk and severity of adverse reactions. If therapy was terminated for WBC counts of less than 2,000/mm³ or granulocyte counts of less than 1,000/mm³, drug shouldn't be reinstated.

Patient monitoring

• Obtain baseline CBC before starting therapy. Don't start drug if WBC count is lower than 3,500/mm³.
• Monitor CBC weekly during treatment, and for at least 4 weeks after drug is discontinued.

• Periodically assess patient for abnormal body movement.
• Some patients experience transient fevers (temperature of more than 100.4° F [38° C]), especially in the first 3 weeks of therapy. Monitor patient closely.

Breast-feeding patients

• Animal studies have shown that drug appears in breast milk. Women taking clozapine shouldn't breast-feed.

Pediatric patients

• Safety in children hasn't been established.

Geriatric patients

• Geriatric patients may require reduced dosages, because they may be more sensitive to adverse reactions, especially orthostatic hypotension, dry mouth, and constipation. Monitor these patients closely.

Patient education

• Warn patient about risk of developing agranulocytosis. Safe use of drug requires blood tests weekly during treatment.
• Advise patient to promptly report flulike symptoms, fever, sore throat, lethargy, malaise, or other signs of infection.
• Advise patient to call before taking OTC drugs or alcohol.
• Tell patient that ice chips or sugarless candy or gum may relieve dry mouth.
• Warn patient to rise slowly to upright position to avoid orthostatic hypotension.

codeine phosphate
codeine sulfate

Pharmacologic classification: opioid
Therapeutic classification: analgesic, antitussive
Controlled substance schedule: II
Pregnancy risk category: C

Indications and dosages

▶*Mild to moderate pain. Adults:* 15 to 60 mg P.O. or 15 to 60 mg (phosphate) S.C. or I.M. q 4 to 6 hours, p.r.n., or around-the-clock. *Children:* 0.5 mg/kg (or 15 mg/m²) P.O. q 4 to 6 hours, or 0.5 mg/kg (or 15 mg/m²) (phosphate) S.C. or I.M. q 4 to 6 hours.
▶*Nonproductive cough. Adults and children age 12 and older:* 10 to 20 mg P.O. q 4 to 6 hours. Maximum dose is 120 mg/24 hours. *Children ages 6 to 11:* 5 to 10 mg P.O. q 4 to 6 hours, not to exceed 60 mg daily. *Children ages 2 to 6:* 1 mg/kg P.O. daily divided into four equal doses, administered q 4 to 6 hours, not to exceed 30 mg in 24 hours.

How supplied
Available by prescription only
Injection: 15 mg/ml, 30 mg/ml, 60 mg/ml
codeine phosphate
Oral solution: 15 mg/5 ml codeine phosphate
Tablets: 15 mg, 30 mg, 60 mg; 30 mg, 60 mg
(soluble)

Pharmacodynamics
Analgesic action: Codeine (methylmorphine)
has analgesic properties that result from its agonist activity at the opiate receptors.
Antitussive action: Codeine has a direct suppressant action on the cough reflex center.

Pharmacokinetics
Absorption: Well absorbed after oral or parenteral administration. It's about two-thirds as
potent orally as parenterally.
Distribution: Distributed widely throughout the
body; it crosses the placenta and enters breast
milk.
Metabolism: Metabolized mainly in the liver, by
demethylation or by conjugation with glucuronic acid.
Excretion: Excreted mainly in the urine as nor-
codeine and free and conjugated morphine.

Route	Onset	Peak	Duration
P.O.	½-¾ hr	1-2 hr	4-6 hr
I.V.	Immediate	Immediate	4-6 hr
I.M.	10-30 min	½-1 hr	4-6 hr
S.C.	10-30 min	Unknown	4-6 hr

Contraindications and precautions
Contraindicated in patients hypersensitive to drug.
Use cautiously in geriatric or debilitated patients
and in patients with impaired renal or hepatic
function, head injuries, increased intracranial
pressure, increased CSF pressure, hypothyroidism,
Addison's disease, acute alcoholism, CNS depression, bronchial asthma, COPD, respiratory
depression, or shock.

Interactions
Drug-drug. *Anticholinergics:* Concurrent use
may cause paralytic ileus. Monitor patient closely.
*Antihistamines, barbiturates, benzodiazepines,
CNS depressants, general anesthetics, MAO inhibitors, muscle relaxants, narcotic analgesics,
phenothiazines, sedative-hypnotics, tricyclic
antidepressants:* Potentiate drug's respiratory
and CNS depression, sedation, and hypotensive
effects. Use together with extreme caution.
Cimetidine: Increases respiratory and CNS depression. Avoid using together.
Digitoxin, phenytoin, rifampin: Drug accumulation and enhanced effects may result. Monitor patient closely.
Drug-lifestyle. *Alcohol use:* Potentiates respiratory and CNS depression, sedation, and hypotensive effects of drug. Discourage alcohol use.

Adverse reactions
CNS: *sedation, clouded sensorium, euphoria,
dizziness, light-headedness.*
CV: *hypotension,* flushing, **bradycardia.**
GI: *nausea, vomiting, constipation, dry mouth,*
ileus, increased plasma amylase and lipase levels.
GU: *urine retention.*
Respiratory: *respiratory depression.*
Skin: pruritus, *diaphoresis.*
Other: physical dependence.

Overdose and treatment
The most common signs and symptoms of overdose are CNS depression, respiratory depression,
and miosis (pinpoint pupils). Other acute toxic
effects include hypotension, bradycardia, hypothermia, shock, apnea, cardiopulmonary arrest, circulatory collapse, pulmonary edema, and
seizures.

To treat acute overdose, first establish adequate respiratory exchange via a patent airway
and ventilation as needed; administer narcotic
antagonist (naloxone) to reverse respiratory depression. (Because the duration of action of
codeine is longer than that of naloxone, repeated naloxone dosing is necessary.) Naloxone
shouldn't be given unless the patient has clinically significant respiratory or CV depression.
Monitor vital signs closely.

If patient shows signs and symptoms within 2
hours of ingestion of an oral overdose, empty the
stomach immediately by inducing emesis with
ipecac syrup or using gastric lavage. Use caution
to avoid risk of aspiration. Administer activated
charcoal via nasogastric tube for further removal
of drug in an oral overdose.

Provide symptomatic and supportive treatment (continued respiratory support, correction
of fluid or electrolyte imbalance). Monitor laboratory parameters, vital signs, and neurologic
status closely.

Special considerations
Consider the recommendations relevant to all
opioids as well as the following.
⚠ ALERT Don't mix with other solutions because codeine phosphate is incompatible with
many drugs.
● Codeine and aspirin have additive analgesic effects. Give together for maximum pain relief.
● Codeine has a much lower abuse potential than
morphine.
● Patients who become physically dependent on
drug may experience acute withdrawal syndrome
if given a narcotic antagonist.
● Drug may delay gastric emptying, increase biliary tract pressure resulting from contraction of
the sphincter of Oddi, and may interfere with
hepatobiliary imaging studies.

Patient monitoring
● Monitor cough type and frequency.
● Monitor respiratory and circulatory status.

Reactions may be *common*, uncommon, *life-threatening*, or COMMON AND LIFE-THREATENING.

Breast-feeding patients
• Drug appears in breast milk; assess risk-to-benefit ratio before administering.

Pediatric patients
• Administer cautiously to children. Codeine-containing cough preparations may be hazardous in young children. Use a calibrated measuring device and don't exceed the recommended daily dose.

Geriatric patients
• Lower doses are usually indicated for geriatric patients, who may be more sensitive to the therapeutic and adverse effects of drug.

Patient education
• Inform patient that codeine may cause drowsiness, dizziness, or blurred vision; tell him to use caution while driving or performing tasks that require mental alertness.
• Instruct patient to ask for or to take drug before pain is intense.
• Advise patient that GI distress from oral medication can be lessened when drug is taken with milk.

colchicine

Pharmacologic classification: colchicum autumnale alkaloid
Therapeutic classification: antigout
Pregnancy risk category: C (oral), D (parenteral)

Indications and dosages
➤ **To prevent acute attacks of gout as prophylactic or maintenance therapy.** *Adults:* 0.5 or 0.6 mg P.O. one to four times weekly.
➤ **To prevent attacks of gout in patients undergoing surgery.** *Adults:* 0.5 to 0.6 mg P.O. t.i.d. 3 days before and 3 days after surgery.
➤ **Acute gout, acute gouty arthritis.** *Adults:* Initially, 0.5 to 1.2 mg P.O., followed by 0.5 to 1.2 mg P.O. q 1 to 2 hours; total daily dose is usually 4 to 8 mg P.O.; give until pain is relieved or until nausea, vomiting, or diarrhea ensues. Or, 2 mg I.V. followed by 0.5 mg I.V. q 6 hours if necessary. Total I.V. dose over 24 hours (one course of treatment) not to exceed 4 mg.
➤ **Familial Mediterranean fever** ◇. *Adults:* 1 to 2 mg P.O. daily in divided doses.
➤ **Amyloidosis suppressant** ◇. *Adults:* 500 to 600 mcg P.O. once daily to b.i.d.
➤ **Dermatitis herpetiformis suppressant** ◇. *Adults:* 600 mcg P.O. b.i.d. or t.i.d.
➤ **Hepatic cirrhosis** ◇. *Adults:* 1 mg P.O. 5 days weekly.
➤ **Primary biliary cirrhosis** ◇. *Adults:* 0.6 mg b.i.d.

How supplied
Available by prescription only
Injection: 0.5 mg/ml
Tablets: 0.5 mg, 0.6 mg

Pharmacodynamics
Antigout action: Colchicine's exact mechanism of action is unknown, but it's involved in leukocyte migration inhibition; reduction of lactic acid production by leukocytes, resulting in decreased deposits of uric acid; and interference with kinin formation.
Anti-inflammatory action: Colchicine reduces the inflammatory response to deposited uric acid crystals and diminishes phagocytosis.

Pharmacokinetics
Absorption: When administered P.O., rapidly absorbed from the GI tract. Unchanged drug may be reabsorbed from the intestine by biliary processes.
Distribution: Distributed rapidly into various tissues after reabsorption from the intestine. It's concentrated in leukocytes and distributed into the kidneys, liver, spleen, and intestinal tract, but is absent in the heart, skeletal muscle, and brain.
Metabolism: Metabolized partially in the liver and also slowly metabolized in other tissues.
Excretion: Excreted primarily in the feces, with lesser amounts excreted in urine.

Route	Onset	Peak	Duration
P.O.	Unknown	Unknown	Unknown
I.V.	6-12 hr	Unknown	Unknown

Contraindications and precautions
Contraindicated in patients hypersensitive to drug and in those with blood dyscrasias or serious CV, renal, or GI disease. Use cautiously in geriatric or debilitated patients and in those with early signs of CV, renal, or GI disease.

Interactions
Drug-drug. *Erythromycin:* Increased serum colchicine levels. May need to reduce colchicine dosage.
Loop diuretics: May decrease efficacy of colchicine prophylaxis. Avoid use together.
Phenylbutazone: May increase risk of leukopenia or thrombocytopenia. Avoid use together.
Vitamin B: Impaired absorption. Avoid use together.
Drug-lifestyle. *Alcohol use:* May inhibit drug action. Discourage alcohol use.

Adverse reactions
CNS: peripheral neuritis.
GI: *nausea, vomiting, abdominal pain, diarrhea.*
GU: reversible azoospermia.
Hematologic: *aplastic anemia, thrombocytopenia, and agranulocytosis* (with long-term use); nonthrombocytopenic purpura.

◇ Unlabeled clinical use

Hepatic: increased alkaline phosphatase, AST, and ALT levels.
Skin: alopecia, urticaria, dermatitis.
Other: severe local irritation if extravasation occurs, myopathy, *hypersensitivity reactions.*

Overdose and treatment

Signs and symptoms of overdose include nausea, vomiting, abdominal pain, and diarrhea. Diarrhea may be severe and bloody from hemorrhagic gastroenteritis. Burning sensations in the throat, stomach, and skin also may occur. Extensive vascular damage may result in shock, hematuria, and oliguria, indicating kidney damage. Patient develops severe dehydration, hypotension, and muscle weakness with an ascending paralysis of the CNS. Patient usually remains conscious, but delirium and convulsions may occur. Death may result from respiratory depression.

There's no known antidote. Treatment begins with gastric lavage and preventive measures for shock. Recent studies support the use of hemodialysis and peritoneal dialysis; atropine and morphine may relieve abdominal pain; paregoric usually is administered to control diarrhea and cramps. Respiratory assistance may be needed.

Special considerations

- To avoid cumulative toxicity, a course of oral colchicine shouldn't be repeated for at least 3 days; a course of I.V. colchicine shouldn't be repeated for several weeks.
- Don't administer I.M. or S.C.; severe local irritation occurs.
- Give colchicine by slow I.V. push over 2 to 5 minutes by direct I.V. injection or into tubing of a free-flowing I.V. with compatible I.V. fluid. Avoid extravasation. Don't dilute colchicine injection with bacteriostatic normal saline solution, D_5W, or any other fluid that might change pH of colchicine solution. If lower concentration of colchicine injection is needed, dilute with sterile water or normal saline solution. However, if diluted solution becomes turbid, don't inject.
- Drug must be discontinued if weakness, anorexia, nausea, vomiting, or diarrhea occurs. First sign of acute overdose may be GI symptoms, followed by vascular damage, muscle weakness, and ascending paralysis. Delirium and convulsions may occur without loss of consciousness.
- Store drug in a tightly closed, light-resistant container, away from moisture and heat.
- Colchicine may cause false-positive results of urine tests for RBCs or hemoglobin.

Patient monitoring

- Obtain baseline laboratory studies, including CBC, before starting therapy and periodically thereafter.

Breast-feeding patients

- Safety hasn't been established in breast-feeding women. It isn't known if drug appears in breast milk.

Pediatric patients

- Safety and efficacy in children haven't been established.

Geriatric patients

- Administer with caution to geriatric or debilitated patients, especially those with renal, GI, or heart disease or hematologic disorders. Reduce dosage if weakness, anorexia, nausea, vomiting, or diarrhea occurs.

Patient education

- Advise patient to report rash, sore throat, fever, unusual bleeding, bruising, tiredness, weakness, numbness, or tingling.
- Tell patient to discontinue drug as soon as gout pain is relieved or at the first sign of nausea, vomiting, stomach pain, or diarrhea, and to report persistent symptoms.

colesevelam hydrochloride
Welchol

Pharmacologic classification: polymeric bile acid sequestrant
Therapeutic classification: antilipemic
Pregnancy risk category: B

Indications and dosages

➤ *Adjunct to diet and exercise, either alone or with an HMG-CoA reductase inhibitor, for the reduction of elevated low-density lipoprotein (LDL) cholesterol in patients with primary hypercholesterolemia (Frederickson Type IIa).* Adults: Three tablets (1,875 mg) P.O. twice daily with meals and liquid or six tablets (3,750 mg) once daily with a meal and liquid. Daily dosage can be increased to seven tablets (4,375 mg) for added effect.

How supplied

Available by prescription only
Tablets: 625 mg

Pharmacodynamics

Colesevelam binds bile acids in the intestinal tract, impeding their absorption and causing their elimination in feces. In response to this bile acid depletion, serum LDL levels decrease as the liver uses LDL cholesterol to replenish reduced bile acid stores.

Pharmacokinetics

Absorption: Not absorbed.
Distribution: None.
Metabolism: None.
Excretion: Colesevelam is excreted in feces as a complex bound to bile acids.

Route	Onset	Peak	Duration
P.O.	Unknown	2 wk	Unknown

Adverse reactions

CNS: headache, pain, asthenia.
EENT: pharyngitis, rhinitis, sinusitis.
GI: abdominal pain, *constipation*, diarrhea, dyspepsia, *flatulence,* nausea.
Musculoskeletal: myalgia, back pain.
Respiratory: increased cough.
Other: accidental injury, *infection,* flu syndrome.

Interactions

None reported.

Overdose and treatment

The risk of systemic toxicity is low because drug isn't systemically absorbed. Doses as high as 4.5 g daily have been well tolerated. There's no experience with higher doses.

Contraindications and precautions

Colesevelam is contraindicated in patients hypersensitive to any of its components and in patients with bowel obstruction. Use cautiously in patients susceptible to vitamin K deficiency and in patients with dysphagia, swallowing disorders, severe GI motility disorders, major GI tract surgery, or deficiencies of fat soluble vitamins. Also use cautiously in patients with serum triglyceride levels above 300 mg/dl.

Special considerations

• Rule out secondary causes of hypercholesterolemia before starting drug, such as poorly controlled diabetes, hypothyroidism, nephrotic syndrome, dysproteinemias, obstructive liver disease, other drug therapy, and alcoholism.
• Give drug with a meal and a liquid.
• Store tablets at room temperature and protect them from moisture.

Patient monitoring

• Monitor patient's bowel habits. If severe constipation develops, decrease dosage, add a stool softener, or discontinue drug.
• Monitor the effects of concurrent drug therapy to identify possible drug interactions.
• Monitor total cholesterol, LDL, and triglyceride levels periodically during therapy.

Breast-feeding patients

• Use only when clearly necessary because there are no studies in breast-feeding women.

Pediatric patients

• Safety and efficacy haven't been established.

Patient education

• Instruct patient to take drug with a meal and a liquid.
• Teach patient to monitor bowel habits. Encourage a diet high in fiber and fluids. Instruct patient to notify prescriber promptly if severe constipation develops.
• Encourage patient to follow prescribed diet, exercise, and monitoring of serum lipid levels.

• Tell patient to notify prescriber if she is pregnant or breast-feeding.

colestipol hydrochloride
Colestid

Pharmacologic classification: anion exchange resin
Therapeutic classification: antilipemic
Pregnancy risk category: C

Indications and dosages

➤ **Primary hypercholesterolemia and xanthomas. Tablets.** *Adults:* Initially, 2 g P.O. once daily or b.i.d., then increase in 2-g increments at 1- to 2-month intervals. Usual dosage is 2 to 16 g P.O. daily given as a single dose or in divided doses.
Granules
Initially, 5 g P.O. once daily or b.i.d.; then increase in 5-g increments at 1- to 2-month intervals. Usual dosage is 5 to 30 g P.O. daily given as a single dose or in divided doses.
Children: 10 to 20 g or 500 mg/kg P.O. daily in two to four divided doses (lower doses of 125 to 250 mg/kg have been used when serum cholesterol levels were 15% to 20% above normal after only dietary management).
➤ **Digitoxin overdose**◇. *Adults:* Initially, 10 g P.O. followed by 5 g P.O. q 6 to 8 hours.

How supplied

Available by prescription only
Granules for oral suspension: 5 g/packet, 300 g and 500 g multidose with calibrated scoop
Tablets: 1 g

Pharmacodynamics

Antilipemic action: Bile is normally excreted into the intestine to facilitate absorption of fat and other lipid materials. Colestipol binds with bile acid, forming an insoluble compound that is excreted in feces. With less bile available in the digestive system, less fat and lipid materials in food are absorbed, more cholesterol is used by the liver to replace its supply of bile acids, and the serum cholesterol level decreases.

Pharmacokinetics

Absorption: Not absorbed. Cholesterol levels may decrease in 24 to 48 hours, with peak effect occurring at 1 month. In some patients, the initial decrease is followed by a return to baseline cholesterol levels (or higher) on continued therapy.
Distribution: None.
Metabolism: None.
Excretion: Excreted in feces; cholesterol levels return to baseline within 1 month after therapy stops.

Route	Onset	Peak	Duration
P.O.	Unknown	Unknown	Unknown

Contraindications and precautions

Contraindicated in patients hypersensitive to bile-acid sequestering resins. Use cautiously in patients prone to constipation and in those with conditions aggravated by constipation, such as symptomatic coronary artery disease.

Interactions

Drug-drug. *Cardiac glycosides, chenodiol, digitoxin, digoxin, penicillin G, tetracycline, thiazide diuretics:* Colestipol impairs absorption, thus decreasing their therapeutic effect. Other drugs should be given 1 hour before or 4 hours after colestipol.

Oral drugs: May require adjustment to compensate for possible binding with colestipol; readjustment also must be made when colestipol is withdrawn to prevent high-dose toxicity.

Adverse reactions

CNS: headache, dizziness, anxiety, vertigo, insomnia, fatigue, syncope.
EENT: tinnitus.
GI: constipation, *fecal impaction,* hemorrhoids, abdominal discomfort, flatulence, nausea, vomiting, steatorrhea, *GI bleeding,* diarrhea, anorexia, difficulty swallowing, transient esophageal obstruction, irritation of tongue.
GU: dysuria, hematuria.
Hematologic: anemia, ecchymoses, bleeding tendencies.
Hepatic: altered serum levels of alkaline phosphatase, ALT, AST.
Metabolic: altered serum levels of chloride, phosphorus, potassium, and sodium; hyperchloremic acidosis with long-term use or high dosage.
Musculoskeletal: backache, muscle and joint pain, osteoporosis.
Skin: rash, irritation of perianal area.
Other: vitamin A, D, E, and K deficiencies from decreased absorption.

Overdose and treatment

Overdose of colestipol hasn't been reported. Chief potential risk is intestinal obstruction; treatment would depend on location and degree of obstruction and on amount of gut motility.

Special considerations

● To mix, sprinkle granules on surface of preferred beverage or wet food, let stand a few minutes, and stir to obtain uniform suspension; avoid excess foaming by using large glass and mixing slowly. Use at least 90 ml of water or other fluid, soups, milk, or pulpy fruit; rinse container and have patient drink this to be sure he ingests entire dose. Tablets should be swallowed whole.
● Drug effects are most successful if used with a diet and exercise program.

Patient monitoring

● Monitor levels of cardiac glycosides and other drugs to ensure appropriate dosage during and after therapy with colestipol.
● Serum cholesterol levels must be checked frequently during first few months of therapy and periodically thereafter.
● Bowel habits must be monitored; constipation must be treated promptly by decreasing dosage, increasing fluid intake, adding a stool softener, or discontinuing drug.
● Observe patient for signs of vitamin A, D, or K deficiency.

Breast-feeding patients

● Safety in breast-feeding women hasn't been established.

Pediatric patients

● Safety in children hasn't been established. Drug isn't usually recommended; however, it's been used in a limited number of children with hypercholesterolemia.

Geriatric patients

● Geriatric patients are more likely to experience adverse GI effects, as well as adverse nutritional effects.

Patient education

● Explain disease process and rationale for therapy and encourage patient to comply with continued blood testing and special diet; although therapy isn't curative, it helps control serum cholesterol levels.
● Teach patient how to administer drug. To enhance palatability, tell patient to mix and refrigerate the next daily dose the previous evening.

corticotropin (adrenocorticotropic hormone, ACTH)

ACTH, Acthar, H.P. Acthar Gel

Pharmacologic classification: anterior pituitary hormone
Therapeutic classification: diagnostic aid, replacement hormone, multiple sclerosis, and nonsuppurative thyroiditis treatment
Pregnancy risk category: C

Indications and dosages

➤ *Diagnostic test of adrenocortical function.* Adults: Up to 80 units I.M. or S.C. in divided doses; or a single dose of repository form; or 10 to 25 units (aqueous form) in 500 ml of D₅W I.V. over 8 hours, between blood samplings. Individual dosages vary with adrenal glands' sensitivity to stimulation and with the specific disease. Infants and younger children require larger doses per kilogram than do older children and adults.

➤ **Replacement hormone.** *Adults:* 20 units S.C. or I.M. q.i.d.

➤ **Exacerbations of multiple sclerosis.** *Adults:* 80 to 120 units I.M. daily for 2 to 3 weeks.

➤ **Severe allergic reactions, collagen disorders, dermatologic disorders, inflammation.** *Adults:* 40 to 80 units I.M. or S.C. daily. Adjust dosage based upon patient response.

➤ **Infantile spasms.** *Infants:* 20 to 40 units I.M. (of repository injection) daily or 80 units I.M. every other day for 3 months or 1 month after spasm ceases.

How supplied
Available by prescription only
Injection: 25 units/vial, 40 units/vial
Repository injection: 40 units/ml, 80 units/ml

Pharmacodynamics
Diagnostic action: Corticotropin is used to test adrenocortical function. Corticotropin binds with a specific receptor in the adrenal cell plasma membrane, stimulating the synthesis of the entire spectrum of adrenal steroids, one of which is cortisol. The effect of corticotropin is measured by analyzing plasma cortisol before and after drug administration. In patients with primary adrenocortical insufficiency, corticotropin doesn't increase plasma cortisol levels significantly.

Anti-inflammatory action: In nonsuppurative thyroiditis and acute exacerbations of multiple sclerosis, corticotropin stimulates release of adrenal cortex hormones, which combat tissue responses to inflammatory processes.

Pharmacokinetics
Absorption: Absorbed rapidly after I.M. administration.
Distribution: Exact distribution of corticotropin is unknown, but it's removed rapidly from plasma by many tissues.
Metabolism: Unknown.
Excretion: Probably excreted by the kidneys. Half-life is about 15 minutes.

Route	Onset	Peak	Duration
I.V., I.M.	Rapid	1 hr	2-4 hr
Repository (I.M.)	Unknown	Unknown	3 days
S.C.	Unknown	Unknown	Unknown

Contraindications and precautions
Contraindicated in patients with peptic ulcer, scleroderma, osteoporosis, systemic fungal infections, ocular herpes simplex, peptic ulceration, heart failure, hypertension, sensitivity to pork and pork products, adrenocortical hyperfunction or primary insufficiency, or Cushing's syndrome. Also contraindicated in those who have had recent surgery.

Use cautiously in women who are pregnant or of childbearing age. Also use cautiously in patients being immunized and in those with latent tuberculosis, hypothyroidism, cirrhosis, acute gouty arthritis, psychotic tendencies, renal insufficiency, diverticulitis, ulcerative colitis, thromboembolic disorders, seizures, uncontrolled hypertension, or myasthenia gravis.

Use cautiously if surgery or emergency treatment is required.

Interactions
Drug-drug. *Amphotericin B, carbonic anhydrase inhibitors, diuretics:* Increased electrolyte loss from diuretic therapy. Monitor serum blood levels, especially potassium.
Cardiac glycosides: May increase the risk of arrhythmias or digitalis toxicity from hypokalemia. Monitor patient closely.
Cortisone, estrogens, hydrocortisone: May elevate plasma cortisol levels abnormally. Use cautiously.
Hepatic enzyme–inducing drugs: May increase corticotropin metabolism. Monitor patient closely.
Indomethacin, NSAIDs, salicylates: Increased risk of GI bleeding. Avoid use together.
Insulin, oral antidiabetics: Corticotropin may aggravate diabetes mellitus. Patient may need increased antidiabetic dosage. Monitor blood glucose levels closely.

Adverse reactions
CNS: *seizures,* dizziness, vertigo, **increased intracranial pressure with papilledema,** pseudotumor cerebri.
CV: hypertension, **heart failure,** necrotizing vasculitis, **shock.**
EENT: cataracts, glaucoma.
GI: **peptic ulceration with perforation and hemorrhage, pancreatitis,** abdominal distention, ulcerative esophagitis, nausea, vomiting, increased serum amylase level.
GU: menstrual irregularities.
Hematologic: ecchymoses.
Metabolic: activation of latent diabetes mellitus, *sodium and fluid retention,* calcium and potassium loss, hypokalemic alkalosis, negative nitrogen balance.
Musculoskeletal: muscle weakness, steroid myopathy, loss of muscle mass, osteoporosis, suppression of growth in children, vertebral compression fractures.
Respiratory: pneumonia.
Skin: impaired wound healing; thin, fragile skin; petechiae; facial erythema; diaphoresis; acne; hyperpigmentation; allergic reactions; hirsutism.
Other: abscess and septic infection, cushingoid symptoms, progressive increase in antibodies, loss of corticotropin stimulatory effect, **hypersensitivity reactions** (rash, **bronchospasm**).

Overdose and treatment
Specific information unavailable. Treatment is supportive, as appropriate.

Special considerations
● Cosyntropin is less antigenic and less likely to cause allergic reactions than corticotropin. However, allergic reactions occur rarely with corticotropin.
● In patient with suspected sensitivity to porcine proteins, perform skin testing. To decrease the risk of anaphylaxis in patient with limited adrenal reserves, 1 mg of dexamethasone may be given at midnight before the corticotropin test and 0.5 mg at start of test.
● Observe neonates of corticotropin-treated women for signs of hypoadrenalism.
● Counteract edema by low-sodium, high-potassium intake; nitrogen loss by high-protein diet; and psychotic symptoms by reducing corticotropin dosage or administering sedatives.
● Drug may mask signs of chronic disease and decrease host resistance and ability to localize infection.
● If administering gel, it must be warmed to room temperature, drawn into a large needle, and given slowly, deep I.M. with a 22G needle.
● Don't discontinue drug abruptly, especially after prolonged therapy. An addisonian crisis may occur.
● Refrigerate reconstituted product and use within 24 hours.
● Corticotropin therapy alters protein-bound iodine levels; radioactive iodine (^{131}I) uptake and T_3 uptake.

Patient monitoring
● Monitor weight, fluid exchange, and resting blood pressure levels until minimal effective dosage is achieved.

Breast-feeding patients
● Safety hasn't been established. Because the potential for severe adverse reactions exists, benefits and risks must be weighed.

Pediatric patients
● Use with caution because prolonged use of drug inhibits skeletal growth. Intermittent administration is recommended.

Patient education
● Warn patient that injection is painful.
● Tell patient to report marked fluid retention, muscle weakness, abdominal pain, seizures, or headache.
● Instruct patient not to be vaccinated during corticotropin therapy.
● Teach patient how to monitor for edema, and tell him about the need for fluid and salt restriction as appropriate.
● Warn patient not to stop drug except as prescribed. Tell him that abrupt discontinuation may cause severe adverse reactions.

cortisone acetate
Cortone

Pharmacologic classification: glucocorticoid, mineralocorticoid
Therapeutic classification: anti-inflammatory, replacement therapy
Pregnancy risk category: NR

Indications and dosages
➤ *Adrenal insufficiency, allergy, inflammation.* Adults: 25 to 300 mg P.O. or 20 to 300 mg I.M. daily or on alternate days. Dosage is highly individualized, depending on severity of disease.
Children: 20 to 300 mg/m² P.O. daily in four divided doses or 7 to 37.5 mg/m² I.M. once or twice daily. Dosage must be highly individualized.

How supplied
Available by prescription only
Injection (I.M. use): 50 mg/ml suspension
Tablets: 5 mg, 10 mg, 25 mg

Pharmacodynamics
Adrenocorticoid replacement: Cortisone acetate is an adrenocorticoid with both glucocorticoid and mineralocorticoid properties. A weak anti-inflammatory agent, drug has only about 80% of the anti-inflammatory activity of an equal weight of hydrocortisone. It's a potent mineralocorticoid, however, having twice the potency of prednisone. Cortisone (or hydrocortisone) is usually the drug of choice for replacement therapy in patients with adrenal insufficiency. It's usually not used for inflammatory or immunosuppressant activity because of the extremely large doses that must be used and because of the unwanted mineralocorticoid effects. Injectable form has a slow onset but a long duration of action. It's usually used only when the oral dosage form can't be used.

Pharmacokinetics
Absorption: Absorbed readily after oral administration.
Distribution: Distributed rapidly to muscle, liver, skin, intestines, and kidneys. Cortisone is extensively bound to plasma proteins (transcortin and albumin). Only the unbound portion is active. Cortisone is distributed into breast milk and through the placenta.
Metabolism: Metabolized in the liver to the active metabolite hydrocortisone, which in turn is metabolized to inactive glucuronide and sulfate metabolites. Duration of hypothalamic-pituitary-adrenal (HPA) axis suppression is 1 to 1½ days.
Excretion: Inactive metabolites and small amounts of unmetabolized drug are excreted by the kidneys. Insignificant quantities of the drug

---

are also excreted in feces. Biological half-life of cortisone is 8 to 12 hours.

Route	Onset	Peak	Duration
P.O.	Variable	1-2 hr	Variable
I.M.	24-48 hr	Variable	Variable

Contraindications and precautions

Contraindicated in patients hypersensitive to drug or its ingredients and in patients with systemic fungal infections. Use cautiously in patients with renal disease, recent MI, GI ulcer, hypertension, osteoporosis, diabetes mellitus, hypothyroidism, cirrhosis, diverticulitis, ulcerative colitis, recent intestinal anastomosis, thromboembolic disorders, seizures, myasthenia gravis, heart failure, tuberculosis, ocular herpes, emotional instability, or psychotic tendencies.

Interactions

Drug-drug. *Amphotericin B, diuretics:* Enhanced hypokalemia. Monitor serum blood levels closely, especially potassium.

Antacids, cholestyramine, colestipol: Decrease cortisone's effect by adsorbing the corticosteroid, decreasing the amount absorbed. Monitor patient carefully.

Barbiturates, phenytoin, rifampin: Decreased corticosteroid effects. Monitor patient closely.

Cardiac glycosides: Hypokalemia may increase the risk of toxicity in patients concurrently receiving cardiac glycosides. Avoid use together.

Estrogens: May reduce cortisone metabolism and prolong cortisone half-life. Avoid use together.

Inactivated vaccines, toxoids: Cortisone may have a diminished response to toxoids or inactivated vaccines. Avoid use together.

Insulin, oral antidiabetics: Increased risk of hyperglycemia. Adjust antidiabetic dosage as needed.

Isoniazid, salicylates: When used together, cortisone increases the metabolism of isoniazid and salicylates. Use together cautiously.

NSAIDs: May increase the risk of GI ulceration. Avoid use together.

Oral anticoagulants: Cortisone may decrease the effects. PT and INR must be checked.

Drug-lifestyle. *Alcohol use:* Increased risk of gastric irritation and GI ulceration. Advise patient to avoid alcohol.

Adverse reactions

CNS: euphoria, insomnia, psychotic behavior, pseudotumor cerebri, vertigo, headache, paresthesia, *seizures.*

CV: *heart failure,* hypertension, edema, *arrhythmias,* thrombophlebitis, *thromboembolism.*

EENT: cataracts, glaucoma.

GI: *peptic ulcer,* GI irritation, increased appetite, *pancreatitis,* nausea, vomiting.

GU: increased urine glucose and calcium levels, menstrual irregularities.

Metabolic: hypokalemia, hyperglycemia, carbohydrate intolerance, hypercholesterolemia, hypokalemia, hypocalcemia, decreased thyroxine and triiodothyronine levels.

Musculoskeletal: muscle weakness, osteoporosis, growth suppression in children.

Skin: delayed wound healing, acne, various skin eruptions, atrophy at I.M. injection sites, hirsutism.

Other: cushingoid symptoms (moonface, buffalo hump, central obesity).

susceptibility to infections, *acute adrenal insufficiency* may follow increased stress (infection, surgery, trauma) or abrupt withdrawal after long-term therapy.

After abrupt withdrawal: rebound inflammation, fatigue, weakness, arthralgia, fever, dizziness, lethargy, depression, fainting, orthostatic hypotension, dyspnea, anorexia, hypoglycemia. After prolonged use, sudden withdrawal may be fatal.

Overdose and treatment

Acute ingestion, even in massive doses, is rarely a clinical problem. Toxic signs and symptoms rarely occur if the drug is used for less than 3 weeks, even at large dosage ranges. However, long-term use causes adverse physiologic effects.

Special considerations

Most adverse reactions to corticosteroids are dose- or duration-dependent.

⚠ ALERT Check for sensitivity to any other corticosteroid. Drug isn't for I.V. use. For better results and less toxicity, give a once-daily dose in the morning.

● Drug therapy suppresses reactions to skin tests; causes false-negative results in the nitroblue tetrazolium test for systemic bacterial infections; and decreases ^{131}I uptake and protein-bound iodine levels in thyroid function tests.

Patient monitoring

● Monitor serum electrolyte and blood glucose levels.

● Monitor patient for fluid and electrolyte imbalance.

Pediatric patients

● Long-term use of cortisone in children and adolescents may delay growth and maturation.

Geriatric patients

● Use with caution in geriatric patients in whom osteoporosis is more likely to develop.

Patient education

● Inform patient of potential adverse reactions.

● Tell patient not to discontinue drug abruptly or without medical consent.

● Advise patient to avoid exposure to viral infections (such as measles and chicken pox) and to notify prescriber if such exposure occurs.

• Instruct patient to carry a card indicating his need for supplemental glucocorticoids during stress. This card should contain prescriber's name, medication, and dose taken.

---

cosyntropin
Cortrosyn

Pharmacologic classification: anterior pituitary hormone
Therapeutic classification: diagnostic
Pregnancy risk category: C

Indications and dosages
➤ *Diagnostic test of adrenocortical function.* *Adults and children age 2 and older:* 0.25 to 0.75 mg I.M. or I.V. (unless label prohibits I.V. administration) between blood samplings. To administer as I.V. infusion, dilute 0.25 mg in D₅W or normal saline solution, and infuse over 6 hours (40 mcg/hour).
Children under age 2: 0.125 mg I.M. or I.V.

How supplied
Available by prescription only
Injection: 0.25 mg

Pharmacodynamics
Diagnostic action: Cosyntropin is used to test adrenal function. Drug binds with a specific receptor in the adrenal cell plasma membrane to begin synthesis of its entire spectrum of hormones, one of which is cortisol. In patients with primary adrenocortical insufficiency, cosyntropin doesn't increase plasma cortisol levels significantly.

Pharmacokinetics
Absorption: Inactivated by the proteolytic enzymes in the GI tract. After I.M. administration, cosyntropin is absorbed rapidly. After rapid I.V. administration in patients with normal adrenocortical function, plasma cortisol levels begin to increase within 5 minutes and double within 15 to 30 minutes. Peak levels begin to decrease in 2 to 4 hours.
Distribution: Not fully understood, but drug is removed rapidly from plasma by many tissues.
Metabolism: Unknown.
Excretion: Probably excreted by the kidneys.

Route	Onset	Peak	Duration
I.V.	Rapid	45-60 min	Unknown
I.M., S.C.	Unknown	45-60 min	Unknown

Contraindications and precautions
Contraindicated in patients hypersensitive to drug.

Interactions
Drug-drug. *Blood, plasma products:* Inactivate cosyntropin. Avoid administration together.

Cortisone, estrogens, hydrocortisone: May cause abnormally elevated plasma cortisol levels. Avoid use together.

Adverse reactions
CNS: *seizures,* dizziness, vertigo, *increased intracranial pressure with papilledema,* pseudotumor cerebri.
CV: flushing.
EENT: cataracts, glaucoma.
GI: peptic ulcer, *pancreatitis,* abdominal distention, ulcerative esophagitis, nausea, vomiting.
GU: menstrual irregularities.
Hematologic: ecchymoses.
Metabolic: altered blood glucose levels.
Musculoskeletal: fractures, muscle weakness, steroid myopathy, loss of muscle mass, osteoporosis, vertebral compression.
Skin: pruritus; impaired wound healing; thin, fragile skin; petechiae; facial erythema; diaphoresis; acne; hyperpigmentation; hirsutism.
Other: *hypersensitivity reactions,* cushingoid symptoms.

Overdose and treatment
Acute overdose requires no therapy other than symptomatic treatment and supportive care, as appropriate.

Special considerations
• High plasma cortisol levels may be reported erroneously in patients receiving spironolactone, cortisone, or hydrocortisone when fluorometric analysis is used. This doesn't occur with the radioimmunoassay or competitive protein-binding method. However, therapy can be maintained with prednisone, dexamethasone, or betamethasone because these aren't detectable by the fluorometric method.
• More cortisol is secreted if dosage is given slowly, not rapidly I.V.
• Cosyntropin is less antigenic than corticotropin and less likely to produce allergic reactions.
• For rapid screening, plasma cortisol levels are determined before and 30 minutes after administration of 0.25 mg I.M. or I.V. injection over 2 minutes. Some clinicians prefer plasma cortisol concentration determinations at 60 minutes after injection of cosyntropin.
• Reconstitute powder by adding 1 ml of normal saline solution to 0.25-mg vial to yield a solution containing 0.25 mg/ml.
• Reconstituted solution is stable for 24 hours at room temperature or for 21 days if refrigerated at 36° to 46° F (2° to 8° C).

Patient monitoring
A normal response to cosyntropin includes the following values: The control plasma cortisol level exceeds 5 mcg/100 ml plasma; 30 minutes after the injection, cortisol levels increase by 7 mcg/100 ml above control; 30-minute cortisol levels exceed 18 mcg/100 ml.

Reactions may be *common*, uncommon, *life-threatening*, or COMMON AND LIFE-THREATENING.

Patient education
● Inform patient taking spironolactone, cortisone, hydrocortisone, or estrogen that these medications may interfere with test results.
● Tell patient to report adverse effects immediately.

co-trimoxazole (trimethoprim-sulfamethoxazole)
Apo-Sulfatrim*, Bactrim, Bactrim DS, Bactrim I.V., Cotrim, Cotrim D.S., Novo-Trimel*, Roubac*, Septra, Septra DS, Septra I.V., SMZ-TMP, Sulfatrim

Pharmacologic classification: sulfonamide and folate antagonist
Therapeutic classification: antibiotic
Pregnancy risk category: C

Indications and dosages
➤*Urinary tract infections and shigellosis. Adults:* One double-strength or two regular strength tablets P.O. q 12 hours for 10 to 14 days or 5 days for shigellosis. Or, 8 to 10 mg/kg (based on trimethoprim) I.V. daily given in two to four equally divided doses for up to 14 days (5 days for shigellosis). Maximum daily dose is 960 mg.
Children over age 2 months: 8 mg/kg trimethoprim and 40 mg/kg sulfamethoxazole P.O. daily in two divided doses q 12 hours (10 days for urinary tract infections; 5 days for shigellosis).
➤*Primary prophylaxis against toxoplasmosis in HIV-infected patients. Adults and adolescents:* 160 mg (based on trimethoprim) P.O. daily.
Children: 150 mg/m² (based on trimethoprim) P.O. daily in two divided doses.
➤ *Otitis media. Children over age 2 months:* 8 mg/kg trimethoprim and 40 mg/kg sulfamethoxazole P.O. daily, in two divided doses q 12 hours for 10 days.
➤Pneumocystis carinii *pneumonitis. Adults and children over age 2 months:* 15 to 20 mg/kg trimethoprim and 75 to 100 mg/kg sulfamethoxazole P.O. daily, in equally divided doses, q 6 to 8 hours for 14 to 21 days.
➤*Prophylaxis of* P. carinii *pneumonia. Adults:* 160 mg (based on trimethoprim) daily.
Children: 150 mg/m² (based on trimethoprim) daily in two divided doses for 3 consecutive days each week.
➤*Chronic bronchitis. Adults:* One double-strength or two regular-strength tablets P.O. q 12 hours for 14 days.
➤*Traveler's diarrhea. Adults:* One double-strength or two regular-strength tablets P.O. q 12 hours for 5 days.
Note: For the following unlabeled uses, dosages refer to oral trimethoprim (as co-trimoxazole).

➤*Septic agranulocytosis* ◊. *Adults:* 2.5 mg/kg I.V. q.i.d.; for prophylaxis, 80 to 160 mg b.i.d.
➤*Nocardia infection* ◊. *Adults:* 640 mg P.O. daily for 7 months.
➤*Pharyngeal gonococcal infections* ◊. *Adults:* 720 mg P.O. daily for 5 days.
➤*Chancroid* ◊. *Adults:* 160 mg P.O. b.i.d for 7 days.
➤*Pertussis* ◊. *Adults:* 320 mg P.O. daily in two divided doses.
Children: 40 mg/kg P.O. daily in two divided doses.
➤*Cholera* ◊. *Adults:* 160 mg P.O. b.i.d for 3 days.
Children: 5 mg/kg P.O. b.i.d for 3 days.
➤*Isosporiasis* ◊. *Adults:* 160 mg P.O. q.i.d. for 10 days, followed by 160 mg b.i.d. for 3 weeks.
✦ *Dosage adjustment.* In patients with impaired renal function, adjust dose or frequency of administration of parenteral form according to degree of renal impairment, severity of infection, and susceptibility of organism.

Creatinine clearance (ml/min)	Adult dosage
15 to 30	One-half the usual regimen
< 15	Use isn't recommended

How supplied
Available by prescription only
Injection: trimethoprim 16 mg/ml and sulfamethoxazole 80 mg/ml
Suspension: trimethoprim 40 mg and sulfamethoxazole 200 mg/5 ml
Tablets: trimethoprim 80 mg and sulfamethoxazole 400 mg; trimethoprim 160 mg and sulfamethoxazole 800 mg

Pharmacodynamics
Antibacterial action: Co-trimoxazole is generally bactericidal; it acts by sequential blockade of folic acid enzymes in the synthesis pathway. The sulfamethoxazole component inhibits formation of dihydrofolic acid from para-aminobenzoic (PABA), whereas trimethoprim inhibits dihydrofolate reductase. Both drugs block folic acid synthesis, preventing bacterial cell synthesis of essential nucleic acids.

Co-trimoxazole is effective against *Escherichia coli, Klebsiella, Enterobacter, Proteus mirabilis, Haemophilus influenzae, Streptococcus pneumoniae, Staphylococcus aureus, Acinetobacter, Salmonella, Shigella,* and *P. carinii.*

Pharmacokinetics
Absorption: Well absorbed from the GI tract after oral administration.
Distribution: Distributed widely into body tissues and fluids, including middle ear fluid, prostatic fluid, bile, aqueous humor, and CSF. Protein

binding is 44% for trimethoprim, 70% for sulfamethoxazole. Drug crosses the placenta.
Metabolism: Metabolized by the liver.
Excretion: Both components of co-trimoxazole are excreted primarily in urine by glomerular filtration and renal tubular secretion; some appears in breast milk. Trimethoprim's plasma half-life in patients with normal renal function is 8 to 11 hours, extended to 26 hours in patients with severe renal dysfunction; sulfamethoxazole's plasma half-life is 10 to 13 hours, extended to 30 to 40 hours in patients with severe renal dysfunction. Hemodialysis removes some co-trimoxazole.

Route	Onset	Peak	Duration
P.O.	Unknown	1-4 hr	Unknown
I.V.	Immediate	Immediate	Unknown

Contraindications and precautions

Contraindicated in patients hypersensitive to trimethoprim or sulfonamides, those with severe renal impairment (creatinine clearance of less than 15 ml/minute) or porphyria, those with megaloblastic anemia caused by folate deficiency, pregnant women at term, breast-feeding women, and children under age 2 months.

Use cautiously in patients with impaired renal or hepatic function, severe allergies, severe bronchial asthma, G6PD deficiency, or blood dyscrasia.

Interactions

Drug-drug. *Cyclosporine:* Increased risk of nephrotoxicity. Avoid use together.
Digoxin: Increased digoxin levels. Monitor serum levels closely.
Indomethacin: May increase sulfamethoxazole levels. Dosage adjustment may be necessary.
Methotrexate: Increased methotrexate levels. Use together cautiously.
Oral anticoagulants: Co-trimoxazole may inhibit hepatic metabolism, enhancing anticoagulant effects. Observe patient for signs of bleeding.
Oral sulfonylureas: Enhanced hypoglycemic effects. Monitor blood glucose levels.
Para-aminobenzoic acid: Antagonized sulfonamide effects. Monitor patient closely.
Phenytoin: Inhibited phenytoin metabolism. Dosage adjustment may be necessary.
Pyrimethamine: May cause megaloblastic anemia in pyrimethamine doses greater than 25 mg weekly. Avoid use together.
Tricyclic antidepressants: Decreased antidepressant effect. Monitor patient closely.
Zidovudine: Serum zidovudine levels may be increased. Monitor patient carefully.
Drug-lifestyle. *Sun exposure:* Photosensitivity reaction may occur. Advise patient to take precautions.

Adverse reactions

CNS: headache, mental depression, aseptic meningitis, apathy, *seizures*, hallucinations, ataxia, nervousness, fatigue, vertigo, insomnia.

EENT: tinnitus.
GI: *nausea, vomiting, diarrhea,* abdominal pain, anorexia, stomatitis, *pancreatitis,* pseudomembranous colitis.
GU: *toxic nephrosis with oliguria and anuria,* crystalluria, hematuria, interstitial nephritis.
Hematologic: *agranulocytosis, aplastic anemia,* megaloblastic anemia, *thrombocytopenia, leukopenia, hemolytic anemia, pancytopenia.*
Hepatic: jaundice, *hepatic necrosis.*
Musculoskeletal: arthralgia, myalgia, muscle weakness.
Respiratory: pulmonary infiltrates.
Skin: *erythema multiforme (Stevens-Johnson syndrome)*, generalized skin eruptions, epidermal necrolysis, exfoliative dermatitis, photosensitivity, urticaria, pruritus.
Other: *hypersensitivity reactions* (*serum sickness, drug fever, anaphylaxis*), thrombophlebitis, rhabdomyolysis.

Overdose and treatment

Signs and symptoms of overdose include mental depression, drowsiness, anorexia, jaundice, confusion, headache, nausea, vomiting, diarrhea, facial swelling, slight elevations in liver function test results, and bone marrow depression.

Treat by emesis or gastric lavage, followed by supportive care (correction of acidosis, forced oral fluids, and I.V. fluids). Treatment of renal failure may be required; transfuse appropriate blood products in severe hematologic toxicity; use folinic acid to rescue bone marrow. Hemodialysis has limited ability to remove co-trimoxazole. Peritoneal dialysis isn't effective.

Special considerations

Consider the recommendations relevant to all sulfonamides as well as the following.
⚠ ALERT Note that DS means double-strength.
⚠ ALERT Occasionally, dosage is written as trimethoprim component; check it carefully.
⚠ ALERT Drug isn't for I.M. use.
• Co-trimoxazole has been used effectively to treat chronic bacterial prostatitis and as prophylaxis against recurrent urinary tract infection in women and traveler's diarrhea.
• For I.V. use, dilute infusion in D₅W. Don't mix with other drugs. Don't administer by rapid infusion or bolus injection. Infuse slowly over 60 to 90 minutes.
• I.V. infusion must be diluted before use. Each 5 ml should be added to 125 ml D₅W. Don't refrigerate solution; diluted solutions must be used within 6 hours. A dilution of 5 ml per 75 ml D₅W may be prepared for patients requiring fluid restriction, but these solutions should be used within 2 hours.
• Check solution carefully for precipitate before starting infusion. Don't use solution containing a precipitate.
• Shake oral suspension thoroughly before administering.

Reactions may be *common*, uncommon, *life-threatening*, or COMMON AND LIFE-THREATENING.

• Trimethoprim can interfere with serum methotrexate assay as determined by the competitive binding protein technique. No interference occurs if radioimmunoassay is used.

Patient monitoring
• Assess I.V. site for signs of phlebitis or infiltration.
• Monitor renal and liver function tests.

Pregnant patients
• Use only when crucial in pregnant women.

Breast-feeding patients
• Drug isn't recommended for breast-feeding women.

Pediatric patients
• Drug isn't recommended for infants under age 2 months.

Geriatric patients
• In geriatric patients, diminished renal function may prolong half-life. Such patients also have an increased risk of adverse reactions.

Patient education
• Inform patient of potential adverse reactions.
• Tell patient to take drug as prescribed, even if he feels better.
• Instruct patient to take oral dose with 8 oz. (240 ml) of water on an empty stomach.

cromolyn sodium
Gastrocrom, Intal, Intal Inhaler, Intal Nebulizer Solution, Nasalcrom, Opticrom

Pharmacologic classification: chromone derivative
Therapeutic classification: mast cell stabilizer, antiasthmatic
Pregnancy risk category: B

Indications and dosages
➤ *Adjunct in treatment of severe perennial bronchial asthma. Adults and children over age 5:* Two inhalations q.i.d. at regular intervals; aqueous solution administered through a nebulizer, one ampule q.i.d.
➤ *Prevention and treatment of allergic rhinitis. Adults and children age 6 and older:* One spray (5.2 mg) of nasal solution in each nostril t.i.d. or q.i.d. May give up to six times daily.
➤ *Prevention of exercise-induced bronchospasm. Adults and children over age 5:* Two metered sprays using inhaler no more than 1 hour before anticipated exercise.

Inhalation of 20 mg of oral inhalation solution may be used in adults or children age 2 and older. Repeat inhalation as required for protection during long exercise.

➤ *Allergic ocular disorders (giant papillary conjunctivitis, vernal keratoconjunctivitis, vernal keratitis, allergic keratoconjunctivitis). Adults and children over age 4:* Instill one to two drops in each eye 4 to 6 times daily at regular intervals. One drop contains about 1.6 mg cromolyn sodium.
➤ *Systemic mastocytosis. Adults:* 200 mg P.O. q.i.d.
Children ages 2 to 12: 100 mg P.O. q.i.d.
Children under age 2: 20 mg/kg daily P.O. divided in four equal doses.
➤ *Food allergy, inflammatory bowel disease ◇. Adults:* 200 mg P.O. q.i.d. 15 to 20 minutes before meals.

How supplied
Available by prescription only
Aerosol: 800 mcg/metered spray
Ophthalmic solution: 4%
Oral concentrate: 100 mg/5ml
Solution: 20 mg/2 ml for nebulization
Available without a prescription
Nasal solution: 5.2 mg/metered spray (40 mg/ml)

Pharmacodynamics
Antiasthmatic action: Cromolyn prevents release of mediators of type I allergic reactions, including histamine and slow-reacting substance of anaphylaxis (SRS A), from sensitized mast cells after the antigen-antibody union has taken place. Cromolyn doesn't inhibit binding of IgE to mast cells nor the interaction between cell-bound IgE and the specific antigen. It does inhibit the release of substances (such as histamine and SRS-A) in response to IgE binding to mast cells. Main site of action occurs locally on the lung mucosa, nasal mucosa, and eyes.
Bronchodilating action: Besides mast cell stabilization, recent evidence suggests that drug may have a bronchodilating effect by an unknown mechanism. Comparative studies have shown cromolyn and theophylline to be equally efficacious but less effective than orally inhaled beta$_2$-adrenergic agonists in preventing bronchospasm.
Ocular antiallergy action: Cromolyn inhibits degranulation of sensitized mast cells that occurs after exposure to specific antigens, preventing release of histamine and SRS-A.

Cromolyn has no direct anti-inflammatory, vasoconstrictor, antihistamine, antiserotonin, or corticosteroid-like properties.

Cromolyn dissolved in water and given orally has been found to be effective in managing food allergy, inflammatory bowel disease (Crohn's disease, ulcerative colitis), and systemic mastocytosis.

Pharmacokinetics
Absorption: Only 0.5% to 2% of an oral dose is absorbed. The amount reaching the lungs depends on patient's ability to use inhaler correctly, amount of bronchoconstriction, and size or

presence of mucus plugs. The degree of absorption depends on method of administration; most absorption occurs with the aerosol via metered-dose inhaler, and least occurs with the administration of the solution via power-operated nebulizer. Less than 7% of an intranasal dose of cromolyn as a solution is absorbed systemically. Only minimal absorption (0.03%) of an ophthalmic dose occurs after instillation into the eye. Absorption half-life from the lung is 1 hour. A plasma level of 9 ng/ml can be achieved 15 minutes after a 20-mg dose.

Distribution: Cromolyn doesn't cross most biological membranes because it's ionized and lipid-insoluble at the body's pH. Less than 0.1% of a dose crosses to the placenta; it isn't known if drug is distributed into breast milk.

Metabolism: None significant.

Excretion: Excreted unchanged in urine (50%) and bile (about 50%). Small amounts may be excreted in the feces or exhaled. Elimination half-life is 81 minutes.

Route	Onset	Peak	Duration
P.O.	Unknown	Unknown	Unknown
Inhalation, intranasal, ophthalmic	Unknown	Unknown	Unknown

Contraindications and precautions

Contraindicated in patients experiencing acute asthma attacks or status asthmaticus and in patients hypersensitive to drug. Use inhalation form cautiously in patients with cardiac disease or arrhythmias.

Interactions
None reported.

Adverse reactions

CNS: dizziness, headache.
EENT: *irritated throat and trachea*, nasal congestion, pharyngeal irritation, *sneezing*, nasal burning and irritation, epistaxis, lacrimation, swollen parotid gland.
GI: nausea, esophagitis, abdominal pain, bad taste.
GU: dysuria, urinary frequency.
Musculoskeletal: joint swelling and pain.
Respiratory: *bronchospasm* (after inhalation of dry powder), *cough*, wheezing, *eosinophilic pneumonia.*
Skin: rash, urticaria.
Other: *angioedema.*

Overdose and treatment
No information available.

Special considerations
● Therapeutic effects may not occur for 2 to 4 weeks after therapy starts.
● Bronchospasm or cough occasionally occurs after inhalation and may require stopping ther-

apy. Prior bronchodilation may help but it may still be necessary to stop the cromolyn therapy.
● Asthma symptoms may recur if cromolyn dosage is reduced below the recommended dosage.
● Use reduced dosage in patients with impaired renal or hepatic function.
● Eosinophilic pneumonia or pulmonary infiltrates with eosinophilia requires stopping drug.
● Nasal solution may cause nasal stinging or sneezing immediately after instillation of drug, but this reaction rarely requires discontinuation of drug.
● Protect oral solution and ophthalmic solution from direct sunlight.

Patient monitoring
● Monitor pulmonary status before and immediately after therapy.
● Pulmonary function tests are needed to confirm significant bronchodilator-reversible component of airway obstruction in patients considered for cromolyn therapy.
● Watch for recurrence of asthmatic symptoms when corticosteroids are also used. Use only when acute episode has been controlled, airway is cleared, and patient is able to inhale.

Pregnant patients
● Animal studies have shown adverse fetal effects when cromolyn sodium is administered parenterally in high doses with high-dose isoproterenol.

Pediatric patients
● Cromolyn use in children under age 5 is limited to the inhalation route of administration. The safety of the nebulizer solution in children under age 2 hasn't been established. Safety of nasal solution in children under age 6 hasn't been established.

Patient education
● Teach correct use of metered-dose inhaler: Exhale completely before placing mouthpiece between lips; then inhale deeply and slowly with steady, even breath. Remove inhaler from mouth, hold breath for 5 to 10 seconds, and exhale.
● Urge patient to call prescriber if drug causes wheezing or coughing.
● Instruct patient with asthma or seasonal or perennial allergic rhinitis to administer drug at regular intervals to ensure clinical effectiveness.
● Advise patient that gargling and rinsing mouth after administration can help reduce mouth dryness.
● Tell patient taking prescribed adrenocorticoids to continue taking them during therapy, if appropriate.
● Instruct patient who uses a bronchodilator inhaler to administer dose about 5 minutes before taking cromolyn (unless otherwise indicated); explain that this step helps reduce adverse reactions.

Reactions may be *common*, uncommon, *life-threatening*, or COMMON AND LIFE-THREATENING.

cyanocobalamin (vitamin B₁₂)
Bedoz,* Cobex, Crystamine,
Cyanoject, Cyomin, Rubesol-1000,
Rubramin PC, Vibal

hydroxocobalamin (vitamin B₁₂)
Hydrobexan, Hydro-Cobex, LA-12

Pharmacologic classification: water-soluble
vitamin
Therapeutic classification: vitamin, nutrition
supplement
Pregnancy risk category: C (parenteral)

Indications and dosages
➤ *RDA for vitamin B₁₂. Neonates and in-
fants up to age 6 months:* 0.4 mcg
Infants ages 6 months to 1 year: 0.5 mcg
Children ages 1 to 3: 0.9 mcg
Children ages 4 to 8: 1.2 mcg
Children ages 9 to 13: 1.8 mcg
Adults and children age 14 and older: 2.4 mcg
Pregnant women: 2.6 mcg
Breast-feeding women: 2.8 mcg
➤ *Vitamin B₁₂ deficiency from any cause
except malabsorption related to pernicious anemia or other GI disease. Adults:*
30 mcg S.C. or I.M. daily for 5 to 10 days, depending on severity of deficiency. Maintenance
dosage is 100 to 200 mcg I.M. once monthly. For
subsequent prophylaxis, advise adequate nutrition and daily RDA vitamin B₁₂ supplements.
Children: 1 to 5 mg given in single doses of
100 mcg I.M. or S.C. over 2 or more weeks. Maintenance dosage is 60 mcg/month I.M. or S.C.
➤ *Schilling test flushing dose. Adults and
children:* 1,000 mcg I.M. in a single dose.

How supplied
Available by prescription only
Injection: 100 mcg/ml, 1,000 mcg/ml
Tablets: 25 mcg, 50 mcg, 100 mcg, 250 mcg,
500 mcg, 1,000 mcg

Pharmacodynamics
Nutritional action: Vitamin B₁₂ can be converted to coenzyme B₁₂ in tissues and, as such,
is essential for conversion of methyl-malonate to
succinate and synthesis of methionine from ho-
mocystine, a reaction that also requires folate.
Without coenzyme B₁₂, folate deficiency occurs.
Vitamin B₁₂ also facilitates fat and carbohydrate
metabolism and protein synthesis. Cells characterized by rapid division (epithelial cells, bone
marrow, and myeloid cells) appear to have the
greatest requirement for vitamin B₁₂.
   Vitamin B₁₂ deficiency may cause megaloblastic anemia, GI lesions, and neurologic damage; it begins with an inability to produce myelin
followed by gradual degeneration of the axon and
nerve. Parenteral administration of vitamin B₁₂

completely reverses the megaloblastic anemia
and GI symptoms of vitamin B₁₂ deficiency.

Pharmacokinetics
Absorption: After oral administration, vitamin
B₁₂ is absorbed irregularly from the distal small
intestine. Vitamin B₁₂ is protein-bound, and this
bond must be split by proteolysis and gastric acid
before absorption. Absorption depends on sufficient intrinsic factor and calcium. Vitamin B₁₂ is
inadequate in malabsorptive states and in pernicious anemia. After oral administration of doses
of less than 3 mcg, peak plasma levels aren't
reached for 8 to 12 hours.
Distribution: Distributed into the liver, bone
marrow, and other tissues, including the placenta.
At birth, the vitamin B₁₂ level in neonates is three
to five times that in the mother. Vitamin B₁₂ is
distributed into breast milk in levels about equal
to the maternal vitamin B₁₂ level. Unlike cyanocobalamin, hydroxocobalamin is absorbed more
slowly parenterally and may be taken up by the
liver in larger quantities; it also produces a greater
increase in serum cobalamin levels and less urinary excretion.
Metabolism: Cyanocobalamin and hydroxocobalamin are metabolized in the liver.
Excretion: In healthy persons receiving only dietary vitamin B₁₂, about 3 to 8 mcg of the vitamin is secreted into the GI tract daily, mainly from
bile, and all but about 1 mcg is reabsorbed; less
than 0.25 mcg is usually excreted in the urine
daily. When vitamin B₁₂ is administered in
amounts that exceed the binding capacity of plasma, the liver, and other tissues, it's free in the
blood for urinary excretion.

Route	Onset	Peak	Duration
P.O.	Unknown	8-12 hr	Unknown
I.M., S.C.	Unknown	1 hr	Unknown

Contraindications and precautions
Contraindicated in patients hypersensitive to vitamin B₁₂ or cobalt and in patients with early
Leber's disease. Use cautiously in anemic patients
with cardiac, pulmonary, or hypertensive disease
and in those with severe vitamin B₁₂–dependent
deficiencies.

Interactions
Drug-drug. *Aminoglycosides, aminosalicylic
acid and its salts, anticonvulsants, cobalt
irradiation of the small bowel, colchicine,
extended-release potassium preparations:* Decreased vitamin B₁₂ absorption from the GI tract.
Don't use together.
Ascorbic acid: May destroy vitamin B₁₂. Don't
administer within 1 hour of giving vitamin B₁₂.
Chloramphenicol: Antagonized hematopoietic
response. Don't give together.
Colchicine: Increased neomycin-induced malabsorption of vitamin B₁₂. Don't use together.

Drug-lifestyle. *Alcohol use:* Decreased vitamin B_{12} absorption from the GI tract. Advise patient to avoid alcohol use.

Smoking: Increased vitamin B_{12} requirement. Tell patient to avoid smoking.

Adverse reactions

CV: peripheral vascular thrombosis, *heart failure.*
GI: transient diarrhea.
Respiratory: pulmonary edema.
Skin: itching, transitory exanthema, urticaria.
Other: *anaphylaxis* (with parenteral administration), pain and burning at S.C. or I.M. injection site.

Overdose and treatment

Not applicable. Even in large doses, vitamin B_{12} isn't usually toxic.

Special considerations

● Determine patient's diet and drug history, including patterns of alcohol use, to identify poor nutritional habits.
● Administer oral solution promptly after mixing with fruit juice. Ascorbic acid causes instability of vitamin B_{12}. Protect oral solution from light.
● Administer oral vitamin B_{12} with meals to increase absorption.
● Don't mix the parenteral form with dextrose solutions, alkaline or strongly acidic solutions, or oxidizing and reducing agents, because anaphylaxis may occur with I.V. use.
● Parenteral therapy is preferred for patients with pernicious anemia because oral administration may be unreliable. In patients with neurologic complications, prolonged inadequate oral therapy may lead to permanent spinal cord damage. Oral therapy is appropriate for mild conditions without neurologic signs and for patients who refuse or are sensitive to the parenteral form.
● Patients with a history of sensitivities and those suspected of being sensitive to vitamin B_{12} should receive an intradermal test dose before therapy begins. Sensitization to vitamin B_{12} may develop after as many as 8 years of treatment.
● Expect therapeutic response to occur within 48 hours; it's measured by laboratory values and effect on fatigue, GI symptoms, anorexia, pallid or yellow complexion, glossitis, distaste for meat, dyspnea on exertion, palpitations, neurologic degeneration (paresthesia, loss of vibratory and position sense and deep reflexes, incoordination), psychotic behavior, anosmia, and visual disturbances.
● Therapeutic response to vitamin B_{12} may be impaired by concurrent infection, uremia, folic acid or iron deficiency, or drugs having bone marrow suppressant effects. Large doses of vitamin B_{12} may improve folate-deficient megaloblastic anemia.
● Patients with mild peripheral neurologic defects may respond to concomitant physical therapy. Usually, neurologic damage that doesn't improve after 12 to 18 months of therapy is considered irreversible. Severe vitamin B_{12} deficiency that persists for 3 months or longer may cause permanent spinal cord degeneration.
● Vitamin B_{12} therapy may cause false-positive results for intrinsic factor antibodies, which are present in the blood of half of all patients with pernicious anemia.
● Methotrexate, pyrimethamine, and most anti-infectives invalidate diagnostic blood assays for vitamin B_{12}.

Patient monitoring

● Monitor bowel function because regularity is essential for consistent absorption of oral preparations.
● Monitor vital signs in patients with cardiac disease and in those receiving parenteral vitamin B_{12}. Watch for symptoms of pulmonary edema, which tend to develop early in therapy.
● Expect reticulocyte level to rise in 3 to 4 days, peak in 5 to 8 days, and then gradually decline as erythrocyte count and hemoglobin rise to normal levels (in 4 to 6 weeks).
● Monitor potassium levels during the first 48 hours, especially in patients with pernicious anemia or megaloblastic anemia. Potassium supplements may be required. Conversion to normal erythropoiesis increases erythrocyte potassium requirement and can result in fatal hypokalemia in these patients.
● Continue periodic hematologic evaluations throughout patient's lifetime.

Breast-feeding patients

● Vitamin B_{12} appears in breast milk in levels that approximate the maternal vitamin B_{12} level. The Food and Nutrition Board of the National Academy of Sciences-National Research Council recommends that breast-feeding women consume 2.8 mcg of vitamin B_{12} daily.

Pediatric patients

● Safety and efficacy of vitamin B_{12} for use in children haven't been established. Intake for children should be 0.5 to 2 mcg daily, as recommended by the Food and Nutrition Board of the National Academy of Sciences, National Research Council.
● Some of these products contain benzyl alcohol, which has been linked to a fatal "gasping syndrome" in premature infants.

Patient education

● Emphasize importance of a well-balanced diet. To prevent progression of subacute combined degeneration, don't use folic acid instead of vitamin B_{12} to prevent anemia.
● Instruct patient to report infection or disease in case his condition requires increased dosage of vitamin B_{12}.
● Tell patient with pernicious anemia that he must have lifelong treatment with vitamin B_{12} to pre-

vent recurring symptoms and the risk of incapacitating and irreversible spinal cord damage.
● Instruct patient to store tablets in a tightly closed container at room temperature.

cyclizine hydrochloride
Marezine

cyclizine lactate
Marezine, Marzine*

Pharmacologic classification: piperazine-derivative antihistamine
Therapeutic classification: antiemetic, antivertigo
Pregnancy risk category: B

Indications and dosages
➤**Motion sickness (prophylaxis and treatment).** *Adults and children over age 12:* 50 mg P.O. (hydrochloride) 30 minutes before travel, then q 4 to 6 hours, p.r.n., to maximum of 200 mg daily; or 50 mg I.M. (lactate) q 4 to 6 hours, p.r.n.
Children ages 6 to 12: 25 mg P.O. up to t.i.d. under medical supervision.

How supplied
Available with or without a prescription
cyclizine hydrochloride
Tablets: 50 mg
cyclizine lactate
Injection: 50 mg/ml

Pharmacodynamics
Antiemetic action: Probably inhibits nausea and vomiting by centrally depressing sensitivity of the labyrinth apparatus that relays stimuli to the chemoreceptor trigger zone and thus stimulates the vomiting center in the brain.
Antivertigo action: Depresses conduction in vestibular-cerebellar pathways and reduces labyrinth excitability.

Pharmacokinetics
Absorption: Not well characterized; onset of action between 30 and 60 minutes.
Distribution: Well distributed throughout body.
Metabolism: Metabolized in liver.
Excretion: No information available; drug effect lasts 4 to 6 hours.

Route	Onset	Peak	Duration
P.O., I.M.	30-60 min	Unknown	Unknown

Contraindications and precautions
Contraindicated in patients hypersensitive to drug. Use cautiously in patients with heart failure, BPH, asthma, or recent surgery.

Interactions
Drug-drug. *Aminoglycosides, cisplatin, loop diuretics, salicylates, vancomycin:* May mask signs of ototoxicity. Don't give concurrently.
CNS depressants (such as antianxiety drugs, barbiturates, sleeping aids, tranquilizers): Additive sedative and CNS depressant effects. Monitor patient closely.
Drug-lifestyle. *Alcohol use:* Additive sedative and CNS depressant effects. Discourage use of alcohol.

Adverse reactions
CNS: *drowsiness,* auditory and visual hallucinations, restlessness, excitation, nervousness.
CV: hypotension, palpitations, tachycardia.
EENT: blurred vision, diplopia, tinnitus, dry nose and throat.
GI: constipation, dry mouth, anorexia, nausea, vomiting, diarrhea, cholestatic jaundice.
GU: urine retention, urinary frequency.
Skin: urticaria, rash.

Overdose and treatment
Signs and symptoms of overdose may include either CNS depression (sedation, reduced mental alertness, apnea, and CV collapse) or CNS stimulation (insomnia, hallucinations, tremors, or seizures). Anticholinergic symptoms, such as dry mouth, flushed skin, fixed and dilated pupils, and GI symptoms, are common, especially in children.

Treat overdose with gastric lavage to empty stomach contents; inducing emesis with ipecac syrup may be ineffective. Treat hypotension with vasopressors, and control seizures with diazepam or phenytoin. Don't give stimulants.

Special considerations
Consider the recommendations relevant to all antihistamines as well as the following.
● Injectable cyclizine is for I.M. use only. When giving I.M., aspirate and check carefully for blood return; inadvertent I.V. administration can cause anaphylaxis.
● Injectable solution is incompatible with many drugs; check compatibility before mixing in same syringe.
● Store in a cool place; at room temperature, injection may turn slightly yellow but doesn't lose its potency.
● Cyclizine may prevent, reduce, or mask response to diagnostic skin testing. Stop cyclizine 4 days before diagnostic skin testing to avoid altered test response.

Patient monitoring
● Monitor patient for adverse effects.
● Closely monitor patients with history of heart failure when using this drug.

Breast-feeding patients
● Antihistamines such as cyclizine shouldn't be used during breast-feeding. Most appear in breast milk, exposing infant to risks of unusual ex-

citability; premature infants are at particular risk for seizures. Cyclizine also may inhibit lactation.

Pediatric patients
• Drug isn't indicated for use in children under age 6; they may experience paradoxical hyperexcitability. Safety and efficacy of I.M. administration in children haven't been established and use isn't recommended.

Geriatric patients
• Elderly patients are usually more sensitive to adverse effects of antihistamines and are more likely than younger patients to experience dizziness, sedation, hyperexcitability, dry mouth, and urine retention.

Patient education
• Instruct patient to stay in places of minimal motion (such as in middle, not front or back, of ship), avoid excessive intake of food or drink, and not to read while in motion.
• Tell patient to avoid hazardous activities requiring mental alertness until CNS reaction is determined.

cyclobenzaprine hydrochloride
Flexeril

Pharmacologic classification: tricyclic antidepressant derivative
Therapeutic classification: skeletal muscle relaxant
Pregnancy risk category: B

Indications and dosages
➤ *Adjunct in acute, painful musculoskeletal conditions. Adults:* 20 to 40 mg P.O. divided b.i.d. to q.i.d.; maximum dose is 60 mg daily. Drug shouldn't be administered for more than 2 weeks.
➤ *Fibrositis ◇. Adults:* 10 to 40 mg P.O. daily.

How supplied
Available by prescription only
Tablets: 10 mg

Pharmacodynamics
Skeletal muscle relaxant action: Cyclobenzaprine relaxes skeletal muscles through an unknown mechanism of action. Cyclobenzaprine is a CNS depressant.

Drug also potentiates the effects of norepinephrine and exhibits anticholinergic effects similar to those of tricyclic antidepressants, including central and peripheral antimuscarinic actions, sedation, and an increase in heart rate.

Pharmacokinetics
Absorption: Almost completely absorbed during first pass through GI tract.

Distribution: About 93% is plasma protein–bound.
Metabolism: During first pass through GI tract and liver, drug and metabolites undergo enterohepatic recycling. The half-life of cyclobenzaprine is 1 to 3 days.
Excretion: Excreted primarily in urine as conjugated metabolites; also excreted in feces via bile as unchanged drug.

Route	Onset	Peak	Duration
P.O.	1 hr	3-8 hr	12-24 hr

Contraindications and precautions
Contraindicated in patients who have received MAO inhibitors within 14 days; patients in acute recovery phase of MI; and patients with hyperthyroidism, hypersensitivity to drug, heart block, arrhythmias, conduction disturbances, or heart failure. Use cautiously in geriatric or debilitated patients and in those with increased intraocular pressure, glaucoma, or urine retention.

Interactions
Drug-drug. *Antidyskinetics, antimuscarinics:* Potentiated antimuscarinic effects. Use together cautiously.
CNS depressants: May potentiate CNS depression. Avoid use together.
Guanadrel, guanethidine: Decreased or blocked antihypertensive effects. Avoid use together.
MAO inhibitors: Hyperpyretic crisis, seizures, and death have occurred with concomitant administration of MAO inhibitors and tricyclics; the potential for this interaction with cyclobenzaprine also exists. Allow 14 days to elapse after stopping MAO inhibitor therapy before starting cyclobenzaprine, and allow 5 to 7 days after stopping cyclobenzaprine therapy before starting MAO inhibitor.
Drug-lifestyle. *Alcohol use:* May potentiate CNS-depressant effects when used together. Advise patient to avoid alcohol use.

Adverse reactions
CNS: *drowsiness,* headache, syncope, insomnia, fatigue, asthenia, nervousness, confusion, paresthesia, *dizziness,* depression, visual disturbances, *seizures.*
CV: tachycardia, *arrhythmias,* palpitations, hypotension, vasodilation.
EENT: blurred vision.
GI: dyspepsia, abnormal taste, constipation, nausea, *dry mouth.*
GU: urine retention, urinary frequency.
Skin: rash, urticaria, pruritus.
Other: with high doses, adverse reactions similar to those of other tricyclic antidepressants.

Overdose and treatment
Signs and symptoms of overdose include severe drowsiness, troubled breathing, syncope, seizures, tachycardia, arrhythmias, hallucinations, changes in body temperature, and vomiting.

Reactions may be *common,* uncommon, *life-threatening,* or COMMON AND LIFE-THREATENING.

To treat overdose, induce emesis or perform gastric lavage. As ordered, give 20 to 30 g activated charcoal every 4 to 6 hours for 24 to 48 hours. Take ECG and monitor cardiac functions for arrhythmias. Monitor vital signs, especially body temperature and ECG. Maintain adequate airway and fluid intake. If needed, 1 to 3 mg I.V. physostigmine may be given to combat severe life-threatening antimuscarinic effects. Provide supportive therapy for arrhythmias, cardiac failure, circulatory shock, seizures, and metabolic acidosis as necessary.

Special considerations
● Drug may cause effects and adverse reactions similar to those of other tricyclic antidepressants.
● Note that the antimuscarinic effect of the drug may inhibit salivary flow, resulting in development of dental caries, periodontal disease, oral candidiasis, and mouth discomfort.
● Drug is intended for short-term (2 or 3 weeks) treatment, because risk-benefit ratio with prolonged use isn't known. Additionally, muscle spasm accompanying acute musculoskeletal conditions is usually transient.
● Spasmolytic effect usually begins within 1 or 2 days and may be manifested by lessening of pain and tenderness and an increase in range of motion and ability to perform activities of daily living.

Patient monitoring
● Monitor patient for GI problems.
● Be alert for nausea, headache, and malaise, which may occur if drug is stopped abruptly after long-term therapy.

Pediatric patients
● Drug isn't recommended for children under age 15.

Geriatric patients
● Geriatric patients are more sensitive to the effects of the drug.

Patient education
● Warn patient about possible drowsiness and dizziness. Tell him to avoid hazardous activities that require alertness until reaction to drug is known.
● Advise patient to relieve dry mouth (anticholinergic effect) with frequent clear water rinses, extra fluid intake, or with sugarless gum or candy.
● Tell patient to report discomfort immediately.
● Advise patient to use cough and cold preparations cautiously because some products contain alcohol.
● Instruct patient to check with dentist to minimize risk of dental disease (tooth decay, fungal infections, or gum disease) if treatment lasts longer than 2 weeks.

cyclopentolate hydrochloride
AK-Pentolate, Cyclogyl, Minims Cyclopentolate*, Pentolair

Pharmacologic classification: anticholinergic
Therapeutic classification: cycloplegic, mydriatic
Pregnancy risk category: C

Indications and dosages
➤ *Diagnostic procedures requiring mydriasis and cycloplegia.* Adults: Instill 1 drop of 1% solution in eye, followed by another drop in 5 minutes, 40 to 50 minutes before procedure. Use 2% solution in heavily pigmented irises.
Children: Instill 1 drop of 0.5%, 1%, or 2% solution in each eye, followed by 1 drop of 0.5% or 1% solution in 5 minutes, if necessary, 40 to 50 minutes before procedure.

How supplied
Available by prescription only
Ophthalmic solution: 0.5%, 1%, 2%

Pharmacodynamics
Cycloplegic and mydriatic action: Anticholinergic action prevents the sphincter muscle of the iris and the muscle of the ciliary body from responding to cholinergic stimulation. This results in unopposed adrenergic influence, producing pupillary dilation (mydriasis) and paralysis of accommodation (cycloplegia).

Pharmacokinetics
Absorption: Rapid onset of action and shorter duration of action than atropine or homatropine.
Distribution: Unknown.
Metabolism: Unknown.
Excretion: Recovery from mydriasis usually occurs in about 24 hours; recovery from cycloplegia may occur in 6 to 24 hours.

Route	Onset	Peak	Duration
Oph-thalmic	Rapid	½-1¼ hr	6-24 hr

Contraindications and precautions
Contraindicated in patients hypersensitive to drug or belladonna alkaloid and in patients with glaucoma or adhesions between the iris and lens. Use cautiously in children, elderly patients, and patients with increased intraocular pressure.

Interactions
Drug-drug. *Carbachol, cholinesterase inhibitors, pilocarpine:* Interference with antiglaucoma action. Avoid use together.
Drug-lifestyle. *Sun exposure:* Photophobia may occur. Advise patient to take precautions.

Adverse reactions

CNS: irritability, confusion, somnolence, hallucinations, ataxia, *seizures,* behavioral disturbances in children.
CV: tachycardia.
EENT: eye burning on instillation, blurred vision, eye dryness, *photophobia,* ocular congestion, contact dermatitis in eye, conjunctivitis, increased intraocular pressure, transient stinging and burning, irritation, hyperemia.
GU: urine retention.
Skin: dryness.

Overdose and treatment

Signs and symptoms of overdose include flushing, warm dry skin, dry mouth, dilated pupils, delirium, hallucinations, tachycardia, bladder distention, ataxia, hypotension, respiratory depression, coma, and death.

Induce emesis or give activated charcoal. Use physostigmine to antagonize cyclopentolate's anticholinergic activity, and in severe toxicity; propranolol may be used to treat symptomatic tachyarrhythmias unresponsive to physostigmine.

Special considerations

● Superior to homatropine hydrobromide, cyclopentolate has a shorter duration of action.
● Recovery usually occurs within 24 hours; however, 1 to 2 drops of a 1% or 2% pilocarpine solution instilled into the eye may reduce recovery time to 3 to 6 hours.
● To minimize systemic absorption, apply light finger-pressure to lacrimal sac during and for 1 to 2 minutes following topical instillation especially in children and when the 2% solution is used.

Patient monitoring

● Assess patient's CNS status.

Breast-feeding patients

● No data are available; however, use drug with extreme caution in breast-feeding women because of potential for CNS and cardiopulmonary effects in infants.

Pediatric patients

● Avoid getting preparation in child's mouth while administering. Infants and young children may experience an increased sensitivity to the cardiopulmonary and CNS effects of drug. Young infants shouldn't be given solution more concentrated than 0.5%.

Geriatric patients

● Use drug cautiously in geriatric patients because undiagnosed angle-closure glaucoma may be present.

Patient education

● Warn patient that drug will cause burning sensation when instilled.

● Advise patient to protect eyes from bright light; dark glasses may reduce sensitivity.
● Teach patient to instill drug. Warn him not to touch tip of dropper to eye or surrounding tissue.

cyclophosphamide
Cytoxan, Neosar

Pharmacologic classification: alkylating agent (not specific to cell cycle phase)
Therapeutic classification: antineoplastic
Pregnancy risk category: D

Indications and dosages

Dosages and indications may vary. Check literature for recommended protocols.
➤ *Breast, head, neck, lung, and ovarian carcinoma; Hodgkin's disease; chronic lymphocytic or myelocytic and acute lymphoblastic leukemia; neuroblastoma; retinoblastoma; malignant lymphomas; multiple myeloma; mycosis fungoides; sarcomas◇; severe rheumatoid disorders◇; immunosuppression after transplants◇. Adults:* 40 to 50 mg/kg I.V. in divided doses over 2 to 5 days. Oral dosing for initial and maintenance dosage is 1 to 5 mg/kg P.O. daily.
➤ *Polymyositis◇. Adults:* 1 to 2 mg/kg P.O. daily.
➤ *Rheumatoid arthritis◇. Adults:* 1.5 to 3 mg/kg P.O. daily.
➤ *Wegener's granulomatosis◇. Adults:* 1 to 2 mg/kg P.O. daily (usually administered with prednisone).
➤ *Nephrotic syndrome in children. Children:* 2.5 to 3 mg/kg P.O. daily for 60 to 90 days.
✦ *Dosage adjustment.* Adjust dosage of cyclophosphamide in patients with renal impairment.

How supplied

Available by prescription only
Injection: 100-mg, 200-mg, 500-mg, 1-g, 2-g vials
Tablets: 25 mg, 50 mg

Pharmacodynamics

Antineoplastic action: Cytotoxic action of cyclophosphamide is mediated by its two active metabolites. These metabolites function as alkylating agents, preventing cell division by cross-linking DNA strands. This results in an imbalance of growth within the cell, leading to cell death. Cyclophosphamide also has significant immunosuppressive activity.

Pharmacokinetics

Absorption: Almost completely absorbed from the GI tract at doses of 100 mg or less. Higher doses (300 mg) are about 75% absorbed.
Distribution: Distributed throughout the body, although only minimal amounts have been found in saliva, sweat, and synovial fluid. The level in

---

CSF is too low for treatment of meningeal leukemia. The active metabolites are about 50% bound to plasma proteins.

Metabolism: Metabolized to its active form by hepatic microsomal enzymes. The activity of these metabolites is terminated by metabolism to inactive forms.

Excretion: Eliminated primarily in urine, with 15% to 30% excreted as unchanged drug. The elimination half-life ranges from 3 to 12 hours.

Route	Onset	Peak	Duration
P.O., I.V.	Unknown	Unknown	Unknown

Contraindications and precautions

Contraindicated in patients hypersensitive to drug and in those with severe bone marrow suppression. Use cautiously in patients with impaired renal or hepatic function, leukopenia, thrombocytopenia, or malignant cell infiltration of bone marrow and in those who have recently undergone radiation therapy or chemotherapy.

Interactions

Drug-drug. *Allopurinol, chloramphenicol, chloroquine, imipramine, phenothiazines, potassium iodide, vitamin A:* May inhibit cyclophosphamide metabolism. Monitor patient closely.

Barbiturates, chloral hydrate, phenytoin: Increased cyclophosphamide metabolism. Use cautiously.

Corticosteroids: Inhibited cyclophosphamide metabolism, reducing its effect. Eventual reduction of dose or discontinuation of corticosteroids may increase cyclophosphamide metabolism to a toxic level. Use with extreme caution.

Doxorubicin: Potentiated cardiotoxic effects. Avoid use together.

Succinylcholine: Prolonged respiratory distress and apnea. Use succinylcholine with caution or not at all.

Adverse reactions

CV: *cardiotoxicity* (with very high doses and with doxorubicin).

GI: anorexia, *nausea, vomiting* (within 6 hours), abdominal pain, stomatitis, mucositis.

GU: hemorrhagic cystitis, fertility impairment.

Hematologic: *leukopenia* (nadir between days 8 to 15, recovery in 17 to 28 days), *thrombocytopenia, anemia.*

Hepatic: *hepatotoxicity.*

Metabolic: increased serum uric acid levels.

Respiratory: *pulmonary fibrosis* (with high doses).

Skin: *reversible alopecia.*

Other: *secondary malignant disease, anaphylaxis, hypersensitivity reactions,* decreased serum pseudocholinesterase levels.

Overdose and treatment

Signs and symptoms of overdose include myelosuppression, alopecia, nausea, vomiting, and anorexia.

Treatment is generally supportive and includes antiemetics and transfusion of blood components. Drug is dialyzable.

Special considerations

• Follow institutional guidelines for safe preparation, administration, and disposal of chemotherapeutic drugs.

• Reconstitute vials with appropriate volume of bacteriostatic or sterile water for injection to give a concentration of 20 mg/ml.

• Reconstituted solution is stable 6 days if refrigerated or 24 hours at room temperature.

• Drug can be given by direct I.V. push into a running I.V. line or by infusion in normal saline solution or D_5W.

• I.M. injections shouldn't be given when platelet counts are low.

• Oral form should be taken with or after a meal. Higher oral doses (400 mg) may be tolerated better if divided into smaller doses.

• Administration with cold foods such as ice cream may improve toleration of oral dose.

• Push fluid (3 L daily) to prevent hemorrhagic cystitis. Some clinicians use uroprotectant agents such as mesna. Drug shouldn't be given at bedtime, because voiding afterward is too infrequent to avoid cystitis. If hemorrhagic cystitis occurs, discontinue drug. Cystitis can occur months after therapy has been discontinued.

• Reduced drug dosage is warranted if patient is also receiving corticosteroid therapy and develops viral or bacterial infections.

• Nausea and vomiting are most common with high doses of I.V. cyclophosphamide.

• Drug has been used successfully to treat many nonmalignant conditions, for example, multiple sclerosis, because of its immunosuppressive activity.

• Drug may suppress positive reaction to *Candida,* mumps, trichophytin, and tuberculin TB skin tests. A false-positive result for the Papanicolaou test may occur.

Patient monitoring

• Monitor uric acid, CBC, and renal and hepatic functions.

• Observe for hematuria and dysuria.

• Monitor for cyclophosphamide toxicity if patient's corticosteroid therapy is discontinued.

Pregnant patients

• Advise both men and women to practice contraception while taking drug and for 4 months after because drug has teratogenic properties.

Breast-feeding patients

• Drug appears in breast milk; woman should discontinue breast-feeding because of risk of serious adverse reactions, mutagenicity, and carcinogenicity in the infant.

Patient education
• Emphasize importance of continuing medication despite nausea and vomiting.
• Advise patient to report vomiting that occurs shortly after an oral dose.
• Warn patient that alopecia is likely to occur, but that it's reversible.
• Encourage adequate fluid intake to prevent hemorrhagic cystitis and to facilitate uric acid excretion.
• Tell patient to promptly report unusual bleeding or bruising.
• Advise patient to avoid individuals with infections and to call immediately if fever, chills, or signs of infection occur.

cycloserine
Seromycin

Pharmacologic classification: isoxizolidone, d-alanine analogue
Therapeutic classification: antitubercular
Pregnancy risk category: C

Indications and dosages
➤ **Adjunctive treatment in pulmonary or extrapulmonary tuberculosis.** *Adults:* Initially, 250 mg P.O. q 12 hours for 2 weeks; then, if blood levels are below 25 to 30 mcg/ml and there are no clinical signs of toxicity, dosage is increased to 250 mg P.O. q 8 hours for 2 weeks. If optimum blood levels are still not achieved, and there are no signs of clinical toxicity, then dosage is increased to 250 mg P.O. q 6 hours. Maximum dose is 1 g daily. If CNS toxicity occurs, drug is discontinued for 1 week, then resumed at 250 mg daily for 2 weeks. If no serious toxic effects occur, dosage is increased by 250-mg increments q 10 days until blood levels reach 25 to 30 mcg/ml.
Children: 10 to 20 mg/kg (maximum, 750 to 1,000 mg) P.O. daily administered in two equally divided doses.
➤ **Urinary tract infections.** *Adults:* 250 mg P.O. q 12 hours for 2 weeks.

How supplied
Available by prescription only
Capsules: 250 mg

Pharmacodynamics
Antibiotic action: Cycloserine inhibits bacterial cell utilization of amino acids, thereby inhibiting cell wall synthesis. Its action is bacteriostatic or bactericidal, depending on organism susceptibility and drug concentration at infection site. Cycloserine is active against *Mycobacterium tuberculosis, M. bovis,* and some strains of *M. kansasii, M. marinum, M. ulcerans, M. avium, M. smegmatis,* and *M. intracellulare.* It's also active against some gram-negative and gram-positive bacteria, including *Staphylococcus aureus, Enterobacter,* and *Escherichia coli.* Cycloserine is considered adjunctive therapy in tuberculosis and is combined with other antitubercular agents to prevent or delay development of drug resistance by *M. tuberculosis.*

Pharmacokinetics
Absorption: About 80% of oral dose is absorbed from the GI tract.
Distribution: Distributed widely into body tissues and fluids, including CSF. Drug crosses the placenta; it doesn't bind to plasma proteins.
Metabolism: May be metabolized partially.
Excretion: Excreted primarily in urine by glomerular filtration. Small amounts of drug are excreted in feces and breast milk. Elimination plasma half-life in adults is 10 hours. Drug is hemodialyzable.

Route	Onset	Peak	Duration
P.O.	Unknown	4-8 hr	Unknown

Contraindications and precautions
Contraindicated in patients hypersensitive to drug and in those with seizure disorders, depression or severe anxiety, psychosis, severe renal insufficiency, or excessive concurrent use of alcohol. Use cautiously in patients with impaired renal function.

Interactions
Drug-drug. *Ethionamide, isoniazid:* Increased hazard of CNS toxicity, drowsiness, and dizziness. Use with extreme caution.
Phenytoin: Inhibited phenytoin metabolism and risk of toxic blood levels. Dosage adjustment may be required.
Drug-lifestyle. *Alcohol use:* Increased risk of seizures. Discourage alcohol use.

Adverse reactions
CNS: *seizures,* drowsiness, somnolence, headache, tremor, dysarthria, vertigo, confusion, memory loss, *suicidal tendencies,* psychosis, hyperirritability, character changes, aggression, paresthesia, paresis, hyperreflexia, *coma.*
CV: *sudden-onset heart failure.*
Hepatic: elevated transaminase level.
Skin: rash.
Other: *hypersensitivity reactions* (allergic dermatitis).

Overdose and treatment
Signs and symptoms of overdose include CNS depression accompanied by dizziness, hyperreflexia, confusion, or seizures.

    Treat with gastric lavage and supportive care, including oxygen, I.V. fluids, pressor agents (for circulatory shock), and body temperature stabilization. Treat seizures with anticonvulsants and pyridoxine.

Special considerations
• Drug should be taken after meals to avoid gastric irritation.

Reactions may be *common,* uncommon, **life-threatening,** or COMMON AND LIFE-THREATENING.

- Specimens for culture and sensitivity testing will be done before first dose, but therapy can begin pending test results; repeat testing periodically to detect drug resistance.
- Pyridoxine (200 to 300 mg daily) may be used to treat or prevent neurotoxic effects.
- Anticonvulsants, tranquilizers, or sedatives may be prescribed to relieve adverse reactions.

Patient monitoring
- Monitor hematologic, renal, and liver function studies before and periodically during therapy to minimize toxicity; toxic reactions may occur at blood levels above 30 mcg/ml.
- Assess level of consciousness and neurologic function; monitor patient for personality changes and other early signs of CNS toxicity.

Breast-feeding patients
- Drug appears in breast milk; use cautiously in breast-feeding women.

Geriatric patients
- Because geriatric patients commonly have renal impairment, which decreases excretion of drugs, use drug with caution.

Patient education
- Explain rationale for long-term therapy
- Teach signs and symptoms of hypersensitivity and other adverse reactions, and emphasize need to report unusual effects and rash promptly.
- Warn patient to avoid hazardous tasks that require mental alertness because drug may cause drowsiness or dizziness.
- Advise patient to take drug after meals to avoid gastric irritation.
- Urge patient to complete entire prescribed regimen, to comply with instructions for around-the-clock dosage, and not to discontinue drug without medical approval.
- Explain importance of follow-up appointments.

cyclosporine
Neoral, Sandimmune

cyclosporine, modified
Gengraf

Pharmacologic classification: polypeptide antibiotic
Therapeutic classification: immunosuppressant
Pregnancy risk category: C

Indications and dosages
➤ **Prophylaxis of organ rejection in kidney, liver, heart, bone marrow, pancreas◇, cornea transplants◇.** *Adults and children:* 15 mg/kg P.O. daily 4 to 12 hours before transplantation. Continue daily dose postoperatively for 1 to 2 weeks. Then, gradually reduce dosage

by 5% weekly to maintenance level of 5 to 10 mg/kg daily. Or, administer an I.V. concentrate of 5 to 6 mg/kg 4 to 12 hours before transplantation.

Postoperatively, administer 5 to 6 mg/kg daily as an I.V. dilute solution infusion (50 mg per 20 to 100 ml infused over 2 to 6 hours) until patient can tolerate oral forms.

Note: Sandimmune and Neoral aren't bioequivalent and can't be used interchangeably without prescriber supervision. When converting to Neoral from Sandimmune, start with same daily dose (1:1) and follow serum trough levels frequently.
➤ **Prophylaxis of organ rejection in kidney, liver, and heart allogeneic transplants.** Gengraf. *Adults:* same intial dosage as Sandimmune.
➤ **Treatment of severe, active rheumatoid arthritis that hasn't adequately responded to methotrexate.** Gengraf. *Adults:* 2.5 mg/kg P.O. daily taken b.i.d. May be increased by 0.5 to 0.75 mg/kg daily after 8 weeks and again after 12 weeks to a maximum of 4 mg/kg daily.
➤ **Nonimmunocomprimised patients with severe, recalcitrant plaque psoriasis who have failed to respond to at least one systemic therapy or in patients for whom other systemic therapies are contraindicated or can't be tolerated.** Gengraf. *Adults:* 2.5 mg/kg P.O. daily given b.i.d for at least 4 weeks. If no improvement, increase dosage at 2-week intervals by 0.5 mg/kg daily to a maximum of 4 mg/kg daily.
➤ **Conversion from Sandimmune to Gengraf.** *Adults:* Use same daily dose as previously used on Sandimmune. Monitor blood levels every 4 to 7 days after conversion, and monitor blood pressure and serum creatinine every 2 weeks during the first 2 months.

How supplied
Available by prescription only
Capsules: 25 mg, 50 mg, 100 mg
Capsules for microemulsion: 25 mg, 100 mg
Emulsion solution: 100 mg
Injection: 50 mg/ml
Oral solution: 100 mg/ml

Pharmacodynamics
Immunosuppressant action: Exact mechanism is unknown; its action is thought to be related to the inhibition of induction of interleukin-2, which plays a role in both cellular and humoral immune responses.

Pharmacokinetics
Absorption: Absorption after oral administration varies widely between patients and in the same individual. Only 30% of an oral dose reaches systemic circulation. Neoral has a greater bioavailability than Sandimmune. Cyclosporine modified (Gengraf) has an increased bioavailability compared to non-modified, peaking in 1½ to 2 hours.

Distribution: Distributed widely outside the blood volume. About 33% to 47% is found in plasma; 4% to 9%, in leukocytes; 5% to 12%, in granulocytes; and 41% to 58%, in erythrocytes. In plasma, about 90% is bound to proteins, primarily lipoproteins. Cyclosporine crosses the placenta; cord blood levels are about 60% those of maternal blood. Cyclosporine enters breast milk.
Metabolism: Metabolized extensively in the liver.
Excretion: Primarily excreted in the feces (biliary excretion) with only 6% of drug found in urine.

Route	Onset	Peak	Duration
P.O.	Unknown	3½ hr	Unknown
I.V.	Unknown	Unknown	Unknown

Contraindications and precautions
Contraindicated in patients hypersensitive to drug or to polyoxyethylated castor oil (found in injectable form). Gengraf is contraindicated in patients with rheumatoid arthritis or psoriasis with abnormal renal function, uncontrolled hypertension, or malignancies. Psoriasis patients shouldn't receive PUVA or UVB therapy, methotrexate, other immunosuppressants, coal tar, or radiation.

Interactions
Drug-drug. *Allopurinol, bromocriptine, clarithromycin, danazol, diltiazem, erythromycin, fluconazole, itraconazole, ketoconazole, methylprednisolone, metoclopramide, nicardipine, verapamil:* Increased Gengraf levels. Monitor levels.
Aminoglycosides, amphotericin B: Increased nephrotoxicity and cyclosporine blood levels. Avoid use together.
Amphotericin B, cimetidine, diclofenac, gentamycin, ketoconazole, melphalan, naproxen, ranitidine, sulfamethoxazole/trimethoprim, sulindac, tacrolimus, tobramycin, vancomycin: May potentiate renal dysfunction when used with Gengraf. Use cautiously.
Carbamazepine, nafcillin, octreotide, phenobarbital, phenytoin, rifampin, ticlopidine: Decreased Gengraf levels. Monitor levels.
Co-trimoxazole, phenobarbital, phenytoin, rifampin: Lower plasma levels of cyclosporine. Monitor patient closely.
Digoxin, lovastatin, prednisolone: Decreased clearance of these drugs when used with Gengraf. Use cautiously.
Diltiazem, erythromycin, fluconazole, itraconazole, ketoconazole, possibly corticosteroids, verapamil: Increased plasma cyclosporine levels. Reduced dosage of cyclosporine may be necessary.
Immunosuppressants (except corticosteroids): Increased risk of malignancy (lymphoma) and susceptibility to infection. Avoid use together.
Potassium-sparing diuretics: Increased risk for hyperkalemia when used with Gengraf. Avoid use together.

Vaccines: Decreased effectiveness when given with Gengraf. Avoid use of live attenuated vaccines.
Drug-herb. *Alfalfa sprouts, astragalus, echinacea, licorice:* Possible interference with immunosuppressive effect of the drug. Discourage concomitant use.
St. John's wort: May reduce cyclosporine levels, decreasing efficacy. Discourage concurrent use.
Drug-food. *Grapefruit juice:* May increase trough levels. Discourage use together.

Adverse reactions
CNS: *tremor, headache, seizures,* confusion, paresthesia.
CV: hypertension, flushing.
EENT: *gum hyperplasia,* oral candidiasis, sinusitis.
GI: *nausea, vomiting,* diarrhea, abdominal discomfort.
GU: *nephrotoxicity.*
Hematologic: anemia, *leukopenia, thrombocytopenia,* hemolytic anemia.
Hepatic: *hepatotoxicity.*
Skin: acne, hirsutism.
Other: *anaphylaxis,* gynecomastia, increased low-density lipoprotein levels, *infections.*

Overdose and treatment
Signs and symptoms of overdose include extensions of common adverse effects. Hepatotoxicity and nephrotoxicity often accompany nausea and vomiting; tremor and seizures may occur.

Up to 2 hours after ingestion, empty stomach by induced emesis or lavage; thereafter, treat supportively. Monitor vital signs and fluid and electrolyte levels closely. Drug isn't removed by hemodialysis or charcoal hemoperfusion.

Special considerations
● Cyclosporine can cause nephrotoxicity and hepatotoxicity.
● Cyclosporine usually is prescribed with corticosteroids.
● Consider possible kidney rejection before discontinuation of drug for suspected nephrotoxicity.
● Give dose at the same time each day. Measure oral solution carefully in oral syringe and mix with plain or chocolate milk or fruit juice to improve palatability; serve in a glass to minimize drug adherence to container walls. Drug can be taken with food to minimize nausea.
● Neoral capsules and oral solution are bioequivalent. Sandimmune capsules and oral solution have decreased bioavailability compared with Neoral.
⚡ **ALERT** Gengraf and Sandimmune aren't bioequivalent and can't be interchanged. Conversion from Gengraf to Sandimmune should be done with increased monitoring to prevent underdosing.
● Gengraf is bioequivalent to and interchangeable with Neoral capsules.

Reactions may be *common,* uncommon, *life-threatening,* or COMMON AND LIFE-THREATENING.

• Psoriasis patients previously treated with PUVA, methotrexate, immunosuppressants, UVB, coal tar, or radiation therapy are at increased risk for developing skin malignancies when taking Gengraf.

• Changes in cyclosporine formulation should be made cautiously under medical supervision.

Patient monitoring

• Monitor hepatic and renal function tests routinely; hepatotoxicity may occur in first month after transplantation, but renal toxicity may be delayed for 2 to 3 months.

• **Rheumatoid arthritis patients:** Before starting treatment, measure blood pressure and creatinine levels at least twice to obtain baseline. Evaluate blood pressure and serum creatinine every 2 weeks during first 3 months, then monthly if the patient is stable. Monitor blood pressure and serum creatinine after an increase in dose of NSAIDs or introduction of a new NSAID. Monitor CBC and liver function test monthly if receiving methotrexate concomitantly. If hypertension occurs, decrease dosage of Gengraf by 25% to 50%. If hypertension persists, decrease dosage further or control blood pressure with antihypertensives.

• **Psoriasis patients:** Initially, measure blood pressure at least twice. Evaluate patient for occult infection and tumors initially and throughout treatment. Obtain baseline serum creatinine (on two occasions), CBC, BUN, serum magnesium, uric acid, potassium, and lipids. Evaluate serum creatinine and BUN every 2 weeks during first 3 months and then monthly thereafter if patient is stable. If the serum creatinine is greater than or equal to 25% above pretreatment, repeat serum creatinine within 2 weeks. If it remains greater than or equal to 25% to 50% above baseline, reduce dose by 25% to 50%. If at any time the serum creatinine is greater than or equal to 50% above baseline, reduce dosage by 25% to 50%. Discontinue if reversibility of serum creatine isn't achieved after two dosage modifications. Monitor serum creatinine after dose increase of NSAID or after initiation of new NSAID.

• Evalaute blood pressure, CBC, uric acid, potassium, lipids, and magnesium every 2 weeks for the first 3 months, then monthly if patient is stable or more frequently when dosage adjustments are made. Dosage should be reduced by 25% to 50% for an abnormality of clinical concern.

Breast-feeding patients

• Safety hasn't been established; avoid use in breast-feeding women.

Pediatric patients

• Safety and efficacy haven't been established; however, drug has been used in children as young as age 6 months. Use with caution.

Patient education

• Teach patient about rationale for therapy; explain possible adverse effects and importance of reporting them—especially fever, sore throat, mouth sores, abdominal pain, unusual bleeding or bruising, pale stools, or dark urine.

• Encourage compliance with therapy and follow-up visits.

• Teach patient how and when to take medication for optimal benefit and minimal discomfort; caution against discontinuing drug without medical approval.

• Advise patient to improve palatability of oral solution by diluting with room temperature milk, chocolate milk, or orange juice. Don't take Neoral with grapefruit juice or food.

• Tell patient not to rinse syringe with water.

• Warn patient to wear protection when in the sun and to avoid excessive sun exposure.

• Advise patient of the potential risk during pregnancy and the increased risk of neoplasia, hypertension, and renal dysfunction.

• Warn patient that during the use of cyclosporine, vaccination may be less effective.

• Tell patient to take Gengraf on a consistent schedule with regard to time of day and relation to meals.

cyproheptadine hydrochloride
Periactin

Pharmacologic classification: piperidine-derivative antihistamine
Therapeutic classification: antihistamine (H_1-receptor antagonist), antipruritic
Pregnancy risk category: B

Indications and dosages

➤ *Allergy symptoms, pruritus, cold urticaria, allergic conjunctivitis, appetite stimulant, vascular cluster headaches.*
Adults: 4 mg P.O. t.i.d. or q.i.d. Maximum dose is 0.5 mg/kg daily.
Children ages 7 to 14: 4 mg P.O. b.i.d. or t.i.d. Maximum dose is 16 mg daily.
Children ages 2 to 6: 2 mg P.O. b.i.d. or t.i.d. Maximum dose is 12 mg daily.
➤ *Cushing's syndrome◇. Adults:* 8 to 24 mg P.O. daily in divided doses.

How supplied

Available by prescription only
Syrup: 2 mg/5 ml
Tablets: 4 mg

Pharmacodynamics

Antihistamine action: Antihistamines compete with histamine for H_1-receptor sites on smooth muscle of the bronchi, GI tract, uterus, and large blood vessels; they bind to cellular receptors, preventing access of histamine, thereby suppressing histamine-induced allergic symptoms.

They don't directly alter histamine or its release. Drug also displays significant anticholinergic and antiserotonin activity.

Pharmacokinetics
Absorption: Well absorbed from the GI tract.
Distribution: Unknown.
Metabolism: Appears to be almost completely metabolized in the liver.
Excretion: Drug's metabolites are excreted primarily in urine; unchanged drug isn't excreted in urine. Small amounts of unchanged cyproheptadine and metabolites are excreted in feces.

Route	Onset	Peak	Duration
P.O.	15-60 min	6-9 hr	Unknown

Contraindications and precautions
Contraindicated in patients hypersensitive to drug or other drugs of similar chemical structure; in those with acute asthma, angle-closure glaucoma, stenosing peptic ulcer, symptomatic prostatic hyperplasia, bladder neck obstruction, and pyloroduodenal obstruction; in concurrent therapy with MAO inhibitors; in neonates or premature infants; in geriatric or debilitated patients; and in breast-feeding women.

Use cautiously in patients with increased intraocular pressure, hyperthyroidism, CV disease, hypertension, or bronchial asthma.

Interactions
Drug-drug. *CNS depressants:* Additive sedative effects. Avoid use together.
MAO inhibitors: Prolonged and intensified central depressant and anticholinergic effects. Avoid use together.
Thyrotropin-releasing hormone: Serum amylase and prolactin levels may be increased. Monitor patient closely.
Drug-lifestyle. *Alcohol use:* Additive sedative effects. Discourage alcohol use.
Sun exposure: Photosensitivity reactions may occur. Advise patient to take precautions.

Adverse reactions
CNS: *drowsiness,* dizziness, headache, fatigue, sedation, sleepiness, incoordination, confusion, restlessness, insomnia, nervousness, tremor, *seizures,* toxic psychosis.
CV: hypotension, palpitations, tachycardia.
GI: nausea, vomiting, epigastric distress, *dry mouth,* diarrhea, constipation.
GU: urine retention, urinary frequency.
Hematologic: hemolytic anemia, *leukopenia, agranulocytosis, thrombocytopenia.*
Metabolic: weight gain.
Skin: rash, urticaria, photosensitivity.
Other: *anaphylaxis.*

Overdose and treatment
Signs and symptoms of overdose may include either CNS depression (sedation, reduced mental alertness, apnea, and CV collapse) or CNS

stimulation (insomnia, hallucinations, tremors, or seizures). Anticholinergic symptoms, such as dry mouth, flushed skin, fixed and dilated pupils, and GI symptoms, are common, especially in children.

Treat overdose by inducing emesis with ipecac syrup (in conscious patient), followed by activated charcoal to reduce further drug absorption. Use gastric lavage if patient is unconscious or ipecac fails. Treat hypotension with vasopressors, and control seizures with diazepam and phenytoin. Don't give stimulants.

Special considerations
Consider the recommendations relevant to all antihistamines as well as the following.
● Drug also has been used experimentally to stimulate appetite and increase weight gain in children.
● In some patients, sedative effect disappears within 3 or 4 days.
● Discontinue drug 4 days before diagnostic skin tests. Antihistamines can prevent, reduce, or mask positive skin test response.

Patient monitoring
● Drug can cause weight gain. Monitor patient's weight.
● Assess patient's CNS status.

Breast-feeding patients
● Antihistamines such as cyproheptadine shouldn't be used during breast-feeding. Many of these drugs appear in breast milk, exposing the infant to risks of unusual excitability; premature infants are at particular risk for seizures.

Pediatric patients
● CNS stimulation (agitation, confusion, tremors, hallucinations) is more common in children and may require dosage reduction. Drug isn't indicated for use in newborn or premature infants.

Geriatric patients
● Geriatric patients are more susceptible to the sedative effect of drug. Instruct patient to change positions slowly and gradually. Geriatric patients may experience dizziness or hypotension more readily than younger patients.

Patient education
● Inform patient about potential adverse reactions.
● Tell patient that GI distress can be reduced by taking drug with food or milk.
● Instruct patient to report if tolerance to drug develops, because a different antihistamine may need to be prescribed.

Reactions may be *common,* uncommon, *life-threatening,* or COMMON AND LIFE-THREATENING.

cytarabine (ara-C, cytosine arabinoside)
Cytosar-U

Pharmacologic classification: antimetabolite (specific to S phase of cell cycle)
Therapeutic classification: antineoplastic
Pregnancy risk category: D

Indications and dosages
Dosages and indications may vary. Check literature for recommended protocols.
►*Acute myelocytic and other acute leukemias.* Adults and children: 200 mg/m² I.V. daily by continuous I.V. infusion for 5 days at about 2-week intervals for remission induction. Or, 30 mg/m² intrathecally (range, 5 to 75 mg/m²) q 4 days until CSF findings are normal; then followed by one additional dose. Dosages up to 3 g/m² q 12 hours for up to 12 doses have been given by continuous infusion for refractory acute leukemias.

How supplied
Available by prescription only
Injection: 100-mg, 500-mg, 1-g, 2-g vials; 20 mg/ml (100 mg); 20 mg/ml pharmacy bulk package (1g)

Pharmacodynamics
Antineoplastic action: Cytarabine requires conversion to its active metabolite within the cell. This metabolite acts as a competitive inhibitor of the enzyme DNA polymerase, disrupting the normal synthesis of DNA.

Pharmacokinetics
Absorption: Poorly absorbed (less than 20%) across the GI tract because of rapid deactivation in the gut lumen. After I.M. or S.C. administration, peak plasma levels are less than after I.V. administration.
Distribution: Rapidly distributed widely through the body. About 13% of the drug is bound to plasma proteins. Drug penetrates the blood-brain barrier only slightly after a rapid I.V. dose; however, when administered by continuous I.V. infusion, CSF levels achieve a level 40% to 60% of that of plasma levels.
Metabolism: Metabolized primarily in the liver but also in the kidneys, GI mucosa, and granulocytes.
Excretion: Biphasic elimination of drug, with an initial half-life of 8 minutes and a terminal phase half-life of 1 to 3 hours. Cytarabine and its metabolites are excreted in urine. Less than 10% of a dose is excreted as unchanged drug in urine.

Route	Onset	Peak	Duration
I.V., intra-thecal	Unknown	Unknown	Unknown
S.C.	Unknown	20-60 min	Unknown

Contraindications and precautions
Contraindicated in patients hypersensitive to drug. Use cautiously in patients with impaired hepatic function.

Interactions
Drug-drug. *Digoxin*: Combination chemotherapy (including cytarabine) may decrease digoxin absorption even several days after chemotherapy stops. Digoxin capsules and digitoxin don't appear to be affected. Patient effect and serum digoxin levels must be evaluated.
Gentamicin: Antagonized gentamicin activity. Use cautiously.
Methotrexate: Decreased cellular uptake of methotrexate, reducing its effectiveness. Avoid use together.

Adverse reactions
CNS: neurotoxicity, malaise, dizziness, headache.
CV: edema, thrombophlebitis.
EENT: conjunctivitis.
GI: *nausea, vomiting,* diarrhea, anorexia, anal ulcer, abdominal pain, oral ulcers in 5 to 10 days, projectile vomiting from large I.V. dose given rapidly.
GU: renal dysfunction.
Hematologic: *leukopenia,* with initial WBC count nadir 7 to 9 days after drug is stopped and a second (more severe) nadir 15 to 24 days after drug is stopped; anemia; reticulocytopenia; *thrombocytopenia,* with platelet count nadir occurring between days 12 to 15; *megaloblastosis.*
Hepatic: *hepatotoxicity* (usually mild and reversible), jaundice.
Metabolic: hyperuricemia.
Musculoskeletal: myalgia, bone pain.
Skin: rash, pruritus.
Other: flu syndrome, infection, fever, *anaphylaxis.*

Overdose and treatment
Signs and symptoms of overdose include myelosuppression, nausea, vomiting, and megaloblastosis. Treatment is usually supportive and includes transfusion of blood components and antiemetics.

Special considerations
• To reconstitute the 100-mg vial for I.V. administration, use 5 ml bacteriostatic water for injection (20 mg/ml); for the 500-mg vial, use 10 ml bacteriostatic water for injection (50 mg/ml).
• Drug may be further diluted with D₅W or normal saline solution for continuous I.V. infusion.
• For intrathecal injection, dilute drug in 5 to 15 ml of lactated Ringer's solution, Elliot's B solution, or normal saline solution with no preservative, and administer after withdrawing an equivalent volume of CSF.
• Don't reconstitute drug with bacteriostatic diluent for intrathecal administration because the

preservative, benzyl alcohol, has been linked to a higher risk of neurologic toxicity.
• Reconstituted solutions are stable for 48 hours at room temperature. Infusion solutions up to a concentration of 5 mg/ml are stable for 7 days at room temperature. Discard cloudy reconstituted solution.
• Dose modification may be required in thrombocytopenia, leukopenia, renal or hepatic disease, and after other chemotherapy or radiation therapy.
• Excellent mouth care can help prevent adverse oral reactions.
• Nausea and vomiting are more frequent when large doses are administered rapidly by I.V. push. These reactions are less frequent with infusion. To reduce nausea, give antiemetic before administering.
• Corticosteroid eyedrops (dexamethasone) may be prescribed to prevent drug-induced keratitis.
• Avoid I.M. injections of any drugs in patient with severely depressed platelet count (thrombocytopenia) to prevent bleeding.
• Pyridoxine supplements may be administered to prevent neuropathies; however, prophylactic use of pyridoxine may not prevent cytarabine neurotoxicity.

Patient monitoring
• Watch for signs of infection (cough, fever, sore throat). Monitor CBC.
• Monitor intake and output carefully. Maintain high fluid intake and give allopurinol, if ordered, to avoid urate nephropathy in leukemia induction therapy. Monitor uric acid and plasma digoxin levels.
• Monitor hepatic function.
• Monitor patients receiving high doses for cerebellar dysfunction.

Pregnant patients
• Caution women of childbearing age to avoid becoming pregnant during therapy and to consult with prescriber before becoming pregnant. Drug may harm fetus.

Breast-feeding patients
• It isn't known if drug appears in breast milk. However, because of the risk of serious adverse reactions, mutagenicity, and carcinogenicity in the infant, breast-feeding isn't recommended.

Patient education
• Encourage adequate fluid intake to increase urine output and facilitate excretion of uric acid.
• Advise patient to avoid exposure to people with infections. Tell him to call prescriber immediately if signs of infection or unusual bleeding occurs.

cytomegalovirus immune globulin intravenous, human, (CMV-IGIV)
CytoGam

Pharmacologic classification: immune globulin
Therapeutic classification: immune serum
Pregnancy risk category: C

Indications and dosages
➤ **To attenuate primary cytomegalovirus (CMV) disease in seronegative kidney transplant recipients who receive a kidney from a CMV-seropositive donor.** *Adults:* Maximum total dosage per infusion is 150 mg/kg I.V. administered as follows:
Within 72 hours of transplant: 150 mg/kg
2 weeks posttransplant: 100 mg/kg
4 weeks posttransplant: 100 mg/kg
6 weeks posttransplant: 100 mg/kg
8 weeks posttransplant: 100 mg/kg
12 weeks posttransplant: 50 mg/kg
16 weeks posttransplant: 50 mg/kg.
Administer initial dose I.V. at 15 mg/kg/hour. If no adverse reactions occur after 30 minutes, increase to 30 mg/kg/hour. If no adverse reactions occur after a subsequent 30 minutes, infusion may be increased to 60 mg/kg/hour. Volume shouldn't exceed 75 ml/hour. Subsequent doses may be administered at 15 mg/kg/hour for 15 minutes, increasing as with initial dose at 15-minute intervals, if no adverse reactions occur to a maximum rate of 60 mg/kg/hour.
➤ **Prophylaxis of CMV disease related to lung, liver, pancreas, and heart transplants.** *Adults:* Used with ganciclovir in organ transplants from CMV seropositive donors into seronegative recipients. Maximum total dosage per infusion is 150 mg/kg I.V. administered as follows:
Within 72 hours of transplant: 150 mg/kg
2 weeks posttransplant: 150 mg/kg
4 weeks posttransplant: 150 mg/kg
6 weeks posttransplant: 150 mg/kg
8 weeks posttransplant: 150 mg/kg
12 weeks posttransplant: 100 mg/kg
16 weeks posttransplant: 100 mg/kg.
Administer initial dose at 15 mg/kg/hour. If no adverse reactions occur after 30 minutes, increase to 30 mg/kg/hour. If no adverse reactions occur after a subsequent 30 minutes, infusion may be increased to 60 mg/kg/hour (volume shouldn't exceed 75 ml/hour). Subsequent doses may be given at 15 mg/kg/hour for 15 minutes, increasing every 15 minutes in a stepwise fashion to a maximum rate of 60 mg/kg/hour (volume shouldn't exceed 75 ml/hour). Monitor patient closely during and after each rate change.

How supplied
Available by prescription only
Injection: 2.5 g as lyophilized powder with 50 ml sterile water (diluent supplied)

Pharmacodynamics
Immune action: Contains a relatively high concentration of immunoglobulin G (IgG) antibodies against CMV and can raise relevant antibodies in CMV-exposed patients to levels sufficient to attenuate or reduce the risk of serious CMV disease.

Pharmacokinetics
Absorption: Administered I.V.
Distribution: No information available; other immune globulins are distributed between intravascular and extravascular spaces.
Metabolism: No information available.
Excretion: No information available.

Route	Onset	Peak	Duration
I.V.	Unknown	Unknown	Unknown

Contraindications and precautions
Contraindicated in patients with sensitivity to other human immunoglobulin preparations or with selective immunoglobulin A (IgA) deficiency. An aseptic meningitis syndrome (AMS) has been reported infrequently with IGIV treatment. Syndrome usually begins within several hours to 2 days following IGIV treatment. Characterized by severe headache, nuchal rigidity, drowsiness, fever, photophobia, painful eye movements, nausea, and vomiting.

CSF studies are frequently positive with pleocytosis up to several thousand cells per cubic millimeter, predominately from the granulocytic series, and elevated protein levels up to several hundred mg/dl. Patients exhibiting signs and symptoms should receive a thorough neurological examination (including CSF studies) to rule out other causes of meningitis. Ending IGIV treatment has resulted in remission of AMS within several days without sequelae.

Interactions
Drug-drug. *Live-virus vaccines:* Potential for interference with the immune response to live virus vaccines; vaccination should be deferred for at least 3 months after CMV immune globulin administration.

Adverse reactions
CV: hypotension, flushing.
GI: nausea, vomiting.
Musculoskeletal: muscle cramps, back pain.
Respiratory: wheezing.
Other: *anaphylaxis,* chills, fever.

Overdose and treatment
Presumed major signs and symptoms of overdose would be related to volume overload.

If anaphylaxis or drop in blood pressure occurs, stop infusion and administer supportive therapy, including drugs such as diphenhydramine and epinephrine.

Special considerations
• CMV immune globulin provides passive immunity.
• Infusion should begin within 6 hours and finish within 12 hours of reconstitution.
• Administer through a separate I.V. line using a constant infusion pump. Filters aren't necessary.
• If unable to administer through separate line, piggyback into line of saline solution or one of the following dextrose solutions with or without saline solution: $D_{2.5}W$, D_5W, $D_{10}W$, or $D_{20}W$. Don't dilute more than 1:2 with any of the above solutions.
• Reconstitute drug as follows: Remove tab portion of vial cap and clean rubber stopper with 70% alcohol or equivalent. Add 50 ml sterile water for injection. Don't shake vial; avoid foaming. After adding water, release residual vacuum in vial to hasten dissolving process. Rotate vial gently to wet all undissolved powder. Allow 30 minutes for powder to dissolve before administration. Inspect vial for clarity and particles.
• Store drug in refrigerator at 35.6° to 46.4° F (2° to 8° C).

Patient monitoring
• Monitor vital signs before infusion, midway through infusion, after infusion, and before increase in infusion rate.
• Monitor patient closely during each change of infusion rate.

Pregnant patients
• It isn't known whether CMV-IGIV can cause fetal harm when given during pregnancy. Use during pregnancy only if necessary.

Breast feeding patients
• It isn't known whether CMV-IGIV appears in breast milk or whether transmission to a nursing infant poses any risk.

Pediatric patients
• CMV-IGIV has been used in neonates and children in clinical trials.

Patient education
• Inform patient of potential adverse reactions.

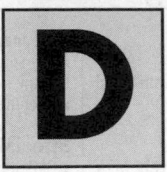

dacarbazine (DTIC)
DTIC-Dome

Pharmacologic classification: alkylating agent
(not specific to cell cycle)
Therapeutic classification: antineoplastic
Pregnancy risk category: C

Indications and dosages
Dosage and indications may vary. Check current
literature for recommended protocols.
➤**Metastatic malignant melanoma.**
Adults: 2 to 4.5 mg/kg I.V. daily for 10 days, then
repeat q 4 weeks as tolerated; or 250 mg/m² I.V.
daily for 5 days, repeated at 3-week intervals.
➤**Hodgkin's disease.** *Adults:* 150 mg/m² I.V.
(with other agents) for 5 days, repeat q 4 weeks;
or 375 mg/m² on day 1 of a combination regimen, repeated q 15 days.
✦ **Dosage adjustment.** Reduce dosage when
giving repeated doses to patients with severely
impaired renal function. Use lower dose if renal
function or bone marrow is impaired.

How supplied
Available by prescription only
Injection: 100 mg, 200 mg

Pharmacodynamics
Antineoplastic action: Three mechanisms have
been proposed to explain the cytotoxicity of dacarbazine: alkylation, in which DNA and RNA synthesis are inhibited; antimetabolite activity as a
false precursor for purine synthesis; and binding with protein sulfhydryl groups.

Pharmacokinetics
Absorption: Administered I.V.
Distribution: Believed to localize in body tissues, especially the liver. It crosses the blood-brain barrier to a limited extent and is minimally
bound to plasma proteins.
Metabolism: Rapidly metabolized in the liver to
several compounds, some of which may be active.
Excretion: Eliminated in a biphasic manner, with
an initial phase half-life of 19 minutes and terminal phase of 5 hours in patients with normal
renal and hepatic function. About 30% to 45%
of a dose is excreted unchanged in urine.

Route	Onset	Peak	Duration
I.V.	Unknown	Unknown	Unknown

Contraindications and precautions
Contraindicated in patients hypersensitive to drug.
Use cautiously in patients with impaired bone
marrow function.

Interactions
Drug-drug. *Amphotericin B:* Increased risk of
nephrotoxicity. Monitor patient carefully.
Anticoagulants, aspirin: Increased risk of bleeding. Avoid use together.
Bone marrow suppressants: Additive toxicity.
Monitor patient carefully.
Phenobarbital, phenytoin: Increased risk of toxicity. Monitor patient carefully.
Drug-lifestyle. *Sun exposure:* Photosensitivity
reactions may occur, especially during the first
2 days of therapy. Advise patient to take precautions.

Adverse reactions
CNS: facial paresthesia.
GI: *severe nausea and vomiting, anorexia.*
GU: increased serum BUN level.
Hematologic: *leukopenia, thrombocytopenia.*
Hepatic: transient increase in liver enzyme levels.
Skin: phototoxicity, rash, facial flushing, alopecia.
Other: *flu syndrome* (fever, malaise, myalgia
beginning 7 days after treatment ends and lasting possibly 7 to 21 days), *anaphylaxis*, severe pain (if I.V. solution infiltrates or if solution
is too concentrated), tissue damage.

Overdose and treatment
Signs and symptoms of overdose include myelo-suppression and diarrhea.
Treatment is supportive and includes trans-fusion of blood components and monitoring of
hematologic parameters.

Special considerations
● Follow all procedures for safe handling, administration, and disposal of chemotherapeutic
drugs.
● To reconstitute drug for I.V. administration, use
a volume of sterile water for injection that yields
10 mg/ml (9.9 ml for 100-mg vial, 19.7 ml for
200-mg vial).
● Drug may be diluted further with D_5W or normal saline solution to a volume of 100 to 200 ml
for I.V. infusion over 30 minutes. Increase volume or slow the infusion to decrease pain at infusion site.
● Drug may be administered by I.V. push over 1
to 2 minutes.

Reactions may be *common*, uncommon, *life-threatening*, or COMMON AND LIFE-THREATENING.

• A change in solution color from ivory to pink indicates some drug degradation. During infusion, protect solution from light to avoid possible drug breakdown.

• Treating extravasation with hot packs may relieve burning, local pain, and irritation.

• Discard refrigerated solution after 72 hours and room temperature solution after 8 hours.

• Nausea and vomiting may be minimized by administering dacarbazine by I.V. infusion and by hydrating patient 4 to 6 hours before therapy.

• Avoid all I.M. injections when platelet count is less than 100,000/mm³.

Patient monitoring
• Monitor uric acid levels.

• Monitor CBC. Stop drug if WBC count reaches 3,000/mm³ or platelet count reaches 100,000/mm³.

• Monitor daily temperature. Observe patient for signs and symptoms of infection.

Pregnant patients
• Counsel patient to avoid pregnancy. Advise her to inform prescriber immediately if she suspects she's pregnant.

Breast-feeding patients
• It isn't known whether drug appears in breast milk. However, because of risk of serious adverse reactions, mutagenicity, and carcinogenicity in the infant, breast-feeding isn't recommended during therapy.

Patient education
• Instruct patient to avoid contact with people who have infections and to report signs and symptoms of infection or unusual bleeding immediately.

• Reassure patient that hair growth should resume 4 to 8 weeks after treatment has ended, but hair is usually of a different texture and its color will be lost as therapy continues.

• Reassure patient that flu syndrome may be treated with mild antipyretics such as acetaminophen.

• Teach the patient the signs and symptoms of bleeding, and instruct him to report them promptly.

---

daclizumab
Zenapax

Pharmacologic classification: humanized immunoglobulin G1 monoclonal antibody
Therapeutic classification: immunosuppressive agent
Pregnancy risk category: C

Indications and dosages
➤ **Prophylaxis of acute organ rejection in patients receiving renal transplants.**
Adults: 1 mg/kg in 50 ml normal saline solution I.V., given over 15 minutes via a central or pe-

ripheral line. The standard course of therapy is five doses. Administer first dose no more than 24 hours before transplantation; remaining four doses are given at 14-day intervals. Drug is used as part of an immunosuppressive regimen that includes corticosteroids and cyclosporine.

How supplied
Available by prescription only
Injection (for I.V. use): 25 mg/5 ml

Pharmacodynamics
Immunosuppressive action: An interleukin (IL)-2 receptor antagonist that binds to the 1-alpha Tac subunit of the IL-2 receptor complex and inhibits IL-2 binding. This effect prevents IL-2 mediated activation of lymphocytes, a critical pathway in the cellular immune response against allografts. Once in circulation, drug impairs the response of the immune system to antigenic challenges. Following drug administration, the Tac subunit of the IL-2 receptor is saturated for about 120 days post-transplant.

Pharmacokinetics
Absorption: Serum levels increase between first and fifth doses.
Distribution: Unknown.
Metabolism: Unknown, but given a known relationship between body weight and systemic clearance, dosing is based on mg/kg.
Excretion: Estimated terminal elimination half-life is 20 days (480 hours).

Route	Onset	Peak	Duration
I.V.	Unknown	Unknown	Unknown

Contraindications and precautions
Contraindicated in patients hypersensitive to drug or its components. It isn't known whether drug has a long-term effect on the immune response to antigens first encountered during therapy. Readministration of drug after initial course of treatment hasn't been studied. The possible risks of prolonged immunosuppression, anaphylaxis, or anaphylactoid reactions haven't been identified.

Interactions
None reported.

Adverse reactions
CNS: *tremor, headache, dizziness, insomnia,* generalized weakness, prickly sensation, *fever, pain, fatigue,* depression, anxiety.
CV: tachycardia, hypertension, **pulmonary edema,** hypotension, aggravated hypertension, edema, fluid overload, chest pain.
EENT: blurred vision, pharyngitis, rhinitis.
GI: constipation, nausea, diarrhea, vomiting, abdominal pain, dyspepsia, pyrosis, abdominal distention, epigastric pain, flatulence, gastritis, hemorrhoids.
GU: *oliguria,* dysuria, **renal tubular necrosis, renal damage,** urine retention, hydro-

---

nephrosis, urinary tract bleeding, urinary tract disorder, *renal insufficiency*.
Hematologic: *lymphocele*.
Metabolic: diabetes mellitus, dehydration.
Musculoskeletal: *musculoskeletal or back pain,* arthralgia, myalgia, leg cramps.
Respiratory: dyspnea, cough, atelectasis, congestion, *hypoxia,* rales, abnormal breath sounds, pleural effusion.
Skin: *acne, impaired wound healing without infection,* pruritus, hirsutism, rash, night sweats, increased sweating.
Other: *posttraumatic pain,* shivering, extremity edema.

Overdose and treatment
No information available. Maximum tolerated dosage hasn't been determined. Doses up to 1.5 mg/kg have been administered to bone marrow transplant recipients without adverse effects.

Special considerations
● Only clinicians experienced in immunosuppressive therapy, management, and follow up of organ transplant patients should use drug. Patients receiving drug should be managed in facilities equipped and staffed with adequate laboratory and supportive medical care.
● Drug isn't for direct injection. Dilute in 50 ml of sterile normal saline solution before administration. To avoid foaming, don't shake. Inspect for particulates or discoloration before use. If there are particulates or discoloration, don't use.
● Administer over 15 minutes via a central or peripheral line. Don't add to or infuse other drugs simultaneously through the same I.V. line.
● Drug may be refrigerated at 36° to 46° F (2° to 8° C) for 24 hours, and is stable at room temperature for 4 hours. Discard solution if not used within 24 hours.

Patient monitoring
● Monitor patient for response.
● Monitor patient for adverse effects.
● Lipoproliferative disorders and opportunistic infections were no more common when compared with placebo in clinical trials. However, patients undergoing immunosuppressive therapy are at increased risk; monitor them carefully.

Breast-feeding patients
● It isn't known whether drug appears in breast milk. Because of risks, either the drug or breast-feeding should be discontinued.

Pediatric patients
● No adequate or well-controlled clinical trial exists involving children. The immune response to vaccines, infection, or other antigenic stimuli during or after therapy is unknown.

Geriatric patients
● Use drug cautiously in elderly patients.

Patient education
● Tell patient to consult prescriber before taking other medications during drug therapy.
● Advise patient to practice infection prevention measures.
● Inform patient that neither he nor any household member should receive vaccinations unless medically approved.
● Tell patient to immediately report wounds that fail to heal, unusual bruising or bleeding, or fever.
● Urge patient to drink plenty of fluids during drug therapy and to report painful urination, blood in the urine, or a decreased urine volume.

dactinomycin (actinomycin D)
Cosmegen

Pharmacologic classification: antibiotic antineoplastic (not specific to cell cycle phase)
Therapeutic classification: antineoplastic
Pregnancy risk category: C

Indications and dosages
Dosage and indications may vary. Check current literature for recommended protocols.
➤ *Uterine cancer, testicular cancer, Wilms' tumor, rhabdomyosarcoma, Ewing's sarcoma, sarcoma botryoides, Kaposi's sarcoma ◇, acute organ (kidney or heart) rejection ◇, malignant melanoma ◇, acute lymphocytic leukemia ◇, advanced tumors of breast or ovary ◇, Paget's disease of bone ◇. Adults:* 500 mcg (0.5 mg) I.V. daily for a maximum of 5 days. Maximum dose is 15 mcg/kg/day or 400 to 600 mcg/m²/day for 5 days. After bone marrow recovery, course may be repeated.
Children: 15 mcg/kg (0.015 mg/kg) I.V. daily for a maximum of 5 days. Or, give a total dosage of 2,500 mcg/m² I.V. over a 1-week period. Maximum dose is 15 mcg/kg/day or 400 to 600 mcg/m²/day. After bone marrow recovery, course may be repeated.
    For isolation-perfusion, use 50 mcg/kg for leg or pelvis; 35 mcg/kg for arm. Dose should be based on body surface area in obese or edematous patients.

How supplied
Available by prescription only
Injection: 500-mcg vial

Pharmacodynamics
Antineoplastic action: Dactinomycin exerts its cytotoxic activity by intercalating between DNA base pairs and uncoiling the DNA helix. The result is inhibition of DNA synthesis and DNA-dependent RNA synthesis.

Pharmacokinetics
Absorption: Administered I.V.

Distribution: Widely distributed into body tissues, with highest levels found in the bone marrow and nucleated cells. Drug doesn't cross the blood-brain barrier to a significant extent.
Metabolism: Only minimally metabolized in the liver.
Excretion: Excreted in the urine and bile. Plasma elimination half-life of drug is 36 hours.

Route	Onset	Peak	Duration
I.V.	Unknown	Unknown	Unknown

Contraindications and precautions
Contraindicated in patients with chickenpox or herpes zoster.

Interactions
Drug-drug. *Bone marrow suppressants*: May cause additive toxicity. Monitor patient closely.
Vitamin K derivatives: Decreased drug effectiveness. Monitor patient closely.

Adverse reactions
CNS: malaise, fatigue, lethargy.
GI: *anorexia, nausea, vomiting,* abdominal pain, diarrhea, *stomatitis,* ulceration, proctitis.
Hematologic: *anemia, leukopenia, thrombocytopenia, pancytopenia, aplastic anemia, agranulocytosis.*
Hepatic: *hepatotoxicity.*
Metabolic: increased blood and urine levels of uric acid, hypocalcemia.
Musculoskeletal: myalgia.
Skin: *erythema,* desquamation; *hyperpigmentation of skin,* especially in previously irradiated areas; *acnelike eruptions;* reversible alopecia.
Other: phlebitis and severe damage to soft tissue at injection site, fever.

Overdose and treatment
Signs and symptoms of overdose include myelosuppression, nausea, vomiting, glossitis, and oral ulceration.
   Treatment is generally supportive and includes antiemetics and transfusion of blood components.

Special considerations
• To reduce nausea, give an antiemetic before administering. Nausea usually occurs within 30 minutes of a dose.
• Use body surface area calculation in obese or edematous patients.
• Use gloves when preparing and administering this drug.
• To reconstitute for I.V. administration, add 1.1 ml of preservative-free sterile water for injection to drug to yield 0.5 mg/ml. Don't use a preserved diluent, because precipitation may occur.
• Drug may be diluted further with D_5W or normal saline solution for administration by I.V. infusion.
• Discard unused solution because it doesn't contain preservatives.

• Drug may be administered by I.V. push injection into the tubing of a freely flowing I.V. infusion. Don't administer through an in-line I.V. filter.
• Drug is a vesicant; treatment of extravasation includes topical administration of dimethyl sulfoxide and cold compresses.
• Patients who have received other cytotoxic drugs or radiation within 6 weeks of dactinomycin may exhibit erythema followed by hyperpigmentation, edema, or both; desquamation; vesiculation; and, rarely, necrosis.

Patient monitoring
• Monitor CBC daily and platelet counts every third day. Leukocyte and platelet nadirs usually occur 14 to 21 days after completion of course of therapy. Observe for signs of bleeding.
• Monitor renal and hepatic functions.

Breast-feeding patients
• It isn't known whether drug appears in breast milk. However, because of risks of serious adverse reactions, mutagenicity, and carcinogenicity in infants, breast-feeding isn't recommended.

Pediatric patients
• Restrict use of drug in infants age 6 months or younger; adverse reactions are more frequent in infants under age 6 months.

Patient education
• Advise patient to avoid exposure to people with infections.
• Warn patient that alopecia may occur but is usually reversible.
• Tell patient to report sore throat, fever, or signs of bleeding promptly.

dalteparin sodium
Fragmin

Pharmacologic classification: low-molecular-weight heparin derivative
Therapeutic classification: anticoagulant
Pregnancy risk category: B

Indications and dosages
➤ *Prophylaxis against deep vein thrombosis (DVT) in patients undergoing abdominal surgery who are at risk for thromboembolic complications (including those who are over age 40, obese, undergoing general anesthesia lasting longer than 30 minutes, and with history of DVT or pulmonary embolism). Adults:* 2,500 IU S.C. daily, starting 1 to 2 hours before surgery and repeated once daily for 5 to 10 days postoperatively. In abdominal surgery patients at high risk for thromboembolic complications (such as those with malignant disease), 5,000 IU S.C. daily starting on the evening before surgery and repeated once daily for 5 to 10 days postoperatively. Or, 2500 IU S.C. within 1 to 2 hours

before surgery, followed 12 hours later by a second dose of 2,500 IU S.C. and then 5,000 IU S.C. once daily for 5 to 10 days postoperatively.

➤ *Prophylaxis of DVT in patients undergoing hip replacement surgery. Adults:* 2,500 IU S.C. within 2 hours before surgery and second dose 2,500 IU S.C. in the evening of surgery (at least 6 hours after first dose). If surgery is performed in the evening, omit second dose on day of surgery. Starting on first postoperative day, administer 5,000 IU S.C. once daily for 5 to 10 days. Or, 5,000 IU S.C. on the evening before surgery, followed by 5,000 IU S.C. once daily starting in the evening of surgery for 5 to 10 days postoperatively.

How supplied

Available by prescription only

Injection: 2,500 anti-factor Xa IU/0.2 ml, 5,000 anti-factor Xa IU/0.2 ml

Pharmacodynamics

Anticoagulant action: Drug acts by enhancing the inhibition of factor Xa and thrombin by antithrombin.

Pharmacokinetics

Absorption: Absolute bioavailability measured in anti-factor Xa activity is about 87%.

Distribution: Volume of distribution for dalteparin anti-factor Xa activity is 40 to 60 ml/kg.

Metabolism: Unknown.

Excretion: Unknown.

Route	Onset	Peak	Duration
S.C.	Unknown	4 hr	Unknown

Contraindications and precautions

Contraindicated in patients hypersensitive to drug, heparin, or pork products and in those with active major bleeding or thrombocytopenia with positive in vitro tests for antiplatelet antibody in the presence of drug.

Use with extreme caution in patients with a history of heparin-induced thrombocytopenia and in those with increased risk of hemorrhage, such as those with severe uncontrolled hypertension, bacterial endocarditis, congenital or acquired bleeding disorders, active ulceration, angiodysplastic GI disease, or hemorrhagic CVA. Also use cautiously if patient has had recent brain, spinal, or ophthalmic surgery or if patient has bleeding diathesis, thrombocytopenia, platelet defects, severe liver or kidney insufficiency, hypertensive or diabetic retinopathy, or recent GI bleeding.

Interactions

Drug-drug. *Oral anticoagulants, platelet inhibitors:* May increase risk of bleeding. Use together cautiously.

Adverse reactions

Hematologic: *thrombocytopenia, hemorrhage,* ecchymoses, bleeding complications.

Hepatic: elevated AST and ALT levels.

Skin: pruritus, rash, *hematoma.*

Other: fever.

Overdose and treatment

Overdose may cause hemorrhagic complications. Usually, they may be stopped by slow I.V. injection of protamine sulfate (1% solution), at a dose of 1 mg protamine for every 100 anti-factor Xa IU of dalteparin given. A second infusion of 0.5 mg protamine sulfate per 100 anti-factor Xa IU of dalteparin may be administered if the aPTT measured 2 to 4 hours after the first infusion remains prolonged. Even with these additional doses of protamine sulfate, the aPTT may remain more prolonged than would usually be found following administration of conventional heparin.

Special considerations

⚠ ALERT Don't give drug I.M.

⚠ ALERT Drug isn't interchangeable (unit for unit) with unfractionated heparin or other low-molecular-weight heparins.

● Patients receiving dalteparin who need neuraxial anesthesia or spinal puncture may be at increased risk for an epidural or spinal hematoma, which can result in long-term or permanent paralysis.

● Patient should assume a sitting or lying position when drug is administered. Inject dalteparin S.C. deeply. Injection sites include a U-shaped area around the navel, the upper outer side of the thigh, or the upper outer quadrangle of the buttock. Rotate sites daily. When the area around the navel or the thigh is used, use the thumb and forefinger to lift up a fold of skin while the injection is being given. Insert the entire length of the needle at a 45- to 90-degree angle.

● Don't mix drug with other injections or infusions unless specific compatibility data are available that support such mixing.

Patient monitoring

● Periodic CBC (including platelet count) and stool occult blood tests are recommended in patients receiving dalteparin. Patients don't need regular monitoring of PT, INR, or aPTT.

● Monitor patient closely for thrombocytopenia.

● Stop drug if a thromboembolic event occurs despite dalteparin prophylaxis.

Breast-feeding patients

● It isn't known whether drug appears in breast milk; use cautiously in breast-feeding women.

Pediatric patients

● Safety and effectiveness in children haven't been established.

Patient education
• Instruct patient and his family to watch for evidnce of bleeding and report them immediately.
• Tell patient to avoid OTC medications containing aspirin or other salicylates.

danaparoid sodium
Orgaran

Pharmacologic classification: glycosaminoglycan
Therapeutic classification: antithrombotic
Pregnancy risk category: B

Indications and dosages
➤ *Prophylaxis against postoperative deep vein thrombosis (DVT), which may lead to pulmonary embolism in patients undergoing elective hip replacement surgery.* Adults: 750 anti-Xa units S.C. b.i.d. beginning 1 to 4 hours preoperatively; then no sooner than 2 hours after surgery. Continue treatment for 7 to 10 days postoperatively or until risk of DVT has diminished.

How supplied
Available by prescription only
Ampule: 750 anti-Xa units/0.6 ml
Syringe: 750 anti-Xa units/0.6 ml

Pharmacodynamics
Antithrombotic action: Prevents fibrin formation by inhibiting generation of thrombin by anti-Xa and anti-IIa. Because of its predominant anti-Xa activity, danaparoid injection has little effect on clotting assays such as PT, INR, and aPTT. Drug has only minor effect on platelet function and platelet aggregability.

Pharmacokinetics
Pharmacokinetics have been described by monitoring of biologic activity (plasma anti-Xa activity) because no specific chemical assay methods are currently available.
Absorption: S.C. administration is about 100% bioavailable, compared with same dose administered I.V. Onset and duration are unknown.
Distribution: Not reported.
Metabolism: Not reported.
Excretion: Mainly eliminated through the kidneys. Mean value for the terminal half-life is about 24 hours. In patients with severely impaired renal function, elimination half-life of plasma anti-Xa activity may be prolonged.

Route	Onset	Peak	Duration
S.C.	Unknown	2-5 hr	Unknown

Contraindications and precautions
Contraindicated in patients hypersensitive to drug or to pork products and in patients with severe hemorrhagic diathesis (such as hemophilia or idiopathic thrombocytopenic purpura), active

major bleeding (including hemorrhagic stroke in the acute phase), or type II thrombocytopenia with positive in vitro tests for antiplatelet antibody in the presence of drug.

Use with extreme caution in patients who have had recent brain, spinal, or ophthalmic surgery and patients at increased risk of hemorrhage, such as those with severe uncontrolled hypertension, acute bacterial endocarditis, congenital or acquired bleeding disorders, active ulcerative and angiodysplastic GI disease, nonhemorrhagic CVA, or postoperative use of indwelling epidural catheter.

Use cautiously in patients with impaired renal function and in those receiving oral anticoagulants or platelet inhibitors.

Interactions
Drug-drug. *Oral anticoagulants, platelet inhibitors:* May increase the risk of bleeding. Use together cautiously.

Adverse reactions
CNS: insomnia, headache, asthenia, dizziness.
CV: peripheral edema, ***hemorrhage.***
GI: *nausea, constipation,* vomiting.
GU: urinary tract infection, urine retention.
Hematologic: anemia.
Musculoskeletal: joint disorder, pain.
Skin: rash, pruritus.
Other: *fever,* pain at injection site, infection.

Overdose and treatment
Signs and symptoms of acute toxicity after I.V. dosing are respiratory depression, prostration, and twitching. Overdose may lead to bleeding complications.

The effects of danaparoid on anti-Xa activity can't be currently antagonized with other drugs. Although protamine sulfate partially neutralizes the anti-Xa activity of danaparoid and can be safely coadministered, there's no evidence that protamine sulfate can reduce severe nonsurgical bleeding during treatment with danaparoid. If serious bleeding occurs, stop drug and administer blood or blood products as needed.

Special considerations
◼ **ALERT** Drug isn't interchangeable (unit for unit) with heparin or low-molecular-weight heparin.
◼ **ALERT** Don't give drug I.M.
• Drug contains sodium sulfite, which may cause allergic-type reactions, including anaphylactoid symptoms and life-threatening or less severe asthmatic episodes in certain patients. The presence of sulfite allergy in the general population is unknown and probably low. Sulfite sensitivity is seen more frequently in asthmatic than in nonasthmatic patients.
• Risks and benefits of danaparoid injection should be carefully considered before use in patients with severely impaired renal function or hemorrhagic disorders.

• To administer drug, have patient lie down. Give S.C. injection deeply, using a 25G to 26G needle. Alternate injection sites between the left and right anterolateral and posterolateral abdominal wall. Gently pull up a skin fold with thumb and forefinger and insert entire length of the needle into tissue. Don't rub or pinch afterward.

Patient monitoring

• Periodic CBC (including platelet count) and fecal occult blood tests are recommended during therapy. Patients don't need regular monitoring of PT, INR, or aPTT.
• Drug has little effect on PT, INR, aPTT, fibrinolytic activity, or bleeding time.
• Monitor patient's hematocrit and blood pressure closely; a decrease in either may signal hemorrhage. If serious bleeding occurs, stop drug and transfuse blood products if needed.

Breast-feeding patients

• It isn't known whether drug appears in breast milk; use cautiously in breast-feeding women.

Pediatric patients

• Safety and effectiveness in children haven't been established.

Patient education

• Instruct patient and family to watch for and report signs of bleeding.
• Tell patient to avoid OTC drugs containing aspirin or other salicylates.

---

danazol
Cyclomen*, Danocrine

Pharmacologic classification: androgen
Therapeutic classification: antiestrogen, androgen
Pregnancy risk category: X

Indications and dosages

➤ *Mild endometriosis. Adults:* Initially, 100 to 200 mg P.O. b.i.d. uninterrupted for 3 to 6 months; may continue for 9 months. Subsequent dosage based on patient response.
➤ *Moderate to severe endometriosis. Adults:* 400 mg P.O. b.i.d. uninterrupted for 3 to 6 months; may continue for 9 months.
➤ *Fibrocystic breast disease. Adults:* 100 to 400 mg P.O. daily in two divided doses uninterrupted for 2 to 6 months.
➤ *Prevention of hereditary angioedema. Adults:* 200 mg P.O. b.i.d. or t.i.d., continued until favorable response is achieved. Then, decrease dosage by half at 1- to 3-month intervals.

How supplied

Available by prescription only
Capsules: 50 mg, 100 mg, 200 mg

Pharmacodynamics

Antiestrogenic action: The antiestrogenic actions of danazol cause regression and atrophy of normal and ectopic endometrial tissue. Drug also decreases the growth and nodularity of abnormal breast tissue in fibrocystic breast disease.
Androgenic action: The androgenic effects of danazol increase levels of the C1 and C4 components of complement, which reduces the frequency and severity of attacks caused by hereditary angioedema.

Pharmacokinetics

Absorption: Amount absorbed isn't proportional to dose; doubling the dose produces an increase of only 35% to 40% in absorption.
Distribution: Unknown.
Metabolism: Metabolized to 2-hydroxymethylethisterone.
Excretion: Unknown.

Route	Onset	Peak	Duration
P.O.	1 mo	6-8 wk	Variable

Contraindications and precautions

Contraindicated in pregnant patients, breast-feeding patients, and patients with undiagnosed abnormal genital bleeding, porphyria, or impaired renal, cardiac, or hepatic function. Use cautiously in patients with seizure disorders or migraine headaches.

Interactions

Drug-drug. *Carbamazepine:* May increase plasma carbamazepine levels. Evaluate patient carefully.
Cyclosporine: Increased cyclosporine levels and increased risk of nephrotoxicity. Monitor patient closely.
Warfarin-type anticoagulants: Prolonged PT and INR. Monitor PT and INR.

Adverse reactions

CNS: dizziness, headache, sleep disorders, fatigue, tremor, irritability, excitation, lethargy, mental depression, chills, paresthesia.
CV: elevated blood pressure.
EENT: visual disturbances.
GI: gastric irritation, nausea, vomiting, diarrhea, constipation, change in appetite.
GU: hematuria; *hypoestrogenic effects, such as flushing, diaphoresis, vaginitis (including itching, dryness, and burning), vaginal bleeding, nervousness, emotional lability, menstrual irregularities.*
Hematologic: prolonged PT and INR (especially during anticoagulant therapy).
Hepatic: reversible jaundice, elevated liver enzyme levels, hepatic dysfunction.
Musculoskeletal: muscle cramps or spasms.
Other: androgenic effects in women, including *weight gain, hirsutism,* hoarseness, clitoral enlargement, *decreased breast size,* acne, edema, altered libido, *oily skin or hair,* voice deepening.

Reactions may be *common*, uncommon, *life-threatening*, or COMMON AND LIFE-THREATENING.

Overdose and treatment
No information available. Empty stomach by induced emesis or gastric lavage; follow with activated charcoal to reduce absorption. Treatment is supportive.

Special considerations
• To treat endometriosis and fibrocystic breast disease, begin danazol therapy during menstruation.
• Danazol provides alternative therapy for patients who can't tolerate or fail to respond to other therapy. (It isn't indicated when surgery is the best choice.)

Patient monitoring
• Because drug may cause hepatic dysfunction, obtain periodic liver function studies.

Breast-feeding patients
• Because of the risk of serious adverse reactions in the infant, a decision should be made to discontinue breast-feeding or the drug, depending on the importance of drug to patient.

Pediatric patients
• Use cautiously because of possible androgenic effects.
• Use danazol with extreme caution in children to avoid precocious puberty and premature closure of the epiphyses. Obtain X-ray examinations every 6 months to assess skeletal maturation.

Geriatric patients
• Use cautiously. Assess elderly men for the development of prostatic hypertrophy; symptomatic prostatic hypertrophy or prostatic carcinoma mandates discontinuation of danazol.

Patient education
• Advise patient taking danazol for fibrocystic disease to examine breasts regularly. Tell patient to immediately report a breast nodule that enlarges during treatment.
• Tell patient desiring birth control to use a nonhormonal contraceptive; during danazol treatment, ovulation may not be suppressed by hormonal contraceptives.
• Advise patient to report voice changes or other signs of virilization promptly. Some androgenic effects such as deepening of the voice may not be reversed by stopping drug.
• Instruct patient to immediately report nausea, vomiting, headache, and visual disturbances, which may suggest pseudotumor cerebri.
• Advise women that amenorrhea usually occurs after 6 to 8 weeks of therapy.
• Advise men that periodic evaluation of semen may be indicated.

dantrolene sodium
Dantrium

Pharmacologic classification: hydantoin derivative
Therapeutic classification: skeletal muscle relaxant
Pregnancy risk category: C

Indications and dosages
➤ **Spasticity from upper motor neuron disorders.** *Adults:* 25 mg P.O. daily, increased gradually in increments of 25 mg at 4- to 7-day intervals, up to 100 mg b.i.d. to q.i.d., to maximum of 400 mg daily.
Children over age 5: 0.5 mg/kg P.O. b.i.d., increased to t.i.d. and then q.i.d. Increase dosage further, p.r.n., by 0.5 mg/kg up to 3 mg/kg b.i.d. to q.i.d. Maximum dose is 100 mg q.i.d.
➤ **Prevention of malignant hyperthermia in susceptible patients who need surgery.** *Adults:* 4 to 8 mg/kg/day P.O. in three to four divided doses for 1 to 2 days before procedure; administer last dose 3 to 4 hours before procedure. Or, give 2.5 mg/kg I.V. over 1 hour about 75 minutes before anesthesia.
➤ **Management of malignant hyperthermia crisis.** *Adults and children:* Initially, 1 mg/kg I.V. Continued until symptoms subside or maximum cumulative dose of 10 mg/kg has been reached.
➤ **Prevention of recurrence of malignant hyperthermia after crisis.** *Adults:* 4 to 8 mg/kg/day P.O. given in four divided doses for up to 3 days after crisis. Or, 1 mg/kg or more I.V. based on clinical situation.
➤ **To reduce succinylcholine-induced muscle fasciculations and postoperative muscle pain** ◇. *Adults who weigh more than 45 kg (99 lb):* 150 mg P.O. 2 hours before succinylcholine.
Adults who weigh less than 45 kg: 100 mg P.O. 2 hours before succinylcholine.

How supplied
Available by prescription only
Capsules: 25 mg, 50 mg, 100 mg
Injection: 20 mg parenteral (contains 3 g mannitol)

Pharmacodynamics
Skeletal muscle relaxant action: A hydantoin derivative, dantrolene is chemically and pharmacologically unrelated to other skeletal muscle relaxants. It directly affects skeletal muscle, reducing muscle tension. It interferes with the release of calcium ions from the sarcoplasmic reticulum, resulting in decreased muscle contraction. This mechanism is of particular importance in malignant hyperthermia when increased myoplasmic calcium ion concentrations activate acute catabolism in the skeletal muscle cell. Dantrolene prevents or reduces the increase in

◇ Unlabeled clinical use

myoplasmic calcium levels related to malignant hyperthermia crises.

Pharmacokinetics
Absorption: 35% of oral dose is absorbed through GI tract, with serum half-life reached within 8 or 9 hours after oral administration. Therapeutic effect in patients with upper motor neuron disorders may take 1 week or more.
Distribution: Substantially plasma protein–bound, mainly to albumin.
Metabolism: Metabolized in the liver to its less active 5-hydroxy derivatives, and to its amino derivative by reductive pathways.
Excretion: Excreted in urine as metabolites.

Route	Onset	Peak	Duration
P.O.	Unknown	5 hr	Unknown
I.V.	Unknown	Unknown	3 hr after infusion ends

Contraindications and precautions
Contraindicated in patients with upper motor neuron disorders who use spasticity to maintain motor function, patients with spasms in rheumatic disorders, patients with active hepatic disease, and breast-feeding women. Contraindicated in combination with verapamil in management of malignant hyperthermia. Use cautiously in women (especially those taking estrogen), patients over age 35, and patients with severely impaired cardiac or pulmonary function or preexisting hepatic disease.

Interactions
Drug-drug. *CNS depressant drugs:* Increased CNS depression. Avoid use together.
Estrogen: increased risk of hepatotoxicity. Use together cautiously.
Verapamil: Has resulted in cardiac collapse. Don't use together.
Drug-lifestyle. *Alcohol use:* Increases CNS depression. Advise patient to avoid alcohol.

Adverse reactions
CNS: *muscle weakness, drowsiness, dizziness, light-headedness, malaise, fatigue, headache, confusion, nervousness, insomnia, seizures.*
CV: tachycardia, blood pressure changes.
EENT: excessive lacrimation, speech disturbance, altered taste, diplopia, visual disturbances.
GI: anorexia, constipation, cramping, dysphagia, metallic taste, severe diarrhea, GI bleeding.
GU: urinary frequency, hematuria, incontinence, nocturia, dysuria, crystalluria, difficult erection, urine retention.
Hepatic: altered liver function test results, *hepatitis.*
Musculoskeletal: myalgia, back pain.
Respiratory: pleural effusion with pericarditis.
Skin: eczematous eruption, pruritus, urticaria, abnormal hair growth, diaphoresis.
Other: chills, fever.

Overdose and treatment
Signs and symptoms of overdose include nausea, vomiting, and exaggeration of adverse reactions, particularly CNS depression.

Treatment includes supportive measures, gastric lavage, and observation of symptoms. Maintain adequate airway, have emergency ventilation equipment on hand, monitor ECG, and administer large quantities of I.V. solutions to prevent crystalluria. Monitor vital signs closely. The benefit of dialysis isn't known.

Special considerations
● Before therapy begins, check patient's baseline neuromuscular functions—posture, gait, coordination, range of motion, muscle strength and tone, presence of abnormal muscle movements, and reflexes—and document them for later comparison.
● Drug may weaken muscles and impair walking ability. Use cautiously, and carefully supervise patients receiving drug for prevention of malignant hyperthermia.
● Because of the risk of hepatic injury, discontinue drug if improvement isn't evident within 45 days.
● Risk of hepatotoxicity may be greater in women, patients over age 35, and patients taking other medications (especially estrogen) or large dantrolene doses (400 mg or more daily) for prolonged periods.
● Clinical signs of malignant hyperthermia include skeletal muscle rigidity (often the first sign), sudden tachycardia, cardiac arrhythmias, cyanosis, tachypnea, severe hypercarbia, unstable blood pressure, rapidly rising temperature, acidosis, and shock.
● In malignant hyperthermia crisis, give drug by rapid I.V. injection as soon as reaction is recognized.
● To reconstitute, add 60 ml sterile water for injection to 20-mg vial. Don't use bacteriostatic water, D_5W, or normal saline for injection. Store reconstituted solution away from direct sunlight at room temperature, and discard after 6 hours.
● To prepare suspension for single oral dose, dissolve contents of appropriate number of capsules in fruit juice or other suitable liquid.

Patient monitoring
● Perform baseline and regularly scheduled liver function tests (alkaline phosphatase, ALT, AST, and total bilirubin), blood cell counts, and renal function tests.

Breast-feeding patients
● Contraindicated for use in breast-feeding women.

Pediatric patients
● Drug isn't recommended for long-term use in children under age 5.

Reactions may be *common,* uncommon, *life-threatening,* or COMMON AND LIFE-THREATENING.

Geriatric patients

• Use drug with extreme caution in geriatric patients.

Patient education

• Instruct patient to report promptly the onset of jaundice: yellow skin or sclerae, dark urine, clay-colored stools, itching, and abdominal discomfort. Hepatotoxicity occurs more frequently between the third and twelfth month of therapy.
• Advise patient susceptible to malignant hyperthermia to carry or wear medical identification that indicates diagnosis, prescriber's name and telephone number, drug causing reaction, and treatment used.
• Advise patient to avoid excessive or unnecessary exposure to sunlight and to wear protective clothing and a sunscreen because photosensitivity reactions may occur.
• Warn patient to avoid hazardous activities that require alertness until CNS depressant effects are determined. Drug may cause drowsiness.
• Advise patient to report adverse reactions immediately.
• Tell patient to store drug away from heat and direct light (not in bathroom medicine cabinet) and to keep out of reach of children.
• If patient misses a dose, tell him to take it within 1 hour; otherwise, he should omit the dose and return to regular dosing schedule. Tell him not to double the dose.

dapsone
Avlosulfon*

Pharmacologic classification: synthetic sulfone
Therapeutic classification: antileprotic, antimalarial
Pregnancy risk category: C

Indications and dosages

➤*Multibacillary leprosy. Adults:* 100 mg P.O. daily plus rifampin and clofazimine for 12 months.
Children ages 10 to 14: 50 mg daily P.O. plus rifampin and clofazimine for 12 months.
Children under age 10: Give appropriately adjusted dosage plus rifampin and clofazimine for 12 months.
➤*Paucibacillary leprosy. Adults:* 100 mg P.O. daily plus rifampin for 6 months.
Children ages 10 to 14: 50 mg daily P.O. plus rifampin for 6 months.
Children under age 10: Give appropriately adjusted dosage plus rifampin for 6 months.
➤*Prophylaxis for people in close contact with leprosy patient. Adults and children age 12 and older:* 50 mg P.O. daily.
Children ages 6 to 12: 25 mg P.O. daily.
Children ages 2 to 5: 25 mg P.O. three times weekly.

Infants ages 6 months to 23 months: 12 mg P.O. three times weekly.
Infants under age 6 months: 6 mg P.O. three times weekly.
➤*Dermatitis herpetiformis. Adults:* Initially, 50 mg P.O. daily; may increase dose, p.r.n., to obtain full control.
✦*Dosage adjustment.* Dapsone levels are influenced by acetylation rates. Patients with high acetylation rates may need dose adjustments.
➤*Malaria suppression or prophylaxis. Adults:* 100 mg P.O. weekly with pyrimethamine 12.5 mg P.O. weekly. Continue prophylaxis throughout exposure and 6 months after exposure.
Children: 2 mg/kg P.O. weekly with pyrimethamine 0.25 mg/kg weekly. Continue prophylaxis throughout exposure and 6 months after exposure.
➤*Treatment of* Pneumocystis carinii *pneumonia* ◇. *Adults:* 100 mg P.O. daily. Usually given with trimethoprim, 20 mg/kg daily, for 21 days.
➤*Prophylaxis of* P. carinii *pneumonia* ◇. *Adults:* 50 mg b.i.d or 100 mg daily P.O.
➤*Prophylaxis of toxoplasmosis in HIV-infected patients* ◇. *Adults and adolescents:* 50 mg daily with pyrimethamine 50 mg once weekly and leucovorin 25 mg once weekly. *Children age 1 month and older:* 2 mg/kg or 15 mg/m² (maximum 25 mg) P.O. once daily plus pyrimethamine and leucovorin.

How supplied
Available by prescription only
Tablets: 25 mg, 100 mg

Pharmacodynamics
Antibiotic action: Drug is bacteriostatic and bactericidal; like sulfonamides, it probably acts mainly by inhibiting folic acid. It acts against *Mycobacterium leprae* and *Mycobacterium tuberculosis* and has some activity against *P. carinii* and *Plasmodium.*

Pharmacokinetics
Absorption: When given orally, drug is rapidly and almost completely absorbed.
Distribution: Distributed widely into most body tissues and fluids; 70% to 90% is protein-bound.
Metabolism: Undergoes acetylation by liver enzymes; rate varies and is genetically determined. Almost 50% of blacks and whites are slow acetylators, and more than 80% of Chinese, Japanese, and Inuits are fast acetylators.
Excretion: Excreted primarily in urine. Small amounts are excreted in feces. Substantial amounts appear in breast milk. Dapsone undergoes enterohepatic circulation; half-life in adults ranges from 10 to 50 hours (average 28 hours). Orally administered charcoal may enhance excretion. Dapsone is dialyzable.

Route	Onset	Peak	Duration
P.O.	Unknown	4-8 hr	Unknown

Contraindications and precautions

Contraindicated in patients hypersensitive to drug. Use cautiously in patients with impaired renal, hepatic, or CV disease; refractory types of anemia; and G6PD deficiency.

Interactions

Drug-drug. *Activated charcoal*: Decreases GI absorption of dapsone. Monitor patient carefully.
Didanosine: May cause dapsone to fail, leading to an increase in infection. Avoid use together.
Folic acid antagonists such as methotrexate: Increased risk of adverse hematologic reactions. Avoid use together.
Para-aminobenzoic acid: May antagonize the effect of dapsone by interfering with the primary mechanism of action. Monitor patient for lack of efficacy.
Probenecid: Reduces urinary excretion of dapsone metabolites, increasing plasma levels. Monitor patient closely.
Rifampin: Increased hepatic metabolism of dapsone. Monitor patient for lack of efficacy.
Trimethoprim: Serum levels of both drugs may increase, possibly increasing their pharmacologic and toxic effects. Monitor patient carefully.
Drug-lifestyle. *Sun exposure:* Photosensitivity reactions may occur. Tell patient to take precautions.

Adverse reactions

CNS: insomnia, psychosis, headache, paresthesia, peripheral neuropathy, vertigo.
CV: tachycardia.
EENT: tinnitus, blurred vision.
GI: anorexia, abdominal pain, nausea, vomiting, *pancreatitis.*
GU: albuminuria, nephrotic syndrome, renal papillary necrosis, male infertility.
Hematologic: hemolytic anemia, *agranulocytosis, aplastic anemia.*
Respiratory: pulmonary eosinophilia.
Skin: lupus erythematosus, phototoxicity, *exfoliative dermatitis, toxic erythema, erythema multiforme, toxic epidermal necrolysis, morbilliform and scarlatiniform reactions, urticaria, erythema nodosum.*
Other: fever, infectious mononucleosis-like syndrome, *sulfone syndrome (fever, malaise, jaundice [with hepatic necrosis], exfoliative dermatitis, lymphadenopathy, methemoglobinemia, hemolytic anemia), leprosy reactional states.*

Overdose and treatment

Signs and symptoms of overdose include nausea, vomiting, and hyperexcitability occurring within minutes or up to 24 hours after ingestion; methemoglobin-induced depression, cyanosis, and seizures may occur. Hemolysis is a late complication (up to 14 days after ingestion).

Treatment is by gastric lavage, followed by activated charcoal. Patients with dapsone-induced methemoglobinemia (without G6PD deficiency) can be given methylene blue. Hemodialysis also may be used to enhance elimination.

Special considerations

• Give drug with or after meals to avoid gastric irritation. Ensure adequate fluid intake.
• Specimens for culture and sensitivity testing should be obtained before first dose, but therapy may begin before test results are complete; repeat tests periodically to detect drug resistance.
• Isolation of patient with inactive leprosy isn't required; however, be sure to disinfect surfaces that contact discharge from nose or skin lesions.
• Therapeutic effect on leprosy may not be evident for 3 to 6 months after therapy starts.
• Because drug is dialyzable, patients undergoing hemodialysis may need dosage adjustments.
• During therapy for leprosy, two types of leprosy reactional states related to the effectiveness of dapsone therapy may occur. Type I, reversal reaction, includes erythema followed by swelling of skin and nerve lesions in tuberculoid patients. Skin lesions may ulcerate and multiply, and acute neuritis may cause neural dysfunction. Severe cases require hospitalization, analgesics, corticosteroids, and nerve trunk decompression while dapsone therapy is continued. Type II, erythema nodosum leprosum, occurs mainly in lepromatous leprosy and occurs about 50% of the time during the first year of therapy. Signs and symptoms include tender erythematous skin nodules, fever, malaise, orchitis, neuritis, albuminuria, iritis, joint swelling, epistaxis, and depression; skin lesions may ulcerate. Treatment includes one or more of the following drugs while dapsone is continued: corticosteroids, analgesics, and thalidomide. Additional treatment guidelines are available from National Hansen's Disease Center at the U.S. Public Health Service at Carville, LA, 1-800-642-2477.

Patient monitoring

• Monitor dapsone serum levels periodically to maintain effective levels. Levels of 0.1 to 7 mcg/ml (average 2.3 mcg/ml) are usually effective and safe.
• Monitor vital signs frequently during early weeks of drug therapy. Frequent or high fever may require reduced dosage or discontinuation of drug.
• Patient requires observation for adverse effects and monitoring of hematologic and liver function studies to minimize toxicity.
• Watch skin and mucous membranes for early signs of allergic reactions or leprosy reactional states.

Breast-feeding patients

• Dapsone appears in breast milk and is tumorigenic in animals. An alternative feeding method is recommended during therapy.

Pediatric patients

• Use drug cautiously in children.

Reactions may be *common,* uncommon, *life-threatening,* or COMMON AND LIFE-THREATENING.

Geriatric patients
● These patients commonly have decreased renal function, which decreases drug excretion. Use cautiously.

Patient education
● Explain disease process and rationale for long-term therapy to patient and family; emphasize that improvement may not occur for 3 to 6 months and that treatment must continue for 1 to 2 years or more.
● Teach signs and symptoms of hypersensitivity and other adverse reactions, and emphasize need to report these promptly. Explain possibility of cumulative effects. Urge patient to report any unusual effects or reactions and to report loss of appetite, nausea, or vomiting promptly.
● Teach patient how to take drug. Emphasize the need to comply with prescribed regimen. Encourage patient to report symptoms that worsen or that don't improve after 3 months of treatment. Urge patient not to stop drug without medical approval.
● Explain the importance of follow-up visits and the need to monitor close contacts at 6- to 12-month intervals for 10 years.
● Teach sanitary disposal of secretions from nose or skin lesions.
● Assure patient and family that inactive leprosy is no barrier to employment or school attendance.
● New mothers need not be separated from infant during therapy; teach signs of cyanosis and methemoglobinemia.

daunorubicin citrate liposomal
DaunoXome

Pharmacologic classification: anthracycline
Therapeutic classification: antineoplastic
Pregnancy risk category: D

Indications and dosages
➤ *First-line cytotoxic therapy for advanced HIV-related Kaposi's sarcoma.*
Adults: 40 mg/m² I.V. over 60 minutes once every 2 weeks. Continue treatment until there's evidence of progressive disease or until other HIV complications preclude continuation of therapy.
✦ *Dosage adjustment.* In patients with impaired hepatic and renal function, reduce dosage as follows: If serum bilirubin is 1.2 to 3 mg/dl, give three-fourths the normal dose; if serum bilirubin or creatinine is greater than 3 mg/dl, give one-half the normal dose.

How supplied
Available by prescription only
Injection: 2 mg/ml (equivalent to 50 mg daunorubicin base)

Pharmacodynamics
Antineoplastic action: Daunorubicin exerts cytotoxic activity by intercalating between DNA base pairs and uncoiling the DNA helix. This inhibits DNA synthesis and DNA-dependent RNA synthesis. The drug may also inhibit polymerase activity. The liposomal preparation of daunorubicin maximizes the selectivity of daunorubicin for solid tumors in situ. After penetrating the tumor, daunorubicin is released over time to exert antineoplastic activity.

Pharmacokinetics
Absorption: Administered I.V.
Distribution: Thought to be distributed primarily in the vascular fluid volume.
Metabolism: Metabolized by the liver into active metabolites.
Excretion: Apparent elimination half-life is 4½ hours.

Route	Onset	Peak	Duration
I.V.	Unknown	Unknown	Unknown

Contraindications and precautions
Contraindicated in patients who have experienced a severe hypersensitivity reaction to daunorubicin citrate liposomal or any of its components. Use cautiously in patients with myelosuppression, cardiac disease, previous radiotherapy encompassing the heart, previous anthracycline use (doxorubicin more than 300 mg/m² or equivalent), or hepatic or renal dysfunction.

Interactions
None reported.

Adverse reactions
CNS: *headache, neuropathy,* depression, dizziness, syncope, insomnia, amnesia, anxiety, ataxia, confusion, *seizures,* hallucination, tremor, hypertonia, meningitis, *fatigue,* malaise, emotional lability, abnormal gait, hyperkinesia, somnolence, abnormal thinking.
CV: *cardiomyopathy,* chest pain, hypertension, palpitations, *arrhythmias, pericardial effusion, pericardial tamponade, cardiac arrest,* angina pectoris, *pulmonary hypertension,* flushing, edema, tachycardia, *MI.*
EENT: *rhinitis,* stomatitis, sinusitis, abnormal vision, conjunctivitis, tinnitus, eye pain, deafness, earache.
GI: taste disturbances, gingival bleeding, dry mouth, *nausea, diarrhea, abdominal pain, vomiting, anorexia,* constipation, *GI hemorrhage,* gastritis, dysphagia, stomatitis, increased appetite, melena, hemorrhoids, tenesmus.
GU: dysuria, nocturia, polyuria.
Hematologic: neutropenia.
Hepatic: *hepatomegaly.*
Metabolic: dehydration, thirst.
Musculoskeletal: *rigors, back pain,* arthralgia, myalgia.

Respiratory: *cough, dyspnea,* hemoptysis, hiccups, pulmonary infiltration, increased sputum.
Skin: alopecia, pruritus, *increased sweating,* dry skin, seborrhea, folliculitis, local tissue necrosis with extravasation.
Other: tooth caries, *fever,* splenomegaly, lymphadenopathy, *opportunistic infections, allergic reactions,* flulike symptoms, injection site inflammation.

Overdose and treatment

Acute overdose increases the severity of adverse effects such as myelosuppression, fatigue, nausea, and vomiting. Treatment is usually supportive.

Special considerations

• Administer only under the supervision of clinicians specializing in chemotherapy.
• **ALERT** Daunorubicin citrate liposomal exhibits unique pharmacokinetic properties compared to conventional daunorubicin hydrochloride and shouldn't be substituted on a milligram per milligram basis.
• Dilute drug with D_5W before administration. Withdraw the calculated volume of drug from the vial and transfer it into an equivalent amount of D_5W. The recommended concentration after dilution is 1 mg/ml.
• Don't mix daunorubicin citrate liposomal with other drugs, saline solution, bacteriostatic agents, or any other solution.
• After dilution, immediately administer I.V. over 60 minutes. If unable to use immediately, refrigerate at 36° to 46° F (2° to 8° C) for a maximum of 6 hours.
• Don't use in-line filters for the I.V. infusion.
• A triad of back pain, flushing and chest tightness may occur within the first 5 minutes of the infusion. This triad subsides after stopping the infusion and generally doesn't recur when the infusion is administered at a slower rate.
• Drug is a vesicant.
• Follow procedures for proper handling and disposal of antineoplastics.

Patient monitoring

• Monitor and assess cardiac function regularly before administering each dose because of the potential risk for cardiac toxicity and heart failure. Determine left ventricular ejection fraction at total cumulative dose of 320 mg/m² and every 160 mg/m² thereafter.
• Because local tissue necrosis is possible, monitor I.V. site closely to avoid extravasation.
• Careful hematologic monitoring is required because severe myelosuppression may occur. Repeat blood counts before each dose. Withhold treatment if absolute granulocyte count is less than 750 cells/mm³.
• Monitor patient closely for signs of opportunistic infections, especially because HIV-infected patients are immunocompromised.

Pregnant patients

• Drug causes severe maternal toxicity and embryolethality; advise patient to avoid becoming pregnant during treatment.

Breast-feeding patients

• Safety during breast-feeding hasn't been established. Because of the risk of serious adverse effects in the nursing infant, avoid breast-feeding.

Pediatric patients

• Safety and efficacy haven't been established in children.

Geriatric patients

• Safety and efficacy haven't been established in geriatric patients.

Patient education

• Inform patient that alopecia may occur but that it is usually reversible.
• Instruct patient to report sore throat, fever, or any other signs of infection; tell patient to avoid exposure to people with infections.
• Advise patient to report suspected or confirmed pregnancy while receiving drug.
• Tell patient to report back pain, flushing, and chest tightness during the infusion.

daunorubicin hydrochloride
Cerubidine

Pharmacologic classification: antibiotic antineoplastic (not specific to cell cycle phase)
Therapeutic classification: antineoplastic
Pregnancy risk category: D

Indications and dosages

Dosage and indications may vary. Check current literature for recommended protocols.
➤ *Remission induction in acute non-lymphocytic leukemia (myelogenous, monocytic, erythroid). Adults under age 60:* 45 mg/m² I.V. daily on days 1 to 3 of first course and on days 1 and 2 of subsequent courses. Give all courses with cytosine arabinoside infusions.
Adults age 60 and older: 30 mg/m² I.V. daily on days 1 to 3 of first course and on days 1 and 2 of subsequent courses. Give all courses with cytosine arabinoside infusions.
➤ *Remission induction in acute lymphocytic leukemia. Adults:* 45 mg/m² I.V. daily on days 1 to 3; give with vincristine, prednisone, and L-asparaginase.
Children age 2 and older: 25 mg/m² I.V. on day 1 weekly for up to 6 weeks, if needed; give with vincristine and prednisone.
Children under age 2 or with a body surface area of less than 0.5 m²: Calculate dose based on body weight (1 mg/kg) rather than body surface area.
✦ *Dosage adjustment.* Reduce dosage if patient has hepatic or renal impairment. If serum

bilirubin level is 1.2 to 3 mg/dl, reduce dose by 25%. If serum bilirubin or creatinine level is more than 3 mg/dl, reduce dose by 50%.

How supplied
Available by prescription only
Injection: 20-mg vials (with 100 mg of mannitol)

Pharmacodynamics
Antineoplastic action: Drug exerts cytotoxic activity by intercalating between DNA base pairs and uncoiling the DNA helix. The result is inhibition of DNA synthesis and DNA-dependent RNA synthesis. Drug may also inhibit polymerase activity.

Pharmacokinetics
Absorption: Administered I.V.
Distribution: Widely distributed into body tissues, with the highest levels in the spleen, kidneys, liver, lungs, and heart. Drug doesn't cross the blood-brain barrier.
Metabolism: Extensively metabolized in the liver by microsomal enzymes. One of the metabolites has cytotoxic activity.
Excretion: Primarily excreted in bile, with a small portion in urine. Plasma elimination is biphasic, with an initial phase half-life of 45 minutes and a terminal phase half-life of 18½ hours.

Route	Onset	Peak	Duration
I.V.	Unknown	Unknown	Unknown

Contraindications and precautions
No known contraindications. Use cautiously in patients with myelosuppression or impaired cardiac, renal, or hepatic function.

Interactions
Drug-drug. *Dexamethasone phosphate, heparin sodium:* Admixture of these drugs results in precipitate formation. Don't mix daunorubicin with either of these drugs.
Doxorubicin: Additive cardiotoxicity. Monitor patient closely.
Hepatotoxic drugs: Increased risk of hepatotoxicity. Monitor patient closely.

Adverse reactions
CV: *irreversible cardiomyopathy,* ECG changes.
GI: *nausea, vomiting,* diarrhea, *mucositis.*
GU: red urine.
Hematologic: *bone marrow suppression* (lowest blood counts 10 to 14 days after administration).
Hepatic: *hepatotoxicity.*
Metabolic: hyperuricemia.
Skin: *alopecia,* rash.
Other: *severe cellulitis and tissue sloughing* (if drug extravasates), fever, chills.

Overdose and treatment
Signs and symptoms of overdose include myelosuppression, nausea, vomiting, and stomatitis. Treatment is usually supportive and includes transfusion of blood components and antiemetics.

Special considerations
⚠ ALERT Reddish color of drug looks similar to that of doxorubicin (Adriamycin). Don't confuse the two drugs.
● Erythematous streaking along the vein or flushing in the face indicates that the drug is being administered too rapidly.
● To reconstitute drug for I.V. administration, add 4 ml of sterile water for injection to a 20-mg vial to give a concentration of 5 mg/ml.
● Drug may be diluted further into 100 ml of D_5W or normal saline solution and infused over 30 to 45 minutes.
● For I.V. push administration, reconstituted drug is withdrawn into a syringe containing 10 to 15 ml of normal saline or D_5W and injected over 2 to 3 minutes into the tubing of a freely flowing I.V. infusion. Reconstituted solution is stable for 24 hours at room temperature and 48 hours refrigerated.
● Drug is a vesicant; extravasation may be treated with topical application of dimethyl sulfoxide and ice packs at the site.
● Antiemetics may be used to prevent or treat nausea and vomiting.
● Skin may darken or redden in previous radiation fields.
● To prevent cardiomyopathy, limit cumulative dose in adults to 500 to 600 mg/m² (400 to 450 mg/m² if patient has been receiving other cardiotoxic agents, such as cyclophosphamide, or radiation therapy that encompasses the heart).
● Don't use a scalp tourniquet or apply ice to prevent alopecia because doing so may compromise drug effectiveness.

Patient monitoring
● ECG monitoring or monitoring of systolic injection fraction may help to identify early changes from drug-induced cardiomyopathy. An ECG or determination of systolic ejection fraction should be performed before each course of therapy.
● Monitor CBC and hepatic function.
● Monitor heart rate. A high resting pulse rate may indicate an adverse cardiac reaction.

Breast-feeding patients
● It isn't known whether drug appears in breast milk. However, because of risk for serious adverse reactions, mutagenicity, and carcinogenicity in the infant, breast-feeding isn't recommended.

Pediatric patients
● Children have an increased risk of drug-induced cardiotoxicity, which may occur at lower doses. Total lifetime dosage for children over age 2 is 300 mg/m²; for children under age 2, 10 mg/kg.

Geriatric patients
• These patients have an increased risk of drug-induced cardiotoxicity.
• Monitor elderly patients for hematologic toxicity because some have poor bone marrow reserve.

Patient education
• Warn patient that urine may turn red for 1 to 2 days and that this is a drug effect, not bleeding.
• Advise patient that alopecia may occur, but that it's usually reversible.
• Tell patient to avoid exposure to people with infections.
• Encourage adequate fluid intake to increase urine output and facilitate excretion of uric acid.
• Warn patient that nausea and vomiting may be severe and may last 24 to 48 hours.
• Instruct patient to report a sore throat, fever, or signs of bleeding.

deferoxamine mesylate
Desferal

Pharmacologic classification: chelating agent
Therapeutic classification: heavy metal antagonist
Pregnancy risk category: C

Indications and dosages
➤ *Acute iron intoxication. Adults and children:* 1 g I.M. or I.V. (I.M. injection is preferred route for all patients in shock), followed by 500 mg I.M. or I.V. q 4 hours for two doses; then 500 mg I.M. or I.V. q 4 to 12 hours, if needed. I.V. infusion rate shouldn't exceed 15 mg/kg/hour for the first 1 g. Subsequent rate shouldn't exceed 125 mg/hour. Don't exceed 6 g in 24 hours. (Reserve I.V. infusion for patients in CV collapse.)
➤ *Chronic iron overload from multiple transfusions. Adults and children:* 500 mg to 1 g I.M. daily and 2 g slow I.V. infusion in separate solution along with each unit of blood transfused. I.V. infusion rate shouldn't exceed 15 mg/kg/hour. Or, give 1 to 2 g via an S.C. infusion pump over 8 to 24 hours.

How supplied
Available by prescription only
Injectable powder for injection: 500-mg vial

Pharmacodynamics
Chelating action: Deferoxamine chelates iron by binding ferric ions to the 3 hydroxamic groups of the molecule, preventing it from entering into further chemical reactions. It also chelates aluminum to a lesser extent.

Pharmacokinetics
Absorption: Absorbed poorly after oral administration; however, absorption may occur in patients with acute iron toxicity.

Distribution: Distributed widely into the body after parenteral administration.
Metabolism: Small amounts are metabolized by plasma enzymes.
Excretion: Excreted in urine as unchanged drug or as ferrioxamine, the deferoxamine-iron complex.

Route	Onset	Peak	Duration
I.V., I.M., S.C.	Unknown	Unknown	Unknown

Contraindications and precautions
Contraindicated in patients with severe renal disease or anuria. Use cautiously in patients with impaired renal function.

Interactions
Drug-drug. *Ascorbic acid:* Increases availability of iron for chelation. Administer together except for patients with cardiac failure.

Adverse reactions
CV: tachycardia.
EENT: blurred vision, cataracts, hearing loss, visual field defects.
GI: diarrhea, abdominal discomfort, nausea, vomiting.
GU: dysuria.
Musculoskeletal: leg cramps.
Other: *hypersensitivity reactions* (cutaneous wheal formation, pruritus, rash, *anaphylaxis*); pain and induration at injection site; fever; *erythema, urticaria, hypotension, shock* after too-rapid I.V. administration; susceptibility to infection.

Overdose and treatment
Acute intoxication may extend and worsen adverse reactions. Treat symptomatically. Drug can be removed by hemodialysis.

Special considerations
• Use I.M. route for acute iron intoxication if patient isn't in shock. If patient is in shock, administer I.V. slowly; avoid S.C. route.
• Drug has been used to treat iron overload from congenital anemias and in the diagnosis and treatment of primary hemochromatosis. It's been applied topically to remove corneal rust rings and has been used I.V. or intraperitoneally to promote aluminum excretion or removal.
• Drug has also been used experimentally as a chelator to reduce aluminum levels in bones of patients with renal failure and in patients with dialysis-induced encephalopathy. It also slows cognitive deterioration by 50%.

Patient monitoring
🔌 **ALERT** Observe patient closely, and be prepared to treat hypersensitivity reactions. Keep epinephrine 1:1,000 available.
• Monitor fluid intake and output carefully.

• Monitor renal, vision, and hearing function throughout therapy.

Pregnant patients
• Drug can cause fetal anomalies. Don't give to pregnant patient unless benefits outweigh risks.

Pediatric patients
• Drug is safe and effective in children over age 3. Monitor child's growth.

Geriatric patients
• Use drug cautiously because these patients are more likely to have visual or hearing impairment and renal dysfunction than younger patients.

Patient education
• Advise patient that ophthalmic and, possibly, audiometric examinations are needed every 3 to 6 months during continuous therapy; stress importance of reporting changes in vision or hearing.
• Explain that drug may turn urine red.

delavirdine mesylate
Rescriptor

Pharmacologic classification: non-nucleoside reverse-transcriptase inhibitor of HIV-1
Therapeutic classification: antiviral
Pregnancy risk category: C

Indications and dosages
➤ **HIV infection.** *Adults:* 400 mg P.O. t.i.d. with other antiretrovirals as appropriate.

How supplied
Available by prescription only
Tablets: 100 mg, 200 mg

Pharmacodynamics
Antiviral action: Delavirdine is a non-nucleoside reverse transcriptase inhibitor of HIV-1. It binds directly to reverse transcriptase and blocks RNA- and DNA-dependent DNA polymerase activities.

Pharmacokinetics
Absorption: Rapidly absorbed following oral administration.
Distribution: 98% bound to plasma proteins, primarily albumin. Distribution into CSF, saliva, and semen is about 0.4%, 6%, and 2% of plasma levels, respectively.
Metabolism: Converted to several inactive metabolites; primarily metabolized in liver by cytochrome P-450 3A (CYP3A) enzyme system; however, CYP2D6 may also be involved. Delavirdine can reduce CYP3A activity and can inhibit its own metabolism; this is usually reversed within 1 week after discontinuation of the drug. CYP2C9 and CYP2C19 activity may also be reduced by delavirdine.
Excretion: About 44% of dose is recovered in feces and 51% is excreted in urine. Less than 5%

appears unchanged in urine. Mean elimination half-life is 5.8 hours.

Route	Onset	Peak	Duration
P.O.	Unknown	1 hr	Unknown

Contraindications and precautions
Contraindicated in patients hypersensitive to drug formulation. Use cautiously in patients with impaired hepatic function. Non-nucleoside reverse transcriptase inhibitors, used alone or in combination, may confer cross-resistance to other drugs in that class.

Interactions
Drug-drug. *Amphetamines, benzodiazepines, calcium channel blockers, clarithromycin, dapsone, ergot alkaloid preparations, indinavir, nonsedating antihistamines, quinidine, rifabutin, saquinavir, sedative hypnotics, warfarin:* Increased or prolonged therapeutic and adverse effects. Avoid use together; however, reduced doses of indinavir with delavirdine may be used.
Antacids: Reduced delavirdine absorption. Separate doses by at least 1 hour.
Carbamazepine, phenobarbital, phenytoin, rifabutin, rifampin: Decreased plasma delavirdine levels. Use cautiously.
Clarithromycin, fluoxetine, ketoconazole: 50% increase in delavirdine bioavailability. Monitor patient.
Didanosine: 20% decrease in absorption of both drugs. Separate doses by at least 1 hour.
H₂-receptor antagonists: Increased gastric pH reduces absorption of delavirdine. Long-term use of these drugs with delavirdine isn't recommended.
Indinavir: Increased plasma levels. Consider a lower indinavir dose when given with delavirdine.
Saquinavir: Five-fold increase in bioavailability. Monitor AST and ALT levels frequently during concurrent use.

Adverse reactions
CNS: asthenia, *fatigue,* headache, abnormal coordination, agitation, amnesia, anxiety, change in dreams, lethargy, malaise, cognitive impairment, confusion, depression, disorientation, emotional lability, hallucinations, hyperesthesia, hyperreflexia, hypesthesia, impaired concentration, insomnia, manic symptoms, muscle cramps, nervousness, neuropathy, nightmares, nystagmus, paralysis, paranoid symptoms, paresthesia, restlessness, somnolence, tingling, tremor, vertigo, weakness, pallor.
CV: *bradycardia,* peripheral edema, palpitations, orthostatic hypotension, syncope, tachycardia, vasodilation, chest pain.
EENT: epistaxis, laryngismus, pharyngitis, rhinitis, sinusitis, blepharitis, diplopia, conjunctivitis, dry eyes, ear pain, photophobia, tinnitus.
GI: taste perversion, *nausea,* vomiting, diarrhea, anorexia, aphthous stomatitis, bloody stools, co-

---

* Canada only   ◇ Unlabeled clinical use

litis, constipation, decreased appetite, diverticulitis, duodenitis, dry mouth, dyspepsia, dysphagia, enteritis, esophagitis, fecal incontinence, flatulence, gagging, gastritis, gastroesophageal reflux, *GI bleeding,* gingivitis, gum hemorrhage, increased thirst and appetite, increased saliva, mouth ulcer, *pancreatitis,* sialadenitis, stomatitis, tongue edema or ulceration, abdominal cramps, distention, pain (generalized or localized).

GU: renal calculi, epididymitis, hematuria, hemospermia, impotence, renal pain, metrorrhagia, nocturia, polyuria, proteinuria, vaginal candidiasis.

Hematologic: bruises, *anemia,* ecchymoses, eosinophilia, *granulocytosis, neutropenia, pancytopenia,* petechia, prolonged aPTT, purpura, spleen disorder, *thrombocytopenia.*

Hepatic: *hepatitis, increased ALT and AST levels.*

Metabolic: alcohol intolerance; bilirubinemia; hyperkalemia; hyperuricemia; hypocalcemia; hyponatremia; hypophosphatemia; increased GGT, lipase, serum alkaline phosphatase, serum amylase, and serum CK levels; weight changes.

Musculoskeletal: flank pain, back pain, pain (generalized or localized), neck rigidity, arthralgia or arthritis of single and many joints, bone pain, leg cramps, muscle weakness, myalgia, tendon disorder, tenosynovitis, tetany.

Respiratory: upper respiratory tract infection, bronchitis, chest congestion, cough, dyspnea.

Skin: sebaceous cyst, epidermal cyst, *rash, pruritus,* dermal leukocytoblastic vasculitis, dermatitis, desquamation, diaphoresis, dry skin, erythema multiforme, folliculitis, fungal dermatitis, alopecia, nail disorder, petechial rash, seborrhea, skin nodule, *Stevens-Johnson syndrome,* urticaria.

Other: *angioedema, allergic reaction,* breast enlargement, decreased libido, chills, edema (generalized or localized), fever, flu syndrome, lip edema, trauma.

Overdose and treatment
No information is available. Provide supportive treatment. Remove drug by gastric lavage or emesis, if needed. Dialysis is unlikely to be effective because drug is highly protein-bound.

Special considerations
• Rash is more common in patients with lower CD4+ cell counts and usually occurs within the first 3 weeks of treatment. Severe rash has occurred in 3.6% of patients. In most cases, rash lasted less than 2 weeks and didn't need dose reduction or drug discontinuation. Most patients resumed therapy after it was interrupted by rash.
• Rash occurs mainly on the upper body and proximal arms, with decreasing intensity on the neck and face and less on the rest of the trunk and limbs. Erythema multiforme and Stevens-Johnson syndrome are rare and have resolved after drug was stopped. Occurrence of drug-related rash after 1 month of therapy is uncommon except in prolonged interruption of drug treatment.
• Symptomatic relief may be obtained by using diphenhydramine, hydroxyzine, or topical corticosteroids.

Patient monitoring
• Neutropenia (absolute neutrophil count less than 750/mm³), anemia (hemoglobin less than 7 g/dl), thrombocytopenia (platelet count less than 50,000/mm³), increased ALT and AST levels (more than five times upper limit of normal), increased bilirubin levels (more than 2½ times upper limit of normal), and increased amylase levels (more than twice upper limit of normal) may occur during delavirdine therapy. Monitor patient carefully.
• Monitor patients with hepatic or renal impairment because effect of drug hasn't been studied.

Breast-feeding patients
• Advise HIV-infected women not to breast-feed.

Pediatric patients
• Safety and effectiveness haven't been studied in patients under age 16.

Geriatric patients
• Safety and effectiveness haven't been studied in patients over age 65.

Patient education
• Instruct patient to discontinue drug and report severe rash or such symptoms as fever, blistering, oral lesions, conjunctivitis, swelling, or muscle or joint aches occur.
• Tell patient that drug doesn't cure HIV-1 infection and that he may continue to develop HIV-related illnesses, including opportunistic infections. Therapy doesn't affect such illnesses.
• Advise patient to remain under medical supervision when taking drug because long-term effects aren't known.
• Inform patient to take drug as prescribed and not to alter doses without medical approval. If he misses a dose, tell him to take the next dose as soon as possible; he shouldn't double the next dose.
• Inform patient that drug may be dispersed in water before ingestion. Tell patient to add tablets to at least 3 oz (90 ml) of water, let stand for a few minutes, and stir until a uniform dispersion occurs. Tell patient to drink dispersion promptly, rinse glass, and swallow the rinse to make sure entire dose is consumed.
• Advise patient with achlorhydria to take drug with an acidic beverage such as orange or cranberry juice.
• Advise patient to report the use of other prescription or OTC medications.

Reactions may be *common,* uncommon, *life-threatening,* or COMMON AND LIFE-THREATENING.

demeclocycline hydrochloride
Declomycin

Pharmacologic classification: tetracycline antibiotic
Therapeutic classification: antibiotic
Pregnancy risk category: D

Indications and dosages
➤ *Infections caused by susceptible organisms.* *Adults:* 150 mg P.O. q 6 hours or 300 mg P.O. q 12 hours.
Children over age 8: 6.6 to 13.2 mg/kg P.O. daily, divided q 6 to 12 hours.
➤ *Gonorrhea.* *Adults:* 600 mg P.O. initially; then 300 mg P.O. q 12 hours for 4 days (total, 3 g).
➤ *SIADH secretion (a hypo-osmolar state)* ◊. *Adults:* 600 to 1,200 mg P.O. daily in three or four divided doses.

How supplied
Available by prescription only
Tablets (film-coated): 150 mg, 300 mg

Pharmacodynamics
Antibacterial action: Demeclocycline is bacteriostatic. Tetracyclines bind reversibly to ribosomal subunits, thereby inhibiting bacterial protein synthesis. Demeclocycline is active against many gram-negative and gram-positive organisms, *Mycoplasma, Rickettsia, Chlamydia,* and spirochetes.

Pharmacokinetics
Absorption: About 60% to 80% is absorbed from the GI tract after oral administration; peak serum levels occur at 3 to 4 hours. Food or milk reduces absorption by 50%; antacids chelate with tetracyclines and further reduce absorption. Drug has the greatest affinity of all tetracyclines for calcium ions.
Distribution: Distributed widely into body tissues and fluids, including synovial, pleural, prostatic, and seminal fluids; bronchial secretions; saliva; and aqueous humor. CSF penetration is poor. Drug crosses the placenta. About 36% to 91% is protein-bound.
Metabolism: Not metabolized.
Excretion: Excreted primarily unchanged in urine by glomerular filtration; some drug may appear in breast milk. Plasma half-life is 10 to 17 hours in adults with normal renal function. Hemodialysis and peritoneal dialysis remove minimal amounts of demeclocycline.

Route	Onset	Peak	Duration
P.O.	Unknown	3-4 hr	Unknown

Contraindications and precautions
Contraindicated in patients hypersensitive to drug or other tetracyclines. Use cautiously in women during second half of pregnancy, children under age 8, and patients with impaired renal or hepatic function.

Interactions
Drug-drug. *Antacids containing aluminum, calcium, or magnesium; antidiarrheals; iron products; laxatives containing aluminum, magnesium, or calcium; sodium bicarbonate; zinc:* Impaired absorption of oral tetracycline. Avoid use together.
Digoxin: Lowered dosages of digoxin because of increased bioavailability. Monitor serum digoxin levels.
Methoxyflurane: Increased risk of nephrotoxicity. Avoid use together.
Oral anticoagulants: Increased anticoagulant effect. Monitor INR and PT, and adjust dosage as needed.
Oral contraceptives: Decreased contraceptive effectiveness. Breakthrough bleeding has been reported. Recommend a nonhormonal birth control method.
Penicillin: May interfere with bactericidal action of penicillin. Give penicillin 2 to 3 hours before tetracycline.
Drug-food. *Food, milk, other dairy products:* May impair tetracycline absorption. Give antibiotic 1 hour before or 2 hours after these food products.
Drug-lifestyle. *Sun exposure:* May potentiate photosensitivity reactions. Advise patient to take precautions.

Adverse reactions
CNS: *intracranial hypertension (pseudotumor cerebri),* dizziness.
CV: pericarditis.
EENT: dysphagia, glossitis, tinnitus, visual disturbances.
GI: anorexia, *nausea, vomiting, diarrhea,* enterocolitis, anogenital inflammation, *pancreatitis.*
GU: *increased BUN level.*
Hematologic: *neutropenia,* eosinophilia, *thrombocytopenia,* hemolytic anemia.
Hepatic: elevated liver enzyme levels.
Skin: *maculopapular and erythematous rash, photosensitivity, increased pigmentation, urticaria.*
Other: *hypersensitivity reactions (anaphylaxis),* diabetes insipidus syndrome (polyuria, polydipsia, weakness), permanent tooth discoloration or bone growth retardation in children under age 8.

Overdose and treatment
Signs and symptoms of overdose are usually limited to the GI tract. Treatment may include antacids or gastric lavage if ingestion occurred within 4 hours.

Special considerations
⚠ **ALERT** Check expiration date. Outdated or deteriorated tetracyclines have been linked to reversible nephrotoxicity (Fanconi's syndrome).

• As an anti-infective, drug is usually reserved for patients intolerant of other antibiotics.
• Drug causes false-negative results in urine tests using glucose oxidase reagent (Diastix, Chemstrip uG, or glucose enzymatic test strip). It also causes false elevations in fluorometric tests for urinary catecholamines.

Patient monitoring
• A reversible diabetes insipidus syndrome has been reported with long-term use of demeclocycline; monitor patient for this disorder (weakness, polyuria, polydipsia).
• Monitor renal and liver function tests.
• Monitor fluid balance and daily weights in patients with impaired renal or liver function.

Pregnant patients
• Advise women taking oral contraceptives to use barrier contraception during drug treatment.

Breast-feeding patients
• Avoid use of drug in breast-feeding women.

Pediatric patients
• Don't use drug in children under age 8.

Patient education
• Instruct patient to take entire amount of medication exactly as prescribed, even if he feels better.
• Tell patient to report signs and symptoms of superinfection.
• Advise patient not to expose drug to light or heat; store in tightly capped container.
• Stress good oral hygiene.

desipramine hydrochloride
Norpramin

Pharmacologic classification: dibenzazepine tricyclic antidepressant
Therapeutic classification: antidepressant
Pregnancy risk category: NR

Indications and dosages
➤ *Depression. Adults:* 100 to 200 mg P.O. daily in divided doses, increasing to maximum of 300 mg daily. Or, the entire dose can be given once daily, usually h.s.
Elderly patients and adolescents: 25 to 100 mg P.O. daily, increasing gradually to a maximum of 100 mg daily (maximum 150 mg daily only for the severely ill in these age groups).

How supplied
Available by prescription only
Tablets: 10 mg, 25 mg, 50 mg, 75 mg, 100 mg, 150 mg
Tablets (film-coated): 10 mg, 25 mg, 50 mg, 75 mg, 100 mg, 150 mg

Pharmacodynamics
Antidepressant action: Drug is thought to exert antidepressant effects by inhibiting reuptake of norepinephrine and serotonin in CNS nerve terminals (presynaptic neurons), which results in increased levels and enhanced activity of these neurotransmitters in the synaptic cleft. Desipramine inhibits reuptake of norepinephrine more strongly than serotonin; it has a lesser risk of sedative effects and less anticholinergic and hypotensive activity than its parent compound, imipramine.

Pharmacokinetics
Absorption: Absorbed rapidly from the GI tract after oral administration.
Distribution: Distributed widely into the body, including the CNS and breast milk. Drug is 90% protein-bound. Proposed therapeutic plasma levels (parent drug and metabolite) range from 125 to 300 ng/ml.
Metabolism: Metabolized by the liver; a significant first-pass effect may explain variability of serum levels in different patients taking the same dosage.
Excretion: Excreted primarily in urine.

Route	Onset	Peak	Duration
P.O.	Unknown	4-6 hr	2-4 wk

Contraindications and precautions
Contraindicated in patients hypersensitive to drug, in those who have taken MAO inhibitors within the previous 14 days, and in patients in the acute recovery phase of MI.

Use with extreme caution in patients taking thyroid medication and in those with a history of seizure disorders, urine retention, CV or thyroid disease, or glaucoma. Use cautiously in patients who are depressed with suicidal ideation; dispense minimal quantities.

Interactions
Drug-drug. *Antiarrhythmics, pimozide, thyroid medication:* Increased risk of cardiac arrhythmias and conduction defects. Avoid use together.
Barbiturates: Induced desipramine metabolism and decreased therapeutic efficacy. Monitor patient carefully.
Beta blockers, cimetidine, methylphenidate, oral contraceptives, propoxyphene: May inhibit desipramine metabolism, increasing plasma levels and toxicity. Avoid use together.
Cimetidine, fluoxetine, fluvoxamine, paroxetine, sertraline: May increase serum desipramine levels. Monitor patient carefully.
Clonidine, ephedrine, epinephrine, norepinephrine, phenylephrine: May increase blood pressure; use together cautiously.
Clonidine, guanabenz, guanadrel, guanethidine, methyldopa, reserpine: Decreased hypotensive effects. Avoid use together.

Reactions may be *common*, uncommon, ***life-threatening***, or COMMON AND LIFE-THREATENING.

CNS depressants: Additive effects. Avoid use together.

Disulfiram, ethchlorvynol: May cause delirium and tachycardia. Avoid use together.

Haloperidol, phenothiazines: Decreased metabolism and increased levels of desipramine. Adjust dosages of both drugs.

MAO inhibitors: May cause severe excitation, hyperpyrexia, or seizures, usually with high dosage. Avoid use together.

Selective serotonin-reuptake inhibitors: Patient may become toxic to tricyclic antidepressant at much lower dosages. Dosage reduction may be needed.

Warfarin: May increase PT and risk of bleeding. Monitor PT and INR.

Drug-herb. *Evening primrose oil:* Possible additive or synergistic effect, resulting in lower seizure threshold and increased risk of seizure. Discourage concomitant use.

Drug-lifestyle. *Alcohol use:* May enhance CNS depression. Encourage patient to avoid alcohol use.

Heavy smoking: May lower plasma levels of desipramine. Discourage smoking.

Sun exposure: May increase risk of photosensitivity. Advise patient to take precautions.

Adverse reactions
CNS: *drowsiness, dizziness,* excitation, tremor, weakness, confusion, anxiety, restlessness, agitation, headache, nervousness, EEG changes, *seizures,* extrapyramidal reactions.
CV: orthostatic hypotension, *tachycardia, ECG changes,* hypertension.
EENT: *blurred vision,* tinnitus, mydriasis.
GI: *dry mouth, constipation,* nausea, vomiting, anorexia, paralytic ileus.
GU: *urine retention.*
Hematologic: decreased WBC counts.
Hepatic: elevated liver function test results.
Metabolic: hyperglycemia, hypoglycemia.
Skin: *diaphoresis,* rash, urticaria, photosensitivity.
Other: *hypersensitivity reaction.*
After abrupt withdrawal of long-term therapy: nausea, headache, malaise (doesn't indicate addiction).

Overdose and treatment
The first 12 hours after acute ingestion are a stimulatory phase characterized by excessive anticholinergic activity (agitation, irritation, confusion, hallucinations, parkinsonian symptoms, hyperthermia, seizures, urine retention, dry mucous membranes, pupillary dilatation, constipation, and ileus). This is followed by CNS depressant effects, including hypothermia, decreased or absent reflexes, sedation, hypotension, cyanosis; and cardiac irregularities, including tachycardia, conduction disturbances, and quinidine-like effects on the ECG.

Severity of overdose is best indicated by widening of the QRS complex, which usually represents a serum level in excess of 1,000 ng/ml; serum levels are generally not helpful. Metabolic acidosis may follow hypotension, hypoventilation, and seizures.

Treatment is symptomatic and supportive, including maintaining airway, stable body temperature, and fluid and electrolyte balance. Induce emesis with ipecac if patient is conscious; follow with gastric lavage and activated charcoal to prevent further absorption. Dialysis is of little use. Physostigmine may be used cautiously to reverse CV abnormalities or coma; too rapid administration may cause seizures. Treat seizures with parenteral diazepam or phenytoin; arrhythmias, with parenteral phenytoin or lidocaine; and acidosis, with sodium bicarbonate. Don't give barbiturates; these may enhance CNS and respiratory depressant effects.

Special considerations
Consider the recommendations relevant to all tricyclic antidepressants as well as the following.
● Dispense drug in the smallest possible quantities to depressed outpatients because drug has been used to commit suicide.
● Drug has a lesser risk of sedative effects and fewer anticholinergic and hypotensive effects than its parent compound imipramine.
● Tolerance usually develops to sedative effects of drug during early weeks of therapy.
● Drug shouldn't be withdrawn abruptly; rather, it should be tapered gradually over 3 to 6 weeks.
● Discontinue drug at least 48 hours before surgical procedures.
● In patients with bipolar illness, drug may induce a hypomanic state.

Patient monitoring
● Check standing and sitting blood pressure to assess orthostasis before giving desipramine.

Breast-feeding patients
● Drug appears in breast milk in levels equal to those in maternal serum. The potential benefit to the woman should outweigh the possible adverse reactions in the infant.

Pediatric patients
● Drug isn't recommended for patients under age 12. Sudden death has been reported in children using drug.

Geriatric patients
● Geriatric patients may be more susceptible to adverse CV and anticholinergic effects.

Patient education
● Tell patient to take the full dose at bedtime to alleviate daytime sedation.
● Explain that full effects of drug may not become apparent for 4 weeks and some after therapy starts.
● Tell patient to take drug exactly as prescribed and not to double the dose for missed ones.

• To prevent dizziness, advise patient to lie down for about 30 minutes after each dose at start of therapy and to avoid sudden orthostatic changes, especially when rising to upright position.

• Warn patient not to stop taking drug suddenly.

• Encourage patient to report unusual or troublesome effects, especially confusion, movement disorders, rapid heartbeat, dizziness, fainting, or difficulty urinating.

• Tell patient sugarless chewing gum or hard candy or ice may alleviate dry mouth.

• Stress importance of regular dental hygiene to avoid caries.

---

desmopressin acetate
DDAVP, Stimate

Pharmacologic classification: posterior pituitary hormone
Therapeutic classification: antidiuretic, hemostatic
Pregnancy risk category: B

Indications and dosages
➤ *Central cranial diabetes insipidus, temporary polyuria, polydipsia related to pituitary trauma. Adults:* 0.1 to 0.4 ml (10 to 40 mcg) intranasally in one to three divided doses daily. Adjust morning and evening doses separately for adequate diurnal rhythm of water turnover. Use the lowest effective dosage. Or, 0.05 mg P.O. b.i.d. initially. Adjust individual dosage in increments of 0.1 mg to 1.2 mg daily, divided into two or three doses. Optimal dosage range is 0.1 to 0.8 mg daily in divided doses. Or give 0.5 ml (2 mcg) to 1 ml (4 mcg) I.V. or S.C. daily, usually in two divided doses.
Children ages 3 months to 12 years: 0.05 to 0.3 ml (5 to 30 mcg) intranasally daily in one or two doses.
➤ *Hemophilia A, von Willebrand's disease. Adults and children:* 0.3 mcg/kg diluted in normal saline solution and infused I.V. slowly over 15 to 30 minutes. May repeat dosage, if necessary, as indicated by laboratory response and patient's condition. Or, give one spray per nostril.
➤ *Primary nocturnal enuresis. Children age 6 and older:* 20 mcg (two to four metered sprays), intranasally h.s. Dosage adjusted according to response. Maximum recommended dose is 40 mcg daily.

How supplied
Available by prescription only
Injection: 4 mcg/ml in 1-ml single-dose ampules and 10-ml multiple-dose vials
Nasal solution: 0.1 mg/ml, 1.5 mg/ml
Tablets: 0.1 mg, 0.2 mg

Pharmacodynamics
Antidiuretic action: Drug is used to control or prevent signs and complications of neurogenic diabetes insipidus. The site of action is primari-

ly at the renal tubular level. Desmopressin increases water permeability at the renal tubule and collecting duct, resulting in increased urine osmolality and decreased urinary flow rate.
Hemostatic action: Desmopressin increases factor VIII activity by releasing endogenous factor VIII from plasma storage sites.

Pharmacokinetics
Absorption: Destroyed in the GI tract. After intranasal administration, 10% to 20% of dose is absorbed through nasal mucosa.
Distribution: Not fully understood.
Metabolism: Unknown.
Excretion: Plasma levels decline in two phases: Half-life of fast phase is about 8 minutes; slow phase, 75 minutes. Duration of action after intranasal administration is 8 to 20 hours; after I.V. administration, 12 to 24 hours for mild hemophilia and about 3 hours for von Willebrand's disease.

Route	Onset	Peak	Duration
P.O.	1 hr	1-1½ hr	8-12 hr
I.V.	15-30 min	Unknown	4-12 hr
Nasal	1 hr	1-5 hr	8-12 hr

Contraindications and precautions
Contraindicated in patients hypersensitive to drug and in patients with type IIB von Willebrand's disease. Use cautiously in patients with coronary artery insufficiency or hypertensive CV disease and in those with conditions related to fluid and electrolyte imbalances, such as cystic fibrosis, because these patients are susceptible to hyponatremia.

Interactions
Drug-drug. *Carbamazepine, chlorpropamide, clofibrate:* May potentiate the antidiuretic action of desmopressin. Avoid use together.
Demeclocycline, epinephrine, heparin, lithium, norepinephrine: May decrease antidiuretic effect. Use together cautiously.
Drug-lifestyle. *Alcohol use:* May increase risk of adverse effects. Discourage use together.

Adverse reactions
CNS: headache.
CV: flushing, slight rise in blood pressure at high dosage.
EENT: rhinitis, epistaxis, sore throat, cough.
GI: nausea, abdominal cramps.
GU: vulvar pain.
Other: local erythema, swelling, burning (after injection).

Overdose and treatment
Signs and symptoms of overdose include drowsiness, listlessness, headache, confusion, anuria, and weight gain (water intoxication).

Treatment requires water restriction and temporary withdrawal of desmopressin until polyuria occurs. Severe water intoxication may require

---

Reactions may be *common,* uncommon, *life-threatening,* or COMMON AND LIFE-THREATENING.

osmotic diuresis with mannitol, hypertonic dextrose, or urea—alone or with furosemide.

Special considerations
Consider the recommendations relevant to all posterior pituitary hormones as well as the following.
● Desmopressin may be administered intranasally through a flexible catheter called a rhinyle. A measured quantity is drawn up into the catheter, one end is inserted into patient's nose, and patient blows on the other end to deposit drug into nasal cavity. Drug is also available in nasal spray, which may be easier for some patients.
● Patients may be switched from intranasal to S.C. desmopressin (such as during episodes of rhinorrhea). They should receive ⅒ of their usual dosage parenterally.
● Desmopressin isn't indicated for hemophilia A patients with factor VIII levels up to 5% or in patients with severe von Willebrand's disease.
● Drug therapy may enable some patients to avoid the hazards of contaminated blood products.

Patient monitoring
● Monitor patient for early signs of water intoxication—drowsiness, listlessness, headache, confusion, anuria, and weight gain—to prevent seizures, coma, and death.
● Especially in young or elderly patients, adjust fluid intake to reduce risk of water intoxication and sodium depletion.
● Weigh patient daily and observe for edema.

Pediatric patients
● Drug isn't recommended for infants under age 3 months because of their increased tendency to develop fluid imbalance.
● Use cautiously in infants because of risk of hyponatremia and water intoxication.
● Safety and efficacy of parenteral desmopressin haven't been established for management of diabetes insipidus in children under age 12.

Geriatric patients
● These patients have an increased risk of hyponatremia and water intoxication; therefore, restriction of their fluid intake is recommended.
● Because geriatric patients are more sensitive to effects of drug, they may need a lower dosage.

Patient education
● Teach patient correct administration technique. Evaluate patient's proficiency at drug administration and accurate measurement on return visits; some patients have trouble measuring drug and inhaling it into nostrils.
● Emphasize that patient shouldn't increase or decrease dosage unless prescribed.
● Assist patient in planning a schedule for fluid intake if oral fluids must be reduced to decrease the possibility of water intoxication and hyponatremia. A diuretic may be administered if excessive fluid retention occurs.

● Tell patient to store drug away from heat and direct light, not in bathroom, where heat and moisture can cause drug to deteriorate.

desonide
DesOwen, Tridesilon

Pharmacologic classification: topical adrenocorticoid
Therapeutic classification: anti-inflammatory
Pregnancy risk category: C

Indications and dosages
► **Adjunctive therapy for inflammation in acute and chronic corticosteroid-responsive dermatoses.** *Adults and children:* Apply sparingly to affected area b.i.d. to q.i.d.

How supplied
Available by prescription only
Cream, lotion, ointment: 0.05%

Pharmacodynamics
Anti-inflammatory action: Desonide stimulates the synthesis of enzymes needed to decrease the inflammatory response. Desonide is a group IV nonfluorinated glucocorticoid with a potency similar to that of alclometasone dipropionate 0.05% and fluocinolone acetonide 0.01%.

Pharmacokinetics
Absorption: Amount absorbed depends on the amount applied and on the nature of the skin at the application site. It ranges from about 1% in areas with a thick stratum corneum (such as the palms, soles, elbows, and knees) to as much as 36% in areas of the thinnest stratum corneum (face, eyelids, and genitals). Absorption increases in areas of skin damage, inflammation, or occlusion. Some systemic absorption of topical steroids occurs, especially through the oral mucosa.
Distribution: After topical application, desonide is distributed throughout the local skin layer. Any drug that's absorbed into circulation is removed rapidly from the blood and distributed into muscle, liver, skin, intestines, and kidneys.
Metabolism: After topical administration, drug is metabolized primarily in the skin. The small amount that's absorbed into systemic circulation is metabolized primarily in the liver to inactive compounds.
Excretion: Inactive metabolites are excreted by the kidneys, primarily as glucuronides and sulfates, but also as unconjugated products. Small amounts of metabolites are excreted in feces.

Route	Onset	Peak	Duration
Topical	Unknown	Unknown	Unknown

Contraindications and precautions
Contraindicated in patients hypersensitive to drug.

Interactions
None significant.

Adverse reactions
Metabolic: hyperglycemia, glucosuria.
Skin: burning, pruritus, irritation, dryness, erythema, folliculitis, perioral dermatitis, allergic contact dermatitis, hypertrichosis, hypopigmentation, acneiform eruptions; *maceration of skin, secondary infection, atrophy, striae, and miliaria* with occlusive dressings.
Other: *hypothalamic-pituitary-adrenal axis suppression,* Cushing's syndrome.

Overdose and treatment
No information available.

Special considerations
• Gently wash skin before applying. Rub drug in gently, leaving a thin coat. When treating hairy sites, part hair and apply directly to lesions.

Patient monitoring
• Monitor patient for skin infection, striae, or atrophy; if these develop, stop drug.

Pediatric patients
• Children may be more susceptible to systemic absorption and hypothalamic-pituitary-adrenal axis suppression.
• Avoid using plastic pants or tight-fitting diapers on treated area in young child.

Patient education
• Teach patient to apply drug.
• If patient uses an occlusive dressing, advise against leaving dressing in place longer than 12 hours each day or using occlusive dressing on infected or exudative lesions.
• Tell patient to report adverse effects immediately.

dexamethasone (ophthalmic suspension)
Maxidex

dexamethasone sodium phosphate
AK-Dex, Decadron, Dexair, I-Methasone, Ocu-Dex

Pharmacologic classification: corticosteroid
Therapeutic classification: ophthalmic anti-inflammatory
Pregnancy risk category: C

Indications and dosages
➤ *Uveitis; iridocyclitis; inflammation of eyelids, conjunctiva, cornea, anterior segment of globe; corneal injury from burns or penetration by foreign bodies; allergic conjunctivitis; suppression of* *graft rejection after keratoplasty. Adults and children:* Instill 1 to 2 drops of suspension or solution or apply 1.25 to 2.5 cm of ointment into conjunctival sac. For initial therapy of severe cases, instill solution or suspension into conjunctival sac every hour. Gradually discontinue dose as patient's condition improves. In mild condition, instill drops up to four to six times daily or apply ointment t.i.d. or q.i.d. As patient's condition improves, taper dose to b.i.d. and then once daily. Treatment may extend from a few days to several weeks.

How supplied
Available by prescription only
dexamethasone
Ophthalmic suspension: 0.1%
dexamethasone sodium phosphate
Ophthalmic ointment: 0.05%
Ophthalmic solution: 0.1%

Pharmacodynamics
Anti-inflammatory action: Corticosteroids stimulate the synthesis of enzymes needed to decrease the inflammatory response. Dexamethasone, a long-acting fluorinated synthetic adrenocorticoid with strong anti-inflammatory activity and minimal mineralocorticoid activity, is 25 to 30 times more potent than an equal weight of hydrocortisone.
Drug is poorly soluble and therefore has a slower onset but a longer duration of action when applied in a liquid suspension. Sodium phosphate salt is highly soluble and has a rapid onset but short duration of action.

Pharmacokinetics
Absorption: After ophthalmic administration, drug is absorbed through the aqueous humor. Because doses are low, little if any systemic absorption occurs.
Distribution: Distributed throughout local tissue layers. Drug absorbed into circulation is rapidly removed from blood and distributed into muscle, liver, skin, intestines, and kidneys.
Metabolism: Primarily metabolized locally. The small amount absorbed into systemic circulation is metabolized mainly in the liver to inactive compounds.
Excretion: Inactive metabolites are excreted by the kidneys, primarily as glucuronides and sulfates, but also as unconjugated products. Small amounts of metabolites are also excreted in feces.

Route	Onset	Peak	Duration
Oph-thalmic	Unknown	Unknown	Unknown

Contraindications and precautions
Contraindicated in patients with acute superficial herpes simplex (dendritic keratitis), vaccinia, varicella, or other fungal or viral diseases of cornea and conjunctiva; ocular tuberculosis; or acute, purulent, untreated infections of the eye.

Use cautiously in patients with corneal abrasions that may be infected (especially with herpes). Also use cautiously in patients with glaucoma because intraocular pressure may increase. Glaucoma medications may need to be increased to compensate.

Interactions
None reported.

Adverse reactions
EENT: increased intraocular pressure, thinning of cornea, interference with corneal wound healing, increased susceptibility to viral or fungal corneal infection, corneal ulceration, glaucoma exacerbation, cataracts, defects in visual acuity and visual field, optic nerve damage, mild blurred vision, burning eyes, stinging eyes, red eyes, watery eyes, discharge, discomfort, ocular pain, foreign body sensation (with excessive or long-term use).
Other: systemic effects and adrenal suppression with excessive or long-term use.

Overdose and treatment
None reported.

Special considerations
● Shake suspension well before use.
● Drug isn't recommended for long-term use.

Patient monitoring
● Monitor patient for signs of corneal ulceration; if they appear, patient may need to stop drug.

Patient education
◪ ALERT Warn patient to call immediately and stop drug if visual acuity changes or visual field diminishes.
● Teach patient how to instill drops or ointment. Advise him to wash hands before and after administering, and warn him not to touch tip of dropper to eye or surrounding tissue.
● Tell patient to apply light finger pressure on lacrimal sac for 1 minute after installation.
● Warn patient not to share medication.

dexamethasone (systemic)
Decadron, Deronil*, Dexasone*, Dexone, Hexadrol

dexamethasone acetate
Dalalone D.P., Decadron-LA, Decaject-L.A., Dexasone L.A., Dexone L.A., Solurex LA

dexamethasone sodium phosphate
AK-Dex, Dalalone, Decadrol, Decadron, Decaject, Dexameth, Dexasone, Dexone, Hexadrol Phosphate, Oradexon*, Solurex

Pharmacologic classification: glucocorticoid
Therapeutic classification: anti-inflammatory, immunosuppressant
Pregnancy risk category: NR

Indications and dosages
➤ *Cerebral edema.* dexamethasone sodium phosphate. *Adults:* Initially, 10 mg I.V.; then 4 mg I.M. q 6 hours for 2 to 4 days. Then taper over 5 to 7 days.
➤ *Inflammatory conditions, allergic reactions, neoplasias. Adults:* 0.75 to 9 mg P.O. daily divided b.i.d., t.i.d., or q.i.d.
Children: 0.024 to 0.34 mg/kg P.O. daily in four divided doses.
dexamethasone acetate
Adults: 4 to 16 mg intra-articularly or into soft tissue q 1 to 3 weeks. Or, 0.8 to 1.6 mg into lesions q 1 to 3 weeks. Or, 8 to 16 mg I.M. q 1 to 3 weeks, p.r.n.
dexamethasone sodium phosphate
Adults: 0.2 to 6 mg intra-articularly, intralesionally, or into soft tissue. Or, 0.5 to 9 mg I.M.
➤ *Shock (other than adrenal crisis). Dexamethasone sodium phosphate. Adults:* 1 to 6 mg/kg I.V. daily as a single dose; or 40 mg I.V. q 2 to 6 hours, p.r.n.
➤ *Dexamethasone suppression test. Adults:* 0.5 mg P.O. q 6 hours for 48 hours.
➤ *Adrenal insufficiency. Adults:* 0.75 to 9 g P.O. daily in divided doses.
Children: 0.024 to 0.34 mg/kg P.O. daily in four divided doses.
dexamethasone sodium phosphate
Adults: 0.5 to 9 mg I.M. or I.V. daily.
Children: 0.235 to 1.25 mg/m2 I.M. or I.V. once daily or b.i.d.
➤ *Tuberculous meningitis. Adults:* 8 to 12 mg daily tapered over 6 to 8 weeks.
➤ *Prevention of hyaline membrane disease in premature infants◇. Adults:* 5 mg (phosphate) I.M. t.i.d. to mother for 2 days before delivery.
➤ *Prevention of chemotherapy-induced nausea and vomiting◇. Adults:* 10 to 20 mg I.V. before chemotherapy. Additional doses (individualized and usually lower than initial dose) may be given I.V. or P.O. for 24 to 72 hours after chemotherapy, if needed.

How supplied
Available by prescription only
dexamethasone
Elixir: 0.5 mg/5 ml
Oral solution: 0.5 mg/0.5 ml, 0.5 mg/5 ml
Tablets: 0.25 mg, 0.5 mg, 0.75 mg, 1 mg, 1.5 mg, 2 mg, 4 mg, 6 mg
dexamethasone acetate
Injection: 8 mg/ml, 16 mg/ml suspension

dexamethasone sodium phosphate
Injection: 4 mg/ml, 10 mg/ml
Injection (I.V. use only): 24 mg/ml

Pharmacodynamics
Anti-inflammatory action: Dexamethasone stimulates the synthesis of enzymes needed to decrease the inflammatory response. It causes suppression of the immune system by reducing activity and volume of the lymphatic system, producing lymphocytopenia (primarily T-lymphocytes), decreasing passage of immune complexes through basement membranes, and possibly by depressing reactivity of tissue to antigen-antibody interactions.

Drug is a long-acting synthetic adrenocorticoid with strong anti-inflammatory activity and minimal mineralocorticoid properties. It's 25 to 30 times more potent than an equal weight of hydrocortisone.

The acetate salt is a suspension and shouldn't be used I.V. It's particularly useful as an anti-inflammatory agent in intra-articular, intradermal, and intralesional injections.

The sodium phosphate salt is highly soluble and has a more rapid onset and a shorter duration of action than does the acetate salt. It's most commonly used for cerebral edema and unresponsive shock. It can also be used in intra-articular, intralesional, or soft tissue inflammation. Dexamethasone is also used as a treatment for chemotherapy-induced nausea and bronchial asthma symptoms and as a diagnostic test for Cushing's syndrome.

Pharmacokinetics
Absorption: After oral use, drug is absorbed readily. The suspension for injection has a variable onset and duration of action, depending on whether it's injected into an intra-articular space, a muscle, or the blood supply to the muscle. After I.V. injection, dexamethasone is rapidly and completely absorbed into the tissues.
Distribution: Removed rapidly from blood and distributed to muscle, liver, skin, intestines, and kidneys. Dexamethasone is bound weakly to plasma proteins (transcortin and albumin). Only the unbound portion is active. Adrenocorticoids appear in breast milk and the placenta.
Metabolism: Metabolized in the liver to inactive glucuronide and sulfate metabolites.
Excretion: Inactive metabolites and small amounts of unmetabolized drug are excreted by the kidneys. Insignificant quantities are also excreted in feces; biologic half-life is 36 to 54 hours.

Route	Onset	Peak	Duration
P.O.	1-2 hr	1-2 hr	2½ days
I.V.	1 hr	1 hr	Variable
I.M.			
acetate	1 hr	8 hr	Unknown
phosphate	1 hr	1 hr	6 days

Contraindications and precautions
Contraindicated in patients hypersensitive to any component of drug and in those with systemic fungal infections.

Use cautiously in patients with recent MI, GI ulcer, renal disease, hypertension, osteoporosis, diabetes mellitus, hypothyroidism, cirrhosis, diverticulitis, nonspecific ulcerative colitis, recent intestinal anastomoses, thromboembolic disorders, seizures, myasthenia gravis, heart failure, tuberculosis, ocular herpes simplex, emotional instability, and psychotic tendencies. Because some formulations contain sulfite preservatives, also use cautiously in patients sensitive to sulfites.

Interactions
Drug-drug. *Amphotericin B, diuretics:* Increased risk of hypokalemia. Monitor serum potassium levels.
Antacids, cholestyramine, colestipol: Decreased corticosteroid effect. Monitor patient closely, and adjust dosage as needed.
Aspirin, NSAIDs: May increase the risk of GI ulceration. Use together cautiously.
Barbiturates, phenytoin, rifampin: May cause decreased corticosteroid effects. Adjust dosage as needed.
Cardiac glycosides: Hypokalemia may increase the risk of toxicity. Adjust dosage as needed.
Estrogens: May reduce dexamethasone metabolism by increasing transcortin levels. Monitor patient carefully.
Insulin, oral antidiabetics: Increased risk of hyperglycemia. Adjust dosage as needed.
Isoniazid, salicylates: Increased metabolism of these drugs. Monitor patient carefully.
Oral anticoagulants: Decreased anticoagulant effects. Monitor PT and INR closely.
Skin-test antigens: Decreased response. Defer skin testing until therapy is completed.
Toxoids, vaccines: Decreased antibody response and increased risk of neurologic complications. Avoid concurrent use.
Drug-lifestyle. *Alcohol use:* Increased risk of gastric irritation and GI ulceration. Advise patient to avoid alcohol.

Adverse reactions
Most adverse reactions to corticosteroids are dose- or duration-dependent.
CNS: *euphoria, insomnia,* psychotic behavior, pseudotumor cerebri, vertigo, headache, paresthesia, *seizures.*
CV: *heart failure,* hypertension, edema, *arrhythmias,* thrombophlebitis, *thromboembolism.*
EENT: cataracts, glaucoma.
GI: *peptic ulceration,* GI irritation, increased appetite, *pancreatitis,* nausea, vomiting.
GU: menstrual irregularities.
Metabolic: hypokalemia, hypocalcemia, hyperglycemia, carbohydrate intolerance, decreased levels of thyroxine and triiodothyronine, increased urine glucose and calcium levels.

Reactions may be *common,* uncommon, *life-threatening,* or COMMON AND LIFE-THREATENING.

Musculoskeletal: muscle weakness, osteoporosis, growth suppression in children.

Skin: hirsutism, delayed wound healing, acne, skin eruptions, atrophy at I.M. injection sites, cushingoid state (moonface, buffalo hump, central obesity).

Other: susceptibility to infections, *acute adrenal insufficiency following increased stress (infection, surgery, or trauma) or abrupt withdrawal after long-term therapy.*

Overdose and treatment

Acute ingestion, even in massive doses, rarely poses a clinical problem. Toxic signs and symptoms rarely occur if drug is used for less than 3 weeks, even at large dosage ranges. However, long-term use causes adverse physiologic effects, including suppression of the hypothalamic-pituitary-adrenal axis, cushingoid appearance, muscle weakness, and osteoporosis.

Special considerations

⚠ ALERT After abrupt withdrawal, patient may experience rebound inflammation, fatigue, weakness, arthralgia, fever, dizziness, lethargy, depression, fainting, orthostatic hypotension, dyspnea, anorexia, or hypoglycemia. After prolonged use, sudden withdrawal may be fatal.

● Determine whether patient is sensitive to other corticosteroids.

● For better results and less toxicity, consider a once-daily dose in the morning.

● Give drug by I.M. injection deep into gluteal muscle. Rotate sites. Avoid S.C. injection.

● Drug is being used investigationally to prevent hyaline membrane disease (respiratory distress syndrome) in premature infants. The suspension (phosphate salt) is given I.M. to the mother two or three times daily for 2 days before delivery.

● Dexamethasone causes false-negative results in the nitroblue tetrazolium test for systemic bacterial infections and decreases ^{131}I uptake and protein-bound iodine levels in thyroid function tests.

Patient monitoring

● Patient's weight, blood pressure, and serum electrolyte levels must be checked frequently.

● Monitor patient for depression or psychotic episodes.

Pediatric patients

● Long-term use of drug in children and adolescents may delay growth and maturation.

Patient education

● Tell patient not to stop drug abruptly or without prescriber's consent.

● Instruct patient to take drug with food or milk.

● Teach patient signs of early adrenal insufficiency: fatigue, muscle weakness, joint pain, fever, anorexia, nausea, dyspnea, dizziness, and fainting.

dexamethasone sodium phosphate
Decadron Phosphate

Pharmacologic classification: corticosteroid
Therapeutic classification: anti-inflammatory
Pregnancy risk category: C

Indications and dosages

➤ *Inflammation from corticosteroid-responsive dermatoses. Adults and children:* Apply sparingly t.i.d. or q.i.d. For aerosol use on scalp, shake can well and apply to dry scalp after shampooing. Hold can upright. Slide applicator tube under hair so it touches scalp. Spray while moving tube to all affected areas, keeping tube under hair and in contact with scalp throughout spraying, which should take about 2 seconds. Inadequately covered areas may be spot sprayed. Slide applicator tube through hair to touch scalp, press and immediately release spray button. Don't massage medication into scalp or spray forehead or eyes.

How supplied

Available by prescription only
Aerosol: 0.01%, 0.04%

Pharmacodynamics

Anti-inflammatory action: Dexamethasone is a synthetic fluorinated corticosteroid. It's usually classed as a group VII potency anti-inflammatory. Occlusive dressings may be used in severe cases. The aerosol spray is usually used for scalp conditions.

Pharmacokinetics

Absorption: Absorption depends on the potency of the preparation, the amount applied, the vehicle used, and the skin at the application site. It ranges from about 1% in areas with a thick stratum corneum (such as the palms, soles, elbows, and knees) to 25% in areas of the thinnest stratum corneum (face, eyelids, and genitals). Inflamed or damaged skin may absorb more than 33%. Absorption increases in areas of skin damage, inflammation, or occlusion. Some systemic absorption occurs, especially through the oral mucosa.

Distribution: After topical administration, dexamethasone is distributed throughout the local skin layer. If absorbed into circulation, drug is distributed rapidly into muscle, liver, skin, intestines, and kidneys.

Metabolism: After topical administration, dexamethasone is metabolized primarily in the skin. The small amount absorbed into systemic circulation is metabolized mainly in the liver to inactive compounds.

Excretion: Inactive metabolites are excreted by the kidneys, primarily as glucuronides and sulfates, but also as unconjugated products. Small amounts of the metabolites are also excreted in feces.

Route	Onset	Peak	Duration
Topical	Unknown	Unknown	Unknown

Contraindications and precautions
Contraindicated in patients hypersensitive to drug.

Interactions
None significant.

Adverse reactions
Metabolic: hyperglycemia, glucosuria.
Skin: burning, pruritus, irritation, dryness, erythema, folliculitis, hypertrichosis, acneiform eruptions, perioral dermatitis, hypopigmentation, allergic contact dermatitis; *maceration, secondary infection, atrophy, striae, miliaria* (with occlusive dressings).
Other: *hypothalamic-pituitary-adrenal axis suppression,* Cushing's syndrome.

Overdose and treatment
Topical corticosteroids can be absorbed in sufficient amounts to produce systemic effects.

Special considerations
• Gently wash skin before applying.
• To prevent skin damage, rub cream in gently, leaving a thin coat.
• When treating hairy sites, part hair and apply directly to lesions.
• Continue treatment for a few days after lesions clear.

Patient monitoring
• Stop drug if skin infection, striae, or atrophy occurs.

Patient education
• Teach patient and family how to apply drug.
• If occlusive dressing is ordered, tell patient to remove dressing and notify prescriber if a fever develops.
• Advise patient not to leave occlusive dressing on more than 12 hours each day.
• Tell patient not to use occlusive dressing on infected or exudative lesions.

---

dexmedetomidine hydrochloride
Precedex

Pharmacologic classification: selective alpha$_2$-adrenoceptor agonist with sedative properties
Therapeutic classification: sedative
Pregnancy risk category: C

Indications and dosages
➤ *Sedation of initially intubated and mechanically ventilated patients in ICU*

setting. Adults: Loading infusion of 1 mcg/kg I.V. over 10 minutes; then a maintenance infusion of 0.2 to 0.7 mcg/kg/hr for up to 24 hours, adjusted to achieve the desired level of sedation.
✦ *Dosage adjustment.* Consider dosage adjustment in elderly patients and those with renal or hepatic failure.

How supplied
Available by prescription only
Injection: 100 mcg/ml in 2-ml vials and 2-ml ampules

Pharmacodynamics
Sedative action: Thought to produce sedation by selective stimulation of alpha$_2$-adrenoceptors in the CNS.

Pharmacokinetics
Absorption: Administered I.V.
Distribution: After I.V. administration, drug is rapidly and widely distributed. It is 94% protein-bound.
Metabolism: Almost completely hepatically metabolized to inactive metabolites.
Excretion: Inactive metabolites are 95% eliminated by kidneys and 4% in feces. Elimination half-life is about 2 hours.

Route	Onset	Peak	Duration
I.V.	Unknown	Unknown	Unknown

Contraindications and precautions
Use cautiously in elderly patients and patients with advanced heart block or renal or hepatic impairment.

Interactions
Drug-drug. *Anesthetics, hypnotics, opioids, sedatives:* Possible enhanced effects of these drugs. Reduce their dosages if needed.

Adverse reactions
CV: *hypotension, **bradycardia, arrhythmias**.*
GI: nausea, thirst.
GU: oliguria.
Hematologic: anemia, leukocytosis.
Respiratory: *hypoxia,* pleural effusion, ***pulmonary edema.***
Other: pain, infection.

Overdose and treatment
Bradycardia, hypotension, and first- and second degree AV block have been reported in patients receiving doses of dexmedetomidine substantially higher than the recommended dose.
   These have resolved spontaneously. Stopping the infusion and providing supportive care and resuscitation, if necessary, are the primary treatments for overdose.

Special considerations
• Drug should be administered only by persons skilled in managing patients in the ICU setting

---

Reactions may be *common*, uncommon, *life-threatening*, or COMMON AND LIFE-THREATENING.

and where the patient's cardiac status can be monitored continuously.

ALERT Administer using a controlled infusion device at the rate calculated for body weight.

ALERT Don't administer infusion for longer than 24 hours.

• Dexmedetomidine has been continuously infused in mechanically ventilated patients before extubation, during extubation, and after extubation. It isn't necessary to discontinue dexmedetomidine before extubation.

• Dexmedetomidine must be diluted in saline solution before administration. To prepare the infusion, withdraw 2 ml of dexmedetomidine and add to 48 ml of saline solution injection to a total of 50 ml. Shake gently to mix well.

• Don't co-administer through the same I.V. catheter with blood or plasma because physical compatibility hasn't been established. Dexmedetomidine infusion is compatible with lactated Ringer's solution, D5W, saline solution, and 20% mannitol. It's also compatible with thiopental sodium, etomidate, vecuronium bromide, pancuronium bromide, succinylcholine, atracurium besylate, mivacurium chloride, glycopyrrolate bromide, phenylephrine hydrochloride, atropine sulfate, midazolam, morphine sulfate, fentanyl citrate, and plasma-substitute.

Patient monitoring

• Continuously monitor cardiac status.

• Renal and hepatic function should be determined before administration, particularly in elderly patients.

• Some patients receiving dexmedetomidine are arousable and alert when stimulated. This alone shouldn't be considered evidence of lack of efficacy in the absence of other clinical signs and symptoms.

Breast-feeding patients

• It isn't known whether drug appears in breast milk. Because many drugs do, use caution when administering drug to breast-feeding women.

Pediatric patients

• Safety and effectiveness haven't been established in patients younger than age 18.

Geriatric patients

• Bradycardia and hypotension have occurred in patients over age 65. Consider a dosage reduction in this group.

Patient education

• Tell patient he will be sedated while the drug is administered, but that he may arouse when stimulated.

• Tell patient he will be closely monitored and attended while sedated.

dexpanthenol
Ilopan, Panthoderm

Pharmacologic classification: vitamin B complex analogue
Therapeutic classification: GI stimulant, emollient
Pregnancy risk category: C

Indications and dosages

➤ *Emollient and protectant over colostomy area or other surgical site.*
Adults and children: Apply thin layer q.d. to b.i.d., p.r.n.

➤ *Itching, wounds, insect bites, poison ivy, poison oak, diaper rash, chafing, mild eczema, decubitus ulcers, dry lesions.*
Adults and children: Apply thin layer topically q.d. to b.i.d., p.r.n.

➤ *Prevention of postoperative adynamic ileus. Adults:* 250 to 500 mg I.M.; repeat in 2 hours. Then give q 6 hours, p.r.n.

➤ *Treatment of adynamic ileus. Adults:* 500 mg I.M., repeat in 2 hours. Then give q 6 hours, p.r.n.

How supplied
Available by prescription only
Injection: 250 mg/ml in vials, ampules, and prefilled syringes
Topical cream: 2%

Pharmacodynamics
Emollient action: By stimulating granulation and epithelialization, dexpanthenol promotes healing and relieves itching.
GI stimulant action: Dexpanthenol is an analogue of pantothenic acid, a precursor of coenzyme A, which serves as a cofactor in the synthesis of acetylcholine. Dexpanthenol stimulates the acetylation of choline to acetylcholine, which increases peristalsis.

Pharmacokinetics
Absorption: Dexpanthenol is absorbed from I.M. sites.
Distribution: After conversion to pantothenic acid, drug is distributed widely, mainly as coenzyme A. Levels are highest in liver, adrenal glands, heart, and kidneys.
Metabolism: Conversion to pantothenic acid occurs readily.
Excretion: Most metabolites are excreted in urine; remainder in feces.

Route	Onset	Peak	Duration
I.M., topical	Unknown	Unknown	Unknown

Contraindications and precautions
Contraindicated in patients with ileus caused by obstruction because of risk for severe cramping and worsening of condition. Contraindicated on

◇ Unlabeled clinical use

wounds in patients with hemophilia because of risk for severe bleeding.

Interactions
Drug-drug. *Antibiotics, barbiturates:* Allergic responses to dexpanthenol may occur (very rare). Monitor patient for adverse effects.
Succinylcholine: Prolonged succinylcholine action. Give these drugs at least 1 hour apart.

Adverse reactions
CV: slight decreases in blood pressure.
GI: intestinal colic, vomiting, diarrhea.
Respiratory: breathing difficulties.
Skin: itching, red patches, dermatitis, tingling.

Overdose and treatment
No information available.

Special considerations
● Avoid use with drugs that decrease GI motility.

Patient monitoring
● Monitor patient for adverse reactions; stop drug if hypersensitivity reaction occurs.
● Monitor fluid and electrolytes (especially potassium) in patients with adynamic ileus. Anemia, hypoproteinemia, and infection may contribute to the condition.

Pediatric patients
● Safety of parenteral form hasn't been established.

Geriatric patients
● Use cautiously; agitation has been reported.

Patient education
● Review adverse reactions.

dexrazoxane
Zinecard

Pharmacologic classification: intracellular chelating agent
Therapeutic classification: cardioprotective
Pregnancy risk category: C

Indications and dosages
➤ *Reduction of occurrence and severity of doxorubicin-induced cardiomyopathy in women with metastatic breast cancer who have received a cumulative doxorubicin dose of 300 mg/m² but would benefit from continued doxorubicin therapy.*
Adults: Dosage ratio of dexrazoxane to doxorubicin must be 10:1, such as 500 mg/m² dexrazoxane and 50 mg/m² doxorubicin. After reconstitution, give dexrazoxane by slow I.V. push or rapid drip I.V. infusion. After completion and before a total elapsed time of 30 minutes from the beginning of the dexrazoxane administration, give doxorubicin dose by I.V. injection.

How supplied
Available by prescription only
Injection: 250 mg, 500 mg in single-dose vials

Pharmacodynamics
Cardioprotective action: Specific mechanism is unknown. Drug is a cyclic derivative of EDTA that readily penetrates cell membranes. It may be converted intracellularly to a ring-opened chelating agent that interferes with iron-mediated free radical generation believed to be responsible, in part, for anthracycline-induced cardiomyopathy.

Pharmacokinetics
Absorption: Administered I.V.
Distribution: Unknown. Drug isn't bound to plasma proteins.
Metabolism: Not believed to be metabolized.
Excretion: Primarily excreted in urine.

Route	Onset	Peak	Duration
I.V.	Unknown	Unknown	Unknown

Contraindications and precautions
Contraindicated in patients who aren't receiving doxorubicin as part of the chemotherapy regimen. Use cautiously in all patients because additive effects of immunosuppression may occur from concomitant administration of cytotoxic drugs.

Interactions
None significant.

Adverse reactions
The following reactions (except for pain on injection) may be attributed to the FAC regimen (fluorouracil, doxorubicin, cyclophosphamide) given shortly after dexrazoxane.
CNS: *fatigue, malaise, neurotoxicity.*
GI: *nausea, vomiting, anorexia, stomatitis, diarrhea,* esophagitis, dysphagia.
Hematologic: *hemorrhage.*
Skin: *alopecia,* urticaria.
Other: *fever, infection, pain on injection, sepsis,* streaking at I.V. insertion site, erythema, phlebitis, extravasation.

Overdose and treatment
There are no known reports of overdose, although myelosuppression is most likely to occur.
Because dexrazoxane isn't bound to plasma protein, peritoneal dialysis or hemodialysis may be effective in removing drug from body. Manage suspected overdose with good supportive care until resolution of myelosuppression and related conditions is complete. Management of overdose should include treatment of infections, fluid regulation, and maintenance of nutritional requirements.

Reactions may be *common*, uncommon, *life-threatening*, or COMMON AND LIFE-THREATENING.

Special considerations

⚠ ALERT Doxorubicin shouldn't be given before dexrazoxane. Also, dexrazoxane isn't recommended for use at the start of doxorubicin therapy but only after a cumulative dosage of doxorubicin of 300 mg/m² has been reached and continuation of doxorubicin is desired.

• Drug must be diluted with the diluent supplied with drug (0.167 M sodium lactate injection) to give 10 mg dexrazoxane for each milliliter of sodium lactate. Give reconstituted solution by slow I.V. push or rapid drip I.V. infusion from a bag.

• Reconstituted solution, when transferred to an empty infusion bag, is stable for 6 hours from the time of reconstitution when stored at controlled room temperature (36° to 46° F [2° to 8° C]) or refrigerated. Discard unused solution.

• Reconstituted drug may be diluted with either normal saline solution or D₅W injection to 1.3 to 5.0 mg/ml in I.V. infusion bags. The resulting solution is stable for 6 hours under the same storage conditions as the diluted drug.

• Don't mix dexrazoxane with other drugs because of possible incompatibility.

• Use caution when handling and preparing the reconstituted solution; follow same precautions as handling antineoplastics. Wear gloves. If drug powder or solution contacts skin or mucosa, immediately wash thoroughly with soap and water.

Patient monitoring

• Monitor CBC closely because drug is always used with other cytotoxic drugs and it may add to the myelosuppressive effects cytotoxic drugs.

• Administering Zinecard with doxorubicin doesn't eliminate the possibility of cardiac toxicity. Carefully monitor cardiac function.

Breast-feeding patients

• Because of the potential for serious adverse effects in breast-fed infants, breast-feeding isn't recommended.

Pediatric patients

• Safety and effectiveness in children haven't been established.

Patient education

• Inform patient of need for drug during continued doxorubicin therapy.

• Warn patient to watch for signs of infection (fever, sore throat, fatigue) and bleeding (easy bruising, nose bleeds, bleeding gums, melena). Tell patient to take temperature daily and teach him infection control and bleeding precautions.

• Inform patient that alopecia may occur but that it's usually reversible.

dextran 1
Promit

dextran, low-molecular-weight (dextran 40)
Gentran 40, LMD 10%, Rheomacrodex

dextran, high-molecular-weight (dextran 70, dextran 75)
Gendex 75, Gentran 70, Macrodex

Pharmacologic classification: glucose polymer
Therapeutic classification: plasma volume expander
Pregnancy risk category: C

Indications and dosages

➤ **Prevention of severe anaphylactoid reaction caused by low- or high-molecular-weight dextran.** *Adults:* 20 ml dextran 1 by rapid I.V. push 1 to 2 minutes before dextran infusion.
Children: 0.3 ml/kg dextran 1 by rapid I.V. push 1 to 2 minutes before dextran infusion.

➤ **Plasma volume expansion.** Dosage depends on amount of fluid loss. *Adults:* Initially, 500 ml of dextran 40 with CVP monitoring. Infuse remaining dose slowly. Total daily dose shouldn't exceed 2 g/kg (20 ml/kg) body weight. If therapy continues past 24 hours, don't exceed 1 g/kg daily. Continue for no more than 5 days.

Usual dose of dextran 70 or 75 solution is 30 g (500 ml of 6% solution) I.V. In emergencies, may be administered at 1.2 to 2.4 g/minute (20 to 40 ml/minute). Total dose during the first 24 hours isn't to exceed 1.2 g/kg; actual dose depends on amount of fluid loss and resultant hemoconcentration and must be determined individually. In normovolemic patients, the administration shouldn't exceed 240 mg/minute (4 ml/minute). *Children:* Total dosage of dextran 70 or 75 shouldn't exceed 1.2 g/kg (20 ml/kg), with the dose based on body weight or surface area. If therapy is continued, dosage shouldn't exceed 0.6 g/kg (10 ml/kg) daily.

➤ **Priming pump oxygenators.** *Adults:* Dextran 40 can be used as the only priming fluid or as an additive to other primers in pump oxygenators. Dextran 40 is added to the perfusion circuit as the 10% solution in a dose of 1 to 2 g/kg (10 to 20 ml/kg); total dose shouldn't exceed 2 g/kg (20 ml/kg).

➤ **Prophylaxis of venous thrombosis and pulmonary embolism.** *Adults:* Dextran 40 therapy usually should be given during the surgical procedure. On the day of surgery, dextran 40 (10% solution) is given at the dose of 50 to 100 g (500 to 1,000 ml or about 10 ml/kg). Treatment is continued for 2 to 3 days at a dose of 50 g (500 ml) daily. Then, if needed, 50 g (500 ml) may be given q 2 or 3 days for up to 2 weeks to reduce the risk of thromboembolism (deep venous thrombosis) or pulmonary embolism.

How supplied
Available by prescription only
dextran 1
Injection: 150 mg/ml in 20-ml vials
low-molecular-weight dextran
Injection: 10% dextran 40 in D_5W or normal saline solution
high-molecular-weight dextran
Injection: 6% dextran 70 in normal saline solution or D_5W; 6% dextran 75 in normal saline solution or D_5W

Pharmacodynamics
Plasma-expanding action: Dextran 40 (10%) has an average molecular weight of 40,000, the osmotic equivalent of twice the volume of plasma. Dextran 40 has a duration of action of 2 to 4 hours. Dextran 70 has an average molecular weight of 70,000. I.V. infusion results in an expansion of the plasma volume slightly in excess of the volume infused. This effect, useful in treating shock, lasts for about 12 hours. Dextran 40, 70, and 75 enhance blood flow, particularly in microcirculation.
Prophylaxis of venous thrombosis and pulmonary embolism: Dextran 40 inhibits vascular stasis and platelet adhesiveness and alters the structure and lysability of fibrin clots. Dextran 40 increases cardiac output and arterial, venous, and microcirculatory flow and reduces mean transit time, mainly by expanding plasma volume and by reducing blood viscosity through hemodilution and reducing red cell aggregation.

Pharmacokinetics
Absorption: Dextran 40 and 70 given by I.V. infusion. Plasma level depends on rate of infusion and rate of disappearance of drug from plasma.
Distribution: Distributed throughout vascular system.
Metabolism: Dextran molecules with molecular weights above 50,000 are enzymatically degraded by dextrinase to glucose at about 70 to 90 mg/kg daily. Process is variable.
Excretion: Dextran molecules with molecular weights below 50,000 are eliminated by renal excretion, with 40% of dextran 70 appearing in urine within 24 hours. About 50% of dextran 40 excreted in urine within 3 hours, 60% within 6 hours, and 75% within 24 hours. Remaining 25% is hydrolyzed partially and excreted in urine, excreted partially in feces, and partially oxidized.

Route	Onset	Peak	Duration
I.V.	Immediate	Immediate	Unknown

Contraindications and precautions
Low-molecular-weight dextran is contraindicated in patients hypersensitive to drug and in those with marked hemostatic defects, marked cardiac decompensation, and renal disease with severe oliguria or anuria. High-molecular-weight dextran is also contraindicated in patients with hypervolemic conditions and severe bleeding disorders.

Use low-molecular-weight dextran cautiously in patients with active hemorrhage, thrombocytopenia, or diabetes mellitus. High-molecular-weight dextran should be used cautiously in patients with active hemorrhage, thrombocytopenia, impaired renal clearance, chronic liver disease, and abdominal conditions or in those undergoing bowel surgery.

Interactions
Drug-drug. *Anticoagulants, antiplatelet drugs:* Abnormally prolonged bleeding times can occur with either high- or low-molecular-weight dextran. Monitor patient closely.

Adverse reactions
CV: thrombophlebitis.
EENT: nasal congestion (with high-molecular-weight dextran).
GI: nausea, vomiting.
GU: tubular stasis and blocking, increased urine viscosity, oliguria, anuria, increased specific gravity of urine (with high-molecular-weight dextran).
Hematologic: *decreased hemoglobin level and hematocrit,* increased bleeding time (with higher doses of low-molecular-weight dextran), increased bleeding time and significant suppression of platelet function (with high-molecular-weight dextran in doses of 15 ml/kg body weight).
Hepatic: increased AST and ALT levels.
Musculoskeletal: arthralgia.
Other: *hypersensitivity reactions* (urticaria, *anaphylaxis*), fever.

Overdose and treatment
Rapidly cleared by the kidneys so effects are short-lived with minimal consequences.

Special considerations
● Dehydrated patients should be well hydrated before dextran infusion.
● Dextran in saline solution is hazardous when given to patients with heart failure, severe renal failure, and clinical states in which edema exists with sodium restriction. Use D_5W solution.
● Drug works as plasma expander via colloidal osmotic effect, drawing fluid from interstitial to intravascular space. Provides plasma expansion slightly greater than volume infused. Observe for circulatory overload or rise in CVP readings.
● Dextran 1 should be given just before infusing low- or high-molecular-weight dextran. Repeat dosage of dextran 1 if more than 15 minutes elapses during infusion.

Reactions may be *common*, uncommon, *life-threatening*, or COMMON AND LIFE-THREATENING.

● Avoid doses that exceed recommendations, because dose-related increases in wound hematoma, wound seroma, wound bleeding, occult bleeding (such as hematuria and melena), and pulmonary edema have been observed.

● Store at constant temperature of 77° F (25° C). Solution may precipitate in storage. Discard any solution that isn't clear.

● Falsely elevated blood glucose levels may occur in patients receiving dextran 40 or 70 if test uses high levels of acid. Dextran may cause turbidity, which interferes with bilirubin assays that use alcohol, total protein levels using biuret reagent, and blood glucose levels using orthotoluidine method. Blood typing and cross-matching using enzyme techniques may give unreliable readings if samples are taken after dextran infusion.

Patient monitoring

● Monitor urine output during administration. If oliguria or anuria occurs or isn't reversed by initial infusion (500 ml), stop administration.
● Monitor urine or serum osmolarity; urine specific gravity will be increased by urine dextran concentration.
● Monitor CVP when dextran is given by rapid I.V. infusion. A precipitous rise in CVP or other signs of fluid overload indicate need to stop infusion.
● Monitor hemoglobin level and hematocrit; don't allow to fall below 30% by volume.
● Monitor patient closely during early phase of infusion; check for infiltration, phlebitis, and anaphylactoid reactions.

Breast-feeding patients

● It isn't known whether dextran appears in breast milk. A decision should be made to stop either breast-feeding or drug.

Geriatric patients

● Use dextran cautiously in elderly patients; they may be at increased risk for fluid overload.

Patient education

● Explain use and administration of dextran to patient and family.
● Tell patient to report adverse effects.

dextranomer
Debrisan

Pharmacologic classification: synthetic polysaccharide
Therapeutic classification: topical debriding agent
Pregnancy risk category: NR

Indications and dosages

➤ **Cleaning of exudative wounds.** *Adults and children:* Apply to affected area once or twice daily or more often if drainage is heavy. Apply to at least ¼" thickness, and cover with sterile gauze.

How supplied
Available by prescription only
Beads: 4 g, 25 g, 60 g, 120 g
Paste: 10 g

Pharmacodynamics
Debriding action: Dextranomer cleans wound surfaces by capillary action, drawing wound exudate, bacteria, and contaminants into the beads and therefore enhancing formation of granulative tissue and promoting wound healing.

Pharmacokinetics
Absorption: Drug absorption is limited with topical use.
Distribution: None.
Metabolism: None.
Excretion: None.

Route	Onset	Peak	Duration
Topical	Unknown	Unknown	Unknown

Contraindications and precautions
Contraindicated in deep fistulas, sinus tracts, or any area where complete removal isn't assured and in dry wounds because it's ineffective.

Interactions
None reported.

Adverse reactions
Skin: transient pain at site, bleeding, erythema, contact dermatitis.

Overdose and treatment
No information available.

Special considerations
● Use strict aseptic technique when applying dextranomer.
● Dextranomer isn't an enzyme and can't be used for dry wounds.
● Clean wound before applying, leaving area moist; cover wound to a thickness of at least ¼". Then bandage lightly to hold beads in place. Be sure to leave room for expansion (1 g of beads absorbs 4 ml of exudate).
● When product is saturated and grayish yellow, irrigate wound and remove beads or paste; beads must be removed thoroughly, especially before any surgical treatment, and vigorous irrigation or soaking may be necessary.
● If dressing becomes dry, don't remove it without prior wetting to loosen bandage and beads.
● Don't use in areas where complete removal can't be ensured—for example, in fistulas or sinus tracts.
● Drug should be discontinued if sensitization develops.

Patient monitoring
● Monitor patient for adverse reactions; discontinue drug if sensitization develops.

• Monitor patient's wound. Stop treatment when area is free of exudate.

Breast-feeding
• Women should avoid breast-feeding if drug is used in breast area.

Patient education
• Teach patient how to perform sterile dressing changes before discharge.
• Advise patient to avoid drug contact with eyes and to wash hands well after application.

---

dextroamphetamine sulfate
Dexedrine, DextroStat

Pharmacologic classification: amphetamine
Therapeutic classification: CNS stimulant, short-term adjunctive anorexigenic agent, sympathomimetic amine
Controlled substance schedule: II
Pregnancy risk category: C

Indications and dosages
➤ **Narcolepsy.** *Adults:* 5 to 60 mg P.O. daily in divided doses. Long-acting dosage forms allow once-daily dosing.
Children over age 12: 10 mg P.O. daily, increased in 10-mg increments weekly, as indicated.
Children ages 6 to 12: 5 mg P.O. daily, increased in 5-mg increments weekly, as indicated.
➤ **Short-term adjunct in exogenous obesity** ◇. *Adults:* 5 to 30 mg P.O. daily 30 to 60 minutes before meals in divided doses of 5 to 10 mg. Or, give one 10- or 15-mg sustained-release capsule daily as a single dose in the morning.
➤ **Attention deficit hyperactivity disorder (ADHD).** *Children age 6 and older:* 5 mg P.O. once daily or b.i.d., increased by 5-mg increments weekly, p.r.n. Total daily dose should rarely exceed 40 mg.
Children ages 3 to 5: 2.5 mg P.O. daily, increased by 2.5-mg increments weekly, as necessary; not recommended for children under age 3.

How supplied
Available by prescription only
Capsules (sustained-release): 5 mg, 10 mg, 15 mg
Tablets: 5 mg, 10 mg

Pharmacodynamics
CNS stimulant action: Amphetamines are sympathomimetic amines with CNS stimulant activity. In hyperactive children, they have a paradoxical calming effect.
Anorexigenic action: Anorexigenic effects are thought to occur in the hypothalamus, where decreased smell and taste acuity decreases appetite. They may be tried for short-term control of refractory obesity, with caloric restriction and behavior modification.

The cerebral cortex and reticular activating system appear to be the primary sites of activity; amphetamines release nerve terminal stores of norepinephrine, promoting nerve impulse transmission. At high dosages, effects are mediated by dopamine.

Amphetamines are used to treat narcolepsy and as adjuncts to psychosocial measures in ADHD in children. Their precise mechanism of action in these conditions is unknown.

Pharmacokinetics
Absorption: Rapidly absorbed from the GI tract.
Distribution: Distributed widely throughout the body.
Metabolism: Unknown.
Excretion: Excreted in urine.

Route	Onset	Peak	Duration
P.O.			
Regular	Unknown	2 hr	Unknown
Extended	Unknown	8-10 hr	Unknown

Contraindications and precautions
Contraindicated in patients hypersensitive to sympathomimetic amines, patients with idiosyncratic reactions to them, patients who have taken an MAO inhibitor within 14 days, and patients with hyperthyroidism, moderate to severe hypertension, symptomatic CV disease, glaucoma, advanced arteriosclerosis, or a history of drug abuse. Use cautiously in patients with motor and phonic tics, Tourette syndrome, and agitated states.

Interactions
Drug-drug. *Acetazolamide, alkalizing agents, antacids, sodium bicarbonate:* Enhanced renal reabsorption of dextroamphetamine. Monitor patient for enhanced amphetamine effects.
Acidifying agents, ammonium chloride, ascorbic acid: Enhanced dextroamphetamine excretion and shortened duration of action. Monitor patient for decreased amphetamine effects.
Adrenergic blockers: Inhibited by amphetamines. Avoid use together.
Antihypertensives: May antagonize antihypertensive effects. Avoid use together.
Barbiturates: Antagonize dextroamphetamine by CNS depression. Avoid use together.
Chlorpromazine: Inhibits the central stimulant effects of amphetamines. Can be used to treat amphetamine poisoning.
CNS stimulants, haloperidol, phenothiazines, theophylline, tricyclic antidepressants: Increased CNS effects. Avoid use together.
Insulin, oral antidiabetic: Possible altered need for these drugs. Monitor blood glucose levels.
Lithium carbonate: May inhibit antiobesity and stimulating effects of amphetamines. Monitor patient closely.
MAO inhibitors: May cause hypertensive crisis. Don't use within 14 days of MAO inhibitor.

Reactions may be *common*, uncommon, *life-threatening*, or COMMON AND LIFE-THREATENING.

Meperidine: Amphetamines potentiate analgesic effect. Use together cautiously.

Methenamine therapy: Increases urinary excretion of amphetamines and reduces efficacy. Monitor patient closely.

Norepinephrine: Amphetamines enhance the adrenergic effect. Monitor patient closely.

Phenobarbitol, phenytoin: May produce a synergistic anticonvulsant action. Monitor patient closely.

Drug-food. *Caffeine:* May increase amphetamine and related amine effects. Tell patient to use cautiously.

Adverse reactions

CNS: *restlessness,* tremor, *insomnia,* dizziness, headache, chills, overstimulation, dysphoria, euphoria.

CV: *tachycardia, palpitations,* hypertension, *arrhythmias.*

GI: dry mouth, unpleasant taste, diarrhea, constipation, anorexia, weight loss, other GI disturbances.

GU: impotence.

Skin: urticaria.

Other: altered libido.

Overdose and treatment

Individual responses vary widely. Toxic symptoms may occur at 15 and 30 mg and can cause severe reactions; however, doses of 400 mg or more haven't always proved fatal. Symptoms of overdose include restlessness, tremor, hyperreflexia, tachypnea, confusion, aggressiveness, hallucinations, and panic; fatigue and depression usually follow excitement stage. Other symptoms may include arrhythmias, shock, alterations in blood pressure, nausea, vomiting, diarrhea, and abdominal cramps; death is usually preceded by seizures and coma.

Treat overdose symptomatically and supportively. If ingestion was recent (within 4 hours), use gastric lavage or emesis and sedate with a barbiturate; monitor vital signs and fluid and electrolyte balance. Urinary acidification may enhance excretion. Saline catharsis (magnesium citrate) may hasten GI evacuation of unabsorbed sustained-release drug.

Special considerations

● Drug may elevate plasma corticosteroid levels and may interfere with urinary steroid determinations.

● Give dextroamphetamine 30 to 60 minutes before meals when using as an anorexigenic agent. To minimize insomnia, avoid giving drug within 6 hours of bedtime.

● For narcolepsy, patient should take first dose on awakening.

● When tolerance to anorexigenic effect develops, dosage should be discontinued, not increased.

Patient monitoring

● Take vital signs regularly, and observe patient for signs of excessive stimulation.

● Monitor blood and urine glucose levels. Drug may alter daily insulin requirement in patients with diabetes.

Breast-feeding patients

● Safety hasn't been established. Alternative feeding method is recommended during therapy with dextroamphetamine sulfate.

Pediatric patients

● Drug isn't recommended for treatment of obesity in children under age 12.

Geriatric patients

● Use lower doses. Avoid using drug in elderly patients with CV, CNS, or GI disturbances.

Patient education

● Teach parents about drug-free periods for children with ADHD, especially during periods of reduced stress.

● Warn patient to avoid hazardous activities that require alertness until CNS response is determined.

● Instruct patient to take drug early in the day to minimize insomnia.

● Tell patient not to crush sustained-release forms or to increase dosage.

dextromethorphan hydrobromide

Balminil D.M.*, Benylin DM, Broncho-Grippol-DM*, Delsym, DM Syrup*, Hold, Koffex*, Mediquell, Neo-DM*, Robidex*, Sedatuss*, St. Joseph Cough Suppressant for Children, Sucrets Cough Control Formula, Suppress, Trocal, Vicks Formula 44

Pharmacologic classification: levorphanol derivative (dextrorotatory methyl ether)
Therapeutic classification: antitussive (nonnarcotic)
Pregnancy risk category: C

Indications and dosages

► *Nonproductive cough (chronic).* Adults and children age 12 and older: 10 to 20 mg P.O. q 4 hours. Or, 30 mg q 6 to 8 hours. Or, controlled-release liquid b.i.d. (60 mg b.i.d.). Maximum dose is 120 mg daily.

Children ages 6 to 12: 5 to 10 mg P.O. q 4 hours. Or, 15 mg q 6 to 8 hours. Or, controlled-release liquid b.i.d. (30 mg b.i.d.). Maximum dose is 60 mg daily.

Children ages 2 to 6: 2.5 to 5 mg P.O. q 4 hours. Or, 7.5 mg q 6 to 8 hours. Or, sustained-action liquid 15 mg b.i.d. Maximum dose is 30 mg daily.

How supplied
Available without a prescription
Capsules (liquid-filled): 30 mg
Lozenges: 5 mg, 7.5 mg, 15 mg
Solution: 3.5 mg/5 ml, 5 mg/5 ml, 7.5 mg/5 ml, 10 mg/5 ml, 12.5 mg/5 ml, 15 mg/5 ml
Syrup: 10 mg/5 ml, 15 mg/15 ml
Tablets: 200 mg

Pharmacodynamics
Antitussive action: Dextromethorphan suppresses the cough reflex by direct action on the cough center in the medulla. Dextromethorphan is almost equal in antitussive potency to codeine but causes no analgesia or addiction and little or no CNS depression and has no expectorant action; it also produces fewer subjective and GI adverse effects than codeine. Treatment is intended to relieve cough frequency without abolishing protective cough reflex. In therapeutic doses, drug doesn't inhibit ciliary activity.

Pharmacokinetics
Absorption: Absorbed readily from the GI tract.
Distribution: Unknown.
Metabolism: Metabolized extensively by the liver. Plasma half-life is about 11 hours.
Excretion: Little is excreted unchanged. Metabolites are excreted primarily in urine; about 7% to 10% is excreted in feces.

Route	Onset	Peak	Duration
P.O.	< ½ hr	Unknown	3-6 hr

Contraindications and precautions
Contraindicated in patients currently taking MAO inhibitors or within 2 weeks of stopping an MAO inhibitor. Use cautiously in atopic children, sedated or debilitated patients, and patients confined to the supine position. Also use cautiously in patients sensitive to aspirin.

Interactions
Drug-drug. *MAO inhibitors:* May cause nausea, hypotension, excitation, hyperpyrexia, and coma. Don't give dextromethorphan within 2 weeks after stopping an MAO inhibitor.
Selegiline: May cause confusion, coma, or hyperpyrexia. Avoid use together.
Drug-herb. *Parsley:* May promote or produce serotonin syndrome. Tell patient to avoid use together.

Adverse reactions
CNS: drowsiness, dizziness.
GI: nausea, vomiting, stomach pain.

Overdose and treatment
Signs and symptoms of overdose may include nausea, vomiting, drowsiness, dizziness, blurred vision, nystagmus, shallow respirations, urine retention, toxic psychosis, stupor, and coma.

Treatment of overdose involves administering activated charcoal to reduce drug absorption and I.V. naloxone to support respiration. Other symptoms are treated supportively.

Special considerations
● Treatment is intended to relieve cough intensity and frequency without abolishing the protective cough reflex.
● May be used with percussion and chest vibration.

Patient monitoring
● Note nature and frequency of coughing.

Breast-feeding patients
● Safety hasn't been established.

Pediatric patients
● Don't use syrup, tablets, or lozenges in children under age 2. Sustained-action liquid may be used in children under age 2, but dosage must be individualized.

Patient education
● Tell patient to report persistent cough lasting more than 7 days.
● Instruct patient to use sugarless throat lozenges for throat irritation and resulting cough.
● Recommend a humidifier to filter out dust, smoke, and air pollutants.

dextrose (d-glucose)
$D_{2.5}W$, D_5W, $D_{10}W$, $D_{20}W$, $D_{25}W$, $D_{30}W$, $D_{38}W$, $D_{40}W$, $D_{50}W$, $D_{60}W$, $D_{70}W$

Pharmacologic classification: carbohydrate
Therapeutic classification: total parenteral nutrition component, caloric product, fluid volume replacement
Pregnancy risk category: C

Indications and dosages
➤*Fluid replacement and calorie supplementation in patients who can't maintain adequate oral intake or who are restricted from doing so. Adults and children:* Dosage depends on fluid and caloric requirements. Use peripheral I.V. infusion of 2.5% or 5% solution or central I.V. infusion of 10% or 20% solution for minimal fluid needs. Use 50% solution to treat insulin-induced hypoglycemia. Solutions from 10% to 70% are used diluted in admixtures, normally with amino acid solutions, and administered via a central vein.

How supplied
Available by prescription only
Injection: 1,000 ml (2.5%, 5%, 10%, 20%, 30%, 40%, 50%, 60%, 70%); 500 ml (5%, 10%, 20%, 30%, 40%, 50%, 60%, 70%); 400 ml (5%); 250 ml (5%, 10%); 100 ml (5%); 70-ml pin-top vial (70% for additive use only); 50 ml (5% and 50% available in vial, ampule, and Bristoject);

10 ml (25%); 5-ml ampule (10%); 3-ml ampule (10%)

Pharmacodynamics
Metabolic action: A rapidly metabolized source of calories and fluids in patients with inadequate oral intake. While increasing blood glucose levels, dextrose may decrease body protein and nitrogen losses, promote glycogen deposition, and decrease or prevent ketosis if sufficient doses are given. Dextrose also may induce diuresis. Parenterally injected doses of dextrose undergo oxidation to carbon dioxide and water. A 5% solution is isotonic and is administered peripherally. Concentrated dextrose infusions provide increased caloric intake with less fluid volume; they may be irritating if given by peripheral infusion. Solutions above 10% should be given only by central venous catheter.

Pharmacokinetics
Absorption: Administered I.V.
Distribution: As a source of calories and water for hydration, dextrose solutions expand plasma volume.
Metabolism: Metabolized to carbon dioxide and water.
Excretion: In some patients, dextrose solutions may produce diuresis.

Route	Onset	Peak	Duration
I.V.	Immediate	Immediate	Unknown

Contraindications and precautions
Contraindicated in patients in diabetic coma while blood glucose level remains excessively high. Concentrated solutions are contraindicated in patients with intracranial or intraspinal hemorrhage, dehydrated patients with alcohol withdrawal syndrome, and patients with severe dehydration, anuria, hepatic coma, or glucose-galactose malabsorption syndrome.

Use cautiously in patients with cardiac or pulmonary disease, hypertension, renal insufficiency, urinary obstruction, or hypovolemia.

Interactions
Drug-drug. *Additives:* Possible incompatibility. Must be introduced aseptically, mixed thoroughly, and not stored.
Blood: Possible pseudoagglutination of RBCs. Don't give with blood through same infusion set.
Corticosteroids, corticotropin: May cause increased serum glucose levels. Administer cautiously; monitor patient closely.
Insulin, oral hypoglycemics: May alter drug requirements and cause vitamin B complex deficiency. Monitor serum glucose levels.

Adverse reactions
CNS: confusion, *unconsciousness in hyperosmolar hyperglycemic nonketotic syndrome.*

CV: *pulmonary edema, exacerbated hypertension, heart failure in susceptible patients (with fluid overload);* phlebitis, venous sclerosis, tissue necrosis (with prolonged or concentrated infusions, especially when administered peripherally).
GI: glycosuria, osmotic diuresis.
Metabolic: hyperglycemia, hypervolemia, hypovolemia, dehydration, hyperosmolarity (with rapid infusion of concentrated solution or prolonged infusion); hypoglycemia from rebound hyperinsulinemia.
Skin: sloughing and tissue necrosis, if extravasation occurs with concentrated solutions.
Other: fever, vitamin B complex deficiency (with rapid termination of long-term infusion).

Overdose and treatment
If fluid or solute overload occurs during I.V. therapy, reevaluate the patient's condition and institute appropriate corrective treatment. Decrease infusion rate or adjust insulin dosage as needed.

Special considerations
• Monitor infusion rate for maximum dextrose infusion of 0.5 g/kg/hour, using largest available peripheral vein and well-placed needle or catheter. However, hypertonic dextrose solutions may cause thrombosis if infused via peripheral vein; therefore, administer via central venous catheter.
• Avoid rapid administration, which may cause hyperglycemia, hyperosmolar syndrome, or glycosuria.
• Infuse concentrated solutions slowly; rapid infusion can cause hyperglycemia and fluid shifts.
• Hypertonic solutions are more likely than isotonic or hypotonic solutions to cause irritation; they should be administered into larger central veins.
• Depletion of pancreatic insulin production and secretion can occur. To avoid an adverse effect on insulin production, patient may need to have insulin added to infusions.
• Excessive administration of potassium-free solutions may result in hypokalemia. Potassium should be added to dextrose solutions and administered to fasting patients with good renal function; special precautions should be taken with patients receiving a cardiac glycoside.
• Infuse concentrated solutions via central venous catheter with meticulous aseptic technique because bacteria thrive in high-glucose environments.
• D_5W or $D_{10}W$ solution is advisable upon discontinuation of concentrated dextrose infusions to avoid rebound hypoglycemia.

Patient monitoring
• Monitor serum glucose levels during long-term treatment.
• Monitor fluid imbalance or changes in electrolyte levels and acid-base balance by periodic laboratory determinations during prolonged ther-

apy. Additional electrolyte supplementation may be needed.

• Carefully monitor patient's intake, output, and body weight, especially in patients with renal dysfunction.

• If fluid or solute overload occurs during I.V. therapy, reevaluate patient's condition and institute appropriate corrective treatment. Decrease infusion rate or adjust insulin dosage as needed.

Pediatric patients
• Use cautiously in infants of diabetic women, except as may be indicated for newborn infants who are hypoglycemic.

Patient education
• Explain need for drug.
• Tell patient to report adverse effects promptly.

diazepam
Apo-Diazepam*, Diastat, Novodipam*, Valium, Vivol*, Zetran

Pharmacologic classification: benzodiazepine
Therapeutic classification: antianxiety, skeletal muscle relaxant, amnesic, anticonvulsant, sedative-hypnotic
Controlled substance schedule: IV
Pregnancy risk category: D

Indications and dosages
➤ *Anxiety. Adults:* Depending on severity, 2 to 10 mg P.O. b.i.d. to q.i.d. or 15 to 30 mg extended-release capsules P.O. once daily. Or, 2 to 10 mg I.M. or I.V. q 3 to 4 hours, p.r.n.
Children age 6 months and older: 1 to 2.5 mg P.O. t.i.d. or q.i.d.; increase dose gradually, as needed and tolerated.
➤ *Acute alcohol withdrawal. Adults:* 10 mg P.O. t.i.d. or q.i.d. for the first 24 hours; reduce to 5 mg t.i.d. or q.i.d., p.r.n. Or, 10 mg I.M. or I.V. initially, followed by 5 to 10 mg q 3 to 4 hours, p.r.n.
➤ *Muscle spasm. Adults:* 2 to 10 mg P.O. b.i.d. to q.i.d. or 15 to 30 mg extended-release capsules once daily. Or, give 5 to 10 mg I.M. or I.V. q 3 to 4 hours, p.r.n.
➤ *Tetanus. Infants over age 30 days to children age 5:* 1 to 2 mg I.M. or I.V. slowly, repeated q 3 to 4 hours.
Children age 5 and older: 5 to 10 mg I.M. or I.V. slowly q 3 to 4 hours, p.r.n.
➤ *Adjunct to convulsive disorders. Adults:* 2 to 10 mg P.O. b.i.d. to q.i.d.
Children age 6 months and older: Initially, 1 to 2.5 mg P.O. t.i.d. or q.i.d.; increase dose as tolerated and needed.
➤ *Adjunct to anesthesia, endoscopic procedures. Adults:* 5 to 10 mg I.M. before surgery. Or, administer I.V. slowly just before procedure, adjusting dose to effect. Usually, less than 10 mg is used, but up to 20 mg may be given.

➤ *Cardioversion. Adults:* Administer 5 to 15 mg I.V. 5 to 10 minutes before procedure.
➤ *Status epilepticus. Adults:* 5 to 10 mg I.V. (preferred) or I.M. initially, repeated at 10- to 15-minute intervals up to a maximum dose of 30 mg. Repeat q 2 to 4 hours, p.r.n.
Children age 5 and older: 1 mg I.V. q 2 to 5 minutes up to a maximum dose of 10 mg; repeat in 2 to 4 hours, p.r.n.
Infants over age 30 days to children age 5: 0.2 to 0.5 mg I.V. q 2 to 5 minutes up to a maximum dose of 5 mg.
➤ *Control of acute repetitive seizure activity in patients already taking antiepileptic drugs. Children age 12 and older:* 0.2 mg/kg P.R. using applicator. A second dose may be given 4 to 12 hours after the first dose, if needed.
Children ages 6 to 11: 0.3 mg/kg P.R. using applicator. A second dose may be given 4 to 12 hours after the first dose, if needed.
Children ages 2 to 5: 0.5 mg/kg P.R. using applicator. A second dose may be given 4 to 12 hours after the first dose, if needed.

How supplied
Available by prescription only
Capsules (extended-release): 15 mg
Injection: 5 mg/ml in ampules, vials, and disposable syringes
Oral solution: 5 mg/ml; 5 mg/5 ml, 10 mg/10 ml
Rectal gel: 2.5 mg, 5 mg, 10 mg, 15 mg, 20 mg twin packs
Tablets: 2 mg, 5 mg, 10 mg

Pharmacodynamics
Anxiolytic and sedative-hypnotic actions: Diazepam depresses the CNS at the limbic and subcortical levels of the brain. It produces an antianxiety effect by influencing the effect of the neurotransmitter gamma-aminobutyric acid on its receptor in the ascending reticular activating system, which increases inhibition and blocks cortical and limbic arousal.
Anticonvulsant action: Diazepam suppresses the spread of seizure activity produced by epileptogenic foci in the cortex, thalamus, and limbic structures by enhancing presynaptic inhibition.
Amnesic action: The exact mechanism of action is unknown.
Skeletal muscle relaxant action: The exact mechanism is unknown, but drug may inhibit polysynaptic afferent pathways.

Pharmacokinetics
Absorption: When administered orally, drug is absorbed through the GI tract. I.M. administration yields erratic absorption. Drug is well absorbed rectally and reaches peak plasma levels in 1½ hours.
Distribution: Distributed widely throughout the body. About 85% to 95% of an administered dose is bound to plasma protein.

Metabolism: Metabolized in the liver to the active metabolite desmethyldiazepam.

Excretion: Most metabolites of diazepam are excreted in urine, with only small amounts excreted in feces. Half-life of desmethyldiazepam is 30 to 200 hours. Duration of sedative effect is 3 hours; this may be prolonged up to 90 hours in elderly patients and in patients with hepatic or renal dysfunction. Anticonvulsant effect is 30 to 60 minutes after I.V. administration.

Route	Onset	Peak	Duration
P.O.	½ hr	2 hr	3-8 hr
I.V.	1-5 min	Immediate	15-60 min
I.M.	Unknown	2 hr	Unknown
P.R.	Unknown	1-5 hr	Unknown

Contraindications and precautions

Contraindicated in patients hypersensitive to drug; patients with angle-closure glaucoma; patients experiencing shock, coma, or acute alcohol intoxication (parenteral form); and children under age 6 months (oral form). Use cautiously in elderly patients, debilitated patients, and patients with impaired hepatic or renal function, depression, or chronic open-angle glaucoma. Avoid use in pregnant women, especially during the first trimester.

Interactions

Drug-drug. *Antacids:* Decrease the absorption of diazepam. Avoid use together.

Antidepressants, antihistamines, barbiturates, general anesthetics, MAO inhibitors, narcotics, phenothiazines: Potentiated CNS depressant effects. Avoid use together.

Cimetidine and possibly disulfiram: Diminished hepatic metabolism of diazepam, which increases its plasma level. Monitor patient closely.

Digoxin: Possible decreased digoxin clearance. Monitor patient for digoxin toxicity.

Haloperidol: May alter seizure pattern. Benzodiazepines also may reduce serum haloperidol levels. Avoid use together.

Levodopa: Diazepam may inhibit the therapeutic effect of levodopa. Monitor patient carefully.

Nondepolarizing neuromuscular blocking agents, such as pancuronium and succinylcholine: Intensified and prolonged respiratory depression. Don't use together.

Oral contraceptives: May impair the metabolism of diazepam. Monitor patient closely.

Drug-lifestyle. *Alcohol use:* Diazepam potentiates the CNS depressant effects of alcohol. Advise patient to avoid use together.

Heavy smoking: Accelerates metabolism of diazepam, lowering clinical effectiveness. Advise patient to avoid use together.

Adverse reactions

CNS: *drowsiness,* slurred speech, tremor, transient amnesia, fatigue, ataxia, headache, insomnia, paradoxical anxiety, hallucinations, changes in EEG patterns.

CV: hypotension, *CV collapse, bradycardia.*

EENT: diplopia, blurred vision, nystagmus.

GI: nausea, constipation.

GU: incontinence, urine retention.

Hematologic: *neutropenia.*

Hepatic: elevated liver function test results, *jaundice.*

Musculoskeletal: *dysarthria.*

Respiratory: *respiratory depression.*

Skin: rash.

Other: physical or psychological dependence, altered libido, *acute withdrawal syndrome* after sudden discontinuation in physically dependent persons, *pain, phlebitis* (at injection site).

Overdose and treatment

Signs and symptoms of overdose include somnolence, confusion, coma, hypoactive reflexes, dyspnea, labored breathing, hypotension, bradycardia, slurred speech, and unsteady gait or impaired coordination.

Support blood pressure and respiration until drug effects subside; monitor vital signs. Mechanical ventilatory assistance via endotracheal tube may be required to maintain a patent airway and support adequate oxygenation. Flumazenil, a specific benzodiazepine antagonist, may be useful, but shouldn't be administered during status epilepticus. Use I.V. fluids and vasopressors such as dopamine and phenylephrine to treat hypotension as needed. If the patient is conscious, induce emesis; use gastric lavage if ingestion was recent, but only if an endotracheal tube is present to prevent aspiration. After emesis or lavage, administer activated charcoal with a cathartic as a single dose. Dialysis is of limited value.

Special considerations

● Don't discontinue drug suddenly; decrease dosage slowly over 8 to 12 weeks after long-term therapy.

● To enhance taste, oral solution can be mixed with liquids or semisolid foods, such as applesauce or pudding, immediately before administration.

● Extended-release capsule should be swallowed whole; don't let patient crush or chew it.

● Shake oral suspension well before administering.

● When prescribing with opiates for endoscopic procedures, reduce opiate dose by at least one-third.

● Parenteral forms of diazepam may be diluted in normal saline solution; a slight precipitate may form, but the solution can still be used.

● Diazepam interacts with plastic. Don't store it in plastic syringes or use plastic administration sets because doing so decreases drug availability.

● I.V. route is preferred because of rapid and more uniform absorption.

• For I.V. administration, infuse drug slowly, directly into a large vein, at no more than 5 mg/minute for adults or 0.25 mg/kg of body weight over 3 minutes for children. Don't inject diazepam into small veins to avoid extravasation into S.C. tissue. Observe infusion site for phlebitis. If direct I.V. administration isn't possible, inject diazepam directly into I.V. tubing at point closest to vein insertion site to prevent extravasation.

• Administration by continuous I.V. infusion isn't recommended.

• Inject I.M. dose deep into deltoid muscle. Aspirate for backflow to prevent inadvertent intra-arterial administration. Use I.M. route only if I.V. or oral routes are unavailable.

• Patient should remain in bed under observation for at least 3 hours after parenteral administration of diazepam to prevent potential hazards; keep resuscitation equipment nearby.

• Lower doses are effective in patients with renal or hepatic dysfunction.

• Anticipate possible transient increase in frequency or severity of seizures when diazepam is used as adjunctive treatment of convulsive disorders. Impose seizure precautions.

• Don't mix diazepam with other drugs in a syringe or infusion container.

• Use Diastat rectal gel to treat no more than five episodes per month and no more than one episode every 5 days.

Patient monitoring

• During prolonged therapy, periodically monitor blood counts and liver function studies.

• Assess gag reflex postendoscopy and before resuming oral intake to prevent aspiration.

Pregnant patients

• Warn woman to call prescriber immediately if she becomes pregnant.

Breast-feeding patients

• Diazepam appears in breast milk. The breastfed infant of a woman who uses diazepam may become sedated, have feeding difficulties, or lose weight. Avoid use of drug in breast-feeding women.

Pediatric patients

• Safe use of oral diazepam in infants under age 6 months hasn't been established. Safe use of parenteral diazepam in infants under age 30 days hasn't been established.

• Closely observe neonates whose mothers took diazepam for a prolonged period during pregnancy; the infants may show withdrawal symptoms.

• Use of rectal diazepam during labor may cause neonatal flaccidity.

• Safety and efficacy of rectal diazepam haven't been established in children under age 2.

Geriatric patients

• These patients are more sensitive to the CNS depressant effects of diazepam. Use cautiously.

• Lower doses are usually effective because of decreased elimination.

• Elderly patients who receive this drug need assistance with walking and activities of daily living when therapy starts or dosage increases.

• Parenteral administration of this drug is more likely to cause apnea, hypotension, and bradycardia in geriatric patients.

Patient education

• Advise patient about risk of physical and psychological dependence with long-term use.

• Warn patient that sudden position changes can cause dizziness. Advise patient to dangle legs for a few minutes before getting out of bed to prevent falls and injury.

• Caution patient to avoid alcohol while taking diazepam.

• Advise patient not to discontinue drug suddenly.

• Teach patient's caregiver when to use rectal gel (to control bouts of increased seizure activity) and how to monitor and record patient's clinical response.

• Teach patient's caregiver how to administer rectal gel.

diazoxide
Hyperstat IV, Proglycem

Pharmacologic classification: peripheral vasodilator
Therapeutic classification: antihypertensive, antihypoglycemic
Pregnancy risk category: C

Indications and dosages

➤ *Hypertensive crisis. Adults and children:* 1 to 3 mg/kg I.V. (up to a maximum of 150 mg) q 5 to 15 minutes until blood pressure is reduced adequately.

➤ *Hypoglycemia from hyperinsulinism. Adults and children:* Usual dosage is 3 to 8 mg/kg P.O. daily divided into two or three equal doses. *Infants and newborns:* Usual dosage is 8 to 15 mg/kg P.O. daily divided into two or three equal doses.

How supplied
Available by prescription only
Capsules: 50 mg
Injection: 15 mg/ml in 20-ml ampule
Oral suspension: 50 mg/ml in 30-ml bottle

Pharmacodynamics
Antihypertensive action: Diazoxide directly relaxes arteriolar smooth muscle, causing vasodilation and reducing peripheral vascular resistance, thus reducing blood pressure.
Antihypoglycemic action: Diazoxide increases blood glucose levels by inhibiting pancreatic

secretion of insulin, by stimulating catecholamine release, or by increasing hepatic release of glucose.

Pharmacokinetics

Absorption: After I.V. administration, blood pressure should decrease promptly, with maximum decrease in less than 5 minutes. After oral administration, hyperglycemic effect begins in 1 hour.

Distribution: Distributed throughout the body; highest level is found in kidneys, liver, and adrenal glands; diazoxide crosses placenta and blood-brain barrier. Drug is about 90% protein-bound.

Metabolism: Metabolized partially in the liver.

Excretion: Excreted slowly by the kidneys. Duration of antihypertensive effect varies widely, ranging from 30 minutes to 72 hours (average 3 to 12 hours) after I.V. administration; after oral administration, antihypoglycemic effect persists for about 8 hours. Antihypertensive and antihypoglycemic effects may be prolonged in patients with renal dysfunction.

Route	Onset	Peak	Duration
P.O.	Unknown	Unknown	Unknown
I.V.	1 min	2-5 min	2-12 hr

Contraindications and precautions

Parenteral form is contraindicated in patients hypersensitive to drug, other thiazides, or sulfonamide-derived drugs, and in the treatment of compensatory hypertension (such as that linked to coarctation of the aorta or arteriovenous shunt). Oral form is contraindicated in patients with functional hypoglycemia.

Use cautiously in patients with uremia or impaired cerebral or cardiac function.

Interactions

Drug-drug. *Antihypertensives:* Diazoxide may potentiate antihypertensive effects; especially if given I.V. within 6 hours after patient has received another antihypertensive. Use together cautiously.

Diuretics: May potentiate antihypoglycemic, hyperuricemic, or antihypertensive effects of diazoxide. Monitor patient closely.

Insulin, oral antidiabetics: Insulin and oral antidiabetic requirements may change in previously stable diabetic patients. Monitor blood glucose levels.

Phenytoin: May increase metabolism and decrease plasma protein–binding of phenytoin. Monitor patient closely.

Thiazides: May enhance diazoxide effects. Use together cautiously.

Warfarin: Diazoxide may displace warfarin, bilirubin, or other highly protein-bound substances from protein-binding sites. Avoid use together.

Adverse reactions

CNS: dizziness, weakness; headache, malaise, anxiety, insomnia, paresthesia (with oral form); headache, *seizures, paralysis, cerebral is-*

chemia, light-headedness, euphoria (with parenteral form).

CV: *arrhythmias,* tachycardia, hypotension, hypertension (with oral form); *sodium and water retention, orthostatic hypotension,* diaphoresis, flushing, warmth, angina, myocardial ischemia, ECG changes, *shock, MI* (with parenteral form).

EENT: diplopia, transient cataracts, blurred vision, lacrimation (with oral administration); optic nerve infarction (with parenteral form).

GI: abdominal discomfort, diarrhea; nausea, vomiting, anorexia, taste alteration (with oral form); *nausea, vomiting,* dry mouth, constipation (with parenteral form).

GU: azotemia, reversible nephrotic syndrome, decreased urine output, hematuria, albuminuria (with oral form).

Hematologic: *leukopenia, thrombocytopenia,* anemia, eosinophilia, excessive bleeding (with oral form).

Metabolic: *sodium and fluid retention, ketoacidosis and hyperosmolar nonketotic syndrome, hyperuricemia, hyperglycemia.*

Skin: hirsutism; rash, pruritus (with oral form).

Other: fever (with oral form); inflammation and pain from extravasation.

Overdose and treatment

Overdose causes mainly hyperglycemia; ketoacidosis and hypotension may occur.

Treat acute overdose supportively and symptomatically. If hyperglycemia develops, give insulin and replace fluid and electrolyte losses; use vasopressors if hypotension fails to respond to conservative treatment. Prolonged monitoring may be necessary because of the long half-life of diazoxide.

Special considerations

● Diazoxide is used to treat only hypoglycemia resulting from hyperinsulinism; it isn't used to treat functional hypoglycemia. It may be used temporarily to control preoperative or postoperative hypoglycemia in patients with hyperinsulinism.

● I.V. use of diazoxide is seldom necessary for more than 4 or 5 days. The use of 300-mg I.V. bolus push is no longer recommended. Switch to therapy with oral antihypertensives as soon as possible.

● Significant hypotension doesn't occur after oral administration in doses used to treat hypoglycemia.

● Drug may be given by constant I.V. infusion (at 7.5 to 30 mg/minute) until adequate blood pressure reduction occurs.

● Diazoxide inhibits glucose-stimulated insulin release and may cause false-negative insulin response to glucagon.

Patient monitoring

● Monitor blood pressure and ECG continuously. Keep norepinephrine available.

• After I.V. injection, monitor blood pressure every 5 minutes for 15 to 30 minutes, then hourly when patient is stable. Discontinue if severe hypotension develops or if blood pressure continues to decrease 30 minutes after drug infusion; keep patient recumbent during this time and have norepinephrine available. Monitor I.V. site for infiltration or extravasation.

• Intake and output must be monitored carefully. If fluid or sodium retention develops, diuretics may be given 30 to 60 minutes after diazoxide. Patient must be recumbent for 8 to 10 hours after diuretic administration.

• Monitor daily blood glucose and electrolyte levels, watching diabetic patients closely for severe hyperglycemia or hyperglycemic hyperosmolar nonketotic coma; also monitor daily urine glucose and ketone levels, intake and output, and weight. Check serum uric acid levels frequently.

Breast-feeding patients
• It isn't known whether drug appears in breast milk; an alternative feeding method is recommended during therapy.

Pediatric patients
• Use cautiously in children.

Geriatric patients
• Geriatric patients may have a more pronounced hypotensive response.

Patient education
• Explain that orthostatic hypotension can be minimized by rising slowly and avoiding sudden position changes.

• Tell patient to report adverse effects immediately, including pain and redness at injection site, which may indicate infiltration.

• Instruct patient to check weight daily and report gains of more than 5 lb/week; diazoxide causes sodium and water retention.

• Reassure patient that excessive hair growth is a common reaction that subsides when drug treatment is completed.

dibucaine
Nupercainal

Pharmacologic classification: local anesthetic (amide)
Therapeutic classification: local amide anesthetic
Pregnancy risk category: B

Indications and dosages
➤ *Temporary relief of pain and itching from abrasions, sunburn, minor burns, insect bites, and other minor skin conditions.* Adults and children: Apply to affected areas, p.r.n. Maximum daily dose of 1% ointment is 30 g for adults and 7.5 g for children.

➤ *Temporary relief of pain, itching, and burning caused by hemorrhoids.* Adults: Instill 1% ointment into rectum using a rectal applicator each morning and evening and after each bowel movement, p.r.n. Apply additional ointment topically to anal tissues. Maximum daily dose is 30 g.

How supplied
Available without a prescription
Cream (topical): 0.5%
Ointment (rectal or topical): 1%

Pharmacodynamics
Anesthetic action: Dibucaine inhibits conduction of nerve impulses and decreases cell membrane permeability to ions, anesthetizing local nerve endings.

Pharmacokinetics
Absorption: Dibucaine has limited absorption.
Distribution: None.
Metabolism: None.
Excretion: None.

Route	Onset	Peak	Duration
Topical, P.R.	Unknown	Unknown	Unknown

Contraindications and precautions
Contraindicated in patients hypersensitive to drug, sulfites, or other amide-type local anesthetics and for use on large skin areas, on broken skin or mucous membranes, and in eyes.

Interactions
None reported.

Adverse reactions
Skin: irritation, inflammation, contact dermatitis, cutaneous lesions.
Other: *hypersensitivity reactions* (urticaria, edema, burning, stinging, tenderness).

Overdose and treatment
Clean area thoroughly with mild soap and water.

Special considerations
• Use dibucaine topically only for short periods.
• Don't use in or near the eye.
• Discontinue drug if sensitization occurs or condition worsens.

Patient monitoring
• If rectal bleeding, rash, pain, swelling, or other symptoms develop, notify prescriber immediately and discontinue drug.

Breast-feeding patients
• Drug shouldn't be used in breast-feeding women.

Reactions may be *common*, uncommon, *life-threatening*, or COMMON AND LIFE-THREATENING.

Pediatric patients
● Adjust dosage to patient's age, size, and physical condition.

Geriatric patients
● Adjust dosage to patient's age, size, and physical condition.

Patient education
● Advise patient to call if condition worsens or if symptoms persist for more than 7 days after use.
● Explain correct use of drug.
● Emphasize need to wash hands thoroughly after use.
● Caution patient to apply drug sparingly to minimize untoward effects.
● Tell patient to keep drug out of reach of children.

diclofenac potassium
Cataflam

diclofenac sodium
Voltaren, Voltaren-XR

Pharmacologic classification: NSAID
Therapeutic classification: antiarthritic, anti-inflammatory
Pregnancy risk category: B

Indications and dosages
➤ *Osteoarthritis.* **diclofenac sodium.** *Adults:* 50 mg P.O. b.i.d. or t.i.d. Or, 75 mg P.O. b.i.d..
➤ *Ankylosing spondylitis.* *Adults:* 25 mg P.O. q.i.d. Another 25 mg dose may be needed h.s.
➤ *Rheumatoid arthritis.* **diclofenac sodium.** *Adults:* 50 mg P.O. t.i.d. or q.i.d. Or, 75 mg P.O. b.i.d.
➤ *Analgesia and primary dysmenorrhea.* **diclofenac potassium.** *Adults:* 50 mg diclofenac potassium P.O. t.i.d. Or, 100 mg P.O. initially, followed by 50-mg doses, up to a maximum dose of 200 mg in first 24 hours. Subsequent dosing should follow 50 mg t.i.d. regimen.

How supplied
Available by prescription only
diclofenac potassium
Tablets: 50 mg
diclofenac sodium
Tablets (delayed-release): 25 mg, 50 mg, 75 mg
Tablets (extended-release): 100 mg
Ophthalmic drops: 0.1%

Pharmacodynamics
Anti-inflammatory and antipyretic actions: Diclofenac exerts anti-inflammatory and antipyretic actions through an unknown mechanism that may involve inhibition of prostaglandin synthesis.

Pharmacokinetics
Absorption: After oral administration, diclofenac is rapidly and almost completely absorbed. Absorption is delayed by food.
Distribution: Highly (nearly 100%) protein-bound.
Metabolism: Undergoes first-pass metabolism, with 60% of unchanged drug reaching systemic circulation. The principal active metabolite, 48-hydroxydiclofenac, has about 3% of the activity of the parent compound. Mean terminal half-life is about 1¼ to 1¾ hours after an oral dose.
Excretion: About 40% to 60% is excreted in the urine; the balance is excreted in the bile. The 4´-hydroxy metabolite accounts for 20% to 30% of the dose excreted in the urine; the other metabolites account for 10% to 20%; 5% to 10% is excreted unchanged in the urine. More than 90% is excreted within 72 hours. Moderate renal impairment doesn't alter the elimination of unchanged diclofenac but may slow the elimination of the metabolites. Hepatic impairment doesn't appear to affect the pharmacokinetics of diclofenac.

Route	Onset	Peak	Duration
P.O.			
Regular	10 min	1 hr	8 hr
Enteric	30 min	2-3 hr	8 hr
Extended	Unknown	Unknown	Unknown

Contraindications and precautions
Oral form is contraindicated in patients hypersensitive to drug and in those with hepatic porphyria or a history of asthma, urticaria, or other allergic reactions after taking aspirin or other NSAIDs. Avoid use during late pregnancy or while breast-feeding. Ophthalmic solution is contraindicated in patients hypersensitive to any component of the drug and in those wearing soft contact lenses; also avoid use during late pregnancy.

Use oral form cautiously in patients with history of peptic ulcer disease, hepatic or renal dysfunction, cardiac disease, hypertension, or conditions related to fluid retention.

Use ophthalmic solution cautiously in patients hypersensitive to aspirin, phenylacetic acid derivatives, and other NSAIDs and in surgical patients with known bleeding tendencies or in those receiving medications that may prolong bleeding time.

Interactions
Drug-drug. *Aspirin:* Decreased diclofenac levels. Concurrent use isn't recommended.
Beta blockers: May blunt antihypertensive effects. Don't use together.
Cyclosporine, digoxin, methotrexate: Increased toxicity of these drugs. Monitor patient and serum levels closely.
Diuretics: Diuretic action may be inhibited. Monitor patient closely.

Insulin, oral antidiabetics: May alter patient's response to these drugs. Monitor blood glucose levels closely.

Lithium: Decreased renal clearance of lithium and increased plasma levels; may lead to lithium toxicity. Monitor serum levels closely.

Potassium-sparing diuretics: May increase serum potassium levels. Monitor serum potassium levels closely.

Warfarin: Altered platelet function. Monitor anticoagulant dosage closely.

Drug-lifestyle. *Sun exposure:* May cause photosensitivity reactions. Advise patient to take precautions.

Adverse reactions

Unless otherwise noted, the following adverse reactions refer to oral administration of drug:

CNS: anxiety, depression, dizziness, drowsiness, insomnia, irritability, headache.

CV: *heart failure,* hypertension, edema.

EENT: *tinnitus,* laryngeal edema, swelling of the lips and tongue, blurred vision, eye pain, night blindness, epistaxis, taste disorder, reversible hearing loss; *transient stinging and burning, increased intraocular pressure, keratitis,* anterior chamber reaction, ocular allergy (with ophthalmic solution).

GI: *abdominal pain or cramps, constipation, diarrhea, indigestion, nausea,* vomiting, abdominal distention, flatulence, peptic ulceration, *bleeding,* melena, bloody diarrhea, appetite change, colitis.

GU: proteinuria, *acute renal failure,* oliguria, interstitial nephritis, papillary necrosis *nephrotic syndrome,* fluid retention.

Hematologic: increased platelet aggregation time.

Hepatic: elevated liver enzyme levels, jaundice, *hepatitis, hepatotoxicity.*

Metabolic: hypoglycemia, hyperglycemia.

Musculoskeletal: back, leg, or joint pain.

Respiratory: asthma.

Skin: rash, pruritus, urticaria, eczema, dermatitis, alopecia, photosensitivity, bullous eruption, *Stevens-Johnson syndrome,* allergic purpura.

Other: *anaphylaxis, anaphylactoid reactions, angioedema,* viral infection (with ophthalmic solution).

Overdose and treatment

No information available. There's no special antidote. Supportive and symptomatic treatment may include induction of vomiting or gastric lavage. Treatment with activated charcoal or dialysis may also be appropriate.

Special considerations

● Administration with other drugs, such as glucocorticoids, that produce adverse GI effects may aggravate such effects.

● Because the anti-inflammatory, antipyretic, and analgesic effects of diclofenac may mask the usual signs of infection, monitor carefully for infection.

Patient monitoring

● Monitor renal function during treatment. Use cautiously and at reduced dosage in patients with renal impairment.

● Periodic ophthalmologic examinations are recommended during prolonged therapy.

● Monitor liver function during therapy. Abnormal liver function test results and severe hepatic reactions may occur.

● Periodic evaluation of hematopoietic function is recommended because bone marrow abnormalities have occurred. Regular check of hemoglobin level is important to detect toxic effects on the GI tract.

Breast-feeding patients

● Low levels of diclofenac have been measured in breast milk. Risk-to-benefit ratio must be considered.

Pediatric patients

● Drug isn't recommended for use in children.

Geriatric patients

● Use cautiously in geriatric patients; they may be more susceptible to adverse reactions, especially GI toxicity and nephrotoxicity. Reduce dosage to lowest level that controls symptoms.

Patient education

● Advise patient to take drug with meals or milk to avoid GI upset.

● Teach patient to restrict salt intake, as diclofenac may cause edema, especially if patient is hypertensive.

● Instruct patient to report symptoms that may be related to GI ulceration, such as epigastric pain and black or tarry stools, as well as other unusual symptoms such as skin rash, pruritus or significant edema or weight gain.

dicloxacillin sodium
Dycill, Dynapen, Pathocil

Pharmacologic classification: penicillinase-resistant penicillin
Therapeutic classification: antibiotic
Pregnancy risk category: B

Indications and dosages

➤ *Systemic infections caused by penicillinase-producing staphylococci. Adults and children who weigh 40 kg (88 lb) or more:* 125 to 250 mg P.O. q 6 hours.

Infants and children over age 1 month who weigh less than 40 lg: 12.5 to 50 mg/kg P.O. daily, divided into doses given q 6 hours. Serious infection may warrant higher dosage (75 to 100 mg/kg daily in divided doses q 6 hours).

How supplied
Available by prescription only
Capsules: 125 mg, 250 mg, 500 mg
Oral suspension: 62.5 mg/5 ml (after reconstitution)

Pharmacodynamics
Antibiotic action: Dicloxacillin is bactericidal; it adheres to bacterial penicillin-binding proteins, thus inhibiting bacterial cell wall synthesis. Dicloxacillin resists the effects of penicillinases—enzymes that inactivate penicillin—and is thus active against many strains of penicillinase-producing bacteria; this activity is most important against penicillinase-producing staphylococci; some strains may remain resistant. Dicloxacillin is also active against a few gram-positive aerobic and anaerobic bacilli but has no significant effect on gram-negative bacilli.

Pharmacokinetics
Absorption: Absorbed rapidly but incompletely (35% to 76%) from the GI tract; it's relatively acid stable. Food may decrease both rate and extent of absorption.
Distribution: Distributed widely into bone, bile, and pleural and synovial fluids. CSF penetration is poor but is enhanced by meningeal inflammation. Drug crosses the placenta, and is 95% to 99% protein-bound.
Metabolism: Metabolized only partially.
Excretion: Excreted in urine by renal tubular secretion and glomerular filtration; also excreted in breast milk. Elimination half-life in adults is ½ to 1 hour, extended minimally to 2¼ hours in patients with renal impairment.

Route	Onset	Peak	Duration
P.O.	Unknown	2 hr	6 hr

Contraindications and precautions
Contraindicated in patients hypersensitive to drug or other penicillins. Use cautiously in patients with other drug allergies, especially to cephalosporins, or in those with mononucleosis.

Interactions
Drug-drug. *Aminoglycosides:* Dicloxacillin may falsely decrease serum aminoglycoside levels. Monitor patient carefully.
Oral contraceptives: May decrease contraceptive efficacy. Recommend additional form of contraceptive during penicillin therapy.
Probenecid: Blocked renal tubular secretion of dicloxacillin, raising its serum levels. Probenecid may be used for this purpose.
Drug-food. *Any food:* Interference with drug absorption. Give drug 1 hour before or 2 hours after meals.

Adverse reactions
CNS: neuromuscular irritability, *seizures,* lethargy, hallucinations, anxiety, confusion, agitation, depression, dizziness, fatigue.

GI: *nausea,* vomiting, *epigastric distress,* flatulence, *diarrhea,* enterocolitis, pseudomembranous colitis, black "hairy" tongue, abdominal pain.
GU: interstitial nephritis, nephropathy.
Hematologic: eosinophilia, anemia, *thrombocytopenia, leukopenia,* hemolytic anemia, *agranulocytosis.*
Hepatic: transient elevations in liver function test results, cholestasis, *hepatitis.*
Other: *hypersensitivity reactions* (pruritus, urticaria, rash, *anaphylaxis*), overgrowth of nonsusceptible organisms.

Overdose and treatment
Overdose may cause neuromuscular irritability or seizures.
    Treatment is supportive. After recent ingestion (4 hours or less), empty the stomach by induced emesis or gastric lavage; follow with activated charcoal to reduce absorption. Drug isn't appreciably dialyzable.

Special considerations
Consider the recommendations relevant to all penicillins as well as the following.
● Aminoglycosides produce synergistic bactericidal effects against *Staphylococcus aureus.* However, the drugs are physically and chemically incompatible and are inactivated when mixed or given together. Dicloxacillin may falsely decrease serum aminoglycoside levels.
● Give drug with water only; acid in fruit juice or carbonated beverage may inactivate drug.
● Give dose on empty stomach; food decreases absorption.

Patient monitoring
● Regularly assess renal, hepatic, and hematopoietic function during prolonged therapy.

Breast-feeding patients
● Dicloxacillin appears in breast milk; use drug cautiously in breast-feeding women.

Pediatric patients
● Elimination of dicloxacillin is reduced in neonates; safety in neonates hasn't been established.

Geriatric patients
● Half-life may be prolonged because of impaired renal function.

Patient education
● Tell patient to report severe diarrhea promptly. He should also report rash or itching.
● Instruct patient to complete full course of therapy as prescribed, even if he feels better.

---

* Canada only   ◇ Unlabeled clinical use

dicyclomine hydrochloride
Antispas, A-Spas, Bentyl, Bentylol*,
Byclomine, Dibent, Formulex*,
Lomine*, Neoquess, Or-Tyl,
Spasmoban*, Spasmoject

Pharmacologic classification: anticholinergic
Therapeutic classification: antimuscarinic, GI
antispasmodic
Pregnancy risk category: B

Indications and dosages
➤ *Irritable bowel syndrome and other
functional GI disorders.* Adults: Initially,
20 mg P.O. q.i.d.; then increase to 40 mg P.O.
q.i.d. during first week of therapy unless precluded by adverse reactions. Or, 20 mg I.M. q 4
to 6 hours.
Children age 2 and older: 10 mg P.O. t.i.d. or
q.i.d.
Infants ages 6 months to 23 months: 5 to 10 mg
P.O. t.i.d. or q.i.d.
➤ *Infant colic◇.* Infants age 6 months and
older: 5 to 10 mg P.O. t.i.d. or q.i.d. Adjust dosage
according to patient's needs and response.

How supplied
Available by prescription only
Capsules: 10 mg
Injection: 10 mg/ml in 2-ml vials, 10-ml vials,
2-ml ampules
Syrup: 10 mg/5 ml
Tablets: 20 mg

Pharmacodynamics
Antispasmodic action: Dicyclomine exerts a
nonspecific, direct spasmolytic action on smooth
muscle. It also has some local anesthetic properties that may contribute to spasmolysis in the
GI and biliary tracts.

Pharmacokinetics
Absorption: About 67% of an oral dose is ab-
sorbed from the GI tract.
Distribution: Largely unknown.
Metabolism: Unknown.
Excretion: After oral administration, 80% of a
dose is excreted in urine and 10% in feces.

Route	Onset	Peak	Duration
P.O., I.M.	Unknown	1-1½ hr	Unknown

Contraindications and precautions
Contraindicated in patients with obstructive uropathy, obstructive disease of the GI tract, reflux
esophagitis, severe ulcerative colitis, myasthenia
gravis, hypersensitivity to anticholinergics, unstable CV status in acute hemorrhage, or glaucoma. Also contraindicated in breast-feeding
patients and in children under age 6 months.

Use cautiously in patients with autonomic neuropathy, hyperthyroidism, coronary artery disease, arrhythmias, heart failure, hypertension,

hiatal hernia, hepatic or renal disease, prostatic
hyperplasia, and ulcerative colitis.

Interactions
Drug-drug. *Amantadine, antihistamines, antiparkinsonians, disopyramide, glutethimide,
meperidine, phenothiazines, procainamide,
quinidine, tricyclic antidepressants:* May cause
additive adverse effects. Avoid use together.
Antacids: Decreased oral absorption of anticholinergics. Give dicyclomine at least 1 hour before antacids.
Digoxin (slow-dissolving tablets): Increased
digoxin levels. Monitor digoxin levels closely.
Levodopa and ketoconazole: Decreased GI absorption. Avoid use together.
Methotrimeprazine: May enhance risk of extrapyramidal reactions. Avoid use together.
*Oral potassium supplements (especially wax-
matrix forms):* Potassium-induced GI ulcerations may be increased. Use together cautiously.

Adverse reactions
CNS: *headache; dizziness;* insomnia; light-
headedness; drowsiness; nervousness, confusion,
and excitement in elderly patients.
CV: *palpitations,* tachycardia.
EENT: blurred vision, increased intraocular pressure, mydriasis.
GI: nausea, vomiting, *constipation, dry mouth,*
abdominal distention, heartburn, paralytic ileus.
GU: *urinary hesitancy, urine retention,* impotence.
Skin: urticaria, decreased sweating or possible
anhidrosis, other dermal manifestations, local irritation.
Other: fever, allergic reactions, dependence.

Overdose and treatment
Signs and symptoms of overdose include curare-
like CNS stimulation followed by depression, and
such psychotic symptoms as disorientation, confusion, hallucinations, delusions, anxiety, agitation, and restlessness. Peripheral effects may include dilated, nonreactive pupils; hot, flushed,
dry skin; tachycardia; hypertension; and increased
respiration.
    Treatment is primarily symptomatic and sup-
portive, as necessary. Maintain patent airway. If
patient is alert, induce emesis (or use gastric
lavage) and follow with a saline cathartic and activated charcoal to prevent further drug absorption. In severe cases, physostigmine may be administered to block the antimuscarinic effects of
dicyclomine. Give fluids, as needed, to treat shock;
diazepam to control psychotic symptoms; and pilocarpine (instilled into the eyes) to relieve mydriasis. If urine retention occurs, catheterization
may be necessary.

Special considerations
⚠ ALERT High environmental temperatures may
induce heatstroke during drug use. If symptoms
occur, discontinue drug.

Reactions may be *common*, uncommon, *life-threatening*, or COMMON AND LIFE-THREATENING.

• Never give dicyclomine I.V. or S.C.
• Be prepared to adjust dose based on patient's needs and response.

Patient monitoring
• Monitor vital signs and urine output carefully.

Breast-feeding patients
• Dicyclomine may appear in breast milk; it also may decrease milk production. Breast-feeding women should avoid it.

Pediatric patients
• Safety and effectiveness in children haven't been established. Administer cautiously to infants age 6 months or over; seizures have been reported.
• Drug is contraindicated in infants under age 6 months.

Geriatric patients
• Administer drug cautiously and in reduced doses.

Patient education
• Tell patient that syrup form may be diluted with water.
• Warn patient that high environmental temperatures may induce heatstroke during therapy; tell patient to avoid such temperatures.
• Advise patient to avoid driving and other hazardous activities if drowsiness or blurred vision occurs; and report rash or other skin eruption.

didanosine (ddI)
Videx, Videx EC

Pharmacologic classification: purine analogue
Therapeutic classification: antiviral
Pregnancy risk category: B

Indications and dosages
➤ *Treatment of HIV infection when antiretroviral therapy is warranted.* Adults who weigh 60 kg *(132 lb) or more:* 200 mg (tablets) P.O. b.i.d. Or, 400 mg (as two 200-mg chewable tablets or one 400-mg delayed-release capsule) once daily. Or, 250 mg buffered powder P.O. b.i.d.
Adults who weigh less than 60 kg: 125 mg (tablets) P.O. b.i.d. Or, 250 mg (as chewable tablets or delayed-release capsule) once daily. Or, 167 mg buffered powder P.O. b.i.d.
Children: 120 mg/m² P.O. b.i.d. To prevent gastric acid degradation, children over age 1 should receive a 2-tablet dose, and children under age 1 should receive a 1-tablet dose. Videx EC isn't for use in children.
✦ *Dosage adjustment.* Patients with renal or hepatic impairment may need their dosage adjusted.

How supplied
Available by prescription only
Capsules (delayed-release): 125 mg, 200 mg, 250 mg, 400 mg
Powder for oral solution (buffered): 100 mg/packet, 167 mg/packet, 250 mg/packet
Powder for oral solution (pediatric): 2 g and 4 g in 4- and 8-ounce bottles, respectively
Tablets (chewable): 25 mg, 50 mg, 100 mg, 150 mg, 200 mg

Pharmacodynamics
Antiviral actions: Didanosine is a synthetic purine analogue of deoxyadenosine. After it enters the cell, it's converted to its active form dideoxyadenosine triphosphate (ddATP), which inhibits replication of HIV by preventing DNA replication. In addition, ddATP inhibits the enzyme HIV-RNA dependent DNA polymerase (reverse transcriptase).

Pharmacokinetics
Absorption: Degrades rapidly in gastric acid. Commercially available preparations contain buffers to raise stomach pH. Bioavailability averages about 33%; tablets may exhibit better bioavailability than buffered powder for oral solution. Food can decrease absorption by 50%.
Distribution: Widely distributed; drug penetration into the CNS varies, but CSF levels average 46% of concurrent plasma levels.
Metabolism: Metabolism isn't fully understood, but is probably similar to that of endogenous purines.
Excretion: Excreted in urine as allantoin, hypoxanthine, xanthine, and uric acid. Serum half life averages 0.8 hours.

Route	Onset	Peak	Duration
P.O.	Unknown	¼- 1½ hr	Unknown

Contraindications and precautions
Contraindicated in patients with history of hypersensitivity to any drug component. Use very cautiously in patients with history of pancreatitis. Also use cautiously in patients with peripheral neuropathy, impaired renal or hepatic function, or hyperuricemia.

Interactions
Drug-drug. *Allopurinol:* increased didanosine concentration. Concomitant use isn't recommended.
Antacids that contain magnesium or aluminum hydroxides: May produce enhanced adverse effects, such as diarrhea or constipation. Avoid use together.
Dapsone, drugs that need gastric acid for adequate absorption, ketoconazole: Decreased buffering action of didanosine. Give such drugs 2 hours before didanosine.
Fluoroquinolones, tetracyclines: Decreased antibiotic absorption from buffering agents in di-

danosine tablets or antacids in pediatric suspension. Separate administration times.

Ganciclovir: Increased didanosine level. Monitor patient for toxicity.

Itraconazole: May decrease serum itraconazole levels. Avoid use together.

Methadone: Decreased didanosine level. Monitor patient closely for clinical effect if this combination can't be avoided. Dosage adjustment may be necessary.

Drug-food. *Any food:* Decreased absorption. Give drug on an empty stomach at least 30 minutes before a meal.

Drug-lifestyle. *Alcohol use:* Increased risk of pancreatitis. Discourage concomitant use.

Adverse reactions

CNS: *headache, seizures,* confusion, anxiety, nervousness, asthenia, abnormal thinking, twitching, depression, *peripheral neuropathy.*

EENT: blurred vision, retinal changes, optic neuritis.

GI: *diarrhea, nausea, vomiting, abdominal pain, pancreatitis,* dry mouth, anorexia.

Hematologic: *leukopenia,* granulocytosis, *thrombocytopenia,* anemia.

Hepatic: *hepatic failure,* elevated liver enzyme levels, hepatomegaly.

Metabolic: increased serum uric acid levels, *lactic acidosis.*

Musculoskeletal: myopathy.

Respiratory: pneumonia, dyspnea.

Skin: *rash,* pruritus, sarcoma.

Other: pain, infection, *allergic reactions, chills, fever.*

Overdose and treatment

Possible effects of overdose include diarrhea, pancreatitis, peripheral neuropathy, hyperuricemia, and hepatic dysfunction.

Treatment is supportive. No specific antidote is known, and it's unknown whether drug is dialyzable.

Special considerations

⚠ ALERT Didanosine shouldn't be used as monotherapy.

● The 200-mg chewable tablet should be used only as a component of a once-daily regimen.

⚠ ALERT Pediatric powder for oral solution must be prepared by the pharmacist before dispensing. It must be constituted with water and then diluted with antacid (manufacturer recommends either Mylanta Double Strength Liquid or Maalox TC) to a final concentration of 10 mg/ml. Admixture is stable for 30 days if kept at 36° to 46° F (2° to 8° C). Shake well before measuring the dose.

⚠ ALERT Don't confuse drug with other antivirals that use abbreviations for identification.

● Most patients over age 1 should receive two tablets per dose. Tablets contain buffers that raise stomach pH to levels that prevent degradation of the active drug. Tablets should be thoroughly chewed before swallowing, and the patient should drink at least 1 oz of water with each dose. If tablets are manually crushed, mix drug in 1 oz (30 ml) water; stir to disperse uniformly and have patient drink it immediately. Single-dose packets containing buffered powder for oral solution are available.

● To administer buffered powder for oral solution, carefully open the packet and pour the contents into 4 oz (120 ml) water. Don't use fruit juice or other acidic beverages. Stir for 2 or 3 minutes until the powder dissolves completely. Administer immediately.

● When preparing powder or crushing tablets, avoid excessive dispersal of drug particles into the air.

● Consider substituting the chewable tablets if diarrhea occurs.

● The major toxicity of drug use is pancreatitis, which has been fatal in some cases. It must be considered when abdominal pain, nausea, and vomiting develop or biochemical markers are elevated. Discontinue use of drug until pancreatitis is excluded. If pancreatitis is confirmed, don't use the drug again.

Patient monitoring

● Monitor liver and renal function test results.

● Monitor patient for signs of lactic acidosis and hepatotoxicity including weakness, lethargy, abdominal pain, feeling cold, dizziness, lightheadedness, and a slow, irregular heartbeat. Most cases of lactic acidosis have affected women.

Pregnant patients

● Fatal lactic acidosis has occurred in women who have taken didanosine alone or with stavudine or other antiretrovirals. This combination should only be used in pregnant women if the benefit outweighs the potential risk.

Breast-feeding patients

● It isn't known whether drug appears in breast milk. Because of risk of serious adverse effects in the infant, breast-feeding isn't recommended.

Pediatric patients

● Retinal depigmentation has occurred in some children receiving drug. Children should receive dilated retinal examinations at least every 6 months or if vision changes. Videx EC isn't for use in children.

Patient education

● Tell patient to take drug on an empty stomach to ensure adequate absorption, to chew tablets thoroughly before swallowing, and to drink at least 1 oz (30 ml) water with each dose.

● Remind patient using buffered powder for oral solution not to use fruit juice or other acidic beverages, to allow 3 minutes for powder to dissolve completely, and to take immediately. Be sure he understands how to mix the solution.

Reactions may be *common,* uncommon, *life-threatening,* or COMMON AND LIFE-THREATENING.

diflorasone diacetate
Florone, Florone E, Maxiflor, Psorcon

Pharmacologic classification: topical adrenocorticoid
Therapeutic classification: anti-inflammatory
Pregnancy risk category: C

Indications and dosages
➤ *Inflammation from corticosteroid-responsive dermatoses. Adults and children:* Apply sparingly in a thin film once daily to q.i.d., as determined by severity of condition.

How supplied
Available by prescription only
Cream, ointment: 0.05%

Pharmacodynamics
Anti-inflammatory action: Stimulates synthesis of enzymes needed to decrease the inflammatory response. A group I-II potency anti-inflammatory.

Pharmacokinetics
Absorption: Amount of drug absorbed depends on amount applied and on nature and condition of skin at application site. Ranges from about 1% in areas with thick stratum corneum (palms, soles, elbows, knees) to as high as 36% in areas of thinnest stratum corneum (face, eyelids, genitals). Absorption increases in areas of skin damage, inflammation, or occlusion. Some systemic absorption of topical steroids occurs, especially through oral mucosa.
Distribution: After topical application, drug is distributed throughout local skin. Absorbed into circulation and is distributed rapidly into muscle, liver, skin, intestines, and kidneys.
Metabolism: After topical administration, metabolized primarily in skin. Small amount absorbed into systemic circulation is metabolized primarily in liver to inactive compounds.
Excretion: Inactive metabolites are excreted by kidneys, primarily as glucuronides and sulfates but also as unconjugated products. Small amounts of metabolites also excreted in feces.

Route	Onset	Peak	Duration
Topical	Unknown	Unknown	Unknown

Contraindications and precautions
Contraindicated in patients hypersensitive to drug.

Interactions
None reported.

Adverse reactions
GU: glycosuria.
Metabolic: hyperglycemia, *hypothalamic-pituitary-adrenal (HPA) axis suppression,* Cushing's syndrome.

Skin: burning, pruritus; irritation; dryness; erythema; folliculitis; perioral dermatitis; hypertrichosis; hypopigmentation; acneiform eruptions; *maceration, secondary infection, atrophy, striae, miliaria* (with occlusive dressings).

Overdose and treatment
No information available.

Special considerations
● Thoroughly clean area before application to reduce risk of infection.
● Occlusive dressings usually should be avoided but may be used cautiously for severe or persistent dermatoses.
● Stop therapy if skin irritation or contact dermatitis develops.

Patient monitoring
● Monitor patient's response to treatment.
● Monitor patient for adverse effects.

Pregnant patients
● Safe use hasn't been established. Topical corticosteroids should be used only if potential benefits to mother outweigh risk to fetus.

Pediatric patients
● Children may be more susceptible to HPA-axis suppression and Cushing's syndrome than adults. Monitor patient for delayed weight gain, growth retardation, and lack of response.

Patient education
● Tell patient to use drug only as instructed, to use it externally, and to keep it away from eyes.
● Instruct patient not to bandage or wrap treated area without medical approval.
● Tell parents not to put tight clothes or diapers over treated areas in infants.

diflunisal
Dolobid

Pharmacologic classification: NSAID, salicylic acid derivative
Therapeutic classification: nonnarcotic analgesic, antipyretic, anti-inflammatory
Pregnancy risk category: C

Indications and dosages
➤ *Mild to moderate pain. Adults:* Initially, 1 g. Then 500 mg P.O. daily in two or three divided doses, usually q 8 to 12 hours. Maximum, 1,500 mg daily.
✦ *Dosage adjustment.* In adults over age 65, start with half the usual adult dosage.
➤ *Rheumatoid arthritis, osteoarthritis. Adults:* 500 to 1,000 mg P.O. daily in two divided doses, usually q 12 hours. Maximum, 1,500 mg daily.
✦ *Dosage adjustment.* In adults over age 65, start with half the usual dose.

How supplied
Available by prescription only
Tablets (film-coated): 250 mg, 500 mg

Pharmacodynamics
Analgesic, antipyretic, and anti-inflammatory actions: Mechanisms of action are unknown, but are probably related to inhibition of prostaglandin synthesis. Diflunisal is a salicylic acid derivative, but isn't hydrolyzed to free salicylate in vivo.

Pharmacokinetics
Absorption: Absorbed rapidly and completely via the GI tract.
Distribution: Highly protein-bound.
Metabolism: Metabolized in the liver; it isn't metabolized to salicylic acid.
Excretion: Excreted in urine. Half-life is 8 to 12 hours.

Route	Onset	Peak	Duration
P.O.	1 hr	2-3 hr	8-12 hr

Contraindications and precautions
Contraindicated in patients hypersensitive to the drug or in whom acute asthmatic attacks, urticaria, or rhinitis is precipitated by aspirin or other NSAIDs. Use cautiously in patients with GI bleeding, history of peptic ulcer disease, renal impairment, and compromised cardiac function, hypertension, or other conditions predisposing patient to fluid retention.

Because of the epidemiologic link with Reye's syndrome, the Centers for Disease Control and Prevention recommend not giving salicylates to children and teenagers with chickenpox or flulike illness.

Interactions
Drug-drug. *Acetaminophen:* May increase serum acetaminophen levels by as much as 50%, raising the risk of hepatotoxicity. This interaction may also be nephrotoxic. Avoid use together.
Antacids, aspirin: Delayed and decreased diflunisal absorption. Monitor patient for decreased therapeutic effect.
Antibiotics, corticosteroids, NSAIDs: May potentiate the adverse GI effects of diflunisal.Use together cautiously.
Anticoagulants, thrombolytics: Potentiated anticoagulant effects. Use together cautiously.
Antihypertensives: Decreased effect on blood pressure. Monitore blood pressure closely.
Cyclosporine, diuretics, gold compounds: May increase nephrotoxic potential. Avoid use together.
Furosemide: Decreased hyperuricemic effect of furosemide. Monitor patient carefully.
Highly protein-bound drugs, such as phenytoin, sulfonylureas, and warfarin: May cause displacement of either drug and adverse effects. Monitor patient closely for both drugs.
Hydrochlorothiazide: Increased hydrochlorothiazide level and decreased hyperuricemic, di-

uretic, antihypertensive, and natriuretic effects. Avoid use together.
Indomethacin: Decreased renal clearance of indomethacin. Fatal GI hemorrhage has also been reported. Avoid use together.
Lithium: Possible increased lithium levels. Monitor lithium levels closely.
Methotrexate, nifedipine, verapamil: Decreased renal excretion of these drugs. Monitor patient carefully.
Probenecid: Decreased renal clearance of diflunisal. Monitor patient closely.
Sulindac: Decreased levels of sulindac's active metabolite. Monitor patient carefully for reduced effect.
Drug-lifestyle. *Alcohol use:* May potentiate adverse GI effects. Advise patient to avoid alcohol consumption.

Adverse reactions
CNS: *dizziness,* somnolence, insomnia, *headache,* fatigue.
EENT: *tinnitus.*
GI: *nausea, dyspepsia, GI pain, diarrhea,* vomiting, constipation, flatulence.
GU: increased serum BUN and creatinine levels, renal impairment, hematuria, interstitial nephritis.
Hematologic: prolonged bleeding time.
Hepatic: increased liver function test results.
Metabolic: hyperkalemia, hypouricemia.
Skin: *rash,* pruritus, sweating, stomatitis, *erythema multiforme, Stevens-Johnson syndrome.*

Overdose and treatment
Signs and symptoms of overdose include drowsiness, nausea, vomiting, hyperventilation, tachycardia, sweating, tinnitus, disorientation, stupor, and coma.

To treat diflunisal overdose, empty stomach immediately by inducing emesis with ipecac syrup, if patient is conscious, or by performing gastric lavage. Give activated charcoal via nasogastric tube. Provide symptomatic and supportive measures (respiratory support and correction of fluid and electrolyte imbalances). Monitor laboratory parameters and vital signs closely. Hemodialysis has little effect.

Special considerations
⚠ ALERT Don't give salicylates to children and teenagers with chickenpox or flulike symptoms because of the risk of Reye's syndrome.
● Diflunisal is recommended for twice-daily dosing for added patient convenience and compliance.
● Don't break, crush, or allow patient to chew diflunisal. Patient should swallow it whole.
● Give diflunisal with water, milk, or meals to minimize GI upset.
● Don't give with aspirin or acetaminophen.
● Institute safety measures to prevent injury if patient experiences CNS effects.

Patient monitoring

• Monitor results of laboratory tests, especially renal and liver function studies. Assess presence and amount of peripheral edema. Monitor weight frequently.

• Evaluate patient's response to diflunisal therapy as evidenced by a reduction in pain or inflammation. Monitor vital signs frequently, especially temperature.

• Assess patient for signs and symptoms of hemorrhage, such as bruising, petechiae, coffee ground emesis, and black, tarry stools.

Breast-feeding patients

• Because drug appears in breast milk, breast-feeding isn't recommended.

Pediatric patients

• Don't use long-term diflunisal therapy in children under age 14; safety hasn't been established.

Geriatric patients

• Patients over age 60 may be more susceptible to the toxic effects (particularly GI toxicity) of this drug. The effects of this drug on renal prostaglandins may cause fluid retention and edema, a significant drawback for geriatric patients, especially those with heart failure or hypertension.

Patient education

• Instruct patient in diflunisal regimen and need for compliance. Advise him to report adverse reactions.

• Tell patient to take diflunisal with foods to minimize GI upset and to swallow capsule whole.

• Caution patient to avoid activities requiring alertness or concentration, such as driving, until CNS effects are known.

• Instruct patient in safety measures to prevent injury.

digoxin
Lanoxicaps, Lanoxin, Novodigoxin*

Pharmacologic classification: cardiac glycoside
Therapeutic classification: antiarrhythmic, inotropic
Pregnancy risk category: C

Indications and dosages

➤ *Heart failure, atrial fibrillation and flutter, paroxysmal atrial tachycardia.*
Tablets, elixir. *Adults:* For rapid digitalization, give 0.75 to 1.25 mg P.O. over 24 hours in two or more divided doses q 6 to 8 hours. For slow digitalization, give 0.125 to 0.5 mg daily for 5 to 7 days. Maintenance dosage is 0.125 to 0.5 mg daily.
Children age 10 and older: 10 to 15 mcg/kg P.O. over 24 hours in two or more divided doses q 6

to 8 hours. Maintenance dosage is 25% to 35% of total digitalizing dose.
Children ages 5 to 10: 20 to 35 mcg/kg P.O. over 24 hours in two or more divided doses q 6 to 8 hours. Maintenance dosage is 25% to 35% of total digitalizing dose.
Children ages 2 to 5: 30 to 40 mcg/kg P.O. over 24 hours in two or more divided doses q 6 to 8 hours. Maintenance dosage is 25% to 35% of total digitalizing dose.
Infants ages 1 month to 2 years: 35 to 60 mcg/kg P.O. over 24 hours in two or more divided doses q 6 to 8 hours. Maintenance dosage is 25% to 35% of total digitalizing dose.
Neonates: 25 to 35 mcg/kg P.O. over 24 hours in two or more divided doses q 6 to 8 hours. Maintenance dosage is 25% to 35% of total digitalizing dose.
Premature infants: 20 to 30 mcg/kg P.O. over 24 hours in two or more divided doses q 6 to 8 hours. Maintenance dosage is 20% to 30% of total digitalizing dose.
Capsules
Adults: For rapid digitalization, give 0.4 to 0.6 mg P.O. initially, followed by 0.1 to 0.3 mg q 6 to 8 hours, as needed and tolerated, for 24 hours. For slow digitalization, give 0.05 to 0.35 mg daily in two divided doses for 7 to 22 days, as needed, until therapeutic serum levels are reached. Maintenance dosage is 0.05 to 0.35 mg daily in one or two divided doses.
Children: Digitalizing dose is based on child's age and is administered in three or more divided doses over the first 24 hours. Initial dose should be 50% of the total dose; subsequent doses are given q 4 to 8 hours as needed and tolerated.
Children age 10 and older: For rapid digitalization, give 8 to 12 mcg/kg P.O. over 24 hours, divided as above. Maintenance dosage is 25% to 35% of total digitalizing dose, given daily as a single dose.
Children ages 5 to 10: For rapid digitalization, give 15 to 30 mcg/kg P.O. over 24 hours, divided as above. Maintenance dosage is 25% to 35% of total digitalizing dose, divided and given in two or three equal portions daily.
Children ages 2 to 5: For rapid digitalization, give 25 to 35 mcg/kg P.O. over 24 hours, divided as above. Maintenance dosage is 25% to 35% of total digitalizing dose, divided and given in two or three equal portions daily.
Injection
Adults: For rapid digitalization, give 0.4 to 0.6 mg I.V. initially, followed by 0.1 to 0.3 mg I.V. q 4 to 8 hours, as needed and tolerated, for 24 hours. For slow digitalization, give appropriate daily maintenance dosage for 7 to 22 days as needed until therapeutic serum levels are reached. Maintenance dosage is 0.125 to 0.5 mg I.V. daily in one or two divided doses.
Children: Digitalizing dose is based on child's age and is administered in three or more divided doses over the first 24 hours. Initial dose

should be 50% of total dose; subsequent doses are given q 4 to 8 hours as needed and tolerated.
Children age 10 and older: For rapid digitalization, give 8 to 12 mcg/kg I.V. over 24 hours, divided as above. Maintenance dosage is 25% to 35% of total digitalizing dose, given daily as a single dose.
Children ages 5 to 10: For rapid digitalization, give 15 to 30 mcg/kg I.V. over 24 hours, divided as above. Maintenance dosage is 25% to 35% of total digitalizing dose, divided and given in two or three equal portions daily.
Children ages 2 to 5: For rapid digitalization, give 25 to 35 mcg/kg I.V. over 24 hours, divided as above. Maintenance dosage is 25% to 35% of total digitalizing dose, divided and given in two or three equal portions daily.
Infants ages 1 month to 2 years: For rapid digitalization, give 30 to 50 mcg/kg I.V. over 24 hours, divided as above. Maintenance dosage is 25% to 35% of total digitalizing dose, divided and given in two or three equal portions daily.
Neonates: For rapid digitalization, give 20 to 30 mcg/kg I.V. over 24 hours, divided as above. Maintenance dosage is 25% to 35% of the total digitalizing dose, divided and given in two or three equal portions daily.
Premature infants: For rapid digitalization, give 15 to 25 mcg/kg I.V. over 24 hours, divided as above. Maintenance dosage is 20% to 30% of the total digitalizing dose, divided and given in two or three equal portions daily.
✦ *Dosage adjustment.* Reduce dosage in patients with impaired renal function. Hypothyroid patients are highly sensitive to glycosides; hyperthyroid patients may need larger doses.

How supplied
Available by prescription only
Capsules: 0.05 mg, 0.10 mg, 0.20 mg
Elixir: 0.05 mg/ml
Injection: 0.1 mg/ml (pediatric), 0.25 mg/ml, 0.5 mg/2 ml
Tablets: 0.125 mg, 0.25 mg

Pharmacodynamics
Inotropic action: The effect of digoxin on the myocardium is dose related and involves both direct and indirect mechanisms. It directly increases the force and velocity of myocardial contraction, AV node refractory period, and total peripheral resistance; at higher doses, it also increases sympathetic outflow. It indirectly depresses the SA node and prolongs conduction to the AV node. In patients with heart failure, increased contractile force boosts cardiac output, improves systolic emptying, and decreases diastolic heart size. It also reduces ventricular end-diastolic pressure and, consequently, pulmonary and systemic venous pressures. Increased myocardial contractility and cardiac output reflexively reduce sympathetic tone in patients with heart failure. This compensates for the direct vasoconstrictive action of the drug, thereby reducing total periph-

eral resistance. It also slows increased heart rate and causes diuresis in edematous patients.
Antiarrhythmic action: Digoxin-induced heart-rate slowing in patients without heart failure is negligible and stems mainly from vagal (cholinergic) and sympatholytic effects on the SA node; however, with toxic doses, heart-rate slowing results from direct depression of SA node automaticity. Therapeutic doses produce little effect on the action potential, but toxic doses increase the automaticity (spontaneous diastolic depolarization) of all cardiac regions except the SA node.

Pharmacokinetics
Absorption: With tablet or elixir, 60% to 85% of dose is absorbed. With capsule form, bioavailability increases. About 90% to 100% of a dose is absorbed. With I.M. administration, about 80% of dose is absorbed.
Distribution: Distributed widely in body tissues. Highest levels occur in the heart, kidneys, intestine, stomach, liver, and skeletal muscle; lowest levels are in the plasma and brain. Digoxin crosses both the blood-brain barrier and the placenta; fetal and maternal digoxin levels are equivalent at birth. About 20% to 30% of drug is bound to plasma proteins. Usual therapeutic range for steady state serum levels is 0.5 to 2 ng/ml. In treatment of atrial tachyarrhythmias, higher serum levels (such as 2 to 4 ng/ml) may be needed. Because of long half-life of drug, achievement of steady state levels may take 7 days or longer, depending on patient's renal function. Toxic symptoms may appear within the usual therapeutic range; however, these are more frequent and serious with levels above 2.5 ng/ml.
Metabolism: In most patients, a small amount of digoxin apparently is metabolized in the liver and gut by bacteria. This metabolism varies and may be substantial in some patients. Drug undergoes some enterohepatic recirculation (also variable). Metabolites have minimal cardiac activity.
Excretion: Most of dose is excreted by the kidneys as unchanged drug. Some patients excrete a substantial amount of metabolized or reduced drug. In patients with renal failure, biliary excretion is a more important excretion route. In healthy patients, terminal half-life is 30 to 40 hours. In patients lacking functioning kidneys, half-life increases to at least 4 days.

Route	Onset	Peak	Duration
P.O.	1½-2 hr	2-6 hr	3-4 days
I.M.	30 min	4-6 hr	Unknown
I.V.	5-30 min	1-4 hr	3-4 days

Contraindications and precautions
Contraindicated in patients hypersensitive to drug and in those with digitalis-induced toxicity, ventricular fibrillation, or ventricular tachycardia unless caused by heart failure.

Use very cautiously in elderly patients and in patients with acute MI, incomplete AV block, sinus bradycardia, PVCs, chronic constrictive pericarditis, hypertrophic cardiomyopathy, renal insufficiency, severe pulmonary disease, hypothyroidism, or in patients with hypokalemia or hypomagnesemia.

Interactions
Drug-drug. *Amiloride:* Inhibited digoxin effect and increased digoxin excretion. Monitor patient for altered digoxin effect.

Amiodarone, diltiazem, nifedipine, quinidine, verapamil: Increased serum digoxin levels, predisposing the patient to toxicity. Avoid use together.

Aminosalicylic acid, antacids, kaolin-pectin, magnesium trisilicate, sulfasalazine: Decreased absorption of orally administered digoxin. Monitor for altered digoxin effect. Separate administration times as far as possible from each other.

Amphotericin B, carbenicillin, corticosteroids, corticotropin, edetate disodium, laxatives, sodium polystyrene sulfonate, ticarcillin: Possible digoxin toxicity. Monitor digoxin levels closely.

Antibiotics: Increased digoxin bioavailability and serum levels. Monitor digoxin levels closely; separate administration times.

Anticholinergics: May increase digoxin absorption of oral digoxin tablets. Monitor blood levels and observe patient for toxicity.

Cholestyramine, colestipol, metoclopramide: Impaired absorption. Monitor digoxin levels closely. Space doses by giving digoxin 1¼ hours before or 2 hours after other drugs.

Cytotoxic agents, radiation therapy: Decreased digoxin absorption if the intestinal mucosa is damaged. Use of digoxin elixir or capsules is recommended in this situation.

Diuretics, such as ethacrynic acid, furosemide, bumetanide: May cause hypokalemia and hypomagnesemia. Monitor blood levels closely.

Glucagon, dextrose-insulin infusions, large dextrose doses: Digitalis toxicity. Avoid use together.

I.V. calcium: Synergistic effects that precipitate arrhythmias. Avoid use together.

Rauwolfia alkaloids, sympathomimetics (such as ephedrine, epinephrine, isoproterenol): Increased risk of arrhythmias. Avoid use together.

Parenteral calcium, thiazides: May cause hypercalcemia. Monitor serum calcium levels.

Procainamide, propranolol, verapamil: Additive cardiac effects. Avoid use together.

Succinylcholine: May precipitate cardiac arrhythmias by potentiating digoxin effects. Avoid use together.

Drug-herb. *Betel palm, fumitory, goldenseal, lily-of-the-valley, motherwort, rue, shepherd's purse:* Enhanced cardiac effects. Monitor patient closely.

Gossypol, hawthorn, licorice, oleander, Siberian ginseng, squill: May enhance toxicity. Discourage use together.

Plantain, St. John's wort: Decreased digoxin level and decreased efficacy. Discourage use together.

Adverse reactions
The following signs of toxicity may occur with all cardiac glycosides.

CNS: *fatigue, generalized muscle weakness, agitation, hallucinations,* headache, malaise, dizziness, vertigo, stupor, paresthesia.

CV: ***arrhythmias*** (most commonly, conduction disturbances with or without AV block, PVCs, and supraventricular arrhythmias) that may lead to increased severity of ***heart failure*** and hypotension.

EENT: *yellow-green halos around visual images, blurred vision,* light flashes, photophobia, diplopia.

GI: *anorexia, nausea,* vomiting, diarrhea.

Overdose and treatment
Overdose primarily causes GI, CNS, and cardiac reactions. Severe intoxication may cause hyperkalemia, which may develop rapidly into life threatening cardiac changes. Cardiac signs and symptoms of digoxin toxicity may occur with or without other evidence of toxicity and commonly precede other toxic effects. Because toxic cardiac effects also can occur as effects of heart disease, determining whether these effects result from underlying heart disease or digoxin toxicity may be difficult. Digoxin has caused almost every kind of arrhythmia; various combinations of arrhythmias may occur in the same patient. Patients with chronic digoxin toxicity commonly have ventricular arrhythmias or AV conduction disturbances. Patients with digoxin-induced ventricular tachycardia have a high risk of mortality because ventricular fibrillation or asystole may result.

If toxicity is suspected, discontinue drug and measure serum drug levels. Usually, drug takes at least 6 hours to distribute between plasma and tissue and reach equilibrium; plasma levels drawn earlier may show higher digoxin levels than those present after drug is distributed into the tissues.

Other treatment measures include immediate emesis induction, gastric lavage, and administration of activated charcoal to reduce absorption of drug remaining in the gut. Repeated doses of activated charcoal (such as 50 g q 6 hours) may help reduce further absorption, especially of any drug undergoing enterohepatic recirculation. Some clinicians advocate cholestyramine administration if digoxin was recently ingested; however, it may not be useful if the ingestion is life threatening. Interacting drugs probably should be discontinued. Ventricular arrhythmias may be treated with I.V. potassium (replacement dose; but not in patients with significant AV block), I.V. phenytoin, I.V. lidocaine, or I.V. propranolol. Refractory ventricular tachyarrhythmias may be controlled with overdrive pacing. Procainamide may be used for ventricular arrhythmias that don't respond to the above treatments. In severe AV block, asystole, and hemodynamically significant sinus bradycardia, atropine restores a normal rate.

Administration of digoxin-specific antibody fragments (digoxin immune Fab, or Digibind) is a treatment for life-threatening digoxin toxicity. Each 40 mg of digoxin immune Fab binds about 0.6 mg of digoxin in the bloodstream. The complex is then excreted in the urine, rapidly decreasing serum levels and therefore cardiac drug levels.

Special considerations

● Digoxin is the most widely used cardiac glycoside. Many oral forms and a parenteral form are available, facilitating use of the drug in both acute and long-term clinical settings.

● **ALERT** Don't confuse digoxin with doxepin, desoxyn, or digitoxin.

● **ALERT** Excessive slowing of heart rate (60 beats/minute or less) may be a sign of digitalis toxicity. Withhold drug and check serum levels.

● Drug may cause ECG changes, including increased PR interval and depression of ST segment.

● Ask patient about use of cardiac glycosides within the previous 2 to 3 weeks before administering a loading dose. Always divide loading dose over first 24 hours unless clinical situation indicates otherwise.

● GI absorption may be reduced in patients with heart failure, especially right heart failure.

● Because digoxin may predispose patients to postcardioversion asystole, most clinicians withhold digoxin 1 or 2 days before elective cardioversion in patients with atrial fibrillation. (However, consider consequences of increased ventricular response to atrial fibrillation if drug is withheld.)

● Calcium must not be given rapidly I.V. to patient receiving digoxin. Calcium affects cardiac contractility and excitability in much the same way that digoxin does and may lead to serious arrhythmias.

● Digoxin solution is enclosed in a soft capsule (Lanoxicaps). Because these capsules are better absorbed than tablets, dose is usually slightly less. Lanoxicaps contain 8% alcohol.

Patient monitoring

● Obtain baseline heart rate and rhythm, blood pressure, and serum electrolyte levels before giving first dose.

● Monitor clinical status. Take apical pulse for a full minute. Watch for significant changes (sudden rate increase or decrease, pulse deficit, irregular beats, and especially regularization of a previously irregular rhythm). Check blood pressure and obtain 12-lead ECG if these changes occur.

● Adjust dose to patient's condition and renal function; monitor ECG and serum levels of digoxin, calcium, potassium, magnesium, and creatinine. Therapeutic digoxin levels range from 0.5 to 2 ng/ml. Take corrective action before hypokalemia develops.

Pregnant patients

● Safety isn't known. Only use if clearly needed.

Breast-feeding patients

● Serum levels and milk levels are similar; however, the amount a breastfed infant would be exposed to is far below the usual infant maintenance dose. Caution is recommended when drug is used in a breast-feeding mother.

Pediatric patients

● Children have a poorly defined range of serum levels; however, toxicity apparently doesn't occur at same levels considered toxic in adults. Divided daily dosing is recommended for infants and children under age 10; older children need adult doses proportional to body weight.

Geriatric patients

● Use digoxin cautiously (especially in renally compromised patients), and adjust dosage to prevent systemic accumulation.

Patient education

● Inform patient and responsible family member about drug action, medication regimen, ways to take pulse, reportable signs, and follow-up plans. Patient must understand importance of follow-up laboratory tests and have access to outpatient laboratory facilities.

● Instruct patient not to take an extra dose of digoxin if dose is missed.

● Tell patient to report severe nausea, vomiting, or diarrhea because these conditions may make patient more susceptible to toxicity.

● Advise patient to use the same brand consistently.

● Tell patient to notify prescriber before using OTC or herbal preparations, especially those high in sodium.

digoxin immune Fab (ovine)
Digibind

Pharmacologic classification: antibody fragment
Therapeutic classification: cardiac glycoside antidote
Pregnancy risk category: C

Indications and dosages

➤ *Potentially life-threatening digoxin or digitoxin intoxication.* Adults and children: Administered I.V. over 30 minutes or as a bolus if cardiac arrest is imminent. Dosage varies based on amount of drug to be neutralized; average dose for adults is 6 vials (228 mg). However, if toxicity resulted from acute digoxin ingestion and neither a serum digoxin level nor an estimated ingestion amount is known, 10 to 20 vials (380 to 760 mg) should be administered. See package insert for complete, specific dosage instructions.

How supplied
Available by prescription only
Injection: 38-mg vial

Pharmacodynamics
Cardiac glycoside antidote: Specific antigen-binding fragments bind to free digoxin in extracellular fluid and intravascularly to prevent and reverse pharmacologic and toxic effects of the cardiac glycoside. This binding is preferential for digoxin and digitoxin; preliminary evidence suggests some binding to other digoxin derivatives and cardioactive metabolites.

Once free digoxin is bound and removed from serum, tissue-bound digoxin is released into the serum to maintain efflux-influx balance. As digoxin is released, it's bound and removed by digoxin immune Fab, resulting in a reduction of serum and tissue digoxin. Cardiac glycoside toxicity begins to subside within 30 minutes after completion of a 15- to 30-minute I.V. infusion of digoxin immune Fab. The onset of action and response is variable and appears to depend on rate of infusion, dose administered relative to body load of glycoside, and possibly other, as yet unidentified, factors. Reversal of toxicity, including hyperkalemia, is usually complete within 2 to 6 hours after administration of digoxin immune Fab.

Pharmacokinetics
Absorption: Serum levels peak at the completion of I.V. infusion. Digoxin immune Fab has a serum half-life of 15 to 20 hours. The association reaction between Fab fragments and glycoside molecules appears to occur rapidly; data are limited.
Distribution: Distribution isn't fully characterized. After I.V. administration, drug appears to be distributed rapidly throughout extracellular space, into both plasma and interstitial fluid. It isn't known whether digoxin immune Fab crosses the placental barrier or is distributed into breast milk.
Metabolism: Unknown.
Excretion: Excreted in urine via glomerular filtration.

Route	Onset	Peak	Duration
I.V.	30 min	End of infusion	15-20 hr

Contraindications and precautions
No known contraindications. Use cautiously in patients known to be allergic to ovine proteins. In these high-risk patients, skin testing is recommended because drug is derived from digoxin-specific antibody fragments obtained from immunized sheep.

Interactions
Drug-drug. *Cardiac glycosides, including digoxin, digitoxin, and lanatoside C:* When used together, digoxin immune Fab binds cardiac glycosides. This also occurs if redigitalization is attempted before elimination of digoxin immune Fab is complete (several days with normal renal function; 1 week or longer with renal impairment). Drug is used for this effect.

Adverse reactions
CV: *heart failure,* rapid ventricular rate (both caused by reversal of cardiac glycoside's therapeutic effects).
Metabolic: hypokalemia.
Other: *hypersensitivity reactions (anaphylaxis).*

Overdose and treatment
Limited information is available; however, administration of doses larger than needed for neutralizing the cardiac glycoside may subject the patient to increased risk of allergic or febrile reaction or delayed serum sickness. Large doses may also prolong the time span required before redigitalization.

Special considerations
● Digoxin immune Fab therapy alters standard cardiac glycoside determinations by radioimmunoassay procedures. Results may be falsely increased or decreased, depending on separation method used. Serum potassium levels may decrease rapidly.
● Measure serum digoxin or digitoxin levels before giving antidote because serum levels may be difficult to interpret after therapy with antidote.
● Give I.V. using a 0.22-micron filter needle over 30 minutes or as a bolus injection when cardiac arrest is imminent. Dose depends on amount of digoxin to be neutralized. Each 38-mg vial binds about 0.5 mg of digoxin or digitoxin. Reconstitute vial with 4 ml of sterile water for injection, mix gently, and use immediately. May be stored in refrigerator up to 4 hours.
● To determine appropriate dose, divide the total digitalis body load by 0.5; the resultant number estimates the number of vials required for appropriate dose. Or, in cases of acute ingestion of known quantity of digitalis, multiply the amount of digitalis ingested in milligrams by 0.80 (to account for incomplete absorption).
● Skin testing may be appropriate for high-risk patients. One of two methods may be used:
Intradermal test—dilute 0.1 ml of reconstituted solution in 9.9 ml of sterile saline for injection; then withdraw and inject 0.1 ml of this solution intradermally. Inspect site after 20 minutes for signs of erythema or urticaria.

Scratch test—dilute as for intradermal test. Place one drop of diluted solution on skin and make a ¼" scratch through the drop with a sterile needle. Inspect site after 20 minutes for signs of erythema or urticaria. If results are positive, avoid use of digoxin immune Fab unless necessary. If systemic reaction occurs, treat symptomatically.
• Pretreat patients with sensitivity or allergy to sheep or ovine products, or when skin test results are positive, with an antihistamine such as diphenhydramine and a corticosteroid before administering digoxin immune Fab.

⚠ **ALERT** Keep drugs and equipment for resuscitation readily available during administration of digoxin immune Fab for patients who respond poorly to withdrawal of inotropic effects of digoxin. Dopamine or dobutamine, or other cardiac load-reducing agents, may be used. Catecholamines may aggravate arrhythmias induced by digitalis toxicity; use cautiously.

Patient monitoring
• Closely monitor temperature, blood pressure, ECG, and potassium level before, during, and after administration of antidote.
• Potassium levels must be checked repeatedly because severe digitalis intoxication can cause life-threatening hyperkalemia, and reversal by digoxin immune Fab may lead to rapid hypokalemia.

Breast-feeding patients
• It isn't known whether digoxin immune Fab appears in breast milk; use cautiously in breast-feeding women.

Pediatric patients
• Consider the risk-to-benefit ratio. Adverse effects haven't occurred in infants and small children. Monitor for volume overload in small children. Very small doses may require diluting reconstituted solution with 36 ml of sterile saline for injection to produce a 1 mg/ml solution.
• Infants may require smaller doses; manufacturer recommends reconstituting as directed and administering with a tuberculin syringe.

Patient education
• Explain use and administration to patient and family.
• Instruct patient to report adverse effects immediately.

---

dihydroergotamine mesylate
D.H.E. 45, Migranal

Pharmacologic classification: ergot alkaloid
Therapeutic classification: vasoconstrictor
Pregnancy risk category: X

Indications and dosages
➤ *To prevent or abort vascular headaches, including migraine headaches.* Adults: 1 mg

I.M. or I.V., repeated at 1-hour intervals, up to total of 3 mg I.M. or 2 mg I.V. Maximum weekly dose is 6 mg.
➤ *To treat acute migraine headaches with or without aura.* Adults: 1 spray (0.5 mg) administered in each nostril, then another spray in each nostril in 15 minutes for a total of 4 sprays (2 mg).

How supplied
Available by prescription only
Injection: 1 mg/ml
Nasal spray: 4 mg/ml

Pharmacodynamics
Vasoconstrictor action: By stimulating alpha-adrenergic receptors, drug causes peripheral vasoconstriction (if vascular tone is low). However, it causes vasodilation in hypertonic blood vessels. At high doses, it's a competitive alpha-adrenergic blocker. In therapeutic doses, drug inhibits the reuptake of norepinephrine. A weak antagonist of serotonin, drug slows the increased platelet aggregation caused by serotonin.

In treatment of vascular headaches, drug probably causes direct vasoconstriction of the dilated carotid artery bed while decreasing the amplitude of pulsations. Its serotoninergic and catecholamine effects also appear to be involved.

Effects on blood pressure are minimal. The vasoconstrictor effect is more pronounced on veins and venules than on arteries and arterioles.

Pharmacokinetics
Absorption: Incompletely and irregularly absorbed from GI tract. Onset of action depends on how quickly after headache drug is given. After I.M. injection or intranasal administration, onset of action occurs within 15 to 30 minutes, and after I.V. injection, within a few minutes. Duration of action persists 3 to 4 hours after I.M. injection.
Distribution: 90% of dose is plasma protein-bound.
Metabolism: Extensively metabolized, probably in liver.
Excretion: 10% of dose excreted in urine within 72 hours as metabolites; rest in feces.

Route	Onset	Peak	Duration
I.V.	5 min	15 min	8 hr
I.M.	15-30 min	30 min	3-4 hr
Intranasal	Rapid	½-1 hr	Unknown

Contraindications and precautions
Contraindicated in patients hypersensitive to drug, in pregnant or breast-feeding women, and in those with peripheral and occlusive vascular disease, coronary artery disease, uncontrolled hypertension, sepsis, hemiplegic or basilar migraine, and severe hepatic or renal dysfunction. Avoid use of drug in patients with uncontrolled hyper-

tension or within 24 hours of 5-HT$_1$ agonists, ergotamine-containing or ergot type drugs, or methysergide.

Interactions

Drug-drug. *Antihypertensives:* Antagonized antihypertensive effects. Monitor blood pressure closely.
Erythromycin, other macrolides: Possible ergot toxicity. Monitor patient for drug effects.
Propranolol, other beta blockers: Blocked natural pathway for vasodilation in patients receiving ergot alkaloids; may result in excessive vasoconstriction and cold limbs. Monitor patient closely.
Vasodilators: May result in pressor effects and dangerous hypertension. Monitor blood pressure closely.

Adverse reactions

CV: numbness and tingling in fingers and toes, transient tachycardia or ***bradycardia***, precordial distress and pain, increased arterial pressure, localized edema.
GI: *nausea, vomiting.*
Musculoskeletal: weakness in legs, muscle pain in limbs.
Skin: itching.

Overdose and treatment

Overdose may cause signs and symptoms of ergot toxicity, including peripheral ischemia, paresthesia, headache, nausea, and vomiting.

Treatment requires prolonged and careful monitoring. Provide respiratory support, treat seizures, if necessary, and apply warmth (not direct heat) to ischemic extremities if vasospasm occurs. Administer vasodilators (nitroprusside, prazosin, or tolazoline) if needed.

Special considerations

● Drug is most effective when used at first sign of migraine or as soon after onset as possible.
● If severe vasospasm occurs, keep limbs warm. Provide supportive treatment to prevent tissue damage. Give vasodilators if needed.
● Protect ampules from heat and light. Don't use if discolored.
● For short-term use only. Don't exceed recommended dose.
● Ergotamine rebound or an increase in frequency or duration of headaches may occur when drug is stopped.

Patient monitoring

● If patient is of childbearing age, rule out pregnancy before therapy.
● Monitor blood pressure if drug is used for orthostatic hypotension.
● Monitor patient for signs of illness or infection.

Pregnant patients

● Drug possesses oxytocic properties. Women of child-bearing potential should be informed of fetal risk.

Breast-feeding patients

● Because it's likely that drug appears in breast milk and may cause vomiting, diarrhea, faint pulse, and unstable blood pressure in breast-fed infant, breast-feeding isn't recommended while the mother is taking drug.

Geriatric patients

● Use drug cautiously in elderly patients. Safety and efficacy haven't been established.

Patient education

● Advise patient to lie down and relax in a quiet, darkened room after dose is administered.
● Urge patient to report immediately feelings of numbness or tingling in fingers and toes or red or violet blisters on hands or feet.
● Warn patient to avoid alcoholic beverages during drug therapy.
● Caution patient to avoid smoking during therapy because the adverse effects of drug may be increased.
● Tell patient to avoid prolonged exposure to very cold temperatures while taking drug. Cold may increase adverse reactions.
● Advise patient to report illness or infection, which may increase sensitivity to drug reactions.
● Instruct patient to prime the pump before using nasal spray.
● Instruct patient to discard nasal spray applicator once it has been prepared and unused drug after 8 hours.

dihydrotachysterol
DHT, DHT Intensol, Hytakerol

Pharmacologic classification: vitamin D analogue
Therapeutic classification: antihypocalcemic
Pregnancy risk category: C

Indications and dosages

➤ ***Hypocalcemia with hypoparathyroidism and pseudohypoparathyroidism; treatment of acute, chronic and latent forms of tetany.*** *Adults:* Initially, 0.8 to 2.4 g P.O. daily for several days. Maintenance dosage is 0.2 to 1 mg daily, as required for normal serum calcium levels. Average dose is 0.6 mg daily.
Children: Initially, 1 to 5 mg P.O. daily for 4 days; then continue dosage or reduce to one-fourth the initial amount. Usual maintenance dosage is 0.5 to 1.5 mg daily, as required for normal serum calcium levels.
➤ ***Prevention of thyroidectomy-induced hypocalcemia*** ◇. *Adults:* 0.25 mg P.O. daily given with calcium supplements until danger of hypocalcemic tetany has passed.

▶**Familial hypophosphatemia** ◇. *Adults and children:* 0.5 to 2 mg P.O. daily (until healing of bones occurs). Maintenance dosage is 0.2 to 1.5 mg daily.
▶**Renal osteodystrophy in chronic uremia** ◇. *Adults:* 0.1 to 0.6 mg P.O. daily.
Children: 0.1 to 0.5 mg P.O. daily.
▶**Osteoporosis** ◇. *Adults:* 0.6 mg P.O. daily given with calcium and fluoride.

How supplied
Available by prescription only
Capsules: 0.125 mg
Solution: 0.2 mg/ml (Intensol)
Tablets: 0.125 mg, 0.2 mg, 0.4 mg

Pharmacodynamics
Antihypocalcemic action: Once activated to its 25-hydroxy form, drug works with parathyroid hormone to regulate levels of calcium. It appears to have little activity as the parent compound.

Pharmacokinetics
Absorption: Absorbed readily from the small intestine.
Distribution: Distributed widely; it is largely protein-bound.
Metabolism: Metabolized in the liver, and has a duration of action up to 9 weeks.
Excretion: Excreted in urine and bile.

Route	Onset	Peak	Duration
P.O.	Several hr	1-2 wk	9 wk

Contraindications and precautions
Contraindicated in patients with hypercalcemia or vitamin D toxicity. Use cautiously in those with a history of renal calculi. Drug isn't recommended in breast-feeding women.

Interactions
Drug-drug. *Barbiturates, phenytoin, primidone:* May increase metabolism and therefore reduce activity of dihydrotachysterol. Avoid use together.
Magnesium-containing antacids: May alter dihydrotachysterol absorption. Avoid use together.
Mineral oil, orlistat: May interfere with intestinal absorption of vitamin D analogues. Avoid use together.
Cardiac glycosides: Increased risk of arrhythmias. Avoid use together.
Cholestyramine, colestipol: Decreased absorption of vitamin D analogues. Avoid use together.
Corticosteroids: Counteract vitamin D analogue effects. Don't use together.
Thiazide diuretics: May cause hypercalcemia. Use together cautiously.
Vitamin D analogues: Increase toxicity. Avoid use together.

Adverse reactions
CNS: headache, somnolence, irritability.

CV: hypertension, **arrhythmias.**
EENT: conjunctivitis, photophobia, rhinorrhea.
GI: nausea, vomiting, constipation, polydipsia, **pancreatitis,** metallic taste, dry mouth, anorexia, diarrhea.
GU: polyuria, nocturia, nephrocalcinosis.
Hepatic: altered serum alkaline phosphatase level.
Metabolic: weight loss; alterations in cholesterol levels and electrolytes, such as magnesium, phosphate, and calcium, in serum and urine.
Musculoskeletal: weakness, bone and muscle pain.
Other: decreased libido, thirst, hyperthermia.

Overdose and treatment
Hypercalcemia is the only sign of overdose. Treatment involves stopping therapy, starting a low-calcium diet, increasing fluid intake, and providing supportive measures. In severe cases, death from cardiac and renal failure has occurred. Calcitonin administration may help reverse hypercalcemia.

Special considerations
● Adequate dietary calcium intake is necessary; usually supplemented with 10 to 15 g oral calcium lactate or gluconate daily.
● 1 mg of dihydrotachysterol is equivalent to 120,000 units ergocalciferol (vitamin D_2).
● Store in tightly closed, light-resistant container. Don't refrigerate.

Patient monitoring
● Monitor serum and urine calcium levels. Observe patient for signs and symptoms of hypercalcemia.
● There's some evidence that monitoring urine calcium and urine creatinine is helpful in screening for hypercalciuria. The ratio of urine calcium to urine creatinine should be less than or equal to 0.18. A value of more than 0.2 suggests hypercalciuria, and the dose should be decreased regardless of serum calcium level.

Breast-feeding patients
● Don't use in breast-feeding women.

Pediatric patients
● Some infants may be hyperreactive to drug.

Patient education
● Explain importance of a calcium-rich diet.
● Tell patient to report early signs of hypercalcemia; thirst, headache, vertigo, tinnitus, or anorexia promptly.

Reactions may be *common*, uncommon, *life-threatening*, or COMMON AND LIFE-THREATENING.

diltiazem hydrochloride
Cardizem, Cardizem CD, Cardizem SR, Dilacor XR, Tiazac

Pharmacologic classification: calcium channel blocker
Therapeutic classification: antianginal
Pregnancy risk category: C

Indications and dosages
➤ *Management of Prinzmetal's or variant angina or chronic stable angina pectoris.* *Adults:* 30 mg P.O. q.i.d. before meals and h.s. Increase dose gradually to maximum of 360 mg daily divided into three to four doses, as indicated. Or, 120 or 180 mg (extended-release) P.O. once daily. Adjust over a 7- to 14-day period as needed and tolerated up to a maximum dose of 480 mg daily.
➤ *Hypertension.* *Adults:* 60 to 120 mg P.O. b.i.d. (sustained-release). Adjust up to maximum recommended dose of 360 mg daily, as necessary. Or, give 180 to 240 mg (extended-release) P.O. once daily. Adjust dose based on patient response to a maximum dose of 480 mg daily.
➤ *Atrial fibrillation or flutter; paroxysmal supraventricular tachycardia.* *Adults:* 0.25 mg/kg I.V. as a bolus injection over 2 minutes. Repeat after 15 minutes if response isn't adequate with a dose of 0.35 mg/kg I.V. over 2 minutes. Follow bolus with continuous I.V. infusion at 5 to 15 mg/hour (for up to 24 hours).

How supplied
Available by prescription only
Capsules (extended-release): 60 mg, 90 mg, 120 mg, 180 mg, 240 mg, 300 mg, 360 mg
Capsules (extended-release, containing multiple 60-mg beads): 120 mg, 180 mg, 240 mg
Injection: 5 mg/ml (25 mg and 50 mg)
Injection: 25 mg
Injection (for I.V. infusion only): 100 mg
Tablets: 30 mg, 60 mg, 90 mg, 120 mg

Pharmacodynamics
Antianginal and antihypertensive actions: By dilating systemic arteries, diltiazem decreases total peripheral resistance and afterload, slightly reduces blood pressure, and increases cardiac index when given in high doses (more than 200 mg). Afterload reduction, which occurs at rest and with exercise, and the resulting decrease in myocardial oxygen consumption account for the effectiveness of diltiazem in controlling chronic stable angina.

Diltiazem also decreases myocardial oxygen demand and cardiac work by reducing heart rate, relieving coronary artery spasm (through coronary artery vasodilation), and dilating peripheral vessels. These effects relieve ischemia and pain. In patients with Prinzmetal's angina, diltiazem inhibits coronary artery spasm, increasing myocardial oxygen delivery.
Antiarrhythmic action: By impeding the slow inward influx of calcium at the AV node, diltiazem decreases conduction velocity and increases refractory period, thereby decreasing the impulses transmitted to the ventricles in atrial fibrillation or flutter. The end result is a decreased ventricular rate.

Pharmacokinetics
Absorption: About 80% of a dose is absorbed rapidly from the GI tract. However, only about 40% of drug enters systemic circulation because of a significant first-pass effect in the liver.
Distribution: About 70% to 85% of circulating drug is bound to plasma proteins.
Metabolism: Metabolized in the liver.
Excretion: About 35% is excreted in the urine and about 65% in the bile as unchanged drug and inactive and active metabolites. Elimination half-life is 3 to 9 hours. Half-life may increase in geriatric patients; however, renal dysfunction doesn't appear to affect half-life.

Route	Onset	Peak	Duration
P.O.			
Regular	½-1 hr	2-3 hr	6-8 hr
Extended	2-3 hr	10-14 hr	12-24 hr
I.V.	3 min	Immediate	1-10 hr

Contraindications and precautions
Contraindicated in patients with sick sinus syndrome or second- or third-degree AV block in the absence of an artificial pacemaker; in patients with supraventricular tachycardias linked to a bypass tract such as in Wolfe-Parkinson-White syndrome or Lown-Ganong-Levine syndrome; and in patients with left ventricular failure, hypotension (systolic blood pressure less than 90 mm Hg), hypersensitivity to the drug, acute MI, and pulmonary congestion (documented by X-ray). Use cautiously in elderly patients and patients with heart failure or impaired hepatic or renal function.

Interactions
Drug-drug. *Anesthetics:* Effects may be potentiated. Monitor patient.
Beta blockers: Combined effects that result in heart failure, conduction disturbances, arrhythmias, and hypotension. Use together cautiously.
Cimetidine: May increase diltiazem level. Carefully monitor patient.
Cyclosporine: Increased serum cyclosporine levels and cyclosporine-induced nephrotoxicity. If used together, monitor cyclosporine levels.
Digoxin: Increased digoxin levels. Monitor patient for toxicity.
Furosemide: Forms a precipitate when mixed with diltiazem injection. Give drugs through separate I.V. lines.

Adverse reactions

CNS: *headache,* dizziness, asthenia, somnolence.
CV: *edema,* **arrhythmias,** flushing, **brady-
cardia,** hypotension, conduction abnormalities,
heart failure, AV block, abnormal ECG.
GI: *nausea, constipation,* abdominal discom-
fort.
Hepatic: acute hepatic injury.
Skin: *rash.*

Overdose and treatment

Effects of overdose primarily are extensions of
adverse reactions of drug. Heart block, asystole,
and hypotension are the most serious effects and
require immediate attention.

Treatment may involve I.V. isoproterenol, norepinephrine, epinephrine, atropine, or calcium
gluconate administered in usual doses. Adequate
hydration must be ensured. Inotropic agents, including dobutamine and dopamine, may be used,
if necessary. If severe conduction disturbances
(such as heart block and asystole) with hypotension that doesn't respond to drug therapy develops, initiate cardiac pacing immediately with
cardiopulmonary resuscitation measures, as indicated.

Special considerations

● S.L. nitroglycerin may be administered concomitantly, as needed, if patient has acute angina symptoms.
● Diltiazem has been used investigationally to prevent reinfarction after non-Q-wave MI; as an adjunct in the treatment of peripheral vascular disorders; and in the treatment of several spastic
smooth muscle disorders, including esophageal
spasm.

Patient monitoring

● Monitor blood pressure and heart rate during
initiation of therapy and dosage adjustments.
● If systolic blood pressure is less than 90 mm
Hg or heart rate is less than 60 beats/minute,
dose should be withheld until patient is further
evaluated.

Breast-feeding patients

● Drug appears in breast milk; therefore, patients
should discontinue breast-feeding during diltiazem therapy.

Geriatric patients

● Use drug cautiously in geriatric patients because the half-life may be prolonged.

Patient education

● Tell patient that nitrate therapy prescribed during titration of diltiazem dosage may cause dizziness. Urge patient to continue compliance.
● Inform patient of proper use, dose, and adverse
effects of diltiazem.
● Instruct patient to continue taking drug even
when feeling better.

● Tell patient to report feelings of lightheadedness or dizziness and to avoid sudden position
changes.

dimenhydrinate
Apo-Dimenhydrinate*, Calm-X,
Dimetabs, Dinate, Dommanate,
Dramamine, Dramocen, Dramoject,
Dymenate, Gravol*, Hydrate, PMS-
Dimenhydrinate*

Pharmacologic classification: ethanolamine-
derivative antihistamine
Therapeutic classification: antihistamine (H_1-
receptor antagonist), antiemetic, antivertigo
Pregnancy risk category: B

Indications and dosages

➤ **Prophylaxis and treatment of nausea,
vomiting, dizziness from motion sickness.** *Adults and children age 12 and older:*
50 to 100 mg q 4 to 6 hours P.O., I.V., or I.M. For
I.V. administration, dilute each 50-mg dose in
10 ml of normal saline solution and inject slowly over 2 minutes.
Children: 1.25 mg/kg daily or 37.5 mg/m² daily
P.O. or I.M. q.i.d. not to exceed 300 mg daily, or
according to the following schedule:
Children ages 6 to 12: 25 to 50 mg P.O. q 6 to 8
hours. Maximum, 150 mg daily.
Children ages 2 to 6: 12.5 to 25 mg P.O. q 6 to
8 hours. Maximum, 75 mg daily.
➤ **Meniere's disease ◇.** *Adults:* 50 mg I.M. for
acute attack. Maintenance, 25 to 50 mg P.O. t.i.d.

How supplied

Available with or without a prescription
Injection: 50 mg/ml
Solution: 12.5 mg/5 ml
Tablets: 50 mg
Tablets (chewable): 50 mg
Tablets (film-coated): 50 mg

Pharmacodynamics

Antiemetic and antivertigo actions: Dimenhydrinate probably inhibits nausea and vomiting
by centrally depressing sensitivity of the labyrinth
apparatus that relays stimuli to the chemoreceptor trigger zone and stimulates the vomiting center in the brain.

Pharmacokinetics

Absorption: Well absorbed.
Distribution: Well distributed throughout the
body and crosses the placenta.
Metabolism: Metabolized in the liver.
Excretion: Metabolites are excreted in urine.

Route	Onset	Peak	Duration
P.O.	15-30 min	Unknown	3-6 hr
I.V.	Immediate	Unknown	3-6 hr
I.M.	20-30 min	Unknown	3-6 hr

Reactions may be *common,* uncommon, *life-threatening,* or COMMON AND LIFE-THREATENING.

Contraindications and precautions
Contraindicated in patients hypersensitive to drug or its components. The I.V. product contains benzyl alcohol, which has been linked to a fatal "gasping syndrome" in premature infants and low-birth-weight infants. Use cautiously in patients receiving ototoxic drugs and those with seizures, acute angle-closure glaucoma, or an enlarged prostate gland.

Interactions
Drug-drug. *Aminoglycosides, cisplatin, loop diuretics, salicylates, vancomycin:* Dimenhydrinate may mask the signs of ototoxicity, which can be caused by these drugs. Monitor patient closely.
CNS depressants, such as anxiolytics, barbiturates, sleeping agents, and tranquilizers: Additive CNS sedation and depression. Avoid use together.
Drug-lifestyle. *Alcohol use:* May cause additive CNS depression. Advise patient to avoid alcohol use.

Adverse reactions
CNS: *drowsiness,* headache, dizziness, confusion, nervousness, insomnia, vertigo, tingling and weakness of hands, lassitude, excitation.
CV: palpitations, hypotension, tachycardia, tightness of chest.
EENT: blurred vision, dry respiratory passages, diplopia, nasal congestion.
GI: dry mouth, nausea, vomiting, diarrhea, epigastric distress, constipation, anorexia.
Respiratory: wheezing, thickened bronchial secretions.
Skin: photosensitivity, urticaria, rash.
Other: *anaphylaxis.*

Overdose and treatment
Signs and symptoms of overdose may include either CNS depression (sedation, reduced mental alertness, apnea, and CV collapse) or CNS stimulation (insomnia, hallucinations, tremors, or seizures). Anticholinergic symptoms, such as dry mouth, flushed skin, fixed and dilated pupils, and GI symptoms, are likely to occur, especially in children.

Use gastric lavage to empty stomach contents; emetics may be ineffective. Diazepam or phenytoin may be used to control seizures. Provide supportive treatment.

Special considerations
⚠ **ALERT** Most I.V. products contain benzyl alcohol, which has been linked to a fatal gasping syndrome in premature infants and low-birth-weight infants.
● Incorrectly administered or undiluted I.V. solution is irritating to veins and may cause sclerosis.
● Parenteral solution is incompatible with many drugs; don't mix other drugs in the same syringe.
● Antiemetic effect may diminish with prolonged use.

● Dimenhydrinate may alter or confuse test results for xanthines (caffeine, aminophylline) because of its 8-chlorotheophylline content; discontinue dimenhydrinate 4 days before diagnostic skin tests to avoid preventing, reducing, or masking test response.

Patient monitoring
● Monitor patient for drowsiness. Tolerance to CNS depressant effects usually develops within a few days.

Breast-feeding patients
● Avoid use of antihistamines in breast-feeding patients. Many, including dimenhydrinate, appear in breast milk, exposing the infant to risks of unusual excitability; premature infants are at particular risk for seizures.

Pediatric patients
● Safety in neonates hasn't been established. Infants and children under age 6 may experience paradoxical hyperexcitability. I.V. dosage for children hasn't been established.

Geriatric patients
● Geriatric patients are usually more sensitive to adverse effects of antihistamines than younger patients and are especially likely to experience a greater degree of dizziness, sedation, hyperexcitability, dry mouth, and urine retention.

Patient education
● Tell patient to avoid hazardous activities, such as driving or operating heavy machinery, until adverse CNS effects of drug are known.

● To prevent motion sickness, patient should take medication 30 minutes before traveling and again before meals and at bedtime.

dimercaprol
BAL in Oil

Pharmacologic classification: chelating agent
Therapeutic classification: heavy metal antagonist
Pregnancy risk category: C

Indications and dosages
➤ *Severe arsenic or gold poisoning. Adults and children:* 3 mg/kg deep I.M. q 4 hours for 2 days and then q.i.d. on day 3. Then b.i.d. for 10 days.
➤ *Mild arsenic or gold poisoning. Adults and children:* 2.5 mg/kg deep I.M. q.i.d. for 2 days and then b.i.d. on day 3. Then once daily for 10 days.
➤ *Severe gold dermatitis. Adults and children:* 2.5 mg/kg deep I.M. q 4 hours for 2 days and then b.i.d. for 7 days.
➤ *Gold-induced thrombocytopenia. Adults and children:* 100 mg deep I.M. b.i.d. for 15 days.

➤*Mercury poisoning. Adults and children:* Initially, 5 mg/kg deep I.M. and then 2.5 mg/kg daily or b.i.d. for 10 days.

➤*Acute lead encephalopathy or blood lead level above 100 mcg/dl. Adults and children:* 4 mg/kg (or 75 to 83 mg/m²) deep I.M. injection, then give simultaneously with edetate calcium disodium (250 mg/m²) q 4 hours for 3 to 5 days. Use separate injection sites.

How supplied
Available by prescription only
Injection: 100 mg/ml

Pharmacodynamics
Chelating action: The sulfhydryl groups of dimercaprol form heterocyclic ring complexes with heavy metals, particularly arsenic, mercury, and gold, preventing or reversing their binding to body ligands.

Pharmacokinetics
Absorption: Absorbed slowly through the skin.
Distribution: Distributed to all tissues, mainly the intracellular space, with the highest levels of dimercaprol occurring in the liver and kidneys.
Metabolism: Uncomplexed dimercaprol is metabolized rapidly to inactive products.
Excretion: Most dimercaprol-metal complexes and inactive metabolites are excreted in urine and feces.

Route	Onset	Peak	Duration
I.M.	Unknown	30-60 min	4 hr

Contraindications and precautions
Contraindicated in patients with hepatic dysfunction (except postarsenical jaundice). Use cautiously in patients with hypertension or oliguria. Avoid use in pregnant women unless required to treat a life-threatening acute poisoning.

Interactions
Drug-drug. *Cadmium, iron, selenium, uranium:* Toxic complexes form with these drugs. Delay iron therapy for 24 hours after stopping dimercaprol.

Adverse reactions
CNS: pain or tightness in throat, chest, or hands; headache; paresthesia; muscle pain or weakness, anxiety.
CV: *transient increase in blood pressure* (returns to normal in 2 hours), *tachycardia.*
EENT: blepharospasm, conjunctivitis, lacrimation, rhinorrhea, excessive salivation.
GI: *nausea; vomiting; burning sensation in lips, mouth, and throat; abdominal pain.*
Other: *fever.*

Overdose and treatment
Signs and symptoms of overdose include vomiting, seizures, stupor, coma, hypertension, and tachycardia; they subside in 1 to 6 hours. Support CV and respiratory status; control seizures with diazepam.

Special considerations
🔔 **ALERT** Administer drug by deep I.M. injection only.
● Treat patient as soon as possible after poisoning for optimal therapeutic effect.
● Adverse effects of dimercaprol are usually mild and transitory and occur in about half of the patients who receive an I.M. dose of 5 mg/kg. In patients who receive doses in excess of 5 mg/kg, adverse effects usually occur within 30 minutes after injection and subside in 1 to 6 hours.
● Dimercaprol therapy blocks thyroid uptake of ¹³¹I, causing decreased values.

Patient monitoring
● Monitor vital signs and intake and output during therapy, and keep urine alkaline to prevent renal failure.

Pregnant patients
● Safety in pregnancy hasn't been established, and drug shouldn't be used unless judged by a prescriber to be necessary to treat a life-threatening acute poisoning.

Pediatric patients
● Fever is common, usually appearing after the second or third dose, and may persist throughout therapy.
● Acrodynia in infants and children has been treated with 3 mg/kg of dimercaprol I.M. every 4 hours for 2 days, then every 6 hours for 1 day, followed by every 12 hours for 7 to 8 days.

Geriatric patients
● Use drug cautiously.

Patient education
● Advise patient that drug may cause a bad taste in the mouth or bad breath. It also may cause a burning sensation of the lips, mouth, throat, eyes, and penis, and pain in the teeth.

dinoprostone
(prostaglandin E₂)
Cervidil, Prepidil, Prostin E₂

Pharmacologic classification: prostaglandin
Therapeutic classification: oxytocic
Pregnancy risk category: C

Indications and dosages
➤*Abort second-trimester pregnancy, evacuate uterus in cases of missed abortion, intrauterine fetal deaths up to 28 weeks of gestation, benign hydatidiform mole. Adults:* Insert 20-mg suppository high into posterior vaginal fornix. Repeat q 3 to 5 hours until abortion is complete. Don't exceed 240 mg.

▶ *Ripening of an unfavorable cervix in pregnant patients at or near term (gel or insert).* *Adults:* Insert one applicator (0.5 mg) of gel into vagina. May repeat dose in 6 hours if no response. Maximum recommended dose in 24 hours is 1.5 mg. Or one 10-mg insert into posterior vaginal fornix. Have patient remain supine for 2 hours. Remove insert upon onset of active labor or 12 hours after insertion.

How supplied
Available by prescription only
Vaginal gel: 0.5 mg
Vaginal insert: 10 mg
Vaginal suppositories: 20 mg

Pharmacodynamics
Oxytocic action: Exact mechanism unknown. Stimulates myometrial contractions in the gravid uterus similar to the contractions of term labor. Its action may result from one or more of the following: direct stimulation, regulation of cellular calcium transport, or regulation of intracellular levels of cyclic 3,5-adenosine monophosphate. Reductions in plasma estrogen and progesterone levels play a role in drug's uterine action, but this effect doesn't occur consistently. Drug facilitates cervical dilations by directly softening the cervix.

Pharmacokinetics
Absorption: Following vaginal insertion, drug diffuses slowly into maternal blood. Some local absorption into uterus through cervix or local vascular and lymphatic channels, but accounts for only small portion of dose. Contractions appear within 10 minutes of dosing, with peak effect in 17 hours. No correlation of activity with plasma levels.
Distribution: Distributed widely in mother.
Metabolism: Metabolized in lungs, liver, kidneys, spleen, and other maternal tissues. At least nine inactive metabolites.
Excretion: Drug and metabolites excreted primarily in urine, with small amounts in feces.

Route	Onset	Peak	Duration
Intravaginal			
Gel	15-30 min	Unknown	Unknown
Insert	Unknown	Unknown	Unknown
Suppository	10 min	Unknown	2-6 hr

Contraindications and precautions
Gel form is contraindicated when prolonged contractions of the uterus are considered inappropriate and in patients hypersensitive to prostaglandins or constituents of the gel. Also contraindicated in patients with placenta previa or unexplained vaginal bleeding during this pregnancy and in whom vaginal delivery isn't indicated (because of vasa previa or active herpes genitalia).

Suppository form is contraindicated in patients hypersensitive to the drug and in those with acute pelvic inflammatory disease or active cardiac, pulmonary, renal, or hepatic disease.

Vaginal insert is contraindicated in patients hypersensitive to prostaglandins or when there's suspicion or definite evidence of marked cephalopelvic disproportion or fetal distress where delivery isn't imminent. The insert is also contraindicated in patients with unexplained vaginal bleeding during pregnancy, multiparity with six or more previous term pregnancies, and when oxytocics are contraindicated or the patient is already receiving I.V. oxytocic drugs.

Use suppository form cautiously in patients with asthma, seizure disorders, anemia, diabetes, hypertension or hypotension, jaundice, scarred uterus, cervicitis, acute vaginitis, and CV, renal, or hepatic disease. Use gel form cautiously in patients with asthma or history of asthma, glaucoma or raised intraocular pressure, or renal or hepatic dysfunction and in those with ruptured membranes. Insert should be used cautiously in patients with nonvertex presentation and in those with ruptured membranes or history of previous uterine hypertonia, glaucoma, or childhood asthma.

Interactions
Drug-drug. *Oxytocics (oxytocin):* Enhanced effects of these drugs. When using gel for cervical ripening, concomitant use isn't recommended because cervical laceration and trauma have been reported. Dosing interval of 6 to 12 hours should be allowed before starting oxytocin treatment.
Drug-lifestyle. *Alcohol use:* Inhibits effectiveness of drug with high doses. Discourage use.

Adverse reactions
CNS: *headache, dizziness,* anxiety, hot flashes, paresthesia, weakness, syncope.
CV: chest pain, *arrhythmias.*
EENT: blurred vision, eye pain.
GI: *nausea, vomiting, diarrhea.*
GU: vaginal pain, vaginitis, endometritis, breast tenderness.
Musculoskeletal: *nocturnal leg cramps,* backache, muscle cramps.
Respiratory: cough, dyspnea.
Skin: diaphoresis, rash.
Other: *fever, shivering, chills.*

Overdose and treatment
Overdose causes extensions of adverse reactions. Because drug is rapidly metabolized, treatment involves discontinuing the drug and providing supportive treatment.

Special considerations
● Store suppositories in freezer at –4° F (–20°C); warm to room temperature (in foil) just before use.

- To prevent absorption through skin, use gloves and keep drug handling to a minimum.
- Premedicate patient with an antiemetic and antidiarrheal to minimize GI effects.
- Abortion should be complete within 30 hours.
- Drug-induced fever is self-limiting and transient. Sponge baths or increased fluid intake usually corrects problem.

Patient monitoring
- Confirmation of fetal death is imperative before administration when used for missed abortion or intrauterine fetal death.
- Monitor patient adverse effects.

Patient education
- Advise patient of expected adverse reactions, especially fever, nausea, vomiting (occurs in two-thirds of all patients), or diarrhea (occurs in about half of all patients), all of which are self-limiting.
- Instruct patient to remain in prone position for 10 minutes after insertion of drug.

diphenhydramine hydrochloride
Benadryl, Benadryl Allergy, Benylin, Compoz, Diphen AF, Diphen Cough, Diphenadryl, Hydramine, Nervine Nighttime Sleep-Aid, Nytol, Sleep-Eze 3, Sominex, Tusstat, Twilite

Pharmacologic classification: ethanolamine-derivative antihistamine
Therapeutic classification: antihistamine (H₁-receptor antagonist), antiemetic, antivertigo, antitussive, sedative-hypnotic, topical anesthetic, antidyskinetic (anticholinergic)
Pregnancy risk category: B

Indications and dosages
➤**Rhinitis, allergy symptoms, motion sickness, Parkinson's disease.** *Adults and children age 12 and older:* 25 to 50 mg P.O. t.i.d. or q.i.d. Or, 10 to 50 mg I.V. or deep I.M. Maximum I.M. or I.V. dose is 400 mg daily.
Children under age 12: 5 mg/kg daily P.O., deep I.M., or I.V. in divided doses q.i.d. Maximum, 300 mg daily.
➤**Nonproductive cough.** *Adults and children age 12 and older:* 25 mg P.O. q 4 to 6 hours. Maximum, 150 mg daily.
Children ages 6 to 12: 12.5 mg P.O. q 4 to 6 hours. Maximum, 75 mg daily.
Children ages 2 to 6: 6.25 mg P.O. q 4 to 6 hours. Maximum, 25 mg daily.
➤**Insomnia.** *Adults:* 50 mg P.O. h.s.
➤**Sedation.** *Adults:* 25 to 50 mg P.O., or deep I.M., p.r.n.

How supplied
Available with or without a prescription
Capsules: 25 mg, 50 mg

Capsules (liquid-filled): 25 mg, 50 mg
Cream (topical): 1%, 2%
Elixir: 12.5 mg/5 ml
Gel (topical): 1%, 2%
Injection: 10 mg/ml, 50 mg/ml
Solution: 12.5 mg/5 ml
Solution (topical): 1%, 2%
Spray: 1%, 2%
Stick (Topical): 2%
Tablets: 25 mg, 50 mg
Tablets (chewable): 12.5 mg
Tablets (film-coated): 25 mg, 50 mg

Pharmacodynamics
Antihistamine action: Antihistamines compete for H₁-receptor sites on the smooth muscle of the bronchi, GI tract, uterus, and large blood vessels; by binding to cellular receptors, they prevent access of histamine and suppress histamine-induced allergic symptoms, even though they don't prevent its release.
Antivertigo, antiemetic, and antidyskinetic actions: Central antimuscarinic actions of antihistamines probably are responsible for these effects of diphenhydramine.
Antitussive action: Drug suppresses the cough reflex by a direct effect on the cough center.
Sedative action: Mechanism of the CNS depressant effects of diphenhydramine is unknown.
Anesthetic action: Drug is structurally related to local anesthetics, which prevent initiation and transmission of nerve impulses; this is the probable source of its topical and local anesthetic effects.

Pharmacokinetics
Absorption: Well absorbed from the GI tract.
Distribution: Distributed widely throughout the body, including the CNS; drug crosses the placenta and appears in breast milk. Drug is about 82% protein-bound.
Metabolism: About 50% to 60% of an oral dose of diphenhydramine is metabolized by the liver before reaching the systemic circulation (first-pass effect); virtually all available drug is metabolized by the liver within 24 to 48 hours.
Excretion: Plasma elimination half-life of drug is about 2½ to 9 hours; drug and metabolites are excreted primarily in urine.

Route	Onset	Peak	Duration
P.O.	15 min	1-4 hr	6-8 hr
I.V.	Immediate	1-4 hr	6-8 hr
I.M.	Unknown	1-4 hr	6-8 hr
Topical	Unknown	Unknown	Unknown

Contraindications and precautions
Contraindicated in patients hypersensitive to drug, patients having acute asthmatic attacks, and neonates, premature neonates, and breast-feeding patients.

Use with extreme caution in patients with angle-closure glaucoma, prostatic hyperplasia, pyloroduodenal and bladder neck obstruction, asthma or COPD, increased intraocular pressure, hyperthyroidism, CV disease, hypertension, and stenosing peptic ulcer.

Interactions

Drug-drug. *CNS depressants, such as anxiolytics, barbiturates, sleeping aids, and tranquilizers:* Additive CNS depression. Use together cautiously.

Epinephrine: Enhanced effects. Monitor patient closely.

Heparin: Partially counteracts the anticoagulant effects of heparin. Monitor PT and INR.

MAO inhibitors: Increased anticholinergic effects. Don't use together.

Sulfonylureas: Diphenhydramine may diminish the effects of sulfonylureas. Monitor patient closely.

Drug-lifestyle. *Alcohol use:* May cause additive CNS depression. Tell patient to use cautiously.

Sun exposure: May cause photosensitivity reactions. Advise patient to take precautions.

Adverse reactions

CNS: *drowsiness,* confusion, insomnia, headache, vertigo, *sedation, sleepiness, dizziness, incoordination,* fatigue, restlessness, tremor, nervousness, *seizures.*

CV: palpitations, hypotension, tachycardia.

EENT: diplopia, blurred vision, tinnitus.

GI: *nausea,* vomiting, diarrhea, *dry mouth,* constipation, *epigastric distress,* anorexia.

GU: dysuria, urine retention, urinary frequency.

Hematologic: hemolytic anemia, *thrombocytopenia, agranulocytosis.*

Respiratory: nasal congestion, *thickening of bronchial secretions.*

Skin: urticaria, photosensitivity, rash.

Other: *anaphylaxis.*

Overdose and treatment

Drowsiness is the usual symptom of overdose. Seizures, coma, and respiratory depression may occur with profound overdose. Anticholinergic symptoms, such as dry mouth, flushed skin, fixed and dilated pupils, and GI symptoms, are common, especially in children.

Treat overdose by inducing emesis with ipecac syrup (in conscious patient), followed by activated charcoal to reduce further drug absorption. Use gastric lavage if patient is unconscious or ipecac fails. Treat hypotension with vasopressors and control seizures with diazepam or phenytoin. Don't give stimulants.

Special considerations

● Stop drug 4 days before diagnostic skin tests; antihistamines can prevent, reduce, or mask positive skin test response.

● Diphenhydramine injection is compatible with most I.V. solutions but is incompatible with some drugs; check compatibility before mixing in the same I.V. line.

● Alternate injection sites to prevent irritation. Administer deep I.M. into large muscle.

● Drowsiness is the most common adverse effect during initial therapy but usually disappears with continued use of drug.

● Injectable and elixir solutions are light-sensitive; protect them from light.

Patient monitoring

● Make sure the I.V. site is patent. Drug given perivascularly causes tissue irritation.

Breast-feeding patients

● Avoid use of antihistamines during breast-feeding. Many of these drugs appear in breast milk, exposing the infant to risks of unusual excitability; premature infants are at particular risk for seizures.

Pediatric patients

● Drug shouldn't be used in premature infants or neonates. Infants and children, especially those under age 6, may experience paradoxical hyperexcitability.

Geriatric patients

● These patients are usually more sensitive to adverse effects of antihistamines than younger patients and are especially likely to experience a greater degree of dizziness, sedation, hyperexcitability, dry mouth, and urine retention. Symptoms usually respond to a decrease in medication dosage.

Patient education

● Advise patient that drowsiness is very common initially, but may be reduced with continued use of drug.

● Advise patient undergoing skin testing for allergies to notify prescriber of current drug therapy.

diphenoxylate hydrochloride and atropine sulfate
Lofene, Logen, Lomanate, Lomotil, Lonox

Pharmacologic classification: opiate
Therapeutic classification: antidiarrheal
Controlled substance schedule: V
Pregnancy risk category: C

Indications and dosages

➤ *Acute, nonspecific diarrhea. Adults:* 5 mg diphenoxylate component P.O. q.i.d.; then adjust, p.r.n.

Children age 2 and older: 0.3 to 0.4 mg/kg diphenoxylate component P.O. daily in four divided doses using the liquid form; or administer according to diphenoxylate component, as follows:

Children ages 8 to 12: 2 mg P.O. five times daily.
Children ages 5 to 8: 2 mg P.O. q.i.d.
Children ages 2 to 5: 2 mg P.O. t.i.d.

How supplied
Available by prescription only
Liquid: 2.5 mg diphenoxylate hydrochloride and 0.025 mg atropine sulfate/5 ml
Tablets: 2.5 mg diphenoxylate hydrochloride and 0.025 mg atropine sulfate per tablet

Pharmacodynamics
Antidiarrheal action: Diphenoxylate is a meperidine analogue that inhibits GI motility locally and centrally. In high doses, it may produce an opiate effect. Atropine is added in subtherapeutic doses to prevent abuse by deliberate overdose.

Pharmacokinetics
Absorption: About 90% of an oral dose is absorbed.
Distribution: Distributed in breast milk.
Metabolism: Metabolized extensively by the liver.
Excretion: Metabolites are excreted mainly in feces via the biliary tract, with lesser amounts excreted in urine.

Route	Onset	Peak	Duration
P.O.	45-60 min	3 hr	3-4 hr

Contraindications and precautions
Contraindicated in patients hypersensitive to diphenoxylate or atropine and in patients with acute diarrhea caused by poison (until toxic material is eliminated from GI tract), acute diarrhea caused by organisms that penetrate intestinal mucosa, or diarrhea resulting from antibiotic-induced pseudomembranous enterocolitis or enterotoxin-producing bacteria. Also contraindicated in patients with obstructive jaundice and in children under age 2.

Use cautiously in children age 2 and older; in patients with hepatic disease, narcotic dependence, or acute ulcerative colitis; and in pregnant women. Stop therapy immediately if abdominal distention or other signs of toxic megacolon develop.

Interactions
Drug-drug. *CNS depressants such as barbiturates, narcotic agents, tranquilizers:* Increased depressant effect. Avoid use together.
MAO inhibitors: Increased risk of hypertensive crisis. Avoid use together.
Drug-lifestyle. *Alcohol use:* May enhance CNS depression. Tell patient to avoid use together.

Adverse reactions
CNS: *sedation, dizziness,* headache, drowsiness, lethargy, restlessness, depression, euphoria, malaise, confusion, numbness in limbs.
CV: tachycardia.
EENT: mydriasis.
GI: *dry mouth,* nausea, vomiting, abdominal discomfort or distention, ***paralytic ileus,*** anorexia, fluid retention in bowel or megacolon, increased serum amylase, ***pancreatitis,*** swollen

gums, possible physical dependence with long-term use.
GU: urine retention.
Respiratory: *respiratory depression.*
Skin: pruritus, rash, dry skin.
Other: ***angioedema, anaphylaxis.***

Overdose and treatment
Effects of overdose include drowsiness, low blood pressure, marked seizures, apnea, blurred vision, miosis, flushing, dry mouth and mucous membranes, and psychotic episodes.

Treatment is supportive; maintain airway and support vital functions. A narcotic antagonist, such as naloxone, may be given. Gastric lavage may be performed. Monitor patient for 48 to 72 hours.

Special considerations
● Fluid retention in the bowel or megacolon may mask depletion of extracellular fluid and electrolytes, especially in young children treated for acute gastroenteritis.
● Drug is usually ineffective in treating antibiotic-induced diarrhea.
● Reduce dosage as soon as symptoms are controlled.

Patient monitoring
● Monitor vital signs and intake and output; observe patient for adverse reactions, especially CNS reactions.
● Monitor bowel function.

Breast-feeding patients
● Drug appears in breast milk; drug effects have been reported in breast-fed infants of women taking drug.

Pediatric patients
● Drug is contraindicated in children under age 2; some children may experience respiratory depression.
● Children, especially those with Down syndrome, appear to be particularly sensitive to atropine content of drug.

Geriatric patients
● Geriatric patients may be more susceptible to respiratory depression and to exacerbation of glaucoma.

Patient education
● Warn patient to take drug exactly as ordered and not to exceed recommended dose.
● Advise patient to maintain adequate fluid intake during course of diarrhea and teach him about diet and fluid replacement.
● Caution patient to avoid driving during drug therapy because drowsiness and dizziness may occur.
● Advise patient to call prescriber if drug isn't effective within 48 hours.

Reactions may be *common*, uncommon, *life-threatening*, or COMMON AND LIFE-THREATENING.

• Warn patient that prolonged use may result in tolerance and that use of larger-than-recommended doses may result in drug dependence.

diphtheria and tetanus toxoids, adsorbed

Pharmacologic classification: toxoid
Therapeutic classification: diphtheria and tetanus prophylaxis
Pregnancy risk category: C

Indications and dosages

➤ **Primary immunization.** Adults and children age 7 and older: Use adult strength. Give 0.5 ml I.M. 4 to 8 weeks apart for two doses and a third dose 6 to 12 months later. Booster dose is 0.5 ml I.M. q 10 years.

Children ages 1 to 7: Use pediatric strength. Give two 0.5-ml doses I.M. 4 to 8 weeks apart. Give a third dose 6 to 12 months after the second injection. If final immunizing dose is given after the 7th birthday, use the adult strength.

Infants ages 6 weeks to 1 year: Use pediatric strength. Give three 0.5-ml doses I.M. 4 to 8 weeks apart. Give a fourth dose 6 to 12 months after third injection.

How supplied

Available by prescription only in pediatric (DT) and adult (Td) strengths
Injection (pediatric use): 6.6 limit flocculation (Lf) units of diphtheria toxoid and 5 Lf units of tetanus toxoid per 0.5 ml, in 5-ml vials; 7.5 Lf units diphtheria toxoid and 7.5 Lf units tetanus toxoid per 0.5 ml, in multidose vials; 10 Lf units diphtheria toxoid and 5 Lf units tetanus toxoid per 0.5 ml in single-dose and 5-ml vials; 12.5 Lf units diphtheria toxoid and 5 Lf units tetanus toxoid per 0.5 ml, in 5-ml vials
Injection (adult use): 2 Lf units of diphtheria toxoid and 2 Lf units of tetanus toxoid per 0.5 ml in multidose vials; 2 Lf units of diphtheria toxoid and 5 Lf units of tetanus toxoid per 0.5 ml in single-dose and multidose vials

Pharmacodynamics

Diphtheria and tetanus prophylaxis actions: Diphtheria and tetanus toxoids promote active immunization to diphtheria and tetanus by inducing production of antitoxins.

Pharmacokinetics

No information available.

Route	Onset	Peak	Duration
I.M.	Unknown	Unknown	10 yr

Contraindications and precautions

Contraindicated in immunosuppressed patients and in those receiving radiation or corticosteroid therapy. Defer vaccination in patients with respiratory illness and during polio outbreaks; also defer in those with acute illness except during emergency. When polio is a risk, a single antigen is used. In children under age 6, use only when diphtheria, tetanus, and pertussis combination is contraindicated because of pertussis component. DT shouldn't be used in children age 7 or older because of an increased risk of adverse reactions. Drug is also contraindicated in patients with history of adverse reactions to constituents of drug.

Interactions

Drug-drug. *Corticosteroids, immunosuppressants:* May impair the immune response to diphtheria and tetanus toxoids. Avoid elective immunization under these circumstances.

Adverse reactions

CNS: malaise, headache.
CV: flushing, tachycardia, hypotension.
Skin: *pain, stinging, edema, erythema, induration at injection site,* urticaria, pruritus.
Other: *anaphylaxis,* chills, fever, *shock.*

Overdose and treatment

No information available.

Special considerations

• Obtain a thorough history of allergies and reactions to immunizations.
• Epinephrine solution 1:1,000 should be available to treat allergic reactions.
• Diphtheria and tetanus toxoids are used primarily when pertussis vaccine is contraindicated or used separately.
• These toxoids aren't used to treat active tetanus or diphtheria infections.
• To prevent sciatic nerve damage, avoid administration in gluteal muscle. During primary immunization, don't inject same site more than once.

Patient monitoring

• Document manufacturer, lot number, date of injection, and name and title of person administering injection on permanent record or log.

Pregnant patients

• Teratogenicity hasn't been reported. Immunization during pregnancy is recommended when needed.

Pediatric patients

• Children age 7 and older have an increased risk of development of adverse reactions when preparations containing more than 7 Lf units of diphtheria toxoid are administered; therefore, children age 7 and older should receive Td (adult) preparations, not the pediatric (DT) preparation.

Patient education

• Inform patient that he may experience discomfort at the injection site and that a nodule may develop there and persist for several weeks after immunization. Fever, headache, upset stomach, general malaise, or body aches and pains may also develop. Tell patient to relieve such effects with acetaminophen.

• Tell patient to report distressing adverse reactions.

diphtheria and tetanus toxoids and pertussis vaccine, adsorbed (DTP)

Acel-Imune, diphtheria and tetanus toxoids and acellular pertussis vaccine adsorbed (DTaP), DTwP, Tri-Immunol, Tripedia

Pharmacologic classification: combination toxoid and vaccine
Therapeutic classification: diphtheria, tetanus, and pertussis prophylaxis
Pregnancy risk category: C

Indications and dosages

➤ **Primary immunization.** *Children age 6 weeks to 7 years:* Give 0.5 ml I.M. 4 to 8 weeks apart for three doses and a fourth dose at least 6 months after the third dose (recommended at 15 to 20 months of age). Children 4 to 6 years of age (up to the seventh birthday), who received all 4 doses by the fourth birthday, including one or more doses of whole-cell pertussis DPT, should receive a single dose of Tripedia vaccine before entering kindergarten or elementary school. This dose isn't needed if the fourth dose was given on or after the fourth birthday.

How supplied

Available by prescription only
Whole-cell vaccine
Injection: 6.7 limit flocculation (Lf) units inactivated diphtheria, 5 Lf units inactivated tetanus, and 4 protective units pertussis per 0.5 ml in 2.5-, 5-, and 7.5-ml vials
Acellular vaccine
Injection: 6.7 Lf units inactivated diphtheria, 5 Lf units inactivated tetanus, and 46.8 mcg acellular pertussis antigens per 0.5 ml in single-dose and 7.5-ml vials; 7.5 Lf units inactivated diphtheria, 5 Lf units inactivated tetanus, and 40 mcg acellular pertussis antigen per 0.5 ml in 5-ml vials; 15 Lf units of inactivated diphtheria, 6 Lf units inactivated tetanus, and 40 mcg acellualr pertussis antigens per 0.5 ml in 7.5-ml vials; 25 Lf units of inactivated diphtheria, 10 Lf units inactivated tetanus, and 58 mcg acellular pertussis vaccine per 0.5 ml in 0.5-ml vials

Pharmacodynamics

Diphtheria, tetanus, and pertussis (whooping cough) prophylaxis: Vaccine promotes active immunity to diphtheria, tetanus, and pertussis by inducing production of antitoxin and antibodies.

Pharmacokinetics

No information available.

Route	Onset	Peak	Duration
I.M.	2 wk after last dose	Unknown	4-6 yr

Contraindications and precautions

Contraindicated in immunosuppressed patients and in those on corticosteroid therapy or with history of seizures. Defer vaccination in patients with acute febrile illness. Children with neurologic disorders shouldn't receive pertussis component. Also, children who exhibit neurologic signs after injection shouldn't receive pertussis component in any succeeding injections. Give diphtheria and tetanus toxoids (called DT) instead.

Interactions

Drug-drug. *Corticosteroids, immunosuppressants:* May impair the immune response to the toxoids and vaccine. Patient shouldn't have elective immunization under these circumstances.

Adverse reactions

CNS: *encephalopathy, seizures,* peripheral neuropathy.
Hematologic: thrombocytopenic purpura.
Skin: soreness, redness, expected nodule remaining several weeks at injection site, urticaria.
Other: *anaphylaxis, fever, hypersensitivity reactions, shock.*

Overdose and treatment

No information available.

Special considerations

■ **ALERT** Vaccine isn't routinely given to people age 7 and older; it is given only in special circumstances.
• Obtain history of allergies and reactions to immunizations, especially to pertussis vaccine.
• Epinephrine solution 1:1,000 should be available to treat allergic reactions.
• Don't use to treat active tetanus, diphtheria, or pertussis infections.

Patient monitoring

• Acellular vaccine may cause less local pain and fever.
• Monitor patient for hypersensitivity reactions including anaphylaxis.

Patient education

• Explain to parents that child may experience discomfort at the injection site after immunization and that a nodule may develop there and persist for several weeks. Fever, upset stomach, or general malaise may also develop. Recommend acetaminophen liquid to relieve such discomfort.
• Tell parents to report worrisome or intolerable reactions promptly.

---

dipyridamole 451

• Stress importance of keeping scheduled appointments for subsequent doses. Full immunization requires a series of injections.

dipivefrin hydrochloride
Propine

Pharmacologic classification: sympathomimetic
Therapeutic classification: antiglaucoma
Pregnancy risk category: B

Indications and dosages
➤ *To reduce intraocular pressure in chronic open-angle glaucoma.* Adults: For initial glaucoma therapy, 1 drop in eye q 12 hours. Adjust dose based on patient response as determined by tonometric readings.

How supplied
Available by prescription only
Ophthalmic solution: 0.1%

Pharmacodynamics
Antiglaucoma action: Dipivefrin is a prodrug converted to epinephrine in the eye. It decreases aqueous humor production and enhances outflow. It's often used with a miotic agent.

Pharmacokinetics
Absorption: Absorbed quickly.
Distribution: Unknown.
Metabolism: Unknown.
Excretion: Unknown.

Route	Onset	Peak	Duration
Oph-thalmic	½ hr	1 hr	>12 hr

Contraindications and precautions
Contraindicated in patients with angle-closure glaucoma or hypersensitivity to drug. Use cautiously in patients with asthma, hypersensitivity to epinephrine, and aphakia or CV disease.

Interactions
Drug-drug. *Anesthetics, digoxin, tricyclic antidepressants:* Increased risk of cardiac arrhythmias. Monitor patient closely.
Ophthalmic anhydrase inhibitors, beta blockers, osmotic agents: Enhanced lowering of intraocular pressure. Use together cautiously.
Sympathomimetics: Possible additive effects if significant systemic absorption occurs. Monitor patient closely.

Adverse reactions
CV: tachycardia, hypertension, *arrhythmias.*
EENT: eye burning or stinging, conjunctival injection, conjunctivitis, mydriasis, allergic reaction, photophobia.

Overdose and treatment
Overdose is rare with ophthalmic use but may cause the following effects after accidental ingestion: hypertension with tachycardia or bradycardia, arrhythmias, precordial pain, anxiety, nervousness, insomnia, muscle tremor, cerebral hemorrhage, seizures, altered mental status, anorexia, nausea and vomiting, and acute renal failure.

To treat oral overdose, dilute immediately then initiate emesis followed by activated charcoal and a cathartic, unless patient is comatose or obtunded. Monitor urine output. As ordered, treat seizures with I.V. diazepam and hypertension with nitroprusside; treat arrhythmias appropriately, depending on the type of arrhythmia. Preparations containing sulfites may cause GI or cardiac toxicities and hypotension.

Special considerations
• Drug may cause fewer adverse reactions than conventional epinephrine therapy; it's often used with other antiglaucoma drugs.
• Protect from heat and light.

Patient monitoring
• Monitor patient for hypertension.

Geriatric patients
• Use cautiously to avoid precipitating angle-closure glaucoma.

Patient education
• Teach patient the correct way to instill drops, and caution against touching eye with dropper.
• Tell patient that instillation of drug may cause transient burning or stinging.
• Instruct patient not to blink more than usual and not to close his eyes tightly after instillation.
• If patient uses other eye drops, tell him to instill dipivefrin first and wait at least 5 minutes before using the other drops.

dipyridamole
Persantine

Pharmacologic classification: pyrimidine analogue
Therapeutic classification: coronary vasodilator, platelet aggregation inhibitor
Pregnancy risk category: B

Indications and dosages
➤ *Alternative to exercise in thallium myocardial perfusion imaging.* Adults: 0.142 mg/kg/minute I.V. infused over 4 minutes (0.57 mg/kg total).
➤ *Inhibition of platelet adhesion in patients with prosthetic heart valves, in combination with warfarin or aspirin.* Adults: 75 to 100 mg P.O. q.i.d.
➤ *Chronic angina pectoris.* Adults: 50 mg P.O. t.i.d. at least 1 hour before meals; 2 to 3

months of therapy may be required to achieve a clinical response.

➤*Prevention of thromboembolic complications in patients with various thromboembolic disorders other than prosthetic heart valves◇. Adults:* 150 to 400 mg P.O. daily (with warfarin or aspirin).

How supplied
Available by prescription only
Injection: 10 mg/2 ml
Tablets: 25 mg, 50 mg, 75 mg

Pharmacodynamics
Coronary vasodilating action: Dipyridamole increases coronary blood flow by selectively dilating the coronary arteries. Coronary vasodilator effect follows inhibition of serum adenosine deaminase, which allows accumulation of adenosine, a potent vasodilator. Dipyridamole inhibits platelet adhesion by increasing effects of prostacyclin or by inhibiting phosphodiesterase.

Pharmacokinetics
Absorption: Absorption is variable and slow; bioavailability ranges from 27% to 59%.
Distribution: Animal studies indicate wide distribution in body tissues; small amounts cross the placenta. Protein-binding ranges from 91% to 97%.
Metabolism: Metabolized by the liver.
Excretion: Elimination occurs via biliary excretion of glucuronide conjugates. Some dipyridamole and conjugates may undergo enterohepatic circulation and fecal excretion; a small amount is excreted in urine. Half-life varies from 1 to 12 hours.

Route	Onset	Peak	Duration
P.O.	Unknown	75 min	Unknown

Contraindications and precautions
No known contraindications. Use cautiously in patients with hypotension.

Interactions
Drug-drug. *Aminophylline:* Inhibits dipyridamole action. Avoid use together.
Heparin, oral anticoagulants: Enhance anticoagulant effects. Monitor patient closely.

Adverse reactions
CNS: *headache, dizziness.*
CV: flushing, fainting, *hypotension;* angina, chest pain, *blood pressure lability, hypertension* (with I.V. infusion).
GI: *nausea,* vomiting, diarrhea, abdominal distress.
Hematologic: increased bleeding time.
Skin: rash, irritation (with undiluted injection), pruritus.

Overdose and treatment
Effects of overdose include peripheral vasodilation and hypotension. Maintain blood pressure and treat symptomatically.

Special considerations
● Give drug at least 1 hour before meals.
● When used as a pharmacologic stress test, total doses beyond 60 mg appear to be unnecessary.
● Dilute I.V. form to at least a 1:2 ratio with 0.45% saline injection, normal saline injection, or D_5W to a total volume of 20 to 50 ml. Inject thallium within 5 minutes of dipyridamole.

Patient monitoring
● Monitor blood pressure.
● Be alert for adverse reactions, including signs of bleeding and prolonged bleeding time, especially at high doses and during long-term therapy.

Breast-feeding patients
● Safety in breast-feeding women hasn't been established.

Pediatric patients
● Dosage hasn't been established in children.

Patient education
● Explain that clinical response may require 2 to 3 months of continuous therapy; encourage patient compliance.
● Discuss adverse reactions and how to manage therapy.

---

dirithromycin
Dynabac

Pharmacologic classification: macrolide
Therapeutic classification: antibiotic
Pregnancy risk category: C

Indications and dosages
➤*Acute bacterial exacerbations of chronic bronchitis caused by* Moraxella catarrhalis *or* Streptococcus pneumoniae; *secondary bacterial infection of acute bronchitis caused by* M. catarrhalis *or* S. pneumoniae; *uncomplicated skin and skin structure infections caused by* Staphylococcus aureus *(methicillin susceptible). Adults and children age 12 and older:* 500 mg P.O. daily with food for 7 days.
➤*Community-acquired pneumonia caused by* Legionella pneumophila, Mycoplasma pneumoniae, *or* S. pneumoniae. *Adults and children age 12 and older:* 500 mg P.O. daily with food for 14 days.
➤*Pharyngitis or tonsillitis caused by* Streptococcus pyogenes. *Adults and children age 12 and older:* 500 mg P.O. daily with food for 10 days.

How supplied
Available by prescription only
Tablets: 250 mg

Pharmacodynamics
Antibiotic action: Dirithromycin inhibits bacterial RNA-dependent protein synthesis by binding to the 50S subunit of the ribosome. Its spectrum of activity includes gram-positive aerobes such as *S. aureus* (methicillin-susceptible strains only), *S. pneumoniae, S. pyogenes;* gram-negative aerobes such as *L. pneumophila* and *M. catarrhalis;* and other bacteria such as *M. pneumoniae.*

Pharmacokinetics
Absorption: Rapidly absorbed from GI tract and converted by nonenzymatic hydrolysis to the microbiologically active compound erythromycylamine. Food slightly increases bioavailability of drug.
Distribution: Widely distributed throughout the body. The protein-binding of erythromycylamine ranges from 15% to 30%.
Metabolism: Undergoes little to no hepatic metabolism.
Excretion: Primarily eliminated in bile or feces with a small amount in urine. Mean half-life of erythromycylamine is about 8 hours.

Route	Onset	Peak	Duration
P.O.	Unknown	4 hr	Unknown

Contraindications and precautions
Contraindicated in patients hypersensitive to dirithromycin, erythromycin, or other macrolide antibiotics.

Use cautiously in patients with hepatic insufficiency and in pregnant women.

Interactions
Drug-drug. *Alfentanil, anticoagulants, bromocriptine, carbamazepine, cyclosporine, digoxin, disopyramide, ergotamine, hexobarbital, lovastatin, phenytoin, triazolam, valproate:* These drugs interact with erythromycin products; it isn't known whether these same drug interactions occur with dirithromycin. Use caution during coadministration.
Antacids, H₂-receptor antagonists: Absorption may be slightly enhanced when dirithromycin is administered immediately after these drugs.
Theophylline: Dirithromycin may alter steady state plasma level of theophylline. Monitor theophylline plasma levels. Dosage adjustments may be needed.
Drug-food. *Any food:* Increases absorption; administer drug with food.

Adverse reactions
CNS: headache, dizziness, vertigo, insomnia, asthenia.
GI: abdominal pain, nausea, diarrhea, vomiting, dyspepsia, GI disorder, flatulence.
Hematologic: increased platelet, eosinophil, and neutrophil counts.
Metabolic: hyperkalemia, decreased bicarbonate levels, increased CK levels.
Respiratory: increased cough, dyspnea.
Skin: rash, pruritus, urticaria.
Other: pain (nonspecific).

Overdose and treatment
Signs and symptoms of a macrolide antibiotic overdose may include nausea, vomiting, epigastric distress, and diarrhea.

Treatment should be supportive because forced diuresis, dialysis, and hemoperfusion haven't been established to be helpful for an overdose of dirithromycin.

Special considerations
● Obtain culture and sensitivity tests before starting treatment. Therapy may begin pending results.
● Don't use drug in patients with known, suspected, or potential bacteremias because serum levels are inadequate to provide antibacterial coverage of the bloodstream.

Patient monitoring
● Monitor patient for superinfection. Drug may cause overgrowth of nonsusceptible bacteria or fungi.

Breast-feeding patients
● It isn't known whether dirithromycin appears in breast milk; administer cautiously to breast-feeding women.

Pediatric patients
● Safety and effectiveness in children under age 12 haven't been established.

Patient education
● Tell patient to take all of drug as prescribed, even after he feels better.
● Instruct patient to take drug with food or within 1 hour of having eaten. Tell him not to cut, chew, or crush the tablet.

disopyramide phosphate
Norpace, Norpace CR, Rythmodan*, Rythmodan-LA*

Pharmacologic classification: pyridine derivative antiarrhythmic, group IA antiarrhythmic
Therapeutic classification: ventricular antiarrhythmic, supraventricular antiarrhythmic, atrial antitachyarrhythmic
Pregnancy risk category: C

Indications and dosages
➤ *PVCs (unifocal, multifocal, or coupled); ventricular tachycardia; conversion of atrial fibrillation, atrial flutter, and paroxysmal atrial tachycardia to normal sinus rhythm. Adults:* Initially, 200 to 300 mg

loading dose. Usual maintenance dosage is 150 mg P.O. q 6 hours or 300 mg (extended-release) P.O. q 12 hours. If patient weighs less than 50 kg (110 lb), give 100 mg P.O. q 6 hours or 200 mg (extended-release) P.O. q 12 hours. For patients with cardiomyopathy or possible cardiac decompensation, give 100 mg P.O. q 6 to 8 hours initially and then adjust as indicated.

Children ages 12 to 18: 6 to 15 mg/kg P.O. daily.
Children ages 4 to 12: 10 to 15 mg/kg P.O. daily.
Children ages 1 to 4: 10 to 20 mg/kg P.O. daily.
Children younger than 1: 10 to 30 mg/kg P.O. daily.

All children's doses should be divided equally and given q 6 hours. Extended-release capsules not recommended for use in children.

✦ *Dosage adjustment.* Geriatric patients may need dosage reduction. Adults with hepatic insufficiency or moderately impaired renal function should receive 100 mg P.O. q 6 hours or 200 mg (extended-release) q 12 hours. Patients with severely impaired renal function should receive only 100 mg (regular-release) at the following intervals.

Creatinine clearance (ml/min)	Dosage interval
30-40	q 8 hr
15-30	q 12 hr
< 15	q 24 hr

How supplied
Available by prescription only
Capsules: 100 mg, 150 mg
Capsules (extended-release): 100 mg, 150 mg

Pharmacodynamics
Antiarrhythmic action: A class IA antiarrhythmic agent, disopyramide depresses phase 0 of the action potential. It's considered a myocardial depressant because it decreases myocardial excitability and conduction velocity and may depress myocardial contractility. It also possesses anticholinergic activity that may modify the direct myocardial effects of the drug. In therapeutic doses, disopyramide reduces conduction velocity in the atria, ventricles, and His-Purkinje system. By prolonging the effective refractory period, it helps control atrial tachyarrhythmias (however, this indication is unapproved in the United States). Its anticholinergic action, which is much greater than quinidine's, may increase AV node conductivity.

Disopyramide also has a greater myocardial depressant (negative inotropic) effect than quinidine. It helps manage premature ventricular beats by suppressing automaticity in the His-Purkinje system and ectopic pacemakers. At therapeutic doses, it usually doesn't prolong the QRS segment duration and PR interval but may prolong the QT interval.

Pharmacokinetics
Absorption: Rapidly and well absorbed from the GI tract; about 60% to 80% of drug reaches systemic circulation.

Distribution: Well distributed throughout extracellular fluid but isn't extensively bound to tissues. Plasma protein–binding varies, depending on drug levels, but generally ranges from about 50% to 65%. Usual therapeutic serum level ranges from 2 to 4 mcg/ml, although some patients may require up to 7 mcg/ml. Levels above 9 mcg/ml generally are considered toxic.

Metabolism: Metabolized in the liver to one major metabolite that possesses little antiarrhythmic activity but greater anticholinergic activity than the parent compound.

Excretion: About 90% of an orally administered dose is excreted in the urine as unchanged drug and metabolites; 40% to 60% is excreted as unchanged drug. Usual elimination half-life is about 7 hours but lengthens in patients with renal or hepatic insufficiency. Duration of effect is usually 6 to 7 hours.

Route	Onset	Peak	Duration
P.O.	½-3½ hr	2-2½ hr	1½-8½ hr

Contraindications and precautions
Contraindicated in patients hypersensitive to drug and in those with cardiogenic shock or second- or third-degree heart block in the absence of an artificial pacemaker.

Use very cautiously and, if possible, avoid in patients with heart failure. Use cautiously in patients with underlying conduction abnormalities, urinary tract diseases (especially prostatic hyperplasia), hepatic or renal impairment, myasthenia gravis, or acute angle-closure glaucoma.

Interactions
Drug-drug. *Antiarrhythmics:* May cause additive or antagonistic cardiac effects and additive toxicity. Monitor patient closely.
Anticholinergics: May cause additive anticholinergic effects. Monitor patient closely.
Erythromycin: Increased disopyramide levels, causing arrhythmias and increased QT intervals. Avoid use together.
Insulin, oral antidiabetics: Additive hypoglycemia. Monitor blood glucose levels.
Rifampin: May impair antiarrhythmic activity of disopyramide. Monitor patient closely.
Warfarin: May potentiate anticoagulant effects. Monitor PT and INR closely.
Drug-herb. *Jimson weed:* May adversely affect the function of the CV system. Tell patient to avoid use together.

Adverse reactions
CNS: dizziness, agitation, depression, fatigue, muscle weakness, syncope.
CV: *hypotension, **heart failure, heart block,** edema, **arrhythmias,** chest pain.*
EENT: *blurred vision, dry eyes or nose.*

GI: nausea, vomiting, anorexia, bloating, abdominal pain, diarrhea.
Hepatic: cholestatic jaundice.
Metabolic: weight gain.
Musculoskeletal: aches, pain, muscle weakness.
Respiratory: shortness of breath.
Skin: rash, pruritus, dermatosis.

Overdose and treatment

Signs and symptoms of overdose include anticholinergic effects, severe hypotension, widening of QRS complex and QT interval, ventricular arrhythmias, cardiac conduction disturbances, bradycardia, heart failure, asystole, loss of consciousness, seizures, apnea episodes, and respiratory arrest.

Treatment involves general supportive measures (including respiratory and CV support) and hemodynamic and ECG monitoring. If ingestion was recent, gastric lavage, emesis induction, and administration of activated charcoal may decrease absorption. Isoproterenol or dopamine may be administered to correct hypotension after adequate hydration has been ensured. Digoxin and diuretics may be administered to treat heart failure. Hemodialysis and charcoal hemoperfusion may effectively remove disopyramide. Some patients may require intra-aortic balloon counterpulsation, mechanically assisted respiration, or endocardial pacing.

Special considerations

⚠ ALERT Patients with atrial flutter or fibrillation should be digitalized before disopyramide administration to ensure that enhanced AV conduction doesn't lead to ventricular tachycardia.
• Correct underlying electrolyte abnormalities, especially hypokalemia, before administering drug because disopyramide may be ineffective in patients with these problems.
• Don't give sustained-release capsules for rapid control of ventricular arrhythmias if therapeutic blood drug levels must be attained rapidly, or if patient has cardiomyopathy, possible cardiac decompensation, or severe renal impairment.
• If drug causes constipation, administer laxatives and ensure proper diet.
• Drug is commonly prescribed for patients who can't tolerate quinidine or procainamide.
• Pharmacist may prepare disopyramide suspension; 100-mg capsules are used with cherry syrup to prepare suspension (this may be best form for young children).
• Drug is removed by hemodialysis. Dosage adjustments may be necessary in patients undergoing dialysis.

Patient monitoring

• Patient must be monitored for signs of developing heart block, such as QRS complex widening by more than 25% or QT interval lengthening by more than 25% above baseline.

Breast-feeding patients

• Drug appears in breast milk; recommend alternative infant feeding methods during drug therapy.

Pediatric patients

• Although safety and effectiveness of drug in children haven't been established, current recommendations call for total daily dose given in equally divided doses every 6 hours or at intervals based on individual requirements. Monitor children during initial adjustment period; dose adjustment should begin at lower end of recommended ranges. Monitor serum drug levels and therapeutic response carefully.

Geriatric patients

• Monitor patient closely for signs of toxicity.
• Monitor serum electrolyte and drug levels.

Patient education

• When changing from immediate-release to sustained-release capsules, advise patient to begin taking sustained-release capsule 6 hours after last immediate-release capsule.
• Teach patient importance of taking drug on time, exactly as prescribed. To do this, he may have to use an alarm clock for night doses.
• Advise patient to use sugarless gum or hard candy to relieve dry mouth.

---

disulfiram
Antabuse

Pharmacologic classification: aldehyde dehydrogenase inhibitor
Therapeutic classification: alcoholic deterrent
Pregnancy risk category: C

Indications and dosages

➤ **Adjunct in management of chronic alcoholism.** *Adults:* Give maximum dose of 500 mg P.O. as a single dose in the morning for 1 to 2 weeks. Can be taken in evening if drowsiness occurs. Maintenance dosage is 125 to 500 mg daily (average dose 250 mg) until permanent self-control is established. Treatment may continue for months or years.

How supplied

Available by prescription only
Tablets: 250 mg, 500 mg

Pharmacodynamics

Antialcoholic action: Disulfiram irreversibly inhibits aldehyde dehydrogenase, which prevents the oxidation of alcohol after the acetaldehyde stage. It interacts with ingested alcohol to produce acetaldehyde levels five to ten times higher than are produced by normal alcohol metabolism. Excess acetaldehyde produces a highly unpleasant reaction (nausea and vomiting) to even a small quantity of alcohol. Tolerance to disulfiram doesn't occur; rather, sensitivity to alcohol increases with longer duration of therapy.

Pharmacokinetics

Absorption: Absorbed completely after oral administration, but 3 to 12 hours may be required before effects occur.

Distribution: Highly lipid-soluble and initially localized in adipose tissue.

Metabolism: Mostly oxidized in the liver and excreted in urine as free drug and metabolites (for example, diethyldithiocarbamate, diethylamine, and carbon disulfide).

Excretion: 5% to 20% is unabsorbed and eliminated in feces. A small amount is eliminated through the lungs, but most is excreted in urine. Several days may be needed to eliminate drug entirely.

Route	Onset	Peak	Duration
P.O.	1-2 hr	Unknown	14 days

Contraindications and precautions

Contraindicated in patients intoxicated by alcohol and within 12 hours of alcohol ingestion; in those with psychoses, myocardial disease, coronary occlusion, or hypersensitivity to disulfiram or to other thiuram derivatives used in pesticides and rubber vulcanization; and in patients receiving metronidazole, paraldehyde, alcohol, or alcohol-containing preparations.

Use with extreme caution in patients with diabetes mellitus, hypothyroidism, seizure disorder, cerebral damage, or nephritis or hepatic cirrhosis or insufficiency and with concurrent phenytoin therapy. Drug shouldn't be administered during pregnancy.

Interactions

Drug-drug. *Bacampicillin:* May precipitate disulfiram reaction. Don't use together.

Barbiturates, chlordiazepoxide, CNS depressants, coumarin anticoagulants, diazepam, midazolam, paraldehyde, phenytoin: Increased blood levels of these drugs. Use together cautiously.

Isoniazid: Increased risk of ataxia, unsteady gait, or marked behavioral changes. Don't use together.

Metronidazole: Increased risk of psychosis or confusion. Avoid use together.

Tricyclic antidepressants, especially amitriptyline: May cause transient delirium. Monitor patient closely.

Drug-herb. *Passion flower, pill-bearing spurge, squaw vine, squill, sundew, sweet flag, tormentil, valerian, yarrow, pokeweed:* Disulfiram reaction if herbal form contains alcohol. Discourage use together.

Drug-food. *Caffeine:* Exaggerated or prolonged effects of caffeine may occur. Advise patient to avoid caffeine.

Drug-lifestyle. *Alcohol use (all sources, including cough syrups, liniments, shaving lotions, back-rub preparations):* May precipitate

disulfiram reaction. Alcohol reaction may occur as long as 2 weeks after single disulfiram dose; the longer patient remains on drug, the more sensitive he becomes to alcohol. Advise patient to be alert for and avoid use of these products.

Marijuana use: Synergistic CNS stimulation when used with marijuana. Advise patient to avoid use.

Adverse reactions

CNS: drowsiness, headache, fatigue, delirium, depression, neuritis, peripheral neuritis, polyneuritis, restlessness, psychotic reactions.

EENT: optic neuritis.

GI: metallic or garlic aftertaste.

GU: impotence.

Metabolic: elevated serum cholesterol levels.

Skin: acneiform or allergic dermatitis, occasional eruptions.

Other: *disulfiram reaction* (precipitated by alcohol use), which may include flushing, throbbing headache, dyspnea, nausea, copious vomiting, diaphoresis, thirst, chest pain, palpitations, hyperventilation, hypotension, syncope, anxiety, weakness, blurred vision, confusion, arthropathy. In severe reactions: respiratory depression, CV collapse, arrhythmias, MI, acute heart failure, seizures, unconsciousness, or death.

Overdose and treatment

Overdose may cause GI upset, vomiting, abnormal EEG findings, drowsiness, altered consciousness, hallucinations, speech impairment, incoordination, and coma.

Treat overdose by gastric aspiration or lavage along with supportive therapy.

Treatment of alcohol-induced disulfiram reaction is supportive and symptomatic. These reactions aren't usually life-threatening. Emergency equipment and drugs should be available because arrhythmias and severe hypotension may occur. Treat severe reactions like shock by giving plasma or electrolyte solutions, as needed. Large I.V. doses of ascorbic acid, iron, and antihistamines have been used but are of questionable value. Hypokalemia has been reported; it requires careful monitoring and potassium supplements.

Special considerations

⚠ ALERT Caution patient's family that disulfiram should never be given to the patient without his knowledge; severe reaction or death could result if patient ingests alcohol.

- Disulfiram shouldn't be given for at least 12 hours after alcohol ingestion.
- Drug use requires close medical supervision. Patients should clearly understand consequences of disulfiram therapy and give informed consent before use.
- Use drug only in patients who are cooperative and well motivated, and who are receiving supportive psychiatric therapy.

Patient monitoring
● Complete physical examination and laboratory studies (CBC, electrolytes, transaminases) should precede therapy and be repeated regularly.

Pregnant patients
● Drug shouldn't be administered during pregnancy.

Patient education
● Explain that although disulfiram can help discourage use of alcohol, it isn't a cure for alcoholism.
● Warn patient to avoid all sources of alcohol: sauces or soups made with sherry or other wines or alcohol (even "cooking alcohol"), some herbal preparations, and cough syrups. External applications of after-shave lotion, liniments, or other topical preparations may cause disulfiram reaction (because of the products' alcohol content).
● Warn patient that drug may cause drowsiness.
● Instruct patient to carry identification card stating that disulfiram is being used and including the telephone number of the prescriber or clinic to contact if a reaction occurs.

dobutamine hydrochloride
Dobutrex

Pharmacologic classification: adrenergic, beta$_1$ agonist
Therapeutic classification: inotropic
Pregnancy risk category: B

Indications and dosages
➤ *To increase cardiac output in short-term treatment of cardiac decompensation caused by depressed contractility.*
Adults: 2 to 20 mcg/kg/minute as an I.V. infusion. Rarely, infusion rates up to 40 mcg/kg/minute may be needed. Adjust dosage carefully to patient response.
✦ *Dosage adjustment.* Geriatric patients require lower doses because they may be more sensitive to the effects of the drug.

How supplied
Available by prescription only
Injection: 12.5 mg/ml in 20-ml vials (parenteral)
Premixed: 0.5 mg/ml (125 or 250 mg) in D$_5$W; 1 mg/ml (250 or 500 mg) in D$_5$W; 2 mg/ml (500 mg) in D$_5$W; 4 mg/ml (1,000 mg) in D$_5$W

Pharmacodynamics
Inotropic action: Dobutamine selectively stimulates beta$_1$-adrenergic receptors to increase myocardial contractility and stroke volume, resulting in increased cardiac output (a positive inotropic effect in patients with normal hearts or in heart failure). At therapeutic doses, dobutamine decreases peripheral resistance (afterload), reduces ventricular filling pressure (preload), and may facilitate AV node conduction. Systolic

blood pressure and pulse pressure may remain unchanged or increased from increased cardiac output. Increased myocardial contractility results in increased coronary blood flow and myocardial oxygen consumption. Heart rate usually remains unchanged; however, excessive doses do have chronotropic effects. Dobutamine doesn't appear to affect dopaminergic receptors, nor does it cause renal or mesenteric vasodilation; however, urine flow may increase because of increased cardiac output.

Pharmacokinetics
Absorption: Administered I.V.
Distribution: Widely distributed throughout the body.
Metabolism: Metabolized by the liver and by conjugation to inactive metabolites.
Excretion: Excreted mainly in urine, with minor amounts in feces, as its metabolites and conjugates.

Route	Onset	Peak	Duration
I.V.	1-2 min	10 min	<5 min after infusion ends

Contraindications and precautions
Contraindicated in patients hypersensitive to drug or its formulation and in those with idiopathic hypertrophic subaortic stenosis. Use cautiously in patients with a history of hypertension or after recent MI. Drug may precipitate an exaggerated pressor response.

Interactions
Drug-drug. *Beta blockers:* May antagonize the cardiac effects of dobutamine. Don't use together.
Bretylium: May potentiate actions of vasopressors on adrenergic receptors. Monitor patient closely for arrhythmias.
Guanadrel, guanethidine: May potentiate the pressor effects of dobutamine, possibly resulting in hypertension and cardiac arrhythmias. Monitor patient closely.
Inhaled hydrocarbon anesthetics: May trigger ventricular arrhythmias. Provide careful ECG monitoring.
Nitroprusside: May increase cardiac output and decrease pulmonary wedge pressure. Monitor patient closely.
Rauwolfia alkaloids: May prolong dobutamine action (a denervation supersensitivity response). Monitor patient closely.
Tricyclic antidepressants: May potentiate pressor response. Use cautiously.
Drug-herb. *Rue:* May increase inotropic potential. Tell patient to use cautiously.

Adverse reactions
CNS: headache.
CV: *increased heart rate,* **hypertension, PVCs,** angina, nonspecific chest pain, palpitations, hypotension.

GI: nausea, vomiting.
Respiratory: shortness of breath, *asthmatic episodes.*
Other: phlebitis, *hypersensitivity reactions (anaphylaxis).*

Overdose and treatment
Signs and symptoms of overdose include nervousness and fatigue. No treatment is necessary beyond dosage reduction or withdrawal of drug.

Special considerations
Consider the recommendations relevant to all adrenergics as well as the following.

◪ ALERT Dobutamine is incompatible with alkaline solution (sodium bicarbonate). Also, don't mix with or give through same I.V. line as heparin, hydrocortisone, cefazolin, or penicillin.
● Before administration of dobutamine, correct hypovolemia with appropriate plasma volume expanders.
● Before giving dobutamine, administer a cardiac glycoside if patient has atrial fibrillation (dobutamine increases AV conduction).
● Adjust dose to meet individual needs and achieve desired clinical response. Drug must be administered by I.V. infusion using an infusion pump or other device to control flow rate.
● Concentration of infusion solution shouldn't exceed 5,000 mcg/ml; use the solution within 24 hours. Rate and duration of infusion depend on patient response.

Patient monitoring
● Monitor ECG, blood pressure, cardiac output, and pulmonary wedge pressure. Monitor serum electrolytes, especially potassium.
● Most patients experience an increase of 10 to 20 mm Hg in systolic blood pressure; some show an increase of 50 mm Hg or more. Most also experience an increase in heart rate of 5 to 15 beats/minute; some show increases of 30 or more beats/minute. Premature ventricular arrhythmias may also occur in about 5% of patients. Dosage reduction may be necessary when these occur.

Breast-feeding patients
● It isn't known whether dobutamine appears in breast milk. Administer cautiously to breast-feeding women.

Pediatric patients
● Increases cardiac output and systemic pressure in children. Use cautiously in children.

Geriatric patients
● Use cautiously in geriatric patients.

Patient education
● Advise patient to report adverse reactions, especially dyspnea and drug-induced headache.
● Instruct patient to report pain at I.V. site.

docetaxel
Taxotere

Pharmacologic classification: taxoid
Therapeutic classification: antineoplastic
Pregnancy risk category: D

Indications and dosages
➤ *Treatment of patients with locally advanced or metastatic breast cancer who have progressed during anthracycline-based therapy or have relapsed during anthracycline-based adjuvant therapy.*
Adults: 60 to 100 mg/m² I.V. over 1 hour q 3 weeks.
➤ *Non-small-cell lung carcinoma.* Monotherapy. *Adults:* 100 mg/m² I.V. over 1 hour q 3 weeks.
Combination therapy
Adults: 75 to 100 mg/m² I.V. over 1 hour q 3 weeks.

How supplied
Available by prescription only
Injection: 20 mg, 80 mg

Pharmacodynamics
Antineoplastic action: Docetaxel acts by disrupting the microtubular network in cells that's essential for mitotic and interphase cellular functions.

Pharmacokinetics
Absorption: Administered I.V.
Distribution: About 94% protein-bound.
Metabolism: Undergoes oxidative metabolism.
Excretion: Eliminated primarily in feces with a small amount eliminated in urine.

Route	Onset	Peak	Duration
I.V.	Rapid	Unknown	Unknown

Contraindications and precautions
Contraindicated in patients with history of severe hypersensitivity to drug or other drugs formulated with polysorbate 80. Don't give docetaxel to patients with neutrophil counts below 1,500 cells/mm³.

Interactions
Drug-drug. *Compounds that induce, inhibit, or are metabolized by cytochrome P-450 3A4, such as cyclosporine, erythromycin, ketoconazole, and troleandomycin:* Metabolism of docetaxel may be modified. Use together cautiously.

Adverse reactions
CNS: paresthesia, dysesthesia, pain (including burning sensation), weakness.
CV: flushing, fluid retention, hypotension, chest tightness.
GI: *stomatitis,* nausea, vomiting, diarrhea.

Reactions may be *common,* uncommon, *life-threatening,* or COMMON AND LIFE-THREATENING.

Hematologic: *anemia,* NEUTROPENIA, FEBRILE NEUTROPENIA, *myelosuppression* (dose-limiting), LEUKOPENIA, *thrombocytopenia.*
Hepatic: *increased liver function test results.*
Musculoskeletal: *myalgia,* arthralgia, back pain.
Respiratory: dyspnea.
Skin: *alopecia,* maculopapular eruptions, desquamation, nail pigmentation alteration, onycholysis, nail pain, rash.
Other: *hypersensitivity reactions, infections,* drug fever, chills.

Overdose and treatment
Signs and symptoms of overdose may include bone marrow suppression, peripheral neurotoxicity, and mucositis. There's no known antidote for docetaxel. Closely monitor patient's vital functions.

Special considerations
● Patients with bilirubin values above the upper limit of normal usually shouldn't receive docetaxel. Also, patients with ALT or AST levels more than 1.5 times the upper limit of normal and alkaline phosphatase levels more than 2.5 times the upper limit of normal usually shouldn't receive drug.
● Premedicate patient with oral corticosteroids such as dexamethasone 16 mg daily for 5 days starting 1 day before docetaxel administration, to reduce fluid retention and hypersensitivity reactions.
● Dilute docetaxel before administration using the diluent supplied with drug. Allow drug and diluent to stand at room temperature for about 5 minutes before mixing. After adding the entire contents of diluent to the vial of docetaxel, gently rotate the vial for about 15 seconds. Then allow solution to stand for a few minutes to allow any foam to dissipate.
● To prepare docetaxel infusion solution, aseptically withdraw the required amount of premix solution from the vial and inject into a 250-ml infusion bag or bottle of normal saline solution or D₅W solution to produce a final concentration of 0.3 to 0.9 mg/ml. Doses exceeding 240 mg require a larger volume of infusion solution so a concentration of 0.9 mg/ml of docetaxel isn't exceeded. Thoroughly mix the infusion by manual rotation.
● Use caution during preparation and administration of docetaxel. Use of gloves is recommended. If solution contacts skin, wash skin immediately and thoroughly with soap and water. If docetaxel contacts mucous membranes, flush membranes thoroughly with water. Mark all waste materials with CHEMOTHERAPY HAZARD labels.
● Contact of the undiluted concentrate with plasticized polyvinyl chloride equipment or devices used to prepare solutions for infusion isn't recommended. Prepare and store infusion solutions in bottles (glass, polypropylene) or plastic bags

(polypropylene, polyolefin) and administer through polyethylene-lined administration sets.

Patient monitoring
● Monitor patient closely for hypersensitivity reactions, especially during the first and second infusions. If minor reactions such as flushing or localized skin reactions occur, interruption of therapy isn't required. More severe reactions require the immediate discontinuation of docetaxel and aggressive treatment.
● Bone marrow toxicity is the most frequent and dose-limiting toxicity. Frequent blood count monitoring is necessary during therapy.
● Patients who initially receive 100 mg/m² and who experience febrile neutropenia, a neutrophil count less than 500 cells/mm³ for more than 1 week, severe or cumulative cutaneous reactions, or severe peripheral neuropathy during docetaxel therapy should have dosage adjusted from 100 to 75 mg/m². If the patient continues to experience these reactions, dosage should either be decreased from 75 to 55 mg/m² or the drug discontinued.
● Patients who initially receive 60 mg/m² and who don't experience febrile neutropenia, a neutrophil count less than 500 cells/mm³ for more than 1 week, severe or cumulative cutaneous reactions, or severe peripheral neuropathy during docetaxel therapy may tolerate higher doses.

Pregnant patients
● Advise patient of childbearing age to avoid becoming pregnant during therapy because of potential harm to fetus.

Breast-feeding patients
● Because of risk of serious adverse reactions in breast-fed infants, it's recommended that breast-feeding be discontinued during docetaxel therapy.

Pediatric patients
● Safety and effectiveness in children under age 16 haven't been established.

Patient education
● Explain that alopecia occurs in almost 80% of patients.
● Tell patient to promptly report a sore throat, fever, unusual bruising, or bleeding.

docosanol
Abreva

Pharmacologic classification: antiviral
Therapeutic classification: antiviral
Pregnancy risk category: B

Indications and dosages
➤ *Recurrent oral-facial herpes simplex.*
Adults and children age 12 and over: Applied topically five times daily starting with first indi-

cation of an episode and continuing until lesion is healed. Rub in gently but completely.

How supplied
Available without a prescription
Cream: 10%

Pharmacodynamics
The main mechanism of anti-herpes simplex virus activity appears to be inhibition of fusion between the cell's plasma membrane and the herpes simplex virus envelope, which blocks the entry and subsequent replication of the virus.

Pharmacokinetics
Absorption: Not absorbed.
Distribution: Not applicable.
Metabolism: Not applicable.
Excretion: Not applicable.

Route	Onset	Peak	Duration
Topical	Unknown	Unknown	Unknown

Adverse reactions
CNS: *headache.*
Skin: reaction at application site.

Interactions
None reported.

Overdose and treatment
Adverse reactions caused by overdose are unlikely because topical application leads to limited absorption and because absorption is poor following oral administration.

Contraindications and precautions
Contraindicated in patients hypersensitive to drug or any of its components.

Special considerations
• Use drug only to treat oral-facial herpes simplex.
• Start treatment as early as possible after symptoms start.
• Avoid application in or near patient's eyes.

Patient monitoring
• Monitor patient for drug effect, and continue treatment until lesion has healed.

Breast-feeding patients
• It isn't known whether docosanol appears in breast milk. Because many drugs do, use caution when giving this drug to a breast-feeding woman.

Pediatric patients
• Safety and efficacy in children under age 12 haven't been established.

Geriatric patients
• Adverse reactions in elderly patients seem similar in nature and frequency to those in younger patients.

Patient education
• Advise patient to start treatment as soon as symptoms appear.
• Tell patient to use cream only on lips or face.
• Caution patient not to apply drug in or near the eyes because it may cause irritation.
• Tell patient to continue treatment until the lesion has healed.
• Notify patient that lesions are considered contagious until completely healed.
• Urge patient to report worsening condition.
• Caution patient that drug should be used during pregnancy only if clearly needed.
• Advise patient to store drug at room temperature and not to freeze it.

docusate calcium
Pro-Cal-Sof, Surfak

docusate potassium
Dialose, Diocto-K, Kasof

docusate sodium
Colace, Diocto, Dioeze, Diosuccin, DOK, D.O.S., Doxinate, D-S-S, Duosol, Modane Soft, Pro-Sof, Regulax SS, Regulex*, Regutol

Pharmacologic classification: surfactant
Therapeutic classification: emollient laxative
Pregnancy risk category: C

Indications and dosages
➤ **Stool softener. docusate sodium.** *Adults and children age 12 and older:* 50 to 200 mg P.O. daily until bowel movements are normal. Alternatively, add 50 to 100 mg to saline or oil retention enema to treat fecal impaction.
Children ages 6 to 12: 40 to 120 mg P.O. daily.
Children ages 3 to 6: 20 to 60 mg P.O. daily.
Children under age 3: 10 to 40 mg P.O. daily.
docusate calcium or potassium
Adults: 240 mg (calcium) or 100 to 300 mg (potassium) P.O. daily until bowel movements are normal. Higher doses are for initial therapy. Adjust dose to individual response.
Children age 6 and older: 50 to 150 mg (calcium) or 100 mg (potassium) P.O. daily.

How supplied
Available without a prescription
Capsules: 50 mg, 100 mg, 240 mg, 250 mg
Solution: 10 mg/ml
Syrup: 16.7 mg/5 ml, 20 mg/5 ml
Tablets: 100 mg

Pharmacodynamics
Laxative action: Docusate salts act as detergents in the intestine, reducing surface tension of interfacing liquids; this promotes incorporation of fat and additional liquid, softening the stool.

Reactions may be *common*, uncommon, *life-threatening*, or COMMON AND LIFE-THREATENING.

Pharmacokinetics

Absorption: Absorbed minimally in the duodenum and jejunum.
Distribution: Distributed primarily locally, in the gut.
Metabolism: None.
Excretion: Excreted in feces.

Route	Onset	Peak	Duration
P.O.	24-72 hr	24-72 hr	24-72 hr

Contraindications and precautions

Contraindicated in patients hypersensitive to drug and in those with intestinal obstruction, undiagnosed abdominal pain, vomiting or other signs of appendicitis, fecal impaction, or acute surgical abdomen.

Interactions

Drug-drug. *Mineral oil:* Docusate salts may increase absorption of mineral oil and cause toxicity. Separate administration times.

Adverse reactions

GI: bitter taste, mild abdominal cramping, diarrhea, laxative dependence.

Overdose and treatment

No information available.

Special considerations

● Liquid or syrup must be given in 6 to 8 oz (180 to 240 ml) of milk or fruit juice or in infant's formula to prevent throat irritation.
● Avoid using docusate sodium in sodium-restricted patients.
● Docusate salts are available with casanthranol (Peri-Colace), senna (Senokot, Gentlax), and phenolphthalein (Ex-Lax, Feen-a-Mint, Correctol).
● Docusate salts are the preferred laxative for most patients who must avoid straining at stool, such as those recovering from MI or rectal surgery. Docusate salts also are used commonly to treat patients with postpartum constipation.

Patient monitoring

● Before giving for constipation, determine whether patient has adequate fluid intake, exercise, and diet.
● Discontinue drug if severe cramping occurs.

Breast-feeding patients

● Because absorption of docusate salts is minimal, they presumably pose no risk to breast-feeding infants.

Geriatric patients

● Docusate salts are good choices for geriatric patients because they rarely cause laxative dependence, cause fewer adverse effects, and are gentler than some other laxatives.

Patient education

● Docusate salts lose their effectiveness over time; advise patient to report failure of medication.
● Teach patient about dietary sources of bulk, which include bran and other cereals, fresh fruit, and vegetables.

---

dofetilide
Tikosyn

Pharmacologic classification: antiarrhythmic
Therapeutic classification: class III antiarrhythmic
Pregnancy risk category: C

Indications and dosages

➤ *Maintenance of normal sinus rhythm in patients with symptomatic atrial fibrillation or atrial flutter for more than 1 week; conversion of atrial fibrillation and atrial flutter to normal sinus rhythm.*
Adults: Dosage is individualized and based on creatinine clearance and QT interval, which must be determined before first dose. Usual recommended dose is 500 mcg P.O. b.i.d. for patients with creatinine clearance greater than 60 ml/minute.
✦ *Dosage adjustment.* Adjust dosage based on the following schedule.

Creatinine clearance (ml/min)	Starting dose
40-60	250 mcg P.O. b.i.d.
20-39	125 mcg P.O. b.i.d.

At 2 to 3 hours after first dose, determine QT interval. If it has increased by more than 15% over baseline, or if it's more than 500 msec (550 msec in patients with ventricular conduction abnormalities), adjust dosage as follows: If starting dose based on creatinine clearance was 500 mcg P.O. b.i.d., give 250 mcg P.O. b.i.d. If starting dose based on creatinine clearance was 250 mcg P.O. b.i.d., give 125 mcg P.O. b.i.d. If starting dose based on creatinine clearance was 125 mcg P.O. b.i.d., give 125 mcg P.O. once daily.
Determine QT interval 2 to 3 hours after each subsequent dose while patient is hospitalized. If at any time after second dose QT interval is more than 500 msec (550 msec in patients with ventricular conduction abnormalities), stop drug.

How supplied

Available by prescription only
Capsules: 125 mcg (0.125 mg), 250 mcg (0.25 mg), 500 mcg (0.5 mg)

Pharmacodynamics

Antiarrhythmic action: Prolongs repolarization without affecting conduction velocity by block-

---

◇ Unlabeled clinical use

ing the cardiac ion channel carrying potassium current. No effect is seen on sodium channels, alpha-adrenergic receptors, or beta-adrenergic receptors.

Pharmacokinetics
Absorption: Bioavailability after oral administration is greater than 90% with plasma levels peaking in 2 to 3 hours. Steady state plasma levels are achieved in 2 to 3 days. Absorption unaffected by food or antacid.
Distribution: Widely distributed throughout body; has a distribution volume of 3 L/kg. Plasma protein–binding is 60% to 70%.
Metabolism: Metabolized to a small extent by CYP3A4 isoenzyme of cytochrome P-450 system of the liver.
Excretion: About 80% is excreted in urine, of which 80% is excreted as unchanged drug with remaining 20% as inactive or minimally active metabolites.

Route	Onset	Peak	Duration
P.O.	Unknown	2-3 hr	Unknown

Contraindications and precautions
Contraindicated in patients with creatinine clearance less than 20 ml/minute and in those with congenital or acquired long QT interval syndrome. Don't use drug in patients with baseline QT interval greater than 440 msec (500 msec in patients with ventricular conduction abnormalities). Use cautiously in patients with severe hepatic impairment.

Drug is distributed only to hospitals and other institutions confirmed to have received applicable dosing and treatment initiation programs. Such confirmation is also needed for inpatient and subsequent outpatient discharge and refill prescriptions.

Interactions
Drug-drug. *Amiloride, amiodarone, diltiazem, macrolide antibiotics, metformin, nefazodone, norfloxacin, protease inhibitors, quinine, serotonin reuptake inhibitors, triamterene, zafirlukast:* Possible increased plasma dofetilide levels. Use together cautiously.
Class I, Class III antiarrhythmics: Effect hasn't been studied; concomitant use not recommended. Hold antiarrhythmics for at least three half-lives before giving dofetilide.
Drugs that inhibit renal cation transport system (cimetidine, ketoconazole, megestrol, prochlorperazine, sulfamethoxazole, trimethoprim), verapamil: Decreased dofetilide metabolism and excretion and increased plasma levels. Don't use together.
Drugs that prolong QT interval (bepridil, oral macrolides, phenothiazines, tricyclic antidepressants): May enhance QT interval prolongation. Don't use concomitantly.
Potassium-wasting diuretics: Increased risk of torsades de pointes. Maintain potassium levels

within normal range before and throughout drug therapy.
Drug-food. *Grapefruit juice:* Possible decreased hepatic metabolism and increased plasma levels. Tell patient not to use together.

Adverse reactions
CNS: *headache,* dizziness, syncope, paresthesia, insomnia, anxiety, migraine, cerebral ischemia, facial paralysis, ***CVA.***
CV: ***ventricular fibrillation, ventricular tachycardia, torsades de pointes, AV block,*** chest pain, ***bradycardia,*** edema, ***cardiac arrest, sudden death, MI.***
GI: nausea, diarrhea, abdominal pain.
GU: urinary tract infection.
Hepatic: liver damage.
Musculoskeletal: back pain, arthralgia, flaccid paralysis.
Respiratory: respiratory tract infection, dyspnea, increased cough.
Skin: rash.
Other: flulike syndrome, accidental injury, ***angioedema.***

Overdose and treatment
The most likely effect of overdose is excessive prolongation of the QT interval. There's no known antidote. Treatment is symptomatic and supportive. Start cardiac monitoring. Charcoal slurry may be given and is useful especially within first 15 minutes after administration. Treatment of torsades de pointes or overdose may include isoproterenol, with or without cardiac pacing. Magnesium sulfate also may be effective.

Special considerations
• Patients in atrial fibrillation should be anticoagulated according to usual practice before electrical or pharmacologic cardioversion. Anticoagulation therapy may be continued after cardioversion according to usual medical practice.
🚩 ALERT For at least 3 days, patient must be in a facility equipped with ECG monitoring and a staff trained in managing ventricular arrhythmias.
• If a dose is missed, patient shouldn't double next dose. Instead, patient should skip that dose and wait until the next administration time for regularly scheduled dose.

Patient monitoring
• Monitor patient for prolonged diarrhea, sweating, or vomiting. These symptoms may indicate an electrolyte imbalance that may increase potential for arrhythmia.
• Monitor renal function routinely (at least every 3 months) and creatinine clearance.
• Withhold Class I or III antiarrhythmics for at least 3 half-lives before starting drug.

Breast-feeding patients
• Because there's no information on dofetilide use in breast-feeding mothers, advise women not to breast-feed while taking drug.

Reactions may be *common,* uncommon, ***life-threatening***, or COMMON AND LIFE-THREATENING.

Pediatric patients
• Safety and effectiveness in patients under age 18 haven't been established.

Geriatric patients
• There's no change in elimination based on age when dosage is adjusted for renal function.

Patient education
• Urge patient to report any change in OTC, prescription, or supplement/herb use.
• Tell patient not to use OTC Tagamet-HB for ulcers or heartburn. Antacids, Zantac 75 mg, and other acid-reduction drugs, such as Pepcid, Prilosec, Axid, and Prevacid, can be used.
• Inform patient that dofetilide can be taken without regard to meals or antacid administration.
• Inform patient that grapefruit juice can decrease metabolism of drug and lead to toxicity.
• Instruct woman to call if she becomes pregnant.
• Advise woman not to breast-feed while taking drug.

---

dolasetron mesylate
Anzemet

Pharmacologic classification: selective serotonin (5-HT$_3$) receptor antagonist
Therapeutic classification: antinauseant, antiemetic
Pregnancy risk category: B

Indications and dosages
➤**Prevention of nausea and vomiting caused by chemotherapy.** *Adults:* 100 mg P.O. as a single dose 1 hour before chemotherapy. Or, 1.8 mg/kg as a single I.V. dose 30 minutes before chemotherapy. Or, a fixed dose of 100 mg I.V. 30 minutes before chemotherapy.
Children ages 2 to 16: 1.8 mg/kg P.O. 1 hour before chemotherapy. Or, 1.8 mg/kg as a single I.V. dose 30 minutes before chemotherapy. Injectable form can be mixed with apple and apple-grape juice and administered P.O. 1 hour before chemotherapy. Maximum daily dose is 100 mg.
➤**Prevention of postoperative nausea and vomiting.** *Adults:* 100 mg P.O. within 2 hours before surgery; 12.5 mg as a single I.V. dose about 15 minutes before anesthesia stops.
Children ages 2 to 16: 1.2 mg/kg P.O. given within 2 hours before surgery, to maximum of 100 mg. Or, 0.35 mg/kg (up to 12.5 mg) as a single I.V. dose about 15 minutes before anesthesia stops. Injectable form (1.2 mg/kg up to 100-mg dose) can be mixed with apple and apple-grape juice and administered P.O. 2 hours before surgery.
➤**Treatment of postoperative nausea and vomiting. I.V. form.** *Adults:* 12.5 mg as a single I.V. dose as soon as nausea or vomiting occurs.

Children ages 2 to 16: 0.35 mg/kg, to maximum dose of 12.5 mg, as a single I.V. dose as soon as nausea or vomiting occurs.

How supplied
Available by prescription only
Injection: 20 mg/ml as 12.5 mg/0.625-ml ampules or 100 mg/5-ml vials
Tablets: 50 mg, 100 mg

Pharmacodynamics
Antinauseant and antiemetic actions: A selective serotonin (5-HT$_3$) receptor antagonist that blocks the action of serotonin receptors located on the nerve terminals of the vagus nerve in the periphery and in the central chemoreceptor trigger zone. By doing so, drug prevents serotonin from stimulating the vomiting reflex.

Pharmacokinetics
Absorption: Orally administered drug, injection, I.V. solution, and tablets are bioequivalent. Oral dolasetron is well absorbed, although parent drug is rarely detected in plasma because of rapid and complete metabolism to most clinically relevant metabolite, hydrodolasetron.
Distribution: Widely distributed in body, with mean apparent distribution volume of 5.8 L/kg; 69% to 77% of hydrodolasetron bound to plasma protein.
Metabolism: A ubiquitous enzyme, carbonyl reductase, mediates reduction to hydrodolasetron. Cytochrome P-450 (CYP) 2D6 and CYP3A are responsible for subsequent hydroxylation and N-oxidation of hydrodolasetron, respectively.
Excretion: Two-thirds of dose excreted in urine and one-third in feces. Mean elimination half-life is 8 hours.

Route	Onset	Peak	Duration
P.O.	Rapid	1 hr	8 hr
I.V.	Rapid	30 min	7 hr

Contraindications and precautions
Contraindicated in patients hypersensitive to drug. Use cautiously in patients with or at risk for prolonged cardiac conduction intervals, particularly QTc interval. These include patients taking antiarrhythmics or other drugs that prolong the QT interval; those with hypokalemia or hypomagnesemia; those at risk for electrolyte abnormalities, including those receiving diuretics; those with congenital QT syndrome; and those who have received cumulative high-dose anthracycline therapy.

Interactions
Drug-drug. *Antiarrhythmics:* Administration with drugs that prolong ECG intervals can increase risk of arrhythmias. Monitor patient closely.
Cimetidine: Drugs that inhibit P-450 enzymes can increase hydrodolasetron levels. Monitor patient for adverse effects.

◇ Unlabeled clinical use

Rifampin: Drugs that induce P-450 enzymes may decrease hydrodolasetron levels. Monitor patient for decreased antiemetic efficacy.

Adverse reactions
CNS: *headache,* dizziness, drowsiness, fatigue.
CV: *arrhythmias,* ECG changes, hypotension, hypertension, tachycardia, **bradycardia.**
GI: *diarrhea,* dyspepsia, abdominal pain, constipation, anorexia.
GU: oliguria, urine retention.
Hepatic: elevated liver function test results.
Skin: pruritus, rash.
Other: fever, chills, pain at injection site.

Overdose and treatment
There's no specific antidote for overdose. Provide supportive care. It's not known whether drug is removed by hemodialysis or peritoneal dialysis.

Special considerations
• Safety and efficacy of multiple doses haven't been evaluated.
• Injection can be infused as rapidly as 100 mg/30 seconds or diluted in 50 ml compatible solution and infused over 15 minutes.
• Injection for oral administration is stable in apple or apple-grape juice for 2 hours at room temperature.

Patient monitoring
• Monitor patient for evidence of arrhythmias.
• Monitor therapeutic effect.

Breast-feeding patients
• It isn't known whether drug appears in breast milk. Use cautiously in breast-feeding women.

Pediatric patients
• There's no information on drug use in children under age 2.
• Efficacy in children ages 2 to 17 who receive chemotherapy is consistent with that seen in adults.
• Efficacy in children with postoperative nausea and vomiting is unknown.

Geriatric patients
• Dosage adjustment isn't needed in patients over age 65.
• Effectiveness in prevention of nausea and vomiting in elderly patients is similar to that in younger patients.

Patient education
• Inform patient that oral doses of drug must be taken 1 to 2 hours before surgery or 1 hour before chemotherapy to be effective.
• Inform patient about possible adverse effects.
• Instruct patient not to mix injection in juice for oral administration until just before dosing.
• Tell patient to report nausea or vomiting.

donepezil hydrochloride
Aricept

Pharmacologic classification: acetylcholinesterase inhibitor
Therapeutic classification: cholinomimetic
Pregnancy risk category: C

Indications and dosages
➤ *Mild to moderate dementia of the Alzheimer's type. Adults:* Initially, 5 mg P.O. daily h.s. After 4 to 6 weeks, dosage may be increased to 10 mg daily.

How supplied
Available by prescription only
Tablets: 5 mg, 10 mg

Pharmacodynamics
Anticholinesterase action: Drug is believed to inhibit the enzyme acetylcholinesterase in the CNS, increasing the concentration of acetylcholine and temporarily improving cognitive function in patients with Alzheimer's disease. Drug doesn't alter the course of the underlying disease process.

Pharmacokinetics
Absorption: Well absorbed with a relative bioavailability of 100%. Steady state is reached within 15 days.
Distribution: Steady state volume of distribution is 12 L/kg. Donepezil is about 96% bound to plasma proteins, mainly to albumins (about 75%) and α1-acid glycoprotein (about 21%) over the concentration range of 2 to 1,000 ng/ml.
Metabolism: Extensively metabolized to four major metabolites (two are known to be active) and several minor metabolites (not all have been identified). Donepezil is metabolized by CYP-450 isoenzymes 2D6 and 3A4 and undergoes glucuronidation.
Excretion: Both excreted in the urine intact and extensively metabolized by the liver. Elimination half-life is about 70 hours and mean apparent plasma clearance is 0.13 L/hour/kg. About 17% of drug is eliminated by the kidneys as unchanged drug.

Route	Onset	Peak	Duration
P.O.	Unknown	3-4 hr	Unknown

Contraindications and precautions
Contraindicated in patients hypersensitive to drug or piperidine derivatives. Use very cautiously in patients with sick sinus syndrome or other supraventricular cardiac conduction conditions because drug may cause bradycardia. Use cautiously in patients with CV disease, asthma, or history of ulcer disease and in those taking NSAIDs.

Interactions
Drug-drug. *Anticholinergics:* May interfere with anticholinergic activity. Monitor patient.

Reactions may be *common*, uncommon, **life-threatening**, or COMMON AND LIFE-THREATENING.

Bethanechol, succinylcholine: May produce additive effects. Monitor patient closely.
Carbamazepine, dexamethasone, phenobarbital, phenytoin, rifampin: May speed donepezil elimination. Monitor patient.
Cholinomimetics, cholinesterase inhibitors: May produce synergistic effect. Monitor patient closely.
Drug-herb. *Jaborandi, pill-bearing spurge:* Additive effect may occur and the risk of toxicity may increase. Tell patient to use together cautiously.

Adverse reactions

CNS: abnormal dreams or crying, aggression, aphasia, ataxia, dizziness, syncope, fatigue, depression, *headache, insomnia,* irritability, nervousness, paresthesia, restlessness, somnolence, *seizures,* tremor, vertigo.
CV: *atrial fibrillation,* chest pain, hypertension, vasodilation, hypotension.
EENT: blurred vision, cataract, eye irritation, sore throat.
GI: anorexia, bloating, *diarrhea,* epigastric pain, fecal incontinence, GI bleeding, *nausea,* vomiting.
GU: frequent urination, nocturia.
Hematologic: ecchymoses.
Metabolic: dehydration, weight loss.
Musculoskeletal: arthritis, bone fracture, muscle cramps.
Respiratory: bronchitis, dyspnea.
Skin: diaphoresis, pruritus, urticaria.
Other: influenza, toothache, increased libido, hot flashes, pain.

Overdose and treatment

Overdose can result in cholinergic crisis characterized by severe nausea, vomiting, salivation, sweating, bradycardia, hypotension, respiratory depression, collapse, and seizures. Increasing muscle weakness may also occur and may result in death if respiratory muscles are involved.

Tertiary anticholinergics such as atropine may be used as an antidote for drug overdose. I.V. atropine sulfate titrated to effect is recommended; give an initial dose of 1 to 2 mg I.V. and base subsequent doses on response. Atypical responses in blood pressure and heart rate have been reported with other cholinomimetics when coadministered with quaternary anticholinergics such as glycopyrrolate. It isn't known whether donepezil or its metabolites can be removed by dialysis.

Special considerations

• Diarrhea, nausea, and vomiting occur more frequently with the 10-mg dose than with the 5-mg dose. These effects are mostly mild and transient, sometimes lasting 1 to 3 weeks, and resolve during continued drug therapy.
• Although not observed in clinical trials, drug may cause bladder outflow obstruction.
• Cholinomimetics have potential to cause generalized seizures. However, seizure activity also may be due to Alzheimer's disease.

Patient monitoring

• Drug may increase gastric acid secretion. Closely monitor patients at increased risk for development of ulcers for symptoms of active or occult GI bleeding.

Breast-feeding patients

• It isn't known whether donepezil appears in breast milk. Avoid use of donepezil in breast-feeding women.

Pediatric patients

• Safety and efficacy in children haven't been established.

Geriatric patients

• Mean plasma drug levels of geriatric patients with Alzheimer's disease are comparable with those observed in young healthy volunteers.

Patient education

• Explain to patient and caregiver that drug doesn't alter disease but can stabilize or alleviate symptoms. Effects of therapy depend on drug administration at regular intervals.
• Tell caregiver to give drug in the evening, just before bedtime.
• Advise patient and caregiver to immediately report significant adverse effects or changes in overall health status.
• Tell patient to inform his prescriber that he's using this drug before he receives anesthesia.

dopamine hydrochloride
Intropin

Pharmacologic classification: adrenergic
Therapeutic classification: inotropic, vasopressor
Pregnancy risk category: C

Indications and dosages

➤ *Adjunct in shock to increase cardiac output, blood pressure, and urine flow.*
Adults and children: 2 to 5 mcg/kg/minute I.V. infusion, up to 20 to 50 mcg/kg/minute. Infusion rate may be increased by 1 to 4 mcg/kg/minute at 10- to 30-minute intervals until optimum response is achieved. In severely ill patient, infusion may begin at 5 mcg/kg/minute and gradually increased by increments of 5 to 10 mcg/kg/minute until optimum response is achieved, up to 20-50 mcg/kg/minute.
➤ *Short-term treatment of severe, refractory, chronic heart failure. Adults:* Initially, 0.5 to 2 mcg/kg/minute I.V. infusion. Dosage may be increased until desired renal response occurs. Average dosage, 1 to 3 mcg/kg/minute.

How supplied

Available by prescription only
Injection: 40 mg/ml, 80 mg/ml, and 160 mg/ml parenteral concentrate for injection for I.V. in-

fusion; 0.8 mg/ml (200 or 400 mg) in D_5W, 1.6 mg/ml (400 or 800 mg) in D_5W, and 3.2 mg/ml (800 mg) in D_5W parenteral injection for I.V. infusion

Pharmacodynamics
Vasopressor action: An immediate precursor of norepinephrine, dopamine stimulates dopaminergic, beta-adrenergic, and alpha-adrenergic receptors of the sympathetic nervous system. The main effects produced are dose dependent. It has a direct stimulating effect on $beta_1$ receptors (in I.V. doses of 2 to 10 mcg/kg/minute) and little or no effect on $beta_2$ receptors. In I.V. doses of 0.5 to 2 mcg/kg/minute it acts on dopaminergic receptors, causing vasodilation in the renal, mesenteric, coronary, and intracerebral vascular beds; in I.V. doses of more than 10 mcg/kg/minute, it stimulates alpha receptors.

Low to moderate doses result in cardiac stimulation (positive inotropic effects) and renal and mesenteric vasodilation (dopaminergic response). High doses result in increased peripheral resistance and renal vasoconstriction.

Pharmacokinetics
Absorption: Administered I.V.
Distribution: Widely distributed throughout the body; however, it doesn't cross the blood-brain barrier.
Metabolism: Metabolized to inactive compounds in the liver, kidneys, and plasma by MAO and catechol-O-methyltransferase. About 25% is metabolized to norepinephrine within adrenergic nerve terminals.
Excretion: Excreted in urine, mainly as its metabolites.

Route	Onset	Peak	Duration
I.V.	5 min	Unknown	< 10 min after infusion ends

Contraindications and precautions
Contraindicated in patients with uncorrected tachyarrhythmias, pheochromocytoma, or ventricular fibrillation.

Use cautiously in patients with occlusive vascular disease, cold injuries, diabetic endarteritis, and arterial embolism; in those taking MAO inhibitors; and in pregnant women.

Interactions
Drug-drug. *Alpha blockers:* Antagonize the peripheral vasoconstriction caused by high doses of dopamine. Don't use together.
Beta blockers: Antagonize the cardiac effects of dopamine. Don't use together.
Diuretics: Increased diuretic effects of both agents. Don't use together.
Ergot alkaloids: Extreme elevations in blood pressure. Don't use together.

General anesthetics, especially halothane and other halogenated hydrocarbons: Ventricular arrhythmias and hypertension. Don't use together.
MAO inhibitors: May prolong and intensify dopamine effects. Avoid use together.
Oxytocics: Advanced vasoconstriction. Dosage adjustments may be needed.
Phenytoin: Hypotension and bradycardia. Monitor blood pressure and heart rate closely.

Adverse reactions
CNS: headache.
CV: ectopic beats, tachycardia, anginal pain, palpitations, *hypotension,* **bradycardia,** conduction disturbances, hypertension, vasoconstriction, widening of QRS complex (less frequently).
GI: nausea, vomiting.
GU: azotemia.
Metabolic: hyperglycemia, decreased thyroid-stimulating hormone, growth hormone, and prolactin levels.
Respiratory: dyspnea, *asthma attacks.*
Other: necrosis and tissue sloughing with extravasation, piloerection, *anaphylactic reactions.*

Overdose and treatment
Signs and symptoms of overdose include excessive, severe hypertension. No treatment is necessary beyond dosage reduction or withdrawal of drug. If that fails to lower blood pressure, a short-acting alpha blocker may be helpful.

Special considerations
Consider the recommendations relevant to all adrenergics as well as the following.
⚠ ALERT Severe hypotension may result with abrupt withdrawal of infusion; therefore, reduce dose gradually. Expand blood volume with I.V. fluids, if necessary.
● Correct hypovolemia with plasma volume expanders before administration of dopamine.
● Dopamine is administered by I.V. infusion using an infusion device to control flow.
● Don't mix other drugs in dopamine solutions. Discard solutions after 24 hours.
● Give drug into a large vein to prevent the possibility of extravasation. If necessary to administer in hand or ankle veins, change injection site to larger vein as soon as possible. Monitor continuously for free flow. Central venous access is recommended.
● Dose may require adjustment to meet individual needs of patient and to achieve desired clinical response. If dose required to obtain desired systolic blood pressure exceeds optimum renal response, reduce dose as soon as hemodynamic condition is stabilized.
● If extravasation occurs, stop infusion and infiltrate site promptly with 10 to 15 ml saline injection containing 5 to 10 mg of phentolamine. Use syringe with a fine needle, and infiltrate area liberally with phentolamine solution. In children,

---

0.1 to 0.2 mg/kg up to 10 mg per dose is recommended.

Patient monitoring
● During infusion monitor ECG, blood pressure, cardiac output, central venous pressure, pulmonary artery wedge pressure, pulse rate, urine output, and color and temperature of limbs.

Pregnant patients
● Use only when potential benefits outweigh the risks to the fetus.

Breast-feeding patients
● It isn't known whether drug appears in breast milk; use drug cautiously in breast-feeding women.

Pediatric patients
● No increase in adverse effects has been noted in children.

Geriatric patients
● Lower doses are indicated because geriatric patients may be more sensitive to effects of the drug.

Patient education
● Advise patient to report adverse reactions.
● Inform patient of need for frequent monitoring of his vital signs and condition.

---

dornase alfa
Pulmozyme

Pharmacologic classification: recombinant human deoxyribonuclease I, mucolytic enzyme
Therapeutic classification: respiratory inhalant
Pregnancy risk category: B

Indications and dosages
➤ *To improve pulmonary function and reduce frequency of moderate to severe respiratory infections in patients with cystic fibrosis (CF). Adults and children ages 5 and over:* One ampule (2.5 mg/2.5 ml) inhaled once daily. Treatment usually takes 10 to 15 minutes. Use drug only with an approved nebulizer. Patients over age 21 and those with a baseline forced vital capacity greater than 85% may need twice-daily dosing.

How supplied
Available by prescription only
Inhalation solution: 2.5-ml ampule containing 1 mg/ml dornase alfa

Pharmacodynamics
Respiratory inhalant action: A purified solution of recombinant human deoxyribonuclease I, an enzyme that selectively breaks down DNA. Patients with CF retain thick, purulent pulmonary

secretions rich in extracellular DNA. Dornase alfa hydrolyzes the excess DNA, reducing sputum viscosity.

Pharmacokinetics
Absorption: After inhalation, drug achieves mean sputum level of 3 mcg/ml within 15 minutes, declining to an average of 0.6 mcg/ml within 2 hours.
Distribution: No information available.
Metabolism: No information available.
Excretion: No information available.

Route	Onset	Peak	Duration
Inhalation	3-7 days	9 days	Unknown

Contraindications and precautions
Contraindicated in patients hypersensitive to drug or Chinese hamster ovary cell–derived products.

Interactions
None reported.

Adverse reactions
CV: *chest pain.*
EENT: *pharyngitis, voice alteration,* laryngitis, conjunctivitis.
Skin: *rash,* urticaria.

Overdose and treatment
CF patients have received up to 20 mg twice daily for up to 6 days and 10 mg twice daily intermittently (2 weeks on, 2 weeks off) for 168 days. These doses were well tolerated.

Special considerations
● Mixing dornase alfa with another drug in nebulizer could cause adverse changes in one or both drugs.
● Drug should be used with standard therapies prescribed for CF.
● Safety and efficacy of daily administration haven't been demonstrated in patients with forced vital capacity less than 40% of predicted value or for longer than 12 months.

Patient monitoring
● Monitor patient's response to treatment.
● Monitor patient for adverse effects.

Breast-feeding patients
● It's unknown whether drug appears in breast milk. Use cautiously when administering to breast-feeding women.

Pediatric patients
● Safety and efficacy of daily administration haven't been demonstrated in patients under age 5.

Patient education
● Advise patient to store drug in refrigerator at 36° to 46° F (2° to 8° C), protect from strong light, refrigerate during transport, and avoid exposing to room temperatures for more than 24 hours.

• Tell patient to discard solution if cloudy or discolored.
• Inform patient that drug contains no preservative and that entire ampule must be used or discarded once opened.
• Instruct patient in proper use and maintenance of nebulizer and compressor system.

dorzolamide hydrochloride
Trusopt

Pharmacologic classification: sulfonamide
Therapeutic classification: anti-glaucoma
Pregnancy risk category: C

Indications and dosages
➤ *Treatment of increased intraocular pressure in patients with ocular hypertension or open-angle glaucoma. Adults:* Instill 1 drop in the conjunctival sac of affected eye t.i.d.

How supplied
Available by prescription only
Ophthalmic solution: 2%

Pharmacodynamics
Antiglaucoma action: Dorzolamide inhibits carbonic anhydrase in the ciliary processes of the eye, which decreases aqueous humor secretion, presumably by slowing the formation of bicarbonate ions with subsequent reduction in sodium and fluid transport. The result is a reduction in intraocular pressure.

Pharmacokinetics
Absorption: Reaches the systemic circulation when applied topically.
Distribution: Accumulates in RBCs during chronic dosing as a result of binding to carbonic anhydrase II.
Metabolism: Unknown.
Excretion: Primarily excreted unchanged in urine.

Route	Onset	Peak	Duration
Oph-thalmic	Unknown	Unknown	Unknown

Contraindications and precautions
Contraindicated in patients hypersensitive to any component of drug or in those with impaired renal function. Use cautiously in patients with impaired hepatic function.

Interactions
Drug-drug. *Oral carbonic anhydrase inhibitors:* May cause additive effects. Don't administer together.

Adverse reactions
CNS: asthenia, headache, fatigue.

EENT: *ocular burning and stinging, ocular discomfort, superficial punctate keratitis, ocular allergic reactions, blurred vision, lacrimation, dryness, photophobia,* iridocyclitis, redness, eyelid crusting, ocular pain.
GI: *bitter taste,* nausea.
GU: urolithiasis.
Skin: rash.

Overdose and treatment
Overdose may result in electrolyte imbalance, acidosis, and possible CNS effects. Monitor serum electrolyte levels (especially potassium) and blood pH levels. Treatment is supportive.

Special considerations
• Because dorzolamide is a sulfonamide and is absorbed systemically, the same types of adverse reactions that are attributable to sulfonamides may occur with topical administration of dorzolamide.
• If more than one topical ophthalmic drug is being used, administer drugs at least 10 minutes apart.

Patient monitoring
• Inform patient to report ocular reactions, particularly conjunctivitis and lid reactions, and discontinue drug.

Breast-feeding patients
• It isn't known whether drug appears in breast milk. Because of the risk for serious adverse reactions to the breast-fed infant, use in breast-feeding women isn't recommended.

Pediatric patients
• Safety and effectiveness in children haven't been established.

Geriatric patients
• Use cautiously because greater sensitivity to drug may occur in older adults.

Patient education
• Teach patient how to instill drops. Advise him to wash hands before and after instilling solution, and warn him not to touch dropper or tip to eye or surrounding tissue.
• Advise patient to apply light finger pressure on lacrimal sac for 1 minute after instillation to minimize systemic absorption of drug.
• Tell patient not to wear soft contact lenses while using drug.
• Stress importance of compliance with recommended therapy.

Reactions may be *common*, uncommon, *life-threatening*, or COMMON AND LIFE-THREATENING.

doxacurium chloride
Nuromax

Pharmacologic classification: nondepolarizing neuromuscular blocker
Therapeutic classification: skeletal muscle relaxant
Pregnancy risk category: C

Indications and dosages
➤ *To provide skeletal muscle relaxation for endotracheal intubation and during surgery as an adjunct to general anesthesia. Adults:* Dosage is highly individualized; 0.05 mg/kg rapid I.V. produces adequate conditions for endotracheal intubation in 5 minutes in about 90% of patients when used as part of a thiopental-narcotic induction technique. Lower doses may require longer delay before intubation is possible. Neuromuscular blockade at this dose lasts an average of 100 minutes.
Children over age 2: Dosage is highly individualized; an initial dose of 0.03 mg/kg I.V. administered during halothane anesthesia produces effective blockade in 7 minutes and has a duration of 30 minutes. Under the same conditions, 0.05 mg/kg produces a blockade in 4 minutes and lasts 45 minutes.
➤ *Maintenance of neuromuscular blockade during long procedures. Adults and children over age 2:* After initial dose of 0.05 mg/kg I.V., maintenance dosages of 0.005 and 0.01 mg/kg prolong neuromuscular blockade for an average of 30 minutes and 45 minutes, respectively. Children usually require more frequent administration of maintenance dosages.
✦ *Dosage adjustment.* Adjust dosage to ideal body weight in obese patients (patients whose weight is 30% or more above their ideal weight) to avoid prolonged neuromuscular blockade.

How supplied
Available by prescription only
Injection: 1 mg/ml

Pharmacodynamics
Skeletal muscle relaxant action: Doxacurium binds competitively to cholinergic receptors on the motor end-plate to antagonize the action of acetylcholine, resulting in a block of neuromuscular transmission.

Pharmacokinetics
Absorption: Administered I.V.
Distribution: Plasma protein–binding of drug is about 30% in human plasma.
Metabolism: Not metabolized.
Excretion: Primarily eliminated as unchanged drug in urine and bile.

Route	Onset	Peak	Duration
I.V.	2 min	3-6 min	Variable

Contraindications and precautions
Contraindicated in patients hypersensitive to drug and in neonates. Drug contains benzyl ethanol, which has been linked to death in newborns.

Use cautiously, perhaps at a reduced dose, in debilitated patients; in patients with metastatic cancer, severe electrolyte disturbances, or neuromuscular diseases; and in those in whom potentiation or difficulty in reversal of neuromuscular blockade is anticipated. Patients with myasthenia gravis or myasthenic syndrome (Eaton-Lambert syndrome) are particularly sensitive to the effects of nondepolarizing relaxants. Shorter-acting agents are recommended for use in such patients.

Interactions
Drug-drug. *Alkaline solutions:* Drug is physically incompatible with alkaline solutions; precipitate may form. Don't give these drugs through the same I.V. line.
Antibiotics (aminoglycosides, such as gentamycin, kanamycin, neomycin, and streptomycin, tetracyclines, bacitracin, polymyxins, lincomycin, clindamycin, colistin, and colistimethate sodium), lithium, local anesthetics, magnesium salts, procainamide, quinidine: Neuromuscular blocking action of doxacurium may be enhanced. Use together cautiously. Monitor patient for excessive weakness.
Carbamazepine, phenytoin: Delayed onset of neuromuscular blockade and shortened duration. Monitor patient.
Enflurane, halothane, isoflurane: Decrease in dose needed to produce 50% suppression of response to ulnar nerve stimulation of doxacurium by 30% to 45%. May also prolong the clinically effective duration of action of doxacurium by up to 25%. Don't use together.

Adverse reactions
Respiratory: dyspnea, *respiratory depression, respiratory insufficiency or apnea.*
Musculoskeletal: prolonged muscle weakness.

Overdose and treatment
Overdose with neuromuscular blocking agents such as doxacurium may result in neuromuscular block beyond the time needed for surgery and anesthesia.

The primary treatment is maintenance of a patent airway and controlled ventilation until recovery of normal neuromuscular function is assured. Once initial evidence of recovery is observed, further recovery may be facilitated by administration of an anticholinesterase agent (such as neostigmine or edrophonium) with an appropriate anticholinergic agent.

Special considerations
● All times of onset and duration of neuromuscular blockade are averages; considerable individual variation in dosages is normal.

• As with other nondepolarizing neuromuscular blocking agents, a reduction in dosage of doxacurium must be considered in cachectic or debilitated patients; in patients with neuromuscular diseases, severe electrolyte abnormalities, or carcinomatosis; and in other patients in whom potentiation of neuromuscular block or difficulty with reversal is anticipated. Increased doses of doxacurium may be required in burn patients.

• Drug has no effect on consciousness or pain threshold. To avoid distress to the patient, it shouldn't be administered until patient's consciousness is obtunded by general anesthetic.

• Drug may prolong neuromuscular block in patients undergoing renal transplantation, and onset and duration of the block may vary with patients undergoing liver transplantation.

• Use drug only under direct medical supervision by caregivers familiar with use of neuromuscular blocking agents and in airway management. Don't use unless facilities and equipment for mechanical ventilation, oxygen therapy, and intubation and an antagonist are within reach.

• Use of a peripheral nerve stimulator will permit the most advantageous use of doxacurium, minimize the possibility of overdose or underdose, and assist in the evaluation of recovery.

• Doxacurium is acidic (pH 3.9 to 5.0) and may not be compatible with alkaline solutions having a pH above 8.5 (such as barbiturate solutions).

• Doxacurium diluted up to 1:10 in D_5W injection, USP or normal saline injection, USP, is physically and chemically stable when stored in polypropylene syringes at 41° to 77° F (5° to 25° C) for up to 24 hours. Because dilution reduces preservative effectiveness of benzyl alcohol, use aseptic technique to prepare diluted product. Use diluted product immediately; discard any unused portion after 8 hours.

Patient monitoring
• Monitor ECG, especially for bradycardia.
• Monitor respirations until patient is fully recovered from neuromuscular blockade, as evidenced by tests of muscle strength (such as hand grips, head lift, and ability to cough).

Breast-feeding patients
• It isn't known whether drug appears in breast milk. Use cautiously when administrating to breast-feeding women.

Pediatric patients
• Drug use hasn't been studied in children under age 2.

Geriatric patients
• Geriatric patients may be more sensitive to the effects of the drug. They may experience a slower onset of the blockade and a longer duration.

Patient education
• Reassure patient and family that he will be monitored at all times.

doxapram hydrochloride
Dopram

Pharmacologic classification: analeptic
Therapeutic classification: CNS and respiratory stimulant
Pregnancy risk category: B

Indications and dosages
➤ *Postanesthesia respiratory stimulation.* *Adults:* 0.5 to 1 mg/kg of body weight as a single I.V. injection (not to exceed 1.5 mg/kg) or as several injections q 5 minutes, not to exceed 2 mg/kg total dosage. Or, 250 mg in 250 ml of normal saline solution or D_5W infused at 5 mg/minute I.V. until a satisfactory response is achieved. Maintain at 1 to 3 mg/minute. Recommended total dose for infusion shouldn't exceed 4 mg/kg.

➤ *Drug-induced CNS depression.* *Adults:* For injection, priming dose of 2 mg/kg I.V. repeated in 5 minutes and again q 1 to 2 hours until patient awakens (and if relapse occurs). Maximum daily dose is 3 g.

For infusion, priming dose of 2 mg/kg I.V., repeated in 5 minutes and again in 1 to 2 hours if needed. If response occurs, give I.V. infusion (1 mg/ml) at 1 to 3 mg/minute until patient awakens. Don't infuse for longer than 2 hours or administer more than 3 g/day. May resume I.V. infusion after a rest period of 30 minutes to 2 hours, if needed.

➤ *Chronic pulmonary disease related to acute hypercapnia.* *Adults:* Infusion of 1 to 2 mg/minute (using 2 mg/ml solution). Maximum dose is 3 mg/minute for a maximum duration of 2 hours. Don't use drug with mechanical ventilation. Use infusion pump to regulate rate.

How supplied
Available by prescription only
Injection: 20 mg/ml (benzyl alcohol 0.9%)

Pharmacodynamics
Respiratory stimulant action: Doxapram increases respiratory rate by direct stimulation of the medullary respiratory center and possibly by indirect action on chemoreceptors in the carotid artery and aortic arch. Doxapram causes increased release of catecholamines.

Pharmacokinetics
Absorption: Administered I.V.
Distribution: Distributed throughout the body.
Metabolism: 99% metabolized by the liver.
Excretion: Metabolites are excreted in urine.

Route	Onset	Peak	Duration
I.V.	20-40 sec	1-2 min	5-12 min

Contraindications and precautions
Contraindicated in patients with seizure disorders; head injury; CV disorders; frank, uncom-

pensated heart failure; severe hypertension; CVA; respiratory failure or incompetence secondary to neuromuscular disorders; muscle paresis; flail chest; obstructed airway; pulmonary embolism; pneumothorax; restrictive respiratory disease; acute bronchial asthma or extreme dyspnea; or hypoxia not related to hypercapnia. Drug also contraindicated in neonates because product contains benzyl alcohol.

Use cautiously in patients with bronchial asthma, severe tachycardia or arrhythmias, cerebral edema or increased CSF pressure, hyperthyroidism, pheochromocytoma, or metabolic disorders.

Interactions
Drug-drug. *Anesthetics such as cyclopropane, enflurane, and halothane:* Sensitize the myocardium to catecholamines. Discontinue at least 10 minutes before giving doxapram.
MAO inhibitors, sympathomimetic drugs: Added pressor effects. Use together cautiously.
Neuromuscular blockers: Doxapram temporarily may mask residual effects of neuromuscular blockers used after anesthesia. Monitor patient closely.

Adverse reactions
CNS: *seizures, headache,* dizziness, apprehension, disorientation, hyperactivity, bilateral Babinski's signs, paresthesia.
CV: flushing, *chest pain and tightness, variations in heart rate, hypertension,* lowered T waves, *arrhythmias.*
EENT: sneezing, *laryngospasm.*
GI: nausea, vomiting, diarrhea.
GU: urine retention, bladder stimulation with incontinence, increased BUN levels, albuminuria.
Hematologic: decreased erythrocyte and leukocyte counts, reduced hemoglobin and hematocrit levels.
Musculoskeletal: muscle spasms.
Respiratory: hiccups, cough, *bronchospasm,* dyspnea, rebound hypoventilation.
Skin: diaphoresis, pruritus.

Overdose and treatment
Signs and symptoms of overdose include hypertension, tachycardia, arrhythmias, skeletal muscle hyperactivity, and dyspnea.

Treatment is supportive. Keep oxygen and resuscitative equipment available, but use oxygen cautiously because rapid increase in partial pressure of oxygen can suppress carotid chemoreceptor activity. Keep I.V. anticonvulsants available to treat seizures.

Special considerations
● Use of doxapram as an analeptic is strongly discouraged; use only in surgery or emergency room.
● Establish adequate airway before administering drug; prevent aspiration of vomitus by placing patient on his side.

● For I.V. infusion, dilute to 1 mg/ml. Doxapram shouldn't be infused faster than recommended rate because hemolysis may occur. Use only on an intermittent basis; maximum infusion period is 2 hours.
● Avoid repeated injections in the site for long periods because of risk of thrombophlebitis or local skin irritation.
● Don't combine doxapram, which is acidic, with alkaline solutions, such as thiopental sodium; solution is compatible with D_5W or $D_{10}W$ and normal saline solution.
● Give oxygen cautiously to patients with COPD who are narcotized or those who have just undergone surgery; doxapram-stimulated respiration increases oxygen demand.

Patient monitoring
● Monitor blood pressure, heart rate, deep tendon reflexes, and arterial blood gas (ABG) levels before giving drug and every 30 minutes afterward. Discontinue drug if ABG levels deteriorate or mechanical ventilation is started.

Breast-feeding patients
● Safety in breast-feeding women hasn't been established. Distribution into breast milk is unknown.

Pediatric patients
● Safety in children under age 12 hasn't been established.

Geriatric patients
● No specific recommendations exist for use in geriatric patients. However, geriatric patients may be predisposed to one of several illnesses that preclude its use.

Patient education
● Inform patient (if alert) and family of need for drug; answer questions and address concerns.

doxazosin mesylate
Cardura

Pharmacologic classification: alpha blocker
Therapeutic classification: antihypertensive
Pregnancy risk category: C

Indications and dosages
➤ *Essential hypertension.* **Adult:** Dosage must be individualized. Initially, give 1 mg P.O. daily and determine effect on standing and supine blood pressure at 2 to 6 hours and 24 hours after dosing. If necessary, increase dose to 2 mg daily. To minimize adverse reactions, adjust dose slowly (dosage typically increased only q 2 weeks). If necessary, increase dose to 4 mg daily, then 8 mg. Maximum daily dose is 16 mg, but doses exceeding 4 mg daily are more likely to cause adverse reactions.

▶*BPH. Adults:* Initially, 1 mg P.O. once daily in the morning or evening; increase to 2 mg and, thereafter, to 4 mg and 8 mg once daily. Recommended adjustment interval is 1 to 2 weeks.

How supplied
Available by prescription only
Tablets: 1 mg, 2 mg, 4 mg, 8 mg

Pharmacodynamics
Hypotensive action: Doxazosin selectively blocks postsynaptic alpha$_1$-adrenergic receptors, dilating both resistance (arterioles) and capacitance (veins) vessels. It lowers both supine and standing blood pressure, producing more pronounced effects on diastolic pressure. Maximum reductions occur 2 to 6 hours after dosing and are linked to a small increase in standing heart rate. Doxazosin has a greater effect on blood pressure and heart rate in the standing position.
Benign prostatic hyperplasia: Doxazosin improves urine flow related to relaxation of smooth muscles produced by blockade of alpha adrenoreceptors in the bladder neck and prostate.

Pharmacokinetics
Absorption: Readily absorbed from the GI tract after oral administration.
Distribution: 98% protein-bound. It's distributed in breast milk in levels about 20 times greater than in maternal plasma.
Metabolism: Extensively metabolized in the liver by *O*-demethylation or hydroxylation. Secondary peaking of plasma levels suggests enterohepatic recycling.
Excretion: 63% is excreted in bile and feces (4.8% as unchanged drug); 9% is excreted in urine.

Route	Onset	Peak	Duration
P.O.	1-2 hr	2-3 hr	24 hr

Contraindications and precautions
Contraindicated in patients hypersensitive to drug and quinazoline derivatives (including prazosin and terazosin). Use cautiously in patients with impaired hepatic function.

Interactions
Drug-drug. *Clonidine:* Antihypertensive effects of clonidine may be decreased. Monitor patient closely.
Drug-herb. *Butcher's broom:* Possible reduced doxazosin effects. Tell patient to avoid use together.

Adverse reactions
CNS: *dizziness,* vertigo, somnolence, drowsiness, *asthenia, headache.*
CV: *orthostatic hypotension,* hypotension, edema, palpitations, **arrhythmias,** tachycardia.
EENT: rhinitis, pharyngitis, abnormal vision.
GI: nausea, vomiting, diarrhea, constipation.

Hematologic: mean WBC and neutrophil counts may be decreased.
Musculoskeletal: arthralgia, myalgia, pain.
Respiratory: dyspnea.
Skin: rash, pruritus.

Overdose and treatment
Keep patient supine to restore blood pressure and heart rate. If necessary, treat shock with volume expanders. Administer vasopressors and monitor and support renal function.

Special considerations
● Tolerance to antihypertensive effects of doxazosin hasn't been observed.
● No apparent differences exist in the hypotensive response of whites and blacks or of geriatric patients.
● First-dose effect (orthostatic hypotension) occurs with doxazosin but is less pronounced than with prazosin or terazosin.

Patient monitoring
● Orthostatic effects are most likely to occur 2 to 6 hours after dose. Monitor blood pressure during this time after the first dose and after subsequent increases in dosage. Daily doses above 4 mg increase the potential of excessive orthostatic effects.

Breast-feeding patients
● Drug accumulates in breast milk at levels about 20 times greater than in maternal plasma.

Pediatric patients
● Safety and efficacy in children haven't been established.

Geriatric patients
● Use drug cautiously in geriatric patients with underlying autonomic dysfunction or arrhythmias.

Patient education
● Tell patient that orthostatic hypotension and syncope may occur, especially after first few doses and with dosage changes. Patient should rise slowly to prevent orthostatic hypotension.
● Caution patient that drug may cause drowsiness and somnolence. Patient should avoid driving and other hazardous tasks that require alertness for 12 to 24 hours after first dose, after dosage increases, and after resumption of interrupted therapy.
● Tell patient to report bothersome palpitations or dizziness.
● Inform patient drug may be taken with food if nausea occurs. Tell patient that nausea should improve as therapy continues.

---

doxepin hydrochloride
Sinequan, Triadapin*

Pharmacologic classification: tricyclic antidepressant (TCA)
Therapeutic classification: antidepressant
Pregnancy risk category: NR

Indications and dosages
➤ **Depression or anxiety.** *Adults:* Initially, 25 to 75 mg P.O. daily in divided doses, to a maximum of 300 mg daily. Or, give entire maintenance dosage once daily with a maximum dose of 150 mg P.O.
✦ **Dosage adjustment.** Reduce dosage in geriatric, debilitated, or adolescent patients and in those receiving other medications (especially anticholinergics).

How supplied
Available by prescription only
Capsules: 10 mg, 25 mg, 50 mg, 75 mg, 100 mg, 150 mg
Oral concentrate: 10 mg/ml

Pharmacodynamics
Antidepressant action: Doxepin is thought to exert antidepressant effects by inhibiting reuptake of norepinephrine and serotonin in CNS nerve terminals (presynaptic neurons), which results in increased levels and enhanced activity of these neurotransmitters in the synaptic cleft. Doxepin more actively inhibits reuptake of serotonin than norepinephrine. Anxiolytic effects of this drug usually precede antidepressant effects. Doxepin also may be used as an anxiolytic. Doxepin has the greatest sedative effect of all tricyclic antidepressants; tolerance to this effect usually develops in a few weeks.

Pharmacokinetics
Absorption: Absorbed rapidly from the GI tract after oral administration.
Distribution: Distributed widely into the body, including the CNS and breast milk. Drug is 90% protein-bound. Steady state is achieved within 7 days.
Metabolism: Metabolized by the liver to the active metabolite desmethyldoxepin. A significant first-pass effect may explain variability of serum levels in different patients taking the same dosage.
Excretion: Mostly excreted in urine.

Route	Onset	Peak	Duration
P.O.	Unknown	2 hr	Unknown

Contraindications and precautions
Contraindicated in patients hypersensitive to drug and in those with glaucoma or a tendency to retain urine. Use cautiously in patients with CV disease because of the increased risk of arrhythmias, patients with suicidal ideation, patients with renal or hepatic impairment, and patients with seizure or thyroid disorders.

Interactions
Drug-drug. *Antiarrhythmics such as disopyramide, procainamide, and quinidine; pimozide; thyroid medication:* May increase risk of cardiac arrhythmias and conduction defects. Monitor ECG closely.
Atropine, other anticholinergics: Increased risk of oversedation, paralytic ileus, visual changes, and severe constipation. Monitor patient closely.
Barbiturates: Increased doxepin metabolism and decreased therapeutic efficacy. Monitor patient closely; dosage adjustment may be necessary.
Beta blockers, cimetidine, fluoxetine, methylphenidate, oral contraceptives, propoxyphene, sertraline: May inhibit doxepin metabolism, increasing plasma levels and toxicity. Monitor serum level closely.
Centrally acting antihypertensives: Decreased hypotensive effects. Monitor blood pressure closely.
Clonidine: Increased hypertensive effect. Monitor blood pressure closely.
CNS depressants: Additive effects are likely. Avoid use together.
Disulfiram, ethchlorvynol: Increased risk of delirium and tachycardia. Monitor patient closely.
Haloperidol, phenothiazines: Decreased metabolism and increased doxepin levels. Adjust dosages of both drugs.
MAO inhibitors: Increased risk of severe excitation, hyperpyrexia, or seizures, usually with high dose. Monitor patient closely.
Metrizamide: Increased risk of seizures. Avoid use together.
Sympathomimetics, such as ephedrine, epinephrine, and norepinephrine: May increase blood pressure. Use cautiously.
Warfarin: May increase PT and INR and risk of bleeding. Monitor PT and INR.
Drug-herb. *Evening primrose oil:* Possible additive or synergistic effect resulting in lower seizure threshold and increased risk of seizure. Discourage concomitant use.
Drug-food. *Carbonated beverages, grape juice:* Incompatible. Don't give together.
Drug-lifestyle. *Alcohol use:* Enhanced CNS depression. Advise patient to avoid use together.
Heavy smoking: Increased doxepin metabolism and decreased efficacy. Advise patient to avoid use together.
Sun exposure: Increased risk of photosensitivity reactions. Advise patient to take precautions.

Adverse reactions
CNS: *drowsiness, dizziness,* confusion, numbness, hallucinations, paresthesia, ataxia, weakness, headache, ***seizures,*** extrapyramidal reactions.
CV: *orthostatic hypotension, tachycardia,* ECG changes.
EENT: *blurred vision,* tinnitus.

◇ Unlabeled clinical use

GI: *dry mouth, constipation,* nausea, vomiting, anorexia.
GU: urine retention.
Hematologic: eosinophilia, *bone marrow depression.*
Hepatic: elevated liver function test results.
Metabolic: hyperglycemia, hypoglycemia.
Skin: *diaphoresis,* rash, urticaria, photosensitivity.
Other: *hypersensitivity reaction.*

Overdose and treatment

The first 12 hours after acute ingestion are a stimulatory phase characterized by excessive anticholinergic activity (agitation, irritation, confusion, hallucinations, hyperthermia, parkinsonian symptoms, seizures, urine retention, dry mucous membranes, pupillary dilatation, constipation, and ileus). This is followed by CNS depressant effects, including hypothermia, decreased or absent reflexes, sedation, hypotension, cyanosis, and cardiac irregularities, including tachycardia, conduction disturbances, and quinidine-like effects on the ECG. Severity of overdose is best indicated by widening of QRS complex. Metabolic acidosis may follow hypotension, hypoventilation, and seizures.

Treatment is symptomatic and supportive, including maintaining airway, stable body temperature, and fluid and electrolyte balance. Induce emesis with ipecac if patient is conscious; follow with gastric lavage and activated charcoal to prevent further absorption. Dialysis is of little use. Physostigmine may be cautiously used to reverse central anticholinergic effects. Treat seizures with parenteral diazepam or phenytoin; arrhythmias with parenteral phenytoin or lidocaine; and acidosis with sodium bicarbonate. Don't give barbiturates: these may enhance CNS and respiratory depressant effects.

Special considerations

⚑ **ALERT** Because hypertensive episodes have occurred during surgery in patients receiving TCAs, drug should be gradually discontinued several days before surgery.
● After abrupt withdrawal of long-term therapy patient may experience nausea, headache, and malaise. This doesn't indicate addiction.

Patient monitoring
● If signs of psychosis occur or increase, expect dosage to be reduced.
● Record mood changes. Monitor patient for suicidal tendencies, and provide a minimum supply of drug.

Breast-feeding patients
● Drug appears in breast milk. Avoid use of drug in breast-feeding women, especially if high doses are used.

Pediatric patients
● Doxepin is rarely used to treat anxiety in children.

Geriatric patients
● Adverse CNS reactions, orthostatic hypotension, and GI and GU disturbances are more likely to develop in geriatric patients.

Patient education
● Teach patient to dilute oral concentrate with 4 oz (120 ml) of water, milk, or juice (grapefruit, orange, pineapple, prune, or tomato). Drug is incompatible with carbonated beverages.
● Tell patient to use ice chips, sugarless gum or hard candy, or saliva substitutes to treat dry mouth.
● Warn patient to avoid taking other drugs while taking doxepin unless they've been prescribed.
● Instruct patient to take full dose at bedtime.

doxercalciferol
Hectorol

Pharmacologic classification: synthetic vitamin D analogue
Therapeutic classification: parathyroid hormone antagonist
Pregnancy risk category: B

Indications and dosages

➤ *Reduction of elevated intact parathyroid hormone (PTH) levels in the management of secondary hyperparathyroidism in patients undergoing long-term renal dialysis.* **Adults:** Initially, 10 mcg P.O. three times weekly or 4.0 mcg I.V. bolus three times weekly at dialysis. Dosage adjusted as needed to lower intact PTH levels to 150 to 300 pg/ml. Dosage may be increased by 2.5 mcg (P.O.) or 1.0 to 2.0 mcg (I.V.) at 8-week intervals if the intact PTH level isn't decreased by 50% and fails to reach target range. Maximum dose is 20 mcg P.O. three times weekly or 6 mcg I.V. three times weekly. If intact PTH levels go below 100 pg/ml, suspend drug for 1 week, then resume at a dose that's at least 2.5 mcg (P.O.) or 1.0 mcg (I.V.) lower than the last administered dose.

How supplied
Available by prescription only
Capsules: 2.5 mcg
Injection: 2 mcg/ml; 4 mcg/2 ml ampules.

Pharmacodynamics
PTH antagonist action: Once activated, doxercalciferol and other biologically active vitamin D metabolites regulate blood calcium levels required for essential body functions. Doxercalciferol acts directly on the parathyroid glands to suppress PTH synthesis and secretion.

Pharmacokinetics
Absorption: Absorbed from the GI tract or administered I.V.
Distribution: No information available.
Metabolism: Metabolized to its active forms in the liver via CYP 27.

Excretion: The major metabolite of doxercalciferol attains peak blood levels at 11 to 12 hours after repeated oral doses and 2 to 14 hours after a single I.V. dose of 5 mcg . Elimination half-life after an oral dose is 32 to 37 hours, with a range of up to 96 hours.

Route	Onset	Peak	Duration
P.O.	Unknown	11-12 hr	Unknown
I.V.	Unknown	2-14 hr	Unknown

Contraindications and precautions
Contraindicated in patients with a recent history of hypercalcemia, hyperphosphatemia, or vitamin D toxicity. Use cautiously in patients with hepatic insufficiency and frequently monitor calcium, phosphorus, and intact PTH levels in these patients.

Interactions
Drug-drug. *Calcium-containing or non-aluminum-containing phosphate binders:* May cause hypercalcemia or hyperphosphatemia and decrease effectiveness of doxercalciferol. Use cautiously together and adjust dose of phosphate binders as appropriate.

Cholestyramine, mineral oil: Reduce intestinal absorption of doxercalciferol. Avoid use together.

Glutethimide, phenobarbital, and other enzyme inducers; phenytoin and other enzyme inhibitors: May affect the metabolism of doxercalciferol. Adjust dosage as appropriate.

Magnesium-containing antacids: May cause hypermagnesemia. Avoid use together.

Orlistat: May interfere with intestinal absorption of vitamin D analogues. Avoid use together.

Vitamin D supplements: May cause additive effects and hypercalcemia. Avoid use together.

Adverse reactions
CNS: *dizziness, headache, malaise,* sleep disorder.
CV: *bradycardia, edema.*
GI: anorexia, dyspepsia, *nausea, vomiting,* constipation.
Metabolic: weight gain.
Musculoskeletal: arthralgia.
Respiratory: *dyspnea.*
Skin: pruritus.
Other: abscess.

Overdose and treatment
Excessive doses of doxercalciferol can cause hypercalcemia, hypercalciuria, hyperphosphatemia, and oversuppression of PTH secretion.

For hypercalcemia of greater than 1 mg/dl above the upper limit of normal, suspend doxercalciferol therapy immediately, institute a low-calcium diet, and withdraw calcium supplements. Check serum calcium levels weekly until levels return to normal, usually in 2 to 7 days. Dialysis, using a low-calcium or calcium-free dialysate, may correct persistently or markedly elevated serum calcium levels. When serum calcium levels have returned to within normal limits, drug can be restarted at a dose that's at least 2.5 mcg lower than prior therapy.

For acute overdose, treatment should consist of general supportive measures. Within 10 minutes of ingestion, induce vomiting or perform gastric lavage to prevent further absorption. If postingestion time is more than 10 minutes, administer mineral oil to promote fecal elimination. Monitor serum calcium levels, urinary calcium excretion, and ECG findings. If serum calcium levels are persistently and markedly elevated, consider drugs, such as corticosteroids or phosphates, or therapeutic measures, such as dialysis or forced diuresis.

Special considerations
● Management of secondary hyperparathyroidism may prevent bone disease in patients with renal failure.

● Doxercalciferol is administered with dialysis (about every other day). Dosing must be individualized and based on intact PTH levels, with monitoring of serum calcium and phosphorus levels before doxercalciferol therapy and weekly thereafter.

● Calcium-based or nonaluminum-containing phosphate binders and a low-phosphate diet are used to control serum phosphorus levels in dialysis patients. Expect adjustments in doses of doxercalciferol and therapies such as dietary phosphate binders in order to sustain PTH suppression and maintain serum calcium and phosphorus levels within acceptable ranges.

● Progressive hypercalcemia secondary to vitamin D overdose may require emergency attention. Acute hypercalcemia may exacerbate arrhythmias and seizures and affect the action of digoxin. Chronic hypercalcemia can lead to vascular and soft-tissue calcification.

● Discard unused I.V. portion of drug.

Patient monitoring
● Serum levels of intact PTH, calcium and phosphorus should be obtained before treatment. Obtain weekly during the first 12 weeks and periodically thereafter.

● If the patient has hypercalcemia or hyperphosphatemia, or if the product of serum calcium times serum phosphorus (Ca × P) is greater than 70, administration of doxercalciferol must be stopped, as ordered, until these parameters are lowered.

Breast-feeding patients
● It's unknown whether doxercalciferol appears in breast milk, but other vitamin D derivatives do and the potential for serious adverse reactions in nursing infants exists. Based on importance of drug to the woman, it should be decided whether breast-feeding or drug should be discontinued.

Pediatric patients
• Safety and efficacy in children haven't been established.

Patient education
• Inform patient that dose must be adjusted over several months to achieve satisfactory PTH suppression.
• Instruct patient to adhere to a low-phosphorus diet and to follow instructions regarding calcium supplementation.
• Tell patient to obtain prescriber's approval before using OTC drugs, including antacids and vitamin preparations containing calcium or vitamin D.
• Inform patient that early signs and symptoms of hypercalcemia include weakness, headache, somnolence, nausea, vomiting, dry mouth, constipation, muscle pain, bone pain, and metallic taste. Late signs and symptoms include polyuria, polydipsia, anorexia, weight loss, nocturia, conjunctivitis, pancreatitis, photophobia.

---

doxorubicin hydrochloride
Adriamycin PFS, Adriamycin RDF, Rubex

Pharmacologic classification: antineoplastic antibiotic (not specific to phase of cell cycle)
Therapeutic classification: antineoplastic
Pregnancy risk category: D

Indications and dosages
Dosage and indications may vary. Check current literature for recommended protocol or for information on liposomal doxorubicin.
➤ *Bladder, breast, lung, ovarian, stomach, and thyroid cancers; Hodgkin's disease; acute lymphoblastic and myeloblastic leukemia; Wilms' tumor; neuroblastoma; lymphoma; sarcoma.* Adults: 60 to 75 mg/m² I.V. as a single dose q 21 days; or 25 to 30 mg/m² I.V. as a single daily dose on days 1 to 3 of 4-week cycle. Or, 20 mg/m² I.V. once weekly. Maximum cumulative dosage is 550 mg/m² (450 mg/m² in patients who have received chest irradiation).

How supplied
Available by prescription only
Injection: 10-mg, 20-mg, 50-mg, 100-mg, 150-mg vials
Injection (preservative-free): 2 mg/ml (10 mg, 20 mg, 50 mg, 75 mg, and 200 mg)

Pharmacodynamics
Antineoplastic action: Doxorubicin exerts its cytotoxic activity by intercalating between DNA base pairs and uncoiling the DNA helix. The result is inhibition of DNA synthesis and DNA-dependent RNA synthesis. Doxorubicin also inhibits protein synthesis.

Pharmacokinetics
Absorption: Administered I.V.
Distribution: Distributed widely into body tissues, with the highest levels found in the liver, heart, and kidneys. It doesn't cross the blood-brain barrier.
Metabolism: Extensively metabolized by hepatic microsomal enzymes to several metabolites, one of which possesses cytotoxic activity.
Excretion: Excreted primarily in bile. A minute amount is eliminated in urine. The plasma elimination of doxorubicin is described as biphasic with a half-life of about 15 to 30 minutes in the initial phase and 16½ hours in the terminal phase.

Route	Onset	Peak	Duration
I.V.	Unknown	Unknown	Unknown

Contraindications and precautions
Contraindicated in patients with marked myelosuppression induced by previous treatment with other antitumor agents or by radiotherapy and in those who have received lifetime cumulative dosage of 550 mg/m².

Interactions
Drug-drug. *Aminophylline, cephalosporins, dexamethasone phosphate, fluorouracil, heparin sodium, hydrocortisone, sodium phosphate:* Result in a precipitate when mixed with doxorubicin. Administer through separate I.V. lines.
Cyclophosphamide, daunorubicin: Potentiate the cardiotoxicity of doxorubicin through additive effects on the heart. Avoid use together.
Cyclophosphamide: Doxorubicin may worsen induced hemorrhagic cystitis. Monitor patient closely.
Digoxin: Levels may be decreased if used with doxorubicin. Monitor serum digoxin levels closely.
Mercaptopurine: Hepatotoxicity. Don't use together.
Phenytoin: Decreased phenytoin levels. Monitor serum phenytoin levels.
Streptozocin: Increases the plasma half-life of doxorubicin, increasing the activity of doxorubicin. Dosage may have to be adjusted.
Verapamil: Increased doxorubicin levels. Monitor patient for signs of toxicity.
Drug-herb. *Green tea:* May enhance the antitumor activity of doxorubicin. Monitor patient closely.

Adverse reactions
CV: cardiac depression, seen in such ECG changes as sinus tachycardia, T-wave flattening, ST-segment depression, voltage reduction; *arrhythmias; acute left ventricular failure; irreversible cardiomyopathy.*
EENT: conjunctivitis.
GI: *nausea, vomiting,* diarrhea, *stomatitis,* esophagitis, anorexia, necrotizing colitis.
GU: red urine.

Reactions may be *common,* uncommon, ***life-threatening,*** or COMMON AND LIFE-THREATENING.

Hematologic: *leukopenia during days 10 to 15 with recovery by day 21,* ***thrombocytopenia,*** myelosuppression.
Metabolic: hyperuricemia.
Skin: urticaria, facial flushing.
Other: *severe cellulitis or tissue sloughing* (with extravasates), *alopecia,* fever, chills, ***anaphylaxis.***

Overdose and treatment

Signs and symptoms of overdose include myelosuppression, nausea, vomiting, mucositis, and irreversible myocardial toxicity.

Treatment is usually supportive and includes transfusion of blood components, antiemetics, antibiotics for infections which may develop, symptomatic treatment of mucositis, and cardiac glycoside preparations.

Special considerations

⚠ ALERT Reddish color is similar to that of daunorubicin. Don't confuse the two drugs.
● If signs of heart failure occur, stop drug and reevaluate patient.
● The alternative dosage schedule (once-weekly dosing) has been found to cause a lower risk of cardiomyopathy.
● To reconstitute, add 5 ml of normal saline injection, USP, to the 10-mg vial, 10 ml to the 20-mg vial, and 25 ml to the 50-mg vial, to yield a concentration of 2 mg/ml.
● Drug may be further diluted with normal saline solution or D₅W and administered by I.V. infusion.
● Drug may be administered by I.V. push injection over 5 to 10 minutes into the tubing of a freely flowing I.V. infusion.
● If cumulative dose exceeds 550 mg/m² body surface area, cardiac adverse reactions, which begin 2 weeks to 6 months after stopping drug, develop in 30% of patients. With high doses of doxorubicin, consider concomitant dosing with the cardioprotective agent dexrazoxane.
● The occurrence of streaking along a vein or facial flushing indicates that drug is being administered too rapidly.
● Applying a scalp tourniquet or ice may decrease alopecia. However, don't use these if treating leukemias or other neoplasms in which stem cells may be present in scalp.
● Discontinue drug or slow infusion if tachycardia develops. Drug is a vesicant; treat extravasation with topical application of dimethyl sulfoxide and ice packs.
● Esophagitis is very common in patients who have also received radiation therapy.

Patient monitoring
● Monitor CBC and hepatic function.
● Decrease dosage as follows if serum bilirubin level increases: 50% of dose when bilirubin level is 1.2 to 3 mg/100 ml; 25% of dose when bilirubin level exceeds 3 mg/100 ml.

Breast-feeding patients
● It isn't known whether doxorubicin appears in breast milk. However, because of the risk of serious adverse reactions, mutagenicity, and carcinogenicity in the infant, breast-feeding isn't recommended.

Pediatric patients
● Children under age 2 have a higher risk of drug-induced cardiotoxicity.

Geriatric patients
● Patients over age 70 have an increased risk of drug-induced cardiotoxicity. Take caution in geriatric patients with low bone marrow reserve to prevent serious hematologic toxicity.

Patient education
● Encourage adequate fluid intake to increase urine output and facilitate excretion of uric acid.
● Advise patient to avoid exposure to people with infections.
● Warn patient that alopecia will occur. Explain that hair growth should resume 2 to 5 months after drug is stopped.
● Advise patient that urine will appear red for 1 to 2 days after the dose and doesn't indicate bleeding. The urine may stain clothes.
● Instruct patient not to receive immunizations during therapy and for several weeks after. Other members of the patient's household should also not receive immunizations during the same period.
● Tell patient to call prescriber if unusual bruising or bleeding or signs of an infection occur.

doxorubicin hydrochloride liposomal
Doxil

Pharmacologic classification: anthracycline
Therapeutic classification: antineoplastic
Pregnancy risk category: D

Indications and dosages
➤ *Metastatic carcinoma of the ovary in patients with disease that is refractory to both paclitaxel- and platinum-based chemotherapy regimens. Adults:* 50 mg/m² (doxorubicin hydrochloride equivalent) I.V. at 1 mg/minute once every 4 weeks for a minimum of 4 courses. Continue treatment as long as the patient doesn't progress, shows no evidence of cardiotoxicity, and continues to tolerate treatment. If no infusion-related adverse events are observed, increase infusion rate to complete administration over 1 hour.
➤ *AIDS-related Kaposi's sarcoma in patients with disease that has progressed on prior combination chemotherapy or in patients who are intolerant to such therapy. Adults:* 20 mg/m² (doxorubicin hydrochloride equivalent) I.V. over 30 minutes,

once every 3 weeks, for as long as patients respond satisfactorily and tolerate treatment.

✦ *Dosage adjustment.* For patients with impaired hepatic function, reduce dosage as follows: If serum bilirubin is 1.2 to 3 mg/dl give ½ normal dose; if serum bilirubin is over 3 mg/dl give ¼ normal dose.

The dose modifications shown in the tables on the next page are recommended for managing palmar-plantar erythrodysesthesia, hematologic toxicity, and stomatitis.

How supplied
Available by prescription only
Injection: 2 mg/ml

Pharmacodynamics
Antineoplastic action: Doxorubicin hydrochloride liposomal is doxorubicin hydrochloride encapsulated in liposomes which, due to their small size and persistence in the circulation, are able to penetrate the altered vasculature of tumors. The mechanism of action of doxorubicin hydrochloride is thought to be related to its ability to bind DNA and inhibit nucleic acid synthesis.

The mechanism of action of the drug, which consists of doxorubicin hydrochloride encapsulated in liposomes, is thought to be related to its ability to bind DNA and inhibit nucleic acid synthesis.

Pharmacokinetics
Absorption: Administered I.V.
Distribution: Distributed mostly to vascular fluid. Plasma protein–binding hasn't been determined; however, the plasma protein–binding of doxorubicin is about 70%.
Metabolism: Doxorubicinol, the major metabolite of doxorubicin, is detected at very low levels in the plasma.
Excretion: Plasma elimination is slow and is described as biphasic, with a half-life of about 5 hours in the first phase and 55 hours in the second phase at doses of 10 to 20 mg/m².

Route	Onset	Peak	Duration
I.V.	Unknown	Unknown	Unknown

Contraindications and precautions
Contraindicated in patients with a history of hypersensitivity reactions to the conventional formulation of doxorubicin hydrochloride or any component in the liposomal formulation. Also, contraindicated in patients with marked myelosuppression or those who have received a lifetime cumulative dosage of 550 mg/m² or 400 mg/m² who have received radiotherapy to the mediastinal area or concomitant therapy with other cardiotoxic agents, such as cyclophosphamide. Use in patients with a history of cardiovascular disease only when the benefit of the drug outweighs the risk to the patient.

Use cautiously in patients who have received other anthracyclines. The total dose of doxorubicin hydrochloride administered to the individual patient should also take into account any previous or concomitant therapy with related compounds such as daunorubicin. Heart failure and cardiomyopathy may be encountered after discontinuation of therapy.

Interactions
None reported; however, doxorubicin hydrochloride liposomal may interact with drugs known to interact with the conventional formulation of doxorubicin hydrochloride.

Adverse reactions
CNS: *asthenia,* paresthesia, headache, somnolence, dizziness, depression, insomnia, anxiety, malaise, emotional lability, fatigue.
CV: chest pain, hypotension, tachycardia, peripheral edema, cardiomyopathy, *heart failure, arrhythmias,* pericardial effusion.
EENT: pharyngitis, rhinitis, conjunctivitis, retinitis, optic neuritis.
GI: *mucous membrane disorder,* mouth ulceration, *nausea, vomiting, constipation, anorexia, diarrhea,* abdominal pain, dyspepsia, oral candidiasis, enlarged abdomen, esophagitis, dysphagia, *stomatitis,* taste perversion, glossitis.
GU: albuminuria.
Hematologic: LEUKOPENIA, NEUTROPENIA, THROMBOCYTOPENIA, *anemia,* increased PT.
Hepatic: hyperbilirubinemia.
Metabolic: dehydration, weight loss, hypocalcemia, hyperglycemia.
Musculoskeletal: myalgia, back pain.
Respiratory: dyspnea, increased cough, pneumonia.
Skin: *rash, alopecia,* dry skin, pruritus, skin discoloration, skin disorder, exfoliative, sweating, *palmar-plantar erythrodysesthesia,* alopecia.
Other: dermatitis, herpes zoster, fever, allergic reaction, chills, infection, infusion-related reactions.

Overdose and treatment
Acute overdose with doxorubicin hydrochloride increases mucositis, leukopenia, and thrombocytopenia.

Treatment of acute overdose consists of treatment of the severely myelosuppressed patient with hospitalization, antibiotics, platelet and granulocyte transfusions, and symptomatic treatment of mucositis.

Special considerations
● Patient's hepatic function must be evaluated before therapy, and dosage adjusted accordingly.
⚑ **ALERT** Doxorubicin hydrochloride liposomal exhibits unique pharmacokinetic properties compared to conventional doxorubicin hydrochloride and shouldn't be substituted on a mg per mg basis.
● Follow procedures for proper handling and disposal of antineoplastic drugs.

Managing palmar-plantar erythrodysesthesia

Grade	Symptoms	Dosage adjustment
1	Mild erythema, swelling, or desquamation not interfering with daily activities	No change needed unless patient has experienced a previous grade 3 or 4 skin toxicity. If so, delay up to 2 weeks and decrease dose by 25%. Return to original dose interval.
2	Erythema, desquamation, or swelling interfering with, but not precluding, normal physical activities; small blisters or ulcerations less than 2 cm in diameter	Delay dosing up to 2 weeks or until resolved to grade 0-1. If after 2 weeks there's no resolution, discontinue drug.
3	Blistering, ulceration, or swelling interfering with walking or normal daily activities; can't wear regular clothing	Delay dosing up to 2 weeks or until resolved to grade 0-1. Decrease dose by 25% and return to original dose interval. If after 2 weeks there's no resolution, discontinue drug.
4	Diffuse or local process causing infectious complications, or a bedridden state or hospitalization	Delay dosing up to 2 weeks or until resolved to grade 0-1. Decrease dose by 25% and return to original dose interval. If after 2 weeks there's no resolution, discontinue drug.

Managing hematologic toxicity

Grade	ANC (cells/mm³)	Platelets (cells/mm³)	Dosage adjustment
1	1500 - 1900	75,000 - 150,000	Resume treatment with no dose reduction.
2	1000 - < 1500	50,000 - < 75,000	Wait until ANC > 1,500 and platelets > 75,000; redose with no dose reduction.
3	500 - 999	25,000 - < 50,000	Wait until ANC ≥ 1,500 and platelets ≥ 75,000; redose with no dose reduction.
4	< 500	< 25,000	Wait until ANC ≥ 1,500 and platelets ≥ 75,000; redose at 25% dose reduction or continue full dose with cytokine support.

Managing stomatitis

Grade	Symptoms	Dosage adjustment
1	Painless ulcers, erythema, or mild soreness	No change needed unless patient has experienced previous grade 3 or 4 toxicity. If so, delay up to 2 weeks and decrease dose by 25%. Return to original dose interval.
2	Painful erythema, edema, or ulcers, but can eat	Delay dosing up to 2 weeks or until resolved to grade 0-1. If after 2 weeks there's no resolution, discontinue drug.
3	Painful erythema, edema, or ulcers, and can't eat	Delay dosing up to 2 weeks or until resolved to grade 0-1. Decrease dose by 25% and return to original dose interval. If after 2 weeks there's no resolution, discontinue drug.
4	Requires parenteral or enteral support	Delay dosing up to 2 weeks or until resolved to grade 0-1. Decrease dose by 25% and return to original dose interval. If after 2 weeks there's no resolution, discontinue drug.

• Dilute appropriate dose (up to a maximum of 90 mg) in 250 ml of D₅W using aseptic technique. Refrigerate diluted solution at 36° to 46° F (2° to 8° C) and administer within 24 hours.

⚠ **ALERT** Carefully check the label on the I.V. bag before administering. Accidental substitution of doxorubicin hydrochloride liposomal for conventional doxorubicin hydrochloride has resulted in severe side effects.

• Don't use with in-line filters.

• Infuse drug I.V. over 30 to 60 minutes depending on the dose; carefully monitor the patient during infusion. Acute infusion-associated reactions (flushing, shortness of breath, facial swelling, headache, chills, back pain, tightness in the chest or throat, or hypotension) may occur. These reactions resolve over several hours to a day once the infusion is stopped. The reaction may resolve by slowing the infusion rate.

• Don't give I.M. or S.C. Avoid extravasation. If signs or symptoms of extravasation occur, stop the I.V. infusion immediately and restart in another vein. The application of ice over the site of extravasation for about 30 minutes may be helpful in alleviating the local reaction.

Patient monitoring

• Drug may potentiate the toxicity of other antineoplastic therapies.

• Monitor cardiac function closely by endomyocardial biopsy, echocardiography, or gated radionuclide scans. If results indicate possible cardiac injury, the benefit of continued therapy must be weighed against the risk of myocardial injury.

• Monitor CBC, including platelets, before each dose and frequently throughout therapy. Leukopenia is usually transient. Hematologic toxicity may require dose reduction or suspension or delay of therapy. Persistent severe myelosuppression may result in superinfection or hemorrhage. Patient may require G-CSF (or GM-CSF) to support blood counts.

Breast-feeding patients

• It isn't known whether drug appears in breast milk. Because many drugs are excreted in breast milk and because of the potential for serious adverse reactions in nursing infants, women should discontinue nursing before taking this drug.

Pediatric patients

• Safety and effectiveness in children haven't been established.

Geriatric patients

• No overall differences were observed between elderly and younger subjects, but greater sensitivity in some older individuals can't be ruled out.

Patient education

• Tell patient to report symptoms of hand-foot syndrome such as tingling or burning, redness, flaking, bothersome swelling, small blisters, or small sores on the palms of hands or soles of feet.

• Advise patient to report symptoms of stomatitis such as painful redness, swelling, or sores in the mouth.

• Advise patient to avoid exposure to people with infections. Tell patient to report temperature of 100.5° F (38° C) or higher.

• Inform patient to report nausea, vomiting, tiredness, weakness, rash, or mild hair loss.

• Advise women of childbearing age to avoid pregnancy during therapy.

---

doxycycline
Vibramycin

doxycycline calcium
Vibramycin

doxycycline hyclate
Doryx, Doxy 100, Doxy 200, Doxy Caps, Vibramycin, Vibra-Tabs

doxycycline monohydrate
Monodox, Vibramycin

Pharmacologic classification: tetracycline
Therapeutic classification: antibiotic
Pregnancy risk category: D

Indications and dosages

➤ *Infections caused by sensitive organisms.* **Adults and children who weigh 45 kg (99 lb) and over:** 100 mg P.O. q 12 hours on day 1; then 100 mg P.O. daily. Or, 200 mg I.V. on day 1 in one or two infusions; then 100 to 200 mg I.V. daily.

Children over age 8 who weigh less than 45 kg: 4.4 mg/kg P.O. or I.V. daily, divided q 12 hours day 1; then 2.2 to 4.4 mg/kg daily.

➤ *Gonorrhea in patients allergic to penicillin.* **Adults:** 100 mg P.O. b.i.d. for 7 days; or 300 mg P.O. initially and repeat dose in 1 hour.

➤ *Syphilis in patients allergic to penicillin.* **Adults:** 100 mg P.O. b.i.d. for 2 weeks (early detection) or 4 weeks (if more than 1 year's duration).

➤ **Chlamydia trachomatis,** *nongonococcal* *urethritis,* **and** *uncomplicated urethral,* *endocervical, or rectal infections.* **Adults:** 100 mg P.O. b.i.d. for at least 7 days.

➤ *Acute pelvic inflammatory disease (PID).* **Adults:** 250 mg I.M. ceftriaxone, followed by 100 mg doxycycline P.O. b.i.d. for 10 to 14 days.

➤ *Acute epididymoorchitis caused by* C. **trachomatis** *or* **Neisseria gonorrhoeae.** **Adults:** 100 mg P.O. b.i.d for at least 10 days.

➤ *Prevention of traveler's diarrhea commonly caused by enterotoxigenic* **Esche-**

---

richia coli. *Adults:* 100 mg P.O. daily for up to 3 days.

➤ *Prophylaxis for rape victims*◊. *Adults and adolescents:* 100 mg P.O. b.i.d. for 7 days after a single 2-g oral dose of metronidazole is given in conjunction with a single 125-mg I.M. dose of ceftriaxone.

➤ *Chemoprophylaxis for malaria in travelers to areas where chloroquine-resistant Plasmodium falciparum is endemic and mefloquine is contraindicated*◊. *Adults:* 100 mg P.O. once daily. Begin prophylaxis 1 to 2 days before travel to malarious areas; continue daily while in affected area, and continue for 4 weeks after return from malarious area.
Children over age 8: Give 2 mg/kg P.O. daily as a single dose; don't exceed 100 mg daily. Use the same dosage schedule as for adults.

➤ *Lyme disease*◊. *Adults and children age 9 and older:* 100 mg P.O. b.i.d. or t.i.d. for 10 to 30 days.

➤ *Pleural effusions related to cancer*◊. *Adults:* 500 mg of doxycycline diluted in 250 ml of normal saline and instilled into pleural space via a chest tube.

➤ *Trachoma. Adults:* 2.5 to 4 mg/kg P.O. once daily for 36 to 40 days.

How supplied
Available by prescription only
doxycycline calcium
Oral suspension: 50 mg/5 ml
doxycycline hyclate
Capsules: 50 mg
Capsules (delayed-release): 100 mg
Injection: 100 mg, 200 mg
Tablets (film-coated): 100 mg
doxycycline monohydrate
Capsules: 50 mg, 100 mg
Oral suspension: 25 mg/5 ml

Pharmacodynamics
Antibacterial action: Doxycycline is bacteriostatic; it binds reversibly to ribosomal units, thereby inhibiting bacterial protein synthesis.

Spectrum of activity of the drug includes many gram-negative and gram-positive organisms, *Mycoplasma, Rickettsia, Chlamydia,* and spirochetes.

Pharmacokinetics
Absorption: About 90% to 100% is absorbed after oral administration. Doxycycline has the least affinity for calcium of all tetracyclines; its absorption is insignificantly altered by milk or other dairy products.
Distribution: Distributed widely into body tissues and fluids, including synovial, pleural, prostatic, and seminal fluids; bronchial secretions; saliva; and aqueous humor. CSF penetration is poor. Doxycycline readily crosses the placenta, and is 25% to 93% protein-bound.
Metabolism: Insignificantly metabolized; some hepatic degradation occurs.

Excretion: Excreted primarily unchanged in urine by glomerular filtration; some may be excreted in breast milk. Plasma half-life is 22 to 24 hours after multiple dosing in adults with normal renal function; 20 to 30 hours in patients with severe renal impairment. Some drug is excreted in feces.

Route	Onset	Peak	Duration
P.O.	Unknown	1½-4 hr	Unknown
I.V.	Immediate	Unknown	Unknown

Contraindications and precautions
Contraindicated in patients hypersensitive to drug or other tetracyclines. Use cautiously in patients with impaired renal or hepatic function. Use during last half of pregnancy and in children under age 8 may cause permanent discoloration of teeth, enamel defects, and bone growth retardation.

Interactions
Drug-drug. *Antacids containing aluminum, calcium, or magnesium or laxatives containing magnesium; oral iron products, sodium bicarbonate, zinc:* Decreased absorption of oral doxycycline. Give antibiotic 1 hour before or 2 hours after these drugs.
Carbamazepine, phenobarbital: Decreased antibiotic effect. Avoid use together.
Digoxin: Increased bioavailability. Monitor serum digoxin levels. Lowered dosages of digoxin may be needed.
Methoxyflurane: Nephrotoxicity with tetracyclines. Monitor serum levels carefully.
Oral anticoagulants: Increased anticoagulant effect. Monitor PT and INR and adjust dose as needed.
Oral contraceptives: Decreased contraceptive effectiveness and increased risk of breakthrough bleeding. Advise a nonhormonal form of birth control.
Penicillin: May antagonize bactericidal effects. Administer penicillin 2 to 3 hours before tetracycline.
Drug-lifestyle. *Alcohol use:* May decrease antibiotic effect. Discourage use together.
Sun exposure: May cause photosensitivity reactions. Patient should take precautions.

Adverse reactions
CNS: *intracranial hypertension (pseudotumor cerebri).*
CV: pericarditis, thrombophlebitis.
EENT: glossitis, dysphagia.
GI: anorexia, *epigastric distress, nausea,* vomiting, *diarrhea,* oral candidiasis, enterocolitis, anogenital inflammation.
Hematologic: *neutropenia,* eosinophilia, *thrombocytopenia,* hemolytic anemia.
Hepatic: elevated liver enzyme levels.
Skin: *maculopapular and erythematous rashes, photosensitivity, increased pigmentation, urticaria.*

Other: *hypersensitivity reactions (anaphylaxis)*, permanent discoloration of teeth, enamel defects, bone growth retardation if used in children under age 8, superinfection.

Overdose and treatment
Signs and symptoms of overdose are usually limited to the GI tract; give antacids or empty stomach by gastric lavage if ingestion occurred within the preceding 4 hours.

Special considerations
● Doxycycline causes false-negative results in urine tests using glucose oxidase reagent (Diastix, Chemstrip uG, or glucose enzymatic test strip); parenteral dosage form may cause false-negative Clinitest results.
● Doxycycline also causes false elevations in fluorometric tests for urinary catecholamines.
ALERT Don't confuse doxycycline with doxylamine or dicyclomine.
ALERT Check expiration date. Outdated or deteriorated tetracyclines have been linked to reversible nephrotoxicity (Fanconi's syndrome).
● Reconstitute powder for injection with sterile water for injection. Use 10 ml in a 100-mg vial and 20 ml in a 200-mg vial. Dilute solution to 100 to 1,000 ml for I.V. infusion. Don't infuse solutions more concentrated than 1 mg/ml.
● Reconstituted solution is stable for 72 hours if refrigerated and protected from light.
● Give I.V. infusion slowly (minimum 1 hour). Infusion must be completed within 12 hours (within 6 hours in lactated Ringer's solution or D₅W in lactated Ringer's solution).
● Drug may not be given S.C. or I.M.
● Drug may be used in patients with impaired renal function; it doesn't accumulate or cause a significant rise in BUN levels.

Patient monitoring
● With larger doses or prolonged therapy, watch for superinfection, especially in high-risk patients.
● Tell patient to check tongue for fungal infection. Stress good oral hygiene.

Breast-feeding patients
● Avoid use in breast-feeding women.

Pediatric patients
● Avoid use of drug in children under age 8 unless other drugs prove ineffective or are contraindicated.

Patient education
● Instruct patient to take entire amount of medication as prescribed, even if he feels better.
● Tell patient to take oral form of medication with food or milk if GI upset occurs.

dronabinol
Marinol

Pharmacologic classification: cannabinoid
Therapeutic classification: antiemetic, appetite stimulant
Controlled substance schedule: III
Pregnancy risk category: C

Indications and dosages
➤ *Nausea and vomiting caused by chemotherapy.* Adults and children: 5 mg/m² P.O. 1 to 3 hours before chemotherapy; then same dose q 2 to 4 hours after chemotherapy for a total of 4 to 6 doses daily. Dose may be increased in increments of 2.5 mg/m² to maximum of 15 mg/m² per dose.
➤ *Appetite stimulation in treatment of anorexia caused by AIDS-related weight loss.* Adults: 2.5 mg P.O. b.i.d. before lunch and supper, increased, if necessary, to a maximum of 20 mg daily.

How supplied
Available by prescription only
Capsules: 2.5 mg, 5 mg, 10 mg

Pharmacodynamics
Antiemetic action: A synthetic cannabinoid that inhibits vomiting centers in the brain and possibly in the chemoreceptor trigger zone and other sites.

Pharmacokinetics
Absorption: 90% to 95% of dose absorbed; action begins in 30 to 60 minutes, with peak action in 2 to 4 hours.
Distribution: Distributed rapidly into many tissue sites. 97% to 99% protein-bound.
Metabolism: Extensive metabolism in liver. Metabolite activity unknown.
Excretion: Excreted primarily in feces via biliary tract. Drug effect may persist for several days after treatment ends; duration varies considerably among patients.

Route	Onset	Peak	Duration
P.O.	30-60 min	2-4 hr	Unknown

Contraindications and precautions
Contraindicated in patients hypersensitive to sesame oil or cannabinoids. Use cautiously in elderly, pregnant, or breast-feeding patients and in those with heart disease, psychiatric illness, or history of drug abuse.

Interactions
Drug-drug. *Anticholinergics:* May cause tachycardia. Monitor patient closely.
Psychotomimetic drugs, sedatives: Concomitant use may have additive sedative effect. Use cautiously; monitor patient closely.

Drug-lifestyle. *Alcohol use:* May cause additive sedative effect. Discourage use.

Adverse reactions

CNS: *dizziness, drowsiness, euphoria, ataxia,* depersonalization, hallucinations, somnolence, headache, muddled thinking, asthenia, amnesia, confusion, *paranoia.*
CV: tachycardia, orthostatic hypotension, palpitations, vasodilation.
EENT: visual disturbances.
GI: *dry mouth, nausea, vomiting,* diarrhea.

Overdose and treatment

Treat overdose with symptomatic and supportive therapy. Observe patient in quiet environment and provide supportive measures including reassurance.

Special considerations

● Drug is used only in patients with nausea and vomiting resulting from cancer chemotherapy who don't respond to other treatment; give drug before chemotherapy infusion.
● Drug is major active ingredient of *Cannabis sativa* (marijuana); has potential for abuse.

Patient monitoring

● Monitor frequency and degree of vomiting.
● Monitor pulse, blood pressure, and fluid intake and output to help prevent dehydration; observe for signs of confusion.

Breast-feeding patients

● Because drug appears in breast milk and is absorbed by breast-feeding infants, it shouldn't be given to breast-feeding women.

Geriatric patients

● Elderly patients may be more susceptible to adverse reactions. Use cautiously.

Patient education

● Warn patient to avoid driving and other activities requiring sound judgment until extent of CNS depressant effects are known.
● Urge family to ensure that patient is supervised by a responsible person during and immediately after treatment.
● Caution patient and family to anticipate drug's mood-altering effects.

---

droperidol
Inapsine

Pharmacologic classification: butyrophenone derivative
Therapeutic classification: tranquilizer
Pregnancy risk category: C

Indications and dosages
➤ *Delirium. Adults:* 5 mg I.M., p.r.n. It's given for its quick onset and sedative quality.

➤ *Anesthetic premedication. Adults:* 2.5 to 10 mg I.M. 30 to 60 minutes before induction of general anesthesia.
Children ages 2 to 12: 0.088 to 0.165 mg/kg I.V. or I.M.
➤ *Adjunct for induction of general anesthesia. Adults:* 0.22 to 0.275 mg/kg I.V. (preferably) or I.M. with an analgesic or general anesthetic.
Children: 0.088 to 0.165 mg/kg I.V. or I.M.
➤ *Adjunct for maintenance of general anesthesia. Adults:* 1.25 to 2.5 mg I.V.
➤ *For use without a general anesthetic during diagnostic procedures. Adults:* 2.5 to 10 mg I.M. 30 to 60 minutes before the procedure. Additional doses of 1.25 to 2.5 mg I.V. are given, p.r.n.
➤ *Adjunct to regional anesthesia. Adults:* 2.5 to 5 mg I.M. or slow I.V. injection.
➤ *Antiemetic in conjunction with chemotherapy* ◇. *Adults:* 6.25 mg I.M. or by slow I.V. injection.

How supplied
Available by prescription only
Injection: 2.5 mg/ml

Pharmacodynamics
Tranquilizer action: Droperidol produces marked sedation by directly blocking subcortical receptors. Droperidol also blocks CNS receptors at the chemoreceptor trigger zone, producing an antiemetic effect.

Pharmacokinetics
Absorption: Well absorbed after I.M. injection. Some alteration of consciousness may persist for 12 hours.
Distribution: Not well understood; drug crosses the blood-brain barrier and is distributed in the CSF. It also crosses the placenta.
Metabolism: Metabolized by the liver to *p*-fluorophenylacetic acid and *p*-hydroxypiperidine.
Excretion: Excreted in urine and feces.

Route	Onset	Peak	Duration
I.V., I.M.	3-10 min	½ hr	2-4 hr

Contraindications and precautions
Contraindicated in patients hypersensitive to drug or intolerant of it. Use cautiously in patients with hypotension and other CV disease because of its vasodilatory effects, in patients with hepatic or renal disease in whom drug clearance may be impaired, and in patients taking other CNS depressants, including alcohol, opiates, and sedatives, because droperidol may potentiate the effects of these drugs.

Interactions
Drug-drug. *Fentanyl citrate:* May cause hypertension and respiratory depression. Avoid use together if possible.

Opiates, other analgesics, other CNS depressants, such as barbiturates, tranquilizers, and sedative-hypnotics: Additive CNS depression. When used together, reduce dosage of both drugs.
Drug-lifestyle. *Alcohol use:* Drug potentiates CNS depressant effects. Advise patient to avoid alcohol.

Adverse reactions

CNS: *sedation,* altered consciousness, postoperative hallucinations, extrapyramidal reactions, temporarily altered EEG pattern.
CV: *hypotension* with rebound tachycardia, **bradycardia**, decreased pulmonary artery pressure.
Respiratory: *respiratory depression.*

Overdose and treatment

Signs and symptoms of overdose include extensions of the pharmacologic actions of the drug. Treat an overdose symptomatically and supportively.

Special considerations

◤ **ALERT** Discontinue drug if patient shows signs of hypersensitivity, severe persistent hypotension, respiratory depression, paradoxical hypertension, or dystonia.
● Have fluids and other measures to manage hypotension readily available.
● Droperidol has been used for its antiemetic effects in preventing or treating chemotherapy-induced nausea and vomiting, especially that produced by cisplatin.

Patient monitoring

● Vital signs must be monitored and patient observed for extrapyramidal reactions. Droperidol is related to haloperidol and is more likely than other antipsychotics to cause extrapyramidal symptoms.
● Observe patient for postoperative hallucinations or emergence delirium and drowsiness.

Breast-feeding patients

● It isn't known whether droperidol appears in breast milk.

Pediatric patients

● Safety and efficacy in children under age 2 haven't been established.

Geriatric patients

● Use drug cautiously. Geriatric patients are more prone to extrapyramidal reactions, CNS disturbances, and CV side effects.

Patient education

● Advise patient of possible postoperative effects.
● Warn patient to rise slowly to prevent orthostatic hypotension.

Reactions may be *common,* uncommon, *life-threatening,* or COMMON AND LIFE-THREATENING.

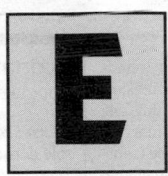

echothiophate iodide
Phospholine Iodide

Pharmacologic classification: cholinesterase inhibitor
Therapeutic classification: miotic
Pregnancy risk category: NR

Indications and dosages
➤ *Open-angle glaucoma, conditions obstructing aqueous outflow.* Adults and children: 1 drop of 0.03% to 0.125% solution into conjunctival sac daily. Maximum, 1 drop b.i.d. Use lowest possible dosage to continuously control intraocular pressure.
➤ *Diagnosis of convergent strabismus.* Adults: 1 drop of 0.125% solution daily h.s. for 2 to 3 weeks.
➤ *Treatment of convergent strabismus.* Adults: 1 drop of 0.03% to 0.125% solution daily or every other day h.s. Or, 1 drop of 0.06% solution daily.

How supplied
Available by prescription only
Ophthalmic: powder for reconstitution to make 0.03%, 0.06%, 0.125%, 0.25% solutions

Pharmacodynamics
Miotic action: Echothiophate reduces the enzymatic degradation of acetylcholine by inhibiting cholinesterase. Acetylcholine acts on the effector cells of the iridic sphincter and ciliary muscles, causing pupillary constriction and accommodation spasm.

Pharmacokinetics
Absorption: Unknown.
Distribution: Unknown.
Metabolism: Unknown.
Excretion: Duration of effect can be up to 1 week or longer.

Route	Onset	Peak	Duration
Oph-thalmic	10 min-8 hr	½-24 hr	Days-4 wk

Contraindications and precautions
Contraindicated in patients hypersensitive to drug or iodine and in patients with acute angle-closure glaucoma (before iridectomy) and other forms of glaucoma (except primary open-angle glaucoma). Use with extreme caution, if at all, in patients with seizure disorders, vasomotor insta-

bility, parkinsonism, bronchial asthma, spastic GI conditions, urinary tract obstruction, peptic ulcer, severe bradycardia or hypotension, vascular hypertension, MI, or history or risk of retinal detachment. Use cautiously in patients with corneal abrasion.

Interactions
Drug-drug. *Anticholinergics, belladonna alkaloids (such as atropine), cyclopentolate:* Antagonized miotic effects. Avoid concomitant use.
Cholinesterase inhibitors: Possible additive effect causing sytemic effects. Monitor patient closely.
Local anesthetics, ophthalmic tetracaine: May cause increased systemic toxicity and prolonged ocular anesthesia. Monitor patient closely.
Ophthalmic adrenocorticoids: May cause increased intraocular pressure and decreased antiglaucoma effectiveness. Avoid concomitant use.
Pilocarpine, systemic anticholinesterase drugs used for myasthenia gravis: Effects may be additive. Watch for signs of toxicity.
Succinylcholine: Respiratory and CV collapse. Don't use together.
Drug-lifestyle. *Cocaine use:* May increase risk of cocaine toxicity. Advise patient to avoid concomitant use.
Organophosphate insecticides (parathion, malathion): May have additive effects causing systemic effects. Tell at-risk patient to protect himself from exposure.

Adverse reactions
CNS: fatigue, muscle weakness, paresthesia, headache.
CV: *bradycardia,* flushing, hypotension.
EENT: ciliary spasm or spasm of eye accommodation, ciliary or circumcorneal injection, nonreversible cataract formation (time- and dose-related), reversible iris cysts, pupillary block, blurred or dimmed vision, eye or brow pain, twitching of eyelids, hyperemia, photophobia, lens opacities, lacrimation, retinal detachment.
GI: diarrhea, nausea, vomiting, abdominal pain, intestinal cramps, salivation.
GU: frequent urination.
Respiratory: *bronchoconstriction.*
Skin: diaphoresis.
Other: decreased plasma cholinesterase activity.

Overdose and treatment
Signs and symptoms of overdose include tremor, syncope, headache, bradycardia, hypotension, arrhythmias, diarrhea, nausea, vomiting, abdominal pain, excessive salivation, urinary incontinence, and dyspnea. Toxicity can be cumulative, with symptoms appearing weeks to months after initiating therapy.

To treat accidental overdose after ingestion, employ general measures, such as emesis, cathartics, or lavage to remove drug from the GI tract. Treat dermal exposure by washing the area twice with soap and water. The extent of echothiophate's potential toxicity isn't well known; observe patient closely for signs and symptoms, and treat symptomatically and supportively. Atropine sulfate (S.C., I.M., or I.V.) has been suggested as the antidote of choice.

Special considerations
• Echothiophate iodide is a potent, long-acting, irreversible drug.
• Reconstitute powder carefully to avoid contamination; use only diluent provided. Discard refrigerated, reconstituted solution after 6 months; discard room temperature solution after 1 month.
• Stop drug at least 2 weeks before surgery if succinylcholine will be used in surgery. Inform anesthesiologist.

Patient monitoring
• Monitor patient for evidence of toxicity. Toxicity is cumulative; toxic sytemic symptoms may not appear for weeks or months after start of therapy. Atropine sulfate S.C., I.M., or I.V. is antidote of choice.

Pediatric patients
• Safety and efficacy haven't been established; iris cysts have been reported, but they usually resolve spontaneously when drug is discontinued. Many ophthalmologists avoid using drug in children because of reports of lens opacities in adults.

Geriatric patients
• Elderly patients may have an increased risk of adverse reactions.

Patient education
• Warn patient that transient brow ache or dimmed or blurred vision is common at first but usually disappears in 5 to 10 days; advise instillation at bedtime to minimize effects of blurred vision.
• Tell patient or family to inform prescriber or anesthesiologist about use of drug before general anesthesia is administered.
• Teach patient correct use, storage, and reconstitution of product.

econazole nitrate
Spectazole

Pharmacologic classification: synthetic imidazole derivative
Therapeutic classification: antifungal
Pregnancy risk category: C

Indications and dosages
➤ *Cutaneous candidiasis. Adults and children:* Gently rub sufficient quantity into affected areas b.i.d. in the morning and evening.
➤ *Tinea pedis, tinea cruris, tinea corporis, and tinea versicolor. Adults and children:* Gently rub into affected area once daily.

How supplied
Available by prescription only
Cream: 1% (water-soluble base)

Pharmacodynamics
Antifungal action: Although exact mechanism of action is unknown, drug is thought to alter cellular membranes and interfere with intracellular enzymes. Econazole is active against many fungi, including dermatophytes and yeasts, as well as some gram-positive bacteria.

Pharmacokinetics
Absorption: Minimal but rapid percutaneous absorption.
Distribution: Minimal.
Metabolism: Unknown.
Excretion: Unknown.

Route	Onset	Peak	Duration
Topical	Unknown	Unknown	Unknown

Contraindications and precautions
Contraindicated in patients hypersensitive to drug.

Interactions
Drug-drug. *Corticosteroids:* May inhibit antifungal activity of econazole nitrate, in a concentration-dependent manner, in the treatment of *Saccharomyces cerevisiae* and *Candida albicans.* Avoid use together.

Adverse reactions
Skin: burning, pruritus, stinging, erythema.

Overdose and treatment
No information available. If a reaction suggesting sensitivity or chemical irritation occurs, discontinue therapy.

Special considerations
• Wash affected area with soap and water, and dry thoroughly before applying drug.

Patient monitoring
• Relief of symptoms usually occurs within 1 to 2 weeks of therapy.

Reactions may be *common*, uncommon, *life-threatening*, or COMMON AND LIFE-THREATENING.

Breast-feeding patients
● It isn't known whether drug appears in breast milk. Use cautiously in breast-feeding women.

Patient education
● Tell patient to wash hands well after application.
● Caution patient to use medication as directed for the entire period of treatment, even though symptoms may lessen.
● Instruct patient with tinea pedis to wear well-fitting, well-ventilated shoes, and to change all-cotton socks daily.

---

edetate calcium disodium (calcium EDTA)
Calcium Disodium Versenate

Pharmacologic classification: chelating drug
Therapeutic classification: heavy metal antagonist
Pregnancy risk category: NR

Indications and dosages
➤ *Acute lead encephalopathy or blood lead levels above 70 mcg/dl.* Adults and children: 1.5 g/m² I.V. or I.M. daily in divided doses q 12 hours for 3 to 5 days, usually with dimercaprol. Give second course in 5 to 7 days, if necessary.
➤ *Lead poisoning without encephalopathy or asymptomatic with blood levels below 70 mcg/dl.* Children: 1 g/m² I.V. or I.M. daily in divided doses.
➤ *Other heavy metal poisonings* ◇ *Adults:* 1 g in 500 ml of D₅W or normal saline injection infused I.V. over a 5-hour period once daily for 3 days.

How supplied
Available by prescription only
Injection: 200 mg/ml

Pharmacodynamics
Chelating action: Calcium in edetate calcium disodium is displaced by divalent and trivalent heavy metals and forms a soluble complex that is excreted in urine, thus removing the heavy metal.

Pharmacokinetics
Absorption: Well absorbed after I.M. or S.C. injection. After I.V. administration, chelated lead appears in urine within 1 hour; excretion of lead peaks in 24 to 48 hours.
Distribution: Distributed primarily in extracellular fluid.
Metabolism: None.
Excretion: Excreted rapidly in urine. After I.V. administration, 50% of drug excreted in urine unchanged or as a metal chelate in 1 hour; 95% of drug excreted in 24 hours.

Route	Onset	Peak	Duration
I.V., I.M.	1 hr	24-48 hr	Unknown

Contraindications and precautions
Contraindicated in patients with anuria, hepatitis, and acute renal disease. Use with extreme caution in patients with mild renal disease.

Interactions
Drug-drug. *Zinc insulin:* Interference with action of insulin by binding with zinc. Monitor glucose levels; insulin dose may need adjustment.

Adverse reactions
CNS: tremor, headache, numbness, tingling, malaise, fatigue.
CV: hypotension, cardiac rhythm irregularities.
GI: cheilosis, nausea, vomiting, anorexia, thirst.
GU: proteinuria, hematuria, *nephrotoxicity with renal tubular necrosis leading to fatal nephrosis.*
Hematologic: transient bone marrow depression.
Hepatic: *mild increases in ALT and AST levels.*
Musculoskeletal: myalgia, arthralgia.
Other: pain at I.M. injection site, fever, chills.

Overdose and treatment
Signs and symptoms of overdose include acute renal failure with anuria and altered consciousness consistent with increased intracranial pressure in patients with lead encephalopathy.
Reduce intracranial pressure with hyperventilation and furosemide or mannitol; monitor vital signs and ECG closely. Barbiturate infusion may be needed in severe cases; hemodialysis may be needed in acute renal failure.

Special considerations
● Add 1% procaine or lidocaine to solution before I.M. injection to decrease pain at site.
● Avoid rapid I.V. infusion and infusions of large fluid volumes in patients with lead encephalopathy.
● Hydrate patients before giving drug to ensure adequate urine flow; monitor renal status frequently.
● Parenterally administered edetate calcium disodium has been used in poisoning by radioactive and nuclear fusion products and other heavy metals except mercury, gold, or arsenic poisoning. Has also been used to aid diagnosis of lead poisoning.
● For I.V. infusion, dilute drug with D₅W solution or normal saline solution; give one-half the daily dose over at least 1 hour in asymptomatic patients, 2 hours in symptomatic patients. The second daily infusion should be given 6 or more hours after the first. If administered as a single dose, infuse over 12 to 24 hours.
● If drug is given as a continuous I.V. infusion, interrupt infusion for at least 1 hour before a blood lead level reading to avoid a falsely elevated value.

Patient monitoring

● Monitor infusion site closely. Extravasation severely irritates tissue; rotate infusion sites with multiple doses or long-term therapy.

● Monitor calcium levels, and observe patient for seizures or altered vital signs and ECG during infusion. Administer infusion over at least 3 hours; have patient remain supine for 20 to 30 minutes after infusion because of possible orthostatic hypotension. Drug also exerts a negative inotropic effect on the heart.

● Monitor hepatic and renal function before treatment and periodically throughout.

● Monitor intake and output, urinalysis, BUN level, and ECG throughout treatment; interrupt I.V. for 1 hour before drawing blood.

Pediatric patients

● I.M. route is recommended for children.

Patient education

● Explain measures as needed to avoid future heavy metal poisoning.

---

edetate disodium (EDTA)
Disotate, Endrate

Pharmacologic classification: chelating drug
Therapeutic classification: heavy metal antagonist
Pregnancy risk category: NR

Indications and dosages

➤ *Hypercalcemia. Adults:* 50 mg/kg daily by slow I.V. infusion to a maximum of 3 g in 24 hours. Dilute in 500 ml of D_5W or normal saline solution. Give over 3 or more hours.
Children: 40 mg/kg by slow I.V. infusion, diluted to a maximum of 30 mg/ml in D_5W or normal saline solution and given over 3 or more hours. Maximum, 70 mg/kg daily.
➤ *Cardiac glycoside–induced ventricular arrhythmias. Adults and children:* I.V. infusion of 15 mg/kg/hour. Maximum, 60 mg/kg daily. Dilute in D_5W.

How supplied

Available by prescription only
Injection: 150 mg/ml

Pharmacodynamics

Chelating action: Binds many divalent and trivalent ions but has the strongest affinity for calcium, with which it forms a stable complex readily excreted by the kidneys. Also chelates magnesium, zinc, and other trace metals, increasing their excretion in urine; doesn't decrease CSF calcium levels.

Pharmacokinetics

Absorption: Administered I.V.

Distribution: Doesn't enter CSF in significant amounts but is distributed widely throughout rest of body.
Metabolism: None.
Excretion: After I.V. administration, is excreted rapidly in urine; 95% of dose excreted within 24 hours.

Route	Onset	Peak	Duration
I.V.	Unknown	Unknown	Unknown

Contraindications and precautions

Contraindicated in patients hypersensitive to drug and in those with anuria, known or suspected hypocalcemia, significant renal disease, active or healed tubercular lesions, or history of seizures or intracranial lesions.

Use cautiously in patients with limited cardiac reserve, heart failure, or hypokalemia.

Interactions

Drug-drug. *Cardiac glycosides:* Drug indirectly interferes with cardiac effects of cardiac glycosides by decreasing intracellular calcium via chelation and urinary excretion of extracellular calcium. Monitor patient.
Insulin: Requirements may be decreased by chelation of zinc in exogenous insulin. Monitor serum glucose levels.

Adverse reactions

CNS: circumoral paresthesia, numbness, headache, *seizures*.
CV: hypotension, thrombophlebitis.
GI: nausea, vomiting, diarrhea.
GU: *nephrotoxicity* with urinary urgency, nocturia, dysuria, polyuria, proteinuria, renal insufficiency, *acute renal failure, acute tubular necrosis*.
Hepatic: decreased serum alkaline phosphatase levels.
Metabolic: *severe hypocalcemia,* decreased magnesium level, hypoglycemia.
Skin: exfoliative dermatitis, erythema.
Other: pain at infusion site, extravasation.

Overdose and treatment

Effects of overdose include hypotension, arrhythmias, and cardiac arrest.

Treat hypotension with fluids, if necessary. Treat arrhythmias with lidocaine and seizures and tetany with calcium replacement. Use I.V. diazepam for refractory seizures. Replace magnesium and potassium as necessary.

Special considerations

● Don't exceed recommended rate of infusion or dosage; rapid infusion or high levels of edetate disodium may greatly decrease serum calcium levels, causing seizures and death. Have I.V. calcium replacement readily available whenever drug is given.

● Drug also has been used topically or by iontophoresis to treat corneal calcium deposits.

Reactions may be *common,* uncommon, *life-threatening*, or COMMON AND LIFE-THREATENING.

Patient monitoring
• Monitor serum calcium and potassium levels before treatment.
• Monitor infusion site closely. Extravasation severely irritates tissue; rotate infusion sites with multiple doses or long-term therapy.
• Monitor infusion rate. Don't exceed recommended rate of infusion or dosage.
• Monitor serum calcium level, ECG, and vital signs continuously throughout therapy.
• Monitor serum glucose level if patient is diabetic.

Pediatric patients
• Give recommended dose slowly, over at least 3 hours.

Geriatric patients
• Elderly patients with renal or cardiac failure are at increased risk; lower doses are recommended.

Patient education
• Explain possible adverse reactions; stress importance of reporting signs and symptoms promptly.
• Tell diabetic patient that insulin dosage may need adjustment.

---

edrophonium chloride
Enlon, Reversol, Tensilon

Pharmacologic classification: cholinesterase inhibitor
Therapeutic classification: cholinergic agonist, diagnostic
Pregnancy risk category: NR

Indications and dosages
➤ **Curare antagonist (to reverse neuromuscular blocking action).** *Adults:* 10 mg I.V. over 30 to 45 seconds, repeated p.r.n. to 40-mg maximum dose. Larger doses may potentiate rather than antagonize effect of curare.
➤ **Diagnostic aid in myasthenia gravis.** *Adults:* 2 mg I.V. within 15 to 30 seconds; then 8 mg if no response (increased muscular strength) occurs. Or, 10 mg I.M. If cholinergic reaction occurs, 2 mg I.M. 30 minutes later to rule out false-negative response.
Children who weigh more than 34 kg (75 lb): 2 mg I.V. If no response within 45 seconds, give 1 mg q 45 seconds to maximum dose of 10 mg. Or, 5 mg I.M.
Children who weigh 34 kg or less: 1 mg I.V. If no response within 45 seconds, give 1 mg q 45 seconds to maximum dose of 5 mg. Or, 2 mg I.M.
Infants: 0.5 mg I.V.
➤ **To differentiate myasthenic crisis from cholinergic crisis.** *Adults:* 1 mg I.V. If no response in 1 minute, repeat dose once. Increased muscle strength confirms myasthenic crisis; no increase or exaggerated weakness confirms cholinergic crisis.

➤ **Tensilon test for evaluating treatment requirements in myasthenia gravis.** *Adults:* 1 to 2 mg I.V. 1 hour after oral intake of drug being used in treatment. Response will be myasthenic in the undertreated patient, adequate in the controlled patient, and cholinergic in the overtreated patient.
➤ **To terminate paroxysmal atrial tachycardia or as an aid in diagnosing supraventricular tachyarrhythmias and evaluating the function of demand pacemakers** ◊. *Adults:* 10 mg I.V. over 5 minutes.
✦ **Dosage adjustment.** In elderly or digitalized adults, 5 to 7 mg I.V. over 5 minutes.
➤ **To slow supraventricular tachyarrhythmias unresponsive to a cardiac glycoside** ◊. *Adults:* 2 mg/minute I.V. test dose, followed by 2 mg q minute until a total dose of 10 mg is given. If heart rate decreases in response to this dose, infusion of 0.25 mg/minute may be started; infusion may be increased to 2 mg/minute if necessary.

How supplied
Available by prescription only
Injection: 10 mg/ml in 1-ml ampule, 10-ml vial, 15-ml vial

Pharmacodynamics
Cholinergic action: Edrophonium blocks hydrolysis of acetylcholine by cholinesterase, resulting in acetylcholine accumulation at cholinergic synapses. This leads to increased cholinergic receptor stimulation at the neuromuscular junction and vagal sites. Edrophonium is a short-acting drug, which makes it particularly useful for diagnosing myasthenia gravis.

Pharmacokinetics
Absorption: No information available.
Distribution: Not clearly identified.
Metabolism: Exact metabolic fate is unknown; drug isn't hydrolyzed by cholinesterases.
Excretion: Exact excretion mode is unknown.

Route	Onset	Peak	Duration
I.V.	< 1 min	Unknown	5-20 min
I.M.	2-10 min	Unknown	10-30 min

Contraindications and precautions
Contraindicated in patients hypersensitive to anticholinesterase agents and in those with mechanical obstruction of the intestine or urinary tract. Use cautiously in patients with bronchial asthma or arrhythmias.

Interactions
Drug-drug. *Aminoglycosides, anesthetics:* Prolonged or enhanced muscle weakness. Use together cautiously.
Cardiac glycosides: Increased cardiac sensitivity to edrophonium. Use together cautiously.
Cholinergic drugs: Additive toxicity. Avoid use together.

◊ Unlabeled clinical use

Corticosteroids: Decreased cholinergic effects of edrophonium; when corticosteroids are stopped, cholinergic effects may increase, possibly affecting muscle strength. Watch for lack of drug effect.

Ganglionic blockers such as mecamylamine: May lead to a critical blood pressure decrease. Avoid use together.

Magnesium: Direct depressant effect on skeletal muscle. Avoid use together.

Procainamide, quinidine: May reverse cholinergic effect of edrophonium on muscle. Use together cautiously.

Succinylcholine: Prolonged respiratory depression from plasma esterase inhibition. Avoid use together.

Drug-herb. *Jaborandi tree, pill-bearing spurge:* Additive effect and increased risk of toxicity. Tell patient to use cautiously.

Adverse reactions

CNS: *seizures,* weakness.
CV: hypotension, ***bradycardia, AV block, cardiac arrest***.
EENT: excessive lacrimation, diplopia, miosis, conjunctival hyperemia.
GI: nausea, vomiting, *diarrhea, abdominal cramps,* dysphagia, excessive salivation.
GU: urinary frequency, incontinence.
Musculoskeletal: dysarthria, muscle cramps, muscle fasciculation.
Respiratory: ***paralysis of muscles of respiration, central respiratory paralysis, bronchospasm, laryngospasm,*** increased bronchial secretions.
Skin: diaphoresis.

Overdose and treatment

Signs and symptoms of overdose include muscle weakness, nausea, vomiting, diarrhea, blurred vision, miosis, excessive tearing, bronchospasm, increased bronchial secretions, hypotension, incoordination, excessive sweating, cramps, fasciculations, paralysis, bradycardia or tachycardia, excessive salivation, and restlessness or agitation. Muscles first weakened by overdose include neck, jaw, and pharyngeal muscles, followed by muscle weakening of the shoulder, arms, pelvis, outer eye, and legs.

Discontinue drug immediately. Support respiration; bronchial suctioning may be performed. Atropine may be given to block the muscarinic effects of edrophonium but won't counter the paralytic effects of the drug on skeletal muscle. Avoid atropine overdose, because it may lead to bronchial plug formation.

Special considerations

● When giving edrophonium to differentiate myasthenic crisis from cholinergic crisis, evaluate patient's muscle strength closely.
● For easier administration, use a tuberculin syringe with an I.V. needle.

● Atropine sulfate injection should always be readily available as an antagonist for the muscarinic effects of edrophonium.

Patient monitoring
● Monitor patient for adverse reactions and for therapeutic effects.

Pregnant patients
● Drug may cause uterine irritability and induce premature labor when given I.V. to patients near term.

Breast-feeding patients
● Safety hasn't been established. Breast-feeding women should avoid edrophonium.

Pediatric patients
● Children may require I.M. administration; with this route, drug effects may be delayed for 2 to 10 minutes.

Geriatric patients
● Geriatric patients may be more sensitive to effects of this drug. Use cautiously.

Patient education
● Tell patient that the adverse effects of the drug will be transient because of its short duration of effect.

---

efavirenz
Sustiva

Pharmacologic classification: nonnucleoside, reverse transcriptase inhibitor
Therapeutic classification: antiretroviral
Pregnancy risk category: C

Indications and dosages
➤**Treatment of HIV-1 infection.** *Adults:* 600 mg P.O. once daily with a protease inhibitor or with nucleoside analogue reverse transcriptase inhibitors.
Children age 3 and older who weigh 40 kg (88 lb) or more: 600 mg P.O. once daily with a protease inhibitor or with nucleoside analogue reverse transcriptase inhibitors.
Children age 3 and older who weigh 10 to 39 kg (22 to 87 lb): Give the following doses with a protease inhibitor or with nucleoside analogue reverse transcriptase inhibitors.
Children who weigh 10 to 14 kg (22 to 32 lb): 200 mg P.O. once daily.
Children who weigh 15 to 19 kg (33 to 43 lb): 250 mg P.O. once daily.
Children who weigh 20 to 24 kg (44 to 54 lb): 300 mg P.O. once daily.
Children who weigh 25 to 32 kg (55 to 71 lb): 350 mg P.O. once daily.
Children who weigh 33 to 39 kg (72 to 87 lb): 400 mg P.O. once daily.

How supplied
Available by prescription only
Capsules: 50 mg, 100 mg, 200 mg

Pharmacodynamics
Antiretroviral action: Efavirenz inhibits the transcription of HIV 1 RNA to DNA, a critical step in the viral replication process. Therefore, drug lowers the amount of HIV in the blood (the viral load) and increases CD4 lymphocytes.

Pharmacokinetics
Absorption: Relative bioavailability increased by about 50% when taken with a high-fat meal.
Distribution: Highly bound to plasma proteins (about 99.5% to 99.75%); also distributed into the cerebrospinal fluid.
Metabolism: Metabolized primarily by cytochrome P-450 3A4 and cytochrome P-450 2B6 to hydroxylated inactive metabolites.
Excretion: 14% to 34% is excreted in urine (less than 1% is excreted unchanged), and 16% to 61% is excreted in feces. Terminal elimination half-life is 52 to 76 hours.

Route	Onset	Peak	Duration
P.O.	Unknown	3-5 hr	Unknown

Contraindications and precautions
Contraindicated in patients hypersensitive to efavirenz or its components. Use cautiously in patients with hepatic impairment or in those concurrently receiving hepatotoxic medications.

Interactions
Drug-drug. *Clarithromycin, indinavir:* May decrease plasma levels. Consider alternative therapy or dosage adjustment.
Drugs that induce the cytochrome P-450 enzyme system (such as phenobarbital, rifabutin, rifampin): Increased efavirenz clearance and lower plasma levels. Avoid use together.
Ergot derivatives, midazolam, triazolam: Competition for cytochrome P-450 enzyme system may inhibit metabolism of these drugs and cause serious or life-threatening adverse events (such as arrhythmias, prolonged sedation, or respiratory depression). Avoid use together.
Oral contraceptives: Potential interaction hasn't been determined. Advise use of barrier contraception in addition to oral contraceptive.
Psychoactive drugs: May cause additive CNS effects. Avoid use together.
Ritonavir: Increased risk of adverse effects. Monitor patient.
Saquinavir: Decreased levels of both drugs. Don't use with saquinavir as sole protease inhibitor.
Warfarin: Altered warfarin levels and effects. Monitor INR.
Drug-food. *High-fat meals:* May increase absorption of drug. Instruct patient to follow a low-fat diet.
Drug-lifestyle. *Alcohol use:* Enhanced CNS effects. Discourage concurrent use.

Adverse reactions
CNS: abnormal dreams or thinking, agitation, amnesia, confusion, depersonalization, depression, *dizziness,* euphoria, fatigue, hallucinations, delusions, headache, hypoesthesia, impaired concentration, insomnia, somnolence, nervousness.
GI: abdominal pain, anorexia, *diarrhea,* dyspepsia, flatulence, *nausea,* vomiting, *pancreatitis.*
GU: hematuria, kidney stones.
Hepatic: increased AST, ALT, and total cholesterol levels.
Skin: increased sweating, *erythema multiforme, Stevens-Johnson syndrome, toxic epidermal necrolysis, rash,* pruritus.
Other: fever.

Overdose and treatment
Overdose may cause CNS symptoms and involuntary muscle contractions.

Treatment should involve supportive care, including frequent monitoring of vital signs and observation of clinical status. Activated charcoal may be given to aid in the removal of unabsorbed drug. Efavirenz is unlikely to be removed by hemodialysis.

Special considerations
● Give drug with other antiretrovirals because resistant viruses emerge rapidly when drug is used alone. Don't use drug as monotherapy or add it as a single agent to a failing regimen.
● Giving drug with ritonavir is more likely to cause adverse effects (such as dizziness, nausea, paresthesia) and laboratory abnormalities (elevated liver enzyme levels).

Patient monitoring
● Monitor liver function and cholesterol levels.
● Monitor patient for adverse reactions.

Pregnant patients
● Pregnancy must be ruled out before starting therapy in women of childbearing age.

Breast-feeding patients
● HIV-infected women shouldn't breast-feed their infants to avoid risking transmitting the disease. The drug appears in breast milk of animals. Instruct affected women not to nurse their infants.

Pediatric patients
● Children may be more prone to adverse reactions, especially diarrhea, nausea, vomiting, and rash.

Geriatric patients
● Geriatric patients may be more susceptible to CNS effects of drug.

Patient education
● Tell patient drug may be taken without regard to meals but should not be taken with high-fat foods.

---

* Canada only   ◇ Unlabeled clinical use

• Inform patient that drug doesn't cure HIV infection and that it won't deter development of opportunistic infections and other complications of HIV disease or transmission of HIV to others through sexual contact or blood contamination.
• Instruct patient to take drug at the same time daily and always with other antiretrovirals.
• Tell patient to take drug exactly as prescribed and not to stop without medical approval.
• Instruct patient to report adverse reactions.
• Inform patient that rash is the most common adverse effect. If this occurs, tell patient to report it immediately, because it may be serious in rare cases.
• Advise patient that dizziness, difficulty sleeping or concentrating, drowsiness, or unusual dreams may occur the first few days of therapy. Reassure him that these symptoms generally resolve after 2 to 4 weeks and may be less problematic if drug is taken at bedtime.
• Tell patient to avoid alcoholic beverages, driving, or operating machinery until the effects of the drug are known.

eflornithine hydrochloride
Vaniqa

Pharmacologic classification: ornithine decarboxylase (ODC) inhibitor
Therapeutic classification: hair growth retardant
Pregnancy risk category: C

Indications and dosages
➤ *Reduction of unwanted facial hair in women. Adults and children older than age 12:* Thin layer applied to affected areas of the face and adjacent areas under chin and rubbed in thoroughly twice daily, at least 8 hours apart.

How supplied
Available by prescription only
Cream: 13.9 %

Pharmacodynamics
Thought to irreversibly inhibit skin ODC activity. This enzyme is necessary in the synthesis of polyamines. Animal data indicate that inhibition of ODC affects cell division and synthetic functions, which affect hair growth. Drug retards hair growth in nonclinical and clinical studies.

Pharmacokinetics
Absorption: Less than 1% of the radioactive dose is absorbed after single or multiple doses under conditions of clinical use that included shaving within 2 hours before radiolabeled dose application in addition to other forms of cutting, plucking, and tweezing to remove facial hair.
Distribution: Time to reach steady state is 4 days of twice-daily application.
Metabolism: Not known to be metabolized.

Excretion: Unchanged in urine. The steady state plasma half-life of eflornithine is about 8 hours.

Route	Onset	Peak	Duration
Topical	Unknown	8 hr	Unknown

Adverse reactions
CNS: headache, dizziness, asthenia, vertigo.
GI: dyspepsia, anorexia, nausea.
Skin: *acne, pseudofolliculitis barbae,* stinging or burning sensation, dry skin, pruritus, erythema, skin irritation, rash, alopecia, folliculitis, ingrown hair, facial edema.

Interactions
No known interactions.

Overdose and treatment
Information unavailable. Given the low percutaneous penetration of this drug, overdose through the topical route isn't expected. However, with very high topical doses (e.g., multiple tubes per day) or oral ingestion, monitor patient and provide appropriate supportive measures as needed.

Contraindications and precautions
Contraindicated in patients with a history of sensitivity to any component of the preparation.

Special considerations
• Drug has only been studied on the face and adjacent involved areas under the chin. Application of the cream should be limited to these areas.
• Drug isn't expected to cause contact sensitization, phototoxicty, or photosensitization reactions.
• If adverse effects become bothersome, instruct the patient to limit use of drug to once a day. If adverse effects persist, tell patient to consult prescriber.
• Drug is available as a cream in a 30-g tube or two 30-g tubes for a total of 60 g. Drug should be stored at 59° to 86° F (15° to 30° C).

Breast-feeding patients
• It isn't known whether drug appears in human milk. Use cautiously when administering to nursing women.

Pediatric patients
• Don't use drug in children younger than age 12.

Patient education
• Tell patient that drug is intended to reduce unwanted facial and chin hair in women. Urge patient to limit use to these areas.
• Advise patient that drug isn't a depilatory, but rather is believed to retard hair growth. Patient will likely need to continue using a hair removal method along with drug.
• Tell patient that improvement may occur in 4 to 8 weeks and that the condition may return to pretreatment levels 8 weeks after stopping drug.

Reactions may be *common*, uncommon, *life-threatening*, or COMMON AND LIFE-THREATENING.

• Instruct patient to apply drug in a thin layer to affected areas twice daily, at least 8 hours apart. If skin irritation or intolerance develops, tell patient to temporarily reduce the frequency of application to once a day. If irritation continues, patient should stop using drug.
• Tell patient to store drug at 59° to 86° F (15° to 30° C) and not to freeze it.

enalaprilat
Vasotec I.V.

enalapril maleate
Vasotec

Pharmacologic classification: ACE inhibitor
Therapeutic classification: antihypertensive
Pregnancy risk category: C (D in second and third trimesters)

Indications and dosages
➤ *Hypertension. Adults:* If patient doesn't take a diuretic, 5 mg P.O. once daily initially, adjusted according to response. Usual dosage range is 10 to 40 mg daily as a single dose or two divided doses. Or, 1.25-mg I.V. infusion q 6 hours over 5 minutes. If patient takes a diuretic, 2.5 mg P.O. once daily initially. Or, 0.625 mg I.V. over 5 minutes; repeat in 1 hour, if needed, and then follow with 1.25 mg I.V. q 6 hours.
➤ *To convert from I.V. to P.O. therapy. Adults:* If patient didn't receive diuretics and did receive 1.25 mg I.V. q 6 hours, then give 5 mg P.O. once daily initially. If patient did receive diuretics and received 0.625 mg I.V. q 6 hours, then give 2.5 mg P.O. once daily. Adjust dose according to response.
➤ *To convert from P.O. to I.V. therapy. Adults:* 1.25 mg I.V. over 5 minutes q 6 hours.
✦ *Dosage adjustment.* In hypertensive patients with renal impairment and a creatinine clearance less than 30 ml/minute, begin therapy at 2.5 mg daily. Gradually adjust dosage according to response. Patients undergoing hemodialysis should receive a supplemental dose of 2.5 mg on dialysis days.
➤ *Heart failure. Adults:* Initially, 2.5 mg P.O. once or twice daily. Usual maintenance dose is 5 to 20 mg P.O. daily, given in two divided doses. Maximum daily dose is 40 mg P.O. in two divided doses.
➤ *Asymptomatic left ventricular dysfunction. Adults:* Initially, 2.5 mg P.O. b.i.d.; adjust to targeted daily dose of 20 mg (in divided doses) as tolerated.
✦ *Dosage adjustment.* In patients with heart failure and renal impairment or hyponatremia (serum sodium below 130 mEq/L or serum creatinine above 1.6 mg/dl), start with 2.5 mg P.O. daily. Increase to 2.5 mg b.i.d. and then 5 mg b.i.d. and higher as indicated, usually at intervals of 4 days or more.

How supplied
Available by prescription only
Injection: 1.25 mg/ml in 2-ml vials
Tablets: 2.5 mg, 5 mg, 10 mg, 20 mg

Pharmacodynamics
Antihypertensive action: Enalapril inhibits ACE, preventing conversion of angiotensin I to angiotensin II, a potent vasoconstrictor. Reduced angiotensin II levels decrease peripheral arterial resistance, thus lowering blood pressure, and decrease aldosterone secretion, thus reducing sodium and water retention.

Pharmacokinetics
Absorption: About 60% of dose is absorbed from the GI tract.
Distribution: Full distribution pattern is unknown; drug doesn't appear to cross the blood-brain barrier.
Metabolism: Metabolized extensively to the active metabolite enalaprilat.
Excretion: About 94% is excreted in urine and feces as enalaprilat and enalapril.

Route	Onset	Peak	Duration
P.O.	1 hr	4-6 hr	24 hr
I.V.	15 min	1-4 hr	6 hr

Contraindications and precautions
Contraindicated in patients hypersensitive to drug and in those with a history of angioedema related to previous treatment with an ACE inhibitor. Use cautiously in patients with impaired renal function. Avoid use in patients at high risk for cardiogenic shock.

Interactions
Drug-drug. *Antihypertensives, diuretics, phenothiazines:* Increased antihypertensive effects. Use together cautiously.
Aspirin, NSAIDs: Decreased antihypertensive effect. Use together cautiously.
Insulin, oral antidiabetics: Increased risk of hypoglycemia, especially at the start of enalapril therapy. Monitor glucose level closely.
Lithium: Decreased lithium clearance. Monitor lithium level.
Potassium-sparing diuretics, potassium supplements: Enhanced diuretic effects and possible hyperkalemia. Use together cautiously.
Rifampin: Decreased rifampin effects. Monitor patient closely.
Drug-herb. *Capsaicin:* Increased risk of cough. Discourage concomitant use.
Drug-food. *Salt substitutes:* May enhance effects, thereby causing hyperkalemia. Tell patient to use together cautiously.

Adverse reactions
CNS: *headache, dizziness, fatigue,* vertigo, asthenia, syncope.
CV: *hypotension,* chest pain, ***bradycardia.***
GI: diarrhea, nausea, abdominal pain, vomiting.

GU: elevated BUN and serum creatinine levels, decreased renal function in patients with bilateral renal artery stenosis or heart failure.
Hematologic: *neutropenia, thrombocytopenia, agranulocytosis.*
Hepatic: increased liver enzyme and bilirubin levels.
Respiratory: *dry, persistent, tickling, nonproductive cough;* dyspnea.
Skin: rash.
Other: *angioedema.*

Overdose and treatment
The most likely effect is hypotension. After acute ingestion, empty stomach by induced emesis or gastric lavage. Follow with activated charcoal to reduce absorption. Consider hemodialysis in severe cases. Subsequent treatment is usually symptomatic and supportive.

Special considerations
• Stop diuretic therapy 2 to 3 days before starting enalapril therapy to reduce risk of hypotension; if drug doesn't control blood pressure adequately, reinstate diuretic.
• Give drug without regard to meals; food doesn't appear to affect absorption.

Patient monitoring
• Proteinuria and nephrotic syndrome may occur in patients receiving enalapril.
• Obtain WBC and differential counts before treatment, every 2 weeks for 3 months, and periodically thereafter.

Pregnant patients
• Neonatal and fetal death may occur when drug is given during second and third trimesters.

Breast-feeding patients
• It isn't known whether drug appears in breast milk; an alternative feeding method is recommended during therapy.

Pediatric patients
• Safety and efficacy of enalapril in children haven't been established; use only if potential benefit outweighs risk.

Geriatric patients
• Geriatric patients may need lower doses because of impaired drug clearance.

Patient education
• Tell patient to report light-headedness, especially in first few days, so dosage can be adjusted; signs of infection, such as sore throat and fever, because drug may decrease WBC count; facial swelling or difficulty breathing, because drug may cause angioedema; and loss of taste, which may necessitate discontinuing drug.
• Advise patient to avoid sudden position changes to minimize orthostatic hypotension.

• Warn patient to seek medical approval before taking herbal or OTC cold preparations, particularly cough medications.

enoxacin
Penetrex

Pharmacologic classification: fluoroquinolone, antibacterial
Therapeutic classification: antibiotic
Pregnancy risk category: C

Indications and dosages
➤ *Uncomplicated urinary tract infections (cystitis) caused by* Escherichia coli, Staphylococcus epidermidis, *or* Staphylococcus saprophyticus. *Adults:* 200 mg P.O. q 12 hours for 7 days.
➤ *Complicated urinary tract infections caused by* E. coli, Klebsiella pneumoniae, Proteus mirabilis, Pseudomonas aeruginosa, Staphylococcus epidermidis, *or* Enterobacter cloacae. *Adults:* 400 mg P.O. q 12 hours for 14 days.
➤ *Uncomplicated urethral or endocervical gonorrhea caused by* Neisseria gonorrhoeae. *Adults:* 400 mg P.O. as a single dose.
✦ *Dosage adjustment.* In patients with renal impairment, if creatinine clearance is 30 ml/minute or less, start therapy with the usual initial dose and reduce subsequent doses by 50%.

How supplied
Available by prescription only
Tablets (film-coated): 200 mg, 400 mg

Pharmacodynamics
Antibiotic action: Bactericidal. Inhibits the bacterial enzyme DNA gyrase, which is necessary for DNA replication. Active against most strains of gram-positive aerobes, such as *S. epidermidis* and *S. saprophyticus,* and against many gram-negative aerobes, such as *Escherichia cloacae, E. coli, K. pneumoniae, N. gonorrhoeae, P. mirabilis,* and *P. aeruginosa.*

Pharmacokinetics
Absorption: After oral administration, plasma levels may peak within 1 to 3 hours. Absolute oral bioavailability is about 90%.
Distribution: About 40% bound to plasma proteins in healthy people and 14% bound to plasma proteins in people with impaired renal function.
Metabolism: Five metabolites identified in urine; account for 15% to 20% of administered dose.
Excretion: Excreted primarily by kidneys. Plasma half-life is 3 to 6 hours.

Route	Onset	Peak	Duration
P.O.	Unknown	1-3 hr	Unknown

Reactions may be *common*, uncommon, *life-threatening*, or COMMON AND LIFE-THREATENING.

Contraindications and precautions

Contraindicated in patients hypersensitive to drug or other fluoroquinolone antibiotics. Use cautiously in patients with CNS disorders, such as severe cerebral arteriosclerosis or seizure disorders, and in those at increased risk for seizures. Drug may cause CNS stimulation. Use cautiously and with dosage adjustments in patients with impaired renal or hepatic function.

Interactions

Drug-drug. *Aminophylline, cyclosporine, theophylline:* Possible increased levels of these drugs because of decreased metabolism. Use together cautiously.

Bismuth subsalicylate: Decreased enoxacin bioavailability (by about 25%) when given within 60 minutes after enoxacin. Avoid concomitant use.

Digoxin: May raise serum digoxin levels. If signs and symptoms of digoxin toxicity occur, obtain serum digoxin levels and adjust digoxin doses appropriately.

Oral anticoagulants: Increased anticoagulant effect. Monitor PT and INR.

Quinolones with antacids containing aluminum, calcium, magnesium; with divalent or trivalent cations (such as iron); with multivitamins containing zinc; with sucralfate: May substantially interfere with drug absorption and result in insufficient plasma and tissue quinolone levels. Give 8 hours before or 2 hours after enoxacin.

Ranitidine: Oral bioavailability of enoxacin is reduced by 60%. Give ranitidine 8 hours before or 2 hours after enoxacin.

Drug-food. *Any food:* Altered absorption. Give drug on an empty stomach.

Caffeine: Drug interferes with caffeine metabolism, resulting in decrease in caffeine clearance of up to 80%; increases caffeine-related adverse effects. Discourage use.

Drug-lifestyle. *Sun exposure:* Increased risk of photosensitivity reactions. Tell patient to avoid excessive exposure.

Adverse reactions

CNS: headache, restlessness, light-headedness, tremor, confusion, hallucinations, *seizures*.

GI: *nausea, diarrhea*, vomiting, abdominal pain or discomfort, oral candidiasis.

GU: crystalluria.

Hematologic: eosinophilia.

Hepatic: elevated liver enzyme levels.

Musculoskeletal: tendon pain, tendon rupture.

Respiratory: dyspnea, cough.

Skin: *rash*, pruritus, photosensitivity.

Other: *hypersensitivity*.

Overdose and treatment

In acute overdose, stomach should be emptied by inducing vomiting or by gastric lavage; watch patient closely and give supportive treatment. Enoxacin is poorly removed (less than 5% over 4 hours) by hemodialysis.

Special considerations

● Moderate to severe phototoxicity reactions have been observed in patients exposed to direct sunlight while receiving drug.

● Stop therapy if hypersensitivity or phototoxicity occurs.

Patient monitoring

● Obtain specimen for culture and sensitivity tests before giving first dose. Therapy may begin pending results.

● Monitor patient for diarrhea. Pseudomembranous colitis has been reported and may range in severity from mild to life-threatening. Consider this diagnosis in patients who have diarrhea after drug administration.

Pregnant patients

● Safety and efficacy in pregnant women haven't been established.

Breast-feeding patients

● Safety and effectiveness in breast-feeding patients haven't been established.

Pediatric patients

● Safety and effectiveness in children haven't been established.

Patient education

● Advise patient to avoid excessive sunlight and to take other precautions as necessary to prevent phototoxicity.

● Instruct patient to call immediately if pregnancy is suspected.

● Tell patient to avoid antacids containing aluminum, calcium, or magnesium; bismuth subsalicylate; products containing iron; or multivitamins that contain zinc for 8 hours before taking enoxacin.

● Instruct patient to drink fluids liberally but to avoid consumption of products containing caffeine during enoxacin therapy.

● Caution patient that enoxacin may cause dizziness and light-headedness.

● Advise patient that enoxacin may raise the risk of a hypersensitivity reaction, even after first dose. Tell patient to stop drug and call at first sign of rash or other allergic reactions.

● Instruct patient to take enoxacin at least 1 hour before or 2 hours after a meal.

enoxaparin sodium
Lovenox

Pharmacologic classification: low-molecular-weight heparin
Therapeutic classification: anticoagulant
Pregnancy risk category: B

Indications and dosages

➤ *Prevention of deep vein thrombosis (DVT), which may lead to pulmonary em-*

bolism, following hip or knee replacement surgery. Adults: 30 mg S.C. q 12 hours for 7 to 10 days. Give first dose 12 to 24 hours postoperatively provided hemostasis has been established.

➤ *Prevention of DVT, which may lead to pulmonary embolism, following abdominal surgery. Adults:* 40 mg S.C. once daily for 7 to 10 days. Give first dose 2 hours before surgery.

➤ *Prevention of ischemic complications of unstable angina and non-Q-wave MI, when administered with aspirin. Adults:* 1 mg/kg S.C. q 12 hours for 2 to 8 days in conjunction with oral aspirin therapy (100 to 325 mg once daily). To minimize risk of bleeding after vascular instrumentation during the treatment of unstable angina, adhere precisely to the intervals recommended between enoxaparin doses.

➤ *Inpatient treatment of acute DVT with and without pulmonary embolism when administered with warfarin sodium. Adults:* 1 mg/kg S.C. every 12 hours; or, 1.5 mg/kg S.C. once daily (at the same time every day) for 5 to 7 days until therapeutic oral anticoagulant effect (INR 2 to 3) has been achieved. Warfarin sodium therapy usually starts within 72 hours of enoxaparin injection.

➤ *Outpatient treatment of acute DVT without pulmonary embolism when administered with warfarin sodium. Adults:* 1 mg/kg S.C. every 12 hours for 5 to 7 days until therapeutic oral anticoagulant effect (INR 2 to 3) has been achieved. Warfarin sodium therapy usually starts within 72 hours of enoxaparin injection.

How supplied
Available by prescription only
Ampules: 30 mg/0.3 ml
Syringes (graduated prefilled): 60 mg/0.6 ml, 80 mg/0.8 ml, 100 mg/1 ml
Syringes (prefilled): 30 mg/0.3 ml, 40 mg/0.4 ml

Pharmacodynamics
Anticoagulant action: Enoxaparin is a low-molecular-weight heparin that accelerates formation of antithrombin III-thrombin complex and deactivates thrombin, preventing conversion of fibrinogen to fibrin. It has a higher anti-factor Xa to anti-factor IIa activity than unfractionated heparin.

Pharmacokinetics
Absorption: Bioavailability is 92%
Distribution: Volume of distribution of anti-factor Xa activity is about 6 L.
Metabolism: Information not available.
Excretion: Elimination half-life based on anti-factor Xa activity is about 4½ hours after S.C. administration.

Route	Onset	Peak	Duration
S.C.	Unknown	3-5 hr	24 hr

Contraindications and precautions
Contraindicated in patients hypersensitive to drug, heparin, or pork products; in patients with active, major bleeding or thrombocytopenia; and in those who demonstrate antiplatelet antibodies in the presence of drug.

Use with extreme caution in patients with history of heparin-induced thrombocytopenia. Use cautiously in patients with conditions that put them at increased risk for hemorrhage, such as bacterial endocarditis; congenital or acquired bleeding disorders; ulcer disease; angiodysplastic GI disease; hemorrhagic stroke; or recent spinal, eye, or brain surgery; or in those treated concomitantly with NSAIDs, platelet inhibitors, or other anticoagulants that affect hemostasis.

Use with extreme caution in patients with postoperative indwelling epidural catheters. Cases of epidural or spinal hematomas have been reported with the use of enoxaparin and spinal or epidural anesthesia or spinal puncture, resulting in long-term or permanent paralysis.

Also use cautiously in patients with a bleeding diathesis, uncontrolled arterial hypertension, or history of recent GI ulceration, diabetic retinopathy, and hemorrhage.

Use carefully in elderly patients and patients with renal insufficiency who may show delayed elimination of enoxaparin.

Interactions
Drug-drug. *Anticoagulants, antiplatelet drugs, NSAIDs:* Increased risk of bleeding. May also lead to spinal or epidural hematomas in patients with spinal punctures or epidural or spinal anesthesia. Monitor patient carefully.
Plicamycin, valproic acid: May cause hypoprothrombinemia and inhibit platelet aggregation. Monitor patient closely.

Adverse reactions
CNS: confusion, *neurologic injury* when used with spinal or epidural puncture.
CV: edema, peripheral edema, CV toxicity (chest pain, dizziness, irregular heartbeat).
GI: nausea.
Hematologic: hypochromic anemia, *thrombocytopenia, hemorrhage,* ecchymoses, bleeding complications.
Hepatic: elevated liver enzyme levels.
Skin: *rash, urticaria.*
Other: irritation, pain, hematoma, erythema (at injection site); fever; pain; *angioedema.*

Overdose and treatment
Accidental overdose may lead to hemorrhagic complications. This may be largely neutralized by the slow I.V. injection of protamine sulfate (1%) solution. The dose of protamine sulfate should be equal to the dose of enoxaparin injection (1 mg of protamine neutralizes 1 mg of enoxaparin).

Reactions may be *common,* uncommon, *life-threatening,* or COMMON AND LIFE-THREATENING.

Special considerations
● Enoxaparin isn't intended for I.M. administration.
✛ ALERT Drug can't be used interchangeably (unit for unit) with unfractionated heparin or other low-molecular-weight heparins.
● Don't mix drug with other injections or infusions.
● Screen all patients before prophylactic use of enoxaparin to rule out a bleeding disorder.
● Don't expel air bubble from syringe before injecting drug because drug may be lost.

Patient monitoring
● Monitor patient for adverse reactions, including angioedema.

Breast-feeding patients
● It isn't known whether drug appears in breast milk. Use cautiously when administering drug to breast-feeding women.

Pediatric patients
● Safety and efficacy of enoxaparin in children haven't been established.

Patient education
● Explain risk of adverse reactions.
● Instruct patient to watch for signs of bleeding.
● Caution patient against use of aspirin or other salicylates.

entacapone
Comtan

Pharmacologic classification: catechol-O-methyltransferase (COMT) inhibitor
Therapeutic classification: antiparkinsonian
Pregnancy risk category: C

Indication and dosages
➤ *Adjunct to levodopa and carbidopa for treatment of idiopathic Parkinson's disease in patients with signs and symptoms of end-of-dose wearing off. Adults:* 200 mg P.O. with each dose of levodopa and carbidopa to maximum of eight times daily. Maximum recommended daily dose of entacapone is 1,600 mg/day. Reducing daily levodopa dose or extending the interval between doses may be necessary to optimize patient's response.

How supplied
Available by prescription only
Tablets: 200 mg

Pharmacodynamics
Antiparkinsonian action: A reversible inhibitor of peripheral COMT, which is responsible for elimination of various catecholamines, including dopamine. Blocking this pathway when administering levodopa and carbidopa should increase serum levodopa levels, thereby allowing greater dopaminergic stimulation in the CNS and a greater effect in treating parkinsonian symptoms.

Pharmacokinetics
Absorption: Rapid, with serum levels peaking in about 1 hour. Food doesn't affect absorption.
Distribution: About 98% protein-bound, mainly to albumin; isn't distributed widely into tissues. Duration is about 6 hours.
Metabolism: Almost completely metabolized by glucuronidation before elimination. No active metabolites identified.
Excretion: About 10% excreted in urine; remainder excreted in bile and feces. Biphasic half-life: 0.4 to 0.7 hours for first phase; 2.4 hours for second phase.

Route	Onset	Peak	Duration
P.O.	1 hr	1 hr	6 hr

Contraindications and precautions
Contraindicated in patients hypersensitive to drug. Use cautiously in patients with hepatic impairment, biliary obstruction, or orthostatic hypotension.

Interactions
Drug-drug. *Ampicillin, chloramphenicol, cholestyramine, erythromycin, probenecid:* May block biliary excretion, resulting in higher serum levels of entacapone. Use cautiously.
CNS depressants: Additive effect. Use cautiously.
Drugs metabolized by COMT (bitolterol, dobutamine, dopamine, epinephrine, isoetharine, isoproterenol, norepinephrine): May cause higher serum levels of these drugs, resulting in increased heart rate, changes in blood pressure or, possibly, arrhythmias. Use cautiously.
Nonselective MAO inhibitors (such as phenelzine, tranylcypromine): May inhibit normal catecholamine metabolism. Avoid concomitant use.
Drug-lifestyle. *Alcohol use:* May cause additive CNS effects. Discourage use.

Adverse reactions
CNS: *dyskinesia, hyperkinesia,* hypokinesia, dizziness, anxiety, somnolence, agitation, fatigue, asthenia, hallucinations.
GI: *nausea, diarrhea,* abdominal pain, constipation, vomiting, dry mouth, dyspepsia, flatulence, gastritis, taste perversion.
GU: *urine discoloration.*
Hematologic: purpura.
Musculoskeletal: back pain.
Respiratory: dyspnea.
Skin: sweating.
Other: bacterial infection.

Overdose and treatment
Management of overdose is symptomatic; hemodialysis isn't effective because of high protein-binding. In acute stages of overdose, gastric lavage or activated charcoal may be helpful to limit GI absorption.

Special considerations
• Drug should only be used with levodopa and carbidopa; no antiparkinsonian effects will occur when drug is given as monotherapy.
• Levodopa and carbidopa dosage requirements are usually lower when given with entacapone; the levodopa and carbidopa dose should be lowered or dosing interval increased to avoid adverse effects.
• Drug may cause or worsen dyskinesia despite reduction of levodopa dose.
• Hallucinations may occur or worsen when taking this drug.
• Diarrhea most commonly begins within 4 to 12 weeks, but may begin as early as first week or as late as many months after starting treatment.
• Drug may discolor urine.
• Rarely, rhabdomyolysis has occurred with drug use.
◨ **ALERT** Rapid withdrawal or abrupt reduction in drug dose could lead to signs and symptoms of Parkinson's disease; it may also lead to hyperpyrexia and confusion, a symptom complex resembling neuroleptic malignant syndrome. Discontinue drug slowly and monitor patient closely. Adjust other dopaminergic treatment, as needed.
• Drug can be given with immediate or sustained-release levodopa and carbidopa and can be taken with or without food.

Patient monitoring
• Monitor blood pressure closely. Observe for orthostatic hypotension.
• Monitor patient for adverse effects.

Breast-feeding patients
• It isn't known whether drug appears in breast milk. Because many drugs do, use cautiously when giving drug to breast-feeding women.

Pediatric patients
• No identified potential use in children.

Patient education
• Instruct patient not to crush or break tablet and to take it at same time as levodopa and carbidopa.
• Warn patient to avoid potentially hazardous activities, such as driving or operating heavy machinery, until CNS effects of drug are known.
• Advise patient to avoid alcohol during treatment.
• Instruct patient to be careful when standing after prolonged period of sitting or lying down because dizziness may occur. This effect is more common during initial therapy.
• Warn patient that hallucinations, increased dyskinesia, nausea, and diarrhea may occur.
• Inform patient that drug may cause urine to turn brownish orange.
• Advise patient to report if she is pregnant or breast-feeding or if she plans to become pregnant.

ephedrine
ephedrine hydrochloride
ephedrine sulfate
Pretz-D

Pharmacologic classification: adrenergic
Therapeutic classification: bronchodilator, vasopressor (parenteral form), nasal decongestant
Pregnancy risk category: C

Indications and dosages
➤ *To correct hypotensive states. Adults:* 25 to 50 mg I.M. or S.C. Or, 10 to 25 mg via slow I.V. bolus. If necessary, a second I.M. dose of 50 mg or I.V. dose of 25 mg may be administered. Additional I.V. doses may be given in 5 to 10 minutes. Maximum dose is 150 mg daily.
Children: 3 mg/kg or 100 mg/m^2 S.C. or I.V. daily, divided into four to six doses.
➤ *Orthostatic hypotension. Adults:* 25 mg P.O. once daily to q.i.d.
Children: 3 mg/kg P.O. daily, divided into four to six doses.
➤ *Bronchodilator or nasal decongestant. Adults and children older than 12:* 12.5 to 50 mg P.O. q 3 to 4 hours, p.r.n., not to exceed 150 mg in 24 hours. *As nasal decongestant:* 2 to 3 sprays in each nostril not more often than q 4 hours.
Children ages 6 to 12: 6.25 to 12.5 mg P.O. q 4 hours, not to exceed 75 mg in 24 hours. *As nasal decongestant:* 1 to 2 sprays in each nostril, not more often than q 4 hours.
Alternatively, children age 2 and older: 2 to 3 mg/kg or 100 mg/m^2 P.O. daily in four to six divided doses.
➤ *Severe, acute bronchospasm. Adults:* 12.5 to 50 mg I.M., S.C., or I.V.
➤ *Enuresis. Adults:* 25 to 50 mg P.O. h.s.
➤ *Myasthenia gravis. Adults:* 25 mg P.O. t.i.d. or q.i.d.

How supplied
Available with and without a prescription
Capsules: 25 mg, 50 mg
Injection: 25 mg/ml, 50 mg/ml (parenteral)
Nasal spray: 0.25%

Pharmacodynamics
Direct- and indirect-acting sympathomimetic action: Ephedrine stimulates alpha- and beta-adrenergic receptors. Release of norepinephrine from its storage sites is one of its indirect effects. In therapeutic doses, ephedrine relaxes bronchial smooth muscle and produces cardiac stimulation with increased systolic and diastolic blood pressure when norepinephrine stores aren't depleted.
Bronchodilator action: Ephedrine relaxes bronchial smooth muscle by stimulating beta$_2$-adrenergic receptors, resulting in increased vital

---

Reactions may be *common*, uncommon, *life-threatening*, or COMMON AND LIFE-THREATENING.

capacity, relief of mild bronchospasm, improved air exchange, and decreased residual volume.

Vasopressor action: Drug produces positive inotropic effects with low doses by action on $beta_1$-receptors in the heart. Vasodilation results from its effect on $beta_2$-adrenergic receptors; vasoconstriction results from its alpha-adrenergic effects. Pressor effects may result from vasoconstriction or cardiac stimulation; however, when peripheral vascular resistance is decreased, blood pressure elevation results from increased cardiac output.

Nasal decongestant action: Ephedrine stimulates alpha-adrenergic receptors in blood vessels of nasal mucosa, producing vasoconstriction and nasal decongestion.

Pharmacokinetics
Absorption: Rapidly and completely absorbed after oral, S.C., or I.M. administration.
Distribution: Widely distributed throughout the body.
Metabolism: Slowly metabolized in the liver by oxidative deamination, demethylation, aromatic hydroxylation, and conjugation.
Excretion: Dose is mostly excreted unchanged in urine; rate of excretion depends on urine pH.

Route	Onset	Peak	Duration
P.O.	15-60 min	Unknown	3-5 hr
I.V.	5 min	Unknown	1 hr
I.M., S.C.	10-20 min	Unknown	½-1 hr
Nasal spray	Unknown	Unknown	Unknown

Contraindications and precautions
Contraindicated in patients hypersensitive to drug and other sympathomimetics; in those with porphyria, severe coronary artery disease, arrhythmias, angle-closure glaucoma, psychoneurosis, angina pectoris, substantial organic heart disease, or CV disease; and in those taking MAO inhibitors.

Nasal solution is contraindicated in patients with angle-closure glaucoma, psychoneurosis, angina pectoris, substantial organic heart disease, CV disease, and hypersensitivity to drug or other sympathomimetics.

Use extremely cautiously in elderly men and in patients with hypertension, hyperthyroidism, nervous or excitable states, diabetes, and prostatic hyperplasia. Use nasal solution cautiously in patients with hyperthyroidism, hypertension, diabetes mellitus, or prostatic hyperplasia.

Interactions
Drug-drug. *Acetazolamide:* May increase serum ephedrine levels. Monitor patient for toxicity.
Alpha blockers: Unopposed beta-adrenergic effects, resulting in hypotension. Avoid use together.
Antihypertensives: Decreased antihypertensive effects. Monitor blood pressure.

Atropine: Blocks reflex bradycardia and enhances pressor effects. Monitor patient carefully.
Beta blockers: Unopposed alpha-adrenergic effects, resulting in hypertension. Monitor blood pressure.
Cardiac glycosides, general anesthetics (especially cyclopropane, halothane): May sensitize myocardium to effects of ephedrine, causing arrhythmias. Monitor patient closely.
Diuretics, methyldopa, reserpine: Decrease pressor effects of ephedrine. Monitor patient carefully.
Ergot alkaloids: May enhance vasoconstrictor activity. Monitor patient cautiously.
Guanadrel, guanethidine: Enhanced pressor effects of ephedrine. Monitor patient and blood pressure closely.
Levodopa: Enhanced risk of ventricular arrhythmias. Monitor patient closely.
MAO inhibitors, tricyclic antidepressants: Enhanced pressor effects; may cause hypertensive crisis. Allow 14 days after stopping MAO inhibitor before using ephedrine.
Sympathomimetics: Increased effects and toxicity. Avoid use together.
Theophylline: More adverse reactions than either drug when used alone. Use together cautiously.

Adverse reactions
CNS: *insomnia, nervousness,* dizziness, headache, euphoria, confusion, delirium, nervousness and excitation with nasal solution.
CV: *palpitations,* tachycardia, hypertension, precordial pain, *tachycardia* with nasal solution, **arrhythmias.**
EENT: dry nose and throat, rebound nasal congestion with long-term or excessive use, mucosal irritation with nasal solution.
GI: nausea, vomiting, anorexia.
GU: urine retention, painful urination from visceral sphincter spasm.
Musculoskeletal: muscle weakness.
Skin: diaphoresis.

Overdose and treatment
Signs and symptoms of overdose include exaggeration of common adverse reactions, especially arrhythmias, extreme tremor or seizures, nausea and vomiting, fever, and CNS and respiratory depression.

Treatment requires supportive and symptomatic measures. If patient is conscious, induce emesis with ipecac followed by activated charcoal. If patient is depressed or hyperactive, perform gastric lavage. Maintain airway and blood pressure. Don't administer vasopressors. Monitor vital signs closely.

A beta blocker (such as propranolol) may be used to treat arrhythmias. A cardioselective beta blocker is recommended in asthmatic patients. Phentolamine may be used for hypertension, paraldehyde or diazepam for seizures, and dexamethasone for pyrexia.

Special considerations
• As a pressor agent, ephedrine isn't a substitute for blood, plasma, fluids, or electrolytes. Correct fluid volume depletion before administration.

Patient monitoring
• Tolerance may develop after prolonged or excessive use; increased dose may be needed. Also, if drug is discontinued for a few days and readministered, effectiveness may be restored.
• With parenteral dosing, monitor vital signs closely during infusion. Tachycardia is common.

Pregnant patients
• It isn't known whether drug is safe for use during pregnancy. Use drug during pregnancy only when clearly indicated.

Breast-feeding patients
• Avoid use in breast-feeding women.

Pediatric patients
• Use cautiously in children.

Geriatric patients
• Administer cautiously because geriatric patients may be more sensitive to effects of the drug. Lower doses may be recommended.

Patient education
• Instruct patient to clear nose before instilling nasal solutions.
• Tell patient using OTC product to follow directions on label, to take last dose a few hours before bedtime to reduce possibility of insomnia, to take only as directed, and not to increase dose or frequency.
• Advise patient to store drug away from heat and light (not in bathroom medicine cabinet) and to keep out of reach of children.
• Instruct patient who misses a dose to take it as soon as remembered if within 1 hour. If beyond 1 hour, patient should skip dose and return to regular schedule.
• Teach patient to be aware of palpitations and significant pulse rate changes.

epinephrine
Bronkaid Mist, Bronkaid Mistometer*, EpiPen, EpiPen Jr., Primatene Mist, Sus-Phrine

epinephrine bitartrate
AsthmaHaler

epinephrine hydrochloride
Adrenalin Chloride, AsthmaNefrin, Epifrin, Glaucon, microNefrin, Vaponefrin

epinephryl borate
Epinal

Pharmacologic classification: adrenergic
Therapeutic classification: bronchodilator, vasopressor, cardiac stimulant, local anesthetic (adjunct), topical antihemorrhagic, antiglaucoma
Pregnancy risk category: C

Indications and dosages
➤ *Bronchospasm, hypersensitivity reactions, anaphylaxis. Adults:* Initially, 0.1 to 0.5 mg (0.1 to 0.5 ml of a 1:1,000 solution) S.C. or I.M.; may be repeated at 10- to 15-minute intervals, p.r.n. Or, 0.1 to 0.25 mg (1 to 2.5 ml of a 1:10,000 solution) I.V. slowly over 5 to 10 minutes. May be repeated q 5 to 15 minutes if needed or followed by a 1 to 4 mcg/minute I.V. infusion.
Children: 0.01 mg/kg (0.01 ml/kg of a 1:1,000 solution) or 0.3 mg/m^2 (0.3 ml/ m^2 of a 1:1,000 solution) S.C. Dose not to exceed 0.5 mg. May be repeated at 20-minute to 4-hour intervals, p.r.n. Or, 0.02 to 0.025 mg/kg (0.004 to 0.005 ml/kg) or 0.625 mg/m^2 (0.125 ml/m^2) of a 1:200 solution. May be repeated but not more often than q 6 hours. Or, 0.1 mg (10 ml of a 1:100,000 dilution) I.V. slowly over 5 to 10 minutes followed by a 0.1 to 1.5 mcg/kg/minute I.V. infusion.
➤ *Bronchodilator. Adults and children:* 1 inhalation via metered aerosol, repeated once if needed after 1 minute; subsequent doses shouldn't be repeated for at least 3 hours. Or, 1 or 2 deep inhalations via hand-bulb nebulizer of a 1% (1:100) solution; may be repeated at 1- to 2-minute intervals. Or, 0.03 ml (0.3 mg) of a 1% solution via intermittent positive pressure breathing.
➤ *To restore cardiac rhythm in cardiac arrest. Adults:* Initially, 0.5 to 1 mg (range, 0.1 to 1 mg to 10 ml of a 1:10,000 solution) I.V. bolus; may be repeated q 3 to 5 minutes, p.r.n. Or, initial dose followed by 0.3 mg S.C. or 1 to 4 mcg/minute I.V. infusion. Or, 1 mg (10 ml of a 1:10,000 solution) intratracheally, or 0.1 to 1 mg (1 to 10 ml of a 1:10,000 solution) by intracardiac injection.
Children: Initially, 0.01 mg/kg (0.1 ml/kg of a 1:10,000 solution) I.V. bolus or intratracheally; may be repeated q 5 minutes, p.r.n.
Or, initially, 0.1 mcg/kg/minute; may increase in increments of 0.1 mcg/kg/minute to a maximum of 1 mcg/kg/minute. Or, 0.005 to 0.01 mg/kg (0.05 to 0.1 ml/kg of a 1:10,000 solution) by intracardiac injection.
Infants: Initially, 0.01 to 0.03 mg/kg (0.1 to 0.3 ml/kg of a 1:10,000 solution) I.V. bolus or by intratracheal injection. May be repeated q 5 minutes, p.r.n.
➤ *Hemostatic use. Adults:* 1:50,000 to 1:1,000, applied topically.
➤ *To prolong local anesthetic effect. Adults and children:* 1:500,000 to 1:50,000 mixed with local anesthetic.

Reactions may be *common*, uncommon, *life-threatening*, or COMMON AND LIFE-THREATENING.

➤ *Open-angle glaucoma. Adults:* 1 or 2 drops of 1% to 2% solution daily or b.i.d.
➤ *Nasal congestion, local superficial bleeding. Adults and children:* Instill 1 or 2 drops of solution.

How supplied
Available by prescription only
Injection: 0.01 mg/ml (1:100,000), 0.1 mg/ml (1:10,000), 0.5 mg/ml (1:2,000), 1 mg/ml (1:1,000) parenteral; 5 mg/ml (1:200) parenteral suspension
Ophthalmic: 0.1%, 0.25%, 0.5%, 1%, 2% solution
Available without a prescription
Aerosol inhaler: 160 mcg, 200 mcg, 250 mcg/metered spray
Nasal solution: 0.1%
Nebulizer inhaler: 1% (1:100), 1.25%, 2.25%

Pharmacodynamics
Epinephrine acts directly by stimulating alpha- and beta-adrenergic receptors in the sympathetic nervous system. Its main therapeutic effects include relaxation of bronchial smooth muscle, cardiac stimulation, and dilation of skeletal muscle vasculature.

Bronchodilator action: Epinephrine relaxes bronchial smooth muscle by stimulating beta$_2$-adrenergic receptors. Epinephrine constricts bronchial arterioles by stimulating alpha-adrenergic receptors, resulting in relief of bronchospasm, reduced congestion and edema, and increased tidal volume and vital capacity. By inhibiting histamine release, it may reverse bronchiolar constriction, vasodilation, and edema.

CV and vasopressor actions: As a cardiac stimulant, epinephrine produces positive chronotropic and inotropic effects by action on beta$_1$-receptors in the heart, increasing cardiac output, myocardial oxygen consumption, and force of contraction and decreasing cardiac efficiency. Vasodilation results from its effect on beta$_2$-receptors; vasoconstriction results from alpha-adrenergic effects.

Local anesthetic (adjunct) action: Epinephrine acts on alpha receptors in skin, mucous membranes, and viscera; it produces vasoconstriction, which reduces absorption of local anesthetic, thus prolonging its duration of action, localizing anesthesia, and decreasing risk of anesthetic's toxicity.

Local vasoconstriction action: Epinephrine's effect results from action on alpha receptors in skin, mucous membranes, and viscera, which produces vasoconstriction and hemostasis in small vessels.

Antiglaucoma action: Epinephrine's exact mechanism of lowering intraocular pressure is unknown. When applied topically to the conjunctiva or injected into the interior chamber of the eye, epinephrine constricts conjunctival blood vessels, contracts the dilator muscle of the pupil, and may dilate the pupil.

Pharmacokinetics
Absorption: Well absorbed after S.C. or I.M. injection; epinephrine has a rapid onset of action and short duration of action.
Distribution: Distributed widely throughout the body.
Metabolism: Metabolized at sympathetic nerve endings, liver, and other tissues to inactive metabolites.
Excretion: Excreted in urine, mainly as its metabolites and conjugates.

Route	Onset	Peak	Duration
I.V.	Immediate	5 min	Short
I.M.	Variable	Unknown	1-4 hr
S.C.	5-15 min	½ hr	1-4 hr
Inhalation	1-5 min	Unknown	1-3 hr

Contraindications and precautions
Contraindicated in patients with angle-closure glaucoma, shock (other than anaphylaxis), organic brain damage, cardiac dilation, arrhythmias, coronary insufficiency, or cerebral arteriosclerosis. Also contraindicated in patients during general anesthesia with halogenated hydrocarbons or cyclopropane and in patients in labor (may delay second stage).

Some commercial products contain sulfites; contraindicated in patients with sulfite allergies except when epinephrine is being used for treatment of serious allergic reactions or other emergencies.

In conjunction with local anesthetics, epinephrine is contraindicated for use on fingers, toes, ears, nose, and genitalia.

Ophthalmic preparation is contraindicated in patients with angle-closure glaucoma or when nature of the glaucoma hasn't been established and in patients hypersensitive to the drug and in those with organic mental syndrome or cardiac dilation and coronary insufficiency. Nasal solution is contraindicated in patients hypersensitive to drug.

Use extremely cautiously in patients with long-standing bronchial asthma and emphysema in whom degenerative heart disease has developed. Also use cautiously in geriatric patients and in those with hyperthyroidism, CV disease, hypertension, psychoneurosis, and diabetes.

Use ophthalmic preparation cautiously in elderly patients and in patients with diabetes, hypertension, Parkinson's disease, hyperthyroidism, aphakia (eye without lens), cardiac disease, cerebral arteriosclerosis, or bronchial asthma.

Interactions
Drug-drug. *Alpha blockers:* Antagonized vasoconstriction and hypertension. Avoid use together. *Antidiabetics:* Decreased blood glucose effects. Dosage adjustments may be necessary. *Antihistamines, thyroid hormones, tricyclic antidepressants:* May potentiate adverse cardiac effects of epinephrine. Avoid use together.

Beta blockers, such as propranolol: Antagonized cardiac and bronchodilating effects of epinephrine. Monitor patient carefully.

Carbonic anhydrase inhibitors, osmotic agents, topical beta blockers, topical miotics: May cause additive lowering of intraocular pressure. Avoid use together.

Cardiac glycosides, general anesthetics (especially cyclopropane, halothane): May sensitize the myocardium to effects of epinephrine, causing arrhythmias. Provide ECG monitoring.

Doxapram, mazindol, methylphenidate: May enhance CNS stimulation or pressor effects. Monitor patient closely.

Ergot alkaloids, oxytocics: May cause severe hypertension. Avoid use together.

Guanadrel, guanethidine: Decreased hypotensive effects and potentiated effects of epinephrine, resulting in hypertension and arrhythmias. Monitor patient and blood pressure closely.

Levodopa: Increased risk of cardiac arrhythmias. Monitor patient carefully.

MAO inhibitors: Increased risk of hypertensive crisis. Monitor blood pressure closely.

Miotics: Decreased ciliary spasm, mydriasis, blurred vision and increased intraocular pressure. May be used for this reason.

Phenothiazines: Reversal of pressor effects. Avoid use together.

Sympathomimetics: Additive effects and toxicity. Avoid use together.

Adverse reactions

CNS: *nervousness, tremor,* vertigo, *headache,* disorientation, agitation, *drowsiness,* fear, pallor, dizziness, weakness, ***cerebral hemorrhage, CVA.*** In patients with Parkinson's disease, drug increases rigidity, tremor, brow ache, headache, light-headedness with ophthalmic form, nervousness and excitation with nasal form.

CV: *palpitations;* widened pulse pressure; *hypertension; tachycardia; **ventricular fibrillation; shock;*** anginal pain; ECG changes, including a decreased T-wave amplitude; palpitations; tachycardia; ***arrhythmias;*** hypertension with ophthalmic preparation; *tachycardia with nasal solution.*

EENT: corneal or conjunctival pigmentation or corneal edema in long-term use; follicular hypertrophy; chemosis; conjunctivitis; iritis; hyperemic conjunctiva; maculopapular rash; eye pain; allergic lid reaction; ocular irritation; eye stinging, burning, and tearing on instillation of ophthalmic form; rebound nasal congestion; slight sting upon application of nasal solution.

GI: *nausea, vomiting.*

GU: increased BUN levels.

Metabolic: increased blood glucose and serum lactic acid levels.

Respiratory: dyspnea.

Skin: urticaria, pain, hemorrhage (at injection site).

Overdose and treatment

Signs and symptoms of overdose may include a sharp increase in systolic and diastolic blood pressure, increase in venous pressure, severe anxiety, irregular heartbeat, severe nausea or vomiting, severe respiratory distress, unusually large pupils, unusual paleness and coldness of skin, pulmonary edema, renal failure, and metabolic acidosis.

Treatment includes symptomatic and supportive measures, because epinephrine is rapidly inactivated in the body. Monitor vital signs closely. Phentolamine may be needed for hypotension; beta blockers (such as propranolol) may be needed for arrhythmias.

Special considerations

● After S.C. or I.M. injection, massaging the site may hasten absorption.

● Epinephrine is destroyed by oxidizing agents, alkalis (including sodium bicarbonate), halogens, permanganates, chromates, nitrates, and salts of easily reducible metals such as iron, copper, and zinc.

● Avoid I.M. injection into buttocks. Epinephrine-induced vasoconstriction favors growth of the anaerobe *Clostridium perfringens.*

● Intracardiac administration requires external cardiac massage to move drug into coronary circulation.

● Breathing treatment should start with first symptoms of bronchospasm. Patient should use the fewest number of inhalations that provide relief. To prevent excessive dosage, at least 1 or 2 minutes should elapse before taking additional inhalations of epinephrine. Dosage requirements vary.

● Ophthalmic preparation may cause mydriasis with blurred vision and sensitivity to light in some patients being treated for glaucoma. Drug is usually administered at bedtime or after prescribed miotic to minimize these symptoms.

● When using separate solutions of epinephrine and a topical miotic, instill the miotic 2 to 10 minutes before epinephrine.

Patient monitoring

● Blood pressure, pulse, respirations, and urine output must be monitored, and the patient observed closely. Epinephrine may widen pulse pressure. If arrhythmias occur, discontinue epinephrine immediately. Watch for changes in intake and output ratio.

● Make sure patients, especially elderly ones, receive regular tonometry readings during continuous therapy.

Pregnant patients

● Drug inhibits spontaneous or oxytocin-induced labor. With dose sufficient to reduce uterine contractions, drug may cause a prolonged uterine atony with hemorrhage. Drug should be used during pregnancy only if potential benefits outweigh possible risks to fetus.

Reactions may be *common,* uncommon, *life-threatening,* or COMMON AND LIFE-THREATENING.

Breast-feeding patients
• Drug appears in breast milk. Patient should avoid breast-feeding during therapy.

Pediatric patients
• Safety and efficacy of ophthalmic epinephrine in children haven't been established. Use cautiously.

Geriatric patients
• These patients may be more sensitive to effects of epinephrine; lower doses are indicated.

Patient education
• Urge patient to report diminishing effect. Repeated or prolonged use of epinephrine can cause tolerance to effects of drug. Continuing to take epinephrine despite tolerance can be hazardous. Interrupting drug therapy for 12 hours to several days may restore responsiveness to drug.

Inhalation therapy
• Instruct patient in correct use of inhaler.
• Warn patient that overuse or too-frequent use can cause severe adverse reactions.
• Tell patient to save applicator; refills may be available.
• Advise patient to contact prescriber immediately if he receives no relief within 20 minutes or if condition worsens.

Nasal therapy
• Tell patient to contact prescriber if symptoms aren't relieved in 20 minutes or if they become worse, and to report bronchial irritation, nervousness, or sleeplessness, which require dosage reduction.
• Warn patient that intranasal applications may sting slightly and cause rebound congestion or drug-induced rhinitis after prolonged use. Nose drops should be used for 3 or 4 days only. Encourage patient to use drug exactly as prescribed.
• Tell patient to rinse nose dropper or spray tip with hot water after each use to avoid contaminating the solution.
• Instruct patient to gently press finger against nasolacrimal duct for at least 1 or 2 minutes immediately after drug instillation to avoid excessive systemic absorption.

Ophthalmic therapy
• To minimize systemic absorption, tell patient to press finger to lacrimal sac during and for 1 to 2 minutes after instillation of eye drops.
• To prevent contamination, tell patient not to touch applicator tip to any surface and to keep container tightly closed.
• Tell patient not to use epinephrine solution if it's discolored or contains a precipitate.
• Advise patient to remove soft contact lenses before instilling eye drops to avoid staining or damaging them.
• Tell patient to apply a missed dose as soon as possible. If it's close to time for next dose, the patient should wait and apply at regularly scheduled time.

• Tell patient to store drug away from heat and light (not in bathroom medicine cabinet where heat and moisture can cause drug to deteriorate) and out of reach of children.

---

epirubicin hydrochloride
Ellence

Pharmacologic classification: anthracycline
Therapeutic classification: antineoplastic
Pregnancy risk category: D

Indications and dosages
►*Adjuvant therapy in patients with evidence of axillary node tumor involvement following resection of primary breast cancer. Adults:* 100 to 120 mg/m² I.V. infusion over 3 to 5 minutes via a free-flowing I.V. solution on day 1 of each cycle q 3 to 4 weeks, or divided equally in two doses on days 1 and 8 of each cycle. Maximum cumulative (lifetime) dose is 900 mg/m².

Dosage modification after the first cycle is based on toxicity. For patients experiencing platelet counts less than 50,000/mm³, absolute neutrophil count (ANC) less than 250/mm³, neutropenic fever, or grade 3 or 4 nonhematologic toxicity, reduce the day-1 dose in subsequent cycles to 75% of the day-1 dose given in the current cycle. Delay day-1 therapy in subsequent cycles until platelets are at least 100,000/mm³, ANC is at least 1,500/mm³, and nonhematologic toxicities recover to grade 1.

For patients receiving divided doses (days 1 and 8), the day-8 dose should be 75% of the day-1 dose if platelet counts are 75,000 to 100,000/mm³ and ANC is 1,000 to 1,499/mm³. If day-8 platelet counts are less than 75,000/mm³, ANC is less than 1000/mm³, or grade 3 or 4 nonhematologic toxicity has occurred, the day-8 dose should be omitted.

✦*Dosage adjustment.* In patients with bone marrow dysfunction (heavily pretreated patients, patients with bone marrow depression, or those with neoplastic bone marrow infiltration), start at lower doses of 75 to 90 mg/m². In hepatic dysfunction, if bilirubin is 1.2 to 3 mg/dl or AST is two to four times upper limit of normal, give one-half the recommended starting dose. If bilirubin is greater than 3 mg/dl or AST is greater than four times upper limit of normal, give one-fourth the recommended starting dose. Effects in patients with severe hepatic impairment haven't been evaluated, so epirubicin shouldn't be used in these patients. In patients with severe renal dysfunction (serum creatinine over 5 mg/dl), consider lower dosages.

How supplied
Available by prescription only
Injection: 2 mg/ml

◇ Unlabeled clinical use

Pharmacodynamics

Antineoplastic action: The precise mechanisms of cytotoxic effects of epirubicin aren't completely known. Epirubicin is thought to form a complex with DNA by intercalation between nucleotide base pairs; thereby inhibiting DNA, RNA, and protein synthesis; DNA cleavage occurs, resulting in cytocidal activity. The drug may also generate cytotoxic free radicals as well as interfere with replication and transcription of DNA.

Pharmacokinetics

Absorption: Administered I.V.
Distribution: Rapidly and widely distributed into tissues. It binds to plasma proteins, predominantly albumin, and appears to concentrate in RBCs.
Metabolism: Extensively and rapidly metabolized by the liver. Several metabolites form with little to no cytotoxic activity.
Excretion: Eliminated mostly by biliary excretion and, to a lesser extent, urinary excretion.

Route	Onset	Peak	Duration
I.V.	Unknown	Unknown	Unknown

Contraindications and precautions

Contraindicated in patients hypersensitive to this drug, other anthracyclines, or anthracenediones. Also contraindicated in patients with baseline neutrophil counts of less than 1,500 cells/mm³, patients with severe myocardial insufficiency or recent MI, patients whose previous treatment with anthracyclines reached total cumulative doses, and patients with severe hepatic dysfunction.

Use cautiously in patients with active or dormant cardiac disease, patients with previous or current radiotherapy to the mediastinal and pericardial area, previous therapy with other anthracyclines or anthracenediones, or with other cardiotoxic drugs.

Interactions

Drug-drug. *Cardioactive compounds, calcium channel blockers:* May increase risk of heart failure. Monitor cardiac function closely.
Cimetidine: Increased epirubicin level by 50%. Avoid use together.
Cytotoxic drugs: Additive toxicities (especially hematologic and GI) may occur. Monitor patient closely.
Radiation therapy: Effects may be enhanced. Monitor patient carefully.
Drug-lifestyle. *Sun exposure:* Increased risk of photosensitivity reactions. Tell patient to avoid prolonged sun exposure.

Adverse reactions

CNS: lethargy.
CV: cardiomyopathy, *heart failure, cardiotoxicity,* sinus tachycardia, ECG changes, *AV block, ventricular tachycardia.*
EENT: conjunctivitis, keratitis.
GI: nausea, vomiting, diarrhea, anorexia, mucositis.
GU: *amenorrhea.*
Hematologic: LEUKOPENIA, NEUTROPENIA, *febrile neutropenia, anemia,* THROMBOCYTOPENIA.
Skin: alopecia, rash, itch, skin changes, photosensitivity, urticaria.
Other: infection, fever, hot flashes, local toxicity, *anaphylaxis.*

Overdose and treatment

Signs and symptoms of overdose are similar to known toxicities of drug. Provide supportive treatment as needed until recovery. Monitor patient for signs of heart failure, which may occur months after therapy, and provide supportive therapy as appropriate.

Special considerations

● Drug is a vesicant; don't give it I.M. or S.C.
● Patients receiving 120 mg/m² of epirubicin should also receive prophylactic antibiotic therapy with co-trimoxazole or a fluoroquinolone.
● Use of antiemetics before epirubicin may be necessary to reduce nausea and vomiting.
● Anthracycline-induced leukemia may occur.
● Administration of drug after previous radiation therapy may induce an inflammatory cell reaction at the site of irradiation.
● Administer epirubicin under the supervision of a prescriber who is experienced in the use of cancer chemotherapy.
● Pregnant health care providers shouldn't handle this drug.
● Contraceptive methods should be used by both men and women.

Patient monitoring

● Monitor left ventricular ejection fraction (LVEF) regularly during therapy; discontinue drug at the first sign of impaired cardiac function. Early signs of cardiac toxicity may include sinus tachycardia, ECG abnormalities, tachyarrhythmias, bradycardia, AV block, and bundle branch block.
● Obtain baseline total bilirubin level, AST level, creatinine level, and CBC including ANC. Evaluate cardiac function by measuring LVEF before therapy.
● Obtain total and differential WBC, RBC, and platelet counts before and during each cycle of therapy.
● WBC nadir is usually reached 10 to 14 days after drug administration, returning to normal by day 21.
● Recommend monitoring serum uric acid, potassium, calcium phosphate, and creatinine immediately after initial chemotherapy administration in patients susceptible to tumor lysis syndrome. Hydration, urine alkalinization, and prophylaxis with allopurinol may prevent hyperuricemia and minimize potential complications of tumor lysis syndrome.

Reactions may be *common,* uncommon, *life-threatening,* or COMMON AND LIFE-THREATENING.

• Delayed cardiac toxicity may occur 2 to 3 months after completion of treatment and is dependent upon the cumulative dose of epirubicin. Don't exceed a cumulative dose of 900 mg/m².

Breast-feeding patients
• It isn't known whether drug appears in breast milk. Because many drugs do, including anthracyclines, and because of possible serious adverse reactions to epirubicin in nursing infants, women should stop nursing before taking this drug.

Pediatric patients
• Safety and efficacy haven't been established in children. They may be at greater risk for anthracycline-induced cardiotoxicity and heart failure.

Geriatric patients
• Plasma clearance is decreased in elderly women.
• Watch closely for toxicity in elderly patients, especially women over age 70.

Patient education
• Advise patient to report nausea, vomiting, stomatitis, dehydration, fever, evidence of infection, or symptoms of heart failure (tachycardia, dyspnea, edema).
• Inform patient of the risk of cardiac damage and treatment-related leukemia with use of drug.
• Advise men to use effective contraception during treatment.
• Advise women that irreversible amenorrhea or premature menopause may occur.
• Tell patient that hair regrowth usually occurs within 2 to 3 months after therapy is discontinued.

epoetin alfa (erythropoietin)
Epogen, Procrit

Pharmacologic classification: glycoprotein
Therapeutic classification: antianemic
Pregnancy risk category: C

Indications and dosages
➤ **Anemia related to chronic renal failure.** *Adults:* Initially, 50 to 100 units/kg I.V. or S.C. three times weekly. Patients receiving dialysis should receive drug I.V.; patients with chronic renal failure who aren't on dialysis may receive drug S.C. or I.V. Reduce dosage when target hematocrit is reached or if hematocrit increases more than 4 points within a 2-week period. Increase dosage if hematocrit doesn't increase by 5 to 6 points after 8 weeks of therapy and hematocrit is below target range. Maintenance dosage is highly individualized.
➤ **Anemia related to zidovudine therapy in patients infected with HIV.** *Adults:* Before therapy, determine endogenous serum epoetin alfa levels. Patients with levels of 500 milliunits/ml or more are unlikely to respond to therapy.

Initial dose for patients with levels of less than 500 milliunits/ml who are receiving 4,200 mg weekly or less of zidovudine is 100 units/kg I.V. or S.C. three times weekly for 8 weeks. If response is inadequate after 8 weeks, increase dose by increments of 50 to 100 units/kg three times weekly and reevaluate response q 4 to 8 weeks. Individualize maintenance dosage to maintain response, which may be influenced by zidovudine dose or infection or inflammation.
➤ **Anemia secondary to cancer chemotherapy.** *Adults:* 150 units/kg S.C. three times weekly for 8 weeks or until target hemoglobin level is reached. If response isn't satisfactory after 8 weeks, increase dose up to 300 units/kg S.C. three times weekly.
➤ **Reduction of need for allogeneic blood transfusion in anemic patients scheduled to undergo elective, noncardiac, nonvascular surgery.** *Adults:* 300 units/kg S.C. daily for 10 days before surgery, on day of surgery, and for 4 days after surgery. Or, 600 units/kg S.C. in once-weekly doses (21, 14, and 7 days before surgery), plus a fourth dose on day of surgery. Before initiating treatment, establish that hemoglobin level is above 10 g/dl and less than or equal to 13 g/dl.

How supplied
Available by prescription only
Injection: 2,000 units, 3,000 units, 4,000 units, 10,000 units, 20,000 units, 40,000 units

Pharmacodynamics
Antianemic action: Epoetin alfa is a glycoprotein consisting of 165 amino acids synthesized using recombinant DNA technology. It mimics naturally occurring erythropoietin, which is produced by the kidneys. It stimulates the division and differentiation of cells within bone marrow to produce RBCs.

Pharmacokinetics
Absorption: May be given S.C. or I.V.
Distribution: Unknown.
Metabolism: Unknown.
Excretion: Unknown.

Route	Onset	Peak	Duration
I.V.	Unknown	Immediate	Unknown
S.C.	Unknown	5-24 hr	Unknown

Contraindications and precautions
Contraindicated in patients with uncontrolled hypertension and hypersensitivity to mammal cell–derived products or albumin (human).

Interactions
None reported.

Adverse reactions
CNS: *headache, seizures,* paresthesia, *fatigue,* asthenia, dizziness.
CV: *hypertension, edema.*

GI: *nausea, vomiting, diarrhea.*
GU: increased BUN and creatinine.
Metabolic: hyperuricemia, hyperphosphatemia, hyperkalemia.
Musculoskeletal: *arthralgia.*
Respiratory: *cough, shortness of breath.*
Skin: *rash,* urticaria.
Other: increased clotting of arteriovenous grafts, *pyrexia, injection site reactions.*

Overdose and treatment
Maximum safe dose hasn't been established. Doses up to 1,500 units/kg have been administered three times weekly for 3 weeks without direct toxic effects. The drug can cause polycythemia; phlebotomy may be used to bring hematocrit within appropriate levels.

Special considerations
• For HIV-infected patients treated with zidovudine, measure hematocrit once weekly until stabilized and then periodically.
• Most patients eventually require supplemental iron therapy. Before and during therapy, monitor patient's iron stores, including serum ferritin and transferrin saturation.
• If a patient fails to respond to epoetin alfa therapy, consider the following possible causes: vitamin deficiency, iron deficiency, underlying infection, occult blood loss, underlying hematologic disease, hemolysis, aluminum intoxication, osteitis fibrosa cystica, or increased dosage of zidovudine.

Patient monitoring
• Routine monitoring of CBC with differential and platelet counts is recommended.
• Measure hematocrit twice weekly until it has stabilized and during adjustment to a maintenance dosage in patients with chronic renal failure. An interval of 2 to 6 weeks may elapse before a dosage change is reflected in the hematocrit level.
• Monitor blood pressure closely.

Pregnant patients
• Use drug during pregnancy only when benefits outweigh risks to fetus.

Breast-feeding patients
• It isn't known whether drug appears in breast milk. Use cautiously in breast-feeding women.

Pediatric patients
• Safety and efficacy in children haven't been established.

Patient education
• Explain importance of regularly monitoring blood pressure in light of potential drug effects.
• Advise patient to adhere to dietary restrictions during therapy. Make sure he understands that drug won't influence disease process.

epoprostenol sodium
Flolan

Pharmacologic classification: naturally occurring prostaglandin
Therapeutic classification: vasodilator, antiplatelet aggregator
Pregnancy risk category: B

Indications and dosages
➤ *Long-term I.V. treatment of primary pulmonary hypertension and pulmonary hypertension related to the scleroderma spectrum of disease in New York Heart Association class III and class IV patients who don't respond adequately to conventional therapy. Adults:* Initially for acute dose ranging, 2 ng/kg/minute as an I.V. infusion; increase in increments of 2 ng/kg/minute q 15 minutes or longer until dose-limiting pharmacologic effects occur. Begin maintenance dosing with 4 ng/kg/minute less than the maximum tolerated infusion rate as determined during acute dose ranging. If the maximum tolerated infusion rate is less than 5 ng/kg/minute, begin maintenance infusion at one-half the maximum tolerated infusion rate. Base subsequent dosage adjustments on persistence, recurrence, or worsening of patient's symptoms of primary pulmonary hypertension and the occurrence of adverse events because of excessive doses of drug. Increases in dose from the initial maintenance dosage are common and usually are done in increments of 1 to 2 ng/kg/minute at intervals of at least 15 minutes.

How supplied
Available by prescription only
Injection: 0.5 mg/17-ml vial, 1.5 mg/17-ml vial

Pharmacodynamics
Vasodilator and antiplatelet actions: Epoprostenol causes direct vasodilation of pulmonary and systemic arterial vascular beds and inhibits platelet aggregation.

Pharmacokinetics
Absorption: Administered I.V.
Distribution: Unknown.
Metabolism: Extensively metabolized.
Excretion: Excreted primarily in urine with a small amount excreted in feces.

Route	Onset	Peak	Duration
I.V.	Unknown	Unknown	Unknown

Contraindications and precautions
Contraindicated in patients hypersensitive to drug or structurally related compounds. Long-term use of drug is also contraindicated in patients with heart failure because of severe left ventricular systolic dysfunction or in those in whom

---

Reactions may be *common,* uncommon, *life-threatening,* or COMMON AND LIFE-THREATENING.

pulmonary edema develops during initial dose ranging.

Interactions

Drug-drug. *Anticoagulants, antiplatelet drugs:* May increase risk of bleeding. Watch closely for bleeding.
Antihypertensives, diuretics, vasodilators: May cause additional reduction in blood pressure. Monitor blood pressure closely.

Adverse reactions

CNS: *headache, anxiety, nervousness, agitation, dizziness, hyperesthesia, paresthesia.*
CV: *tachycardia, flushing, hypotension, chest pain, bradycardia.*
GI: *nausea, vomiting,* abdominal pain, dyspepsia; *diarrhea.*
Hematologic: *thrombocytopenia.*
Musculoskeletal: back pain, *jaw pain, myalgia, nonspecific musculoskeletal pain.*
Respiratory: dyspnea.
Skin: sweating.
Other: *flulike symptoms, chills, fever, sepsis.*

Overdose and treatment

Overdose may result in flushing, headache, hypotension, tachycardia, nausea, vomiting, and diarrhea.

Treatment usually requires reduction of epoprostenol dosage.

Special considerations

• Drug should be used only by clinicians experienced in the diagnosis and treatment of primary pulmonary hypertension. Determining the appropriate dose for the patient must be done in a setting with adequate personnel and equipment for physiologic monitoring and emergency care.
• Before use, protect reconstituted solutions of the drug from light and refrigerate at 36° to 46° F (2° to 8° C) if not used immediately. Don't freeze reconstituted solutions of drug. Discard reconstituted solution that's been frozen. Discard reconstituted solution if it's been refrigerated for more than 48 hours.
• Avoid abrupt withdrawal or sudden large reductions in infusion rates.
• Administer anticoagulant therapy during long-term use of drug, unless contraindicated. Monitor PT and INR closely.

Patient monitoring

• During maintenance infusion, dose-related effects similar to those observed during startup dosing may necessitate a decrease in infusion rate, but the adverse event may occasionally resolve without dosage adjustment.
• Monitor for adverse reactions.

Breast-feeding patients

• It isn't known whether drug appears in breast milk. Use cautiously in breast-feeding women.

Pediatric patients

• Safety and efficacy in children haven't been established.

Geriatric patients

• In general, dose selection should be cautious because these patients are more likely to have decreased hepatic, renal, or cardiac function; concomitant disease; and multi-drug therapy.

Patient education

• Make sure patient and family understand before starting therapy that I.V. therapy with epoprostenol commonly is needed for prolonged periods, possibly years. Also, make sure patient and family accepts and can care for a permanent I.V. catheter and infusion pump.
• Teach patient and family how to reconstitute drug and give drug via infusion pump using sterile technique. Explain how to use infusion pump. Stress importance of maintaining continuous drug therapy. Provide patient and family with instructions on how to switch to a new infusion pump in the event of pump failure. Also instruct patient and family on how to store drug.
• Instruct patient to report adverse reactions regarding drug therapy immediately because dosage adjustments may be necessary.
• Provide patient with telephone number to obtain assistance for 24-hour support.

eprosartan mesylate
Teveten

Pharmacologic classification: angiotensin II receptor antagonist
Therapeutic classification: antihypertensive
Pregnancy risk category: C (D in second and third trimesters)

Indications and dosages

➤ **Hypertension, alone or with other antihypertensives.** *Adults:* Initially, 600 mg P.O. daily. Daily dose ranges from 400 to 800 mg given as single daily dose or two divided doses.

How supplied

Available by prescription only
Tablets: 400 mg, 600 mg

Pharmacodynamics

Antihypertensive action: An angiotensin II receptor that blocks vasoconstrictor and aldosterone-secreting effects of angiotensin II by selectively blocking binding of angiotensin II to its receptor sites found in many tissues, such as vascular smooth muscle and the adrenal gland.

Pharmacokinetics

Absorption: Absolute bioavailability of single oral dose is about 13%. Onset of action occurs in about 1 to 2 hours, with plasma levels peaking in 1 to 3 hours.

Distribution: Plasma protein–binding about 98%. Duration about 24 hours.
Metabolism: No active metabolites.
Excretion: Eliminated by biliary and renal excretion, primarily as unchanged drug. Following oral administration, about 90% recovered in feces and about 7% in urine. Terminal elimination half-life typically 5 to 9 hours.

Route	Onset	Peak	Duration
P.O.	1-2 hr	1-3 hr	24 hr

Contraindications and precautions
Contraindicated in patients hypersensitive to drug or its components. Use cautiously in patients with an activated renin-angiotensin system, such as volume- or salt-depleted patients, and patients whose renal function may depend on the activity of the renin-angiotensin-aldosterone system, such as patients with severe heart failure. Also use cautiously in patients with renal artery stenosis.

Interactions
None reported.

Adverse reactions
CNS: depression, fatigue, headache, dizziness.
CV: chest pain.
EENT: pharyngitis, rhinitis, sinusitis.
GI: abdominal pain, dyspepsia, diarrhea.
GU: urinary tract infection, increased BUN level.
Hematologic: *neutropenia.*
Metabolic: hypertriglyceridemia.
Musculoskeletal: arthralgia, myalgia.
Respiratory: cough, upper respiratory tract infection, bronchitis.
Other: injury, viral infection, dependent edema, facial edema, *angioedema.*

Overdose and treatment
In case of overdose, give symptomatic and supportive therapy. Drug is poorly removed by hemodialysis.

Special considerations
• Correct hypovolemia and hyponatremia before therapy to reduce risk of symptomatic hypotension.
• A transient episode of hypotension isn't a contraindication to continued treatment. Drug may be restarted once patient's blood pressure has stabilized.
• Use drug alone or with other antihypertensives, such as diuretics and calcium channel blockers. Maximal blood pressure response may take 2 to 3 weeks.

Patient monitoring
• Monitor blood pressure closely for 2 hours during start of therapy. If hypotension occurs, place patient in supine position and, if necessary, give I.V. infusion of normal saline solution.

• Monitor patient for facial or lip swelling; angioedema has occurred with other angiotensin II antagonists.
• Closely observe neonates exposed to eprosartan in utero for hypotension, oliguria, and hyperkalemia.
• Monitor renal function before treatment and periodically throughout.

Pregnant patients
• Drugs that act directly on the renin-angiotensin system can cause fetal and neonatal morbidity and death when administered to pregnant women. If pregnancy is detected, stop drug as soon as possible. These adverse effects haven't occurred when intrauterine drug exposure has been limited to first trimester.

Breast-feeding patients
• It isn't known whether drug appears in breast milk. Because of potential for serious adverse reactions in breast-feeding infants, a decision should be made to stop drug or breast-feeding.

Pediatric patients
• Safety and effectiveness in children haven't been established.

Geriatric patients
• There's a slightly decreased response to drug in elderly patients. No initial dose adjustment necessary.

Patient education
• Advise woman of childbearing age to use reliable form of contraception and to call immediately if pregnancy is suspected. Drug may need to be stopped under medical supervision.
• Advise patient to report facial or lip swelling and signs and symptoms of infection, such as fever or sore throat.
• Tell patient to obtain medical approval before taking OTC product for dry cough.
• Inform patient that drug may be taken without regard to meals.
• Tell patient to store drug at a controlled room temperature (68° to 77° F [20 to 25° C]).

eptifibatide
Integrilin

Pharmacologic classification: glycoprotein IIb/IIIa (GP IIb/IIIa) inhibitor
Therapeutic classification: antiplatelet agent
Pregnancy risk category: B

Indications and dosages
➤*Acute coronary syndrome (unstable angina or non-Q-wave MI) in patients being managed medically and in those undergoing percutaneous coronary intervention.* Adults: 180 mcg/kg (up to maximum dose of 22.6 mg) I.V. bolus as soon as pos-

---

sible following diagnosis, followed by a continuous I.V. infusion of 2 mcg/kg/minute (up to maximum infusion rate of 15 mg/hour) for up to 72 hours. Infusion rate may be decreased to 0.5 mcg/kg/minute during percutaneous coronary intervention. Infusion should then be continued for another 20 to 24 hours after the procedure for up to 96 hours of therapy.

► *Treatment in patients without signs and symptoms of acute coronary syndrome who are undergoing percutaneous coronary intervention. Adults:* I.V. bolus of 135 mcg/kg immediately before procedure, followed by a continuous infusion of 0.5 mcg/kg/minute for 20 to 24 hours.

How supplied
Available by prescription only
Injection: 2 mg /ml, 10-ml vial, 0.75 mg/ml, 100-ml vials

Pharmacodynamics
Antiplatelet action: Reversibly inhibits platelet aggregation by preventing the binding of fibrinogen, von Willebrand factor, and other adhesion molecules to the GP IIb/IIIa receptor on human platelets.

Pharmacokinetics
Absorption: Administered I.V.
Distribution: 25% bound to plasma proteins.
Metabolism: Not reported. No major metabolites have been detected in human plasma.
Excretion: Elimination half-life is 2½ hours. Most of drug appears in urine.

Route	Onset	Peak	Duration
I.V.	Immediate	Immediate	4-6 hr after infusion ends

Contraindications and precautions
Contraindicated in patients hypersensitive to drug or its ingredients. Contraindicated in patients with a history of bleeding diathesis or evidence of active abnormal bleeding within previous 30 days; severe hypertension (systolic blood pressure exceeding 200 mm Hg or diastolic blood pressure of more than 110 mm Hg) not adequately controlled on antihypertensive therapy; major surgery within previous 6 weeks; history of CVA within 30 days; history of hemorrhagic stroke; current or planned use of another parenteral GP IIb/IIIa inhibitor; or a platelet count of less than 100,000/mm³.

Contraindicated in patients whose serum creatinine is 2 mg/dl or higher (for the 180 mcg/kg bolus and 2 mcg/kg/minute infusion) or 4 mg/dl or higher (for the 135 mcg/kg bolus and 0.5 mcg/kg/minute infusion); or in patients who are dependent on renal dialysis.

Use cautiously in patients at increased risk of bleeding and patients weighing more than 143 kg (315 lb).

Interactions
Drug-drug. *Clopidogrel, dipyridamole, NSAIDs, oral anticoagulants, thrombolytics, ticlopidine:* Increased risk of bleeding. Monitor patient closely.
Inhibitors of platelet receptor GP IIb/IIIa: May potentiate serious bleeding. Don't administer together.

Adverse reactions
CV: hypotension.
GU: hematuria.
Hematologic: *bleeding, thrombocytopenia.*
Other: bleeding at femoral artery access site.

Overdose and treatment
Limited data exist. Few patients received doses greater than or equal to two times the recommended dose.

Special considerations
• Drug may be administered in same I.V. line as alteplase, atropine, dobutamine, heparin, lidocaine, meperidine, metoprolol, midazolam, morphine, nitroglycerin, or verapamil.
• Drug may be administered in same I.V. line with normal saline or normal saline solution D₅W, and solution may contain up to 60 mEq/L of potassium chloride.
• Don't administer drug in same I.V. line as furosemide.
• Use drug in conjunction with heparin and aspirin.
• If patient's platelet count is less than 100,000/mm³, discontinue eptifibatide and heparin.
• Discontinue eptifibatide and heparin and achieve sheath hemostasis by standard compressive techniques at least 4 hours before hospital discharge. The arterial access site is the most common site of bleeding.
• If patient is to undergo coronary artery bypass graft surgery, stop infusion before surgery.
• Minimize use of arterial and venous punctures, I.M. injections, and use of urinary catheters, nasotracheal tubes, and nasogastric tubes.

Patient monitoring
• Perform baseline laboratory tests before start of drug therapy: hematocrit, hemoglobin, and platelet count, serum creatinine level, PT, INR, and PTT.
• Monitor patient for bleeding.

Breast-feeding patients
• It isn't known whether drug appears in breast milk. Administer cautiously to breast-feeding women.

Pediatric patients
• Safety in children hasn't been established.

Geriatric patients
● Drug has been used in patients as old as age 94. No significant difference shown compared to younger population.

Patient education
● Advise patient of potential adverse reactions.
● Instruct patient to report chest discomfort or other adverse events immediately.
● Caution patient to avoid activities that might cause bleeding or bruising.

ergocalciferol (vitamin D₂)
Calciferol, Drisdol, Vitamin D

Pharmacologic classification: vitamin
Therapeutic classification: antihypocalcemic
Pregnancy risk category: C

Indications and dosages
➤ *Nutritional rickets or osteomalacia.*
Adults: 25 to 125 mcg P.O. daily if patient has normal GI absorption. With severe malabsorption, 250 mcg to 7.5 mg P.O. or 250 mcg I.M. daily.
Children: 25 to 125 mcg P.O. daily if patient has normal GI absorption. With malabsorption, 250 to 625 mcg P.O. daily.
➤ *Familial hypophosphatemia. Adults:* 250 mcg to 1.5 mg P.O. daily with phosphate supplements.
Children: 1 to 2 mg P.O. daily with phosphate supplements. Increase daily dose in 250- to 500-mcg increments at 3- to 4-month intervals until adequate response is obtained.
➤ *Vitamin D-dependent rickets. Adults:* 250 mcg to 1.5 mg P.O. daily.
Children: 75 to 125 mcg P.O. daily.
➤ *Anticonvulsant-induced rickets and osteomalacia. Adults:* 50 mcg to 1.25 mg P.O. daily.
➤ *Hypoparathyroidism and pseudohypoparathyroidism. Adults:* 625 mcg to 5 mg P.O. daily with calcium supplements.
Children: 1.25 to 5 mg P.O. daily with calcium supplements.
➤ *Fanconi's syndrome◇. Adults:* 1.25 to 5 mg. P.O. daily.
Children: 625 mcg to 1.25 mg P.O. daily.
➤ *Osteoporosis◇. Adults:* 25 to 250 mcg P.O. daily or 1.25 mg P.O. weekly with calcium and fluoride supplements.

How supplied
Available by prescription only
Capsules: 1.25 mg (50,000 units)
Injection: 12.5 mg (500,000 units)/ml
Available without a prescription
Liquid: 8,000 units/ml in 60-ml dropper bottle

Pharmacodynamics
Antihypocalcemic action: Once activated, ergocalciferol acts to regulate the serum levels of calcium by regulating absorption from the GI tract and resorption from bone.

Pharmacokinetics
Absorption: Absorbed readily from the small intestine.
Distribution: Distributed widely and bound to proteins stored in the liver.
Metabolism: Metabolized in the liver and kidneys. It has an average half-life of 24 hours and a duration of up to 6 months.
Excretion: Bile (feces) is the primary excretion route. A small percentage appears in urine.

Route	Onset	Peak	Duration
P.O., I.M.	2-24 hr	4-12 hr	2 days-6 mo

Contraindications and precautions
Contraindicated in patients with hypercalcemia, hypervitaminosis A, or renal osteodystrophy with hyperphosphatemia. Use extremely cautiously, if at all, in patients with impaired renal function, heart disease, renal stones, or arteriosclerosis.

Interactions
Drug-drug. *Cardiac glycosides:* Increased risk of arrhythmias. Monitor patient closely.
Cholestyramine, colestipol, excessive use of mineral oil: Disrupted absorption of ergocalciferol. Avoid use together.
Corticosteroids: Counteract effects of ergocalciferol. Monitor patient carefully.
Magnesium-containing antacids: Increased risk of hypermagnesemia. Monitor magnesium level.
Orlistat: Decreased absorption of vitamin D analogues. Separate drugs by 2 hours.
Phenobarbital, phenytoin: Increased metabolism of ergocalciferol to inactive metabolites. Use together cautiously.
Thiazide diuretics: May cause hypercalcemia in patients with hypoparathyroidism. Monitor patient closely.
Verapamil: Atrial fibrillation may occur when supplemental calcium and calciferol have induced hypercalcemia. Monitor patient carefully.

Adverse reactions
Adverse reactions listed usually occur only in vitamin D toxicity.
CNS: headache, weakness, somnolence, overt psychosis, irritability.
CV: *calcifications of soft tissues, including the heart,* hypertension, **arrhythmias.**
EENT: rhinorrhea, conjunctivitis (calcific), photophobia.
GI: anorexia, nausea, vomiting, constipation, dry mouth, metallic taste, polydipsia.
GU: polyuria, albuminuria, hypercalciuria, nocturia, **impaired renal function,** reversible azotemia.

Hepatic: elevated liver enzyme levels (falsely or actually).
Metabolic: *hypercalcemia,* hyperthermia, increased serum cholesterol levels, weight loss.
Musculoskeletal: bone and muscle pain, bone demineralization.
Skin: pruritus.
Other: decreased libido.

Overdose and treatment

Signs and symptoms of overdose include hypercalcemia, hypercalciuria, and hyperphosphatemia, which may be treated by stopping therapy, starting a low-calcium diet, and increasing fluid intake. A loop diuretic, such as furosemide, may be given with saline I.V. infusion to increase calcium excretion. Provide supportive measures. In severe cases, death from cardiac or renal failure may occur. Calcitonin may decrease hypercalcemia.

Special considerations

• I.M. injection of ergocalciferol dispersed in oil is preferable in patients who are unable to absorb the oral form.
• Patients with hyperphosphatemia require dietary phosphate restrictions and binding agents to avoid metastatic calcifications and renal calculi.
• Doses of 60,000 IU daily can cause hypercalcemia.

Patient monitoring

• Monitor eating and bowel habits; dry mouth, nausea, vomiting, metallic taste, and constipation can be early signs of toxicity.
• Check serum and urine calcium, potassium, and urea levels frequently when patient receives large doses.
• Malabsorption caused by inadequate bile or hepatic dysfunction may require addition of exogenous bile salts.

Breast-feeding patients

• Very little drug appears in breast milk; however, effect on infants of amounts exceeding RDA levels of vitamin D isn't known.

Pediatric patients

• Some infants may be hyperreactive to drug.

Patient education

• Caution patient not to increase daily dose.
• Tell patient to avoid magnesium-containing antacids and mineral oil.
• Instruct patient to swallow tablets whole without crushing or chewing.

ergonovine maleate
Ergotrate Maleate

Pharmacologic classification: ergot alkaloid
Therapeutic classification: oxytocic
Pregnancy risk category: NR

Indications and dosages

➤ *Prevention or treatment of postpartum and postabortion hemorrhage caused by uterine atony or subinvolution.* Adults: 0.2 mg I.M. q 2 to 4 hours, maximum five doses. Or, 0.2 mg I.V. (only for severe uterine bleeding or other life-threatening emergency) over 1 minute while blood pressure and uterine contractions are monitored. I.V. dose may be diluted to 5 ml with normal saline injection.
➤ *Diagnosis of coronary artery spasm (Prinzmetal's angina)* ◊. Adults: 0.1 to 0.4 mg I.V. for one dose.

How supplied

Available by prescription only
Injection: 0.2-mg/ml ampules

Pharmacodynamics

Oxytocic action: Ergonovine maleate stimulates contraction of uterine and vascular smooth muscle. It produces intense uterine contractions followed by periods of relaxation. The drug produces vasoconstriction of primarily capacitance blood vessels, causing an increased CVP and elevated blood pressure. The clinical effect is secondary to contraction of the uterine wall around bleeding vessels, producing hemostasis.

Pharmacokinetics

Absorption: Absorption is rapid following I.M. administration.
Distribution: Unknown.
Metabolism: Metabolized in the liver.
Excretion: Probably primarily nonrenal elimination in feces.

Route	Onset	Peak	Duration
I.V.	Immediate	Unknown	Unknown
I.M.	2-5 min	Unknown	Unknown

Contraindications and precautions

Contraindicated in patients sensitive to ergot preparations; in threatened spontaneous abortion, induction of labor, or before delivery of placenta because captivation of placenta may occur; and in those with history of allergic or idiosyncratic reactions to drug.

Because of the potential for adverse CV effects, use cautiously in patients with hypertension, toxemia, sepsis, occlusive vascular disease, and hepatic, renal, and cardiac disease.

Interactions

Drug-drug. *Cardiac glycosides:* Enhanced vasoconstriction. Avoid use together.

Local anesthetics with vasoconstrictors (lidocaine with epinephrine): Enhanced vasoconstriction. Use cautiously.
Other ergot alkaloids and sympathomimetic amines: Enhanced vasoconstrictor potential. Monitor patient carefully.
Drug-lifestyle. *Smoking:* Enhances vasoconstriction. Advise patient not to smoke.

Adverse reactions
CNS: headache, confusion, dizziness, ringing in ears.
CV: chest pain, weakness in legs (peripheral vasospasm), hypertension, thrombophlebitis.
GI: nausea, vomiting, diarrhea, cramping.
Metabolic: decreased serum prolactin.
Musculoskeletal: pain in arms, legs, or lower back.
Respiratory: shortness of breath.
Other: itching; sweating; *hypersensitivity reactions, signs of shock.*

Overdose and treatment
Signs and symptoms of overdose include seizures, nausea, vomiting, diarrhea, dizziness, fluctuations in blood pressure, weak pulse, chest pain, tingling, and numbness and coldness in the limbs. Rarely, gangrene has occurred.
   Treat seizures with anticonvulsants and hypercoagulability with heparin; give vasodilators to improve blood flow. Gangrene may require amputation.

Special considerations
● Contractions begin immediately after I.V. injection. May continue for 45 minutes after I.V. injection.
● Discontinue drug if hypertension or allergic reactions occur.
● Hypocalcemia may decrease patient response; I.V. administration of calcium salts is necessary.
⚠ ALERT High doses during delivery may cause uterine tetany and possible infant hypoxia or intracranial hemorrhage.
● Drug has been used as a diagnostic agent for angina pectoris.

Patient monitoring
● Monitor blood pressure, pulse rate, uterine response, and character and amount of vaginal bleeding. Watch for sudden changes in vital signs and frequent periods of uterine relaxation.

Pregnant patients
● High doses during delivery may cause uterine tetany and possible infant hypoxia or intracranial hemorrhage.

Breast-feeding patients
● Ergot alkaloids inhibit lactation. Drug appears in breast milk, and ergotism has been reported in breast-fed infants of women given other ergot alkaloids. Use cautiously.

Patient education
● Tell patient not to smoke while taking drug.
● Advise patient of possible adverse reactions.

ergotamine tartrate
Cafergot, Ergomar, Ergostat, Gynergen, Medihaler Ergotamine, Wigraine

Pharmacologic classification: ergot alkaloid
Therapeutic classification: vasoconstrictor
Pregnancy risk category: X

Indications and dosages
➤ *To prevent or abort vascular headache, including migraine and cluster headaches.* Adults: Initially, 2 mg S.L. or P.O., then 1 to 2 mg S.L. or P.O. q 30 minutes, to maximum 6 mg per attack or in 24 hours, and 10 mg weekly. Or, initially 1 inhalation; if not relieved in 5 minutes, repeat 1 inhalation. May repeat inhalations at least 5 minutes apart up to maximum of 6 inhalations per 24 hours or 15 inhalations weekly. Patient may also use rectal suppositories. Initially, 2 mg P.R. at onset of attack; repeat in 1 hour, p.r.n. Maximum dose is 2 suppositories per attack or 5 suppositories weekly.
Children: 1 mg S.L. in older children and adolescents; if no improvement, additional 1-mg dose may be given in 30 minutes.

How supplied
Available by prescription only
Aerosol inhaler: 360 mcg/metered spray
Suppositories: 2 mg (with caffeine 100 mg)
Tablets: 1 mg* (with or without caffeine 100 mg)
Tablets (S.L.): 2 mg

Pharmacodynamics
Vasoconstricting action: By stimulating alpha-adrenergic receptors, ergotamine in therapeutic doses causes peripheral vasoconstriction (if vascular tone is low); however, if vascular tone is high, it produces vasodilation. In high doses, it's a competitive alpha blocker. In therapeutic doses, it inhibits the reuptake of norepinephrine, which increases the vasoconstricting activity of ergotamine. A weaker serotonin antagonist, it slows the increased platelet aggregation caused by serotonin.
   In the treatment of vascular headaches, ergotamine probably causes direct vasoconstriction of dilated carotid artery beds while decreasing the amplitude of pulsations. Its serotoninergic and catecholamine effects also seem to be involved.

Pharmacokinetics
Absorption: Rapidly absorbed after inhalation and variably absorbed after oral administration. Levels peak in ½ to 3 hours. Caffeine may increase rate and extent of absorption. Drug un-

---

dergoes first-pass metabolism after oral administration.
Distribution: Widely distributed throughout the body.
Metabolism: Extensively metabolized in the liver.
Excretion: Part of dose (4%) is excreted in urine within 96 hours; remainder is presumed to be excreted in feces. Ergotamine is dialyzable. Onset of action depends on how promptly drug is given after onset of headache.

Route	Onset	Peak	Duration
P.O.	Variable	½-3 hr	Variable
S.L., inhalation	Variable	Unknown	Variable
P.R.	Unknown	Unknown	Unknown

Contraindications and precautions
Contraindicated in pregnant patients, patients hypersensitive to ergot alkaloids, and patients with peripheral and occlusive vascular diseases, coronary artery disease, hypertension, hepatic or renal dysfunction, severe pruritus, or sepsis.

Interactions
Drug-drug. *Erythromycin, other macrolides:* May cause symptoms of ergot toxicity. Vasodilators (nifedipine, nitroprusslde, or prazosin) may be ordered to treat ergot toxicity.
Propranolol, other beta blockers: Increased vasoconstrictor effects. Monitor patient carefully.
Drug-food. *Caffeine:* May increase rate and extent of absorption. Advise patient to avoid caffeine.
Drug-lifestyle. *Alcohol use:* May worsen headache. Advise patient to avoid alcohol use.
Smoking: May increase adverse effects. Caution patient to avoid smoking.

Adverse reactions
CNS: numbness and tingling in fingers and toes.
CV: transient tachycardia or ***bradycardia***, precordial distress and pain, increased arterial pressure, angina, peripheral vasoconstriction.
GI: nausea, vomiting.
Musculoskeletal: weakness in legs, muscle pain in limbs.
Skin: pruritus, localized edema.

Overdose and treatment
Signs and symptoms of overdose include adverse vasospastic effects, nausea, vomiting, lassitude, impaired mental function, delirium, severe dyspnea, hypotension or hypertension, rapid pulse, weak pulse, unconsciousness, spasms of the limbs, seizures, and shock.

Treatment is supportive and symptomatic, with prolonged and careful monitoring. If patient is conscious and ingestion is recent, empty stomach by emesis or gastric lavage; if comatose, perform gastric lavage after placement of endotracheal tube with cuff inflated. Activated charcoal and a saline (magnesium sulfate) cathartic may be used. Provide respiratory support. Apply warmth (not direct heat) to ischemic extremities if vasospasm occurs. As needed, administer vasodilators (nitroprusside, prazosin, or tolazoline) and, if necessary, I.V. diazepam to treat seizures. Dialysis may be helpful.

Special considerations
● Drug is most effective when used in prodromal stage of headache or as soon as possible after onset. Provide quiet, low-light environment to relax patient after dose is administered.
● S.L. tablet is preferred during early stage of attack because of its rapid absorption.
● Drug isn't effective for muscle contraction headaches.

Patient monitoring
● Rebound headache or increased duration or frequency of headache may occur when drug is stopped.
● If patient experiences severe vasoconstriction with tissue necrosis, administer I.V. sodium nitroprusside or intra-arterial tolazoline. I.V. heparin and 10% dextran 40 in D₅W injection also may be administered to prevent vascular stasis and thrombosis.

Pregnant patients
● Drug is contraindicated in women who are or may become pregnant.

Breast-feeding patients
● Drug appears in breast milk; therefore, use cautiously in breast-feeding women. Excessive drug use may inhibit lactation.

Pediatric patients
● Safety and efficacy of ergotamine in children haven't been established.

Geriatric patients
● Administer cautiously to geriatric patients.

Patient education
● Instruct patient in correct use of drug.
● Urge patient to immediately report to prescriber feelings of numbness or tingling in fingers or toes or red or violet blisters on hands or feet.
● Caution patient to avoid alcoholic beverages and smoking.
● Warn patient to avoid prolonged exposure to very cold temperatures, which may increase adverse effects of drug.
● Advise patient who uses an inhaler to call prescriber promptly if mouth, throat, or lung infection occurs or if condition worsens. Cough, hoarseness, or throat irritation may occur. Patient should gargle and rinse mouth after each dose to help prevent hoarseness and irritation.
● Advise patient not to exceed recommended dosage.

erythromycin base
Apo-Erythro base*, E-Base, E-Mycin, Erybid*, ERYC, Ery-Tab, Erythromycin Base/Filmtabs, Ilotycin, PCE

erythromycin estolate
Ilosone, Novo-rythro*

erythromycin ethylsuccinate
E.E.S., E.E.S. Granules, EryPed, EryPed Drops, Pediazole

erythromycin gluceptate
Ilotycin Gluceptate

erythromycin lactobionate
Erythrocin Lactobionate

erythromycin stearate
Apo-Erythro-S*, Erythrocin Stearate Filmtab, Novo-rythro*

erythromycin (topical)
Akne-Mycin, A/T/S, Del-Mycin, Erycette, EryDerm, Erygel, Erymax, Ery-Sol, Erythra-Derm, Staticin, Theramycin Z, T-Stat

erythromycin (ophthalmic)
Ilotycin

Pharmacologic classification: macrolide
Therapeutic classification: antibiotic
Pregnancy risk category: B

Indications and dosages
➤ *Acute pelvic inflammatory disease caused by* **Neisseria gonorrhoeae.** *Adults:* 500 mg I.V. (gluceptate, lactobionate) q 6 hours for 3 days; then 250 mg (base, estolate, stearate) or 400 mg (ethylsuccinate) P.O. q 6 hours for 7 days.
➤ *Intestinal amebiasis in patients who can't receive metronidazole. Adults:* 250 mg (base, estolate, stearate) or 400 mg (ethylsuccinate) P.O. q 6 hours for 10 to 14 days.
Children: 30 to 50 mg/kg (base, estolate, ethylsuccinate, stearate) P.O. daily, divided q 6 hours for 10 to 14 days.
➤ *Mild to moderately severe respiratory tract, skin, and soft-tissue infections caused by susceptible organisms. Adults:* 250 to 500 mg (base, estolate, stearate) P.O. q 6 hours. Or, 333 mg (base) P.O. q 8 hours. Or, 400 to 800 mg (ethylsuccinate) P.O. q 6 hours. Or, 15 to 20 mg/kg (gluceptate, lactobionate) I.V. daily, in divided doses q 6 hours.
Children: 30 mg/kg to 50 mg/kg (oral erythromycin salts) P.O. daily, in divided doses q 6

hours. Or, 15 to 20 mg/kg I.V. daily in divided doses q 4 to 6 hours.
➤ *Syphilis. Adults:* 500 mg (base, estolate, stearate) P.O. q.i.d. for 14 days.
➤ *Legionnaire's disease. Adults:* 500 mg to 1 g I.V. or P.O. (base, estolate, stearate) or 800 mg to 1,600 mg (ethylsuccinate) P.O. q 6 hours for 21 days.
➤ *Uncomplicated urethral, endocervical, or rectal infections when tetracyclines are contraindicated. Adults:* 500 mg (base, estolate, stearate) or 800 mg (ethylsuccinate) P.O. q.i.d. for at least 7 days.
➤ *Urogenital* Chlamydia trachomatis *infections during pregnancy. Adults:* 500 mg (base, estolate, stearate) P.O. q.i.d. for at least 7 days or 250 mg (base, estolate, stearate) or 400 mg (ethylsuccinate) P.O. q.i.d. for at least 14 days.
➤ *Conjunctivitis caused by* **C. trachomatis** *in neonates. Neonates:* 50 mg/kg P.O. daily in four divided doses for at least 2 weeks.
➤ *Pneumonia of infancy caused by* **C. trachomatis.** *Infants:* 50 mg/kg P.O. daily in four divided doses for at least 3 weeks.
➤ *Topical treatment of acne vulgaris. Adults and children:* Apply to the affected area b.i.d.
➤ *Prophylaxis of ophthalmia neonatorum. Neonates:* Apply 1-cm long ribbon ointment in the lower conjunctival sac of each eye no later than 1 hour after birth. Use new tube for each infant and don't flush after instillation.
➤ *Acute and chronic conjunctivitis, trachoma, other eye infections. Adults and children:* Apply 1-cm long ribbon ointment directly into infected eye up to six times daily, depending on severity of infection.

How supplied
Available by prescription only
erythromycin base
Capsules (delayed-release): 250 mg
Tablets (enteric-coated): 250 mg, 333 mg, 500 mg
erythromycin estolate
Capsules: 250 mg
Suspension: 125 mg/5 ml, 250 mg/5 ml
Tablets: 500 mg
erythromycin ethylsuccinate
Granules for oral suspension: 200 mg/5 ml (after reconstitution)
Oral suspension: 200 mg/5 ml, 400 mg/5 ml
Powder for oral suspension: 100 mg/2.5 ml, 200 mg/5 ml, 400 mg/5 ml (after reconstitution)
Tablets: 400 mg
Tablets (chewable): 200 mg
erythromycin gluceptate
Injection: 500-mg, 1-g vials
erythromycin lactobionate
Injection: 500-mg, 1-g vials
erythromycin stearate
Tablets (film-coated): 250 mg, 500 mg

Reactions may be *common*, uncommon, *life-threatening*, or COMMON AND LIFE-THREATENING.

erythromycin (topical)
Pledgets: 2%
Topical gel: 2%
Topical ointment: 2%
Topical solution: 1.5%, 2%
erythromycin (ophthalmic)
Ointment: 0.5%

Pharmacodynamics
Antibacterial action: Erythromycin inhibits bacterial protein synthesis by binding to the ribosomal 50S subunit. It's used in the treatment of infection with *Haemophilus influenzae, Entamoeba histolytica, Mycoplasma pneumoniae, Corynebacterium diphtheriae, Corynebacterium minutissimum, Legionella pneumophila,* and *Bordetella pertussis.* It may be used as an alternative to penicillins or tetracycline in the treatment of infection with *Streptococcus pneumoniae, Streptococcus viridans, Listeria monocytogenes, Staphylococcus aureus, C. trachomatis, N. gonorrhoeae,* and *Treponema pallidum.*

Pharmacokinetics
Absorption: Because base salt is acid-sensitive, it must be buffered or have enteric coating to prevent destruction by gastric acids. Acid salts and esters (estolate, ethylsuccinate, and stearate) aren't affected by gastric acidity and therefore are well absorbed. Give base and stearate preparations on an empty stomach. Absorption of estolate and ethylsuccinate preparations is unaffected or possibly even enhanced by presence of food. When administered topically, drug is absorbed minimally.
Distribution: Distributed widely to most body tissues and fluids except CSF, where it's distributed only in low levels. Drug crosses the placenta. About 80% of base and 96% of erythromycin estolate are protein-bound.
Metabolism: Metabolized partially in the liver to inactive metabolites.
Excretion: Excreted mainly unchanged in bile. Only small drug amounts (less than 5%) are excreted in urine; some drug appears in breast milk. In patients with normal renal function, plasma half-life is about 1½ hours. Drug isn't dialyzable.

Route	Onset	Peak	Duration
P.O.	Unknown	1-4 hr	Unknown
I.V.	Unknown	Immediate	Unknown
Topical	Unknown	Unknown	Unknown

Contraindications and precautions
Contraindicated in patients hypersensitive to drug or other macrolides. Erythromycin estolate is contraindicated in patients with hepatic disease. Use erythromycin salts cautiously in patients with impaired hepatic function.

Interactions
Drug-drug. *Carbamazepine:* Increased carbemazepine levels and increased risk of toxicity. Monitor patient and carbemazepine levels closely.
Clindamycin, lincomycin: May be antagonistic. Avoid use together.
Cyclosporine: Increased cyclosporine levels and possible nephrotoxicity. Monitor patient closely.
Digoxin: Increased digoxin levels. Monitor patient for digitalis toxicity.
Disopyramide: Increased disopyramide levels and increased risk of arrhythmias and lengthened QT intervals. Monitor patient's ECG.
Isotretinoin: May cause cumulative dryness and excessive skin irritation. Monitor patient carefully.
Midazolam, triazolam: Increased effects of these drugs. Use together cautiously.
Oral anticoagulants: Excessive anticoagulant effect. Monitor PT and INR closely.
Theophylline: Increased theophylline levels and decreased erythromycin levels. Use together cautiously.
Drug-herb. *Pill-bearing spurge:* Inhibition of CYP3A enzymes and altered drug metabolism. Discourage use together.
Drug-lifestyle. *Abrasive or medicated soaps or cleansers, acne preparations or other preparations containing peeling agents (benzoyl peroxide, resorcinol, salicylic acid, sulfur, tretinoin), alcohol-containing products (aftershave, perfumed toiletries, cosmetics, shaving creams or lotions), astringent soaps or cosmetics, medicated cosmetics or cover-ups:* May cause cumulative dryness, resulting in excessive dryness. Tell patient to use together cautiously.

Adverse reactions
CV: *ventricular arrhythmias.*
EENT: bilateral reversible hearing loss (with high systemic or oral doses in patients with renal or hepatic insufficiency); slowed corneal wound healing, blurred vision (with ophthalmic administration).
GI: *abdominal pain, cramping, nausea, vomiting, diarrhea* (with oral or systemic administration).
Hepatic: cholestatic jaundice (with estolate).
Skin: urticaria, rash, eczema (with oral or systemic administration); urticaria, dermatitis (with ophthalmic administration); sensitivity reactions, erythema, burning, *dryness, pruritus,* irritation, peeling, oily skin (with topical application).
Other: overgrowth of nonsusceptible bacteria or fungi; *anaphylaxis;* fever (with oral or systemic administration); *venous irritation, thrombophlebitis* (after I.V. injection); overgrowth of nonsusceptible organisms (with long-term use); *hypersensitivity reactions,* including itching and burning eyes (with ophthalmic administration).

Overdose and treatment
No information available.

Special considerations

• Base and stearate forms aren't available as liquid.

• Absorption of estolate and ethylsuccinate preparations is unaffected or possibly even enhanced by presence of food.

• Erythromycin estolate may cause serious hepatotoxicity (reversible cholestatic jaundice) in adults.

• Don't administer erythromycin lactobionate with other drugs because of chemical instability. Reconstituted solutions are acidic and should be completely administered within 8 hours of preparation.

• Drug may cause overgrowth of nonsusceptible bacteria or fungi.

• Although drug is bacteriostatic, it may be bactericidal in high levels or against highly susceptible organisms.

Patient monitoring

• Perform culture and sensitivity tests before treatment starts and then as needed.

• Monitor liver function tests for increased serum bilirubin, AST, and alkaline phosphatase levels. Other erythromycin salts can cause less severe hepatotoxicity. (Patients who develop hepatotoxicity from erythromycin estolate may react similarly to any erythromycin preparation.)

Pregnant patients

• Use drug during pregnancy only when clearly indicated.

Breast-feeding patients

• Although drug appears in breast milk, no adverse reactions have been reported. Administer cautiously to breast-feeding women.

Patient education

• Instruct patient to take oral form with full glass of water 1 hour before or 2 hours after meals; enteric-coated tablets may be taken with meals.

• Advise patient not to take drug with fruit juice. If patient takes chewable tablets, tell him not to swallow them whole.

• If patient uses topical solution, instruct patient to wash, rinse, and dry affected areas before applying it. Warn patient not to apply solution near eyes, nose, mouth, or other mucous membranes.

• Instruct patient to wash hands before and after applying ophthalmic ointment. Instruct him to clean eye area of excess exudate before applying ointment. Warn him not to allow tube to touch the eye or surrounding tissue. Instruct him to promptly report signs of sensitivity, such as itching eyelids and constant burning.

• Tell patient to take drug exactly as directed and to continue taking it for prescribed period, even after he feels better.

• Instruct patient to report adverse reactions promptly.

esmolol hydrochloride
Brevibloc

Pharmacologic classification: beta blocker
Therapeutic classification: antiarrhythmic
Pregnancy risk category: C

Indications and dosages

➤ *Supraventricular tachycardia (SVT).*
Adults: Dosage range is 50 to 200 mcg/kg/minute; average dose is 100 mcg/kg/minute. Individual dosage adjustment requires stepwise titration in which each step consists of a loading dose followed by a maintenance infusion.

To begin treatment, administer a loading infusion of 500 mcg/kg/minute for 1 minute followed by a 4-minute maintenance infusion of 50 mcg/kg/minute. If tachycardia doesn't subside within 5 minutes, repeat loading dose and follow with maintenance infusion increased to 100 mcg/kg/minute. Continue titration, repeating loading infusion and increasing each maintenance infusion by 50 mcg/kg/minute. As patient's heart rate or blood pressure reaches a safety endpoint, omit loading infusion and reduce the increase in maintenance infusion from 50 to 25 mcg/kg/minute or less; also, increase the interval between titration steps from 5 to 10 minutes.

➤ *Intraoperative and postoperative tachycardia and hypertension.* *Adults:* For immediate control, 80 mg (about 1 mg/kg) I.V. bolus dose over 30 seconds followed by a 150-mcg/kg/minute infusion, if necessary; for gradual control, a loading I.V. infusion of 500 mcg/kg/minute for 1 minute, followed by a 4-minute maintenance infusion of 50 mcg/kg/minute. If an adequate therapeutic effect isn't observed within 5 minutes, repeat the same loading dose and follow with a maintenance infusion increased to 100 mcg/kg/minute (see SVT, above).

➤ *Acute myocardial ischemia◇.* *Adults:* Initially, 500 mcg/kg/minute I.V. for 1 minute followed by a maintenance infusion of 50 mcg/kg/minute for 4 minutes. If necessary, dosage may be gradually adjusted upward using a regimen similar to SVT until the desired response occurs, maximum dose of 300 mcg/kg/minute is reached, or systolic blood pressure is below 90 mm Hg.

How supplied

Available by prescription only
Injection: 10 mg/ml in 10-ml vials; 250 mg/ml in 10-ml ampules

Pharmacodynamics

Antiarrhythmic action: Esmolol, a beta blocker with rapid onset and very short duration of action, decreases blood pressure and heart rate in a dose-related, adjustable manner. Hemodynamic effects are similar to those of propranolol, but drug doesn't increase vascular resistance.

Pharmacokinetics
Absorption: Administered I.V.
Distribution: Distributed rapidly throughout the plasma. Distribution half-life is about 2 minutes. Esmolol is 55% protein-bound.
Metabolism: Hydrolyzed rapidly by plasma esterases.
Excretion: Excreted by the kidneys as metabolites. Elimination half-life is about 9 minutes.

Route	Onset	Peak	Duration
I.V.	Immediate	10-30 min	30 min after infusion

Contraindications and precautions
Contraindicated in patients with sinus bradycardia, heart block greater than first-degree, cardiogenic shock, or overt heart failure. Use cautiously in patients with impaired renal function, diabetes, bronchospasm, or those with hemodynamic compromise.

Interactions
Drug-drug. *Antihypertensives:* May potentiate hypotensive effects. Dosage adjustments may be necessary.
Catecholamine-depleting drugs, such as res erpine: Additive and possibly excessive beta-adrenergic blockade with bradycardia and hypotension. Observe patient closely.
Insulin, oral antidiabetics: May mask symptoms of developing hypoglycemia. Monitor patient closely.
I.V. digoxin: Increased digoxin levels (10% to 20%). Dosage adjustment may be required.
I.V. morphine: Increased esmolol steady state levels (by 50%). Monitor patient carefully.
Nondepolarizing neuromuscular blockers, such as gallamine, metocurine, pancuronium, succinylcholine, or tubocurarine: May potentiate and prolong the action of these drugs; careful postoperative monitoring is necessary after concurrent or sequential use, especially if there's a possibility of incomplete reversal of neuromuscular blockade.
Sympathomimetic amines with beta-adrenergic stimulant activity: Mutual but transient inhibition of therapeutic effects. Use together cautiously.
Xanthines, especially aminophylline, theophylline: Mutual inhibition of therapeutic effects and (except for dyphylline) decreased theophylline clearance, especially in patients with increased theophylline clearance induced by smoking. Concurrent use requires careful monitoring to prevent toxic accumulation of theophylline.

Adverse reactions
CNS: dizziness, somnolence, headache, agitation, fatigue, confusion.
CV: hypotension (sometimes with diaphoresis), peripheral ischemia.
GI: *nausea*, vomiting.

Respiratory: *bronchospasm,* wheezing, dyspnea, nasal congestion.
Other: inflammation, induration (at infusion site).

Overdose and treatment
Limited information is available. Hypotension would be the most likely effect. Effects of esmolol overdose usually disappear quickly after esmolol is withdrawn.

In addition to immediate discontinuation of esmolol infusion, treatment is supportive and symptomatic. Glucagon has been reported to effectively combat the CV effects (bradycardia, hypotension) of overdose with beta blockers. An I.V. dose of 2 to 3 mg is administered over 30 seconds and repeated if necessary, followed by infusion at 5 mg/hour until patient's condition has stabilized. For symptomatic bradycardia, I.V. atropine may be considered.

Special considerations
• I.V. infusion concentrations exceeding 10 mg/ml may produce irritation.
• Drug isn't compatible with 5% sodium bicarbonate injection USP.
• Diluted solutions of esmolol hydrochloride are stable for at least 24 hours at room temperature.
• To convert to other antiarrhythmic therapy after control has been achieved with esmolol, reduce esmolol infusion rate by half 30 minutes after giving first dose of other drug. If after the second dose of the other drug a satisfactory response is maintained for 1 hour, discontinue esmolol.

Patient monitoring
• Monitor patient's pulse and blood pressure.

Pregnant patients
• Use in third trimester may cause fetal bradycardia. Use drug during pregnancy only when benefits to patient outweigh potential risk to fetus.

Breast-feeding patients
• It isn't known whether drug appears in breast milk; however, no problems have been reported by breast-feeding women.

Pediatric patients
• Adequate and well-controlled studies haven't been done. Safety and efficacy in children haven't been established.

Geriatric patients
• Geriatric patients may be less sensitive to some effects of beta blockers. However, reduced metabolic and excretory capabilities in many geriatric patients may lead to increased myocardial depression and require dosage reduction of beta blockers. Base dosage adjustment on clinical response.

Patient education
• Advise patient to report adverse events including pain at I.V. site.

esomeprazole magnesium
Nexium

Pharmacologic classification: proton pump inhibitor, s-isomer of omeprazole
Therapeutic classification: gastroesophageal agent
Pregnancy risk category: B

Indications and dosages
➤ *Gastroesopageal reflux disease (GERD), healing of erosive esophagitis. Adults:* 20 or 40 mg P.O. q.d. for 4 to 8 weeks.
➤ *Maintenance of healing in erosive esophagitis. Adults:* 20 mg P.O. q.d. for no more than 6 months.
➤ *Symptomatic GERD. Adults:* 20 mg P.O. q.d. for 4 weeks. If symptoms continue, treatment may continue 4 more weeks.
➤ *Eradication of* Helicobacter pylori *(with other drugs) to reduce duodenal ulcer recurrence. Adults:* esomeprazole magnesium 40 mg P.O. q.d. plus amoxicillin 1,000 mg P.O. b.i.d. plus clarithromycin 500 mg P.O. b.i.d., all for 10 days.
✦ *Dosage adjustment.* In patients with severe hepatic failure, the maximum daily dose is 20 mg.

How supplied
Available by prescription only
Capsules (delayed-release containing enteric-coated pellets): 20 mg or 40 mg (supplied as 22.3 or 44.5 mg esomeprazole magnesium).

Pharmacodynamics
Gastric secretion inhibitor action: Suppresses gastric secretion through proton pump inhibition. Inhibits the H+-K+-ATPase pump in gastric parietal cells, reducing gastric acidity by blocking the final step in acid production. Esomeprazole magnesium is the s-isomer of omeperazole.

Pharmacokinetics
Absorption: Esomeprazole is formulated as enteric-coated pellets in a gelatin capsule. Plasma levels peak 1½ hours after oral administration. The plasma level following a 40-mg dose is threefold higher than after a 20-mg dose. Repeated once-daily dosing of 40 mg yields systemic bioavailability of 90% compared to a single 40-mg dose, which yields 64%. This may result from reduced hepatic metabolism and clearance with continued dosing. Giving esomeprazole with food reduces mean plasma level by 33% to 53%.
Distribution: Esomeprazole is about 97% protein-bound. The volume of distribution in healthy patients at steady state is 16 L.
Metabolism: Esomeprazole is extensively metabolized by cytochrome P-450-2C19 to form

hydroxy and desmethyl metabolites that have no secretory activity. CYP2C19 exhibits polymorphism and people who are poor metabolizers have increased esomeprazole plasma levels. About 3% of Whites and 15% to 20% of Asians lack cytochrome P-450-2C19. Cytochrome P450-3A4 metabolizes the remaining amount of esomeprazole.
Excretion: Plasma elimination half-life is about 1 to 1½ hours. Less than 1% of active parent drug is excreted in urine. About 80% of an oral dose is excreted as inactive metabolites in urine. Remaining inactive metabolites are excreted in feces. Systemic clearance of esomeprazole decreases with multiple dose administration.

Route	Onset	Peak	Duration
P.O.	Unknown	1½ hr	13-17 hr

Adverse reactions
CNS: headache.
GI: diarrhea, abdominal pain, nausea, flatulence, dry mouth, vomiting, constipation.

Interactions
Drug-drug. *Amoxicillin, clarithromycin:* Increased esomeprazole levels. Monitor patient for toxicity.
Diazepam: Decreased diazepam clearance. Monitor patient for diazepam toxicity.
Other drugs metabolized by cytochrome P-450-2C19: Altered esomeprazole clearance. Monitor patient closely, especially elderly patient or patient with hepatic insufficiency.
Drug-food. *Any food:* Reduced bioavailability. Advise patient to take drug 1 hour before eating.

Overdose and treatment
No antidote is known. Drug is highly protein-bound and therefore probably isn't removed by dialysis. Supportive care is recommended.

Contraindications and precautions
Contraindicated in patients hypersensitive to any component of esomeprazole or omeprazole. Use cautiously when giving drug to pregnant patients, breast-feeding patients, or patients with hepatic insufficiency. Dosage adjustments are required in patients with severe disease.

Special considerations
• Symptomatic response to esomeprazole doesn't rule out the presence of a gastric malignancy.
• Long-term therapy with omeprazole has caused atrophic gastritis.
• Food decreases the extent of absorption; give esomeprazole at least 1 hour before meals.
• Antacids won't interfere with the absorption of esomeprazole.

Patient monitoring
• Monitor liver function test results because drug is extensively metabolized by cytochrome P-450-

---

Reactions may be *common*, uncommon, **life-threatening**, or COMMON AND LIFE-THREATENING.

2C19. Patients with hepatic insufficiency have a risk of increased liver function test results.

Breast-feeding patients
● It isn't known whether drug appears in breast milk. Use it cautiously, however, because omeprazole does appear in breast milk.

Patient education
● Tell patient to take drug exactly as prescribed and at least one hour before meals.
● Inform patient that antacids may be used while taking this drug.
● If patient has trouble swallowing the capsule, suggest that he open it, sprinkle contents into applesauce, and swallow applesauce immediately. Warn against crushing or chewing the drug pellets.
● Urge patient to store capsules at room temperature in a tight container.
● Tell patient to report continued or worsened symptoms; rash or other allergy symptoms; intended, suspected, or confirmed pregnancy; and breast-feeding or the intention to breast-feed.

estazolam
ProSom

Pharmacologic classification: benzodiazepine
Therapeutic classification: hypnotic
Controlled substance schedule: IV
Pregnancy risk category: X

Indications and dosages
➤ *Short-term management of insomnia characterized by difficulty in falling asleep, frequent nocturnal awakenings, or early-morning awakenings. Adults:* Initially, 1 mg P.O. h.s.; may increase to 2 mg as needed and tolerated.
✦ *Dosage adjustment.* In small or debilitated older adults, 0.5 mg P.O. h.s. initially. May increase carefully to 1 mg if needed.

How supplied
Available by prescription only
Tablets: 1 mg, 2 mg

Pharmacodynamics
Hypnotic action: Estazolam depresses the CNS at the limbic and subcortical levels of the brain. It produces a sedative-hypnotic effect by potentiating the effect of the neurotransmitter gamma-aminobutyric acid on its receptor in the ascending reticular activating system, which increases inhibition and blocks both cortical and limbic arousal. Benzodiazepines decrease sleep latency, increase total sleep time, and decrease rapid-eye-movement sleep.

Pharmacokinetics
Absorption: Rapidly and completely absorbed through the GI tract.
Distribution: 93% protein-bound.

Metabolism: Extensively metabolized in the liver.
Excretion: Metabolites are excreted primarily in the urine. Less than 5% is excreted in urine as unchanged drug; 4% of a 2-mg dose is excreted in feces. Elimination half-life ranges from 10 to 24 hours; clearance is accelerated in smokers.

Route	Onset	Peak	Duration
P.O.	Unknown	1-3 hr	Unknown

Contraindications and precautions
Contraindicated in pregnant women or patients hypersensitive to drug. Use cautiously in patients with depression, suicidal tendencies, and hepatic, renal, or pulmonary disease.

Interactions
Drug-drug. *Antihistamines, barbiturates, general anesthetics, MAO inhibitors, narcotics, phenothiazines, tricyclic antidepressants:* Increased CNS effects. Avoid use together.
Cimetidine, disulfiram, isoniazid, oral contraceptives: May decrease hepatic metabolism, increasing estazolam levels. Monitor patient for increased CNS depression.
Digoxin, phenytoin: Increased level of these drugs, with possible toxicity. Monitor patient closely
Probenecid: Increased benzodiazepine effect. Monitor patient carefully.
Rifampin: Increased clearance and decreased half-life of estazolam. Monitor patient for decreased drug effect.
Theophylline: Antagonized estazolam effects. Monitor patient for drug effectiveness.
Drug-lifestyle. *Alcohol use.* May cause excessive respiratory and CNS depression. Advise patient to avoid alcohol.
Heavy smoking: Accelerates estazolam metabolism, resulting in diminished clinical efficacy. Advise patient to avoid smoking.
Caffeine: May enhance CNS effects. Discourage use.

Adverse reactions
CNS: fatigue, dizziness, *daytime drowsiness, somnolence, asthenia, hypokinesia, abnormal thinking.*
GI: dyspepsia, abdominal pain.
Hepatic: AST levels may be increased.
Musculoskeletal: back pain, stiffness.

Overdose and treatment
Overdose may cause somnolence, confusion with reduced or absent reflexes, respiratory depression, apnea, hypotension, impaired coordination, slurred speech, seizures, or coma.

If excitation occurs, don't use barbiturates. Several agents may have been ingested. Perform gastric evacuation and lavage immediately. Monitor respiration, pulse rate, and blood pressure. Use symptomatic and supportive measures. Maintain airway and administer fluids. Flumazenil, a specific benzodiazepine antagonist, may be useful.

Special considerations
Consider the recommendations relevant to all benzodiazepines as well as the following.
● Withdraw drug slowly after prolonged use.

Patient monitoring
● Perform blood counts, urinalysis, and blood chemistry analyses regularly during prolonged therapy.

Pregnant patients
● Drug can cause harm to fetus when given during pregnancy. Safety during labor and delivery hasn't been established.

Breast-feeding patients
● It isn't known whether drug appears in breast milk. Avoid use in breast-feeding women.

Pediatric patients
● Safety and efficacy in children haven't been established.

Geriatric patients
● Elderly patients may be more susceptible to CNS depressant effects of estazolam. Use cautiously. Lower dosage may be required.
● To prevent injury from dizziness and falls, assist elderly patients with activities of daily living, especially when treatment starts or dosage increases.

Patient education
● Urge patient to avoid caffeine or other stimulants.
● Tell patient to avoid alcohol and other CNS depressants.
● Advise patient to immediately report suspected or intended pregnancy during therapy.
● Warn patient that drug may cause drowsiness. Advise special caution.
● Caution patient not to stop drug abruptly after taking it daily for prolonged period and not to vary or increase dosage unless prescribed. Drug should be taken until sleep pattern is established and then slowly tapered as prescribed.
● Inform patient that nocturnal sleep may be disturbed for 1 or 2 nights after drug is stopped.

---

esterified estrogens
Estratab, Menest

Pharmacologic classification: estrogen
Therapeutic classification: estrogen replacement, antineoplastic
Pregnancy risk category: X

Indications and dosages
➤ *Palliative treatment of advanced inoperable prostatic cancer. Adults:* 1.25 to 2.5 mg P.O. q.d. to t.i.d.

➤ *Breast cancer. Men and postmenopausal women:* 10 mg P.O. t.i.d. for 3 or more months.
➤ *Female hypogonadism. Adults:* 2.5 mg P.O. daily to t.i.d. in cycles of 20 days on, 10 days off.
➤ *Castration, primary ovarian failure. Adults:* 2.5 mg P.O. daily to t.i.d. in cycles of 3 weeks on, 1 week off.
➤ *Vasomotor menopausal symptoms. Adults:* 0.3 to 1.25 mg P.O. daily in cycles of 3 weeks on, 1 week off. Dosage may be increased to 2.5 or 3.75 mg P.O. daily, if necessary.
➤ *Atrophic vaginitis and atrophic urethritis. Adults:* 0.3 to 1.25 mg P.O. daily in cycles of 3 weeks on, 1 week off.
➤ *Osteoporosis prevention. Adults:* 0.3 mg P.O. daily; increase to maximum dose of 1.25 mg/day if needed to control concurrent menopausal symptoms.

How supplied
Available by prescription only
Tablets: 0.3 mg, 0.625 mg, 1.25 mg, 2.5 mg

Pharmacodynamics
Estrogenic action: Esterified estrogen mimics the action of endogenous estrogen in treating female hypogonadism, menopausal symptoms, and atrophic vaginitis. It inhibits growth of hormone-sensitive tissue in advanced, inoperable prostatic cancer and in certain carefully selected cases of breast cancer in men and postmenopausal women.

Pharmacokinetics
Absorption: After oral administration, esterified estrogens are well absorbed from the GI tract.
Distribution: About 50% to 80% plasma protein–bound, particularly the estradiol-binding globulin. Distribution occurs throughout the body with highest levels appearing in fat.
Metabolism: Metabolized primarily in the liver, where estrogens are conjugated with sulfate and glucuronide. Large amounts of free estrogen are distributed into the bile, reabsorbed from the GI tract, and recirculated through the liver.
Excretion: Eliminated through the kidneys in the form of sulfate or glucuronide conjugates.

Route	Onset	Peak	Duration
P.O.	Unknown	Unknown	Unknown

Contraindications and precautions
Contraindicated in patients with breast cancer (except metastatic disease), estrogen-dependent neoplasia, active thrombophlebitis or thromboembolic disorders, undiagnosed abnormal genital bleeding, hypersensitivity to drug, history of thromboembolic disease, during pregnancy or breast-feeding.
    Use cautiously in patients with history of hypertension, mental depression, liver impairment, or cardiac or renal dysfunction and in those with

---

bone diseases, migraine, seizures, or diabetes mellitus.

Interactions

Drug-drug. *Anticoagulants:* Decreased anticoagulant effects. Monitor patient closely.

Corticosteroids: Enhanced corticosteroid effects. Monitor patient's fluid and electrolyte status and mental status.

Cyclosporine: Increased risk of toxicity. Monitor patient closely.

Dantrolene, other hepatotoxic drugs: Increased risk of hepatotoxicity. Monitor patient carefully.

Drugs that induce hepatic metabolism, such as carbamazepine, barbiturates, phenytoin, primidone, rifampin: Decreased estrogenic effects. Use together cautiously.

Insulin, oral antidiabetics: Increased blood glucose levels. Adjust dosage as needed.

Phenytoin: Decreased seizure control. Monitor patient for loss of seizure control.

Tamoxifen: Decreased tamoxifen effectiveness. Monitor patient for drug effects.

Drug-food. *Caffeine:* Increased serum caffeine levels. Advise patient to avoid caffeine.

Drug-lifestyle. *Smoking:* Increased risk of adverse CV effects. Advise patient to avoid smoking.

Adverse reactions

CNS: headache, dizziness, chorea, depression, *seizures.*

CV: thrombophlebitis; *thromboembolism;* hypertension; edema; *increased risk of CVA, pulmonary embolism, and MI.*

EENT: worsening of myopia or astigmatism, intolerance of contact lenses.

GI: *nausea,* vomiting, abdominal cramps, bloating, anorexia, increased appetite, weight changes, *pancreatitis,* gallbladder disease.

GU: in women, breakthrough bleeding, altered menstrual flow, dysmenorrhea, amenorrhea, *increased risk of endometrial cancer, possibility of increased risk of breast cancer,* cervical erosion, altered cervical secretions, enlargement of uterine fibromas, vaginal candidiasis; in men, testicular atrophy and impotence.

Hematologic: increased PT and INR and clotting factors VII to X and norepinephrine-induced platelet aggregability.

Hepatic: cholestatic jaundice, *hepatic adenoma.*

Metabolic: decreased serum folate, pyridoxine, and antithrombin III levels; increased triglyceride, glucose, and phospholipid levels; hypercalcemia.

Skin: melasma, rash, hirsutism or hair loss, erythema nodosum, dermatitis.

Other: breast changes (tenderness, enlargement, secretion), gynecomastia in men.

Overdose and treatment

Serious toxicity after overdose of these drugs hasn't been reported. Nausea may occur. Provide appropriate supportive care.

Special considerations

● Make sure patient has physical examination before therapy. Patients receiving long-term therapy should be examined yearly.

● Because of risk of thromboembolism, therapy should be discontinued at least 1 month before procedures that cause prolonged immobilization or raise the risk of thromboembolism, such as knee or hip surgery.

● Notify pathologist about estrogen therapy when sending specimens to laboratory for evaluation.

Patient monitoring

● Monitor serum lipid levels, blood pressure, body weight, and hepatic function.

● Monitor results of yearly breast exam and Pap test.

Pregnant patients

● Drug is contraindicated during pregnancy.

Breast-feeding patients

● Esterified estrogens are contraindicated in breast-feeding women.

Patient education

● Tell patient to read package insert describing estrogen's adverse effects; also give verbal explanation.

● Emphasize importance of regular physical examinations. Postmenopausal women who use estrogen replacement for more than 5 years for menopausal symptoms may be at increased risk for endometrial cancer. This risk is reduced by using cyclic rather than continuous therapy and the lowest possible estrogen dosage. Adding progestins to the regimen decreases risk of endometrial hyperplasia; however, it isn't known whether progestins affect risk of endometrial cancer. No increased risk of breast cancer has been reported.

⊟ ALERT Warn patient to immediately report abdominal pain; pain, numbness, or stiffness in legs or buttocks; pressure or pain in chest or shortness of breath; severe headaches; visual disturbances, such as blind spots, flashing lights, or blurriness; vaginal bleeding or discharge; breast lumps; swelling of hands or feet; yellow skin or sclera; dark urine; and light-colored stools.

● Tell diabetic patient to report elevated blood glucose level test results so that antidiabetic dosage can be adjusted.

● Explain to patient on cyclic therapy for postmenopausal symptoms that, although she may experience withdrawal bleeding during week off drug, fertility isn't restored. Pregnancy can't occur because patient doesn't ovulate.

● Teach woman to perform routine breast self-examination.

- Advise woman of childbearing age to consult prescriber before taking drug and to advise prescriber immediately if she becomes pregnant.
- Teach patient methods to decrease risk of thromboembolism.

estradiol
Alora, Climara, Estrace, Estrace Vaginal Cream, Estraderm, Estring, FemPatch, Vivelle, Vivelle-Dot

estradiol cypionate
depGynogen, Depo-Estradiol Cypionate, DepoGen, Estro-Cyp, Estrofem

estradiol valerate
Delestrogen*, Dioval 40, Dioval XX, Estra-L 40, Gynogen L.A. 20, Valergen 20

Pharmacologic classification: estrogen
Therapeutic classification: estrogen replacement, antineoplastic
Pregnancy risk category: X

Indications and dosages
➤ *Atrophic vaginitis, atrophic dystrophy of the vulva, vasomotor menopausal symptoms, hypogonadism, female castration, primary ovarian failure.* estradiol (tablets). *Adults:* 1 to 2 mg P.O. daily, in cycles of 21 days on and 7 days off or cycles of 5 days on and 2 days off.
estradiol cypionate
Adults: 1 to 5 mg I.M. once q 3 to 4 weeks.
estradiol valerate
Adults: 10 to 20 mg I.M. once a month.
estradiol (transdermal)
Adults: Start with lowest possible dose (0.025 to 0.05 mg/24 hours). Place one transdermal patch (Alora, Estraderm, Vivelle, Vivelle Dot) on trunk of body, preferably abdomen, twice weekly. Climara and FemPatch are applied once weekly. Administer on a cyclic schedule (3 weeks on and 1 week off).
➤ *Atrophic vaginitis.* estradiol (vaginal cream). *Adults:* 2 to 4 g daily for 1 to 2 weeks. When vaginal mucosa is restored, begin maintenance dosage of 1 g one to three times weekly.
estradiol (vaginal ring)
Adults: Insert ring as deeply as possible into the upper third of the vaginal vault. The ring should remain in place for 3 months.
➤ *Female hypogonadism.* estradiol cypionate. *Adults:* 1.5 to 2 mg I.M. at monthly intervals.
estradiol valerate
Adults: 10 to 20 mg I.M. q 4 weeks as needed.
➤ *Inoperable breast cancer.* estradiol (tablets). *Adults:* 10 mg P.O. t.i.d. for 3 months.

➤ *Inoperable prostatic cancer.* estradiol valerate. *Adults:* 30 mg I.M. q 1 to 2 weeks.
estradiol (tablets)
Adults: 1 to 2 mg P.O. t.i.d.
➤ *Prevention of postmenopausal osteoporosis.* estradiol (transdermal). *Adults:* Place one Vivelle 0.025 mg/day or one Estraderm 0.05 mg/24 hours transdermal system on trunk of body, preferably abdomen, twice weekly in a continuous regimen for women who have had a hysterectomy or cyclic regimen for those with an intact uterus. Or, Climara 0.025 mg/24 hours once weekly in a continuous regimen. Adjust dose as needed.
estradiol (tablets)
Adults: 0.5 mg P.O. daily in a cyclic regimen (21 days on and 7 days off).

How supplied
Available by prescription only
estradiol
Ring: 2 mg
Tablets: 0.5 mg, 1 mg, 2 mg
Transdermal: 0.025 mg/24 hours; 0.037 mg/24 hours; 0.05 mg/24 hours; 0.075 mg/24 hours; 0.1 mg/24 hours
Vaginal: 0.1 mg/g cream (in nonliquefying base)
estradiol cypionate
Injection: 5 mg/ml (in oil)
estradiol valerate
Injection: 10 mg/ml, 20 mg/ml, 40 mg/ml (in oil)

Pharmacodynamics
Estrogenic action: Estradiol mimics the action of endogenous estrogen in treating female hypogonadism, menopausal symptoms, and atrophic vaginitis. It inhibits growth of hormone-sensitive tissue in advanced, inoperable prostatic cancer and in certain carefully selected cases of breast cancer in men and postmenopausal women.

Pharmacokinetics
Absorption: After oral administration, estradiol and other natural unconjugated estrogens are well absorbed but substantially inactivated by the liver. Therefore, unconjugated estrogens are usually administered parenterally. After I.M. administration, absorption begins rapidly and continues for days. The cypionate and valerate esters administered in oil have prolonged durations of action because of their slow absorption characteristics. Topically applied estradiol is absorbed readily into the systemic circulation.
Distribution: Estradiol and other natural estrogens are about 50% to 80% plasma protein–bound, particularly the estradiol-binding globulin. Distribution occurs throughout the body, with highest levels appearing in fat.
Metabolism: Steroidal estrogens, including estradiol, are metabolized primarily in the liver, where they are conjugated with sulfate and glucuronide. Because of the rapid metabolism, nonesterified

forms of estrogen, including estradiol, must usually be administered daily.

Excretion: Most estrogen elimination occurs through the kidneys in the form of sulfate or glucuronide conjugates.

Route	Onset	Peak	Duration
P.O., I.M., transdermal, intravaginal	Unknown	Unknown	Unknown

Contraindications and precautions

Contraindicated in pregnant patients and patients with thrombophlebitis or thromboembolic disorders, estrogen-dependent neoplasia, breast or reproductive organ cancer (except for palliative treatment), or undiagnosed abnormal genital bleeding. Also contraindicated in patients with history of thrombophlebitis or thromboembolic disorders from previous estrogen use (except for palliative treatment of breast and prostate cancer).

Use cautiously in patients with cerebrovascular or coronary artery disease, hypertension, asthma, bone diseases, gallbladder disease, migraine, seizures, or cardiac, hepatic, or renal dysfunction. Also use cautiously in women with a strong family history of breast cancer or who have breast nodules, fibrocystic disease, or abnormal mammographic findings.

Interactions

Drug-drug. *Corticosteroids:* May enhance corticosteroid effects. Monitor patient closely.

Cyclosporine: May increase risk of toxicity. Monitor patient and cyclosprine levels frequently.

Dantrolene, other hepatotoxic drugs: May increase risk of hepatotoxicity. Monitor patient closely.

Drugs that induce hepatic metabolism, such as carbamazepine, barbiturates, phenytoin, primidone, rifampin: Decreased estrogenic effects and increased metabolism of certain other drugs. Monitor patient closely.

Insulin, oral antidiabetics: Altered blood glucose levels. Adjust dosage if needed.

Tamoxifen: Decreased tamoxifen effects. Monitor patient closely.

Warfarin-type anticoagulants: Decreased anticoagulant effect. Adjust dosage if needed.

Drug-food. *Caffeine:* May increase serum caffeine levels. Advise patient to avoid caffeine.

Grapefruit juice: Elevated estrogen levels. Advise patient to take drug with liquid other than grapefruit juice.

Drug-lifestyle. *Smoking:* Increased risk of adverse CV effects. Advise patient to avoid smoking.

Adverse reactions

CNS: headache, dizziness, chorea, depression, *seizures.*

CV: thrombophlebitis; *thromboembolism;* hypertension; edema; *increased risk of CVA, pulmonary embolism, and MI.*

EENT: worsening of myopia or astigmatism, intolerance of contact lenses.

GI: *nausea,* vomiting, abdominal cramps, bloating, anorexia, increased appetite, weight changes, *pancreatitis,* gallbladder disease.

GU: in women, breakthrough bleeding, altered menstrual flow, dysmenorrhea, amenorrhea, *increased risk of endometrial cancer, possibility of increased risk of breast cancer,* cervical erosion, altered cervical secretions, enlargement of uterine fibromas, vaginal candidiasis; in men, testicular atrophy and impotence.

Hematologic: increased PT and INR and clotting factors VII to X and norepinephrine-induced platelet aggregability.

Hepatic: cholestatic jaundice, *hepatic adenoma.*

Metabolic: decreased serum folate, pyridoxine, and antithrombin III levels; increased triglyceride, glucose, and phospholipid levels; hypercalcemia.

Skin: melasma, rash, hirsutism or hair loss, erythema nodosum, dermatitis.

Other: breast changes (tenderness, enlargement, secretion), gynecomastia in men.

Overdose and treatment

Serious toxicity hasn't been reported after overdose. Nausea may occur. Provide appropriate supportive care.

Special considerations

● Make sure patient has physical examination before therapy. Patients receiving long-term therapy should be examined yearly.

● Ask patient about allergies, especially to foods and plants. Estradiol is available as an aqueous solution or as a solution in peanut oil; estradiol cypionate, as a solution in cottonseed oil; estradiol valerate, as a solution in castor oil or sesame oil.

● To administer I.M. injection, make sure drug is well dispersed in solution by rolling vial between palms. Inject deeply into large muscle. Rotate injection sites to prevent muscle atrophy. Never give drug I.V.

● Apply transdermal patch to clean, dry, hairless, intact skin on abdomen or buttocks. Don't apply it to breasts, waistline, or other areas where clothing can loosen patch. When applying, ensure thorough contact between patch and skin, especially around edges, and hold in place for about 10 seconds. Rotate application sites.

● In women also taking oral estrogen, treatment with the Estraderm transdermal patch can begin 1 week after withdrawal of oral therapy, sooner if menopausal symptoms appear before the end of the week.

● Transdermal systems are sometimes used on a continuous basis (not cyclic). Other alternatives are 1 to 5 mg (cypionate) I.M. q 3 to 4 weeks; or 10 to 20 mg (valerate) I.M. q 4 weeks, p.r.n.

• Because of risk of thromboembolism, therapy should be discontinued at least 1 month before procedures that cause prolonged immobilization or raise the risk of thromboembolism, such as knee or hip surgery.

• Notify pathologist about estrogen therapy when sending specimens to laboratory for evaluation.

Patient monitoring

• Monitor serum lipid levels, blood pressure, body weight, and hepatic function.

• Monitor patch site for skin reactions when using transdermal form.

Pregnant patients

• Drug is contraindicated in pregnant women.

Breast-feeding patients

• Drug is contraindicated in breast-feeding women.

Geriatric patients

• Frequent physical examinations are recommended in postmenopausal women taking estrogen.

Patient education

• Tell patient not to apply patch to breast area.

• Remind patient not to use the same skin site for at least 1 week after removal of the transdermal system.

• Tell patient to read package insert describing estrogen's adverse effects; however, also give patient verbal explanation.

• Emphasize importance of regular physical examinations. Postmenopausal women who use estrogen replacement for more than 5 years to treat menopausal symptoms may be at increased risk for endometrial cancer. This risk is reduced by using cyclic rather than continuous therapy and the lowest possible estrogen dosage. Adding progestins to the regimen decreases risk of endometrial hyperplasia; however, it isn't known whether progestins affect risk of endometrial cancer. No increased risk of breast cancer has been reported.

⚠ **ALERT** Warn patient to immediately report abdominal pain; pain, numbness, or stiffness in legs or buttocks; pressure or pain in chest or shortness of breath; severe headaches; visual disturbances, such as blind spots, flashing lights, or blurriness; vaginal bleeding or discharge; breast lumps; swelling of hands or feet; yellow skin or sclera; dark urine; and light-colored stools.

• Tell diabetic patient to report elevated blood glucose level test results so that antidiabetic dosage can be adjusted.

• Teach woman to perform routine breast self-examination.

• Advise woman of childbearing age to consult prescriber before taking drug and to advise prescriber immediately if she becomes pregnant.

• Teach patient methods to decrease risk of thromboembolism.

estradiol/norethindrone acetate
Activella, Combipatch

Pharmacologic classification: estrogen/progestin
Therapeutic classification: postmenopausal agent
Pregnancy risk category: X

Indications and dosages

➤ *Moderate-to-severe vasomotor symptoms of menopause, vulvar and vaginal atrophy, hypoestrogenemia from hypogonadism, castration, primary ovarian failure in women with an intact uterus.*
Continuous combined regimen. *Adults:* 9-cm² patch worn continuously on the lower abdomen. Remove old system and apply new system twice weekly during a 28-day cycle. May increase to 16-cm² patch if more progestin is desired.
Continuous sequential regimen
Adults: Patch can be applied as a sequential regimen with an estradiol-only transdermal system (such as Alora, Esclim, Estraderm, Vivelle). A 0.05-mg estradiol-only transdermal patch is worn for first 14 days of a 28-day cycle; replace system twice weekly according to product directions. For remainder of 28-day cycle, apply the 9-cm² patch system to the lower abdomen and replace twice weekly. May increase to 16-cm² patch if more progestin is desired.

➤ *Moderate to severe vasomotor symptoms of menopause, vulvar and vaginal atrophy, prevention of postmenopausal osteoporosis in women with an intact uterus.* *Adults:* 1 tablet (Activella) P.O. daily.

How supplied

Available by prescription only
Tablet: 1 mg estradiol and 0.5 mg norethindrone
Transdermal: 9-cm² system (0.05 mg estradiol and 0.14 mg norethindrone), 16-cm² system (0.05 mg estradiol and 0.25 mg norethindrone)

Pharmacodynamics

Hormone action: Estrogen replacement therapy can reduce the frequency of menopausal symptoms by replacing the naturally declining levels that occur in postmenopausal women.

Pharmacokinetics

Absorption: Estradiol and norethindrone are well absorbed transdermally and via the GI tract.
Distribution: Estradiol is primarily bound to sex hormone–binding protein (SHBG) and norethindrone is primarily bound to albumin and SHBG.
Metabolism: Estradiol is minimally metabolized. Norethindrone is metabolized primarily by the liver.
Excretion: Elimination half-life of estradiol is 2 to 3 hours. Norethindrone has an elimination

half-life of 6 to 8 hours (transdermal system) or 12 to 24 hours (tablet).

Route	Onset	Peak	Duration
P.O.	Unknown	½-8 hr	Unknown
Trans-dermal	12-24 hr	Unknown	Unknown

Contraindications and precautions
Contraindicated in women who may be pregnant; women hypersensitive to estrogen, progestin, or any component of the patch; and women with known or suspected breast cancer, known or suspected estrogen-dependent neoplasia, undiagnosed abnormal genital bleeding, active thrombophlebitis, thromboembolic disorders, or CVA.

Use cautiously in patients with impaired liver function, gallbladder disease, hypertension, asthma, epilepsy, migraine, and cardiac or renal dysfunction.

Interactions
None reported.

Adverse reactions
CNS: *asthenia,* depression, insomnia, nervousness, dizziness, *headache.*
EENT: *pharyngitis, rhinitis, sinusitis.*
GI: *abdominal pain, diarrhea,* dyspepsia, flatulence, *nausea,* constipation.
GU: *dysmenorrhea, leukorrhea, menstrual disorder,* suspicious Papanicolaou smear, *vaginitis,* menorrhagia, vaginal hemorrhage.
Hematologic: altered INR, activated partial thromboplastin time, and platelet aggregation times; increased platelet count and fibrinogen activity.
Musculoskeletal: arthralgia, *back pain.*
Respiratory: *respiratory disorder,* bronchitis.
Skin: application site reactions, acne.
Other: tooth disorder, *accidental injury, flu syndrome, pain, breast pain,* peripheral edema, breast enlargement, infection.

Overdose and treatment
Nausea and withdrawal bleeding are the most common consequences of overdose. Discontinue treatment or remove patch.

Special considerations
• Combination estrogen/progestin regimens are indicated for women with an intact uterus.
• Women not currently receiving continuous estrogen or estrogen/progestin therapy may start therapy at any time.
• Women receiving continuous hormone replacement should complete the current cycle before starting therapy. Women commonly have withdrawal bleeding at the end of the cycle; first day of withdrawal bleeding would be an appropriate time to start therapy.
• Progestins taken with estrogen drugs significantly reduce, but don't eliminate, the risk of endometrial cancer from estrogen use.

• Drug may reduce response to the metyrapone test and sulfobromophthalein retention. Increased thyroid-binding globulin may lead to increased total T_3 and T_4 levels and decreased T_3 resin uptake. Free T_4 and T_3 levels are unaffected.
• Store norethindrone patches in refrigerator before dispensing. Once dispensed, system may be stored at a temperature under 77° F (25° C) for up to 3 months.

Patient monitoring
• Reevaluate hormonal therapy every 3 to 6 months.
• Blood pressure increases may be linked to estrogen use. Monitor patient's blood pressure regularly.
• Monitor patient for signs of endometrial cancer, including persistent or recurring abnormal vaginal bleeding.

Pregnant patients
• Contraindicated during pregnancy.

Breast-feeding patients
• Estrogen and progestin appear in breast milk. The patch shouldn't be used during breast-feeding.

Patient education
• Instruct patient to apply patch system to a smooth (fold-free), clean, dry, nonirritated area of skin on the lower abdomen, avoiding the waistline. Application sites should be rotated, with an interval of at least 1 week between applications to the same site.
• Tell patient not to apply patch on or near the breasts.
• Advise patient of potential for adverse events.
• Tell patient she may store patches at room temperature for up to 3 months.

estramustine phosphate sodium
Emcyt

Pharmacologic classification: estrogen, alkylating agent
Therapeutic classification: antineoplastic
Pregnancy risk category: NR

Indications and dosages
Dosage and indications may vary. Check literature for recommended protocols.
➤ *Palliative treatment of metastatic or progressive cancer of the prostate. Adults:* 10 to 16 mg/kg P.O. in three or four divided doses. Usual dose is 14 mg/kg daily. Therapy should continue for up to 3 months and, if successful, be maintained as long as patient responds.

How supplied
Available by prescription only
Capsules: 140 mg

Pharmacodynamics

Antineoplastic action: Exact mechanism of action is unclear. However, the estrogenic portion of the molecule may act as a carrier of the drug to facilitate selective uptake by tumor cells with estradiol hormone receptors, such as those in the prostate gland. At that point, the nitrogen mustard portion of the drug acts as an alkylating agent.

Pharmacokinetics

Absorption: After oral administration, about 75% of a dose is absorbed across the GI tract.
Distribution: Estramustine is distributed widely into body tissues.
Metabolism: Extensively metabolized in the liver.
Excretion: Drug and its metabolites are eliminated primarily in feces, with a small amount excreted in urine. Terminal phase of plasma elimination has a half-life of 20 hours.

Route	Onset	Peak	Duration
P.O.	Unknown	Unknown	Unknown

Contraindications and precautions

Contraindicated in patients hypersensitive to estradiol and nitrogen mustard and in those with active thrombophlebitis or thromboembolic disorders, except when the actual tumor mass is the cause of the thromboembolic phenomenon. Contraindicated in pregnant and breast-feeding women.

Use cautiously in patients with history of thrombophlebitis or thromboembolic disorders and cerebrovascular or coronary artery disease.

Interactions

Drug-drug. *Anticoagulants:* Decreased anticoagulant effect. Increase anticoagulant dosage as needed.
Calcium-containing drugs, such as antacids: Impaired estramustine absorption. Avoid use together.
Drug-food. *Calcium-rich foods, such as milk and dairy products:* May impair estramustine absorption. Drug shouldn't be taken with these foods.

Adverse reactions

CNS: lethargy, insomnia, headache, anxiety.
CV: chest pain, *MI*, sodium and fluid retention, flushing, thrombophlebitis, hypertension, *heart failure, CVA.*
GI: *nausea, vomiting,* diarrhea, anorexia, flatulence, GI bleeding, thirst.
Hematologic: *leukopenia, thrombocytopenia,* increased norepinephrine-induced platelet aggregability.
Hepatic: elevated liver enzyme and bilirubin levels.
Metabolic: decreased serum folate, pyridoxine, phosphate, and pregnanediol levels; increased ceruloplasmin, cortisol, prolactin PT, sodium, triglyceride, and phospholipid levels; decreased testosterone levels.

Musculoskeletal: leg cramps.
Respiratory: *edema, pulmonary embolism,* dyspnea.
Skin: rash, pruritus, dry skin, thinning of hair.
Other: *painful gynecomastia and breast tenderness.*

Overdose and treatment

Signs and symptoms of overdose include headache, nausea, vomiting, and myelosuppression.

Treatment is usually supportive and includes induction of emesis, gastric lavage, transfusion of blood components, and appropriate symptomatic therapy. Hematologic monitoring should continue for at least 6 weeks after the ingestion.

Special considerations

• Store capsules in refrigerator.
• Phenothiazines can be used to treat nausea and vomiting.
• Estramustine may cause hypertension.
• Drug may exaggerate peripheral edema or heart failure.
• Patients may continue estramustine as long as they're responding favorably. Some patients have taken drug for more than 3 years.

Patient monitoring

• Monitor blood pressure at baseline and routinely during therapy.
• Monitor glucose tolerance periodically during therapy.
• Monitor weight gain regularly in these patients.

Pregnant patients

• Drug is contraindicated during pregnancy.

Breast-feeding patients

• Drug is contraindicated in breast-feeding women.

Geriatric patients

• Use cautiously in elderly patients, who are more likely to have vascular disorders, because estrogen is linked to vascular complications.

Patient education

• Emphasize importance of continuing drug despite nausea and vomiting.
• Tell patient to take drug at least 1 hour before or 2 hours after a meal with a full glass of water.
• Instruct patient not to take milk, milk products, and calcium-rich foods simultaneously with estramustine.
• Advise patient to immediately report vomiting that occurs shortly after a dose is taken.
• Because of possible mutagenic effects, advise patients of childbearing age to use contraceptive measures.

Reactions may be *common,* uncommon, *life-threatening,* or COMMON AND LIFE-THREATENING.

estrogen and progestin

Alesse-28, Brevicon, Demulen 1/35,
Demulen 1/35-28, Demulen 1/50,
Desogen 28, Estrostep 21, Estrostep
Fe, Jenest-28, Levlen, Levora 21,
Levora 28, Loestrin 21-1/20, Loestrin
21-1.5/30, Loestrin Fe 1/20, Loestrin
Fe 1.5/30, Lo/Ovral, Lo/Ovral-28,
Mircette, Modicon 21, Modicon 28,
Necon 1/35-21, Necon 1/35-28, Necon
1/50-21, Necon 1/50-28, Nelova 0.5/35
E 28, Nelova 1/35 E, Nordette-21,
Nordette-28, Norinyl 1+35 21-Day,
Norinyl 1+35 28-Day, Norinyl 1+50
21-Day, Norinyl 1+50 28-Day, Norinyl
1+80 28-Day, Ortho-Cept, Ortho-
Cyclen, Ortho-Novum 1/35-21,
Ortho-Novum 1/35-28, Ortho-Novum
1/50-21, Ortho-Novum 1/50-28,
Ortho-Novum 7/7/7-21, Ortho-
Novum 7/7/7-28, Ortho-Novum 10/11-
21, Ortho-Novum 10/11-28, Ovcon-
35, Ovcon-50, Ovral, Ovral-28, Tri-
Norinyl-21, Tri-Norinyl-28, Triphasil-
21, Triphasil-28, Zovia 1/35 E

Pharmacologic classification: estrogen with
progestin
Therapeutic classification: contraceptive
(hormonal)
Pregnancy risk category: X

Indications and dosages
➤ *Contraception.* **Monophasic therapy.**
Adults: One tablet P.O. daily beginning on day 5
of menstrual cycle (first day of menstrual flow is
day 1), or on the first Sunday after onset of menstruation, or on day 1 of menstrual cycle depending on specific contraceptive. With 20- and
21-tablet packages, new dosing cycle begins 7
days after last tablet taken. With 28-tablet packages, dosage is one tablet daily without interruption; extra tablets are placebos or contain
iron. If next menstrual period doesn't begin on
schedule, rule out pregnancy before starting new
dosing cycle. If menstrual period begins, start
new dosing cycle 7 days after last tablet was tak-
en. If all doses have been taken on schedule and
one menstrual period is missed, continue dosing cycle. If two consecutive menstrual periods
are missed, pregnancy test is required before new
dosing cycle is started.
Biphasic therapy
Adults: One color tablet P.O. daily (Ortho-Novum
10/11) for 10 days, then next color tablet for 11
days.
Triphasic therapy
Adults: One tablet P.O. daily (Ortho-Novum 7/7/7,
Tri-Norinyl, Triphasil) in the sequence specified
by the manufacturer.
➤ *Hypermenorrhea. Adults:* Use only high-
dose combinations. Dosage is same as for contraception.

➤ *Endometriosis.* **Cyclic therapy.** *Adults:*
One 10-mg tablet P.O. daily (Ortho-Novum) for
20 days from day 5 to day 24 of menstrual cycle.
Suppressive therapy
Adults: One 5- or 10-mg tablet P.O. daily (En-
ovid) for 2 weeks, starting on day 5 of menstrual cycle. Continue without interruption for 6 to 9
months, increasing dose by 5 to 10 mg q 2 weeks,
up to 20 mg daily. Up to 40 mg daily may be needed if breakthrough bleeding occurs.

How supplied
Available by prescription only
Tablets—monophasic type
Mestranol 0.1 mg and norethynodrel 2.5 mg
Mestranol 0.1 mg and norethindrone 1 mg
Mestranol 0.1 mg and ethynodiol diacetate 1 mg
Mestranol 0.08 mg and norethindrone 1 mg
Mestranol 0.05 mg and norethindrone 1 mg
Ethinyl estradiol 0.02 mg and levonorgestrel
0.1 mg
Ethinyl estradiol 0.05 mg and norethindrone 1 mg
Ethinyl estradiol 0.05 mg and norethindrone ac-
etate 1 mg
Ethinyl estradiol 0.05 mg and ethynodiol diac-
etate 1 mg
Ethinyl estradiol 0.05 mg and norethindrone ac-
etate 2.5 mg
Ethinyl estradiol 0.05 mg and norgestrel 0.5 mg
Ethinyl estradiol 0.035 mg and norethindrone
1 mg
Ethinyl estradiol 0.035 mg and norethindrone
0.5 mg
Ethinyl estradiol 0.035 mg and norethindrone
0.4 mg
Ethinyl estradiol 0.035 mg and ethynodiol diacetate 1 mg
Ethinyl estradiol 0.03 mg and norethindrone acetate 1.5 mg
Ethinyl estradiol 0.03 mg and norgestrel 0.3 mg
Ethinyl estradiol 0.03 mg and levonorgestrel
0.15 mg
Ethinyl estradiol 0.02 mg and norethindrone 1 mg
Tablets—biphasic type
10 tablets ethinyl estradiol 0.035 mg and norethindrone 0.5 mg; 11 tablets ethinyl estradiol
0.035 mg and norethindrone 1 mg
21 tablets 0.050 mg ethinyl estradiol and 0.15 mg
desogestrel; 5 tablets 0.01 mg ethinyl estradiol
Tablets—triphasic type
7 tablets ethinyl estradiol 0.035 mg and norethindrone 0.5 mg; 9 tablets ethinyl estradiol
0.035 mg and norethindrone 1 mg; 5 tablets
ethinyl estradiol 0.035 mg and norethindrone
0.5 mg
7 tablets ethinyl estradiol 0.035 mg and norethindrone 0.5 mg; 7 tablets ethinyl estradiol
0.035 mg and norethindrone 0.75 mg; 7 tablets
ethinyl estradiol 0.035 mg and norethindrone
1 mg
6 tablets ethinyl estradiol 0.03 and levonorgestrel
0.05 mg; 5 tablets ethinyl estradiol 0.04 mg and
levonorgestrel 0.075 mg; 10 tablets ethinyl estradiol 0.03 mg and levonorgestrel 0.125 mg

---

7 tablets 0.035 ethinyl estradiol and 0.18 mg norgestimate; 7 tablets 0.035 mg ethinyl estradiol and 0.215 norgestimate; 7 tablets 0.035 mg ethinyl estradiol and 0.25 mg norgestimate
5 tablets 0.020 mg ethinyl estradiol and 1 mg norethindrone acetate; 7 tablets 0.030 mg ethinyl estradiol and 1 mg norethindrone acetate; 9 tablets 0.035 mg ethinyl estradiol and 1 mg norethindrone acetate

Pharmacodynamics
Contraceptive action: Estrogen components of oral contraceptives inhibit the release of follicle-stimulating hormone, thereby stopping follicular development and suppressing ovulation.

Progestin components of oral contraceptives inhibit the release of luteinizing hormone, preventing ovulation even in the event of incomplete suppression of follicular development. Progestins also change the endometrial environment to inhibit nidation (implantation of the fertilized egg into the endometrium) and cause thickening of the cervical mucus, blocking the upward migration of sperm.

Pharmacokinetics
Absorption: Most components of oral contraceptives are absorbed relatively well from the GI tract. Bioavailabilities range from 40% to 70%; considerable individual variation exists in extent of absorption.
Distribution: Protein-binding of the various drugs used in oral contraceptives is high, ranging from 80% to 98%. These agents are distributed extensively into virtually all body tissues.
Metabolism: These drugs undergo metabolic transformation before excretion; their rates of metabolism may thus be affected by agents that induce or inhibit metabolism.
Excretion: Very little, if any, is excreted unchanged in urine or feces. They appear primarily as sulfate and glucuronide conjugates.

Route	Onset	Peak	Duration
P.O.	Unknown	1-2 hr	Unknown

Contraindications and precautions
Oral contraceptives are contraindicated in patients with thromboembolic disorders, cerebrovascular or coronary artery disease, or MI because of the link between contraceptives and thromboembolic disease; in patients with known or suspected cancer of the breast or reproductive organs or with benign or malignant liver tumors because of the link between contraceptives and tumorigenesis; in patients with undiagnosed abnormal vaginal bleeding; in women known or suspected to be pregnant; in breast-feeding women; in adolescents with incomplete epiphyseal closure; and in women smokers over age 35.

Use oral contraceptives cautiously in patients with systemic lupus erythematosus, hypertension, mental depression, migraine, epilepsy, asthma, diabetes mellitus, amenorrhea, scanty or irregular periods, fibrocystic breast disease, family history (mother, grandmother, sister) of breast or genital tract cancer, or renal or gallbladder disease. Advise patient to report development or worsening of any of these conditions. Prolonged therapy may be inadvisable in women who plan to become pregnant.

Interactions
Drug-drug. *Aminoglutethimide, ampicillin, antihistamines, barbiturates, carbamazepine, chloramphenicol, felbamate, griseofulvin, isoniazid, neomycin, nitrofurantoin, phenylbutazone, phenytoin, primidone, protease inhibitors, penicillin V, rifampin, sulfonamides, and tetracycline:* Increased metabolism of oral contraceptives, resulting in reduced efficacy, breakthrough bleeding, and occasionally contraceptive failure. Monitor patient for drug effects. *Anticonvulsants, antihypertensives, beta blockers, corticosteroids, oral warfarin-type anticoagulants, tricyclic antidepressants:* Oral contraceptives may interfere with hepatic metabolism of these drugs and cause toxicity or decreased effects. Monitor patient for toxicity and decreased effects.
Insulin, oral antidiabetics: Serum glucose may be affected. Adjust dosage as needed.
Drug-herb. *Red clover:* May interfere with hormonal therapies. Discourage concomitant use.
St. John's wort: possible decreased efficacy of the oral contraceptive due to increased hepatic metabolism. Discourage concomitant use. If concomitant use can't be avoided, encourage use of an additional method of contraception.
Drug-food. *Caffeine:* May increase serum caffeine levels. Advise patient to avoid caffeine.
Drug-lifestyle. *Smoking:* Increases risk of CV effects. Advise patient not to smoke.

Adverse reactions
CNS: headache, dizziness, depression, lethargy, migraine.
CV: ***thromboembolism,*** hypertension, edema, increase in varicosities.
EENT: worsening of myopia or astigmatism, intolerance of contact lenses, unexplained loss of vision, optic neuritis, diplopia, retinal thrombosis, papilledema.
GI: *nausea, vomiting,* abdominal cramps, bloating, diarrhea, constipation, changes in appetite, weight gain, bowel ischemia.
GU: breakthrough bleeding, granulomatous colitis, dysmenorrhea, amenorrhea, cervical erosion or abnormal secretions, enlargement of uterine fibromas, vaginal candidiasis, urinary tract infections,.
Hematologic: increased prothrombin and clotting factors VII to X, plasminogen, norepinephrine-induced platelet aggregation, fibrinogen; decreased antithrombin III.
Hepatic: gallbladder disease, cholestatic jaundice, ***liver tumors.***

Reactions may be *common,* uncommon, *life-threatening,* or COMMON AND LIFE-THREATENING.

Metabolic: hyperglycemia, hypercalcemia, folic acid deficiency; increased sulfobromophthalein retention, thyroid-binding globulin, triglycerides, phospholipids, transcortin and corticosteroids, transferrin, prolactin, renin, and vitamin A; decreased metyrapone, pregnanediol excretion, free T_3 resin uptake, glucose tolerance, zinc, and vitamin B_{12}.

Skin: rash, acne, seborrhea, oily skin, erythema multiforme, hyperpigmentation.

Other: breast tenderness, enlargement, or secretion, libido changes, possible increased risk of congenital anomalies.

Overdose and treatment
Serious toxicity after drug overdose hasn't been reported. Nausea and vomiting, as well as withdrawal bleeding, may occur.

Special considerations
● Astigmatic error and myopic refractive error may be increased twofold to threefold, usually after 6 months of oral contraceptive therapy.
● If patient becomes hypersensitive, discontinue the drug.
● Changes in ocular contour and lubricant quality of tears may necessitate change in size and shape of contact lenses.

Patient monitoring
● Patient monitoring considerations are the same as those relevant to all estrogens and progestins.
● Breakthrough bleeding in patients taking high-dose estrogen-progestin combinations for menstrual disorders may necessitate dosage adjustment.

Pregnant patients
● Drug is contraindicated during pregnancy.

Breast-feeding patients
● Oral contraceptives are contraindicated in breast-feeding women.

Pediatric patients
● To avoid later fertility and menstrual problems, hormonal contraception isn't advised for the adolescent until after at least 2 years of well-established menstrual cycles and completion of physiologic maturation. An estrogen-dominant agent is the best choice for the adolescent with scanty menses, moderate or severe acne, or candidiasis. A progestin-dominant agent is the best choice for the adolescent with dysmenorrhea, hypermenorrhea, fibrocystic breast disease, or cyclic premenstrual weight gain.

Patient education
● Advise patient of potential adverse reactions and inform her that these should diminish after 3 to 6 dosing cycles (months).
● Advise patient to use an additional method of birth control for the first week of administration in the initial cycle (unless using day-1 start).

● Instruct patient to take drug at the same time each day at 24-hour intervals for efficacy of medication, to keep tablets in original container, and to take them in correct (color-coded) sequence.
● Tell patient that night-time dosing may reduce nausea and headaches.
● Suggest taking drug with or immediately after food to reduce nausea.
● Stress importance of annual Papanicolaou smears and gynecologic examinations while taking estrogen-progestin combinations.
● Advise patient of increased risks linked to simultaneous use of cigarettes and oral contraceptives, especially the risk of serious cardiovascular side effects. Strongly advise women who use oral contraceptives not to smoke.
● Instruct patient as follows regarding missed doses.

Monophasic or biphasic cycles
For 20-, 21-, or 24-day dosing schedule:
● If one regular dose is missed, take tablet as soon as possible; if remembered on the next day, take two tablets, then continue regular dosing schedule.
● If two consecutive days are missed, take two tablets a day for next 2 days, then resume regular dosing schedule.
● If 3 consecutive days are missed, discontinue drug and substitute other contraceptive method until period begins or pregnancy is ruled out. Then start new cycle of tablets.
For 28-day dosing schedule:
● Follow instructions for 21-day dosing schedule; if one of the last seven tablets is missed, be sure to take first tablet of next month's cycle on regularly scheduled day.

Triphasic cycle
For 21-day dosing schedule:
● If 1 day is missed, take dose as soon as possible; if remembered on the next day, take two tablets, then continue regular dosing schedule while using additional method of contraception for remainder of cycle.
● If 2 consecutive days are missed, take two tablets daily for next 2 days, then continue regular schedule while using additional contraceptive method for remainder of cycle.
● If 3 consecutive days are missed, discontinue drug and use other contraceptive method until period begins or pregnancy is ruled out. Then start new cycle of tablets.
For 28-day dosing schedule:
● Follow instructions for 21-day dosing schedule; if one of the last seven tablets was missed, be sure to take first tablet of next month's cycle on regularly scheduled day.

◇ Unlabeled clinical use

estrogenic substances, conjugated
Premarin

Pharmacologic classification: estrogen
Therapeutic classification: estrogen replacement, antineoplastic, antiosteoporotic
Pregnancy risk category: X

Indications and dosages
➤ *Abnormal uterine bleeding (hormonal imbalance).* *Adults:* 25 mg I.V. or I.M. Repeat dose in 6 to 12 hours, if necessary.
➤ *Castration and primary ovarian failure.* *Adults:* Initially, 1.25 mg P.O. daily in cycles of 3 weeks on, 1 week off. Adjust dose p.r.n.
➤ *Prevention of osteoporosis.* *Adults:* 0.625 mg P.O. daily given continuously, or cyclically, 25 days on, 5 days off.
➤ *Female hypogonadism.* *Adults:* 0.3 to 0.625 mg P.O. daily, given cyclically 3 weeks on, 1 week off.
➤ *Vasomotor menopausal symptoms.* *Adults:* 0.625 mg P.O. daily, or cyclically 25 days on, 5 days off.
➤ *Atrophic vaginitis or kraurosis vulvae.* *Adults:* 0.3 to 1.25 mg or more P.O. daily. Or, 0.5 to 2 g intravaginally or topically once daily in cycles of 3 weeks on, 1 week off.
➤ *Palliative treatment of inoperable prostatic cancer.* *Adults:* 1.25 to 2.5 mg P.O. t.i.d.
➤ *Palliative treatment of breast cancer.* *Adults:* 10 mg P.O. t.i.d. for 3 months or more.

How supplied
Available by prescription only
Injection: 25 mg/5 ml
Tablets: 0.3 mg, 0.625 mg, 0.9 mg, 1.25 mg, 2.5 mg
Vaginal cream: 0.0625%

Pharmacodynamics
Estrogenic action: Conjugated estrogenic substances mimic the action of endogenous estrogen in treating female hypogonadism, menopausal symptoms, and atrophic vaginitis. They inhibit growth of hormone-sensitive tissue in advanced, inoperable prostatic cancer and in certain carefully selected cases of breast cancer in men and postmenopausal women; they also retard progression of osteoporosis by enhancing calcium and phosphate retention and limiting bone decalcification.

Pharmacokinetics
Absorption: Not well characterized. After I.M. administration, absorption begins rapidly and continues for days.
Distribution: Conjugated estrogens are about 50% to 80% plasma protein–bound and distributed throughout the body, with highest levels appearing in fat.

Metabolism: Conjugated estrogens are metabolized primarily in the liver, where they are conjugated with sulfate and glucuronide. Because of the rapid metabolism, nonesterified forms of estrogen, including estradiol, must usually be administered daily.
Excretion: The majority of estrogen elimination occurs through the kidneys, in the form of sulfate or glucuronide conjugates, or both.

Route	Onset	Peak	Duration
P.O., I.V., I.M., intravaginal	Unknown	Unknown	Unknown

Contraindications and precautions
Contraindicated in patients with thrombophlebitis or thromboembolic disorders, estrogen-dependent neoplasia, breast or reproductive organ cancer (except for palliative treatment), or undiagnosed abnormal genital bleeding and during pregnancy.

Use cautiously in patients with cerebrovascular or coronary artery disease, gallbladder disease, hypertension, asthma, bone disease, migraine, seizures, or cardiac, hepatic, or renal dysfunction or in women with family history (mother, grandmother, sister) of breast or genital tract cancer or who have breast nodules, fibrocystic disease, or abnormal mammographic findings.

Interactions
Drug-drug. *Corticosteroids:* Enhanced corticosteroid effects. Use together cautiously.
Drugs that induce hepatic metabolism (such as barbiturates, carbamazepine, phenytoin, primidone, and rifampin): May decrease estrogenic effects and accelerate the metabolism of certain other agents. Use together cautiously.
Insulin, oral antidiabetics: May alter blood glucose level. Adjust dosage as needed.
Tamoxifen: Decreased tamoxifen effects. Monitor patient closely.
Warfarin-type anticoagulants: Decreased anticoagulant effect. Adjust dosage as needed.
Drug-herb. *Red clover:* May interfere with hormonal therapies. Discourage concomitant use.
Drug-food. *Caffeine:* May increase serum caffeine levels. Advise patient to avoid caffeine.
Drug-lifestyle. *Smoking:* Increases risk of adverse CV effects. Advise patient to avoid smoking.

Adverse reactions
CNS: headache, dizziness, chorea, depression, *seizures.*
CV: thrombophlebitis; *thromboembolism;* hypertension; edema; *increased risk of CVA, pulmonary embolism, and MI.*
EENT: worsening of myopia or astigmatism, intolerance of contact lenses.
GI: *nausea,* vomiting, abdominal cramps, bloating, anorexia, increased appetite, *pancreatitis,* gallbladder disease.

Reactions may be *common,* uncommon, *life-threatening,* or COMMON AND LIFE-THREATENING.

GU: in women, breakthrough bleeding, altered menstrual flow, dysmenorrhea, amenorrhea, *increased risk of endometrial cancer, possibility of increased risk of breast cancer,* cervical erosion, altered cervical secretions, enlargement of uterine fibromas, vaginal candidiasis; in men, testicular atrophy and impotence.

Hematologic: increased PT, INR, clotting factors VII to X, and norepinephrine-induced platelet aggregability.

Hepatic: cholestatic jaundice, *hepatic adenoma.*

Metabolic: decreased serum folate, pyridoxine, and antithrombin III levels; increased triglyceride, glucose, and phospholipid levels; hypercalcemia, weight changes.

Skin: melasma, urticaria, flushing (with rapid I.V. administration), hirsutism or hair loss, erythema nodosum, dermatitis.

Other: breast changes (tenderness, enlargement, secretion), gynecomastia in men.

Overdose and treatment
Serious toxicity after drug overdose hasn't been reported. Nausea may occur. Provide appropriate supportive care.

Special considerations
• Therapy with estrogens increases sulfobromophthalein retention. Thyroid-binding globulin levels may increase, resulting in increased total thyroid levels (measured by protein-bound iodine or total T_4) and decreased uptake of free T_3 resin. Glucose tolerance may be impaired. Pregnanediol excretion may decrease.
• For rapid treatment of dysfunctional uterine bleeding or reduction of surgical bleeding, parenteral administration is preferred.
• Refrigerate before reconstitution. Reconstituted drug may be safely stored in refrigeration for up to 60 days.

Patient monitoring
• Patients receiving long-term therapy should be examined yearly. Monitor serum lipid levels, blood pressure, body weight, and hepatic function.
• Monitor results of yearly breast exam and Pap test.

Pregnant patients
• Drug is contraindicated during pregnancy.

Breast-feeding patients
• Estrogens are contraindicated in breast-feeding women.

Geriatric patients
• Long-term use for menopausal symptoms may increase the risk of certain types of cancer. Frequent physical examinations are recommended.

Patient education
• Advise patient to report adverse reactions.

estropipate
Ogen, Ortho-Est

Pharmacologic classification: estrogen
Therapeutic classification: estrogen replacement
Pregnancy risk category: X

Indications and dosages
➤*Atrophic vaginitis, kraurosis vulvae, vasomotor menopausal symptoms.* Adults: 0.625 to 5 mg P.O. daily for 21 days, followed by 7 days off therapy.
➤*Female hypogonadism, primary ovarian failure, or after castration.* Adults: 1.25 to 7.5 mg P.O. daily for 3 weeks, followed by 8 to 10 days off therapy. Cycle may be repeated if no withdrawal bleeding occurs within 10 days of discontinuing therapy.
➤*Prevention of osteoporosis.* Adults: 0.625 mg P.O. daily for 25 days of a 31-day cycle.

How supplied
Estropipate is available as estrone sodium sulfate. Available by prescription only.
Tablets: 0.625 mg, 1.25 mg, 2.5 mg

Pharmacodynamics
Estrogenic action: Estropipate mimics the action of endogenous estrogen in treating female hypogonadism, menopausal symptoms, and atrophic vaginitis.

Pharmacokinetics
Absorption: After oral administration, estropipate and other synthetic derivatives of the natural estrogens are rapidly absorbed.
Distribution: About 50% to 80% bound to plasma protein. Distribution occurs throughout the body, with highest levels appearing in fat.
Metabolism: Steroidal estrogens are metabolized primarily in the liver, where they are conjugated with sulfate and glucuronide. Because of the rapid metabolism, many forms of estrogen must be administered daily.
Excretion: Mostly eliminated through the kidneys in the form of sulfate or glucuronide conjugates.

Route	Onset	Peak	Duration
P.O.	Unknown	Unknown	Unknown

Contraindications and precautions
Contraindicated in patients with thrombophlebitis or thromboembolic disorders, estrogen-dependent neoplasia, breast or reproductive organ cancer (except for palliative treatment), or undiagnosed abnormal genital bleeding and during pregnancy.

Use cautiously in patients with cerebrovascular or coronary artery disease, gallbladder disease, hypertension, asthma, bone diseases, mental depression, migraine, seizures, or cardiac, hepatic, or renal dysfunction. Also use cautiously in women with family history (mother, grandmother, sister) of breast or genital tract cancer or who have breast nodules, fibrocystic disease, or abnormal mammographic findings.

Interactions

Drug-drug. *Drugs that induce hepatic metabolism, such as rifampin, barbiturates, primidone, carbamazepine, phenytoin:* May result in decreased estrogenic effects from a given dose. These drugs are known to accelerate the metabolism of certain other agents. Use together cautiously.

Insulin, oral antidiabetics: May alter blood glucose level. Adjust dosage as needed.

Tamoxifen: Decreased tamoxifen effects. Monitor patient closely.

Warfarin-type anticoagulants: Decreased anticoagulant effect. Dosage adjustment may be necessary.

Drug-herb. *Red clover:* May interfere with hormonal therapies. Discourage concomitant use.

Drug-food. *Caffeine:* May increase serum caffeine levels. Advise patient to avoid caffeine.

Drug-lifestyle. *Smoking:* Increases risk of adverse CV effects. Advise patient to avoid smoking.

Adverse reactions

CNS: headache, dizziness, depression, migraine, *seizures.*

CV: *increased risk of CVA, pulmonary embolism, MI, thromboembolism,* thrombophlebitis, edema.

EENT: worsening of myopia or astigmatism, intolerance of contact lenses.

GI: vomiting, abdominal cramps, bloating, gallbladder disease.

GU: in women, breakthrough bleeding, increased size of uterine fibromas, dysmenorrhea, amenorrhea, vaginal candidiasis, *increased risk of endometrial cancer, possibility of increased risk of breast cancer,* altered menstrual flow, cervical erosion, altered cervical secretions, cystitis-like syndrome (which resembles premenstrual syndrome); in men, testicular atrophy.

Hematologic: increased PT, clotting factors VII to X, and norepinephrine-induced platelet aggregability.

Hepatic: cholestatic jaundice, *hepatic adenoma.*

Metabolic: decreased serum folate, pyridoxine, and antithrombin III levels; increased triglyceride, glucose, and phospholipid levels; hypercalcemia, weight changes.

Skin: *erythema multiforme,* erythema nodosum, hair loss, hemorrhagic eruption, hirsutism, melasma.

Other: libido changes; in women, aggravation of porphyria, breast changes (tenderness, enlargement, secretion); gynecomastia in men.

Overdose and treatment

Serious toxicity caused by overdose of this drug hasn't been reported. Nausea may occur. Provide appropriate supportive care.

Special considerations

● Therapy with estrogens increases sulfobromophthalein retention. Thyroid-binding globulin levels may increase, resulting in increased total thyroid levels (measured by protein-bound iodine or total T_4) and decreased uptake of free T_3 resin. Glucose tolerance may be impaired. Pregnanediol excretion may decrease.

● When used for progressive, inoperable prostate cancer, remission should be apparent within 3 weeks of therapy.

● When submitting specimens to pathologist for evaluation, note that patient is taking estrogens.

Patient monitoring

● Patient monitoring is the same as for all estrogens.

Pregnant patients

● Drug is contraindicated during pregnancy.

Breast-feeding patients

● Drug is contraindicated in breast-feeding women.

Geriatric patients

● Frequent physical examinations are recommended for postmenopausal women taking estrogens.

Patient education

● Tell patient to read package insert describing adverse estrogen effects; also give verbal explanation.

● Tell diabetic patient to report elevated glucose levels.

● Stress importance of regular physical examinations. Postmenopausal women who use estrogen replacement for more than 5 years may have increased risk of endometrial cancer. Using cyclic therapy and lowest possible estrogen dosage reduces risk. Adding progestins to regimen decreases risk of endometrial hyperplasia; however, it isn't known whether progestins affect risk of endometrial cancer. No increased risk of breast cancer has been reported.

⚠ ALERT Warn patient to immediately report abdominal pain; pain, stiffness, or numbness in legs or buttocks; pressure or pain in chest; shortness of breath; severe headaches; visual disturbances, such as blind spots or flashing lights; vaginal bleeding or discharge; breast lumps; swelling of hands or feet; yellow skin or sclera; dark urine; and light-colored stools.

● Teach woman how to perform routine breast self-examination.

● Advise patient not to become pregnant while on estrogen therapy.

Reactions may be *common*, uncommon, *life-threatening*, or COMMON AND LIFE-THREATENING.

• Advise woman of childbearing age to consult prescriber before taking drug, and to tell prescriber immediately if she becomes pregnant.

etanercept
Enbrel

Pharmacologic classification: tumor necrosis factor (TNF) blocker
Therapeutic classification: antirheumatic
Pregnancy risk category: B

Indications and dosages
➤ *Reduction in signs and symptoms and delaying of structural damage in moderately to severely active rheumatoid arthritis in patients with demonstrated inadequate response to one or more disease-modifying antirheumatic drugs; or with methotrexate in patients who don't respond adequately to methotrexate alone. Adults:* 25 mg S.C. twice weekly given at least 72 to 96 hours apart.
Children ages 4 to 17: 0.4 mg/kg (maximum dose is 25 mg) S.C. twice weekly given at least 72 to 96 hours apart.

How supplied
Available by prescription only
Injection: 25 mg single-use vial

Pharmacodynamics
Antirheumatic action: Binds specifically to TNF and blocks its action with cell-surface TNF receptors, reducing the inflammatory and immune responses of rheumatoid arthritis.

Pharmacokinetics
Absorption: Not reported.
Distribution: Not reported.
Metabolism: Not reported.
Excretion: Elimination half-life is 115 hours.

Route	Onset	Peak	Duration
S.C.	Unknown	72 hr	Unknown

Contraindications and precautions
Contraindicated in patients hypersensitive to etanercept or any of its components and in patients with sepsis. Live vaccines are contraindicated during therapy.
    Use cautiously in patients with underlying diseases that predispose them to infection, such as diabetes, heart failure, or previous active or chronic infection. Use cautiously if rheumatoid arthritis patient has pre-existing or recent onset of demyelinating disorders, including multiple sclerosis, myelitis, and optic neuritis.

Interactions
None reported.

Adverse reactions
CNS: asthenia, *headache,* dizziness.
EENT: *rhinitis,* pharyngitis, sinusitis.
GI: abdominal pain, dyspepsia.
Respiratory: *upper respiratory tract infections,* cough, respiratory disorder.
Skin: *injection site reaction,* rash.
Other: *infections,* malignancies.

Special considerations
• Anti-TNF therapies, including etanercept, may affect defenses against infection.
• Live vaccines shouldn't be given concurrently during drug therapy.
• Don't add other drugs or diluents to reconstituted solution.
• Injection sites should be at least 1" apart; never use areas where skin is tender, bruised, red, or hard. Recommended sites include the thigh, abdomen, and upper arm. Rotate sites regularly.
• Methotrexate, glucocorticoids, salicylates, NSAIDs, and analgesics may be continued during etanercept therapy.

Patient monitoring
• Positive antinuclear antibodies or positive anti-double stranded DNA antibodies may develop as measured by radioimmunoassay.
• Monitor patient for infections.

Breast-feeding patients
• Advise breast-feeding women to stop nursing during therapy.

Pediatric patients
• Juvenile rheumatoid arthritis patients should, if possible, be brought up-to-date with all immunizations in compliance with current immunization guidelines before starting treatment.
• Children with juvenile rheumatoid arthritis are more susceptible to the adverse effects of abdominal pain and vomiting than adults with rheumatoid arthritis.
• Concurrent use with methotrexate and higher doses of etanercept haven't been studied in this population.
• Safety and efficacy haven't been studied in children under age 4.

Geriatric patients
• No overall differences in safety and efficacy have been noted between elderly and younger adults; however, greater sensitivity to drug effects by elderly patients can't be ruled out.

Patient education
• Teach patient how to mix drug, inject drug, and rotate injection sites.
• Tell patient that injection site reactions usually occur within the first month of therapy and decrease thereafter.
• Urge patient to avoid live vaccines while receiving drug.

• Stress importance of alerting all health care providers about etanercept use.
• Instruct patient to promptly report signs and symptoms of infection.
• Teach patient the signs and symptoms of pancytopenia.

ethacrynate sodium
ethacrynic acid
Edecrin

Pharmacologic classification: loop diuretic
Therapeutic classification: diuretic
Pregnancy risk category: B

Indications and dosages
➤ *Acute pulmonary edema. Adults:* 50 mg or 0.5 to 1 mg/kg I.V. to a maximum dose of 100 mg of ethacrynate sodium I.V. slowly over several minutes.
➤ *Edema. Adults:* 50 to 200 mg P.O. daily. Refractory cases may require up to 200 mg b.i.d.
Children: Initially, 25 mg P.O., given cautiously and increased in 25-mg increments daily until desired effect is achieved.
➤ *Hypertension ◇. Adults:* Initially, 25 mg P.O. daily. Adjust dose, as necessary. Maximum maintenance dosage is 200 mg P.O. daily in two divided doses.

How supplied
Available by prescription only
Injectable: 50 mg (with 62.5 mg of mannitol and 0.1 mg of thimerosal)
Tablets: 25 mg, 50 mg

Pharmacodynamics
Diuretic action: Ethacrynic acid inhibits sodium and chloride reabsorption in the proximal part of the ascending loop of Henle, promoting the excretion of sodium, water, chloride, and potassium.

Pharmacokinetics
Absorption: Absorbed rapidly from the GI tract.
Distribution: Ethacrynic acid accumulates in the liver of animals. Ethacrynic acid doesn't enter the CSF, and its distribution into breast milk or the placenta is unknown.
Metabolism: Metabolized by the liver to a potentially active metabolite.
Excretion: 30% to 65% is excreted in urine and 35% to 40% is excreted in bile as the metabolite. Duration of action is 6 to 8 hours after oral administration and about 2 hours after I.V. administration.

Route	Onset	Peak	Duration
P.O.	30 min	2 hr	6-8 hr
I.V.	5 min	15-30 min	2 hr

Contraindications and precautions
Contraindicated in infants, patients hypersensitive to drug, and patients with anuria, hypotension, dehydration with hyponatremia, and metabolic alkalosis with hypokalemia. Also contraindicated if azotemia, oliguria, electrolyte imbalance, or severe watery diarrhea occurs during therapy. Use cautiously in patients with electrolyte abnormalities or impaired hepatic function.

Interactions
Drug-drug. *Aminoglycosides, some cephalosporins, or other ototoxic drugs, such as cisplatin:* May increase risk of deafness. Avoid concurrent use.
Antihypertensives: Increased antihypertensive effect. Reduce dosage if needed.
Cardiac glycosides: Increased risk of digitalis toxicity from ethacrynate-induced hypokalemia. Monitor digitalis and potassium levels.
Diuretics, such as metolazone: May increase diuretic effect. Reduce dosage when adding ethacrynic acid to a diuretic regimen.
Insulin, oral antidiabetics: Increased blood glucose levels. Increased dosage if needed.
Lithium: Reduced renal clearance of lithium. Monitor lithium levels. Dosage adjustment may be necessary.
NSAIDs: Decreased diuretic effectiveness and possible risk of renal failure. Use together cautiously.
Potassium-depleting drugs, such as corticosteroids and amphotericin B: Severe potassium loss may occur. Monitor patient closely.
Potassium-sparing diuretics, such as spironolactone, triamterene, and amiloride: Decreased potassium loss induced by ethacrynic acid. May be used as a therapeutic advantage.
Warfarin: May potentiate anticoagulant effects. Use together cautiously.
Drug-herb. *Dandelion:* Possible interference with diuretic activity. Discourage concomitant use.

Adverse reactions
CNS: confusion, fatigue, vertigo, headache, malaise.
CV: volume depletion and dehydration, orthostatic hypotension.
EENT: transient deafness (with too-rapid I.V. injection), blurred vision, tinnitus, hearing loss.
GI: diarrhea, anorexia, nausea, vomiting, GI bleeding, ***pancreatitis.***
GU: oliguria, hematuria, nocturia, polyuria, frequent urination, azotemia.
Hematologic: ***agranulocytosis,*** neutrope-*nia,* ***thrombocytopenia.***
Metabolic: hypokalemia; hypochloremic alkalosis; asymptomatic hyperuricemia; fluid and electrolyte imbalances, including dilutional hyponatremia, hypocalcemia, hypomagnesemia; hyperglycemia; impaired glucose tolerance.
Other: fever, chills.

Reactions may be *common*, uncommon, *life-threatening*, or COMMON AND LIFE-THREATENING.

Overdose and treatment
Signs and symptoms of overdose include profound electrolyte and volume depletion, which may precipitate circulatory collapse.

Treatment of ethacrynic acid overdose is primarily supportive; empty stomach by inducing emesis or gastric lavage. Replace fluid and electrolytes as needed.

Special considerations
● Give drug slowly over 20 to 30 minutes, by I.V. infusion or by direct I.V. injection over several minutes; rapid injection may cause hypotension.
● Drug shouldn't be given with whole blood or blood products; hemolysis may occur.
● I.V. ethacrynate sodium has been used to treat hypercalcemia and to manage ethylene glycol poisoning and bromide intoxication.

Patient monitoring
● Periodically assess hearing function in patients receiving high-dose therapy. Ethacrynic acid may potentiate ototoxicity of other drugs.

Pregnant patients
● Use drug only when clearly indicated.

Breast-feeding patients
● Don't use drug in breast-feeding women.

Pediatric patients
● Ethacrynate sodium and ethacrynic acid shouldn't be administered to infants. Safety in children hasn't been established.

Geriatric patients
● Elderly and debilitated patients need close observation because they're more susceptible to drug-induced diuresis. Excessive diuresis promotes rapid dehydration, leading to hypovolemia, hypokalemia, hyponatremia, and circulatory collapse. Reduced dosages may be indicated.

Patient education
● Advise patient receiving I.V. form of drug to report pain or irritation at I.V. site immediately.
● Notify diabetic patient that antidiabetic dosage may need to be increased.

ethambutol hydrochloride
Myambutol

Pharmacologic classification: semisynthetic antitubercular
Therapeutic classification: antitubercular
Pregnancy risk category: NR

Indications and dosages
➤ *Adjunctive treatment of pulmonary tuberculosis.* Adults and children age 13 and older: Initial treatment for patients who haven't received previous antitubercular therapy, 15 mg/kg P.O. daily single dose. Retreatment: 25 mg/kg P.O. daily single dose for 60 days with at least one other antitubercular drug; then decrease to 15 mg/kg P.O. daily single dose.

How supplied
Available by prescription only
Tablets: 100 mg, 400 mg

Pharmacodynamics
Antitubercular action: Ethambutol is bacteriostatic; it interferes with mycolic acid incorporation into the mycobacterial cell wall. Ethambutol is active against *Mycobacterium tuberculosis, M. bovis,* and *M. marinum,* some strains of *M. kansasii, M. avium, M. fortuitum,* and *M. intracellulare,* and the combined strain of *M. avium* and *M. intracellulare.* Ethambutol is considered adjunctive therapy in tuberculosis and is combined with other antituberculars to prevent or delay development of drug resistance by *M. tuberculosis.*

Pharmacokinetics
Absorption: Absorbed rapidly from the GI tract.
Distribution: Distributed widely into body tissues and fluids, especially into lungs, erythrocytes, saliva, and kidneys; lesser amounts distribute into brain, ascitic, pleural, and cerebrospinal fluids. Ethambutol is 8% to 22% protein-bound.
Metabolism: Undergoes partial hepatic metabolism.
Excretion: After 24 hours, about 50% of unchanged ethambutol and 8% to 15% of its metabolites are excreted in urine; 20% to 25% is excreted in feces. Small amounts of drug may be excreted in breast milk. Plasma half-life in adults is about 3¼ hours; half-life is prolonged in decreased renal or hepatic function. Ethambutol can be removed by peritoneal dialysis and, to a lesser extent, by hemodialysis.

Route	Onset	Peak	Duration
P.O.	Unknown	2-4 hr	Unknown

Contraindications and precautions
Contraindicated in children under age 13, patients hypersensitive to drug, and patients with optic neuritis. Use cautiously in patients with impaired renal function, cataracts, recurrent eye inflammations, gout, and diabetic retinopathy.

Interactions
Drug-drug. *Aluminum salts:* May delay and reduce the absorption of ethambutol. Separate administration times by several hours.
Drugs that produce neurotoxicity: Increased neurotoxic effects. Avoid use together.

Adverse reactions
CNS: headache, malaise, dizziness, mental confusion, possible hallucinations, peripheral neuritis (numbness and tingling of limbs).
EENT: optic neuritis.

GI: anorexia, nausea, vomiting, abdominal pain, GI upset.
Hematologic: *thrombocytopenia.*
Hepatic: abnormal liver function test results.
Metabolic: elevated uric acid level.
Musculoskeletal: joint pain, precipitation of acute gout.
Respiratory: bloody sputum.
Skin: dermatitis, pruritus, toxic epidermal necrolysis.
Other: *anaphylactoid reactions,* fever.

Overdose and treatment

No specific recommendation is available. Treatment is supportive. After recent ingestion (4 hours or less), empty stomach by induced emesis or gastric lavage. Follow with activated charcoal to decrease absorption.

Special considerations

• Drug can be given with food if necessary to prevent gastric irritation; food doesn't interfere with absorption.
• Specimens for culture and sensitivity testing should be collected before first dose, but therapy can begin before test results are complete; repeat periodically to detect drug resistance.

Patient monitoring

• Assess visual status before therapy; test visual acuity and color discrimination monthly in patients taking more than 15 mg/kg/day. Visual disturbances are dose-related and reversible if detected in time.
• Monitor blood (including serum uric acid) and liver function studies before and periodically during therapy to minimize toxicity.
• Monitor patient for change in renal function. Dosage reduction may be necessary.

Pregnant patients

• Use drug during pregnancy only when benefits outweigh risk to fetus.

Breast-feeding patients

• Drug appears in breast milk. Use cautiously in breast-feeding women.

Pediatric patients

• Drug isn't recommended for use in children under age 13.

Patient education

• Inform patient about risk of hypersensitivity and other adverse reactions, and emphasize need to report these reactions. Urge patient to report any unusual effects, especially blurred vision, red-green color blindness, or changes in urine elimination.
• Assure patient that visual changes will disappear within several weeks or months after drug is discontinued.
• Urge patient to complete the prescribed regimen, to comply with instructions for daily dosage, to avoid missing doses, and not to discontinue drug without medical approval. Explain importance of keeping follow-up appointments.

ethinyl estradiol
Estinyl

Pharmacologic classification: estrogen
Therapeutic classification: estrogen replacement, antineoplastic
Pregnancy risk category: X

Indications and dosages

➤*Palliative treatment of metastatic breast cancer (at least 5 years after menopause).* Adults: 1 mg P.O. t.i.d. for at least 3 months.
➤*Female hypogonadism.* Adults: 0.05 mg P.O. daily to t.i.d. for 2 weeks monthly, followed by 2 weeks progesterone therapy; continue for three to six monthly dosing cycles, followed by 2 months off.
➤*Vasomotor menopausal symptoms.* Adults: 0.02 to 0.05 mg P.O. daily for cycles of 3 weeks on, 1 week off.
➤*Palliative treatment of metastatic inoperable prostatic cancer.* Adults: 0.15 to 2 mg P.O. daily.

How supplied

Available by prescription only
Tablets: 0.02 mg, 0.05 mg, 0.5 mg

Pharmacodynamics

Estrogenic action: Ethinyl estradiol mimics the action of endogenous estrogen in treating female hypogonadism and menopausal symptoms. It inhibits growth of hormone-sensitive tissue in advanced, inoperable prostatic cancer and in certain carefully selected cases of breast cancer in men and postmenopausal women.

Pharmacokinetics

Absorption: After oral administration, estradiol is well absorbed but substantially inactivated by the liver.
Distribution: About 50% to 80% plasma protein–bound, particularly estradiol-binding globulin. Distribution occurs throughout the body, with highest levels appearing in fat.
Metabolism: Steroidal estrogens, including estradiol, are metabolized primarily in the liver, where they are conjugated with sulfate and glucuronide. Because of the rapid metabolism, nonesterified forms of estrogen, including estradiol, must usually be administered daily.
Excretion: The majority of estrogen elimination occurs through the kidneys in the form of sulfate or glucuronide conjugates.

Route	Onset	Peak	Duration
P.O.	Unknown	Unknown	Unknown

Reactions may be *common,* uncommon, *life-threatening,* or COMMON AND LIFE-THREATENING.

Contraindications and precautions

Contraindicated in pregnant patients and patients with thrombophlebitis or thromboembolic disorders, estrogen-dependent neoplasia, breast or reproductive organ cancer (except for palliative treatment), and undiagnosed abnormal genital bleeding.

Use cautiously in patients with cerebrovascular or coronary artery disease, gallbladder disease, hypertension, asthma, mental depression, bone disease, or cardiac, hepatic, or renal dysfunction. Also use cautiously in women who have a family history (mother, grandmother, sister) of breast or genital tract cancer or who have breast nodules, fibrocystic disease, or abnormal mammographic findings.

Interactions

Drug-drug. *Drugs that induce hepatic metabolism (such as barbiturates, carbamazepine, primidone, and rifampin):* May decrease estrogenic effects and accelerate the metabolism of certain other drugs. Use together cautiously.

Insulin, oral antidiabetics: Altered blood glucose levels. Adjust dosage if needed.

Tamoxifen: Decreased tamoxifen effects. Monitor patient closely.

Warfarin-type anticoagulants: Decreased anticoagulant effect. Dosage adjustment may be necessary.

Drug-food. *Caffeine:* May increase serum caffeine levels. Advise patient to avoid caffeine.

Grapefruit juice. Elevated estrogen levels. Advise patient to take drug with liquid other than grapefruit juice.

Drug-lifestyle. *Smoking:* Increases risk of adverse CV effects. Advise patient to avoid smoking.

Adverse reactions

CNS: headache, dizziness, chorea, depression, *seizures.*

CV: thrombophlebitis; ***thromboembolism;*** hypertension; edema; ***increased risk of CVA, pulmonary embolism, and MI.***

EENT: worsening of myopia or astigmatism, intolerance of contact lenses.

GI: *nausea,* vomiting, abdominal cramps, bloating, anorexia, increased appetite, gallbladder disease.

GU: in women, breakthrough bleeding, altered menstrual flow, dysmenorrhea, amenorrhea, ***increased risk of endometrial cancer, possibility of increased risk of breast cancer,*** cervical erosion, altered cervical secretions, enlargement of uterine fibromas, vaginal candidiasis, testicular atrophy, impotence.

Hematologic: increased PT, INR, clotting factors VII to X, and norepinephrine-induced platelet aggregability.

Hepatic: cholestatic jaundice, ***hepatic adenoma.***

Metabolic: decreased serum folate, pyridoxine, and antithrombin III levels; increased triglyceride, glucose, and phospholipid levels; hypercalcemia; weight changes.

Skin: melasma, urticaria, flushing (with rapid I.V. administration), hirsutism or hair loss, erythema nodosum, dermatitis.

Other: breast changes (tenderness, enlargement, secretion), gynecomastia in men.

Overdose and treatment

Serious toxicity after overdose of this drug hasn't been reported. Nausea may occur. Provide appropriate supportive care.

Special considerations

● Make sure patient has thorough physical examination before starting estrogen therapy. Patients receiving long-term therapy should have examinations yearly.

● Because of risk of thromboembolism, therapy should be discontinued at least 1 month before procedures that cause prolonged immobilization or raise the risk of thromboembolism, such as knee or hip surgery.

● Notify pathologist about estrogen therapy when sending specimens to laboratory for evaluation.

Patient monitoring

● Monitor patient for adverse reactions.

● Periodically monitoring serum lipid levels, blood pressure, body weight, and hepatic function.

Pregnant patients

● Drug is contraindicated for use during pregnancy.

Breast-feeding patients

● Drug is contraindicated in breast-feeding women.

Geriatric patients

● Use cautiously in patients whose condition may be aggravated by fluid retention.

Patient education

● Provide patient with a package insert describing adverse reactions of estrogen as well as a verbal explanation.

● Emphasize importance of regular physical examinations.

● Warn patient to immediately report abdominal pain; pain, numbness, or stiffness in legs or buttocks; pressure or pain in chest; shortness of breath; severe headaches; visual disturbances such as blind spots, flashing lights, or blurriness; vaginal bleeding or discharge; breast lumps; swelling of hands or feet; yellow skin or sclera; dark urine; or light-colored stools.

● Tell diabetic patient to report elevated blood glucose test results; antidiabetic medication dosage may be adjusted.

ethosuximide
Zarontin

Pharmacologic classification: succinimide
derivative
Therapeutic classification: anticonvulsant
Pregnancy risk category: C

Indications and dosages
➤ *Absence seizures. Adults and children age
6 and older:* Initially, 250 mg P.O. b.i.d. May increase by 250 mg q 4 to 7 days up to 1.5 g daily.
Children age 3 to 6: 250 mg P.O. daily. Optimal
dose is 20 mg/kg/day.

How supplied
Available by prescription only
Capsules: 250 mg
Syrup: 250 mg/5 ml

Pharmacodynamics
Anticonvulsant action: Ethosuximide raises the
seizure threshold; it suppresses characteristic
spike-and-wave pattern by depressing neuronal
transmission in the motor cortex and basal ganglia. It's indicated for absence seizures refractory to other drugs.

Pharmacokinetics
Absorption: Absorbed from the GI tract; steady
state plasma levels occur in 4 to 7 days.
Distribution: Distributed widely throughout the
body; protein-binding is minimal.
Metabolism: Metabolized extensively in the liver to several inactive metabolites.
Excretion: Excreted in urine, with small
amounts in bile and feces. Plasma half-life is
about 60 hours in adults and about 30 hours in
children.

Route	Onset	Peak	Duration
P.O.	Unknown	3-7 hr	Unknown

Contraindications and precautions
Contraindicated in patients hypersensitive to
succinimide derivatives. Use extremely cautiously in patients who have hepatic or renal disease.

Interactions
Drug-drug. *CNS depressants (anxiolytics, antidepressants, antipsychotics, other anticonvulsants, narcotics):* Additive CNS depression and sedation. Monitor patient closely.
Phenytoin: Increased serum phenytoin levels.
Monitor patient carefully.
Valproic acid: Altered serum ethosuximide levels. Monitor patient closely.
Drug-lifestyle. *Alcohol use:* Additive CNS
depression and sedation. Advise patient to avoid
alcohol.

Adverse reactions
CNS: *drowsiness, headache, fatigue, dizziness,
ataxia, irritability, hiccups, euphoria, lethargy, depression, psychosis.*
EENT: myopia, tongue swelling, gingival hyperplasia.
GI: *nausea, vomiting, diarrhea, weight loss,
cramps, anorexia, epigastric and abdominal
pain.*
GU: vaginal bleeding, urinary frequency, abnormal renal function test results.
Hematologic: *leukopenia,* eosinophilia,
agranulocytosis, pancytopenia.
Hepatic: elevated liver enzyme levels.
Skin: urticaria, pruritic and erythematous rash,
hirsutism, *Stevens-Johnson syndrome.*

Overdose and treatment
Signs and symptoms of ethosuximide overdose,
given alone or with other anticonvulsants, include
CNS depression, ataxia, stupor, and coma. Treatment is symptomatic and supportive. Carefully
monitor vital signs and fluid and electrolyte balance.

Special considerations
● Administer ethosuximide with food to minimize
GI distress.
● Ethosuximide may cause false-positive Coombs'
test results. It also may cause abnormal results
in renal function tests.
● Abrupt discontinuation of drug may precipitate
petit mal seizures.

Patient monitoring
● Observe patient for skin reactions, joint pain,
unexplained fever, or unusual bruising or bleeding (which may signal hematologic or other severe adverse reactions).
● Perform CBC, liver function tests, and urinalysis periodically.
● Therapeutic plasma levels range from 40 to
100 mcg/ml.

Pregnant patients
● Safety hasn't been established.

Breast-feeding patients
● Safety hasn't been established. Advise nursing
women to use an alternative feeding method during ethosuximide therapy.

Pediatric patients
● Don't use drug in children under age 3.

Geriatric patients
● Use cautiously in geriatric patients.

Patient education
● Advise patient to take drug with food or milk
to prevent GI distress, to avoid use with alcoholic
beverages, and to avoid hazardous tasks that re-

Reactions may be *common,* uncommon, *life-threatening,* or COMMON AND LIFE-THREATENING.

quire alertness if drug causes drowsiness, dizziness, or blurred vision.
● Tell patient to report to prescriber the following effects: rash, joint pain, fever, sore throat, or unusual bleeding or bruising.
● Advise patient to contact prescriber immediately if pregnancy is suspected.

etidronate disodium
Didronel

Pharmacologic classification: pyrophosphate analogue
Therapeutic classification: antihypercalcemic
Pregnancy risk category: C

Indications and dosages
➤**Symptomatic Paget's disease.** *Adults:* 5 mg/kg P.O. daily as a single dose 2 hours before a meal with water or juice. Patient shouldn't eat, consume milk or milk products, or take antacids or vitamins with mineral supplements for 2 hours after dose. May give up to 10 mg/kg daily in severe cases, not to exceed 6 months. Maximum dose is 20 mg/kg daily, not to exceed 3 months. May retreat patient only after a drug-free period of 90 days or more.
➤**Heterotopic ossification in spinal cord injuries.** *Adults:* 20 mg/kg P.O. daily for 2 weeks; then 10 mg/kg daily for 10 weeks. Total treatment period is 12 weeks.
➤**Heterotopic ossification after total hip replacement.** *Adults:* 20 mg/kg P.O. daily for 1 month before total hip replacement and for 3 months afterward.
➤**Hypercalcemia related to malignancy.** *Adults:* 7.5 mg/kg I.V. daily for 3 days. May repeat up to 7 days. Then wait 7 days before beginning a second course of treatment.

How supplied
Available by prescription only
Injection: 50 mg/ml (300-mg ampule)
Tablets: 200 mg, 400 mg

Pharmacodynamics
Bone-metabolism inhibitor action: Although the exact mechanism isn't known, etidronate adsorbs to hydroxyapatite crystals in bones, thereby inhibiting their growth and dissolution. It also decreases the number of osteoclasts in bone, thereby slowing excessive remodeling of pagetic or heterotopic bone.

Pharmacokinetics
Absorption: Absorption of oral dose is variable and decreased in the presence of food. Absorption also may be dose-related.
Distribution: About half the dose is distributed to bone.
Metabolism: Not metabolized.

Excretion: About 40% to 60% of drug is excreted within 24 hours in urine.

Route	Onset	Peak	Duration
P.O.	1 mo (in Paget's)	Unknown	Unknown
I.V.	24 hr	After 3rd infusion	Unknown

Contraindications and precautions
Contraindicated in those hypersensitive to drug and in those with clinically overt osteomalacia. Use cautiously in patients with impaired renal function.

Interactions
Drug-drug. *Antacids that contain calcium, magnesium, or aluminum; mineral supplements that contain calcium, iron, magnesium, or aluminum:* May inhibit absorption. Avoid use within 2 hours of dose.
Drug-food. *Foods that contain large amounts of calcium, such as milk and dairy products:* May prevent oral absorption. Tell patient to avoid use within 2 hours of dose.

Adverse reactions
CNS: *seizures.*
GI: diarrhea, increased frequency of bowel movements, nausea, constipation, stomatitis, metallic or altered taste.
Hepatic: abnormal hepatic function.
Metabolic: *elevated serum phosphate level.*
Musculoskeletal: increased or recurrent bone pain, pain at previously asymptomatic sites, increased risk of fracture.
Respiratory: dyspnea.
Other: fever, fluid overload, *hypersensitivity reactions.*

Overdose and treatment
Signs and symptoms of overdose include diarrhea, nausea, and hypocalcemia. Treat with gastric lavage and emesis. Administer calcium if required.

Special considerations
● Drug should be taken in a single dose. However, if nausea occurs, dosage may be divided.
● Adverse reactions occur most frequently at dosage of 20 mg/kg daily.
● I.V. etidronate is administered by slow infusion over at least 2 hours regardless of the dose given or the volume of I.V. fluid in which the drug is diluted. Etidronate for injection must be diluted in at least 250 ml of normal saline solution before administration.

Patient monitoring
● Monitor drug effect by serum alkaline phosphate and urinary hydroxyproline excretion; both are lowered by effective therapy.

Pregnant patients
• Use drug during pregnancy only when clearly indicated.

Breast-feeding patients
• Use drug cautiously in breast-feeding women.

Pediatric patients
• Safety and efficacy for use in children haven't been established.

Patient education
• Instruct patient to take drug on an empty stomach with water or juice and to avoid food, milk or milk products, antacids, and vitamins with mineral supplements for 2 hours.
• Remind patient that improvement may take at least 3 months and may continue even after the drug is stopped.

etodolac
Lodine, Lodine XL

Pharmacologic classification: NSAID
Therapeutic classification: antiarthritic
Pregnancy risk category: C

Indications and dosages
➤ *Acute and long-term management of osteoarthritis, rheumatoid arthritis, and pain. Adults:* For acute pain, 200 to 400 mg P.O. q 6 to 8 hours, p.r.n., not to exceed 1,200 mg daily. For patients who weigh 60 kg (132 lb) or less, total daily dose shouldn't exceed 20 mg/kg.

For osteoarthritis or rheumatoid arthritis, give 800 to 1,200 mg P.O. daily in divided doses initially, followed by adjustments of 600 to 1,200 mg in divided doses: 200 mg P.O. t.i.d. or q.i.d.; 300 mg P.O. b.i.d., t.i.d., or q.i.d.; 400 mg P.O. b.i.d. or t.i.d. Total daily dose shouldn't exceed 1,200 mg. For patients who weigh 60 kg or less, total daily dose shouldn't exceed 20 mg/kg, or 400 to 1,000 mg P.O. daily (extended-release form). Adjust dosage to lowest effective dose based on patient response. Don't exceed maximum dose of 1,000 mg daily.

How supplied
Available by prescription only
Capsules: 200 mg, 300 mg
Tablets: 400 mg, 500 mg
Tablets (extended-release): 400 mg, 500 mg, 600 mg

Pharmacodynamics
Antiarthritic action: Mechanism of action is unknown but probably relates to inhibition of prostaglandin biosynthesis.

Pharmacokinetics
Absorption: Well-absorbed from GI tract. The extent of the effect of food on etodolac absorption is minimal.

Distribution: Found in liver, lungs, heart, and kidneys. Etodolac is 99% bound to plasma proteins.
Metabolism: Extensively metabolized in the liver.
Excretion: Excreted in urine primarily as metabolites; 16% is excreted in feces.

Route	Onset	Peak	Duration
P.O.			
Regular	30 min	1-2 hr	4-12 hr
Extended	Unknown	3-12 hr	6-12 hr

Contraindications and precautions
Contraindicated in patients hypersensitive to drug and in those with history of aspirin- or NSAID-induced asthma, rhinitis, urticaria, or other allergic reactions.

Use cautiously in patients with impaired renal or hepatic function, history of peptic ulcer disease, cardiac disease, hypertension, or conditions associated with fluid retention.

Interactions
Drug-drug. *Antacids:* Decreased peak drug levels. Monitor patient for decreased etodolac effects.
Aspirin: Reduces protein-binding of etodolac without altering its clearance, and may increase GI toxicity. Avoid use together.
Beta blockers, diuretics: May blunt effects of drug. Monitor patient carefully.
Cyclosporine: Impaired elimination and increased risk of nephrotoxicity. Avoid use together.
Digoxin, lithium, methotrexate: Increased levels of these drugs. Monitor drug levels.
Phenytoin: Increased serum phenytoin levels. Monitor patient for signs of toxicity.
Warfarin: Decreased protein-binding of warfarin (clearance unchanged). No dosage adjustment is necessary, but monitor INR and watch for bleeding.
Drug-lifestyle. *Alcohol use:* Increased risk of adverse effects. Advise patient to avoid alcohol.
Sun exposure: Photosensitivity reactions may result from sun exposure. Advise patient to take precautions.

Adverse reactions
CNS: *asthenia, malaise, dizziness,* depression, drowsiness, syncope, nervousness, insomnia.
CV: hypertension, *heart failure,* flushing, palpitations, edema, fluid retention.
EENT: blurred vision, tinnitus, photophobia, dry mouth.
GI: *dyspepsia, flatulence, abdominal pain, diarrhea, nausea,* constipation, gastritis, melena, vomiting, anorexia, peptic ulceration with or without *GI bleeding* or perforation, ulcerative stomatitis, thirst.
GU: dysuria, urinary frequency, *renal failure.*
Hematologic: *leukopenia, thrombocytopenia,* hemolytic anemia, *agranulocytosis.*
Hepatic: elevated liver function test results, *hepatitis.*

Reactions may be *common,* uncommon, *life-threatening*, or COMMON AND LIFE-THREATENING.

Metabolic: decreased serum uric acid levels, weight gain.
Respiratory: asthma.
Skin: pruritus, rash, *Stevens-Johnson syndrome*.
Other: chills, fever.

Overdose and treatment

Signs and symptoms of overdose include lethargy, drowsiness, nausea, vomiting, and epigastric pain. Rare symptoms include GI bleeding, coma, renal failure, hypertension, and anaphylaxis. Treatment is symptomatic and supportive, including stomach decontamination.

Special considerations

● Use concurrent diuretics cautiously in patients with cardiac, renal, or hepatic failure.
● Etodolac 1,200 mg causes less GI bleeding than ibuprofen 2,400 mg daily, indomethacin 200 mg daily, naproxen 750 mg daily, or piroxicam 20 mg daily.

Patient monitoring

● Monitor patient for signs and symptoms of GI ulceration and bleeding.
● In chronic conditions, a therapeutic response to therapy is seen most often within 2 weeks.

Pregnant patients

● Avoid using drug during third trimester.

Breast-feeding patients

● It isn't known whether drug appears in breast milk. Use cautiously.

Pediatric patients

● Safety and efficacy haven't been established in children under age 18.

Geriatric patients

● Drug is well tolerated in older and younger adults and generally doesn't require age-related dosage adjustments. No age-related differences have been reported.

Patient education

● Advise patient of the potential for adverse events and instruct him to report to prescriber any GI effects of drug.
● Tell patient that drug may be taken with food.

etoposide
Toposar, VePesid

Pharmacologic classification: podophyllotoxin (specific to G2 and late S phases of cell cycle)
Therapeutic classification: antineoplastic
Pregnancy risk category: D

Indications and dosages

Dosage and indications may vary. Check literature for current protocol.

▶ *Small-cell carcinoma of the lung.*
Adults: 70 mg/m² P.O. daily (rounded to the nearest 50 mg) for 4 days. Or, 100 mg/m² P.O. (rounded to the nearest 50 mg) daily for 5 days. Repeat q 3 to 4 weeks. Or, 35 mg/m² I.V. daily for 4 days or 50 mg/m² I.V. daily for 5 days. Repeat q 3 to 4 weeks.
▶ *Testicular carcinoma. Adults:* 50 to 100 mg/m² I.V. daily on days 1 to 5. Or, 100 g/m² daily on days 1, 3, and 5 of a regimen repeated q 3 or 4 weeks.
▶ *AIDS-related Kaposi's sarcoma* ◇. *Adults:* 150 mg/m² daily I.V. for 3 consecutive days every 4 weeks. Repeat cycles as necessary.
✦ *Dosage adjustment.* Dosage reduction may be required in patients with impaired renal function.

How supplied

Available by prescription only
Capsules: 50 mg
Injection: 20 mg/ml multiple-dose vials

Pharmacodynamics

Antineoplastic action: Etoposide exerts cytotoxic action by arresting cells in the metaphase portion of cell division. Drug also inhibits cells from entering mitosis and depresses DNA and RNA synthesis.

Pharmacokinetics

Absorption: Only moderately absorbed across the GI tract after oral administration. Etoposide's bioavailability ranges from 25% to 75%, with an average of 50% of the dose being absorbed.
Distribution: Distributed widely into body tissues; the highest levels are found in the liver, spleen, kidneys, healthy brain tissue, and brain tumor tissue. It crosses the blood-brain barrier to a limited and variable extent. Etoposide is about 94% bound to serum albumin.
Metabolism: Only a small portion of a dose of etoposide is metabolized. Metabolism occurs in the liver.
Excretion: Excreted primarily in the urine as unchanged drug. A smaller portion of a dose is excreted in the feces. The plasma elimination of etoposide is described as biphasic, with an initial phase half-life of about ½ to 2 hours and a terminal phase of about 5¼ to 11 hours.

Route	Onset	Peak	Duration
P.O., I.V.	Unknown	Unknown	Unknown

Contraindications and precautions

Contraindicated in patients hypersensitive to drug. Use cautiously in patients who have had cytotoxic or radiation therapy.

Interactions

Drug-drug. *Cisplatin:* Etoposide increases cytotoxicity of cisplatin against certain tumors. May be used for this purpose.

Warfarin: Concurrent administration may cause elongation of PT and INR. Monitor patient closely.

Adverse reactions
CNS: peripheral neuropathy.
CV: hypotension (from too-rapid infusion).
GI: *nausea and vomiting, anorexia, diarrhea,* abdominal pain, *stomatitis.*
Hematologic: *anemia, myelosuppression,* LEUKOPENIA, THROMBOCYTOPENIA.
Skin: *reversible alopecia.*
Other: *anaphylaxis.*

Overdose and treatment
Signs and symptoms of overdose include myelosuppression, nausea, and vomiting. Treatment is usually supportive and includes transfusion of blood components, antiemetics, and appropriate symptomatic therapy.

Special considerations
• Pretreatment with antiemetics may reduce frequency and duration of nausea and vomiting.
• At doses below 200 mg, extent of absorption after oral administration isn't affected by food.
• Have diphenhydramine, hydrocortisone, epinephrine, and airway available in case of an anaphylactoid reaction.
• Etoposide has produced complete remissions in small-cell lung cancer and testicular cancer.
• Use of gloves is recommended when handling etoposide. If solution contacts skin or mucosa, immediately wash the area with soap and water.
• For I.V. administration, dilute etoposide in either D_5W or normal saline solution to 0.2 or 0.4 mg/ml. Higher concentrations may crystallize. Give etoposide by slow I.V. infusion (over at least 30 minutes) to prevent severe hypotension.

Patient monitoring
• Monitor blood pressure before and at 30-minute intervals during infusion. If systolic blood pressure goes below 90 mm Hg, stop infusion.
• Monitor CBC. Drug shouldn't be given if platelet count is less than $50,000/mm^3$ or absolute neutrophil count is less than $500/mm^3$.
• GI toxicity occurs more frequently after oral administration.

Pregnant patients
• High risk for fetal harm. During pregnancy, use drug only for life-threatening conditions or severe disease when much safer drugs aren't available or are ineffective.

Breast-feeding patients
• Because drug appears in breast milk, its use in breast-feeding women isn't recommended.

Pediatric patients
• Safety and effectiveness in children haven't been established.

Geriatric patients
• Elderly patients may be particularly susceptible to the hypotensive effects of etoposide.

Patient education
• Advise patient about potential adverse reactions, and instruct patient to immediately report vomiting that occurs shortly after a dose.
• Advise patient to report sore throat, fever, or unusual bruising or bleeding.
• Advise patient to avoid exposure to people with infections.
• Tell patient not to receive immunizations during therapy with etoposide. Tell other family members to avoid immunizations during this time as well.
• Advise patient to use contraceptive measures during therapy.

etoposide phosphate
Etopophos

Pharmacologic classification: semisynthetic derivative of podophyllotoxin
Therapeutic classification: antineoplastic
Pregnancy risk category: D

Indications and dosages
➤ *Adjunct treatment of refractory testicular cancer. Adults:* Etoposide phosphate doses equivalent to 50 to 100 mg/m² daily of etoposide I.V. on days 1 through 5 of each cycle and given with other approved chemotherapeutic agents. Cycle is repeated when adequate recovery from drug toxicity has occurred (usually at 3- to 4-week intervals). Or, etoposide phosphate doses equivalent to 100 mg/m² daily of etoposide I.V. on days 1, 3, and 5 of each cycle and given in conjunction with other approved chemotherapeutic agents. Cycle is repeated at 3- to 4-week intervals if adequate recovery from drug toxicity has occurred. Infusion rate may range from 5 minutes to 210 minutes, or VePesid may be given P.O. Recommended dose is two times the I.V. dose rounded to the nearest 50 mg.
➤ *Adjunct treatment of small-cell lung cancer. Adults:* Dosage is individualized but may range from etoposide phosphate doses equivalent to 35 mg/m² daily etoposide I.V. for 4 days to etoposide phosphate doses equivalent to 50 mg/m² daily etoposide I.V. for 5 days and given with other approved chemotherapeutic agents. Cycle is repeated when adequate recovery from drug toxicity has occurred (usually at 3- to 4-week intervals). Infusion rate may range from 5 minutes to 210 minutes.
➤ *AIDS-related Kaposi's sarcoma* ◇. *Adults:* 150 mg/m² daily I.V. for 3 consecutive days every 4 weeks. Repeat cycles as necessary.
✦ *Dosage adjustment.* In patients with renal impairment and creatinine clearance above 50 ml/minute, give usual dosage; for creatinine clearance between 15 and 50 ml/minute, give 75% of usual dosage.

How supplied
Available by prescription only
Capsules: 50 mg
Injection: Vials containing etoposide phosphate equivalent to 100 mg etoposide/5 ml

Pharmacodynamics
Antineoplastic action: Although action of drug is unknown, it's believed to exert cytotoxicity by arresting cells in the metaphase portion of cell division. Drug may also inhibit cells from entering mitosis and depressing DNA and RNA synthesis.

Pharmacokinetics
Absorption: Only administered as an I.V. infusion.
Distribution: Distribution is believed to be similar to etoposide. Etoposide crosses the blood-brain barrier to a limited and variable extent and is about 97% bound to serum albumin.
Metabolism: Rapidly and completely converted to etoposide in plasma.
Excretion: After etoposide phosphate is converted to etoposide, etoposide is excreted primarily in the urine as unchanged drug. A smaller portion of a dose is excreted in the feces. The plasma elimination of etoposide is described as biphasic, with an initial phase half-life of about ½ to 2 hours and a terminal phase of about 5¼ to 11 hours.

Route	Onset	Peak	Duration
P.O., I.V.	Unknown	Unknown	Unknown

Contraindications and precautions
Contraindicated in patients with history of hypersensitivity to etoposide phosphate, etoposide, or other components of the formulation.

Interactions
Drug-drug. *High-dose cyclosporine:* May increase the toxic effects of etoposide phosphate because of delayed excretion of the drug. Monitor patient closely for drug effects.
Levamisole hydrochloride: Inhibited phosphatase activities. Avoid using any drug known to inhibit phosphatase activities.
Warfarin: Prolonged PT and INR. Monitor patient carefully.

Adverse reactions
CNS: *asthenia, malaise,* dizziness, peripheral neurotoxicity.
CV: hypertension, hypotension.
GI: *nausea, vomiting, anorexia, mucositis,* constipation, abdominal pain, diarrhea, taste alteration.
Hematologic: *anemia, myelosuppression,* LEUKOPENIA, THROMBOCYTOPENIA, NEUTROPENIA.
Skin: facial flushing, *reversible alopecia,* rash.
Other: *chills, fever,* phlebitis, ***anaphylaxis.***

Overdose and treatment
Because etoposide phosphate is rapidly converted to etoposide, signs and symptoms of overdose would be expected to be similar. Signs and symptoms of etoposide overdose include myelosuppression, nausea, and vomiting.

Treatment is usually supportive and includes transfusion of blood components, use of antiemetics, and appropriate symptomatic therapy.

Special considerations
● Use of gloves is recommended when handling etoposide phosphate. If etoposide phosphate solution comes into contact with the skin or mucosa, immediately and thoroughly wash the skin with soap and water and flush the mucosa with water.
● After reconstitution, solution may be administered without further dilution or it can be further diluted to levels as low as 0.1 mg/ml etoposide with either D_5W injection or normal saline solution.
● If an anaphylactic reaction occurs, stop infusion immediately and administer pressor agents, corticosteroids, antihistamines, or volume expanders, as needed.
● Patients with low serum albumin may be at an increased risk for etoposide-related toxicities.

Patient monitoring
● Monitor CBC. Observe patient for signs of bone marrow depression. Withhold drug if platelet count is less than 50,000/mm³ or absolute neutrophil count is less than 500/mm³ until the blood counts have sufficiently recovered.

Pregnant patients
● High risk for fetal harm. During pregnancy, use drug only for life-threatening conditions or severe disease when much safer drugs aren't available or are ineffective.

Breast-feeding patients
● Drug isn't contraindicated in breast-feeding women.

Pediatric patients
● Safety and efficacy in children haven't been established. Anaphylactoid reactions have been reported in children who received etoposide.

Geriatric patients
● Geriatric patients may be particularly susceptible to the hypotensive effects of etoposide.

Patient education
● Advise patient to avoid exposure to people with infections.
● Tell patient to promptly report a sore throat, fever, unusual bruising, or bleeding.
● Reassure patient that hair should grow back after treatment has ended.
● Tell patient to store capsules in refrigerator.

exemestane
Aromasin

Pharmacologic classification: aromatase inactivator
Therapeutic classification: antineoplastic
Pregnancy risk category: D

Indications and dosages
➤*Advanced breast cancer in postmenopausal women whose disease has progressed following treatment with tamoxifen.* *Adults:* 25 mg P.O. once daily after a meal.

How supplied
Available by prescription only
Tablets: 25 mg

Pharmacodynamics
Antineoplastic action: An irreversible, steroidal aromatase inactivator that acts as a false substrate for the aromatase enzyme, the main enzyme that converts androgens to estrogens in premenopausal and postmenopausal women. Drug is then processed to an intermediate that binds irreversibly to the enzyme's active site, causing inactivation. This effect is known as "suicide inhibition," and results in lower levels of circulating estrogens. Deprivation of estrogen is an effective and selective way to treat estrogen-dependent breast cancer in postmenopausal women.

Pharmacokinetics
Absorption: Rapidly absorbed, with about 42% of dose absorbed from GI tract following oral administration. Actions peak in 1 to 2 hours.
Distribution: Extensively distributed in tissues; is 90% bound to plasma proteins. Duration is about 24 hours.
Metabolism: Extensively metabolized by liver. Isoenzyme involved is cytochrome P-450 A4 (CYP3A4).
Excretion: Excreted equally in urine and feces. Less than 1% excreted unchanged in urine. Elimination half-life is about 24 hours.

Route	Onset	Peak	Duration
P.O.	Unknown	1-2 hr	24 hr

Contraindications and precautions
Contraindicated in patients hypersensitive to drug or its components. Ingestion may cause fetal harm if patient is pregnant.

Interactions
Drug-drug. *Drugs that induce CYP3A4:* May decrease exemestane plasma levels. Monitor patient closely.
Estrogens: May inactivate exemestane. Avoid concomitant use.

Adverse reactions
CNS: *depression, insomnia, anxiety, fatigue, pain,* dizziness, headache, paresthesia, generalized weakness, asthenia, confusion, hypoesthesia.
CV: hypertension, edema, chest pain.
EENT: sinusitis, rhinitis, pharyngitis.
GI: nausea, vomiting, abdominal pain, anorexia, constipation, diarrhea, increased appetite, dyspepsia.
GU: urinary tract infection.
Musculoskeletal: pathologic fractures, arthritis, arthralgia, back pain, skeletal pain.
Respiratory: *dyspnea,* bronchitis, coughing, upper respiratory tract infection.
Skin: rash, increased sweating, alopecia, itching.
Other: fever, infection, flulike syndrome, *hot flashes,* lymphedema.

Overdose and treatment
No known antidote for overdose. Treatment is supportive, with frequent monitoring of vital signs and close observation.

Special considerations
● Don't administer with estrogen-containing drugs because doing so could interfere with intended action.
● Drug should be used only in postmenopausal women.
● Treatment should continue until tumor progression is apparent.

Patient monitoring
● Monitor hepatic and renal function before therapy starts and periodically throughout.
● Monitor CBC periodically.

Breast-feeding patients
● Exemestane shouldn't be administered to premenopausal women. Because many drugs appear in breast milk, use cautiously if a breast-feeding woman is inadvertently exposed to drug.

Pediatric patients
● Safety and effectiveness in children haven't been studied.

Geriatric patients
● No special adjustments are needed in elderly patients.

Patient education
● Advise patient to take drug after a meal.
● Tell patient that she may need to take drug for a long period of time.
● Advise patient to report adverse effects.

Reactions may be *common*, uncommon, *life-threatening*, or COMMON AND LIFE-THREATENING.

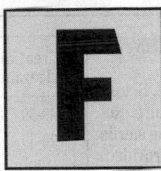

factor IX complex
Hemonyne, Konyne 80, Profilnine SD, Proplex T

factor IX (human)
AlphaNine SD, Mononine

factor IX (recombinant)
BeneFix

Pharmacologic classification: blood derivative
Therapeutic classification: systemic hemostatic
Pregnancy risk category: C

Indications and dosages
➤ *Factor IX deficiency (hemophilia B or Christmas disease), anticoagulant overdose.* factor IX complex and factor IX (human). *Adults and children:* Determine units required by multiplying 0.8 to 1 by body weight (in kg) and then by percent of desired factor IX level increase; administer by slow I.V. infusion or I.V. push. Dosage is highly individualized, depending on degree of deficiency, desired level of factor IX, body weight, and severity of bleeding.

Factor IX complex can also be used to reverse Coumadin anticoagulation when emergencies such as surgery preclude less hazardous therapy.
➤ *Factor IX deficiency (hemophilia B or Christmas disease).* BeneFix. *Adults and children:* Determine units required by multiplying 1.2 by body weight (in kg) and then multiply that result by the percent of factor IX increase desired. Administer I.V. over several minutes. Repeat q 12 to 24 hours adjusting dose to clinical response.
➤ *Hemostasis in patients with factor VIII inhibitors.* factor IX complex. *Adults and children:* Usual dose is 75 IU/kg I.V. Repeat q 12 hours, p.r.n.
➤ *Hemostasis in factor VII deficiency.* Proplex T. *Adults and children:* Determine units required by multiplying 0.5 by body weight (kg) and then multiply that result by percent of factor VII increase desired. Administer I.V. and repeat q 4 to 6 hours.

How supplied
Available by prescription only
Injection: Vials, with diluents. Units specified on label.

Pharmacodynamics
Hemostatic action: Factor IX complex directly replaces deficient clotting factor.

Pharmacokinetics
Absorption: Factor IX complex must be given parenterally for systemic effect.
Distribution: Equilibration within extravascular space takes 4 to 6 hours.
Metabolism: Factor IX complex is rapidly cleared by plasma.
Excretion: Factor IX half-life is about 24 hours.

Route	Onset	Peak	Duration
I.V.	Immediate	10-30 min	Unknown

Contraindications and precautions
Contraindicated in patients with hepatic disease in whom there's any suspicion of intravascular coagulation or fibrinolysis. Mononine is contraindicated in patients hypersensitive to murine (mouse) protein. BeneFix is produced in a Chinese hamster ovary cell line so it is contraindicated in patients with a known sensitivity to hamster protein. Use cautiously in infants.

Interactions
Drug-drug. *Aminocaproic acid:* Increased risk of thrombosis. Avoid concomitant use.

Adverse reactions
CNS: headache, tingling.
CV: *flushing, thromboembolic reactions, MI, disseminated intravascular coagulation, pulmonary embolism,* increased coagulation assays (PT, INR), changes in blood pressure.
GI: nausea, vomiting.
Skin: urticaria.
Other: *transient fever, chills.*

Overdose and treatment
Signs and symptoms of overdose include a risk of disseminated intravascular coagulation on repeated use because of increased levels of factors II, IX, and X.

Special considerations
● Refrigerate vials until needed; before reconstituting, warm to room temperature. Use 20 ml sterile water for injection of each vial of lyophilized drug. To mix, gently roll vial between hands; don't shake or mix with other I.V. solutions. Keep product away from heat (but don't refrigerate, be-

cause this may cause precipitation of active ingredient), and use within 3 hours.

• BeneFix: Refrigerate vials until needed. Before reconstituting, warm to room temperature. Reconstitute per package instructions using sterile double-ended needle and filter spike provided. Administer within 3 hours.

• Adverse reactions are usually related to too-rapid infusion. Take baseline pulse rate before I.V. administration; if pulse rate increases significantly during infusion, reduce flow rate or stop drug. If patient complains of tingling sensation, fever, chills, or headache, decrease flow rate. A rate of 100 units/minute is usually well-tolerated; don't give drug faster than 3 ml/minute.

• Human derivative forms of drug may contain the causative agents of hepatitis and other viral diseases (HIV). The risk of infection with use of these agents cannot be eliminated. The DNA-recombinant form of factor IX is inherently free from the risk of blood-borne pathogens, but is only indicated for the treatment of Factor IX deficiency.

• Immunize patient with hepatitis B vaccine to decrease risk of transmission of hepatitis.

Patient monitoring

• Monitor coagulation studies before and during therapy.

• Monitor vital signs regularly, and be alert for allergic reactions.

Pediatric patients

• Administer human forms of this drug cautiously to neonates and other infants because of increased risk of hepatitis; only heat-treated products are now available, thus decreasing the risk. The DNA-recombinant form is the treatment of choice in children.

Patient education

• Teach or review proper storage, preparation, and injection technique for the specific product that the patient uses.

---

famciclovir
Famvir

Pharmacologic classification: synthetic acyclic guanine derivative
Therapeutic classification: antiviral
Pregnancy risk category: B

Indications and dosages

➤ *Management of acute herpes zoster in immunocompetent patients. Adults:* 500 mg P.O. q 8 hours for 7 days.

✦ *Dosage adjustment.* In adults with reduced renal function, adjust dosage using the table at the top of the next column.

Creatinine clearance (ml/min)	Dosage regimen
40-59	500 mg q 12 hr
20-39	500 mg q 24 hr
< 20	250 mg q 48 hr

➤ *Recurrent genital herpes in immunocompetent patients. Adults:* 125 mg P.O. b.i.d. for 5 days.

➤ *Chronic suppressive therapy for recurrent episodes of genital herpes in immunocompetent patients. Adults:* 250 mg P.O. q. 12 hours for up to 1 year.

✦ *Dosage adjustment.* In adults with reduced renal function, adjust dosage using this table.

Creatinine clearance (ml/min)	Dosage regimen
40-59	125 mg q 12 hr
20-39	125 mg q 24 hr
< 20	125 mg q 48 hr

➤ *Chronic suppression or maintenance prophylaxis of HSV infection in HIV-infected patients. Adults:* 500 mg P.O. b.i.d. for 7 days.

How supplied

Available by prescription only
Tablets: 125 mg, 250 mg, 500 mg

Pharmacodynamics

Antiviral action: Famciclovir, a prodrug, changes to an active antiviral compound, penciclovir. It enters viral cells (herpes simplex types 1 and 2, varicella zoster), where it inhibits DNA polymerase, viral DNA synthesis, and, thus, viral replication.

Pharmacokinetics

Absorption: Absolute bioavailability of famciclovir is 77%. Because bioavailability isn't affected by food intake, the drug can be taken without regard to meals.
Distribution: Less than 20% protein-bound.
Metabolism: Extensively metabolized in the liver to the active drug penciclovir (98.5%) and other inactive metabolites.
Excretion: Primarily eliminated in the urine.

Route	Onset	Peak	Duration
P.O.	Unknown	1 hr	Unknown

Contraindications and precautions

Contraindicated in patients hypersensitive to drug. Use cautiously in patients with impaired renal or hepatic function.

Interactions
Drug-drug. *Probenecid or other drugs significantly eliminated by active renal tubular secretion:* May increase penciclovir levels. Monitor patient for increased adverse effects.

Adverse reactions
CNS: *headache,* fatigue, dizziness, paresthesia, somnolence.
EENT: pharyngitis, sinusitis.
GI: diarrhea, *nausea,* vomiting, constipation, anorexia, abdominal pain.
Hepatic: increased liver function test results, increased total bilirubin.
Musculoskeletal: back pain, arthralgia.
Skin: pruritus; zoster-related signs, symptoms, and complications.
Other: fever, injury, pain, rigors.

Overdose and treatment
No acute overdose reported. Give symptomatic and supportive therapy. It isn't known whether hemodialysis removes famciclovir from the blood. However, hemodialysis enhances elimination of acyclovir, a related nucleoside analogue.

Special considerations
• Drug may be given without regard to meals.

Patient monitoring
• Monitor renal and liver function tests.

Pregnant patients
• Use drug during pregnancy only when clearly indicated.

Breast-feeding patients
• It isn't known whether drug appears in breast milk. Use drug cautiously in breast-feeding women.

Pediatric patients
• Safety and effectiveness haven't been established in children under age 18.

Patient education
• Explain that treatment is more effective when started within 48 hours of rash onset.
• Inform patient that drug isn't a cure for genital herpes but can decrease the duration and severity of symptoms.
• Advise patient of potential adverse reactions.

famotidine
Pepcid, Pepcid AC, Pepcid AC Acid Controller, Pepcid RPD

Pharmacologic classification: H_2-receptor antagonist
Therapeutic classification: antiulcer
Pregnancy risk category: B

Indications and dosages
➤ *Duodenal and gastric ulcer. Adults:* For acute therapy, 40 mg P.O. h.s. for 4 to 8 weeks; for maintenance therapy, 20 mg P.O. h.s.
➤ *Pathologic hypersecretory conditions (such as Zollinger-Ellison syndrome). Adults:* 20 mg P.O. q 6 hours. As much as 160 mg q 6 hours may be administered.
➤ *Short-term treatment of gastroesophageal reflux disease. Adults:* 20 to 40 mg P.O. b.i.d. for up to 12 weeks.
➤ *Hospitalized patients with intractable ulcers or hypersecretory conditions or patients who can't take oral drugs; patients with GI bleeding; to control gastric pH in critically ill patients. Adults:* 20 mg I.V. q 12 hours.
➤ *Prevention or treatment of heartburn. Adults and children age 12 and older:* 1 tablet (Pepcid AC) P.O. when symptoms occur; or 10 mg P.O. 1 hour before meals to prevent symptoms. Drug can be used b.i.d. if necessary.
✦ *Dosage adjustment.* In patients with severe renal insufficiency (creatinine clearance less than 10 ml/minute), dosage may be reduced to 20 mg h.s., or the dosing interval may be prolonged to 36 to 48 hours to avoid excess accumulation of drug.

How supplied
Available by prescription only
Injection: 10 mg/ml
Injection, premixed: 20 mg/50 ml normal saline solution
Suspension: 40 mg/5 ml
Tablets: 20 mg, 40 mg
Tablets (orally disintegrating): 20 mg, 40 mg
Available without a prescription (Pepcid AC)
Gelcaps: 10 mg
Tablets: 10 mg
Tablets (chewable): 10 mg

Pharmacodynamics
Antiulcer action: Famotidine competitively inhibits action of histamine at H_2-receptors in gastric parietal cells. This inhibits basal and nocturnal gastric acid secretion from stimulation by such factors as caffeine, food, and pentagastrin.

Pharmacokinetics
Absorption: When administered orally, about 40% to 45% of dose is absorbed.
Distribution: Distributed widely to many body tissues.

◇ Unlabeled clinical use

Metabolism: About 30% to 35% of an administered dose is metabolized by the liver.
Excretion: Most is excreted unchanged in urine. Famotidine has a longer duration of effect than its 2½- to 4-hour half-life suggests.

Route	Onset	Peak	Duration
P.O.	1 hr	½-3 hr	10-12 hr
I.V.	1 hr	1-4 hr	10-15 hr

Contraindications and precautions
Contraindicated in patients hypersensitive to drug.

Interactions
Drug-drug. *Enteric-coated drugs:* Enteric coatings may dissolve too rapidly because of increased gastric pH. Use together cautiously.
Ketoconazole: Decreased ketoconazole absorption. Increase ketoconazole dosage if needed.

Adverse reactions
CNS: *headache,* dizziness, vertigo, malaise, paresthesia.
CV: palpitations, flushing.
EENT: tinnitus, orbital edema.
GI: taste disorder, diarrhea, constipation, anorexia, dry mouth.
GU: increased BUN and creatinine levels.
Hepatic: elevated liver enzyme levels.
Musculoskeletal: musculoskeletal pain.
Skin: acne, dry skin.
Other: transient irritation at I.V. site, fever.

Overdose and treatment
Overdose hasn't been reported. Treatment should include gastric lavage or induced emesis, followed by activated charcoal to prevent further absorption and supportive and symptomatic therapy. Hemodialysis doesn't remove famotidine.

Special considerations
● Drug isn't recommended for use longer than 8 weeks in patients with uncomplicated duodenal ulcer.
● After administration via nasogastric tube, flush tube to clear it and ensure passage of drug to stomach.
● Antacids may be administered concurrently.
● Drug appears to cause fewer adverse reactions and drug interactions than cimetidine.
● Drug may antagonize pentagastrin during gastric acid secretion tests. In skin tests using allergen extracts, drug may cause false-negative results.
⚠ ALERT Don't confuse drug with drugs of similar names, such as felodipine.

Patient monitoring
● Monitor patient as needed for all H$_2$-receptor antagonists.

Pregnant patients
● Use drug during pregnancy only when clearly indicated.

Breast-feeding patients
● Drug may appear in breast milk. Use cautiously in breast-feeding women.

Geriatric patients
● Use drug cautiously in elderly patients because of increased risk of adverse reactions, particularly those affecting the CNS.

Patient education
● Caution patient to take drug only as directed and to continue taking doses, even after pain subsides, to ensure adequate healing.
● Instruct patient to take dose at bedtime.
● Tell patient to open RPD tablet blisters with dry hands; place tablet on tongue and let melt. Swallow with saliva.

fat emulsions
Intralipid 10%, Intralipid 20%, Intralipid 30%, Liposyn II 10%, Liposyn II 20%, Liposyn III 10% and 20%

Pharmacologic classification: lipid
Therapeutic classification: total parenteral nutrition (TPN)
Pregnancy risk category: C

Indications and dosages
➤ **Source of calories adjunctive to TPN.**
Intralipid. *Adults:* 1 ml/minute I.V. for 15 to 30 minutes (10% emulsion). Or, 0.5 ml/minute I.V. for 15 to 30 minutes (20% emulsion). If no adverse reactions occur, increase rate to deliver 500 ml over 4 to 8 hours. Total daily dose shouldn't exceed 2.5 g/kg (10% emulsion) and 3 g/kg (20% emulsion).
Children: 0.1 ml/minute for 10 to 15 minutes (10% emulsion). Or, 0.05 ml/minute I.V. for 10 to 15 minutes (20% emulsion). If no adverse reactions occur, increase rate to deliver 1 g/kg over 4 hours. Daily dose shouldn't exceed 4 g/kg, which equals 60% of daily caloric intake. Protein-carbohydrate TPN should supply remaining 40%.
➤ **Fatty acid deficiency. Intralipid.** *Adults and children:* 8% to 10% of total caloric intake I.V.

How supplied
Available by prescription only
Injection: 50 ml (10%, 20%), 100 ml (10%, 20%, 30%), 200 ml (10%, 20%), 250 ml (10%, 20%), 500 ml (10%, 20%)

Pharmacodynamics
Metabolic action: I.V. fat emulsions are prepared from soybean or safflower oil and provide a mixture of neutral triglycerides, predominantly fatty acids. Besides fatty acids (linoleic, oleic, palmitic, stearic, and linolenic), these preparations also contain 1.2% egg yolk phospholipids (an emulsifier) and glycerol (to adjust tonicity).

I.V. fat emulsions are isotonic and may be given centrally or peripherally.

Linoleic, linolenic, and arachidonic acids are essential in humans. Signs of essential fatty acid deficiency (EFAD) include scaly dermatitis, alopecia, growth retardation, poor wound healing, thrombocytopenia, and fatty liver. I.V. fat emulsions prevent or reverse the biochemical and clinical signs of EFAD and provide 1.1 kcal/ml (10%) or 2 kcal/ml (20%).

Pharmacokinetics
Absorption: Administered I.V. (peripheral or central).
Distribution: Distributed through plasma compartment.
Metabolism: Metabolized and used as energy source, causing increased heat production, decreased respiratory quotient, and increased oxygen consumption.
Excretion: Infused fat particles cleared from bloodstream in manner similar to chylomicrons.

Route	Onset	Peak	Duration
I.V.	Immediate	Immediate	Unknown

Contraindications and precautions
Contraindicated in patients with hyperlipidemia, lipid nephrosis, acute pancreatitis accompanied by hyperlipidemia, or severe egg allergies. Use cautiously in patients with severe hepatic disease, pulmonary disease, anemia, or blood coagulation disorders (especially thrombocytopenia) and in those at risk for fat embolism.

Interactions
None reported.

Adverse reactions
Early reactions to fat overload
CNS: headache, sleepiness, dizziness.
CV: flushing.
EENT: pressure over eyes.
GI: nausea, vomiting.
Hematologic: *hypercoagulability.*
Hepatic: transient abnormalities in liver function test results, altered results of serum bilirubin tests (especially in infants).
Metabolic: hyperlipidemia.
Musculoskeletal: chest and back pain.
Respiratory: dyspnea, cyanosis.
Skin: diaphoresis, irritation (at infusion site).
Other: *hypersensitivity reactions.*
Delayed reactions to fat overload
CNS: *focal seizures.*
Hematologic: *thrombocytopenia, leukopenia,* leukocytosis.
Hepatic: transient increases in liver function test results, altered results of serum bilirubin tests (especially in infants), hepatomegaly.
Other: fever, splenomegaly.

Overdose and treatment
Signs and symptoms of overdose or "overloading syndrome" include focal seizures, splenomegaly, leukocytosis, fever, and shock.

The infusion should be discontinued until visual inspection of plasma, determination of triglyceride levels, or nephelometric measurement of plasma light-scattering activity confirms lipid clearance. Reevaluate patient and institute appropriate corrective measures.

Special considerations
● Some brands of fat emulsion can be mixed with amino acid solution and dextrose in the same I.V. container. The order of mixing is important; see package insert for further information.
● Don't use an in-line filter when administering drug; fat particles (0.5 mcg) are larger than 0.22-mcg cellulose filter.
● Fat emulsions may extract small amounts of plasticizers from I.V. administration sets made of polyvinyl chloride. Nonphthalate administration sets are available; however, phthalate extraction can be minimized from regular I.V. tubing by not storing primed administration sets.
● Discard fat emulsion if it separates or becomes oily.
● Change all I.V. tubing at each infusion because lipids support bacterial growth.
● Avoid rapid infusion by using infusion pump to regulate rate.
● Abnormally high mean corpuscular hemoglobin and mean corpuscular hemoglobin concentration values may be found in blood samples drawn during or shortly after fat emulsion infusion.

Patient monitoring
● Monitor lipid levels before and during treatment.
● Monitor hepatic function with long-term use.
● Check injection site daily for signs of inflammation or infection.
● Watch closely for adverse effects, especially during the first half hour of infusion.
● Monitor patient for allergic reactions.
● In neonates, monitor platelet count frequently; these patients tend to develop thrombocytopenia.
● In jaundiced infants, monitor bilirubin levels.
● In premature infants, monitor bilirubin level and triglycerides or serum free fatty acid levels daily; free fatty acids displace bilirubin bound to albumin.

Pediatric patients
● Because premature and small-for-gestational-age infants have poor clearance of I.V. fat emulsions, lower doses are needed to reduce likelihood of fat overload.
● Cautiously administer fat emulsions to jaundiced or premature infants. Deaths in preterm infants have been reported from intravascular fat accumulation in lungs.

Patient education
- Explain the need for fat emulsion therapy and answer questions.
- Tell patient to report adverse reactions promptly.

---

felodipine
Plendil

Pharmacologic classification: calcium channel blocker
Therapeutic classification: antihypertensive
Pregnancy risk category: C

Indications and dosages
➤ **Hypertension.** *Adults:* 5 mg P.O. daily. Adjust dosage based on patient response, typically at intervals of at least 2 weeks. Usual dose is 2.5 to 10 mg P.O. daily; doses exceeding 10 mg daily increase peripheral edema and vasodilatory adverse effects.
✦ **Dosage adjustment.** Elderly patients or patients with impaired hepatic function should receive a starting dose of 2.5 mg daily. Doses of more than 10 mg shouldn't be considered.

How supplied
Available by prescription only
Tablets (extended-release): 2.5 mg, 5 mg, 10 mg

Pharmacodynamics
Antihypertensive action: A dihydropyridine-derivative calcium channel blocker, felodipine blocks the entry of calcium ions into vascular smooth muscle and cardiac cells. This type of calcium channel blocker shows some selectivity for smooth muscle as compared with cardiac muscle. Effects on vascular smooth muscle are relaxation and vasodilation.

Pharmacokinetics
Absorption: Almost completely absorbed, but extensive first-pass metabolism reduces absolute bioavailability to about 20%.
Distribution: Over 99% bound to plasma proteins.
Metabolism: Metabolism probably hepatic; at least 6 inactive metabolites known.
Excretion: Over 70% of a dose appears in urine, and 10% appears in feces as metabolites.

Route	Onset	Peak	Duration
P.O.	2-5 hr	2½-5 hr	24 hr

Contraindications and precautions
Contraindicated in patients hypersensitive to drug. Use cautiously in patients with impaired hepatic function or heart failure, especially those receiving beta blockers. Use cautiously in elderly patients.

Interactions
Drug-drug. *Anticonvulsants:* May decrease plasma felodipine level. Monitor patient for clinical effects.
Cimetidine: Decreased felodipine clearance. Use lower doses of felodipine.
CYP 3A4 inhibitors (cimetidine, erythromycin, itraconazole, ketoconazole): Increased felodipine effects. Monitor patient for hypotension and increased heart rate.
Digoxin: Decreased peak serum levels of digoxin, but total absorbed drug is unchanged. Clinical significance is unknown.
Theophylline: May slightly decrease theophylline levels. Monitor patient for drug effects.
Drug-food. *Grapefruit juice:* May increase bioavailability and effect of drug when taken together. Avoid use together.

Adverse reactions
CNS: *headache,* dizziness, paresthesia, asthenia.
CV: *flushing, peripheral edema,* chest pain, palpitations.
EENT: rhinorrhea, pharyngitis, gingival hyperplasia.
GI: abdominal pain, nausea, constipation, diarrhea.
Musculoskeletal: muscle cramps, back pain.
Respiratory: upper respiratory tract infection, cough.
Skin: rash.

Overdose and treatment
Expected signs and symptoms include peripheral vasodilation, bradycardia, and hypotension. Provide supportive care. I.V. fluids or sympathomimetics may be useful in treating hypotension, and atropine (0.5 to 1 mg I.V.) may treat bradycardia. It isn't known whether drug may be removed by dialysis.

Special considerations
Consider the recommendations relevant to all calcium channel blockers as well as the following.
- Peripheral edema appears to be both dose- and age-dependent. It's more common in patients taking higher doses, especially those age 60 and older.
- Drug may be given without regard to meals. However, a small study reported a more than twofold increase of bioavailability when drug was taken with doubly concentrated grapefruit juice compared with water or orange juice.

Patient monitoring
- Monitor patient as for all calcium channel blockers.

Pregnant patients
- Use drug in pregnancy only when benefits justify risk to fetus.

Breast-feeding patients
• It isn't known whether drug appears in breast milk. Because of risk of serious adverse effects to the infant, breast-feeding isn't recommended.

Pediatric patients
• Safety and efficacy in children haven't been established.

Geriatric patients
• Elderly patients have higher blood levels of drug. Mean drug clearance from elderly hypertensive patients (average age 74) is less than half of that observed in young patients (average age 26). Check blood pressure closely during dosage adjustment. Maximum daily dose is 10 mg.

Patient education
• Tell patient to maintain good oral hygiene and to see a dentist regularly because drug may increase the risk of mild gingival hyperplasia.
• Remind patient to swallow tablet whole and not to crush or chew it.
• Inform patient that he should continue taking drug even when feeling better, watch his diet, and call before taking other drugs, including OTC medicines.

fenofibrate (micronized)
TriCor

Pharmacologic classification: fibric acid derivative
Therapeutic classification: antihyperlipidemic
Pregnancy risk category: C

Indications and dosages
➤ *Adjunct to diet for treatment of patients with very high serum triglyceride levels (type IV and V hyperlipidemia) who are at high risk of pancreatitis and who don't respond adequately to diet alone.* Adults: 67 to 200 mg P.O. daily. Based on response, increase dose if necessary following repeat triglyceride levels at 4- to 8-week intervals to maximum dose of 200 mg daily.
➤ *Adjunct to diet for the reduction of low-density lipoprotein (LDL) cholesterol, total cholesterol, triglycerides, and apolipoprotein B in patients with primary hypercholesterolemia or mixed dyslipidemia (Frederickson types IIa and IIb).* Adults: 200 mg P.O. daily.
✦ *Dosage adjustment.* Minimize dose in renally impaired patients and elderly patients. Start with 67 mg daily and increase only after effects on renal function and triglyceride levels have been evaluated at this dose.

How supplied
Available by prescription only
Capsules: 67 mg, 134 mg, 200 mg

Pharmacodynamics
Antihyperlipidemic action: Exact mechanism of action isn't known; drug is thought to lower triglyceride levels by inhibiting triglyceride synthesis, resulting in a decrease in the amount of very-low-density lipoprotein released into the circulation. Fenofibrate may stimulate the breakdown of triglyceride-rich protein.

Pharmacokinetics
Absorption: Well absorbed. Food increases drug absorption by 35%.
Distribution: Steady state plasma levels are achieved within 5 days after therapy starts. Drug is almost entirely bound to plasma protein.
Metabolism: Rapidly hydrolyzed by esterases to fenofibric acid, an active metabolite. Fenofibric acid is primarily conjugated with glucuronic acid and excreted in urine.
Excretion: Primarily excreted in the urine; 25% is excreted in the feces; elimination half-life is 20 hours.

Route	Onset	Peak	Duration
P.O.	Unknown	6-8 hr	Unknown

Contraindications and precautions
Contraindicated in patients hypersensitive to drug and those with gallbladder disease, hepatic dysfunction (including primary biliary cirrhosis), severe renal dysfunction, and unexplained persistent liver function abnormalities.

Interactions
Drug-drug. *Bile acid resins:* May bind with and inhibit absorption of fenofibrate. Fenofibrate should be taken 1 hour before or 4 to 6 hours after taking these agents.
Coumarin-type anticoagulants: Protein-binding displacement of the anticoagulant and potentiation of its effects. Use extremely cautiously; reduce dose of anticoagulant to keep PT and INR in desired range.
Cyclosporine: Cyclosporine-induced renal dysfunction may compromise fenofibrate elimination. Use cyclosporine and fenofibrate together cautiously.
HMG-CoA inhibitors (statins): No data are available on use of statins with fenofibrate; however, because of risk of myopathy, rhabdomyolysis, and acute renal failure reported with combined use of statins and gemfibrozil (another fibrate derivative), determine whether the benefit of further alterations in lipid levels outweighs the risk of adverse effects.

Adverse reactions
CNS: dizziness, pain, asthenia, fatigue, paresthesia, insomnia, headache.
CV: *arrhythmias.*
EENT: eye irritation, eye floaters, earache, conjunctivitis, blurred vision, rhinitis, sinusitis.

GI: dyspepsia, eructation, flatulence, increased appetite, nausea, vomiting, abdominal pain, constipation, diarrhea.
GU: polyuria, vaginitis, increased creatinine and BUN levels.
Hematologic: decreased hemoglobin levels.
Hepatic: elevated liver enzyme levels.
Metabolic: decreased uric acid levels.
Musculoskeletal: arthralgia.
Respiratory: cough.
Skin: urticaria, pruritus, rash.
Other: *infections,* decreased libido, flu syndrome.

Overdose and treatment
No cases of overdose have been reported. If overdose does occur, initiate supportive measures. Because drug is highly protein-bound, hemodialysis is unlikely to help.

Special considerations
● Fenofibrate lowers serum uric acid levels in normal patients as well as hyperuricemic patients by increasing uric acid excretion.
● Drug shouldn't be used for primary or secondary prevention of coronary artery disease.
● If possible, change or discontinue the use of beta blockers, estrogens, and thiazide diuretics because they may increase plasma triglyceride levels.
● Pancreatitis may occur in patients receiving fenofibrate; myositis and rhabdomyolysis may occur in those with renal failure. Assess creatine kinase levels in patients with myalgia, muscle tenderness, or weakness.
● Withdraw therapy in patients who don't achieve an adequate response after 2 months of treatment with the maximum daily dose.

Patient monitoring
● Drug may cause excretion of cholesterol into the bile leading to cholelithiasis. If suspected, perform appropriate tests and discontinue drug.
● Mild to moderate decreases in hemoglobin, hematocrit, and WBC count may occur at start of therapy but stabilize with long-term administration.
● Monitor liver function periodically for the duration of therapy. Discontinue therapy if liver enzyme levels are more than three times the patient's baseline.

Breast-feeding patients
● Don't use drug in breast-feeding patients; either the drug or breast-feeding should be discontinued.

Pediatric patients
● Drug isn't indicated for use in children. Safety and efficacy haven't been established.

Geriatric patients
● Drug acts similarly in elderly patients (ages 77 to 87) as in young adults; similar dosing regimens can be used. Start with 67 mg daily.

Patient education
● Advise patient to promptly report unexplained muscle weakness, pain, or tenderness, especially if accompanied by malaise or fever.
● Instruct patient to take drug with meals to optimize drug absorption.

fenoldopam mesylate
Corlopam

Pharmacologic classification: dopamine D_1-like receptor agonist
Therapeutic classification: antihypertensive
Pregnancy risk category: B

Indications and dosages
➤ *Short-term (up to 48 hours) in-hospital management of severe hypertension when rapid but quickly reversible reduction of blood pressure is indicated, including malignant hypertension with deteriorating end-organ function. Adults:* Administer by continuous I.V. infusion. Infusion rate starts at 0.025 to 0.3 mcg/kg/minute and is adjusted upward or downward at no more than q 15 minutes to achieve desired blood pressure. Recommended increments are 0.05 to 0.1 mcg/kg/minute.

How supplied
Available by prescription only
Ampules: 10 mg/ml in single-dose 1-ml, 2-ml, 5-ml ampules

Pharmacodynamics
Antihypertensive action: Rapid-acting vasodilator. Fenoldopam is an agonist for D_1-like dopamine receptors and binds with moderate affinity to alpha$_2$-adrenoreceptors. No significant affinity for D_2-like receptors, alpha$_1$ or beta adrenoreceptors, 5HT, 5HT$_2$, or muscarinic receptors has been noted. In addition, fenoldopam has no effect on ACE activity, although it may increase norepinephrine plasma levels.

Pharmacokinetics
Absorption: Administered I.V.
Distribution: Steady state plasma levels of 3.2 to 4 ng/ml were reported with infusion rates of 0.1 mcg/kg/minute.
Metabolism: Principal routes of conjugation are methylation, glucuronidation, and sulfation.
Excretion: Elimination is largely by conjugation, without participation of cytochrome P-450 enzymes. Elimination half-life is reported to be about 5 minutes. Following I.V. administration, 90% of drug is excreted in urine and 10% in feces. Only 4% of drug is excreted unchanged.

Route	Onset	Peak	Duration
I.V.	15 min	20 min	Unknown

Reactions may be *common*, uncommon, *life-threatening*, or COMMON AND LIFE-THREATENING.

Contraindications and precautions
No contraindications are known. Use cautiously because drug is a rapid-acting, potent vasodilator that may precipitate severe hypotension.

Use cautiously in patients with glaucoma or ocular hypertension because dose-dependent increases in intraocular pressure may occur. Drug may cause symptomatic hypotension; use particularly cautiously when administering to patients who have sustained an acute cerebral infarction or hemorrhage.

Fenoldopam contains sodium metabisulfite, which may cause allergic-type reactions (including anaphylactoid symptoms and severe asthmatic episodes in certain susceptible individuals). Sulfite sensitivity is more frequent in asthmatic than in nonasthmatic people.

Interactions
Drug-drug. *Beta blockers:* Unexpected hypotension could result from beta-blocker inhibition of the reflex response to fenoldopam. Avoid use together.

Adverse reactions
CNS: dizziness, headache, insomnia.
CV: hypotension, orthostatic hypotension, palpitations, *bradycardia*, tachycardia, angina, *MI*, *heart failure*, T wave inversion, flushing.
EENT: nasal congestion.
GI: nausea, vomiting, abdominal pain, constipation, diarrhea.
GU: oliguria, urinary tract infection.
Hematologic: leukocytosis, bleeding.
Metabolic: increased BUN, creatinine, serum glucose, LD, and transaminase levels; hypokalemia.
Musculoskeletal: limb cramp, back pain.
Respiratory: dyspnea.
Other: pyrexia, nonspecific chest pain, injection site reaction.

Overdose and treatment
Intentional overdose hasn't been reported. The most likely reaction would be excessive hypotension, which should be treated by stopping drug and providing supportive measures.

Special considerations
• Drug causes a dose-related tachycardia that diminishes over time but remains substantial at higher doses.
• Diluted solution is stable at room temperature for at least 24 hours.
• Drug may be abruptly discontinued or infusion gradually tapered. Oral antihypertensives can be added once blood pressure is stable during infusion or after its discontinuation.

Patient monitoring
• Monitor blood pressure frequently during infusions; monitor blood pressure and heart rate every 15 minutes until patient is stable.

• Monitor serum electrolytes and watch for hypokalemia.

Pregnant patients
• Use during pregnancy only if clearly needed.

Breast-feeding patients
• Drug may appear in breast milk; use cautiously in breast-feeding women.

Pediatric patients
• Safety and efficacy in children haven't been established.

Patient education
• Advise patient that drug causes dose-related decreases in blood pressure and increases in heart rate.
• Encourage patient to report adverse reactions promptly.

fenoprofen calcium
Nalfon

Pharmacologic classification: NSAID
Therapeutic classification: nonnarcotic analgesic, antipyretic, anti-inflammatory
Pregnancy risk category: NR

Indications and dosages
➤ *Rheumatoid arthritis, osteoarthritis.*
Adults: 300 to 600 mg P.O. t.i.d. or q.i.d. Maximum, 3.2 g daily.
➤ *Mild to moderate pain. Adults:* 200 mg P.O. q 4 to 6 hours, p.r.n.
➤ *Fever* ◇. *Adults:* Single oral doses up to 400 mg P.O.
➤ *Acute gouty arthritis* ◇. *Adults:* 800 mg P.O. q 6 hours; decrease dose based on patient response.

How supplied
Available by prescription only
Capsules: 200 mg, 300 mg
Tablets: 600 mg

Pharmacodynamics
Analgesic, anti-inflammatory, and antipyretic actions: Mechanisms of action unknown, but drug is thought to inhibit prostaglandin synthesis.

Pharmacokinetics
Absorption: Absorbed rapidly and completely from the GI tract.
Distribution: About 99% is protein-bound.
Metabolism: Metabolized in the liver.
Excretion: Excreted chiefly in urine with a serum half-life of 2½ to 3 hours. A small amount is excreted in feces.

Route	Onset	Peak	Duration
P.O.	15-30 min	2 hr	4-6 hr

Contraindications and precautions

Contraindicated in pregnant patients, patients hypersensitive to drug, and patients with significantly impaired renal function or history of aspirin- or NSAID-induced asthma, rhinitis, or urticaria.

Use cautiously in elderly patients and patients with history of GI events, peptic ulcer disease, compromised cardiac function, or hypertension.

Interactions

Drug-drug. *Acetaminophen, gold compounds:* Increased nephrotoxicity may occur. Use together cautiously.

Anticoagulants, thrombolytics (coumarin derivatives, heparin, streptokinase, urokinase): May potentiate anticoagulant effects. Use together cautiously.

Anti-inflammatory drugs: May increase risk of nephrotoxicity, bleeding, and adverse GI reactions. Use together cautiously or not at all.

Aspirin: May decrease fenoprofen bioavailability and increase risk of bleeding problems. Avoid use together.

Cefamandole, cefoperazone, drugs that inhibit platelet aggregation (such as dextran, dipyridamole, mezlocillin, piperacillin, sulfinpyrazone, ticarcillin, valproic acid), plicamycin, salicylates: Increased risk of bleeding problems. Avoid use together.

Corticosteroids, corticotropin, salicylates: May increase adverse GI reactions, including ulceration and hemorrhage. Avoid use together.

Coumarin derivatives, nifedipine, phenytoin, verapamil: Toxicity may occur. Use together cautiously.

Diuretics: Increased nephrotoxic potential. Use together cautiously.

Insulin, oral antidiabetics: Increased hypoglycemic effects. Dosage may need adjustment.

Lithium, methotrexate: May decrease renal clearance of fenoprofen. Use cautiously together and monitor patient for signs of toxicity.

Drug-lifestyle. *Alcohol use:* May increase adverse GI reactions. Discourage use together.

Adverse reactions

CNS: *headache,* dizziness, *somnolence,* fatigue, nervousness, asthenia, tremor, confusion.

CV: peripheral edema, palpitations.

EENT: tinnitus, blurred vision, decreased hearing.

GI: *epigastric distress, nausea,* **GI bleeding,** vomiting, occult blood loss, peptic ulceration, constipation, anorexia, *dyspepsia,* flatulence.

GU: oliguria, interstitial nephritis, proteinuria, reversible **renal failure,** papillary necrosis, cystitis, hematuria, increased BUN and creatinine levels.

Hematologic: prolonged bleeding time, anemia, **aplastic anemia, agranulocytosis, thrombocytopenia, hemorrhage,** bruising, hemolytic anemia.

Hepatic: elevated enzyme levels, **hepatitis.**

Metabolic: hyperkalemia.

Respiratory: dyspnea, upper respiratory tract infections, nasopharyngitis.

Skin: *pruritus,* rash, urticaria, increased diaphoresis.

Other: *anaphylaxis, angioedema.*

Overdose and treatment

Little is known about fenoprofen overdose. Nonoliguric renal failure, tachycardia, and hypotension have been observed. Other symptoms include drowsiness, dizziness, confusion and lethargy, nausea, vomiting, headache, tinnitus, and blurred vision. Elevations in serum creatinine and BUN levels have been reported.

To treat an overdose of fenoprofen, empty stomach immediately by inducing emesis with ipecac syrup or by gastric lavage. Administer activated charcoal via nasogastric tube. Provide symptomatic and supportive measures (respiratory support and correction of fluid and electrolyte imbalances). Monitor laboratory parameters and vital signs closely. Dialysis is of little value.

Special considerations

● Fenoprofen has been used to treat fever, acute gouty arthritis, and juvenile arthritis.

● Drug may cause false elevations in free and total serum T_3, but thyroid-stimulating hormone and T_4 are unaffected.

⚠ ALERT Don't confuse Nalfon with Naldecon.

● Because NSAIDs impair synthesis of renal prostaglandins, they can decrease renal blood flow and lead to reversible renal impairment, especially in elderly patients, patients who take diuretics, and patients with renal failure, heart failure, or liver dysfunction.

Patient monitoring

● Monitor patient for CNS effects. Institute safety measures to prevent injury.

● Monitor renal, hepatic, and auditory function in patients receiving long-term therapy. Stop drug if abnormalities occur.

Pregnant patients

● Safety during pregnancy hasn't been evaluated; use in pregnant patients isn't recommended.

Breast-feeding patients

● Drug appears in breast milk; avoid use in breast-feeding women.

Pediatric patients

● Safe use of fenoprofen in children hasn't been established. Drug isn't recommended for use in children under age 14.

Geriatric patients

● Patients over age 60 may be more susceptible to toxic effects of fenoprofen, especially adverse GI reactions. Use cautiously.

Reactions may be *common,* uncommon, *life-threatening,* or COMMON AND LIFE-THREATENING.

• Effects of drug on renal prostaglandins may cause fluid retention and edema, a significant drawback for elderly patients and those with heart failure.

Patient education
• Tell patient to avoid activities that require alertness or concentration until CNS effects of drug are known.
• Advise patient to call prescriber for specific instruction before taking OTC analgesics.

fentanyl citrate
Sublimaze

fentanyl transdermal system
Duragesic-25, Duragesic-50, Duragesic-75, Duragesic-100

fentanyl transmucosal
Actiq, Fentanyl Oralet

Pharmacologic classification: opioid agonist
Therapeutic classification: analgesic, adjunct to anesthesia, anesthetic
Controlled substance schedule: II
Pregnancy risk category: C

Indications and dosages
➤ *Preoperatively. Adults:* 50 to 100 mcg I.M. 30 to 60 minutes before surgery.
Children and adults who weigh less than 15 kg (33 lb): 5 mcg/kg as lozenge (Oralet only) P.O. for patient to suck until dissolved, 20 to 40 minutes before surgery.
➤ *Adjunct to general anesthetic.* Low-dose regimen for minor procedures. *Adults:* 2 mcg/kg I.V.
Moderate-dose regimen for major procedures
Adults: Initial dose is 2 to 20 mcg/kg I.V. May give additional doses of 25 to 100 mcg I.V. or I.M., p.r.n.
High-dose regimen for complicated procedures
Adults: Initial dose is 20 to 50 mcg/kg I.V. May give additional doses of 25 mcg to one-half the initial dose, p.r.n.
➤ *Adjunct to anesthesia (lozenge). Adults and children older than age 2:* 5 mcg/kg lozenge (Oralet only) P.O.
➤ *Adjunct to regional anesthesia. Adults:* 50 to 100 mcg I.M. or slow I.V. over 1 to 2 minutes.
➤ *Induction and maintenance of anesthesia. Children age 2 to 12:* Reduced dose as low as 1.7 to 3.3 mcg/kg.
➤ *Postoperative analgesic. Adults:* 50 to 100 mcg I.M. q 1 to 2 hours, p.r.n.
➤ *Management of chronic pain in patients who can't be managed by lesser means. Adults:* Apply one transdermal patch to a portion of the upper torso on an area of skin that isn't irritated and hasn't been irradiated. Start with the 25-mcg/hour system; adjust dosage as needed and tolerated. Each system may be worn for 72 hours.
➤ *Management of breakthrough cancer pain.* Actiq. *Adults:* Initial dose is 200 mcg. Give second dose 15 minutes after the previous dose (unit) has been completed. Don't give more than 2 units for each breakthrough pain episode while the patient is in the adjustment phase. Evaluate each new dose used in the adjustment period over 1 to 2 days. Once an effective dose is established, limit patient to 4 units/day or less. Discontinue Actiq via gradual downward adjustment.
✦ *Dosage adjustment.* Lower doses are usually indicated for elderly patients who may be more sensitive to the therapeutic and adverse effects of drug.

How supplied
Available by prescription only
Injection: 50 mcg/ml
Transdermal system: Patches designed to release 25 mcg, 50 mcg, 75 mcg, or 100 mcg of fentanyl/hour.
Transmucosal: 100 mcg, 200 mcg, 300 mcg, 400 mcg (Oralet); 200 mcg, 400 mcg, 600 mcg, 800 mcg, 1200 mcg, 1600 mcg (Actiq)

Pharmacodynamics
Analgesic action: Fentanyl binds to the opiate receptors as an agonist to alter the patient's perception of painful stimuli, thus providing analgesia for moderate to severe pain. Its CNS and respiratory depressant effects are similar to those of morphine. Drug has little hypnotic activity and rarely causes histamine release.

Pharmacokinetics
Absorption: Varies with form administered.
Distribution: Redistribution has been suggested as the main cause of the brief analgesic effect of fentanyl.
Metabolism: Metabolized in the liver.
Excretion: Excreted in urine as metabolites and unchanged drug. Elimination half-life is about 7 hours after parenteral use, 5 to 15 hours after transmucosal use, and 18 hours after transdermal use.

Route	Onset	Peak	Duration
I.V.	1-2 min	3-5 min	½-1 hr
I.M.	7-15 min	20-30 min	1-2 hr
Trans-dermal	12-24 hr	1-3 days	Variable
Trans-mucosal	5-15 min	20-50 min	Unknown

Contraindications and precautions
Contraindicated in patients intolerant of drug. Use cautiously in elderly or debilitated patients and in those with head injuries, increased CSF pressure, COPD, decreased respiratory reserve,

compromised respirations, arrhythmias, or hepatic, renal, or cardiac disease.

Interactions

Drug-drug. *Cimetidine:* May increase respiratory and CNS depression. Reduce fentanyl dosage by one-quarter to one-third as needed.

CNS depressants (antihistamines, barbiturates, benzodiazepines, general anesthetics, muscle relaxants, narcotic analgesics, phenothiazines, sedative-hypnotics, tricyclic antidepressants): Potentiated respiratory and CNS depression, sedation, and hypotensive effects of drug. Use together cautiously.

Diazepam, general anesthetics: Severe CV depression may result. Avoid use together.

Droperidol: Hypotension and decreased pulmonary artery pressure. Use together cautiously.

Drugs extensively metabolized in the liver (digitoxin, phenytoin, rifampin): Drug accumulation and enhanced effects. Use together cautiously.

MAO inhibitors: Increased CNS effects. Don't give fentanyl to patient who has taken an MAO inhibitor within 14 days.

Narcotic antagonists: May cause acute withdrawal syndrome. Use cautiously.

Spinal anesthesia and some peridural anesthetics: Fentanyl can alter respiration by blocking intercostal nerves. Avoid use together.

Drug-lifestyle. *Alcohol use:* May cause additive effects. Advise patient to avoid alcohol.

Adverse reactions

CNS: *sedation, somnolence, clouded sensorium, euphoria,* dizziness, headache, *confusion, asthenia,* nervousness, hallucinations, anxiety, depression.

CV: *hypotension,* hypertension, ***arrhythmias,*** chest pain.

GI: *nausea, vomiting, constipation,* ileus, abdominal pain, *dry mouth,* anorexia, diarrhea, dyspepsia, increased plasma amylase and lipase levels.

GU: *urine retention.*

Respiratory: ***respiratory depression,*** hypoventilation, dyspnea, ***apnea.***

Skin: reaction at application site (erythema, papules, edema), *pruritus, diaphoresis.*

Other: physical dependence.

Overdose and treatment

The most common signs and symptoms are extensions of drug action. They include CNS depression, respiratory depression, and miosis. Other acute toxic effects include hypotension, bradycardia, hypothermia, shock, apnea, cardiopulmonary arrest, circulatory collapse, pulmonary edema, and seizures.

To treat acute overdose, first establish adequate respiratory exchange via a patent airway and ventilation as needed; administer a narcotic antagonist (naloxone) to reverse respiratory depression. (Because the duration of action of fentanyl is longer than that of naloxone, repeated dosing may be necessary.) Naloxone shouldn't be given unless the patient has clinically significant respiratory or CV depression. Monitor vital signs closely.

Provide symptomatic and supportive treatment. Monitor laboratory values, vital signs, and neurologic status closely.

Special considerations

• Fentanyl may cause bradycardia. Pretreatment with an anticholinergic (such as atropine or glycopyrrolate) may minimize this effect.

• High doses can produce muscle rigidity. This effect can be reversed by naloxone.

• Many anesthesiologists use epidural and intrathecal fentanyl as a potent adjunct to epidural anesthesia.

Transmucosal form

• The fentanyl Oralet is used as an adjunct to anesthesia; Actiq is used for breakthrough cancer pain.

⚠ ALERT Amount of drug in lozenges can be fatal to a child.

Transdermal form

• Transdermal fentanyl isn't recommended for postoperative pain.

• Dosage adjustments in patients using the transdermal system should be made gradually. Reaching steady state levels of a new dose may take up to 6 days; delay dose adjustment until after at least two applications.

• Most patients experience good control of pain for 3 days while wearing the transdermal system, although a few may need a new application after 48 hours. Because serum fentanyl level increases for the first 24 hours after application, analgesic effect can't be evaluated for the first day.

• When reducing opiate therapy or switching to a different analgesic, withdraw the transdermal system gradually. Because the serum level of fentanyl decreases very gradually after removal, give half of the equianalgesic dose of the new analgesic 12 to 18 hours after removal.

Patient monitoring

• Observe patient for delayed onset of respiratory depression.

• Monitor patient's heart rate.

• Monitor patient for at least 12 hours for adverse reactions to transdermal system. Serum fentanyl levels decrease very gradually and may take as long as 17 hours to decline by 50%.

Pregnant patients

• Drug use is contraindicated during pregnancy unless benefits outweigh risks to fetus.

Breast-feeding patients

• Drug appears in breast milk; don't administer to breast-feeding women.

Pediatric patients

• Safe use in children under age 2 hasn't been established for parenteral or transmucosal (buccal) use.

• Safe use in children under age 12 hasn't been established for transdermal system.

• Transdermal system shouldn't be used in children under age 18 who weigh less than 50 kg (110 lb).

• Buccal form shouldn't be used in any child who weighs less than 15 kg (33 lb).

Geriatric patients

• Use cautiously in elderly patients.

Patient education

• Teach proper application of transdermal patch.

• Tell patient to apply a replacement patch to a new site if another patch is needed after 72 hours.

• Warn patient to keep lozenges out of reach of children.

• Advise patient on proper disposal of lozenges.

ferrous fumarate

Femiron, Feostat, Fumasorb, Fumerin, Hemocyte, Ircon, Ircon-FA, Neo-Fer*, Nephro-Fer, Novofumar*, Palafer*, Span-FF

Pharmacologic classification: oral iron supplement
Therapeutic classification: hematinic
Pregnancy risk category: A

Indications and dosages

➤ *Iron-deficiency states. Adults:* 50 to 100 mg P.O. of elemental iron, t.i.d. Adjust dose gradually, as needed and as tolerated.
Children: 4 to 6 mg/kg P.O. daily divided into three doses.

✦ *Dosage adjustment.* Elderly patients may need higher doses because reduced gastric secretions and achlorhydria may lower capacity for iron absorption.

How supplied

Available without a prescription. Ferrous fumarate is 30% elemental iron.
Capsules (extended-release): 325 mg
Drops: 45 mg/0.6 ml
Suspension: 100 mg/5 ml
Tablets: 63 mg, 195 mg, 200 mg, 324 mg, 325 mg, 350 mg
Tablets (chewable): 100 mg

Pharmacodynamics

Hematinic action: Ferrous fumarate replaces iron, an essential component in the formation of hemoglobin.

Pharmacokinetics

Absorption: Absorbed from the entire length of the GI tract, but primary absorption sites are the duodenum and proximal jejunum. Up to 10% of iron is absorbed by healthy individuals; patients with iron-deficiency anemia may absorb up to 60%. Enteric coating and some extended-release formulas have decreased absorption because they're designed to release iron past the points of highest absorption; food may decrease absorption by 40 to 60%.

Distribution: Transported through GI mucosal cells directly into the blood, where it's immediately bound to a carrier protein, transferrin, and transported to the bone marrow for incorporation into hemoglobin. Iron is highly protein-bound.

Metabolism: Liberated by the destruction of hemoglobin, but is conserved and reused by the body.

Excretion: Healthy people lose only small amounts of iron daily. Men and postmenopausal women lose about 1 mg daily, and premenopausal women about 1.5 mg daily. The loss usually occurs in nails, hair, feces, and urine; trace amounts are lost in bile and sweat.

Route	Onset	Peak	Duration
P.O.	4 days	7-10 days	4-6 mo

Contraindications and precautions

Contraindicated in patients receiving repeated blood transfusions and patients with primary hemochromatosis or hemosiderosis, hemolytic anemia unless iron-deficiency anemia is also present, peptic ulcer disease, regional enteritis, and ulcerative colitis. Use cautiously on long-term basis.

Interactions

Drug-drug. *Antacids, aluminum-containing phosphate binders, cholestyramine, cimetidine, vitamin E:* Decreased ferrous fumarate absorption. Separate doses by 1- to 2-hour intervals.
Chloramphenicol: Delayed response to iron therapy. Monitor patient carefully.
Doxycycline: May interfere with ferrous fumarate absorption even when doses are separated. Avoid use together.
L-thyroxine: May decrease L-thyroxine absorption. Separate doses by at least 2 hours. Monitor thyroid function.
Levodopa, methyldopa: May decrease absorption of these drugs. Monitor patient carefully.
Penicillamine: Decreased penicillamine absorption; separate doses by at least 2 hours.
Quinolones: Decreased quinolone absorption. Monitor patient closely.
Tetracycline: Inhibited absorption of both drugs; give tetracycline 3 hours after or 2 hours before iron supplement.
Vitamin C: Increased iron absorption. May be used as a beneficial drug interaction.
Drug-herb. *Black cohosh, chamomile, feverfew, gossypol, hawthorn, nettle, plantain, St.*

John's wort: Decreased iron absorption. Discourage concomitant use.
Drug-food. *Cereals, cheese, coffee, eggs, milk, tea, whole-grain breads, yogurt:* May impair oral iron absorption. Tell patient to avoid use together.

Adverse reactions
GI: *nausea,* epigastric pain, vomiting, *constipation,* diarrhea, black stools, anorexia.
Other: temporary staining of teeth (with suspension and drops).

Overdose and treatment
The lethal dose of iron is between 200 and 250 mg/kg; fatalities have occurred with lower doses. Signs and symptoms may follow ingestion of 20 to 60 mg/kg. Between 30 minutes and 8 hours after ingestion, patient may experience lethargy, nausea, vomiting, green and then tarry stools, weak and rapid pulse, hypotension, dehydration, acidosis, and coma. If death doesn't immediately ensue, symptoms may clear for about 24 hours. At 12 to 48 hours, symptoms may return, accompanied by diffuse vascular congestion, pulmonary edema, shock, seizures, anuria, and hyperthermia. Death may follow.

Treatment requires immediate support of airway, breathing, and circulation. In conscious patient with intact gag reflex, induce emesis with ipecac; otherwise, empty stomach by gastric lavage. Follow emesis with lavage, using a 1% sodium bicarbonate solution, to convert iron to the less irritating, poorly absorbed form (phosphate solutions have been used, but carry hazard of other adverse effects). X-ray abdomen to determine continued presence of excess iron; if serum iron levels exceed 350 mg/dl, deferoxamine may be used for systemic chelation.

Survivors are likely to sustain organ damage, including pyloric or antral stenosis, hepatic cirrhosis, CNS damage, and intestinal obstruction.

Special considerations
● Ferrous fumarate blackens feces and may interfere with tests for occult blood in the stool; the guaiac test and orthotoluidine test may yield false-positive results, but the benzidine test usually isn't affected.
● Iron overload may decrease uptake of technetium 99m and thus interfere with skeletal imaging.
● Drug may cause dark-colored stools.
● Drug may stain teeth.

Patient monitoring
● Monitor patient for adverse reactions and therapeutic effects.

Breast-feeding patients
● Iron supplements are commonly recommended for breast-feeding women; no adverse effects have been documented.

Pediatric patients
● Iron overdose may be fatal in children; treat immediately.

Geriatric patients
● Because iron-induced constipation is common in elderly patients, stress proper diet.

Patient education
● Instruct patient to take tablets with orange juice or water, but not with milk or antacids.
● Explain that patient may mix liquid forms in water or juice.
● Instruct patient not to crush or chew sustained-release forms.
● Tell patient to take suspension with straw to direct drops to back of throat.

ferrous gluconate
Apo-Ferrous Gluconate*, Fergon, Ferralet, Fertinic*, Novoferrogluc*, Simron

Pharmacologic classification: oral iron supplement
Therapeutic classification: hematinic
Pregnancy risk category: A

Indications and dosages
➤ *Iron deficiency. Adults:* 100 to 200 mg elemental iron P.O. t.i.d
Children ages 2 to 12: 3 mg/kg P.O. daily in three or four divided doses.
Children ages 6 months to 2 years: Up to 6 mg/kg P.O. daily in three or four divided doses.
Infants: 10 to 25 mg P.O. daily divided into three or four doses.
✦ *Dosage adjustment.* Elderly patients may need higher doses because reduced gastric secretions and achlorhydria may lower their capacity for iron absorption.

How supplied
Available without a prescription. Ferrous gluconate is 11.6% elemental iron.
Capsules: 86 mg (contains 10 mg Fe+), 325 mg (contains 38 mg Fe+)
Elixir: 300 mg/5 ml (contains 35 mg Fe+)
Tablets: 300 mg (contains 35 mg Fe+), 320 mg, 325 mg (320-mg tablet contains 37 mg Fe+)

Pharmacodynamics
Hematinic action: Ferrous gluconate replaces iron, an essential component in the formation of hemoglobin.

Pharmacokinetics
Absorption: Absorbed from the entire length of the GI tract, but primary absorption sites are the duodenum and proximal jejunum. Up to 10% of iron is absorbed by healthy individuals; patients with iron-deficiency anemia may absorb up to

60%. Food may decrease absorption by 33% to 50%.

Distribution: Transported through GI mucosal cells directly into the blood, where it is immediately bound to a carrier protein, transferrin, and transported to the bone marrow for incorporation into hemoglobin. Iron is highly protein-bound.

Metabolism: Liberated by the destruction of hemoglobin, but is conserved and reused by the body.

Excretion: Healthy people lose only small amounts of iron daily. Men and postmenopausal women lose about 1 mg/day, premenopausal women about 1.5 mg/day. Loss usually occurs in nails, hair, feces, and urine; trace amounts are lost in bile and sweat.

Route	Onset	Peak	Duration
P.O.	4 days	7-10 days	2-4 mo

Contraindications and precautions

Contraindicated in patients receiving repeated blood transfusions and those with peptic ulceration, regional enteritis, ulcerative colitis, hemosiderosis, primary hemochromatosis, or hemolytic anemia unless iron deficiency anemia is also present. Use cautiously on long-term basis.

Interactions

Drug-drug. *Antacids, aluminum-containing phosphate binders, cholestyramine, cimetidine, vitamin E:* Decreased ferrous fumarate absorption. Separate doses by 1- to 2-hour intervals.

Chloramphenicol: Delayed response to iron therapy. Monitor patient carefully.

Doxycycline: May interfere with ferrous fumarate absorption even when doses are separated. Avoid use together.

ʟ-thyroxine: May decrease ʟ-thyroxine absorption. Separate doses by at least 2 hours. Monitor thyroid function.

Levodopa, methyldopa: May decrease absorption of these drugs. Monitor patient carefully.

Penicillamine: Decreased penicillamine absorption. Separate doses by at least 2 hours.

Quinolones: May decrease quinolone absorption. Monitor patient closely.

Tetracycline: Inhibits absorption of both drugs; give tetracycline 3 hours after or 2 hours before iron supplement.

Vitamin C: Increased iron absorption. May be used as a beneficial drug interaction.

Drug-herb. *Black cohosh, chamomile, feverfew, gossypol, hawthorn, nettle, plantain, St John's wort.* Decreased iron absorption. Discourage concomitant use.

Drug-food. *Cereals, cheese, coffee, eggs, milk, tea, whole-grain breads, yogurt:* May impair oral iron absorption. Tell patient to avoid use together.

Adverse reactions

GI: *nausea,* epigastric pain, vomiting, *constipation,* diarrhea, *black stools,* anorexia.

Other: temporary staining of teeth (with elixir).

Overdose and treatment

The lethal dose of iron is between 200 and 250 mg/kg; fatalities have occurred with lower doses. Signs and symptoms may follow ingestion of 20 to 60 mg/kg. Between 30 minutes and 8 hours after ingestion, patient may experience lethargy, nausea, vomiting, green and then tarry stools, weak and rapid pulse, hypotension, dehydration, acidosis, and coma. If death doesn't immediately ensue, symptoms may clear for about 24 hours. At 12 to 48 hours, symptoms may return, accompanied by diffuse vascular congestion, pulmonary edema, shock, seizures, anuria, and hyperthermia. Death may follow.

Treatment requires immediate support of airway, breathing, and circulation. In conscious patient with intact gag reflex, induce emesis with ipecac; otherwise, empty stomach by gastric lavage. Follow emesis with lavage, using a 1% sodium bicarbonate solution, to convert iron to less irritating, poorly absorbed form (phosphate solutions have been used, but carry hazard of other adverse effects). Take abdominal X-ray to determine continued presence of excess iron; if serum iron levels exceed 350 mg/dl, deferoxamine may be used for systemic chelation.

Survivors are likely to sustain organ damage, including pyloric or antral stenosis, hepatic cirrhosis, CNS damage, and intestinal obstruction.

Special considerations

● Ferrous gluconate blackens feces and may interfere with test for occult blood in the stools; the guaiac test and orthotoluidine test may yield false-positive results, but the benzidine test is usually not affected.

● Iron overload may decrease uptake of technetium 99m and thus interfere with skeletal imaging.

● Drug can be given between meals or with some food, but absorption may be decreased.

Patient monitoring

● Monitor patient for adverse reactions and therapeutic effects.

Breast-feeding patients

● Iron supplements are commonly recommended for breast-feeding women; no adverse effects have been documented.

Pediatric patients

● Overdose may be fatal in children; treat immediately.

Geriatric patients

● Iron-induced constipation is common in elderly patients; stress proper diet.

Patient education
• To promote absorption, tell patient to take tablets with orange juice.

⚠ ALERT Inform parents that as few as three tablets can cause poisioning in children.

• Caution patient not to substitute one iron salt for another because the amounts of elemental iron vary.

---

ferrous sulfate
Apo-Ferrous Sulfate*, ED-IN-SOL, Feosol, Feratab, Fer-In-Sol, Fer-Iron, Fero-Grad-500*, Fero-Gradumet, Ferospace, Ferralyn Lanacaps, Ferra-TD, Mol-Iron, Novoferrosulfa*, PMS Ferrous Sulfate*, Slow FE

Pharmacologic classification: oral iron supplement
Therapeutic classification: hematinic
Pregnancy risk category: A

Indications and dosages
➤*Iron deficiency. Adults:* 100 to 200 mg elemental iron P.O. t.i.d . For extended-release capsules, 150 to 250 mg P.O. once or twice daily. For extended-release tablets, 160 to 525 mg once or twice daily.

Children ages 2 to 12: 3 mg/kg P.O. daily in three or four divided doses.

Children ages 6 months to 2 years: up to 6 mg/kg P.O. daily in three or four divided doses.

Infants: 10 to 25 mg/day P.O. in three or four divided doses.

✦ *Dosage adjustment.* Geriatric patients may need higher doses because reduced gastric secretions and achlorhydria may lower capacity for iron absorption.

How supplied
Available without a prescription. Ferrous sulfate is 20% elemental iron. Dried and powdered form (exsiccated), is about 30% elemental iron.
Capsules: 150 mg, 190 mg, 250 mg
Capsules (extended-release): 150 mg, 159 mg, 250 mg
Elixir: 220 mg/5 ml
Liquid: 75 mg/0.6 ml, 125 mg/ml
Syrup: 90 mg/5 ml
Tablets(exsiccated): 195 mg, 200 mg, 300 mg, 324 mg, 325 mg
Tablets (exsiccated, extended-release): 160 mg
Tablets (timed-release): 525 mg

Pharmacodynamics
Hematinic action: Ferrous sulfate replaces iron, an essential component in the formation of hemoglobin.

Pharmacokinetics
Absorption: Absorbed from the entire length of the GI tract, but primary absorption sites are the duodenum and proximal jejunum. Up to 10% of iron is absorbed by healthy individuals; patients with iron-deficiency anemia may absorb up to 60%. Enteric coating and some extended-release formulas have decreased absorption because they're designed to release iron past the points of highest absorption; food may decrease absorption by 33% to 50%.

Distribution: Transported through GI mucosal cells directly into the blood, where it's immediately bound to a carrier protein, transferrin, and transported to the bone marrow for incorporation into hemoglobin. Iron is highly protein-bound.

Metabolism: Liberated by the destruction of hemoglobin, but is conserved and reused by the body.

Excretion: Healthy people lose very little iron each day. Men and postmenopausal women lose about 1 mg/day, and premenopausal women about 1.5 mg/day. The loss usually occurs in nails, hair, feces, and urine; trace amounts are lost in bile and sweat.

Route	Onset	Peak	Duration
P.O.	4 days	7-10 days	2-4 mo

Contraindications and precautions
Contraindicated in patients receiving repeated blood transfusions and in those with hemosiderosis, primary hemochromatosis, hemolytic anemia unless iron deficiency anemia is also present, peptic ulceration, ulcerative colitis, or regional enteritis. Use cautiously on long-term basis.

Interactions
Drug-drug. *Antacids, aluminum-containing phosphate binders, cholestyramine, cimetidine, vitamin E:* Decreased ferrous fumarate absorption. Separate doses by 1- to 2-hour intervals.

Chloramphenicol: Delayed response to iron therapy. Monitor patient carefully.

Doxycycline: May interfere with ferrous fumarate absorption even when doses are separated. Avoid use together.

L-thyroxine: May decrease L-thyroxine absorption. Separate doses by at least 2 hours. Monitor thyroid function.

Levodopa, methyldopa: May decrease absorption of these drugs. Monitor patient carefully.

Penicillamine: Decreased penicillamine absorption. Separate doses by at least 2 hours.

Quinolones: Drug may decrease quinolone absorption. Monitor patient closely.

Tetracycline: Inhibits absorption of both drugs. Give tetracycline 3 hours after or 2 hours before iron supplement.

Vitamin C: Increased iron absorption. May be used as a beneficial drug interaction.

Drug-herb. *Black cohosh, chamomile, feverfew, gossypol, hawthorn, nettle, plantain, St.*

John's wort: Decreased iron absorption. Discourage concomitant use.

Drug-food. *Cereals, cheese, coffee, eggs, milk, tea, whole-grain breads, yogurt:* May impair oral iron absorption. Tell patient to avoid use together.

Adverse reactions
GI: *nausea,* epigastric pain, vomiting, *constipation, black stools,* diarrhea, anorexia.
Other: temporary staining of teeth (with liquid forms).

Overdose and treatment
The lethal dose of iron is 200 to 250 mg/kg; fatalities have occurred with lower doses. Signs and symptoms may follow ingestion of 20 to 60 mg/kg. Between 30 minutes and 8 hours after ingestion, patient may experience lethargy, nausea, vomiting, green and then tarry stools, weak and rapid pulse, hypotension, dehydration, acidosis, and coma. If death doesn't immediately ensue, symptoms may clear for about 24 hours. At 12 to 48 hours, symptoms may return, accompanied by diffuse vascular congestion, pulmonary edema, shock, seizures, anuria, and hyperthermia. Death may follow.

Treatment requires immediate support of airway, breathing, and circulation. In conscious patient with intact gag reflex, induce emesis with ipecac; otherwise, empty stomach by gastric lavage. Follow emesis with lavage, using a 1% sodium bicarbonate solution, to convert iron to less irritating, poorly absorbed form (phosphate solutions have been used, but carry hazard of other adverse effects). Take abdominal X-ray to determine continued presence of excess iron; if serum iron levels exceed 350 mg/dl, deferoxamine may be used for systemic chelation.

Survivors are likely to sustain organ damage, including pyloric or antral stenosis, hepatic cirrhosis, CNS damage, and intestinal obstruction.

Special considerations
● Drug may be taken with meals to minimize GI effects; maximum absorption will occur if drug is taken between meals.
● Ferrous sulfate blackens feces and may interfere with tests for occult blood in the stool; the guaiac test and orthotoluidine test may yield false-positive results, but the benzidine test is usually not affected.
● Iron overload may decrease uptake of technetium 99m and thus interfere with skeletal imaging.
● Drug may cause dark-colored stools.
● Drug may stain teeth.

Patient monitoring
● Monitor patient for adverse reactions and therapeutic effects.

Breast-feeding patients
● Iron supplements are commonly recommended for breast-feeding women; no adverse effects have been documented.

Pediatric patients
● Extended-release iron capsules or tablets usually aren't recommended for children. Overdose may be fatal; treat immediately.

Geriatric patients
● Iron-induced constipation is common in elderly patients; stress proper diet.

Patient education
● Instruct patient not to crush or chew extended-release forms.
● Explain that patient may mix liquid forms in water or juice and may drink through a straw.
● Inform parents that as few as three tablets can cause serious iron poisoning in children.

fexofenadine hydrochloride
Allegra

Pharmacologic classification: H₁-receptor antagonist
Therapeutic classification: antihistaminic
Pregnancy risk category: C

Indications and dosages
➤ **Seasonal allergic rhinitis.** *Adults and children age 12 and older:* 60 mg P.O. b.i.d. or 180 mg P.O. daily.
✦ **Dosage adjustment.** In patients with impaired renal function, 60 mg P.O. once daily.
Children ages 6 to 11: 30 mg P.O. b.i.d.
➤ **Chronic idiopathic urticaria.** *Adults and children age 12 and older:* 60 mg P.O. b.i.d.
✦ **Dosage adjustment.** In patients with impaired renal function, 60 mg P.O. once daily.
Children ages 6 to 11: 30 mg P.O. b.i.d.
✦ **Dosage adjustment.** In pediatric patients with impaired renal function, 30 mg P.O. once daily.

How supplied
Available by prescription only
Capsules: 60 mg
Tablets: 30 mg, 60 mg, 180 mg

Pharmacodynamics
Antihistaminic action: Principal effects of fexofenadine are mediated through selective inhibition of peripheral H₁ receptors.

Pharmacokinetics
Absorption: Rapidly absorbed.
Distribution: 60% to 70% bound to plasma protein.
Metabolism: About 5% of drug is metabolized.

Excretion: Mainly excreted in feces; less so in urine. Mean elimination half-life of drug is 14½ hours.

Route	Onset	Peak	Duration
P.O.	Unknown	3 hr	14 hr

Contraindications and precautions

Contraindicated in patients hypersensitive to drug or its components. Use cautiously in patients with impaired renal function.

Interactions

None reported.

Adverse reactions

CNS: fatigue, drowsiness.
GI: nausea, dyspepsia.
GU: dysmenorrhea.
Other: viral infection.

Overdose and treatment

Overdose of up to 800 mg doesn't cause significant adverse reactions. Treatment should be symptomatic and supportive. Fexofenadine isn't effectively removed by hemodialysis.

Special considerations

● No data exists to indicate a risk of abuse or dependency with fexofenadine.
● Drub may interfere with antigen skin-testing procedures. Discontinue drug 24 to 48 hours before test.

Patient monitoring

● Monitor patient for adverse reactions.

Pregnant patients

● Use drug only during pregnancy when potential benefit outweighs risk to fetus.

Breast-feeding patients

● It isn't known whether drug appears in breast milk. Use cautiously when administering drug to breast-feeding women.

Pediatric patients

● Safety and efficacy in children under age 6 haven't been established.

Patient education

● Caution patient not to perform hazardous activities if drug causes drowsiness.
● Instruct patient not to exceed prescribed dosage and to take drug only when needed.

filgrastim (granulocyte colony-stimulating factor, G-CSF)
Neupogen

Pharmacologic classification: hematopoietic agent
Therapeutic classification: colony-stimulating factor
Pregnancy risk category: C

Indications and dosages

➤ *To decrease occurrence of infection after chemotherapy for nonmyeloid malignancies, chronic severe neutropenia, and after bone marrow transplantation in cancer patients; to treat agranulocytosis, pancytopenia with colchicine overdose, acute leukemia myelodysplastic syndrome, and hematologic toxicity with zidovudine antiviral therapy.* *Adults:* Initially, 5 mcg/kg S.C. or I.V. as a single daily dose. May increase dose incrementally by 5 mcg/kg for each course of chemotherapy according to duration and severity of absolute neutrophil count (ANC) nadir.

Don't administer earlier than 24 hours after or within 24 hours before chemotherapy.

Give filgrastim daily for up to 2 weeks until ANC nadir reaches 10,000/mm³ after the anticipated chemoinduced ANC nadir. Duration of treatment depends on the myelosuppressive potential of the chemotherapy used. Discontinue if ANC nadir surpasses 10,000/mm³.
➤ *AIDS ◊. Adults:* 0.3 to 3.6 mcg/kg S.C. or I.V. daily.
➤ *Aplastic anemia ◊. Adults:* 800 to 1,200 mcg/m² S.C. or I.V. daily.
➤ *Hairy cell leukemia, myelodysplasia ◊. Adults:* 15 to 500 mcg/m² S.C. or I.V. daily.

How supplied

Available by prescription only
Injection: 300 mcg/ml in 1-ml and 1.6-ml single-dose vials

Pharmacodynamics

Immunostimulant action: Filgrastim is a naturally occurring cytokine glycoprotein that stimulates proliferation, differentiation, and functional activity of neutrophils, causing a rapid increase in WBC counts within 2 to 3 days in patients with normal bone marrow function or 7 to 14 days in patients with bone marrow suppression. Blood counts return to pretreatment levels, usually within 1 week after therapy ends.

Pharmacokinetics

Absorption: After S.C. bolus dose, blood levels suggest rapid absorption.
Distribution: Unknown.
Metabolism: Unknown.

Excretion: Elimination half-life is about 3½ hours.

Route	Onset	Peak	Duration
I.V.	5-60 min	24 hr	1-7 days
S.C.	5-60 min	2-8 hr	1-7 days

Contraindications and precautions
Contraindicated in patients hypersensitive to proteins derived from *Escherichia coli* or to drug or its components.

Interactions
Drug-drug. *Chemotherapy drugs:* May cause rapidly dividing myeloid cells to be sensitive to cytotoxic drugs. Don't give filgrastim within 24 hours before or after a chemotherapy drug.
Lithium: May potentiate myeloproliferative effects of filgrastim. Use cautiously in patients taking lithium.

Adverse reactions
CNS: headache, weakness, *fatigue*.
CV: *MI, arrhythmias,* chest pain, transient hypotension.
GI: *nausea, vomiting, diarrhea, mucositis,* stomatitis, constipation.
GU: increased serum creatinine levels.
Hematologic: *thrombocytopenia,* leukocytosis, transient increases in neutrophil levels.
Hepatic: elevated liver enzyme levels.
Metabolic: elevated uric acid levels.
Musculoskeletal: *skeletal pain.*
Respiratory: dyspnea, cough.
Skin: *alopecia,* rash, cutaneous vasculitis.
Other: *fever, hypersensitivity reactions.*

Overdose and treatment
Maximum tolerated dose hasn't been determined. Overdose hasn't been reported.

Special considerations
● Drug may interfere with antigen skin-testing procedures. Discontinue drug 24 to 48 hours before test.
● Store drug in refrigerator, but don't freeze it.
● Filgrastim isn't compatible with normal saline solution.

Patient monitoring
● Obtain CBC and platelet counts before and twice weekly during therapy.
● Regular monitoring of hematocrit and platelet counts is recommended.
● Adult respiratory distress syndrome may occur in septic patients because of the influx of neutrophils at the site of inflammation.
● MI and arrhythmias have occurred; if patient has a cardiac condition, watch closely.
● Bone pain is the most frequent adverse reaction and may be controlled with nonnarcotic analgesics if mild to moderate or may require narcotic analgesics if severe.

Breast-feeding patients
● It isn't known whether drug appears in breast milk. Risk-to-benefit ratio must be assessed.

Pediatric patients
● Efficacy hasn't been established, but there's no evidence of greater toxicity in children than in adults.

Geriatric patients
● No age-related problems have been reported.

Patient education
● Review package insert information with patient. Thorough instruction is essential if home use is prescribed.
● If patient has questions about insurance reimbursement, provide manufacturer's hotline number: 800-272-9376.

finasteride
Propecia, Proscar

Pharmacologic classification: steroid (synthetic 4-azasteroid) derivative
Therapeutic classification: androgen synthesis inhibitor
Pregnancy risk category: X

Indications and dosages
➤ *Symptomatic BPH.* Adult men: 5 mg P.O. daily, usually for 6 to 12 months.
➤ *Male pattern baldness (androgenetic alopecia).* Adult men: 1 mg P.O. daily, usually for 3 months or more. Continued use is recommended to sustain benefit. Withdrawal of treatment leads to reversal of effect within 12 months.

How supplied
Available by prescription only
Tablets: 1 mg, 5 mg

Pharmacodynamics
Androgen synthesis inhibition action: Finasteride competitively inhibits steroid 5α-reductase, an enzyme responsible for formation of the potent androgen 5α-dihydrotestosterone (DHT) from testosterone. Finasteride has a greater affinity for Type II 5α-reductase than Type I and lacks affinity for the androgen receptor. Because DHT influences development of the prostate gland, decreasing levels of this hormone in adult men should relieve the symptoms associated with BPH. In men with male pattern baldness, the balding scalp contains miniaturized hair follicles and increased amounts of DHT. Finasteride decreases scalp and serum DHT levels in these men.

Pharmacokinetics
Absorption: Average bioavailability of drug was 63% in one study.
Distribution: About 90% bound to plasma proteins. Drug crosses the blood-brain barrier.

Metabolism: Extensively metabolized by the liver; at least 2 metabolites have been identified. Metabolites are responsible for less than 20% of total activity of the drug.
Excretion: Part of oral dose (39%) is excreted in urine as metabolites; 57% is excreted in feces. No unchanged drug is found in urine.

Route	Onset	Peak	Duration
P.O.	Unknown	1-2 hr	Unknown

Contraindications and precautions
Contraindicated in patients hypersensitive to drug and in women (pregnant and not pregnant) and children.

Interactions
Drug-drug. *Theophylline:* Clinically insignificant increases in theophylline clearance and decreased half-life (10%). Use together cautiously.

Adverse reactions
GU: impotence, decreased ejaculate volume.
CV: nonbeneficial decreased prostate-specific antigen (PSA) serum levels.
Other: decreased libido.

Overdose and treatment
Experience with overdose is limited. Patients have received single doses of 400 mg and doses of up to 80 mg daily for 3 months without adverse effects.

Special considerations
● Closely evaluate patient for conditions that might mimic BPH before therapy, including hypotonic bladder, prostate cancer, infection, stricture, or other neurologic conditions.
◼ **ALERT** All women of childbearing age should avoid exposure to drug and semen of patient receiving this drug. Exposure to broken or crushed tablets or to semen of treated patient during pregnancy presents hazard to male fetus.
● Because it isn't possible to identify prospectively which patients will respond to finasteride, a minimum of 6 months of therapy may be necessary.
● Long-term effects of drug on the complications of BPH, including acute urinary obstruction or the need for surgery, aren't known.
● Current investigations aim to determine effectiveness of drug as adjuvant therapy after radical prostatectomy; as adjunctive treatment of prostate cancer; acne, and hirsutism.
● PSA levels are decreased by 50% in patients with BPH who are taking finasteride.

Patient monitoring
● Carefully monitor patients who have large residual urine volumes or severely diminished urine flows. Not all patients respond to drug, and these patients may not be candidates for finasteride therapy.
● Recommend carefully evaluating sustained increases in serum PSA. In patients receiving

finasteride therapy, this could indicate noncompliance to therapy.

Pregnant patients
● Not indicated for use in women; potential hazard to male fetus when pregnant women come in contact with broken or crushed tablet or semen of male patient receiving drug.

Breast-feeding patients
● It isn't known whether drug appears in breast milk; however, it isn't indicated for use in women.

Pediatric patients
● Drug isn't indicated for use in children.

Geriatric patients
● Although elimination of drug is decreased in elderly patients, dosage adjustments aren't necessary.

Patient education
● Advise patient that anyone who is or may become pregnant must not handle crushed tablets or have contact with patient's semen because of risk of adverse effects on a male fetus.
● Explain that drug may decrease the volume of ejaculate but doesn't appear to impair normal sexual function. However, impotence and decreased libido have occurred in less than 4% of patients treated with drug.

flavoxate hydrochloride
Urispas

Pharmacologic classification: flavone derivative
Therapeutic classification: urinary tract spasmolytic
Pregnancy risk category: B

Indications and dosages
➤ *Symptomatic relief of dysuria, frequency, urgency, nocturia, incontinence, and suprapubic pain from urologic disorders.* Adults and children over age 12: 100 to 200 mg P.O. t.i.d. or q.i.d.

How supplied
Available by prescription only
Tablets (film-coated): 100 mg

Pharmacodynamics
Spasmolytic action: Flavoxate exerts a direct spasmolytic effect on smooth muscle, primarily in the urinary tract. Acting on the detrusor muscle, this agent increases bladder capacity in patients with bladder spasticity; by cholinergic blockade, drug also has local anesthetic and analgesic effects.

Pharmacokinetics
Absorption: Drug is absorbed well from the GI tract; levels peak in about 2 hours.
Distribution: Unknown.
Metabolism: Unknown.
Excretion: Drug is excreted in urine; 10% to 30% appears in urine within 6 hours.

Route	Onset	Peak	Duration
P.O.	Unknown	2 hr	Unknown

Contraindications and precautions
Contraindicated in patients with pyloric or duodenal obstruction, obstructive intestinal lesions or ileus, achalasia, GI hemorrhage, or obstructive uropathies of lower urinary tract. Use cautiously in patients with or suspected of having glaucoma.

Interactions
Drug-drug. *CNS depressants:* Potentiated effects of these agents. Monitor patient closely.
Drug-lifestyle. *Exercise, hot weather:* Increased risk of heatstroke. Advise patient to take precautions.

Adverse reactions
CNS: *confusion,* nervousness, dizziness, headache, drowsiness.
CV: tachycardia, palpitations.
EENT: *blurred vision,* disturbed eye accommodation, increased ocular tension.
GI: dry mouth, nausea, vomiting.
GU: dysuria.
Hematologic: eosinophilia, *leukopenia.*
Skin: urticaria, dermatoses.
Other: fever.

Overdose and treatment
Signs and symptoms of overdose include clumsiness, dizziness, drowsiness, fever, flushing, hallucinations, shortness of breath, nervousness, restlessness, or irritability.

Treatment begins with gastric lavage or emesis and may include physostigmine rarely in cases of otherwise refractory life-threatening emergencies.

Special considerations
● Dosage may be reduced when symptoms improve.

Patient monitoring
● Check patient history for other drug use before giving drugs with anticholinergic adverse reactions. Such reactions may be intensified by flavoxate.
● Monitor patient for clinical effectiveness.
● Monitor patient for adverse effects.

Breast-feeding patients
● It isn't known whether drug appears in breast milk. Use cautiously in breast-feeding women.

Pediatric patients
● Safety hasn't been established in children under age 12.

Geriatric patients
● Warn family members that elderly patients are more likely to become confused.

Patient education
● Warn patient to avoid driving or other hazardous activities because of risk of drowsiness, blurred vision, and confusion.

---

flecainide acetate
Tambocor

Pharmacologic classification: benzamide derivative local anesthetic (amide)
Therapeutic classification: antiarrhythmic
Pregnancy risk category: C

Indications and dosages
➤ *Sustained ventricular tachycardia.* *Adults:* 100 mg P.O. q 12 hours. May increase in increments of 50 mg b.i.d. q 4 days until efficacy is achieved. Maximum dose is 400 mg daily.
➤ *Paroxysmal supraventricular tachycardia, paroxysmal atrial fibrillation or flutter in patients without structural heart disease.* *Adults:* 50 mg P.O. q 12 hours. May increase in increments of 50 mg b.i.d. q 4 days until efficacy is achieved. Maximum dose is 300 mg daily.
✦ *Dosage adjustment.* Reduce dosage in patients with renal impairment (creatinine clearance of less than 35 ml/minute) beginning at 100 mg/day (50 mg b.i.d.); increase dosage cautiously at intervals longer than 4 days. For patients with less severe renal impairment, initial dose is 100 mg q 12 hours, increasing cautiously at intervals longer than 4 days.

How supplied
Available by prescription only
Tablets: 50 mg, 100 mg, 150 mg

Pharmacodynamics
Antiarrhythmic action: A class IC antiarrhythmic, flecainide suppresses SA node automaticity and prolongs conduction in the atria, AV node, ventricles, accessory pathways, and His-Purkinje system. It has the most pronounced effect on the His-Purkinje system, as shown by QRS-complex widening; this leads to a prolonged QT interval. The drug has relatively little effect on action potential duration except in Purkinje's fibers, where it shortens it. A proarrhythmic (arrhythmogenic) effect may result from the potent effects of the drug on the conduction system. Effects on the sinus node are strongest in patients with sinus node disease (sick sinus syndrome). Flecainide also exerts a moderate negative inotropic effect.

Pharmacokinetics

Absorption: Rapidly and almost completely absorbed from the GI tract; bioavailability of commercially available tablets is 85% to 90%.

Distribution: Apparently well distributed throughout the body. Only about 40% binds to plasma proteins. Trough serum levels ranging from 0.2 to 1 mcg/ml provide the greatest therapeutic benefit. Trough serum levels higher than 0.7 to 1 mcg/ml have been associated with increased adverse effects.

Metabolism: Metabolized in the liver to inactive metabolites. About 30% of an orally administered dose escapes metabolism and is excreted in the urine unchanged.

Excretion: Elimination half-life averages about 20 hours. Plasma half-life may be prolonged in patients with heart failure and renal disease.

Route	Onset	Peak	Duration
P.O.	Immediate	1-6 hr	Unknown

Contraindications and precautions

Contraindicated in patients hypersensitive to drug and in those with cardiogenic shock, second- or third-degree AV block, or right bundle branch block with a left hemiblock (in the absence of an artificial pacemaker). Drug has proarrhythmic effects in patients with atrial fibrillation or flutter; therefore it isn't recommended for these patients.

Use cautiously in patients with heart failure, cardiomyopathy, severe renal or hepatic disease, prolonged QT interval, sick sinus syndrome, or blood dyscrasia.

Interactions

Drug-drug. *Acidifying and alkalizing agents:* Alkalization decreases renal flecainide excretion; acidification increases it. Monitor patient carefully.

Amiodarone, quinidine: May increase plasma flecainide levels. Monitor drug levels and patient for toxicity; dosage adjustment may be necessary.

Beta blockers: May cause additive negative inotropic effects. Monitor patient carefully.

Carbonic anhydrase inhibitors, high-dose antacids, sodium bicarbonate: Marked effect on urine acidity. Monitor patient for subtherapeutic or toxic levels and effects.

Cimetidine: May decrease renal and nonrenal flecainide clearance. Monitor patient carefully.

Digoxin: Increased serum digoxin levels. Monitor digoxin levels.

Disopyramide, verapamil: Negative inotropic effects. Don't give these drugs with flecainide unless risks outweigh benefits.

Drug-lifestyle. *Smoking:* May lower serum flecainide levels. Encourage patient to quit smoking.

Adverse reactions

CNS: *dizziness, headache,* fatigue, tremor, anxiety, insomnia, depression, malaise, paresthesia, ataxia, vertigo, *light-headedness, syncope,* asthenia.

CV: *new or worsened arrhythmias,* chest pain, flushing, edema, *heart failure, cardiac arrest,* palpitations.

EENT: *blurred vision and other visual disturbances.*

GI: nausea, constipation, abdominal pain, dyspepsia, vomiting, diarrhea, anorexia.

Respiratory: *dyspnea.*

Skin: rash.

Other: fever.

Overdose and treatment

Effects of overdose include increased PR and QT intervals, increased QRS complex duration, decreased myocardial contractility, conduction disturbances, and hypotension.

Treatment usually involves symptomatic and supportive measures along with ECG, blood pressure, and respiratory monitoring. Inotropic agents, including dopamine and dobutamine, may be used. Hemodynamic support, including use of an intra-aortic balloon pump and transvenous pacing, may be needed. Because of long half-life of drug, supportive measures may need to be continued for extended periods. Hemodialysis is ineffective in reducing serum drug levels.

Special considerations

⚡ ALERT Drug has been linked to excessive mortality or nonfatal cardiac arrest rate in national multi-center trials. Its use should be restricted to those patients in whom benefits outweigh risks.

• Tambocor is a strong negative inotrope and may cause or worsen heart failure, especially in those with cardiomyopathy, heart failure, or low ejection fraction.

• Hypokalemia or hyperkalemia may alter drug effects and should be corrected before giving drug.

• Therapy should begin in the hospital with careful monitoring of patient with symptomatic heart failure, sinus node dysfunction, sustained ventricular tachycardia, or underlying structural heart disease and in patient changing from another antiarrhythmic in whom discontinuation of current antiarrhythmic is likely to cause life-threatening arrhythmias.

• Loading doses may worsen arrhythmias and therefore aren't recommended. Dosage adjustments should be made at intervals of at least 4 days because of long half-life.

• Most patients can be maintained on an every-12-hour dosage schedule, but some need drug every 8 hours.

• Twice-daily dosing improves patient compliance.

• Full therapeutic effect of drug may take 3 to 5 days.

• Flecainide is a class IC antiarrhythmic. Adverse effects increase when trough serum levels exceed 0.7 mcg/ml. Periodically monitor blood levels, especially in patients with renal failure or heart

---

Reactions may be *common*, uncommon, *life-threatening*, or COMMON AND LIFE-THREATENING.

failure. Therapeutic levels range from 0.2 to 1 mcg/ml.

• Drug may increase acute and chronic endocardial pacing thresholds and may suppress ventricular escape rhythms. Determine pacing threshold before giving drug, after 1 week of therapy, and regularly thereafter. It shouldn't be given to patients with poor thresholds or nonprogrammable artificial pacemakers unless pacing rescue is available.

• In heart failure and myocardial dysfunction, initial dose shouldn't exceed 100 mg every 12 hours; common initial dose is 50 mg every 12 hours.

• Use in hepatic impairment hasn't been fully evaluated; however, because flecainide is metabolized extensively (probably in the liver), use it in patients with significant hepatic impairment only when benefits clearly outweigh risks. Dosage reduction may be necessary; monitor patient carefully for signs of toxicity. Serum levels also must be monitored.

Patient monitoring
• Monitor patient for signs of toxicity.
• Monitor patient's cardiac status.
• Monitor drug compliance.

Breast-feeding patients
• Limited data indicate that drug appears in breast milk. Breast-feeding isn't recommended during flecainide therapy because of the risk of adverse effects in infant.

Pediatric patients
• Safety and efficacy haven't been established in children under age 18. Limited data suggest usefulness in management of paroxysmal reentrant supraventricular tachycardia.

Geriatric patients
• Geriatric patients are more susceptible to adverse effects. Monitor patient carefully.

Patient education
• Advise patient to closely follow administration instruction.
• Warn patient of potential adverse drug effects.

---

floxuridine
FUDR

Pharmacologic classification: antimetabolite (specific to S phase of cell cycle)
Therapeutic classification: antineoplastic
Pregnancy risk category: D

Indications and dosages
Dosage and indications may vary. Check current literature for recommended protocol.

➤ *Palliative management of GI adenocarcinoma metastatic to the liver; cancer of the brain◇, head◇, neck◇, gall-*
bladder◇, or bile duct◇. Adults: 0.1 to 0.6 mg/kg daily by intra-arterial infusion; or 0.4 to 0.6 mg/kg daily into hepatic artery.

➤ *Solid tumors◇. Adults:* 0.5 to 1 mg/kg daily by I.V. infusion for 6 to 15 days or until toxicity occurs. Or, 30 mg/kg daily by single injection for 5 days; then 15 mg/kg every other day for up to 11 days or until toxicity occurs.

How supplied
Available by prescription only
Injection: 500-mg vials

Pharmacodynamics
Antineoplastic action: Floxuridine exerts its cytotoxic activity after conversion to its active form, by competitively inhibiting the enzyme thymidylate synthetase; this halts DNA synthesis and leads to cell death.

Pharmacokinetics
Absorption: Not administered orally.
Distribution: Crosses the blood-brain barrier to a limited extent.
Metabolism: Metabolized to fluorouracil in the liver after intra-arterial infusions and rapid I.V. injections.
Excretion: About 60% of a dose is excreted through the lungs as carbon dioxide. A small amount is excreted by the kidneys as unchanged drug and metabolites.

Route	Onset	Peak	Duration
Intra-arterial	Unknown	Unknown	Unknown

Contraindications and precautions
Contraindicated in patients with poor nutritional state, bone marrow suppression, or serious infection. Use in pregnancy only if the potential benefits justify the potential risk to the fetus.

Use cautiously in patients following high-dose pelvic radiation therapy or use of alkylating agents and in those with impaired renal or hepatic function.

Interactions
Drug-lifestyle. *Sun exposure:* May increase skin reaction. Advise patient to take precautions.

Adverse reactions
CNS: cerebellar ataxia, malaise, weakness, headache, lethargy, disorientation, confusion, euphoria.
CV: myocardial ischemia, angina.
EENT: blurred vision, nystagmus, photophobia, epistaxis.
GI: *anorexia, stomatitis, nausea, vomiting, diarrhea, bleeding, enteritis,* GI ulceration.
Hematologic: *leukopenia, anemia, thrombocytopenia, agranulocytosis.*
Hepatic: elevated liver enzymes levels, increased bilirubin levels, *drug-induced hepatotoxicity.*

Skin: *erythema*, dermatitis, pruritus, rash, alopecia, photosensitivity.
Other: thrombophlebitis, *anaphylaxis*, fever.

Overdose and treatment
Signs and symptoms of overdose include myelosuppression, diarrhea, alopecia, dermatitis, and hyperpigmentation.

Treatment is usually supportive and includes transfusion of blood components and antidiarrheal agents.

Special considerations
• Reconstituted solutions are stable for 14 days when refrigerated.
• Therapeutic effect may take 1 to 6 weeks.
• Drug is commonly given via hepatic arterial infusion for hepatic metastases.

Patient monitoring
• Discontinue drug if severe skin and GI adverse reactions occur.
• Monitor patient's intake and output, CBC, and renal and hepatic function.

Pregnant patients
• Women of childbearing age should avoid this drug to avoid toxicity to fetus. Use only when potential benefits to pregnant woman justify risks to fetus.

Breast-feeding patients
• It isn't known whether drug appears in breast milk. However, because of risk of serious adverse reactions, mutagenicity, and carcinogenicity in the infant, breast-feeding isn't recommended.

Patient education
• Advise patient to report nausea, vomiting, stomach pain, signs of infection, or unusual bruising or bleeding.

---

fluconazole
DiFlucan

Pharmacologic classification: bis-triazole derivative
Therapeutic classification: antifungal
Pregnancy risk category: C

Indications and dosages
➤ **Oropharyngeal and esophageal candidiasis.** *Adults:* 200 mg P.O. or I.V. on day 1 followed by 100 mg P.O. or I.V. once daily. As much as 400 mg daily has been used for esophageal disease. Continue for at least 2 weeks after symptoms resolve.
Children: 6 mg/kg on day 1, followed by 3 mg/kg for at least 2 weeks.
➤ **Systemic candidiasis.** *Adults:* Up to 400 mg P.O. or I.V. once daily. Continue for at least 2 weeks after symptoms resolve.
Children: 6 to 12 mg/kg/day I.V. or P.O.

➤ **Cryptococcal meningitis.** *Adults:* 400 mg I.V. or P.O. on day 1, followed by 200 mg once daily. Continue treatment for 10 to 12 weeks after CSF culture becomes negative. For suppression of relapse in patients with AIDS, give 200 mg once daily.
Children: 12 mg/kg I.V. or P.O. on the first day, followed by 6 mg/kg once daily for 10 to 12 weeks.
➤ **Vaginal candidiasis.** *Adults:* 150 mg P.O. as a single dose.
➤ **Urinary tract infection or peritonitis.** *Adults:* 50 to 200 mg P.O. or I.V. daily.
➤ **Prophylaxis in patients undergoing bone marrow transplantation.** *Adults:* 400 mg P.O. or I.V. daily for several days before transplantation and 7 days after neutrophil count rises above 1,000 cells/mm³.
➤ **Candidal infection, long-term suppression in patients with HIV infection.** *Adults:* 100 to 200 mg P.O. or I.V. daily.
➤ **Prophylaxis against mucocutaneous candidiasis, cryptococcosis, coccidioidomycosis, or histoplasmosis in patients with HIV infection** ◇. *Adults:* 200 to 400 mg P.O. or I.V. daily.
Children and infants: 2 to 8 mg/kg P.O. daily.
✦ **Dosage adjustment.** Patients with renal impairment should have their dosages adjusted based on this table:

Creatinine clearance (ml/min)	Percentage of usual adult dose
21-49	50
11-20	25

Patients receiving hemodialysis should receive one full dose after each session.

How supplied
Available by prescription only
Injection: 200 mg/100 ml, 400 mg/200 ml
Suspension: 10 mg/ ml, 40 mg/ml
Tablets: 50 mg, 100 mg, 150 mg, 200 mg

Pharmacodynamics
Antifungal action: Fluconazole exerts its fungistatic effects by inhibiting fungal cytochrome P-450. The spectrum of activity includes *Cryptococcus neoformans, Candida* (including systemic *C. albicans*), *Aspergillus flavus, Aspergillus fumigatus, Coccidioides immitis,* and *Histoplasma capsulatum.*

Pharmacokinetics
Absorption: After oral administration, absorption is rapid and complete.
Distribution: Well distributed to various sites, including CNS, saliva, sputum, blister fluid, urine, normal skin, nails, and blister skin. CNS levels of drug approach 50% to 90% of that of serum. Fluconazole is 12% protein-bound.

Metabolism: Fluconazole is primarily metabolized hepatically.
Elimination: Primarily excreted via the kidneys. More than 80% of an administered dose is excreted unchanged in the urine. Excretion rate diminishes as renal function decreases.

Route	Onset	Peak	Duration
P.O.	Unknown	1-2 hr	30 hr
I.V.	Immediate	Unknown	Unknown

Contraindications and precautions
Contraindicated in patients hypersensitive to drug and other drugs in same class.

Interactions
Drug-drug. *Amitriptyline, carbamazepine, I.V. midazolam:* Increased serum levels of these drugs. Monitor patient for increased adverse reactions or toxicity.
Cimetidine: Decreased fluconazole levels. Monitor patient carefully.
Cyclosporine: Increased cyclosporine levels. Monitor cyclosporine levels.
Glipizide, glyburide, sulfonylureas, tolbutamide: Increased hypoglycemic effects. Use together cautiously and monitor blood glucose.
Hydrochlorothiazide: Decreased fluconazole clearance and elevating serum levels. Use together cautiously.
Isoniazid, phenytoin, rifampin, sulfonylureas, valproic acid: Elevated hepatic transaminase levels. Monitor patient carefully.
Phenytoin: May significantly increase phenytoin levels. Monitor phenytoin levels.
Rifampin: Can lower fluconazole levels. Monitor patient for drug effects.
Tacrolimus: Increased tacrolimus levels. Monitor patient carefully.
Theophylline: Increased theophylline levels. Monitor theophylline levels.
Warfarin: Enhanced hypoprothrombinemic effects. Monitor PT and INR closely.
Zidovudine: Increased zidovine activity. Monitor patient carefully.
Drug-food. *Caffeine:* May increase caffeine levels. Advise avoiding caffeine.

Adverse reactions
CNS: headache.
GI: *nausea,* vomiting, abdominal pain, diarrhea.
Hepatic: *hepatotoxicity,* elevated liver enzyme levels.
Skin: rash, *Stevens-Johnson syndrome,* alopecia.
Other: *anaphylaxis.*

Overdose and treatment
Treatment is largely supportive.

Special considerations
● Adjust dose in those with renal dysfunction.
● Fluconazole isn't compatible with other I.V. drugs.

● Bioavailability of oral drug is comparable to I.V. dosing.
● Adverse reactions (including transaminase elevations) are more frequent and more severe in patients with severe underlying illness (including AIDS and malignancies).

Patient monitoring
● Monitor patient for anaphylaxis and other adverse reactions.

Pregnant patients
● Fluconazole shouldn't be given to pregnant HIV-infected women and should be discontinued if pregnancy occurs. Use in pregnancy only if potential benefits outweigh the risk to the fetus.

Breast-feeding patients
● Drug appears in breast milk at levels similar to those of plasma. Therefore, use in breast-feeding women isn't recommended.

Pediatric patients
● Safety and efficacy in children under age 6 months aren't established.

Patient education
● Warn patient of potential adverse reactions and urge patient to promptly report adverse drug events.

flucytosine (5-FC)
Ancobon

Pharmacologic classification: fluorinated pyrimidine
Therapeutic classification: antifungal
Pregnancy risk category: C

Indications and dosages
➤ **Severe fungal infections caused by susceptible strains of Candida and Cryptococcus.** *Adults:* 50 to 150 mg/kg daily P.O., administered in divided doses q 6 hours.
➤ **Chromomycosis ◇.** *Adults:* 150 mg/kg P.O. daily.
✦ **Dosage adjustment.** In patients with renal impairment who have a creatinine clearance of 50 ml/minute or less, reduce dosage by 20% to 80%. Or, increase the dosing interval as follows.

Creatinine clearance (ml/min)	Dosage interval (hr)
20-40	12
10-20	24
< 10	24-48

Monitor serum levels. Flucytosine is removed by hemodialysis and peritoneal dialysis. Dosage of 20 to 50 mg/kg P.O. immediately after hemodialysis q 2 to 3 days ensures therapeutic blood levels.

How supplied
Available by prescription only
Capsules: 250 mg, 500 mg

Pharmacodynamics
Antifungal action: Flucytosine penetrates fungal cells, where it's converted to fluorouracil, which interferes with pyrimidine metabolism; it also may be converted to fluorodeoxyuredylic acid, which interferes with DNA synthesis. Because human cells lack the enzymes needed to convert drug to these toxic metabolites, flucytosine is selectively toxic to fungal, not host cells. It's active against some strains of *Cryptococcus* and *Candida*.

Pharmacokinetics
Absorption: About 75% to 90% of an oral dose is absorbed. Food decreases absorption.
Distribution: Distributed widely into the liver, kidneys, spleen, heart, bronchial secretions, joints, peritoneal fluid, and aqueous humor. CSF levels vary from 60% to 100% of serum levels. It's 2% to 4% bound to plasma proteins.
Metabolism: Only small amounts are metabolized.
Excretion: About 75% to 95% of a dose is excreted unchanged in urine; less than 10% is excreted unchanged in feces. Serum half-life is 2½ to 6 hours with normal renal function; as long as 1,160 hours with creatinine clearance less than 2 ml/minute.

Route	Onset	Peak	Duration
P.O.	Unknown	2-6 hr	Unknown

Contraindications and precautions
Contraindicated in patients hypersensitive to drug. Use cautiously in patients with impaired renal or hepatic function and bone marrow suppression.

Interactions
Drug-drug. *Amphotericin B:* Synergistic effects and possible enhanced toxicity. Monitor patient carefully.
Drug-lifestyle. *Sun exposure:* Increased risk of photosensitivity reactions. Advise patient to take precautions.

Adverse reactions
CNS: headache, vertigo, sedation, fatigue, weakness, confusion, hallucinations, psychosis, ataxia, hearing loss, paresthesia, parkinsonism, peripheral neuropathy.
CV: *cardiac arrest, myocardial toxicity, ventricular dysfunction.*
GI: nausea, vomiting, diarrhea, abdominal pain, emesis, dry mouth, duodenal ulcer, *hemorrhage,* ulcerative colitis.
GU: azotemia, elevated creatinine and BUN levels, crystalluria, *renal failure.*

Hematologic: anemia, *leukopenia, bone marrow suppression, thrombocytopenia,* eosinophilia, *agranulocytosis, aplastic anemia.*
Hepatic: elevated liver enzyme levels, elevated serum alkaline phosphatase levels, jaundice.
Metabolic: hypoglycemia, hypokalemia.
Respiratory: *respiratory arrest,* chest pain, dyspnea.
Skin: occasional rash, pruritus, urticaria, photosensitivity, allergic reactions, *toxic epidermal necrolysis.*

Overdose and treatment
Flucytosine overdose may affect CV and pulmonary function.

Treatment is largely supportive. Induced emesis or lavage may be useful within 4 hours after ingestion. Activated charcoal and osmotic cathartics also may be helpful. Flucytosine is readily removed by either hemodialysis or peritoneal dialysis.

Special considerations
● Hematologic studies and renal and hepatic function studies should precede therapy and should be repeated frequently thereafter.
● Giving capsules over 15-minute period helps reduce nausea, vomiting, and GI distress.

Patient monitoring
● Monitor intake and output to ensure adequate renal function.
● Prolonged serum levels in excess of 100 mcg/ml may be related to toxicity; monitor serum levels, especially in patients with renal insufficiency.

Pregnant patients
● Use drug only when potential benefits justify risk to fetus.

Breast-feeding patients
● Safety hasn't been established in breast-feeding women.

Pediatric patients
● Safety and efficacy in children haven't been established.

Patient education
● Advise patient of adverse reactions and the need to report them.
● Tell patient to call prescriber promptly if urine output decreases or signs of bleeding or bruising occur.
● Explain that adequate response may take several weeks or months.
● Advise patient to adhere to medical regimen and to return as instructed for follow-up visits.

Reactions may be *common,* uncommon, *life-threatening,* or COMMON AND LIFE-THREATENING.

fludarabine phosphate
Fludara

Pharmacologic classification: antimetabolite
Therapeutic classification: antineoplastic
Pregnancy risk category: D

Indications and dosages
➤ **Treatment of B-cell chronic lymphocytic leukemia (CLL) in patients who
haven't responded or have responded inadequately to at least one standard alkylating agent regimen.** *Adults:* Usually,
25 mg/m² I.V. over 30 minutes (or by rapid I.V.
injection or continuous I.V. infusion ◊) for 5 consecutive days q 28 days. Therapy based on patient response and tolerance.
➤ **Mycosis fungoides, hairy-cell leukemia, Hodgkin's and malignant lympho-
ma** ◊. *Adults:* Usually, 18 to 30 mg/m² I.V. over
30 minutes (or by rapid I.V. injection or continuous I.V. infusion ◊) for 5 consecutive days q 28
days. Therapy based on patient response and tolerance.

How supplied
Available by prescription only
Injection: 50 mg as lyophilized powder

Pharmacodynamics
Antineoplastic action: After rapid conversion
of fludarabine to its active metabolite, the metabolite appears to inhibit DNA synthesis by inhibiting DNA polymerase alpha, ribonucleotide reductase, and DNA primase. The exact mechanism
of action isn't fully established.

Pharmacokinetics
Absorption: Administered I.V.
Distribution: Widely distributed with a volume
of distribution of 96 to 98 L/m² at steady state.
Metabolism: Rapidly dephosphorylated and then
phosphorylated intracellularly to its active metabolite.
Excretion: 23% is excreted in urine as unchanged active metabolite. Half-life is about 10
hours.

Route	Onset	Peak	Duration
I.V.	7-21 wk	Unknown	Unknown

Contraindications and precautions
Contraindicated in patients hypersensitive to drug
or its components. Use cautiously in patients with
renal insufficiency.

Interactions
Drug-drug. *Other myelosuppressive agents:*
Additive toxicity. Don't use with other myelosup-
presive agents.
Pentostatin: Increased risk of pulmonary tox-
icity. Avoid use together.

Adverse reactions
CNS: *fatigue, malaise, weakness, paresthesia,*
peripheral neuropathy, headache, sleep disorder, depression, cerebellar syndrome, **CVA,** agitation, *confusion,* **coma.**
CV: *edema,* angina, transient ischemic attack,
phlebitis, **arrhythmias, heart failure,**
supraventricular tachycardia, deep venous thrombosis, **aneurysm, hemorrhage.**
EENT: *visual disturbances,* hearing loss, delayed blindness (with high doses), sinusitis,
pharyngitis, epistaxis.
GI: *nausea, vomiting, diarrhea,* constipation,
anorexia, stomatitis, **GI bleeding,** esophagitis,
mucositis.
GU: dysuria, *urinary infection* or hesitancy, proteinuria, hematuria, **renal failure.**
Hematologic: hemolytic anemia, MYELO-
SUPPRESSION.
Hepatic: *liver failure,* cholelithiasis.
Metabolic: hypocalcemia, hyperkalemia, hyperglycemia, dehydration, hyperuricemia, hyperphosphatemia.
Musculoskeletal: *myalgia.*
Respiratory: *cough, pneumonia, dyspnea, upper respiratory tract infection,* allergic pneu-
monitis, hemoptysis, hypoxia, bronchitis.
Skin: alopecia, diaphoresis, *rash,* pruritus,
seborrhea.
Other: *fever, chills, infection, pain,* tumor ly-
sis syndrome, **anaphylaxis.**

Overdose and treatment
High doses may cause irreversible CNS toxicity
characterized by delayed blindness, coma, and
death. Severe thrombocytopenia and neutropenia secondary to bone marrow suppression also
occur.
    There's no specific antidote, and treatment
consists of discontinuing therapy and taking supportive measures.

Special considerations
● Drug has been used investigationally for treating malignant lymphoma, macroglobulinemic
lymphoma, prolymphocytic leukemia, prolym-
phocytoid variant of CLL, mycosis fungoides, hairy
cell leukemia, and Hodgkin's disease.
● Administer drug under the direct supervision
of clinician experienced in antineoplastic therapy.
● Tumor lysis syndrome (hyperuricemia, hyperphosphatemia, hypocalcemia, metabolic acidosis, hyperkalemia, hematuria, urate crystalluria,
and renal failure) has occurred in CLL patients
with large tumors.
● Severe neurologic effects, including blindness,
may occur when high doses are used to treat
acute leukemia.
● Advanced age, renal insufficiency, and bone
marrow impairment may predispose patient to
severe toxicity; toxic effects are dose-dependent.
● Optimal duration of therapy hasn't been established; three additional cycles after achieving

---

◊ Unlabeled clinical use

maximal response are recommended before discontinuing drug.

Patient monitoring
● Careful hematologic monitoring is required, especially of neutrophil and platelet counts.

Breast-feeding patients
● It isn't known whether drug appears in breast milk. Risk-benefit ratio must be determined.

Pediatric patients
● Safety and efficacy in children haven't been established.

Geriatric patients
● Advanced age may increase toxicity potential.

Patient education
● Tell patient to avoid contact with infected persons and report signs of infection or unusual bleeding immediately.

---

fludrocortisone acetate
Florinef

Pharmacologic classification: mineralocorticoid, glucocorticoid
Therapeutic classification: mineralocorticoid replacement therapy
Pregnancy risk category: C

Indications and dosages
➤ **Adrenal insufficiency (partial replacement), salt-losing adrenogenital syndrome.** *Adults:* 0.1 to 0.2 mg P.O. daily.
Children: 0.05 to 0.1 mg P.O. daily.
➤ **Orthostatic hypotension in diabetic patients** ◇. *Adults:* 0.1 to 0.4 mg P.O. daily.
➤ **Orthostatic hypotension from levodopa therapy** ◇. *Adults:* 0.05 to 0.2 mg P.O. daily.

How supplied
Available by prescription only
Tablets: 0.1 mg

Pharmacodynamics
Adrenal hormone replacement: Fludrocortisone, a synthetic glucocorticoid with potent mineralocorticoid activity, is used for partial replacement of steroid hormones in adrenocortical insufficiency and in salt-losing forms of congenital adrenogenital syndrome. In treating adrenocortical insufficiency, an exogenous glucocorticoid must also be administered for adequate control. (Cortisone or hydrocortisone are usually the drugs of choice for replacement because they produce both mineralocorticoid and glucocorticoid activity.) Fludrocortisone is administered on a variable schedule ranging from three times weekly to twice daily, depending on individual requirements.

Pharmacokinetics
Absorption: Absorbed readily from the GI tract.
Distribution: Removed rapidly from blood and distributed to muscle, liver, skin, intestines, and kidneys. It has a plasma half-life of about 3.5 hours. It's extensively bound to plasma proteins (transcortin and albumin). Only the unbound portion is active. Adrenocorticoids are distributed into breast milk and through the placenta.
Metabolism: Metabolized in the liver to inactive glucuronide and sulfate metabolites.
Excretion: Inactive metabolites and small amounts of unmetabolized drug are excreted by the kidneys. Insignificant quantities of drug are also excreted in feces. Biologic half-life is 18 to 36 hours.

Route	Onset	Peak	Duration
P.O.	Variable	2 hr	1-2 days

Contraindications and precautions
Contraindicated in patients hypersensitive to drug and those with systemic fungal infections.

Use cautiously in patients with hypothyroidism, cirrhosis, ocular herpes simplex, emotional nstability, psychotic tendencies, nonspecific ulcerative colitis, diverticulitis, fresh intestinal anastamoses, peptic ulcer, renal insufficiency, hypertension, osteoporosis, and myasthenia gravis.

Interactions
Drug-drug. *Amphotericin B, thiazide diuretics:* Concurrent use may enhance hypokalemia. Monitor electrolytes.
Barbiturates, phenytoin, rifampin: Decreased corticosteroid effects. Monitor patient carefully.
Cardiac glycosides: Increased risk of toxicity if hypokalemia occurs. Monitor patient closely.
Isoniazid, salicylates: Increased metabolism of these drugs. Monitor patient for drug effects.
Drug-food. *Sodium-containing drugs or foods:* May increase blood pressure. Sodium intake may need to be adjusted.

Adverse reactions
CV: *sodium and water retention,* hypertension, cardiac hypertrophy, edema, **heart failure**.
Metabolic: increased serum sodium levels, hypokalemia.
Skin: bruising, diaphoresis, urticaria, allergic rash.

Overdose and treatment
Acute toxicity occurs as an extension of the therapeutic effect, such as disturbances in fluid and electrolyte balance, hypokalemia, edema, hypertension, and cardiac insufficiency.

In acute toxicity, administer symptomatic treatment and correct fluid and electrolyte imbalance.

Special considerations
● Severe hypoglycemia tends to develop in addisonian patients within 3 hours of glucose tol-

---

erance tests. Perform only if necessary in these patients.

• Use only with other supplemental measures, such as glucocorticoids, control of electrolytes, and control of infection.

• Supplemental dosages may be required in times of physiologic stress from serious illness, trauma, or surgery.

Patient monitoring

• Monitor patient for significant weight gain, edema, hypertension, or severe headaches.

Pediatric patients

• Long-term use in children and adolescents may delay growth and maturation.

Patient education

• Teach patient to recognize signs of electrolyte imbalance: muscle weakness, paresthesia, numbness, fatigue, anorexia, nausea, altered mental status, increased urination, altered heart rhythm, severe or continuing headaches, unusual weight gain, or swelling of the feet.

• Tell patient to take missed doses as soon as possible, unless it's almost time for the next dose, and not to double the dose.

---

flumazenil
Romazicon

Pharmacologic classification: benzodiazepine antagonist
Therapeutic classification: antidote
Pregnancy risk category: C

Indications and dosages

➤ *Complete or partial reversal of sedative effects of benzodiazepines after anesthesia or short diagnostic procedures (conscious sedation).* *Adults:* Initially, 0.2 mg I.V. over 15 seconds. If patient doesn't reach desired level of consciousness after 45 seconds, repeat dose. Repeat at 1-minute intervals until a cumulative dose of 1 mg has been given (initial dose plus four additional doses). Most patients respond after 0.6 to 1 mg of drug. If resedation occurs, dose may be repeated after 20 minutes, but no more than 1 mg should be given at one time, and patient shouldn't receive more than 3 mg/hour.

➤ *Management of suspected benzodiazepine overdose.* *Adults:* Initially, 0.2 mg I.V. over 30 seconds. If patient doesn't reach desired level of consciousness after 30 seconds, administer 0.3 mg over 30 seconds. If patient still doesn't respond adequately, give 0.5 mg over 30 seconds, then repeat 0.5-mg doses at 1-minute intervals until a cumulative dose of 3 mg has been given. Most patients with benzodiazepine overdose respond to cumulative doses between 1 and 3 mg; rarely, patients who respond partially after 3 mg may require additional doses. Don't give more than 5 mg over 5 minutes initially; sedation that persists after this dose is unlikely to be caused by benzodiazepines. If resedation occurs, dose may be repeated after 20 minutes, but no more than 1 mg should be given at one time, and patient shouldn't receive more than 3 mg/hour.

How supplied

Available by prescription only
Injection: 0.1 mg/ml in 5-ml and 10-ml multiple-dose vials

Pharmacodynamics

Antidote action: Flumazenil competitively inhibits the actions of benzodiazepines on the gamma-aminobutyric acid–benzodiazepine receptor complex.

Pharmacokinetics

Absorption: Administered I.V.
Distribution: After administration, drug is redistributed rapidly (initial distribution half-life is 7 to 15 minutes). It's about 50% bound to plasma proteins.
Metabolism: Rapidly extracted from the blood and metabolized by the liver. Metabolites that have been identified are inactive. Ingestion of food during an I.V. infusion enhances extraction of drug from plasma, probably by increasing hepatic blood flow.
Excretion: About 90% to 95% is excreted in urine as metabolites; the remainder is excreted in feces. Plasma half-life is about 54 minutes.

Route	Onset	Peak	Duration
I.V.	1-2 min	6-10 min	Variable

Contraindications and precautions

Contraindicated in patients hypersensitive to drug or benzodiazepines, patients who show evidence of serious tricyclic antidepressant overdose, and patients who received a benzodiazepine to treat a potentially life-threatening condition such as status epilepticus or increased intracranial pressure.

Use cautiously in alcohol-dependent or psychiatric patients, in those at high risk for seizures, and in those with head injuries, signs of seizures, or recent high intake of benzodiazepines, such as patients in the intensive care unit.

Interactions

Drug-drug. *Antidepressants, drugs that can cause seizures or arrhythmias:* May cause seizures or arrhythmias after flumazenil removes the effects of the benzodiazepine overdose. Flumazenil shouldn't be used in mixed overdose, especially when seizures (from any cause) are likely to occur.
Drug-food. *Any food:* Ingestion of food during I.V. flumazenil infusion increases drug clearance by 50%. Be aware of this interaction.

Adverse reactions
CNS: *dizziness, abnormal or blurred vision, headache, seizures,* agitation, emotional lability, tremor, insomnia.
CV: *arrhythmias,* cutaneous vasodilation, palpitations.
GI: nausea, vomiting.
Respiratory: dyspnea, hyperventilation.
Skin: *diaphoresis.*
Other: *pain* at injection site.

Overdose and treatment
In clinical trials, large doses of flumazenil were administered I.V. to volunteers in the absence of a benzodiazepine agonist. No serious adverse reactions, clinical signs or symptoms, or altered laboratory tests were noted.

In patients with benzodiazepine overdose, large doses of flumazenil may produce agitation or anxiety, hyperesthesia, increased muscle tone, or seizures. Seizures may be treated with barbiturates, phenytoin, or benzodiazepines.

Special considerations
● Because flumazenil has a duration of action shorter than that of benzodiazepines, monitor patient carefully and administer additional drug as needed. Duration and degree of effect depend on plasma levels of the sedating benzodiazepine and the dose of flumazenil.
● Resedation may occur after reversal of benzodiazepine effect.
● Flumazenil can be given by direct injection or diluted with a compatible solution.

Patient monitoring
● Monitor patient for resedation according to duration of drug being reversed. Usually, serious resedation is unlikely in patient who fails to show signs of resedation 2 hours after a 1-mg dose of flumazenil.

Breast-feeding patients
● It isn't known whether drug appears in breast milk. Use cautiously in breast-feeding women.

Pediatric patients
● Because no clinical data exist regarding risks, benefits, or dosage range in children, manufacturer doesn't recommend its use.

Patient education
● Because of risk of resedation, advise patient to avoid hazardous activities (such as driving a car), alcohol, CNS depressants, and OTC drugs within 24 hours of the procedure.

---

flunisolide
Nasal inhalant
Nasalide, Nasarel

Oral inhalant
AeroBid, AeroBid-M

Pharmacologic classification: glucocorticoid
Therapeutic classification: anti-inflammatory, antiasthmatic
Pregnancy risk category: C

Indications and dosages
➤ *Corticosteroid-dependent asthma. Adults:* 2 inhalations b.i.d. for a total daily dose of 1 mg. Maximum, 8 inhalations (2 mg) daily.
Children age 6 and older: 2 inhalations b.i.d. Maximum, 4 inhalations daily.
➤ *Seasonal or perennial rhinitis. Adults:* 2 sprays (50 mcg) in each nostril b.i.d. (total dose 200 mcg daily). If needed, increase to 2 sprays in each nostril t.i.d. (total dose 300 mcg daily). Maximum, 8 sprays in each nostril daily (400 mcg daily).
Children ages 6 to 14: 1 spray (25 mcg) in each nostril t.i.d. or 2 sprays (50 mcg) in each nostril b.i.d. (total dose 150 to 200 mcg daily). Maximum dose is 4 sprays in each nostril daily (200 mcg/day).

How supplied
Available by prescription only
Nasal inhalant: 25 mcg/metered spray; 200 doses/bottle
Oral inhalant: 250 mcg/metered spray; at least 100 doses/inhaler

Pharmacodynamics
Anti-inflammatory action: Flunisolide stimulates synthesis of enzymes needed to decrease the inflammatory response. The anti-inflammatory and vasoconstrictor potency of topically applied flunisolide is several hundred times greater than that of hydrocortisone and about equal to that of an equal weight of triamcinolone; the metabolite, 6-beta-hydroxyflunisolide, has about three times the activity of hydrocortisone.
Antiasthmatic action: The nasal inhalant form is used in the symptomatic treatment of seasonal or perennial rhinitis. In patients who require corticosteroids to control symptoms, the oral inhalant form is used to treat bronchial asthma.

Pharmacokinetics
Absorption: About 50% of a nasally inhaled dose is absorbed systemically. After oral inhalation, about 40% of dose is absorbed from the lungs and GI tract; only about 20% of an orally inhaled dose reaches systemic circulation unmetabolized because of extensive metabolism in the liver. Onset of action usually occurs in a few days but may take as long as 4 weeks.

Reactions may be *common,* uncommon, *life-threatening,* or COMMON AND LIFE-THREATENING.

Distribution: Distribution following intranasal administration or oral inhalation hasn't been described. No evidence exists of tissue storage of flunisolide or its metabolites.

Metabolism: When swallowed, undergoes rapid metabolism in the liver or GI tract to several metabolites, one of which has glucocorticoid activity. Flunisolide and its 6-beta-hydroxy metabolite are eventually conjugated in the liver, by glucuronic acid or surface sulfate, to inactive metabolites.

Excretion: Excretion pathway is unknown when drug is given as inhalant; however, when it's given systemically, metabolites are excreted in roughly equal portions in feces and urine. Biologic half-life of drug averages about 2 hours.

Route	Onset	Peak	Duration
Inhalation	Variable	10-30 min	Unknown

Contraindications and precautions

Contraindicated in patients hypersensitive to drug. Nasal inhalant is contraindicated in the presence of untreated localized infection involving nasal mucosa. Oral inhalant shouldn't be used by patients with status asthmaticus or respiratory infections.

Use nasal inhalant cautiously in patients with tuberculosis; untreated fungal, bacterial, or systemic viral or ocular herpes simplex infections; or septal ulcers, trauma, or surgery in the nasal region. Oral inhalant isn't recommended for patients with asthma controlled by bronchodilators or other noncorticosteroids alone or patients with nonasthma bronchial diseases.

Interactions

None reported.

Adverse reactions

CNS: headache with nasal inhalant; dizziness, irritability, and nervousness with oral inhalant.
CV: chest pain, edema with oral inhalant.
EENT: nasopharyngeal fungal infection; *mild, transient nasal burning and stinging;* stinging, dryness, sneezing, epistaxis, and watery eyes with nasal inhalant.
GI: nausea and vomiting with nasal inhalant; dry mouth, abdominal pain, decreased appetite, *nausea, vomiting, diarrhea, and upset stomach* with oral inhalant.
Respiratory: *upper respiratory tract infection* with oral inhalant.
Skin: rash, pruritus with oral inhalant.
Other: *cold symptoms, flu,* fever with oral inhalant.

Overdose and treatment

No information available.

Special considerations

• Recommendations for use of flunisolide and for care and teaching of the patient during ther-

apy are the same as those for all inhalant adrenocorticoids.

Patient monitoring
• Monitor patient for adverse reactions.
• Monitor patient for development of oral fungal infections.

Pregnant patients
• Use drug during pregnancy only if potential benefits justify risk to fetus.

Breast-feeding patients
• Use drug cautiously in breast-feeding patients.

Pediatric patients
• Safety and efficacy haven't been established in children under age 6 months.

Patient education
• Inform patient that drug doesn't relieve emergency asthma attacks.
• Advise patient of proper administration method.

fluocinonide
Fluocinonide-E Emollient Cream, Lidemol*, Lidex, Lidex-E, Lyderm*

Pharmacologic classification: topical adrenocorticoid
Therapeutic classification: anti-inflammatory
Pregnancy risk category: C

Indications and dosages
➤ **Inflammation from corticosteroid-responsive dermatoses.** *Adults and children:* Apply sparingly b.i.d. or t.i.d. Occlusive dressings may be used for severe or resistant dermatoses.

How supplied
Available by prescription only
Cream, gel, ointment, solution: 0.05%

Pharmacodynamics
Anti-inflammatory action: Fluocinonide stimulates synthesis of enzymes needed to decrease the inflammatory response. Fluocinonide is a high-potency fluorinated glucocorticoid categorized as a group II topical corticosteroid.

Pharmacokinetics
Absorption: Amount absorbed depends on amount applied and on nature of skin at application site. It ranges from about 1% in areas of thick stratum corneum (such as the palms, soles, elbows, and knees) to as high as 36% in areas of thin stratum corneum (face, eyelids, and genitals). Absorption increases in areas of skin damage, inflammation, or occlusion. Some systemic absorption of corticosteroids occurs, especially through the oral mucosa.

◊ Unlabeled clinical use

Distribution: After topical application, is distributed throughout the local skin. Any drug absorbed into circulation is removed rapidly from the blood and distributed into muscle, liver, skin, intestines, and kidneys.

Metabolism: After topical administration, is metabolized primarily in the skin. The small amount absorbed into systemic circulation is metabolized primarily in the liver to inactive compounds.

Excretion: Inactive metabolites are excreted by the kidneys, primarily as glucuronides and sulfates, but also as unconjugated products. Small amounts of metabolites are excreted in feces.

Route	Onset	Peak	Duration
Topical	Unknown	Unknown	Unknown

Contraindications and precautions

Contraindicated in patients hypersensitive to drug. Also contraindicated as monotherapy in bacterial infections such as impetigo or cellulites. Contraindicated for use on the face, groin, or axilla.

Interactions

None significant.

Adverse reactions

Metabolic: hyperglycemia, glucosuria.

Skin: burning; pruritus; irritation; dryness; erythema; folliculitis; hypertrichosis; hypopigmentation; acneiform eruptions; perioral dermatitis; allergic contact dermatitis; *maceration, secondary infection, atrophy, striae, and miliaria* with occlusive dressings.

Other: *hypothalamic-pituitary-adrenal axis suppression,* Cushing's syndrome.

Overdose and treatment

No information available.

Special considerations

• Gently wash skin before applying. To prevent skin damage, rub in gently, leaving a thin coat. When treating hairy sites, part hair and apply directly to lesion.

• Avoid applying near eyes or mucous membranes, or in ear canal.

• For patients with eczematous dermatitis whose skin may be irritated by adhesive material, hold dressing in place with gauze, elastic bandages, stockings, or stockinette.

• If an occlusive dressing has been applied and a fever develops, remove dressing.

• If antifungals or antibiotics are used concurrently, stop drug until infection is controlled.

• Avoid using plastic pants or tight-fitting diapers on treated areas in young children. Children may absorb larger amounts of drug and be more prone to systemic toxicity.

• Continue treatment for a few days after lesions clear.

⚕ ALERT Don't confuse fluocinolone with fluocinonide.

Patient monitoring

• Monitor patient for skin infection, striae, and atrophy. Discontinue drug if they occur.

• Systemic absorption is likely with use of occlusive dressings, prolonged treatment, or extensive body surface treatment. Watch for symptoms.

Patient education

• Teach patient and family how to apply drug using gloves, sterile applicator, or careful hand washing.

• If an occlusive dressing is used, advise patient to leave in place no more than 12 hours each day and not to use occlusive dressings on infected or exudative lesions.

• Tell patient to stop drug and report signs of systemic absorption, skin irritation or ulceration, hypersensitivity, or infection.

fluorometholone

Eflone, Flarex, Fluor-Op, FML Forte, FML Liquifilm, FML S.O.P., FML-S Liquifilm

Pharmacologic classification: corticosteroid
Therapeutic classification: ophthalmic anti-inflammatory
Pregnancy risk category: C

Indications and dosages

➤ *Inflammatory and allergic conditions of cornea, conjunctiva, sclera, anterior uvea.* *Adults and children:* In severe cases, instill 2 drops of suspension in conjunctival sac q 1 to 2 hours or ½" ointment q 4 hours during the first 1 to 2 days of therapy. In mild to moderate cases, 1 to 2 drops of suspension may be used b.i.d. to q.i.d. or ½" ointment daily to t.i.d.

How supplied

Available by prescription only
Ophthalmic ointment: 0.1%
Ophthalmic suspension: 0.1%, 0.25%

Pharmacodynamics

Anti-inflammatory action: Fluorometholone stimulates synthesis of enzymes needed to decrease the inflammatory response. Fluorometholone is a synthetic fluorinated corticosteroid that is less likely than hydrocortisone, prednisolone, or dexamethasone to cause intraocular hypertension.

Pharmacokinetics

Absorption: After ophthalmic administration, drug is absorbed mainly into the aqueous humor. Slight systemic absorption typically occurs.

Distribution: Drug is distributed throughout the local tissue layers. Any drug absorbed into circulation is removed rapidly from the blood and distributed into muscle, skin, intestines, and kidneys.

Metabolism: Drug is primarily metabolized locally. The small amount absorbed into systemic circulation is metabolized primarily in liver to inactive compounds.

Excretion: Inactive metabolites are excreted by the kidneys, primarily as glucuronides and sulfates, but also as unconjugated products. Small amounts of the metabolites are also excreted in the feces.

Route	Onset	Peak	Duration
Oph-thalmic	Unknown	Unknown	Unknown

Contraindications and precautions

Contraindicated in patients with vaccinia, varicella, acute superficial herpes simplex (dendritic keratitis), or other fungal or viral eye diseases; ocular tuberculosis; or any acute, purulent, untreated eye infection.

Use cautiously in patients with corneal abrasions that may be contaminated (especially with herpes).

Interactions

None reported.

Adverse reactions

EENT: increased intraocular pressure, thinning of cornea, interference with corneal wound healing, corneal ulceration, increased susceptibility to viral or fungal corneal infections; with excessive or long-term use, glaucoma exacerbation, discharge, discomfort, ocular pain, foreign body sensation, cataracts, decreased visual acuity, diminished visual field, optic nerve damage.

Other: systemic effects and adrenal suppression in excessive or long-term use.

Overdose and treatment

No information available.

Special considerations

● Drug is less likely to cause increased intraocular pressure with long-term use than other ophthalmic anti-inflammatory drugs (except medrysone).
● In chronic conditions, withdraw treatment by gradually decreasing frequency of applications.
● Shake well before use.

Patient monitoring

● Monitor patient for clinical effect.
● Duration of treatment may range from a few days to several weeks; however, long-term use should be avoided. Monitor intraocular pressure.

Pediatric patients

● Safety and efficacy in children under age 2 haven't been established.

Patient education

● Teach patient how to instill drops or apply ointment. Advise him to wash hands before and af-

ter application, and warn him not to touch tip of applicator to eye or surrounding tissue.
● Advise patient to apply light finger pressure on lacrimal sac for 1 minute after instillation.
● Warn patient not to use leftover drug for new eye inflammation; it may cause serious problems.
● Instruct patient to consult prescriber if no improvement occurs after 2 days. Warn against stopping treatment prematurely.

---

fluorouracil (5-FU)
Adrucil, Efudex, Fluoroplex

Pharmacologic classification: antimetabolite (specific to S phase of cell cycle)
Therapeutic classification: antineoplastic
Pregnancy risk category: D (injection), X (topical)

Indications and dosages

Dosage and indications may vary. Check current literature for recommended protocol.
➤ *Palliative management of colon, rectal, breast, gastric, pancreatic, ovarian* ◇, *cervical* ◇, *bladder* ◇, *and liver* ◇ *cancers.*
Adults and children: 12 mg/kg I.V. for 4 days. Then, if no toxicity occurs, give 6 mg/kg I.V. on days 6, 8, 10, and 12. Maintenance therapy is a repeated course q 30 days. Don't exceed 800 mg daily (400 mg daily in severely ill patients).
➤ *Actinic or solar keratoses. Adults:* Sufficient cream or lotion to cover lesions b.i.d. for 2 to 4 weeks. Usually, 1% preparations are used on head, neck, and chest, 2% and 5% on hands.
➤ *Superficial basal cell carcinomas.*
Adults: 5% solution or cream in a sufficient amount to cover lesion b.i.d. for 3 to 6 weeks, up to 12 weeks.

How supplied

Available by prescription only
Cream: 1%, 5%
Injection: 50 mg/ml in 10-ml, 20-ml, 50-ml, 100-ml vials
Topical solution: 1%, 2%, 5%

Pharmacodynamics

Antineoplastic action: Fluorouracil exerts cytotoxic activity by acting as an antimetabolite, competing for the enzyme that's important in the synthesis of thymidine, an essential substrate for DNA synthesis. Therefore, DNA synthesis is inhibited. Drug also inhibits RNA synthesis to a lesser extent.

Pharmacokinetics

Absorption: Given parenterally because it's absorbed poorly after oral administration.
Distribution: Distributes widely into all areas of body water and tissues, including tumors, bone marrow, liver, and intestinal mucosa. Fluorouracil crosses the blood-brain barrier to a significant extent.

◇ Unlabeled clinical use

Metabolism: A small amount is converted in the tissues to the active metabolite, with most of drug degraded in the liver.

Excretion: Metabolites are primarily excreted through the lungs as carbon dioxide. A small portion of a dose is excreted in urine as unchanged drug.

Route	Onset	Peak	Duration
I.V., topical	Unknown	Unknown	Unknown

Contraindications and precautions

Contraindicated in patients hypersensitive to drug, patients who are in a poor nutritional state, patients with bone marrow suppression (WBC counts of 5,000/mm³ or less or platelet counts of 100,000/ mm³ or less), patients with potentially serious infections, and patients who have had major surgery within the previous month. Topical 5-FU should be avoided during pregnancy.

Use cautiously in patients who have had high-dose pelvic radiation therapy or have received alkylating agents. Also use cautiously in patients with widespread neoplastic infiltration of bone marrow and impaired renal or hepatic function.

Interactions

Drug-drug. *Leucovorin calcium, previous treatment with alkylating drugs:* May enhance toxicity. Use extremely cautiously.

Drug-lifestyle. *Sun exposure:* May cause photosensitivity reactions. Advise patient to take precautions.

Adverse reactions

CNS: acute cerebellar syndrome, confusion, disorientation, euphoria, ataxia, headache, *weakness, malaise.*

CV: *myocardial ischemia*, angina.

EENT: nystagmus.

GI: *stomatitis, GI ulcer* (may precede leukopenia), *nausea, vomiting, diarrhea, anorexia,* GI bleeding.

Hematologic: leukopenia, thrombocytopenia, agranulocytosis, anemia.

Metabolic: hypoalbuminemia because of drug-induced protein malabsorption.

Skin: *reversible alopecia, dermatitis, erythema, scaling, pruritus,* nail changes, pigmented palmar creases, erythematous contact dermatitis, desquamative rash of hands and feet with long-term use ("hand-foot syndrome").

Other: *pain, burning,* soreness, suppuration, swelling (with topical use), *anaphylaxis,* thrombophlebitis.

Overdose and treatment

Signs and symptoms of overdose include myelosuppression, diarrhea, alopecia, dermatitis, hyperpigmentation, nausea, and vomiting.

Treatment is usually supportive and includes transfusion of blood components, antiemetics, and antidiarrheals.

Special considerations

• Drug may be administered I.V. push over 1 to 2 minutes.

• Drug may be further diluted in D_5W or normal saline solution for infusions up to 24 hours in duration.

• Solution is more stable in plastic I.V. bags than in glass bottles.

• Don't refrigerate fluorouracil.

• Drug can be diluted in 120 ml of water and administered orally; however, this isn't an FDA-approved method of administration, and absorption is erratic.

• Topical application to larger ulcerated areas may cause systemic toxicity.

Patient monitoring

• WBC count nadir occurs 9 to 14 days after first dose; platelet count nadir occurs in 7 to 14 days.

• General photosensitivity occurs for 2 to 3 months after a dose.

• Monitor intake and output, CBC, and renal and hepatic function.

Pregnant patients

• During pregnancy, use drug only for life-threatening or serious situations when no other safe alternatives are available.

Breast-feeding patients

• It isn't known whether drug appears in breast milk. However, because of potential for serious adverse reactions, mutagenicity, and carcinogenicity in the infant, breast-feeding isn't recommended.

Pediatric patients

• Safety and efficacy in children haven't been established.

Patient education

• Warn patient to avoid strong sunlight or ultraviolet light because it will intensify the skin reaction. Encourage use of sunscreens.

• Tell patient to avoid exposure to people with infections. Advise patient to promptly report signs of infection or unusual bleeding.

• Reassure patient that hair should grow back after treatment is discontinued.

• Advise patient to apply topical fluorouracil with gloves and wash hands thoroughly after application.

• Warn patient that treated area may be unsightly during therapy and for several weeks after therapy is stopped. Complete healing may not occur until 1 or 2 months after treatment is stopped.

Reactions may be *common,* uncommon, *life-threatening,* or COMMON AND LIFE-THREATENING.

fluoxetine
Prozac, Prozac Pulvules, Sarafem

Pharmacologic classification: selective serotonin reuptake inhibitor
Therapeutic classification: antidepressant
Pregnancy risk category: C

Indications and dosages
➤ *Depression, panic disorder ◇, bipolar disorder ◇, alcohol dependence ◇, cataplexy ◇, myoclonus ◇. Adults:* (Prozac) 20 mg P.O. daily in the morning. Increase dosage, p.r.n., after several weeks to 40 mg daily with a dose morning and midday. Don't exceed 80 mg daily.
➤ *Obsessive-compulsive disorder. Adults:* (Prozac) Initially, 20 mg P.O. daily. Gradually increase dosage after several weeks as needed and tolerated to 60 to 80 mg daily.
➤ *Bulimia nervosa. Adults:* (Prozac) 60 P.O. daily in the morning.
➤ *Premenstrual dysphoric disorder (PMDD). Adults:* (Sarafem) 20 mg P.O. daily. Maximum dose is 80 mg P.O. daily.

How supplied
Available by prescription only
Capsules: 10 mg, 20 mg (Prozac and Sarafem), 40 mg (Prozac)
Oral solution: 20 mg/5 ml
Tablets: 10 mg

Pharmacodynamics
Antidepressant action: The antidepressant action of fluoxetine is purportedly related to its inhibition of CNS neuronal uptake of serotonin. Fluoxetine blocks uptake of serotonin, but not of norepinephrine, into human platelets. Animal studies suggest that it's a much more potent uptake inhibitor of serotonin than of norepinephrine.

Pharmacokinetics
Absorption: Well absorbed after oral administration. Absorption isn't altered by food.
Distribution: Apparently highly protein-bound (about 95%).
Metabolism: Metabolized primarily in the liver to active metabolites.
Excretion: Excreted by the kidneys. Elimination half-life is 2 to 3 days. Norfluoxetine (the primary active metabolite) has an elimination half-life of 7 to 9 days.

Route	Onset	Peak	Duration
P.O.	Unknown	6-8 hr	Unknown

Contraindications and precautions
Contraindicated in patients hypersensitive to drug and in patients who took an MAO inhibitor within 14 days of starting therapy. MAO inhibitors and thioridazine shouldn't be given with fluoxetine or within 5 weeks after fluoxetine has been discontinued. Use cautiously in patients at high risk of suicide or in those with a history of seizures, diabetes mellitus, or renal, hepatic, or CV disease.

Interactions
Drug-drug. *Benzodiazepines (such as alprazolam), lithium, tricyclic antidepressants:* Increased adverse CNS effects. Increased tricyclic antidepressant and lithium levels. Monitor patient closely for adverse effects and toxicity. Dosage adjustments may be necessary.
Carbamazepine, flecainide, vinblastine: Increased serum levels of these drugs. Monitor serum levels and the patient for adverse effects.
Cyproheptadine: May reverse or decrease fluoxetine effects. Monitor patient closely.
Insulin, oral antidiabetics: Altered blood glucose levels. May alter requirements for antidiabetic medication.
Phenytoin: Increased phenytoin levels and risk of toxicity. Monitor phenytoin levels; dosage adjustment may be needed.
Tryptophan: Increased adverse CNS effects (agitation, restlessness) and GI distress. Use cautiously.
Warfarin: Increased risk of bleeding. Monitor PT and INR.
Warfarin and other highly protein-bound drugs: Increased levels of fluoxetine or other highly protein-bound drugs. Monitor patient closely.
Drug-herb. *St. John's wort:* Increased risk of serotonin syndrome. Discourage concomitant use.
Drug-lifestyle. *Alcohol use:* May increase CNS depression. Advise patient to avoid alcohol.

Adverse reactions
CNS: *nervousness, anxiety, insomnia, headache, drowsiness, tremor, dizziness, asthenia,* fatigue.
CV: palpitations, hot flashes.
EENT: nasal congestion, pharyngitis, sinusitis.
GI: *nausea, diarrhea, dry mouth, anorexia, dyspepsia,* constipation, abdominal pain, vomiting, flatulence, increased appetite.
GU: sexual dysfunction.
Metabolic: *weight loss,* SIADH.
Musculoskeletal: muscle pain.
Respiratory: cough, upper respiratory infection, respiratory distress.
Skin: *rash, pruritus,* diaphoresis.
Other: flu syndrome, fever.

Overdose and treatment
Signs and symptoms of overdose include agitation, restlessness, hypomania, other signs of CNS excitation and, in patients who took higher doses of fluoxetine, nausea and vomiting.

To treat fluoxetine overdose, establish and maintain an airway; ensure adequate oxygenation and ventilation. Activated charcoal, which may be used with sorbitol, may be as effective as emesis or lavage. Monitor cardiac and vital signs, and provide usual supportive measures. Fluoxetine-

---

◇ Unlabeled clinical use

induced seizures that don't subside spontaneously may respond to diazepam. Forced diuresis, dialysis, hemoperfusion, and exchange transfusion are unlikely to be of benefit.

Special considerations
● Consider the patient to have a risk of suicide until depressive state improves considerably. Supervise high-risk patients closely during early therapy. To reduce risk of intentional overdose, give the smallest quantity of pulvules consistent with good management.
● Full antidepressant effect may take 4 weeks or longer.
● Treatment of acute depression usually requires at least several months of continuous drug therapy; optimal duration of therapy hasn't been established.
● Because of its long elimination half-life, changes in fluoxetine dosage won't be reflected in plasma for several weeks, affecting titration to final dose and withdrawal from treatment.
● Fluoxetine therapy may activate mania or hypomania.
● Prescribe lower or less frequent doses in patients with renal or hepatic impairment. Consider lower or less frequent dosages in elderly patients and others with concurrent disease or multiple drug therapy.

Patient monitoring
● Monitor patient closely for improvement of depressive state and decreased risk of suicide.
● If patient takes Sarafem for PMDD, reevaluate patient for long-term effectiveness of therapy. Clinical effectiveness hasn't been studied beyond 6 months.

Pregnant patients
● Avoid using drug during pregnancy. Because of its long half-life, patient planning to become pregnant should consult prescriber to ascertain when risk to fetus has passed.

Breast-feeding patients
● Drug appears in breast milk and shouldn't be used by breast-feeding patients.

Pediatric patients
● Safety and efficacy in children haven't been established.

Geriatric patients
● No overall differences in safety and efficacy were observed in elderly patients; however, elderly patients may have increased sensitivity to drug.

Patient education
● Inform patient that drug may cause dizziness or drowsiness. Advise patient to avoid hazardous tasks that require alertness until CNS response to drug is established.

● Caution patient to avoid ingestion of alcohol and to seek medical approval before taking other drugs.
● Tell patient to promptly report rash or hives, anxiety, nervousness, anorexia (especially if underweight), suspicion of pregnancy, or intent to become pregnant.

fluoxymesterone
Halotestin

Pharmacologic classification: androgen
Therapeutic classification: androgen replacement, antineoplastic
Controlled substance schedule: III
Pregnancy risk category: X

Indications and dosages
➤ *Male hypogonadism. Adults:* 5 to 20 mg P.O. daily in a single dose or in three or four divided doses.
➤ *Palliation of breast cancer in women. Adults:* 10 to 40 mg P.O. daily in three or four divided doses.
➤ *Postpartum breast engorgement. Adults:* 2.5 mg P.O. shortly after parturition; then 5 to 10 mg daily for 4 to 5 days in divided doses.
➤ *Vasomotor symptoms related to menopause. Adults:* 1 to 2 mg P.O. b.i.d. combined with ethinyl estradiol 0.02 or 0.04 mg P.O. b.i.d. for 21 days; then 7 days without drug. Repeat regimen when necessary.
➤ *Delayed puberty. Males:* 2.5 to 20 mg daily. Most patients respond to dosages of 2.5 to 10 mg daily.

How supplied
Available by prescription only
Tablets: 2 mg, 5 mg, 10 mg

Pharmacodynamics
Androgenic action: Mimics action of the endogenous androgen testosterone by stimulating receptors in androgen-responsive organs and tissues. Exerts inhibitory, antiestrogenic effects on hormone-responsive breast tumors and metastases.
Antianemic action: Enhances production of erythropoietic stimulating factors, thereby increasing production of RBCs.

Pharmacokinetics
Absorption: No information available.
Distribution: No information available.
Metabolism: Eliminated primarily by hepatic metabolism.
Excretion: No information available.

Route	Onset	Peak	Duration
P.O.	Unknown	Unknown	9 hr

Contraindications and precautions

Contraindicated in pregnant patients, breast-feeding women, patients hypersensitive to drug, men with breast cancer or prostate cancer, and patients with cardiac, hepatic, or renal decompensation

Use cautiously in prepubertal boys and patients with benign prostatic hyperplasia or aspirin sensitivity.

Interactions

Drug-drug. *Anticoagulants:* Concomitant use may potentiate action. Monitor INR.

Hepatotoxic drugs: May increase risk of hepatotoxicity. Monitor patient closely.

Insulin, oral antidiabetics: Decreased blood glucose levels may need dosage adjustment. Monitor serum glucose levels.

Adverse reactions

CNS: headache, anxiety, depression, paresthesia, sleep apnea syndrome.

CV: edema.

GI: nausea.

Hematologic: polycythemia, elevated serum lipid levels, suppression of clotting factors, prolonged PT and INR.

Hepatic: reversible jaundice, peliosis, *cholestatic hepatitis,* elevated liver enzyme levels, *liver cell tumors.*

Metabolic: elevated serum sodium, potassium, calcium, phosphate, and cholesterol levels.

Skin: *hypersensitivity skin manifestations.*

Other: *hypoestrogenic effects in women* (flushing; diaphoresis; vaginitis, including itching, dryness, and burning; vaginal bleeding; nervousness; emotional lability; menstrual irregularities); excessive hormonal effects in men (prepubertal—*premature epiphyseal closure, acne,* priapism, *growth of body and facial hair,* phallic enlargement; postpubertal—testicular atrophy, oligospermia, decreased ejaculatory volume, impotence, gynecomastia, epididymitis), androgenic effects in women (acne, edema, weight gain, hirsutism, hoarseness, clitoral enlargement, deepening voice, decreased breast size, changes in libido, male-pattern baldness, oily skin or hair).

Overdose and treatment

No information available.

Special considerations

Consider the recommendations relevant to all androgens as well as the following.

• Observe women carefully for signs of excessive virilization. If possible, stop drug at first sign of virilization because some adverse effects (deepening of voice, clitoral enlargement) aren't reversible.

• Patients with metastatic breast cancer should have regular determinations of serum calcium levels to identify potential for serious hypercalcemia.

• When drug is used in breast cancer, subjective effects may not appear for about 1 month; objective improvement not for 3 months.

• Drug contains tartrazine. Watch for signs of allergic reactions in patients sensitive to aspirin or tartrazine.

• Women with an intact uterus receiving ethinyl estradiol must be monitored closely for endometrial carcinoma. Rule out malignancy if recurrent vaginal bleeding occurs.

• Fluoxymesterone may cause abnormal results of glucose tolerance test. Thyroid function test results (protein-bound iodine ^{131}I uptake, thyroid-binding capacity) may decrease.

Patient monitoring

• Monitor hepatic function and serum calcium level before therapy starts and periodically during therapy.

• Monitor serum blood glucose level if patient takes oral antidiabetics.

• Monitor serum coagulation studies if patient takes oral anticoagulants.

• In children, monitor X-rays frequently to evaluate closure of epiphyses.

Breast-feeding patients

• It isn't known whether drug appears in breast milk. Because of potential adverse effects in infant, a decision should be made to stop either breast-feeding or drug, depending on patient's need for drug.

Pediatric patients

• Use with extreme caution in children to avoid precocious puberty and premature closure of epiphyses. X-ray examinations every 6 months are recommended to assess skeletal maturation.

Geriatric patients

• Use cautiously. Observe elderly men for prostatic hyperplasia. Development of symptomatic prostatic hyperplasia or prostatic cancer requires stopping drug.

Patient education

• Explain to patient taking drug for palliation of breast cancer that virilization usually occurs at dosage used. Tell patient to report androgenic effects immediately. Stopping drug will prevent further androgenic changes but probably won't reverse those already present.

• Tell woman to report menstrual irregularities and to stop therapy pending etiologic determination.

• Advise man to report overly frequent or persistent penile erections.

• Advise patient to report persistent GI distress, diarrhea, or onset of jaundice.

fluphenazine decanoate
Modecate*, Prolixin Decanoate

fluphenazine enanthate
Moditen Enanthate*, Prolixin
Enanthate

fluphenazine hydrochloride
Permitil, Prolixin

Pharmacologic classification: phenothiazine
(piperazine derivative)
Therapeutic classification: antipsychotic
Pregnancy risk category: C

Indications and dosages
➤ *Psychotic disorders.* *Adults:* Initially, 0.5 to
10 mg fluphenazine hydrochloride P.O. daily in
divided doses q 6 to 8 hours; may increase cautiously to 20 mg. Maintenance dosage is 1 to 5 mg
P.O. daily. I.M. doses are one-third to one-half
that of oral doses; the usual starting dose is
1.25 mg I.M. The initial total daily dose is 2.5 to
10 mg divided and given every 6 to 8 hours. For
the enanthate and decanoate formulations, 12.5 to
25 mg I.M. q. 3 to 6 weeks.
✦ *Dosage adjustment.* Use lower doses for
geriatric patients (1 to 2.5 mg P.O. daily).

How supplied
Available by prescription only
fluphenazine decanoate
Depot injection: 25 mg/ml
fluphenazine enanthate
Depot injection: 25 mg/ml
fluphenazine hydrochloride
Elixir: 2.5 mg/5 ml (with 14% alcohol)
I.M. injection: 2.5 mg/ml
Oral concentrate: 5 mg/ml (Prolixin contains
14% alcohol and Permitil contains 1% alcohol)
Tablets: 1 mg, 2.5 mg, 5 mg, 10 mg

Pharmacodynamics
Antipsychotic action: Fluphenazine is thought
to exert antipsychotic effects by postsynaptic
blockade of CNS dopamine receptors, thereby inhibiting dopamine-mediated effects.

Fluphenazine has many other central and peripheral effects; it produces both alpha and ganglionic blockade and counteracts histamine- and
serotonin-mediated activity. Its most prominent
adverse reactions are extrapyramidal.

Pharmacokinetics
Absorption: Rate and extent of absorption vary
with route of administration; oral tablet absorption is erratic and variable.
Distribution: Distributed widely into the body,
including breast milk. CNS levels of drug are usually higher than those in plasma. Drug is 91% to
99% protein-bound.

Metabolism: Metabolized extensively by the
liver, but no active metabolites are formed;
duration of action is about 6 to 8 hours after oral
administration; 1 to 6 weeks (average, 2 weeks)
after I.M. depot administration.
Excretion: Mostly excreted in urine via the kidneys; some is excreted in feces via the biliary
tract.

Route	Onset	Peak	Duration
P.O.	< 1 hr	½ hr	6-8 hr
I.M. (HCl)	< 1hr	1½-2 hr	6-8 hr
I.M.	24-72 hr	Unknown	1-6 wk
S.C.	Unknown	Unknown	Unknown

Contraindications and precautions
Contraindicated in patients hypersensitive to drug
and patients experiencing coma, CNS depression,
bone marrow suppression, other blood dyscrasia, subcortical damage, or liver damage.

Use cautiously in elderly or debilitated patients and in those with pheochromocytoma,
severe CV disease, peptic ulcer disease, exposure to extreme hot or cold (including antipyretic
therapy), exposure to phosphorus insecticides,
respiratory or seizure disorders, hypocalcemia,
severe reaction to insulin or electroconvulsive
therapy, mitral insufficiency, glaucoma, or prostatic hyperplasia. Use parenteral form cautiously in patients with asthma and those allergic to
sulfites.

Interactions
Drug-drug. *Aluminum- and magnesium-
containing antacids and antidiarrheals:* Decreased absorption. Monitor patient.
*Antiarrhythmics, disopyramide, procainamide,
quinidine:* Increased risk of arrhythmias and
conduction defects. Avoid use together.
*Anticholinergics, including antidepressants,
antihistamines, antiparkinsonians, atropine,
MAO inhibitors, meperidine, phenothiazines:*
Oversedation, paralytic ileus, visual changes, and
severe constipation. Avoid use together.
Beta blockers: Increased plasma levels and toxicity. Monitor patient closely.
Bromocriptine: Antagonized therapeutic effect
of bromocriptine on prolactin secretion. Monitor patient for drug effect.
*Centrally acting antihypertensives, such as
clonidine, guanabenz, guanadrel, guanethidine, methyldopa, and reserpine:* Inhibition
of blood pressure response. Monitor patient
closely.
*CNS depressants, including analgesics, barbi-
turates, narcotics, parenteral magnesium sulfate, tranquilizers, and general, spinal, or
epidural anesthetics:* Additive effects of oversedation, respiratory depression, and hypotension
are likely. Avoid use together.
Dopamine: Decreased vasoconstricting effects.
Monitor patient carefully.

Reactions may be *common*, uncommon, *life-threatening*, or COMMON AND LIFE-THREATENING.

Levodopa: Decreased effectiveness and increased toxicity of levodopa. Monitor patient carefully.

Lithium: May result in severe neurologic toxicity with an encephalitis-like syndrome and a decreased therapeutic response to fluphenazine. Monitor patient closely.

Metrizamide: Increased risk of seizures. Observe patient closely.

Nitrates: May result in hypotension. Check blood pressure frequently.

Phenobarbital: Enhanced renal excretion. Monitor patient closely.

Phenytoin, tricyclic antidepressants: Inhibited metabolism and increased toxicity of these drugs. Monitor patient closely.

Propylthiouracil: Increased risk of agranulocytosis. Monitor patient carefully.

Sympathomimetics including ephedrine, epinephrine, and phenylephrine (common in nasal sprays) and appetite suppressants: Decreased stimulatory and pressor effects of these drugs. Use together cautiously.

Drug-food. *Caffeine:* Increased fluphenazine metabolism. Advise patient to avoid caffeine.

Drug-lifestyle. *Alcohol use:* May increase CNS depression. Advise patient not to drink alcohol.

Smoking: Increased fluphenazine metabolism. Advise patient to avoid smoking.

Sun exposure: Increased risk of photosensitivity. Advise patient to take precautions.

Adverse reactions

CNS: *extrapyramidal reactions, tardive dyskinesia, sedation, pseudoparkinsonism, EEG changes, drowsiness, seizures,* dizziness.

CV: *orthostatic hypotension,* tachycardia, ECG changes.

EENT: ocular changes, *blurred vision,* nasal congestion.

GI: *dry mouth, constipation.*

GU: *urine retention,* dark urine, menstrual irregularities, inhibited ejaculation.

Hematologic: *leukopenia, agranulocytosis,* eosinophilia, hemolytic anemia, *aplastic anemia, thrombocytopenia.*

Hepatic: cholestatic jaundice, abnormal liver function test results.

Metabolic: elevated protein-bound iodine level, weight gain, increased appetite.

Skin: mild photosensitivity, allergic reactions.

Other: gynecomastia, *neuroleptic malignant syndrome.*

Overdose and treatment

CNS depression is characterized by deep, unarousable sleep and possible coma, hypotension or hypertension, extrapyramidal symptoms, dystonia, abnormal involuntary muscle movements, agitation, seizures, arrhythmias, ECG changes, hypothermia or hyperthermia, and autonomic nervous system dysfunction.

Treatment is symptomatic and supportive, including maintaining vital signs, airway, stable body temperature, and fluid and electrolyte balance. Don't induce vomiting: Drug inhibits cough reflex, and aspiration may occur. Use gastric lavage and then activated charcoal and saline cathartics; dialysis doesn't help. Regulate body temperature as needed. Treat hypotension with I.V. fluids. Don't give epinephrine. Treat seizures with parenteral diazepam or barbiturates, arrhythmias with parenteral phenytoin (1 mg/kg with rate adjusted to blood pressure), and extrapyramidal reactions with benztropine 1 to 2 mg or parenteral diphenhydramine at 10 to 50 mg.

Special considerations

● Fluphenazine causes false-positive test results for urinary porphyrins, urobilinogen, amylase, and 5-hydroxyindoleacetic acid, because of darkening of urine by metabolites; it also causes false-positive urine pregnancy test results using human chorionic gonadotropin.

● Fluphenazine elevates test results for liver enzymes and causes quinidine-like ECG effects.

● Depot injection (25 mg/ml) and I.M. injection (2.5 mg/ml) aren't interchangeable.

● Depot injection isn't recommended for patients who aren't stabilized on a phenothiazine. This form has a prolonged elimination; its action couldn't be terminated in case of adverse reactions.

● After abrupt withdrawal of long-term therapy, patient may experience gastritis, nausea, vomiting, dizziness, tremor, feeling of warmth or cold, diaphoresis, tachycardia, headache, or insomnia.

Patient monitoring

● Recommendations are the same as for all phenothiazines.

Pregnant patients

● Recommendations are the same as for all phenothiazines.

Breast-feeding patients

● Drug appears in breast milk. Use cautiously; potential benefits to the woman should outweigh the potential harm to the infant.

Pediatric patients

● Safety and efficacy in children under age 12 haven't been established.

Geriatric patients

● Recommendations are the same as for all phenothiazines.

Patient education

● Inform patient that drug may cause dizziness or drowsiness. Advise patient to avoid hazardous tasks that require alertness until CNS response to drug is established.

● Tell patient to avoid ingestion of alcohol and to seek medical approval before taking other drugs.

● Instruct patient to promptly report rash or hives, anxiety, nervousness, anorexia (especially in underweight patients), suspicion of pregnancy, or intent to become pregnant.

flurandrenolide
Cordran, Cordran SP, Drenison*

Pharmacologic classification: topical adreno-corticoid
Therapeutic classification: anti-inflammatory
Pregnancy risk category: C

Indications and dosages
➤ *Inflammation from corticosteroid-responsive dermatoses. Adults and children:* Apply cream, lotion, or ointment sparingly daily to q.i.d. Apply tape q 12 hours.

How supplied
Available by prescription only
Cream: 0.025%, 0.05%
Lotion: 0.05%
Ointment: 0.025%, 0.05%
Tape: 4 mcg/cm^2

Pharmacodynamics
Anti-inflammatory action: Stimulates synthesis of enzymes needed to decrease the inflammatory response. A group III (0.05%, 0.025%) fluorinated glucocorticoid.

Pharmacokinetics
Absorption: Amount absorbed depends on strength of preparation, amount applied, and nature and condition of skin at application site. Ranges from about 1% in areas with thick stratum corneum (such as palms, soles, elbows, and knees) to as high as 36% in areas of thinnest stratum corneum (face, eyelids, and genitals). Absorption increases in areas of skin damage, inflammation, or occlusion. Some systemic absorption may occur, especially through oral mucosa.
Distribution: After topical application, distributed throughout local skin. Any drug absorbed into circulation is removed rapidly from blood and distributed into muscle, liver, skin, intestines, and kidneys.
Metabolism: After topical administration, metabolized primarily in skin. Small amount absorbed into systemic circulation metabolized primarily in liver to inactive compounds.
Excretion: Inactive metabolites excreted by kidneys, primarily as glucuronides and sulfates, but also as unconjugated products. Small amounts of metabolites also excreted in feces.

Route	Onset	Peak	Duration
Topical	Unknown	Unknown	Unknown

Contraindications and precautions
Contraindicated in patients hypersensitive to drug.

Interactions
None reported.

Adverse reactions
Metabolic: hyperglycemia, glucosuria, *hypothalamic-pituitary-adrenal axis suppression,* Cushing's syndrome.
Skin: burning; pruritus; irritation; dryness; erythema; folliculitis; hypertrichosis; hypopigmentation; acneiform eruptions; allergic contact dermatitis; *maceration, secondary infection, atrophy, striae, and miliaria with occlusive dressings;* purpura, stripping of epidermis, and furunculosis with tape.

Overdose and treatment
No information available.

Special considerations
● Gently wash skin before applying. To prevent skin damage, rub in gently, leaving a thin coat. When treating hairy sites, part hair and apply directly to lesions.
⚠ **ALERT** Don't use tape for exudative lesions or lesions in intertriginous areas.
● Occlusive dressings may be used for severe or resistant dermatoses. The tape is usually applied as an occlusive dressing to clean, dry, affected areas.
● Don't tear Cordran tape; cut it with scissors. Make sure skin is dry for 1 hour before applying tape.
● Replace tape every 12 hours or, if well tolerated and adherence is satisfactory, every 24 hours.
● For patients with eczematous dermatitis whose skin may be irritated by adhesive material, hold dressings in place with gauze, elastic bandages, stockings, or stockinette.
● Treatment should be continued for a few days after lesions clear.

Patient monitoring
● Monitor patient for fever; remove occlusive dressing if fever develops.
● Monitor patient for adverse effects; stop drug if patient develops skin infection, striae, or atrophy.
● Watch for signs of systemic absorption, which is likely with use of occlusive dressings, prolonged treatment, or extensive body surface treatment.

Pediatric patients
● Avoid using plastic pants or tight-fitting diapers on treated areas in young children. Children may absorb larger amounts of drug and be more prone to systemic toxicity.

Patient education
● Teach patient and family how to apply drug.
● Instruct patient not to leave occlusive dressing in place for more than 12 hours each day.
● Tell patient to report signs of systemic absorption, skin irritation, hypersensitivity, or infection.

Reactions may be *common*, uncommon, *life-threatening*, or COMMON AND LIFE-THREATENING.

flurazepam hydrochloride
Apo-Flurazepam*, Dalmane, Novoflupam*

Pharmacologic classification: benzodiazepine
Therapeutic classification: sedative-hypnotic
Controlled substance schedule: IV
Pregnancy risk category: X

Indications and dosages
➤ *Insomnia. Adults:* 15 to 30 mg P.O. h.s.
✦ *Dosage adjustment.* In patients over age 65, 15 mg P.O. h.s.

How supplied
Available by prescription only
Capsules: 15 mg, 30 mg

Pharmacodynamics
Sedative action: Flurazepam depresses the CNS at the limbic and subcortical levels of the brain. It produces a sedative effect by potentiating the effect of the neurotransmitter gamma-aminobutyric acid on its receptor in the ascending reticular activating system, which increases inhibition and blocks both cortical and limbic arousal.

Pharmacokinetics
Absorption: When administered orally, flurazepam is absorbed rapidly through the GI tract.
Distribution: Distributed widely throughout the body. About 97% of administered dose is bound to plasma protein.
Metabolism: Metabolized in the liver to the active metabolite desalkylflurazepam.
Excretion: Desalkylflurazepam is excreted in urine; half-life is 50 to 100 hours.

Route	Onset	Peak	Duration
P.O.	< 20 min	1-2 hr	7-10 hr

Contraindications and precautions
Contraindicated in pregnant patients and patients hypersensitive to drug.

Use cautiously in patients with impaired renal or hepatic function, chronic pulmonary insufficiency, mental depression, suicidal tendencies, or history of drug abuse.

Interactions
Drug-drug. *Antidepressants, antihistamines, barbiturates, general anesthetics, MAO inhibitors, narcotics, phenothiazines:* Increased CNS depressant effects of these drugs. Use together cautiously.
Cimetidine, disulfiram, isoniazid, oral contraceptives, ritonavir: May decrease benzodiazepine metabolism, leading to toxicity. Monitor patient carefully.
Digoxin: Serum levels may increase, resulting in toxicity. Monitor patient closely.
Levodopa: Decreased levodopa effect. Monitor patient for drug effects.

Phenytoin: Increased phenytoin levels. Monitoring phenytoin levels.
Rifampin: Enhanced benzodiazepine metabolism. Monitor patient closely.
Theophylline: May act as an antagonist with flurazepam. Monitor patient closely.
Drug-lifestyle. *Alcohol use:* Excessive CNS and respiratory depression. Advise patient to avoid alcohol.
Heavy smoking: Accelerates flurazepam metabolism. Monitor patient for drug effect.

Adverse reactions
CNS: *daytime sedation, dizziness, drowsiness, disturbed coordination,* lethargy, confusion, *headache,* light-headedness, nervousness, hallucinations, staggering, ataxia, disorientation, changes in EEG patterns, *coma.*
GI: nausea, vomiting, heartburn, diarrhea, abdominal pain.
Hepatic: elevated liver enzyme levels.
Other: physical or psychological dependence.

Overdose and treatment
Signs and symptoms of overdose include somnolence, confusion, hypoactive reflexes, dyspnea, labored breathing, hypotension, bradycardia, slurred speech, unsteady gait or impaired coordination, and, eventually, coma.

Support blood pressure and respiration until drug effects subside; monitor vital signs. Mechanical ventilatory assistance via endotracheal (ET) tube may be required to maintain a patent airway and support adequate oxygenation. Use I.V. fluids to promote diuresis and vasopressors such as dopamine and phenylephrine to treat hypotension, as needed. Flumazenil, a specific benzodiazepine antagonist, may be useful as an adjunct to supportive therapy.

If patient is conscious, induce emesis. Use gastric lavage if ingestion was recent, but only if an ET tube is present to prevent aspiration. After emesis or lavage, administer activated charcoal with a cathartic as a single dose. Dialysis is of limited value. Don't use barbiturates if excitation occurs to avoid exacerbation of excitatory state or potentiation of CNS depressant effects.

Special considerations
Consider the recommendations relevant to all benzodiazepines as well as the following.
• Studies have demonstrated a carryover effect. Drug is most effective after 3 or 4 nights of use because of long half-life. Don't increase dose more frequently than every 5 days.
• Drug is useful for patients who have trouble falling asleep and who awaken frequently at night and early in the morning.
• Although prolonged use isn't recommended, this drug has proven effective for up to 4 weeks of continuous use.
• Rapid withdrawal after prolonged use can cause withdrawal symptoms.

● Lower doses are effective in patients with renal or hepatic dysfunction.

Patient monitoring
● Monitor hepatic function and AST, ALT, bilirubin, and alkaline phosphatase levels for changes.
● Recommendations are the same as for all benzodiazepines.

Pregnant patients
● Drug is contraindicated during pregnancy.

Breast-feeding patients
● Drug appears in breast milk. A breast-fed infant may become sedated, have feeding difficulties, or lose weight. Avoid use in breast-feeding women.

Pediatric patients
● Closely observe a neonate for withdrawal symptoms if the mother took flurazepam during pregnancy.
● Use of flurazepam during labor may cause neonatal flaccidity.
● Drug isn't for use in children under age 15.
● Neonates are more sensitive to flurazepam because of slower metabolism. The possibility of toxicity is greatly increased.

Geriatric patients
● Elderly patients are more susceptible to CNS depressant effects of flurazepam. They may need assistance and supervision with walking and daily activities when therapy starts or dosage increases.
● Lower doses usually are effective in elderly patients because of decreased elimination.

Patient education
● Warn patient to avoid alcohol while taking drug.
● Emphasize the risk for excessive CNS depression if drug is taken with alcohol, even if taken the evening before ingestion of alcohol.
● Advise patient that rebound insomnia may occur after stopping drug.
● Tell patient not to discontinue drug abruptly after prolonged therapy and not to exceed prescribed dosage.

flurbiprofen
Ansaid

Pharmacologic classification: NSAID, phenylalkanoic acid derivative
Therapeutic classification: antiarthritic
Pregnancy risk category: B

Indications and dosages
➤ **Rheumatoid arthritis, osteoarthritis.**
Adults: 200 to 300 mg P.O. daily, divided b.i.d., t.i.d., or q.i.d.
✦ **Dosage adjustment.** Patients with end-stage renal disease may accumulate flurbiprofen

metabolites, but half-life of parent compound is unchanged. Monitor patient closely and adjust dosage accordingly.

How supplied
Available by prescription only
Tablets: 50 mg, 100 mg

Pharmacodynamics
Anti-inflammatory action: An NSAID, flurbiprofen interferes with the synthesis of prostaglandins.

Pharmacokinetics
Absorption: Well absorbed after oral administration. Administering drug with food alters rate, but not extent, of absorption.
Distribution: Highly bound (more than 99%) to plasma proteins.
Metabolism: Metabolized primarily in the liver. The major metabolite shows little anti-inflammatory activity.
Excretion: Excreted primarily in urine. Average elimination half-life is 6 to 10 hours.

Route	Onset	Peak	Duration
P.O.	Unknown	1½ hr	Unknown

Contraindications and precautions
Contraindicated in patients hypersensitive to drug and patients with a history of aspirin- or NSAID-induced asthma, urticaria, or other allergic-type reactions.

Use cautiously in elderly or debilitated patients and those with history of peptic ulcer disease, herpes simplex keratitis, impaired renal or hepatic function, cardiac disease, or conditions that cause fluid retention.

Interactions
Drug-drug. *Aspirin:* May decrease flurbiprofen levels and increase GI toxicity. Avoid use together.
Beta blockers: Antihypertensive effect of beta blockers may be impaired. Monitor patient carefully.
Cyclosporine: Increased risk of nephrotoxicity. Use together extremely cautiously.
Diuretics: Decreased diuretic effect. Monitor patient carefully.
Lithium: Lithium levels may be increased. Monitor serum levels.
Methotrexate: Increased risk of methotrexate toxicity. Avoid use together.
Oral anticoagulants: Increased bleeding tendencies. Avoid use together.
Drug-lifestyle. *Alcohol use:* Increased risk of adverse GI reactions. Advise patient to avoid alcohol.
Sun exposure: May potentiate photosensitivity reactions. Advise patient to take precautions.

Reactions may be *common*, uncommon, *life-threatening*, or COMMON AND LIFE-THREATENING.

Adverse reactions

CNS: *headache,* anxiety, insomnia, dizziness, increased reflexes, tremors, amnesia, asthenia, drowsiness, malaise, depression.
CV: *edema,* **heart failure,** hypertension, vasodilation.
EENT: rhinitis, tinnitus, visual changes, epistaxis.
GI: *dyspepsia, diarrhea, abdominal pain, nausea,* constipation, *bleeding,* flatulence, vomiting.
GU: *symptoms suggesting urinary tract infection,* hematuria, interstitial nephritis, *renal failure.*
Hematologic: *thrombocytopenia, neutropenia,* anemia, *aplastic anemia.*
Hepatic: *elevated liver enzyme levels, jaundice.*
Metabolic: weight changes.
Respiratory: asthma.
Skin: rash, photosensitivity, urticaria, *angioedema.*

Overdose and treatment

Overdose has resulted in lethargy, coma, respiratory depression, epigastric pain, and distress.

Treatment should be supportive. Emptying the stomach by emesis or lavage would be of little use if the ingestion took place more than an hour before treatment, but is still recommended.

Special considerations

Consider the recommendations relevant to all NSAIDs as well as the following.

Patient monitoring

• Closely monitor patient with impaired hepatic or renal function and elderly or debilitated patients; they may need lower doses. These patients may be at risk for renal toxicity.
• Periodically monitor renal function.
• Patients receiving long-term therapy should have periodic liver function studies, ophthalmologic and auditory examinations, and hematocrit determinations.

Pregnant patients

• Recommendations are the same as for all NSAIDs.

Breast-feeding patients

• A breast-feeding woman taking 200 mg of flurbiprofen daily could deliver as much as 0.1 mg to the infant daily. Breast-feeding isn't recommended while using the drug.

Pediatric patients

• Safety in children hasn't been established.

Patient education

• Advise patient to discontinue drug and contact prescriber promptly if GI bleeding occurs.
• Tell patient to take drug with food, milk, or antacid to minimize GI upset.

• Advise patient to avoid hazardous activities that require alertness until the adverse CNS effects of the drug are known.
• Tell patient to immediately report to prescriber edema, substantial weight gain, black stools, rash, itching, or visual disturbances.

flurbiprofen sodium
Ocufen

Pharmacologic classification: NSAID
Therapeutic classification: ophthalmic anti-inflammatory, antimiotic
Pregnancy risk category: C

Indications and dosages

➤ *Inhibition of intraoperative miosis.*
Adults: Instill 1 drop into the eye undergoing surgery about q 30 minutes, beginning 2 hours before surgery. Give a total of 4 drops.

How supplied

Available by prescription only
Ophthalmic solution: 0.03%

Pharmacodynamics

Anti-inflammatory action: Acts by inhibiting the cyclooxygenase enzyme essential in converting arachidonic acid to prostaglandin. When applied topically, it inhibits prostaglandin synthesis in the iris, ciliary body, and conjunctiva. Doesn't affect intraocular pressure or tonographic aqueous outflow resistance.
Antimiotic action: Inhibits or reduces miosis and possibly some manifestations of ocular inflammation induced by ocular trauma. When administered prophylactically, topical flurbiprofen inhibits intraoperative trauma-induced miosis. However, drug has little, if any, effect if administered after trauma-induced miosis is present. Doesn't inhibit or reduce light-induced miosis.

Pharmacokinetics

Absorption: No information available on absorption after ophthalmic administration.
Distribution: At least 99% bound to plasma proteins. Unknown whether drug crosses placenta or is distributed into breast milk.
Metabolism: After ophthalmic administration, absorbed systemically; metabolized primarily in liver where converted mainly to inactive glucuronide and sulfate compounds.
Excretion: Inactive metabolites excreted by kidneys, primarily as glucuronides and sulfates. Biological half-life of orally administered flurbiprofen is 6 to 10 hours.

Route	Onset	Peak	Duration
Oph-thalmic	Unknown	Unknown	Unknown

Contraindications and precautions
Contraindicated in patients hypersensitive to drug. Use cautiously in patients with history of herpes simplex keratitis, aspirin or NSAID allergy, bleeding tendencies, and those receiving drug that may prolong clotting times.

Interactions
Drug-drug. *Acetylcholine, carbachol:* May be rendered ineffective. Avoid use together.
Anticoagulants: May increase risk of bleeding if systemic absorption is significant. Monitor patient closely.

Adverse reactions
EENT: transient burning and stinging on instillation, ocular irritation.

Overdose and treatment
Overdose ordinarily won't cause acute complications. After accidental ingestion, fluids are recommended to dilute the drug.

Special considerations
• Wound healing may be delayed with drug use.
• Store away from heat in a dark, tightly closed container; protect drug from freezing.

Patient monitoring
• Monitor patient for adverse effects.

Pediatric patients
• Safety and efficacy in children haven't been established.

Patient education
• Teach patient not to touch eye dropper to eye.
• Remind patient to keep drug container closed tightly.
• Advise patient not to use more drug than amount prescribed or to use flurbiprofen for other eye problems unless prescribed.
• Instruct patient to discard drug when outdated or no longer needed.

flutamide
Eulexin

Pharmacologic classification: nonsteroidal antiandrogen
Therapeutic classification: antineoplastic
Pregnancy risk category: D

Indications and dosages
➤ *Treatment of metastatic prostatic carcinoma (stage D2) in combination with luteinizing hormone-releasing hormone analogues, such as leuprolide acetate.*
Adult men: 250 mg P.O. q 8 hours.

How supplied
Available by prescription only
Capsules: 125 mg

Pharmacodynamics
Antitumor action: Flutamide inhibits androgen uptake or prevents binding of androgens in nucleus of cells within target tissues. Prostatic carcinoma is known to be androgen-sensitive.

Pharmacokinetics
Absorption: Rapidly and completely absorbed after oral administration.
Distribution: Concentrates in the prostate in animals. Drug and its active metabolite are about 95% protein-bound.
Metabolism: Metabolism is rapid, with at least six metabolites identified. More than 97% of drug is metabolized within 1 hour of administration.
Excretion: More than 95% is excreted in urine.

Route	Onset	Peak	Duration
P.O.	Unknown	2 hr	Unknown

Contraindications and precautions
Contraindicated in patients hypersensitive to drug and patients with severe hepataic impairment.

Interactions
Drug-drug. *Anticoagulants:* Increased risk of bleeding. Monitor PT and INR.

Adverse reactions
CNS: *drowsiness, confusion, depression, anxiety, nervousness.*
CV: *peripheral edema, hypertension.*
GI: *diarrhea, nausea, vomiting.*
GU: *impotence.*
Hematologic: anemia, **leukopenia, thrombocytopenia,** hemolytic anemia.
Hepatic: elevated liver enzyme levels, **hepatitis.**
Skin: rash, photosensitivity.
Other: *hot flashes, loss of libido,* gynecomastia.

Overdose and treatment
No overdose has been reported. Dosage as high as 1,500 mg daily for 36 weeks has been reported without serious adverse effects.

Special considerations
• Flutamide must be taken continuously with the agent used for medical castration (such as leuprolide acetate) to produce full benefit of therapy. Leuprolide suppresses testosterone production, while flutamide inhibits testosterone action at the cellular level. Together they can impair the growth of androgen-responsive tumors.

Patient monitoring
• Monitor patient for adverse reactions.
• Monitor liver function test results, CBC, and prostate-specific antigen levels closely.

Pediatric patients
• Safety in children hasn't been established.

Reactions may be *common,* uncommon, *life-threatening,* or COMMON AND LIFE-THREATENING.

Patient education
• Tell patient not to discontinue either leuprolide or flutamide without medical approval.
• Explain that some symptoms may worsen initially before they improve.

---

fluticasone propionate
Cutivate, Flonase, Flovent

Pharmacologic classification: corticosteroid
Therapeutic classification: topical and inhaled anti-inflammatory
Pregnancy risk category: C

Indications and dosages
➤ *Relief of inflammation and pruritus from corticosteroid-responsive dermatoses. Adults:* Apply sparingly to affected area b.i.d. and rub in gently and completely.
➤ *Allergic rhinitis. Adults:* 2 sprays in each nostril once daily or 1 spray b.i.d.
➤ *Management of nasal symptoms of seasonal and perennial allergic rhinitis in children. Adolescents and children age 4 and older:* Initially, 1 spray (50 mcg) in each nostril once daily. If patient doesn't respond or symptoms are severe, increase to 2 sprays in each nostril daily. Once adequate control is achieved, decrease dose to 1 spray in each nostril daily. Maximum dose is 2 sprays in each nostril daily.
➤ *Maintenance treatment of asthma as prophylactic therapy. Inhalation aerosol. Adults and children age 12 and older:* For patients previously on bronchodilator therapy alone, 88 mcg inhalation aerosol b.i.d.; highest recommended dose is 440 mcg b.i.d. For patients previously on inhaled corticosteroids, 88 to 220 mcg inhalation aerosol b.i.d.; highest recommended dose is 440 mcg b.i.d. For patients previously on oral corticosteroids, 880 mcg inhalation aerosol b.i.d.; highest recommended dose is 880 mcg b.i.d.
Inhalation powder
Adults and adolescents: For patients previously on bronchodilators alone, 100 mcg inhalation powder b.i.d.; highest recommended dose is 500 mcg b.i.d. For patients previously on inhaled corticosteroids, 100 to 250 mcg inhalation powder b.i.d.; highest recommended dose is 500 mcg b.i.d. For patients previously on oral corticosteroids, 1,000 mcg inhalation powder b.i.d.; highest recommended dose is 1,000 mcg b.i.d.
Children ages 4 to 11: For patients previously on bronchodilators alone, 50 mcg inhalation powder b.i.d.; highest recommended dose is 100 mcg b.i.d. For patients previously on inhaled corticosteroids, 50 mcg inhalation powder b.i.d.; highest recommended dose is 100 mcg b.i.d.

How supplied
Available by prescription only
Cream: 0.05%
Inhalation aerosol: 44 mcg/actuation, 110 mcg/actuation, 220 mcg/actuation
Inhalation powder: 50-mcg, 100-mcg, 250-mcg Rotadisk
Metered nasal spray: 50 mcg/actuation
Ointment: 0.005%

Pharmacodynamics
Anti-inflammatory action: Fluticasone stimulates synthesis of enzymes needed to decrease inflammation.

Pharmacokinetics
Absorption: Amount absorbed depends on the amount applied, application site, vehicle used, use of occlusive dressing, and integrity of epidermal barrier. Some systemic absorption does occur.
Distribution: Distributed throughout the local skin.
Metabolism: Metabolized primarily by the skin. Absorbed drug is extensively metabolized by the liver.
Excretion: Less than 5% is excreted in urine as metabolites; rest is excreted in feces as parent drug and metabolites.

Route	Onset	Peak	Duration
Topical, inhalation	Unknown	Unknown	Unknown

Contraindications and precautions
Contraindicated in patients hypersensitive to drug or its components and in patients with viral, fungal, herpetic, or tubercular skin lesions. Flovent inhalation aerosol and powder are contraindicated as the primary treatment in status asthmaticus or other acute episodes of asthma where intensive measures are required.

Use care when transferring patients from systemically active corticosteroids to Flovent inhalation aerosol or powder; deaths have occurred in asthmatic patients during and after transfer from systemic corticosteroids to less systemically available inhalation corticosteroids. During periods of stress or severe asthma attack, instruct patients who have been withdrawn from systemic corticosteroids to resume oral corticosteroids in large doses immediately and contact their prescribers for further assistance.

Interactions
Drug-drug. *Ketoconazole:* Increased mean fluticasone levels. Use care when giving fluticasone with long-term ketoconazole and other cytochrome P-450 3A4 inhibitors.

Adverse reactions
CNS: dizziness, giddiness.
GU: dysmenorrhea.
Metabolic: hyperglycemia, glucosuria.
Musculoskeletal: pain in joints, sprain or strain aches and pains, pain in limbs.
Respiratory: bronchitis, chest congestion.

Skin: stinging, burning, pruritus, irritation, dryness, erythema, folliculitis, skin atrophy, leukoderma, vesicles, numbness of fingers, rash, hypertrichosis, acneiform eruptions, hypopigmentation, perioral dermatitis, allergic contact dermatitis, secondary infection, striae, miliaria.
Other: *hypothalamic-pituitary-adrenal axis suppression,* Cushing's syndrome, fever.

Special considerations
● Not used for treatment of rosacea, perioral dermatitis, or acne.
● Mixing with other bases or vehicles may affect potency far beyond expectations.
● Flovent inhalation aerosol and powder aren't indicated for relief of acute bronchospasm.
● The Rotadisk device eliminates the need for hand-breath coordination because it is breath-activated.

Patient monitoring
● During withdrawal from oral corticosteroids, some patients may experience symptoms of systemically active corticosteroid withdrawal, such as joint or musculoskeletal pain, malaise, and depression, despite maintenance or improvement of respiratory function.
● Because of the possibility of systemic absorption of inhalation corticosteroids, carefully observe patients treated with these drugs for any evidence of systemic corticosteroid effects. Take special care during periods of stress or postoperatively for adrenal insufficiency.

Pregnant patients
● Use drug during pregnancy only when potential benefits justify risks to fetus.

Breast-feeding patients
● Use cautiously in breast-feeding women because it isn't known whether topical or inhaled corticosteroids undergo sufficient absorption to produce systemic effects in the infant.

Pediatric patients
● Safety and efficacy of topical form haven't been established in children.
● Safety and efficacy of nasal form haven't been established in children under age 12; use of drug isn't recommended in these patients.
● Growth velocity may be reduced in children or teenagers from use of corticosteroids for treatment or from inadequate control of chronic disease such as asthma. The benefits of asthma control from corticosteroid therapy must be weighed against the possibility of growth suppression in these patients.

Patient education
● Advise patient that proper application includes washing area before application and applying agent sparingly and rubbing it in lightly.
● Instruct patient to report burning, irritation, or persistent or worsened condition.

● Tell patient to avoid prolonged use, contact with eyes, or use around genital area, rectal area, on face, and in skin creases.
● Urge patient to rinse mouth well after corticosteroid inhalation.
● Urge patient receiving inhaled corticosteroids to avoid exposure and to consult prescriber immediately if he has been exposed to chickenpox or measles.
● Explain proper administration using the nasal spray pump, including the need to prime the pump.

fluticasone propionate and salmeterol inhalation powder
Advair Diskus 100/50, Advair Diskus 250/50, Advair Diskus 500/50

Pharmacologic classification: corticosteroid, long-acting beta$_2$-adrenergic agonist
Therapeutic classification: anti-inflammatory, bronchodilator
Pregnancy risk category: C

Indications and dosages
➤ *Long-term maintenance of asthma.*
Adults and children over age 12: 1 oral inhalation twice daily, morning and evening, at least 12 hours apart.
Adults and children over age 12 not currently taking an inhaled corticosteroid: 1 oral inhalation of Advair Diskus 100/50 twice daily.
Adults and children over age 12 currently taking beclomethasone dipropionate: If daily dose of beclomethasone dipropionate is 420 mcg or less, start with 1 oral inhalation of Advair Diskus 100/50 twice daily. If beclomethasone dipropionate daily dose is 462 to 840 mcg, start with one oral inhalation of Advair Diskus 250/50 twice daily.
Adults and children over age 12 currently taking budesonide: If daily dose of budesonide is 400 mcg or less, start with 1 oral inhalation of Advair Diskus 100/50 twice daily. If budesonide daily dose is 800 to 1,200 mcg, start with 1 oral inhalation of Advair Diskus 250/50 twice daily. If budesonide daily dose is 1,600 mcg, start with 1 oral inhalation of Advair Diskus 500/50 twice daily.
Adults and children over age 12 currently taking flunisolide: If daily dose of flunisolide is 1,000 mcg or less, start with 1 oral inhalation of Advair Diskus 100/50 twice daily. If flunisolide daily dose is 1,250 to 2,000 mcg, start with 1 oral inhalation of Advair Diskus 250/50 twice daily.
Adults and children over age 12 currently taking fluticasone propionate inhalation aerosol: If daily dose of fluticasone propionate inhalation aerosol is 176 mcg or less, start with 1 oral inhalation of Advair Diskus 100/50 twice daily. If fluticasone propionate inhalation aerosol daily dose is 440 mcg, start with 1 oral inhalation of Advair Diskus 250/50 twice daily. If fluticasone

propionate inhalation aerosol daily dose is 660 to 880 mcg, start with 1 oral inhalation of Advair Diskus 500/50 twice daily.

Adults and children over age 12 currently taking fluticasone propionate inhalation powder: If fluticasone propionate inhalation powder daily dose is 200 mcg or less, start with 1 oral inhalation of Advair Diskus 100/50 twice daily. If fluticasone propionate inhalation powder daily dose is 500 mcg, start with 1 oral inhalation of Advair Diskus 250/50 twice daily. If fluticasone propionate inhalation powder daily dose is 1,000 mcg, start with 1 oral inhalation of Advair Diskus 500/50 twice daily.

Adults and children over age 12 currently taking triamcinolone acetonide: If triamcinolone acetonide daily dose is 1,000 mcg or less, start with 1 oral inhalation of Advair Diskus 100/50 twice daily. If triamcinolone acetonide daily dose is 1,100 to 1,600 mcg, start with 1 oral inhalation of Advair Diskus 250/50 twice daily.

For patients already using an inhaled corticosteriod, maximum oral inhalation of Advair Diskus is 500/50 twice daily.

How supplied
Available by prescription only
Inhalation powder: 100 mcg fluticasone/50 mcg salmeterol, 250 mcg fluticasone/50 mcg salmeterol, 500 mcg fluticasone/50 mcg salmeterol

Pharmacodynamics
Anti-inflammatory action: Fluticasone is a synthetic corticosteroid with potent anti-inflammatory activity, although precise mechanisms of action in asthma are unknown. Corticosteroids inhibit mast cells, eosinophils, basophils, lymphocytes, macrophages, and neutrophils, and they inhibit production or secretion of histamine, eicosanoids, leukotrienes, and cytokines.

Salmeterol xinafoate is a long-acting beta-adrenergic agonist selective for $beta_2$-adrenoceptors. Pharmacologic effects are at least in part attributable to stimulation of intracellular adenyl cyclase, the enzyme that catalyzes conversion of ATP to cAMP. Increased cAMP levels relax bronchial smooth muscle and inhibit release of mediators of immediate hypersensitivity from cells, especially mast cells. In vitro tests show that salmeterol is a potent and long-lasting inhibitor of the release of mast cell mediators, such as histamine, leukotrienes, and prostaglandin D_2, from human lung.

Pharmacokinetics
Absorption: Most of the fluticasone propionate delivered to the lung is systemically absorbed. Salmeterol acts locally in the lung; therefore, plasma levels don't predict therapeutic effect. Because of the small therapeutic dose, systemic levels of salmeterol are low and undetectable after inhalation of recommended doses. Following long-term administration of an inhaled dose of 50 mcg of salmeterol inhalation twice daily, sal-

meterol was detected in plasma within 5 to 45 minutes and peaked at 20 minutes.

Distribution: Drug is 91% bound to plasma proteins, is weakly and reversibly bound to erythrocytes, and isn't significantly bound to human transcortin. Binding of salmeterol to human plasma proteins averages 96%.

Metabolism: The total clearance of fluticasone propionate is high, with renal clearance accounting for less than 0.02% of the total. The only circulating metabolite is the 17 beta-carboxylic acid derivative, which is formed via the cytochrome P-450 3A4 pathway. Salmeterol base is extensively metabolized by hydroxylation, with subsequent elimination predominantly in the feces. No significant amount of unchanged salmeterol base was detected in either urine or feces.

Excretion: Following I.V. dosing, fluticasone had a terminal elimination half-life of about 7.8 hours. Less than 5% of a dose is excreted in urine as metabolites, with the remainder excreted in feces as parent drug and metabolite. Salmeterol xinafoate is about 25% to 60% eliminated in urine and feces, respectively, over a period of 7 days. Terminal elimination half-life is about 5.5 hours.

Route	Onset	Peak	Duration
Inhalation			
fluti-casone	Unknown	1-2 hr	Unknown
salme-terol	Unknown	5 min	Unknown

Adverse reactions
CNS: sleep disorders, tremors, hypnagogic effects, compressed nerve syndromes, *headache.*
CV: palpitations.
EENT: *pharyngitis,* sinusitis, hoarseness/dysphonia, oral candidiasis, rhinorrhea, rhinitis, sneezing, nasal irritation, blood in nasal mucosa, keratitis, conjunctivitis, eye redness, viral eye infections, congestion.
GI: nausea, vomiting, abdominal pain and discomfort, diarrhea, gastroenteritis, oral discomfort and pain, constipation, oral ulcerations, oral erythema and rashes, appendicitis, dental discomfort and pain, unusual taste.
Musculoskeletal: muscle pain, arthralgia, articular rheumatism, muscle stiffness, tightness, rigidity, bone and cartilage disorders.
Hepatic: abnormal liver function test results.
Respiratory: *upper respiratory tract infection,* upper respiratory tract inflammation, lower viral respiratory tract infections, bronchitis, cough, pneumonia.
Skin: viral skin infections, urticaria, skin flakiness, disorders of sweat and sebum, sweating.
Other: viral infections, pain, chest symptoms, fluid retention, bacterial infections, allergies, allergic reactions.

Interactions
Drug-drug. *Beta blockers:* Blocked pulmonary effect of salmeterol may produce severe bron-

chospasm in patients with asthma. Avoid concurrent use. If necessary, use a cardioselective beta blocker extremely cautiously.

Ketoconazole, other inhibitors of cytochrome P-450: May increase fluticasone levels and adverse effects. Use together cautiously.

Loop diuretics, thiazide diuretics: ECG changes or hypokalemia may result from or be worsened by potassium-wasting diuretics. Use together cautiously.

MAO inhibitors, tricyclic antidepressants: May potentiate the action of salmeterol on the vascular system. Avoid use within 2 weeks of these drugs.

Overdose and treatment

Chronic overdose of fluticasone may cause signs and symptoms of hypercorticism. Salmeterol overdose may cause seizures, angina, hypertension, hypotension, tachycardia, arrhythmias, nervousness, headache, tremor, muscle cramps, dry mouth, palpitations, nausea, prolonged QTc interval, ventricular arrhythmia, hypokalemia, hyperglycemia, cardiac arrest, and death.

Treatment consists of discontinuing drug and possibly using a cardioselective beta blocker. Cardiac monitoring is necessary.

Contraindications and precautions

Contraindicated in patients hypersensitive to any component of the drug. Also, contraindicated as primary treatment of status asthmaticus or other acute asthmatic episodes. Use extremely cautiously, if at all, in patients with active or quiescent respiratory tuberculosis infection; untreated systemic fungal, bacterial, viral, or parasitic infection; or ocular herpes simplex. Use cautiously in patients with CV disorders, especially coronary insufficiency, cardiac arrhythmias, and hypertension; in patients with seizure disorders or thyrotoxicosis; in patients unusually responsive to sympathomimetic amines; and in patients with hepatic impairment (because salmeterol is metabolized mainly in the liver).

Special considerations

● Don't switch from systemic corticosteroids to Advair Diskus because of hypothalamic-pituitary-adrenal axis suppression. Death can occur from adrenal insufficiency.

● Don't start Advair Diskus therapy during rapidly deteriorating or potentially life-threatening episodes of asthma. Serious acute respiratory events, including fatality, can occur.

● Don't use Advair Diskus to treat status asthmaticus. When prescribing Advair Diskus, make sure the patient has an inhaled, short-acting beta₂-agonist (such as albuterol) for acute symptoms.

● Don't use an inhaled long-acting beta₂-agonist with Advair Diskus for prevention of exercise-induced bronchospasm or maintenance treatment of asthma.

● Advair Diskus can produce paradoxical bronchospasm. If it does, treat immediately with a short-acting inhaled bronchodilator (such as albuterol), and discontinue Advair Diskus therapy.

● If patient is exposed to chickenpox, consider prophylaxis with varicella zoster immune globulin. If chickenpox develops, consider antiviral treatment.

● If patient is exposed to measles, consider prophylaxis with pooled I.M. immunoglobulin.

● Store at 68° to 78° F (20° to 25° C) in a dry place away from direct heat or sunlight. Discard the device 1 month after removal from the moisture-protective overwrap pouch or after every blister has been used, whichever comes first. Don't attempt to take the device apart.

Patient monitoring

● Monitor patient for urticaria, angioedema, rash, bronchospasm, or other signs of hypersensitivity, which may occur immediately after a dose of Advair Diskus.

● Monitor patient for increased use of inhaled short-acting beta₂-agonist. The dose of Advair Diskus may need to be increased.

● Monitor patient for hypercorticism and adrenal suppression. If these occur, reduce dosage slowly.

● Monitor patient for eosinophilia, vasculitic rash, worsening pulmonary symptoms, cardiac complications, or neuropathy, which may be signs of a serious eosinophilic condition.

Breast-feeding patients

● It isn't known whether the components of Advair Diskus appear in breast milk.

Pediatric patients

● Closely monitor growth in children because growth suppression may occur. Maintain child on lowest effective dose to minimize potential for growth suppression.

● Safety and efficacy in children less than age 12 haven't been established.

Geriatric patients

● No dose adjustments necessary.

Patient education

● Instruct patient on proper use of Diskus device to provide effective treatment.

● Tell patient to avoid exhaling into the Diskus and to activate and use the Diskus in a level, horizontal position.

● Instruct patient to keep the Diskus in a dry place, to avoid washing the mouthpiece or other parts of the device, and to avoid taking the Diskus apart.

● Tell patient to stop taking an oral or inhaled short-acting beta₂-agonist regularly when beginning treatment with Advair Diskus, and to use the short-acting beta₂-agonist for relief of acute symptoms.

● Instruct patient to rinse mouth after inhalation to prevent oral candidiasis.

Reactions may be *common*, uncommon, *life-threatening*, or COMMON AND LIFE-THREATENING.

• Inform patient that improvement may be seen within 30 minutes after an Advair dose; however, the full benefit may not occur for 1 week or more.

• Instruct patient not to exceed recommended prescribing dose under any circumstances.

• Instruct patient not to relieve acute symptoms with Advair Diskus. Acute symptoms should be treated with an inhaled short-acting beta$_2$-agonist (such as albuterol).

• Instruct patient to report decreasing effects or use of increasing doses of their short-acting inhaled beta$_2$-agonist.

• Instruct patient not to use Advair Diskus with a spacer device.

• Tell patient to report palpitations, chest pain, rapid heart rate, tremor, or nervousness.

• Instruct patient to contact prescriber before using Advair Diskus if she is pregnant or breast-feeding.

• Instruct patient to contact prescriber immediately if exposed to chickenpox or measles.

---

fluvastatin sodium
Lescol, Lescol XL

Pharmacologic classification: hydroxy-methylglutaryl-coenzyme A (HMG-CoA) reductase inhibitor
Therapeutic classification: cholesterol-lowering antilipemic
Pregnancy risk category: X

Indications and dosages
➤ *To reduce low-density lipoprotein (LDL) cholesterol, total cholesterol, triglyceride, and apolipoprotein B levels and to increase high density lipoprotein (HDL) cholesterol levels in patients with primary hypercholesterolemia (types IIa and IIb) when response to diet and other nondrug measures has been inadequate; to slow progression of coronary atherosclerosis in patients with coronary artery disease. Adults:* 20 mg to 40 mg P.O. h.s. Increase dose as necessary to a maximum of 80 mg daily (in divided doses). For patients who need LDL-C reduction to a goal of greater than or equal to 25%, the recommended starting dose is 40 mg as one capsule, 80 mg as one Lescol XL tablet P.O. as a single dose in the evening, or 80 mg in divided doses of the 40-mg capsule given b.i.d. For patients who need LDL-C reduction to a goal of less than 25%, a starting dose of 20 mg may be used. The recommended dosing range is 20 mg to 80 mg daily.

✦ *Dosage adjustment.* With a persistent increase in ALT or AST levels of at least three times the upper limit of normal, withdrawal of fluvastatin is recommended. Because fluvastatin is cleared hepatically, with less than 5% of the dose excreted into urine, dosage adjustments for mild to moderate renal impairment aren't necessary. Use cautiously with severe impairment.

How supplied
Available by prescription only
Capsules: 20 mg, 40 mg
Tablet (extended-release): 80 mg

Pharmacodynamics
Antilipemic action: Fluvastatin is a competitive inhibitor of HMG-CoA reductase, which is responsible for the conversion of HMG-CoA to mevalonate, a precursor of sterols, including cholesterol. This enzyme is an early (and rate-limiting) step in the synthetic pathway of cholesterol. Fluvastatin increases HDL and decreases LDL, very-low-density lipoproteins, and plasma triglycerides.

Pharmacokinetics
Absorption: Absorbed rapidly and virtually completely (98%) after oral administration on an empty stomach.
Distribution: Over 98% of circulating drug is bound to plasma proteins.
Metabolism: Completely metabolized in the liver. It has no active metabolites.
Excretion: About 5% is excreted in urine and 90% in feces.

Route	Onset	Peak	Duration
P.O.			
Regular	Unknown	1 hr	Unknown
Extended	Unknown	3 hr	Unknown

Contraindications and precautions
Contraindicated in patients hypersensitive to drug; in those with active liver disease or conditions that cause unexplained persistent elevations of serum transaminase levels; in pregnant and breast-feeding women; and in women of childbearing age unless they have no risk of pregnancy.

Use cautiously in patients with impaired renal function and history of hepatic disease or heavy alcohol consumption.

Interactions
Drug-drug. *Cholestyramine, colestipol:* May bind fluvastatin in the GI tract and decrease absorption. Administer fluvastatin at bedtime, at least 2 hours after the resin, to avoid significant interaction from the drug binding to the resin.
Cimetidine, omeprazole, ranitidine: Decreased fluvastatin metabolism. Monitor patient closely.
Cyclosporine and other immunosuppressants, erythromycin, gemfibrozil, niacin: Increased risk of polymyositis and rhabdomyolysis when given with fluvastatin. Avoid use together.
Digoxin: Altered digoxin pharmacokinetics. Monitor patient's serum digoxin levels carefully.
Rifampin: Increased fluvastatin metabolism and decreased plasma levels. Monitor patient closely for lack of effect.

Warfarin: Increased anticoagulant effect with bleeding. Monitor patient closely.
Drug-lifestyle. *Alcohol use:* Increased risk of hepatotoxicity. Encourage patient to avoid alcohol.

Adverse reactions
CNS: headache, fatigue, dizziness, insomnia.
EENT: sinusitis, rhinitis, pharyngitis.
GI: dyspepsia, diarrhea, nausea, vomiting, abdominal pain, constipation, flatulence.
Hepatic: increased liver enzyme levels, increased bilirubin levels.
Hematologic: *thrombocytopenia, leukopenia,* hemolytic anemia.
Metabolic: abnormal thyroid function test results.
Musculoskeletal: arthropathy, muscle pain.
Respiratory: *upper respiratory tract infection,* cough, bronchitis.
Other: *hypersensitivity reactions* (rash, pruritus), tooth disorder.

Overdose and treatment
No specific information on overdose is available. If an accidental overdose occurs, treat symptomatically and provide supportive treatment as needed. The dialyzability of fluvastatin and its metabolites in humans is unknown.

Special considerations
• Start fluvastatin therapy only after diet and other nondrug therapies have proven ineffective.
• Drug may be taken without regard to meals; however, efficacy is enhanced if drug is taken in the evening.

Patient monitoring
• Monitor patient closely for signs of myopathy and rhabdomyolysis.
• Liver function tests should be performed at the start of therapy, and at 12 weeks after start of therapy or increase in dose.

Pregnant patients
• Drug shouldn't be used during pregnancy.

Breast-feeding patients
• Preclinical data suggest that drug appears in breast milk at twice the level of plasma. The potential for serious adverse reactions in nursing infants indicates that breast-feeding women shouldn't take fluvastatin.

Pediatric patients
• Safety and efficacy in patients under age 18 haven't been established. Use in children isn't recommended.

Patient education
• Instruct patient to take fluvastatin at bedtime to enhance effectiveness.
• Warn patient to restrict alcohol intake because of potentially serious adverse effects.
• Tell patient to report to prescriber adverse reactions, particularly muscle aches and pains.

fluvoxamine maleate
Luvox

Pharmacologic classification: selective serotonin reuptake inhibitor
Therapeutic classification: anticompulsive
Pregnancy risk category: C

Indications and dosages
➤ *Obsessive-compulsive disorder.* *Adults:* Initially, 50 mg P.O. daily h.s. Increase in 50-mg increments q 4 to 7 days until maximum benefit occurs. Maximum daily dose is 300 mg. Give total daily doses exceeding 100 mg in two divided doses.
Children ages 8 to 17: 25 mg P.O. h.s. Increase in 25-mg increments q 4 to 7 days until maximum benefit occurs. Maximum daily dose is 200 mg. Give total daily doses exceeding 50 mg in two divided doses.
✦ *Dosage adjustment.* Because elderly patients and patients with hepatic impairment may have decreased clearance of fluvoxamine maleate, dosage adjustment may be appropriate.

How supplied
Available by prescription only
Tablets: 25 mg, 50 mg, 100 mg

Pharmacodynamics
Anticompulsive action: The exact mechanism of action is unknown. Fluvoxamine is a potent selective inhibitor of the neuronal uptake of serotonin, which is thought to reduce obsessive-compulsive behavior.

Pharmacokinetics
Absorption: Absolute bioavailability of drug is 53%.
Distribution: Mean apparent volume of distribution is about 25 L/kg. About 80% of drug is bound to plasma protein (mostly albumin).
Metabolism: Extensively metabolized in the liver mostly by oxidative demethylation and deamination.
Excretion: Metabolites are primarily excreted in urine.

Route	Onset	Peak	Duration
P.O.	Unknown	3-8 hr	Unknown

Contraindications and precautions
Contraindicated in patients hypersensitive to drug or to other phenylpiperazine antidepressants and patients who have taken an MAO inhibitor within 14 days. Use cautiously in patients with hepatic dysfunction, conditions that may affect hemodynamic responses or metabolism, or a history of mania or seizures.

Reactions may be *common,* uncommon, *life-threatening,* or COMMON AND LIFE-THREATENING.

Interactions
Drug-drug. *Benzodiazepines, theophylline, warfarin:* Reduced clearance of these drugs. Use together cautiously.

Carbamazepine, clozapine, methadone, metoprolol, propranolol, tricyclic antidepressants: Increased fluvoxamine levels. Use together cautiously, and monitor patient closely for adverse reactions. Dosage adjustments may be necessary.

Diazepam: Decreased diazepam clearance. Diazepam shouldn't be coadministered with fluvoxamine.

Diltiazem: May cause bradycardia. Monitor patient's heart rate.

Lithium, tryptophan: May enhance fluvoxamine effects. Use together cautiously.

MAO inhibitors: May cause severe excitation, hyperpyrexia, myoclonus, delirium, and coma. Avoid use together or within 2 weeks of each other.

Drug-lifestyle. *Smoking:* May decrease drug effectiveness. Advise patient to avoid smoking.

Adverse reactions
CNS: headache, asthenia, somnolence, insomnia, nervousness, dizziness, tremor, anxiety, hypertonia, agitation, depression, CNS stimulation.
CV: palpitations, vasodilation.
EENT: amblyopia.
GI: *nausea, diarrhea, constipation, dyspepsia,* anorexia, *vomiting,* flatulence, dysphagia, *dry mouth,* taste perversion.
GU: abnormal ejaculation, urinary frequency, impotence, anorgasmia, urine retention.
Metabolic: SIADH, hyponatremia.
Respiratory: upper respiratory tract infection, dyspnea, yawning.
Skin: sweating.
Other: decreased libido, flulike syndrome, chills, tooth disorder.

Overdose and treatment
Common signs and symptoms of fluvoxamine overdose include drowsiness, vomiting, diarrhea, and dizziness. Coma, tachycardia, bradycardia, hypotension, ECG abnormalities, liver function abnormalities, and seizures may also occur. Symptoms such as aspiration pneumonitis, respiratory difficulties, or hypokalemia may occur because of loss of consciousness or vomiting.

Treatment is supportive. Besides maintaining an open airway and monitoring vital signs and ECG, administration of activated charcoal may be as effective as emesis or lavage. Because absorption with overdose may be delayed, measures to minimize absorption may be necessary for up to 24 hours after ingestion. Dialysis isn't believed to be beneficial.

Special considerations
• Allow at least 14 days after stopping fluvoxamine before starting an MAO inhibitor.
• Allow at least 14 days after stopping MAO inhibitor therapy before starting fluvoxamine.

Patient monitoring
• Monitor patient for suicidal tendencies, and provide a minimum supply of drug.

Pregnant patients
• Drug shouldn't be used during pregnancy.

Breast-feeding patients
• Drug appears in breast milk and shouldn't be given to breast-feeding women.

Pediatric patients
• Safety and efficacy in children under age 8 haven't been established.

Geriatric patients
• Drug clearance is decreased by about 50% in elderly patients compared with younger patients. Administer drug cautiously in this age group and adjust dosage slowly during initiation of therapy.

Patient education
• Warn patient not to engage in hazardous activities that require mental alertness and coordination until CNS effects are known.
• Urge patient to avoid alcoholic beverages.
• Alert patient that smoking may decrease drug effectiveness.
• Inform patient that several weeks of therapy may be needed to obtain full antidepressant effect. Once improvement is seen, advise patient not to stop drug until directed.
• Advise patient to report use of herbal remedies or OTC medications because of possible drug interactions.

folic acid
Folvite

Pharmacologic classification: folic acid derivative
Therapeutic classification: vitamin supplement
Pregnancy risk category: A

Indications and dosages
➤ **Megaloblastic or macrocytic anemia secondary to folic acid deficiency, hepatic disease, alcoholism, intestinal obstruction, excessive hemolysis.** *Pregnant and breast-feeding patients:* 0.8 mg P.O., S.C., or I.M. daily.
Adults and children age 4 and older: 0.4 mg P.O., S.C., or I.M. daily for 4 to 5 days. After anemia secondary to folic acid deficiency is corrected, proper diet and RDA supplements are necessary to prevent recurrence.
Children under age 4: Up to 0.3 mg P.O., S.C., or I.M. daily.
➤ **Prevention of megaloblastic anemia of pregnancy and fetal damage.** *Adults:* 1 mg P.O., S.C., or I.M. daily during pregnancy.

➤ *Nutritional supplement. Adults:* 0.15 to 0.2 mg P.O., S.C., or I.M. daily for men; 0.15 to 0.18 mg P.O., S.C., or I.M. daily for women.
Children: 0.05 mg P.O. daily.
➤ *Tropical sprue. Adults:* 3 to 15 mg P.O. daily.

How supplied
Available by prescription only
Injection: 10-ml vials (folic acid 5 mg/ml contains 1.5% benzyl alcohol and EDTA; Folvite 5 mg/ml contains 1.5% benzyl alcohol)
Tablets: 1 mg
Available without a prescription
Tablets: 0.4 mg, 0.8 mg

Pharmacodynamics
Nutritional action: Exogenous folate is required to maintain normal erythropoiesis and to perform nucleoprotein synthesis. Folic acid stimulates production of RBCs, WBCs, and platelets in certain megaloblastic anemias.

Dietary folic acid is present in foods, primarily as reduced folate polyglutamate. This vitamin may be absorbed only after hydrolysis, reduction, and methylation occur in the GI tract. Conversion to active tetrahydrofolate may require vitamin B_{12}.

Oral synthetic form of folic acid is a monoglutamate and is absorbed completely after administration, even in malabsorption syndromes.

Pharmacokinetics
Absorption: Absorbed rapidly from the GI tract, mainly from the proximal part of the small intestine. Normal serum folate levels range from 0.005 to 0.015 mcg/ml. Usually, serum levels less than 0.005 mcg/ml indicate folate deficiency; those less than 0.002 mcg/ml usually result in megaloblastic anemia.
Distribution: The active tetrahydrofolic acid and its derivatives are distributed into all body tissues; the liver contains about half of the total body folate stores. Folate is actively concentrated in the CSF. Folic acid is distributed into breast milk.
Metabolism: Metabolized in the liver to N-methyltetrahydrofolic acid, the main form of folate storage and transport.
Excretion: A single 0.1-mg to 0.2-mg dose usually results in only a trace amount of drug in urine. After administering large doses, excessive folate is excreted unchanged in urine. Small amounts of folic acid have been recovered in feces. About 0.05 mg/day of normal body folate stores is lost by a combination of urinary and fecal excretion and oxidative cleavage of the molecule.

Route	Onset	Peak	Duration
P.O.	20-30 min	2-3 hr	Unknown
I.V.	5 min	10 min	Unknown
I.M.	10-20 min	< 1 hr	Unknown

Contraindications and precautions
Contraindicated in patients with undiagnosed anemia (because it may mask pernicious anemia)

and in those with pernicious anemia and other megaloblastic anemias where vitamin B_{12} is deficient.

Interactions
Drug-drug. *Aminosalicylic acid, chloramphenicol, methotrexate, oral contraceptives, pyrimethamine, sulfasalazine, triamterene, trimethoprim:* May act as antagonists to folic acid. Monitor patient for decreased drug effect.
Anticonvulsants, such as phenobarbital and phenytoin: Increased anticonvulsant metabolism and decreased anticonvulsant levels. Monitor serum blood levels.
Phenytoin, primidone: Decreased serum folate levels; symptoms of folic acid deficiency in long-term therapy. Monitor patient closely.
Pyrimethamine: Interference with antimicrobial actions of pyrimethamine against toxoplasmosis. Avoid use together.

Adverse reactions
CNS: general malaise.
Respiratory: *bronchospasm.*
Skin: allergic reactions (rash, pruritus, erythema).

Overdose and treatment
Folic acid is relatively nontoxic. Adverse GI and CNS effects have been reported rarely in patients receiving 15 mg of folic acid daily for 1 month.

Special considerations
● The RDA for folic acid is 25 to 200 mcg in children and 180 to 200 mcg in adults; 100 mcg daily is considered an adequate oral supplement. Pregnant women need 400 mcg daily. During the first 6 months of breast-feeding, women need 280 mcg daily. During the second 6 months, this requirement decreases to 260 mcg daily.
● The preferred route of administration for folic acid is P.O. The manufacturer recommends deep I.M., S.C., or I.V. only when P.O. treatment isn't feasible or when malabsorption is suspected.
● Patients undergoing renal dialysis are at risk for folate deficiency.
● Protect folic acid injections from light.

Patient monitoring
● Monitor CBC to measure effectiveness of drug treatment.

Pregnant patients
● Starting therapy before pregnancy may reduce risk of fetal neural tube defects.

Breast-feeding patients
● Folic acid appears in breast milk. Daily doses of 0.8 mg are sufficient to maintain a normoblastic bone marrow after clinical symptoms have subsided and blood components have returned to normal.

Patient education

● Advise patient of potential adverse reactions.

---

fomivirsen sodium
Vitravene

Pharmacologic classification: phosphoro-
thioate oligonucleotide
Therapeutic classification: antiviral
Pregnancy risk category: C

Indications and dosages

➤*Local treatment of cytomegalovirus
(CMV) retinitis in patients with AIDS,
who are intolerant of or have a contraindication to other treatments, or who
were insufficiently responsive to previous treatments. Adults:* Induction dose is
330 mcg (0.05 ml) by intravitreal injection every
other week for two doses. Subsequent maintenance dosage is 330 mcg (0.05 ml) by intravitreal injection once every 4 weeks after induction.

How supplied

Available by prescription only
Intravitreal injection: Preservative-free, single-
use vials containing 0.25 ml, 6.6 mg/ml

Pharmacodynamics

Antiviral action: Drug inhibits human CMV replication by binding to the target mRNA and subsequently inhibiting virus replication.

Pharmacokinetics

No information available.

Route	Onset	Peak	Duration
Intravitreal	Within hrs	Unknown	Unknown

Contraindications and precautions

Contraindicated in patients hypersensitive to drug
or its components and in those who have been
treated within 2 to 4 weeks with either I.V. or intravitreal cidofovir because of an increased risk
of exaggerated ocular inflammation.

Interactions

None reported.

Adverse reactions

CNS: asthenia, headache, abnormal thinking, depression, dizziness, neuropathy, pain.
CV: chest pain.
EENT: abnormal or blurred vision, anterior chamber inflammation, cataract, conjunctival hemorrhage, decreased visual acuity, desaturation of
color vision, eye pain, floaters, increased intraocular pressure, *ocular inflammation, iritis,* photophobia, retinal detachment, retinal edema, retinal hemorrhage, retinal pigment changes,
uveitis, vitritis, application site reaction, conjunctival hyperemia, conjunctivitis, corneal edema, decreased peripheral vision, eye irritation,

hypotony, keratic precipitates, optic neuritis, pho-
topsia, retinal vascular disease, visual field defect, vitreous hemorrhage, vitreous opacity, si-
nusitis.
GI: abdominal pain, anorexia, diarrhea, nausea,
vomiting, oral candidiasis, *pancreatitis.*
GU: catheter infection, *kidney failure.*
Hematologic: anemia, lymphoma-like reaction,
neutropenia, thrombocytopenia.
Hepatic: abnormal liver function test results, in-
creased GGT levels.
Metabolic: decreased weight, dehydration.
Musculoskeletal: back pain.
Respiratory: bronchitis, dyspnea, increased
cough, pneumonia.
Skin: rash, sweating.
Other: allergic reactions, cachexia, fever, flulike
syndrome, infection, *sepsis,* systemic CMV.

Overdose and treatment

None reported.

Special considerations

⚠ **ALERT** Drug is for ophthalmic use only by
intravitreal injection.
● Drug provides localized therapy limited to the
treated eye and doesn't provide treatment for systemic CMV disease.
● Ocular inflammation (uveitis) is most common
during induction dosing.

Patient monitoring

● Monitor light perception and optic nerve head
perfusion postinjection.
● Monitor patient for increased intraocular pressure. This is usually transient and returns to normal without treatment or with temporary use of
topical medications.
● Monitor patient for extraocular CMV disease or
disease in the contralateral eye.

Pregnant patients

● Safety and efficacy in pregnant women haven't
been reported.

Breast-feeding patients

● It isn't known whether drug appears in breast
milk. Discontinue drug or nursing.

Pediatric patients

● Safety and efficacy in children haven't been
established.

Geriatric patients

● Safety and efficacy in patients over age 65 haven't
been established.

Patient education

● Inform patient that drug doesn't cure CMV retinitis and that some patients continue to experience progression of retinitis during and following treatment.
● Tell patient that drug treats only the eye in which
it has been injected and that CMV may also exist

---

in the body. Stress importance of follow-up visits to monitor progress and to check for additional infections.
● Advise HIV-infected patient to continue taking antiretroviral therapy as indicated.

formoterol fumarate inhalation powder
Foradil Aerolizer

Pharmacologic classification: long-acting selective beta$_2$-adrenergic agonist
Therapeutic classification: bronchodilator
Pregnancy risk category: C

Indications and dosages
➤ *Prevention and maintenance treatment of bronchospasm in patients with reversible obstructive airway disease or nocturnal asthma, who usually need treatment with short-acting inhaled beta$_2$-adrenergic agonists. Adults and children age 5 and older:* One 12-mcg capsule by inhalation via Aerolizer inhaler every 12 hours. Total daily dose shouldn't exceed one capsule twice daily (24 mcg/day). If symptoms are present between doses, use a short-acting beta$_2$-adrenergic agonist for immediate relief.
➤ *Prevention of exercise-induced bronchospasm. Adults and children age 12 and older:* One 12-mcg capsule by inhalation via Aerolizer inhaler at least 15 minutes before exercise given occasionally, p.r.n. Avoid giving additional doses within 12 hours of first dose.

How supplied
Available by prescription only.
Capsules for inhalation: 12 mcg

Pharmacodynamics
Formoterol fumarate acts locally in the lung to cause bronchodilation via long-acting selective beta$_2$-adrenergic receptor agonist activity. Because some beta$_2$-adrenergic receptors are also present in the heart, adrenergic stimulation may occur in the CV system with use of formoterol. At a cellular level, formoterol stimulates intracellular adenyl cyclase, the enzyme responsible for catalyzing the conversion of ATP to cAMP. This increase in cAMP leads to relaxation of bronchial smooth muscle and inhibition of mediator release from mast cells.

Pharmacokinetics
Absorption: Rapidly absorbed into plasma. Drug levels peak within 5 minutes after a 120-mcg dose. Similar to other products for oral inhalation, most of inhaled dose is probably swallowed and absorbed from the GI tract.
Distribution: 61% to 64% bound to human plasma proteins.
Metabolism: Occurs primarily via direct glucuronidation and O-demethylation (involving

cytochrome P-450 isoenzymes 2D6, 2C19, 2C9, and 2A6). Doesn't appear to inhibit CYP-450 enzymes at therapeutic levels.
Excretion: 59% to 62% eliminated in urine and 32% to 34% eliminated in feces over 104 hours. When 12 to 24 mcg formoterol was administered to asthma patients, about 10% of total dose was excreted in urine as unchanged drug and about 15% to 18% was eliminated in urine as direct glucuronide conjugates of formoterol.

Route	Onset	Peak	Duration
Oral inhalation	≤15 min	1-3 hr	12 hr

Adverse reactions
CNS: tremor, dizziness, insomnia, nervousness, headache, fatigue, malaise.
CV: chest pain, angina, hypertension, hypotension, tachycardia, *arrhythmias,* palpitations.
EENT: dry mouth, tonsillitis, dysphonia.
GI: nausea.
Metabolic: hypokalemia, hyperglycemia, metabolic acidosis.
Musculoskeletal: muscle cramps.
Respiratory: bronchitis, chest infection, dyspnea.
Skin: rash.
Other: viral infection.

Interactions
Drug-drug. *Adrenergics:* Possible potentiation of sympathetic effects of formoterol. Use cautiously.
Beta blockers: Possible antagonized effects of beta agonists, causing bronchospasm in asthmatic patients. Avoid use except when benefit outweighs risks. Use cardioselective beta blockers with caution to minimize risk of bronchospasm.
Corticosteroids, diuretics, xanthine derivatives: Possible potentiation of hypokalemic effect of formoterol. Use cautiously.
MAO inhibitors, tricyclic antidepressants, and other drugs that prolong QT interval: Possible increased risk of ventricular arrhythmias. Use cautiously.
Non-potassium-sparing diuretics (such as loop or thiazide diuretics): Possible worsening of ECG changes or hypokalemia with beta agonists. Use cautiously and monitor patient closely.

Overdose and treatment
Signs and symptoms of overdose include excessive beta-adrenergic stimulation and exaggeration of adverse effects. Cardiac arrest and death may result.
    Treatment of overdose should include discontinuation of drug, cardiac monitoring, appropriate symptomatic relief or supportive therapy, and possibly judicious use of cardioselective beta blockers. It's unknown whether dialysis is beneficial.

Reactions may be *common,* uncommon, *life-threatening,* or COMMON AND LIFE-THREATENING.

Contraindications and precautions
Contraindicated in patients hypersensitive to drug or its components.

Use cautiously in patients with CV disease, particularly coronary insufficiency, cardiac arrhythmias, and hypertension, and in those who are unusually responsive to sympathomimetic amines. Also use cautiously in patients with diabetes mellitus because hyperglycemia and ketoacidosis have occurred rarely with use of beta agonists. Also use cautiously in patients with seizure disorders or thyrotoxicosis.

Special considerations
● Drug isn't indicated for patients able to control asthma symptoms with occasional use of inhaled, short-acting beta$_2$ agonists or for treatment of acute bronchospasm that needs immediate reversal with short-acting beta$_2$ agonists.
● Drug may be used with short-acting beta$_2$ agonists, inhaled corticosteroids, and theophylline therapy to manage asthma.
● Patients using drug twice daily shouldn't take additional doses to prevent exercise-induced bronchospasm.
● Don't use as a substitute for short-acting beta$_2$ agonists for immediate relief of bronchospasm, or as a substitute for inhaled or oral corticosteroids.
● Don't begin use in patients with rapidly deteriorating or significantly worsening asthma.
● If usual dose doesn't control symptoms of bronchoconstriction, and the patient's short-acting beta$_2$ agonist becomes less effective, reevaluate patient and treatment regimen.
● For patients formerly using regularly scheduled short-acting beta$_2$ agonists, use of the short-acting drug should be decreased to an as needed basis when long-acting formoterol therapy starts.
● Capsules should be given only by oral inhalation and used only with the Aerolizer inhaler. They aren't for oral ingestion. The patient shouldn't exhale into the device. Capsules should remain in the unopened blister until administration time and should be removed immediately before use.
● Before dispensing, drug should be stored in refrigerator. Once dispensed to patient, drug may be stored at room temperature.
● Don't use Foradil Aerolizer with a spacer device.
● Pierce capsules only once. In rare instances, the gelatin capsule may break into small pieces and enter the patient's mouth or throat with inhalation. However, the Aerolizer contains a screen that should catch any broken pieces before they leave the device. To minimize the possibility of shattering the capsule, strictly follow storage and use instructions.
● As with all beta$_2$ agonists, drug may produce life-threatening paradoxical bronchospasm. If this occurs, discontinue formoterol immediately and use an alternative drug.

Patient monitoring
● Monitor patient for tachycardia, hypertension, and other adverse CV effects. If they occur, drug may need to be discontinued.
● Watch for immediate hypersensitivity reactions, such as anaphylaxis, urticaria, angioedema, rash, and bronchospasm.

Breast-feeding patients
● It isn't known whether drug appears in breast milk. Use cautiously in breast-feeding women.

Pediatric patients
● Safety and efficacy in children under age 5 haven't been established.

Geriatric patients
● No overall differences in safety or efficacy have been observed in elderly patients. However, increased sensitivity of some elderly patients is possible.

Patient education
● Tell patient not to increase the dose or frequency of use without medical advice.
● Warn patient not to stop or reduce other medication taken for asthma.
● Advise patient that drug isn't for acute asthmatic episodes. A short-acting beta$_2$ agonist should be prescribed for this use.
● Advise patient to report worsening symptoms, less effective treatment, or increasing use of short-acting beta$_2$ agonist.
● Tell patient to report nausea, vomiting, shakiness, headache, fast or irregular heartbeat, or sleeplessness.
● Warn patient not to exceed the recommended daily dose.
● Tell patient being treated for exercise-induced bronchospasm to take drug at least 15 minutes before exercise. Additional doses can't be taken for 12 hours.
● Tell patient that adverse effects, such as palpitations, chest pain, rapid heart rate, tremor, and nervousness, may occur.
● Tell patient not to use the Foradil Aerolizer with a spacer device or to exhale or blow into the Aerolizer inhaler.
● Advise patient to avoid washing the Aerolizer and to always keep it dry. A new device comes with each refill. The new device should replace the old one.
● Tell patient to avoid exposing capsules to moisture and to handle them only with dry hands.
● Advise woman to notify prescriber if she becomes pregnant or is breast-feeding.

---

foscarnet sodium
(phosphonoformic acid)
Foscavir

Pharmacologic classification: pyrophosphate analogue
Therapeutic classification: antiviral
Pregnancy risk category: C

Indications and dosages
➤ *Cytomegalovirus (CMV) retinitis in patients with AIDS. Adults:* Initially, 90 mg/kg as an I.V. infusion (over 1.5 to 2 hours) q 12 hours or 60 mg/kg as an I.V. infusion (over 1 hour) q 8 hours for 2 to 3 weeks as an induction treatment in patients with normal renal function. Follow with a maintenance infusion of 90 to 120 mg/kg daily administered over 2 hours; increase as needed and tolerated to 120 mg/kg daily if disease shows signs of progression. Dose should be individualized based upon renal function.
➤ *Mucocutaneous acyclovir-resistant herpes simplex virus (HSV) infection. Adults:* 40 mg/kg I.V. Administer as an I.V. infusion over 1 hour q 8 to 12 hours for 2 to 3 weeks, depending on response.
✦ *Dosage adjustment.* For adult patients with renal impairment, calculate weight-adjusted creatinine clearance (ml/minute/kg):
For men:

$$\frac{\text{creatinine}}{\text{clearance}} = \frac{(140 - \text{age})}{(\text{serum creatinine} \times 72)};$$

For women: Multiply the above value by 0.85. Administer the drug according to the tables on the next page.

How supplied
Available by prescription only
Injection: 24 mg/ml in 250-ml and 500-ml vials

Pharmacodynamics
Antiviral action: An analogue of pyrophosphate (important in enzymatic reactions), drug inhibits known herpes viruses in vitro by blocking the pyrophosphate binding site on DNA polymerases and reverse transcriptases.

Pharmacokinetics
Absorption: Unknown.
Distribution: About 14% to 17% bound to plasma proteins; drug is deposited in bone.
Metabolism: Unknown.
Excretion: About 80% to 90% appears in urine unchanged. Drug clearance is dependent on renal function. Plasma half-life is about 3 hours.

Route	Onset	Peak	Duration
I.V.	Unknown	Immediate	Unknown

Contraindications and precautions
Contraindicated in patients hypersensitive to drug. Use extremely cautiously in patients with impaired renal function.

Interactions
Drug-drug. *Nephrotoxic drugs, such as amphotericin B and aminoglycosides:* Increased risk of nephrotoxicity. Avoid use together.
Pentamidine: Increased risk of nephrotoxicity; severe hypocalcemia has also been reported. Don't use together.
Zidovudine: Increased occurrence and severity of anemia. Monitor blood counts.

Adverse reactions
CNS: *headache, seizures,* fatigue, malaise, asthenia, paresthesia, dizziness, hypoesthesia, neuropathy, tremor, ataxia, generalized spasms, dementia, stupor, sensory disturbances, meningitis, aphasia, abnormal coordination, EEG abnormalities, depression, confusion, anxiety, insomnia, somnolence, nervousness, amnesia, agitation, aggressive reaction, hallucinations.
CV: *hypertension, palpitations, ECG abnormalities, sinus tachycardia,* cerebrovascular disorder, *first-degree AV block, hypotension, flushing,* edema.
EENT: sinusitis, pharyngitis, rhinitis, visual disturbances, eye pain, conjunctivitis.
GI: taste perversion, *nausea, diarrhea, vomiting, abdominal pain, anorexia,* constipation, dysphagia, rectal hemorrhage, dry mouth, dyspepsia, melena, flatulence, ulcerative stomatitis, *pancreatitis.*
GU: *abnormal renal function, decreased creatinine clearance and increased serum creatinine levels, albuminuria, dysuria, polyuria, urethral disorder, urine retention, urinary tract infections, acute renal failure,* candidiasis.
Hematologic: *anemia, granulocytopenia, leukopenia, bone marrow suppression, thrombocytopenia,* platelet abnormalities, thrombocytosis, WBC count abnormalities.
Hepatic: abnormal hepatic function, increased liver enzyme levels.
Metabolic: hypokalemia, hypomagnesemia, hypophosphatemia or hyperphosphatemia, hypocalcemia.
Musculoskeletal: leg cramps, back or chest pain, arthralgia, myalgia.
Respiratory: *cough, dyspnea,* pneumonitis, respiratory insufficiency, pulmonary infiltration, stridor, pneumothorax, *bronchospasm,* hemoptysis, flulike symptoms.
Skin: *rash, increased sweating,* pruritus, skin ulceration, erythematous rash, seborrhea, skin discoloration, facial edema.
Other: *fever,* lymphadenopathy, pain, infection, sepsis, rigors, inflammation and pain at infusion site, lymphoma-like disorder, sarcoma, bacterial or fungal infections, abscess.

Reactions may be *common,* uncommon, *life-threatening,* or COMMON AND LIFE-THREATENING.

Managing herpes simplex virus infection

Induction dose		
Creatinine clearance (ml/min/kg)	**Equivalent to 80 mg/kg/ day (40 mg/kg q 12 hr)**	**Equivalent to 120 mg/kg/ day (40 mg/kg q 8 hr)**
> 1.4	40 q 12 hr	40 q 8 hr
> 1.0 – 1.4	30 q 12 hr	30 q 8 hr
> 0.8 – 1.0	20 q 12 hr	35 q 12 hr
> 0.6 – 0.8	35 q 24 hr	25 q 12 hr
> 0.5 – 0.6	25 q 24 hr	40 q 24 hr
≥ 0.4 – 0.5	20 q 24 hr	35 q 24 hr
< 0.4	Not recommended	Not recommended

Managing cytomegalovirus infection

Induction dose		
Creatinine clearance (ml/min/kg)	**Equivalent to 180 mg/kg/ day (60 mg/kg q 8 hr)**	**Equivalent to 180 mg/kg/ day (90 mg/kg q 12 hr)**
> 1.4	60 q 8 hr	90 q 12 hr
> 1.0 – 1.4	45 q 8 hr	70 q 12 hr
> 0.8 – 1.0	50 q 12 hr	50 q 12 hr
> 0.6 – 0.8	40 q 12 hr	80 q 24 hr
> 0.5 – 0.6	60 q 24 hr	60 q 24 hr
≥ 0.4 – 0.5	50 q 24 hr	50 q 24 hr
< 0.4	Not recommended	Not recommended

Maintenance dose		
Creatinine clearance (ml/min/kg)	**Equivalent to 90 mg/kg/ day (Once daily)**	**Equivalent to 120 mg/kg/ day (Once daily)**
> 1.4	90 q 24 hr	120 q 24 hr
> 1.0 – 1.4	70 q 24 hr	90 q 24 hr
> 0.8 – 1.0	50 q 24 hr	65 q 24 hr
> 0.6 – 0.8	80 q 48 hr	105 q 48 hr
> 0.5 – 0.6	60 q 48 hr	80 q 48 hr
≥ 0.4 – 0.5	50 q 48 hr	65 q 48 hr
< 0.4	Not recommended	Not recommended

Special considerations

● Anemia is common (up to 33% of patients treated with drug) and may be severe enough to require transfusions.
● Don't exceed the recommended dosage, infusion rate, or frequency of administration. All doses must be individualized according to patient's renal function.
● An infusion pump must be used to administer foscarnet.
● Foscarnet may be active against certain CMV strains resistant to ganciclovir.

Patient monitoring

● Monitor renal function, and assess patient for anemia.

Breast-feeding patients

● It isn't known whether drug appears in breast milk; however, animal studies indicate that drug may concentrate in breast milk when given at high doses. Use cautiously.

Pediatric patients

● Safety and efficacy in children haven't been established. In animals, up to 40% of a dose is deposited in the teeth and bones; similar deposition may be seen in growing children.

Geriatric patients

● It isn't known whether age alters drug response. However, elderly patients are likely to have renal insufficiency, which requires alterations in dosage.

Patient education
• Warn patient of the high frequency of adverse reactions and the need for ongoing laboratory studies.
• Advise patient to report to prescriber perioral tingling, numbness in the limbs, and paresthesia.

fosfomycin tromethamine
Monurol

Pharmacologic classification: phosphonic acid derivative
Therapeutic classification: antibiotic
Pregnancy risk category: B

Indications and dosages
➤ *Uncomplicated urinary tract infections (acute cystitis) in women caused by susceptible strains of* Escherichia coli *and* Enterococcus faecalis. *Women over age 18:* 1 sachet P.O. mixed with 3 to 4 oz (½ cup) of cold water just before ingestion.

How supplied
Available by prescription only
Single-dose sachet: 3 g

Pharmacodynamics
Bactericidal action: Inhibits bacterial cell wall synthesis. It's effective in the urinary tract because it reduces adherence of bacteria to uroepithelial cells.

Pharmacokinetics
Absorption: Rapidly absorbed following oral administration and converted to free acid, fosfomycin. When drug is taken on empty stomach, levels peak within 2 hours; within 4 hours when taken with food.
Distribution: Mean apparent steady state volume of distribution is 136 L following oral administration. Not bound to plasma proteins; distributed to kidneys, bladder wall, prostate, and seminal vesicles. Crosses placenta.
Metabolism: Not reported.
Excretion: Excreted unchanged in both urine and feces.

Route	Onset	Peak	Duration
P.O.	Unknown	2-4 hr	Unknown

Contraindications and precautions
Contraindicated in patients hypersensitive to drug. Use cautiously in patients with renal impairment.

Interactions
Drug-drug. *Metoclopramide:* Lowers serum level and urinary excretion of fosfomycin. Avoid concomitant use.
Other drugs that increase GI motility: May increase GI effects. Monitor patient.

Adverse reactions
CNS: asthenia, dizziness, *headache.*
EENT: pharyngitis, rhinitis.
GI: abdominal pain, *diarrhea,* dyspepsia, nausea.
GU: dysmenorrhea, vaginitis.
Musculoskeletal: back pain.
Skin: rash.

Overdose and treatment
No cases of overdose have been reported. If overdose occurs, provide supportive and symptomatic treatment.

Special considerations
• Using more than one single-dose sachet to treat a single episode of acute cystitis won't improve success and may cause adverse reactions.

Patient monitoring
• Obtain urine specimens for culture and sensitivity before therapy and after completion.
• Monitor therapeutic response.

Breast-feeding patients
• It isn't known whether drug appears in breast milk. Because many drugs do, a decision should be made to either stop breast-feeding or drug.

Pediatric patients
• Safety and effectiveness in children age 12 and under haven't been established in well-controlled studies.

Geriatric patients
• There are no significant differences in drug effectiveness or safety in women age 65 or under compared with those over age 65.

Patient education
• Show patient how to properly take drug. The entire contents of a single-dose sachet should be mixed with 3 to 4 oz (½ cup) cold water, stirred to dissolve, and drunk immediately.
• Tell patient to call if symptoms don't improve in 2 to 3 days.
• Inform patient that drug may be taken without regard to food.

fosinopril sodium
Monopril

Pharmacologic classification: angiotensin-converting enzyme (ACE) inhibitor
Therapeutic classification: antihypertensive
Pregnancy risk category: C (D in second and third trimesters)

Indications and dosages
➤ *Treatment of hypertension. Adults:* Initially, 10 mg P.O. daily. Adjust dose based on blood pressure response at peak and trough levels. Usual dosage is 20 to 40 mg daily. Maximum, up to 80 mg daily. Dose may be divided.

➤ *Treatment of heart failure. Adults:* Initially, 10 mg P.O. daily. Maximum, up to 40 mg daily. Dose may be divided.

How supplied
Available by prescription only
Tablets: 10 mg, 20 mg, 40 mg

Pharmacodynamics
Antihypertensive action: Fosinopril is believed to lower blood pressure primarily by suppressing the renin-angiotensin-aldosterone system, although it also has been effective in patients with low-renin hypertension.

Pharmacokinetics
Absorption: Absorbed slowly through GI tract, primarily via proximal small intestine.
Distribution: More than 95% is protein-bound.
Metabolism: Hydrolyzed primarily in the liver and gut wall by esterases.
Excretion: Part of drug (50%) is excreted in urine, the remainder in feces.

Route	Onset	Peak	Duration
P.O.	1 hr	3 hr	24 hr

Contraindications and precautions
Contraindicated in patients hypersensitive to drug or other ACE inhibitors and in breast-feeding women. Use cautiously in those patients with impaired renal or hepatic function and in those with history of angioedema, hypotension, or hyperkalemia.

Interactions
Drug-drug. *Antacids:* May impair fosinopril absorption; separate administration by at least 2 hours.
Diuretics and other antihypertensives: Excessive hypotension may occur. Effect may be minimized by stopping diuretic.
Lithium: Increased serum lithium levels and possible lithium toxicity. Monitor lithium levels frequently.
Potassium supplements, potassium-sparing diuretics: Increased risk of hyperkalemia. Monitor potassium levels.
Drug-herb. *Capsaicin:* Increased risk of cough. Discourage concomitant use.
Drug-food. *Salt substitutes containing potassium:* Risk of hyperkalemia. Advise patient to avoid use of potassium salt substitutes.

Adverse reactions
CNS: headache, dizziness, fatigue, syncope, paresthesia, sleep disturbance, *CVA.*
CV: chest pain, angina, *MI,* rhythm disturbances, palpitations, hypotension, orthostatic hypotension.
EENT: tinnitus, sinusitis.
GI: nausea, vomiting, diarrhea, *pancreatitis,* dry mouth, abdominal distention, abdominal pain, constipation.

GU: sexual dysfunction, increased BUN and serum creatinine levels, renal insufficiency.
Hematologic: decreased hematocrit or hemoglobin levels, *neutropenia, agranulocytosis.*
Hepatic: elevated liver function test results, *hepatitis.*
Metabolic: hyperkalemia.
Musculoskeletal: arthralgia, musculoskeletal pain, myalgia, gout.
Respiratory: *dry, persistent, tickling, nonproductive cough; bronchospasm.*
Skin: urticaria, rash, photosensitivity, pruritus.
Other: decreased libido, *angioedema.*

Overdose and treatment
Overdose hasn't been reported; however, the most common sign of overdose is likely to be hypotension.

Treat with infusion of normal saline. Hemodialysis and peritoneal dialysis aren't effective in removing the drug.

Special considerations
● Diuretic therapy is usually discontinued 2 to 3 days before ACE inhibitor therapy starts to reduce risk of hypotension. If fosinopril doesn't adequately control blood pressure, diuretic may resume with care.
● Risk of orthostatic hypotension is low.
● Blood pressure is lowered within 1 hour of a single dose of 10 to 40 mg.
● False low measurements of digoxin levels may result with the DIGI TAB radioimmunoassay kit for digoxin; other kits may be used.

Patient monitoring
● Monitor potassium levels and renal function.
● Perform CBC with differential counts before therapy, and then every 2 weeks for 3 months and periodically thereafter.

Breast-feeding patients
● Avoid drug in breast-feeding patients; significant levels appear in breast milk.

Pediatric patients
● Safety and efficacy in children haven't been established.

Geriatric patients
● No age-related differences have been observed.

Patient education
● Tell patient to take dose 1 hour before or 2 hours after food or antacids.
● Advise patient to report light-headedness in the first few days of therapy and signs of infection such as fever or sore throat. Tell patient to stop drug immediately and notify prescriber about swelling of tongue, lips, face, mucous membranes, eyes, or limbs; difficulty swallowing or breathing; or hoarseness.
● Advise patient to maintain the same salt intake as before therapy, because salt restriction can

lead to precipitous decrease in blood pressure with initial doses. Large reductions in blood pressure may also occur with excessive perspiration and dehydration.

● Warn patient to avoid sudden position changes until effect of drug is known; however, orthostatic hypotension is infrequent.

---

fosphenytoin sodium
Cerebyx

Pharmacologic classification: hydantoin derivative
Therapeutic classification: anticonvulsant
Pregnancy risk category: D

Indications and dosages
➤ *Status epilepticus. Adults:* 15 to 20 mg phenytoin sodium equivalent (PE)/kg I.V. at 100 to 150 PE/minute as a loading dose and then 4 to 6 mg PE/kg I.V. daily as a maintenance dosage. (Phenytoin may be used instead of fosphenytoin as maintenance using the appropriate dose.)
➤ *Prevention and treatment of seizures during neurosurgery. Adults:* 10 to 20 mg PE/kg I.M. or I.V. at an I.V. infusion rate not exceeding 150 mg PE/minute as a loading dose. Maintenance dosage is 4 to 6 mg PE/kg I.V. daily.
➤ *Short-term substitution for oral phenytoin therapy. Adults:* Same total daily dose as oral phenytoin sodium therapy given as a single daily dose I.M. or I.V. at an I.V. infusion rate not exceeding 150 mg PE/minute. (Some patients may need more frequent dosing.)

How supplied
Available by prescription only
Injection: 2 ml (150 mg fosphenytoin sodium equivalent to 100 mg phenytoin sodium), 10 ml (750 mg fosphenytoin sodium equivalent to 500 mg phenytoin sodium)

Pharmacodynamics
Anticonvulsant action: Because fosphenytoin is a prodrug of phenytoin, its anticonvulsant action is that of phenytoin. Phenytoin stabilizes neuronal membranes and limits seizure activity by modulating voltage-dependent sodium channels of neurons, inhibiting calcium flux across neuronal membranes, modulating voltage-dependent calcium channels of neurons, and enhancing sodium-potassium adenosine triphosphatase activity of neurons and glial cells.

Pharmacokinetics
Absorption: No information available.
Distribution: About 95% to 99% is bound to plasma proteins, primarily albumin. Volume of distribution increases with dose and rate and ranges from 4.3 to 10.8 L.
Metabolism: Conversion half-life of fosphenytoin to phenytoin is about 15 minutes. Phosphatases are believed to play a major role in the conversion.
Excretion: Unknown, although it isn't excreted in urine.

Route	Onset	Peak	Duration
I.V.	Unknown	End of infusion	Unknown
I.M.	Unknown	30 min	Unknown

Contraindications and precautions
Contraindicated in patients hypersensitive to drug, its components, phenytoin, or other hydantoins. Also contraindicated in patients with sinus bradycardia, SA block, second- and third-degree AV block, and Adams-Stokes syndrome because of the effect of parenteral phenytoin on ventricular automaticity.

Use cautiously in patients with hypotension, severe myocardial insufficiency, impaired renal or hepatic function, hypoalbuminemia, porphyria, diabetes mellitus, and history of hypersensitivity to similarly structured drugs, such as barbiturates and succinimides.

Interactions
Drug-drug. *Amiodarone, chloramphenicol, chlordiazepoxide, cimetidine, diazepam, dicumarol, disulfiram, estrogens, ethosuximide, fluoxetine, H₂-receptor antagonists, halothane, isoniazid, methylphenidate, phenothiazines, phenylbutazone, salicylates, succinimides, sulfonamides, tolbutamide, trazodone:* Increased plasma phenytoin levels. Monitor patient carefully.
Carbamazepine, reserpine: Plasma phenytoin levels may be decreased. Use together cautiously.
Coumarin, digitoxin, doxycycline, estrogens, furosemide, oral contraceptives, rifampin, quinidine, theophylline, vitamin D: Efficacy may be decreased by phenytoin because of increased hepatic metabolism. Monitor patient carefully.
Phenobarbital, sodium valproate, valproic acid: Altered phenytoin levels. Monitor patient closely.
Tricyclic antidepressants: Lower seizure threshold. Adjust phenytoin dosage as needed.
Drug-lifestyle. *Acute alcohol use:* Increased phenytoin levels. Advise patient to avoid alcohol.
Long-term alcohol use: Decreased phenytoin levels. Advise patient to avoid alcohol.

Adverse reactions
CNS: increased or decreased reflexes, speech disorders, dysarthria, asthenia, *intracranial hypertension, cerebral hemorrhage,* thinking abnormalities, nervousness, hypesthesia, extrapyramidal syndrome, brain edema, headache, *nystagmus, dizziness, somnolence, ataxia,* stupor, incoordination, paresthesia, agitation, tremor, vertigo.
CV: hypertension, *cardiac arrest,* palpitations, *bradycardia,* atrial flutter, *bundle branch block,* cardiomegaly, orthostatic hypotension,

---

Reactions may be *common,* uncommon, *life-threatening,* or COMMON AND LIFE-THREATENING.

pulmonary embolus, QT interval prolongation, thrombophlebitis, ventricular extrasystoles, *heart failure*, vasodilation, tachycardia, hypotension.

EENT: epistaxis, pharyngitis, sinusitis, deafness, visual field defect, eye pain, conjunctivitis, photophobia, hyperacusis, mydriasis, parosmia, ear pain, tinnitus, diplopia, amblyopia.

GI: taste loss, taste perversion, constipation, dyspepsia, diarrhea, anorexia, GI hemorrhage, increased salivation, tenesmus, tongue edema, dysphagia, flatulence, gastritis, ileus, nausea, dry mouth, vomiting.

GU: urine retention, oliguria, dysuria, vaginitis, albuminuria, genital edema, kidney failure, polyuria, urethral pain, urinary incontinence, vaginal candidiasis.

Hematologic: *thrombocytopenia,* anemia, leukocytosis, hypochromic anemia, *leukopenia, agranulocytosis, granulocytopenia, pancytopenia,* ecchymoses.

Hepatic: elevated liver enzyme levels.

Metabolic: diabetes insipidus, hypokalemia, hyperglycemia, hypophosphatemia, alkalosis, acidosis, dehydration, hyperkalemia, ketosis, decreased serum levels of T_4.

Musculoskeletal: myasthenia, myopathy, leg cramps, arthralgia, myalgia, pelvic pain, back pain.

Respiratory: cyanosis, pneumonia, hyperventilation, rhinitis, *apnea,* aspiration pneumonia, asthma, dyspnea, atelectasis, increased cough, increased sputum, hypoxia, pneumothorax, hemoptysis, bronchitis.

Skin: petechia, rash, maculopapular rash, urticaria, sweating, skin discoloration, contact dermatitis, pustular rash, skin nodule, *pruritus.*

Other: lymphadenopathy.

Overdose and treatment

There have been no reports of fosphenytoin overdose. However, because it is a prodrug of phenytoin, overdose may be similar. Early signs and symptoms of phenytoin overdose may include drowsiness, nausea, vomiting, nystagmus, ataxia, dysarthria, tremor, and slurred speech; hypotension, respiratory depression, and coma may follow. Death is caused by respiratory and circulatory depression. Estimated lethal dose of phenytoin in adults is 2 to 5 g.

Formate and phosphate are metabolites of fosphenytoin and, therefore, may contribute to evidence of toxicity following overdose. Signs and symptoms of formate toxicity are similar to those of methanol toxicity and are associated with severe anion-gap metabolic acidosis. Large amounts of phosphate, delivered rapidly, could potentially cause hypocalcemia with paresthesia, muscle spasms, and seizures. Ionized free calcium levels can be measured and, if low, used to guide treatment.

Treatment is with gastric lavage or emesis and followed by supportive treatment. Monitor vital signs and fluid and electrolyte balance. Forced diuresis is of little or no value. Hemodialysis or peritoneal dialysis may be helpful.

Special considerations

● Always prescribe and dispense fosphenytoin in PE units. Don't make adjustments in the recommended doses when substituting fosphenytoin for phenytoin and vice versa.

● Administer dose of I.V. fosphenytoin used to treat status epilepticus at a maximum of 150 mg PE/minute. The typical infusion for a 50-kg (110-lb) patient takes 5 to 7 minutes, whereas that of an identical molar dose of phenytoin can't be accomplished in less than 15 to 20 minutes because of the untoward CV effects that accompany the direct I.V. administration of phenytoin at rates of more than 50 mg/minute.

● If rapid phenytoin loading is a primary goal, I.V. administration of fosphenytoin is preferred because the time to achieve therapeutic plasma phenytoin levels is greater following I.M. than that following I.V. administration.

● Patients receiving fosphenytoin at doses of 20 mg PE/kg at 150 mg PE/minute are expected to experience some sensory discomfort, with the groin being the most common location. The occurrence and intensity of the discomfort can be lessened by slowing or temporarily stopping the infusion.

● The phosphate load provided by fosphenytoin (0.0037 mmol phosphate/mg PE fosphenytoin) must be taken into consideration when treating patients who require phosphate restriction, such as those with severe renal impairment.

● Discontinue drug in patients with acute hepatotoxicity and don't readminister to these patients.

● I.M. drug administration generates systemic phenytoin levels similar enough to oral phenytoin sodium to allow essentially interchangeable use.

● A dose of 15 to 20 mg PE/kg of fosphenytoin infused I.V. at 100 to 150 mg PE/minute yields plasma-free phenytoin levels over time that approximate those achieved when an equivalent dose of phenytoin sodium (such as parenteral dilantin) is administered at 50 mg/minute I.V.

● Interpretation of total phenytoin plasma levels should be made cautiously in patients with renal or hepatic disease or hypoalbuminemia due to an increased fraction in unbound phenytoin. Unbound phenytoin levels may be more useful in these patients. Also, these patients are at increased risk for both the frequency and severity of adverse reactions when fosphenytoin is administered I.V.

● Fosphenytoin may produce artificially low results in dexamethasone or metyrapone tests.

Patient monitoring

● Monitor patient's ECG, blood pressure, and respiration continuously throughout the period of maximum serum phenytoin levels, about 10 to 20 minutes after the end of fosphenytoin infusion. Severe CV complications are most common in elderly or gravely ill patients. Reduction in rate of administration or discontinuation of dosing may be needed.

• Discontinue drug if rash appears. If rash is exfoliative, purpuric, or bullous or if lupus erythematosus, Stevens-Johnson syndrome, or toxic epidermal necrolysis is suspected, don't resume drug use; seek alternative therapy. If rash is mild (measles-like or scarlatiniform), therapy may be resumed after rash has disappeared. If rash recurs when therapy resumes, further fosphenytoin or phenytoin administration is contraindicated.

• Following drug use, phenytoin levels shouldn't be monitored until conversion to phenytoin is essentially complete; about 2 hours after the end of an I.V. infusion or 4 hours after I.M. administration.

Breast-feeding patients
• Because it isn't known whether fosphenytoin appears in breast milk, breast-feeding isn't recommended.

Pediatric patients
• Safety and efficacy in children haven't been established.

Geriatric patients
• Geriatric patients metabolize and excrete phenytoin slowly; therefore, administer fosphenytoin cautiously to older adults.

Patient education
• Warn patient that sensory disturbances may occur with I.V. drug administration.
• Tell patient to report adverse reactions, especially rash, immediately.

furosemide
Apo-Furosemide*, Lasix, Lasix Special*, Novosemide*, Uritol*

Pharmacologic classification: loop diuretic
Therapeutic classification: diuretic, antihypertensive
Pregnancy risk category: C

Indications and dosages
➤ *Acute pulmonary edema. Adults:* 40 mg I.V. injected slowly; then 80 mg I.V. within 1 hour, p.r.n.
Infants and children: 1 mg/kg I.M. or I.V. q 2 hours until response is achieved; maximum dose is 6 mg/kg daily.
➤ *Edema. Adults:* 20 to 80 mg P.O. daily in morning, with second dose given in 6 to 8 hours, carefully adjusted up to 600 mg daily, p.r.n. Or, 20 to 40 mg I.M. or I.V. Increased by 20 mg q 2 hours until desired response is achieved. I.V. dosage should be given slowly over 1 to 2 minutes.

Infants and children: 2 mg/kg daily P.O., increased by 1 to 2 mg/kg in 6 to 8 hours, p.r.n., carefully adjusted not to exceed 6 mg/kg daily.
➤ *Hypertension. Adults:* 40 mg P.O. b.i.d. Adjust dosage according to response.
➤ *Hypercalcemia ◇. Adults:* 80 to 100 mg I.V. q 1 to 2 hours. Or, 120 mg P.O. daily.
✦ *Dosage adjustment.* Reduced dosages may be indicated in elderly patients.

How supplied
Available by prescription only
Injection: 10 mg/ml
Solution: 10 mg/ml, 40 mg/5 ml
Tablets: 20 mg, 40 mg, 80 mg

Pharmacodynamics
Diuretic action: Loop diuretics inhibit sodium and chloride reabsorption in the proximal part of the ascending loop of Henle, promoting the excretion of sodium, water, chloride, and potassium.
Antihypertensive action: This drug effect may be the result of renal and peripheral vasodilatation and a temporary increase in glomerular filtration rate and a decrease in peripheral vascular resistance.

Pharmacokinetics
Absorption: About 60% of a dose is absorbed from the GI tract after oral administration. Food delays oral absorption but doesn't alter diuretic response. Diuresis begins in 30 to 60 minutes and peaks 1 to 2 hours after oral administration. Diuresis follows I.V. administration within 5 minutes and peaks in 20 to 60 minutes.
Distribution: About 95% is plasma protein–bound. It crosses the placenta and appears in breast milk.
Metabolism: Metabolized minimally by the liver.
Excretion: About 50% to 80% of a dose is excreted in urine; plasma half-life is about 30 minutes. Duration of action is 6 to 8 hours after oral administration and about 2 hours after I.V. administration.

Route	Onset	Peak	Duration
P.O.	20-30 min	1-2 hr	6-8 hr
I.V.	5 min	½ hr	2 hr

Contraindications and precautions
Contraindicated in patients hypersensitive to drug and patients with anuria, hepatic coma, or severe electrolyte depletion. Contraindicated if increased azotemia, oliguria, or progressive renal disease occur during therapy. Use cautiously in pregnant patients and those with hepatic cirrhosis.

Interactions
Drug-drug. *Aminoglycoside antibiotics, cisplatin, ethacrynic acid:* May potentiate ototoxicity. Don't use together.

Reactions may be *common*, uncommon, **life-threatening**, or COMMON AND LIFE-THREATENING.

Amphotericin B, corticosteroids, corticotropin, metolazone: Increased risk of hypokalemia. Monitor potassium levels.

Antidiabetics: Decreased hypoglycemic effects. Monitor glucose levels.

Antihypertensives: Increased risk of hypotension. Check blood pressure frequently.

Cardiac glycosides, lithium, neuromuscular blockers: Increased risk of toxicity. Monitor potassium levels.

NSAIDs: May inhibit diuretic response. Use together cautiously.

Salicylates: May cause salicylate toxicity. Use together cautiously.

Sucralfate: May reduce diuretic and antihypertensive effect. Separate administration by 2 hours.

Drug-herb. *Aloe:* May increase drug effects. Tell patient to use together cautiously.

Dandelion: Possible interference with diuretic activity. Discourage concomitant use.

Ginseng: Decreased effect of the loop diuretic. Discourage concomitant use.

Drug-lifestyle. *Sun exposure:* Potentiates photosensitivity reactions. Advise patient to take precautions.

Adverse reactions

CNS: vertigo, headache, dizziness, paresthesia, restlessness.

CV: volume depletion and dehydration, orthostatic hypotension.

EENT: transient deafness with too-rapid I.V. injection, blurred vision.

GI: abdominal discomfort and pain, diarrhea, anorexia, nausea, vomiting, constipation, *pancreatitis.*

GU: nocturia, polyuria, frequent urination, altered renal function test results, oliguria.

Hematologic: *agranulocytosis, leukopenia, thrombocytopenia,* azotemia, anemia, *aplastic anemia.*

Hepatic: altered liver function test results.

Metabolic: hypokalemia; hypochloremic alkalosis; asymptomatic hyperuricemia; fluid and electrolyte imbalances, including dilutional hyponatremia, hypocalcemia, hypomagnesemia; hyperglycemia; impaired glucose tolerance.

Musculoskeletal: muscle spasm, weakness.

Skin: dermatitis, purpura.

Other: fever, transient pain at I.M. injection site, thrombophlebitis with I.V. administration.

Overdose and treatment

Signs and symptoms of overdose include profound electrolyte and volume depletion, which may precipitate circulatory collapse.

Treatment is chiefly supportive; replace fluids and electrolytes.

Special considerations

Consider the recommendations relevant to all loop diuretics as well as the following.

● Give I.V. furosemide slowly, over 1 to 2 minutes. For I.V. infusion, dilute furosemide in D_5W,

normal saline solution, or lactated Ringer's solution, and use within 24 hours. If high-dose furosemide therapy is needed, administer as a controlled infusion not exceeding 4 mg/minute.

● Sorbitol content of oral preparations may cause diarrhea, especially at high doses.

Patient monitoring

● Monitor serum potassium and CBC before treatment and periodically throughout therapy.

● Monitor patient for adverse effects.

Pregnant patients

● Use cautiously during pregnancy.

Breast-feeding patients

● Drug shouldn't be used by breast-feeding women.

Pediatric patients

● Use drug cautiously in neonates. The usual pediatric dosage can be used, but extend dosing intervals.

Geriatric patients

● Elderly and debilitated patients need close observation because they're more susceptible to drug-induced diuresis. Excessive diuresis promotes rapid dehydration, leading to hypovolemia, hypokalemia, hyponatremia, and circulatory collapse.

Patient education

● Warn patient that photosensitivity reaction may occur. Explain that reaction is a photoallergy in which ultraviolet radiation alters drug structure, causing allergic reactions in some people.

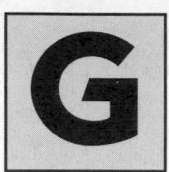

gabapentin
Neurontin

Pharmacologic classification: 1-amino-methyl cyclohexoneacetic acid
Therapeutic classification: anticonvulsant
Pregnancy risk category: C

Indications and dosages
➤*Adjunctive treatment of partial seizures with and without secondary generalization.* *Adults and children age 13 and older:* 300 mg P.O. on day 1, 300 mg P.O. b.i.d. on day 2, and 300 mg P.O. t.i.d. on day 3. Increased as needed and tolerated to 1,800 mg daily, given in three divided doses. Usual dose is 300 to 600 mg P.O. t.i.d., although doses up to 3,600 mg daily have been well tolerated.
Children ages 3 to 12: 10 to 15 mg/kg daily P.O. in three divided doses. Effective dose in children age 5 and older is 25 to 35 mg/kg daily P.O. in three divided doses. Effective dose in children ages 3 to 4 is 40 mg/kg daily P.O. in three divided doses. Doses up to 50 mg/kg daily have been well tolerated.
✦*Dosage adjustment.* In patients age 12 and older with compromised renal function and in patients receiving hemodialysis, use the following dosage guide.

Creatinine clearance (ml/min)	Dosage
> 60	400 mg P.O. t.i.d.
30-60	300 mg P.O. b.i.d.
15-30	300 mg P.O. daily
< 15	300 mg P.O. every other day

Hemodialysis patients who have never received gabapentin should receive a loading dose of 300 to 400 mg P.O. and 200 mg to 300 mg P.O. after each 4 hours of hemodialysis.
➤*Neuropathic pain ◊.* *Adults and children age 12 and older:* 300 mg P.O. t.i.d. titrated weekly to maximum dose of 1800 mg/day.

How supplied
Available by prescription only
Capsules: 100 mg, 300 mg, 400 mg
Oral solution: 250 mg/5 ml
Tablets: 600 mg, 800 mg

Pharmacodynamics
Anticonvulsant action: Mechanism of action is unknown. Although it's structurally related to gamma-aminobutyric acid (GABA), drug doesn't interact with GABA receptors, isn't converted metabolically into GABA or a GABA agonist, and doesn't inhibit GABA uptake or degradation. Gabapentin exhibits no affinity for other common receptor sites.

Pharmacokinetics
Absorption: Bioavailability isn't dose proportional. A 400-mg dose, for example, is about 25% less bioavailable than a 100-mg dose. Over the recommended dose range of 300 to 600 mg t.i.d., however, differences in bioavailability aren't large, and bioavailability is about 60%. Food has no effect on the rate or extent of absorption.
Distribution: Drug circulates largely unbound (less than 3%) to plasma protein. It crosses the blood-brain barrier with about 20% of the corresponding plasma levels found in CSF.
Metabolism: Not appreciably metabolized in humans.
Excretion: Eliminated from systemic circulation by renal excretion as unchanged drug. Elimination half-life is 5 to 7 hours. Drug can be removed from plasma by hemodialysis.

Route	Onset	Peak	Duration
P.O.	Unknown	Unknown	Unknown

Contraindications and precautions
Contraindicated in patients hypersensitive to drug. Use cautiously in patients with altered renal function due to drug accumulation.

Interactions
Drug-drug. *Antacids:* Decreased gabapentin absorption. Separate administration by at least 2 hours.

Adverse reactions
CNS: *fatigue, somnolence, dizziness, ataxia, tremor,* nervousness, dysarthria, amnesia, depression, abnormal thinking, twitching, incoordination.
CV: peripheral edema, vasodilation.
EENT: *diplopia, rhinitis,* pharyngitis, dry throat, coughing, dental abnormalities, *amblyopia, nystagmus.*
GI: nausea, vomiting, dyspepsia, dry mouth, constipation, increased appetite.
GU: impotence.

Reactions may be *common*, uncommon, *life-threatening*, or COMMON AND LIFE-THREATENING.

Hematologic: *leukopenia,* decreased WBC count.
Metabolic: weight gain.
Musculoskeletal: back pain, myalgia, fractures.
Skin: pruritus, abrasion.

Overdose and treatment

Acute gabapentin overdose may cause double vision, slurred speech, drowsiness, lethargy, and diarrhea.

Supportive care is recommended. Gabapentin can be removed by hemodialysis and may be indicated by the patient's clinical state or by presence of significant renal impairment.

Special considerations

• Don't withdraw other anticonvulsants suddenly in patients starting gabapentin therapy. Discontinue drug therapy or substitute alternative drug gradually over at least 1 week to minimize risk of seizures.
• Drug can be taken without regard to meals.

Patient monitoring

• Routine monitoring of plasma drug levels isn't necessary. Drug doesn't appear to alter plasma levels of other anticonvulsants.
• Gabapentin causes false-positive results on Ames N-Multistix SG dipstick test for urinary protein when added to other antiepileptic drugs. The more specific sulfosalicylic acid precipitation procedure is recommended to determine the presence of urine protein.

Pregnant patients

• Data concerning use during pregnancy is inadequate; however, gabapentin is teratogenic in mice and rats.

Breast-feeding patients

• It isn't known whether drug appears in breast milk. Discontinue breast-feeding if gabapentin therapy starts because of potential for serious adverse reactions.

Pediatric patients

• Safety and efficacy in children under age 12 haven't been established.

Patient education

• Instruct patient to take first dose at bedtime to minimize effects of drowsiness, dizziness, fatigue, and ataxia.
• Warn patient to avoid driving or operating heavy machinery until adverse CNS effects of drug are known.
• Inform patient that drug can be taken without regard to meals.

galantamine hydrobromide
Reminyl

Pharmacologic classification: reversible, competitive acetylcholinesterase inhibitor
Therapeutic classification: cholinomimetic
Pregnancy risk category: B

Indications and dosages

➤ *Mild to moderate dementia of Alzheimer's type.* Adults: Initially, 4 mg twice daily, preferably with morning and evening meals. If dose is well tolerated after minimum of 4 weeks of therapy, increase dose to 8 mg twice daily. A further increase to 12 mg twice daily may be attempted but only after at least 4 weeks of therapy at the previous dose. Recommended dosage range is 16 to 24 mg daily in two divided doses.
✦ *Dosage adjustment.* For patients with moderately impaired hepatic function (Child-Pugh score of 7 to 9), dose usually shouldn't exceed 16 mg daily. For patients with severe hepatic impairment (Child-Pugh score of 10 to 15), drug isn't recommended. For patients with moderate renal impairment, dose usually shouldn't exceed 16 mg daily. For patients with severe renal impairment (creatinine clearance < 9 ml/minute), drug isn't recommended.

How supplied

Available by prescription only
Tablets: 4 mg, 8 mg, 12 mg

Pharmacodynamics

Exact mechanism of action is unknown. Drug is a competitive and reversible inhibitor of acetylcholinesterase, which is believed to enhance cholinergic function by increasing the level of acetylcholine in the brain.

Pharmacokinetics

Absorption: Rapidly and well absorbed, with an oral bioavailability of about 90%. Levels peak in about 1 hour. In elderly patients, drug levels are 30% to 40% higher than in young healthy people.
Distribution: Primarily distributed to blood cells. Protein-binding isn't significant.
Metabolism: Metabolized in the liver by cytochrome P-450 enzymes (CYP2D6 and CYP3A4) and glucuronidated. Concurrent therapy with inhibitors of these enzyme systems may result in modest increases in bioavailability of galantamine.
Excretion: Excreted in urine unchanged, as the glucuronide, and as metabolites. Terminal half-life is about 7 hours.

Route	Onset	Peak	Duration
P.O.	Unknown	1 hr	Unknown

Adverse reactions

CNS: dizziness, headache, tremor, depression, insomnia, somnolence, fatigue, syncope.

CV: *bradycardia.*
EENT: rhinitis.
GI: *nausea, vomiting,* anorexia, *diarrhea,* abdominal pain, dyspepsia, anorexia.
GU: urinary tract infection, hematuria.
Hematologic: anemia.
Metabolic: weight loss.

Interactions
Drug-drug. *Amitriptyline, fluoxetine, fluvoxamine, quinidine:* Decreased galantamine clearance. Monitor patient closely.
Anticholinergics: Possible antagonized anticholinerigic activity. Monitor patient.
Cholinergics (such as bethanechol, succinylcholine): Synergistic effect. Monitor patient closely. May need to avoid use before procedures using general anesthesia with succinylcholine-type neuromuscular blockers.
Cimetidine, erythromycin, ketoconazole, paroxetine: Increased galantamine bioavailability. Monitor patient closely.

Overdose and treatment
Signs and symptoms of overdose are similar to those of other cholinergics and generally involve the CNS, parasympathetic nervous system, and neuromuscular junctions. In addition to muscle weakness or fasciculations, some or all of the following signs of cholinergic crisis may be present: severe nausea, vomiting, GI cramping, salivation, lacrimation, urination, defecation, sweating, bradycardia, hypotension, respiratory depression, collapse, and seizures. Increasing muscle weakness is possible and may result in death if respiratory muscles are involved.

Contact a poison control center for the latest recommendations for the management of a drug overdose. Treatment is supportive and symptomatic. Atropine I.V. may be used as an antidote for galantamine overdose. An initial dose of 0.5 to 1 mg is recommended, with subsequent doses based on clinical response. It's unknown whether drug is removed by dialysis.

Contraindications and precautions
Contraindicated in patients hypersensitive to drug or its components.

Use cautiously in patients with supraventricular cardiac conduction disorders and in those taking other drugs that significantly slow heart rate. Use cautiously during or before procedures involving anesthesia using succinylcholine-type or similar neuromuscular blockers. Also use cautiously in patients with history of peptic ulcer disease and in those taking NSAIDs. Because of the potential for cholinomimetic effects, use cautiously in patients with bladder outflow obstruction, seizures, asthma, or COPD.

Special considerations
• Bradycardia and heart block have been reported in patients with and without underlying cardiac

conduction abnormalities. Consider all patients at risk for adverse effects on cardiac conduction.
• Give drug with food and antiemetics and ensure adequate fluid intake to decrease the risk of nausea and vomiting.
• If drug is stopped for several days or longer, it should be restarted at the lowest dose and increased, at 4-week intervals or longer, to the previous dosage level.

Patient monitoring
• Because of the risk of increased gastric acid secretion, monitor patients closely for symptoms of active or occult GI bleeding, especially those with an increased risk of developing ulcers.

Breast-feeding patients
• It isn't known whether drug appears in breast milk. There's no indication for use in breast-feeding mothers.

Pediatric patients
• Safety and efficacy in children haven't been established.

Geriatric patients
• No specific dosage adjustments are needed for elderly patients.

Patient education
• Advise patient to take drug with morning and evening meals.
• Tell patient that dosage increases should occur no more often than every 4 weeks.
• Inform patient that nausea and vomiting are common adverse effects.
• Advise patient that the most common adverse effects can be minimized by following the recommended dosing and administration schedule.
• Tell patient that, if therapy is interrupted for several days or longer, drug should be restarted at the lowest dose and increased based on the recommended dosing schedule.
• Urge patient to report bradycardia immediately.
• Advise patient that drug is believed to enhance cognitive function, but there's no evidence that it alters the underlying disease process.

ganciclovir (DHPG)
Cytovene

Pharmacologic classification: synthetic nucleoside
Therapeutic classification: antiviral
Pregnancy risk category: C

Indications and dosages
➤ *Treatment of cytomegalovirus (CMV) retinitis.* **Adults:** Initially, 5 mg/kg I.V. (given at a constant rate over 1 hour) q 12 hours for 14 to 21 days; followed by a maintenance dosage of 5 mg/kg I.V. once daily for 7 days weekly or 6 mg/kg I.V. once daily for 5 days weekly. These

I.V. infusions should be given at a constant rate over 1 hour. Or, a maintenance dosage of 1,000 mg P.O. t.i.d. or 500 mg P.O. q 3 hours while awake (six times daily) may be used.

➤ *Prevention of CMV in transplant recipients.* Adults: 5 mg/kg I.V. over 1 hour q 12 hours for 7 to 14 days, followed by a maintenance dosage of 5 mg/kg once daily for 7 days weekly or 6 mg/kg once daily for 5 days weekly.

➤ *Other CMV infections*◇. Adults: 5 mg/kg I.V. over 1 hour q 12 hours for 14 to 21 days. Or, 2.5 mg/kg I.V. q 8 hours for 14 to 21 days.

✦ *Dosage adjustment.* Adjust dosage in patients with renal impairment. Consider a dosage reduction for patients with neutropenia, anemia, or thrombocytopenia.

Creatinine clearance (ml/min)	Dosage
50-69	2.5 mg/kg q 12 hr
25-49	2.5 mg/kg q 24 hr
10-24	1.25 mg/kg q 24 hr

How supplied
Available by prescription only
Capsules: 250 mg, 500 mg
Injection: 500-mg vial

Pharmacodynamics
Antiviral action: Ganciclovir is a synthetic nucleoside analogue of 2′-deoxyguanosine. It competitively inhibits viral DNA polymerase and may be incorporated into viral DNA to cause early termination of DNA replication. It is active against CMV, herpes simplex virus type 1 and type 2 (HSV-1 and HSV-2), varicella zoster virus, Epstein-Barr virus, and hepatitis B virus.

Pharmacokinetics
Absorption: About 5% of oral ganciclovir is absorbed under fasting conditions and 6% to 9% following food.
Distribution: Only 1% to 2% protein-bound. It preferentially concentrates in CMV-infected cells because cellular kinases convert it to ganciclovir triphosphate.
Metabolism: Most (more than 90%) is excreted unchanged.
Excretion: Elimination half-life is about 3 hours in patients with normal renal function; it can be as long as 30 hours in patients with severe renal failure. The primary route of excretion is through the kidneys by glomerular filtration and some renal tubular secretion.

Route	Onset	Peak	Duration
P.O.	Unknown	1¾-3 hr	Unknown
I.V.	Unknown	Immediate	Unknown

Contraindications and precautions
Contraindicated in patients hypersensitive to ganciclovir or acyclovir and with an absolute neutrophil count less than 500 mm³ or a platelet count below 25,000 mm³. Use cautiously in patients with impaired renal function.

Interactions
Drug-drug. *Cytotoxic drugs:* Additive toxicity (bone marrow depression, stomatitis, alopecia). Monitor patient closely.
Imipenem-cilastatin: Increased risk of seizures. Monitor patient closely.
Immunosuppressants, such as azathioprine, corticosteroids, cyclosporine: Enhanced immune and bone marrow suppression. Use together cautiously.
Nephrotoxic drugs (amphotericin B, cyclosporine): Increased risk of renal impairment. Monitor renal function closely.
Probenecid: Decreased renal clearance of ganciclovir. Monitor patient closely.
Zidovudine: Higher risk of neutropenia. Monitor patient closely.
Drug-lifestyle. *Sun exposure:* Photosensitivity reactions may occur. Urge patient to take precautions.

Adverse reactions
CNS: altered dreams, confusion, ataxia, headache, *seizures, coma,* dizziness, somnolence, tremor, abnormal thinking, agitation, amnesia, anxiety, neuropathy, paresthesia, asthenia.
EENT: retinal detachment (in CMV retinitis patients).
GI: *nausea, vomiting, diarrhea, anorexia, abdominal pain,* flatulence, dyspepsia, dry mouth.
GU: increased serum creatinine levels.
Hematologic: *granulocytopenia, thrombocytopenia, leukopenia,* anemia.
Hepatic: abnormal liver function test results.
Respiratory: pneumonia.
Skin: *rash; sweating;* pruritus, inflammation, pain (at injection site), photosensitivity.
Other: phlebitis, chills, *sepsis, fever,* infection.

Overdose and treatment
Overdose may result in emesis, neutropenia, or GI disturbances.

Treatment should be symptomatic and supportive. Hemodialysis may be useful. Hydrate the patient to reduce plasma levels.

Special considerations
● Drug has a high potential for toxicity; use only when the potential for benefit outweighs risk.
● Reconstitute with sterile water for injection. Don't reconstitute with bacteriostatic water for injection because this may lead to the formation of a precipitate. Reconstituted solutions are stable for 12 hours.
● Don't refrigerate.
▐ **ALERT** Don't administer by S.C. or I.M. routes or as rapid I.V. bolus.

• Administer drug over 1 hour because of its high risk of toxicity.

Patient monitoring

• Monitor CBC to detect neutropenia, which may occur in as many as 40% of patients. It usually appears after about 10 days of therapy and may be more likely with a higher dosage (15 mg/kg daily). Neutropenia is reversible but may necessitate discontinuation of therapy. Patient may resume drug therapy when blood counts return to normal.

• Adverse reactions occur frequently, can be reduced with reduction of dose, and generally resolve when drug therapy is discontinued.

Breast-feeding patients

• Don't use drug in breast-feeding women. Instruct women to discontinue breast-feeding until at least 72 hours after last treatment.

Pediatric patients

• Few data are available on use in children under age 12. Use extremely cautiously, keeping in mind the potential for carcinogenic and reproductive toxicity.

Geriatric patients

• Use cautiously in elderly patients with compromised renal function.

Patient education

• Inform patient that maintenance infusions are necessary to prevent recurrence of disease.

• Instruct patient to have regular eye examinations to monitor retinitis.

• Advise patient to immediately report evidence of infection (fever, sore throat) or easy bruising or bleeding.

• Instruct patient to take oral dose with food.

• Advise patient to take precautions with sun exposure.

• Advise patient that drug may cause infertility.

• Advise women of childbearing age to use reliable birth control during treatment because drug can be harmful to fetus.

• Advise men to use barrier contraception during treatment and for at least 90 days after treatment.

---

gatifloxacin
Tequin

Pharmacologic classification: fluoroquinolone antibiotic
Therapeutic classification: antibiotic
Pregnancy risk category: C

Indications and dosages

➤ *Acute bacterial exacerbation of chronic bronchitis caused by* Streptococcus pneumoniae, Haemophilus influenzae, Haemophilus parainfluenzae, Moraxella catarrhalis, *or* Staphylococcus aureus; com-

plicated urinary tract infection caused by Escherichia coli, Klebsiella pneumoniae, *or* Proteus mirabilis; *acute pyelonephritis caused by* E. coli. *Adults:* 400 mg I.V. or P.O. daily for 7 to 10 days.

➤ *Acute sinusitis caused by* S. pneumoniae *or* H. influenzae. *Adults:* 400 mg I.V. or P.O. daily for 10 days.

➤ *Community-acquired pneumonia caused by* S. pneumoniae, H. influenzae, H. parainfluenzae, M. catarrhalis, S. aureus, Mycoplasma pneumoniae, Chlamydia pneumoniae, *or* Legionella pneumophila. *Adults:* 400 mg I.V. or P.O. daily for 7 to 14 days.

➤ *Uncomplicated urethral gonorrhea in men and cervical gonorrhea or acute uncomplicated rectal infections in women caused by* Neisseria gonorrhoeae. *Adults:* 400 mg P.O. or I.V. as single dose.

➤ *Uncomplicated urinary tract infection caused by* E. coli, K. pneumoniae, *or* P. mirabilis. *Adults:* 400 mg I.V. or P.O. as single dose, or 200 mg I.V. or P.O. daily for 3 days.

✦ *Dosage adjustment*
For patients with creatinine clearance less than 40 ml/minute, those on hemodialysis, and those on continuous peritoneal dialysis, initial dose is 400 mg I.V. or P.O. daily, and subsequent doses are 200 mg I.V. or P.O. daily. For patients on hemodialysis, administer after hemodialysis session is complete.

How supplied

Available by prescription only
Injection: 200 mg/20-ml vial, 400 mg/40-ml vial, 200 mg in 100 ml D₅W, 400 mg in 200 ml D₅W
Tablets: 200 mg, 400 mg

Pharmacodynamics

Antibiotic action: Gatifloxacin inhibits DNA gyrase and topoisomerase, preventing cell replication and division. It is active against gram-positive and gram-negative organisms, including: *S. aureus, S. pneumoniae, E. coli, H. influenzae, H. parainfluenzae, K. pneumoniae, M. catarrhalis, N. gonorrhoeae, P. mirabilis, C. pneumoniae, L. pneumophilia,* and *M. pneumoniae.*

Pharmacokinetics

Absorption: 96% of gatifloxacin is absorbed after oral administration; levels peak in 1 to 2 hours.
Distribution: Gatifloxacin is 20% protein-bound. It is widely distributed into many tissues and fluids.
Metabolism: Limited biotransformation.
Excretion: More than 70% of gatifloxacin is excreted unchanged by the kidneys. Serum half-life is 7 to 14 hours.

Route	Onset	Peak	Duration
P.O.	Unknown	1-2 hr	Unknown
I.V.	Unknown	Unknown	Unknown

Reactions may be *common,* uncommon, **life-threatening,** or COMMON AND LIFE-THREATENING.

Contraindications and precautions

Contraindicated in patients hypersensitive to fluoroquinolones. Don't use in patients with prolongation of QTc interval or in patients with uncorrected hypokalemia.

Use cautiously in patients with clinically significant bradycardia, acute myocardial ischemia, known or suspected CNS disorders, or renal insufficiency.

Interactions

Drug-drug. *Antacids that contain aluminum or magnesium, ferrous sulfate; didanosine buffered tablets, buffered powder, or buffered solution; products that contain zinc, magnesium or iron:* Decreased gatifloxacin absorption. Give gatifloxacin 4 hours before these products.
Antidiabetics (glyburide, insulin): Possible symptomatic hypoglycemia or hyperglycemia. Monitor blood glucose level.
Antipsychotics, erythromycin, tricyclic antidepressants: Possible prolonged QTc interval. Use cautiously.
Class IA antiarrhythmics (procainamide, quinidine), class III antiarrhythmics (amiodarone, sotalol): Possible prolonged QTc interval. Avoid concomitant use.
Digoxin: Possible increase in digoxin levels. Watch for signs of digoxin toxicity.
NSAIDs: Increased risk of CNS stimulation and seizures. Use together cautiously.
Probenecid: Increased gatifloxacin levels and prolonged half-life. Monitor patient closely.
Warfarin: Possible enhanced effects of warfarin. Monitor PT and INR.
Drug-lifestyle. *Sun exposure:* Photosensitivity reactions may occur. Urge patient to take precautions.

Adverse reactions

CNS: headache, dizziness, abnormal dreams, insomnia, paresthesia, tremor, vertigo.
CV: palpitations, chest pain.
EENT: tinnitus, abnormal vision, pharyngitis.
GI: nausea, diarrhea, abdominal pain, constipation, dyspepsia, oral candidiasis, glossitis, stomatitis, mouth ulcer, vomiting, taste perversion.
GU: dysuria, hematuria, vaginitis.
Musculoskeletal: back pain.
Respiratory: dyspnea.
Skin: rash, sweating.
Other: allergic reaction, redness at injection site, chills, fever, peripheral edema.

Overdose and treatment

Signs and symptoms of overdose include decreased respiratory rate, vomiting, tremors, and convulsions.

To treat an overdose of oral gatifloxacin, empty the stomach by inducing vomiting or performing gastric lavage. Provide symptomatic and supportive treatment, monitor ECG, and maintain hydration. Gatifloxacin isn't removed by hemodialysis or peritoneal dialyisis.

Special considerations

● In patients being treated for gonorrhea, test for syphilis at time of diagnosis.
● Dilute drug in single-use vials with D₅W or normal saline solution to a final concentration of 2 mg/ml before administration. Diluted solutions are stable for 14 days at room temperature or refrigerated. Frozen solutions are stable up to 6 months except for 5% sodium bicarbonate solutions. Thaw at room temperature. After thawing, solutions are stable for 14 days when stored at room temperature or under refrigeration. Don't mix with other drugs. Infuse over 60 minutes.
● Discard any unused portion of the single dose vials.
● Pseudomembranous colitis may occur in patients taking antibiotics.
● Discontinue drug if patient experiences convulsions, increased intracranial pressure, psychosis, or CNS stimulation leading to tremors, restlessness, light-headedness, confusion, hallucinations, paranoia, depression, nightmares, and insomnia.
● Discontinue drug if patient experiences pain, inflammation, or rupture of a tendon.
● Discontinue drug for skin rash or other sign of hypersensitivity.

Patient monitoring

● Monitor blood glucose in patients with diabetes.
● Monitor patients concurrently receiving digoxin for signs and symptoms of digoxin toxicity.
● Monitor kidney function in patients with renal insufficiency.

Breast-feeding patients

● It isn't known whether gatifloxacin appears in breast milk. Use cautiously when giving gatifloxacin to a breast-feeding woman.

Pediatric patients

● Safety and effectiveness of gatifloxacin haven't been established in patients under age 18.

Geriatric patients

● No dosage adjustment is necessary based on age.

Patient education

● Tell patient to take drug as prescribed and to finish all of it even if symptoms disappear.
● Advise patient to take drug 4 hours before products that contain aluminum, magnesium, zinc, or iron.
● Urge patient to use sunblock and wear protective clothing when exposed to excessive sunlight.
● Warn patient to avoid hazardous tasks until adverse CNS effects of drugs are known.
● Advise diabetic patient to monitor blood glucose levels and notify prescriber if hypoglycemia occurs.
● Urge patient to immediately report symptoms of allergic reaction, such as palpitations, fainting spells, rash, hives, difficulty swallowing or

breathing, tightness in throat, hoarseness, and swelling of the lips, tongue, or face.
• Advise patient to stop drug, refrain from exercise, and notify prescriber if pain, inflammation, or rupture of a tendon occur.

gemcitabine hydrochloride
Gemzar

Pharmacologic classification: pyrimidine nucleoside analogue
Therapeutic classification: antitumor
Pregnancy risk category: D

Indications and dosages
➤ *Locally advanced (nonresectable stage II or stage III) or metastatic pancreatic adenocarcinoma (stage IV) and in patients previously treated with fluorouracil.* Adults: 1,000 mg/m² I.V. over 30 minutes once weekly for up to 7 weeks or until toxicity necessitates reducing or holding a dose. Treatment course of 7 weeks is followed by 1 week rest. Subsequent dosage cycles consist of one infusion weekly for 3 out of 4 consecutive weeks.
✦ *Dosage adjustment.* Adjust dosage if bone marrow suppression is detected. Give full dose if absolute granulocyte count (AGC) is 1,000/mm³ or more and platelet count is 100,000/mm³ or more. If AGC is 500/mm³ to 999/mm³, or if platelet count is 50,000/mm³ to 99,000/mm³, give 75% of dose. Hold dose if AGC is less than 500/mm³ or platelet count is less than 50,000/mm³. Adjust dosage for subsequent cycles based on AGC and platelet count nadirs and degree of nonhematologic toxicity.
➤ *Advanced non-small-cell lung cancer.* Adults: 1,000 mg/m² I.V. over 30 minutes once weekly for up to 7 weeks or until toxicity necessitates reducing or holding a dose. Treatment course of 7 weeks is followed by 1 week rest. Subsequent dosage cycles consist of one infusion weekly for 3 out of 4 consecutive weeks.
➤ *Inoperable, locally advanced (stage IIIA or IIIB) or metastatic (stage IV) non-small cell lung carcinoma as initial treatment in combination with cisplatin.* 4-week schedule. Adults: 1,000 mg/m² I.V. over 30 minutes on days 1, 8, and 15 of each 28-day cycle. Cisplatin is administered on day 1 after gemcitabine administration is completed.
3-week schedule
Adults: 1,250 mg/m² I.V. over 30 minutes on days 1 and 8 of each 21-day cycle. Cisplatin is administered on day 1 after gemcitabine administration is completed.
✦ *Dosage adjustment.* When used in combination with cisplatin, reduce dosage by 50% in the occurrence of severe nonhematologic toxicity.
➤ *Advanced or metastatic bladder cancer◊.* Adults: 1,200 mg/m² to 1,250 mg/m² I.V.
over 30 minutes, once a week for 3 weeks of a 4-week cycle.

How supplied
Available by prescription only
Powder for injection: 200 mg/10-ml vial, 1 g/50-ml vial

Pharmacodynamics
Cytotoxic action: Drug inhibits DNA synthesis and blocks progression of cells through G1/S-phase boundary.

Pharmacokinetics
Absorption: Administered I.V.
Distribution: Volume of distribution (Vd) increases with increased infusion time. Following an infusion lasting less than 70 minutes, Vd was 50 L/m², suggesting that drug isn't extensively distributed. The Vd increased to 370 L/m² for longer infusions, reflecting slow equilibration of gemcitabine with the tissue compartment. Plasma protein–binding is negligible. Longer infusion time results in longer drug half-life.
Metabolism: Metabolized to an inactive uracil metabolite.
Excretion: Drug clearance decreases with increasing age; it is also less in women than men. This results in an increased half-life with increased age and in women.

Route	Onset	Peak	Duration
I.V.	Unknown	Unknown	Unknown

Contraindications and precautions
Contraindicated in patients hypersensitive to drug.

Interactions
None reported.

Adverse reactions
CNS: *paresthesia, somnolence.*
CV: *edema, peripheral edema.*
GI: *constipation, diarrhea, nausea, stomatitis, vomiting.*
GU: *elevated BUN* and creatinine levels, *hematuria, proteinuria.*
Hematologic: *anemia, **leukopenia, neutropenia, thrombocytopenia, hemorrhage.***
Hepatic: *elevated liver enzyme levels.*
Respiratory: ***bronchospasm,** dyspnea.*
Skin: *alopecia, rash.*
Other: *fever, flulike symptoms,* INFECTION, *pain.*

Overdose and treatment
There's no known antidote for drug overdose. If overdose is suspected, monitor patient with appropriate blood counts and provide supportive therapy.

Special considerations
⚠ **ALERT** Preparation and administration of parenteral form of drug causes mutagenic, teratogenic, and carcinogenic risks for personnel.

Reactions may be *common*, uncommon, *life-threatening*, or COMMON AND LIFE-THREATENING.

• Prolonging infusion time beyond 60 minutes and giving drug more frequently than weekly increase drug toxicity.
• Age, gender, and renal impairment may predispose patient to toxicity.
• Use caution when giving drug to patients with renal and hepatic impairment.

Patient monitoring
• Monitor renal and hepatic function tests before treatment and periodically thereafter.
• Monitor CBC, differential, and platelet count before giving each dose. Drug can suppress bone marrow function and cause leukopenia, thrombocytopenia, and anemia.
• When drug is used with cisplatin, monitor serum creatinine, potassium, calcium, and magnesium levels.

Breast-feeding patients
• It isn't known whether drug appears in breast milk. Avoid use in breast-feeding women.

Pediatric patients
• Drug hasn't been studied in children

Geriatric patients
• Drug clearance is affected by age; however, dosage adjustment isn't indicated.

Patient education
• Advise patient to take temperature daily and to watch for signs of infection (fever, sore throat, fatigue) and bleeding (easy bruising, nosebleeds, bleeding gums, melena).

gemfibrozil
Lopid

Pharmacologic classification: fibric acid derivative
Therapeutic classification: antilipemic
Pregnancy risk category: C

Indications and dosages
➤ *Type IV hyperlipidemia (hypertriglyceridemia) and severe hypercholesterolemia unresponsive to diet and other drugs; to reduce risk of cardiac disease in type IIb patients without history of disease.* Adults: 1,200 mg P.O. administered in two divided doses 30 minutes before morning and evening meals.

How supplied
Available by prescription only
Tablets: 600 mg

Pharmacodynamics
Antilipemic action: Gemfibrozil decreases serum triglyceride and very-low-density lipoprotein (VLDL) cholesterol levels while increasing serum high-density lipoprotein cholesterol. It also inhibits lipolysis in adipose tissue and reduces hepatic triglyceride synthesis. Drug is closely related to clofibrate pharmacologically.

Pharmacokinetics
Absorption: Well absorbed from GI tract. Plasma VLDL levels decrease in 2 to 5 days with decreases continuing for several months.
Distribution: 95% protein-bound.
Metabolism: Metabolized by the liver.
Excretion: Eliminated mostly in urine but some is excreted in feces. After a single dose, half-life is 1½ hours.

Route	Onset	Peak	Duration
P.O.	2-5 days	4 wk	Unknown

Contraindications and precautions
Contraindicated in patients hypersensitive to drug and in those with hepatic or severe renal dysfunction (including primary biliary cirrhosis) or gallbladder disease.

Interactions
Drug-drug. *Lovastatin, pravastatin, simvastatin:* Myopathy with rhabdomyolysis can occur. Avoid use together.
Oral anticoagulants: Enhanced effect of oral anticoagulants, increasing risk of hemorrhage. Adjust anticoagulant dose to maintain the desired PT and INR, and monitor patient frequently.

Adverse reactions
CNS: headache, fatigue, vertigo.
CV: atrial fibrillation.
GI: abdominal and epigastric pain, diarrhea, nausea, vomiting, *dyspepsia*, constipation, acute appendicitis.
Hematologic: anemia, *leukopenia*, eosinophilia, *thrombocytopenia*.
Hepatic: bile duct obstruction, elevated liver enzyme levels.
Metabolic: hypokalemia.
Skin: rash, dermatitis, pruritus, eczema.

Overdose and treatment
In overdose, immediately induce emesis or perform gastric lavage.

Special considerations
• Because drug is pharmacologically related to clofibrate, adverse reactions linked to clofibrate may occur with gemfibrozil as well. Clofibrate may increase the risk of death from cancer, postcholecystectomy complications, and pancreatitis. These hazards haven't been studied in gemfibrozil, however.
• Before starting gemfibrozil, aggressively attempt treatment through behavioral changes (diet and exercise) as well as identification and treatment of possible underlying causes of hyperlipoproteinemia.

Patient monitoring

• Monitor serum lipoprotein levels and liver function tests regularly; discontinue drug if a substantial lipid response isn't obtained.
• Monitor periodic CBC during the first 12 months of therapy.

Breast-feeding patients

• Safety in breast-feeding women hasn't been established.

Pediatric patients

• Safety and efficacy in children under age 18 haven't been established.

Patient education

• Instruct patient to report adverse reactions promptly, and to comply with prescribed regimen, diet, and exercise.
• Warn patient not to exceed prescribed dose.
• Instruct patient to inform prescriber about muscle soreness or dark urine.

---

gemtuzumab ozogamicin
Mylotarg

Pharmacologic classification: antibody-cytotoxic antitumor antibiotic conjugate
Therapeutic classification: chemotherapy agent
Pregnancy risk category: D

Indications and dosage

➤ *Treatment of patients with CD33-positive acute myeloid leukemia in first relapse and who aren't considered candidates for cytotoxic chemotherapy.* Adults age 60 and older: 9 mg/m^2 I.V. infusion over 2 hours every 14 days for a total of two doses. Premedicate with diphenhydramine 50 mg P.O., and acetaminophen 650 to 1,000 mg P.O. 1 hour before infusion.

How supplied

Available by prescription only
Powder for injection: 5mg

Pharmacodynamics

CD33-binding action: Thought to bind to the CD33 antigen expressed on the surface of leukemic blasts in more than 80% of patients with acute myeloid leukemia. This results in formation of a complex that is internalized by the cell. The calicheamicin derivative is then released inside the cell, causing DNA double-strand breaks and cell death.

Pharmacokinetics

Absorption: Administered I.V.
Distribution: Unknown.
Metabolism: Unknown. Studies suggest that liver microsomal enzymes are involved.

Excretion: The elimination half-lives of total and unconjugated calicheamicin are about 45 and 100 hours, respectively, after the first dose. After the second dose, the elimination half-life of total calicheamicin is increased to 60 hours.

Route	Onset	Peak	Duration
I.V.	Unknown	Unknown	Unknown

Contraindications and precautions

Contraindicated in patients hypersensitive to gemtuzumab ozogamicin or any of its components. Use cautiously in patients with hepatic impairment.

Interactions

None known.

Adverse reactions

CNS: *asthenia, depression, dizziness, headache, insomnia, pain.*
CV: *hypertension, hypotension, tachycardia.*
EENT: *epistaxis, pharyngitis, rhinitis.*
GI: *enlarged abdomen, abdominal pain, anorexia, constipation, diarrhea, dyspepsia, nausea, stomatitis, vomiting.*
GU: *hematuria, vaginal hemorrhage.*
Hematologic: *ecchymoses, anemia,* HEMORRHAGE, LEUKOPENIA, NEUTROPENIA, NEUTROPENIC FEVER, THROMBOCYTOPENIA.
Hepatic: *hepatotoxicity, increased liver enzyme levels.*
Metabolic: hyperglycemia, *hypokalemia, hypomagnesemia, increased LD level.*
Musculoskeletal: *arthralgia, back pain.*
Respiratory: *increased cough, dyspnea, hypoxia, pneumonia.*
Skin: *local reaction, peripheral edema, petechiae, rash.*
Other: *herpes simplex, chills, fever, pain,* **sepsis.**

Overdose and treatment

Signs and symptoms of overdose are unknown. Provide general supportive measures. Blood pressure and blood counts should be carefully monitored. Gemtuzumab isn't dialyzable.

Special considerations

• Drug should be used only under the supervision of a clinician experienced in the use of chemotherapy drugs.
• Gemtuzumab can produce a postinfusion symptom complex of chills, fever, hypotension, hypertension, hyperglycemia, hypoxia, and dyspnea that may occur during the first 24 hours after administration.
• Premedicate with diphenhydramine and acetaminophen. Additional doses of acetaminophen 650 to 1,000 mg P.O. can be given every 4 hours, as needed.
• Tumor lysis syndrome may occur. Provide adequate hydration and treat with allopurinol to prevent hyperuricemia.

Reactions may be *common*, uncommon, *life-threatening*, or COMMON AND LIFE-THREATENING.

⚠ ALERT Drug is light sensitive and must be protected from direct and indirect sunlight and unshielded fluorescent light during preparation and administration of the infusion.

• Administer in 100 ml of saline solution injection. Place the 100-ml I.V. bag into a UV protectant bag. The resulting drug solution in the I.V. bag should be used immediately.

• A separate I.V. line equipped with a low protein-binding 1.2-micron terminal filter must be used to administer drug. May be infused by central or peripheral line.

⚠ ALERT Don't give as an I.V. push or bolus.

Patient monitoring

• Monitor vital signs during infusion and for 4 hours after infusion.

• Severe myelosuppression will occur in all patients given the recommended dose of this drug. Careful hematologic monitoring is required.

• Monitor electrolytes, hepatic function, CBC, and platelets during therapy.

Breast-feeding patients

• It isn't known whether gemtuzumab ozogamicin appears in breast milk. Because of the potential for serious adverse reactions in nursing infants, a decision should be made whether to discontinue nursing or to discontinue drug, taking into account the importance of the drug to the mother.

Pediatric patients

• Safety and effectiveness haven't been established.

Patient education

• Advise patient about postinfusion symptoms. Tell patient to continue taking acetaminophen 650 to 1,000 mg every 4 hours as needed.

• Advise patient to watch for signs of infection, including fever, sore throat, fatigue, and bleeding (easy bruising, nosebleeds, bleeding gums, and melena). Tell patient to take temperature daily.

---

gentamicin sulfate
Cidomycin*, G-myticin, Garamycin, Genoptic, Genoptic S.O.P., Gentacidin, Gentafair, Gentak, Gentasol, Jenamicin

Pharmacologic classification: aminoglycoside
Therapeutic classification: antibiotic
Pregnancy risk category: D

Indications and dosages
➤ *Serious infections caused by susceptible organisms. Adults with normal renal function:* 3 mg/kg I.M. or I.V. infusion (in 50 to 100 ml of normal saline solution or D_5W infused over 30 minutes to 2 hours) daily in divided doses q 8 hours. May be given by direct I.V. push if

necessary. For life-threatening infections, patient may receive up to 5 mg/kg daily in three to four divided doses.
Children with normal renal function: 2 to 2.5 mg/kg I.M. or I.V. infusion q 8 hours.
Infants and neonates over age 1 week with normal renal function: 2.5 mg/kg I.M. or I.V. infusion q 8 hours.
Neonates under age 1 week: 2.5 mg/kg I.M. or I.V. infusion q 12 hours. For I.V. infusion, dilute in normal saline solution or D_5W and infuse over 30 minutes to 2 hours.
➤ *Meningitis. Adults:* Systemic therapy as above; may also use 4 to 8 mg intrathecally daily.
Children: Systemic therapy as above; may also use 1 to 2 mg intrathecally daily.
➤ *Endocarditis prophylaxis for GI or GU procedure or surgery. Adults:* 1.5 mg/kg I.M. or I.V. 30 minutes before procedure or surgery and 6 hours after. Give with ampicillin.
Children: 2 mg/kg I.M. or I.V. 30 minutes before procedure or surgery and 6 hours after. Give with ampicillin.
➤ *External ocular infections caused by susceptible organisms. Adults and children:* Instill 1 to 2 drops in eye q 4 hours. In severe infections, may use up to 2 drops q hour. Apply ointment to lower conjunctival sac b.i.d. or t.i.d.
➤ *Primary and secondary bacterial infections; superficial burns; skin ulcers; infected lacerations, abrasions, insect bites, or minor surgical wounds. Adults and children over age 1:* Rub in small amount gently t.i.d. or q.i.d., with or without gauze dressing.
➤ *Pelvic inflammatory disease. Adults:* Initially, 2 mg/kg I.M. or I.V. Then 1.5 mg/kg q 8 hours.
✦ *Dosage adjustment.* In patients with renal impairment, initial dose is the same as for those with normal renal function. Subsequent doses and frequency are determined by renal function studies and blood levels; keep peak serum levels between 4 and 10 mcg/ml and trough serum levels between 1 and 2 mcg/ml. One method is to administer 1-mg/kg doses and adjust the dosing interval based on steady state serum creatinine using the following formula:

$$\frac{\text{Creatinine}}{\text{(mg/100 ml)}} \times 8 = \frac{\text{dosing interval}}{\text{(hours)}}$$

➤ *Posthemodialysis to maintain therapeutic blood levels. Adults:* 1 to 1.7 mg/kg I.M. or by I.V. infusion after each dialysis.
Children: 2 to 2.5 mg/kg I.M. or by I.V. infusion after each dialysis.

How supplied
Available by prescription only
Injection: 40 mg/ml (adult), 10 mg/ml (pediatric), 2 mg/ml (intrathecal)
Ophthalmic ointment: 3 mg/g
Ophthalmic solution: 3 mg/ml
Topical cream or ointment: 0.1%

Pharmacodynamics
Antibiotic action: Gentamicin is bactericidal; it binds directly to the 30S ribosomal subunit, thus inhibiting bacterial protein synthesis. Its spectrum of activity includes many aerobic gram-negative organisms (including most strains of *Pseudomonas aeruginosa*) and some aerobic gram-positive organisms. Gentamicin may act against some bacterial strains resistant to other aminoglycosides; bacterial strains resistant to gentamicin may be susceptible to tobramycin, netilmicin, or amikacin.

Pharmacokinetics
Absorption: Absorbed poorly after oral administration.
Distribution: Distributed widely after parenteral administration; intraocular penetration is poor. CSF penetration is low even in patients with inflamed meninges. Intraventricular administration produces high levels throughout the CNS. Protein-binding is minimal. Gentamicin crosses the placenta.
Metabolism: Not metabolized.
Excretion: Excreted primarily in urine by glomerular filtration; small amounts may be excreted in bile and breast milk. Elimination half-life in adults is 2 to 3 hours. In patients with severe renal damage, half-life may extend to 24 to 60 hours.

Route	Onset	Peak	Duration
I.V.	Immediate	30-90 min	Unknown
I.M.	Unknown	30-90 min	Unknown
Intra-thecal	Unknown	Unknown	Unknown
Topical	Unknown	Unknown	Unknown
Oph-thalmic	Unknown	Unknown	Unknown

Contraindications and precautions
Contraindicated in patients hypersensitive to drug or in those with cross-sensitivity to other aminoglycosides such as neomycin.

Use systemic treatment cautiously in neonates, infants, elderly patients, and patients with renal disorders, neuromuscular disorders, or hearing dysfunction.

Interactions
Drug-drug. *Acyclovir, aminoglycosides, amphotericin B, capreomycin, cephalosporins, cisplatin, methoxyflurane, polymyxin B, vancomycin:* May increase the risk of nephrotoxicity, ototoxicity, or neurotoxicity. Use together cautiously.
Bumetanide, ethacrynic acid, furosemide, mannitol, urea: Increased risk of ototoxicity. Use cautiously.
Dimenhydrinate, other antiemetic and antivertigo drugs: May mask gentamicin-induced ototoxicity. Use cautiously.

General anesthetics, neuromuscular blockers such as succinylcholine and tubocurarine: Increased neuromuscular blockade. Monitor patient closely.
Indomethacin (I.V.): Increased peak and trough gentamicin levels. Monitor serum gentamicin levels closely.
Penicillin: Synergistic bactericidal effect against *P. aeruginosa, Escherichia coli, Klebsiella, Citrobacter, Enterobacter, Serratia,* and *Proteus mirabilis*; however, drugs are physically and chemically incompatible and are inactivated when mixed or given together. Don't mix drugs.

Adverse reactions
CNS: headache, lethargy, encephalopathy, confusion, dizziness, *seizures,* numbness, peripheral neuropathy (with injected form).
CV: hypotension (with injected form).
EENT: *ototoxicity,* blurred vision (with injected form); burning, stinging, blurred vision (with ophthalmic ointment); transient irritation (with ophthalmic solution); conjunctival hyperemia (with ophthalmic form).
GI: vomiting, nausea (with injected form).
GU: *nephrotoxicity* (with injected form).
Hematologic: anemia, eosinophilia, *leukopenia, thrombocytopenia, granulocytopenia* (with injected form).
Musculoskeletal: muscle twitching, myasthenia gravis–like syndrome.
Respiratory: *apnea* (with injected form).
Skin: rash, urticaria, pruritus, tingling (with injected form); minor skin irritation, possible photosensitivity, allergic contact dermatitis (with topical administration).
Other: fever, *anaphylaxis,* pain at injection site (with injected form); *hypersensitivity reactions,* overgrowth of nonsusceptible organisms (with ophthalmic form and long-term use).

Overdose and treatment
Signs and symptoms of overdose include ototoxicity, nephrotoxicity, and neuromuscular toxicity. Drug can be removed by hemodialysis or peritoneal dialysis. Treatment with calcium salts or anticholinesterases reverses neuromuscular blockade.

Special considerations
Consider the recommendations relevant to all aminoglycosides as well as the following.
⚡ ALERT Use preservative-free form for intrathecal route.
● Because drug is dializable, patients undergoing hemodialysis may need dosage adjustments.
● Systemic absorption from excessive use may cause systemic toxicities.

Patient monitoring
● Monitor serum drug levels. Prolonged peak serum level above 10 mcg/ml and trough serum level above 2 mcg/ml increases risk of toxicity.

Reactions may be *common,* uncommon, *life-threatening,* or common and life-threatening.

Patient education
● Inform patient of the proper administration technique.
● Instruct patient to promptly report worsened lesions or skin irritation.

glatiramer acetate
(formerly copolymer-1)
Copaxone

Pharmacologic classification: acetate salts of synthetic peptides containing four naturally occurring amino acids (L-alanine, L-glutamic acid, L-lysine, L-tyrosine)
Therapeutic classification: immune response modifier
Pregnancy risk category: B

Indications and dosages
➤ *To reduce frequency of relapses in patients with relapsing-remitting multiple sclerosis.* *Adults:* 20 mg S.C. daily.

How supplied
Available by prescription only
Injection for S.C. use: sterile lyophilized material containing 20 mg glatiramer acetate and 40 mg mannitol, USP, in a single-use 2-ml vial (amber glass); 1-ml vials of sterile water for injection (in clear glass) are included for reconstitution

Pharmacodynamics
Immune response modifier action: Mechanism unknown. Thought to act by modifying immune processes responsible for the pathogenesis of multiple sclerosis.

Pharmacokinetics
Pharmacokinetics in patients with impaired renal function aren't known.
Absorption: A substantial fraction of dose injected S.C. may be hydrolyzed locally. Some is presumed to enter lymphatic circulation and regional lymph nodes; some may enter systemic circulation.
Distribution: No information available.
Metabolism: No information available.
Excretion: No information available.

Route	Onset	Peak	Duration
S.C.	Unknown	Unknown	Unknown

Contraindications and precautions
Contraindicated in patients hypersensitive to drug or mannitol.

Interactions
None reported.

Adverse reactions
CNS: abnormal dreams, agitation, *anxiety, asthenia,* confusion, emotional lability, *hyperto-*
nia, migraine, nervousness, speech disorder, stupor, tremor, syncope, vertigo.
CV: edema, peripheral edema, *chest pain,* hypertension, *palpitations, vasodilation,* tachycardia.
EENT: ear pain, eye disorder, laryngismus, nystagmus, *rhinitis.*
GI: anorexia, *diarrhea,* gastroenteritis, GI disorder, *nausea,* oral candidiasis, salivary gland enlargement, tooth caries, ulcerative stomatitis, vomiting.
GU: amenorrhea, bowel urgency, dysmenorrhea, hematuria, impotence, menorrhagia, suspicious Papanicolaou smear, *urinary urgency,* vaginal candidiasis, vaginal hemorrhage.
Hematologic: ecchymoses, *lymphadenopathy.*
Metabolic: weight gain.
Musculoskeletal: arthralgia, *back pain,* neck pain, foot drop.
Respiratory: bronchitis, *dyspnea,* hyperventilation.
Skin: eczema, erythema, herpes simplex and zoster, *pruritus, rash,* skin atrophy, skin nodule, *sweating,* urticaria, warts.
Other: bacterial infection, chills, cyst, facial edema, fever, *flu syndrome, infection, injection site reaction* or hemorrhage, *pain.*

Special considerations
● Administer drug by S.C. injection only.
● Store drug in refrigerator (36° to 46° F [2° to 8° C]); diluent can be kept at room temperature.
● Use immediately after reconstitution because drug doesn't contain preservatives. Discard unused drug.
● About 26% of patients experienced at least one episode of transient chest pain which usually began at least 1 month after treatment began; it wasn't accompanied by other symptoms and appeared not to be significant.

Patient monitoring
● Monitor patient for immediate postinjection reactions. Such reactions have occurred in 10% of patients with multiple sclerosis; signs and symptoms include flushing, chest pain, palpitations, anxiety, dyspnea, throat constriction, and urticaria. Reactions are transient, self-limited, and need no specific treatment. Onset may occur several months after therapy starts; patients may have more than one episode.
● Monitor patient for adverse effects.

Breast-feeding patients
● It isn't known whether drug appears in breast milk. Use cautiously in breast-feeding women.

Pediatric patients
● Safety and efficacy haven't been established in children under age 18.

Geriatric patients
● Drug hasn't been studied specifically in elderly patients.

Patient education
- Explain need for aseptic injection techniques and warn patient against reuse of needles and syringes.
- Instruct patient to report planned, suspected, or known pregnancy.
- Tell patient to call if she is breast-feeding.
- Advise patient not to change drug or dosing schedule or to stop drug without medical approval.
- Urge patient to call immediately if dizziness, hives, sweating, chest pain, difficulty breathing, or severe pain occurs following drug injection.

---

glimepiride
Amaryl

Pharmacologic classification: sulfonylurea
Therapeutic classification: antidiabetic
Pregnancy risk category: C

Indications and dosages
➤ *Adjunct to diet and exercise to lower blood glucose level in patients with type 2 (non-insulin-dependent) diabetes mellitus whose hyperglycemia can't be managed by diet and exercise alone.* Adults: Initially, 1 to 2 mg P.O. once daily with first main meal of the day; usual maintenance dosage is 1 to 4 mg P.O. once daily. Maximum recommended dose is 8 mg once daily. After dose of 2 mg is reached, increase dosage in increments not exceeding 2 mg at 1- to 2-week intervals based on patient's blood glucose response.
➤ *Adjunct to insulin therapy in patients with type 2 (non-insulin-dependent) diabetes mellitus whose hyperglycemia can't be managed by diet and exercise in conjunction with an oral hypoglycemic agent.* Adults: 8 mg P.O. once daily with first main meal of the day with low-dose insulin. Increase weekly as needed and guided by patient's blood glucose response.
➤ *Adjunct to metformin therapy in patients with type 2 (non-insulin-dependent) diabetes mellitus whose hyperglycemia can't be managed by diet, exercise, and glimepiride or metformin alone.* Adults: 8 mg P.O. once daily with first main meal of the day, with metformin if patient responds inadequately to glimepiride monotherapy. Adjust dosages based on patient's blood glucose response to determine minimum effective dosage of each drug.
✦ *Dosage adjustment.* Patients with renal impairment need cautious dosing. Give 1 mg P.O. once daily with first main meal of the day, followed by appropriate dosage adjustment as necessary.

How supplied
Available by prescription only
Tablets: 1 mg, 2 mg, 4 mg

Pharmacodynamics
Antidiabetic action: Drug appears to lower blood glucose level by stimulating insulin release from functioning pancreatic beta cells. Also, drug can lead to increased sensitivity of peripheral tissues to insulin.

Pharmacokinetics
Absorption: Completely absorbed from the GI tract.
Distribution: Protein-binding exceeds 99.5%.
Metabolism: Completely metabolized by oxidative biotransformation.
Excretion: Metabolites are excreted in urine (about 60%) and feces (about 40%).

Route	Onset	Peak	Duration
P.O.	Unknown	2-3 hr	> 24 hr

Contraindications and precautions
Contraindicated in patients hypersensitive to drug and in those with diabetic ketoacidosis (with or without coma) because this condition should be treated with insulin. Also contraindicated as sole therapy for type 1 diabetes or diabetes complicated by pregnancy.

Use cautiously in debilitated or malnourished patients and in those with adrenal, pituitary, hepatic, or renal insufficiency because these patients are more susceptible to the hypoglycemic action of glucose-lowering drugs.

Interactions
Drug-drug. *Beta blockers:* May mask symptoms of hypoglycemia. Monitor patient carefully.
Corticosteroids, estrogens, isoniazid, nicotinic acid, oral contraceptives, phenothiazines, phenytoin, sympathomimetics, thiazide and other diuretics, thyroid products: Increased risk of hyperglycemia. May require dosage adjustment.
Insulin: Increased risk of hypoglycemia. May require dosage adjustment.
NSAIDs and other drugs that are highly protein-bound, such as beta blockers, chloramphenicol, coumarins, MAO inhibitors, probenecid, salicylates, and sulfonamides: May potentiate hypoglycemic action. May require dosage adjustment.
Drug-lifestyle. *Alcohol use:* Alters glycemic control (hypoglycemia most common). May also cause disulfiram-like reaction. Advise patient to avoid alcohol.

Adverse reactions
CNS: dizziness, asthenia, headache.
EENT: changes in accommodation, blurred vision.
GI: vomiting, abdominal pain, nausea, diarrhea.
Hematologic: *leukopenia,* hemolytic anemia, *agranulocytosis, thrombocytopenia, aplastic anemia, pancytopenia.*
Hepatic: cholestatic jaundice, elevated transaminase levels.

Reactions may be *common*, uncommon, *life-threatening*, or COMMON AND LIFE-THREATENING.

Metabolic: hypoglycemia.
Skin: allergic skin reactions (pruritus, erythema, urticaria, morbilliform or maculopapular eruptions).

Overdose and treatment

Sulfonylurea overdose can produce hypoglycemia. Mild hypoglycemic symptoms without loss of consciousness or neurologic findings should be treated aggressively with oral glucose and adjustments in drug dosage and meal patterns. Monitor patient closely until he's out of danger.

Severe hypoglycemic reactions with coma, seizure, or other neurologic impairment occur infrequently but constitute medical emergencies requiring immediate hospitalization. If hypoglycemic coma occurs or is suspected, give a rapid I.V. injection of concentrated (50%) glucose solution followed by continuous infusion of a more dilute (10%) glucose solution at a rate that will maintain the blood glucose at a level of more than 100 mg/dl. Monitor patient closely for at least 24 to 48 hours because hypoglycemia may recur after apparent clinical recovery.

Special considerations

Consider the recommendations relevant to all sulfonylureas as well as the following.
● In elderly, debilitated, or malnourished patients or in patients with renal or hepatic insufficiency, the initial dose, dose increments, and maintenance dosage should be conservative to avoid hypoglycemic reactions.
● Oral hypoglycemics may increase the risk of CV mortality compared with diet or diet and insulin therapy.

Patient monitoring

● Monitor fasting blood glucose level periodically to determine therapeutic response. Also monitor glycosylated hemoglobin, usually every 3 to 6 months, to more precisely assess long-term glycemic control.
● During maintenance therapy, stop glimepiride if satisfactory lowering of blood glucose level is no longer achieved. Secondary failures to glimepiride monotherapy can be treated with glimepiride-insulin combination therapy.

Breast-feeding patients

● It isn't known whether drug appears in breast milk. Because of the risk of hypoglycemia in nursing infants, avoid giving drug to breast-feeding women.

Pediatric patients

● Safety and efficacy in children haven't been established.

Geriatric patients

● These patients may be more sensitive to drug effects because of reduced metabolism and elimination.

Patient education

● Instruct patient to take drug with first meal of the day.
● Make sure patient understands that therapy relieves symptoms but doesn't cure disease.
● Stress importance of adhering to specific diet, weight reduction, exercise, and personal hygiene programs. Explain how and when to monitor blood glucose level.
● Teach patient how to recognize and manage hyperglycemia and hypoglycemia.
● Advise patient to wear or carry medical identification regarding diabetic status.

glipizide
Glucotrol, Glucotrol XL

Pharmacologic classification: sulfonylurea
Therapeutic classification: antidiabetic
Pregnancy risk category: C

Indications and dosages

➤ *Adjunct to diet to lower blood glucose levels in patients with non-insulin-dependent diabetes mellitus.* Tablets. *Adults:* Initially, 5 mg P.O. daily 30 minutes before breakfast. Adjust dose in increments of 2.5 to 5 mg. Usual maintenance dosage is 10 to 15 mg daily. Maximum recommended daily dose is 40 mg. Divide total daily doses of more than 15 mg except when using extended-release tablets.
✦ *Dosage adjustment.* Initial dosage in elderly patients or those with hepatic disease may be 2.5 mg.
Extended-release tablets
Adults: Initially, 5 mg P.O. daily. May increase to 10 mg after 3 months based on glycosylated hemoglobin measurement. Subsequent dose adjustments should be based on glycosylated hemoglobin measurements at 3-month intervals. If no response after 3 months on higher dose, previous dose should be resumed. Maximum daily dose is 20 mg.
➤ *To replace insulin therapy. Adults:* If insulin dose is more than 20 units daily, patient may be started at usual dose of glipizide (5 mg daily) plus 50% of insulin dosage. If insulin dose is less than 20 units, insulin may be discontinued.

How supplied

Available by prescription only
Tablets: 5 mg, 10 mg
Tablets (extended-release): 2.5 mg, 5 mg, 10 mg

Pharmacodynamics

Antidiabetic action: Glipizide decreases blood glucose levels by stimulating insulin release from functioning beta cells in the pancreas. After prolonged administration, hypoglycemic effects of drug appear to reflect extrapancreatic effects, possibly including reduction of basal hepatic glucose production and enhanced peripheral sensitivity to insulin.

Pharmacokinetics
Absorption: Absorbed rapidly and completely from the GI tract.
Distribution: Probably distributed in the extracellular fluid. Drug is about 92% to 99% protein-bound.
Metabolism: Metabolized almost completely by the liver to inactive metabolites.
Excretion: Excreted primarily in urine; small amounts are excreted in feces. Renal clearance of unchanged glipizide increases with increasing urinary pH. Duration of action is 10 to 24 hours; half-life is 2 to 4 hours.

Route	Onset	Peak	Duration
P.O.			
Regular	15-30 min	1-3 hr	4 hr
Extended	2-3 hr	6-12 hr	24 hr

Contraindications and precautions
Contraindicated in pregnant patients, breast-feeding women, patients hypersensitive to drug, and patients with diabetic ketoacidosis with or without coma. Also contraindicated as sole therapy for type 1 diabetes.

Use cautiously in patients with impaired renal or hepatic function and in geriatric, malnourished, or debilitated patients.

Interactions
Drug-drug. *Adrenocorticoids, amphetamines, baclofen, corticotropin, epinephrine, estrogens, ethacrynic acid, furosemide, glucocorticoids, oral contraceptives, phenytoin, thiazide diuretics, thyroid hormones, triamterene:* May increase glucose levels. Dosage adjustments may be required.
Anabolic steroids, chloramphenicol, clofibrate, guanethidine, insulin, MAO inhibitors, probenecid, salicylates, sulfonamides: Enhanced hypoglycemic effect from displacement of glipizide from protein-binding sites. Monitor patient.
Antifungal antibiotics such as miconazole, fluconazole: Increased glipizide levels and hypoglycemia. Monitor patient.
Beta blockers, including ophthalmics: May mask symptoms of hypoglycemia. Monitor patient closely.
Cimetidine: Potentiated hypoglycemic effects from prevention of hepatic metabolism. Monitor patient closely.
Corticosteroids, glucagon, rifampin, thiazide diuretics: May decrease hypoglycemic response. Monitor patient closely.
Hydantoins: Increased hydantoin levels. Monitor blood levels.
Drug-food. *Any food:* Delayed absorption. Tell patient to take drug 30 minutes before meals.
Drug-lifestyle. *Alcohol use:* Altered glycemic control. May also cause a disulfiram-like reaction. Advise patient to avoid alcohol.

Smoking: Increased corticosteroid release, requiring higher dosages. Discourage smoking.

Adverse reactions
CNS: *asthenia,* dizziness, drowsiness, headache, pain, tremor, nervousness, insomnia, anxiety, depression, hypesthesia, paresthesia.
GI: nausea, constipation, diarrhea, flatulence, dyspepsia, vomiting.
GU: altered BUN level.
Hematologic: *leukopenia,* hemolytic anemia, *agranulocytosis, thrombocytopenia, aplastic anemia.*
Hepatic: cholestatic jaundice, altered liver enzyme levels.
Metabolic: altered cholesterol level, SIADH, *hypoglycemia.*
Skin: rash, pruritus.

Overdose and treatment
Signs and symptoms include low blood glucose levels, tingling of lips and tongue, hunger, nausea, decreased cerebral function, increased sympathetic activity, and, ultimately, seizures, stupor, and coma.

Mild hypoglycemia responds to treatment with oral glucose and dosage adjustments. If patient loses consciousness or experiences other neurologic changes, he should receive a rapid injection of dextrose 50%, followed by continuous infusion of dextrose 10% at a rate to maintain blood glucose levels more than 100 mg/dl. Monitor patient for 24 to 48 hours.

Special considerations
Consider the recommendations relevant to all sulfonylureas as well as the following.
● To improve glucose control in patients who receive 15 mg/day or more, doses can be divided and given 30 minutes before the morning and evening meals.
● Some patients taking glipizide can be controlled on a once-daily regimen; others show better response with divided doses.
● Drug has a mild diuretic effect that may be useful in patients with heart failure or cirrhosis.
● Patients who may be more sensitive to drug, such as elderly, debilitated, or malnourished people, should begin therapy with lower doses (2.5 mg once daily).
● Oral antidiabetics may increase the risk of CV mortality as compared with diet or diet and insulin therapy.

Patient monitoring
● When substituting glipizide for chlorpropamide, monitor patient carefully during the first week because of the prolonged retention of chlorpropamide.
● Monitor blood glucose, urine glucose, ketone, and glycosylated hemoglobin levels.

Reactions may be *common*, uncommon, *life-threatening*, or COMMON AND LIFE-THREATENING.

Pregnant patients
• Use in pregnancy usually isn't recommended. If glipizide must be used, manufacturer recommends stopping drug at least 1 month before expected delivery to prevent neonatal hypoglycemia.

Pediatric patients
• Safety and efficacy in children haven't been established.

Geriatric patients
• These patients may be more sensitive to drug effects.
• Hypoglycemia causes increased neurologic symptoms in elderly patients.

Patient education
• Emphasize the importance of following prescribed diet, exercise, and medical regimen.
• Tell patient that, if a dose is missed, it should be taken immediately, unless it's almost time to take the next dose. Patient shouldn't double the dose.
• Advise patient to avoid alcohol and products containing alcohol when taking glipizide.
• Suggest that drug be taken with food if glipizide causes GI upset.
• Teach patient how to monitor blood glucose, urine glucose, and ketone levels, as needed.
• Teach patient how to recognize and manage hyperglycemia and hypoglycemia.

glucagon
Pharmacologic classification: antihypoglycemic
Therapeutic classification: glucose-elevating agent
Pregnancy risk category: B

Indications and dosages
➤ *Severe hypoglycemia. Adults and children who weigh more than 20 kg (44 lb):* 1 mg S.C., I.M., or I.V. May repeat dose after 15 minutes if patient fails to respond. When patient responds, give supplemental carbohydrates.
Children who weigh less than 20 kg: 0.5 mg S.C., I.M., or I.V. Or, 20 to 30 mcg/kg. May repeat dose after 15 minutes if patient fails to respond. When patient responds, give supplemental carbohydrates.
➤ *Diagnostic aid for radiographic examination of stomach, duodenum, and small intestine. Adults:* 1 or 2 mg I.M. or 0.25 to 2 mg I.V. For relaxation of the stomach, use 0.5. mg I.V. or 2 mg I.M.

How supplied
Available by prescription only
Powder for injection: 1 mg (1 unit)/vial, 10 mg (10 units)/vial

Pharmacodynamics
Antihypoglycemic action: Glucagon increases plasma glucose levels and causes smooth muscle relaxation and an inotropic myocardial effect because of the stimulation of adenylate cyclase to produce cAMP. The cAMP initiates a series of reactions that leads to the degradation of glycogen to glucose. Hepatic stores of glycogen are necessary for glucagon to exert an antihypoglycemic effect.
Diagnostic action: The mechanism by which glucagon relaxes smooth muscles of the GI tract hasn't been fully defined.

Pharmacokinetics
Absorption: Glucagon is destroyed in the GI tract; therefore, it must be given parenterally. Administration to comatose hypoglycemic patients (with normal liver glycogen stores) usually produces a return to consciousness within 20 minutes.
Distribution: Not fully understood.
Metabolism: Degraded extensively by the liver, in the kidneys and plasma, and at its tissue receptor sites in plasma membranes.
Excretion: Metabolic products are excreted by the kidneys. Half-life is about 3 to 10 minutes.

Route	Onset	Peak	Duration
I.V.	Immediate	½ hr	60-90 min
I.M., S.C.	Unknown	Unknown	Unknown

Contraindications and precautions
Contraindicated in patients hypersensitive to drug and in those with pheochromocytoma. Use cautiously in patients with insulinoma.

Interactions
Drug-drug. *Anticoagulants:* Enhanced anticoagulant effect. Monitor patient for bleeding.
Epinephrine: Increased and prolonged hyperglycemic effect. Monitor blood glucose levels.
Phenytoin: Appears to inhibit glucagon-induced insulin release. Use cautiously as a diagnostic agent in patients with diabetes mellitus.

Adverse reactions
CV: hypotension.
GI: nausea, vomiting.
Metabolic: hypokalemia.
Respiratory: respiratory distress.
Other: *hypersensitivity reactions (bronchospasm,* rash, dizziness, light-headedness).

Overdose and treatment
Overdose may cause nausea, vomiting, and hypokalemia. Treat symptomatically.

Special considerations
• Glucagon should be used only under direct medical supervision.
• For I.V. drip infusion, glucagon is compatible with dextrose solution but forms a precipitate in chloride solutions.

• Glucagon has a positive inotropic and chrono-tropic action on the heart and may be used to treat beta blocker overdose.

• Mixed solutions with diluent are stable for 48 hours when stored at 41° F (5° C). Following re-constitution with sterile water, use immediately. Discard unused portion.

Patient monitoring
• If patient experiences nausea and vomiting from glucagon administration and can't retain some form of sugar for 1 hour, consider administra-tion of I.V. dextrose.

Breast-feeding patients
• It isn't known whether drug appears in breast milk.

Pediatric patients
• Glucagon has been used safely and effectively for the treatment of hypoglycemia in children. Safety and efficacy in diagnostic procedures haven't been established.

Patient education
• Provide patient with instructions on how to mix and inject medication properly.
• Tell patient to expect response usually within 20 minutes after injection.

---

glyburide
DiaBeta, Glynase PresTab, Micronase

Pharmacologic classification: sulfonylurea
Therapeutic classification: antidiabetic
Pregnancy risk category: C (B for Glynase, Micronase)

Indications and dosages
➤ *Adjunct to diet to lower blood glucose levels in patients with type 2 (non-insulin-dependent) diabetes mellitus.*
Adults: Initially, 2.5 to 5 mg P.O. daily with break-fast. Start patients who are more sensitive to hypo-glycemic drugs at 1.25 mg daily. Usual mainte-nance dosage is 1.25 to 20 mg daily, either as a single dose or in divided doses.

For micronized tablets, initially give 1.5 to 3 mg P.O. with breakfast. Usual maintenance dosage is 0.75 to 12 mg P.O. daily.
✦ *Dosage adjustment.* In elderly, debilitated, or malnourished patients or those with renal or liver dysfunction, start with 1.25 mg once daily.
➤ *To replace insulin therapy. Adults:* If in-sulin dose is more than 40 units daily, patient may be started on 5 mg of glyburide daily plus 50% of the insulin dose. Patients maintained on less than 20 units daily should receive 2.5 to 5 mg daily; those maintained on 20 to 40 units daily should receive 5 mg daily. In all patients, gly-buride is substituted and insulin discontinued abruptly.

For micronized tablets, if insulin dose is more than 40 units daily, give 3 mg P.O. with a 50% re-duction in insulin. Patients maintained on 20 to 40 units daily should receive 3 mg P.O. as a sin-gle daily dose; those maintained on less than 20 units daily should receive 1.5 to 3 mg daily as a single dose.

How supplied
Available by prescription only
Tablets: 1.25 mg, 2.5 mg, 5 mg
Tablets (micronized): 1.5 mg, 3 mg, 6 mg

Pharmacodynamics
Antidiabetic action: Glyburide decreases blood glucose levels by stimulating insulin release from functioning beta cells in the pancreas. After pro-longed administration, hypoglycemic effects ap-pear to be related to extrapancreatic effects, pos-sibly including reduction of basal hepatic glucose production and enhanced peripheral sensitivity to insulin. The latter may result either from an increase in the number of insulin receptors or from changes in events subsequent to insulin binding.

Pharmacokinetics
Absorption: Almost completely absorbed from GI tract. A micronized tablet results in significant absorption; a 3-mg micronized tablet provides blood levels similar to a 5-mg conventional tablet.
Distribution: 99% protein-bound. Distribution isn't fully understood.
Metabolism: Metabolized completely by the liv-er to inactive metabolites.
Excretion: Excreted as metabolites in urine and feces in equal proportions. Duration of action is 24 hours, and half-life is 10 hours.

Route	Onset	Peak	Duration
P.O.	1-4 hr	4 hr	24 hr

Contraindications and precautions
Contraindicated in pregnant patients, breast-feeding women, patients hypersensitive to drug, and patients with diabetic ketoacidosis with or without coma. Use cautiously in patients with im-paired renal or hepatic function and in elderly, malnourished, or debilitated patients.

Interactions
Drug-drug. *Adrenocorticoids, amphetamines, baclofen, corticotropin, diazoxide, epineph-rine, ethacrynic acid, furosemide, glucagon, glucocorticoids, phenytoin, rifampin, thiazide diuretics, thyroid hormones, triamterene:* In-creased blood glucose levels. Dosage adjustments may be required.
Anabolic steroids, chloramphenicol, clofibrate, guanethidine, insulin, MAO inhibitors, probenecid, salicylates, sulfonamides: Enhanced hypoglycemic effect by displacement of glyburide from its protein-binding sites. Monitor glucose levels and patient carefully.

Reactions may be *common*, uncommon, *life-threatening*, or COMMON AND LIFE-THREATENING.

Anticoagulants: May increase plasma levels of both drugs and, after continued therapy, decrease plasma levels and anticoagulant effect. Monitor blood glucose and PT.

Beta blockers, including ophthalmics: Increased risk of hypoglycemia. Use together cautiously.

Hydantoins: May increase hydantoin levels. Monitor blood levels.

Drug-lifestyle. *Alcohol use:* Altered glycemic control, most commonly hypoglycemia. May also cause a disulfiram-like reaction consisting of nausea, vomiting, abdominal cramps, and headaches. Discourage use together.

Smoking: May increase corticosteroid release; patients who smoke may need higher glyburide dosage. Advise patient to stop smoking.

Adverse reactions

EENT: changes in accommodation, blurred vision.

GI: nausea, epigastric fullness, heartburn.

GU: altered BUN levels.

Hematologic: *leukopenia,* hemolytic anemia, *agranulocytosis, thrombocytopenia, aplastic anemia.*

Hepatic: cholestatic jaundice, *hepatitis,* abnormal liver function.

Metabolic: altered cholesterol level, hypoglycemia, SIADH.

Musculoskeletal: arthralgia, myalgia.

Skin: rash, pruritus, other allergic reactions.

Other: *angioedema.*

Overdose and treatment

Signs and symptoms of overdose include low blood glucose levels, tingling of lips and tongue, hunger, nausea, decreased cerebral function (lethargy, yawning, confusion, agitation, and nervousness), increased sympathetic activity (tachycardia, sweating, and tremor) and, ultimately, seizures, stupor, and coma.

Mild hypoglycemia, without loss of consciousness or neurologic findings, responds to treatment with oral glucose and dosage adjustments. Patient with severe hypoglycemia should be hospitalized immediately. If hypoglycemic coma is suspected, patient should receive rapid injection of dextrose 50%, followed by a continuous infusion of dextrose 10% at a rate to maintain blood glucose levels greater than 100 mg/dl. Monitor patient for 24 to 48 hours.

Special considerations

Consider the recommendations relevant to all sulfonylureas as well as the following.

● To improve control in patients receiving 10 mg daily or more, divided doses, usually given before the morning and evening meals, are recommended.

● Some patients taking glyburide may be controlled effectively on a once-daily regimen, whereas others show better response with divided dosing.

● Glyburide is a second generation sulfonylurea oral antidiabetic. It appears to cause fewer adverse reactions than first generation drugs.

● Drug has a mild diuretic effect that may be useful in patients with chronic heart failure or cirrhosis.

● Oral antidiabetics may increase the risk of CV mortality compared with diet or diet and insulin therapy.

Patient monitoring

● When substituting glyburide for chlorpropamide, monitor patient closely during the first week because of the prolonged retention of chlorpropamide in the body.

● Monitor blood glucose, urine glucose, and ketone levels.

Pediatric patients

● Glyburide is ineffective in insulin-dependent (type 1, juvenile-onset) diabetes.

● Safety and efficacy in children haven't been established.

Geriatric patients

● These patients may be more sensitive to drug effects because of reduced metabolism and elimination.

● Hypoglycemia causes more neurologic symptoms in elderly patients

Patient education

● Emphasize importance of following prescribed diet, exercise, and medical regimen.

● Advise patient to avoid alcohol and alcohol-containing products while taking glyburide.

● Suggest that patient take drug with food if GI upset occurs.

● Teach patient how to monitor blood glucose, urine glucose, and ketone levels.

● Inform patient of the signs and symptoms of hyperglycemia and hypoglycemia and what to do if they occur.

glyburide and metformin hydrochloride
Glucovance

Pharmacologic classification: combination sulfonylurea and biguanide
Therapeutic classification: antidiabetic
Pregnancy risk category: B

Indications and dosages

➤ *Adjunct to diet and exercise to improve glycemic control in patients with type 2 diabetes whose hyperglycemia cannot be controlled with diet and exercise alone.*
Adults: initially, 1.25 mg/250 mg P.O. once daily or b.i.d. with meals. In patients whose hyperglycemia can't be managed with diet and exercise alone, start with 1.25 mg/250 mg once daily with meals. In patients with glycosylated hemoglobin above 9% or fasting plasma glucose above 200 mg/dl, start with 1.25 mg/250 mg twice daily with morning and evening meals. Daily dose

may be increased in increments of 1.25 mg/250 mg daily every 2 weeks up to the minimum dose needed to adequately control blood glucose. Maximum 20 mg glyburide and 2,000 mg metformin daily.

➤ *Second-line therapy in patients with type 2 diabetes when diet, exercise, and initial treatment with a sulfonlyurea or metformin don't provide adequate glycemic control. Adults:* initially 2.5 mg/500 mg or 5 mg/500 mg twice daily with meals. Increase in increments of no more than 5 mg/500 mg up to the minimum effective dose needed to adequately control blood glucose. Maximum, 20 mg glyburide and 2,000 mg metformin daily.

✦ *Dosage adjustment*
Initial and maintenance dosing should be conservative in elderly patients because of the likelihood of decreased renal function. Any dosage adjustment requires careful assessment of renal function. Elderly, debilitated, and malnourished patients shouldn't be given the maximum dose to avoid the risk of hypoglycemia.

How supplied
Tablets: 1.25 mg glyburide and 250 mg metformin, 2.5 mg glyburide and 500 mg metformin, 5 mg glyburide and 500 mg metformin.

Pharmacodynamics
Hypoglycemic action: Glyburide appears to lower blood glucose levels by stimulating the release of insulin from the pancreas. The mechanism by which glyburide lowers blood glucose during long-term administration isn't clearly established. Metformin decreases hepatic glucose production and intestinal absorption of glucose and improves insulin sensitivity.

Pharmacokinetics
glyburide
Absorption: Absorbed almost completely from the GI tract.
Distribution: Extensively protein-bound.
Metabolism: Metabolized completely by the liver to weakly active metabolites.
Excretion: Excreted as metabolites in urine and bile in equal proportions. Half-life is 10 hours.
metformin
Absorption: Absorbed from GI tract, with food decreasing extent and slightly delaying rate of absorption.
Distribution: Negligibly bound to plasma proteins.
Metabolism: Not metabolized.
Excretion: Excreted unchanged in urine. Half-life is 6.2 hours.

Route	Onset	Peak	Duration
P.O.			
glyburide	1 hr	4 hr	24 hr
metformin	Unknown	Unknown	Unknown

Contraindications and precautions
Contraindicated in patients hypersensitive to glyburide or metformin and patients with renal disease, renal dysfunction, or metabolic acidosis (including diabetic ketoacidosis). Contraindicated in heart failure that needs pharmacologic treatment.

Use cautiously in elderly, hepatically impaired, debilitated, or malnourished patients and those with adrenal or pituitary insufficiency because of increased risk of hypoglycemia.

Interactions
Drug-drug. *Beta blockers, chloramphenicol, ciprofloxacin, coumarins, highly protein-bound drugs, MAO inhibitors, miconazole, NSAIDs, probenecid, salicylates, sulfonamides:* Increased hypoglycemic activity of glyburide. Monitor blood glucose level.
Calcium channel blockers, corticosteroids, estrogens, isoniazid, nicotinic acid, oral contraceptives, phenothiazines, phenytoin, sympathomimetics, thiazides and other diuretics, thyroid agents: Increased risk of hyperglycemia. Monitor patient's blood glucose level.
Cationic drugs (such as amiloride, cimetidine, digoxin, morphine, procainamide, quinidine, quinine, ranitidine, triamterene, trimethoprim, vancomycin): May increase metformin levels. Monitor patient.
Furosemide: Increased metformin levels and decreased furosemide levels. Monitor patient closely.
Nifedipine: Increased metformin levels. Metformin dosage may need to be decreased.
Drug-lifestyle. *Alcohol use:* Altered glycemic control, most commonly hypoglycemia. May also cause disulfiram-like reaction with glyburide component. Discourage concomitant use.

Adverse reactions
CNS: headache, dizziness.
GI: *diarrhea,* nausea, vomiting, abdominal pain.
Metabolic: *hypoglycemia.*
Respiratory: *upper respiratory infection.*

Overdose and treatment
Glyburide overdose can produce hypoglycemia. Mild hypoglycemic symptoms, without loss of consciousness or neurologic findings, should be treated aggressively with oral glucose and adjustments in drug, dosage, or meal patterns. Severe hypoglycemic reactions with coma, seizure, or other neurologic impairment occur infrequently but demand immediate hospitalization. If hypoglycemic coma is diagnosed or suspected, the patient should be given a rapid I.V. injection of concentrated (50%) glucose solution followed by continuous infusion of a more dilute (10%) glucose solution at a rate that will maintain the blood glucose at a level above 100 mg/dl. Any patient with hypoglycemia should be monitored closely until out of danger and, if the reaction is severe, for a minimum of 24 to 48 hours,

---

Reactions may be *common*, uncommon, *life-threatening*, or COMMON AND LIFE-THREATENING.

since hypoglycemia may recur after apparent clinical recovery.

Metformin overdose hasn't been linked to hypoglycemia, but lactic acidosis may occur. Hemodialysis may remove metformin, but not glyburide.

Special considerations

● Drug should be temporarily discontinued in patients undergoing radiologic studies involving intravascular administration of iodinated contrast materials, because use of such products may result in acute alteration of renal function.
● For patients previously treated with glyburide or metformin, the starting dose of Glucovance shouldn't exceed the daily dose of the glyburide (or equivalent dose of another sulfonylurea) and metformin already being taken.
● Lactic acidosis is a rare, but serious (50% fatal), metabolic complication that can result from metformin accumulation. Reported cases have occurred primarily in diabetic patients with significant renal insufficiency; with multiple medical or surgical problems; and with multiple drug regimens. The risk of lactic acidosis increases with the degree of renal impairment and patient's age.
● Early symptoms of lactic acidosis may include malaise, myalgias, respiratory distress, increasing somnolence, and nonspecific abdominal distress.
● GI symptoms that occur after a patient is stabilized on any dose level of Glucovance are unlikely to be drug-related and could be from lactic acidosis or other serious disease.
● Lactic acidosis should be suspected in any diabetic patient with metabolic acidosis lacking evidence of ketoacidosis.
● Discontinue drug if CV collapse, acute heart failure, acute MI, or other conditions characterized by hypoxemia occur, because these conditions may be related to lactic acidosis and may cause prerenal azotemia.

Patient monitoring

● Assess blood glucose level before therapy and regularly thereafter. Monitor glycosylated hemoglobin to assess long-term therapy.
● Obtain baseline renal function studies and don't start drug if serum creatinine levels are 1.5 mg/dl or more for men or 1.4 mg/dl or more for women. Monitor renal function at least once yearly while the patient takes drug and more often in those with increased risk of renal dysfunction. If renal impairment is detected, drug should be discontinued.
● Monitor patient closely during times of increased stress, such as infection, fever, surgery, or trauma; insulin therapy may be needed. Drug therapy should be temporarily suspended for any surgical procedure that requires restricted intake of food and fluids and shouldn't be restarted until oral intake has resumed.

● Monitor patient's hematologic status for megaloblastic anemia. Patients with inadequate vitamin B_{12} or calcium intake or absorption seem predisposed to developing subnormal vitamin B_{12} levels when taking metformin. They should have serum vitamin B_{12} level determinations every 2 to 3 years.
● Evaluate patient who develops laboratory abnormalities or clinical illness for evidence of ketoacidosis or lactic acidosis, including serum electrolytes, ketones, blood glucose, blood pH, lactate, pyruvate, and metformin levels. Discontinue drug if evidence of acidosis occurs.

Breast-feeding patients

● Drug isn't recommended for breast-feeding women.

Pediatric patients

● Safety and efficacy haven't been established in children.

Geriatric patients

● All patients should have a baseline serum creatinine that indicates normal renal function before starting therapy.
● Treatment shouldn't begin in patients age 80 or older unless creatinine clearance measurement shows that renal function isn't reduced.
● In elderly patients, renal function should be monitored regularly and, generally, Glucovance shouldn't be adjusted to the maximum dose.

Patient education

● Tell patient to take once-daily dose with breakfast and twice-daily dose with breakfast and dinner.
● Teach the patient about diabetes and the importance of following therapeutic regimen; adhering to diet, weight reduction, regular exercise and hygiene programs; and avoiding infection.
● Explain how and when to monitor blood glucose level and how to differentiate between hypoglycemia and hyperglycemia.
● Instruct patient to stop drug and report unexplained hyperventilation, myalgia, malaise, unusual somnolence, or other symptoms of early lactic acidosis.
● Tell patient that GI symptoms are common early in drug therapy. GI symptoms that occur after prolonged therapy may be related to lactic acidosis or other serious disease and should be reported promptly.
● Counsel patient against excessive alcohol intake, either acute or chronic.
● Advise patient not to take any other medications, including OTC drugs, without checking with prescriber.
● Instruct patient to wear or carry medical identification.

glycerin (glycerol)
Fleet Babylax, Ophthalgan,
Osmoglyn, Sani-Supp

Pharmacologic classification: trihydric
alcohol, ophthalmic osmotic vehicle
Therapeutic classification: laxative (osmotic),
ophthalmic osmotic, adjunct in treating
glaucoma, lubricant
Pregnancy risk category: C

Indications and dosages
➤ **Constipation.** *Adults and children age 6
and older:* 3 g as a suppository or 5 to 15 ml as
an enema.
Children under age 6: 1 to 1.5 g as a suppository or 2 to 5 ml as an enema.
➤ **Reduction of intraocular pressure.**
Adults: 1 to 2 g/kg P.O. 60 to 90 minutes preoperatively.
➤ **Reduction of corneal edema.** *Adults:*
1 to 2 drops of ophthalmic solution topically before eye examination; 1 to 2 drops q 3 to 4 hours
for corneal edema.
➤ **To act as an osmotic diuretic.** *Adults:*
1 to 2 g/kg P.O. 1 to 1½ hours before surgery.

How supplied
Available by prescription only
Ophthalmic solution: 7.5-ml containers
Oral solution: 50% (0.6 g/ml), 75% (0.94 g/ml)
Available without a prescription
Rectal solution: 4 ml/applicator
Suppository: 1.5 g (for infants), 3 g (adults)

Pharmacodynamics
Laxative action: Glycerin suppositories produce laxative action by causing rectal distention,
thereby stimulating the urge to defecate; by causing local rectal irritation; and by triggering a hyperosmolar mechanism that draws water into the
colon.
Antiglaucoma action: Orally administered
glycerin helps reduce intraocular pressure by
increasing plasma osmotic pressure, thereby
drawing water into the blood from extravascular spaces. It also reduces intraocular fluid
volume independently of routine flow mechanisms, decreasing intraocular pressure; it may
cause tissue dehydration and decreased CSF
pressure.
   Topically applied glycerin produces a hygro-
scopic (moisture-retaining) effect that reduces
edema and improves visualization in ophthal-
moscopy or gonioscopy. Glycerin reduces fluid
in the cornea via its osmotic action and clears
corneal haze.

Pharmacokinetics
Rectal form
Absorption: Absorbed poorly; after rectal administration, laxative effect occurs in 15 to 30
minutes.

Distribution: Distributed locally.
Metabolism: No information available.
Excretion: Excreted in feces.
Oral form
Absorption: Absorbed rapidly from GI tract, with
serum levels peaking in 60 to 90 minutes with
oral administration; intraocular pressure decreases
in 10 to 30 minutes. Action peaks in 30 minutes
to 2 hours, with effects persisting for 4 to 8 hours.
Intracranial pressure (ICP) decreases in 10 to 60
minutes; effect persists for 2 to 3 hours.
Distribution: Distributed throughout blood but
doesn't enter ocular fluid; drug may enter breast
milk.
Metabolism: About 80% metabolized in liver,
10% to 20% in kidneys.
Excretion: Excreted in feces and urine.

Route	Onset	Peak	Duration
P.O.	Rapid	60-90 min	4-8 hr
P.R., oph-thalmic	Unknown	Unknown	Unknown

Contraindications and precautions
Contraindicated in patients hypersensitive to drug.
Rectal administration of drug is contraindicated
in those with intestinal obstruction. Also contraindicated in patients with undiagnosed abdominal pain, vomiting, or other signs of appendicitis, fecal impaction, or acute surgical
abdomen.
   Use oral form cautiously in elderly or dehydrated patients and in those with diabetes or cardiac, renal, or hepatic disease.

Interactions
Drug-drug. *Diuretics:* Possible additive effects.
Avoid concomitant use.

Adverse reactions
CNS: mild headache, dizziness (with oral administration).
EENT: eye pain, irritation.
GI: cramping pain, thirst, nausea, vomiting, diarrhea (with oral administration); rectal discomfort, hyperemia of rectal mucosa (with rectal administration).
Metabolic: mild hyperglycemia, mild glycosuria.

Overdose and treatment
No information available.

Special considerations
● Drug is useful in acute angle-closure glaucoma; before iridectomy (with carbonic anhydrase
inhibitors or topical miotics); in trauma or disease, such as congenital glaucoma and some secondary glaucoma forms; and before or after
surgery, such as retinal detachment surgery,
cataract extraction, or keratoplasty.
● Drug is used to facilitate ophthalmoscopic and
gonioscopic examination and to differentiate superficial edema and deep corneal edema.

Reactions may be *common*, uncommon, *life-threatening*, or COMMON AND LIFE-THREATENING.

⚠ ALERT Stop drug if hypersensitivity symptoms occur.

• When administering glycerin orally, don't give hypotonic fluids to relieve thirst and headache from glycerin-induced dehydration; these will counteract osmotic effects.

• Use topical tetracaine hydrochloride or proparacaine before ophthalmic instillation to prevent discomfort.

• Don't touch tip of dropper to eye, surrounding tissues, or tear-film; glycerin will absorb moisture.

• To prevent or relieve headache, have patient remain supine during and after oral administration.

• Commercially available solutions may be poured over ice and sipped through a straw.

• Hyperosmolar laxatives are used most commonly to help laxative-dependent patients reestablish normal bowel habits.

• Other uses include reducing ICP in patients with CVA, meningitis, encephalitis, Reye's syndrome, or CNS trauma or tumors. Also used for reducing brain volume during neurosurgical procedures through oral administration, I.V. administration, or both.

• If excess glycerin is administered into eye, irrigate conjunctiva with sterile normal saline solution or water. Systemic effects aren't expected.

Patient monitoring

• Monitor diabetic patient for possible altered serum and urine glucose levels; dosage adjustment may be needed.

• Monitor serum glucose level if patient has diabetes.

• Monitor patient for adverse effects.

Breast-feeding patients

• Safety in breast-feeding women hasn't been established. Possible risks must be weighed against benefits.

Pediatric patients

• Safety and effectiveness of ophthalmic glycerin solutions in children haven't been established.

Geriatric patients

• Dehydrated elderly patients may experience seizures and disorientation.

Patient education

• Instruct patient to report severe headache after oral dose.

• Teach correct way to instill drops, and warn patient not to touch eye with dropper.

• Tell patient to lie down during and after administration to prevent or relieve headache.

glycopyrrolate
Robinul, Robinul Forte

Pharmacologic classification: anticholinergic
Therapeutic classification: antimuscarinic, GI antispasmodic
Pregnancy risk category: B

Indications and dosages

➤ **Blockade of cholinergic effects of anticholinesterase drugs used to reverse neuromuscular blockade.** *Adults and children:* 0.2 mg I.V. for each 1 mg neostigmine or 5 mg of pyridostigmine. May be given I.V. without dilution or may be added to dextrose injection and infused.

➤ **Preoperatively to diminish secretions and block cardiac vagal reflexes.** *Adults and children over age 2:* 0.0044 mg/kg of body weight given I.M. 30 to 60 minutes before anesthesia.

➤ **Adjunctive therapy in peptic ulcers and other GI disorders.** *Adults:* 1 to 2 mg P.O. t.i.d. or 0.1 mg I.M. t.i.d. or q.i.d. Dosage should be individualized.

How supplied

Available by prescription only
Injection: 0.2 mg/ml in 1-ml, 2-ml, 5-ml, 20-ml vials
Tablets: 1 mg, 2 mg

Pharmacodynamics

Anticholinergic action: Glycopyrrolate inhibits muscarinic actions of acetylcholine on autonomic effectors innervated by postganglionic cholinergic nerves. This action blocks adverse muscarinic effects of anticholinesterase agents used to reverse curariform-induced neuromuscular blockade. Glycopyrrolate decreases secretions and GI motility by the same mechanism. Glycopyrrolate blocks cardiac vagal reflexes by blocking vagal inhibition of the SA node.

Pharmacokinetics

Absorption: Poorly absorbed from GI tract (10% to 25%) after oral administration.
Distribution: Rapidly distributed. Because it's a quaternary amine, drug doesn't cross the blood-brain barrier or enter the CNS.
Metabolism: Exact metabolic fate is unknown.
Excretion: Small amount of drug is eliminated in urine as unchanged drug and metabolites. Drug is mostly excreted unchanged in feces or bile.

Route	Onset	Peak	Duration
P.O.	Unknown	Unknown	8-12 hr
I.V.	1 min	Unknown	3-7 hr
I.M., S.C.	15-30 min	30-45 min	3-7 hr

Contraindications and precautions

Contraindicated in patients hypersensitive to drug and in those with glaucoma, obstructive uropathy, obstructive disease of the GI tract, myasthenia gravis, paralytic ileus, intestinal atony, unstable CV status in acute hemorrhage, severe ulcerative colitis, or toxic megacolon.

Use cautiously in patients with autonomic neuropathy, hyperthyroidism, coronary artery disease, arrhythmias, heart failure, hypertension, hiatal hernia, hepatic or renal disease, and ulcerative colitis. Also use cautiously in hot or humid conditions where drug-induced heatstroke may occur.

Interactions

Drug-drug. *Amantadine, antihistamines, antiparkinsonians, disopyramide, glutethimide, meperidine, phenothiazines, procainamide, quinidine, tricyclic antidepressants:* Additive adverse effects. Avoid use together.

Antacids: Decreased oral absorption of anticholinergics. Give glycopyrrolate at least 1 hour before antacids.

Levodopa, ketoconazole: Decreased GI absorption. Separate administration times by 2 to 3 hours.

Oral potassium supplements, especially waxmatrix formulations: Increased risk of potassium-induced GI ulcerations. Use cautiously.

Slowly dissolving digoxin tablets: May yield higher serum digoxin levels when administered with anticholinergics. Use cautiously; dose adjustment may be needed.

Adverse reactions

CNS: weakness, nervousness, insomnia, drowsiness, dizziness, headache, confusion or excitement (in elderly patients).

CV: palpitations, tachycardia.

EENT: *dilated pupils, blurred vision,* photophobia, increased intraocular pressure.

GI: *constipation, dry mouth,* nausea, loss of taste, abdominal distension, vomiting, epigastric distress.

GU: *urinary hesitancy, urine retention,* impotence.

Skin: urticaria, decreased sweating or anhidrosis, other dermal manifestations.

Other: allergic reactions *(anaphylaxis),* fever.

Overdose and treatment

Overdose causes such peripheral effects as dilated, nonreactive pupils; blurred vision; flushed, hot, dry skin; dryness of mucous membranes; dysphagia; decreased or absent bowel sounds; urine retention; hyperthermia; tachycardia; hypertension; and increased respiration.

Treatment is primarily symptomatic and supportive, as needed. If patient is alert, induce emesis (or use gastric lavage) and follow with a saline cathartic and activated charcoal to prevent further drug absorption. In severe life-threatening cases, physostigmine may be administered to block antimuscarinic effects of glycopyrrolate. Give fluids, as needed, to treat shock. If urine retention occurs, catheterization may be necessary.

Special considerations

Consider the recommendations relevant to all anticholinergics as well as the following.
● Even slight overdose can lead to toxicity.
● For immediate treatment of bradycardia, some clinicians prefer atropine over glycopyrrolate.
● Don't mix glycopyrrolate with I.V. solutions containing sodium chloride or bicarbonate.
● Drug may be administered with neostigmine or physostigmine in same syringe.
● Drug is incompatible with thiopental, methohexital, secobarbital, pentobarbital, chloramphenicol, dimenhydrinate, and diazepam.

Patient monitoring

● Monitor patient closely for toxicity.
● Monitor patient for CNS effects and for urinary hesitancy or urine retention.

Breast-feeding patients

● Drug may appear in breast milk, possibly resulting in infant toxicity. Breast-feeding women should avoid this drug.
● Drug may decrease milk production.

Pediatric patients

● Drug isn't recommended for peptic ulcer in children under age 12.
● Manufacturer recommends that drug not be used in neonates under age 1 month because glycopyrrolate injection contains benzyl alcohol.

Geriatric patients

● Administer glycopyrrolate cautiously to elderly patients, even though it may be the preferred anticholinergic in these patients.

Patient education

● Instruct patient to take oral drug 30 to 60 minutes before meals.
● Warn patient to avoid activities that require alertness until CNS effects of drug are known.
● Advise patient to contact prescriber to report signs of urinary hesitancy or urine retention.

gold sodium thiomalate
Aurolate

Pharmacologic classification: gold salt
Therapeutic classification: antiarthritic
Pregnancy risk category: C

Indications and dosages

➤ *Rheumatoid arthritis, psoriatic arthritis◇, Felty's syndrome◇. Adults:* Initially, 10 mg I.M.; then 25 mg in second week and continued for a third dose the following week. Continue until 1 g (cumulative) has been given, unless toxicity occurs. If improvement occurs without toxicity before initial 1-g dose, a maintenance dosage of 25 to 50 mg every other week for 2 to 20 weeks may be started. Then continue to every third and then every fourth week indefinitely.

Weekly injections may be restarted any time, if necessary. If patient doesn't respond after reaching initial 1-g dose, then discontinue therapy, give 25 to 50 mg I.M. for another 10 weeks, or increase dose by 10 mg q 1 to 4 weeks (maximum dose per injection is 100 mg).

Children: 10-mg test dose; then 1 mg/kg weekly. Continue as listed for adults. Maximum single dose for children under age 12 is 50 mg.

➤ *Palindromic rheumatism ◇. Adults:* Initially, 10 to 15 mg I.M. weekly until 1-g dose is reached.

➤ *Pemphigus ◇. Adults:* Initially, 10 mg I.M.; then 25 mg I.M. for second week followed by 50 mg I.M. weekly. When patient is off corticosteroid therapy, maintenance dosage of 25 to 50 mg I.M. q 2 weeks may be administered.

How supplied
Available by prescription only
Injection: 50 mg/ml with benzyl alcohol

Pharmacodynamics
Antiarthritic action: Gold sodium thiomalate is thought to be effective against rheumatoid arthritis by altering the immune system to reduce inflammation. Although the exact mechanism remains unknown, these compounds have reduced serum levels of immunoglobulins and rheumatoid factors in patients with arthritis.

Pharmacokinetics
Absorption: Absorption is rapid.
Distribution: Higher tissue levels occur with parenteral gold salts, with a mean steady state plasma level of 1 to 5 mcg/ml. Drug is distributed widely throughout the body in lymph nodes, bone marrow, kidneys, liver, spleen, and tissues. About 85% to 90% is protein-bound.
Metabolism: Not broken down into its elemental form. The half-life with cumulative dosing is 14 to 40 days.
Excretion: About 70% is excreted in the urine, 30% in feces.

Route	Onset	Peak	Duration
I.M.	Unknown	3-6 hr	Unknown

Contraindications and precautions
Contraindicated in patients hypersensitive to drug; those with hepatitis, exfoliative dermatitis, or a history of severe toxicity from previous exposure to gold or heavy metals; and patients with severe uncontrollable diabetes, renal disease, hepatic dysfunction, uncontrolled heart failure, marked hypertension, systemic lupus erythematosus, colitis, or Sjögren's syndrome. Also contraindicated in patients with urticaria, eczema, hemorrhagic conditions, or severe hematologic disorders and in those who have recently received radiation therapy.

Interactions
Drug-drug. *Drugs known to cause blood dyscrasias:* Additive risk of hematologic toxicity. Avoid use together.
Drug-lifestyle. *Sun or ultraviolet light exposure:* May cause photosensitivity reactions. Advise patient to use precautions.

Adverse reactions
Adverse reactions to gold are considered severe and potentially life-threatening.
CNS: confusion, hallucinations, *seizures.*
CV: *bradycardia,* hypotension.
EENT: corneal gold deposition, corneal ulcers.
GI: *metallic taste, stomatitis, diarrhea,* anorexia, abdominal cramps, nausea, vomiting, ulcerative enterocolitis.
GU: albuminuria, proteinuria, *nephrotic syndrome,* nephritis, acute tubular necrosis, hematuria, *acute renal failure.*
Hematologic: *thrombocytopenia* (with or without purpura), *aplastic anemia, agranulocytosis, leukopenia,* eosinophilia, anemia.
Hepatic: *hepatitis,* jaundice, elevated liver function test results.
Skin: diaphoresis, photosensitivity, *rash, dermatitis,* erythema, exfoliative dermatitis.
Other: *anaphylaxis, angioedema.*

Overdose and treatment
When severe reactions to gold occur, corticosteroids, dimercaprol (a chelating agent), or penicillamine may be given to aid recovery. Prednisone 40 to 100 mg daily in divided doses is recommended to manage severe renal, hematologic, pulmonary, or enterocolitic reactions to gold. Dimercaprol may be used together with corticosteroids to facilitate removal of the gold when corticosteroid treatment alone is ineffective.

Special considerations
● Administer all gold salts I.M., preferably intragluteally. Normal color of drug is pale yellow; don't use it if it darkens.
● Vasomotor adverse effects are more common with gold sodium thiomalate than with other gold salts.
● Most adverse reactions are readily reversible if drug is discontinued immediately.
● If adverse reactions are mild, some rheumatologists order resumption of gold therapy after 2 to 3 weeks' rest.
● Serum protein-bound iodine test, especially when done by the chloric acid digestion method, gives false readings during and for several weeks after gold therapy.

Patient monitoring
● Obtain pregnancy test before starting therapy.
● Obtain patient's urine for analysis for protein and sediment changes before each injection.
● Monitor CBC and platelet count monthly or before every other injection. Stop drug if platelet count drops below 100,000/mm³, hemoglobin

drops from baseline, granulocytes are less than 1,500/mm³, leukocytes are less than 4,000/mm³, or eosinophils are greater than 5%.

● Patient should remain recumbent for 10 to 20 minutes and remain under medical observation for 30 minutes after administration because of possible anaphylactic reaction.

Breast-feeding patients
● Drug isn't recommended for use in breast-feeding women.

Pediatric patients
● Use in children under age 6 isn't recommended.

Geriatric patients
● Administer usual adult dose. Use cautiously in patients with decreased renal function.

Patient education
● Inform patient that beneficial drug effect may take 3 months.
● Explain that vasomotor adverse reactions—faintness, weakness, dizziness, flushing, nausea, vomiting, diaphoresis—may occur immediately after injection. Advise patient to lie down until symptoms subside.
● Tell patient that stomatitis is commonly preceded by a metallic taste; this symptom must be reported to prescriber immediately.
● Advise patient to report rash or other skin problems to prescriber immediately.

gonadorelin acetate
Lutrepulse

Pharmacologic classification: gonadotropin-releasing hormone (GnRH)
Therapeutic classification: fertility
Pregnancy risk category: B

Indications and dosages
➤ **To induce ovulation in women with primary hypothalamic amenorrhea.**
Adults: 5 mcg I.V. q 90 minutes (using a Lutrepulse pump, 0.8 mg solution at 50 microliters/pulse) for 21 days. If no response after three treatment intervals, dosage may be increased. Usual dose is 1 to 20 mcg.

How supplied
Available by prescription only
Injection: 0.8 mg/10 ml, 3.2 mg/10 ml, in 10-ml vials
Supplied as a kit with I.V. supplies and portable infusion pump

Pharmacodynamics
Ovulation-stimulating action: Mimics the action of GnRH, which results in the synthesis and release of luteinizing hormone (LH) from the anterior pituitary. LH subsequently acts on the reproductive organs to regulate hormone synthesis.

Pharmacokinetics
Absorption: Administered I.V. using a portable pump designed to administer the drug in a pulsatile fashion to mimic the endogenous hormone.
Distribution: Low plasma volume of distribution (10 to 15 L) and high rate of clearance from plasma.
Metabolism: Rapidly metabolized. Several biologically inactive peptide fragments have been identified.
Excretion: Excreted primarily in urine. The high initial clearance rate (half-life of 2 to 10 minutes) is followed by a somewhat slower terminal half-life of 10 to 40 minutes.

Route	Onset	Peak	Duration
I.V.	Unknown	Unknown	10-40 min

Contraindications and precautions
Contraindicated in patients hypersensitive to drug, in women with conditions that could be complicated by pregnancy (such as prolactinoma), in those who are anovulatory from any cause other than a hypothalamic disorder, and in those with ovarian cysts.

Interactions
Drug-drug. *Ovary-stimulating drugs:* Risk of ovarian hyperstimulation. Avoid use together.

Adverse reactions
GU: multiple pregnancy, ovarian hyperstimulation.
Skin: hematoma, local infection, inflammation, mild phlebitis.

Overdose and treatment
No harmful effects are expected if the pump were to malfunction and deliver the entire contents of the highest concentration vial (3.2 mg). Bolus doses of up to 3,000 mcg haven't proven harmful in clinical trials; however, continuous exposure (nonpulsatile administration) to gonadorelin may temporarily reduce pituitary responsiveness.

Special considerations
● To mimic the action of the naturally occurring hormone, gonadorelin requires a pulsatile administration with a special portable infusion pump. The pulse period is set at 1 minute (drug is infused over 1 minute); pulse interval is set at 90 minutes.

Patient monitoring
● Close monitoring of dosage and ultrasonography of the ovaries are necessary to monitor drug response. Patients usually need pelvic ultrasound on days 7 and 14 after establishment of a baseline scan, although the interval between scans may be shortened.
● Regular pelvic examinations and midluteal phase serum progesterone determinations are necessary.

Reactions may be *common*, uncommon, *life-threatening*, or COMMON AND LIFE-THREATENING.

• Similar drugs have caused anaphylaxis; monitor patient for signs and symptoms.

Breast-feeding patients
• It isn't known whether drug appears in breast milk; however, there's no reason to administer drug to a breast-feeding woman.

Pediatric patients
• Safety and efficacy in patients under age 18 haven't been established.

Patient education
• Inform patient of the signs and symptoms of hypersensitivity reactions (hives, wheezing, difficulty breathing) and instruct her to report them immediately.
• Stress that a multiple pregnancy is possible (about 12% probability).

---

goserelin acetate
Zoladex, Zoladex 3-month

Pharmacologic classification: synthetic decapeptide
Therapeutic classification: luteinizing hormone–releasing hormone (LHRH) analogue
Pregnancy risk category: X (endometriosis and endometrial thinning); D (advanced breast cancer)

Indications and dosages
➤ *Endometriosis, advanced breast carcinoma, endometrial thinning. Women:* 1 (3.6-mg) implant S.C. q 28 days into the upper abdominal wall for 6 months. Treatment of endometriosis shouldn't exceed 6 months.
➤ *Palliative treatment of advanced carcinoma of the prostate. Men:* 1 (10.8 mg) implant S.C. q 12 weeks into the upper abdominal wall.

How supplied
Available by prescription only
Implant: 3.6 mg, 10.8 mg

Pharmacodynamics
Hormonal action: Long-term administration of goserelin, an LHRH, acts on the pituitary to decrease the release of follicle-stimulating hormone (FSH) and luteinizing hormone. In men, the result is dramatically decreased serum levels of testosterone.

Pharmacokinetics
Absorption: Slowly absorbed from implant site.
Distribution: Administration of the implant results in measurable levels of drug in serum throughout the dosing period.
Metabolism: Clearance of goserelin following S.C. administration of the drug is rapid and occurs via a combination of hepatic metabolism and urinary excretion.

Excretion: Elimination half-life is about 4¼ hours in patients with normal renal function. Substantial renal impairment prolongs half-life, but this doesn't appear to increase the risk of adverse effects.

Route	Onset	Peak	Duration
S.C.	Unknown	12-15 days	Unknown

Contraindications and precautions
Contraindicated in patients hypersensitive to LHRH, LHRH agonist analogues, or goserelin acetate. Also contraindicated in pregnant or breast-feeding women. The 10.8-mg implant is contraindicated for use in women.

Use cautiously in patients who take anticonvulsants or corticosteroids and those at risk for hyperlipidemia, osteoporosis, or chronic alcohol or tobacco abuse.

Interactions
None reported.

Adverse reactions
CNS: lethargy, pain (worsened in the first 30 days), dizziness, *insomnia, asthenia,* anxiety, *depression, headache,* chills, *emotional lability.*
CV: edema, *heart failure, arrhythmias, peripheral edema, CVA,* hypertension, *MI,* peripheral vascular disorder, chest pain.
GI: nausea, vomiting, diarrhea, constipation, ulcer, anorexia, abdominal pain.
GU: *impotence, sexual dysfunction, lower urinary tract symptoms,* renal insufficiency, urinary obstruction, *vaginitis,* urinary tract infection, amenorrhea, increased serum testosterone levels during the first week of therapy.
Hematologic: anemia.
Metabolic: increased serum acid phosphatase initially (will decrease by week 4); hyperglycemia; weight gain; increased low-density lipoprotein, high-density lipoprotein, and triglyceride levels.
Musculoskeletal: gout, back pain.
Respiratory: COPD, upper respiratory tract infection.
Skin: rash, *diaphoresis, acne, seborrhea,* hirsutism.
Other: *changes in libido, hot flashes, infection,* breast swelling and tenderness, *changes in breast size,* breast pain.

Overdose and treatment
No information is available regarding accidental or intentional overdose. In animal studies, doses up to 1 mg/kg daily produced no non endocrine-related symptoms.

Special considerations
• Give drug every 28 days for the 3.6-mg implant and every 12 weeks for the 10.8-mg implant, always under direct medical supervision. Local anesthesia may be used before injection.

• In the unlikely event of the need to surgically remove goserelin, it may be localized by ultrasound.

• Because Zoladex may suppress the pituitary-gonadal system, diagnostic tests of the pituitary-gonadotropic and gonadal functions conducted during treatment and until resumption of menses may show results that are misleading.

Patient monitoring

• Consider periodic monitoring of liver function tests, serum lipid profile and bone mineral density.

• Monitor drug serum levels.

Breast-feeding patients

• It isn't known whether drug appears in breast milk.

Pediatric patients

• Safety and efficacy in children under age 18 haven't been established.

Patient education

• Advise patient to report on time for each new implant.

• Advise patient to immediately report any implant-site reactions or other adverse reactions, such as those related to hypoestrogenism (hot flashes, headache, vaginal dryness, change in libido, depression, sweating, and change in breast size).

granisetron hydrochloride
Kytril

Pharmacologic classification: selective 5-hydroxytryptamine (5-HT$_3$) receptor antagonist
Therapeutic classification: antiemetic, antinausea
Pregnancy risk category: B

Indications and dosages

➤ *Prevention of nausea and vomiting caused by emetogenic cancer chemotherapy.* Adults and children ages 2 to 16: 10 mcg/kg I.V. infused over 5 minutes. Begin infusion within 30 minutes before administration of chemotherapy.

Oral form
Adults: 1 mg P.O. b.i.d. Give the first 1-mg tablet 1 hour before chemotherapy administration and the second tablet 12 hours after the first. Give only on days when chemotherapy is given. Continued treatment while not on chemotherapy isn't useful.

How supplied

Available by prescription only
Injection: 1 mg/ml
Tablets: 1 mg

Pharmacodynamics

Antiemetic action: Granisetron is a selective 5-HT$_3$ receptor antagonist thought to bind to serotonin receptors of the 5-HT$_3$ type located peripherally on vagal nerve terminals and centrally in the chemoreceptor trigger zone of the area postrema. This binding blocks serotonin stimulation and subsequent vomiting after emetogenic stimuli, such as cisplatin administration.

Pharmacokinetics

Absorption: Not determined.
Distribution: Distributed freely between plasma and RBCs. Plasma protein–binding is about 65%.
Metabolism: Metabolized by the liver, possibly mediated by the cytochrome P-450 3A subfamily.
Excretion: About 12% is eliminated unchanged in the urine in 48 hours; the remainder is excreted as metabolites: 48% in the urine and 38% in the feces.

Route	Onset	Peak	Duration
P.O., I. V.	Unknown	Unknown	Unknown

Contraindications and precautions

Contraindicated in patients hypersensitive to drug.

Interactions

Drug-herb. *Horehound:* Enhanced serotonergic effects. Discourage use together.

Adverse reactions

CNS: *headache, asthenia,* somnolence, dizziness, anxiety.
CV: hypertension.
GI: diarrhea, *constipation,* abdominal pain, *nausea,* vomiting, decreased appetite.
Hematologic: *leukopenia,* anemia, *thrombocytopenia.*
Hepatic: elevated liver function test results.
Skin: alopecia.
Other: fever.

Overdose and treatment

No antidote for overdose exists. Give symptomatic treatment. Overdose of up to 38.5 mg of granisetron has been reported without symptoms or only a slight headache.

Special considerations

• Don't mix with other drugs; information about compatibility is limited.

• Diluted solutions are stable for 24 hours at room temperature.

• No dosage adjustment is recommended for patients with renal impairment or hepatic disease.

Patient monitoring

• Monitor patient for decreased symptoms and increased nausea or abdominal pain.

Breast-feeding patients
● It isn't known whether drug appears in breast milk.

Pediatric patients
● Safety and efficacy in children under age 2 haven't been established.
● Safety and efficacy of the oral form haven't been established in children.

Patient education
● Tell patient to watch for signs of an anaphylactoid reaction—local or generalized hives, chest tightness, wheezing, and dizziness or weakness—and to report them immediately.

griseofulvin microsize
Fulvicin-U/F, Grifulvin V, Grisactin

griseofulvin ultramicrosize
Fulvicin P/G, Grisactin Ultra, Gris-PEG

Pharmacologic classification: penicillium antibiotic
Therapeutic classification: antifungal
Pregnancy risk category: C

Indications and dosages
➤ *Tinea corporis, tinea capitis, tinea barbae, or tinea cruris infections. Adults:* 330 mg ultramicrosize P.O. daily, or 500 mg microsize P.O. daily.
Children who weigh 14 to 23 kg (30 to 50 lb): 82.5 to 165 mg ultramicrosize P.O. daily. Or, 125 to 250 mg microsize P.O. daily.
Children who weigh more than 23 kg: 165 to 330 mg ultramicrosize P.O. daily. Or, 250 to 500 mg microsize P.O. daily.
➤ *Tinea pedis or tinea unguium infections. Adults:* 660 mg ultramicrosize P.O. daily. Or, 1 g microsize P.O. daily.
Children who weigh 14 to 23 kg (30 to 50 lb): 82.5 to 165 mg ultramicrosize P.O. daily. Or, 125 to 250 mg microsize P.O. daily.
Children who weigh more than 23 kg: 165 to 330 mg ultramicrosize P.O. daily. Or, 250 to 500 mg microsize P.O. daily.

How supplied
Available by prescription only
microsize
Capsules: 250 mg
Oral suspension: 125 mg/5 ml
Tablets: 250 mg, 500 mg
ultramicrosize
Tablets: 125 mg, 165 mg, 250 mg, 330 mg
Tablets (film-coated): 125 mg, 250 mg

Pharmacodynamics
Antifungal action: Griseofulvin disrupts fungal cell's mitotic spindle, interfering with cell division; it also may inhibit DNA replication. Drug

also enters keratin precursor cells, slowing fungal growth. Active against *Trichophyton, Microsporum,* and *Epidermophyton* species.

Pharmacokinetics
Absorption: Absorbed primarily in the duodenum and varies among individuals. Ultramicrosize preparations are absorbed almost completely; microsize absorption ranges from 25% to 70% and may be increased by giving with a high-fat meal.
Distribution: Concentrates in skin, hair, nails, fat, liver, and skeletal muscle; it's tightly bound to new keratin.
Metabolism: Oxidatively demethylated and conjugated with glucuronic acid to inactive metabolites in the liver.
Excretion: About 50% of drug and its metabolites is excreted in urine and 33% in feces within 5 days. Less than 1% of a dose appears unchanged in urine. Drug is also excreted in perspiration. Elimination half-life is 9 to 24 hours.

Route	Onset	Peak	Duration
P.O.	Unknown	4-8 hr	Unknown

Contraindications and precautions
Contraindicated in those hypersensitive to drug and those with porphyria or hepatocellular failure. Also contraindicated in pregnant women and women who intend to become pregnant during therapy. Use cautiously in penicillin-sensitive patients.

Interactions
Drug-drug. *Barbiturates:* Impaired griseofulvin absorption. Dosage may need to be increased.
Cyclosporine, salicylates: Serum levels of these drugs may be decreased. Monitor patient for decreased therapeutic effects.
Oral contraceptives: Decreased contraceptive efficacy. Suggest alternative method of contraception.
Warfarin: Decreased PT and INR. Dosage adjustment may be needed.
Drug-food. *High-fat meals:* Increased absorption. May be given together.
Drug-lifestyle. *Alcohol use:* Increased alcohol effect, producing tachycardia, diaphoresis, and flushing. Advise patient to avoid alcohol.

Adverse reactions
CNS: headache (in early stages of treatment), transient decrease in hearing, fatigue with large doses, occasional mental confusion, impaired performance of routine activities, psychotic symptoms, dizziness, insomnia, paresthesia of the hands and feet after extended therapy.
EENT: oral thrush.
GI: nausea, vomiting, flatulence, diarrhea, epigastric distress, *bleeding.*
GU: proteinuria, menstrual irregularities.
Hematologic: *leukopenia, granulocytopenia,* porphyria.

Hepatic: *hepatotoxicity.*
Skin: *rash, urticaria,* photosensitivity.
Other: *hypersensitivity reactions,* lupus
erythematosus, *angioedema.*

Overdose and treatment
Signs and symptoms of overdose include headache, lethargy, confusion, vertigo, blurred vision,
nausea, vomiting, and diarrhea.

Treatment is supportive. After recent ingestion (within 4 hours), empty stomach by induced
emesis or gastric lavage. Follow with activated
charcoal to decrease absorption. A cathartic may
also be helpful.

Special considerations
● Confirm identification of organism before therapy begins.
● Give drug with or after meals, consisting of a
high-fat content (if allowed), to minimize GI distress.
● Treatment of tinea pedis may require combined
oral and topical therapy.
◖ ALERT Because griseofulvin ultramicrosize
is dispersed in polyethylene glycol, it's absorbed
more rapidly and completely than microsize and
is effective at one-half to two-thirds the usual gri-
selfulvin dose. Don't interchange preparations.

Patient monitoring
● Assess nutrition and monitor food intake; drug
may alter taste sensation, suppressing appetite.
● Check CBC regularly for possible adverse effects; monitor renal and liver function studies periodically.

Pregnant patients
● Contraindicated in pregnant women and women
who intend to become pregnant during therapy.

Breast-feeding patients
● Safety hasn't been established in breast-feeding
women.

Pediatric patients
● Microsize griseofulvin has been used in children as young as age 3 months.
● Manufacturer states that dosage of ultramicrosize griseofulvin hasn't been established in children age 2 years and younger.

Patient education
● Encourage patient to maintain adequate nutritional intake.
● Stress importance of completing prescribed
regimen to prevent relapse even though symptoms may abate quickly.
● Tell patient to report adverse reactions immediately.
● Advise patient to avoid exposure to intense indoor light and sunlight to reduce the risk of photosensitivity reactions.

● Explain that drug may potentiate alcohol effects, and advise patient to avoid alcohol during
therapy.

guaifenesin
Anti-Tuss, Balminil Expectorant*,
Breonesin, Diabetic Tussin EX,
Duratuss-G, Fenesin, Gee-Gee,
Genatuss, GG-Cen, Glyate,
Glycotuss, Glytuss, Guafenex L.A.,
Humibid L.A., Humibid Sprinkle,
Hytuss, Hytuss 2X, Muco-Fen-LA,
Mytussin, Naldecon Senior EX,
Organidin NR, Respa-GF, Resyl*,
Robitussin, Scot-Tussin, Touro EX,
Tusibron, Uni-tussin

Pharmacologic classification: propanediol
derivative
Therapeutic classification: expectorant
Pregnancy risk category: C

Indications and dosages
➤ *Expectorant. Adults and children age 12
and older:* 100 to 400 mg P.O. q 4 hours. Maxi-
mum, 2.4 g daily.
Children ages 6 to 11: 100 to 200 mg P.O. q 4
hours. Maximum, 1.2 g daily.
Children ages 2 to 5: 50 to 100 mg P.O. q 4 hours.
Maximum, 600 mg daily.
Children under age 2: Individualize dosage.
Extended-release form
Adults and children over age 12: 600 to 1,200 mg
P.O. q 12 hours. Maximum, 2,400 mg in 24 hours.
Children ages 6 to 12: 600 mg P.O. q 12 hours.
Maximum, 1,200 mg in 24 hours.
Children ages 2 to 6: 300 mg P.O. q 12 hours.
Maximum, 600 mg in 24 hours.

How supplied
Available by prescription only
Capsules: 300 mg
Tablets: 1,200 mg
Tablets (extended-release): 600 mg
Available without a prescription
Capsules: 200 mg
Capsules (extended-release): 300 mg
Syrup: 100 mg/5 ml, 200 mg/5 ml
Tablets: 100 mg, 200 mg

Pharmacodynamics
Expectorant action: Guaifenesin increases respiratory tract fluid by reducing adhesiveness and
surface tension, decreasing viscosity of the secretions and thereby facilitating their removal.

Pharmacokinetics
Unknown.

Route	Onset	Peak	Duration
P.O.	Unknown	Unknown	Unknown

Reactions may be *common,* uncommon, *life-threatening,* or **COMMON AND LIFE-THREATENING.**

Contraindications and precautions
Contraindicated in patients hypersensitive to drug.

Interactions
None significant.

Adverse reactions
CNS: dizziness, headache.
GI: vomiting and nausea (with large doses).
Skin: rash.

Overdose and treatment
No information available.

Special considerations
● Efficacy of guaifenesin as an expectorant hasn't been clearly established because of conflicting results of clinical studies.

Patient monitoring
● Patient should be re-evaluated if symptoms persist for more than 1 week, if cough recurs, or if cough is accompanied by fever, rash, or persistent headache.

Breast-feeding patients
● It isn't known whether drug appears in breast milk. Safety in breast feeding women hasn't been established.

Pediatric patients
● Individualize dosage for children under age 2.

Geriatric patients
● No specific recommendations are available. Most liquid forms contain alcohol (3.5% to 10%).

Patient education
● Advise patient to take drug with a glass of water to help loosen mucus in lungs.
● Advise patient to use sugarless throat lozenges to decrease throat irritation and cough and to report cough that persists longer than 7 days.

guanabenz acetate
Wytensin

Pharmacologic classification: centrally acting antiadrenergic
Therapeutic classification: antihypertensive
Pregnancy risk category: C

Indications and dosages
➤ **Hypertension (generally considered a step 2 agent).** *Adults:* Initially, 2 to 4 mg P.O. b.i.d. Dosage may be increased in increments of 4 to 8 mg daily q 1 to 2 weeks. The usual maintenance dosage ranges from 8 to 16 mg daily. Maximum, 32 mg b.i.d.
Children age 12 and older: Initially, 0.5 to 4 mg P.O. daily. Maintenance dosage ranges from 4 to 24 mg daily, administered in two divided doses.

➤ *Management of opiate withdrawal* ◇.
Adults: 4 mg P.O. b.i.d. to q.i.d.

How supplied
Available by prescription only
Tablets: 4 mg, 8 mg

Pharmacodynamics
Antihypertensive action: Guanabenz decreases blood pressure by stimulating central alpha₂-adrenergic receptors, decreasing cerebral sympathetic outflow and thus decreasing peripheral vascular resistance.

Pharmacokinetics
Absorption: After oral administration, 70% to 80% is absorbed from the GI tract.
Distribution: Appears to be distributed widely into the body, and is about 90% protein-bound.
Metabolism: Metabolized extensively in the liver; several metabolites are formed.
Excretion: Guanabenz and its metabolites are excreted primarily in urine; remaining drug is excreted in feces.

Route	Onset	Peak	Duration
P.O.	1 hr	2-5 hr	6-12 hr

Contraindications and precautions
Contraindicated in patients hypersensitive to drug. Use cautiously in elderly patients and patients with impaired renal or hepatic function, severe coronary insufficiency, recent MI, and cerebrovascular disease.

Interactions
Drug-drug. *Antihypertensives, diuretics:* Increased risk of excessive hypotension. Monitor blood pressure frequently.
Barbiturates, benzodiazepines, other sedatives, phenothiazines: Increased CNS depressant effects. Use together cautiously.
MAO inhibitors, tricyclic antidepressants: Inhibited antihypertensive effects of guanabenz. Monitor blood pressure frequently.
Drug-lifestyle. *Alcohol use:* Increased CNS depressant effects. Advise patient to avoid alcohol.

Adverse reactions
CNS: *drowsiness, sedation, dizziness, weakness,* headache.
CV: *rebound hypertension.*
GI: *dry mouth.*
Hepatic: elevations in liver enzyme levels.
Metabolic: may reduce serum cholesterol and total triglyceride levels slightly.

Overdose and treatment
Signs and symptoms of overdose include bradycardia, CNS depression, respiratory depression, hypothermia, apnea, seizures, lethargy, agitation, irritability, diarrhea, and hypotension.

Don't induce emesis; CNS depression occurs rapidly. After adequate respiration is assured,

◇ Unlabeled clinical use

empty stomach by gastric lavage; then give activated charcoal and a saline cathartic to decrease absorption. Follow with symptomatic and supportive care.

Special considerations
• Abrupt discontinuation of guanabenz causes severe rebound hypertension; reduce dosage gradually over 2 to 4 days.
• Reduced dosages may be required in patients with hepatic impairment.

Patient monitoring
• Monitor patient for adverse reactions, including CNS effects.
• Monitor liver enzyme and serum triglyceride levels.

Breast-feeding patients
• It isn't known whether guanabenz appears in breast milk; an alternative feeding method is recommended during therapy.

Pediatric patients
• Drug has been used to treat hypertension in a few children over age 12; safety and efficacy in younger children haven't been established.

Geriatric patients
• These patients may be more sensitive to antihypertensive and sedative effects of guanabenz. Start therapy at lower doses.

Patient education
• Explain signs and symptoms of adverse effects and importance of reporting them.
• Warn patient to avoid hazardous activities that require mental alertness and to avoid alcohol and other CNS depressants.
• Suggest taking drug at bedtime until tolerance develops to sedation, drowsiness, and other CNS effects.
• Warn patient to seek medical approval before taking OTC cold preparations.
• Advise patient not to discontinue drug suddenly; severe rebound hypertension may occur.

guanadrel sulfate
Hylorel

Pharmacologic classification: adrenergic neuron blocker
Therapeutic classification: antihypertensive
Pregnancy risk category: B

Indications and dosages
➤ *Hypertension. Adults:* Initially, 5 mg P.O. b.i.d.; adjust dosage until blood pressure is controlled. Most patients need 20 to 75 mg daily, usually given b.i.d. (400 mg daily is rarely used).
✦ *Dosage adjustment.* For a patient with renal impairment, use the guide at the top of the next column.

Creatinine clearance (ml/min)	Dosage
30 to 60	5 mg q 24 hr
< 30	5 mg q 48 hr

How supplied
Available by prescription only
Tablets: 10 mg, 25 mg

Pharmacodynamics
Antihypertensive action: Guanadrel reduces blood pressure by peripheral inhibition of norepinephrine release in adrenergic nerve endings, thus decreasing arteriolar vasoconstriction.

Pharmacokinetics
Absorption: Absorbed rapidly and almost completely from the GI tract.
Distribution: Distributed widely into the body; about 20% protein-bound. Drug doesn't enter the CNS.
Metabolism: About 40% to 50% of a dose is metabolized by the liver.
Excretion: Drug and its metabolites are eliminated primarily in urine. Plasma half-life is about 10 hours but varies considerably.

Route	Onset	Peak	Duration
P.O.	2 hr	4-6 hr	4-14 hr

Contraindications and precautions
Contraindicated in patients hypersensitive to drug and in those with known or suspected pheochromocytoma or heart failure. Also contraindicated in patients receiving MAO inhibitors or within 1 week of stopping MAO inhibitor therapy.
    Use cautiously in patients with regional vascular disease, bronchial asthma, or peptic ulcer disease.

Interactions
Drug-drug. *Antihypertensives, diuretics:* Enhanced antihypertensive effects. Monitor blood pressure closely.
Amphetamines, ephedrine, MAO inhibitors, methylphenidate, norepinephrine, phenothiazines, tricyclic antidepressants: May antagonize antihypertensive effects of guanadrel. Dosage adjustment may be needed.
Drug-lifestyle. *Alcohol use:* Increased risk of guanadrel-induced orthostatic hypotension. Discourage alcohol use, and monitor blood pressure frequently.

Adverse reactions
CNS: *fatigue, drowsiness, faintness, headache, confusion, paresthesia,* depression.
CV: *palpitations, chest pain, peripheral edema, orthostatic hypotension.*
EENT: glossitis, *visual disturbances.*

Reactions may be *common*, uncommon, ***life-threatening***, or COMMON AND LIFE-THREATENING.

GI: *diarrhea*, dry mouth, *indigestion, constipation, anorexia*, nausea, vomiting, *abdominal pain.*
GU: impotence, *ejaculation disturbances, nocturia, urination frequency.*
Metabolic: *weight gain.*
Musculoskeletal: *aching limbs, leg cramps.*
Respiratory: *shortness of breath, cough.*

Overdose and treatment

Signs and symptoms of overdose include hypotension, dizziness, blurred vision, and syncope. After acute ingestion, empty stomach by induced emesis or gastric lavage. The effect of activated charcoal in absorbing guanadrel hasn't been determined. Further treatment is usually symptomatic and supportive. If excessive hypotension occurs and persists despite conservative treatment, a vasoconstrictor (phenylephrine) may be considered.

Special considerations

● Separate use of guanadrel and MAO inhibitors by at least 1 week.
● Discontinue guanadrel 48 to 72 hours before surgery to minimize risk of vascular collapse during anesthesia.

Patient monitoring

● Monitor supine and standing blood pressure, especially during periods of dosage adjustment.
● Assess patient for signs and symptoms of edema.

Breast-feeding patients

● It isn't known whether drug appears in breast milk. An alternative feeding method is recommended during therapy.

Pediatric patients

● Safety and efficacy in children haven't been established; use drug only if potential benefit outweighs risk.

Geriatric patients

● These patients may be more sensitive to orthostatic hypotension.

Patient education

● Instruct patient to report weight gain of more than 5 lb (2.25 kg) weekly.
● Explain that orthostatic hypotension can be minimized by rising slowly from a supine position and avoiding sudden position changes; it may be aggravated by fever, hot weather, hot showers, prolonged standing, exercise, and alcohol.
● Warn patient to avoid hazardous activities that require mental alertness and to take drug at bedtime until tolerance develops to sedation, drowsiness, and other CNS effects.
● Warn patient to seek medical approval before taking OTC cold preparations.

guanethidine monosulfate
Ismelin

Pharmacologic classification: adrenergic neuron blocker
Therapeutic classification: antihypertensive
Pregnancy risk category: C

Indications and dosages

➤ *Moderate to severe hypertension, signs and symptoms of thyrotoxicosis* ◇ *.* **Adults:** Initially, 10 mg P.O. once daily. Increased by 10 mg at weekly to monthly intervals, as necessary. Usual dose is 25 to 50 mg once daily. Some patients may need up to 300 mg.

How supplied

Available by prescription only
Tablets: 10 mg, 25 mg

Pharmacodynamics

Antihypertensive action: Guanethidine acts peripherally; it decreases arteriolar vasoconstriction and reduces blood pressure by inhibiting norepinephrine release and depleting norepinephrine stores in adrenergic nerve endings.

Pharmacokinetics

Absorption: Absorbed incompletely from the GI tract. Maximal antihypertensive effects usually aren't evident for 1 to 3 weeks.
Distribution: Distributed throughout the body; it isn't protein-bound but demonstrates extensive tissue binding.
Metabolism: Undergoes partial hepatic metabolism to pharmacologically less active metabolites.
Excretion: Drug and metabolites are excreted primarily in urine; small amounts are excreted in feces. Elimination half-life after long-term administration is biphasic.

Route	Onset	Peak	Duration
P.O.	Unknown	8 hr	3-4 days

Contraindications and precautions

Contraindicated in patients hypersensitive to drug, patients receiving an MAO inhibitor, and patients with pheochromocytoma or heart failure. Use cautiously in patients taking other antihypertensives and patients with severe cardiac disease, recent MI, cerebrovascular disease, peptic ulcer, impaired renal function, or bronchial asthma.

Interactions

Drug-drug. *Amphetamines, ephedrine, MAO inhibitors, methylphenidate, norepinephrine, oral contraceptives, phenothiazines, tricyclic antidepressants:* May antagonize the antihypertensive effect of guanethidine. Discontinue MAO inhibitor therapy 1 week before starting guanethidine. Dosage may need adjustment.

◇ Unlabeled clinical use

Antihypertensives, diuretics, levodopa: May potentiate antihypertensive effect of guanethidine. Use together cautiously.

Cardiac glycosides: May result in additive bradycardia. Monitor patient closely.

Metaraminol, norepinephrine, oral sympathomimetic nasal decongestants: Guanethidine potentiates pressor effects of such agents. Monitor blood pressure closely.

Rauwolfia alkaloids (reserpine): May cause excessive orthostatic hypotension, bradycardia, and mental depression. Monitor patient closely.

Drug-lifestyle. *Alcohol use:* Increased hypotensive effect of guanethidine. Advise patient to avoid alcohol.

Adverse reactions
CNS: syncope, *fatigue, headache, drowsiness, paresthesia, confusion,* depression.
CV: *palpitations, chest pain, orthostatic hypotension, peripheral edema, **bradycardia**, **heart failure**.*
EENT: *visual disturbances,* glossitis.
GI: *diarrhea, indigestion, constipation, anorexia,* nausea, vomiting, abdominal pain.
GU: *nocturia, urination frequency, ejaculation disturbances,* impotence.
Metabolic: *weight gain.*
Musculoskeletal: *aching limbs, leg cramps.*
Respiratory: *shortness of breath, cough.*

Overdose and treatment
Signs and symptoms of overdose include hypotension, blurred vision, syncope, bradycardia, and severe diarrhea.

After acute ingestion, empty stomach by induced emesis or gastric lavage and give activated charcoal to reduce absorption. Further treatment is usually symptomatic and supportive.

Special considerations
• When drug is replacing MAO inhibitors, wait at least 1 week before starting guanethidine; if replacing ganglionic blocking agents, withdraw them slowly to prevent a spiking blood pressure response during the transfer period.
• Dosage requirements may be reduced in the presence of fever.
• Discontinue drug 2 to 3 weeks before elective surgery to reduce risk of CV collapse during anesthesia.

Patient monitoring
• Monitor patient for adverse reactions.
• If diarrhea develops, atropine or paregoric may be prescribed.

Breast-feeding patients
• Small amounts of drug appear in breast milk; recommend alternative feeding method during therapy.

Pediatric patients
• Safety and efficacy in children haven't been established.

Geriatric patients
• These patients may be more sensitive to drug's antihypertensive effects.

Patient education
• Tell patient to report persistent diarrhea and weight gain of 5 lb (2.25 kg) weekly. Advise patient not to stop drug but to call for instructions.
• Warn patient to avoid hazardous activities that require mental alertness and to take drug at bedtime until tolerance develops to sedation, drowsiness, and other CNS effects.
• Advise patient to avoid sudden position changes, strenuous exercise, heat, and hot showers, to minimize orthostatic hypotension; and to relieve dry mouth with ice chips, hard candy, or gum.
• Tell patient if a dose is missed not to double the next scheduled dose but to take only the next scheduled dose.
• Advise patient to seek medical approval before taking OTC cold medicines.

guanfacine hydrochloride
Tenex

Pharmacologic classification: centrally acting antiadrenergic
Therapeutic classification: antihypertensive
Pregnancy risk category: B

Indications and dosages
➤ *Mild to moderate hypertension.* Adults: Initially, 0.5 to 1 mg P.O. daily h.s. Average dose is 1 to 3 mg daily.
➤ *Heroin withdrawal* ◇. Adults: 0.03 to 1.5 mg P.O. daily.
➤ *Migraine* ◇. Adults: 1 mg P.O. daily for 12 weeks.

How supplied
Available by prescription only
Tablets: 1 mg, 2 mg

Pharmacodynamics
Antihypertensive action: Centrally acting alpha$_2$-adrenoreceptor agonist whose mechanism of action isn't clearly understood. Appears to stimulate central alpha$_2$-adrenergic receptors that decrease peripheral release of norepinephrine, thus decreasing peripheral vascular resistance and lowering blood pressure. Reduces heart rate by reducing sympathetic nerve impulses from the vasomotor center to the heart. Systolic and diastolic blood pressure are both decreased; cardiac output isn't altered.

Elevated plasma renin activity and plasma catecholamine levels are lowered; however, there's no correlation with individual blood pressure. Single doses of guanfacine stimulate growth hormone secretion, but long-term use has no effect on growth hormone levels.

Pharmacokinetics

Absorption: Absorbed well and completely after oral administration; about 80% bioavailable. Plasma levels peak in 1 to 4 hours.
Distribution: About 70% protein-bound; high distribution to tissues suggested.
Metabolism: Metabolized in liver.
Excretion: About 50% of drug eliminated in urine unchanged, rest as conjugates of metabolites.

Route	Onset	Peak	Duration
P.O.	Unknown	1-4 hr	24 hr

Contraindications and precautions

Contraindicated in patients hypersensitive to drug. Use cautiously in patients with renal or hepatic insufficiency, severe coronary insufficiency, recent MI, or cerebrovascular disease.

Interactions

Drug-drug. *Antihypertensives, diuretic combinations:* Antihypertensive effects may be potentiated; often used to therapeutic advantage.
CNS depressants (such as barbiturates, benzodiazepines, phenothiazines): May enhance depressant effects. Avoid concomitant use.
Estrogens, NSAIDs (especially indomethacin), sympathomimetics: May reduce antihypertensive effects of guanfacine. Indomethacin and other NSAIDs may inhibit renal prostaglandin synthesis or cause sodium and fluid retention, antagonizing antihypertensive activity of guanfacine. Blood pressure may increase via estrogen-induced fluid retention. Monitor patient carefully.
Tricyclic antidepressants: May inhibit antihypertensive effects. Avoid concurrent use.
Drug-lifestyle. *Alcohol:* May enhance CNS depressant effects. Discourage concomitant use.

Adverse reactions

CNS: *dizziness,* fatigue, headache, insomnia, *somnolence,* asthenia.
CV: *bradycardia.*
GI: *constipation,* diarrhea, nausea, *dry mouth.*
Metabolic: altered urinary catecholamine levels and urinary vanillylmandelic acid excretion (may be decreased during therapy but may increase on abrupt withdrawal), increased plasma growth hormone levels.
Skin: dermatitis, pruritus.

Overdose and treatment

Signs and symptoms of overdose include difficulty breathing, extreme dizziness, faintness, slow heartbeat, severe or unusual tiredness or weakness.

Treat symptomatically, with careful cardiac monitoring. Perform gastric lavage and infuse isoproterenol as appropriate.

Special considerations

● Give drug at bedtime to reduce daytime drowsiness.
● Withdrawal syndrome may occur if guanfacine is stopped abruptly or discontinued before surgery; therefore, anesthesiologist must be informed if drug was withdrawn more than 2 days before surgery or if drug hasn't been withdrawn.
● Dry mouth may contribute to development of dental caries, periodontal disease, oral candidiasis, and discomfort.
● Guanfacine is dialyzed poorly.

Patient monitoring

● Monitor blood pressure, especially standing and supine, at regular intervals.
● Monitor pulse rate.

Breast-feeding patients

● It's unknown whether drug appears in breast milk. Use cautiously in breast-feeding women.

Geriatric patients

● Dizziness, drowsiness, hypotension, or faintness occur more frequently in elderly patients, who may be more sensitive to effects of guanfacine.

Patient education

● Stress importance of diet and possible need for sodium restriction and weight reduction.
● Tell patient to take drug as directed even if feeling well and to take daily dose at bedtime to minimize daytime drowsiness.
● Advise patient that drug may cause drowsiness or dizziness. Urge patient to avoid use of alcohol and other CNS depressants, which may add to this effect. Tell patient to avoid driving or performing other tasks that require alertness until effects of drug are known.
● Inform patient to take a missed dose as soon as possible; if taking more than one dose per day when almost time for next dose, skip missed dose and return to regular schedule.
● If patient is to have surgery, including dental surgery, or emergency treatment, advise him to tell medical personnel that he is taking this drug.
● Advise chewing sugarless gum, candy, ice, or saliva substitute for treatment of dry mouth. If condition continues longer than 2 weeks, patient should call for further recommendations.
● Instruct patient not to take other drugs unless prescribed, particularly drugs for cough, cold, asthma, hay fever, or sinus conditions.

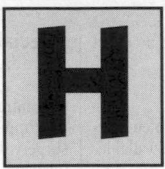

Haemophilus b vaccines

Haemophilus b conjugate vaccine, diphtheria CRM protein conjugate (HbOC)
HibTITER

Haemophilus b conjugate vaccine, meningococcal protein conjugate (PRP-OMP)
PedvaxHIB, Comvax

Haemophilus b polysaccharide conjugate vaccine, tetanus toxoid (PRP-T)
ActHIB, Omnihib

Pharmacologic classification: vaccine
Therapeutic classification: bacterial vaccine
Pregnancy risk category: C

Indications and dosages
➤ *Routine immunization. Haemophilus b conjugate vaccine, diphtheria CRM$_{197}$ protein conjugate. Children ages 2 to 6 months:* 0.5 ml I.M.; repeat in 2 months and again in 4 months (for total of three doses). A booster dose is required at age 15 months.
Previously unvaccinated children ages 7 to 11 months: 0.5 ml I.M.; repeat in 2 months (for total of two doses before age 15 months). A booster dose is required at age 15 months (but no sooner than 2 months after last vaccination).
Previously unvaccinated children ages 12 to 14 months: 0.5 ml I.M. A booster dose is required at age 15 months (but no sooner than 2 months after last vaccination).
Previously unvaccinated children ages 15 to 60 months: 0.5 ml I.M.
Haemophilus b conjugate vaccine, meningococcal protein conjugate
Previously unvaccinated infants ages 2 to 10 months: 0.5 ml I.M. ideally at 2 months. Repeat 2 months later (or as soon as possible thereafter). Administer a booster dose of 0.5 ml I.M. at 12 to 15 months (but no sooner than 2 months after last vaccination).
Previously unvaccinated children ages 11 to 14 months: 0.5 ml I.M.; repeat in 2 months.

Previously unvaccinated children ages 15 to 71 months: 0.5 ml I.M.
Haemophilus b polysaccharide conjugate vaccine, tetanus toxoid
Previously unvaccinated children ages 2 to 6 months: Three 0.5-ml I.M. doses at 8-week intervals, followed by a booster dose at age 15 to 18 months.
Previously unvaccinated children ages 7 to 11 months: Two 0.5-ml I.M. doses at 8-week intervals, followed by a booster dose at age 15 to 18 months.
Previously unvaccinated children ages 12 to 14 months: 0.5 ml I.M., followed by a booster dose at age 15 to 18 months. Administer no earlier than 2 months after previous dose.
Previously unvaccinated children ages 15 to 60 months: 0.5 ml I.M.

How supplied
Available by prescription only
conjugate vaccine, diphtheria CRM$_{197}$
Injection: 10 mcg of purified *Haemophilus* b saccharide and about 25 mcg CRM$_{197}$ protein per 0.5 ml
conjugate vaccine, meningococcal protein conjugate
Injection: 7.5 mcg *Haemophilus* b capsular polysaccharide, 125 mcg *Neisseria meningitidis* OMPC per 0.5 ml.
conjugate vaccine, tetanus toxoid
Powder for injection: 10 mcg *Haemophilu*s b purified capsular polysaccharide, 24 mcg of tetanus toxoid, and 8.5% sucrose

Pharmacodynamics
Prophylactic action: Vaccine promotes active immunity to *H. influenzae* type b.

Pharmacokinetics
Absorption: After I.M. or S.C. administration, increases in *H. influenzae* type b capsular antibody levels in serum are detectable in about 2 weeks and peak within 3 weeks.
Distribution: Limited data indicate that antibodies to *H. influenzae* type b can be detected in fetal blood and in breast milk after administration of the vaccine to pregnant and breast-feeding women.
Metabolism: No information available.
Excretion: The vaccine polysaccharide has been detected in urine for up to 11 days after administration to children.

Reactions may be *common*, uncommon, *life-threatening*, or COMMON AND LIFE-THREATENING.

Route	Onset	Peak	Duration
I.M.	2 wk after dose	Unknown	Several yr after last dose

Contraindications and precautions
Contraindicated in acutely ill patients and those hypersensitive to any component of vaccine, including thimerosal. Don't give drug to patients less than 10 days before or during treatment with immunosuppressive drugs or irradiation.

Interactions
Drug-drug. *Corticosteroids, immunosuppressants:* May impair immune response to the vaccine. Avoid vaccination under these circumstances.

Adverse reactions
CNS: irritability.
GI: diarrhea, vomiting.
Skin: erythema, *pain at injection site.*
Other: *anaphylaxis,* fever.

Overdose and treatment
No information available.

Special considerations
• Epinephrine solution 1:1,000 should be available to treat allergic reactions.
⚠ ALERT Vaccine types are age specific. Check labeling as well as current U.S. Health Service Advisory Committee on Immunization Practices and American Academy of Pediatrics recommendations.
• Vaccine may be given simultaneously with diphtheria, tetanus, and pertussis (DTP) vaccine; measles, mumps, and rubella (MMR) vaccine; poliovirus vaccine, inactivated (IPV); meningococcal vaccine; or pneumococcal vaccine; but it should be given at different sites.
• Administer same vaccine throughout the vaccination series; no data are available to support interchangeability of the vaccines.
• Vaccination shouldn't be used to prevent invasive disease related *H. influenzae* type b disease because of the time required to develop immunity. Instead, use chemoprophylaxis (with drugs such as rifampin) in both vaccinated and unvaccinated individuals because children with immunity may carry and transmit the organism. However, if every child in a household or daycare group has been fully vaccinated, chemoprophylaxis isn't necessary.
• A conjugate vaccine containing meningococcal proteins won't prevent meningococcal disease and one containing the tetanus toxoid conjugate won't produce immunity against tetanus toxoid. Administer DTP vaccine according to the recommended schedule.
• Some vaccine products may contain thimerosal.
• For days or weeks after administration, *Haemophilus* b may interfere with antigen detection tests.

Patient monitoring
• Adverse reactions typically occur within the first 24 hours.
• Monitor patient for anaphylaxis, injection site reactions, and fever.

Pregnant patients
• Drug usually isn't recommended for pregnant women.

Pediatric patients
• Safety and efficacy of PRP-OMP haven't been established for patients under age 2 months. Safety and efficacy of PRP-T haven't been established for patients under age 6 weeks.
• Children under age 24 months in whom invasive *H. influenzae* type b disease develops should be vaccinated because natural immunity may not develop.

Patient education
• *H. influenzae* type b is a cause of meningitis in infants and preschool children. Explain to parents that this vaccine will protect children only against meningitis caused by this organism.
• Tell parents that child may experience swelling and inflammation at injection site and fever. Recommend acetaminophen liquid for fever.
• Tell parents to report worrisome or persistent adverse reactions promptly.

haloperidol
Apo-Haloperidol*, Haldol, Novo-Peridol*, Peridol*

haloperidol decanoate
Haldol Decanoate 50, Haldol Decanoate 100, Haldol LA*

haloperidol lactate
Haldol, Haldol Concentrate, Haloperidol Intensol

Pharmacologic classification: butyrophenone
Therapeutic classification: antipsychotic
Pregnancy risk category: C

Indications and dosages
➤ *Psychotic disorders, alcohol dependence. Adults:* Dosage varies for each patient and symptoms. Initial dosage range is 0.5 to 5 mg P.O. b.i.d. or t.i.d.; or 2 to 5 mg I.M. q 4 to 8 hours, increased rapidly if necessary for prompt control. Maximum dose is 100 mg P.O. daily. Doses of more than 100 mg have been used to treat patients who have severely resistant conditions.
➤ *Psychotic patients who require prolonged therapy. Adults:* 100 mg I.M. of haloperidol decanoate q 4 weeks. Experience with doses of more than 450 mg monthly is limited.

▶*Control of tics, vocal utterances in Tourette syndrome. Adults:* 0.5 to 2 mg P.O. b.i.d. or t.i.d., increased, p.r.n.
Children ages 3 to 12: 0.05 to 0.075 mg/kg daily given b.i.d. or t.i.d.
▶*Delirium. Adults:*1 to 2 mg I.V. every 2 to 4 hours.

How supplied
Available by prescription only
haloperidol
Tablets: 0.5 mg, 1 mg, 2 mg, 5 mg, 10 mg, 20 mg
haloperidol decanoate
Injection: 50 mg/ml, 100 mg/ml
haloperidol lactate
Injection: 5 mg/ml
Oral concentrate: 2 mg/ml

Pharmacodynamics
Antipsychotic action: Haloperidol is thought to exert antipsychotic effects by strong postsynaptic blockade of CNS dopamine receptors, thereby inhibiting dopamine-mediated effects; its pharmacologic effects are most similar to those of piperazine antipsychotics. Its mechanism of action in Tourette syndrome is unknown.

Haloperidol has many other central and peripheral effects; it has weak peripheral anticholinergic effects and antiemetic effects, produces both alpha and ganglionic blockade, and counteracts histamine- and serotonin-mediated activity. Its most prominent adverse reactions are extrapyramidal.

Pharmacokinetics
Absorption: Rate and extent of absorption vary with route of administration. Oral administration yields 60% bioavailability.
Distribution: Distributed widely into body, with high levels in adipose tissue. Drug is 90% to 92% protein-bound.
Metabolism: Metabolized extensively by the liver; there may be only one active metabolite that's less active than parent drug.
Excretion: About 40% of a given dose is excreted in urine within 5 days; about 15% is excreted in feces via the biliary tract.

Route	Onset	Peak	Duration
P.O.	Unknown	3-6 hr	Unknown
I.M.			
decanoate	Unknown	3-9 days	Unknown
lactate	Unknown	10-20 min	Unknown

Contraindications and precautions
Contraindicated in patients hypersensitive to drug and in those experiencing parkinsonism, coma, or CNS depression.

Use haloperidol cautiously in elderly or debilitated patients; in patients with history of seizures, EEG abnormalities, CV disorders, allergies, angle-closure glaucoma, or urine reten-

tion; and in those receiving anticoagulants, anticonvulsants, antiparkinsonians, or lithium.

Interactions
Drug-drug. *Aluminum- and magnesium-containing antacids and antidiarrheals:* Decreased drug absorption. Separate administration times by 2 hours.
Antiarrhythmics, disopyramide, procainamide, quinidine: Increased risk of arrhythmias and conduction defects. Avoid use together.
Anticholinergics, including antidepressants, antihistamines, antiparkinsonians, atropine, MAO inhibitors, meperidine, phenothiazines: Oversedation, paralytic ileus, visual changes, and severe constipation. Use cautiously.
Beta blockers: May inhibit haloperidol metabolism, increasing plasma levels and toxicity. Use cautiously.
Bromocriptine: Haloperidol antagonizes therapeutic effect of bromocriptine on prolactin secretion. Avoid concurrent use.
Centrally acting antihypertensives (such as clonidine, guanabenz, guanadrel, guanethidine, methyldopa, reserpine): Inhibited blood pressure response. Monitor blood pressure carefully.
CNS depressants, including analgesics, barbiturates, narcotics, tranquilizers, and general, spinal, or epidural anesthetics; parenteral magnesium sulfate: Increased CNS depression. Avoid use together.
Dopamine: Decreased vasoconstricting effects. Monitor patient for lack of therapeutic effect.
Levodopa: Decreased effectiveness and increased toxicity of levodopa. Avoid use together.
Lithium: May result in severe neurologic toxicity with an encephalitis-like syndrome and a decreased therapeutic response to haloperidol. Use cautiously; monitor patient.
Metrizamide: Increased risk of seizures. Avoid use together.
Nitrates: Hypotension. Monitor blood pressure frequently.
Phenobarbital: Enhanced renal excretion. Monitor patient closely.
Phenytoin: Inhibited metabolism and increased toxicity of phenytoin. Avoid use together.
Propylthiouracil: Increased risk of agranulocytosis. Avoid use together.
Rifampin: Decreased haloperidol levels and efficacy. Monitor patient carefully.
Sympathomimetics, including ephedrine, epinephrine, and phenylephrine (often found in nasal sprays): May decrease stimulatory and pressor effects of these drugs. Monitor patient carefully.
Drug-herb. *Nutmeg:* Loss of symptom control; interference with psychiatric drug therapy. Discourage use together.
Drug-lifestyle. *Heavy smoking:* Increased haloperidol metabolism. Discourage smoking.

Reactions may be *common*, uncommon, **life-threatening**, or COMMON AND LIFE-THREATENING.

Adverse reactions

CNS: *severe extrapyramidal reactions, tardive dyskinesia, sedation, drowsiness,* lethargy, headache, insomnia, confusion, vertigo, *seizures, neuroleptic malignant syndrome.*
CV: tachycardia, hypotension, hypertension, ECG changes.
EENT: *blurred vision.*
GI: dry mouth, anorexia, constipation, diarrhea, nausea, vomiting, dyspepsia.
GU: urine retention, menstrual irregularities, priapism.
Hematologic: *leukopenia,* leukocytosis.
Hepatic: altered liver function tests, jaundice.
Skin: rash, other skin reactions, diaphoresis.
Other: gynecomastia.

Overdose and treatment

Overdose increases the severity of adverse reactions and can include deep or unarousable sleep, coma, hypotension, hypertension, extrapyramidal symptoms, dystonia, abnormal involuntary muscle movements, agitation, seizures, arrhythmias, ECG changes (may show QT interval prolongation and torsades de pointes), hypothermia, hyperthermia, and autonomic nervous system dysfunction. Overdose with long-acting decanoate requires prolonged recovery time.

Treatment is symptomatic and supportive, including maintaining vital signs, airway, stable body temperature, and fluid and electrolyte balance. Ipecac may be used to induce vomiting, with due regard for antiemetic properties of haloperidol and hazard of aspiration. Gastric lavage also may be used, followed by activated charcoal and saline cathartics; dialysis doesn't help.

Regulate body temperature as needed. Treat hypotension with I.V. fluids; don't give epinephrine. Treat seizures with parenteral diazepam or barbiturates. Treat arrhythmias with parenteral phenytoin, 1 mg/kg I.V., with rate adjusted to blood pressure but not above 50 mg/minute; with ECG monitoring. May repeat every 5 minutes up to 10 mg/kg. Treat extrapyramidal reactions with benztropine at 1 to 2 mg or parenteral diphenhydramine at 10 to 50 mg.

Special considerations

• Drug has few CV adverse effects and may be preferred in patients with cardiac disease.
• Dose of 2 mg is therapeutic equivalent of 100 mg chlorpromazine.
• When changing from tablets to decanoate injection, patient should initially receive 10 to 20 times the oral dose once monthly (not more than 100 mg).

Patient monitoring

• Assess patient periodically for extrapyramidal reactions and tardive dyskinesia.
• Don't withdraw drug abruptly except when required, because abrupt withdrawal may cause severe adverse reaction.

Pediatric patients

• Safety and efficacy of drug injection in children haven't been established, and oral drug isn't recommended for children under age 3.

Geriatric patients

• Drug is especially useful for agitation related to senile dementia. Tardive dyskinesia may occur more often, especially in elderly women.
• Elderly patients usually need lower initial doses and a more gradual dosage adjustment.

Patient education

• Warn patient against activities that require alertness and good psychomotor coordination until CNS response to drug is determined. Drowsiness and dizziness usually subside after a few weeks.
• Tell patient to report adverse effects to prescriber.
• Instruct patient to avoid alcohol or other depressants.

heparin sodium
Heparin Lock Flush, Hep-Lock, Hep-Lock U/P, Liquaemin

Pharmacologic classification: anticoagulant
Therapeutic classification: anticoagulant
Pregnancy risk category: C

Indications and dosages

➤ *Deep vein thrombosis, pulmonary embolism.* Adults: Initially, 5,000 to 10,000 units I.V. push; then adjust dose according to partial thromboplastin time (PTT) results and give dose I.V. q 4 hours (usually 4,000 to 5,000 units); or 5,000 units I.V. bolus, then 20,000 to 40,000 units in 24 hours by I.V. infusion pump. Wait 4 to 6 hours after bolus dose, and adjust hourly rate based on PTT.
Children: Initially, 50 units/kg I.V. bolus. Maintenance dosage is 50 to 100 units/kg I.V. drip q 4 hours. Constant infusion: 20,000 units/m² daily. Adjust dosage based on PTT.
➤ *Embolism prophylaxis, post MI, cerebral thrombosis in evolving CVA, left ventricular thrombi.* Adults: 5,000 units S.C. q 8 to 12 hours.
➤ *Open-heart surgery.* Adults: (total body perfusion) 150 to 400 units/kg continuous I.V. infusion.
➤ *Disseminated intravascular coagulation.* Adults: 50 to 100 units/kg I.V. q 4 hours as a single injection or constant infusion. Discontinue if no improvement in 4 to 8 hours.
Children: 25 to 50 units/kg I.V. q 4 hours, as a single injection or constant infusion. Discontinue if no improvement in 4 to 8 hours.
➤ *To maintain patency of I.V. indwelling catheters.* Adults and children: 10 to 100 units as an I.V. flush (not intended for therapeutic use).
➤ *Unstable angina.* Adults: Keep PTT 1.5 to 2 times control during first week of anginal pain.

► *Anticoagulation in blood transfusion and samples.* *Transfusions and samples:* Mix 7,500 units and 100 ml of normal saline solution and add 6 to 8 ml of mixture to each 100 ml of whole blood or 70 to 150 units to each 10 to 20 ml of blood sample.

Note: Heparin dosing is highly individualized, depending on disease state and patient's age, weight, and renal and hepatic status.

How supplied
Available products are derived from bovine lung or porcine intestinal mucosa. All are injectable and available only by prescription.
heparin sodium
Carpuject: 5,000 units/ml
Disposable syringes: 1,000 units/ml, 2,500 units/ml, 5,000 units/ml, 7,500 units/ml, 10,000 units/ml, 20,000 units/ml
Premixed I.V. solutions: 1,000 units in 500 ml normal saline solution; 2,000 units in 1,000 ml normal saline solution; 12,500 units in 250 ml half-normal saline solution; 25,000 units in 250 ml half-normal saline solution; 25,000 units in 500 ml half-normal saline solution; 10,000 units in 100 ml D_5W; 12,500 units in 250 ml D_5W; 25,000 units in 250 ml D_5W; 25,000 units in 500 ml D_5W
Unit-dose ampules: 1,000 units/ml, 5,000 units/ml, 10,000 units/ml, 20,000 units/ml, 40,000 units/ml
Vials: 1,000 units/ml, 2,000 units/ml, 2,500 units/ml, 5,000 units/ml, 10,000 units/ml, 20,000 units/ml, 40,000 units/ml
heparin sodium flush
Disposable syringes: 10 units/ml, 25 units/ 2.5 ml, 2,500 units/2.5 ml
Vials: 10 units/ml, 100 units/ml

Pharmacodynamics
Anticoagulant action: Heparin accelerates formation of antithrombin III-thrombin complex; it inactivates thrombin and prevents conversion of fibrinogen to fibrin.

Pharmacokinetics
Absorption: Not absorbed from GI tract and must be given parenterally.
Distribution: Extensively bound to lipoprotein, globulins, and fibrinogen; it doesn't cross the placenta.
Metabolism: Although metabolism isn't completely described, drug is thought to be removed by the reticuloendothelial system, with some metabolism occurring in the liver.
Excretion: Little is known; a small fraction is excreted in urine as unchanged drug. Drug doesn't appear in breast milk. Plasma half-life is 1 to 2 hours.

Route	Onset	Peak	Duration
I.V.	Immediate	Unknown	Variable
S.C.	20-60 min	2-4 hr	Variable

Contraindications and precautions
Contraindicated in patients hypersensitive to drug. Conditionally contraindicated in patients with active bleeding; blood dyscrasia; bleeding tendencies, such as hemophilia, thrombocytopenia, or hepatic disease with hypoprothrombinemia; suspected intracranial hemorrhage; suppurative thrombophlebitis; inaccessible ulcerative lesions (especially of GI tract) and open ulcerative wounds; extensive denudation of skin; ascorbic acid deficiency and other conditions that cause increased capillary permeability; subacute bacterial endocarditis; shock; advanced renal disease; threatened abortion; or severe hypertension. Also conditionally contraindicated during or after brain, eye, or spinal cord surgery; during spinal tap or spinal anesthesia; and during continuous tube drainage of stomach or small intestine. Although heparin use is clearly hazardous in these conditions, its risks and its benefits must be evaluated.

Use cautiously in postpartum or menstruating women; patients with mild hepatic or renal disease, alcoholism, or history of asthma, allergies, or GI ulcer; and those with occupations that have a high risk of accidents.

Interactions
Drug-drug. *Cephalosporins, oral anticoagulants, penicillins, platelet inhibitors:* Increased anticoagulant effect. Monitor INR, PT, and PTT. *Antihistamines, cardiac glycosides, nicotine, tetracyclines:* May partially counteract the anticoagulant action of heparin. Dosage adjustment may be needed.
Drug-herb. *Garlic, ginkgo, motherwort, red clover:* Increased risk of bleeding. Discourage use together.

Adverse reactions
Hematologic: *hemorrhage* (with excessive dosage), *overly prolonged clotting time*, *thrombocytopenia*.
Other: irritation, mild pain, hematoma, ulceration, cutaneous or subcutaneous necrosis, *"white clot" syndrome*, *hypersensitivity reactions* (including chills, fever, pruritus, rhinitis, urticaria, *anaphylactoid reactions*).

Overdose and treatment
The major sign of overdose is hemorrhage. Immediate withdrawal of drug usually allows the hemorrhage to resolve; however, severe hemorrhage may require treatment with protamine sulfate. Usually, 1 mg protamine sulfate neutralizes 90 units of bovine heparin or 115 units of porcine heparin.

Heparin administered by I.V. route disappears rapidly from the blood, so the protamine dose depends on when heparin was administered. Give protamine slowly by I.V. injection (over 3 minutes); no more than 50 mg should be given in any 10-minute period.

Reactions may be *common*, uncommon, *life-threatening*, or COMMON AND LIFE-THREATENING.

Heparin administered by S.C. route is slowly absorbed. Give protamine as a 25- to 50-mg loading dose, followed by constant infusion of the remainder of the calculated dose over 8 to 16 hours.

For severe bleeding, transfusions may be required.

Special considerations

• Many I.V. medications are incompatible with heparin and may form precipitates if they come in contact with heparin.
• Avoid I.M. administration of other drugs, if possible, to prevent or minimize hematomas.
• Abrupt withdrawal may increase coagulability; heparin is usually followed by prophylactic oral anticoagulant therapy.
• Heparin interferes with sulfobromophthalein test, causing an upward shift in the absorption peak; heparin also falsely elevates thyroxine level results when competitive protein-binding methods of testing are used. Heparinized blood shouldn't be used for erythrocyte sedimentation rates, platelet counts, fragility tests, or tests involving complement or isoagglutinins.

Patient monitoring

• Obtain baseline INR, PT, and PTT, measure PTT regularly. Anticoagulation is present when PTT values are 1½ to 2 times control values. Valid PT results in the presence of concurrent coumarin or indandione therapy can be obtained only when blood samples are drawn 4 to 6 hours after I.V. heparin dose or 12 to 24 hours after S.C. heparin dose. Continuous I.V. heparin dose doesn't affect reliability of PT result.
• Monitor platelet count and assess patient regularly for signs and symptoms of abnormal bleeding.

Pregnant patients

• Heparin doesn't cross the placental barrier. Use heparin cautiously during pregnancy, especially during the third trimester and postpartum period because of the increased risks of uteroplacental junction bleeding and maternal hemorrhage. Heparin therapy lasting longer than 1 month during pregnancy may result in maternal osteopenia and osteoporosis.

Breast-feeding patients

• Heparin doesn't appear in breast milk.

Pediatric patients

• Because of the risk of overdose, avoid heparin lock flush solutions that contain heparin sodium 100 mg/ml for use in neonates, especially those with a low birth-weight.

Geriatric patients

• At least one manufacturer reports a greater risk of hemorrhage in women over age 60. These patients may have increased heparin plasma levels, and aPTT may be prolonged.

Patient education

• Teach injection technique and methods of record-keeping if patient or family will be giving drug.
• Encourage compliance with medication schedule, follow-up appointments, and need for routine monitoring of blood studies; teach patient and family signs of bleeding, and stress importance of immediately reporting first sign of excess bleeding.
• Caution patient against trying to make up missed doses of heparin and against use of aspirin, motherwort, red clover, and other OTC or herbal medications.
• Instruct patient to inform dentist and other health care providers of his heparin therapy.
• Advise patient to consult prescriber before taking any other drugs, including OTC products.

hepatitis A vaccine, inactivated
Havrix, Vaqta

Pharmacologic classification: vaccine
Therapeutic classification: viral vaccine
Pregnancy risk category: C

Indications and dosages

➤ *Immunization against disease caused by hepatitis A virus. Adults:* 1,440 ELISA units (EL units)/1 ml (Havrix) I.M. as a single dose. Give booster dose of 1,440 EL units/1 ml I.M. 6 to 12 months after initial dose. Or 50 units (Vaqta) I.M. and booster dose 6 months after initial dose.
Children ages 2 to 18: 720 EL units/1 ml (Havrix) I.M. as a single dose and booster dose 6 to 12 months after initial dose.
Children ages 2 to 17: Single dose of 25 units (Vaqta) I.M. and booster dose 6 to 18 months after initial dose.

How supplied
Available by prescription only
Injection: 720 EL units/0.5 ml, 1,440 EL units/1 ml (Havrix); 25 units/0.5 ml, 50 units/0.5 ml (Vaqta)

Pharmacodynamics
Immunostimulant action: Hepatitis A vaccine, inactivated, promotes active immunity to hepatitis A virus. Immunity isn't permanent or completely predictable.

Pharmacokinetics
No information available.

Route	Onset	Peak	Duration
I.M.	1-15 days	Unknown	6 mo

Contraindications and precautions
Contraindicated in patients hypersensitive to any component of vaccine. Use cautiously in patients with thrombocytopenia or bleeding disorders and in those taking anticoagulants; bleeding may occur after I.M. injection.

Interactions
None significant.

Adverse reactions
CNS: malaise, *fatigue, headache,* insomnia, vertigo.
EENT: pharyngitis, photophobia.
GI: *anorexia, nausea,* abdominal pain, diarrhea, dysgeusia, vomiting.
Hepatic: jaundice, hepatitis.
Musculoskeletal: arthralgia, myalgia.
Respiratory: upper respiratory tract infections.
Skin: pruritus, rash, urticaria, *induration, redness, swelling at injection site,* hematoma.
Other: *fever,* lymphadenopathy, hypertonic episode, elevated CK levels.

Overdose and treatment
No information available.

Special considerations
• As with any vaccine, administration of hepatitis A vaccine should be delayed, if possible, in patients with febrile illness.
• Although anaphylaxis is rare, have epinephrine available to treat this reaction.
• If vaccine is administered to immunosuppressed persons or those receiving immunosuppressive therapy, the expected immune response may not be obtained.
• There are no data to support routine vaccination of individuals with chronic hepatitis B or C who lack evidence of chronic liver disease.
• Persons who should receive the vaccine include people traveling to or living in areas of higher endemicity for hepatitis A (Africa, Asia [except Japan], the Mediterranean basin, Eastern Europe, the Middle East, Central and South America, Mexico, and parts of the Caribbean), military personnel, natives of Alaska and the Americas, persons engaging in high-risk sexual activity, and users of illicit injectable drugs. Also, certain institutional workers, child day-care workers, laboratory workers who handle live hepatitis A virus, and handlers of primate animals may benefit from immunization.
• A positive result in the absence of infection may occur in individuals who received hepatitis A vaccine and who are being evaluated by serology to detect IgM anti-HAV.

Patient monitoring
• Serologic confirmation of immunity isn't necessary.

Breast-feeding patients
• It isn't known whether vaccine appears in breast milk. Administer cautiously in breast-feeding women.

Pediatric patients
• Vaccine is well tolerated, highly immunogenic, and effective in children age 2 and older.

Patient education
• Inform patient that vaccine won't prevent hepatitis caused by other agents such as hepatitis B virus, hepatitis C virus, hepatitis E virus, or other pathogens known to infect the liver.

hepatitis B immune globulin, human (HBIG)
BayHep B, Nabi-HB

Pharmacologic classification: immune serum
Therapeutic classification: hepatitis B prophylaxis
Pregnancy risk category: C

Indications and dosages
➤ **Hepatitis B exposure.** *Adults and children:* 0.06 ml/kg I.M. within 7 to 14 days after exposure. Repeat 28 days after exposure.
Neonates born to hepatitis B surface antigen (HBsAg)–positive women: 0.5 ml I.M. within 12 hours of birth. HB vaccination is also indicated.

The American College of Obstetricians and Gynecologists recommends use of HBIG in pregnancy for postexposure prophylaxis. Hepatitis B immune globulin should only be given if clearly needed.

How supplied
Available by prescription only
Injection: 1-ml and 5-ml vials

Pharmacodynamics
Prophylactic action: HBIG provides passive immunity to hepatitis B.

Pharmacokinetics
Absorption: Absorbed slowly after I.M. injection. Antibodies to HBsAG appear in serum within 1 to 6 days, peak within 3 to 11 days, and persist for about 2 to 6 months.
Distribution: Although specific information isn't available, HBIG probably crosses the placenta, as do other immunoglobulins.
Metabolism: No information available.
Excretion: Serum half-life for antibodies to HBsAg is reportedly 25 days.

Route	Onset	Peak	Duration
I.M.	1-6 days	3-9 days	2 mo

Contraindications and precautions
Contraindicated in patients with history of anaphylactic reactions to immune serum or allergic reaction to thimerosal.

Interactions
Drug-drug. *Vaccination with live-virus vaccines, such as measles, mumps, and rubella:* HBIG may interfere with immune response to vaccination. Administer live virus vaccines 2 weeks before or 3 months after HBIG whenever possible.

Reactions may be *common*, uncommon, *life-threatening*, or COMMON AND LIFE-THREATENING.

Adverse reactions

Skin: urticaria, *pain,* tenderness (at injection site).

Other: *anaphylaxis, angioedema.*

Overdose and treatment

Manufacturers report the only evidence of possible overdose would be injection site pain and tenderness. No treatment has been identified.

Special considerations

● Epinephrine solution 1:1,000 should be available to treat allergic reactions.
● Administer drug I.M. only. Severe, even fatal, reactions may occur if administered I.V.
● HBIG may be given simultaneously, but at different sites, with hepatitis B vaccine.
● Store between 36° and 46° F (2° and 8° C). Don't freeze.
● HBIG hasn't been linked to a higher risk of AIDS. The immune globulin is devoid of HIV. Immune globulin recipients don't develop antibodies to HIV.

Patient monitoring

● Monitor patient for adverse reactions.

Pregnant patients

● It's unknown whether drug can harm fetus; use only when potential risk from exposure to hepatitis B infection outweighs potential risk of adverse drug effect.

Breast-feeding patients

● It isn't known whether HBIG appears in breast milk.

Patient education

● Explain that patient's chance of getting AIDS as a result of receiving HBIG is very small.
● Inform patient that HBIG provides temporary protection only against hepatitis B.
● Tell patient what to expect after vaccination: local pain, swelling, and tenderness at the injection site. Recommend acetaminophen to relieve minor discomfort.
● Encourage patient to promptly report headache, skin changes, or difficulty breathing.

---

hepatitis B vaccine, recombinant

Engerix-B, Recombivax HB, Recombivax HB Dialysis Formulation

Pharmacologic classification: vaccine
Therapeutic classification: viral vaccine
Pregnancy risk category: C

Indications and dosages

➤ *Immunization against infection from all known subtypes of hepatitis B; primary preexposure prophylaxis against hepatitis B; postexposure prophylaxis*
(when given with hepatitis B immune globulin). Engerix-B. *Adults age 20 and older:* Initially, give 20 mcg (1-ml adult formulation) I.M., followed by a second dose of 20 mcg I.M. 30 days later. Give a third dose of 20 mcg I.M. 6 months after the initial dose.

Neonates and children up to age 19: Initially, give 10 mcg (0.5-ml pediatric/adolescent formulation) I.M., followed by a second dose of 10 mcg I.M. 30 days later. Give a third dose of 10 mcg I.M. 6 months after the initial dose.

Adults undergoing dialysis or receiving immunosuppressant therapy: Initially, give 40 mcg I.M. (divided into two 20-mcg doses and administered at different sites). Follow with a second dose of 40 mcg I.M. in 30 days, a third dose after 2 months, and a final dose of 40 mcg I.M. 6 months after the initial dose.

Note: Alternative dosing schedule in certain populations (neonates born to infected mothers, persons recently exposed to the virus, and travelers to high-risk areas) who may receive the initial vaccine dose (20 mcg for adults and children over age 10, and 10 mcg for neonates and children up to age 10) followed by a second dose in 1 month and the third dose after 2 months. For prolonged maintenance of protective antibody titers, a booster dose is recommended 12 months after the initial dose.

Recombivax HB

Adults age 20 and older: Initially, give 10 mcg (1-ml adult formulation) I.M., followed by a second dose of 10 mcg I.M. 30 days later. Give a third dose of 10 mcg I.M. 6 months after the initial dose.

Neonates and children up to age 19: Initially, give 5 mcg (0.5 ml pediatric/adolescent formulation) I.M., followed by a second dose of 5 mcg I.M. 30 days later. Give a third dose of 5 mcg I.M. 6 months after the initial dose.

Neonates born to hepatitis B surface antigen (HBsAg)–positive mothers: Initially, give 5 mcg (0.5-ml pediatric/adolescent formulation) I.M. with 0.5 ml hepatitis B immune globulin. Follow with a second dose of 5 mcg I.M. 30 days later. Give a third dose of 5 mcg I.M. 6 months after the initial dose.

Adults undergoing dialysis or receiving immunosuppressant therapy: Initially, give 40 mcg I.M. (1-ml dialysis formulation). Follow with a second dose of 40 mcg I.M. in 30 days, and give a final dose of 40 mcg I.M. 6 months after the initial dose.

How supplied

Available by prescription only
Injection: 5 mcg HBsAg/0.5 ml (Recombivax HB pediatric/adolescent formulation); 10 mcg HBsAg/0.5 ml (Engerix-B, pediatric/adolescent injection); 10 mcg HBsAg/ml (Recombivax HB); 20 mcg HBsAg/ml (Engerix-B); 40 mcg HBsAg/ml (Recombivax HB Dialysis Formulation)

Pharmacodynamics
Prophylactic action: Hepatitis B vaccine promotes active immunity to hepatitis B.

Pharmacokinetics
No information available.

Route	Onset	Peak	Duration
I.M.	2 weeks after last dose	> 6 mo	> 3 yr

Contraindications and precautions
Contraindicated in patients hypersensitive to yeast because recombinant vaccines are derived from yeast cultures.

Use cautiously in patients with active infections or compromised cardiac and pulmonary status and in those to whom a febrile or systemic reaction could pose a risk.

Interactions
Drug-drug. *Corticosteroids, immunosuppressants:* May impair the immune response to hepatitis B vaccine. Larger-than-usual doses of vaccine may be necessary to develop adequate circulating antibody levels.

Adverse reactions
CNS: headache, dizziness, insomnia, paresthesia, neuropathy, transient malaise.
EENT: pharyngitis.
GI: nausea, anorexia, diarrhea, vomiting.
Musculoskeletal: arthralgia, myalgia.
Skin: local inflammation, *soreness* (at injection site).
Other: slight fever, flulike symptoms.

Overdose and treatment
No information available.

Special considerations
● Have epinephrine solution 1:1,000 available.
● The Centers for Disease Control and Prevention report that response to hepatitis B vaccine is significantly better after injection into the deltoid rather than the gluteal muscle.
● Hepatitis B vaccine may be administered S.C., but only to persons, such as hemophiliacs and patients with thrombocytopenia, who are at risk of hemorrhage from I.M. injection. Don't administer I.V.
● Hepatitis B vaccine may be given simultaneously, but at different sites, with hepatitis B immune globulin, influenza virus vaccine, *Haemophilus influenzae* type B conjugate vaccine, polyvalent pneumococcal vaccine, or diphtheria, tetanus, and pertussis vaccine.

Patient monitoring
● Although not necessary for most patients, serologic testing (to confirm immunity to hepatitis B after the three-dose regimen) is recommended for patients over age 50, those at high risk of

needlestick injury (who might require postexposure prophylaxis), hemodialysis patients, immunocompromised patients, and those who inadvertently received one or more injections into the gluteal muscle.

Pregnant patients
● Use drug in pregnant women only when benefits outweigh risks.

Breast-feeding patients
● Use drug cautiously in breast-feeding women.

Pediatric patients
● Routine immunization is recommended for all neonates, regardless of whether the mother tests positive or negative for HBsAg. It's usually well tolerated and highly immunogenic in children and infants of all ages. However, it's most effective in neonates who weigh 2 kg (4.4 lb) or more. To minimize cumulative exposure to mercury in infants under age 6 months, especially neonates and those born prematurely, the use of thimerosal-free hepatitis B vaccine is recommended.

Patient education
● Tell patient that there's no risk of contracting HIV infection or AIDS from hepatitis B vaccine because it's synthetically derived.
● Explain that hepatitis B vaccine provides protection against hepatitis B only, not against hepatitis A or hepatitis C.
● Tell patient to expect some discomfort at injection site and possible fever, headache, or upset stomach. Recommend acetaminophen to relieve such effects. Encourage patient to report distressing adverse reactions.

hetastarch (HES, hydroxyethyl starch)
Hespan

Pharmacologic classification: amylopectin derivative
Therapeutic classification: plasma volume expander
Pregnancy risk category: C

Indications and dosages
➤ *Plasma expander in shock and cardiopulmonary bypass surgery.* **Adults:** 500 to 1,000 ml I.V. dependent on amount of blood lost and resultant hemoconcentration. Total dose usually shouldn't exceed 20 ml/kg, up to 1,500 ml daily. Up to 20 ml/kg (1.2 g/kg)/hour may be used in hemorrhagic shock; in burns or septic shock, rate should be reduced.
➤ *Leukapheresis adjunct.* Hetastarch is an adjunct in leukapheresis to improve harvesting and increase the yield of granulocytes. **Adults:** Hetastarch 250 to 700 ml is infused at a constant fixed ratio, usually 1:8 to venous whole blood during continuous flow centrifugation (CFC) pro-

cedures. Up to 2 CFC procedures weekly, with total of 7 to 10 procedures using hetastarch, have been found safe and effective. Safety of larger numbers of procedures is unknown.

Note: Hetastarch can be used as a priming fluid in pump oxygenators for perfusion during extracorporeal circulation or as a cryoprotective agent for long-term storage of whole blood.

How supplied
Available by prescription only
Injection: 500 ml (6 g/100 ml in normal saline solution)

Pharmacodynamics
Plasma volume expanding action: Hetastarch has an average molecular weight of 450,000 and exhibits colloidal properties similar to human albumin. After an I.V. infusion of hetastarch 6%, the plasma volume expands slightly in excess of the volume infused because of the colloidal osmotic effect. Maximum plasma volume expansion occurs in a few minutes and decreases over 24 to 36 hours. Hemodynamic status may improve for 24 hours or longer.
Leukapheresis adjunctive action: Hetastarch enhances yield of granulocytes obtained by centrifugal means.

Pharmacokinetics
Absorption: Administered I.V.
Distribution: Distributed in blood plasma.
Metabolism: Hetastarch molecules larger than 50,000 molecular weight are slowly enzymatically degraded to molecules that can be excreted.
Excretion: 40% of hetastarch molecules smaller than 50,000 molecular weight are excreted in urine within 24 hours. Hetastarch molecules that aren't hydroxyethylated are slowly degraded to glucose. About 90% of dose is eliminated from the body with an average half-life of 17 days; remainder has a half-life of 48 days.

Route	Onset	Peak	Duration
I.V.	Immediate	Immediate	Unknown

Contraindications and precautions
Contraindicated in patients with severe bleeding disorders, severe heart failure, or renal failure with oliguria and anuria.

Interactions
None reported.

Adverse reactions
CNS: headache.
CV: peripheral edema of the legs.
EENT: periorbital edema.
GI: nausea, vomiting.
Musculoskeletal: muscle pain.
Respiratory: wheezing.
Skin: urticaria, itching.
Other: mild fever, chills, parotid and submaxillary gland enlargement.

Overdose and treatment
Signs and symptoms of overdose include the adverse reactions listed above. Stop infusion if an overdose occurs, and treat supportively.

Special considerations
• When added to whole blood, hetastarch increases the erythrocyte sedimentation rate.
• Don't administer as a substitute for blood or plasma.
• Discard partially used bottle because it doesn't contain a preservative.
• Monitor I.V. site for signs of infiltration and phlebitis.

Patient monitoring
• To avoid circulatory overload, carefully monitor patients with impaired renal function and those at high risk of pulmonary edema or heart failure. Hetastarch 6% in normal saline solution contains 77 mEq sodium and chloride per 500 ml.
• Monitor CBC, total leukocyte and platelet counts, leukocyte differential count, hemoglobin, hematocrit, PT, PTT, electrolyte, BUN, and creatinine levels
• Assess vital signs and cardiopulmonary status to obtain baseline at start of infusion to prevent fluid overload.
• Observe patient for edema.

Pregnant patients
• Hetastarch shouldn't be used in pregnant women, especially during early pregnancy. Drug should be used only when benefit to mother outweighs risk to fetus.

Breast-feeding patients
• Women receiving hetastarch should temporarily discontinue breast-feeding.

Pediatric patients
• Safety and efficacy in children haven't been established.

Geriatric patients
• Use hetastarch cautiously in elderly patients because of the risk of fluid overload; a lower dosage may be sufficient to produce desired plasma volume expansion.

Patient education
• Explain use and administration of drug to patient and family.
• Instruct patient to report adverse reactions promptly.

homatropine hydrobromide
Homatropine*, Isopto Homatropine

Pharmacologic classification: anticholinergic
Therapeutic classification: cycloplegic, mydriatic
Pregnancy risk category: C

Indications and dosages
➤ *Cycloplegic refraction. Adults:* Instill 1 to 2 drops of 2% or 1 drop of 5% solution in eye; repeat in 5 to 10 minutes, p.r.n.
Children: Instill 1 drop of 2% solution in the eye; repeat at 10-minute intervals, p.r.n.
➤ *Uveitis. Adults:* Instill 1 to 2 drops of 2% or 5% solution in eye up to q 3 or 4 hours.
Children: Instill 1 drop of 2% solution b.i.d. or t.i.d.

How supplied
Available by prescription only
Ophthalmic solution: 2%, 5%

Pharmacodynamics
Cycloplegic and mydriatic actions: Anticholinergic action prevents the sphincter muscle of the iris and the muscle of the ciliary body from responding to cholinergic stimulation, resulting in unopposed adrenergic influence and producing pupillary dilation (mydriasis) and paralysis of accommodation (cycloplegia).

Pharmacokinetics
Absorption: Unknown.
Distribution: Unknown.
Metabolism: Unknown.
Excretion: Recovery from cycloplegic and mydriatic effects usually occurs within 1 to 3 days.

Route	Onset	Peak	Duration
Oph-thalmic	Rapid	40-60 min	1-3 days

Contraindications and precautions
Contraindicated in patients hypersensitive to drug or other belladonna alkaloids such as atropine, and in those with glaucoma or those who have adhesions between the iris and lens.

Use cautiously in the elderly and in those with increased ocular pressure.

Interactions
Drug-drug. *Carbachol, cholinesterase inhibitors, pilocarpine:* Interference with the antiglaucoma effects of these drugs. Avoid use together.

Adverse reactions
CNS: confusion, somnolence, headache.
CV: tachycardia.
EENT: eye irritation, *blurred vision, photophobia,* increased intraocular pressure, transient stinging and burning, conjunctivitis, vascular congestion, edema.

GI: dry mouth.
Skin: dryness, rash.

Overdose and treatment
Signs and symptoms of overdose include flushed dry skin, dry mouth, blurred vision, ataxia, dysarthria, hallucinations, tachycardia, and decreased bowel sounds.

Treat accidental ingestion with emesis or activated charcoal. Use physostigmine to antagonize anticholinergic activity of homatropine in severe toxicity; propranolol may be used to treat symptomatic tachyarrhythmias unresponsive to physostigmine.

Special considerations
● Drug may produce symptoms of atropine sulfate poisoning, such as severe mouth dryness and tachycardia.
● Patient may be photophobic and may benefit from wearing dark glasses to minimize discomfort.

Patient monitoring
● Monitor patient for adverse reactions and to ascertain therapeutic result.

Pediatric patients
● Use drug cautiously in young children and infants. There's an increased chance of sensitivity in children with Down syndrome, spastic paralysis, or brain damage. Feeding intolerance may result.

Geriatric patients
● Use drug cautiously in elderly patients because of the risk of undiagnosed glaucoma and increased sensitivity to drug effects.

Patient education
● Provide patient with information on correct method of administration.
● Inform patient that vision will be temporarily blurred after instillation, and advise caution when driving or operating machinery.
● Inform patient that drug may produce drowsiness.

hydralazine hydrochloride
Apresoline

Pharmacologic classification: peripheral vasodilator
Therapeutic classification: antihypertensive
Pregnancy risk category: C

Indications and dosages
➤ *Moderate to severe hypertension. Adults:* Initially, 10 mg P.O. q.i.d. for 2 to 4 days; then increased to 25 mg q.i.d. for remainder of week. If necessary, increase dosage to 50 mg q.i.d. Maximum recommended dose is 200 mg daily, but some patients may require 300 to 400 mg daily.

For severe hypertension, 10 to 50 mg I.M. or 10 to 20 mg I.V. repeated, p.r.n. Switch to oral antihypertensives as soon as possible.

For hypertensive crisis caused by pregnancy, initially 5 mg I.V., followed by 5 to 10 mg I.V. q 20 to 30 minutes until adequate reduction in blood pressure is achieved (usual range, 5 to 20 mg).

Children: Initially, 0.75 mg/kg P.O. daily in four divided doses (25 mg/m² daily); may increase gradually to 7.5 mg/kg daily.

I.M. or I.V. dosage is 0.4 to 1.2 mg/kg or 50 to 100 mg/m² daily in four to six divided doses. Initial parenteral dose shouldn't exceed 20 mg.

➤*Management of severe heart failure.*
Adults: Initially, 50 to 75 mg P.O.; then adjusted according to patient response. Most patients respond to 200 to 600 mg daily, divided q 6 to 12 hours, but doses as high as 3 g daily have been used.

How supplied
Available by prescription only
Tablets: 10 mg, 25 mg, 50 mg, 100 mg
Injection: 20 mg/ml

Pharmacodynamics
Antihypertensive action: Hydralazine has a direct vasodilating effect on vascular smooth muscle, thus lowering blood pressure. The effect of hydralazine on resistance vessels (arterioles and arteries) is greater than that on capacitance vessels (venules and veins).

Pharmacokinetics
Absorption: Absorbed rapidly from GI tract after oral administration; plasma levels peak in 1 hour; bioavailability is 30% to 50%. Antihypertensive effect occurs 20 to 30 minutes after oral dose, 5 to 20 minutes after I.V. administration, and 10 to 30 minutes after I.M. administration. Food enhances absorption.
Distribution: Distributed widely throughout the body; drug is about 88% to 90% protein-bound.
Metabolism: Metabolized extensively in the GI mucosa and the liver. Hydralazine is subject to polymorphic acetylation. Slow acetylators have higher plasma levels, generally requiring lower doses.
Excretion: Mostly excreted in urine, primarily as metabolites; about 10% of an oral dose is excreted in feces. Antihypertensive effect persists 2 to 4 hours after an oral dose and 2 to 6 hours after I.V. or I.M. administration.

Route	Onset	Peak	Duration
P.O.	20-30 min	1-2 hr	2-4 hr
I.V.	5-20 min	10-80 min	2-6 hr
I.M.	10-30 min	1 hr	2-6 hr

Contraindications and precautions
Contraindicated in patients hypersensitive to drug and in those with coronary artery disease or mitral valvular rheumatic heart disease. Use cautiously in patients with suspected cardiac disease, CVA, or severe renal impairment, and in those receiving other antihypertensives.

Interactions
Drug-drug. *Diazoxide, MAO inhibitors:* May cause severe hypotension. Use together cautiously. *Diuretics and other antihypertensives:* Increased effects of these drugs. Use cautiously. *Epinephrine:* Decreased pressor response. Monitor patient closely.

Adverse reactions
CNS: peripheral neuritis, *headache,* dizziness.
CV: orthostatic hypotension, *tachycardia,* edema, angina, *palpitations,* flushing.
EENT: lacrimation, nasal congestion.
GI: *nausea, vomiting, diarrhea, anorexia,* constipation.
Hematologic: *neutropenia, leukopenia, agranulocytosis.*
Musculoskeletal: muscle cramps.
Skin: rash.
Other: *lupus-like syndrome.*

Overdose and treatment
Signs and symptoms of overdose include hypotension, tachycardia, headache, and skin flushing; arrhythmias and shock may occur.

After acute ingestion, empty stomach by emesis or gastric lavage and give activated charcoal to reduce absorption. Follow with symptomatic and supportive care.

Special considerations
● The risk of drug-induced systemic lupus erythematosus (SLE) syndrome is greatest in patients receiving more than 200 mg daily for prolonged periods.
● Food enhances oral absorption and helps minimize gastric irritation.
● Some preparations contain tartrazine, which may cause allergic reactions, especially in aspirin-sensitive patients.
● Inject drug as soon as possible after draining through needle into syringe; drug changes color after contact with metal.
● Patients with renal impairment may respond to lower maintenance dosages of hydralazine.

Patient monitoring
● Recommend performing CBC, lupus erythematosus cell preparation, and ANA titer determinations before therapy and at regular intervals during long-term therapy.
● With I.V. administration, monitor blood pressure every 5 minutes until stable, and then every 15 minutes.
● Headache and palpitations may occur 2 to 4 hours after first oral dose but should subside.
● Sodium retention can occur with long-term use.

Breast-feeding patients
● Drug appears in breast milk but is compatible with breast-feeding according to the American Academy of Pediatrics.

Pediatric patients
● Drug has had limited use in children. Safety and efficacy in children haven't been established; use only if potential benefit outweighs risk.

Geriatric patients
● Geriatric patients may be more sensitive to antihypertensive effects. Use with special caution in patients with history of CVA or impaired renal function; patients with renal impairment may respond to lower maintenance dosages.

Patient education
● Instruct patient that drug should be taken exactly as prescribed, even when feeling well; warn against discontinuing drug suddenly because severe rebound hypertension may occur.
● Explain adverse effects and advise patient to report unusual effects, especially symptoms of SLE (sore throat, fever, rash, and muscle and joint pain).
● Reassure patient that headaches and palpitations occurring 2 to 4 hours after initial dose usually subside.
● Instruct patient to report weight gain that exceeds 5 lb (2.3 kg) weekly.
● Warn patient to seek medical approval before taking OTC cold preparations.

---

hydrochlorothiazide
Apo-Hydro*, Diuchlor H*, Esidrix, Ezide, Hydro-chlor, HydroDIURIL, Hydro-Par, Microzide, Neo-Codema*, Novo-Hydrazide*, Oretic, Urozide*

Pharmacologic classification: thiazide diuretic
Therapeutic classification: diuretic, antihypertensive
Pregnancy risk category: B

Indications and dosages
➤**Edema.** *Adults:* Initially, 25 to 200 mg P.O. daily for several days or until dry weight is attained. Maintenance dosage is 25 to 100 mg P.O. daily or intermittently. A few refractory cases may require up to 200 mg daily.
➤**Hypertension.** *Adults:* 12.5 to 50 mg P.O. once daily. Daily dose increased or decreased based on blood pressure.
Children ages 6 months to 12 years: 2 to 2.2 mg/kg P.O. daily in two divided doses.
Children less than age 6 months: Up to 3.3 mg/kg P.O. daily in two divided doses.

How supplied
Available by prescription only
Capsules: 12.5 mg
Tablets: 25 mg, 50 mg, 100 mg

Solution: 50 mg/5 ml, 100 mg/ml

Pharmacodynamics
Diuretic action: Hydrochlorothiazide increases urinary excretion of sodium and water by inhibiting sodium reabsorption in the cortical diluting tubule of the nephron, thus relieving edema.
Antihypertensive action: Exact mechanism of antihypertensive effect of drug is unknown. It may result partially from direct arteriolar vasodilation and a decrease in total peripheral resistance.

Pharmacokinetics
Absorption: 65% to 75% absorbed from the GI tract.
Distribution: Unknown.
Metabolism: None.
Excretion: Excreted unchanged in urine, usually within 24 hours; half-life is 5½ to 14¼ hours.

Route	Onset	Peak	Duration
P.O.	2 hr	4-5 hr	6-12 hr

Contraindications and precautions
Contraindicated in patients with anuria, hepatic coma, or hypersensitivity to other thiazides or other sulfonamide derivatives. Use cautiously in patients with severely impaired renal or hepatic function or progressive hepatic disease.

Interactions
Drug-drug. *Amphetamine, methenamine compounds (such as methenamine mandelate), quinidine:* Alkaline urine, decreased urinary excretion of some amines, decreased therapeutic efficacy. Monitor patient for drug effect.
Antihypertensives: Increased hypotensive effect; this may be used to therapeutic advantage. Check blood pressure frequently.
Cholestyramine, colestipol: May bind hydrochlorothiazide, preventing its absorption. Give drugs 1 hour apart.
Diazoxide: Increased hyperglycemic, hypotensive, and hyperuricemic effects. Insulin dosage may need adjustment.
Lithium: Reduced renal clearance, elevating serum lithium levels. Reduction in lithium dosage by 50% may be necessary.
Drug-herb. *Dandelion:* Possible interference with diuretic activity. Discourage use together.

Adverse reactions
CNS: dizziness, vertigo, headache, paresthesia, weakness, restlessness.
CV: volume depletion and dehydration, orthostatic hypotension, allergic myocarditis, vasculitis.
GI: anorexia, nausea, *pancreatitis*, epigastric distress, vomiting, abdominal pain, diarrhea, constipation.
GU: polyuria, frequent urination, *renal failure*, interstitial nephritis.

Reactions may be *common*, uncommon, *life-threatening*, or COMMON AND LIFE-THREATENING.

Hematologic: *aplastic anemia, agranulocytosis, leukopenia, thrombocytopenia,* hemolytic anemia.
Hepatic: jaundice.
Metabolism: hypokalemia; asymptomatic hyperuricemia; hyperglycemia and impaired glucose tolerance; fluid and electrolyte imbalances, including dilutional hyponatremia, hypochloremia, metabolic alkalosis, hypercalcemia.
Musculoskeletal: muscle cramps.
Respiratory: respiratory distress, pneumonitis.
Skin: dermatitis, photosensitivity, rash, purpura, alopecia.
Other: *hypersensitivity reactions,* gout, *anaphylaxis.*

Overdose and treatment

Signs and symptoms of overdose include GI irritation and hypermotility, orthostatic hypotension, dizziness, drowsiness, syncope, muscular weakness, diuresis, and lethargy, which may progress to coma.

Treatment is mainly supportive; monitor and assist respiratory, CV, and renal function as indicated. Monitor fluid and electrolyte balance. Induce vomiting with ipecac in conscious patient; otherwise, use gastric lavage to avoid aspiration. Don't give cathartics; these promote additional loss of fluids and electrolytes.

Special considerations

● To prevent nocturia, give drug in the morning.
● Monitor fluid intake and output, weight, blood pressure, and serum electrolyte levels.
● Watch for signs of hypokalemia, such as muscle weakness and cramps. Drug may be used with potassium-sparing diuretic to prevent potassium loss.
● Discontinue thiazides and thiazide-like diuretics before parathyroid function tests.
● In patients with hypertension, therapeutic response may be delayed several weeks.
● Hydrochlorothiazide may interfere with PBI test for thyroid function and should be discontinued before such test.

Patient monitoring

● Drug may cause glucose intolerance. Monitor blood glucose in diabetic patients. May require adjustment of insulin or oral antidiabetic dosage.
● Monitor serum creatinine and BUN levels regularly. Cumulative effects of drug may occur with impaired renal function.
● Monitor blood uric acid levels, especially in patients with history of gout.

Breast-feeding patients

● Drug appears in breast milk; safety and efficacy in breast-feeding women haven't been established.

Pediatric patients

● Drug can be given to children.

Geriatric patients

● Elderly and debilitated patients need close observation and may need reduced dosages. They're more sensitive to excess diuresis because of age-related changes in CV and renal function. Excess diuresis promotes orthostatic hypotension, dehydration, hypovolemia, hyponatremia, hypomagnesemia, and hypokalemia.

Patient education

● Instruct patient to take drug with food to avoid GI upset, to take drug in morning or early afternoon to avoid nocturia, and to avoid sudden postural changes.
● Encourage patient to use sun block to avoid photosensitivity reactions.
● Tell patient to consult prescriber before taking OTC medications.

hydrocortisone (systemic)
Cortef, Hycort*

hydrocortisone acetate
Cortifoam

hydrocortisone cypionate
Cortef

hydrocortisone sodium phosphate
Hydrocortone Phosphate

hydrocortisone sodium succinate
A-hydroCort, Solu-Cortef

Pharmacologic classification: glucocorticoid, mineralocorticoid
Therapeutic classification: adrenocorticoid replacement
Pregnancy risk category: C

Indications and dosages

➤ *Severe inflammation, adrenal insufficiency.* hydrocortisone. *Adults:* 5 to 30 mg P.O. b.i.d., t.i.d., or q.i.d. (as much as 80 mg P.O. q.i.d. may be given in acute situations).
Children: 2 to 8 mg/kg or 16 to 240 mg/m² P.O. daily in three or four divided doses.
hydrocortisone acetate
Adults: 10 to 75 mg into joints or soft tissue at 2- or 3-week intervals. Dose varies with size of joint. In many cases, local anesthetics are injected with dose.
hydrocortisone sodium phosphate
Adults: 15 to 240 mg S.C., I.M., or I.V. daily in divided doses q 12 hours.
hydrocortisone sodium succinate
Adults: Initially, 100 to 500 mg I.M. or I.V., then 50 to 100 mg I.M. as indicated.

➤ *Shock (other than adrenal crisis).* hydrocortisone sodium phosphate. *Children:* 0.16 to 1 mg/kg or 6 to 30 mg/m² I.M. daily or b.i.d.

hydrocortisone sodium succinate
Adults: 100 to 500 mg I.M. or I.V. q 2 to 6 hours. *Children:* 0.16 to 1 mg/kg or 6 to 30 mg/m² I.M. or I.V. daily to b.i.d.

➤ *Life-threatening shock.* hydrocortisone sodium succinate. *Adults:* 0.5 to 2 g I.V. initially, repeated at 2- to 6-hour intervals, p.r.n. High-dose therapy should be continued only until patient's condition has stabilized. Therapy shouldn't continue beyond 72 hours.

➤ *Adjunctive treatment of ulcerative colitis and proctitis.* hydrocortisone. *Adults:* One enema (100 mg) nightly for 21 days.

hydrocortisone acetate (rectal foam)
Adults: 90 mg (1 applicatorful) once or twice daily for 2 or 3 weeks; decrease frequency to every other day thereafter.

How supplied
Available by prescription only
hydrocortisone
Enema: 100 mg/60 ml
Tablets: 5 mg, 10 mg, 20 mg
hydrocortisone acetate
Enema: 10% aerosol foam (provides 90 mg/application)
Injection: 25 mg/ml, 50 mg/ml suspension
hydrocortisone cypionate
Oral suspension: 10 mg/5 ml
hydrocortisone sodium phosphate
Injection: 50 mg/ml solution
hydrocortisone sodium succinate
Injection: 100 mg/vial, 250 mg/vial, 500 mg/vial, 1,000 mg/vial

Pharmacodynamics
Adrenocorticoid replacement action: Hydrocortisone is an adrenocorticoid with both glucocorticoid and mineralocorticoid properties. It's a weak anti-inflammatory but a potent mineralocorticoid, having potency similar to that of cortisone and twice that of prednisone. Hydrocortisone (or cortisone) is usually the drug of choice for replacement therapy in patients with adrenal insufficiency. It's usually not used for immunosuppressant activity because of the extremely large doses necessary and unwanted mineralocorticoid effects.

Hydrocortisone and hydrocortisone cypionate may be given orally. Hydrocortisone sodium phosphate may be given by I.M., S.C., or I.V. injection or by I.V. infusion, usually at 12-hour intervals. Hydrocortisone sodium succinate may be given by I.M. or I.V. injection or I.V. infusion every 2 to 10 hours, depending on the clinical situation. Hydrocortisone acetate is a suspension that may be given by intra-articular, intrasynovial, intrabursal, intralesional, or soft-tissue injection. It has a slow onset but a long duration of action. Injectable forms are usually used only when the oral dosage forms can't be used.

Pharmacokinetics
Absorption: Absorbed readily after oral administration. After oral and I.V. administration, effects peak in about 1 to 2 hours. The acetate suspension for injection has a variable absorption over 24 to 48 hours, depending on whether it's injected into an intra-articular space or a muscle and the blood supply to that muscle.
Distribution: Removed rapidly from the blood and distributed to muscle, liver, skin, intestines, and kidneys. Hydrocortisone is bound extensively to plasma proteins (transcortin and albumin). Only the unbound portion is active. Adrenocorticoids are distributed into breast milk and through the placenta.
Metabolism: Metabolized in the liver to inactive glucuronide and sulfate metabolites.
Excretion: Inactive metabolites and small amounts of unmetabolized drug are excreted by the kidneys. Insignificant quantities of drug are excreted in feces. Biologic half-life of hydrocortisone is 8 to 12 hours.

Route	Onset	Peak	Duration
P.O., I.V., I.M., P.R.	Variable	Variable	Variable

Contraindications and precautions
Contraindicated in patients allergic to any component of the formulation, in those with systemic fungal infections, and in premature infants (with hydrocortisone sodium succinate).

Use hydrocortisone sodium phosphate or succinate cautiously in patients with a recent MI, GI ulcer, renal disease, hypertension, osteoporosis, diabetes mellitus, hypothyroidism, cirrhosis, diverticulitis, ulcerative colitis, recent intestinal anastomosis, thromboembolic disorders, seizures, myasthenia gravis, heart failure, tuberculosis, ocular herpes simplex, emotional instability, and psychotic tendencies.

Interactions
Drug-drug. *Amphotericin B, diuretics:* May result in hypokalemia. Monitor serum potassium levels.
Antacids, cholestyramine, colestipol: Decreased corticosteroid effect from absorption by these drugs. May require dosage adjustment.
Barbiturates, phenytoin, rifampin: May decrease corticosteroid effects because of increased hepatic metabolism. Corticosteroid dosage may need increase.
Cardiac glycosides: Increased risk of toxicity. Monitor patient closely.
Estrogens: Reduced clearance of corticosteroids. Monitor patient for drug effect.
Isoniazid, salicylates: Increased metabolism of these drugs. Monitor patient carefully.
Oral anticoagulants: Decreased anticoagulant effects. Monitor PT and INR.

Reactions may be *common*, uncommon, *life-threatening*, or COMMON AND LIFE-THREATENING.

Ulcerogenic drugs (such as NSAIDs): Increased risk of GI ulceration. Avoid use together.

Adverse reactions

CNS: *euphoria, insomnia,* psychotic behavior, pseudotumor cerebri, vertigo, headache, paresthesia, *seizures.*

CV: *heart failure,* hypertension, edema, *arrhythmias,* thrombophlebitis, *thromboembolism.*

EENT: cataracts, glaucoma.

GI: *peptic ulceration,* GI irritation, increased appetite, *pancreatitis,* nausea, vomiting.

GU: menstrual irregularities.

Metabolic: hypokalemia, hyperglycemia, altered thyroid function tests.

Musculoskeletal: muscle weakness, osteoporosis, growth suppression in children.

Skin: delayed wound healing, acne, various skin eruptions, easy bruising, hirsutism.

Other: susceptibility to infections, cushingoid state (moonface, buffalo hump, central obesity), carbohydrate intolerance, *acute adrenal insufficiency* with increased stress (infection, surgery, trauma) or abrupt withdrawal (after long-term therapy).

Overdose and treatment

Acute ingestion, even in massive doses, is rarely a clinical problem. Toxic signs and symptoms rarely occur if drug is used for less than 3 weeks, even at large doses. However, long-term use causes adverse physiologic effects, including suppression of the hypothalamic-pituitary-adrenal axis, cushingoid appearance, muscle weakness, and osteoporosis.

Special considerations

● Determine whether patient is sensitive to other corticosteroids.
● Most adverse reactions to corticosteroids are dose- or duration-dependent.
● For better results and less toxicity, give a once-daily dose in morning.
● Give oral dose with food when possible. Patient may need medication to prevent GI irritation.
● Salt formulations aren't interchangeable.
● Give I.M. injection deeply into gluteal muscle. Rotate injection sites to prevent muscle atrophy. Avoid S.C. injection because atrophy and sterile abscesses may occur.
● Injectable forms aren't used for alternate-day therapy.
● Always adjust to lowest effective dose.
● Drug may mask or worsen infections, including latent amebiasis.
● Stress (fever, trauma, surgery, and emotional problems) may increase adrenal insufficiency and call for an increase in dosage.
● Watch for depression or psychotic episodes, especially during high-dose therapy.
● Periodic measurement of growth and development may be needed during high-dose or prolonged therapy in children.

● Gradually reduce dosage after long-term therapy. After abrupt withdrawal, patient may experience rebound inflammation, fatigue, weakness, arthralgia, fever, dizziness, lethargy, depression, fainting, orthostatic hypotension, dyspnea, anorexia, and hypoglycemia. After prolonged use, sudden withdrawal may be fatal.

⚠ ALERT Don't confuse Solu-Cortef with Solu-Medrol (methylprednisolone sodium succinate).
● Hydrocortisone suppresses reactions to skin tests, and causes false-negative results in nitro-blue tetrazolium tests for systemic bacterial infections.

Patient monitoring
● Diabetic patient may need increased insulin; monitor blood glucose levels.
● Monitor patient's weight, blood pressure, and serum electrolyte levels.
● Monitor patient for cushingoid effects, including moonface, buffalo hump, central obesity, thinning hair, hypertension, and increased susceptibility to infection.

Pediatric patients
● Long-term use of hydrocortisone in children and adolescents may delay growth and maturation.

Geriatric patients
● Elderly patients may be more susceptible to osteoporosis with prolonged use.

Patient education
● Caution patient to take medication as directed.
● Inform patient of potential adverse effects, and instruct him to contact prescriber immediately to report serious adverse effects.

hydrocortisone (topical)
Acticort 100, Aeroseb-HC, Ala-Cort, Ala-Scalp, Anusol-HC, Bactine, Barriere-HC*, Cetacort, CortaGel, Cortate*, Cort-Dome, Cortizone, Delcort, Dermacort, Dermolate, Dermtex HC, Eldecort, Emo-Cort*, Hi-Cor, Hycort, Hydro-Tex, Hytone, LactiCare-HC, Nutracort, Penecort, Procort, Rectocort*, S-T Cort, Synacort, Tegrin HC, Texacort, Unicort*

hydrocortisone acetate
Anusol-HC, Cortaid, Cort-Dome, Cortef, Corticaine, Corticreme*, Cortoderm*, Gynecort, Hyderm*, Lanacort, Novohydrocort*, Orabase-HCA, Pharma-Cort, Rhulicort

hydrocortisone buteprate
Pandel

---

hydrocortisone butyrate
Locoid

hydrocortisone valerate
Westcort

Pharmacologic classification: glucocorticoid
Therapeutic classification: anti-inflammatory
Pregnancy risk category: C

Indications and dosages
➤ *Inflammation of corticosteroid-responsive dermatoses, including those on face, groin, armpits, and under breasts; seborrheic dermatitis of scalp. Adults and children:* Apply cream, lotion, ointment, foam, or aerosol sparingly once daily to q.i.d.
Aerosol
Shake can well. Direct spray onto affected area from a distance of 15 cm (6 inches). Apply for only 3 seconds (to avoid freezing tissues). Apply to dry scalp after shampooing; no need to massage or rub medication into scalp after spraying. Apply daily until acute phase is controlled, then reduce dosage to once to three times weekly, p.r.n., to maintain control.
Rectal administration
Shake can well. Apply once daily or b.i.d. for 2 to 3 weeks, then every other day, p.r.n.
➤ *Dental lesions. Adults and children:* Apply paste b.i.d. or t.i.d. and h.s.

How supplied
Available by prescription only
hydrocortisone
Aerosol: 1%
Cream: 2.5%
Gel: 1%
Lotion: 0.25%, 0.5%, 1%, 2%, 2.5%
Ointment: 0.5%, 1%, 2.5%
Solution: 1%
Stick, roll-on: 1%
hydrocortisone acetate
Cream: 1%
Lotion: 0.5%
Ointment: 0.5%, 1%
Paste: 0.5%
Rectal foam: 10%
Solution: 1%
Suppositories: 25 mg
hydrocortisone buteprate
Cream: 0.1%, 1%
hydrocortisone butyrate
Cream, ointment, solution: 0.1%
hydrocortisone valerate
Cream, ointment: 0.2%
Available without a prescription
hydrocortisone
Cream: 0.5%, 1%
hydrocortisone acetate
Cream: 0.5%

Pharmacodynamics
Anti-inflammatory action: Hydrocortisone stimulates the synthesis of enzymes needed to decrease the inflammatory response. Hydrocortisone, a corticosteroid secreted by the adrenal cortex, is about 1.25 times more potent an anti-inflammatory agent than equivalent doses of cortisone, but both have twice the mineralocorticoid activity of the other glucocorticoids.

Hydrocortisone 0.5%, 1%, and hydrocortisone acetate 0.5% are available without a prescription for the temporary relief of minor skin irritation, itching, and rashes caused by eczema, insect bites, soaps, and detergents.

Hydrocortisone is also administered rectally as a retention enema for the temporary treatment of acute ulcerative colitis. Hydrocortisone acetate suspension is also available as a rectal suppository or aerosol foam suspension for the temporary treatment of inflammatory conditions of the rectum, such as hemorrhoids, cryptitis, proctitis, and pruritus ani.

Pharmacokinetics
Absorption: Absorption depends on potency of preparation, amount applied, and nature of skin at application site. It ranges from about 1% in areas with a thick stratum corneum (such as the palms, soles, elbows, and knees) to as high as 36% in areas where the stratum corneum is thinnest (face, eyelids, and genitals). Absorption increases in areas of skin damage, inflammation, or occlusion. Some systemic absorption occurs, especially through the oral mucosa.
Distribution: After topical application, drug is distributed throughout the local skin layers. Any drug absorbed into circulation is removed rapidly from the blood and distributed into muscle, liver, skin, intestines, and kidneys.
Metabolism: After topical administration, hydrocortisone is metabolized primarily in the skin. The small amount absorbed into systemic circulation is metabolized primarily in the liver to inactive compounds.
Excretion: Inactive metabolites are excreted by the kidneys, primarily as glucuronides and sulfates, but also as unconjugated products. Small amounts of metabolites are also excreted in feces.

Route	Onset	Peak	Duration
P.R., topical	Unknown	Unknown	Unknown

Contraindications and precautions
Contraindicated in patients hypersensitive to drug.

Interactions
None significant.

Adverse reactions
GU: glucosuria.
Metabolic: hyperglycemia.

Reactions may be *common*, uncommon, *life-threatening*, or COMMON AND LIFE-THREATENING.

Skin: burning, pruritus, irritation, dryness, erythema, folliculitis, hypertrichosis, hypopigmentation, acneiform eruptions, allergic contact dermatitis; maceration, secondary infection, atrophy, striae, miliaria (with occlusive dressings).
Other: *hypothalamic-pituitary-adrenal axis suppression*, Cushing's syndrome.

Overdose and treatment
No information available.

Special considerations
• Gently wash skin before applying. To prevent skin damage, rub in gently, leaving a thin coat. When treating hairy sites, part hair and apply directly to lesions.
• Avoid applying near eyes or mucous membranes or in ear canal; may be safely used on face, groin, and armpits and under breasts.
• If an occlusive dressing is applied and a fever develops, remove dressing.
• Stop drug if skin infection, striae, or atrophy occurs.
• When using aerosol near the face, cover patient's eyes and warn against inhalation of spray. Aerosol contains alcohol and may cause irritation or burning when used on open lesions. Don't spray longer than 3 seconds or from closer than 6 inches (15 cm) to avoid freezing tissues. If spray is applied to dry scalp after shampooing, drug need not be massaged into scalp.
• If antifungals or antibiotics are used concurrently, stop corticosteroid until infection is controlled.
• Continue treatment for a few days after lesions clear.

Patient monitoring
• Systemic absorption is likely with use of occlusive dressings, prolonged treatment, or extensive body surface treatment. Watch for symptoms.
• Monitor patient for fluid or electrolyte disturbances (sodium and fluid retention, potassium loss, hypokalemic alkalosis, negative nitrogen balance from catabolism of protein).
⚠ ALERT Don't confuse hydrocortisone with hydroxychloroquine.

Pediatric patients
• Avoid using plastic pants or tight-fitting diapers on treated areas in young children. Children may absorb larger amounts of drug and be more prone to systemic toxicity.

Patient education
• Teach patient or family member how to apply drug.
• If an occlusive dressing is used, advise patient to leave it in place for no longer than 12 hours each day and not to use the dressing on infected or exudative lesions.
• Tell patient to stop drug and report signs of systemic absorption, skin irritation or ulceration,

hypersensitivity, infection, or lack of improvement.
• For enema administration, tell patient to lie on left side and retain fluid for 1 hour.
• Instruct patient to insert suppositories blunt end first after removing foil wrapper.
• For perianal application, instruct patient to place small amount of drug on a tissue and gently rub in.
• Tell patient to disassemble applicators or aerosol cap and clean with warm water after each use.

hydromorphone hydrochloride
Dilaudid, Dilaudid-HP, Hydrostat IR

Pharmacologic classification: opioid
Therapeutic classification: analgesic, antitussive
Controlled substance schedule: II
Pregnancy risk category: C

Indications and dosages
➤ **Moderate to severe pain.** *Adults:* 2 to 10 mg P.O. q 3 to 6 hours, p.r.n., or around-the-clock. Or, 2 to 4 mg I.M., S.C., or I.V. q 4 to 6 hours, p.r.n., or around-the-clock (give I.V. dose over 3 to 5 minutes). Or, 3 mg rectal suppository q 6 to 8 hours, p.r.n., or around-the-clock. (Give 1 to 14 mg Dilaudid-HP S.C. or I.M. q 4 to 6 hours.)
Note: Give hydromorphone hydrochloride in the smallest effective dose to minimize the development of tolerance and physical dependence. Dose must be individually adjusted based on patient's severity of pain, age, and size.
➤ **Cough.** *Adults:* 1 mg P.O. q 3 to 4 hours, p.r.n. *Children ages 6 to 12:* 0.5 mg P.O. q 3 to 4 hours, p.r.n.

How supplied
Available by prescription only
Injection: 1 mg/ml, 2 mg/ml, 3 mg/ml, 4 mg/ml, 10 mg/ml
Oral liquid: 5 mg/5 ml
Suppository: 3 mg
Tablets: 1 mg, 2 mg, 3 mg, 4 mg, 8 mg

Pharmacodynamics
Antitussive action: Hydromorphone acts directly on the cough center in the medulla, producing an antitussive effect.
Analgesic action: Hydromorphone has analgesic properties related to opiate receptor affinity and is recommended for moderate to severe pain. Unlike other opioids, there's no intrinsic limit to the analgesic effect of hydromorphone.

Pharmacokinetics
Absorption: Well absorbed after oral, rectal, or parenteral administration.
Distribution: Unknown.

Metabolism: Metabolized primarily in the liver, where it undergoes conjugation with glucuronic acid.

Excretion: Excreted primarily in urine as the glucuronide conjugate. Duration of action is 4 to 5 hours.

Route	Onset	Peak	Duration
P.O.	30 min	1½-2 hr	4 hr
I.V.	10-15 min	15-30 min	2-3 hr
I.M.	15 min	½-1 hr	4-5 hr
S.C.	15 min	½-1½ hr	4 hr
P.R.	Unknown	Unknown	4 hr

Contraindications and precautions

Contraindicated in patients hypersensitive to drug; in those with intracranial lesions caused by increased intracranial pressure; and whenever ventilator function is depressed, such as in status asthmaticus, COPD, cor pulmonale, emphysema, and kyphoscoliosis.

Use cautiously in geriatric or debilitated patients and in those with hepatic or renal disease, Addison's disease, hypothyroidism, prostatic hyperplasia, or urethral strictures.

Interactions

Drug-drug. *Anticholinergics:* Increased risk of paralytic ileus. Avoid use together.
Cimetidine: Increased respiratory and CNS depression, causing confusion, disorientation, apnea, or seizures. Reduced dosage of hydromorphone is usually advised.
CNS depressants (antihistamines, barbiturates, benzodiazepines, general anesthetics, muscle relaxants, narcotic analgesics, phenothiazines, sedative-hypnotics, tricyclic antidepressants): Increased respiratory and CNS depression, sedation, and hypotensive effects of drug. Use together with extreme caution.
General anesthetics: Severe CV depression may result. Avoid use together.
Narcotic antagonist: Patients who become physically dependent on drug may experience acute withdrawal syndrome. Avoid use together.
Drug-lifestyle. *Alcohol use:* Increased CNS effects of drug. Discourage use together.

Adverse reactions

CNS: *sedation, somnolence, clouded sensorium,* dizziness, *euphoria.*
CV: *hypotension, bradycardia.*
EENT: blurred vision, diplopia, nystagmus.
GI: *nausea, vomiting, constipation,* ileus.
GU: *urine retention.*
Respiratory: *respiratory depression, bronchospasm.*
Other: induration (with repeated S.C. injections), physical dependence.

Overdose and treatment

The most common signs and symptoms of hydromorphone overdose are CNS depression, respiratory depression, and miosis. Other effects include hypotension, bradycardia, hypothermia, shock, apnea, cardiopulmonary arrest, circulatory collapse, pulmonary edema, and seizures.

To treat an acute overdose, first establish adequate respiratory exchange via a patent airway and ventilation as needed; administer a narcotic antagonist (naloxone) to reverse respiratory depression. (Because the duration of action of hydromorphone is longer than that of naloxone, repeated dosing is necessary.) Naloxone shouldn't be given unless patient has clinically significant respiratory or CV depression. Monitor vital signs closely.

If patient is seen within 2 hours of ingestion of an oral overdose, empty the stomach immediately by inducing emesis with ipecac syrup or using gastric lavage. Use caution to avoid aspiration. Give activated charcoal via nasogastric tube for further removal of an oral overdose.

Provide symptomatic and supportive treatment (continued respiratory support, correction of fluid or electrolyte imbalance). Monitor laboratory values, vital signs, and neurologic status closely.

Contact the local or regional poison control center for further information.

Special considerations

● For a better analgesic effect, give drug before patient has intense pain.
● Dilaudid-HP, a highly concentrated form (10 mg/ml), may be administered in smaller volumes to prevent the discomfort of large-volume I.M. or S.C. injections.
● Rotate injection sites to avoid induration with S.C. injection.
● Keep narcotic antagonist (naloxone) available.
⚠ ALERT Don't confuse hydromorphone with morphine.
● For infusion, drug may be mixed in D₅W, normal saline solution, D₅W in normal saline solution, D₅W in half-normal saline solution, or Ringer's or lactated Ringer's solutions.
● Respiratory depression and hypotension can occur with I.V. administration. Give by direct injection over no less than 2 minutes and monitor patient constantly. Keep resuscitation equipment available.
● Drug may worsen or mask gallbladder pain.
● Increased biliary tract pressure resulting from contraction of the sphincter of Oddi may interfere with hepatobiliary imaging studies.

Patient monitoring

● Monitor patient for adverse reactions and response to dose adjustments.

Breast-feeding patients

● It isn't known whether drug appears in breast milk; use cautiously in breast-feeding women.

Reactions may be *common*, uncommon, *life-threatening*, or COMMON AND LIFE-THREATENING.

Geriatric patients
• Lower doses are usually indicated for elderly patients because they may be more sensitive to therapeutic and adverse effects of drug.

Patient education
• Instruct patient to take or ask for drug before pain becomes intense.
• Warn patient to avoid hazardous activities that require mental alertness.
• Advise patient to avoid alcohol.

hydroxychloroquine sulfate
Plaquenil

Pharmacologic classification: 4-aminoquinoline
Therapeutic classification: antimalarial, anti-inflammatory
Pregnancy risk category: C

Indications and dosages
➤ **Suppressive prophylaxis of malarial attacks.** *Adults:* 400 mg of sulfate (310 mg base) P.O. weekly on exactly the same day each week. (Begin 2 weeks before entering the endemic area and continue for 8 weeks after leaving.)
Infants and children: 5 mg, calculated as base per kilogram of body weight (shouldn't exceed the adult dose regardless of weight) on exactly the same day each week. Start 2 weeks before exposure. If unable to do so, give 10 mg base/kg in two divided doses 6 hours apart.
➤ **Treatment of acute attack of malaria.** *Adults:* 800 mg (620 mg base) followed by 400 mg (310 mg base) in 6 to 8 hours and 400 mg (310 mg base) on each of 2 consecutive days.
Infants and children: Initial dose, 10 mg base/kg (not to exceed a single dose of 620 mg base). Second dose, 5 mg base/kg (not to exceed a single dose of 310 mg base), is given 6 hours after first dose. Third dose, 5 mg base/kg, is given 18 hours after second dose. Fourth dose, 5 mg base/kg, is given 24 hours after third dose.
➤ **Lupus erythematosus (chronic discoid and systemic).** *Adults:* 400 mg P.O. daily or b.i.d., continued for several weeks or months, based on response. Prolonged maintenance dosage is 200 to 400 mg P.O. daily.
➤ **Rheumatoid arthritis.** *Adults:* Initially, 400 to 600 mg P.O. daily. When good response occurs (usually in 4 to 12 weeks), reduce dose by half.

How supplied
Available by prescription only
Tablets: 200 mg (155 mg base)

Pharmacodynamics
Antimalarial action: Hydroxychloroquine binds to DNA, interfering with protein synthesis. It also inhibits DNA and RNA polymerases. It's active against asexual erythrocytic forms of *Plasmodium malariae, P. ovale, P. vivax,* and many strains of *P. falciparum.*
Amebicidal action: Mechanism of action is unknown.
Anti-inflammatory action: Mechanism of action is unknown. Drug may antagonize histamine and serotonin and inhibit prostaglandin effects by inhibiting conversion of arachidonic acid to prostaglandin F2; it may also inhibit chemotaxis of polymorphonuclear leukocytes, macrophages, and eosinophils.

Pharmacokinetics
Absorption: Absorbed readily and almost completely.
Distribution: Bound to plasma proteins. It's concentrated in the liver, spleen, kidneys, heart, and brain and is strongly bound in melanin-containing cells.
Metabolism: Metabolized by the liver to desethylchloroquine and desethyl hydroxychloroquine.
Excretion: Most of an administered dose is excreted unchanged in urine. Drug and its metabolites are excreted slowly in urine; unabsorbed drug is excreted in feces. Small amounts of drug may be present in urine for months after it's discontinued. Drug appears in breast milk.

Route	Onset	Peak	Duration
P.O.	Unknown	2-4½ hr	Unknown

Contraindications and precautions
Contraindicated in patients hypersensitive to drug, in long-term therapy for children, and in patients with retinal or visual field changes or porphyria. Use cautiously in patients with severe GI, neurologic, or blood disorders.

Interactions
Drug-drug. *Digoxin:* May increase serum digoxin levels. Monitor digoxin levels; patient needs close monitoring for signs of digitalis toxicity.
Kaolin, magnesium trisilicate: Decreased hydroxychloroquine absorption. Separate administration times.
Drug-lifestyle. *Prolonged, unprotected sun exposure:* May cause drug-induced dermatoses. Advise patient to take precautions.

Adverse reactions
CNS: irritability, nightmares, ataxia, *seizures*, psychosis, vertigo, nystagmus, dizziness, hypoactive deep tendon reflexes, ataxia, lassitude, headache.
CV: inversion or depression of the T wave, widening of the QRS complex.
EENT: blurred vision; difficulty in focusing; reversible corneal changes; typically irreversible, sometimes progressive or delayed retinal changes, such as narrowing of arterioles; macular lesions; pallor of optic disk; optic atrophy; visual field defects; patchy retinal pigmentation, commonly

leading to blindness; ototoxicity (irreversible nerve deafness, tinnitus, labyrinthitis).
GI: anorexia, abdominal cramps, diarrhea, nausea, vomiting.
Hematologic: *agranulocytosis, leukopenia, thrombocytopenia, hemolysis* (in patients with G6PD deficiency), *aplastic anemia.*
Metabolic: weight loss.
Musculoskeletal: skeletal muscle weakness.
Skin: alopecia, bleaching of hair, pruritus, lichen planus eruptions, skin and mucosal pigmentary changes, pleomorphic skin eruptions.

Overdose and treatment
Symptoms of drug overdose may appear within 30 minutes after ingestion and may include headache, drowsiness, visual changes, CV collapse, and seizures followed by respiratory and cardiac arrest.

Treatment is symptomatic. Empty stomach by emesis or lavage. After lavage, activated charcoal in an amount at least five times the estimated amount of drug ingested may be helpful if given within 30 minutes of ingestion.

Ultra-short-acting barbiturates may help control seizures. Intubation may become necessary. Peritoneal dialysis and exchange transfusions may also be useful. Forced fluids and acidification of the urine are helpful after the acute phase.

Special considerations
⚠ ALERT Dosage may be discussed in mg or mg-base; be aware of the difference.
• Administer drug immediately before or after meals on the same day each week to minimize gastric distress.
• Drug isn't effective for chloroquine-resistant strains of *P. falciparum*.

Patient monitoring
• Monitor patient for blurred vision, increased sensitivity to light, hearing loss, pronounced GI disturbances, or muscle weakness.
• Baseline and periodic ophthalmologic examinations are necessary in prolonged or high-dosage therapy.

Breast-feeding patients
• Safety hasn't been established. Use cautiously in breast-feeding women.

Pediatric patients
• Children are extremely susceptible to toxicity; monitor patient closely for adverse effects. Don't use drug for long-term therapy in children and don't exceed recommended dose.

Patient education
• To prevent drug-induced dermatoses, warn patient to avoid excessive sun exposure.

hydroxyprogesterone caproate
Hylutin

Pharmacologic classification: progestin
Therapeutic classification: progestin, antineoplastic
Pregnancy risk category: X

Indications and dosages
➤ *Amenorrhea and uterine bleeding.*
Adults: 375 mg I.M. May be repeated at 4-week intervals, if needed. After 4 days of desquamation or if there's no bleeding within 21 days after administration, begin cyclic therapy with an estrogen.
➤ *Endometrial cancer. Adults:* 1 g I.M. up to seven times weekly for 12 weeks or as indicated. Therapy is discontinued if relapse occurs or if no objective response is seen after 12 weeks of therapy.

How supplied
Available by prescription only
Injection: 125 mg/ml, 250 mg/ml

Pharmacodynamics
Progestational action: Drug suppresses ovulation, causes thickening of cervical mucus, and induces sloughing of the endometrium. It inhibits growth progression of progestin-sensitive uterine cancer tissue by an unknown mechanism.

Pharmacokinetics
Absorption: Absorbed slowly after I.M. injection.
Distribution: Unknown.
Metabolism: Metabolism is primarily hepatic but isn't well characterized.
Excretion: Excretion is primarily renal, but isn't well characterized.

Route	Onset	Peak	Duration
I.M.	Unknown	Unknown	7-14 days

Contraindications and precautions
Contraindicated during pregnancy, in patients hypersensitive to drug, and in those with thromboembolic disorders, cerebral apoplexy, breast or genital organ cancer, undiagnosed abnormal vaginal bleeding, severe hepatic disease, or missed abortion.

Use cautiously in patients with diabetes mellitus, seizures, migraine, cardiac or renal disease, asthma, mental depression, or impaired liver function.

Interactions
Drug-drug. None reported.

Adverse reactions
CNS: depression.

Reactions may be *common*, uncommon, *life-threatening*, or COMMON AND LIFE-THREATENING.

CV: thrombophlebitis, ***thromboembolism***, *CVA*, ***pulmonary embolism***, edema.
EENT: exophthalmos, diplopia.
GU: breakthrough bleeding, dysmenorrhea, amenorrhea, cervical erosion, abnormal secretions.
Hepatic: cholestatic jaundice.
Metabolic: changes in weight.
Skin: rash, acne, pruritus, melasma; irritation, pain (at injection site).
Other: breast tenderness, enlargement, or secretion.

Overdose and treatment
No information available.

Special considerations
● Endocrine and liver function tests shouldn't be considered reliable until the drug has been discontinued for at least 60 days.

Patient monitoring
● Monitor diabetic patients during therapy for signs of decreased glucose tolerance.
● Patients receiving drug should have a full physical examination, including a gynecologic examination and a Papanicolaou test, every 6 to 12 months.

Pregnant patients
● Drug is contraindicated for use in pregnant women.

Breast-feeding patients
● Drug is contraindicated for use in breast-feeding women.

Patient education
● Warn patient that edema and weight gain are likely.
● Remind patient that normal menstrual cycles may not resume for 2 to 3 months after discontinuing drug therapy.
● Advise patient of potential risks to the fetus if she becomes pregnant during therapy or is inadvertently exposed to drug during the first 4 months of pregnancy.

hydroxyurea
Droxia, Hydrea

Pharmacologic classification: antimetabolite (specific to S phase of cell cycle)
Therapeutic classification: antineoplastic
Pregnancy risk category: D

Indications and dosages
Dosage and indications for hydroxyurea may vary. Check current literature for recommended protocol.
➤ ***Solid tumors.*** *Adults:* 80 mg/kg P.O. as a single dose q 3 days. Or, 20 to 30 mg/kg P.O. as a single daily dose.

➤ ***Head and neck cancers, excluding the lip.*** *Adults:* 80 mg/kg P.O. as a single dose q 3 days.
➤ ***Resistant chronic myelocytic leukemia.*** *Adults:* 20 to 30 mg/kg P.O. as a single daily dose.

How supplied
Available by prescription only
Capsules: 250 mg, 500 mg

Pharmacodynamics
Antineoplastic action: The exact mechanism of the cytotoxic action of hydroxyurea is unclear. However, hydroxyurea inhibits DNA synthesis without interfering with RNA or protein synthesis. Drug may act as an antimetabolite, inhibiting the incorporation of thymidine into DNA, and it may also damage DNA directly.

Pharmacokinetics
Absorption: Well absorbed after oral administration. Higher serum levels are achieved if drug is given as a large, single dose rather than in divided doses.
Distribution: Hydroxyurea crosses the blood brain barrier.
Metabolism: About 50% of an oral dose is degraded in the liver.
Excretion: The remaining 50% is excreted in urine as unchanged drug. The metabolites are excreted through the lungs as carbon dioxide and in urine as urea.

Route	Onset	Peak	Duration
P.O.	Unknown	2 hr	24 hr

Contraindications and precautions
Contraindicated in patients hypersensitive to drug and in those with marked bone marrow depression (leukopenia [less than 2,500 WBCs/mm^3], thrombocytopenia [less than 100,000 platelets/mm^3], or severe anemia).

Use cautiously in patients with impaired renal function. Don't administer to pregnant women or women of childbearing age who may become pregnant unless potential benefit to patient outweighs possible risk to fetus.

Interactions
Drug-drug. *Didanosine, indinavir, stavudine:* Fatal pancreatitis has occurred with concomitant use. Avoid use together.
Fluorouracil: Neurotoxicity may occur. Avoid use together.

Adverse reactions
CNS: hallucinations, headache, dizziness, disorientation, ***seizures***, malaise.
GI: *anorexia, nausea, vomiting, diarrhea*, stomatitis, constipation, ***pancreatitis***.
GU: increased BUN and serum creatinine levels.
Hematologic: ***leukopenia, thrombocytopenia***, anemia, *megaloblastosis*, ***bone mar-***

row suppression with rapid recovery (dose-limiting and dose-related).
Skin: rash, alopecia, erythema.
Other: fever, chills.

Overdose and treatment
Signs and symptoms of overdose include myelo-suppression, ulceration of buccal and GI mucosa, facial erythema, maculopapular rash, disorientation, hallucinations, and impairment of renal tubular function.

Treatment is usually supportive and includes transfusion of blood components.

Special considerations
● Dosage may need adjustment after other chemotherapy or radiation therapy.
● Auditory and visual hallucinations and blood toxicity increase when decreased renal function exists.
● Avoid all I.M. injections when platelet counts are below 100,000/mm³.
● Store capsules in tight container at room temperature. Avoid exposure to excessive heat.
● Drug is currently under investigation for the treatment of sickle cell anemia. Use of drug for this disease isn't recommended because of the potential for toxicity.

Patient monitoring
● Monitor CBC at least weekly throughout therapy.
● Monitor intake and output levels; patient must remain hydrated.
● Recommend obtaining BUN, uric acid, and serum creatinine levels routinely.
● Drug may exacerbate postirradiation erythema.

Pregnant patients
● Don't give drug to pregnant women or women of childbearing age who may become pregnant unless potential benefit to patient outweighs possible risk to fetus.

Breast-feeding patients
● It isn't known whether drug appears in breast milk. However, because of risk of serious adverse reactions, mutagenicity, and carcinogenicity in the infant, breast-feeding isn't recommended.

Pediatric patients
● Children may need a lower dosage.

Geriatric patients
● Elderly patients may be more sensitive to effects of drug, requiring a lower dosage.

Patient education
● Emphasize importance of continuing drug therapy despite nausea and vomiting.
● Encourage daily fluid intake of 10 to 12 8-oz glasses to increase urine output and facilitate excretion of uric acid.

● Advise patient of possible adverse reactions, and instruct him to report immediately post-dose vomiting, and unusual bruising or bleeding.
● Advise patient to avoid exposure to people with infections and to report signs of infection immediately.

hydroxyzine hydrochloride
Anx, Anxanil, Apo-Hydroxyzine*, Atarax, Hydroxacen, Hyzine-50, Multipax*, Neucalm, Novo-Hydroxyzin*, Quiess, QYS, Vistacon, Vistazine-50

hydroxyzine pamoate
Vistaril

Pharmacologic classification: antihistamine (piperazine derivative)
Therapeutic classification: antianxiety, sedative, antipruritic, antiemetic, antispasmodic
Pregnancy risk category: NR

Indications and dosages
➤ *Anxiety, tension, hyperkinesia. Adults:* 50 to 100 mg P.O. q.i.d.
Children age 6 and over: 50 to 100 mg P.O. daily in divided doses.
Children under age 6: 50 mg P.O. daily in divided doses.
➤ *Preoperative and postoperative adjunctive sedation, to control emesis, adjunct to asthma treatment. Adults:* 25 to 100 mg I.M. q 4 to 6 hours.
Children: 1.1 mg/kg I.M. q 4 to 6 hours.
➤ *Pruritus. Adults:* 25 mg P.O. t.i.d. or q.i.d.
Children age 6 and over: 50 to 100 mg P.O. daily in divided doses.
Children under age 6: 50 mg P.O. daily in divided doses.

How supplied
Available by prescription only
hydroxyzine hydrochloride
Injection: 25 mg/ml, 50 mg/ml
Syrup: 10 mg/5 ml
Tablets: 10 mg, 25 mg, 50 mg, 100 mg
Tablets (film-coated): 10 mg, 25 mg, 50 mg
hydroxyzine pamoate
Capsules: 25 mg, 50 mg, 100 mg
Oral suspension: 25 mg/5 ml

Pharmacodynamics
Anxiolytic and sedative actions: Hydroxyzine produces its sedative and antianxiety effects through suppression of activity at subcortical levels; analgesia occurs at high doses.
Antipruritic action: Drug is a direct competitor of histamine for binding at cellular receptor sites.

Reactions may be *common*, uncommon, *life-threatening*, or COMMON AND LIFE-THREATENING.

Other actions: Hydroxyzine is used as a pre-operative and postoperative adjunct for its sedative, antihistaminic, and anticholinergic activity.

Pharmacokinetics
Absorption: Absorbed rapidly and completely after oral administration. Serum levels peak in 2 to 4 hours. Sedation and other clinical effects are usually noticed in 15 to 30 minutes.
Distribution: Not well understood.
Metabolism: Metabolized almost completely in the liver.
Excretion: Metabolites are excreted primarily in urine; small amounts of drug and metabolites are found in feces. Half-life of drug is 3 hours. Sedative effects can last for 4 to 6 hours, and antihistaminic effects can persist for up to 4 days.

Route	Onset	Peak	Duration
P.O.	15-30 min	2 hr	4-6 hr
I.M.	Unknown	Unknown	4-6 hr

Contraindications and precautions
Contraindicated in patients hypersensitive to drug and during early pregnancy.
Use cautiously with adjustments in dosage in geriatric or debilitated patients.

Interactions
Drug-drug. *Anticholinergics:* Additive anticholinergic effects. Monitor patient closely.
Barbiturates, opioids, tranquilizers, other CNS depressants: Increased CNS effects. Reduce dose of CNS depressants by 50%.
Epinephrine: Concurrent use blocks vasopressor action. If a vasoconstrictor is needed, use norepinephrine or phenylephrine.
Drug-lifestyle. *Alcohol use:* Additive effects. Advise patient to avoid alcohol.

Adverse reactions
CNS: *drowsiness,* involuntary motor activity.
GI: *dry mouth.*
Other: marked discomfort at I.M. injection site, *hypersensitivity reactions.*

Overdose and treatment
Signs and symptoms of overdose include excessive sedation and hypotension; seizures may occur.
Treatment is supportive only. For recent oral ingestion, empty gastric contents through emesis or lavage. Correct hypotension with fluids and vasopressors (phenylephrine or metaraminol). Don't give epinephrine because hydroxyzine may counteract its effect.

Special considerations
● Carefully review patient's drug sensitivities and the use of CNS depressants for potential dose adjustments.
● Drug therapy falsely elevates urinary 17-hydroxycorticosteroid levels. It also may cause false-negative skin allergen tests by attenuating

or inhibiting the cutaneous response to histamine.

Patient monitoring
● Observe patient for excessive sedation, especially if he's receiving other CNS depressants.

Pregnant patients
● Drug isn't to be used during early pregnancy because of potential risk to the fetus. Safety and efficacy in pregnant women haven't been determined.

Breast-feeding patients
● It isn't known whether drug appears in breast milk. Safety hasn't been established in breast-feeding women.

Geriatric patients
● These patients may experience greater CNS depression and anticholinergic effects. Lower doses are indicated.

Patient education
● Advise patient to avoid tasks that require mental alertness or physical coordination until CNS effects of drug are known.
● Advise patient against use of other CNS depressants with hydroxyzine unless prescribed. Advise him to avoid alcohol and alcohol-containing products.
● Instruct patient to seek medical approval before taking OTC cold or allergy preparations that contain antihistamine, which may potentiate the effects of hydroxyzine.

hyoscyamine
Cystospaz

hyoscyamine sulfate
A-Spas S/L, Anaspaz, Cystospaz-M, Levsin, Levsin Drops, Levsin/SL, Levsinex Timecaps,

Pharmacologic classification: belladonna alkaloid
Therapeutic classification: anticholinergic
Pregnancy risk category: C

Indications and dosages
➤ *GI tract disorders caused by spasm; adjunctive therapy for peptic ulcers. Adults:* 0.125 to 0.25 mg P.O. or S.L. q.i.d. before meals and h.s.; 0.375 to 0.75 mg P.O. (extended-release form) q 12 hours; or 0.25 to 0.5 mg I.M., I.V., or S.C. q 4 hours b.i.d. to q.i.d. (Substitute oral form when symptoms are controlled.)
Children ages 2 to 12: 0.033 mg at about 10 kg (22 lb); 0.0625 mg at about 20 kg (44 lb); 0.0938 mg at about 40 kg (88 lb); 0.125 mg at about 50 kg (110 lb). May repeat q 4 hours, p.r.n. Maximum dose is 0.75 mg daily.

Children under age 2: 0.0125 mg at about 2.3 kg (5 lb); 0.0167 mg at about 3.4 kg (7.5 lb); 0.02 mg at about 5 kg (11 lb); 0.025 mg at about 6.8 kg (15 lb); 0.033 mg at about 10 kg (22 lb); 0.05 mg at about 15 kg (33 lb). May repeat q 4 hours, p.r.n. Maximum daily doses are 0.075 mg, 0.1 mg, 0.125 mg, 0.15 mg, 0.2 mg, and 0.275 mg, respectively.

➤*Endoscopy or hypotonic duodenography. Adults:* 0.25 to 0.5 mg I.V., I.M., or S.C., 5 to 10 minutes before procedure.

➤*Preoperative medication. Adults and children over age 2:* 5 mcg/kg I.V., I.M., or S.C. 30 to 60 minutes before induction of anesthesia.

How supplied
Available by prescription only
hyoscyamine
Tablets: 0.15 mg
hyoscyamine sulfate
Capsules (extended-release): 0.375 mg
Elixir: 0.125 mg/5 ml
Injection: 0.5 mg/ml
Oral solution: 0.125 mg/ml
Tablets: 0.125 mg
Tablets (extended-release): 0.375 mg
Tablets (sublingual): 0.125 mg

Pharmacodynamics
Antispasmodic and antiulcer actions: Hyoscyamine competitively blocks acetylcholine at cholinergic neuroeffector sites, decreasing GI motility and inhibiting gastric acid secretion.

Pharmacokinetics
Absorption: Well absorbed when taken orally.
Distribution: Well distributed throughout the body and crosses the blood-brain barrier. About 50% of dose binds to plasma proteins.
Metabolism: Metabolized in the liver. Usual duration of effect is up to 4 hours with standard oral and parenteral administration and up to 12 hours for the extended-release preparation.
Excretion: Excreted in the urine.

Route	Onset	Peak	Duration
P.O.			
Regular	20-30 min	½-1 hr	4-12 hr
Extended	20-30 min	40-90 min	12 hr
I.V.	2 min	15-30 min	4 hr
I.M., S.C.	Unknown	15-30 min	4-12 hr
S.L.	5-20 min	½-1 hr	4 hr

Contraindications and precautions
Contraindicated in patients with glaucoma, obstructive uropathy, obstructive disease of the GI tract, severe ulcerative colitis, myasthenia gravis, hypersensitivity to anticholinergics, paralytic ileus, intestinal atony, unstable CV status in acute hemorrhage, or toxic megacolon.

Use cautiously in patients with autonomic neuropathy, hyperthyroidism, coronary artery disease, arrhythmias, heart failure, hypertension, hiatal hernia with reflux esophagitis, hepatic or renal disease, and ulcerative colitis. Also use cautiously in hot or humid environments where drug-induced heat stroke can occur.

Interactions
Drug-drug. *Amantadine:* Increased anticholinergic effects. Avoid use together.
Antacids, antidiarrheals: Decreased hyoscyamine absorption. Give hyoscyamine 1 hour before these drugs.
Antihistamines, phenothiazines, tricyclic antidepressants: Increased adverse anticholinergic effects of hyoscyamine. Avoid use together.
Haloperidol, phenothiazines: Reduced antipsychotic effectiveness. Monitor patient carefully.

Adverse reactions
CNS: headache, insomnia, drowsiness, dizziness, nervousness, weakness, *confusion and excitement* in elderly patients.
CV: *palpitations,* tachycardia.
EENT: *blurred vision,* mydriasis, increased intraocular pressure, cycloplegia, photophobia.
GI: *dry mouth,* dysphagia, *constipation,* heartburn, loss of taste, nausea, vomiting, *paralytic ileus.*
GU: *urinary hesitancy, urine retention,* impotence.
Skin: urticaria, decreased sweating or possible anhidrosis, other dermal manifestations.
Other: fever, allergic reactions.

Overdose and treatment
Signs and symptoms of overdose include curare-like symptoms, such as respiratory paralysis; central stimulation followed by depression; and such psychotic symptoms as disorientation, confusion, hallucinations, delusions, anxiety, agitation, and restlessness. Peripheral effects may include dilated, nonreactive pupils; blurred vision; flushed, hot, dry skin; dryness of mucous membranes; dysphagia; decreased or absent bowel sounds; urine retention, hyperthermia; headache; tachycardia; hypertension; and increased respiration.

Treatment is primarily symptomatic and supportive, as needed. Maintain patent airway. If patient is alert, induce emesis (or use gastric lavage) and follow with a saline cathartic and activated charcoal to prevent further drug absorption. In severe cases, physostigmine may be administered to block antimuscarinic effects. Give fluids, as needed, to treat shock; diazepam to control psychotic symptoms; and pilocarpine (instilled into the eyes) to relieve mydriasis. If urine retention occurs, catheterization may be necessary.

Special considerations
● Consider the recommendations relevant to all anticholinergics.
● Hyoscyamine is administered P.O. Hyoscyamine sulfate usually is administered P.O. or S.L., but may be given I.V., I.M., or S.C. when therapeutic

effect is needed or if oral administration isn't possible.

Patient monitoring
• Drug regimen is adjusted based on patient's response and tolerance.

Breast-feeding patients
• Drug may appear in breast milk, possibly resulting in infant toxicity. Avoid use in breast-feeding women. Drug also may decrease milk production.

Pediatric patients
• Safety and efficacy for use in children haven't been reported.

Geriatric patients
• Use drug cautiously in geriatric patients; lower doses are indicated.

Patient education
• Advise patient to avoid driving or performing other hazardous activities if drowsiness, dizziness, or blurred vision occurs.
• Tell patient to drink fluids to avoid constipation.
• Instruct patient to report rash or other skin eruptions.
• Advise patient that extended-release tablets may not completely disintegrate and tablet fragments may be excreted in stools.
• Tell patient not to crush or chew extended-release tablets.

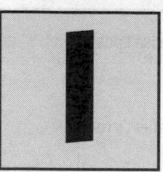

ibuprofen
Advil, Children's Advil, Medipren, Motrin, Motrin IB, Nuprin, Pediacare Fever, Rufen, Trendar

Pharmacologic classification: NSAID
Therapeutic classification: nonnarcotic analgesic, antipyretic, anti-inflammatory
Pregnancy risk category: B (D in third trimester)

Indications and dosages
➤ *Arthritis, gout, and postextraction dental pain. Adults:* 300 to 800 mg P.O. t.i.d. or q.i.d. Don't exceed 3,200 mg daily.
➤ *Primary dysmenorrhea. Adults:* 400 mg P.O. q 4 to 6 hours.
➤ *Mild to moderate pain. Adults:* 400 mg P.O. q 4 to 6 hours.
Children: 10 mg/kg P.O. q 6 to 8 hours; maximum dose is 40 mg/kg.
➤ *Juvenile arthritis. Children:* 20 to 40 mg/kg P.O. daily, divided into three or four doses. For mild disease, 20 mg/kg daily in divided doses.
➤ *Fever reduction. Adults:* 200 to 400 mg P.O. q 4 to 6 hours, p.r.n. Don't exceed 1,200 mg daily or take for more than 3 days.
Children ages 6 months to 12 years: 5 mg/kg P.O. q 6 to 8 hours, p.r.n., if baseline temperature is 102.5° F (39.2° C) or below; 10 mg/kg P.O. q 6 to 8 hours, p.r.n., if baseline temperature is more than 102.5° F. Recommended daily maximum dose is 40 mg/kg.

How supplied
Available without a prescription
Oral drops: 40 mg/ml
Oral suspension: 100 mg/5 ml, 100 mg/2.5 ml
Tablets: 100 mg, 200 mg
Tablets (chewable): 50 mg, 100 mg
Available by prescription only
Tablets: 300 mg, 400 mg, 600 mg, 800 mg

Pharmacodynamics
Analgesic, antipyretic, and anti-inflammatory actions: Mechanisms of action are unknown; ibuprofen is thought to inhibit prostaglandin synthesis.

Pharmacokinetics
Absorption: 80% of oral dose is absorbed from GI tract.
Distribution: Highly protein-bound.

Metabolism: Undergoes biotransformation in the liver.
Excretion: Excreted mainly in urine, with some biliary excretion. Plasma half-life ranges from 2 to 4 hours.

Route	Onset	Peak	Duration
P.O.	Variable	Variable	Variable

Contraindications and precautions
Contraindicated in patients hypersensitive to drug or in those who have the syndrome of nasal polyps, angioedema, and bronchospastic reaction to aspirin or other NSAIDs.

Use cautiously in patients with impaired renal or hepatic function, GI disorders, peptic ulcer disease, cardiac decompensation, hypertension, or coagulation defects. Because chewable tablets contain aspartame, use cautiously in patients with phenylketonuria. Ibuprofen is contraindicated during the last trimester of pregnancy because it may cause problems with the fetus or complications during delivery.

Interactions
Drug-drug. *ACE inhibitors:* Reduced response when used together; may result in acute reduction in renal function. Monitor patient closely.
Acetaminophen, gold compounds, other anti-inflammatories: Increased nephrotoxicity may occur. Use cautiously.
Antacids: May decrease the absorption of ibuprofen. Patient should take drugs at separate times.
Anticoagulants, thrombolytics (coumarin derivatives, heparin, streptokinase, urokinase): Increased anticoagulant effects. Dosage adjustment may be needed. Monitor coagulation studies.
Antihypertensives, diuretics: Concurrent use may decrease effectiveness of these drugs; diuretics may increase nephrotoxicity. Monitor patient closely.
Aspirin, carbenicillin, cefamandole, cefoperazone, corticosteroids, dextran, dipyridamole, mezlocillin, piperacillin, plicamycin, salicylates, sulfinpyrazone, ticarcillin, valproic acid, or other anti-inflammatory agents: Increased risk of bleeding or adverse GI reactions. Avoid use together.
Aspirin: May decrease the bioavailability of ibuprofen. Monitor patient for drug effect.
Insulin, oral antidiabetics: May potentiate hypoglycemic effects. Dosage adjustment may be needed.
Lithium, methotrexate: Decreased renal clearance of these drugs. Use together cautiously.

Reactions may be *common*, uncommon, *life-threatening*, or COMMON AND LIFE-THREATENING.

Nifedipine, phenytoin, verapamil: Toxicity may occur. Avoid use together.

Drug-herb. *Feverfew:* Decreased effectiveness of ibuprofen. Discourage use together.

Ginkgo biloba: Increased risk of bleeding from decreased platelet aggregation. Discourage use together.

Adverse reactions
CNS: headache, dizziness, nervousness, aseptic meningitis.
CV: peripheral edema, fluid retention, edema.
EENT: tinnitus.
GI: epigastric distress, nausea, occult blood loss, peptic ulceration, diarrhea, constipation, dyspepsia, flatulence, heartburn, decreased appetite.
GU: *acute renal failure,* azotemia, cystitis, hematuria.
Hematologic: prolonged bleeding time, anemia, *neutropenia, pancytopenia, thrombocytopenia, aplastic anemia, leukopenia, agranulocytosis.*
Hepatic: elevated liver enzyme levels.
Respiratory: *bronchospasm.*
Skin: pruritus, rash, urticaria, *Stevens-Johnson syndrome.*

Overdose and treatment
Signs and symptoms of overdose include dizziness, drowsiness, paresthesia, vomiting, nausea, abdominal pain, headache, sweating, nystagmus, apnea, and cyanosis.

To treat drug overdose, empty stomach immediately by inducing emesis with ipecac syrup or by gastric lavage. Administer activated charcoal via nasogastric tube. Provide symptomatic and supportive measures (respiratory support and correction of fluid and electrolyte imbalances). Monitor laboratory parameters and vital signs closely. Alkaline diuresis may enhance renal excretion. Dialysis is of minimal value because ibuprofen is strongly protein-bound.

Special considerations
Consider the recommendations relevant to all NSAIDs as well as the following.
• Maximum results in arthritis may require 1 to 2 weeks of continuous therapy with ibuprofen. Improvement may be seen, however, within 7 days.
• Give drug on an empty stomach, 1 hour before or 2 hours after meals, for maximum absorption. However, it may be administered with meals to lessen GI upset.

Patient monitoring
• Monitor auditory and ophthalmic functions periodically during ibuprofen therapy.
• Monitor cardiopulmonary status closely; monitor vital signs, especially heart rate and blood pressure.
• Observe patient for possible fluid retention.

Pregnant patients
• Drug shouldn't be used in third trimester unless specifically directed.

Breast-feeding patients
• Drug doesn't enter breast milk in significant quantities. However, manufacturer recommends alternative feeding methods during ibuprofen therapy.

Pediatric patients
• Safety and efficacy in children under age 6 months haven't been established.

Geriatric patients
• Patients over age 60 may be more susceptible to the toxic effects of ibuprofen, especially adverse GI reactions. Use lowest possible effective dose. The effect of drug on renal prostaglandins may cause fluid retention and edema, a significant drawback for geriatric patients, especially those with heart failure.

Patient education
• Instruct patient to seek medical approval before taking OTC drugs.
• Advise patient not to take ibuprofen for longer than 10 days for analgesic use and not to exceed maximum dose of six tablets (1.2 g) daily. Caution patient not to take drug if fever lasts longer than 3 days, unless prescribed.
• Tell patient to report adverse reactions; they're usually dose-related.
• Instruct patient in safety measures to prevent injury. Caution him to avoid hazardous activities that require mental alertness until CNS effects of drug are known.
• Encourage patient to adhere to prescribed drug regimen and stress importance of medical follow-up.

ibutilide fumarate
Corvert

Pharmacologic classification: ibutilide derivative
Therapeutic classification: class III supraventricular antiarrhythmic
Pregnancy risk category: C

Indications and dosages
➤ *Rapid conversion of atrial fibrillation or atrial flutter of recent onset to sinus rhythm.* Adults who weigh 60 kg (132 lb) or more: 1 mg I.V. over 10 minutes.
Adult who weigh less than 60 kg: 0.01 mg/kg I.V. over 10 minutes. Stop infusion if arrhythmia is terminated or if sustained or nonsustained ventricular tachycardia or marked prolongation of QT interval occurs. If arrhythmia doesn't terminate within 10 minutes after infusion ends, a second 10-minute infusion of equal strength may be administered.

How supplied
Available by prescription only
Injection: 0.1 mg/ml

Pharmacodynamics
Antiarrhythmic action: An antiarrhythmic with predominantly class III properties, ibutilide prolongs action potential duration in isolated cardiac myocytes and increases both atrial and ventricular refractoriness.

Pharmacokinetics
Absorption: Administered I.V.
Distribution: Highly distributed and about 40% protein-bound.
Metabolism: Not clearly defined.
Excretion: Excreted mainly in urine with the rest excreted in feces; half-life of drug is about 6 hours.

Route	Onset	Peak	Duration
I.V.	Unknown	Unknown	Unknown

Contraindications and precautions
Contraindicated in patients hypersensitive to drug or its components and in those with a history of polymorphic ventricular tachycardia, such as torsades de pointes.

Use cautiously in patients with hepatic or renal dysfunction.

Interactions
Drug-drug. *Class Ia antiarrhythmic drugs (disopyramide, procainamide, quinidine) and other class III drugs (amiodarone, sotalol):* Increased potential for prolonged refractoriness. Avoid concurrent administration and for at least five half-lives before administration of ibutilide and for 4 hours after ibutilide dosing.
Digoxin: Supraventricular arrhythmias may mask the cardiotoxicity related to excessive digoxin levels. Use cautiously.
H₁-receptor antagonist antihistamines, phenothiazines, tetracyclic antidepressants, tricyclic antidepressants, and other drugs that prolong QT interval: Increased risk for proarrhythmia. Patient needs ECG monitoring.

Adverse reactions
CNS: headache.
CV: ventricular extrasystoles, nonsustained ventricular tachycardia, hypotension, bundle branch block, **sustained ventricular tachycardia,** AV block, hypertension, QT-interval prolongation, **bradycardia,** palpitations, tachycardia.
GI: nausea.

Overdose and treatment
Overdose could exaggerate the expected prolongation of repolarization seen at usual clinical doses. Treatment should be supportive and appropriate for the condition.

Special considerations
● Proper equipment and facilities, including cardiac monitoring, intracardiac pacing facilities, cardioverter-defibrillator, and medication for treatment of sustained ventricular tachycardia, should be available during and after drug administration.
● Hypokalemia and hypomagnesemia should be corrected before therapy begins to reduce the potential for proarrhythmia.
● Admixtures of the product, with approved diluents, are chemically and physically stable for 24 hours at room temperature and for 48 hours at refrigerated temperatures.

Patient monitoring
◪ **ALERT** Patients with atrial fibrillation of more than 2 to 3 days' duration must be given adequate anticoagulants, usually for at least 2 weeks.
● Monitor patient's ECG continuously throughout drug administration and for at least 4 hours afterward or until QTc interval has returned to baseline because drug can induce or worsen ventricular arrhythmias in some patients. Longer monitoring is required if arrhythmic activity is noted.

Breast-feeding patients
● It isn't known whether drug appears in breast milk; discourage breast-feeding during drug therapy.

Pediatric patients
● Safety and efficacy in children under age 18 haven't been established.

Patient education
● Tell patient to report adverse reactions at once.
● Instruct patient to report discomfort at I.V. injection site.

idarubicin
Idamycin, Idamycin PFS

Pharmacologic classification: antibiotic antineoplastic
Therapeutic classification: antineoplastic
Pregnancy risk category: D

Indications and dosages
➤ *Treatment of acute myelocytic leukemia in adults, including French-American-British classifications M1 through M7, in combination with other approved antileukemic agents.* Adults: 12 mg/m² daily by slow I.V. injection (over 10 to 15 minutes) for 3 days. Administer with cytarabine 100 mg/m² daily by continuous infusion for 7 days, or give cytarabine as a 25-mg/m² bolus followed by 200 mg/m² daily by continuous I.V. infusion for 5 days. A second course may be administered if needed.

✦ **Dosage adjustment**. If patient experiences severe mucositis, delay administration until recovery is complete and reduce dosage by 25%. Also, reduce dosage in patients with hepatic or renal impairment. Idarubicin shouldn't be given if bilirubin level is more than 5 mg/dl.

Dosages and indications may vary. Check current literature for recommended protocol.

How supplied
Available by prescription only
Injection: 5 mg, 10 mg, 20 mg (lyophilized powder) in single-dose vials with 50 mg, 100 mg, or 200 mg lactose; 1 mg/ml preservative free in 5-ml, 10-ml, 20-ml single-use vials

Pharmacodynamics
Antineoplastic action: Idarubicin inhibits nucleic acid synthesis by intercalation and interacts with the enzyme topoisomerase II. It's highly lipophilic, which speeds cellular uptake.

Pharmacokinetics
Absorption: Administered I.V.
Distribution: Highly lipophilic and 97% tissue-bound, with highest levels in nucleated blood and bone marrow cells. Its metabolite, idarubicinol, is detected in CSF; clinical significance of this is under evaluation.
Metabolism: Extensive extrahepatic metabolism is indicated. Metabolite has cytotoxic activity.
Excretion: Excreted predominantly by biliary excretion as its metabolite and, to a lesser extent, by renal elimination. Mean terminal half-life is 22 hours (range, 4 to 46 hours) when used as a single agent and 20 hours (range, 7 to 38 hours) when combined with cytarabine. Plasma levels of metabolite are sustained for longer than 8 days.

Route	Onset	Peak	Duration
I.V.	Unknown	Unknown	Unknown

Contraindications and precautions
No known contraindications. Use cautiously in patients with impaired renal or hepatic function and in those with bone marrow suppression induced by previous drug therapy or radiation therapy and those with cardiac disease.

Interactions
None reported.

Adverse reactions
CNS: *headache, changed mental status,* peripheral neuropathy, *seizures.*
CV: *heart failure,* atrial fibrillation, chest pain, *MI,* asymptomatic decline in left ventricular ejection fraction, *myocardial insufficiency, arrhythmias, myocardial toxicity.*
GI: *nausea, vomiting, cramps, diarrhea, mucositis.*
GU: decreased renal function.

Hematologic: *hemorrhage, myelosuppression.*
Hepatic: changes in hepatic function.
Skin: *alopecia, rash, urticaria, bullous erythrodermatous rash on palms and soles,* hives (at injection site), erythema (at previously irradiated sites), tissue necrosis at injection site (if extravasation occurs).
Other: INFECTION, *fever,* hyperuricemia, *hypersensitivity reactions.*

Overdose and treatment
Severe and prolonged myelosuppression and possibly increased severity of GI toxicity are anticipated. Supportive treatment, including platelet transfusions, antibiotics, and treatment of mucositis, is required. Acute cardiac toxicity with severe arrhythmias and delayed cardiac failure also may occur. Peritoneal dialysis or hemodialysis isn't effective.

Special considerations
• Idarubicin shouldn't be mixed with other drugs unless specific compatibility data are available. Heparin causes precipitation. Degradation occurs with prolonged contact with alkaline solutions.
🛈 ALERT Drug should be given only by a clinician in a facility capable of immediate response and treatment to hemorrhagic condition or overwhelming infection.
• Hyperuricemia may result from rapid lysis of leukemic cells; take appropriate preventive measures (including adequate hydration) before starting treatment.
• Systemic infections should be controlled before therapy begins.
• If extravasation or signs of extravasation occur, discontinue the infusion immediately and restart in another vein. Treat the site with intermittent ice packs for 30 minutes four times daily for 4 days.
• Follow usual chemotherapy mixing precautions. Vial is under negative pressure.
• Reconstituted solutions are stable for 3 days (72 hours) at 59° to 86° F (15° to 30° C); 7 days if refrigerated. Discard unused solutions appropriately.

Patient monitoring
• Frequently monitor CBC and hepatic and renal function.

Breast-feeding patients
• It isn't known whether idarubicin appears in breast milk. To avoid risk of serious adverse reactions in the infant, discontinue breast-feeding before starting therapy with idarubicin.

Pediatric patients
• Safety and efficacy in children haven't been established.

Patient education

• Instruct patient to recognize signs and symptoms of extravasation and to report them if they occur.
• Tell patient to report signs and symptoms of infection, including persistent fever or sore throat.
• Advise patient to minimize dangerous behavior that can cause bleeding and to report bleeding or abnormal bruising.

ifosfamide
Ifex

Pharmacologic classification: alkylating agent (not specific to cell cycle phase)
Therapeutic classification: antineoplastic
Pregnancy risk category: D

Indications and dosages
➤ *Germ cell testicular cancer.* Adults: 1.2 g/m² I.V. daily for 5 days. Regimen is usually repeated q 3 weeks. Drug may be given by slow I.V. push, by intermittent infusion over at least 30 minutes, or by continuous infusion. Dosages and indications may vary. Check current literature for recommended protocol.
➤ *Lung cancer◇, Hodgkin's and malignant lymphoma◇, breast cancer◇, acute and chronic lymphocytic leukemia◇, ovarian cancer◇, gastric cancer◇, pancreatic cancer◇, sarcomas◇.* Adults: 1.2 g/m² I.V. daily for 5 days. Regimen is usually repeated q 3 weeks. Drug may be given by slow I.V. push, by intermittent infusion over at least 30 minutes, or by continuous infusion. Dosage and indications may vary. Check current literature for recommended protocol.

How supplied
Available by prescription only
Injection: 1-g, 3-g vials

Pharmacodynamics
Antineoplastic action: Ifosfamide requires activation by hepatic microsomal enzymes to exert its cytotoxic activity. The active compound cross-links strands of DNA and also breaks the DNA chain.

Pharmacokinetics
Absorption: Administered I.V.
Distribution: Crosses the blood-brain barrier along with its metabolites.
Metabolism: About 50% of a dose is metabolized in the liver.
Excretion: Excreted primarily in the urine. The terminal half-life is about 7 hours at doses of 1.6 to 2.4 g/m² daily and about 15 hours at a single dose of 3.8 to 5 g/m².

Route	Onset	Peak	Duration
I.V.	Unknown	Unknown	Unknown

Contraindications and precautions
Contraindicated in patients with severe bone marrow suppression or hypersensitivity to drug. Use cautiously in patients with renal or hepatic impairment, compromised bone marrow reserve as indicated by granulocytopenia, bone marrow metastases, prior radiation therapy, or therapy with cytotoxic agents. Contraindicated in pregnancy due to possible embryotoxic and teratogenic effects on the fetus.

Interactions
Drug-drug. *Chloral hydrate, phenobarbital, phenytoin:* May increase the activity of ifosfamide by induction of hepatic microsomal enzymes, increasing the conversion of ifosfamide to its active form. Be alert for possible combined drug actions, desirable or undesirable, involving ifosfamide, even though it has been used successfully with other drugs, including other cytotoxic drugs.

Adverse reactions
CNS: *somnolence, confusion,* **coma, seizures,** *ataxia, hallucinations, depressive psychosis,* dizziness, disorientation, cranial nerve dysfunction.
CV: phlebitis.
GI: *nausea, vomiting.*
GU: **hemorrhagic cystitis,** *hematuria,* **nephrotoxicity,** *dysuria, urinary frequency.*
Hematologic: **leukopenia, thrombocytopenia, myelosuppression.**
Hepatic: elevated liver enzyme levels, liver dysfunction.
Metabolic: *metabolic acidosis.*
Skin: *alopecia.*
Other: infection.

Overdose and treatment
Signs and symptoms of overdose include myelosuppression, nausea, vomiting, alopecia, and hemorrhagic cystitis.
    Treatment is usually supportive and includes antiemetics, transfusion of blood components, and bladder irrigation.

Special considerations
• Follow all established procedures for the safe handling, administration, and disposal of chemotherapeutic agents.
• Push fluids (3 L daily) and administer with mesna (Mesnex) to prevent hemorrhagic cystitis. Avoid giving drug at bedtime, because infrequent voiding during the night increases the possibility of cystitis. Bladder irrigation with normal saline solution decreases the possibility of cystitis.
• Drug can be further diluted with D₅W or normal saline solution for I.V. infusion. This solution is stable for 7 days at room temperature and for 6 weeks at 41° F (5° C).
• Drug may be given by I.V. push injection in a minimum of 75 ml normal saline solution over 30 minutes.

Reactions may be *common*, uncommon, *life-threatening*, or COMMON AND LIFE-THREATENING.

• Infusing each dose over 2 hours or longer decreases the possibility of cystitis.

Patient monitoring

• Assess patient for changes in mental status and cerebellar dysfunction. Dose may have to be decreased.
• Monitor CBC, renal finction tests, and liver function tests.
• Sterile phlebitis may occur at the injection site; apply warm compresses.

Pregnant patients

• Patient who becomes pregnant while taking drug should be informed of the risk to fetus.

Breast-feeding patients

• Drug appears in breast milk. Because of the potential for serious adverse reactions, mutagenicity, and carcinogenicity in the infant, breast-feeding isn't recommended.

Pediatric patients

• Safety and efficacy in children haven't been established.

Patient education

• Tell patient to ensure adequate fluid intake to prevent bladder toxicity and to facilitate excretion of uric acid.
• Warn patient to avoid exposure to infections and to report signs of infection or unusual bleeding immediately.
• Reassure patient that hair should grow back after treatment has ended.
• Tell patient to contact prescriber immediately if blood appears in the urine.
• Advise both men and women to use contraceptive measures during therapy.

---

imipenem and cilastatin sodium

Primaxin I.M., Primaxin I.V.

Pharmacologic classification: carbapenem (thienamycin class), beta-lactam antibiotic
Therapeutic classification: antibiotic
Pregnancy risk category: C

Indications and dosages

➤ *Mild to moderate lower respiratory tract, skin and skin-structure, or gynecologic infections.* Adults who weigh at least 70 kg (154 lb): 500 to 750 mg I.M. q 12 hours.
➤ *Mild to moderate intra-abdominal infections.* Adults who weigh at least 70 kg (154 lb): 750 mg I.M. q 12 hours.
➤ *Serious respiratory and urinary tract infections; intra-abdominal, gynecologic, bone, joint, or skin infections; bacterial septicemia; endocarditis.* Adults who weigh at least 70 kg (154 lb): 250 mg to 1 g by

I.V. infusion q 6 to 8 hours. Maximum daily dose is 50 mg/kg or 4 g, whichever is less.
Children: 15 to 25 mg/kg q 6 hours.
✦ *Dosage adjustment.* In patients with renal impairment and creatinine clearance of 6 to 20 ml/minute, 125 to 250 mg I.V. q 12 hours for most pathogens. There may be an increased risk of seizures when doses of 500 mg q 12 hours are administered to these patients. When creatinine clearance is 5 ml/minute or less, imipenem shouldn't be given unless hemodialysis is instituted within 48 hours.

Note: In patients who weigh less than 70 kg (154 lb) or those with impaired renal function, dosages vary. Check current literature for recommended protocol.

How supplied

Available by prescription only
Injection: 250-mg, 500-mg vials, ADD-Vantage, and infusion bottles
Powder (for I.M. injection): 500-mg, 750-mg vial

Pharmacodynamics

Antibacterial action: A bactericidal drug, imipenem inhibits bacterial cell wall synthesis. Its spectrum of antimicrobial activity includes many gram-positive, gram-negative, and anaerobic bacteria, including *Staphylococcus* and *Streptococcus* species, *Escherichia coli, Klebsiella, Proteus, Enterobacter* species, *Pseudomonas aeruginosa,* and *Bacteroides* species, including *B. fragilis.* Resistant bacteria include methicillin-resistant staphylococci, *Clostridium difficile,* and other *Pseudomonas* species.

Cilastatin inhibits the enzymatic breakdown of imipenem in the kidneys, making it effective in treating urinary tract infections.

Pharmacokinetics

Absorption: Following I.M. administration, imipenem blood levels peak within 2 hours; cilastatin levels reach their peak within 1 hour. After I.V. administration, peak levels of both agents appear in about 20 minutes. Imipenem is about 75% bioavailable and cilastatin is about 95% bioavailable after I.M. administration compared with I.V. administration.
Distribution: Distributed rapidly and widely. About 20% of imipenem is protein-bound; 40% of cilastatin is protein-bound.
Metabolism: Imipenem is metabolized by kidney dehydropeptidase I, resulting in low urine levels. Cilastatin inhibits this enzyme, thereby reducing metabolism of imipenem.
Excretion: About 70% of imipenem and cilastatin dose is excreted unchanged by the kidneys (when imipenem is combined with cilastatin) by tubular secretion and glomerular filtration. Imipenem is cleared by hemodialysis; therefore, a supplemental dose is required after this procedure. Half-life of drug is about 1 hour after I.V. administration. The prolonged absorption that

---

occurs after I.M. administration results in a longer half-life (2 to 3 hours).

Route	Onset	Peak	Duration
I.M.	Unknown	1-2 hr	Unknown
I.V.	Unknown	Unknown	Unknown

Contraindications and precautions

Contraindicated in patients hypersensitive to drug. Imipenem and cilastatin sodium reconstituted with lidocaine hydrochloride for I.M. injection is contraindicated in patients hypersensitive to local anesthetics of the amide type and in patients with severe shock or heart block.

Use cautiously in patients with impaired renal function, seizure disorders, or allergy to penicillins or cephalosporins.

Interactions

Drug-drug. *Chloramphenicol:* May impede the bactericidal effects of imipenem. Give chloramphenicol a few hours after imipenem and cilastatin.

Ganciclovir: Generalized seizures have occurred in several patients during combined imipenem and cilastatin and ganciclovir therapy. Monitor patient closely.

Probenecid: May prevent tubular secretion of cilastatin (but not imipenem) and prolong plasma cilastatin half-life. Use together cautiously.

Adverse reactions

CNS: *seizures,* dizziness, somnolence.
CV: thrombophlebitis, hypotension.
GI: nausea, vomiting, diarrhea, *pseudomembranous colitis.*
Hematologic: *agranulocytosis,* thrombocytosis.
Hepatic: transient increases in liver enzyme levels.
Skin: rash, urticaria, pruritus, pain at injection site.
Other: *hypersensitivity reactions (anaphylaxis),* fever.

Overdose and treatment

If overdose occurs, discontinue drug, treat symptomatically, and institute supportive measures as required. Although imipenem and cilastatin sodium are hemodialyzable, use of hemodialysis in treating drug overdose is questionable.

Special considerations

● Culture and sensitivity tests should be done before starting therapy.
● Drug may be physically incompatible with aminoglycosides; avoid mixing together.
● Drug isn't to be administered by direct I.V. bolus injection. Infuse 250- or 500-mg dose over 20 to 30 minutes; infuse 1-g dose over 40 to 60 minutes. If nausea occurs, slow infusion.
● Drug has broadest antibacterial spectrum of any available antibiotic. It's most valuable for empiric treatment of unidentified infections and for mixed infections that would otherwise require

combination of antibiotics, possibly including an aminoglycoside.
● Interferes with urinary glucose determinations using the cupric sulfate method.

Patient monitoring

● Continue use of anticonvulsants in patients with seizure disorders. Patients who exhibit CNS toxicity should receive phenytoin or benzodiazepines. Reduce dosage or discontinue drug if CNS toxicity continues.
● Prolonged use may result in overgrowth of nonsusceptible organisms. In addition, use of imipenem and cilastatin as a sole course of therapy has resulted in resistance during therapy.

Breast-feeding patients

● It's unknown whether drug appears in breast milk. Administer cautiously to breast-feeding women.

Pediatric patients

● Safety and efficacy in children under age 12 haven't been established; however, drug has been used in children ages 3 months to 13 years. Dosage range is 15 to 25 mg/kg every 6 hours.

Geriatric patients

● Administer cautiously to geriatric patients because they may also have renal dysfunction.

Patient education

● Advise patient of potential adverse reactions.
● Instruct patient to report to prescriber immediately any serious adverse drug effects.

imipramine hydrochloride
Apo-Imipramine*, Impril*, Novopramine*, Tofranil

imipramine pamoate
Tofranil-PM

Pharmacologic classification: dibenzazepine tricyclic antidepressant
Therapeutic classification: antidepressant
Pregnancy risk category: D

Indications and dosages

➤**Depression.** *Adults:* Initially, 75 to 100 mg P.O. daily in divided doses, with 25- to 50-mg increments, up to 200 mg. Or, some patients can start with lower doses (25 mg P.O.) and dosage is adjusted slowly in 25-mg increments every other day. Maximum dose is 300 mg daily. Or, entire dosage may be given h.s. Maximum daily dose is 200 mg for outpatients, 300 mg for inpatients, 100 mg for elderly patients.
➤**Childhood enuresis.** *Children age 6 and older:* 25 to 75 mg P.O. daily, 1 hour before bedtime. Usual dose is 1.5 mg/kg daily in three divided doses. Maximum dose is 2.5 mg/kg daily.

How supplied
Available by prescription only
imipramine hydrochloride
Tablets: 10 mg, 25 mg, 50 mg
imipramine pamoate
Capsules: 75 mg, 100 mg, 125 mg, 150 mg

Pharmacodynamics
Antidepressant action: Imipramine is thought to exert its antidepressant effects by inhibiting reuptake of norepinephrine and serotonin in CNS nerve terminals (presynaptic neurons), which results in increased levels and enhanced activity of these neurotransmitters in the synaptic cleft. Drug also has anticholinergic activity and is used to treat nocturnal enuresis in children over age 6.

Pharmacokinetics
Absorption: Absorbed rapidly from GI tract.
Distribution: Distributed widely throughout the body, including the CNS and breast milk. Drug is 90% protein-bound. Steady state is achieved within 2 to 5 days. Therapeutic plasma levels (parent drug and metabolite) range from 150 to 300 ng/ml.
Metabolism: Metabolized by the liver to the active metabolite desipramine. A significant first-pass effect may explain variability of serum levels in different patients taking the same dosage.
Excretion: Mostly excreted in urine.

Route	Onset	Peak	Duration
P.O.	Unknown	½-2 hr	Unknown

Contraindications and precautions
Contraindicated during acute recovery phase of MI, in patients hypersensitive to drug, and in those receiving MAO inhibitors.

Use cautiously in patients at risk for suicide; in those with impaired renal or hepatic function, history of urine retention, angle-closure glaucoma, increased intraocular pressure, CV disease, hyperthyroidism, and in patients receiving thyroid medications.

Interactions
Drug-drug. *Antiarrhythmics (disopyramide, procainamide, quinidine), pimozide, thyroid medication:* May increase risk of arrhythmias and conduction defects. Avoid use together.
Atropine or other anticholinergic drugs, including antihistamines, antiparkinsonian agents, meperidine, and phenothiazines; CNS depressants, including analgesics, anesthetics, barbiturates, narcotics, and tranquilizers: Oversedation, paralytic ileus, visual changes, and severe constipation. Avoid use together.
Barbiturates: Induced imipramine metabolism and decreased therapeutic efficacy. Avoid use together.
Beta blockers, cimetidine, methylphenidate, oral contraceptives, propoxyphene: Inhibited imipramine metabolism, increasing plasma levels and toxicity. Use together cautiously.

Centrally acting antihypertensives, such as clonidine, guanabenz, guanadrel, guanethidine, methyldopa, and reserpine: Decreased hypotensive effects of antihypertensives. Use cautiously.
Disulfiram or ethchlorvynol: May cause delirium and tachycardia. Observe patient closely.
Haloperidol and phenothiazines: Decreased metabolism of imipramine, decreasing therapeutic efficacy. Monitor patient closely.
Metrizamide: Increased risk of seizures. Monitor patient closely.
Sympathomimetics, including ephedrine, epinephrine, and phenylephrine (often found in nasal sprays): May increase blood pressure. Patient needs frequent blood pressure checks.
Warfarin: May prolong PT and cause bleeding. Monitor PT and INR.
Drug-herb. *Evening primrose oil:* Possible additive or synergistic effect resulting in lower seizure threshold and increasing the risk of seizure. Discourage use together.
Drug-lifestyle. *Alcohol use:* Additive CNS depressant effects. Advise patient to avoid alcohol.
Heavy smoking: Induced imipramine metabolism and decreased therapeutic efficacy. Monitor patient for therapeutic effect.

Adverse reactions
CNS: *drowsiness, dizziness,* excitation, tremor, confusion, hallucinations, anxiety, ataxia, paresthesia, nervousness, EEG changes, **seizures,** extrapyramidal reactions.
CV: *orthostatic hypotension, tachycardia, ECG changes,* hypertension, **MI, CVA, arrhythmias, heart block,** *precipitation of heart failure.*
EENT: blurred vision, tinnitus, mydriasis.
GI: *dry mouth, constipation,* nausea, vomiting, anorexia, paralytic ileus, abdominal cramps.
GU: *urine retention,* testicular swelling, impotence.
Metabolic: increased or decreased serum glucose levels.
Skin: *diaphoresis,* rash, urticaria, photosensitivity, pruritus.
Other: gynecomastia, galactorrhea and breast enlargement, altered libido, SIADH, **hypersensitivity reaction.**

Overdose and treatment
Drug overdose is typically life-threatening, particularly when combined with alcohol. The first 12 hours after acute ingestion are a stimulatory phase characterized by excessive anticholinergic activity including agitation, irritation, confusion, hallucinations, hyperthermia, parkinsonian symptoms, seizure, urine retention, dry mucous membranes, pupillary dilatation, constipation, and ileus. This is followed by CNS depressant effects, including hypothermia, decreased or absent reflexes, sedation, hypotension, cyanosis, and cardiac irregularities, including tachycardia, conduction disturbances, and quinidine-like effects on the ECG.

Severity of overdose is best indicated by widening of the QRS complex, which usually represents a serum level in excess of 1,000 ng/ml; serum levels are usually not helpful. Metabolic acidosis may follow hypotension, hypoventilation, and seizures.

Treatment is symptomatic and supportive, including maintaining airway, stable body temperature, and fluid or electrolyte balance. Induce emesis if patient is conscious; follow with gastric lavage and activated charcoal to prevent further absorption. Dialysis is of little use.

Treat seizures with parenteral diazepam or phenytoin and arrhythmias with parenteral phenytoin or lidocaine. Don't use quinidine, procainamide, and atropine during an overdose. Treat acidosis with sodium bicarbonate. Don't give barbiturates; these may enhance CNS and respiratory depressant effects.

Special considerations
● Drug causes a high risk of orthostatic hypotension.
● Discontinue drug at least 48 hours before surgical procedures.
● Drug shouldn't be withdrawn abruptly, but tapered gradually over time. After abrupt withdrawal of long-term therapy, patient may experience nausea, headache, and malaise. These symptoms do not indicate addiction.

Patient monitoring
● Monitor sitting and standing blood pressures after initial dose.
● Tolerance to sedative effects of drug usually develops over several weeks.

Breast-feeding patients
● Drug appears in breast milk in low levels. The potential benefit to the woman should outweigh possible risks to the infant.

Pediatric patients
● Drug isn't recommended for treating depression in patients under age 12. Don't use pamoate salt for enuresis in children.

Geriatric patients
● Recommended dose is 30 to 40 mg P.O. daily, not to exceed 100 mg daily. Start therapy at low doses (10 mg) and adjust slowly. Geriatric patients may be at greater risk for adverse cardiac reactions.

Patient education
● Tell patient to take drug exactly as prescribed.
● Explain that full effects of drug may not become apparent for up to 4 to 6 weeks.
● Warn patient not to discontinue drug abruptly, not to share drug with others, and not to drink alcoholic beverages while taking drug.
● Advise patient to take drug with food or milk if it causes stomach upset.

● Suggest relieving dry mouth with sugarless chewing gum or hard candy. Encourage good dental prophylaxis because persistent dry mouth may lead to dental caries.
● Encourage patient to report unusual or troublesome effects immediately, including confusion, movement disorders, rapid heartbeat, dizziness, fainting, or difficulty urinating.

immune globulin (gamma globulin, IG, immune serum globulin, ISG)

immune globulin for I.M. use (IGIM)
BayGam

immune globulin for I.V. use (IGIV)
Gamimune N (5%, 10%), Gammagard S/D, Gammar-P IV, Iveegam, Polygam S/D, Sandoglobulin, Venoglobulin-I, Venoglobulin-S

Pharmacologic classification: immune serum
Therapeutic classification: antibody production stimulator
Pregnancy risk category: C

Indications and dosages
➤ *Agammaglobulinemia, hypogammaglobulinemia, immune deficiency.* IGIV.
Adults and children: For Gamimune N only, 100 to 200 mg/kg or 2 to 4 ml/kg I.V. infusion monthly. Infusion rate is 0.01 to 0.02 ml/kg/minute for 30 minutes. Rate can then be increased to maximum of 0.08 ml/kg/minute for remainder of infusion.

For Gammagard S/D only, initially 200 to 400 mg/kg I.V., followed by 100 mg/kg monthly. Start infusion at 0.5 ml/kg/hour, gradually increasing to maximum of 4 ml/kg/hour.

For Gammar-P IV only, 200 to 400 mg/kg q 3 to 4 weeks. Infusion rate is 0.01 ml/kg/minute, increasing to 0.02 ml/kg/minute after 15 to 30 minutes, with gradual increase to 0.06 ml/kg/minute.

For Iveegam only, 200 mg/kg I.V. monthly. If response is inadequate, doses may be increased up to 800 mg/kg or the drug may be administered more frequently. Infuse at 1 to 2 ml/minute.

For Polygam S/D only, 100 mg/kg I.V. monthly. An initial dose of 200 to 400 mg/kg may be administered. Start infusion at 0.5 ml/kg/hour, gradually increasing to maximum of 4 ml/kg/hour.

For Sandoglobulin, 200 mg/kg I.V. monthly. Start with 0.5 to 1 ml/minute of a 3% solution; increase up to 2.5 ml/minute gradually after 15 to 30 minutes.

For Venoglobulin-I only, 200 mg/kg I.V. monthly; may be increased to 300 to 400 mg/kg and may be repeated more frequently than once monthly. Infuse at 0.01 to 0.02 ml/kg/minute for 30 minutes, then increase to 0.04 ml/kg/minute or higher, if tolerated.

For Venoglobulin-S only, 200 mg/kg I.V. monthly. Increase dose to 300 to 400 mg/kg monthly or administer more frequently if adequate IgI levels aren't achieved. Start infusion at 0.01 to 0.02 ml/kg/minute for 30 minutes, then increase 5% solutions to 0.04 ml/kg/minute and 10% solutions to 0.05 ml/kg/minute, if tolerated.

► *Hepatitis A exposure.* IGIM. *Adults and children:* 0.02 to 0.04 ml/kg I.M. as soon as possible after exposure. Up to 0.1 ml/kg may be given after prolonged or intense exposure.

► *Measles exposure.* IGIM. *Adults and children:* 0.2 to 0.25 ml/kg within 6 days after exposure.

► *Postexposure prophylaxis of measles for immunosuppressed patients.* IGIM. *Adults and children:* 0.5 ml/kg I.M. within 6 days after exposure.

► *Chickenpox exposure◇.* IGIM. *Adults and children:* 0.6 to 1.2 ml/kg I.M. as soon as exposed.

► *Rubella exposure in first trimester of pregnancy◇.* IGIM. *Women:* 0.55 ml/kg I.M. as soon as exposed

► *Idiopathic thrombocytopenic purpura.* IGIV. *Adults and children:* Initially, 400 mg/kg daily of Sandoglobulin or Gamimune N (5% or 10%) I.V. for 2 to 5 consecutive days depending on platelet count and clinical response. Maintenance dosage is 400 to 1,000 mg/kg I.V. of Gamimune N 5%, 10%, or Sandoglobulin as a single infusion to maintain a platelet count greater than 30,000/mm³. Or 1,000 mg/kg of Gammagard S/D and Polygam S/D as a single dose. May give up to three doses on alternate days if needed.

► *Bone marrow transplantation.* IGIV. *Adults over age 20:* Gamimune N 10%, 500 mg/kg on day 7 and day 2 before transplantation; then weekly through 90 days after transplantation.

How supplied
Available by prescription only
IGIM
Injection: 2-ml, 10-ml vials
IGIV
I.V.: Gamimune N—5% and 10% solution in 10-ml, 50-ml, 100-ml, and 250-ml single-use vials; Gammagard S/D—2.5-g, 5-g, and 10-g single-use vials for reconstitution; Gammar-P IV—1-g, 2.5-g, and 5-g vials with diluent and 10-g vials with administration set and diluent; Iveegam—1-g, 2.5-g, and 5-g vials with diluent; Polygam S/D—2.5 g, 5 g, and 10-g single-use vials with diluent; Sandoglobulin—1-g, 3-g, 6-g, and 12-g vials or kits with diluent or bulk packs without diluent; Venoglobulin-I—2.5-g and 5-g vials with or without reconstitution kits with sterile water, 10-g vials with reconstitution kit and administration set, and 0.5-g vials with reconstitution kit; Venoglobulin-S—5% and 10% in 50-ml, 100-ml, and 200-ml vials.

Pharmacodynamics
Immune action: Immune globulin provides passive immunity by increasing antibody titer. The mechanism by which IGIV increases platelet counts in idiopathic thrombocytopenic purpura isn't fully known.

Pharmacokinetics
Absorption: Slow I.M. absorption.
Distribution: Distributed evenly between intravascular and extravascular spaces.
Metabolism: No information available.
Excretion: Serum half-life is reportedly 21 to 24 days in immunocompetent patients.

Route	Onset	Peak	Duration
I.V.	Unknown	2 days	Unknown

Contraindications and precautions
Contraindicated in patients hypersensitive to drug.

Interactions
Drug-drug. *Live-virus vaccines:* Immune globulin may interfere with the immune response to live virus vaccines (such as measles, mumps, rubella). Live-virus vaccines must not be given within 3 months after administration of immune globulin.

Adverse reactions
CNS: faintness, headache, malaise, aseptic meningitis syndrome.
CV: chest pain, chest tightness.
GI: nausea, vomiting.
GU: increased serum creatinine and BUN, oliguria, anuria, *acute renal failure*, acute tubular necrosis, proximal tubular nephropathy, osmotic nephrosis.
Musculoskeletal: hip pain, joint pain, muscle stiffness (at injection site).
Respiratory: dyspnea, shortness of breath.
Skin: erythema, urticaria.
Other: fever, *anaphylaxis*, chills, infusion reactions.

Overdose and treatment
Excessively rapid I.V. infusion can precipitate an anaphylactoid reaction.

Special considerations
● Obtain a thorough history of allergies and reactions to immunizations.
● Epinephrine solution 1:1,000 should be available to treat allergic reactions.
● Inject I.M. formulation into different sites, preferably into buttocks. Don't inject more than 3 ml per injection site.
● Don't give for hepatitis A exposure if 2 weeks or more have elapsed since exposure or after onset of clinical illness.
● Store Sandoglobulin and Gammagard S/D at room temperature not exceeding 77° F (25° C); Gamimune-N and Iveegam, at 36° to 46° F (2° to 8° C) but don't freeze; Gammar-P IV, at room

temperature below 86° F (30° C) but don't freeze; Venoglobulin-I at room temperature below 86° F (30° C).

• Immune globulin has been studied in the treatment of various conditions, including Kawasaki disease, asthma, allergic disorders, autoimmune neutropenia, myasthenia gravis, and platelet transfusion rejection. It also has been used in the prophylaxis of infections in immunocompromised patients.

• Gamimune N can be diluted with D_5W.

• Reconstitute Gammagard S/D with diluent (sterile water for injection) and transfer device provided by manufacturer. Administration set (provided) contains a 15-micron in-line filter that must be used during administration.

• Reconstitute Sandoglobulin with diluent supplied (normal saline solution).

Patient monitoring

• Closely monitor blood pressure in patient receiving IGIV, especially if it's patient's first infusion of immune globulin.

Pregnant patients

• Although pregnancy isn't a contraindication to use, it's unknown whether immune globulin can cause fetal harm.

Breast-feeding patients

• It isn't known whether immune globulin appears in breast milk. Use cautiously in breast-feeding women.

Patient education

• Explain that the patient's chances of getting AIDS or hepatitis after receiving immune globulin are minute because of stringent government standards that require testing for these viruses.

• Instruct patient to promptly report headache, skin changes, or difficulty breathing; decreased urine output; sudden weight gain; swelling; and shortness of breath.

---

inamrinone lactate
Inocor

Pharmacologic classification: bipyridine derivative
Therapeutic classification: inotropic, vasodilator
Pregnancy risk category: C

Indications and dosages
➤ **Short-term management of heart failure.** *Adults:* Initially, 0.75 mg/kg I.V. bolus over 2 to 3 minutes; then begin maintenance infusion of 5 to 10 mcg/kg/minute. Additional bolus of 0.75 mg/kg may be given 30 minutes after therapy is initiated. Maximum daily dose is 10 mg/kg.
➤ **Cardiac life support in patients in whom other preferred drugs cannot be used for pump failure and acute pul-**
monary edema. *Adults:* 0.75 mg/kg I.V. bolus over 2 to 3 minutes, then 5 to 15 mcg/kg/minute.

How supplied
Available by prescription only
Injection: 5 mg/ml

Pharmacodynamics
Vasodilating action: The primary vasodilating effect of inamrinone seems to stem from a direct effect on peripheral vessels.
Inotropic action: The mechanism of action responsible for the apparent inotropic effect isn't fully understood; however, it may be linked to inhibition of phosphodiesterase activity, resulting in increased cellular levels of adenosine 3',5'-cyclic phosphate; this, in turn, may alter intracellular and extracellular calcium levels. The role of calcium homeostasis hasn't been determined. Clinical effects include increased cardiac output mediated by reduced afterload and, possibly, inotropism.

Pharmacokinetics
Absorption: Rapidly absorbed.
Distribution: Distribution volume is 1.2 L/kg. Distribution sites are unknown. Protein binding ranges from 10% to 49%. Therapeutic steady state serum levels range from 0.5 to 7 mcg/ml (ideal concentration: 3 mcg/ml).
Metabolism: Metabolized in the liver to several metabolites of unknown activity.
Excretion: In normal patients, inamrinone is excreted in the urine, with a terminal elimination half-life of about 4 hours. Half-life may be prolonged slightly in patients with heart failure.

Route	Onset	Peak	Duration
I.V.	2-5 min	10 min	½-2 hr

Contraindications and precautions
Contraindicated in patients hypersensitive to inamrinone or bisulfites. It shouldn't be used in patients with severe aortic or pulmonic valvular disease in place of surgical intervention or during an acute phase of MI.

Interactions
Drug-drug. *Cardiac glycosides:* Increased inotropic effect. This is a benefit in certain conditions.
Disopyramide: May cause severe hypotension. Avoid use together.

Adverse reactions
CV: *arrhythmias,* hypotension, chest pain.
GI: nausea, vomiting, anorexia, abdominal pain.
Hematologic: *thrombocytopenia.*
Hepatic: elevated liver enzyme levels.
Metabolic: decreased serum potassium.
Other: burning at injection site, *hypersensitivity reactions* (pericarditis, ascites, myositis vasculitis, pleuritis), fever.

Reactions may be *common*, uncommon, *life-threatening*, or COMMON AND LIFE-THREATENING.

Overdose and treatment

Overdose may cause severe hypotension. Treatment may include administration of a potent vasopressor, such as norepinephrine, as well as other general supportive measures, including cautious fluid volume replacement.

Special considerations

• Dispense drug as supplied or dilute in normal or half-normal saline solution to concentration of 1 to 3 mg/ml. Don't dilute drug with solutions containing dextrose because a slow chemical reaction occurs over 24 hours. However, amrinone can be injected into running dextrose infusions through Y-connector or directly into tubing. Use diluted solution within 24 hours.

• Don't administer furosemide in I.V. lines containing amrinone because a chemical reaction occurs immediately.

• Inamrinone is prescribed primarily for patients who haven't responded to therapy with cardiac glycosides, diuretics, and vasodilators.

• Store at room temperature and protect from light.

Patient monitoring

• Monitor blood pressure and heart rate throughout infusion. Slow or stop infusion if patient's blood pressure decreases or if arrhythmias (ventricular or supraventricular) occur. Dosage may need to be reduced.

• Monitor platelet counts. A count below 150,000/mm³ usually necessitates dosage reduction. Thrombocytopenia usually occurs after prolonged treatment.

• Monitor electrolyte levels (especially potassium) because drug increases cardiac output, which may cause diuresis.

• Hemodynamic monitoring may be useful in guiding therapy.

• Monitor liver function tests to detect hepatic damage (rare).

• Observe patient for adverse GI effects (such as nausea, vomiting, and diarrhea); reduce dosage or discontinue drug.

Breast-feeding patients

• Drug may appear in breast milk. Safety in breast-feeding women hasn't been established.

Pediatric patients

• Safety and efficacy in children under age 18 haven't been established.

Patient education

• Warn patient that burning may occur at the injection site.

• Tell patient to report adverse reactions promptly.

indapamide
Lozol

Pharmacologic classification: thiazide-like diuretic
Therapeutic classification: diuretic, antihypertensive
Pregnancy risk category: B

Indications and dosages

➤ *Edema of heart failure. Adults:* 2.5 mg P.O. as a single daily dose taken in the morning; increase dose to 5 mg daily after 1 week if response is poor.

➤ *Hypertension. Adults:* 1.25 mg P.O. as a single daily dose taken in the morning; increase dose to 2.5 mg daily after 4 weeks if response is poor. Maximum daily dose is 5 mg.

How supplied

Available by prescription only
Tablets: 1.25 mg, 2.5 mg

Pharmacodynamics

Diuretic action: Indapamide increases urinary excretion of sodium and water by inhibiting sodium reabsorption in the cortical diluting tubule of the nephron, thus relieving edema.

Antihypertensive action: Exact mechanism of antihypertensive effect of indapamide is unknown. This effect may result from direct arteriolar vasodilatation through calcium channel blockade. Drug also reduces total body sodium.

Pharmacokinetics

Absorption: Absorbed completely from the GI tract.

Distribution: Distributed widely into body tissues because of its lipophilicity; drug is 71% to 79% plasma protein-bound.

Metabolism: Indapamide undergoes significant hepatic metabolism. Half-life is about 14 hr.

Excretion: About 60% of drug dose is excreted in urine within 48 hours; about 16% to 23% is excreted in feces.

Route	Onset	Peak	Duration
P.O.	1-2 hr	2-5 hr	36 hr

Contraindications and precautions

Contraindicated in patients with anuria or hypersensitivity to other sulfonamide-derived drugs. Use cautiously in patients with severe impaired renal or hepatic function and progressive hepatic disease.

Interactions

Drug-drug. *Amphetamine, quinidine:* Indapamide turns urine slightly more alkaline and may decrease urinary excretion of some amines, such as alkaline urine. Monitor patient.

Antihypertensives: Indapamide potentiates hypotensive effects. This may be used to therapeutic advantage.

Cholestyramine and colestipol: May bind indapamide, preventing its absorption. Give drugs 1 hour apart.

Diazoxide: Increased hyperglycemic, hypotensive, and hyperuricemic effects of diazoxide. Monitor patient closely; insulin dose may need adjustment.

Lithium: Reduced renal clearance, elevating serum lithium levels. May necessitate reduction in lithium dosage by 50%.

Methenamine compounds (such as methenamine mandelate): Decreased therapeutic efficacy of indapamide. Monitor patient closely.

Adverse reactions

CNS: headache, nervousness, dizziness, lightheadedness, weakness, vertigo, restlessness, drowsiness, fatigue, anxiety, depression, numbness of limbs, irritability, agitation.

CV: volume depletion and dehydration, orthostatic hypotension, palpitations, PVCs, irregular heart rhythm, vasculitis, flushing.

EENT: rhinorrhea.

GI: anorexia, nausea, epigastric distress, vomiting, abdominal pain, diarrhea, constipation.

GU: nocturia, polyuria, frequent urination, impotence.

Metabolic: asymptomatic hyperuricemia; fluid and electrolyte imbalances, including dilutional hyponatremia and hypochloremia, metabolic alkalosis, hypokalemia; gout; weight loss.

Musculoskeletal: muscle cramps and spasms.

Skin: rash, pruritus.

Overdose and treatment

Signs and symptoms of overdose include GI irritation and hypermotility, diuresis, and lethargy, which may progress to coma.

Treatment is mainly supportive; monitor and assist respiratory, CV, and renal function as indicated. Monitor fluid and electrolyte balance. Induce vomiting with ipecac in conscious patient; otherwise, use gastric lavage to avoid aspiration. Don't give cathartics; these promote additional loss of fluids and electrolytes.

Special considerations

● To prevent nocturia, give drug in the morning.

● Consult prescriber and dietitian about a high-potassium diet. Foods rich in potassium include citrus fruits, tomatoes, bananas, apricots, and dates.

● Monitor serum creatinine and BUN levels regularly. Cumulative effects of drug may occur with impaired renal function.

● Discontinue thiazides and thiazide-like diuretics before parathyroid function tests.

● Therapeutic response may be delayed several weeks in hypertensive states. Also, if dose must be increased to 5 mg, additional therapy may be considered.

Patient teaching

● Indapamide therapy may interfere with PBI test for thyroid function and should be discontinued before such test is done.

Patient monitoring

● Monitor fluid intake and output, weight, blood pressure, and serum electrolyte levels.

● Watch for signs of hypokalemia, such as muscle weakness and cramps. Drug may be used with potassium-sparing diuretic to prevent potassium loss.

● Monitor blood uric acid levels, especially in patients with history of gout.

● Monitor blood glucose levels, especially in patients with diabetes.

Breast-feeding patients

● Drug appears in breast milk; its safety and effectiveness in breast-feeding women haven't been established.

Pediatric patients

● Safety and efficacy in children haven't been established.

Geriatric patients

● Geriatric and debilitated patients require close observation and may require reduced dosages. They're more sensitive to excess diuresis because of age-related changes in CV and renal function. Excess diuresis promotes orthostatic hypotension, dehydration, hypovolemia, hyponatremia, hypomagnesemia, and hypokalemia.

Patient education

● Instruct patient to take drug in morning to prevent nocturia and with food if GI upset occurs.

● Advise patient to avoid sudden posture changes and to rise slowly to avoid orthostatic hypotension.

● Tell patient to report muscle weakness, cramps, and irregular heartbeat to prescriber.

indinavir sulfate
Crixivan

Pharmacologic classification: HIV protease inhibitor
Therapeutic classification: antiviral
Pregnancy risk category: C

Indications and dosages

➤ *Treatment of patients with HIV infection when antiretroviral therapy is warranted.* *Adults:* 800 mg P.O. q 8 hours with other antiretroviral agents. Indinavir shouldn't be used as monotherapy.

✦ *Dosage adjustment.* Reduce dosage to 600 mg P.O. q 8 hours in patients with mild to moderate hepatic insufficiency resulting from cirrhosis.

How supplied
Available by prescription only
Capsules: 200 mg, 400 mg

Pharmacodynamics
Antiviral action: Indinavir sulfate inhibits HIV protease, an enzyme required for the proteolytic cleavage of viral polyprotein precursors into individual functional proteins found in infectious HIV. By binding to the protease active site, indinavir prevents cleavage of the viral polyproteins, resulting in formation of immature noninfectious viral particles.

Pharmacokinetics
Absorption: Rapidly absorbed in GI tract when administered on an empty stomach. A meal high in calories, fat, and protein significantly interferes with drug absorption, whereas lighter meals don't.
Distribution: About 60% is plasma protein-bound.
Metabolism: Metabolized to at least seven metabolites. Cytochrome P-450 3A4 (CYP3A4) is the major enzyme responsible for formation of the oxidative metabolites.
Excretion: Less than 20% is excreted unchanged in urine.

Route	Onset	Peak	Duration
P.O.	Unknown	Unknown	Unknown

Contraindications and precautions
Contraindicated in patients hypersensitive to any component of drug. Use cautiously in patients with hepatic insufficiency resulting from cirrhosis.

Interactions
Drug-drug. *Didanosine:* A normal gastric pH may be necessary for optimal absorption of indinavir. Administer these drugs and indinavir at least 1 hour apart on an empty stomach.
HMG-CoA reductase inhibitors, such as atorvastatin, lovastatin, and simvastatin: Increased risk of myopathy, including rhabdomyolysis. Use together cautiously.
Itraconazole, ketoconazole: Increased indinavir levels. Consider a dosage reduction of indinavir when administered together.
Midazolam, triazolam: Competition for CYP3A4 by indinavir could result in inhibition of the metabolism of these drugs and create the potential for serious or life-threatening events, such as arrhythmias or prolonged sedation. These drugs shouldn't be administered with indinavir.
Rifabutin: Increased plasma levels of rifabutin and decreased plasma levels of indinavir. Reduced dosage of rifabutin and increased dosage of indinavir is necessary.
Rifampin: A potent inducer of CYP3A4, which could markedly diminish plasma levels of indinavir. Coadministration of indinavir and rifampin isn't recommended.

Drug-herb. *St. John's wort:* Reduced indinavir levels by more than 50%. Warn patient not to use together.
Drug-food. *Grapefruit juice:* Plasma levels and therapeutic effect of indinavir may be decreased. Tell patient to take with liquid other than grapefruit juice.

Adverse reactions
CNS: malaise, headache, insomnia, dizziness, somnolence, asthenia, fatigue.
GI: abdominal pain, *nausea,* diarrhea, vomiting, acid regurgitation, anorexia, dry mouth, taste perversion.
GU: nephrolithiasis, hematuria.
Hematologic: anemia, ***thrombocytopenia, neutropenia.***
Hepatic: elevations in ALT, AST, and serum amylase levels; hyperbilirubinemia; jaundice.
Musculoskeletal: flank pain, back pain.

Overdose and treatment
Acute or chronic overdose may cause renal and GI effects. Treatment is supportive, and the patient is observed closely. It's not known whether indinavir is removed by hemodialysis or peritoneal dialysis.

Special considerations
● Dosage of indinavir is the same whether drug is used alone or with other antiretroviral agents. However, antiretroviral activity of indinavir may be increased when used with approved reverse transcriptase inhibitors.
● When administering indinavir with rifabutin, reduce the dose of rifabutin by half. However, when administering indinavir with ketoconazole, decrease dose of indinavir to 600 mg q 8 hours.

Patient monitoring
● Periodically measure HIV-RNA, CD4+.
● Drug may cause nephrolithiasis. If signs and symptoms of nephrolithiasis occur, consider stopping drug for 1 to 3 days during the acute phase. To prevent nephrolithiasis, patient should maintain adequate hydration.

Breast-feeding patients
● Drug may appear in breast milk. Because of the potential for indinavir to cause adverse effects in nursing infants and to prevent transmitting the infection to the infant, breast-feeding isn't recommended.

Pediatric patients
● Safety and efficacy in children haven't been established.

Patient education
● Inform patient that indinavir isn't a cure for HIV infection. Opportunistic infections and other complications of HIV disease may continue to develop. Drug also hasn't been shown to reduce risk

of transmitting HIV to others through sexual contact or blood contamination.

• Caution patient not to adjust dosage or discontinue indinavir therapy without medical approval.

• Advise patient that, if a dose of indinavir is missed, therapy should be resumed with the next dose and that a double dose shouldn't be taken.

• Instruct patient to take drug on an empty stomach with water 1 hour before or 2 hours after a meal. Alternatively, he may take it with other liquids (such as skim milk, juice, coffee, or tea) or with a light meal. Inform patient that a meal high in calories, fat, and protein reduces the absorption of indinavir.

• Tell patient to store capsules in the original container and to keep the desiccant in the bottle because the capsules are sensitive to moisture.

• Instruct patient to drink at least 1.5 L of fluid daily.

---

indomethacin, indomethacin sodium trihydrate
Apo-Indomethacin*, Indocid*, Indocin, Indocin IV, Indocin SR, Novomethacin*

Pharmacologic classification: NSAID
Therapeutic classification: nonnarcotic analgesic, antipyretic, anti-inflammatory
Pregnancy risk category: NR

Indications and dosages
➤ *Moderate to severe arthritis, ankylosing spondylitis. Adults:* 25 mg P.O. b.i.d. or t.i.d. with food or antacids; dose may be increased by 25 to 50 mg daily q 7 days up to 200 mg daily. Or, 50 mg P.R. q.i.d. Or, sustained-release capsules may be given: 75 mg to start, in the morning or h.s., followed, if necessary, by 75 mg b.i.d.
➤ *Acute gouty arthritis. Adults:* 50 mg t.i.d. Reduce dose as soon as possible; then stop it. Don't use sustained-release capsules for this condition.
➤ *To close a hemodynamically significant patent ductus arteriosus in premature infants (I.V. form only). Neonates less than 48 hours old:* 0.2 mg/kg I.V. followed by two doses of 0.1 mg/kg at 12- to 24-hour intervals.
Neonates ages 2 to 7 days: 0.2 mg/kg I.V. followed by two doses of 0.2 mg/kg at 12- to 24-hour intervals.
Neonates over age 7 days: 0.2 mg/kg I.V. followed by two doses of 0.25 mg/kg at 12- to 24-hour intervals.
➤ *Acute shoulder pain. Adults:* 75 to 150 mg P.O. daily in three or four divided doses with food or antacids; usual treatment is 7 to 14 days.
➤ *Pericarditis◊. Adults:* 75 to 200 mg P.O. daily in three or four divided doses.
➤ *Dysmenorrhea◊. Adults:* 25 mg P.O. t.i.d. with food or antacids.

➤ *Bartter's syndrome◊. Adults:* 150 mg P.O. daily in divided doses with food or antacids.
Children: 0.5 to 2 mg/kg P.O. daily in divided doses.

How supplied
Available by prescription only
Capsules: 25 mg, 50 mg
Capsules (sustained-release): 75 mg
Injection: 1-mg vials
Suppositories: 50 mg
Suspension: 25 mg/5 ml

Pharmacodynamics
Analgesic, antipyretic, and anti-inflammatory actions: Exact mechanisms of action are unknown; indomethacin is thought to produce its analgesic, antipyretic, and anti-inflammatory effects by inhibiting prostaglandin synthesis and possibly by inhibiting phosphodiesterase.
Closure of patent ductus arteriosus: Mechanism of action is unknown, but is believed to be through inhibition of prostaglandin synthesis.

Pharmacokinetics
Absorption: Absorbed rapidly and completely from the GI tract.
Distribution: Highly protein-bound.
Metabolism: Metabolized in the liver. Half-life is 4½ hr.
Excretion: Excreted mainly in urine, with some biliary excretion.

Route	Onset	Peak	Duration
P.O., I.V., P.R.	Unknown	Unknown	Unknown

Contraindications and precautions
Contraindicated in patients hypersensitive to drug; in patients with history of aspirin- or NSAID-induced asthma, rhinitis, or urticaria; and in pregnant or breast-feeding women. Also contraindicated in infants with untreated infection, active bleeding, coagulation defects or thrombocytopenia, congenital heart disease in those for whom patency of the ductus arteriosus is necessary for satisfactory pulmonary or systemic blood flow, necrotizing enterocolitis, or impaired renal function. Suppositories are contraindicated in patients with a history of proctitis or recent rectal bleeding.

Use cautiously in elderly patients and patients with history of GI disease, impaired renal or hepatic function, epilepsy, parkinsonism, CV disease, infection, mental illness, or depression.

Interactions
Drug-drug. *Acetaminophen, gold compounds, other anti-inflammatories:* Increased nephrotoxicity. Don't use together.
Anticoagulants, thrombolytics (such as coumarin derivatives, heparin, streptokinase, urokinase): May potentiate anticoagulant effects. Monitor PT, PTT, and INR.

Reactions may be *common*, uncommon, *life-threatening*, or COMMON AND LIFE-THREATENING.

Antihypertensives, diuretics: Decreased effectiveness. Avoid concurrent use.

Aspirin: May decrease the bioavailability of indomethacin. Avoid use together.

Aspirin, carbenicillin (parenteral), cefamandole, cefoperazone, corticosteroids, corticotropin, dextran, dipyridamole, mezlocillin, piperacillin, plicamycin, salicylates, sulfinpyrazone, ticarcillin, valproic acid, or other anti-inflammatories: Bleeding problems may occur. Monitor patient closely.

Diflunisal: Decreased indomethacin clearance and increased toxicity. Avoid use together.

Digoxin, nifedipine, phenytoin, verapamil: Toxicity may occur. Monitor patient carefully.

Dipyridamole: May potentiate water retention. Monitor patient closely.

Insulin, oral antidiabetics: May potentiate hypoglycemic effects. Avoid use together.

Lithium, methotrexate: Indomethacin may decrease the renal clearance of these drugs. Monitor patient closely.

Penicillamine: Increased bioavailability and toxicity of penicillamine. Monitor patient closely.

Triamterene and other diuretics: Potential nephrotoxicity. Avoid use together.

Drug-herb. *Senna:* May block diarrheal effects. Discourage use together.

Drug-lifestyle. *Alcohol use:* May increase GI adverse effects. Advise patient to avoid alcohol.

Adverse reactions
Oral and rectal forms
CNS: *headache, dizziness,* depression, drowsiness, confusion, somnolence, fatigue, peripheral neuropathy, *seizures,* psychic disturbances, syncope, vertigo.

CV: hypertension, *edema, heart failure.*

EENT: blurred vision, corneal and retinal damage, hearing loss, tinnitus.

GI: *nausea,* anorexia, *diarrhea, peptic ulceration, GI bleeding,* constipation, dyspepsia, *pancreatitis.*

GU: hematuria, *acute renal failure,* proteinuria, interstitial nephritis.

Hematologic: *hemolytic anemia, aplastic anemia, agranulocytosis, leukopenia, thrombocytopenic purpura,* iron-deficiency anemia.

Metabolic: hyperkalemia.

Skin: pruritus, urticaria, *Stevens-Johnson syndrome.*

Other: *hypersensitivity* (rash, respiratory distress, *anaphylaxis, angioedema*).

I.V. form
GU: proteinuria, interstitial nephritis.

Overdose and treatment
Signs and symptoms of overdose include dizziness, nausea, vomiting, intense headache, mental confusion, drowsiness, tinnitus, sweating, blurred vision, paresthesia, and seizures.

To treat overdose, empty stomach immediately by inducing emesis with ipecac syrup or by gastric lavage. Administer activated charcoal via nasogastric tube. Provide symptomatic and supportive measures (respiratory support and correction of fluid and electrolyte imbalances). Monitor laboratory parameters and vital signs closely. Dialysis may be of little value because indomethacin is strongly protein-bound.

Special considerations
Consider the recommendations relevant to all NSAIDs as well as the following.
● Don't mix oral suspension with liquids or antacids before administering.
● Patient should retain suppository in the rectum for at least 1 hour after insertion to ensure maximum absorption.
● Reconstitute 1 mg vial of I.V. dose with 1 to 2 ml of sterile water for injection or normal saline solution for injection. Prepare solution immediately before use to prevent deterioration. Don't use solution if it's discolored or contains a precipitate.
● Use I.V. administration only for premature neonates with patent ductus arteriosus. Don't administer a second or third I.V. dose if anuria or marked oliguria exists.
● If ductus arteriosus reopens, a second course of one to three doses may be given. If ineffective, surgery may be necessary.
● Drug therapy may interfere with dexamethasone suppression test results. It also may interfere with urinary 5-hydroxyindoleacetic acid determinations.

Patient monitoring
● Monitor patient carefully for bleeding and for reduced urine output.
● Monitor cardiopulmonary status for significant changes. Watch for signs and symptoms of fluid overload. Check weight and intake and output daily.
● Monitor renal function studies before start of therapy and frequently during therapy to prevent adverse effects.
● Severe headache may occur. If headache persists, decrease dose.

Breast-feeding patients
● Drug appears in breast milk in levels similar to those in maternal plasma; avoid use in breast-feeding women.

Pediatric patients
● Safety of long-term drug use in children under age 14 hasn't been established. Use of I.V. indomethacin in premature infants for patent ductus arteriosus is considered an alternative to surgery.

Geriatric patients
● Patients over age 60 may be more susceptible to the toxic effects of indomethacin. The drug's effect on renal prostaglandins may cause fluid

---

retention and edema, a significant drawback for geriatric patients and those with heart failure.

Patient education
• Instruct patient in proper administration of dosage form prescribed, such as suppository, sustained-release capsule, or suspension.
• Advise patient to seek medical approval before taking OTC medications.
• Caution patient to avoid hazardous activities that require alertness or concentration.
• Tell patient to report signs and symptoms of adverse reactions and to adhere to prescribed drug regimen.

infliximab
Remicade

Pharmacologic classification: monoclonal antibody IgG1k
Therapeutic classification: anti-inflammatory
Pregnancy risk category: C

Indications and dosages
➤*Reduction of signs and symptoms in patients with moderately to severely active Crohn's disease with inadequate response to conventional therapy. Adults*: 5 mg/kg single I.V. infusion over a period of not less than 2 hours.
➤*Reduction in the number of draining enterocutaneous fistulas in patients with fistulizing Crohn's disease. Adults*: 5 mg/kg I.V. infused over a period of not less than 2 hours. Give additional doses of 5 mg/kg at 2 and 6 weeks after initial infusion.
➤*Reduction of signs and symptoms and inhibiting progression of structural damage in patients with rheumatoid arthritis with inadequate response to methotrexate alone. Adults*: 3 mg/kg I.V. infusion over a period of not less than 2 hours. Give additional doses of 3 mg/kg at 2 and 6 weeks after initial infusion and every 8 weeks thereafter. Dose may be increased up to 10 mg/kg or doses may be given every 4 weeks if response is inadequate.

How supplied
Available by prescription only
Injection: 100 mg in 20-ml vial

Pharmacodynamics
Anti-inflammatory action: Drug is a monoclonal antibody that binds to tumor necrosis factor (TNF)-alpha to neutralize its activity and inhibit its binding with receptors, reducing the infiltration of inflammatory cells and TNF-alpha production in inflamed areas of the intestine and joints.

Pharmacokinetics
Absorption: Administered I.V.
Distribution: Not reported.

Metabolism: Not reported.
Excretion: Terminal half-life is 9½ days.

Route	Onset	Peak	Duration
I.V.	Unknown	Unknown	Unknown

Contraindications and precautions
Contraindicated in patients hypersensitive to murine proteins or other components of the drug. Use cautiously in elderly patients.

Interactions
None reported.

Adverse reactions
CNS: *headache, fatigue,* dizziness, malaise, insomnia.
CV: hypertension, hypotension, flushing, tachycardia, chest pain.
EENT: pharyngitis, rhinitis, sinusitis, conjunctivitis.
GI: *nausea, abdominal pain,* vomiting, constipation, dyspepsia, flatulence, intestinal obstruction, oral pain, ulcerative stomatitis.
GU: dysuria, increased micturition frequency.
Hematologic: anemia, hematoma, ecchymoses.
Hepatic: elevated liver enzyme levels.
Musculoskeletal: myalgia, arthralgia, arthritis, back pain.
Respiratory: *upper respiratory tract infections,* bronchitis, *cough,* dyspnea, respiratory tract allergic reaction.
Skin: rash, pruritus, candidiasis, acne, alopecia, eczema, erythema, erythematous rash, maculopapular rash, papular rash, dry skin, increased sweating, urticaria.
Other: *fever,* chills, pain, peripheral edema, hot flashes, abscess, flu syndrome, toothache.

Overdose and treatment
Single doses of up to 20 mg/kg have been given without direct toxic effects. If overdose occurs, monitor patient for signs and symptoms of adverse effects and give symptomatic treatment.

Special considerations
• Drug is incompatible with plasticized polyvinyl chloride equipment or devices; prepare only in glass infusion bottles or polypropylene or polyolefin infusion bags. Administer through polyethylene-lined administration sets with an in-line, sterile, nonpyrogenic, low-protein-binding filter (pore size of 1.2 mm or less).
• Vials don't contain antibacterial preservatives.
• Dilute total volume of reconstituted dose to 250 ml with normal saline solution injection. Infusion concentration range is 0.4 to 4 mg/ml. Infusion should begin within 3 hours of preparation and must be administered over a period of not less than 2 hours.
• Drug shouldn't be infused in the same I.V. line with other agents.

Patient monitoring

- Infusion-related reactions such as fever, chills, pruritus, urticaria, dyspnea, hypotension, hypertension, and chest pain may occur. If an infusion reaction occurs, discontinue drug, notify prescriber, and be prepared to give acetaminophen, antihistamines, corticosteroids, and epinephrine, as ordered.
- Monitor patient for development of lymphomas and infection. Patients with long duration of Crohn's disease and long-term exposure to immunosuppressant therapies are more susceptible to development of lymphomas and infections.
- Drug may affect normal immune responses. Autoimmune antibodies and lupus-like syndrome may develop; discontinue drug therapy. Symptoms can be expected to resolve.

Breast-feeding patients

- It isn't known whether infliximab appears in breast milk. Discontinue either drug or breast-feeding.

Pediatric patients

- Safety and efficacy of drug use in children haven't been established.

Geriatric patients

- Use cautiously in patients over age 65.

Patient education

- Tell patient about infusion-reaction symptoms and instruct him to report adverse effects.
- Inform patient of postinfusion side effects and instruct him to report them promptly.

---

influenza virus vaccine, 2000-2001 trivalent types A & B (purified surface antigen)
Fluvirin

influenza virus vaccine, 2000-2001 trivalent types A & B (subvirion or purified subvirion)
Fluogen, FluShield, Fluzone

influenza virus vaccine, 2000-2001 trivalent types A & B (whole virion)
Fluzone

Pharmacologic classification: vaccine
Therapeutic classification: viral vaccine
Pregnancy risk category: C

Indications and dosages

➤ *Annual influenza prophylaxis in high-risk patients. Adults and children age 13 and older:* 0.5 ml I.M. (whole viron or subviron).

Children ages 9 to 12: 0.5 ml I.M. (subviron only).
Children ages 3 to 8: 0.5 ml I.M. (subviron only).
Infants and children ages 6 to 35 months: 0.25 ml I.M. (subviron only).

Note: Second dose may be given in previously unvaccinated children under age 9 at least 1 month after first dose. Check package insert for annual changes and additional dosing recommendations.

How supplied

Available by prescription only
Injection: 0.5-ml prefilled syringe; 5-ml vials

Pharmacodynamics

Influenza prophylaxis: Vaccine promotes active immunity to influenza by inducing antibody production. Protection is provided only against those strains of virus from which the vaccine is prepared (or closely related strains).

Pharmacokinetics

Absorption: Duration of immunity varies widely.
Distribution: No information available.
Metabolism: No information available.
Excretion: No information available.

Route	Onset	Peak	Duration
I.M.	Unknown	Unknown	About 1 yr

Contraindications and precautions

Contraindicated in patients hypersensitive to chicken eggs or any component of the vaccine such as thimersol. Defer vaccination in patients with acute respiratory or other active infection and delay immunization in those with an active neurologic disorder.

Interactions

Drug-drug. *Aminopyrine, phenytoin:* Decreased serum phenytoin and aminopyrine levels. Monitor patient and drug levels.
Corticosteroids, immunosuppressants: May impair the immune response to the vaccine. Avoid use together.
Theophylline: Increased serum theophylline levels. Monitor theophylline levels.
Warfarin: Rare prolonged PT, GI bleeding, transient gross hematuria, and epistaxis. Monitor patient closely.

Adverse reactions

CNS: malaise.
Musculoskeletal: myalgia.
Skin: erythema, induration, and *soreness at injection site.*
Other: *anaphylaxis,* fever.

Overdose and treatment

No information available.

Special considerations

- Fever and malaise reactions occur most often in children and in others not exposed to influenza viruses. Severe reactions in adults are rare.
- Patients with a known or suspected hypersensitivity to egg protein should have a skin test to assess sensitivity to vaccine. Administer a scratch test with 0.05 to 0.1 ml of a 1:100 dilution in normal saline solution for injection. Patients with positive skin test reactions shouldn't receive the influenza virus vaccine.
- Epinephrine solution 1:1,000 should be available to treat allergic reactions.
- Influenza vaccine shouldn't be administered to patients with active influenza infection. Such infection should be treated with amantadine.
- To reduce the frequency of adverse reactions, use only the sub viron or purified sub viron vaccine in children.
- Pneumococcal vaccine, DTP, or live attenuated measles virus vaccine may be given simultaneously but at a different injection site.
- Store vaccine between 36° and 46° F (2° and 8° C). Don't freeze.

Patient monitoring
- Monitor patient for adverse reactions.

Pregnant patients
- If given during pregnancy, the influenza vaccine should be given during the second trimester to avoid a coincidental association with spontaneous abortion, which is common in the first trimester. Recommended for women who will be in their second or third trimester during flu season.

Breast-feeding patients
- Breast-feeding isn't a contraindication for receiving vaccine.

Pediatric patients
- Influenza vaccine is contraindicated in children under age 6 months.

Geriatric patients
- Annual vaccination is highly recommended for patients over age 50.

Patient education
- Advise patient of potential injection site discomfort, fever, malaise, and muscle aches.
- Encourage patient to report distressing adverse reactions promptly.
- Warn patient that many cases of Guillain-Barré syndrome were reported after vaccination for the swine flu of 1976. This condition usually causes reversible paralysis and muscle weakness, but it can be fatal in some individuals. Influenza vaccines made after 1976 have a lower risk of Guillain-Barré syndrome, but the condition still occurs, albeit rarely. Patients with history of Guillain-Barré syndrome have a greater risk for repeat episodes.

insulin (regular)
Humulin-R, Novolin R, Novolin R PenFill, Regular (Concentrated) Iletin II, Regular Insulin, Regular Purified Pork Insulin, Velosulin Human*, Velosulin BR

insulin (lispro)
Humalog

isophane insulin suspension (NPH)
Humulin N, NPH-N, Novolin N, Novolin N PenFill, NPH Iletin II

insulin zinc suspension (lente)
Humulin L, Lente Iletin II, Lente L, Novolin L

extended zinc insulin suspension (ultralente)
Humulin U Ultralente, Ultralente*

isophane insulin suspension and insulin injection (70% isophane insulin and 30% insulin injection)
Humulin 70/30, Novolin 70/30, Novolin 70/30 PenFill

isophane insulin suspension and insulin injection (50% isophane insulin and 50% insulin injection)
Humulin 50/50

Pharmacologic classification: pancreatic hormone
Therapeutic classification: antidiabetic
Pregnancy risk category: B

Indications and dosages
➤ *Diabetic ketoacidosis.* **Regular insulin.**
Adults: Administer loading dose of 0.15 units/kg I.V. followed by 0.1 units/kg/hour as a continuous infusion. Decrease insulin infusion when plasma glucose level reaches 300 mg/dl. Start infusion of D_5W separately from the insulin infusion when plasma glucose reaches 250 mg/dl. Thirty minutes before discontinuing insulin infusion, administer a dose of insulin S.C.; intermediate-acting insulin is recommended.

Alternative dosage schedule is 50 to 100 units I.V. and 50 to 100 units S.C. immediately; base subsequent doses on therapeutic response and glucose, acetone, or ketone levels monitored at

1- to 2-hour intervals, or 2.4 to 7.2 units I.V. loading dose followed by 2.4 to 7.2 units/hour.
Children: 0.5 to 1 unit/kg in two divided doses, one given I.V. and the other S.C., followed by 0.5 to 1 unit/kg I.V. q 1 to 2 hours; or 0.1 unit/kg I.V. bolus, then 0.1 unit/kg/hour continuous I.V. infusion until serum glucose decreases to 250 mg/dl; then start S.C. insulin.

➤ *Ketosis-prone diabetes, type 1 diabetes mellitus, diabetes mellitus inadequately controlled by diet and oral antidiabetics. Adults and children:* Individualized dosage adjusted based on patient's serum and urine glucose levels.

➤ *Hyperkalemia. Adults:* 5 to 10 units of regular insulin with 50 ml of D₅W over 5 minutes. Alternatively, 25 units of regular insulin given S.C. and an infusion of 1,000 ml D₁₀W with 90 mEq sodium bicarbonate; infuse 330 ml over 30 minutes and the remainder over 3 hours.

➤ *Provocative test for growth hormone secretion. Adults:* Rapid I.V. injection of regular insulin 0.05 to 0.15 units/kg.

How supplied
Available without a prescription
insulin (regular)
Injection (pork): 100 units/ml
Injection (human): 100 units/ml
isophane insulin suspension (NPH)
Injection (pork): 100 units/ml
Injection (human): 100 units/ml
insulin zinc suspension (lente)
Injection (pork): 100 units/ml
Injection (human): 100 units/ml
extended zinc insulin suspension (ultralente)
Injection (human): 100 units/ml
Available by prescription only
insulin (lispro)
Injection (human): 100 units/ml
Cartridge (human): 100 units/ml in 3-ml cartridges
regular (concentrated) Iletin II insulin
Injection (human): 500 units/ml

Pharmacodynamics
Antidiabetic action: Insulin is used as a replacement for the physiologic production of endogenous insulin in patients with insulin-dependent diabetes mellitus (type 1) and diabetes mellitus inadequately controlled by diet and oral hypoglycemic agents (type 2). Insulin increases glucose transport across muscle and fat-cell membranes to reduce blood glucose levels. It also promotes conversion of glucose to its storage form, glycogen; triggers amino acid uptake and conversion to protein in muscle cells and inhibits protein degradation; stimulates triglyceride formation and inhibits release of free fatty acids from adipose tissue; and stimulates lipoprotein lipase activity, which converts circulating lipoproteins to fatty acids. Insulin is available in various forms and these differ mainly in onset, peak, and duration of action.

Pharmacokinetics
Absorption: Insulin must be given parenterally because it's destroyed in the GI tract. Commercially available preparations are formulated to differ in onset, peak, and duration after subcutaneous administration. They're classified as rapid-acting (½- to 1-hour onset), intermediate-acting (1- to 2-hour onset), and long-acting (4- to 8-hour onset). The accompanying chart summarizes major pharmacokinetic differences
Distribution: Distributed widely throughout the body.
Metabolism: Some insulin is bound and inactivated by peripheral tissues, but the majority appears to be degraded in the liver and kidneys.
Excretion: Filtered by the renal glomeruli and undergoes some tubular reabsorption. Plasma half-life is about 9 minutes after I.V. administration.

Route	Onset	Peak	Duration
I.V.	Immediate	Unknown	Unknown
S.C.			
Rapid	½-1½ hr	2-3 hr	5-7 hr
Intermediate	1-2½ hr	4-15 hr	12-24 hr
Long-acting	4-8 hr	10-30 hr	36 hr

Contraindications and precautions
No known contraindications.

Interactions
Drug-drug. *Anabolic steroids, beta blockers, clofibrate, fenfluramine, MAO inhibitors, salicylates, tetracycline:* Prolonged hypoglycemic effect. Monitor blood glucose levels carefully.
Corticosteroids, dextrothyroxine sodium, epinephrine, thiazide diuretics: Diminish insulin response. Monitor patient for hyperglycemia.
Drug-herb. *Basil, bay, bee pollen, burdock, ginseng, glucomannian, horehound, marsh mallow, myrrh, sage:* May affect glycemic control. Monitor blood glucose carefully and discourage use together.
Drug-lifestyle. *Alcohol use:* May cause a prolonged hypoglycemic effect. Advise patient to avoid alcohol.
Marijuana use: May increase insulin requirements. Inform patient of this interaction.
Smoking: Decreased absorption of insulin administered S.C. Advise patient to avoid smoking within 30 minutes of insulin injection.

Adverse reactions
Skin: urticaria, pruritus, swelling, redness, stinging, warmth at injection site.
Other: *lipoatrophy, lipohypertrophy, hypersensitivity reactions (anaphylaxis, rash), hypoglycemia,* hyperglycemia (rebound, or Somogyi, effect).

Overdose and treatment
Insulin overdose may produce signs and symptoms of hypoglycemia (tachycardia, palpitations, anxiety, hunger, nausea, diaphoresis, tremors, pallor, restlessness, headache, and speech and motor dysfunction).

Treatment is directed toward treating hypoglycemia and is based on patient's symptoms. If patient is responsive, give 10 to 15 g of a fast-acting oral carbohydrate. If patient's signs and symptoms persist after 15 minutes, give an additional 10 g carbohydrate. If patient is unresponsive, an I.V. bolus of $D_{50}W$ solution should immediately increase blood glucose. Some prefer to use $D_{25}W$ because it's less irritating should extravasation occur. A common infusion rate is based on glucose content: 10 to 20 mg/kg/minute. Parenteral glucagon or epinephrine S.C. also may be given; both drugs elevate blood glucose levels in a few minutes by stimulating glycogenolysis. Fluid and electrolyte imbalance may require I.V. fluids and electrolyte (such as potassium) replacement.

Special considerations
● Human insulin may help non–insulin-dependent patients requiring intermittent or short-term therapy (such as pregnancy, surgery, infection, or total parenteral nutrition therapy), for patients with insulin resistance, or for those with lipoatrophy.
● Lente, ultralente insulins may be mixed in any proportion.
● Regular insulin may be mixed with NPH or lente insulins in any proportion. However, in vitro binding occurs over time until an equilibrium is reached. Administer these mixtures either immediately after preparation or after stability occurs (15 minutes for NPH regular, 24 hours for lente regular) in order to minimize variability in patient response. Switching from separate injections to a prepared mixture also may alter the patient's response. When mixing two insulins, always draw regular insulin into the syringe first.
● Lispro insulin may be mixed with Humulin N or Humulin U and given within 15 minutes before a meal to prevent a hypoglycemic reaction. The effects of mixing lispro insulin with insulins of animal source or insulin preparations produced by other manufacturers haven't been studied and may require a change in dosage.
● Store insulin in cool area. Refrigeration is desirable but not essential, except with regular insulin concentrated.
● Administration route is S.C. because it allows slower absorption and causes less pain than I.M. injections. Ketosis-prone, type 1, severely ill, and newly diagnosed diabetics with very high blood glucose levels may require hospitalization and I.V. treatment with regular fast-acting insulin. Ketosis-resistant diabetics may be treated as outpatients with intermediate-acting insulin after they have received instructions on how to alter dosage according to self-performed urine or blood glucose determinations. Some patients, especially pregnant or brittle diabetics, may use a dextrometer to perform fingerstick blood glucose tests at home.
● Injection sites should be rotated; however, unstable diabetics may achieve better control if injection site is rotated within same anatomic region.
● In pregnant diabetic women, insulin requirements increase, sometimes drastically, then decline immediately postpartum.
● Human insulin may be used in patients allergic to pork forms. Humulin is synthesized by a genetically altered strain of *Escherichia coli*. Novolin brands are derived by enzymatic alteration of pork insulin.
● Some patients may develop insulin resistance and require large insulin doses to control symptoms of diabetes. Iletin II, Regular Purified Pork, 500 units/ml may be used for these patients.
● Patient should notify pharmacist several days before prescription refill is needed in case U-500 is not in stock. Give hospital pharmacy sufficient notice before refill of in-house prescription.
● Never store U-500 insulin in same area with other insulin preparations because of danger of severe overdose if given accidentally to other patients. U-500 insulin must be administered with a U-100 syringe because no syringes are made for this drug.

Patient monitoring
● With regular insulin concentrated, monitor patient for a secondary hypoglycemic reaction that may occur 18 to 24 hours after injection. This may be caused by a repository effect of drug and the high concentration of insulin in the preparation (500 units/ml).

Pregnant patients
● Monitor insulin use during pregnancy.

Breast-feeding patients
● Monitor drug use closely in breast-feeding women.

Geriatric patients
● These patients have an increased risk of CVA, MI, and hypoglycemia.

Patient education
● Instruct patient to strictly adhere to manufacturer's instructions regarding assembly, administration, and care of specialized delivery systems, such as insulin pumps.
● Emphasize importance of regular meal times and that meals must not be omitted.
● Tell patient that insulin can be injected immediately after a meal.
● Teach patient that blood glucose monitoring is an essential guide to correct dosage and to therapeutic success.
● Emphasize importance of recognizing hypoglycemic symptoms because insulin-induced hypo-

glycemia is hazardous and may cause brain damage if prolonged.

• Advise patient to always wear a medical identification bracelet or pendant, to carry ample insulin supply and syringes on trips, to have carbohydrates (sugar or candy) on hand for emergency, and to note time-zone changes for dose schedule when traveling.

• Instruct patient not to change the order of mixing insulins or change the model or brand of syringe or needle. Be sure he knows when mixing two insulins, always to draw regular insulin into the syringe first.

• Inform patient that use of marijuana may increase insulin requirements.

• Inform patient that cigarette smoking decreases absorption of insulin administered S.C. Advise him not to smoke within 30 minutes after insulin injection.

insulin aspart (rDNA origin) injection
NovoLog

Pharmacologic classification: human insulin analogue
Therapeutic classification: antidiabetic
Pregnancy risk category: C

Indications and dosages
➤ *Control of hyperglycemia in patients with diabetes mellitus. Adults:* Dosage is individualized based on the patient's needs. Typical daily insulin requirements are 0.5 to 1 unit/kg daily divided in a meal-related treatment regimen. About 50% to 70% of this dose may be provided with NovoLog and the remainder by an intermediate-acting or long-acting insulin. Give within 5 to 10 minutes of start of meal by S.C. injection in the abdominal wall, thigh, or upper arm.

How supplied
Available by prescription only
10-ml vial for injection: 100 units of insulin aspart per ml (U-100)
3-ml PenFill cartridges

Pharmacodynamics
Antidiabetic action: Thought to bind to insulin receptors on muscle and fat cells to lower blood glucose and by facilitating the cellular uptake of glucose and inhibiting the output of glucose from the liver.

Pharmacokinetics
Absorption: NovoLog is as bioavailable as regular human insulin. It has a faster absorption and onset and shorter duration of action compared to regular human insulin.
Distribution: Low plasma protein–binding (0% to 9%), similar to regular insulin.
Metabolism: No information available.

Excretion: Half-life is shorter than that of regular human insulin (81 minutes compared with 141 minutes, respectively).

Route	Onset	Peak	Duration
S.C.	Rapid	1-3 hr	3-5 hr

Interactions
Drug-drug. *ACE inhibitors, disopyramide, fibrates, fluoxetine, MAO inhibitors, oral antidiabetics, propoxyphene, salicylates, somatostatin analogue (octreotide), sulfonamide antibiotics:* May enhance serum glucose–lowering effects of insulin and may potentiate hypoglycemia. Monitor blood glucose and signs of hypoglycemia. May require insulin dose adjustment.
Beta blockers, clonidine: May potentiate or weaken blood glucose–lowering effect of insulin, causing hypoglycemia or hyperglycemia. May mask signs and symptoms of hypoglycemia (may be reduced or absent). Monitor blood glucose level.
Corticosteroids; danazol; diuretics; estrogens and progestogens such as in oral contraceptives; isoniazid; niacin; phenothiazine derivatives; somatropin; sympathomimetics such as epinephrine, salbutamol, and terbutaline; thyroid hormones: May reduce the blood glucose–lowering effect of insulin and may cause hyperglycemia. Monitor blood glucose. May require insulin dose adjustment.
Guanethidine, reserpine: May mask signs and symptoms of hypoglycemia (may be reduced or absent). Monitor blood glucose level.
Lithium salts, pentamidine: May potentiate or weaken blood glucose–lowering effect of insulin, causing hypoglycemia or hyperglycemia. Pentamidine may cause hypoglycemia, which may sometimes be followed by hyperglycemia. Monitor blood glucose level.
Drug-lifestyle. *Alcohol use:* May potentiate or weaken blood glucose–lowering effect of insulin, resulting in hypoglycemia or hyperglycemia. Monitor blood glucose level.

Adverse reactions
Metabolic: hypoglycemia.
Skin: injection site reactions, lipodystrophy, pruritus, rash.
Other: allergic reactions.

Overdose and treatment
Hypoglycemia may occur as a result of an excess of insulin relative to food intake, energy expenditure, or both. Warning signs and symptoms of hypoglycemia include shaking, sweating, dizziness, fatigue, hunger, irritability, confusion, blurred vision, headaches, or nausea and vomiting. Mild hypoglycemia can be treated with oral glucose. Adjustments in drug dosage, meal patterns, or exercise may be needed. More severe episodes involving coma, seizure, or neurologic impairment may be treated with I.M. or S.C. glucagon or concentrated I.V. glucose. Sustained

carbohydrate intake and observation may be necessary because hypoglycemia may recur after apparent recovery.

Contraindications and precautions
Contraindicated during hypoglycemia and in patients hypersensitive to NovoLog or one of its excipients.

Use cautiously in patients prone to hypoglycemia and hypokalemia, such as those who are fasting, have autonomic neuropathy, or who are using potassium-lowering drugs or drugs sensitive to serum potassium levels.

Special considerations
● NovoLog should be given 5 to 10 minutes before the start of a meal. Because of rapid onset and short duration of action, patients may need the addition of longer-acting insulins to prevent pre-meal hyperglycemia. Drug should be given by S.C. injection into the abdominal wall, thigh, or upper arm. It's important to rotate sites to minimize lipodystrophies.
● Insulin vials should be inspected visually before use. NovoLog should be clear and colorless. It should never contain particulate matter, appear cloudy or viscous, or be discolored. Drug shouldn't be used after its expiration date.
● Store drug between 2° and 8° C (36° to 46° F). Don't freeze. Don't expose vials to excessive heat or sunlight. Open vials of NovoLog are stable at room temperature for 28 days.

Patient monitoring
● Monitor warning signs of hypoglycemia and the patient's glucose levels while patient is receiving NovoLog.
● Monitor serum glucose levels regularly.

Breast-feeding patients
● It isn't known whether insulin aspart appears in human milk. Use caution when giving drug to nursing mother.

Pediatric patients
● Safety and effectiveness haven't been studied.

Geriatric patients
● The effect of age on the pharmacokinetics and pharmacodynamics of NovoLog hasn't been studied.

Patient education
● Inform patient of the possible risks and benefits of NovoLog.
● Teach patient to recognize hypoglycemia and hyperglycemia and how to treat them.
● Instruct patient on injection techniques, timing of dose to meals, adherence to meal planning, importance of regular glucose monitoring and periodic glycosylated hemoglobin testing, and proper storage of insulin.
● Tell woman to notify prescriber about planned, suspected, or known pregnancy because information about drug use during pregnancy and breast-feeding isn't available.

insulin glargine (rDNA) injection
Lantus

Pharmacologic classification: pancreatic hormone
Therapeutic classification: antidiabetic
Pregnancy risk category: C

Indications and dosages
➤ *Management of type 1 diabetes mellitus in patients who need basal (long-acting) insulin for the control of hyperglycemia.* Adults and children older than age 6: Individualize dosage and administer S.C. once daily at bedtime.
➤ *Management of type 2 diabetes mellitus in patients who need basal (long-acting) insulin for control of hyperglycemia.* Adults: Individualize dosage and administer S.C. once daily at bedtime.

How supplied
Available by prescription only
Injection: 100 units/ml

Pharmacodynamics
Antidiabetic action: Regulates glucose metabolism by stimulating peripheral glucose uptake, especially by skeletal muscle and fat, and by inhibiting hepatic glucose production.

Pharmacokinetics
Absorption: After S.C. injection of insulin glargine in healthy subjects and in patients with diabetes, the insulin serum levels indicated a slower, more prolonged absorption and a relatively constant level/time profile over 24 hours with no pronounced peak compared with NPH insulin.
Distribution: No information available.
Metabolism: Partly metabolized to form two active metabolites with in vitro activity similar to that of insulin.
Excretion: No information available.

Route	Onset	Peak	Duration
S.C.	Slow	None	11-24 hr

Contraindications and precautions
Lantus is contraindicated in patients who are hypersensitive to insulin glargine or its excipients. Don't use during episodes of hypoglycemia. Use cautiously in patients with renal or hepatic impairment.

Interactions
Drug-drug. *ACE inhibitors, disopyramide, fibrates, fluoxetine, MAO inhibitors, octreotide, oral antidiabetics, propoxyphene, salicylates,*

---

somatostatin analog, sulfonamide antibiotics: May cause hypoglycemia and increased insulin effect. Monitor blood glucose levels. Dosage adjustments of insulin may be required.

Albuterol, corticosteroids, danazol, diuretics, estrogens, isoniazid, phenothiazine derivatives, progestins (including oral contraceptives), somatropin, sympathomimetics (such as epinephrine), terbutaline, thyroid hormoness: May reduce serum glucose–lowering effect of insulin. Monitor blood glucose levels. Insulin dosage may need adjustment.

Beta blockers, clonidine, guanethidine, reserpine: May mask signs of hypoglycemia. Use cautiously. Monitor blood glucose levels.

Beta blockers, clonidine, lithium: May potentiate or weaken serum glucose–lowering effect of insulin. Monitor blood glucose levels. Insulin dosage may need adjustment.

Pentamidine: May cause hypoglycemia, which may be followed by hyperglycemia. Use cautiously. Monitor blood glucose levels.

Drug-lifestyle: *Alcohol use, emotional stress, exercise:* May potentiate or weaken the blood glucose–lowering effect of insulin. Monitor blood glucose levels. Dosage adjustments of insulin may be required.

Adverse reactions
Metabolic: hypoglycemia.
Skin: lipodystrophy, pruritus, rash.
Other: allergic reactions, injection site reaction (pain).

Overdose and treatment
Hypoglycemia may result from excessive insulin dose or from lower insulin requirements caused by increased work or exercise without eating, food not being absorbed in the usual manner because of postponement or omission of a meal, or illness with vomiting, fever, or diarrhea.

Symptoms may include fatigue, weakness, confusion, headache, seizures, dizziness, hunger, nausea, numbness, and pale skin.

Mild episodes of hypoglycemia can be treated with oral glucose or other carbohydrates. Adjustments in drug dosage, meal patterns, or exercise may be needed. More severe episodes with coma, seizure, or neurologic impairment may be treated with I.M./S.C. glucagon or concentrated I.V. glucose. Sustained carbohydrate intake and observation may be needed because hypoglycemia may recur after apparent clinical recovery.

Special considerations
● Insulin glargine isn't intended for I.V. administration. It is only for S.C. administration.
● Because of the prolonged duration of insulin glargine, it is not the insulin of choice for diabetic ketoacidosis.
● Note that the prolonged duration of activity of insulin glargine is dependent on injection into S.C. space.

● The absorption, onset, and duration of action may be affected by exercise and other variables such as illness and emotional stress.
● Insulin glargine must not be diluted or mixed with any other insulin or solution.
● As with any insulin therapy, lipodystrophy may occur at the site of injection and delay insulin absorption. Continuously rotate the injection site within a given area to reduce lipodystrophy.
● Hypoglycemia is the most common adverse effect of insulin. Early symptoms may be different or less pronounced in patients with long duration of diabetes, diabetic nerve disease, or intensified diabetes control. Monitor serum glucose closely in these patients because severe hypoglycemia may result before the patient develops symptoms.

Patient monitoring
● As with any insulin, the desired blood glucose levels as well as the doses and timing of antidiabetic drugs must be determined individually. Blood glucose monitoring is recommended for all patients with diabetes.

Breast-feeding patients
● It isn't known whether insulin glargine appears in significant amounts in breast milk. Because many drugs do, including human insulin, use caution when giving Lantus to a nursing woman.
● Breast-feeding women may need adjustments in insulin dose and diet.

Pediatric patients
● Safety and effectiveness have been established in 6- to 15-year-olds with type 1 diabetes.
● Administration to children under age 6 hasn't been studied.
● Based on the results of clinical trials, the dose recommendation for children is the same as for adults.

Geriatric patients
● Because hypoglycemia may be difficult to recognize in elderly patients with diabetes, the initial dosing, dose increments, and maintenance dosage should be conservative to avoid hypoglycemic reactions.

Patient education
● Educate patient on proper blood glucose monitoring techniques and proper diabetes management.
◪ **ALERT** Educate diabetic patients on the signs and symptoms of hypoglycemia, such as fatigue, weakness, confusion, headache, and pale skin.
● Advise patient to treat mild episodes of hypoglycemia with oral glucose tablets. Encourage patient to always carry glucose tablets in case of a hypoglycemic episode.
● Teach patient the importance of maintaining a diabetic diet and that adjustments in drug dosage, meal patterns, and exercise may be needed to regulate serum glucose.

▶ **ALERT** Any change of insulin should be made cautiously and only under medical supervision. Changes in insulin, strength, manufacturer, type (e.g., regular, NPH, or insulin analogs), species (animal, human), or method of manufacturer (rDNA versus animal source insulin), may result in the need for a change in dosage. Oral antidiabetic treatment also being taken may need to be adjusted.

• Tell patient to consult prescriber before using OTC drugs.

▶ **ALERT** Warn patient not to dilute or mix any other insulin or solution with insulin glargine. If the solution is cloudy, advise the patient to discard the vial.

• Tell patient to store unopened vials and cartridges in the refrigerator.

---

interferon alfa-2a, recombinant
Roferon-A

interferon alfa-2b, recombinant
Intron A

Pharmacologic classification: biological response modifier
Therapeutic classification: antineoplastic
Pregnancy risk category: C

Indications and dosages
▶ **Hairy cell leukemia.** alfa-2a. *Adults:* For induction, 3 million IU S.C. or I.M. daily for 16 to 24 weeks. For maintenance, 3 million IU S.C. or I.M. three times weekly.
alfa-2b
Adults: For induction and maintenance, 2 million IU/m² I.M. or S.C. three times weekly.
▶ **Condylomata acuminata.** alfa-2b. *Adults:* 1 million IU per lesion, intralesionally, three times weekly for 3 weeks.
▶ **Kaposi's sarcoma.** alfa-2a. *Adults:* For induction, 36 million IU S.C. or I.M. daily for 10 to 12 weeks; for maintenance, 36 million IU three times weekly.
alfa-2b
Adults: 30 million IU/m² S.C. or I.M. three times weekly. Maintain dose unless disease progresses rapidly or intolerance occurs.
▶ **Chronic hepatitis C.** *Adults:* 3 million IU (alfa-2b) S.C. or I.M. three times weekly. If response occurs, continue therapy for 6 months. If no response by 16 weeks, discontinue therapy.
▶ **Chronic hepatitis B.** *Adults:* 30 to 35 million IU (alfa-2b) S.C. or I.M. weekly either as 5 million IU daily or 10 million IU three times weekly for 16 weeks.
▶ **Chronic myelogenous leukemia.** *Adults:* 9 million IU (alfa-2a) daily S.C. or I.M. Maintenance dose not established.

▶ **Malignant melanoma.** *Adults:* 20 million IU (alfa-2b) I.V. infusion on 5 consecutive days/week for 4 weeks. Maintenance dose is 10 million IU/m² S.C. three times weekly for 48 weeks.

How supplied
Available by prescription only
alfa-2a
Powder for injection with diluent: 18 million IU/multidose vial
Prefilled syringes: 6 million IU/0.5 ml, 9 million IU/0.5 ml
Solution for injection: 3 million IU/vial, 6 million IU/vial, 9 million IU/vial, 9 million IU/multidose vial, 18 million IU/multidose vial, 36 million IU/multidose vial
alfa-2b
Powder for injection with diluent: 3 million IU/vial; 5 million IU/vial; 10 million IU/vial; 18 million IU/multidose vial; 25 million IU/vial; 50 million IU/vial
Solution for injection: 3 million IU/vial or syringe, 5 million IU/vial or syringe, 10 million IU/vial, 18 million IU/multidose vial, 25 million IU/vial

Pharmacodynamics
Antineoplastic action: Interferon alfa is a sterile protein product produced by recombinant DNA techniques applied to genetically engineered *Escherichia coli* bacteria. The interferons are naturally occurring small protein molecules produced and secreted by cells in response to viral infections or synthetic and biological inducers. Their exact mechanism of action is unknown but appears to involve direct antiproliferative action against tumor cells or viral cells to inhibit replication and modulation of host immune response by enhancing the phagocytic activity of macrophages and augmenting specific cytotoxicity of lymphocytes for target cells. To date, three major classes of interferons have been identified: alfa, beta, and gamma.

Pharmacokinetics
Absorption: More than 80% of dose is absorbed after I.M. or S.C. injection.
Distribution: Not applicable.
Metabolism: Appears to be metabolized in the liver and kidneys.
Excretion: Reabsorbed from glomerular filtrate with minor biliary elimination.

Route	Onset	Peak	Duration
I.M., S.C.	Unknown	Unknown	Unknown

Contraindications and precautions
Contraindicated in patients hypersensitive to drug or to murine (mouse) immunoglobulin. Use cautiously in patients with CV or pulmonary disease, diabetes mellitus, coagulation disorders, or myelosuppression. Contraindicated in pregnant women and in male partners of pregnant women. Use

---

cautiously in breast-feeding women; it isn't known whether drug appears in breast milk.

Interactions

Drug-drug. *Blood dyscrasia–causing drugs, bone marrow depressant therapy, radiation therapy:* Increased bone marrow depressant effects. Dosage reduction may be required.

CNS depressants: Enhanced CNS depression. Monitor patient closely.

Live-virus vaccine: May potentiate replication of vaccine virus, increase adverse effects, and decrease patient's antibody response. Avoid use together.

Methylxanthines, such as aminophylline and theophylline: Increased half-life of these drugs, perhaps by interfering with cytochrome P-450 drug-metabolizing enzymes. Monitor patient closely.

Adverse reactions

CNS: *dizziness, confusion,* paresthesia, numbness, lethargy, *depression, decreased mental status,* forgetfulness, *coma,* nervousness, insomnia, sedation, apathy, anxiety, irritability, fatigue, vertigo, gait disturbances, incoordination, syncope.

CV: hypotension, chest pain, *arrhythmias,* palpitations, *heart failure,* hypertension, edema, *MI,* flushing.

EENT: *dryness or inflammation of the oropharynx,* rhinorrhea, sinusitis, conjunctivitis, earache, eye irritation.

GI: *anorexia, nausea, diarrhea, vomiting,* abdominal fullness, *abdominal pain,* flatulence, constipation, hypermotility, gastric distress, *change in taste,* excessive salivation, dry mouth, thirst.

GU: transient impotence.

Hematologic: *leukopenia, mild thrombocytopenia.*

Hepatic: *hepatitis.*

Metabolic: *weight loss.*

Respiratory: *cough, dyspnea.*

Skin: diaphoresis, *rash, dryness, pruritus, partial alopecia,* urticaria.

Other: *flu syndrome (fever, fatigue, myalgia, headache, chills, arthralgia),* cyanosis, night sweats, hot flashes.

Overdose and treatment

No information available.

Special considerations

● When preparing antineoplastic agents for injection, take special precautions because of their potential for carcinogenicity and mutagenicity. Use of a biological containment cabinet is recommended. Don't shake vials.

⚠ ALERT Use S.C. administration route in patients whose platelet count is less than 50,000/mm³.

● Different brands of interferons may not be therapeutically interchangeable.

● Administration of drug at bedtime minimizes inconvenience of fatigue.

● When using interferon alfa-2b for condyloma-ta acuminata by intralesional injection, use only the 10 million-IU vial reconstituted with 1 ml of diluent. Using other strengths or more diluent would produce a hypertonic solution. For administration, use a 25G to 30G needle and a tuberculin syringe. Up to five lesions may be treated simultaneously.

● The following indications aren't included in U.S. labeling, but drug may be used for these applications: chronic myelocytic leukemia; treatment of renal carcinoma or superficial bladder carcinoma; treatment of malignant lymphomas, especially nodular, poorly differentiated types; malignant melanoma; multiple myeloma; mycosis fungoides; papillomas; and laryngeal papillomatosis (interferon alfa-2b).

Patient monitoring

● Almost all patients experience flulike symptoms at the beginning of therapy; these effects tend to diminish with continued therapy.

● Dosage reduction may be needed if headaches persist. Hypotension may result from fluid depletion; supportive treatment may be required.

● Monitor blood pressure; BUN level; hematocrit; platelet count; ALT, AST, LD, alkaline phosphatase, serum bilirubin, creatinine, and uric acid levels; total and differential leukocyte count; and ECG.

● Monitor patient for CNS adverse reactions, such as decreased mental status and dizziness. Periodic neuropsychiatric monitoring is recommended.

Pregnant patients

● Contraindicated in pregnancy. Women of childbearing age should use an effective method of contraception during therapy with interferon alpha preparations.

Breast-feeding patients

● Drug has potential for serious adverse effects on breast-fed infants; a decision should be made to discontinue breast-feeding or discontinue drug.

Pediatric patients

● Safety and efficacy in children under age 18 haven't been established.

Geriatric patients

● Neurotoxicity and cardiotoxicity are more common in geriatric patients, especially those with underlying CNS or cardiac impairment.

Patient education

● Tell patient that bone marrow depressant effects of interferon increase the risk of microbial infection, delayed healing, and gingival bleeding. Salivary flow may decrease as well.

● Advise patient not to take a missed dose or to double the next dose, but to call for further instructions.

● Inform patient to store drug in refrigerator and to keep it from freezing.

• Caution patient against driving or performing tasks requiring alertness until response to medication is known.

• Advise patient to seek medical approval before taking OTC medications for colds, coughs, allergies, and similar disorders; explain that interferons commonly cause flulike symptoms and patient may need to take acetaminophen before each dose.

• Tell patient drug may cause temporary loss of some hair. Normal hair growth should return when drug is discontinued.

• Inform patient to avoid use of aspirin and chronic alcohol intake because these may increase risk of GI bleeding.

interferon beta-1a
Avonex

Pharmacologic classification: biological response modifier
Therapeutic classification: antiviral, immunoregulator
Pregnancy risk category: C

Indications and dosages
➤ *To slow progression of physical disability and decrease the frequency of clinical exacerbations in relapsing multiple sclerosis.* Adults: 30 mcg I.M. once weekly.

How supplied
Available by prescription only
Lyophilized powder for injection: 33 mcg (6.6 million IU)

Pharmacodynamics
Antiviral and immunoregulator actions: The mechanisms by which interferon beta-1a exerts its actions in multiple sclerosis aren't clearly understood. However, it's known that the biological response–modifying properties of interferon beta-1a are mediated through its interactions with specific cell receptors found on the surface of cells. The binding to these receptors induces the expression of a number of interferon-induced gene products that are believed to be the mediators of the biological actions of interferon beta-1a.

Pharmacokinetics
Absorption: No information available.
Distribution: No information available.
Metabolism: No information available.
Excretion: Elimination half-life is 10 hours following I.M. administration.

Route	Onset	Peak	Duration
I.M.	Unknown	Unknown	Unknown

Contraindications and precautions
Contraindicated in pregnancy and in patients with history of hypersensitivity to natural or recombi-

nant interferon beta, human albumin, or any other component of the formulation. Use cautiously in patients with depression, seizure disorders, or severe cardiac conditions.

Interactions
None reported.

Adverse reactions
CNS: malaise, *asthenia, headache, sleep disturbances, dizziness,* syncope, suicidal tendency, *seizures,* speech disorder, ataxia.
CV: chest pain, vasodilation.
EENT: otitis media, decreased hearing, *sinusitis.*
GI: *nausea, diarrhea, dyspepsia,* anorexia, abdominal pain.
GU: ovarian cyst, vaginitis.
Hematologic: anemia, elevated eosinophil levels, decreased hematocrit.
Hepatic: elevated AST levels.
Musculoskeletal: *muscle ache,* muscle spasm, arthralgia.
Respiratory: *upper respiratory tract infection,* dyspnea.
Skin: ecchymosis (at injection site), injection site reaction, urticaria, alopecia, nevus.
Other: herpes zoster, herpes simplex, *flulike symptoms, pain, fever, chills, infection, hypersensitivity reaction.*

Overdose and treatment
No information available.

Special considerations
• Exercise caution when administering drug to patients with seizure disorders.

• Store vials of drug in the refrigerator. If refrigeration is unavailable, drug can be stored at 77° F (25° C) for up to 30 days. Don't expose drug to high temperatures or freezing.

Patient monitoring
• Perform the following laboratory tests before starting therapy and at periodic intervals thereafter: complete and differential WBC counts, platelet counts, and blood chemistries, including liver function tests.

• Use of interferon beta-1a may cause depression and suicidal ideation. It isn't known whether these symptoms are related to the underlying neurologic basis of multiple sclerosis, to interferon beta-1a treatment, or to both. Closely monitor patient for these symptoms and consider stopping therapy if they occur.

• Monitor patient with cardiac disease, such as angina, heart failure, or arrhythmia, for worsening of clinical condition during initiation of therapy. Although drug doesn't have any known direct-acting cardiac toxicity, it does cause flulike symptoms, which may be stressful to patients with severe cardiac conditions.

Pregnant patients
• Discontinue therapy if pregnancy occurs.

Reactions may be *common*, uncommon, *life-threatening*, or COMMON AND LIFE-THREATENING.

Breast-feeding patients
• It isn't known whether drug appears in breast milk. Consider risks and benefits before continuing breast-feeding or drug therapy.

Pediatric patients
• Safety and efficacy in children under age 18 haven't been established.

Patient education
• Caution patient not to change dosage or administration schedule. If a dose is missed, tell him to take it as soon as he remembers. The regular schedule may then be resumed, but two injections shouldn't be administered within 2 days of each other.
• Instruct patient how to store drug properly.
• Inform patient that flulike symptoms are common following initiation of therapy. Recommend use of acetaminophen to alleviate these symptoms.
☒ ALERT Advise patient to report depression, suicidal ideation, or other adverse reactions.
• Advise women of childbearing age not to become pregnant while taking interferon beta-1a because of the abortifacient potential of drug. If pregnancy does occur, instruct patient to discontinue treatment and call immediately.

interferon beta-1b
Betaseron

Pharmacologic classification: biological response modifier
Therapeutic classification: antiviral, immunoregulator
Pregnancy risk category: C

Indications and dosages
➤ **Reduction of the frequency of exacerbations in relapsing-remitting multiple sclerosis.** *Adults:* 8 million IU (0.25 mg) S.C. every other day.

How supplied
Available by prescription only
Lyophilized powder for injection: 9.6 million IU (0.3 mg)

Pharmacodynamics
Antiviral and immunoregulator actions: The mechanisms by which interferon beta-1b exerts its actions in multiple sclerosis aren't clearly understood. However, it's known that the biological response–modifying properties of interferon beta-1b are mediated through its interactions with specific cell receptors found on the surface of cells. The binding to these receptors induces the expression of a number of interferon-induced gene products that are believed to be the mediators of the biological actions of interferon beta-1b.

Pharmacokinetics
Absorption: Serum levels are undetectable after the recommended dose.
Distribution: No information available.
Metabolism: No information available.
Excretion: No information available on patients with multiple sclerosis; however, in clinical studies involving healthy patients, elimination half-life ranged from 8 minutes to 4 hours.

Route	Onset	Peak	Duration
S.C.	Unknown	1-8 hr	Unknown

Contraindications and precautions
Contraindicated in patients hypersensitive to interferon beta or human albumin. Use cautiously in women of childbearing age; drug is contraindicated in pregnancy.

Interactions
None significant.

Adverse reactions
CNS: *malaise,* depression, anxiety, emotional lability, depersonalization, **suicidal tendencies,** confusion, somnolence, *hypertonia, asthenia, migraine, seizures, headache, dizziness, myasthenia gravis.*
CV: palpitations, hypertension, tachycardia, peripheral vascular disorder.
EENT: laryngitis, *sinusitis,* conjunctivitis, abnormal vision.
GI: *diarrhea, constipation, abdominal pain, vomiting.*
GU: *menstrual disorders (bleeding or spotting, early or delayed menses, fewer days of menstrual flow, menorrhagia), pelvic pain.*
Hematologic: *decreased WBC and absolute neutrophil counts,* **hemorrhage.**
Hepatic: *elevated ALT levels, elevated bilirubin levels.*
Metabolic: Cushing's syndrome, diabetes insipidus, hypothyroidism, diabetes mellitus.
Respiratory: dyspnea.
Skin: *inflammation, pain, and necrosis at injection site; alopecia; diaphoresis.*
Other: *flulike symptoms (fever, chills, myalgia, diaphoresis),* breast pain, *lymphadenopathy,* generalized edema, SIADH.

Overdose and treatment
No information available.

Special considerations
• Drug is being investigated in the treatment of AIDS, AIDS-related Kaposi's sarcoma, metastatic renal-cell carcinoma, malignant melanoma, cutaneous T-cell lymphoma, and acute hepatitis C as unlabeled uses.
• Inject drug immediately after preparation.
• Refrigerate drug or reconstituted product for up to 3 hours at 36° to 46° F (2° to 8° C). Don't freeze.

Patient monitoring

• Perform the following laboratory tests before starting therapy and at periodic intervals thereafter: hemoglobin, complete and differential WBC counts, platelet counts, and blood chemistries, including liver function tests.

⚠ **ALERT** Drug use may cause depression and suicidal ideation. Other mental disorders have been observed and can include anxiety, emotional lability, depersonalization, and confusion. It's not known whether these symptoms are related to the underlying neurologic basis of multiple sclerosis, to interferon beta-1b treatment, or to both. Closely monitor patient with these symptoms and consider stopping therapy.

Pregnant patients

• Discontinue therapy if pregnancy occurs.

Breast-feeding patients

• It isn't known whether drug appears in breast milk. Consider risks and benefits before continuing breast-feeding or drug therapy.

Pediatric patients

• Safety and efficacy in children under age 18 haven't been established.

Patient education

• Caution patient to take protective measures (such as sunscreens, protective clothing) against exposure to ultraviolet light or sunlight until tolerance is determined.

• Teach patient how to self-administer S.C. injections, including solution preparation, use of aseptic technique, rotation of injection sites, and equipment disposal. Periodically reevaluate patient's technique.

• Instruct patient to rotate injection sites to minimize local reactions.

• Inform patient that flulike symptoms are common following initiation of therapy. Recommend taking drug at bedtime to help minimize the symptoms.

• Caution patient not to change dosage or schedule of administration without medical consultation.

• Advise patient to report depression or suicidal ideation.

• Inform women of childbearing age about abortifacient potential of drug.

---

interferon gamma-1b
Actimmune

Pharmacologic classification: biological response modifier
Therapeutic classification: antineoplastic
Pregnancy risk category: C

Indications and dosages

➤ **To decrease the frequency and severity of serious infection of chronic granu-**
lomatous disease and severe malignant osteopetrosis. Adults with body surface area over 0.5 m²: 50 mcg/m² (1 million IU/m²) S.C. three times weekly (such as Monday, Wednesday, and Friday).
Adults with body surface area of 0.5 m² or less: 1.5 mcg/kg S.C. three times weekly (such as Monday, Wednesday, and Friday).

How supplied
Available by prescription only
Injection: 100 mcg (2 million IU)/0.5 ml in single-dose vials

Pharmacodynamics
Antineoplastic action: Interferon gamma-1b is a single-chain polypeptide containing 140 amino acids, produced by fermentation of genetically engineered *Escherichia coli.* It has potent phagocytic activity not seen with other interferons. Exact mechanism of action is unknown, but growing evidence suggests it interacts functionally with other interleukin molecules and all form part of a complex lymphokine network. A broad range of biological activities has been noted, including enhancement of oxidative metabolism of tissue macrophages, antibody-dependent cellular cytotoxicity, natural killer cell activity, and effects on Fc receptor expression on monocytes and major histocompatibility antigen expression. In chronic granulomatous disease, interferon gamma-1b provides enhancement of phagocyte function, including elevation of superoxide levels and improved killing of *Staphylococcus aureus.*

Pharmacokinetics
Absorption: About 90% is absorbed after S.C. injection.
Distribution: No information available.
Metabolism: No information available.
Excretion: No information available. Mean elimination half-life after S.C. dosing is about 6 hours.

Route	Onset	Peak	Duration
P.O.	Unknown	7 hr	Unknown

Contraindications and precautions
Contraindicated in patients hypersensitive to drug or to genetically engineered products derived from *Escherichia coli.* Use cautiously in patients with CV disease (arrhythmias, heart failure, or ischemia), compromised CNS function, or seizure disorders and in those receiving myelosuppressive agents.

Interactions
Drug-drug. *Drugs that use CYP450 degradation pathway:* Interferon gamma-1b can decrease hepatic microsomal cytochrome P-450 levels, which could lead to decreased metabolism of drug. Use cautiously.
Myelosuppressive agents: Additive effects. Use together cautiously.

Reactions may be *common,* uncommon, *life-threatening,* or COMMON AND LIFE-THREATENING.

Adverse reactions

CNS: *fatigue,* decreased mental status, gait disturbance, dizziness.

GI: *nausea, vomiting, diarrhea,* abdominal pain.

GU: proteinuria.

Hematologic: *neutropenia, thrombocytopenia.*

Hepatic: elevated liver enzyme levels (at high doses).

Metabolic: weight loss.

Musculoskeletal: back pain, arthralgia, myalgia.

Skin: *rash, erythema, tenderness* at injection site.

Other: *flu syndrome (headache, fever, chills, myalgia, arthralgia).*

Overdose and treatment

No information available.

Special considerations

● Store drug in refrigerator immediately; don't freeze. Avoid excessive or vigorous agitation. Don't shake. Unopened or unentered vials shouldn't be left at room temperature longer than 12 hours before use. Don't return vials that exceed these limits to refrigerator; discard them.

● Each vial is designed for single use only.

Patient monitoring

● If acute hypersensitivity reaction occurs, discontinue drug immediately and institute symptomatic and supportive treatment.

● Transient cutaneous rash hasn't required discontinuation of therapy.

● If severe adverse reactions occur, reduce dose by 50% or discontinue therapy until reaction subsides.

Breast-feeding patients

● It isn't known whether drug appears in breast milk. Consider risks and benefits before continuing breast-feeding or drug therapy.

Pediatric patients

● Safety and efficacy haven't been established in children under age 1.

Patient education

● Thoroughly review the patient information package insert with patient.

---

ipecac syrup

Pharmacologic classification: alkaloid emetic
Therapeutic classification: emetic
Pregnancy risk category: C

Indications and dosages

➤ **To induce vomiting in poisoning.** *Adults:* 15 to 30 ml P.O., followed by 200 to 300 ml of water.

Children age 1 or older: 15 ml P.O., followed by about 200 ml of water.

Children under age 1: 5 to 10 ml P.O., followed by 100 to 200 ml of water.

May repeat dose once after 20 minutes, if necessary.

How supplied

Available with and without a prescription

Syrup: 70 mg powdered ipecac/ml

Pharmacodynamics

Emetic action: Ipecac syrup directly irritates the GI mucosa and directly stimulates the chemoreceptor trigger zone through the effects of emetine and cephalin, its two alkaloids.

Pharmacokinetics

Absorption: Absorbed in significant amounts mainly when it doesn't produce emesis.

Distribution: No information available.

Metabolism: No information available.

Excretion: Emetine is excreted in urine slowly, over a period lasting up to 60 days.

Route	Onset	Peak	Duration
P.O.	20 min	Unknown	20-25 min

Contraindications and precautions

Contraindicated in semicomatose or unconscious patients or those with severe inebriation, seizures, shock, or loss of gag reflex. Don't give after ingestion of gasoline, kerosene, volatile oils, or caustic substances (lye).

Interactions

Drug-drug. *Activated charcoal:* May inactivate ipecac syrup and shouldn't be taken together. Activated charcoal may be given after patient vomits.

Antiemetics: Decreased effectiveness of ipecac. Avoid use together.

Drug-food. *Carbonated beverages:* May cause abdominal distention. Tell patient to avoid use together.

Milk (or milk products): May decrease therapeutic effectiveness of ipecac syrup. Tell patient to avoid use together.

Vegetable oil: Delays absorption. Tell patient not to take together.

Adverse reactions

CNS: depression, *drowsiness.*

CV: *arrhythmias, bradycardia,* hypotension; atrial fibrillation, *myocarditis* (with excessive doses).

GI: diarrhea.

Overdose and treatment

Effects of overdose include diarrhea, persistent nausea or vomiting (longer than 30 minutes), stomach cramps or pain, arrhythmias, hypotension, myocarditis, difficulty breathing, and unusual fatigue or weakness.

Toxicity from chronic ipecac overdose usually involves use of the concentrated fluid extract

---

in dosage appropriate for the syrup. Effects of cardiotoxicity include tachycardia, T-wave depression, atrial fibrillation, depressed myocardial contractility, heart failure, and myocarditis. Other toxic effects include bloody stools and vomitus, hypotension, shock, seizures, and coma. Heart failure is the usual cause of death.

Treatment requires discontinuation of drug followed by symptomatic and supportive care, which may include digitalis and pacemaker therapy to treat cardiotoxic effects. However, no antidote exists for the cardiotoxic effects of ipecac, which may be fatal despite intensive treatment.

Special considerations
● Ipecac syrup empties the stomach completely within 30 minutes in over 90% of patients; average emptying time is 20 minutes.
⚠ ALERT Don't confuse ipecac syrup with ipecac fluidextract, which is rarely used but is 14 times more potent. Never store these two drugs together—the wrong drug could cause death.
● In antiemetic toxicity, ipecac syrup is usually effective if less than 1 hour has passed since ingestion of antiemetic.
● Ipecac syrup may be used in small amounts as an expectorant in some cough preparations; however, this use has doubtful therapeutic benefit.

Patient monitoring
● Little if any systemic toxicity occurs with doses of 30 ml or less.
● Drug may be abused by patients with eating disorders such as bulimia or anorexia nervosa.

Breast-feeding patients
● Safety in breast-feeding women hasn't been established; possible risks must be weighed against benefits of drug.

Pediatric patients
● Advise parents to keep ipecac syrup at home at all times but to keep it out of children's reach and to call poison control center before using.

Patient education
● Instruct patient to take syrup with 1 or 2 glasses of water.
● Advise patient to take activated charcoal only after vomiting has stopped.

ipratropium bromide
Atrovent

Pharmacologic classification: anticholinergic
Therapeutic classification: bronchodilator
Pregnancy risk category: B

Indications and dosages
➤ **Bronchospasm in chronic bronchitis and emphysema.** *Adults:* Usually, two inhalations (36 mcg) q.i.d.; patient may take additional inhalations, p.r.n., but shouldn't exceed 12 inhalations in 24 hours or 500 mcg q 6 to 8 hours via oral nebulizer.
➤ **Rhinorrhea caused by allergic and nonallergic perennial rhinitis. 0.03% nasal spray.**
Adults and children age 12 and older: Two sprays (42 mcg) per nostril b.i.d. or t.i.d.
➤ **Rhinorrhea caused by the common cold. 0.06% nasal spray.** *Adults and children age 12 and older:* Two sprays (84 mcg) per nostril t.i.d. or q.i.d.
Children ages 5 to 11: Two sprays (84 mcg) per nostril three times daily.

How supplied
Available by prescription only
Inhalation solution: 0.02%
Inhaler: each metered dose supplies 18 mcg
Nasal spray: 0.03%, 0.06%

Pharmacodynamics
Anticholinergic action: Ipratropium appears to inhibit vagally mediated reflexes by antagonizing the action of acetylcholine. Anticholinergics prevent the increases in intracellular concentration of cyclic guanosine monophosphate (cyclic GMP) that result from the interaction of acetylcholine with the muscarinic receptor on bronchial smooth muscle.

The bronchodilation following inhalation is primarily a local, site-specific effect, not a systemic one.

Pharmacokinetics
Absorption: Not readily absorbed into systemic circulation either from the surface of the lung or from the GI tract as confirmed by blood levels and renal excretion studies. Much of an inhaled dose is swallowed.
Distribution: Not applicable.
Metabolism: Metabolism is hepatic; elimination half-life is about 2 hours.
Excretion: Most of an administered dose is excreted unchanged in feces. Absorbed drug is excreted in urine and bile.

Route	Onset	Peak	Duration
Inhalation, intranasal	Unknown	Unknown	Unknown

Contraindications and precautions
Contraindicated in patients hypersensitive to drug or atropine or its derivatives and in those with a history of hypersensitivity to soya lecithin or related food products, such as soybeans and peanuts. Use cautiously in patients with angle-closure glaucoma, prostatic hyperplasia, and bladder-neck obstruction.

Interactions
Drug-drug. *Antimuscarinics, including ophthalmic preparations:* Concurrent use may produce additive effects. Avoid use together.

Fluorocarbon propellant–containing oral inhalants, such as adrenocorticoids, cromolyn, glucocorticoids, and sympathomimetics: Increased risk of fluorocarbon toxicity may result from too-closely timed administration of ipratropium and other fluorocarbon propellant–containing oral inhalants. A 5-minute interval between administration of such agents is recommended.

Drug-herb. *Jaborandi tree, pill-bearing spurge:* Decreased drug effect. Monitor patient closely and discourage herb usage.

Adverse reactions

CNS: dizziness, headache, nervousness.
CV: palpitations, chest pain.
EENT: cough, blurred vision, rhinitis, pharyngitis, sinusitis.
GI: nausea, GI distress, dry mouth.
Musculoskeletal: back pain.
Respiratory: *upper respiratory tract infection, bronchitis,* cough, dyspnea, *bronchospasm,* increased sputum.
Skin: rash.
Other: pain, flulike symptoms.

Overdose and treatment

Acute overdose by inhalation is unlikely because ipratropium isn't well absorbed systemically after aerosol or oral administration.

Special considerations

● Because of delayed onset of bronchodilation, drug isn't recommended for treating acute respiratory distress.
● Nasal spray pump requires priming with seven actuations of the pump. If used regularly as recommended, no further priming is needed. If not used for more than 24 hours, the pump will require two actuations. If not used for more than 7 days, the pump will require seven actuations to reprime.

Patient monitoring

● Monitor patient for adverse and therapeutic effects.

Breast-feeding patients

● It isn't known whether drug appears in breast milk. Although lipid-insoluble quaternary bases pass into breast milk, ipratropium is unlikely to reach the infant, especially when taken by aerosol. Use caution when administering to breast-feeding women.

Patient education

● Instruct patient on correct method of administration.
● Advise patient to allow 1 minute between inhalations.
● Instruct patient to take a missed dose as soon as possible, unless it's almost time for the next scheduled dose, in which case he should skip the missed dose. Warn him to never double the dose.

● Suggest sugarless hard candy, gum, ice, or saliva substitute to relieve dry mouth. Tell patient to report dry mouth to prescriber if it persists longer than 2 weeks.
● Instruct patient to call prescriber if he experiences no benefits within 30 minutes after administration or if condition worsens.

irbesartan
Avapro

Pharmacologic classification: angiotensin II receptor antagonist
Therapeutic classification: antihypertensive
Pregnancy risk category: C (D in second and third trimesters)

Indications and dosages

➤ *Treatment of hypertension, alone or with other antihypertensives. Adults:* Initially, 150 mg P.O. once daily, increased to maximum of 300 mg once daily if necessary, without regard to food.
✦ *Dosage adjustment.* In volume- and salt-depleted patients, give 75 mg P.O. initially.

How supplied

Available by prescription only
Tablets: 75 mg, 150 mg, 300 mg

Pharmacodynamics

Antihypertensive action: Irbesartan blocks the vasoconstrictor and aldosterone-secreting effects of angiotensin II by selectively blocking the binding of angiotensin II to its receptor sites.

Pharmacokinetics

Absorption: Absorbed rapidly and completely. The average absolute bioavailability is 60% to 80% and isn't affected by food.
Distribution: Drug is widely distributed and 90% bound to plasma proteins. It may cross the blood-brain barrier and placenta. Steady state is achieved within 3 days.
Metabolism: Metabolized by conjugation and oxidation. Cytochrome P-450 2C9 is the major enzyme responsible for formation of the oxidative metabolites. Metabolites don't appear to add appreciably to the pharmacologic activity.
Excretion: Excreted in the bile and urine. 20% is excreted in the urine and the rest in the feces. Drug also may appear in breast milk. Elimination half-life is 11 to 15 hours.

Route	Onset	Peak	Duration
P.O.	Unknown	1½-2 hr	24 hr

Contraindications and precautions

Contraindicated in patients hypersensitive to drug or its components and in pregnant or breast-feeding women.

Use cautiously in volume- or salt-depleted patients, in patients whose renal function may depend on the activity of the renin-angiotensin-aldosterone system (e.g., patients with severe heart failure), and in those with unilateral or bilateral renal artery stenosis.

Interactions
None reported.

Adverse reactions
CNS: fatigue, anxiety, dizziness, headache.
CV: chest pain, edema, tachycardia.
EENT: pharyngitis, rhinitis, sinus abnormality.
GI: diarrhea, dyspepsia, abdominal pain, nausea, vomiting.
GU: urinary tract infection.
Musculoskeletal: musculoskeletal trauma or pain.
Respiratory: upper respiratory tract infection.
Skin: rash.

Overdose and treatment
No information available. The signs and symptoms of an overdose are likely to be hypotension and tachycardia, and possibly bradycardia. Drug isn't removed by hemodialysis. If hypotension occurs, place patient in supine position and, if necessary, give an I.V. infusion of normal saline solution.

Special considerations
• Pharmacokinetics of drug aren't altered in patients with renal impairment or in patients on hemodialysis. Irbesartan isn't removed by hemodialysis. Dosage adjustment isn't necessary in patients with mild to severe renal impairment unless patient with renal impairment is also volume depleted.
• Dosage adjustment isn't necessary in patients with hepatic insufficiency.
• Patients not adequately treated by the maximum 300-mg once-daily dosage are unlikely to derive additional benefit from a higher dose or twice-daily dosing.

Patient monitoring
• Monitor blood pressure regularly. A transient hypotensive response isn't a contraindication to further treatment. Therapy with irbesartan usually can be continued once blood pressure has stabilized.

Pregnant patients
• Contraindicated during pregnancy because of potential danger to the fetus. The patient should immediately call prescriber if pregnancy is suspected.

Breast-feeding patients
• Because of the potential for serious adverse reactions in breast-fed infants, alternative feeding method should be used during drug therapy.

Pediatric patients
• Safety and efficacy in children under age 18 haven't been established.

Patient education
• Instruct patient on the proper administration of the drug and the potential adverse reactions.
• Advise patient that if a dose is missed to take it as soon as possible, but not to double the dose.
• Warn patient about symptoms of hypotension and tell him what to do if they occur.
• Caution patient not to discontinue drug without medical approval.

irinotecan hydrochloride
Camptosar

Pharmacologic classification: topoisomerase inhibitor
Therapeutic classification: antineoplastic
Pregnancy risk category: D

Indications and dosages
➤ *Treatment of metastatic carcinoma of the colon or rectum in which the disease has recurred or progressed following fluorouracil (5-FU)-based therapy. Adults:* Initially, 125 mg/m^2 I.V. infusion over 90 minutes. Recommended treatment regimen is 125 mg/m^2 I.V. administered once weekly for 4 weeks, followed by a 2-week rest period. Thereafter, additional courses of treatment may be repeated q 6 weeks (4 weeks on therapy, followed by 2 weeks off therapy). Subsequent doses may be adjusted to as high as 150 mg/m^2 or to as low as 50 mg/m^2 in 25- to 50-mg/m^2 increments depending on patient's tolerance. Treatment with additional courses may continue indefinitely in patients who attain a response or in those whose disease remains stable, provided intolerable toxicity doesn't occur.
➤ *First-line treatment of carcinoma of the colon or rectum in combination therapy with 5-FU and leucovorin. Adults:* 125 mg/m^2 I.V. infusion over 90 minutes on days 1, 8, 15, and 22, with leucovorin 20 mg/m^2 I.V. bolus immediately following Camptosar and 5-FU 500 mg/m^2 I.V. bolus immediately following leucovorin. Or, 180 mg/m^2 I.V. infusion over 90 minutes on days 1, 15, and 29, with leucovorin 200 mg/m^2 I.V. infusion over 2 hours on days 1, 2, 15, 16, 29, and 30, 5-FU 400 mg/m^2 I.V. bolus on days 1, 2, 15, 16, 29, and 30, and 600 mg/m^2 5-FU I.V. infusion over 22 hours on days 1, 2, 15, 16, 29, and 30.

How supplied
Available by prescription only
Injection: 20 mg/ml

Pharmacodynamics
Antineoplastic action: Irinotecan is a derivative of camptothecin. Camptothecins interact

specifically with the enzyme topoisomerase I, which relieves torsional strain in DNA by inducing reversible single-strand breaks. Irinotecan and its active metabolite bind to the topoisomerase I–DNA complex and prevent religation of these single-strand breaks.

Pharmacokinetics
Absorption: Administered I.V.
Distribution: About 30% to 68% bound to plasma protein; its active metabolite, SN-38, is about 95% protein-bound.
Metabolism: Undergoes metabolic conversion in the liver to its active metabolite SN-38.
Excretion: A small amount of drug and SN-38 are excreted in urine. Terminal half-life of irinotecan is 6 hours in patients age 65 and older and 5½ hours in patients under age 65; mean terminal elimination half-life of SN-38 is about 10 hours.

Route	Onset	Peak	Duration
I.V.	Unknown	Unknown	Unknown

Contraindications and precautions
Contraindicated in patients hypersensitive to drug. Use cautiously in geriatric patients and in those who have previously received pelvic or abdominal irradiation because of increased risk of severe myelosuppression. Because of possible fetal risk, drug shouldn't be used during pregnancy.

Interactions
Drug-drug. *Other antineoplastics:* May cause additive adverse effects such as myelosuppression and diarrhea. Monitor patient closely.

Adverse reactions
CNS: *insomnia, dizziness, asthenia, headache.*
CV: *vasodilation, edema.*
EENT: *rhinitis.*
GI: DIARRHEA, *nausea, vomiting, anorexia, constipation, flatulence, stomatitis, dyspepsia, abdominal cramping and pain, abdominal enlargement.*
Hematologic: LEUKOPENIA, *anemia,* NEUTROPENIA.
Hepatic: *increased alkaline phosphatase and AST levels.*
Metabolic: *weight loss, dehydration.*
Musculoskeletal: *back pain.*
Respiratory: *dyspnea, increased cough.*
Skin: *alopecia, sweating, rash.*
Other: *fever, pain, chills, infection.*

Overdose and treatment
The adverse effects of overdose are similar to those reported with the recommended dosage and regimen. There's no known antidote for drug overdose. Institute maximum supportive care to prevent dehydration because of diarrhea and to treat any infectious complications.

Special considerations
● Irinotecan must be diluted before infusion with D₅W injection (preferred) or normal saline solution injection to a final concentration of 0.12 to 1.1 mg/ml.
● Drug solution is stable for up to 24 hours at 77° F (25° C) and in ambient fluorescent lighting. Store solutions diluted in D₅W in refrigerator (35° to 46° F [2° to 8° C]) and protect from light; these are stable for 48 hours. However, because of possible microbial contamination during dilution, use admixture within 24 hours if refrigerated or within 6 hours if kept at room temperature. Refrigeration of admixtures using normal saline solution isn't recommended because visible particulates may form.
● Avoid freezing of drug and admixtures because drug may precipitate.
● Don't add other drugs to drug infusion.
● Irinotecan can induce severe forms of diarrhea.
● Routine administration of a colony-stimulating factor isn't necessary but may be helpful in patients experiencing significant neutropenia.

Patient monitoring
● Careful monitoring of the WBC count with differential, hemoglobin, and platelet count is recommended before each dose of irinotecan.
● Temporarily discontinue therapy if neutropenic fever occurs or if the absolute neutrophil count drops below 500/mm³. Reduce drug dose if the total WBC count decreases to less than 2,000/mm³, neutrophil count to less than 1,000/mm³, hemoglobin to less than 8 g/dl, or platelet count to less than 100,000/mm³. Consult manufacturer for dosage guidelines in these situations.

Pregnant patients
● Drug may be harmful to fetus.

Breast-feeding patients
● It isn't known whether drug appears in breast milk. Because of the potential for serious adverse reactions in breast-fed infants, discontinue breast-feeding during irinotecan therapy.

Pediatric patients
● Safety and efficacy in children haven't been established.

Geriatric patients
● Use caution when administering drug to geriatric patients, especially those with history of heart failure and hypotension.

Patient education
● Advise women of childbearing age to avoid pregnancy because drug may cause fetal harm.
● Inform patient about risk of diarrhea and when and how to treat it if it occurs.
● Tell patient to call prescriber if vomiting occurs, fever or evidence of infection develops, or symptoms of dehydration (fainting, light-headedness,

---

or dizziness) occur following drug administration.
● Warn patient that alopecia may occur.

iron dextran
DexFerrum, InFeD

Pharmacologic classification: parenteral iron supplement
Therapeutic classification: hematinic
Pregnancy risk category: C

Indications and dosages
➤ *Iron-deficiency anemia. Adults and children:* Dosage is highly individualized and is based on patient's weight and hemoglobin level. Drug is usually given I.M.; preservative-free solution can be given I.V. Check current literature for recommended protocol.

How supplied
Available by prescription only
Injection: 50 mg elemental iron/ml in 2-ml single-dose vials

Pharmacodynamics
Hematinic action: Iron dextran is a complex of ferric hydroxide and dextran in a colloidal solution. After I.M. injection, 10% to 50% remains in the muscle for several months; remainder enters bloodstream, increasing plasma iron level for up to 2 weeks. Iron is an essential component of hemoglobin.

Pharmacokinetics
Absorption: I.M. doses are absorbed in two stages: 60% after 3 days, and up to 90% by 3 weeks. Remainder is absorbed over several months or longer.
Distribution: During first 3 days, local inflammation facilitates passage of drug into the lymphatic system; drug is then ingested by macrophages, which enter lymph and blood.
Metabolism: After I.M. or I.V. administration, iron dextran is cleared from plasma by reticuloendothelial cells of the liver, spleen, and bone marrow.
Excretion: In doses of 500 mg or less, half-life is 6 hours. Traces are excreted in breast milk, urine, bile, and feces. Drug can't be removed by hemodialysis.

Route	Onset	Peak	Duration
I.M., I.V.	Unknown	Unknown	Unknown

Contraindications and precautions
Contraindicated in patients hypersensitive to drug, in those with all types of anemia except iron-deficiency anemia, and in those with acute infectious renal disease. Use cautiously in patients with impaired hepatic function, rheumatoid arthritis, and other inflammatory diseases.

Interactions
None reported.

Adverse reactions
CNS: headache, transitory paresthesia, dizziness, malaise.
CV: *hypotensive reaction, peripheral vascular flushing (with overly rapid I.V. administration), bradycardia.*
GI: nausea, anorexia.
Musculoskeletal: arthralgia, myalgia.
Respiratory: *bronchospasm,* dyspnea.
Skin: rash, urticaria, purpura, *brown skin discoloration* (at I.M. injection site); *local phlebitis* (at I.V. injection site); sterile abscess; necrosis; atrophy; fibrosis.
Other: *soreness, inflammation, anaphylaxis,* delayed sensitivity reactions, fever, chills.

Overdose and treatment
Injected iron has much greater bioavailability than oral iron, but data on acute overdose are limited.

Special considerations
● Discontinue oral iron before giving iron dextran.
● Administer a test dose of 0.5 ml iron dextrose I.M. or I.V. with monitoring for drug reactions, including anaphylaxis. Keep epinephrine (0.5 ml of a 1:1,000 solution) readily available for such an emergency.
● I.V. use is controversial, and some health care facilities don't allow it. I.V. is route of choice if patient has insufficient muscle mass for deep injection, impaired absorption from muscle because of stasis or edema, a risk of uncontrolled I.M. bleeding from trauma (as in hemophilia), or need for massive and prolonged parenteral therapy (as in chronic substantial blood loss). Administer no more than 50 mg of iron/minute (1 ml/minute) if using drug undiluted. Vein must be flushed with 10 ml normal saline solution injection to minimize local irritation.
● Large doses (more than 250 mg iron) may color the serum brown. Iron dextran may cause false elevations of serum bilirubin level and false reductions in serum calcium level. Iron dextran prevents meaningful measurement of serum iron level and total iron binding capacity for up to 3 weeks; I.M. injection may cause dense areas of activity for 1 to 6 days on bone scans using technetium 99m diphosphonate.

Patient monitoring
● Monitor hemoglobin, hematocrit, and reticulocyte count during therapy. An increase of about 1 g/dl weekly in hemoglobin is usual.
● Monitor patient for tissue damage and adverse events.

Breast-feeding patients
● Traces of unmetabolized iron dextran appear in breast milk; impact on infant is unknown.

Reactions may be *common*, uncommon, *life-threatening*, or COMMON AND LIFE-THREATENING.

Pediatric patients
• Drug isn't recommended for use in children under age 4 months.

Patient education
• Warn patient of possibility of skin staining with I.M. injections.

iron sucrose injection
Venofer

Pharmacologic classification: polynuclear iron(III)-hydroxide in sucrose
Therapeutic classification: hematinic
Pregnancy risk category: B

Indications and dosages
➤ **Iron deficiency anemia in patients undergoing long-term hemodialysis who are receiving supplemental erythropoietin therapy.** *Adults:* 100 mg (5 ml) of elemental iron I.V. directly in the dialysis line either by slow injection (1 ml per minute) or by infusion over 15 minutes during the dialysis session one to three times weekly to a total of 1,000 mg in 10 doses. Repeat if needed.

How supplied
Available by prescription only
Injection: 20 mg/ml of elemental iron

Pharmacodynamics
Iron replacement action: Iron is essential to the synthesis of hemoglobin to maintain oxygen transport and to the function and formation of other physiologically important heme and non-heme compounds. Following administration, drug is dissociated by the reticuloendothelial system into iron and sucrose. The released iron component eventually replenishes depleted body iron stores, resulting in significant increases in serum iron and serum ferritin and significant decreases in total iron binding capacity.

Pharmacokinetics
Absorption: No information available.
Distribution: Distributed mainly in blood and somewhat in extravascular fluid. A significant amount of iron is also distributed in the liver, spleen, and bone marrow.
Metabolism: Venofer is dissociated by the reticuloendothelial system into iron and sucrose.
Excretion: About 75% of sucrose and 5% of the iron component are eliminated by urinary excretion in 24 hours. In healthy adults, elimination half-life is 6 hours.

Route	Onset	Peak	Duration
I.V.	Unknown	Unknown	Variable

Adverse reactions
CNS: headache, asthenia, malaise, dizziness.

CV: *hypotension,* chest pain, hypertension, fluid retention.
GI: nausea, vomiting, diarrhea, abdominal pain.
Hepatic: elevated liver enzyme levels.
Musculoskeletal: *leg cramps,* bone and muscle pain.
Respiratory: dyspnea, pneumonia, cough.
Skin: pruritus, application site reaction.
Other: fever, accidental injury, pain.

Interactions
Drug-drug. *Oral iron preparations:* Reduced absorption of these compounds. Avoid concomitant use.

Overdose and treatment
Signs and symptoms of overdose or too-rapid infusion include hypotension, headache, nausea, dizziness, joint aches, paresthesia, abdominal and muscle pain, edema, and CV collapse. Administering the solution more slowly and treating with I.V. fluids, hydrocortisone, or antihistamines may alleviate most symptoms.

Contraindications and precautions
Contraindicated in patients with evidence of iron overload, patients hypersensitive to drug or any of its inactive components, and patients with anemia not caused by iron deficiency.

Special considerations
• Rare but fatal hypersensitivity reactions characterized by anaphylaxis, loss of consciousness, collapse, hypotension, dyspnea, or seizures have been reported.
• For administration by slow injection, administer at 1 ml (20 mg elemental iron) undiluted solution per minute, not exceeding one vial (100 mg elemental iron) per injection.
• For administration by infusion, dilute to a maximum of 100 ml in normal saline solution immediately before infusion, and infuse 100 mg elemental iron over at least 15 minutes.
• Administering by infusion may reduce the risk of hypotension.
• Transferrin saturation values increase rapidly after I.V. administration of iron sucrose. Obtain serum iron values 48 hours after I.V. dosing.
• Monitor hemoglobin, hematocrit, serum ferritin, and transferrin saturation.
• Withhold dose in patients with evidence of iron overload.
• Don't mix with other medications or add to parenteral nutrition solutions of I.V. infusion.
• Inspect for particulate matter and discoloration before administration.

Breast-feeding patients
• It's not known whether drug appears in breast milk. Use cautiously when administering to breast-feeding women.

Pediatric patients
• Safety and efficacy haven't been established.

◊ Unlabeled clinical use

Geriatric patients
• Dose selection in elderly patients should be conservative because of the possibility that they have decreased hepatic, renal, and cardiac function; concomitant disease; and other drug therapy.

Patient education
• Instruct patient to notify prescriber if symptoms of overdose occur, such as headache, nausea, dizziness, joint aches, paresthesia, or abdominal and muscle pain.

isoniazid (INH)
Isotamine*, Laniazid, Nydrazid, PMS Isoniazid*

Pharmacologic classification: isonicotinic acid hydrazine
Therapeutic classification: antitubercular
Pregnancy risk category: C

Indications and dosages
➤ *Primary treatment against actively growing tubercle bacilli.* Adults: 5 mg/kg P.O. or I.M. daily in a single dose, up to 300 mg daily, continued for 9 months to 2 years.
Infants and children: 10 mg/kg P.O. or I.M. daily in a single dose, up to 300 mg daily, continued for 18 months to 2 years. Concomitant administration of at least one other effective antitubercular drug is recommended.
➤ *Prophylaxis against tubercle bacilli of those closely exposed or with positive skin test.* Adults: 300 mg P.O. daily in a single dose, continued for 6 months to 1 year.
Infants and children: 10 mg/kg P.O. daily in a single dose, up to 300 mg daily, continued for 6 months to 1 year.

How supplied
Available by prescription only
Injection: 100 mg/ml
Oral solution: 50 mg/5 ml
Tablets: 100 mg, 300 mg

Pharmacodynamics
Antitubercular action: INH interferes with lipid and DNA synthesis, thus inhibiting bacterial cell wall synthesis. Its action is bacteriostatic or bactericidal, depending on organism susceptibility and drug concentration at infection site. INH is active against *Mycobacterium tuberculosis, M. bovis,* and some strains of *M. kansasii.*

Resistance by *M. tuberculosis* develops rapidly when INH is used to treat tuberculosis, and it's usually combined with another antitubercular agent to prevent or delay resistance. During prophylaxis, however, resistance isn't a problem and isoniazid can be used alone.

Pharmacokinetics
Absorption: Rapidly and completely absorbed from the GI tract after oral administration. INH also is absorbed readily after I.M. injection.
Distribution: Distributed widely into body tissues and fluids, including ascitic, synovial, pleural, and cerebrospinal fluids; lungs and other organs; and sputum and saliva. Drug crosses the placenta and enters breast milk in levels similar to plasma.
Metabolism: Inactivated primarily in the liver by genetically controlled acetylation. Rate of metabolism varies individually; fast acetylators metabolize drug five times as rapidly as others. About 50% of blacks and whites are slow acetylators of INH, whereas more than 80% of Chinese, Japanese, and Eskimos are fast acetylators.
Excretion: About 75% of a dose is excreted in urine as unchanged drug and metabolites in 24 hours; some drug is excreted in saliva, sputum, feces, and breast milk. Plasma half-life in adults is 1 to 4 hours, depending on metabolic rate. Drug is removed by peritoneal dialysis or hemodialysis.

Route	Onset	Peak	Duration
P.O.	Unknown	1-2 hr	Unknown
I.M.	Unknown	Unknown	Unknown

Contraindications and precautions
Contraindicated in patients with acute hepatic disease or drug-related hepatic damage. Use cautiously in the elderly and in patients with severe, non-INH-associated hepatic disease, seizure disorders (especially those taking phenytoin), severe renal impairment, or chronic alcoholism.

Interactions
Drug-drug. *Antacids:* Decreased oral absorption of INH. Give antacid at least one hour before INH.
Anticoagulants: May increase anticoagulant activity. Dosage adjustment may be needed.
Benzodiazepines (such as diazepam), carbamazepine, phenytoin: INH-induced inhibition of metabolism and elevation of serum levels, causing toxicity. Monitor patient closely.
Corticosteroids: May decrease INH efficacy. Monitor patient for drug effects.
Cycloserine: Increased hazard of CNS toxicity, drowsiness, and dizziness. Monitor patient for safety.
Disulfiram: May cause coordination difficulties and psychotic episodes. Patient requires close observation.
Rifampin: May accelerate INH metabolism to hepatotoxic metabolites. Use cautiously.
Drug-lifestyle. *Alcohol use:* Increased risk of INH-induced hepatitis and seizures. Advise patient to avoid alcohol.

Adverse reactions
CNS: *peripheral neuropathy* (dose-related and especially in patients who are malnourished, al-

coholic, diabetic, or slow acetylators), usually preceded by paresthesia of hands and feet, *seizures*, toxic encephalopathy, memory impairment, toxic psychosis.

EENT: optic neuritis, atrophy.

GI: nausea, vomiting, epigastric distress.

Hematologic: *agranulocytosis*, hemolytic anemia, *aplastic anemia*, eosinophilia, *thrombocytopenia*, sideroblastic anemia.

Hepatic: *hepatitis*, jaundice, *elevated serum transaminase levels*, bilirubinemia.

Metabolic: hyperglycemia, metabolic acidosis, pyridoxine deficiency, hypocalcemia, hypophosphatemia.

Skin: irritation at I.M. injection site.

Other: gynecomastia, rheumatic and lupus-like syndromes, *hypersensitivity reactions* (fever, rash, lymphadenopathy, vasculitis).

Overdose and treatment

Early signs and symptoms of overdose include nausea, vomiting, slurred speech, dizziness, blurred vision, and visual hallucinations, occurring 30 minutes to 3 hours after ingestion; gross overdose causes CNS depression progressing from stupor to coma, with respiratory distress, intractable seizures, and death.

To treat, establish ventilation; control seizures with diazepam. Pyridoxine is administered to equal dose of INH. Initial dose is 1 to 4 g pyridoxine I.V., followed by 1 g every 30 minutes thereafter, until the entire dose is given. Clear drug with gastric lavage after seizure control, and correct acidosis with parenteral sodium bicarbonate; force diuresis with I.V. fluids and osmotic diuretics, and, if necessary, enhance clearance of the drug with hemodialysis or peritoneal dialysis.

Special considerations

• At least 12 months of preventive therapy is recommended for patients with previous tuberculosis and patients infected with HIV.

• If compliance is a problem, twice-weekly supervised drug administration may be effective. Recommended twice-weekly dose for adults is 15 mg/kg P.O., not to exceed 900 mg.

• Oral doses should be taken on empty stomach for maximum absorption, or with food if gastric irritation occurs.

• Aluminum-containing antacids or laxatives should be taken 1 hour after oral dose of INH.

• Drug may hinder stabilization of serum glucose level in patients with diabetes mellitus.

• Pyridoxine 50 mg P.O. daily is sometimes recommended to prevent peripheral neuropathy from large doses of INH. It also may be useful in patients at risk of developing peripheral neuropathy (malnourished patients, diabetics, and alcohol abusers). Pyridoxine (50 to 200 mg daily) has been used to treat drug-induced neuropathy.

• Because drug is dialyzable, patients undergoing hemodialysis or peritoneal dialysis may need dosage adjustments.

• INH alters results of urine glucose tests that use cupric sulfate method (Benedict's reagent, Diastix, or Chemstrip uG).

Patient monitoring

• Monitor patient for adverse effects, especially hepatic dysfunction, CNS toxicity, and optic neuritis.

• Monitor blood, renal, and hepatic function studies before and periodically during therapy to minimize toxicity; assess visual function periodically.

• Elevated liver function study results occur in about 15% of cases; most abnormalities are mild and transient, but some persist throughout treatment.

• Hepatotoxicity appears to be age-related and may limit use for prophylaxis. Alcohol consumption and history of alcohol-related liver disease also increases risk of hepatotoxicity.

• Improvement is usually evident after 2 to 3 weeks of therapy.

Pregnant patients

• Safe use of drug during pregnancy hasn't been established. Potential benefits to the woman should be weighed against the risks to the fetus.

Breast-feeding patients

• Drug appears in breast milk; use cautiously in breast-feeding women, and monitor infants for possible INH-induced toxicity.

Pediatric patients

• Infants and children tolerate larger doses of drug.

Geriatric patients

• Use cautiously in elderly patients because risk of hepatic effects increases after age 35. Occasionally severe and sometimes fatal hepatitis has occurred, especially in elderly patients.

• Drug prophylaxis in patients with a positive purified protein derivative test may not be indicated in older patients because of risk of hepatotoxicity.

Patient education

• Instruct patient on the proper administration of drug and the potential for adverse reactions.

• Warn patient to avoid alcohol.

• Urge patient to comply with and complete prescribed regimen.

• Advise patient not to discontinue drug without medical approval.

• Explain importance of follow-up appointments.

---

isoproterenol
Isuprel

isoproterenol hydrochloride
Isuprel, Isuprel Mistometer

isoproterenol sulfate
Medihaler-Iso

Pharmacologic classification: adrenergic
Therapeutic classification: bronchodilator, cardiac stimulant
Pregnancy risk category: C

Indications and dosages
➤ *Complete heart block after closure of ventricular septal defect.* *Adults:* I.V. bolus, 0.02 to 0.06 mg (1 to 3 ml of a 1:50,000 dilution).
Children: I.V. bolus, 0.01 to 0.03 mg (0.5 to 1.5 ml of a 1:50,000 dilution).
➤ *Bronchospasm during mild acute asthma attacks.* isoproterenol hydrochloride.
Adults and children: Via aerosol inhalation, one inhalation initially, repeated, p.r.n., after 1 to 5 minutes, to maximum six inhalations daily. Maintenance dosage is one to two inhalations four to six times daily at 3- to 4-hour intervals. Via hand-bulb nebulizer, 5 to 15 deep inhalations of a 0.5% solution; if needed, may be repeated in 5 to 10 minutes. May be repeated up to five times daily.
Or, three to seven deep inhalations of a 1% solution, repeated once in 5 to 10 minutes if needed. May be repeated up to five times daily.
isoproterenol sulfate
Adults and children: For acute dyspneic episodes, one inhalation initially; repeated if needed after 2 to 5 minutes. Maximum six inhalations daily. Maintenance dosage is one to two inhalations up to six times daily.
➤ *Bronchospasm in COPD.* isoproterenol hydrochloride. *Adults and children:* Via hand-bulb nebulizer: 5 to 15 deep inhalations of a 0.5% solution, or 3 to 7 deep inhalations of a 1% solution no more frequently than q 3 to 4 hours.
➤ *Bronchospasm during mild acute asthma attacks or in COPD.* isoproterenol hydrochloride. *Adults and children:* Oral inhalation of 2 ml of 0.125% solution or 2.5 ml of 0.1% solution up to five times daily.
➤ *Acute asthma attacks unresponsive to inhalation therapy or control of bronchospasm during anesthesia.* isoproterenol hydrochloride. *Adults:* 0.01 to 0.02 mg (0.5 to 1 ml of a 1:50,000 dilution) I.V. Repeat, if needed.
➤ *Emergency treatment of arrhythmias.* isoproterenol hydrochloride. *Adults:* Initially, 0.02 to 0.06 mg I.V. bolus. Subsequent doses 0.01 to 0.2 mg I.V. Or, 5 mcg/minute titrated to pa-

tient's response. Range is 2 to 20 mcg/minute. Or, 0.2 mg I.M. or S.C.; subsequent doses 0.02 to 1 mg I.M. or 0.15 to 0.2 mg S.C. In extreme cases, 0.02 mg (0.1 of 1:5,000) intracardiac injection.
Children: May give half of initial adult dose.
➤ *Immediate temporary control of atropine-resistant hemodynamically significant bradycardia.* isoproterenol hydrochloride. *Adults:* 2 to 10 mcg/minute I.V. infusion, titrated to patient's response.
Children: 0.1 mcg/kg/minute, titrated to patient's response. Maximum rate is 1 mcg/kg/minute.
➤ *Heart block, Stokes-Adams attacks, and shock.* isoproterenol hydrochloride. *Adults and children:* 0.5 to 5 mcg/minute by continuous I.V. infusion titrated to patient's response; or 0.02 to 0.06 mg I.V. boluses with 0.01 to 0.2 mg additional doses; or 0.2 mg I.M. or S.C. with 0.02 to 1 mg I.M. or 0.15 to 0.2 mg additional doses.

How supplied
Available by prescription only
isoproterenol
Nebulizer inhaler: 0.25%, 0.5%, 1%
isoproterenol hydrochloride
Aerosol inhaler: 103 mcg/metered spray
Injection: 20 mcg/ml, 200 mcg/ml
isoproterenol sulfate
Aerosol inhaler: 80 mcg/metered spray

Pharmacodynamics
Bronchodilator action: Isoproterenol relaxes bronchial smooth muscle by direct action on beta$_2$-adrenergic receptors, relieving bronchospasm, increasing vital capacity, decreasing residual volume in lungs, and facilitating passage of pulmonary secretions. It also produces relaxation of GI and uterine smooth muscle via stimulation of beta$_2$ receptors. Peripheral vasodilation, cardiac stimulation, and relaxation of bronchial smooth muscle are the main therapeutic effects.
Cardiac stimulant action: Isoproterenol acts on beta$_1$-adrenergic receptors in the heart, producing a positive chronotropic and inotropic effect; it usually increases cardiac output. In patients with AV block, isoproterenol shortens conduction time and the refractory period of the AV node and increases the rate and strength of ventricular contraction.

Pharmacokinetics
Absorption: After injection or oral inhalation, absorption is rapid; after sublingual or rectal administration, absorption is variable and often unreliable.
Distribution: Distributed widely throughout the body.
Metabolism: Metabolized by conjugation in the GI tract and by enzymatic reduction in liver, lungs, and other tissues.

Excretion: Excreted primarily in urine as unchanged drug and its metabolites.

Route	Onset	Peak	Duration
I.V.	Immediate	Unknown	Few min
S.C.	Immediate	Unknown	2 hr
Oral inhaler	Immediate	Unknown	1-3 hr

Contraindications and precautions

Contraindicated in patients with tachycardia caused by digitalis intoxication, in patients with arrhythmias (other than those that may respond to treatment with isoproterenol), and in those with angina pectoris. Use cautiously in the elderly and in patients with impaired renal function, CV disease, coronary insufficiency, diabetes, hyperthyroidism, or a sensitivity to sympathomimetic amines.

Interactions

Drug-drug. *Beta blockers:* Antagonize cardiac-stimulating, bronchodilating, and vasodilating effects of isoproterenol. Monitor patient closely.
Cardiac glycosides, potassium-depleting drugs, and other drugs that affect cardiac rhythm: Arrhythmias may occur. Monitor patient's ECG.
Cyclopropane or halogenated hydrocarbon general anesthetics: Increased risk of arrhythmias. Avoid use together.
Epinephrine and other sympathomimetics: May cause additive CV reactions. Drugs may be used together if at least 4 hours elapse between administration of the two drugs. Use together cautiously.
Ergot alkaloids: May increase blood pressure. Use cautiously.

Adverse reactions

CNS: *headache, mild tremor,* weakness, dizziness, *nervousness,* insomnia.
CV: palpitations, *tachycardia, anginal pain, arrhythmias, cardiac arrest, rapid increase and decrease in blood pressure, Stokes-Adams attacks.*
GI: *nausea, vomiting, heartburn.*
Metabolic: hyperglycemia.
Respiratory: *bronchospasm,* bronchitis, sputum increase, pulmonary edema.
Skin: diaphoresis.
Other: swelling of parotid glands.

Overdose and treatment

Signs and symptoms of overdose include exaggeration of common adverse reactions, particularly arrhythmias, extreme tremors, nausea, vomiting, and profound hypotension.

Treatment includes symptomatic and supportive measures. Monitor vital signs closely. Sedatives (barbiturates) may be used to treat CNS stimulation. Use cardioselective beta blockers to treat tachycardia and arrhythmias. Use these agents cautiously; they may induce asthmatic attack.

Special considerations

● Drug doesn't replace administration of blood, plasma, fluids, or electrolytes in patients with blood volume depletion.
● Severe paradoxical airway resistance may follow oral inhalations.
● Hypotension must be corrected before isoproterenol is administered.
● Prescribed I.V. infusion rate should include specific guidelines for regulating flow or terminating infusion in relation to heart rate, premature beats, ECG changes, precordial distress, blood pressure, and urine flow. Because of danger of precipitating arrhythmias, infusion is usually decreased or temporarily discontinued if heart rate exceeds 110 beats/minute.
● Isoproterenol also has been used to aid diagnosis of coronary artery disease and mitral regurgitation.
● Isoproterenol may reduce the sensitivity of spirometry in the diagnosis of asthma.

Patient monitoring

● Carefully monitor response to therapy by frequent determinations of heart rate, ECG pattern, blood pressure, and central venous pressure, as well as (for patients in shock) urine volume, blood pH, and Pco_2 levels.
● Monitor patient for rebound bronchospasm when effects of drug end.
● Continuously monitor ECG during I.V. administration.
● If three to five treatments within 6 to 12 hours provide minimal or no relief, reevaluate therapy.

Pregnant patients

● Administer drug during pregnancy only when clearly indicated.

Breast-feeding patients

● It isn't known whether drug appears in breast milk. Use cautiously in breast-feeding women.

Pediatric patients

● Use cautiously in children.

Geriatric patients

● These patients may be more sensitive to therapeutic and adverse effects of drug.

Patient education

● Urge patient to call prescriber if condition persists or worsens.
● Advise patient to store oral forms away from heat and light (not in bathroom medicine cabinet, where heat and moisture will cause deterioration of the drug). Keep drug out of the reach of children.
Inhaled form
● Give patient instructions on proper use of inhaler.
● Tell patient that saliva and sputum may appear red or pink after oral inhalation, because isoproterenol turns red on exposure to air.

- Advise patient to rinse mouth with water after drug is absorbed completely and between doses.

Sublingual form
- Tell patient to allow sublingual tablet to dissolve under tongue, without sucking, and not to swallow saliva (may cause epigastric pain) until drug has been absorbed completely.
- Warn patient that frequent use of sublingual tablets may damage teeth due to acidity of drug.

isosorbide dinitrate
Apo-ISDN*, Coronex*, Dilatrate-SR, Isordil, Isordil Titradose, Novosorbide*, Sorbitrate, Sorbitrate SA

Pharmacologic classification: nitrate
Therapeutic classification: antianginal, vasodilator
Pregnancy risk category: C

Indications and dosages
➤*Treatment or prophylaxis of acute anginal attacks; treatment of chronic ischemic heart disease (by preload reduction).* Adults: S.L. form—2.5 to 10 mg for prompt relief of angina pain, repeated q 2 to 3 hours during acute phase, or q 4 to 6 hours for prophylaxis.

Chewable form—2.5 to 10 mg, p.r.n., for acute attack or q 2 to 3 hours for prophylaxis, but only after initial test dose of 5 mg to determine risk of severe hypotension.

Oral form—10 to 20 mg P.O. t.i.d. or q.i.d. for prophylaxis only (use smallest effective dose).

Extended-release forms—20 to 40 mg P.O. q 6 to 12 hours or 80 mg P.O. q 8 to 12 hours.

➤*Adjunctive treatment of heart failure*◊. Adults: 5 to 10 mg S.L. q 3 to 4 hours. Alternatively, give 20 to 40 mg P.O. (or chewable tablets) q 4 hours. Usually administered with vasodilators.

➤*Diffuse esophageal spasm without gastroesophageal reflux*◊. Adults: 10 to 30 mg P.O. q 4 hours.

How supplied
Available by prescription only
Capsules (extended-release): 40 mg
Tablets: 5 mg, 10 mg, 20 mg, 30 mg, 40 mg
Tablets (chewable): 5 mg, 10 mg
Tablets (extended-release): 40 mg
Tablets (S.L.): 2.5 mg, 5 mg, 10 mg

Pharmacodynamics
Antianginal action: Drug reduces myocardial oxygen demand through peripheral vasodilation, resulting in decreased venous filling pressure (preload) and, to a lesser extent, decreased arterial impedance (afterload). These combined effects result in decreased cardiac work and, consequently, reduced myocardial oxygen demands.

Drug also redistributes coronary blood flow from epicardial to subendocardial regions.

Vasodilating action: Drug dilates peripheral vessels (primarily venous), helping to manage pulmonary edema and heart failure caused by decreased venous return to the heart (preload). Arterial vasodilatory effects also decrease arterial impedance (afterload) and thus left ventricular work, benefiting the failing heart. These combined effects may help some patients with acute MI. (Use of isosorbide dinitrate in patients with heart failure and acute MI is currently unapproved.)

Pharmacokinetics
Absorption: Oral form is well absorbed from the GI tract but undergoes first-pass metabolism, resulting in bioavailability of about 50% (depending on dosage form used).

Distribution: Limited information is available on plasma protein binding and distribution of drug. Like nitroglycerin, it's distributed widely throughout the body.

Metabolism: Metabolized in the liver to active metabolites.

Excretion: Metabolites are excreted in the urine; elimination half-life is about 5 to 6 hours with oral administration; 2 hours with S.L. administration. About 80% to 100% of absorbed dose is excreted in urine within 24 hours. Duration of effect is longer than that of S.L. preparations.

Route	Onset	Peak	Duration
P.O.			
Regular	30 min	Unknown	4-6 hr
Chewable	3 min	Unknown	½-2 hr
Extended	1 hr	Unknown	5-6 hr
S.L.	3 min	Unknown	½-2 hr

Contraindications and precautions
Contraindicated in patients hypersensitive to drug, in patients with idiosyncratic reactions to nitrates, and in patients with severe hypotension, shock, or acute MI with low left ventricular filling pressure.

Use cautiously in patients with hypotension or blood volume depletion (such as from diuretic therapy).

Interactions
Drug-drug. *Antihypertensives, calcium channel blockers, phenothiazines, vasodilators:* Additive hypotensive effects. Use cautiously, and check blood pressure frequently.

Drug-lifestyle. *Alcohol use:* Additive hypotensive effects. Advise patient to avoid alcohol.

Adverse reactions
CNS: *headache* (sometimes with throbbing), dizziness, weakness.

CV: *flushing, orthostatic hypotension, tachycardia, palpitations, ankle edema,* fainting.

GI: nausea, vomiting.

Reactions may be *common,* uncommon, *life-threatening,* or COMMON AND LIFE-THREATENING.

Skin: cutaneous vasodilation, rash.
Other: *hypersensitivity reactions*, sublingual burning.

Overdose and treatment

Effects of overdose result primarily from vasodilation and methemoglobinemia and include hypotension, persistent throbbing headache, palpitations, visual disturbance, flushing of the skin and sweating (with skin later becoming cold and cyanotic), nausea and vomiting, colic and bloody diarrhea, orthostatism, initial hyperpnea, dyspnea, slow respiration, bradycardia, heart block, increased intracranial pressure with confusion, fever, paralysis, and tissue hypoxia, which can lead to cyanosis, metabolic acidosis, coma, clonic seizures, and circulatory collapse. Death may result from circulatory collapse or asphyxia.

Treatment includes gastric lavage followed by administration of activated charcoal to remove remaining gastric contents. Monitor blood gas measurements and methemoglobin levels, as indicated. Supportive care includes respiratory support and oxygen administration, passive movement of limbs to aid venous return, recumbent positioning (Trendelenburg position, if necessary), maintenance of adequate body temperature, and administration of I.V. fluids.

An I.V. adrenergic agonist (such as phenylephrine) may be considered if further treatment is required. For methemoglobinemia, methylene blue (1 to 2 mg/kg I.V.) may be given. (Epinephrine and related compounds are contraindicated in isosorbide dinitrate overdose.)

Special considerations

• Store drug in a cool place, in a tightly closed container away from light.
• Maintenance of continuous 24-hour plasma levels may result in refractory tolerance. Dosing regimens should include dose-free intervals, which vary based on form of drug used.
• Drug may cause orthostatic hypotension. To minimize this, have patient change to upright position slowly, walk up and down stairs carefully, and lie down at first sign of dizziness.
• Don't discontinue drug abruptly because this may cause coronary vasospasm.
• Additional dose may be given before anticipated stress or at bedtime if angina is nocturnal.
• Isosorbide dinitrate may interfere with serum cholesterol determination tests using the Zlatkis-Zak color reaction, causing a falsely decreased value.

Patient monitoring

• Monitor blood pressure and intensity and duration of patient's response to drug.
• Drug may cause headache, especially at first. Dose may need to be reduced temporarily, but tolerance usually develops to this effect. In the interim, patient may relieve headache with aspirin or acetaminophen.

Breast-feeding patients

• It isn't known whether drug appears in breast milk. Use cautiously in breast-feeding women.

Pediatric patients

• Methemoglobinemia may occur in infants receiving large doses of isosorbide dinitrate.

Patient education

• Instruct patient to take drug regularly, as prescribed, and to keep it easily accessible at all times. Drug is physiologically necessary but not addictive.
• Warn patient that headache may occur initially, but may respond to usual headache remedies or dosage reduction. Assure patient that headache usually subsides gradually with continued treatment.
• Tell patient to take oral tablets on an empty stomach, either 30 minutes before or 1 to 2 hours after meals; to swallow oral tablets whole; and to chew chewable tablets thoroughly before swallowing.
• Advise patient to sit when self-administering S.L. tablets. He should lubricate tablet with saliva or place a few milliliters of fluid under tongue with tablet. If patient experiences tingling sensation with drug placed sublingually, he may try to hold tablet in buccal pouch. Dose may be repeated every 10 to 15 minutes for maximum of three doses. If no relief occurs, he should call or go to hospital emergency department.
• Warn patient to make positional changes gradually to avoid excessive dizziness.
• Instruct patient to avoid alcohol while taking drug because severe hypotension and CV collapse may occur.
• Advise patient to report blurred vision, dry mouth, or persistent headache.
• Caution patient not to stop long-term therapy abruptly.

isosorbide mononitrate
Imdur, ISMO, Isotrate ER, Monoket

Pharmacologic classification: nitrate
Therapeutic classification: antianginal
Pregnancy risk category: C

Indications and dosages

➤ *Prevention of angina pectoris caused by coronary artery disease (but not to abort acute anginal attacks).* *Adults:* 20 mg P.O. b.i.d., with doses 7 hours apart and first dose on awakening. For extended-release tablets, 30 to 60 mg P.O. once daily, on arising. After several days, dosage may be increased to 120 mg once daily; rarely, 240 mg may be needed.

How supplied

Available by prescription only
Tablets: 10 mg, 20 mg

Tablets (extended-release): 30 mg, 60 mg, 120 mg

Pharmacodynamics

Antianginal action: Drug is the major active metabolite of isosorbide dinitrate. It relaxes vascular smooth muscle and consequently dilates peripheral arteries and veins. Dilation of the veins promotes peripheral pooling of blood and decreases venous return to the heart, thereby reducing left ventricular end-diastolic pressure and pulmonary capillary wedge pressure (preload). Arteriolar relaxation reduces systemic vascular resistance, systolic arterial pressure, and mean arterial pressure (afterload). Dilation of the coronary arteries also occurs.

Pharmacokinetics

Absorption: Absolute bioavailability is almost 100%.
Distribution: Volume of distribution is about 0.6 L/kg. Less than 4% is bound to plasma proteins.
Metabolism: Drug isn't subject to first-pass metabolism in the liver.
Excretion: Less than 1% of isosorbide mononitrate is eliminated in urine. Overall elimination half-life of drug is about 5 hours.

Route	Onset	Peak	Duration
P.O.	30-60 min	Unknown	Unknown

Contraindications and precautions

Contraindicated in patients with hypersensitivity or idiosyncrasy to nitrates, severe hypotension, shock, or acute MI with low left ventricular filling pressure. Use cautiously in patients with hypotension or blood volume depletion (such as from diuretic therapy).

Interactions

Drug-drug. *Calcium channel blockers, organic nitrates:* Marked symptomatic orthostatic hypotension. Dose adjustments of either class of agents may be necessary.
Drug-lifestyle. *Alcohol use:* Increased vasodilation. Advise patient to avoid alcohol.

Adverse reactions

CNS: *headache* (sometimes with throbbing), dizziness, weakness.
CV: *flushing, orthostatic hypotension, tachycardia, palpitations, ankle edema,* fainting.
GI: nausea, vomiting.
Musculoskeletal: arthralgia.
Respiratory: bronchitis, pneumonia, upper respiratory tract infection.
Skin: cutaneous vasodilation, rash.
Other: *hypersensitivity reactions,* sublingual burning.

Overdose and treatment

Signs and symptoms of overdose may include increased intracranial pressure; persistent, throb-

bing headache; confusion; moderate fever; vertigo; palpitations; visual disturbances; nausea and vomiting (possibly with colic and even bloody diarrhea); syncope (especially with upright position); air hunger; dyspnea, later followed by reduced ventilatory effort; diaphoresis, with skin either flushed or cold and clammy; heart block and bradycardia; paralysis; coma; seizures; and death.

No specific antagonist to vasodilator effects of drug is known. However, drug is significantly removed from the blood during hemodialysis.

If drug is ingested, induce emesis or perform gastric lavage followed by activated charcoal administration. Because drug is rapidly and completely absorbed, however, gastric lavage may be effective only with recent ingestion. Treat severe hypotension and reflex tachycardia by elevating legs and administering I.V. fluids. Epinephrine is ineffective in reversing severe hypotension caused by overdose, and epinephrine and related compounds are contraindicated. Administer oxygen and artificial ventilation if necessary. Monitor methemoglobin levels as indicated.

Special considerations

● Drug-free interval sufficient to avoid tolerance to drug isn't completely defined. The recommended regimen involves two daily doses given 7 hours apart, with a gap of 17 hours between the second dose of 1 day and the first dose of the next day. Considering the relatively long half-life of drug, this result is consistent with those obtained for other organic nitrates.

● The asymmetric twice-daily regimen successfully avoids significant rebound or withdrawal effects. In studies of other nitrates, the occurrence and magnitude of such phenomena appear to be highly dependent on the schedule of nitrate administration.

⚠ ALERT Onset of action of oral drug isn't sufficiently rapid to be useful in aborting an acute anginal episode.

Patient monitoring

● Benefits of drug in patients with acute MI or heart failure have not been established. Because effects of drug are difficult to terminate rapidly, its use isn't recommended in such patients. If it's used, however, careful clinical or hemodynamic monitoring must be performed to avoid the hazards of hypotension and tachycardia.

● Monitor blood pressure, especially in those susceptible to hypotension.

● Methemoglobinemia has occurred in patients receiving other organic nitrates and probably could occur as an adverse reaction. Significant methemoglobinemia has occurred with moderate overdoses of organic nitrates. Suspect methemoglobinemia in patients who exhibit signs of impaired oxygen delivery despite adequate cardiac output and adequate Pao_2. Classically, methemoglobinemic blood is chocolate brown, without color change on exposure to air. Treatment of choice for methemoglobinemia is methylene blue, 1 to 2 mg/kg I.V.

Breast-feeding patients
● It isn't known whether drug appears in breast milk. Use caution when administering to breast-feeding women.

Pediatric patients
● Safety and efficacy in children haven't been established.

Patient education
● Tell patient to follow prescribed dosing schedule carefully (two doses taken 7 hours apart) to maintain antianginal effect and to prevent tolerance.
● Extended-release tablets shouldn't be crushed or chewed.
● Warn patient that daily headaches sometimes accompany treatment with nitrates, including isosorbide mononitrate, and are a marker of drug activity. Patient shouldn't alter treatment schedule, because attempts to reduce headaches also will reduce antianginal efficacy. Tell patient to treat headaches with aspirin or acetaminophen.
● Warn patient to avoid alcohol while taking drug because of increased risk of light-headedness.
● Tell patient to rise slowly from recumbent or seated position to avoid light-headedness caused by sudden decrease in blood pressure.

isotretinoin
Accutane

Pharmacologic classification: retinoic acid derivative
Therapeutic classification: antiacne, keratinization stabilizer
Pregnancy risk category: X

Indications and dosages
➤ **Severe recalcitrant nodular acne.** *Adults and adolescents:* 0.5 to 2 mg/kg P.O. daily given in two divided doses and continued for 15 to 20 weeks.
➤ **Keratinization disorders resistant to conventional therapy** ◇, **prevention of skin cancer** ◇. *Adults:* Dosage varies with specific disease and severity of the disorder; dosages up to 2 to 4 mg/kg P.O. daily have been used. Consult current literature for specific recommendations.
➤ **Squamous cell cancer of the head and neck** ◇. *Adults:* 50 to 100 mg/m².

How supplied
Available by prescription only
Capsules: 10 mg, 20 mg, 40 mg

Pharmacodynamics
Antiacne action: Exact mechanism of action is unknown; isotretinoin decreases the size and activity of sebaceous glands, which decreases secretion and probably explains the rapid clinical improvement. A reduction in *Propionibacterium acnes* in the hair follicles occurs as a secondary result of decreased nutrients.
Keratinizing action: Isotretinoin has anti-inflammatory and keratinizing effects. The mechanism is unknown.

Pharmacokinetics
Absorption: When administered orally, drug is absorbed rapidly from the GI tract. Therapeutic range for isotretinoin hasn't been established.
Distribution: Distributed widely. In animals, it's found in most organs and is known to cross the placenta. In humans, degree of placental transfer and the degree of secretion in breast milk are unknown. Isotretinoin is 99.9% protein-bound, primarily to albumin.
Metabolism: Metabolized in the liver and possibly in the gut wall. The major metabolite is 4-oxo-isotretinoin, with tretinoin and 4-oxo-tretinoin also found in the blood and urine.
Excretion: Elimination process isn't fully known, although renal and biliary pathways are known to be used.

Route	Onset	Peak	Duration
P.O.	Unknown	3 hr	Unknown

Contraindications and precautions
Contraindicated in women of childbearing age unless patient has had a negative serum pregnancy test within 2 weeks before beginning therapy, will begin drug therapy on day 2 or 3 of next menstrual period, and will comply with stringent contraceptive measures for 1 month before therapy, during therapy, and for at least 1 month after therapy. Severe fetal abnormalities may occur if used during pregnancy. Also contraindicated in patients hypersensitive to parabens, which are used as preservatives.

Interactions
Drug-drug. *Alcohol-containing preparations, medicated soaps and cleansers, medicated cover-ups, topical resorcinol peeling agents (benzoyl peroxide):* Cumulative drying effect. Use cautiously.
Carbamazepine: Decreased carbamazepine levels. Monitor patient carefully.
Tetracyclines: May increase the risk of pseudotumor cerebri. Avoid use together.
Vitamin A products: Additive toxic effect. Avoid use together.
Drug-lifestyle. *Alcohol use:* Increased plasma triglyceride levels. Advise patient to avoid alcohol.

Adverse reactions
CNS: headache, fatigue, *pseudotumor cerebri* .
EENT: *conjunctivitis, drying of mucous membranes,* corneal deposits, dry eyes, visual disturbances, *epistaxis, dry nose.*

GI: nonspecific GI symptoms, gum bleeding and inflammation, *nausea, vomiting,* anorexia, *dry mouth, abdominal pain,* inflammatory bowel disease.
Hematologic: *anemia, elevated platelet count, elevated erythrocyte sedimentation rates.*
Hepatic: elevated AST, ALT, and alkaline phosphatase levels.
Metabolic: hyperglycemia, *hypertriglyceridemia.*
Musculoskeletal: *musculoskeletal pain (skeletal hyperostosis).*
Skin: *rash, dry skin, facial skin desquamation,* peeling of palms and toes, skin infection, photosensitivity, *cheilitis, pruritus, fragility, petechiae, nail brittleness,* thinning of hair.

Overdose and treatment

Signs and symptoms of overdose are rare and would be extensions of adverse reactions.

Special considerations

• For women of childbearing age, a negative blood test for pregnancy must be obtained before therapy.
• Administer drug with or shortly after meals.
• Therapy usually lasts 15 to 20 weeks, followed by at least 8 weeks off drug before beginning a second course.
• Contact lenses may become uncomfortable during treatment; recommend use of artificial tears.
• Drug has been used in a limited number of patients to treat psoriasis (combined with psoralen and ultraviolet light); it also has been used to treat cutaneous neoplasms.

Patient monitoring

• Monitor patient for visual problems.
• Pregnancy tests must be repeated monthly to avoid administration of drug during pregnancy.

Pregnant patients

• Drug is a potent teratogen and shouldn't be taken during pregnancy.

Breast-feeding patients

• It isn't known whether drug appears in breast milk. Breast-feeding isn't recommended during drug therapy.

Patient education

• Recommend taking drug with or shortly after meals to ease GI discomfort.
• Caution against alcohol ingestion to reduce risk of hypertriglyceridemia.
• Warn patient to be cautious when driving, particularly at night because drug decreases night vision.
• Advise patient not to take vitamin supplements containing vitamin A while taking drug.
• Instruct patient to avoid prolonged exposure to sunlight or sun lamps to prevent photosensitivity.

isradipine
DynaCirc, DynaCirc CR

Pharmacologic classification: calcium channel blocker
Therapeutic classification: antihypertensive
Pregnancy risk category: C

Indications and dosages

➤ *Management of hypertension. Adults:* Individualize dosage. Initially, 2.5 mg P.O. b.i.d. or 5 mg (controlled-release) once daily alone or with thiazide diuretic. Maximal response may require 2 to 4 weeks; therefore, dose adjustments of 5 mg daily should be made at 2- to 4-week intervals up to maximum of 20 mg daily. Doses of 10 mg or more per day haven't been shown to be more effective but rather to lead to increased risk of adverse reactions. Same starting dose is used in geriatric, hepatic-impaired, and renal-impaired patients.

How supplied

Available by prescription only
Capsules: 2.5 mg, 5 mg
Tablets (controlled-release): 5 mg, 10 mg

Pharmacodynamics

Antihypertensive action: A dihydropyridine calcium channel blocker, isradipine binds to calcium channels and inhibits calcium flux into cardiac and smooth muscle, which results in dilation of arterioles. This dilation reduces systemic resistance and lowers blood pressure while producing small increases in resting heart rate.

Pharmacokinetics

Absorption: About 90% to 95% is absorbed after oral administration.
Distribution: 95% bound to plasma protein.
Metabolism: Completely metabolized before elimination, with extensive first-pass metabolism.
Excretion: About 60% to 65% is excreted in urine; 25% to 30% in feces.

Route	Onset	Peak	Duration
P.O.	2 hr	1½ hr	Unknown

Contraindications and precautions

Contraindicated in patients hypersensitive to drug. Use cautiously in patients with heart failure, especially if combined with a beta blocker.

Interactions

Drug-drug. *Fentanyl anesthesia:* Severe hypotension has been reported with concomitant use of a beta blocker and a calcium channel blocker. Avoid use together.

Adverse reactions

CNS: dizziness, *headache,* fatigue, syncope.
CV: edema, flushing, angina, tachycardia, palpitations.

Reactions may be *common,* uncommon, *life-threatening,* or COMMON AND LIFE-THREATENING.

GI: nausea, diarrhea, abdominal discomfort, vomiting.
Respiratory: dyspnea.
Skin: rash.

Overdose and treatment

No well-documented cases of overdose have been reported; however, presumably excessive peripheral vasodilation with marked and prolonged systemic hypotension may occur. Provide symptomatic and supportive treatment, including active CV support, monitoring of input and output and cardiac and respiratory function, elevation of lower legs, and fluid replacement, as needed. Use vasoconstrictors only when not specifically contraindicated.

Special considerations

● Drug has no significant effect on heart rate and no adverse effects on cardiac contractility, conduction or digitalis clearance, or lipid or renal function.
● Administration with food significantly increases by about 1 hour the time to reach peak levels. However, food has no effect on total bioavailability of drug.

Patient monitoring

● Elevated liver function test results have been reported in some patients.
● Individualize dosage. Allow 2 to 4 weeks between dosage adjustments.

Breast-feeding patients

● It isn't known whether drug appears in breast milk. Consider the risk of serious adverse reactions in the infant.

Pediatric patients

● Safety and efficacy haven't been established in children under age 18.

Geriatric patients

● No age-related problems have been reported.

Patient education

● Instruct patient to report irregular heartbeat, shortness of breath, swelling of hands or feet, pronounced dizziness, constipation, nausea, or hypotension.

---

itraconazole
Sporanox

Pharmacologic classification: synthetic triazole
Therapeutic classification: antifungal
Pregnancy risk category: C

Indications and dosages

➤ *Treatment of blastomycosis (pulmonary and extrapulmonary), histoplasmosis (including chronic cavitary pulmonary disease and disseminated nonmeningeal histoplasmosis).* Adults: 200 mg P.O. once daily. If condition doesn't improve or shows evidence of progressive fungal disease, increase dose in 100-mg increments to maximum of 400 mg daily. Give doses of more than 200 mg daily in two divided doses. Or, 200 mg I.V. b.i.d. for four doses, then decrease to 200 mg I.V. once daily for up to 14 days.

➤ *Aspergillosis (pulmonary and extrapulmonary) in patients who are intolerant of or refractory to amphotericin B therapy.* Adults: 200 to 400 mg P.O. daily, or 200 mg I.V. b.i.d. for four doses; then decrease to 200 mg I.V. daily for up to 14 days.

➤ *Oropharyngeal candidiasis.* Adults: 200 mg (20 ml) oral solution P.O. daily for 1 to 2 weeks.

➤ *Esophageal candidiasis.* Adults: 100 mg (10 ml) oral solution P.O. daily for at least 3 weeks.

➤ *Superficial mycoses (dermatophytoses, pityriasis versicolor, sebopsoriasis, candidiasis [vaginal, oral, or chronic mucocutaneous], onychomycosis)* ◊, *leishmaniasis* ◊, *fungal keratitis* ◊, *alternaria-toxicosis* ◊, *zygomycosis* ◊, *and systemic mycoses (candidiasis, cryptococcal infections [meningitis, disseminated], dimorphic infections [paracoccidioidomycosis, coccidioidomycosis])* ◊, *subcutaneous mycoses (sporotrichosis, cutaneous chromomycosis)* ◊. Adults: 50 to 400 mg P.O. daily. Duration of therapy varies from 1 day to greater than 6 months, depending on the condition and mycologic response.

Note: Discontinue drug if signs and symptoms develop that are consistent with liver disease and may be attributable to itraconazole.

How supplied

Available by prescription only
Capsules: 100 mg
Injection: 10 mg/ml
Oral solution: 10 mg/ml

Pharmacodynamics

Antifungal action: Itraconazole is a synthetic triazole antifungal agent. In vitro, itraconazole inhibits the cytochrome P-450 dependent synthesis of ergosterol, a vital component of fungal cell membranes.

Pharmacokinetics

Absorption: Oral bioavailability of drug is maximal when taken with food; absolute oral bioavailability is 55%.
Distribution: Plasma protein–binding of drug is 99.8%; 99.5% for its metabolite, hydroxyitraconazole.
Metabolism: Extensively metabolized by the liver into a large number of metabolites, including hydroxyitraconazole, the major metabolite.

Excretion: Fecal excretion of parent drug varies between 3% and 18% of the dose. Renal excretion of parent drug is less than 0.03% of dose. About 40% of dose is excreted as inactive metabolites in the urine. Drug isn't removed by hemodialysis.

Route	Onset	Peak	Duration
P.O.	Unknown	Unknown	Unknown

Contraindications and precautions

Contraindicated in patients hypersensitive to drug and in breast-feeding women because drug appears in breast milk.

Use cautiously in patients with hypochlorhydria or HIV infection and in those receiving medications that are highly protein-bound.

Interactions

Drug-drug. *Benzodiazepines (midazolam, triazolam):* Increased plasma levels of these drugs, which may prolong hypnotic and sedative effects. Avoid use together.

Calcium channel blockers: May cause edema. Adjust dosage as needed.

Cyclosporine, tacrolimus: Itraconazole may increase cyclosporine or tacrolimus plasma levels. Reduce dosages of these drugs by 50% when using itraconazole doses greater than 100 mg daily. Monitor cyclosporine or tacrolimus levels.

Digoxin: Increased digoxin levels. Monitor digoxin levels.

H_2-receptor antagonists, isoniazid, phenytoin, rifampin: May reduce plasma itraconazole levels. Monitor patient for drug effect.

HMG-CoA reductase inhibitors: Contraindicated during treatment with itraconazole. Don't use together.

Indinavir, ritonavir: Altered plasma levels of either drug. Use together cautiously.

Nonsedating antihistamines: Rarely, possible life-threatening arrhythmias and death. Don't use together.

Oral hypoglycemic agents: May cause severe hypoglycemia. Monitor blood glucose carefully.

Phenytoin: Altered phenytoin metabolism. Monitor phenytoin levels.

Sulfonylureas: Concurrent use may cause hypoglycemia. Monitor serum glucose levels.

Warfarin: Enhanced anticoagulant effect. Monitor PT.

Drug-food. *Grapefruit juice:* Decreased plasma levels and therapeutic effect of itraconazole. Tell patient to take drug with liquid other than grapefruit juice.

Adverse reactions

CNS: malaise, fatigue, headache, dizziness, somnolence.

CV: edema, hypertension.

GI: *nausea,* vomiting, diarrhea, abdominal pain, anorexia.

GU: albuminuria, impotence.

Hepatic: impaired hepatic function.

Metabolic: hypokalemia.

Skin: rash, pruritus.

Other: fever, decreased libido.

Overdose and treatment

In overdose, employ supportive measures, including gastric lavage with sodium bicarbonate. Itraconazole isn't removed by dialysis.

Special considerations

● In life-threatening situations, the recommended loading dose is 200 mg three times daily (600 mg daily) for first 3 days. Continue treatment for minimum of 3 months and until clinical parameters and laboratory tests indicate that the active fungal infection has subsided. An inadequate period of treatment may lead to recurrence of active infection.

● Instruct prescriber to obtain specimens for fungal cultures and other relevant laboratory studies (wet mount, histopathology, serology) before therapy to isolate and identify causative organisms. Therapy may be instituted before results of cultures and other laboratory studies are known; once results become available, adjust anti-infective therapy accordingly.

● The clinical course of histoplasmosis in HIV-infected patients is more severe and usually requires maintenance therapy to prevent relapse. Because hypochlorhydria has occurred in HIV-infected patients, absorption of itraconazole may be decreased.

● Itraconazole shouldn't be given to a patient with creatinine clearance of less than 30 ml/minute.

Patient monitoring

● Monitor hepatic enzyme test values in patients with hepatic function abnormalities.

Pregnant patients

● Drug shouldn't be administered during pregnancy because of risk to fetus.

Breast-feeding patients

● Because drug appears in breast milk, its use is contraindicated in breast-feeding women.

Pediatric patients

● Safety and efficacy in children haven't been established.

Patient education

● Instruct patient to take drug with food to enhance absorption.

● Tell patient to swish oral solution vigorously before swallowing.

● Tell patient to report signs and symptoms that may suggest liver dysfunction (jaundice, unusual fatigue, anorexia, nausea, vomiting, dark urine, pale stool) so appropriate laboratory tests can be performed.

Reactions may be *common*, uncommon, *life-threatening*, or COMMON AND LIFE-THREATENING.

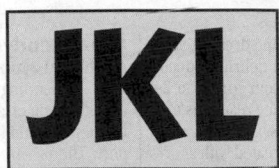

ketamine hydrochloride
Ketalar

Pharmacologic classification: dissociative anesthetic
Therapeutic classification: I.V. anesthetic
Pregnancy risk category: C

Indications and dosages
➤ *Induction of general anesthesia, especially for short diagnostic or surgical procedures not requiring skeletal muscle relaxation; adjunct to other general anesthetics or low-potency agents, such as nitrous oxide.* *Adults and children:* 1 to 4.5 mg/kg I.V. over 60 seconds. Or, 6.5 to 13 mg/kg I.M. To maintain anesthesia, repeat in increments of half to full initial dose.

How supplied
Available by prescription only
Injection: 10 mg/ml, 50 mg/ml, 100 mg/ml

Pharmacodynamics
Anesthetic action: Ketamine induces a profound sense of dissociation from the environment by direct action on the cortex and limbic system.

Pharmacokinetics
Absorption: Absorbed rapidly and well after I.M. injection.
Distribution: Rapidly enters the CNS.
Metabolism: Metabolized by the liver to an active metabolite with one-third the potency of parent drug.
Excretion: Excreted in urine.

Route	Onset	Peak	Duration
I.V.	30 sec	Unknown	5-10 min
I.M.	3-4 min	Unknown	12-25 min

Contraindications and precautions
Contraindicated in patients allergic to drug and in those with CV disease in whom a sudden increase in blood pressure would be harmful.

Interactions
Drug-drug. *Barbiturates, narcotics:* Concurrent use may cause prolonged recovery time. Monitor patient closely.
Enflurane, halothane: Myocardial depression, bradycardia, and hypotension. Avoid use together.
Thyroid hormones: May cause hypertension and tachycardia. Monitor patient closely.

Tubocurarine and other nondepolarizing muscle relaxants: Increased neuromuscular effects; prolonged respiratory depression. Monitor patient closely.

Adverse reactions
CNS: tonic-clonic movements, hallucinations, confusion, excitement, dreamlike states, irrational behavior, psychic abnormalities.
CV: *hypertension, tachycardia,* hypotension, *arrhythmias.*
EENT: diplopia, nystagmus, laryngospasm.
GI: mild anorexia, nausea, vomiting, excessive salivation.
Respiratory: *respiratory depression, apnea.*
Skin: transient erythema, measles-like rash.

Overdose and treatment
Overdose causes respiratory depression. Support respiration, using mechanical ventilation if necessary.

Special considerations
• The effect of ketamine on blood pressure makes it particularly useful in hypovolemic patients as an induction agent that supports blood pressure.
• Barbiturates are incompatible in the same syringe.
• For direct injection, dilute 100 mg/ml concentration with an equal volume of sterile water for injection, normal saline solution, or D_5W. For continuous infusion, prepare a 1-mg/ml solution by adding 5 ml from the 100 mg/ml vial to 500 ml of D_5W or normal saline solution.
• Emergence reactions are less common in patients under age 15 or over age 65 and when drug is given I.M.
• Keep verbal, tactile, and visual stimulation to a minimum during induction and recovery.
• Dissociative and hallucinatory adverse effects have led to drug abuse.

Patient monitoring
• Monitor cardiac function continuously in patients with hypertension or cardiac decompensation.
• Patients need physical support because of rapid induction; monitor vital signs perioperatively. Blood pressure begins to increase shortly after injection, peaks at 10% to 50% above preanesthetic levels, and returns to baseline within 15 minutes. Clinical signs of overdose include respiratory depression.

• Emergence reactions, including dreams, visual imagery, hallucinations, and delirium, occur in 12% of patients and may occur for up to 24 hours postoperatively. Emergence reactions may be reduced by using lower dosage of ketamine with I.V. diazepam and can be treated with short- or ultrashort-acting barbiturates.

Pediatric patients
• Drug is safe and especially useful in managing minor surgical or diagnostic procedures or in repeated procedures that require large amounts of analgesia, such as the changing of burn dressings.

Geriatric patients
• Use drug cautiously, especially in patients with suspected CVA, hypertension, or cardiac disease.

Patient education
• Warn patient to avoid tasks requiring motor coordination and mental alertness for 24 hours after anesthesia.

---

ketoconazole
Nizoral

Pharmacologic classification: imidazole derivative
Therapeutic classification: antifungal
Pregnancy risk category: C

Indications and dosages
➤ *Severe fungal infections caused by susceptible organisms. Adults:* Initially, 200 mg P.O. daily as a single dose. Dose may be increased to 400 mg once daily in patients who don't respond to lower dosage.
Children over age 2: 3.3 to 6.6 mg/kg P.O. daily as a single dose.
➤ *Topical treatment of tinea corporis, tinea cruris, tinea versicolor, and tinea pedis. Adults and children:* Apply daily or b.i.d. for about 2 weeks; for tinea pedis, apply for 6 weeks.
➤ *Seborrheic dermatitis. Adults and children:* Apply b.i.d. for about 4 weeks.
➤ *Dandruff. Adults:* Apply for 1 minute, rinse, then reapply for 3 minutes. Shampoo twice weekly for 4 weeks with at least 3 days between shampoos.
➤ *Prostatic carcinoma◇, disseminated intravascular coagulation related to prostatic cancer◇. Adults:* 400 mg P.O. q 8 hours.

How supplied
Available by prescription only
Cream: 2%
Shampoo: 2%
Tablets: 200 mg

Pharmacodynamics
Antifungal action: Drug is fungicidal and fungistatic, depending on concentrations. It inhibits demethylation of lanosterol, thereby altering membrane permeability and inhibiting purine transport. The in vitro spectrum of activity includes most pathogenic fungi. However, CSF concentrations following oral administration aren't predictable. It shouldn't be used to treat fungal meningitis, and specimens should be obtained for susceptibility testing before therapy. Currently available tests may not accurately reflect in vivo activity, so interpret results cautiously.

Drug is used orally to treat disseminated or pulmonary coccidioidomycosis, paracoccidioidomycosis, or histoplasmosis; oral candidiasis; and candiduria (but low renal clearance may limit its usefulness).

It's also useful in some dermatophytoses, including tinea capitis, tinea cruris, tinea pedis, tinea manus, and tinea unguium (onychomycosis) caused by *Epidermophyton, Microsporum,* or *Trichophyton.*

Pharmacokinetics
Absorption: Converted to the hydrochloride salt before absorption. Absorption is erratic; it's decreased by raised gastric pH and may be increased in extent and consistency by food.
Distribution: Distributed into bile, saliva, cerumen, synovial fluid, and sebum; CSF penetration is erratic and considered minimal. It is 84% to 99% bound to plasma proteins.
Metabolism: Converted into several inactive metabolites in the liver.
Excretion: More than 50% of a dose is excreted in feces within 4 days; drug and metabolites are secreted in bile. About 13% is excreted unchanged in urine. It probably appears in breast milk. Half-life is biphasic, initially 2 hours, with a terminal half-life of 8 hours.

Route	Onset	Peak	Duration
P.O.	Unknown	1-4 hr	Unknown
Topical	Unknown	Unknown	Unknown

Contraindications and precautions
Contraindicated in patients hypersensitive to drug and in those taking oral triazolam because of risk of serious CV adverse events. Use oral form cautiously in patients with hepatic disease. Because CSF levels of ketoconazole are unpredictable after oral use, don't use drug alone to treat fungal meningitis.

Interactions
Drug-drug. *Benzodiazepines:* Increased levels of these drugs, prolonging sedative effect and increasing risk of toxicity. Use together cautiously.
Buspirone, carbamazepine, donepezil, nisoldipine, protease inhibitors, quinidine, zolpidem: Increased levels of these drugs and risk for toxicity. Monitor patient closely.

Reactions may be *common*, uncommon, *life-threatening*, or COMMON AND LIFE-THREATENING.

Corticosteroids: May increase corticosteroid levels. Monitor patient carefully.

Cyclosporine: Drug may raise cyclosporine levels by interfering with metabolism. Monitor patient closely.

Drugs that raise gastric pH (antacids, anti-muscarinic agents, cimetidine, famotidine, ranitidine): Decreased ketoconazole absorption. Give these drugs 2 hours after ketoconazole.

Hepatotoxic drugs: Drug may enhance toxicity. Monitor patient closely.

Oral sulfonylureas: Effects of sulfonylureas may be intensified. Monitor patient closely.

Phenytoin: Serum levels of both drugs may be altered. Monitor patient response to medication; monitor drug levels.

Rifampin: May decrease ketoconazole and rifampin levels to ineffective levels. Avoid use if possible.

Tacrolimus: Increased tacrolimus levels. Use cautiously. Monitor renal function and tacrolimus level.

Warfarin: May enhance anticoagulant effect. Monitor PT and INR.

Drug-herb. *Yew preparations:* Inhibited ketoconazole metabolism. Discourage use together.

Drug-lifestyle. *Alcohol use:* May cause a disulfiram-like reaction. Advise patient to avoid alcohol.

Adverse reactions

CNS: headache, nervousness, dizziness, somnolence, photophobia, *suicidal tendencies,* severe depression (with oral administration).
GI: *nausea, vomiting,* abdominal pain, diarrhea (with oral administration).
GU: impotence (with oral administration).
Hematologic: *thrombocytopenia,* hemolytic anemia, *leukopenia* (with oral administration).
Hepatic: elevated liver enzyme levels, *fatal hepatotoxicity* (with oral administration).
Skin: pruritus; severe irritation, stinging (with topical administration).
Other: gynecomastia with tenderness, fever, chills.

Overdose and treatment

Overdose may cause dizziness, tinnitus, headache, nausea, vomiting, or diarrhea; patients with adrenal hypofunction or patients on long-term corticosteroid therapy may show signs of adrenal crisis.

Treatment includes induced emesis and sodium bicarbonate lavage, followed by activated charcoal and a cathartic; supportive measures as needed.

Special considerations

● Identify organism, but don't delay therapy for laboratory test results.
● Give oral form with citrus juice.
● Oral drug requires acidity for absorption; adjust administration for patients with achlorhydria.

Patient monitoring

● Watch for signs of hepatotoxicity: persistent nausea, unusual fatigue, jaundice, dark urine, and pale stools.

Pregnant patients

● Ketoconazole shouldn't be given to pregnant women.

Breast-feeding patients

● Drug may appear in breast milk. Alternative feeding methods are recommended.

Pediatric patients

● Safe use in children under age 2 hasn't been established. Consider use in children only when the benefits outweigh the risks.

Patient education

● Instruct achlorhydric patient to dissolve each tablet in 4 ml of 0.2 N hydrochloric acid solution or take with 200 ml of 0.1 N hydrochloric acid. Tell patient to use a glass or plastic straw to avoid damaging tooth enamel and to follow each dose with a glass of water.
● Tell patient to avoid driving or performing other hazardous activities if dizziness or drowsiness occur; these often occur early in treatment but abate as treatment continues.
● Caution patient not to alter dose or dosage interval or to discontinue drug without medical approval; to prevent recurrence, therapy must continue until active fungal infection is completely eradicated.
● Reassure patient that nausea will subside; to minimize reaction, patient may take drug with food or may divide dosage into two doses.
● Advise patient to avoid preparations for GI distress (such as antacids); some may alter gastric pH levels and interfere with drug action.
● Caution patient concerning drug-drug and drug-herb interactions.

---

ketoprofen
Orudis, Orudis KT

Pharmacologic classification: NSAID
Therapeutic classification: nonnarcotic analgesic, antipyretic, anti-inflammatory
Pregnancy risk category: B

Indications and dosages

➤ *Rheumatoid arthritis and osteoarthritis. Adults:* 75 mg P.O. t.i.d. or 50 mg q i.d. Maximum dose is 300 mg daily or 200 mg (extended-release capsules) P.O. daily.
➤ *Mild to moderate pain; dysmenorrhea. Adults:* 25 to 50 mg P.O. q 6 to 8 hours, p.r.n.
➤ *Temporary relief of mild aches and pain, fever. Adults:* 12.5 mg q 4 to 6 hours. Don't exceed 75 mg in a 24-hour period.
✦ *Dosage adjustment.* In patients with mildly impaired renal function, maximum total daily

dose is 150 mg. In patients with more severe renal impairment (GFR less than 25 ml/minute) or hepatic dysfunction, the maximum total daily dose is 100 mg.

How supplied
Available by prescription only
Capsules: 25 mg, 50 mg, 75 mg
Capsules (extended-release): 100 mg, 150 mg, 200 mg
Available without a prescription
Tablets: 12.5 mg

Pharmacodynamics
Analgesic, antipyretic, and anti-inflammatory actions: Mechanisms of action are unknown; ketoprofen is thought to inhibit prostaglandin synthesis.

Pharmacokinetics
Absorption: Absorbed rapidly and completely from the GI tract.
Distribution: Highly protein-bound. Extent of body tissue fluid distribution isn't known, but therapeutic levels range from 0.4 to 6 mcg/ml.
Metabolism: Metabolized in the liver.
Excretion: Excreted in urine as parent drug and its metabolites.

Route	Onset	Peak	Duration
P.O.			
Regular	Unknown	1-2 hr	3-4 hr
Extended	Unknown	6-7 hr	Unknown

Contraindications and precautions
Contraindicated in patients hypersensitive to drug and those with a history of aspirin-induced or NSAID-induced asthma, urticaria, or other allergic-type reactions. Use cautiously in patients with impaired renal or hepatic function, peptic ulcer disease, heart failure, hypertension, or fluid retention.

Interactions
Drug-drug. *Acetaminophen, gold compounds, other anti-inflammatories:* Increased nephrotoxicity. Avoid use together.
Antihypertensives, diuretics: Decreased effectiveness of these drugs; increased nephrotoxic potential from diuretics. Don't use together.
Anti-inflammatories, corticosteroids, corticotropin, salicylates: May cause GI ulceration and hemorrhage. Avoid use together.
Aspirin: Decreased bioavailability of ketoprofen. Avoid use together.
Coumarin derivatives, heparin, nifedipine, phenytoin, streptokinase, urokinase, verapamil: Increased risk of bleeding and toxicity. Monitor patient, PT, and INR closely.
Drugs that inhibit platelet aggregation, such as aspirin, parenteral carbenicillin, cefamandole, cefoperazone, dextran, dipyridamole, mezlocillin, piperacillin, plicamycin, salicylates, sulfinpyrazone, ticarcillin, valproic acid, or other anti-inflammatories: Bleeding problems may occur. Monitor patient for signs of bleeding.
Insulin, oral antidiabetics: Because of the influence of prostaglandins on glucose metabolism, concurrent use may potentiate hypoglycemic effects. Monitor blood glucose levels.
Lithium, methotrexate: Decreased renal clearance of lithium and methotrexate. Monitor patient closely
Drug-herb. *Dong quai, feverfew, garlic, ginkgo, ginger, horse chestnut, red clover:* May increase the risk of bleeding. Discourage use together.
Drug-lifestyle: *Alcohol use:* Increased GI adverse effects, including ulceration and hemorrhage. Advise patient to avoid alcohol.
Prolonged sun exposure: Increased risk of photosensitive reaction. Advise patient to take precautions.

Adverse reactions
CNS: headache, dizziness, CNS excitation or depression.
EENT: tinnitus, visual disturbances.
GI: nausea, abdominal pain, diarrhea, constipation, flatulence, *dyspepsia,* anorexia, vomiting, stomatitis, ***peptic ulceration.***
GU: ***nephrotoxicity,*** elevated BUN level.
Hematologic: prolonged bleeding time, ***thrombocytopenia, agranulocytosis.***
Hepatic: elevated liver enzyme levels.
Respiratory: dyspnea, ***bronchospasm, laryngeal edema.***
Skin: rash, photosensitivity, exfoliative dermatitis.
Other: peripheral edema.

Overdose and treatment
Signs and symptoms of overdose include nausea and drowsiness. Induce emesis with ipecac syrup or empty the stomach via gastric lavage; administer activated charcoal via nasogastric tube. Provide symptomatic and supportive measures (respiratory support and correction of fluid and electrolyte imbalances). Monitor laboratory parameters and vital signs closely. Hemodialysis may be useful in removing ketoprofen and assisting in care of renal failure.

Special considerations
Consider the recommendations relevant to all NSAIDs as well as the following.
● Administer tablets on an empty stomach either 30 minutes before or 2 hours after meals to ensure adequate absorption. However, capsules may be taken with foods or antacids to minimize GI distress.
● In vitro interactions with glucose determinations have been reported with glucose oxidase and peroxidase methods resulting in falsely elevated blood glucose concentrations.
● Ketoprofen may interfere with serum iron determination (false increases or decreases depending on method used), and may cause falsely elevated serum bilirubin concentrations.

Reactions may be *common*, uncommon, ***life-threatening***, or COMMON AND LIFE-THREATENING.

Patient monitoring
• Monitor patient for CNS effects and possible photosensitivity reactions.
• Monitor laboratory test results for abnormalities.

Breast-feeding patients
• Most NSAIDs appear in breast milk; however, distribution of ketoprofen is unknown. Avoid use of ketoprofen in breast-feeding women.

Pediatric patients
• Safe use in children under age 12 hasn't been established.

Geriatric patients
• Patients over age 60 may be more susceptible to toxic effects of ketoprofen. Use cautiously. The effects of drug on renal prostaglandins may cause fluid retention and edema, a significant drawback for geriatric patients and those with heart failure. The manufacturer recommends reducing initial dose by 33% to 50% in geriatric patients.

Patient education
• Instruct patient in prescribed drug regimen and proper medication administration, to avoid alcoholic beverages during therapy, and to report adverse reactions.
• Tell patient to seek medical approval before taking OTC medications (especially aspirin and aspirin-containing products).
• Caution patient to avoid activities that require alertness or concentration; stress need for safety measures to prevent injury.
• Advise patient of potential photosensitivity reactions. Recommend use of sunscreen.

ketorolac tromethamine
Toradol

Pharmacologic classification: NSAID
Therapeutic classification: analgesic
Pregnancy risk category: C

Indications and dosages
➤ *Short-term management of severe, acute pain. Adults under age 65:* Dosage should be based on patient response; initially, 60 mg I.M. or 30 mg I.V. as a single dose, or multiple doses of 30 mg I.M. or I.V. q 6 hours. Maximum daily dose shouldn't exceed 120 mg.
✦ *Dosage adjustment.* In patients age 65 or older, renally impaired patients, and those who weigh less than 50 kg (110 lb), 30 mg I.M. or 15 mg I.V. initially as a single dose, or multiple doses of 15 mg I.M. or I.V. q 6 hours. Maximum daily dose shouldn't exceed 60 mg.
➤ *Short-term management of moderately severe, acute pain when switching from parenteral to oral administration. Adults under age 65:* 20 mg P.O. as a single dose fol-

lowed by 10 mg P.O. q 4 to 6 hours, not to exceed 40 mg daily.
✦ *Dosage adjustment.* In patients age 65 or older, renally impaired patients, and those who weigh less than 50 kg (110 lb), 10 mg P.O. as a single dose, followed by 10 mg P.O. q 4 to 6 hours, not to exceed 40 mg daily.

How supplied
Available by prescription only
Injection: 15 mg/ml (1-ml cartridge), 30 mg/ml (1-ml and 2-ml cartridges)
Tablets: 10 mg

Pharmacodynamics
Analgesic action: Ketorolac is an NSAID that acts by inhibiting the synthesis of prostaglandins.

Pharmacokinetics
Absorption: Completely absorbed after I.M. administration. After oral administration, food delays absorption but doesn't decrease total amount of drug absorbed.
Distribution: Mean peak plasma levels occur about 30 minutes after a 50-mg dose and range from 2.2 to 3 mcg/ml. More than 99% of drug is protein-bound.
Metabolism: Metabolism is primarily hepatic; a para-hydroxy metabolite and conjugates have been identified; less than 50% of a dose is metabolized. Liver impairment doesn't substantially alter drug clearance.
Excretion: More than 90% is excreted in urine; the rest in feces. Terminal plasma half-life is 3¾ to 6⅓ hours (average 4½ hours) in young adults; it's substantially prolonged in patients with renal failure.

Route	Onset	Peak	Duration
P.O.	½-1 hr	½-1 hr	6-8 hr
I.V.	Immediate	Immediate	6-8 hr
I.M.	10 min	½-1 hr	6-8 hr

Contraindications and precautions
Contraindicated in patients hypersensitive to drug and those with active peptic ulcer disease, recent GI bleeding or perforation, advanced renal impairment, risk for renal impairment due to volume depletion, suspected or confirmed cerebrovascular bleeding, hemorrhagic diathesis, incomplete hemostasis, or high risk of bleeding.

Also contraindicated in patients with history of peptic ulcer disease or GI bleeding, past allergic reactions to aspirin or other NSAIDs, and during labor and delivery or breast-feeding. In addition, drug is contraindicated as prophylactic analgesic before major surgery or intraoperatively when hemostasis is critical; in patients receiving aspirin, an NSAID, or probenecid; and in those requiring analgesics to be administered epidurally or intrathecally.

Use cautiously in patients with impaired renal or hepatic function.

Interactions
Drug-drug. *Diuretics:* Decreased diuretic efficacy and increased risk of nephrotoxicity. Monitor patient closely.
Lithium: Decreased renal clearance of lithium, increasing lithium levels and risk of lithium toxicity. Avoid use together, if possible. If given together, closely monitor lithium levels.
Methotrexate: Elevated and prolonged methotrexate levels, possibly leading to toxicity. Avoid use together.
NSAIDs: Elevated ketorolac levels with potential for cumulative adverse effects. Avoid use together.
Probenecid: Decreased clearance and increased levels of ketorolac. Avoid use together.
Salicylates, warfarin: Increased blood levels of these drugs. Use with extreme caution; monitor patient closely.
Drug-lifestyle. *Alcohol use:* Increased GI effects, including ulceration and hemorrhage. Advise patient to avoid alcohol.

Adverse reactions
CNS: *drowsiness, sedation,* dizziness, *headache.*
CV: edema, hypertension, palpitations, ***arrhythmias.***
GI: *nausea, dyspepsia, GI pain,* diarrhea, peptic ulceration, vomiting, constipation, flatulence, stomatitis.
GU: *renal failure.*
Hematologic: decreased platelet adhesion, purpura, ***thrombocytopenia.***
Skin: pain at injection site, pruritus, rash, diaphoresis.

Overdose and treatment
Overdose hasn't been reported. Withhold drug and provide supportive treatment.

Special considerations
● Hypovolemia should be corrected before starting therapy with ketorolac.
● The combined duration of ketorolac I.M., I.V., or P.O. shouldn't exceed 5 days. Oral use is only for continuation of I.V. or I.M. therapy.

Patient monitoring
● I.M. injections in patients with coagulopathies or those receiving anticoagulants may cause bleeding and hematoma at the injection site.

Breast-feeding patients
● Because drug appears in breast milk, its use is contraindicated in breast-feeding women.

Pediatric patients
● Drug isn't recommended for children because safety and efficacy haven't been established.

Geriatric patients
● Use lower initial doses (30 mg I.M.) in patients over age 65 or who weigh less than 110 lb. In clinical trials, elderly patients exhibit a longer terminal half-life of drug (average 7 hours compared with 4½ hours in healthy young adults).

Patient education
● Instruct patient to avoid aspirin, aspirin-containing products, and alcoholic beverages during therapy.
● Warn patient that GI ulceration, bleeding, and perforation can occur at any time, with or without warning, in anyone taking NSAIDs on a long-term basis. Inform patient of signs and symptoms of GI bleeding.

ketorolac tromethamine (ophthalmic)
Acular

Pharmacologic classification: NSAID
Therapeutic classification: ophthalmic anti-inflammatory
Pregnancy risk category: C

Indications and dosages
➤ ***Relief of ocular itching caused by seasonal allergic conjunctivitis.*** Adults: Instill 1 drop (0.25 mg) in conjunctival sac q.i.d. Efficacy hasn't been established beyond 1 week of continued use.
➤ ***Treatment of postoperative inflammation following cataract extraction.*** Adults: Instill 1 gtt in the affected eye q.i.d. for 2 weeks beginning 24 hours after surgery.

How supplied
Available by prescription only
Ophthalmic solution: 0.5%

Pharmacodynamics
Anti-inflammatory action: Anti-inflammatory action of ketorolac tromethamine is thought to be a result, in part, of its ability to inhibit prostaglandin biosynthesis. Drug reduces prostaglandin E_2 levels in aqueous humor with ocular administration. It also has demonstrated analgesic and antipyretic activity because of the same mechanism of action.

Pharmacokinetics
No information available.

Route	Onset	Peak	Duration
Oph-thalmic	Unknown	Unknown	Unknown

Contraindications and precautions
Contraindicated in patients hypersensitive to any component of the formulation and in those who wear soft contact lenses. Use cautiously in patients hypersensitive to other NSAIDs or aspirin and in those with bleeding disorders.

Interactions
None reported.

Adverse reactions
EENT: *transient stinging and burning on instillation*, superficial keratitis, superficial ocular infections, ocular irritation, ocular dryness.
Other: *hypersensitivity reactions.*

Overdose and treatment
Overdose ordinarily doesn't cause acute problems. If accidentally ingested, have the patient drink fluids to dilute.

Special considerations
● Ophthalmic solution has been safely administered in conjunction with other ophthalmic medications, such as antibiotics, beta blockers, carbonic anhydrase inhibitors, cycloplegics, and mydriatics.
● Store drug at controlled room temperature and protect from light.

Patient monitoring
● Monitor patient for adverse reactions, including superficial ocular infections and hypersensitivity reactions.

Breast-feeding patients
● Use cautiously in breast-feeding women.

Pediatric patients
● Safety and efficacy in children haven't been established.

Patient education
● Teach patient how to administer eye drops and stress importance of not touching dropper to eye or surrounding area.
● Advise patient not to use more drops than prescribed and to use only as prescribed.

---

ketotifen fumarate
Zaditor

Pharmacologic classification: histamine (H_1-receptor) antagonist and mast cell stabilizer
Therapeutic classification: ophthalmic antihistamine
Pregnancy risk category: C

Indications and dosages
➤ *Temporary prevention of ocular itching caused by allergic conjunctivitis.*
Adults and children age 3 and older: Instill one drop in affected eye q 8 to 12 hours.

How supplied
Available by prescription only
Ophthalmic solution: 0.025%; supplied as 5-ml solution in 7.5-ml bottles

Pharmacodynamics
Antihistamine action: Selective, noncompetitive histamine antagonist (H_1-receptor) and mast cell stabilizer that inhibits release of me-

diators from cells involved in hypersensitivity reactions, thus providing temporary prevention of eye itching.

Pharmacokinetics
Absorption: Effect occurs within minutes after administration.
Distribution: No information available.
Metabolism: No information available.
Excretion: No information available.

Route	Onset	Peak	Duration
Oph-thalmic	Minutes	Unknown	Unknown

Contraindications and precautions
Contraindicated in patients hypersensitive to drug or its component.

Interactions
None reported.

Adverse reactions
CNS: *headache.*
EENT: *conjunctival infection, rhinitis*, ocular allergic reactions, burning or stinging of eyes, conjunctivitis, eye discharge, dry eyes, eye pain, eyelid disorder, itching of eyes, keratitis, lacrimation disorder, mydriasis, photophobia, ocular rash, pharyngitis.
Other: flu syndrome.

Special considerations
● Drug is for ophthalmic use only, and not for injection or oral use.
● Drug isn't indicated for irritation caused by contact lenses.
● Preservative in drug may be absorbed by soft contact lenses. Contact lenses shouldn't be inserted until 10 minutes after drug is instilled.

Patient monitoring
● Monitor patient for sensitivity reactions.
● Monitor patient for signs of infection.

Breast-feeding patients
● It's unknown whether topical ocular product appears in breast milk. Use cautiously in breast-feeding women.

Pediatric patients
● Safety and effectiveness in children below age 3 haven't been established.

Patient education
● Teach patient proper instillation technique. Tell him to avoid contaminating dropper tip and solution and not to touch eyelids or surrounding areas with dropper tip of bottle.
● Tell patient not to wear contact lenses if eyes are red. Warn patient not to use drug to treat irritation related to contact lenses.
● Instruct patient who wears soft contact lenses and whose eyes aren't red to wait at least 10 min-

utes after instilling drug before inserting contact lenses.
• Advise patient to report adverse reactions to drug.
• Advise patient to keep bottle tightly closed when not in use.

labetalol hydrochloride
Normodyne, Trandate

Pharmacologic classification: alpha and beta blocker
Therapeutic classification: antihypertensive
Pregnancy risk category: C

Indications and dosages
➤*Hypertension, pheochromocytoma.*
Adults: 100 mg P.O. b.i.d. with or without a diuretic. Dosage may be increased by 100 mg b.i.d. q 2 or 3 days until optimum response is reached. Usual maintenance dosage is 200 to 600 mg b.i.d.; maximum daily dose is 2,400 mg.
➤*Severe hypertension and hypertensive emergencies, clonidine withdrawal hypertension*◇. *Adults:* Initially, 20 to 80 mg I.V. bolus slowly over 2 minutes; may repeat injections of 40 to 80 mg q 10 minutes to maximum dose of 300 mg. Or, drug may be given as continuous I.V. infusion at 0.5 to 2 mg/minute until satisfactory response is obtained. Usual effective, cumulative dose is 50 to 200 mg, although up to 300 mg may be required.
Oral dose following I.V. therapy: 200 mg P.O. followed by 200 to 400 mg in 6 to 12 hours (depending on blood pressure response); then increase in usual increments at 1-day intervals while patient is hospitalized to achieve desired effects.
➤*Controlled hypotension during anesthesia*◇. *Adults:* Initially, 10 to 30 mg I.V. bolus slowly; may repeat injections of 5 to 10 mg I.V., p.r.n.
✦*Dosage adjustment.* In geriatric patients, use a lower maintenance dosage of 100 to 200 mg P.O. b.i.d.

How supplied
Available by prescription only
Injection: 5 mg/ml in 20-, 40-, and 60-ml vials and 4- and 8-ml disposable syringes
Tablets: 100 mg, 200 mg, 300 mg

Pharmacodynamics
Antihypertensive action: Labetalol inhibits catecholamine access to both beta- and postsynaptic alpha-adrenergic receptor sites. Drug also may have a vasodilating effect.

Pharmacokinetics
Absorption: Oral absorption is high (90% to 100%); however, drug undergoes extensive first-pass metabolism in the liver and only about 25% of an oral dose reaches systemic circulation unchanged.

Distribution: Distributed widely throughout the body; about 50% protein-bound.
Metabolism: Orally administered drug is metabolized extensively in the liver and possibly in GI mucosa.
Excretion: About 5% of a dose is excreted unchanged in urine; remainder is excreted as metabolites in urine and feces (biliary elimination). Plasma half-life is about 5½ hours after I.V. administration or 6 to 8 hours after oral administration.

Route	Onset	Peak	Duration
P.O.	20 min	2-4 hr	8-12 hr
I.V.	2-5 min	5 min	2-4 hr

Contraindications and precautions
Contraindicated in patients hypersensitive to drug, patients with severe and prolonged hypotension, patients with a history of obstructive airway disease such as bronchial asthma, and patients with overt cardiac failure, greater than first-degree heart block, cardiogenic shock, or severe bradycardia.

Use cautiously in patients with heart failure, hepatic failure, chronic bronchitis, emphysema, peripheral vascular disease, and pheochromocytoma.

Interactions
Drug-drug. *Beta-adrenergic agonists:* Labetalol may antagonize bronchodilation produced by these drugs. Avoid use together.
Cimetidine: May increase bioavailability of oral labetalol. If used together, labetalol dosage may need adjustment.
Diuretics and other antihypertensives: Labetalol may potentiate antihypertensive effects of these drugs. Patient requires close monitoring.
Glutethimide: May decrease bioavailability of oral labetalol. Adjust labetalol dosage as needed.
Halothane: Synergistic antihypertensive effect and significant myocardial depression. Monitor patient closely.
Nitroglycerin: Labetalol blunts the reflex tachycardia produced by nitroglycerin without preventing its hypotensive effect. In patients with angina, additional antihypertensive effects may occur. Use cautiously.
Tricyclic antidepressants: May increase risk of labetalol-induced tremor. Avoid use together.

Adverse reactions
CNS: vivid dreams, fatigue, headache, paresthesia, syncope.
CV: *orthostatic hypotension, dizziness, ventricular arrhythmias.*
EENT: nasal stuffiness.
GI: nausea, vomiting, diarrhea.
GU: sexual dysfunction, urine retention.
Hepatic: elevated liver enzyme levels.
Musculoskeletal: muscle spasm, toxic myopathy.
Respiratory: dyspnea, *bronchospasm.*
Skin: rash, transient scalp tingling.

Reactions may be *common*, uncommon, *life-threatening*, or COMMON AND LIFE-THREATENING.

Overdose and treatment

Signs and symptoms of overdose include severe hypotension, bradycardia, heart failure, and bronchospasm.

After acute ingestion, empty stomach by induced emesis or gastric lavage, and give activated charcoal to reduce absorption. Subsequent treatment is usually symptomatic and supportive.

Special considerations

• Unlike other beta blockers, labetalol doesn't decrease resting heart rate or cardiac output.

• Dosage may need to be reduced in patients with hepatic insufficiency and severe renal impairment.

• Dizziness, a troublesome adverse effect, tends to occur in early stages of treatment and in patients taking diuretics or receiving higher doses.

• Ejaculation failure, impotence, and decreased libido have been reported in men.

• It may be more cost-effective for patient to take drug twice daily rather than once daily.

• For I.V. infusion, dilute labetalol injection to an appropriate concentration (such as 200 mg of drug added to 160 ml of solution to provide a concentration of 1 mg/ml). Administer using a controlled infusion device.

• Don't mix labetalol with 5% sodium bicarbonate injection because of incompatibility; avoid giving drug in same infusion line with other alkaline solutions (such as furosemide).

• Patients receiving I.V. labetalol infusion must be kept in the supine position during the infusion and for 3 hours after the infusion.

• Store tablets and injection at 36° to 86° F (2° to 30° C) and protect from light, moisture, and freezing.

• Drug may cause a false-positive increase of urine free and total catecholamine levels when measured by a nonspecific trihydroxindole fluorometric method.

Patient monitoring

• Use specific radioenzyme or high-performance liquid chromatography assay techniques to reduce risk of false-positive urine free and total catecholamine levels.

• Blood pressure must be closely monitored during and after I.V. infusion; after infusion, monitor blood pressure every 5 minutes for 30 minutes, then at 30-minute intervals for 2 hours, then hourly for 6 hours.

• During direct I.V. infusion, monitor blood pressure before and at 5-minute intervals after each injection; maximum hypotensive effect usually occurs in 5 to 15 minutes after each injection.

Pregnant patients

• Labetalol has been effective for managing hypertension related to pregnancy and for reduced proteinuria and prevention of eclampsia. Rarely, transient hypotension, bradycardia, respiratory depression, and hypoglycemia have occurred in neonates.

Breast-feeding patients

• Small amounts of drug appear in breast milk; use cautiously in breast-feeding women.

Pediatric patients

• Safety and efficacy in children haven't been established; use drug only if potential benefit outweighs risk.

Geriatric patients

• These patients may need reduced maintenance dosages because of increased bioavailability or delayed metabolism; they also may experience enhanced adverse effects. Use drug cautiously in elderly patients.

Patient education

• Advise patient that transient scalp tingling may occur at start of therapy but that it usually subsides quickly.

• Tell patient to take drug as prescribed to maintain adequate blood pressure control.

lactulose
Cephulac, Cholac, Chronulac, Constilac, Constulose, Duphalac, Enulose, Heptalac, Kristalose

Pharmacologic classification: disaccharide
Therapeutic classification: laxative
Pregnancy risk category: B

Indications and dosages

➤ **Constipation.** *Adults:* 10 to 20 g P.O. daily (may increase to 40 g if needed).
Children◊: 5 g P.O. daily as single dose after breakfast.

➤ **To prevent and treat portal-systemic encephalopathy, including hepatic precoma and coma in patients with severe hepatic disease.** *Adults:* Initially, 20 to 30 g (30 to 45 ml) P.O. t.i.d. or q.i.d., until two or three soft stools are produced daily. Usual dosage is 60 to 100 g daily in divided doses. Also can be given by retention enema. Mix 200 g of lactulose with 700 ml of water or normal saline solution for retention for 60 minutes. May repeat q 4 to 6 hours. May repeat immediately if retention is less than 30 minutes.
Infants: Initially, 1.67 to 6.67 g P.O. daily in divided doses. Adjust doses q 1 to 2 days to produce two to three loose stools daily.
Older children and adolescents: Initially, 27 to 60 g P.O. daily in divided doses. Adjust doses q 1 to 2 days to produce two to three loose stools daily.

➤ **After barium meal examination◊.** *Adults:* 3.3 to 6.7 g P.O. b.i.d. for 1 to 4 weeks.

➤ **To restore bowel movements after hemorrhoidectomy◊.** *Adults:* 10 g P.O. twice during day before surgery and for 5 days postoperatively.

How supplied
Available by prescription only
Powder: 10 g/packet, 20 g/packet
Rectal solution: 3.33 g/5 ml
Syrup: 10 g/15 ml

Pharmacodynamics
Laxative action: Because lactulose is indigestible, it passes through the GI tract to the colon unchanged; there, it's digested by normally occurring bacteria. The weak acids produced in this manner increase the fluid content of the stool and cause distention, thus promoting peristalsis and bowel evacuation.

Lactulose also is used to reduce serum ammonia levels in patients with hepatic disease. Lactulose breakdown acidifies the colon, which, in turn, converts ammonia (NH_3) to ammonium (NH_4+), which isn't absorbed and is excreted in the stool. Furthermore, this "ion trapping" effect causes ammonia to diffuse from the blood into the colon, where it's excreted as well.

Pharmacokinetics
Absorption: Absorbed minimally.
Distribution: Distributed locally, primarily in the colon.
Metabolism: Metabolized by colonic bacteria (absorbed portion isn't metabolized).
Excretion: Mostly excreted in feces; absorbed portion is excreted in urine.

Route	Onset	Peak	Duration
P.O.	24-48 hr	Variable	Variable
P.R.	Unknown	Unknown	Unknown

Contraindications and precautions
Contraindicated in patients on a low-galactose diet. Use cautiously in patients with diabetes mellitus. Use cautiously in patients who may require electrocautery procedures during proctoscopy or colonoscopy.

Interactions
Drug-drug. *Neomycin and other antibiotics:* May decrease lactulose effectiveness by eliminating bacteria needed to digest it into the active form. Monitor patient for effect.
Nonabsorbable antacids: May decrease lactulose effectiveness by preventing a decrease in the pH of the colon. Avoid use together.

Adverse reactions
GI: *abdominal cramps, belching, gaseous distention, flatulence,* nausea, vomiting, *diarrhea* (with excessive dosage).

Overdose and treatment
No cases of overdose have been reported. Effects would include diarrhea and abdominal cramps.

Special considerations
● After giving drug through nasogastric tube, flush tube with water to clear it and ensure passage of drug to stomach.
● Dilute drug with water or fruit juice to minimize its sweet taste.
● For oral administration, reconstitute powder by dissolving 10- to 20-g packet in 120 ml of water.
● For administration by retention enema, patient should retain drug for 30 to 60 minutes. If retained less than 30 minutes, repeat dose immediately. Begin oral therapy before discontinuing retention enemas.
● Don't administer drug with other laxatives because resulting loose stools may falsely indicate adequate dosage of lactulose.
● Store at 59° to 86° F (15° to 30° C); avoid freezing.

Patient monitoring
● Monitor frequency and consistency of stools.
● Monitor serum potassium, chloride, and carbon dioxide in long-term treatment.

Breast-feeding patients
● It isn't known whether drug appears in breast milk. Use cautiously in breast-feeding women.

Geriatric patients
● Monitor patient's serum electrolyte levels; geriatric patients are more sensitive to possible hypernatremia.

Patient education
● Advise patient to take drug with juice to improve taste.
● Instruct patient to contact prescriber if unusual diarrhea condition occurs.

---

lamivudine (3TC)
Epivir, Epivir-HBV

Pharmacologic classification: synthetic nucleoside analogue
Therapeutic classification: antiviral
Pregnancy risk category: C

Indications and dosages
➤ *Treatment of patients with HIV infection (should be used with other antiretroviral agents).* *Adults who weigh 50 kg (110 lb) or more and children age 16 and older:* 150 mg P.O. b.i.d.
Adults who weigh less than 50 kg (110 lb): 2 mg/kg P.O. b.i.d.
Children ages 3 months to 16 years: 4 mg/kg P.O. b.i.d. Maximum dosage is 150 mg b.i.d.
Neonates age 30 days and younger ◇ : 2 mg/kg P.O. b.i.d.
✦ *Dosage adjustment.* For adults and adolescents with renal impairment, refer to the table on page 725.

Reactions may be *common,* uncommon, *life-threatening,* or COMMON AND LIFE-THREATENING.

Creatinine clearance (ml/min)	Recommended dosage
30-49	150 mg once daily
15-29	150 mg first dose; then 100 mg once daily
5-14	150 mg first dose; then 50 mg once daily
< 5	50 mg first; then 25 mg once daily

In children with renal impairment, consider decreasing the dose or increasing the dosage interval.

▶ *Treatment of chronic hepatitis B with evidence of hepatitis B viral replication and active liver inflammation.* Adults: 100 mg P.O. once daily. Safety and efficacy of treatment beyond 1 year haven't been established; optimum duration of treatment isn't known. Formulation and dosage of lamivudine in Epivir-HBV aren't appropriate for those dually infected with hepatitis B virus (HBV) and HIV; test patients for HIV before starting treatment. If lamivudine is administered to patients with HBV and HIV, use the higher dosage indicated for HIV therapy as part of an appropriate combination regimen.

✦ *Dosage adjustment.* In patients age 16 and older with renal impairment, if creatinine clearance is 30 to 49 ml/minute, 100 mg P.O. on the first day, then 50 mg P.O. once daily thereafter. If clearance is 15 to 29 ml/minute, 100 mg on the first day, then 25 mg P.O. once daily thereafter. If clearance is 5 to 14 ml/minute, 35 mg on the first day, then 15 mg once daily thereafter. If creatinine clearance is less than 5 ml/minute, 35 mg on the first day, then 10 mg P.O. once daily thereafter.

▶ *Post-exposure prophylaxis following occupational exposure to HIV ◇.* Adults: 150 mg P.O. b.i.d. with oral zidovudine (600 mg daily); oral indinavir (800 mg q 8 hours) or oral nelfinavir (750 mg P.O. t.i.d.) is added if risk of transmission is likely. Initiate within a few hours and continue for 28 days.

How supplied
Available by prescription only
Epivir
Oral solution: 10 mg/ml
Tablets: 150 mg
Epivir-HBV
Oral solution: 5 mg/ml
Tablets: 100 mg

Pharmacodynamics
Antiviral action: Lamivudine inhibits HIV reverse transcription via viral DNA chain termination. RNA- and DNA-dependent DNA polymerase activities also are inhibited.

Pharmacokinetics
Absorption: Rapidly absorbed after oral administration in HIV- and HBV-infected patients.
Distribution: Believed to be distributed into extravascular spaces. Volume of distribution is independent of dose and doesn't correlate with body weight. Less than 36% is bound to plasma proteins.
Metabolism: Metabolism is minor route of elimination. The only known metabolite is the trans-sulfoxide metabolite.
Excretion: Primarily eliminated unchanged in urine. Mean elimination half-life is 5 to 7 hours.

Route	Onset	Peak	Duration
P.O.	Unknown	1-3 hr	Unknown

Contraindications and precautions
Contraindicated in patients hypersensitive to drug. Use drug with extreme caution and only if there's no satisfactory alternative therapy in children with history of pancreatitis or other significant risk factors for development of pancreatitis. Stop treatment with lamivudine immediately if clinical signs, symptoms, or laboratory abnormalities suggest pancreatitis.

Use cautiously and reduce dosage in children with a history of prior therapy with nucleoside reverse transcriptase inhibitors and in patients with impaired renal function.

Interactions
Drug-drug. *Co-trimoxazole:* Decreased clearance of lamivudine may cause increased blood levels of lamivudine. Monitor patient closely.

Adverse reactions
Adverse reactions are related to the combination therapy of lamivudine and zidovudine.
CNS: *malaise, headache, fatigue, neuropathy, dizziness, insomnia and other sleep disorders,* depressive disorders.
EENT: *nasal symptoms, sore throat.*
GI: *nausea, diarrhea, vomiting, anorexia,* abdominal pain, abdominal cramps, dyspepsia, *pancreatitis* (in children under age 12).
Hematologic: *neutropenia,* anemia, *thrombocytopenia.*
Hepatic: elevated liver enzyme and bilirubin levels.
Metabolic: lactic acidosis.
Musculoskeletal: *musculoskeletal pain,* myalgia, arthralgia.
Respiratory: *cough.*
Skin: rash.
Other: *fever, chills.*

Overdose and treatment
No information available.

Special considerations
● When used in treatment of HIV infection, drug must be administered with zidovudine. It isn't intended for use as monotherapy.

• Safety and efficacy of treatment of HBV for periods over 1 year or in patients with decompensated liver disease or organ transplant haven't been established.

• Monotherapy with lamivudine in patients with HIV-HBV co-infection in HBV dosage is inadequate and may lead to rapid emergence of HIV resistance. Counseling and testing for HIV infection before and periodically during treatment is recommended. Use higher dosage in combination therapy with other appropriate antiretroviral agents.

Patient monitoring
• Monitor CBC, platelet count, and liver function studies throughout therapy.
• Lactic acidosis and severe hepatomegaly with steatosis have been reported in patients receiving lamivudine. Stop treatment if signs of lactic acidosis or hepatotoxicity develop.

Pregnant patients
• An Antiretroviral Pregnancy Registry has been established to monitor maternal-fetal outcomes of pregnant women exposed to lamivudine. Pregnant patients can be registered by calling 1-800-258-4263.

Breast-feeding patients
• To avoid transmitting HIV to the infant, HIV-positive women shouldn't breast-feed.

Pediatric patients
• Safety and efficacy in treatment of HIV infection haven't been established in children younger than 3 months.

Patient education
• Inform patient that long-term effects of drug are unknown.
• Stress importance of taking drug exactly as prescribed.
• Instruct parents of children receiving drug about signs and symptoms of pancreatitis and tell them to report these immediately if they occur.
• Inform patients receiving dosage of less than therapeutic levels for HIV treatment that HIV testing is recommended.

---

lamivudine/zidovudine
Combivir

Pharmacologic classification: reverse transcriptase inhibitor
Therapeutic classification: antiretroviral
Pregnancy risk category: C

Indications and dosages
➤ *Treatment of HIV infection. Adults and children over age 12 and who weigh 50 kg (110 lb) or more:* One tablet P.O. b.i.d.

How supplied
Available by prescription only
Tablets: Each tablet contains 150 mg lamivudine and 300 mg zidovudine

Pharmacodynamics
Antiretroviral action: Lamivudine and zidovudine are phosphorylated intracellularly to active metabolites that inhibit reverse transcriptase by way of DNA chain termination. Both drugs are also weak inhibitors of mammalian DNA polymerase. Together, they have synergistic antiretroviral activity. Combination therapy with lamivudine and zidovudine aims to suppress or delay emergence of phenotypic and genotypic resistant strains that can occur with retroviral monotherapy, because more mutations are necessary to develop dual resistance.

Pharmacokinetics
Absorption: Both lamivudine and zidovudine are rapidly absorbed following oral administration with oral bioavailability of 86% and 64%, respectively.
Distribution: Both drugs are extensively distributed and exhibit low protein binding.
Metabolism: Only about 5% of lamivudine is metabolized whereas zidovudine is primarily (74%) metabolized in the liver.
Excretion: Lamivudine is primarily eliminated unchanged in the urine. Zidovudine and its major metabolite are primarily eliminated in the urine. Elimination half-lives of lamivudine and zidovudine are 5 to 7 hours and ¼ to 3 hours, respectively. Because renal excretion is a principal route of elimination, dosage adjustments are necessary in patients with compromised renal function, making this fixed ratio combination unsuitable. Hemodialysis and peritoneal dialysis have negligible effect on the removal of zidovudine, but removal of its metabolite, GZDV, is enhanced. The effect of dialysis on lamivudine is unknown.

Route	Onset	Peak	Duration
P.O.	Unknown	Unknown	Unknown

Contraindications and precautions
Contraindicated in patients hypersensitive to components of drug and in those who weigh less than 110 lb, those with creatinine clearance of less than 50 ml/minute, and those experiencing dose-limiting adverse effects.

Use cautiously in patients with bone marrow suppression or renal insufficiency.

Interactions
Drug-drug. *Atovaquone, fluconazole, methadone, probenecid, valproic acid:* Increased bioavailability of zidovudine. Dosage modification isn't needed.
Co-trimoxazole, nelfinavir: Increased lamivudine bioavailability. Dosage modification isn't needed.

Ganciclovir, interferon-alpha, and other bone marrow suppressive or cytotoxic agents: May increase hematologic toxicity of zidovudine. Most drug interaction studies haven't been completed. Use cautiously as with other reverse transcriptase inhibitors.

Nelfinavir, ritonavir: Decreased zidovudine bioavailability. Dosage modification isn't needed.

Adverse reactions
CNS: *headache,* malaise, *fatigue, insomnia, dizziness, neuropathy,* depression.
GI: *nausea, diarrhea, vomiting, anorexia,* abdominal pain, abdominal cramps, dyspepsia, *pancreatitis.*
EENT: *nasal signs and symptoms.*
Hematologic: *neutropenia,* anemia.
Metabolic: lactic acidosis.
Musculoskeletal: *musculoskeletal pain,* myalgia, arthralgia, myopathy, myositis.
Respiratory: *cough.*
Skin: rash.
Other: *fever, chills.*

Overdose and treatment
Overdose (6 g) with lamivudine results in normal hematologic tests and no clinical signs or symptoms. Overdoses of zidovudine, with exposure up to 50 g, results in only nausea and vomiting. No antidote is known for lamivudine/zidovudine overdose.

Special considerations
● Don't use combination drug therapy in patients who need dosage adjustments, such as children or patients with renal dysfunction.
● Combination may be given with or without food.
● Lactic acidosis and severe hepatomegaly with steatosis have been reported in patients receiving lamivudine and zidovudine alone and in combination. Stop treatment if signs of lactic acidosis or hepatotoxicity develop. Hepatotoxic events may be more severe in patients with decompensated liver function due to hepatitis B.
● Myopathy and myositis may result from prolonged use of zidovudine.

Patient monitoring
● Monitor patient for bone marrow toxicity with frequent blood counts, particularly in patients with advanced HIV infection.
● Monitor patient for signs of lactic acidosis and hepatotoxicity.
● Monitor patient's fine motor skills and peripheral sensation for evidence of peripheral neuropathies.

Pregnant patients
● Call 1-800-722-9292 to register patients exposed to Combivir during pregnancy.

Breast-feeding patients
● Although zidovudine appears in breast milk at levels similar to those in serum, it isn't known whether lamivudine/zidovudine appears in breast milk.

Pediatric patients
● Don't use in patients under age 12 because the fixed-dose combination treatment can't be adjusted for this patient group.

Geriatric patients
● Safety and efficacy in patients over age 65 haven't been established.

Patient education
● Advise patient that combination drug therapy isn't a cure for HIV infection, and that he may continue to experience illness including opportunistic infections.
● Warn patient that transmission of HIV virus can still occur with drug therapy.
● Teach patient signs and symptoms of neutropenia and anemia, and instruct him to report such occurrences.
● Advise patient to consult prescriber before taking other medications.
● Warn patient to report abdominal pain immediately.
● Stress importance of taking combination drug therapy exactly as prescribed to reduce the development of resistance.

lamotrigine
Lamictal

Pharmacologic classification: phenyltriazine
Therapeutic classification: anticonvulsant
Pregnancy risk category: C

Indications and dosages
➤ *Adjunct therapy for partial seizures caused by epilepsy and Lennox-Gastaut syndrome.* *Adults and children age 16 and older (12 and older for Lennox-Gastaut syndrome):* 50 mg P.O. daily for 2 weeks, followed by 100 mg daily in two divided doses for 2 weeks. Thereafter, usual maintenance dosage is 300 to 500 mg P.O. daily given in two divided doses. For patients also taking valproic acid, give 25 mg P.O. every other day for 2 weeks, followed by 25 mg P.O. daily for 2 weeks. Thereafter, increase 25 to 50 mg q 1 to 2 weeks. Effective maintenance dosage is 100 to 400 mg daily in one or two divided doses.
➤ *Adjunct treatment of Lennox-Gastaut syndrome in patients receiving hepatic-enzyme-inducing anticonvulsant drugs without concomitant valproic acid therapy.* *Children ages 2 to 12:* 0.6 mg/kg P.O. daily (rounded down to the nearest 5 mg) in two divided doses for 2 weeks. During subsequent 2 weeks, 1.2 mg/kg (rounded down to the nearest 5 mg) daily in two divided doses. Then, increase q 1 to 2 weeks by 1.2 mg/kg (rounded down to the nearest 5 mg) until effective daily dose of

about 5 to 15 mg/kg (maximum of 400 mg daily in two divided doses) is reached.

➤ *Adjunct treatment of Lennox-Gastaut syndrome in patients receiving hepatic-enzyme-inducing anticonvulsant drugs with concomitant valproic acid therapy.* *Children ages 2 to 12:* 0.15 mg/kg P.O. daily (rounded down to the nearest 5 mg) in one or two divided doses for 2 weeks. If the initial calculated daily dose of lamotrigine is 2.5 to 5 mg, then a 5-mg dose should be administered on alternate days for the first 2 weeks. During subsequent 2 weeks, 0.3 mg/kg (rounded down to the nearest 5 mg) daily in one or two divided doses. Then, increase q 1 to 2 weeks by 0.3 mg/kg (rounded down to the nearest 5 mg) until effective daily dose of about 1 to 5 mg/kg (maximum of 200 mg daily in one or two divided doses) is reached.

How supplied
Available by prescription only
Tablets: 25 mg, 100 mg, 150 mg, 200 mg
Tablets (chewable): 5 mg, 25 mg

Pharmacodynamics
Anticonvulsant action: Unknown. Possibly related to inhibition of release of glutamate and aspartate in the brain. This may occur by acting on voltage-sensitive sodium channels.

Pharmacokinetics
Absorption: Rapidly and completely absorbed from the GI tract with negligible first-pass metabolism. Absolute bioavailability is 98%.
Distribution: About 55% is bound to plasma proteins.
Metabolism: Metabolized predominantly by glucuronic acid conjugation; the major metabolite is an inactive 2-N-glucuronide conjugate.
Excretion: Excreted primarily in urine with only a small portion excreted in feces.

Route	Onset	Peak	Duration
P.O.	Unknown	1½-4¾ hr	Unknown

Contraindications and precautions
Contraindicated in patients hypersensitive to drug. Use cautiously in patients with impaired renal, hepatic, or cardiac function.

Interactions
Drug-drug. *Carbamazepine, phenobarbital, phenytoin, primidone:* Decreased lamotrigine steady state levels. Monitor patient carefully.
Folate inhibitors such as cotrimoxazole, methotrexate: May be affected by lamotrigine because it inhibits dihydrofolate reductase, an enzyme involved in the synthesis of folic acid. Patient needs close monitoring because drug may have an additive effect.
Valproic acid: Decreased lamotrigine clearance, which increases steady state levels of drug. Monitor patient closely for toxicity.

Drug-lifestyle. *Sun exposure:* Possible photosensitivity reactions. Advise patient to take precautions.

Adverse reactions
CNS: *dizziness, headache, ataxia, somnolence,* malaise, incoordination, insomnia, tremor, depression, anxiety, *seizures,* irritability, speech disorder, decreased memory, concentration disturbance, sleep disorder, emotional lability, vertigo, mind racing, *suicide attempts.*
CV: palpitations.
EENT: rhinitis, pharyngitis, *diplopia, blurred vision,* vision abnormality, nystagmus, epistaxis.
GI: *nausea,* vomiting, diarrhea, dyspepsia, abdominal pain, constipation, anorexia, dry mouth, rectal hemorrhage, peptic ulcer.
GU: dysmenorrhea, vaginitis, amenorrhea.
Metabolic: weight loss.
Musculoskeletal: dysarthria, muscle spasm, neck pain.
Respiratory: cough, dyspnea, bronchitis.
Skin: *Stevens-Johnson syndrome, rash,* pruritus, alopecia, acne, epidermal neurolyisis, photosensitivity, contact dermatitis, dry skin, sweating.
Other: tooth disorder, flu syndrome, fever, infection, chills, peripheral edema, hot flashes.

Overdose and treatment
Limited information available. Following a suspected overdose, treatment should be supportive. Induce emesis or perform gastric lavage, if necessary. It isn't known whether hemodialysis is effective.

Special considerations
● Drug may be given without regard to meals. Chewable tablets may be swallowed whole, chewed and swallowed with a small amount of water or diluted fruit juice, or dispersed in about 5 ml of liquid for about 1 minute and consumed immediately.
● Don't stop drug abruptly because of increased risk of seizures. Instead, taper drug over at least 2 weeks.
● Stop drug immediately if drug-induced rash appears.
● If lamotrigine is added to a multidrug regimen that includes valproate, reduce dose of lamotrigine and use a lower maintenance dosage in patients with severe renal impairment.

Patient monitoring
● Evaluate patient for reduction in the frequency and duration of seizures.
● Check adjunct serum levels of anticonvulsant.

Breast-feeding patients
● Drug use in breast-feeding women isn't recommended.

Reactions may be *common,* uncommon, *life-threatening,* or COMMON AND LIFE-THREATENING.

Pediatric patients
• Recommended use in children ages 2 to 12 is very limited, and drug must be carefully administered following the detailed guidelines provided with it. The risk of severe, potentially life-threatening rash in children is much higher than that in adults.

Geriatric patients
• Safety and efficacy in patients over age 65 haven't been established.

Patient education
• Inform patient that rash may occur, especially during first 6 weeks of therapy and in children. Combination therapy of valproic acid and lamotrigine is likely to precipitate a serious rash. Although it may resolve with continued therapy, tell patient to report rash immediately in case drug needs to be discontinued.
• Warn patient not to perform potentially hazardous activities until CNS effects are known.
• Advise patient to take protective measures against photosensitivity reactions until tolerance is known.

---

lansoprazole
Prevacid

Pharmacologic classification: acid (proton) pump inhibitor
Therapeutic classification: antiulcer
Pregnancy risk category: B

Indications and dosages
➤ *Short-term treatment of active duodenal ulcer.* Adults: 15 mg P.O. daily before meals for 4 weeks.
➤ *Short-term treatment of erosive esophagitis.* Adults: 30 mg P.O. daily before meals for up to 8 weeks. If healing doesn't occur, an additional 8 weeks of therapy may be needed.
➤ *Long-term treatment of pathologic hypersecretory conditions, including Zollinger-Ellison syndrome.* Adults: Initially, 60 mg P.O. once daily. Increase dosage, p.r.n. Administer daily doses exceeding 120 mg in divided doses.
➤ *Maintenance of healed duodenal ulcer or erosive esophagitis.* Adults: 15 mg P.O. once daily.
➤ *Short-term treatment of gastric ulcer.* Adults: 30 mg P.O. daily for up to 8 weeks.
➤ *Short-term treatment of symptomatic gastroesophageal reflux disease.* Adults: 15 mg P.O. daily for up to 8 weeks.
➤ Helicobacter pylori *eradication to reduce risk of duodenal ulcer recurrence.* Adults: In patients receiving dual therapy, 30 mg P.O. lansoprazole with 1 g P.O. amoxicillin, each given q 8 hours for 14 days. In patients receiving triple therapy, 30 mg P.O. lansoprazole with

1 g P.O. amoxicillin and 500 mg P.O. clarithromycin, all given q 12 hours for 10 to 14 days.
➤ *Healing of NSAID-induced gastric ulcer.* Adults: 30 mg P.O. once daily for 8 weeks.
➤ *Reducing risk of NSAID-related gastric ulcer.* Adults: 15 mg P.O. once daily for up to 12 weeks.

How supplied
Available by prescription only
Capsules (delayed-release): 15 mg, 30 mg

Pharmacodynamics
Antiulcer action: Lansoprazole inhibits activity of the acid (proton) pump and binds to hydrogen-potassium ATPase, located at the secretory surface of the gastric parietal cells, to block the formation of gastric acid.

Pharmacokinetics
Absorption: Rapidly absorbed with absolute bioavailability of more than 80%.
Distribution: 97% bound to plasma proteins.
Metabolism: Extensively metabolized in the liver.
Excretion: About two-thirds of dose is excreted in feces; one-third in urine.

Route	Onset	Peak	Duration
P.O.	Unknown	1¾ hr	Unknown

Contraindications and precautions
Contraindicated in patients hypersensitive to drug.

Interactions
Drug-drug. *Ampicillin esters, iron salts, ketoconazole:* Lansoprazole may interfere with the absorption of these drugs. Separate administration times.
Sucralfate: Delays lansoprazole absorption. Give lansoprazole at least 30 minutes before sucralfate.
Theophylline: May cause mild increase in theophylline excretion. Use together cautiously. Dosage adjustment of theophylline may be necessary.
Drug-herb. *Male fern:* Inactivated in alkaline stomach environment. Discourage concomitant use.

Adverse reactions
CNS: asthenia, headache, agitation, amnesia, anxiety, apathy, confusion, depression, dizziness or syncope, hallucinations, hemiplegia, aggravated hostility, malaise, nervousness, paresthesia, thinking abnormality.
CV: chest pain, edema, angina, *CVA,* hypertension or hypotension, *MI, shock,* palpitations, vasodilation, *cardiospasm.*
EENT: amblyopia, deafness, eye pain, visual field deficits, otitis media, tinnitus.
GI: diarrhea, nausea, abdominal pain, halitosis, melena, anorexia, cholelithiasis, constipation, dry mouth, thirst, dyspepsia, dysphagia, eructation, esophageal stenosis, esophageal ulcer,

---

esophagitis, fecal discoloration, flatulence, gastric nodules, fundic gland polyps, gastroenteritis, GI hemorrhage, hematemesis, increased appetite, increased salivation, rectal hemorrhage, stomatitis, tenesmus, ulcerative colitis, taste perversion.
GU: hematuria, impotence, kidney calculus, albuminuria, abnormal menses, breast tenderness or breast enlargement, candidiasis.
Hematologic: anemia, hemolysis.
Hepatic: abnormal liver function test results.
Metabolic: diabetes mellitus, goiter, hyperglycemia, hypoglycemia, gout, weight changes.
Musculoskeletal: arthritis, arthralgia, musculoskeletal pain, myalgia.
Respiratory: asthma, bronchitis, increased cough, dyspnea, epistaxis, hemoptysis, hiccups, pneumonia, upper respiratory tract inflammation.
Skin: acne, alopecia, pruritus, rash, urticaria.
Other: fever, flu syndrome, infection, gynecomastia, decreased libido.

Overdose and treatment
No adverse effects have been reported with drug overdose. Drug isn't removed by hemodialysis. If required, treatment should be supportive.

Special considerations
• Dosage adjustment isn't necessary in elderly patients or patients with renal insufficiency; however, it may be required for patients with severe liver disease.
• Drug shouldn't be used as maintenance therapy for patients with duodenal ulcer disease or erosive esophagitis.
• Contents of capsule can be mixed with 40 ml of apple juice in a syringe and administered within 3 to 5 minutes via an nasogastric tube. Flush with additional apple juice to administer entire dose and maintain patency of the tube.

Patient monitoring
• Monitor liver function studies in long-term therapy.

Breast-feeding patients
• Because it isn't known whether lansoprazole appears in breast milk, a decision to discontinue breast-feeding or using drug should be made.

Pediatric patients
• Safety and efficacy in children haven't been established.

Geriatric patients
• Although initial dosing regimen need not be altered for geriatric patients, subsequent doses over 30 mg daily shouldn't be administered unless additional gastric acid suppression is necessary.

Patient education
• Instruct patient to take drug before meals.
• Caution patient not to open, chew, or crush capsules; capsules should be swallowed whole.

latanoprost
Xalatan

Pharmacologic classification: prostaglandin analogue
Therapeutic classification: antiglaucoma; ocular antihypertensive
Pregnancy risk category: C

Indications and dosages
➤ *Increased intraocular pressure (IOP) in patients with ocular hypertension or open-angle glaucoma who are intolerant of or insufficiently responsive to other IOP-lowering drugs.* Adults: Instill 1 drop in the conjunctival sac of the affected eyes once daily in the evening.

How supplied
Available by prescription only
Ophthalmic solution: 0.005%

Pharmacodynamics
Antiglaucoma and ocular antihypertensive actions: Exact mechanism of action unknown. Drug may lower IOP by increasing the outflow of aqueous humor.

Pharmacokinetics
Absorption: Absorbed through the cornea.
Distribution: Distribution volume is about 0.16 L/kg. The acid of latanoprost could be measured in aqueous humor during first 4 hours and in plasma only during first hour after local administration.
Metabolism: Hydrolyzed by esterases in the cornea to the biologically active acid. The active acid of drug reaching systemic circulation is primarily metabolized by the liver.
Excretion: Metabolites are mainly eliminated in urine.

Route	Onset	Peak	Duration
Oph-thalmic	2-4 hr	8-12 hr	Unknown

Contraindications and precautions
Contraindicated in patients hypersensitive to drug, benzalkonium chloride, or other ingredients in the product.
    Use cautiously when administering to patients with impaired renal or hepatic function. Use cautiously in patients with active ocular inflammation (iritis, uveitis), patients at risk for macular edema, aphakic patients, and pseudophakic patients.

Interactions
Drug-drug. *Thimerosal:* Precipitation occurs when eyedrops containing thimerosal are mixed with latanoprost. If drugs are used together, administer them at least 5 minutes apart.
Topical beta blockers (betaxolol, carteolol, levobunolol, metipranolol, timolol), topical di-

---

Reactions may be *common*, uncommon, *life-threatening*, or COMMON AND LIFE-THREATENING.

pivefrin, topical epinephrine, an oral carbonic anhydrase inhibitor (acetazolamide), or a topical carbonic anhydrase inhibitor (dorzolamide): IOP-lowering effects of these drugs may be additive. This may be a therapeutic advantage, but if using other topical drugs, separate administration times by 5 minutes.

Adverse reactions
CV: chest pain, angina pectoris.
EENT: *blurred vision; burning; stinging;* itching; conjunctival hyperemia; foreign body sensation; increased pigmentation of iris; punctate epithelial keratopathy; dry eye; excessive tearing; photophobia; conjunctivitis; diplopia; eye pain or discharge; lid crusting, edema, erythema, discomfort, or pain; herpes simplex keratitis.
Musculoskeletal: muscle, joint, or back pain.
Respiratory: upper respiratory tract infection, asthma.
Skin: rash, allergic skin reaction.
Other: cold, flu.

Overdose and treatment
Apart from ocular irritation and conjunctival or episcleral hyperemia, ocular effects of latanoprost at high doses aren't known. Treatment should be symptomatic if overdose occurs.

Special considerations
• Latanoprost may gradually change eye color, increasing the amount of brown pigment in the iris. The change in iris color occurs slowly and may not be noticeable for several months to years. The increased pigmentation may be permanent.
• Protect drug from light; refrigerate unopened bottle.

Patient monitoring
• Monitor IOP-lowering effects of drug.

Breast-feeding patients
• It isn't known whether drug appears in breast milk. Exercise caution when administering drug to breast-feeding women.

Pediatric patients
• Safety and efficacy in children haven't been established.

Patient education
• Tell patient receiving treatment in only one eye about the potential for increased brown pigmentation in the treated eye as well as heterochromia between the eyes.
• Teach patient to instill drops. Advise him to wash hands before and after instilling solution, and warn him not to touch dropper or tip to eye or surrounding tissue.
• Advise patient to apply light finger pressure on lacrimal sac for 1 minute after instillation to minimize systemic absorption of drug.
• Instruct patient to report ocular reactions, especially conjunctivitis and lid reactions.

• Tell patient using contact lenses to remove them before administration of the solution and not to reinsert the contact lenses for 15 minutes after administration.
• Advise patient using more than one topical ophthalmic drug to administer the drugs at least 5 minutes apart.
• Stress importance of compliance with recommended therapy.

leflunomide
Arava

Pharmacologic classification: pyrimidine synthesis inhibitor
Therapeutic classification: antirheumatic agent
Pregnancy risk category: X

Indications and dosages
➤ *To reduce signs and symptoms of active rheumatoid arthritis and to retard structural damage as evidenced by erosions and joint space narrowing seen on X-ray.* Adults: 100 mg P.O. q 24 hours for 3 days, followed by 20 mg (maximum daily dose) P.O. q 24 hours. Dose may be decreased to 10 mg daily if higher dose isn't well tolerated.

How supplied
Available by prescription only
Tablets: 10 mg, 20 mg, 100 mg

Pharmacodynamics
Immunomodulatory action: Drug inhibits dihydroorotate dehydrogenase, an enzyme involved in de novo pyrimidine synthesis, and has antiproliferative activity and anti-inflammatory effects.

Pharmacokinetics
Absorption: Bioavailability is 80%. Without loading dose, peak plasma levels are reached in about 2 months.
Distribution: Over 99% bound to plasma proteins.
Metabolism: Metabolized to an active metabolite (M1), responsible for most of its activity.
Excretion: Leflunomide is eliminated by renal and direct biliary excretion. About 43% is excreted in the urine and 48% in the feces. Half-life of the active metabolite is about 2 weeks.

Route	Onset	Peak	Duration
P.O.	Unknown	6-12 hr	Unknown

Contraindications and precautions
Contraindicated in patients hypersensitive to drug or its components and in women who are or may become pregnant or who are breast-feeding. Drug isn't recommended for patients with hepatic insufficiency, hepatitis B or C, severe immunodeficiency, bone marrow dysplasia, or severe un-

controlled infections. Drug isn't recommended for use by men attempting to father a child.

Vaccination with live-virus vaccines isn't recommended. Consider the long half-life of drug when contemplating administration of a live vaccine after stopping drug treatment.

The risk of malignancy, particularly lymphoproliferative disorders, increases with use of some immunosuppressants, including leflunomide. Use cautiously in patients with renal insufficiency.

Interactions
Drug-drug. *Activated charcoal, cholestyramine:* Decreased leflunomide levels. These drugs are sometimes used for this effect in treating overdose.
Methotrexate, other hepatotoxic drugs: Increased risk of hepatotoxicity. Monitor liver enzyme levels as appropriate.
Rifampin: Increased level of active leflunomide metabolite. Use together cautiously.

Adverse reactions
CNS: asthenia, dizziness, headache, paresthesia, malaise, migraine, sleep disorder, vertigo, neuritis, anxiety, depression, insomnia, neuralgia.
CV: angina pectoris, *hypertension,* chest pain, palpitations, tachycardia, vasculitis, vasodilation, varicose veins, peripheral edema.
EENT: pharyngitis, rhinitis, sinusitis, epistaxis, enlarged salivary glands, blurred vision, cataract, conjunctivitis, eye disorder.
GI: dry mouth, stomatitis, mouth ulcer, oral candidiasis, gingivitis, anorexia, *diarrhea,* dyspepsia, gastroenteritis, nausea, abdominal pain, vomiting, cholelithiasis, colitis, constipation, esophagitis, flatulence, gastritis, melena, taste perversion.
GU: urinary tract infection, albuminuria, cystitis, dysuria, hematuria, menstrual disorder, pelvic pain, vaginal candidiasis, prostate disorder, urinary frequency.
Hematologic: anemia, ecchymoses, hyperlipidemia.
Hepatic: elevated liver enzyme levels.
Metabolic: increased CK levels, diabetes mellitus, hyperglycemia, hyperthyroidism, hypokalemia, weight loss, hypophosphatemia.
Musculoskeletal: arthrosis, back pain, bursitis, muscle cramps, myalgia, bone necrosis, bone pain, arthralgia, leg cramps, joint disorder, neck pain, synovitis, tendon rupture, tenosynovitis.
Respiratory: bronchitis, increased cough, pneumonia, *respiratory tract infection,* asthma, dyspnea, lung disorder.
Skin: *alopecia,* eczema, pruritus, *rash,* dry skin, acne, contact dermatitis, fungal dermatitis, hair discoloration, hematoma, herpes simplex, herpes zoster, nail disorder, skin nodule, subcutaneous nodule, maculopapular rash, skin disorder, skin discoloration, skin ulcer, increased sweating.
Other: *allergic reaction,* fever, flu syndrome, tooth disorder, injury or accident, pain, abscess, cyst, hernia.

Overdose and treatment
No overdose has been reported. If overdose occurs, activated charcoal (50 g every 6 hours for 24 hours) reduces plasma levels. Cholestyramine also may be administered as 8 g P.O. three times daily for 11 days.

Special considerations
● Leflunomide can cause fetal harm when administered to pregnant women; it's recommended that women planning to become pregnant discontinue leflunomide therapy and consult their health care provider.
● Men planning to father a child should discontinue drug therapy and follow recommended leflunomide removal protocol (cholestyramine 8 g, P.O. t.i.d. for 11 days).
● Aspirin, other NSAIDs, and low-dose corticosteroids may be continued during treatment; however, use of drug with antimalarials, intramuscular or oral gold, penicillamine, azathioprine, or methotrexate hasn't been adequately studied.

Patient monitoring
● Monitor liver enzyme (ALT and AST) levels before starting therapy and monthly thereafter until stable. Frequency can then be decreased based on clinical situation.

Breast-feeding patients
● Drug shouldn't be used by breast-feeding women.

Pediatric patients
● Safety in children and adolescents hasn't been established. Not recommended for children under age 18.

Geriatric patients
● No significant differences noted compared with younger population.

Patient education
● Explain the need for and frequency of required blood tests and monitoring.
● Instruct patient to use birth control during treatment and until it has been determined that drug is no longer active.
● Warn woman to immediately notify prescriber if signs or symptoms of pregnancy occur (such as late menses or breast tenderness).

letrozole
Femara

Pharmacologic classification: aromatase inhibitor
Therapeutic classification: hormone
Pregnancy risk category: D

Indications and dosages
➤ *Metastatic breast cancer in postmenopausal women with disease progression*

---

following antiestrogen therapy, hormone receptor positive or hormone receptor unknown advanced or metastatic breast cancer in postmenopausal women. Adults and elderly: 2.5 mg P.O. as a single daily dose, without regard to meals.

How supplied
Available by prescription only
Tablets: 2.5 mg

Pharmacodynamics
Hormone action: Inhibits conversion of androgens to estrogens by competitive inhibition of the aromatase enzyme system. Decreased estrogens are likely to lead to decreased tumor mass or delayed progression of tumor growth in some women.

Pharmacokinetics
Absorption: Rapidly and completely absorbed. Food doesn't affect bioavailability. Steady state plasma levels are reached 2 to 6 weeks after daily dosing.
Distribution: Large volume of distribution (1.9 L/kg). It's weakly protein-bound.
Metabolism: Slowly metabolized to an inactive form. In liver microsomes, letrozole strongly inhibits cytochrome P-450 isozyme 2A6 and moderately inhibits isozyme 2C19.
Excretion: The inactive glucuronide metabolite is eliminated in the urine.

Route	Onset	Peak	Duration
P.O.	Unknown	2 days	Unknown

Contraindications and precautions
Contraindicated in patients hypersensitive to drug or its components. Avoid use in pregnant women because drug may cause fetal harm.
    Use cautiously in patients with severe liver impairment.

Interactions
None reported.

Adverse reactions
CNS: headache, somnolence, dizziness, fatigue, asthenia.
CV: edema, hypertension, ***thromboembolism,*** chest pain.
GI: *nausea,* vomiting, constipation, diarrhea, abdominal pain, anorexia, dyspepsia.
Metabolic: weight gain, hypercholesterolemia.
Musculoskeletal: *bone, limb, and back pain;* arthralgia.
Respiratory: dyspnea, cough.
Skin: rash, pruritus.
Other: hot flashes, viral infections.

Overdose and treatment
There have been no reports of overdose during clinical trials with letrozole. If overdose occurs, consider inducing emesis if patient is alert; provide supportive care and monitor vital signs frequently.

Special considerations
● No dosage adjustment is needed in patients with mild to moderate liver dysfunction or in renally impaired patients with creatinine clearance of 10 ml/minute or more.
● Patients treated with letrozole don't need glucocorticoid or mineralocorticoid replacement therapy. Letrozole significantly lowers serum estrone, estradiol, and estrone sulfate, but hasn't been shown to significantly affect adrenal corticosteroid synthesis, aldosterone synthesis, or synthesis of thyroid hormones.

Patient monitoring
● Monitor patient for decreased tumor progression.

Breast-feeding patients
● It isn't known whether drug appears in breast milk. Use caution when administering letrozole to breast-feeding women.

Patient education
● Instruct patient to take drug exactly as prescribed.
● Tell patient that drug can be taken with or without food.
● Advise patient that drug treatment is long-term, and stress importance of follow-up appointments.
● Tell patient to inform prescriber if pregnancy is suspected or is being planned.

leucovorin calcium (citrovorum factor or folinic acid)
Wellcovorin

Pharmacologic classification: formyl derivative (active reduced form of folic acid)
Therapeutic classification: vitamin, antidote
Pregnancy risk category: C

Indications and dosages
➤ *Overdose of folic acid antagonist. Adults and children:* I.M. or I.V. dose equivalent to weight of antagonist given as soon as possible after the overdose.
➤ *Leucovorin rescue after large methotrexate dose in treatment of cancer. Adults and children:* Administer 24 hours after last dose of methotrexate according to protocol. Initially, 10 mg/m² I.M. or I.V.; then give 10 mg/m² P.O. q 6 hours until serum methotrexate level is less than 5×10^{-8} M (0.05 micromolar). Adjust subsequent doses based upon serum creatinine and methotrexate levels.
➤ *Toxic effects of methotrexate used to treat severe psoriasis. Adults and children:* 4 to 8 mg I.M. 2 hours after methotrexate dose.

◇ Unlabeled clinical use

➤ *Hematologic toxicity from pyrimetha-mine therapy. Adults and children:* Dosage highly individualized depending on dosage of folic acid antagonist and patient's clinical status.

➤ *Prevention of toxicities in* Pneumo-cystis carinii *patients receiving trimetrexate glucuronate. Adults:* 20 mg/m² P.O. or I.V. over 5 to 10 minutes q 6 hours (total daily dose of 80 mg/m²). If administered orally, round up to the next 25-mg dose. Leucovorin should be continued for at least 72 hours after last trimetrexate dose. Adjust doses of both drugs based on patient's hematologic response.

➤ *Advanced colorectal cancer. Adults:* 200 mg/m² by slow I.V. injection over 3 minutes followed by 5-fluorouracil (5-FU) or 20 mg/m² by slow I.V. injection over 3 minutes followed by 5-FU. Repeat treatment for 5 days. May repeat course at 4-week intervals for two courses and then at 4- to 5-week intervals as long as the patient has recovered from toxic effects of previous treatment. Dosage of 5-FU should be individualized.

➤ *Megaloblastic anemia from congenital enzyme deficiency. Adults and children:* 3 to 6 mg I.M. daily.

➤ *Folate-deficient megaloblastic anemias. Adults and children:* Up to 1 mg of leucovorin I.M. daily. Duration of treatment depends on hematologic response.

How supplied
Available by prescription only
Injection: 1-ml ampule (3 mg/ml with 0.9% benzyl alcohol, 5 mg/ml with methyl and propyl parabens); 50-mg, 100-mg, and 350-mg vials for reconstitution (contain no preservatives)
Tablets: 5 mg, 15 mg, 25 mg

Pharmacodynamics
Reversal of folic acid antagonism: Leucovorin is a derivative of tetrahydrofolic acid, the reduced form of folic acid. Leucovorin performs as a cofactor in 1-carbon transfer reactions in the biosynthesis of purines and pyrimidines of nucleic acids. Impairment of thymidylate synthesis in patients with folic acid deficiency may account for defective DNA synthesis, megaloblast formation, and megaloblastic and macrocytic anemias. Leucovorin is a potent antidote for the hematopoietic and reticuloendothelial toxic effects of folic acid antagonists (trimethoprim, pyrimethamine, and methotrexate). Leucovorin rescue is used to prevent or decrease toxicity of massive methotrexate doses. Folinic acid rescues normal cells without reversing the oncolytic effect of methotrexate.

Pharmacokinetics
Absorption: After oral administration, leucovorin is absorbed rapidly. The increase in plasma and serum folate activity after oral administration is mainly from 5-methyltetrahydrofolate

(the major transport and storage form of folate in the body).
Distribution: Tetrahydrofolic acid and its derivatives are distributed throughout the body; the liver contains about half of the total body folate stores.
Metabolism: Metabolized in the liver.
Excretion: Excreted by the kidneys as 10-formyl tetrahydrofolate and 5,10-methenyl tetrahydrofolate.

Route	Onset	Peak	Duration
P.O.	20-30 min	2-3 hr	3-6 hr
I.V.	5 min	10 min	3-6 hr
I.M.	10-20 min	< 1 hr	3-6 hr

Contraindications and precautions
Contraindicated in patients with pernicious anemia and other megaloblastic anemias that result from the lack of vitamin B_{12}.

Interactions
Drug-drug. *Fluorouracil:* Leucovorin increases toxicity of fluorouracil. Use lower doses of fluorouracil.
Phenobarbital, phenytoin, primidone: Decreased serum anticonvulsant levels and increased frequency of seizures. Although this interaction has occurred only in patients receiving folic acid, it should be considered when leucovorin is administered. Adjust anticonvulsant dose.

Adverse reactions
Skin: *hypersensitivity reactions* (urticaria, *anaphylactoid reactions*).

Overdose and treatment
Leucovorin is relatively nontoxic; no specific recommendations for overdose are reported. However, an excessive amount of leucovorin may nullify the chemotherapeutic effect of folic acid antagonists such as methotrexate.

Special considerations
• Drug administration continues until plasma methotrexate levels are less than 5×10^{-8} M.
• Don't use as sole treatment of pernicious anemia or vitamin B_{12} deficiency.
• To treat overdose of folic acid antagonists, use the drug within 1 hour; it isn't effective after a 4-hour delay.
• When giving more than 25 mg, administer drug parenterally.
• Reconstitute drug by adding 5 to 10 ml of sterile water for injection or bacteriostatic water for injection (which contains benzyl alcohol) to vial containing 50 or 100 mg of leucovorin, respectively. Solution will contain 10 mg/ml. Add 17 ml of sterile water for injection or bacteriostatic water for injection to vial containing 350 mg of leucovorin for a resulting concentration of 20 mg/ml. When parenteral doses greater than 10 mg/m² are necessary, only reconstitute with sterile water for injection. If reconstituted with sterile wa-

ter for injection, use immediately. If reconstituted with bacteriostatic water for injection, use within 7 days.
• Leucovorin admixed with $D_{10}W$, normal saline solution, or Ringer's or lactated Ringer's injection is stable for 24 hours when stored at room temperature and protected from light.
• Leucovorin infusion shouldn't exceed 160 mg/minute because of calcium concentration of solution.
• Store at room temperature in a light-resistant container, not in high-moisture areas.

Patient monitoring
• Monitor patient for signs of drug allergy, such as rash, wheezing, pruritus, and urticaria.
• Monitor serum creatinine levels daily to detect possible renal function impairment.
• When used with fluorouracil, monitor CBC and platelet count before each course of therapy and repeat weekly during first two courses of therapy. Also, monitor serum electrolytes and liver function tests before each course of therapy for three courses and then before every other course.

Breast-feeding patients
• It's unknown whether leucovorin appears in breast milk. Use cautiously in breast-feeding women.

Pediatric patients
• Drug may increase frequency of seizures in susceptible children. Don't use diluents containing benzyl alcohol when reconstituting drug for neonates.

Patient education
• Emphasize importance of taking leucovorin only under medical supervision.

leuprolide acetate
Lupron, Lupron Depot, Lupron Depot-Ped, Lupron Depot-3 Month, Lupron Depot-4 month, Viadur

Pharmacologic classification: gonadotropin-releasing hormone
Therapeutic classification: antineoplastic; luteinizing hormone-releasing hormone (LHRH) analogue
Pregnancy risk category: X

Indications and dosages
Dosages and indications vary. Check current literature for recommended protocol. The four different depot preparations aren't interchangeable.
➤ *Management of advanced prostate cancer. Adults:* 7.5 mg I.M. (depot injection) once monthly or 1 mg S.C. daily; or 22.5 mg I.M. (depot injection) q 3 months, 30 mg I.M. q 4 months (depot injection) or 72 mg implanted q 12 months.

➤ *Treatment of endometriosis. Adults:* 3.75 mg I.M. (depot injection) once monthly for a maximum of 6 months or 11.25 mg I.M. every 3 months.
➤ *Correction of anemia related to uterine fibroids before surgery. Adults:* 3.75 mg I.M. once monthly for up to 3 consecutive months with iron therapy.
➤ *Central precocious puberty ◇. Children (girls under age 8 and boys under age 9):* Starting dose is 0.3 mg/kg (minimum 7.5 mg), given as a single I.M. or S.C. dose (depot injection) q 4 weeks. An initial dose of 7.5 mg if weight is 25 kg (55 lb) or less; 11.25 mg if weight is 25 to 37.5 kg (55 to 82¼ lb); and 15 mg if weight is more than 37.5 kg (82½ lb). Adjust upward in increments of 3.75 mg q 4 weeks until clinical or laboratory tests indicate no progression of the disease. If leuprolide acetate injection is used, initial dose is 50 mcg/kg S.C. daily. Adjust upward by 10 mcg/kg daily.

How supplied
Available by prescription only
Implant: 72 mg
Injection: 5 mg/ml in 2.8-ml multiple-dose vials
Suspension for depot injection: 3.75 mg, 7.5 mg, 11.25 mg, 15 mg, 22.5 mg, 30 mg

Pharmacodynamics
Antineoplastic action: Leuprolide is a synthetic analogue of LHRH. It inhibits gonadotropin secretion and androgen or estrogen synthesis. Because of this effect, leuprolide may inhibit the growth of hormone-dependent tumors.
Hormonal action: Because leuprolide lowers levels of sex hormones, it reduces the size of endometrial implants, resulting in decreased dysmenorrhea and pelvic pain in women with endometriosis.

Pharmacokinetics
Absorption: Leuprolide is a polypeptide molecule that's destroyed in the GI tract. After S.C. administration, drug is rapidly and essentially completely absorbed.
Distribution: Distribution hasn't been determined, but high levels may be distributed into kidney, liver, pineal, and pituitary tissue. About 7% to 15% of a dose is bound to plasma proteins.
Metabolism: Metabolism is unclear, but drug may be metabolized in the anterior pituitary and hypothalamus, similar to endogenous gonadotropin-releasing hormone.
Excretion: Plasma elimination half-life is 3 hours.

Route	Onset	Peak	Duration
I.M., S.C.	< 2-4 wk	1-2 mo	2-3 mo

Contraindications and precautions
Contraindicated in patients hypersensitive to drug or other gonadotropin-releasing hormone analogues, during pregnancy or lactation, and in

women with undiagnosed vaginal bleeding. The 30 mg depot form is contraindicated in women. The implant is contraindicated in women and children.

Use cautiously in patients hypersensitive to benzyl alcohol.

Interactions
None reported.

Adverse reactions
CNS: *dizziness, depression, headache, pain,* insomnia, *asthenia.*
CV: *arrhythmias,* angina, **MI,** *peripheral edema, ECG changes,* hypertension, murmur.
GI: *nausea, vomiting,* anorexia, constipation.
GU: *impotence, vaginitis,* urinary frequency, hematuria, urinary tract infection.
Hematologic: anemia.
Hepatic: elevated liver enzyme levels.
Metabolic: *weight changes,* initially increased then decreased with continued therapy serum acid phosphatase and testosterone levels.
Musculoskeletal: transient bone pain during first week of treatment, joint disorder, myalgia, neuromuscular disorder.
Respiratory: dyspnea, sinus congestion, pulmonary fibrosis.
Skin: skin reactions at injection site, dermatitis.
Other: *hot flashes, androgen-like effects,* gynecomastia.

Overdose and treatment
No information available.

Special considerations
● Experimental uses include male contraception, treatment of endocrine disorders, hypogonadism, delayed puberty, oligospermia, anovulation, and amenorrhea.
● When treating endometriosis, administer for a maximum of 6 months. Safety and efficacy of retreatment are unknown.
● To reconstitute suspension containing 3.75, 7.5, 11.25, or 15 mg, add 1 ml of provided diluent to leuprolide acetate powder for injection using a 22G needle; to reconstitute suspension containing 22.5 or 30 mg, add 1.5 ml of provided diluent using a 23G needle. Shake well. Resulting suspension is milky. Use 22.5 and 30 mg concentration immediately.
● Use a 22G needle for monthly injection and a 23G needle for 3-month injection.
● A 0.5 ml low dose, U-100 insulin syringe may be used if necessary to replace manufacturer-provided syringes to inject leuprolide acetate injection; fill syringe to the 20-unit mark.
● Discard solution if particulate matter is visible or if the solution is discolored.
● Erythema or induration may develop at injection site.
● When treating prostate cancer, leuprolide may aggravate signs and symptoms of disease during first 1 to 2 weeks of therapy. Temporary pares-

thesia and weakness may occur during first week of therapy.
● No unusual adverse effects were observed in patients who had received 20 mg daily for 2 years.
● Reversible suppression of fertility in men and women has occurred.
● Refrigerate leuprolide vials for injection until used. Don't freeze. Vial in use may be stored at room temperature. Leuprolide powder for injection suspension may be stored at room temperature. Reconstituted suspension is stable for 24 hours.

Patient monitoring
● Measure serum testosterone and acid phosphatase levels before and during therapy.
● Measure serum testosterone, prostate specific antigen, and prostatic acid phosphatase levels before and during therapy in patients with prostate cancer.
● Monitor liver function tests.

Patient education
● Reassure patient that bone pain is transient and will disappear after about 1 week.
● Inform patient that a temporary reaction of burning, itching, and swelling at injection site may occur. Tell him to report persistent reactions.
● Advise patient to continue taking drug even if feeling well.
● Instruct women of childbearing age to use an effective nonhormonal method of contraception during therapy, and to discontinue drug and notify prescriber if pregnancy occurs.

levalbuterol hydrochloride
Xopenex

Pharmacologic classification: beta$_2$ agonist
Therapeutic classification: bronchodilator
Pregnancy risk category: C

Indications and dosages
➤ *To prevent or treat bronchospasm in patients with reversible obstructive airway disease. Adults and adolescents age 12 and older:* 0.63 mg administered t.i.d. q 6 to 8 hours, by oral inhalation via a nebulizer. Patients with more severe asthma who don't respond adequately may benefit from a dosage of 1.25 mg t.i.d.

How supplied
Available by prescription only
Solution for inhalation: 0.63 mg or 1.25 mg in 3-ml vials

Pharmacodynamics
Bronchodilator action: Levalbuterol activates beta$_2$ receptors on airway smooth muscle, resulting in relaxation of smooth muscle in all airways—from the trachea to the terminal bron-

---

chioles—and subsequent relief of bronchospasm and reduction of airway resistance. Drug also inhibits the release of mediators from mast cells in the airway.

Pharmacokinetics
No information available.

Route	Onset	Peak	Duration
Inhalation	Unknown	12 min	Unknown

Contraindications and precautions
Contraindicated in patients with a history of hypersensitivity to levalbuterol or racemic albuterol.

Use cautiously in patients with cardiovascular disorders, especially coronary insufficiency, hypertension, and arrhythmias. Also use cautiously in patients with seizure disorders, hyperthyroidism, or diabetes mellitus and in patients who are unusually responsive to sympathomimetic amines.

Interactions
Drug-drug. *Beta blockers:* May cause reduced pulmonary effect of the drug and, possibly, severe bronchospasm. Don't use together, if possible. If use together is necessary, consider a cardioselective beta blocker, but administer cautiously.
Digoxin: Decreased digoxin levels (up to 22%). Monitor serum digoxin levels.
Loop or thiazide diuretics: These non–potassium-sparing diuretics may cause ECG changes and hypokalemia. Use together cautiously.
MAO inhibitors, tricyclic antidepressants: Potentiate the action of levalbuterol on the vascular system. Administer with extreme caution in patients being given MAO inhibitors or tricyclic antidepressants, or within 2 weeks of discontinuation of these drugs.
Other short-acting sympathomimetic aerosol bronchodilators or epinephrine: May cause increased adrenergic adverse effects. To avoid serious CV effects, use additional adrenergics cautiously.

Adverse reactions
CNS: dizziness, migraine, nervousness, tremor, anxiety, pain.
CV: tachycardia.
EENT: *rhinitis,* sinusitis, turbinate edema.
GI: dyspepsia.
Musculoskeletal: leg cramps.
Respiratory: increased cough, *viral infection.*
Other: flu syndrome, accidental injury.

Overdose and treatment
Signs and symptoms of overdose are those of excessive beta-receptor stimulation, including seizures, angina, hypertension or hypotension, tachycardia with rates up to 200 beats/minute, arrhythmias, nervousness, headache, tremor, dry mouth, palpitations, nausea, dizziness, fatigue, malaise, and sleeplessness. Hypokalemia also

may occur. As with other sympathomimetics, abuse of levalbuterol may result in cardiac arrest and death.

Treatment consists of stopping the drug and giving symptomatic therapy. A cardioselective beta-receptor blocker may be used, but beta-receptor blockers can cause bronchospasm. It's unknown whether dialysis is beneficial in managing levalbuterol overdose.

Special considerations
● Like other inhaled beta agonists, levalbuterol can produce paradoxical bronchospasm, which may be life-threatening. If this occurs, stop drug immediately and institute alternative therapy.
● Small, transient increases in blood glucose levels may occur after oral inhalation.
● Serum potassium levels may decrease slightly, but potassium supplementation is usually unnecessary.
● Keep unopened vials in foil pouch. Once the foil pouch is opened, use the vials within 2 weeks. If vials are removed from pouch but not used immediately, protect from light and excessive heat and use within 1 week.

Patient monitoring
● Monitor patient for drug effect and for worsening of symptoms.
● Monitor patient for bronchospasm.

Pregnant patients
Use drug only if benefits outweigh risk to the fetus.

Breast-feeding patients
● Plasma levels of levalbuterol are very low following inhalation of therapeutic dosages. It isn't known whether drug appears in breast milk. Administer cautiously to breast-feeding women.

Pediatric patients
● Safety and efficacy of levalbuterol in children under age 12 are unknown.

Geriatric patients
● Safety and efficacy of levalbuterol are unknown in patients age 65 and older. In general, patients in this age group should be started at a dose of 0.63 mg.

Patient education
● Warn patient that he may experience paradoxical bronchospasm (difficulty breathing). Tell him to discontinue drug and contact prescriber immediately if this occurs.
● Inform patient that common adverse effects include palpitations, rapid heart rate, headache, dizziness, tremor, and nervousness.
● Inform patient that the effects of levalbuterol may last up to 8 hours.
● Warn patient not to increase dose or frequency without consulting prescriber.
● Advise patient to seek medical attention immediately if levalbuterol becomes less effective,

if signs and symptoms become worse, or if he's using levalbuterol more frequently than usual.
• Caution patient to use other inhalants and anti-asthma drugs only as directed while taking levalbuterol.
• Advise woman to inform health care provider about the use of levalbuterol if she becomes pregnant or is breast-feeding.
• Instruct patient not to use levalbuterol after the expiration date stamped on the container.
• Inform patient that once the foil pouch is opened, the vials should be used within 2 weeks. If opened pouch isn't used immediately, vials should be protected from light and excessive heat and used within 1 week.
• Tell patient to discard any vials containing discolored solution.

---

levamisole hydrochloride
Ergamisol

Pharmacologic classification: immunomodulator
Therapeutic classification: antineoplastic
Pregnancy risk category: C

Indications and dosages
➤ **Adjuvant treatment with fluorouracil after surgical resection in patients with Dukes' stage C colon cancer.** *Adults:* Initially, 50 mg P.O. q 8 hours for 3 days starting 7 to 30 days after surgery. Repeat q 14 days for 1 year. Administer with fluorouracil 450 mg/m^2 daily by rapid I.V. push for 5 days with a 3-day course of levamisole, starting 21 to 34 days after surgery.

If levamisole therapy begins 7 to 20 days after surgery, start fluorouracil with the second course of levamisole at 21 to 34 days. If levamisole begins 21 to 30 days after surgery, start fluorouracil simultaneously with the first course of therapy.

Maintenance dosage is 50 mg P.O. q 8 hours for 3 days q 2 weeks. Give with fluorouracil 450 mg/m^2.

How supplied
Available by prescription only
Tablets: 50 mg

Pharmacodynamics
Antineoplastic action: An immunomodulator. Mechanism of action with fluorouracil unknown. Its effects on the immune system are complete, but it appears to restore depressed immune function rather than stimulate response to above-normal levels. It also can stimulate antibody formation; enhance T-cell responses by stimulating T-cell activation and proliferation; potentiate monocyte and macrophage formation, including phagocytosis and chemotaxis; increase neutrophil mobility adherence and chemotaxis; and inhibit alkaline phosphatase. Levamisole also has cholinergic activity.

Pharmacokinetics
Absorption: Rapidly absorbed from GI tract; peak plasma levels occur in 1½ to 2 hours.
Distribution: No information available.
Metabolism: Extensively metabolized by liver.
Excretion: 70% of metabolites excreted in urine over 3 days, 5% in feces; less than 5% of unchanged drug excreted in urine; less than 2% in feces.

Route	Onset	Peak	Duration
P.O.	Rapid	1½–2 hr	Unknown

Contraindications and precautions
Contraindicated in patients hypersensitive to drug.

Interactions
Drug-drug. *Phenytoin:* Increased phenytoin levels. Monitor plasma phenytoin levels; decrease dosage as needed.
Warfarin: Possible excessive prolongation of PT and INR. Monitor PT and INR and adjust warfarin dosage as needed.
Drug-lifestyle. *Alcohol:* Disulfiram-like reaction if used together. Discourage use.

Adverse reactions
CNS: *dizziness, headache, paresthesia, somnolence, depression, nervousness, insomnia, anxiety, fatigue, fever.*
CV: chest pain, edema.
EENT: blurred vision, conjunctivitis, *stomatitis, dysgeusia, altered sense of smell.*
GI: *nausea, diarrhea, vomiting, anorexia, abdominal pain, constipation, flatulence, dyspepsia.*
Hematologic: agranulocytosis, leukopenia, thrombocytopenia, anemia.
Hepatic: hyperbilirubinemia.
Musculoskeletal: *arthralgia, myalgia.*
Skin: *alopecia,* dermatitis, **exfoliative dermatitis,** *pruritus, urticaria.*
Other: rigors, *infection.*

Overdose and treatment
Fatalities have been reported after ingestion of 15 mg/kg by a 3-year-old child and of 32 mg/kg by an adult. In case of overdose, gastric lavage is recommended along with symptomatic and supportive measures.

Special considerations
• Don't use drug in higher than recommended dosage or administer more frequently than indicated.
• Before drug therapy begins, patient should be ambulatory, maintain normal oral nutrition, have well-healed wounds, be fully recovered from any postsurgical complications, and not be hospitalized.
• If an acute neurologic syndrome occurs, consider stopping drug immediately.

Reactions may be *common*, uncommon, **life-threatening**, or COMMON AND LIFE-THREATENING.

Patient monitoring

• Obtain CBC with differential, platelet counts, electrolyte levels, and liver function test results before therapy. CBC with differential and platelet counts should be performed weekly before each fluorouracil treatment; electrolyte and liver function tests every 3 months for 1 year. Modify doses as needed.

• If WBC count is 2,500 to 3,500/mm^3, defer fluorouracil dose until count is over 3,500/mm^3. If WBC count is below 2,500/mm^3, defer fluorouracil dose until count is above 3,500/mm^3, and then reduce dose by 20%. If WBC count remains below 2,500/mm^3 for more than 10 days even after deferring fluorouracil, stop drug. Defer both if platelet counts are below 100,000/mm^3.

• If stomatitis or diarrhea develops during initial fluorouracil administration schedule, stop course before full five doses are given. If stomatitis or diarrhea occurs during weekly maintenance therapy, defer next dose of fluorouracil until it subsides. If adverse reactions are moderate to severe, reduce fluorouracil dose by 20% when treatment is resumed.

Pediatric patients

• Safety and efficacy in children haven't been established.

Breast-feeding patients

• Although it's unknown whether drug appears in breast milk, potential for serious adverse reactions in infants must be considered.

Patient education

• Advise patient to use a soft toothbrush and electric razor to avoid trauma and excessive bleeding.

• Tell patient to report unusual bruising or bleeding.

• Flu syndrome frequently accompanies onset of agranulocytosis but may also occur in the absence of agranulocytosis. Instruct patient to report flulike symptoms immediately.

• Advise patient to avoid exposure to persons with infection.

---

levetiracetam
Keppra

Pharmacologic classification: anticonvulsant
Therapeutic classification: anticonvulsant
Pregnancy risk category: C

Indications and dosages

➤ *Adjunctive therapy for partial seizures.*
Adults: Initially, 500 mg b.i.d. Dosage can be increased by 500 mg b.i.d., p.r.n., for seizure control at 2-week intervals to maximum dosage of 1,500 mg b.i.d.

✦ *Dosage adjustment.* For patients with renal impairment, if creatinine clearance is 50 to 80 ml/minute, give 500 to 1,000 mg q 12 hours;

if 30 to 50 ml/minute, give 250 to 750 mg q 12 hours; if less than 30 ml/minute, give 250 to 500 mg q 12 hours. For end-stage renal disease dialysis patients, give 500 to 1,000 mg q 24 hours. A 250- to 500-mg dose should be given after dialysis.

How supplied

Available by prescription only
Tablets: 250 mg, 500 mg, 750 mg

Pharmacodynamics

Anticonvulsant action: Mechanism unknown. Thought to inhibit kindling activity in hippocampus, thus preventing simultaneous neuronal firing that leads to seizure activity.

Pharmacokinetics

Absorption: Rapidly absorbed in GI tract; serum levels peak in about 1 hour. Can be taken with food, but time to reach peak levels is delayed by about 1½ hours with slightly lower serum levels. Steady state serum levels reached in about 2 days.
Distribution: Minimal protein-binding.
Metabolism: No active metabolites; isn't metabolized through cytochrome P-450 system.
Excretion: Elimination half-life is about 7 hours in patients with normal renal function. 66% of drug eliminated unchanged by glomerular filtration and tubular reabsorption.

Route	Onset	Peak	Duration
P.O.	Rapid	1 hr	Unknown

Contraindications and precautions

Contraindicated in patients hypersensitive to drug. Use cautiously in immunocompromised patients and in those with poor renal function.

Interactions

Drug-drug. *Antihistamines, benzodiazepines, narcotics, tricyclic antidepressants, other drugs that cause drowsiness:* Possible severe sedation. Avoid concomitant use.
Drug-lifestyle. *Alcohol use:* Possible severe sedation. Discourage use.

Adverse reactions

CNS: *asthenia, headache, somnolence,* dizziness, depression, vertigo, paresthesia, nervousness, hostility, emotional lability, ataxia, amnesia, anxiety.
EENT: diplopia, sinusitis, pharyngitis, rhinitis.
GI: anorexia.
Hematologic: *leukopenia, neutropenia.*
Musculoskeletal: pain.
Respiratory: cough, infection.

Overdose and treatment

For overdose, emesis or gastric lavage may be helpful in early stages of treatment. Hemodialysis removes about 50% of drug if performed within 4 hours of overdose.

Special considerations
- For patients with poor renal function, dosage reduction is based on creatinine clearance.
- Seizures can occur if drug is stopped abruptly. Tapering is recommended.
- Drug is approved only as an adjunctive drug for partial seizures.
- Drug can be taken with or without food.

Patient monitoring
- Baseline CBC with periodic follow-up may be advisable in immunocompromised patients because of reports of leukopenia and neutropenia.
- Monitor patients closely for such adverse reactions as dizziness, which may lead to falls.

Breast-feeding patients
- It's unknown whether drug appears in breast milk. Determine risks and benefits before administering to breast-feeding women.

Pediatric patients
- Drug isn't recommended for children under age 16.

Geriatric patients
- Inform patient to use extra care when sitting up or standing to avoid falling.

Patient education
- Inform patient to call and not to stop drug suddenly if adverse reactions occur.
- Warn patient to use extra care when sitting or standing to avoid falling.
- Inform patient to take this drug in addition to other prescribed seizure drugs.

levobunolol hydrochloride
AKBeta, Betagan

Pharmacologic classification: beta blocker
Therapeutic classification: antiglaucoma
Pregnancy risk category: C

Indications and dosages
➤ *Chronic open-angle glaucoma and ocular hypertension. Adults:* Instill 1 to 2 drops (0.5% solution) daily or 1 to 2 drops (0.25% solution) b.i.d. in eye.

How supplied
Available by prescription only
Ophthalmic solution: 0.25%, 0.5%

Pharmacodynamics
Antiglaucoma action: Levobunolol is a nonselective beta blocker that reduces intraocular pressure. Exact mechanisms are unknown, but the drug appears to reduce formation of aqueous humor.

Pharmacokinetics
Absorption: Systemic absorption is undetermined but may occur.
Distribution: Unknown.
Metabolism: Unknown.
Excretion: Unknown.

Route	Onset	Peak	Duration
Oph-thalmic	1 hr	2-6 hr	24 hr

Contraindications and precautions
Contraindicated in patients hypersensitive to drug and those with bronchial asthma, history of bronchial asthma or severe COPD, sinus bradycardia, second- or third-degree AV block, cardiac failure, and cardiogenic shock. Use cautiously in patients with chronic bronchitis, emphysema, diabetes mellitus, hyperthyroidism, and myasthenia gravis.

Interactions
Drug-drug. *Carbonic anhydrase inhibitors, epinephrine, pilocarpine:* Increased reductions in intraocular pressure. Use together cautiously.
Catecholamine-depleting drugs, reserpine: Enhanced hypotensive and bradycardiac effects of these drugs. Monitor patient carefully.
Oral beta blockers: Increased systemic effects. Monitor patient carefully.

Adverse reactions
CNS: headache, depression, insomnia.
CV: slight reduction in resting heart rate.
EENT: *transient eye stinging and burning*, tearing, erythema, itching, keratitis, corneal punctate staining, photophobia; decreased corneal sensitivity (with long-term use).
GI: nausea.
Skin: urticaria.
Other: evidence of beta blockade and systemic absorption (*hypotension*, **bradycardia**, *syncope*, **asthmatic attacks in patients with history of asthma, heart failure**).

Overdose and treatment
Overdose is extremely rare with ophthalmic use. However, usual symptoms include bradycardia, hypotension, bronchospasm, heart block, and cardiac failure. After accidental ingestion, emesis is most effective if started within 30 minutes, providing patient isn't obtunded, comatose, or having seizures. Follow with activated charcoal. Treat bradycardia, conduction defects, and hypotension with I.V. fluids, glucagon, atropine, or isoproterenol. Treat bronchoconstriction with I.V. aminophylline, and treat seizures with I.V. diazepam.

Special considerations
⚠ ALERT Drug contains sodium metabisulfite which may precipitate an allergic reaction in susceptible people.
- Levobunolol is faster acting than timolol.

• Because levobunolol has little or no effect on pupil size, don't use drug alone in patients with angle-closure glaucoma; use with a miotic.
• Store at 59° to 86° F (15° to 30° C) in light-resistant container.

Patient monitoring
• Cardiac output is reduced in both healthy patients and those with heart disease. Drug may decrease heart rate and blood pressure and produces beta blockade in bronchi and bronchioles. No effect on pupil size or accommodation has been noted. Monitor patient for these effects.
• In some patients, a few weeks' treatment may be required to stabilize pressure-lowering response; determine intraocular pressure after 4 weeks of treatment.

Geriatric patients
• Use drug cautiously in elderly patients with cardiac or pulmonary disease, whose symptoms may worsen depending on extent of systemic absorption.

Patient education
• Warn patient not to touch dropper to eye or surrounding tissue.
• Show patient how to instill drug. Teach him to press lacrimal sac lightly for 1 minute after drug administration, to decrease chance of systemic absorption.
• Remind patient not to blink more than usual or to close eyes tightly during treatment.
• Tell patient to report severe reaction, although transient stinging and discomfort are common.

levobupivacaine
Chirocaine

Pharmacologic classification: amino amide local anesthetic
Therapeutic classification: local anesthetic
Pregnancy risk category: B

Indications and dosages
➤ **Epidural for surgery.** *Adults:* 50 to 150 mg (10 to 20 ml) 0.5% to 0.75% solution.
➤ **Epidural for cesarean section.** *Adults:* 100 to 150 mg (20 to 30 ml) 0.5% solution.
➤ **Peripheral nerve block.** *Adults:* 75 to 150 mg (30 ml) or 1 to 2 mg/kg (0.4 ml/kg) 0.25% to 0.5% solution.
➤ **Ophthalmic block.** *Adults:* 37.5 to 112.5 mg (5 to 15 ml) 0.75% solution.
➤ **Local infiltration.** *Adults:* 150 mg (60 ml) 0.25% solution.
➤ **Labor analgesia.** *Adults:* 25 to 50 mg (10 to 20 ml) 0.25% solution as epidural bolus.
➤ **Postoperative pain.** *Adults:* 5 to 25 mg/hr (4 to 10 ml/hr) 0.125% to 0.25% solution as epidural infusion.
   Note: Dosage will differ depending on anesthetic procedure, area to be anesthetized, vas-

cularity of area, number of neuronal segments to be blocked, degree of block, duration of anesthesia desired, and individual patient conditions and tolerance. Always use incremental doses.

How supplied
Available by prescription only
Injection: 2.5 mg/ml (0.25%), 5 mg/ml (0.5%), 7.5 mg/ml (0.75%)

Pharmacodynamics
Anesthetic action: Chirocaine blocks the generation and conduction of nerve impulses by increasing the threshold for electrical excitation in the nerve, by slowing propagation of the nerve impulse, and by slowing the action potential.

Pharmacokinetics
Absorption: Depends on dose and route of administration because absorption from the site of administration is affected by vascularity of tissue. Blood levels peak 30 minutes after epidural administration.
Distribution: Plasma protein binding is greater than 97%. Drug is widely distributed to all tissues after parenteral administration.
Metabolism: Is widely metabolized by hepatic enzyme systems with no unchanged drug excreted in the urine or feces. In vitro studies show that CYP 3A4 isoform and CYP 1A2 isoform mediate the metabolism of levobupivacaine.
Excretion: After I.V. administration 71% is recovered from the urine and 24% from the feces. The elimination half-life is 3⅓ hours after I.V. administration with a terminal half-life of 1⅓ hours.

Route	Onset	Peak	Duration
Epidural, local injection	Variable	30 min	80 min

Adverse reactions
CNS: dizziness, *headache*, paresthesia, somnolence, anxiety, hypoesthesia.
CV: hypotension, abnormal ECG, *bradycardia*, tachycardia, hypertension.
EENT: diplopia.
GI: nausea, vomiting, enlarged abdomen, constipation, flatulence, abdominal pain, dyspepsia, diarrhea.
GU: albuminuria, urine incontinence, decreased urine flow, urinary tract infection, hematuria, abnormal urine.
Hematologic: anemia, leukocytosis.
Musculoskeletal: back pain.
Respiratory: cough.
Skin: pruritus, purpura.
Other: postoperative pain, fever, fetal distress, delayed delivery, pain, rigors, hypothermia, hemorrhage in pregnancy, breast pain, increased wound drainage, local anesthesia.

Interactions

Drug-drug. *Calcium channel blockers, clarithromycin, erythromycin, ketoconazole, ritonavir:* Decreased hepatic metabolism and increased effect of levobupivacaine. Consider adjusting levobupivacaine dosage.

Drugs related to amide-type local anesthetics, other local anesthetics: Increased toxic effects of these drugs. Use cautiously.

Omeprazole, phenobarbital, phenytoin, rifampin: Possible increased hepatic metabolism with decreased levobupivacaine effect. Monitor patient closely.

Overdose and treatment

Emergencies are generally related to high plasma levels or high dermatomal level. Toxic reactions may include CNS stimulation, seizures, circulatory depression, apnea, and respiratory depression.

To treat toxic reactions, immediately establish and maintain a patent airway or administer controlled ventilation with 100% oxygen. If necessary, use I.V. barbiturates, anticonvulsants, or muscle relaxants to control convulsions. Supportive treatment of circulatory depression may require the administration of I.V. fluids or appropriate vasopressors. If difficulty is encountered in maintaining a patent airway or prolonged ventilatory support is necessary, endotracheal intubation may be indicated. If maternal hypotension or fetal bradycardia occur in the pregnant patient, maintain the patient in the left lateral decubitus position, if possible, or manually displace the uterus off the great vessels to prevent aortocaval compression of the uterus. Resuscitation in pregnant patients may take longer than in nonpregnant patients. Rapid delivery of the fetus may improve the response to resuscitation efforts.

Contraindications and precautions

Contraindicated in patients hypersensitive to levobupivacaine or to any local anesthetic of the amide type. Don't use in emergency situations in which a fast onset of surgical anesthesia is necessary. Avoid 0.75% levobupivacaine in obstetric patients, and don't use solutions of levobupivacaine for the production of obstetric paracervical block anesthesia. Don't use for I.V. regional anesthesia (Bier block).

Use cautiously when administering large volumes of higher concentrations because cardiac toxicity can occur. Use cautiously in patients with hepatic disease, hypotension, hypovolemia, or impaired CV function, especially heart block.

Special considerations

⚠ ALERT Local anesthetics should be administered only by health care providers experienced in the diagnosis and management of drug-related toxicity and other acute emergencies that may occur.

● Keep resuscitative equipment, drugs, and oxygen immediately available.

● Don't use disinfectants that contain heavy metals, which cause the release of ions, for skin or mucous membrane disinfection because they may cause swelling and edema.

⚠ ALERT Unintended I.V. injection is possible and may result in cardiac arrest.

⚠ ALERT Pregnant women have a high risk of cardiac arrhythmias, cardiac and circulatory arrest, and death if drug is inadvertently administered I.V.

● A test dose of a local anesthetic with a fast onset, preferably a solution containing epinephrine, should be administered before epidural anesthesia with Chirocaine and the patient monitored for CNS and CV toxicity.

● Aspiration for blood or CSF should be performed before injecting any dose of Chirocaine to avoid intravascular or intrathecal injection.

⚠ ALERT An intravascular injection is still possible even if aspirations for blood are negative.

● Administer the smallest dose and concentration required to produce the desired result.

● During epidural administration, administer in incremental volumes of 3 to 5 ml with sufficient time between doses to detect toxicity.

● Small doses of local anesthetics injected into the head and neck area may produce adverse reactions similar to systemic toxicity seen with unintentional intravascular injections of larger doses.

● Local anesthetics rapidly cross the placenta and can cause maternal, fetal, and neonatal toxicity. Adverse reactions may involve alterations in the CNS, peripheral vascular tone, and cardiac function, including maternal hypotension, fetal bradycardia, and fetal decelerations. Monitor the fetal heart rate continuously.

● The 0.75% concentration is indicated for nonobstetrical surgery patients requiring long duration of profound muscle relaxation.

● The 0.125% solution is to be used only as adjunct therapy with fentanyl or clonidine.

● Chirocaine may be incompatible with alkaline solutions having a pH greater than 8.5.

● Levobupivacaine diluted in saline solution is stable when stored in polyvinyl chloride bags at room temperature for up to 24 hours.

Patient monitoring

● Monitor patient for ECG changes, hypotension, and bradycardia.

● Continuously monitor CV and respiratory status and patient's state of consciousness after each injection. Restlessness, anxiety, incoherent speech, lightheadedness, numbness and tingling of mouth and lips, metallic taste, tinnitus, dizziness, blurred vision, tremors, twitching, depression, or drowsiness may be early signs of CNS toxicity.

Breast-feeding patients

● Some local anesthetics appear in breast milk. Use cautiously in breast-feeding women.

Pediatric patients

● Safety and efficacy haven't been established.

Reactions may be *common*, uncommon, *life-threatening*, or COMMON AND LIFE-THREATENING.

Geriatric patients
● No differences in safety and effectiveness have been observed in geriatric patients.

Patient education
● Advise patient that temporary loss of sensation and motor activity in the anesthetized part of the body may occur.

levodopa
Dopar, Larodopa

Pharmacologic classification: dopamine precursor
Therapeutic classification: antiparkinsonian
Pregnancy risk category: C

Indications and dosages
➤**Parkinsonism.** *Adults:* Initially, 0.5 to 1 g P.O. daily, given b.i.d., t.i.d., or q.i.d. with food; increase 100 to 750 mg daily q 3 to 7 days, as tolerated. The usual optimal dosage is 3 to 6 g daily divided into three or more doses. Maximum recommended dose is 8 g daily; some patients may require more. A significant therapeutic response may not be obtained for 6 months. Larger dose requires close supervision.

How supplied
Available by prescription only
Tablets: 100 mg, 250 mg, 500 mg
Capsules: 100 mg, 250 mg, 500 mg

Pharmacodynamics
Antiparkinsonian action: Precise mechanism hasn't been established. A small percentage of each dose crossing the blood-brain barrier is decarboxylated. The dopamine then stimulates dopaminergic receptors in the basal ganglia to enhance the balance between cholinergic and dopaminergic activity, resulting in improved modulation of voluntary nerve impulses transmitted to the motor cortex.

Pharmacokinetics
Absorption: Absorbed rapidly from the small intestine by an active amino acid transport system, with 30% to 50% reaching general circulation.
Distribution: Distributed widely to most body tissues, but not to the CNS, which receives less than 1% of dose because of extensive metabolism in the periphery.
Metabolism: 95% is converted to dopamine by l-aromatic amino acid decarboxylase enzyme in the lumen of the stomach and intestines and on the first pass through the liver.
Excretion: Excreted primarily in urine; 80% of dose is excreted within 24 hours as dopamine metabolites. Half-life is 1 to 3 hours.

Route	Onset	Peak	Duration
P.O.	Unknown	1-3 hr	5 hr

Contraindications and precautions
Contraindicated in patients who have used MAO inhibitors within 14 days; in patients hypersensitive to drug; and in patients with acute angle-closure glaucoma, melanoma, or undiagnosed skin lesions.

Use cautiously in patients with severe renal, CV, hepatic, and pulmonary disorders; peptic ulcer; psychiatric illness; MI with residual arrhythmias; bronchial asthma; emphysema; and endocrine disorders.

Interactions
Drug-drug. *Amantadine, benztropine, procyclidine, trihexyphenidyl:* May increase the efficacy of levodopa. May be used for therapeutic benefit.
Anesthetics, hydrocarbon inhalation: May cause arrhythmias because of increased endogenous dopamine concentration. Stop levodopa 6 to 8 hours before giving anesthetics such as halothane.
Antacids that contain calcium, magnesium, or sodium bicarbonate: May increase levodopa absorption. Give antacids 1 hour after levodopa.
Anticholinergics: May produce mild synergy and increased efficacy. Gradual reduction in anticholinergic dosage is necessary.
Anticonvulsants (such as hydantoins, phenytoin), benzodiazepines, haloperidol, papaverine, phenothiazines, rauwolfia alkaloids, thioxanthenes: May decrease therapeutic effects of levodopa. Monitor patient for decreased effectiveness.
Antihypertensives: Increased hypotensive effect. Monitor blood pressure.
Bromocriptine: May produce additive effects. Reduce levodopa dosage if necessary.
MAO inhibitors: May cause hypertensive crisis. Discontinue MAO inhibitors for 2 to 4 weeks before starting levodopa.
Methyldopa: May alter antiparkinsonian effects of levodopa and produce additive toxic CNS effects. Avoid use together.
Pyridoxine: A small dose (10 mg) reverses antiparkinsonian effects of levodopa. Don't give together.
Sympathomimetics: May increase the risk of arrhythmias. Dosage reduction of the sympathomimetic is recommended; administration of carbidopa with levodopa reduces the tendency of sympathomimetics to cause dopamine-induced arrhythmias. Reduce levodopa dosage.
Tricyclic antidepressants: May increase sympathetic activity, with sinus tachycardia and hypertension. Avoid use together if possible.
Drug-herb. *Jimsonweed:* May adversely affect CV function. Discourage use together.
Kava: May increase parkinsonian symptoms. Discourage use together.
Rauwolfia: May decrease effectiveness of levodopa. Discourage use together.

Adverse reactions

CNS: *aggressive behavior; choreiform, dystonic, and dyskinetic movements; involuntary grimacing; head movements, myoclonic body jerks;* **seizures; neuroleptic malignant syndrome;** ataxia; tremor; muscle twitching; bradykinetic episodes; psychiatric disturbances; mood changes; nervousness; anxiety; disturbing dreams; euphoria; malaise; fatigue; severe depression; **suicidal tendencies;** dementia; delirium; hallucinations.

CV: *orthostatic hypotension,* cardiac irregularities, phlebitis.

EENT: blepharospasm, blurred vision, diplopia, mydriasis or miosis, activation of latent Horner's syndrome, oculogyric crises, excessive salivation.

GI: dry mouth, bitter taste, *nausea, vomiting, anorexia,* constipation, flatulence, diarrhea, abdominal pain.

GU: urinary frequency, urine retention, incontinence, darkened urine, priapism.

Hematologic: *hemolytic anemia, leukopenia, agranulocytosis.*

Hepatic: elevated liver enzyme levels, *hepatotoxicity.*

Metabolic: weight loss.

Respiratory: hyperventilation, hiccups.

Other: dark perspiration.

Overdose and treatment

Signs and symptoms of overdose include spasm or closing of eyelids, irregular heartbeat, or palpitations.

Treatment includes immediate gastric lavage, maintenance of an adequate airway, and judicious administration of I.V. fluids and may include antiarrhythmic drugs, if necessary. Pyridoxine 10 to 25 mg P.O. has been reported to reverse toxic and therapeutic effects of levodopa. (Its usefulness hasn't been established in acute overdose.)

Special considerations

● Levodopa is indicated in treating idiopathic, postencephalitic, arteriosclerotic parkinsonism, and symptomatic parkinsonism that may follow injury to the nervous system by carbon monoxide intoxication and manganese intoxication.

● Give drug between meals and with low-protein snack to maximize drug absorption and minimize GI upset. Foods high in protein appear to interfere with transport of drug.

● Tablets and capsules may be crushed and mixed with applesauce or pureed fruit for patients who have difficulty swallowing pills.

● Maximum effectiveness of drug may not occur for several weeks or months.

● Because of risk of precipitating a symptom complex resembling neuroleptic malignant syndrome, observe patient closely if levodopa dosage is reduced abruptly or discontinued.

● If restarting therapy after a long period of interruption, adjust drug dosage gradually to previous level.

● Patients undergoing surgery should continue levodopa as long as oral intake is permitted, usually 6 to 24 hours before surgery. Resume drug as soon as patient is able to take oral medication.

● Although controversial, a medically supervised period of drug discontinuance may reestablish the effectiveness of a lower dose regimen.

● Combination of levodopa-carbidopa usually reduces amount of levodopa needed, thus reducing risk of adverse reactions.

● Levodopa also has been used to relieve pain of herpes zoster, to manage bone pain in metastatic disease, and to manage hepatic coma.

● Protect drug from heat, light, and moisture. If preparation darkens, it has lost potency and should be discarded.

● Coombs' test occasionally becomes positive during extended therapy. Colorimetric test for uric acid has shown false elevations. False-positive results have been noted on tests for urine glucose using the copper-reduction method; false-negative results have occurred with the glucose oxidase method. Levodopa also may interfere with tests for urine ketones, urine norepinephrine and urine protein determinations.

Patient monitoring

● Monitor patient also receiving antihypertensive medication for possible drug interactions. Discontinue MAO inhibitors at least 2 weeks before levodopa therapy begins.

● Monitor vital signs, especially while adjusting dose.

● Monitor patient for muscle twitching and blepharospasm (twitching of eyelids), which may be an early sign of drug overdose.

● Patients on long-term therapy should be tested regularly for diabetes and acromegaly; check blood tests and liver and kidney function studies periodically for adverse effects. Leukopenia may require cessation of therapy.

● Monitor serum laboratory tests periodically. Coombs' test occasionally becomes positive during extended use. Expect uric acid elevation with colorimetric method but not with uricase method.

● Alkaline phosphatase, AST, ALT, LDH, bilirubin, BUN, and protein-bound iodine levels show transient elevations in patients receiving levodopa; WBC count, hemoglobin level, and hematocrit show occasional reduction.

Breast-feeding patients

● Drug may inhibit lactation and shouldn't be used by breast-feeding women.

Pediatric patients

● Safety of levodopa in children under age 12 hasn't been established.

Geriatric patients

● Smaller doses may be required because of reduced tolerance to effects of drug. Geriatric patients, especially those with osteoporosis, should

---

Reactions may be *common,* uncommon, *life-threatening*, or COMMON AND LIFE-THREATENING.

resume normal activity gradually, because increased mobility may increase risk of fractures. Geriatric patients are more likely to develop adverse effects, such as anxiety, confusion, or nervousness; those with heart disease are more susceptible to cardiac effects of levodopa.

Patient education
● Warn patient and family not to increase drug dose without specific instruction. (They may be tempted to do this as parkinsonian symptoms progress.)
● Explain that therapeutic response may not occur for up to 6 months.
● Advise patient and family that multivitamin preparations, fortified cereals, and certain OTC products may contain pyridoxine (vitamin B_6), which can reverse the effects of levodopa.
● Warn patient of possible dizziness and orthostatic hypotension, especially at start of therapy. Tell patient to change position slowly and dangle legs before getting out of bed. Instruct patient in use of elastic stockings to control this adverse reaction if appropriate.
● Inform patient of signs and symptoms of adverse reactions and therapeutic effects and need to report changes.
● Tell patient to take a missed dose as soon as possible; skip dose if next scheduled dose is within 2 hours, but not to double the dose.
● Advise patient not to take drug with food, and that eating about 15 minutes after administration may help reduce GI upset.
● Warn patient of possible darkening of urine, sweat, and other body fluids.

---

levodopa-carbidopa
Sinemet 10-100, Sinemet 25-100, Sinemet 25-250, Sinemet CR 25-100, Sinemet CR 50-200

Pharmacologic classification: decarboxylase inhibitor/dopamine precursor combination
Therapeutic classification: antiparkinsonian
Pregnancy risk category: C

Indications and dosages
➤ *Parkinsonism. Adults:* Most patients respond to a 25 mg/100 mg combination (1 tablet P.O. t.i.d.). Dose may be increased q 1 or 2 days to maximum of 8 tablets or 1 tablet of 10 mg/100 mg t.i.d. or q.i.d. up to 2 tablets q.i.d.; or 1 sustained-release tablet b.i.d. at intervals at least 6 hours apart. Intervals may be adjusted based on patient response. Usual dose is 2 to 8 tablets daily in divided doses every 4 to 8 hours while awake.
Maintenance therapy must be carefully adjusted based on patient tolerance and desired therapeutic response. Usual maintenance dosage is 3 to 6 tablets of 25 mg carbidopa/250 mg levodopa P.O. daily in divided doses. Don't exceed 8 tablets of 25 mg carbidopa/250 mg levodopa

daily. Optimum daily dose must be determined by careful adjustment for each patient.
Daily dose of carbidopa should be 70 to 100 mg or more to suppress the peripheral metabolism of levodopa.

How supplied
Available by prescription only
Tablets: 10 mg carbidopa with 100 mg levodopa (Sinemet 10-100), 25 mg carbidopa with 100 mg levodopa (Sinemet 25-100), 25 mg carbidopa with 250 mg levodopa (Sinemet 25-250)
Tablets (sustained-release): 50 mg carbidopa with 200 mg levodopa (Sinemet CR 50-200), 25 mg carbidopa with 100 mg levodopa (Sinemet CR 25-100)

Pharmacodynamics
Decarboxylase-inhibiting action: Carbidopa inhibits the peripheral decarboxylation of levodopa, thus slowing its conversion to dopamine in extracerebral tissues. This results in an increased availability of levodopa for transport to the brain, where it undergoes decarboxylation to dopamine.

Pharmacokinetics
Absorption: 40% to 70% of dose is absorbed after oral administration. Plasma levodopa levels increase when carbidopa and levodopa are administered together because carbidopa inhibits the peripheral metabolism of levodopa.
Distribution: Carbidopa is distributed widely in body tissues except the CNS. Levodopa is also distributed into breast milk.
Metabolism: Carbidopa isn't metabolized extensively. It inhibits metabolism of levodopa in the GI tract, thus increasing its absorption from the GI tract and its level in plasma.
Excretion: 30% of the dose is excreted unchanged in urine within 24 hours. When given with carbidopa, the amount of levodopa excreted unchanged in urine increases by about 6%. Half-life is 1 to 2 hours.

Route	Onset	Peak	Duration
P.O.	Unknown	40-150 min	Unknown

Contraindications and precautions
Contraindicated in patients hypersensitive to drug; in those with acute angle-closure glaucoma, melanoma, or undiagnosed skin lesions; and within 14 days of MAO inhibitor therapy.
Use cautiously in patients with severe CV, endocrine, pulmonary, renal, or hepatic disorders; peptic ulcer; psychiatric illness; MI with residual arrhythmias; bronchial asthma; emphysema; and well-controlled chronic open-angle glaucoma.

Interactions
Drug-drug. *Amantadine, benztropine, procyclidine, trihexyphenidyl:* May increase the efficacy of levodopa. May be used for therapeutic benefit.

Anesthetics, hydrocarbon inhalation: May cause arrhythmias because of increased endogenous dopamine concentration. Discontinue levodopa 6 to 8 hours before giving anesthetics such as halothane.

Antacids that contain calcium, magnesium, or sodium bicarbonate: May increase levodopa absorption. Give antacids 1 hour after levodopa.

Anticonvulsants (such as hydantoins, phenytoin), benzodiazepines, haloperidol, papaverine, phenothiazines, rauwolfia alkaloids, or thioxanthenes: May decrease therapeutic effects of levodopa. Monitor patient for decreased effectiveness.

Antihypertensives: Increased hypotensive effect. Monitor blood pressure.

Bromocriptine: May produce additive effects. Reduce levodopa dosage if necessary.

MAO inhibitors: May cause hypertensive crisis. Discontinue MAO inhibitors for 2 to 4 weeks before starting levodopa.

Methyldopa: May alter antiparkinsonian effects of levodopa and produce additive toxic CNS effects. Avoid use together.

Molindone: May inhibit antiparkinsonian effects of levodopa by blocking dopamine receptors in the brain. Avoid use together.

Sympathomimetics: May increase risk of arrhythmias. Dosage reduction of the sympathomimetic is recommended; the administration of carbidopa with levodopa reduces the tendency of sympathomimetics to cause dopamine-induced arrhythmias. Reduce levodopa dose.

Adverse reactions

CNS: *choreiform, dystonic, and dyskinetic movements; involuntary grimacing, head movements, myoclonic body jerks, ataxia,* tremor, and muscle twitching; bradykinetic episodes; psychiatric disturbances; anxiety; disturbing dreams; euphoria; malaise; fatigue; severe depression; ***neuroleptic malignant syndrome; suicidal tendencies;*** dementia; delirium; hallucinations (may necessitate reduction or withdrawal of drug); confusion; insomnia; agitation.

CV: *orthostatic hypotension, **cardiac irregularities,*** phlebitis.

EENT: blepharospasm, blurred vision, diplopia, mydriasis or miosis, oculogyric crises, excessive salivation.

GI: *dry mouth,* bitter taste, *nausea, vomiting, anorexia,* constipation, flatulence, diarrhea, abdominal pain.

GU: urinary frequency, elevated BUN level, urine retention, urinary incontinence, darkened urine, priapism.

Hematologic: ***hemolytic anemia, thrombocytopenia, leukopenia, agranulocytosis.***

Hepatic: elevated levels of ALT, AST, alkaline phosphatase, serum bilirubin, and LD; ***hepatotoxicity.***

Metabolic: weight loss at start of therapy, elevated levels of serum protein–bound iodine, elevated serum gonadotropin levels.

Respiratory: hyperventilation, hiccups.
Other: dark perspiration.

Overdose and treatment

There have been no reports of overdose with carbidopa. Signs and symptoms of levodopa overdose are irregular heartbeat and palpitations, severe continuous nausea and vomiting, spasm or closing of eyelids.

Treatment of overdose includes immediate gastric lavage and antiarrhythmic medication, if necessary. Pyridoxine isn't effective in reversing the actions of carbidopa and levodopa combinations.

Special considerations

● Muscle twitching and blepharospasm (twitching of eyelids) may be an early sign of overdose.

● If patient is being treated with levodopa, discontinue at least 8 hours before starting levodopa-carbidopa. Initial combination therapy should provide no more than 20% to 25% of previous levodopa dosage.

● The combination drug usually reduces the amount of levodopa needed by 75%, thereby reducing the risk of adverse reactions.

● Sustained-release tablets may be split but never crushed or chewed.

● For patients being transferred from conventional levodopa-carbidopa preparation to an extended-release preparation, the extended-release tablet should provide 10% to 30% more levodopa daily.

● Pyridoxine (vitamin B_6) doesn't reverse beneficial effects of levodopa-carbidopa. Multivitamins can be taken without fear of losing control of symptoms.

● If therapy is interrupted temporarily, usual daily dosage may be given as soon as patient resumes oral medications.

● Maximum effectiveness of drug may not occur for several weeks or months.

● Antiglobulin determinations (Coombs' test) are occasionally positive after long-term use. Thyroid function determinations may inhibit thyroid-stimulating hormone response to protirelin.

● Serum and urine uric acid determinations may show false elevations. Urine glucose determinations using copper reduction method may show false-positive results; with the glucose oxidase method, false-negative results. Urine ketone determination using dip-stick method, urine norepinephrine determinations, and urine protein determinations using Lowery test may show false-positive results.

Patient monitoring

● Carefully monitor patients who also receive antihypertensive or hypoglycemic agents. Discontinue MAO inhibitors at least 2 weeks before therapy begins.

● Dosage adjustment is based on patient's response and tolerance to drug. Therapeutic and adverse reactions occur more rapidly with

---

Reactions may be *common,* uncommon, ***life-threatening,*** or **COMMON AND LIFE-THREATENING.**

levodopa-carbidopa combination than with levodopa alone. Observe and monitor vital signs, especially while dosage is being adjusted.
● Test patients on long-term therapy regularly for diabetes and acromegaly; periodically repeat blood test and liver and kidney function studies.

Breast-feeding patients
● Because levodopa may inhibit lactation, don't use drug in breast-feeding women.

Pediatric patients
● Safety of drug in children under age 18 hasn't been established.

Geriatric patients
● Smaller doses may be required in elderly patients because of their reduced tolerance to the effects of levodopa-carbidopa.
● These patients, especially those with osteoporosis, should resume normal activity gradually because increased mobility may increase the risk of fractures.
● Elderly patients are especially vulnerable to adverse CNS effects, such as anxiety, confusion, or nervousness; those with heart disease are more susceptible to cardiac effects.

Patient education
● Instruct patient to report adverse reactions and therapeutic effects.
● Warn patient of possible dizziness or orthostatic hypotension, especially at start of therapy. Tell patient to change position slowly and dangle legs before getting out of bed. Elastic stockings may be helpful in some patients.
● Tell patient to take food shortly after taking drug to relieve gastric irritation.
● Inform patient that drug may cause urine or sweat to darken.
● Tell patient to take a missed dose as soon as possible, to skip a missed dose if next scheduled dose is within 2 hours, and never to double the dose.

levofloxacin
Levaquin, Quixin

Pharmacologic classification: fluorinated carboxyquinolone
Therapeutic classification: broad-spectrum antibacterial
Pregnancy risk category: C

Indications and dosages
➤ *Acute maxillary sinusitis caused by susceptible strains of* Streptococcus pneumoniae, Moraxella catarrhalis, *or* Haemophilus influenzae. *Adults:* 500 mg P.O. or I.V. daily for 10 to 14 days.
➤ *Acute bacterial exacerbation of chronic bronchitis caused by* Staphylococcus aureus, S. pneumoniae, M. catarrhalis, H. in-

fluenzae, *or* H. parainfluenzae. *Adults:* 500 mg P.O. or I.V. daily for 7 days.
➤ *Community-acquired pneumonia caused by* S. aureus, S. pneumoniae, M. catarrhalis, H. influenzae, H. parainfluenzae, Klebsiella pneumoniae, Chlamydia pneumoniae, Legionella pneumoniae, *or* Mycoplasma pneumoniae . *Adults:* 500 mg P.O. or I.V. daily for 7 to 14 days.
➤ *Mild to moderate uncomplicated skin and skin structure infections caused by* S. aureus *or* Streptococcus pyogenes. *Adults:* 500 mg P.O. or I.V. daily for 7 to 10 days.
✦ *Dosage adjustment.* If creatinine clearance is 20 to 49 ml/minute, initial dose is 500 mg and subsequent doses are half the initial dose. If creatinine clearance is 10 to 19 ml/minute, subsequent doses are half the initial dose and the interval is prolonged to q 48 hours.
➤ *Mild to moderate complicated urinary tract infections caused by* Enterococcus faecalis, Enterobacter cloacae, Escherichia coli, K. pneumoniae, Proteus mirabilis, *or* Pseudomonas aeruginosa. *Adults:* 250 mg P.O. or I.V. daily for 10 days.
➤ *Mild to moderate acute pyelonephritis caused by* E. coli. *Adults:* 250 mg P.O. or I.V. daily for 10 days.
✦ *Dosage adjustment.* If creatinine clearance is 10 to 19 ml/minute, dosage interval is increased to q 48 hours.
➤ *Traveler's diarrhea* ◊. *Adults:* 500 mg P.O. as a single dose with loperamide hydrochloride.
➤ *Prophylaxis of traveler's diarrhea* ◊. *Adults:* 500 mg P.O. once daily during period of risk, for up to 3 weeks.
➤ *Complicated skin and skin structure infections due to methicillin-sensitive* S. aureus, E. faecalis, S. pyogenes, *or* P. mirabilis. *Adults:* 750 mg P.O. once daily for 7 to 14 days.
➤ *Bacterial conjunctivitis caused by* S. aureus, S. epidermidis, S. pneumoniae, Streptococcus *(Groups C/F),* Streptococcus *(Group G),* Viridans group streptococci, Acinetobacter iwoffii, H. influenzae, *or* Serratia marcescens. *Adults:* Instill one to two drops in affected eye q 2 hr while awake, up to eight times daily, for the first 2 days, followed by one to two drops in the affected eye q 4 hr while awake, up to four times daily, for days 3 through 7.

How supplied
Available by prescription only
Infusion (premixed): 250 mg in 50 ml D₅W, 500 mg in 100 ml D₅W, 750 mg in 150 ml D₅W
Ophthalmic solution: 0.5%
Single-use vials: 500 mg, 750 mg
Tablets: 250 mg, 500 mg, 750 mg

Pharmacodynamics
Antibacterial action: Drug inhibits bacterial DNA gyrase, an enzyme required for DNA repli-

cation, transcription, repair, and recombination in susceptible bacteria.

Pharmacokinetics

Absorption: The plasma level after I.V. administration is comparable to that observed for equivalent oral doses (on a mg/mg basis). Therefore, oral and I.V. routes are interchangeable.

Distribution: Mean volume of distribution ranges from 89 to 112 L after single and multiple 500-mg doses, indicating widespread distribution into body tissues. Drug also penetrates well into lung tissues, generally two to five times higher than plasma levels.

Metabolism: Undergoes limited metabolism. The only identified metabolites are the desmethyl and *N*-oxide metabolites, which have little relevant pharmacologic activity.

Excretion: Primarily excreted unchanged in the urine. Mean terminal half-life is about 6 to 8 hours.

Route	Onset	Peak	Duration
P.O., I.V.	Unknown	1-2 hr	Unknown

Contraindications and precautions

Contraindicated in patients hypersensitive to drug, its components, or quinolone antimicrobials. Safety and efficacy of levofloxacin in children, adolescents (under age 18), and pregnant and breast-feeding women haven't been established.

Use cautiously in patients with history of seizure disorders or other CNS diseases, such as cerebral arteriosclerosis, because quinolones can cause CNS stimulation and increased intracranial pressure. This may lead to seizures (lowered seizure threshold), toxic psychoses, tremors, restlessness, anxiety, light-headedness, confusion, hallucinations, paranoia, depression, nightmares, insomnia, and, rarely, suicidal thoughts or acts. These can occur after the first dose.

Interactions

Drug-drug. *Antacids that contain aluminum or magnesium, iron salts, products that contain zinc, sucralfate:* May interfere with GI absorption of levofloxacin. Administer these drugs at least 2 hours apart.

Antidiabetics: May alter blood glucose levels. Monitor glucose levels closely.

NSAIDs: May increase CNS stimulation. Monitor patient for seizure activity.

Theophylline: Decreased theophylline clearance. Monitor theophylline levels.

Warfarin and derivatives: Increased effect of oral anticoagulant with some fluoroquinolones. Monitor PT and INR.

Drug-lifestyle. *Sun exposure:* Increased photosensitivity. Advise patient to take precautions.

Adverse reactions

CNS: headache, insomnia, dizziness, encephalopathy, paresthesia, abnormal EEG, *seizures*.
CV: chest pain, palpitations, vasodilation.

EENT: transient decreased vision, foreign body sensation, transient ocular burning, ocular pain or discomfort, photophobia, pharyngitis.
GI: nausea, diarrhea, constipation, vomiting, abdominal pain, dyspepsia, flatulence, pseudomembranous colitis.
GU: vaginitis.
Hematologic: eosinophilia, hemolytic anemia, decreased lymphocyte count.
Metabolic: hypoglycemia.
Musculoskeletal: back pain, tendon rupture.
Respiratory: allergic pneumonitis.
Skin: rash, photosensitivity, pruritus, erythema multiforme, *Stevens-Johnson syndrome*.
Other: pain, *hypersensitivity reactions*, injection site reaction, *anaphylaxis, multisystem organ failure*, fever.

Overdose and treatment

No information available. If acute overdose occurs, empty the stomach, maintain hydration, and observe. Drug isn't effectively removed by hemodialysis or peritoneal dialysis.

Special considerations

• If patient experiences symptoms of excessive CNS stimulation (restlessness, tremor, confusion, hallucinations), stop drug and institute seizure precautions.
• Ruptures of tendons and tendonitis have occurred with quinolone therapy. Discontinue drug if pain, inflammation, or rupture of a tendon occurs. These ruptures can occur after therapy has been stopped.
• For I.V. preparations, single-dose vial must be diluted to concentration of 5 mg/ml. Don't infuse other drugs through the same I.V. line.
• Because a rapid or bolus administration may result in hypotension, I.V. levofloxacin should be administered only by slow infusion over 60 minutes.

Patient monitoring

• Monitor blood glucose and renal, hepatic, and hematopoietic studies as indicated.

Breast-feeding patients

• Based on data about ofloxacin, it can be presumed that levofloxacin will appear in breast milk. Because of potential for serious adverse reactions in breast-fed infants, a decision should be made to discontinue breast-feeding or drug.

Pediatric patients

• Safety and efficacy in children under age 18 haven't been established.

Geriatric patients

• Dosage adjustment based on age alone isn't necessary.

Patient education

• Tell patient to take drug as prescribed, even if symptoms disappear.

Reactions may be *common*, uncommon, *life-threatening*, or COMMON AND LIFE-THREATENING.

• Advise patient to take drug with plenty of fluids and to avoid antacids, sucralfate, and products containing iron or zinc for at least 2 hours before and after each dose.

• Warn patient to avoid hazardous tasks until adverse CNS effects of drug are known.

• Advise patient to use sunblock and wear protective clothing when exposed to excessive sunlight.

• Tell patient to stop drug and report rash or other signs of hypersensitivity.

• Tell patient to report pain or inflammation.

• Tell diabetic patient to monitor blood glucose levels and report a hypoglycemic reaction.

levonorgestrel implants
Norplant System

Pharmacologic classification: progestin
Therapeutic classification: contraceptive
Pregnancy risk category: X

Indications and dosages
➤ **Long-term (up to 5 years) reversible prevention of pregnancy.** *Adults:* Six Silastic capsules containing 36 mg each for a total of 216 mg are surgically implanted in the superficial plane beneath the skin of a woman's upper arm during first 7 days of onset of menses.

How supplied
Available by prescription only
Implants: 36 mg in each of six Silastic capsules; kits also include trocar, scalpel, forceps, syringe, two needles, package of skin closures, three packages of gauze sponges, stretch bandages, and surgical drape

Pharmacodynamics
Contraceptive action: Levonorgestrel is a synthetic, biologically active progestin, exhibiting no significant estrogenic activity. A continuous low dose of levonorgestrel is diffused through the wall of each capsule. Pregnancy is prevented by at least two mechanisms: inhibition of ovulation and thickening of the cervical mucus.

Pharmacokinetics
Absorption: 100% bioavailable. Plasma levels average 0.3 ng/ml over 5 years but are highly variable as a function of individual metabolism and body weight.
Distribution: Bound by the circulating protein sex hormone–binding globulin.
Metabolism: Metabolized by the liver.
Excretion: Metabolites are excreted in the urine.

Route	Onset	Peak	Duration
Subdermal	24 hr	24 hr	Unknown

Contraindications and precautions
Contraindicated in patients with active thrombophlebitis or thromboembolic disorders, undiagnosed abnormal genital bleeding, acute liver disease, malignant or benign liver tumors, known or suspected breast cancer, known or suspected pregnancy, history of idiopathic intracranial hypertension, and hypersensitivity to levonorgestrel or components of the Norplant System.

Use cautiously in diabetic and prediabetic patients and in those with history of depression or hyperlipidemia.

Interactions
Drug-drug. *Carbamazepine, phenytoin:* Reduced efficacy of levonorgestrel. Patient should take additional precautions to avoid pregnancy.

Adverse reactions
CNS: headache, nervousness, dizziness, depression, tingling, numbness.
GI: nausea, *abdominal discomfort,* appetite change.
GU: *amenorrhea, many days of bleeding or prolonged bleeding, spotting, irregular onset of bleeding, frequent onset of bleeding, scanty bleeding, cervicitis, vaginitis, leukorrhea, breast discharge.*
Metabolic: decreased thyroxine levels, increased T_4 uptake, weight gain.
Musculoskeletal: mastalgia, *musculoskeletal pain.*
Skin: dermatitis, acne, hirsutism, hypertrichosis, alopecia; infection, transient pain, itching (at implant site).
Other: adnexal enlargement, *removal difficulty.*

Overdose and treatment
Overdose can occur if more than six Silastic capsules are in situ, resulting in fluid retention with its associated effects and uterine bleeding irregularities. All previously implanted capsules should be removed before insertion of a new set.

Special considerations
• The total implanted dose is 216 mg. Implantation of all six capsules should be performed during the first 7 days of menstrual cycle. Insertion is subdermal in the midportion of the inside of the upper arm, 8 to 10 cm above the elbow crease.
• Each capsule is 2.4 mm in diameter and 34 mm in length.
• Determine whether patient has allergies to the antiseptic or anesthetic to be used, or contraindications to progestin-only contraception.
• During insertion, special attention must be given to asepsis and correct placement of capsules; careful technique minimizes tissue trauma.
• Patients should receive a copy of patient information booklet and should be made aware of potential adverse reactions and of risks and benefits of the system and of other forms of contraception.
• Store at room temperature away from excess heat and moisture.

Patient monitoring
● Patients should be reexamined at least yearly; examinations should focus on implant site, blood pressure, breasts, abdominal and pelvic organs, including cervical cytology, and related laboratory tests.
● Patient should be monitored for recurrent or abnormal vaginal bleeding.
● Patients with strong family history of breast cancer should be monitored for breast nodules.

Patient education
● Tell patient that altered bleeding patterns tend to become more regular after 9 to 12 months.
● Warn patient to report heavy bleeding.
● Advise patient to avoid bumping or wetting the insertion site for at least 3 days after insertion.
● Explain that some tenderness in the implant area may occur for 1 to 2 days.
● Tell patient that insertion usually takes 10 to 15 minutes and causes little or no discomfort because of the local anesthetic.
● Advise patient that, when laboratory studies are ordered, she should inform all health care providers that levonorgestrel implants are being used.
● Tell patient who takes phenytoin or carbamazepine that she may need to use additional contraceptive measures.
● Advise patient to thoroughly review patient information booklet.

---

levothyroxine sodium (T₄ or L-thyroxine sodium)

$(T_4$ or L-thyroxine sodium$)$

Eltroxin, Levo-T, Levothroid, Levoxine, Levoxyl, Synthroid

Pharmacologic classification: thyroid hormone
Therapeutic classification: thyroid hormone replacement
Pregnancy risk category: A

Indications and dosages
➤ *Congenital hypothyroidism.* *Children age 1 and older:* 3 to 5 mcg/kg P.O. daily until adult dose (150 mcg) is reached in early or mid-adolescence.
Children under age 1: Initially, 25 to 50 mcg P.O. daily.
Neonates: 37.5 mcg (25 to 50 mcg) P.O. daily.
Premature neonates under 2 kg (4.4 lb) and those at risk for cardiac failure: 25 mcg P.O. daily initially; dosage may be increased to 50 mcg daily in 4 to 6 weeks.

Alternative dosing schedule
Children over age 12: Over 150 mcg or 2 to 3 mcg/kg daily.
Children ages 6 to 12: 100 to 150 mcg or 4 to 5 mcg/kg daily.
Children ages 1 to 5: 75 to 100 mcg or 5 to 6 mcg/kg daily.

Children ages 6 to 12 months: 50 to 75 mcg or 6 to 8 mcg/kg daily.
Children under age 6 months: 25 to 50 mcg or 8 to 10 mcg/kg daily.
➤ *Myxedema coma.* *Adults:* 300 to 500 mcg I.V. If no response occurs in 24 hours, give an additional 100 to 300 mcg I.V. in 48 hours. A maintenance dosage of 50 to 200 mcg may be given until condition stabilizes and drug can be given orally.
➤ *Thyroid hormone replacement for atrophy of gland, surgical removal, excessive radiation or antithyroid drugs.* *Adults:* For mild hypothyroidism—initially, 50 mcg P.O. daily, increased by 25 to 50 mcg P.O. daily q 2 to 4 weeks until desired response is achieved; may be administered I.V. or I.M. when P.O. ingestion is precluded for long periods. Usual dose is 100 to 200 mcg daily.
    For severe hypothyroidism—12.5 to 25 mcg P.O. daily, increased by 25 to 50 mcg daily q 2 to 4 weeks until desired response is achieved.
Elderly: Start at 12.5 to 50 mcg P.O. daily and increase in 12.5- to 25-mcg increments q 3 to 8 weeks.
✦ *Dosage adjustment.* For patients with CV disease, start at 50 mcg daily and increase in 50-mcg increments at 2- to 4-week intervals.

How supplied
Available by prescription only
Injection: 200 mcg/vial, 500 mcg/vial
Tablets: 25 mcg, 50 mcg, 75 mcg, 88 mcg, 100 mcg, 112 mcg, 125 mcg, 137 mcg, 150 mcg, 175 mcg, 200 mcg, 300 mcg

Pharmacodynamics
Thyroid hormone replacement: Drug affects protein and carbohydrate metabolism, promotes gluconeogenesis, increases the use and mobilization of glycogen stores, stimulates protein synthesis, and regulates cell growth and differentiation.

Pharmacokinetics
Absorption: Between 50% and 80% is absorbed from the GI tract. Full effects don't occur for 1 to 3 weeks after oral therapy begins. After I.M. administration, absorption is variable and poor. After an I.V. dose in patients with myxedema coma, increased responsiveness may occur within 6 to 8 hours, but maximum therapeutic effect may not occur for up to 24 hours.
Distribution: Distribution isn't fully described; however, drug is distributed into most body tissues and fluids. The highest levels are found in the liver and kidneys; 99% is protein-bound.
Metabolism: Metabolized in peripheral tissues, primarily in the liver, kidneys, and intestines. About 85% of metabolized levothyroxine is deiodinated.

Reactions may be *common*, uncommon, *life-threatening*, or COMMON AND LIFE-THREATENING.

Excretion: Fecal excretion eliminates 20% to 40% of levothyroxine. Half-life is 6 to 7 days.

Route	Onset	Peak	Duration
P.O.	24 hr	Unknown	Unknown
I.V., I.M.	Unknown	Unknown	Unknown

Contraindications and precautions

Contraindicated in patients hypersensitive to drug and in patients with acute MI and thyrotoxicosis uncomplicated by hypothyroidism or uncorrected adrenal insufficiency.

Use cautiously in the elderly and in patients with renal impairment, angina pectoris, hypertension, ischemia, or other CV disorders.

Interactions

Drug-drug. *Anticoagulants:* May alter anticoagulant effect. Increased levothyroxine dosage may necessitate decreased anticoagulant dosage.
Beta blockers: May decrease conversion of levothyroxine to liothyronine. Monitor patient.
Cholestyramine: May delay absorption of levothyroxine. Don't administer together.
Corticotropin: Alterations in thyroid status. Monitor patient; dosage adjustments of both medications may be needed.
Estrogens: Increased levothyroxine requirements. Monitor patient for decreased levothyroxine effect.
Hepatic enzyme inducers such as phenytoin: May increase hepatic degradation of levothyroxine and increase dosage requirements. Adjust dosages as needed.
Insulin, oral antidiabetics: Altered serum glucose levels. Adjust doses of these medications as needed.
Somatrem: May accelerate epiphyseal maturation. Avoid concurrent use in children if possible.
Sympathomimetics, tricyclic antidepressants: May increase the effects of these drugs and may lead to coronary insufficiency or arrhythmias. Monitor patient closely if concurrent use is necessary.
Theophylline: Decreased theophylline clearance in hypothyroid patients. Clearance returns to normal when euthyroid state resumes.
Drug-herb. *Horseradish:* Abnormal thyroid function may occur. Discourage use by patients undergoing thyroid function tests.
Kelp: Possible hyperthyroidism. Discourage use together.

Adverse reactions

CNS: *nervousness, insomnia, tremor,* headache.
CV: *tachycardia, palpitations,* **arrhythmias,** *angina pectoris,* **cardiac arrest.**
GI: diarrhea, vomiting.
GU: menstrual irregularities.
Metabolic: weight loss.
Skin: diaphoresis, allergic skin reactions.
Other: heat intolerance, fever.

Overdose and treatment

Evidence of overdose includes signs and symptoms of hyperthyroidism, including weight loss, increased appetite, palpitations, nervousness, diarrhea, abdominal cramps, sweating, tachycardia, increased blood pressure, widened pulse pressure, angina, arrhythmias, tremor, headache, insomnia, heat intolerance, fever, and menstrual irregularities.

Treatment of overdose requires reduction of GI absorption and efforts to counteract central and peripheral effects, primarily sympathetic activity. Use gastric lavage or induce emesis (followed by activated charcoal up to 4 hours after ingestion). If the patient is comatose or is having seizures, inflate cuff on endotracheal tube to prevent aspiration. Treatment may include oxygen and artificial ventilation as needed to support respiration. It also should include appropriate measures to treat heart failure and to control fever, hypoglycemia, and fluid loss. Propranolol (or another beta blocker) may be used to combat many of the effects of increased sympathetic activity. Levothyroxine should be gradually withdrawn over 2 to 6 days, then resumed at a lower dose.

Special considerations

● Levothyroxine has predictable effects because of standard hormonal content; therefore, it's the usual drug of choice for thyroid hormone replacement.
● Administer as a single dose before breakfast.
● Patient with history of lactose intolerance may be sensitive to Levothroid, which contains lactose.
● Synthroid 100- and 300-mcg tablets contain tartrazine, a dye that causes allergic reactions in susceptible individuals.
● When switching from levothyroxine to liothyronine, stop levothyroxine dosage when liothyronine treatment begins. After residual effects of levothyroxine have disappeared, liothyronine dosage can be increased in small increments. When switching from liothyronine to levothyroxine, begin levothyroxine therapy several days before withdrawing liothyronine to avoid relapse.
● Levothroid powder for injection or levothyroxine sodium powder is reconstituted by adding 2 ml or 5 ml of normal saline solution for injection to vial containing 200 or 500 mcg, respectively. Shake until a clear solution is obtained. Concentration is about 100 mcg/ml.
● Synthroid powder for injection is reconstituted by adding 5 ml of normal saline solution for injection or bacteriostatic sodium chloride injection with benzyl alcohol to 200- or 500-mcg vial. Shake until a clear solution is obtained. Concentration is 40 or 100 mcg/ml, respectively. Use reconstituted solutions immediately and don't administer with other I.V. infusion solutions.
● Protect drug from moisture and light.
● Levothyroxine therapy alters radioactive iodine (^{131}I) thyroid uptake, protein-bound iodine levels, and liothyronine uptake.

Patient monitoring

● Carefully observe patient for adverse effects during initial dosage adjustment phase.

● Monitor patient for aggravation of concurrent diseases, such as Addison's disease or diabetes mellitus.

● Patient taking levothyroxine who requires ^{131}I uptake studies must discontinue drug 4 weeks before test.

Breast-feeding patients

● Minimal amounts of drug appear in breast milk. Use cautiously in breast-feeding women.

Pediatric patients

● Partial and temporary hair loss may occur during the first few months of therapy.

Geriatric patients

● Elderly patients are more sensitive to effects of drug. In patients over age 60, initial dosage should be 25% lower than usual recommended dosage.

Patient education

● Advise taking drug at same time each day; encourage morning dosing to avoid insomnia.

● Tell patient to report headache, diarrhea, nervousness, excessive sweating, heat intolerance, chest pain, increased pulse rate, or palpitations.

● Encourage patient to use the same product consistently because all brands don't have equal bioavailability.

● Advise patient to store drug in cool, dry place to prevent deterioration of product.

● Tell patient that replacement therapy is to be taken essentially for life, except in cases of transient hypothyroidism.

lidocaine (lignocaine)
Xylocaine

lidocaine hydrochloride
Anestacon, Dilocaine, L-Caine, Lidoderm Patch, Lidoject, LidoPen Auto-Injector, Nervocaine, Xylocaine, Xylocaine Viscous, Zilactin-L

Pharmacologic classification: amide derivative
Therapeutic classification: ventricular antiarrhythmic, local anesthetic
Pregnancy risk category: B

Indications and dosages

➤ *Ventricular arrhythmias from MI, cardiac manipulation, or cardiac glycosides.* *Adults:* 50 to 100 mg (1 to 1.5 mg/kg) I.V. bolus at 25 to 50 mg/minute. Repeat bolus (e.g., 25 to 50 mg or 0.5 to 0.75 mg/kg) q 5 to 10 minutes until arrhythmia subsides. Don't exceed 300-mg total bolus during a 1-hour period. Simultaneously, begin constant infusion of 1 to 4 mg/

minute. If single bolus has been given, repeat smaller bolus (usually one-half initial bolus) 5 to 10 minutes after start of infusion to maintain therapeutic serum level. After 24 hours of continuous infusion, decrease rate by one half.
Elderly patients: Give half the bolus amount and use slower infusion rate.

✦ *Dosage adjustment.* Give half the bolus amount to lightweight patients and to those with heart failure or hepatic disease. Use slower infusion in those with heart failure or hepatic disease, or patients who weigh less than 50 kg (110 lb)

For I.M. administration in all adults, 300 mg (4.3 mg/kg) in deltoid muscle has been used in early stages of acute MI. If necessary, may be repeated in 60 to 90 minutes.
Children: 0.5 to 1 mg/kg by I.V. bolus; may repeat bolus if needed, not to exceed 3 to 5 mg/kg, followed by infusion of 10 to 50 mcg/kg/minute. In advanced cardiac life support, 1 mg/kg I.V. bolus, followed by an infusion of 20 to 50 mcg/kg/minute if needed after defibrillation or cardioversion.

➤ *Status epilepticus* ◇. *Adults:* 1 mg/kg I.V. bolus; then, if seizure continues, administer 0.5 mg/kg 2 minutes after first dose; infusion at 30 mcg/kg/minute may be used.

➤ *Local anesthesia of skin or mucous membranes, pain from dental extractions, stomatitis.* *Adults and children:* Apply 2% to 5% solution or ointment or 15 ml of Xylocaine Viscous q 3 to 4 hours to oral or nasal mucosa.

➤ *Local anesthesia in procedures involving the male or female urethra.* *Adults:* Instill about 15 ml (male) or 3 to 5 ml (female) into urethra.

➤ *Pain, burning, or itching caused by burns, sunburn, or skin irritation.* *Adults and children:* Apply topical agent liberally.

➤ *Relief of pain caused by post-herpetic neuralgia.* *Adults:* Apply 1 to 3 patches to intact skin, covering most painful area, once daily for up to 12 hours each day. Smaller areas of treatment are recommended in patients who are debilitated or have poor elimination. Excessive dosing by applying patch to larger areas or for longer than recommended wearing time could cause increased absorption of lidocaine and high lidocaine levels, leading to serious adverse effects.

➤ *Lidocaine hydrochloride injection used as procedural anesthetic.* *Adults:* Lidocaine with epinephrine, 7 mg/kg (no more than 500 mg total); lidocaine without epinephrine, 4.4 mg/kg (no more than 300 mg total). For continuous epidural or caudal anesthesia, maximum doses shouldn't be administered at intervals of less than 90 minutes. Maximum recommended dose in paracervical block is 200 mg total. For I.V. regional anesthesia, dose shouldn't exceed 4 mg/kg. See table on page 753.

Children: Dosages are based on age and weight. For I.V. regional anesthesia, use dilute solutions (0.25% to 0.5%) not to exceed 3 mg/kg.

Recommended dosages

Procedure	Injection (without epinephrine)		
	Concentration (%)	Volume (ml)	Total dose (mg)
Infiltration			
Percutaneous	0.5 or 1	1-60	5-300
I.V. regional	0.5	10-60	50-300
Peripheral nerve blocks			
Brachial	1.5	15-20	225-300
Dental	2	1-5	20-100
Intercostal	1	3	30
Paravertebral	1	3-5	30-50
Pudendal (each side)	1	10	100
Paracervical nerve blocks			
Obstetrical analgesia (each side)	1	10	100
Sympathetic nerve blocks			
Cervical (stellate ganglion)	1	5	50
Lumbar	1	5-10	50-100
Central nerve blocks			
Epidural*			
Thoracic	1	20-30	200-300
Lumbar			
Analgesia	1	25-30	250-300
Anesthesia	1.5	15-20	225-300
	2	10-15	200-300
Caudal			
Obstetrical analgesia	1	20-30	200-300
Surgical anesthesia	1.5	15-20	225-300

*Dose determined by number of dermatomes to be anesthetized (2-3 ml/dermatome)

The suggested concentrations and volumes serve only as a guide. Other volumes and concentrations may be used as long as the total maximum recommended dose isn't exceeded.

✦ *Dosage adjustment.* Dosages are reduced for children, geriatric patients, debilitated patients, and patients with cardiac or liver disease.

How supplied
Available by prescription only
Injection: 5 mg/ml, 10 mg/ml, 15 mg/ml, 20 mg/ml, 40 mg/ml, 100 mg/ml, 200 mg/ml
Jelly: 2%
Ointment: 5%
Parenteral injection: 0.5%, 1%, 1.5%, 2%, 4% (lidocaine with epinephrine combinations also available)
Premixed solutions: 2 mg/ml, 4 mg/ml, 8 mg/ml in D_5W
Spray: 10%
Topical solution: 2%, 4%
Available without a prescription
Cream: 0.5%
Gel: 0.5%, 2.5%
Liquid: 2.5%
Ointment: 2.5%
Spray: 0.5%
Transdermal patch: 5%

Pharmacodynamics
Ventricular antiarrhythmic action: One of the oldest antiarrhythmics, lidocaine remains among the most widely used drugs for treating acute ventricular arrhythmias. As a class IB antiarrhythmic, it suppresses automaticity and shortens the effective refractory period and action potential duration of His-Purkinje fibers and suppresses spontaneous ventricular depolarization during diastole. Therapeutic levels don't significantly affect conductive atrial tissue and AV conduction.

Unlike quinidine and procainamide, lidocaine doesn't significantly alter hemodynamics when given in usual doses. Drug seems to act preferentially on diseased or ischemic myocardial tissue; exerting its effects on the conduction system, it inhibits reentry mechanisms and halts ventricular arrhythmias.

Local anesthetic action: As a local anesthetic, lidocaine blocks initiation and conduction of nerve impulses by decreasing the permeability of the nerve cell membrane to sodium ions.

Pharmacokinetics
Absorption: Absorbed after oral administration; however, a significant first-pass effect occurs in the liver and only about 35% of drug reaches systemic circulation. Oral doses high enough to achieve therapeutic blood levels result in an unacceptable toxicity, probably from high levels of lidocaine.
Distribution: Distributed widely throughout the body; it has a high affinity for adipose tissue. After I.V. bolus administration, an early, rapid decline in plasma levels occurs; this is mainly because of distribution into highly perfused tissues, such as the kidneys, lungs, liver, and heart, followed by a slower elimination phase in which metabolism and redistribution into skeletal muscle and adipose tissue occur. The first (early) distribution phase occurs rapidly, calling for a constant infusion after an initial bolus dose. Dis-

tribution volume declines in patients with liver or hepatic disease, resulting in toxic levels with usual doses. About 60% to 80% of circulating drug is bound to plasma proteins. Usual therapeutic drug level is 1.5 to 5 mcg/ml. Although toxicity may occur within this range, levels greater than 5 mcg/ml are considered toxic and warrant dosage reduction.

Metabolism: Metabolized in the liver to two active metabolites. Less than 10% of a parenteral dose escapes metabolism and reaches the kidneys unchanged. Metabolism is affected by hepatic blood flow, which may decrease after MI and with heart failure. Liver disease also may limit metabolism.

Excretion: Half-life undergoes a biphasic process, with an initial phase of 7 to 30 minutes followed by a terminal half-life of 1½ to 2 hours. Elimination half-life may be prolonged in patients with heart failure or liver disease. Continuous infusions of longer than 24 hours also may cause a half-life increase.

Route	Onset	Peak	Duration
I.V.	Immediate	Immediate	10-20 min
I.M.	5-15 min	10 min	2 hr
Peripheral injection	Variable	Variable	Variable
Topical	30-60 sec	Unknown	Variable

Contraindications and precautions

Contraindicated in patients hypersensitive to amide-type local anesthetics, Stokes-Adams syndrome, Wolff-Parkinson-White syndrome, and severe degrees of SA, AV, or intraventricular block in absence of artificial pacemaker. Also contraindicated in patients with inflammation or infection in puncture region, septicemia, severe hypertension, spinal deformities, and neurologic disorders.

Use cautiously in geriatric patients; in patients with renal or hepatic disease, complete or second-degree heart block, sinus bradycardia, or heart failure; and in those who weigh less than 110 lb.

Interactions

Drug-drug. *Antiarrhythmics, including phenytoin, procainamide, propranolol, and quinidine:* May cause additive or antagonist effects as well as additive toxicity. Avoid use together.
Beta blockers: Enhanced sympathomimetic effects. Don't use with lidocaine and epinephrine.
Beta blockers, cimetidine: May cause lidocaine toxicity from reduced hepatic clearance. Avoid use together.
Butyrophenones, phenothiazines: May reduce or reverse the pressor effects of epinephrine. Patient requires monitoring for drug effect.
Cyclic antidepressants, MAO inhibitors: Prolonged and severe hypertension when lidocaine with epinephrine is used. Avoid use together.

Ergot-type oxytoxic drugs, vasopressors: Severe, persistent hypertension or CVA. Avoid using lidocaine with epinephrine.
High-dose lidocaine, succinylcholine: May increase neuromuscular effects of succinylcholine. Use together cautiously.
Drug-herb. *Pareira:* May add to or potentiate neuromuscular blockade. Discourage use together.

Adverse reactions

CNS: seizures; anxiety, nervousness, lethargy, somnolence, paresthesia, muscle twitching; *confusion, tremor, stupor, restlessness, light-headedness,* hallucinations (with systemic form); apprehension, unconsciousness, confusion, tremors, stupor, restlessness, slurred speech, euphoria, depression, light-headedness (with topical use).
CV: *bradycardia,* CARDIAC ARREST; *hypotension, new or worsened arrhythmias* (with systemic form); hypotension, myocardial depression, *arrhythmias* (with topical use); edema, *asystole.*
EENT: *tinnitus, blurred or double vision* (with systemic form); tinnitus, blurred or double vision(with topical use).
GI: nausea, vomiting (with topical use).
Respiratory: *respiratory arrest, status asthmaticus.*
Skin: dermatologic reactions, sensitization; diaphoresis, rash (with topical use).
Other: *anaphylaxis;* soreness at injection site, sensation of cold (with systemic form).

Overdose and treatment

Effects of overdose include signs and symptoms of CNS toxicity, such as seizures or respiratory depression, and CV toxicity (as indicated by hypotension).

Treatment includes general supportive measures and drug discontinuation. A patent airway should be maintained and other respiratory support measures carried out immediately. Diazepam or thiopental may be given to treat any seizures. To treat significant hypotension, vasopressors (including dopamine and norepinephrine) may be administered.

Special considerations

• Drug has been used investigationally to treat refractory status epilepticus.
• Don't administer lidocaine with epinephrine (for local anesthesia) to treat arrhythmias. Use solutions with epinephrine cautiously in CV disorders and in body areas with limited blood supply (ears, nose, fingers, toes).
• Patients receiving lidocaine I.M. show a sevenfold increase in serum CK level. Such CK originates in skeletal muscle, not the heart. Test isoenzyme levels to confirm MI, if using I.M. route.
• When larger volumes are required for local anesthesia, use a solution containing epinephrine.
• For I.V. regional anesthesia, use 50 ml Xylocaine 0.5% injection.

• Preparations used for epidural, spinal, or caudal anesthesia should contain no bacteriostatic agents.

• I.V. infusions are prepared by adding 1 g of lidocaine (using 25 ml of a commercially available 4% or 5 ml of a 20% injection) to 1 L of D₅W injection to provide a concentration of 1 mg/ml. Alternatively, 0.2% or 0.4% is available. In fluid-restricted patients, an 8 mg/ml concentration may be used. Don't add to blood transfusion assemblies.

• In many severely ill patients, seizures may be the first sign of toxicity. However, severe reactions are usually preceded by somnolence, confusion, and paresthesia. Regard all signs and symptoms of toxicity as serious, and promptly reduce dosage or discontinue therapy. Continued infusion could lead to seizures and coma. Give oxygen through nasal cannula, if not contraindicated. Keep oxygen and CPR equipment handy.

• Doses of up to 400 mg I.M. have been advocated in prehospital phase of acute MI.

⚠ ALERT Don't use solutions containing preservatives for spinal, epidural, or caudal block or I.V. injection.

⚠ ALERT Lidocaine injections additive syringes and single-use vials containing 40, 100, or 200 mg/ml are for I.V. infusion preparation and must be diluted before use.

• With epidural use, inject a 2- to 5-ml test dose at least 5 minutes before giving total dose to check for intravascular or subarachnoid injection. Motor paralysis and extensive sensory anesthesia indicate subarachnoid injection.

• Discard partially used vials containing no preservatives.

• Because I.M. lidocaine therapy may increase CK levels, isoenzyme tests should be performed for differential diagnosis of acute MI.

Patient monitoring

• Patient requires constant cardiac monitoring when receiving I.V. lidocaine. Use infusion pump or microdrip system and timer to monitor infusion precisely. Never exceed 4 mg/minute, if possible. A faster infusion greatly increases risk of toxicity.

• Monitor vital signs and serum electrolyte, BUN, and creatinine levels.

• Monitor ECG constantly if administering drug I.V., especially in patients with liver disease, heart failure, hypoxia, respiratory depression, hypovolemia, or shock, because these conditions may affect drug metabolism, excretion, or distribution volume, predisposing patient to drug toxicity.

• Monitor patient for signs of excessive depression of cardiac conductivity (such as sinus node dysfunction, PR-interval prolongation, QRS complex widening, and appearance or exacerbation of arrhythmias). If they occur, reduce dosage or discontinue drug.

• Therapeutic serum levels range from 2 to 5 mcg/ml.

Pediatric patients

• Safety and efficacy in children haven't been established. Use of an I.M. autoinjector device isn't recommended.

Geriatric patients

• Because of concurrent disease states and declining organ system function in geriatric patients, use conservative lidocaine doses.

lindane (gamma benzene hexachloride)
G-well, Kwell, Scabene

Pharmacologic classification: chlorinated hydrocarbon insecticide
Therapeutic classification: scabicide, pediculicide
Pregnancy risk category: B

Indications and dosages

➤ **Scabies.** *Adults and children:* Apply a thin layer of cream or lotion and gently massage it on all skin surfaces, moving from the neck to the toes. For adults and children age 6 and older, 30 to 60 ml; for children under age 6, 30 ml. After 8 to 12 hours, remove drug by bathing and scrubbing well. Treatment may be repeated after 1 week if needed.

➤ **Pediculosis.** *Adults and children:* Apply shampoo to clean, dry, affected area and wait 4 minutes. Then add a small amount of water and lather for 4 to 5 minutes; rinse thoroughly. Comb hair to remove nits. Treatment may be repeated after 1 week if needed.

How supplied

Available by prescription only
Lotion: 1%
Shampoo: 1%

Pharmacodynamics

Scabicide and pediculicide actions: Lindane is toxic to the parasitic mite *Sarcoptes scabiei* and its eggs and to lice (*Pediculus capitis, Pediculus corporis,* and *Phthirus pubis*). Drug is absorbed through the organism's exoskeleton, causing death.

Pharmacokinetics

Absorption: About 10% of topical dose may be absorbed in 24 hours.
Distribution: Stored in body fat.
Metabolism: Metabolism occurs in the liver.
Excretion: Excreted in urine and feces.

Route	Onset	Peak	Duration
Topical	190 min	Unknown	Unknown

Contraindications and precautions

Contraindicated in patients hypersensitive to drug; in patients with raw or inflamed skin or seizure

---

disorders; and in premature infants. Use cautiously in children (including infants).

Interactions
None reported. However, avoid using with other oils or ointments.

Adverse reactions
CNS: *dizziness, seizures.*
Skin: *irritation* (with repeated use).

Overdose and treatment
Ingestion may cause extreme CNS toxicity; symptoms include CNS stimulation, dizziness, and seizures.

To treat lindane ingestion, empty stomach by appropriate measures (emesis or lavage); follow with saline catharsis (don't use oil laxative). Treat seizures with pentobarbital, phenobarbital, or diazepam, as needed.

Special considerations
• No more than 2 oz should be used in one application.
• Make sure patient's body is scrubbed clean and dried before application.
• Avoid applying drug to acutely inflamed skin or raw, weeping surfaces.
• Avoid contact with face, eyes, mucous membranes, and urethral meatus.
• Place hospitalized patient in isolation with linen-handling precautions.

Patient monitoring
• Monitor patient for need of retreatment.
• Monitor patient for signs of systemic toxicity.

Pregnant patients
• The Centers for Disease Control and Prevention (CDC) states that lindane isn't for use in pregnant women.

Breast-feeding patients
• Because drug appears in breast milk in low levels, an alternative method of feeding may be used for 4 days if there's any concern.

Pediatric patients
• Use cautiously, especially in infants and small children, who are much more susceptible to CNS toxicity. Discourage thumb-sucking in children using lindane to prevent ingestion of drug. The CDC recommends other scabicide therapies for children under age 10.

Geriatric patients
• Reduce dosage in geriatric patients because of their increased susceptibility to percutaneous absorption.

Patient education
• Explain correct use of drug.
• The CDC recommends that bathing before application be avoided because toxicity (such as

seizures) has been linked to such application. If the patient does bathe, the skin should be allowed to dry and cool completely before application of lotion. Before application of shampoo, the hair should be washed with plain shampoo and dried.
• Warn patient that itching may continue for several weeks, even if treatment is effective, especially in scabies infestation.
• If drug contacts eyes, tell patient to flush with water and call for further instructions. He should avoid inhaling vapor.
• Explain that reapplication usually isn't necessary unless live mites are found; advise reapplication if drug is accidentally washed off, but caution against overuse.
• Tell patient he may use drug to clean combs and brushes, and to wash them thoroughly afterward; advise patient that all clothing and bed linen that may have been contaminated by him within the past 2 days should be machine-washed in hot water and dried in hot dryer or dry cleaned to avoid reinfestation or transmission of organism.
• Discourage repeated use of drug, which may irritate skin and cause systemic toxicity.
• Caution patient to avoid using with other oils or ointments.
• Advise patient that family and close contacts, including sexual contacts, should be treated at the same time.
• Warn patient not to use if open wounds, cuts, or sores are present on scalp or groin, unless directed.

linezolid
Zyvox

Pharmacologic classification: oxazolidinone
Therapeutic classification: antibiotic
Pregnancy risk category: C

Indications and dosages
➤ *Vancomycin-resistant* Enterococcus faecium *infections, including those with concurrent bacteremia. Adults:* 600 mg I.V. or P.O. q 12 hours for 14 to 28 days.
➤ *Nosocomial pneumonia caused by* Staphylococcus aureus *(methicillin-susceptible [MSSA] and methicillin-resistant [MRSA] strains) or* Streptococcus pneumonia *(penicillin-susceptible strains only); complicated skin and skin-structure infections caused by* S. aureus *(MSSA and MRSA),* Streptococcus pyogenes, *or* Streptococcus agalactiae; *community-acquired pneumonia caused by* S. pneumoniae *(penicillin-susceptible strains only), including those with concurrent bacteremia, or* S. aureus *(MSSA only). Adults:* 600 mg I.V. or P.O. q 12 hours for 10 to 14 days.
➤ *Uncomplicated skin and skin-structure infections caused by* S. aureus *(MSSA only) or* S. pyogenes. *Adults:* 400 mg P.O. q 12 hours for 10 to 14 days.

Reactions may be *common*, uncommon, *life-threatening*, or COMMON AND LIFE-THREATENING.

How supplied
Available by prescription only.
Injection: 2 mg/ml
Powder for oral suspension: 100 mg/5 ml
when constituted
Tablets: 400 mg, 600 mg

Pharmacodynamics
Antibiotic action: Linezolid is bacteriostatic
against enterococci and staphylococci, and
bactericidal against most strains of streptococci. Linezolid exerts its antimicrobial effects
by interfering with bacterial protein synthesis.
Linezolid binds to the 23S ribosomal DNA on the
bacterial 50S ribosomal subunit. This action prevents the formation of a functional 70S ribosomal subunit, thereby blocking the translation step
of bacterial protein synthesis.

Pharmacokinetics
Absorption: Absorption is rapid and complete
after oral dosing. Levels peak in 1 to 2 hours.
Bioavailability is about 100%.
Distribution: Linezolid is distributed readily
into well-perfused tissues. Protein-binding is
about 31%.
Metabolism: Linezolid undergoes oxidative metabolism to two inactive metabolites. It doesn't
appear to be metabolized by the cytochrome P-
450 oxidative system.
Excretion: At steady state, about 30% of a dose
appears in the urine as linezolid and about 50%
as metabolites. Linezolid undergoes significant
renal tubular reabsorption, such that renal clearance is low. Nonrenal clearance accounts for
about 65% of the total clearance.

Route	Onset	Peak	Duration
P.O.	Unknown	1 to 2 hr	Unknown
I.V.	Unknown	½ hr	Unknown

Contraindications and precautions
Contraindicated in patients hypersensitive to linezolid or any inactive components of the formulation.

Use cautiously in patients with uncontrolled
hypertension, pheochromocytoma, carcinoid syndrome, or untreated hyperthyroidism since linezolid wasn't studied in these patients.

Interactions
Drug-drug. *Adrenergics (such as dopamine,
epinephrine, pseudoephedrine):* Hypertension
may occur. Monitor blood pressure and heart
rate. Start continuous infusion of dopamine and
epinephrine at lower doses and adjust to response.
Serotoninergic drugs: Increased risk of serotonin syndrome (confusion, delirium, restlessness, tremors, blushing, diaphoresis, hyperpyrexia). If symptoms develop, consider stopping
serotoninergic drug.
Drug-food. *Foods and beverages high in tyramine, such as aged cheeses, air-dried meats,
red wines, sauerkraut, soy sauce, tap beers:*
Increased blood pressure. Tyramine content of
meals shouldn't exceed 100 mg.

Adverse reactions
CNS: headache, insomnia, dizziness.
GI: diarrhea, nausea, vomiting, constipation, el-
evated amylase, elevated lipase, altered taste,
tongue discoloration, oral candidiasis.
GU: elevated BUN levels, vaginal candidiasis.
Hematologic: anemia, *leukopenia, neu-
tropenia, thrombocytopenia.*
Hepatic: elevated liver enzyme levels.
Skin: rash.
Other: fever, fungal infection.

Overdose and treatment
Limited information is available. Signs and symptoms of overdose have included vomiting, tremors,
decreased activity, and ataxia.

Treatment is supportive, with maintenance of
glomerular filtration. Hemodialysis may be useful in increasing the elimination of linezolid. Peritoneal dialysis and hemoperfusion haven't been
studied.

Special considerations
● Obtain samples for culture and sensitivity testing before starting linezolid therapy. Use results
of sensitivity tests to guide therapy.
● Reconstitute oral suspension according to manufacturer's instructions. Store reconstituted suspension at room temperature and use it within
21 days.
● Linezolid is compatible with D₅W, normal saline
solution for injection, and lactated Ringer's injection.
● Inspect for particulate matter and leaks.
● Infuse drug over 30 to 120 minutes. Don't infuse it in a series connection.
● No dosage adjustment is needed when switching from I.V. to P.O. forms.
● The safety and efficacy of linezolid therapy lasting longer than 28 days haven't been studied.
● Pseudomembranous colitis and superinfection
may occur. Consider these possibilities in patients
who have persistent diarrhea or secondary infections.
● Because inappropriate use of antibiotics may encourage development of resistant organisms, carefully consider alternative agents before starting
linezolid therapy, especially in the outpatient setting.
● Drugs known to be incompatible with linezolid include amphotericin B, chlorpromazine hydrochloride, diazepam, pentamidine isothionate,
erythromycin lactobionate, phenytoin sodium,
trimethoprim sulfamethoxazole, and ceftriaxone
sodium.
● Store drug at room temperature in its protective overwrap. Solution may develop a yellow col-
oration, but this doesn't affect the drug's potency.

Patient monitoring
● Linezolid may cause thrombocytopenia. Monitor platelet count in patients at increased risk of

bleeding, patients with thrombocytopenia, patients receiving other drugs that may cause thrombocytopenia, and patients receiving linezolid for more than 14 days.

Pediatric use
• Safety and effective dosage haven't been determined in children.

Patient education
• Inform patient that tablets and oral suspension may be taken without regard to meals.
• Stress the importance of completing the entire course of therapy, even if the patient feels better.
• Teach patient to alert prescriber about hypertension, use of cough or cold preparations, or treatment with selective serotonin reuptake inhibitors or other antidepressants.
• If patient has phenylketonuria, explain that each 5 ml of linezolid oral suspension contains 20 mg of phenylalanine. Linezolid tablets and injection don't contain phenylalanine.
• Tell patient to limit foods and beverages containing tyramine to less than 100 mg of tyramine per meal. Foods high in tyramine include those that may have undergone protein changes by aging, fermentation, pickling, or smoking to improve flavor (such as aged cheeses, sauerkraut, soy sauce, beer, or red wine).

---

liothyronine sodium (T₃)
Cytomel, Triostat

Pharmacologic classification: thyroid hormone
Therapeutic classification: thyroid hormone replacement
Pregnancy risk category: A

Indications and dosages
➤ *Congenital hypothyroidism. Children:* 5 mcg P.O. daily, increased by 5 mcg q 3 to 4 days until desired response occurs.
➤ *Myxedema. Adults:* Initially, 5 mcg daily, increased by 5 to 10 mcg q 1 to 2 weeks. Maintenance dosage is 50 to 100 mcg daily.
➤ *Myxedema coma, precoma. Adults:* Initially, 25 to 50 mcg I.V.; reassess after 4 to 12 hours, then switch to P.O. as soon as possible. Patients with known or suspected cardiac disease should receive 10 to 20 mcg I.V.
➤ *Nontoxic goiter. Adults:* Initially, 5 mcg P.O. daily; may be increased by 5 to 10 mcg daily at intervals of 1 to 2 weeks until dosage of 25 mcg daily is reached. Thereafter, dosage may be increased by 12.5 to 25 mcg daily at intervals of 1 to 2 weeks until desired response is noted. Usual maintenance dosage is 75 mcg daily.
Adults over age 65: Initially, 5 mcg P.O. daily, increased by 5-mcg increments q 1 to 2 weeks until desired response is obtained.

Children: Initially, 5 mcg P.O. daily, increased by 5-mcg increments at weekly intervals until desired response is achieved.
➤ *Thyroid hormone replacement. Adults:* Initially, 25 mcg P.O. daily, increased by 12.5 to 25 mcg q 1 to 2 weeks until satisfactory response is achieved. Usual maintenance dosage is 25 to 75 mcg daily.
➤ *Liothyronine suppression test to differentiate hyperthyroidism from euthyroidism. Adults:* 75 to 100 mcg daily for 7 days.

How supplied
Available by prescription only
Injection: 10 mcg/ml
Tablets: 5 mcg, 25 mcg, 50 mcg

Pharmacodynamics
Thyroid hormone replacement: Liothyronine is usually a second-line drug in the treatment of hypothyroidism, myxedema, and cretinism. This component of thyroid hormone affects protein and carbohydrate metabolism, promotes gluconeogenesis, increases the utilization and mobilization of glycogen stores, stimulates protein synthesis, and regulates cell growth and differentiation. The major effect of liothyronine is to increase the metabolic rate of tissue. It may be most useful in syndromes of thyroid hormone resistance.

Pharmacokinetics
Absorption: 95% absorbed from the GI tract.
Distribution: Highly protein-bound. Its distribution hasn't been fully described.
Metabolism: Not fully understood.
Excretion: Half-life is 1 to 2 days.

Route	Onset	Peak	Duration
P.O.	Unknown	2-3 days	3 days
I.V.	Unknown	Unknown	Unknown

Contraindications and precautions
Contraindicated in patients hypersensitive to drug and in those with acute MI uncomplicated by hypothyroidism, untreated thyrotoxicosis, or uncorrected adrenal insufficiency.

Use cautiously in the elderly and in patients with angina pectoris, hypertension, ischemia, other CV disorders, renal insufficiency, diabetes, or myxedema.

Interactions
Drug-drug. *Adrenocorticoids, corticotropin:* Altered thyroid status. Change in liothyronine dosage may require change in adrenocorticoid or corticotropin dosage.
Anticoagulants: Altered PT and INR. Monitor patient for potential dosage adjustment.
Estrogens: Increased thyroxine-binding globulin levels. May increase liothyronine requirements. Monitor patient's need for dosage adjustment.

Insulin, oral antidiabetics: May affect dosage requirements of these drugs. Monitor patient for need for dosage adjustment.

Sympathomimetics, tricyclic antidepressants: May increase effects of these drugs, causing coronary insufficiency or arrhythmias. Use together cautiously.

Adverse reactions

CNS: *nervousness, insomnia, tremor,* headache.
CV: *tachycardia, **arrhythmias,*** angina pectoris, ***cardiac decompensation and collapse.***
GI: diarrhea, vomiting.
GU: menstrual irregularities.
Metabolic: weight loss.
Musculoskeletal: accelerated bone maturation in infants and children.
Skin: diaphoresis, skin reactions.
Other: heat intolerance.

Overdose and treatment

Evidence of overdose reflects hyperthyroidism and may include weight loss, increased appetite, palpitations, diarrhea, nervousness, abdominal cramps, sweating, headache, tachycardia, increased blood pressure, widened pulse pressure, angina, arrhythmias, tremor, insomnia, heat intolerance, fever, and menstrual irregularities.

Treatment of overdose reduces GI absorption and counteracts central and peripheral effects, primarily sympathetic activity. Use gastric lavage or induce emesis (followed by activated charcoal up to 4 hours after ingestion). If patient is comatose or having seizures, inflate the cuff on an endotracheal tube to prevent aspiration. Treatment may include oxygen and ventilation to maintain respiration. It also should include appropriate measures to treat heart failure and control fever, hypoglycemia, and fluid loss. Propranolol (or another beta blocker) may be used to counteract many of the effects of increased sympathetic activity. Withdraw liothyronine gradually over 2 to 6 days; then resume at a lower dosage.

Special considerations

● Liothyronine may be preferred when rapid effect is desired or when GI absorption or peripheral conversion of levothyroxine to liothyronine is impaired.
● Oral absorption may be reduced in patients with heart failure.
● When switching from levothyroxine to liothyronine, discontinue levothyroxine and start liothyronine at low dosage, increasing in small increments after residual effects of levothyroxine have disappeared. When switching from liothyronine to levothyroxine, start levothyroxine several days before withdrawing liothyronine to avoid relapse.
● Discontinue drug 7 to 10 days before patient undergoes radioactive iodine uptake studies.

● Liothyronine therapy alters radioactive iodine (^{131}I) uptake, protein-bound iodine levels, and liothyronine uptake.

Patient monitoring

● Monitor thyroid studies to assess response to drug therapy.

Breast-feeding patients

● Minimal amounts of drug appear in breast milk. Use cautiously in breast-feeding women.

Pediatric patients

● Partial hair loss may occur during first few months of therapy. Reassure child and parents that this is temporary. Infants and children may experience accelerated bone maturation.

Geriatric patients

● Elderly patients are more sensitive to effects of drug. In patients over age 60, initial dosage should be 25% lower than usual recommended adult dosage.

Patient education

● Tell patient to report headache, diarrhea, nervousness, excessive sweating, heat intolerance, chest pain, increased pulse rate, or palpitations.
● Advise patient not to store drug in bathroom or other warm, humid areas to prevent deterioration of drug.
● Encourage patient to take drug at the same time each day, preferably in the morning to avoid insomnia.

liotrix
Thyrolar

Pharmacologic classification: thyroid hormone
Therapeutic classification: thyroid hormone replacement
Pregnancy risk category: A

Indications and dosages

➤**Hypothyroidism.** Dosages must be individualized to approximate deficit in patient's thyroid secretion. *Adults:* Initially, 12.5 to 30 mg thyroid equivalent (usually, Thyrolar-1/4 or Thyrolar-1/2) P.O. daily; increased q 1 to 2 weeks until desired response is achieved.
Children over age 12: 2 to 3 mcg/kg daily.
Children ages 6 to 12: 4 to 5 mcg/kg daily.
Children ages 1 to 5: 5 to 6 mcg/kg daily.
Children ages 6 to 12 months: 6 to 8 mcg/kg daily.
Children under age 6 months: 8 to 10 mcg/kg daily.

How supplied

Available by prescription only
Tablets: Thyrolar-1/4—levothyroxine sodium 12.5 mcg and liothyronine sodium 3.1 mcg

Thyrolar-1/2—levothyroxine sodium 25 mcg and liothyronine sodium 6.25 mcg
Thyrolar-1—levothyroxine sodium 50 mcg and liothyronine sodium 12.5 mcg
Thyrolar-2—levothyroxine sodium 100 mcg and liothyronine sodium 25 mcg
Thyrolar-3—levothyroxine sodium 150 mcg and liothyronine sodium 37.5 mcg

Pharmacodynamics

Thyroid stimulant and replacement: Liotrix affects protein and carbohydrate metabolism, promotes gluconeogenesis, increases the use and mobilization of glycogen stores, stimulates protein synthesis, and regulates cell growth and differentiation. The major effect of liotrix is to increase the metabolic rate of tissue. It's used to treat hypothyroidism (myxedema, cretinism, and thyroid hormone deficiency).

Liotrix is a synthetic preparation combining levothyroxine sodium and liothyronine sodium in a 4-to-1 ratio by weight. Such combination products were developed because circulating T_3 was assumed to result from direct release from the thyroid gland. About 80% of T_3 is known to be derived from deiodination of T_4 in peripheral tissues, and patients receiving only T_4 have normal serum T_3 and T_4 levels. Therefore, there's no clinical advantage to combining thyroid agents; such combination could result in excessive T_3 concentration.

Pharmacokinetics

Absorption: About 50% to 95% is absorbed from the GI tract.
Distribution: Distribution isn't fully understood.
Metabolism: Metabolized partially in peripheral tissues (liver, kidneys, and intestines).
Excretion: Excreted partially in feces.

Route	Onset	Peak	Duration
P.O.	Unknown	Unknown	Unknown

Contraindications and precautions

Contraindicated in patients hypersensitive to drug and in those with acute MI uncomplicated by hypothyroidism, untreated thyrotoxicosis, or uncorrected adrenal insufficiency.

Use cautiously in the elderly and in patients with impaired renal function, ischemia, angina pectoris, hypertension, other CV disorders, myxedema, and diabetes mellitus or insipidus.

Interactions

Drug-drug. *Adrenocorticoids, corticotropin:* Altered thyroid status. Changes in liothyronine dosages may require dosage changes in the adrenocorticoid or corticotropin.
Anticoagulants: Altered PT and INR. Monitor patient's need for potential dosage adjustment.
Beta blockers: May decrease conversion of T_4 to T_3. Monitor patient for effect.
Cholestyramine: May delay absorption of T_4. Separate doses by 4 to 5 hours.

Estrogens: Increased thyroxine-binding globulin levels. May increase liothyronine requirements.
Hepatic enzyme inducers such as phenytoin: May increase hepatic degradation of T_4, resulting in increased T_4 requirement. Monitor patient for drug effect.
Insulin, oral antidiabetics: Drug may affect dosage requirements of these agents. Monitor patient's need for potential dosage adjustment.
Somatrem: May accelerate epiphyseal maturation. Monitor patient for effect.
Sympathomimetics, tricyclic antidepressants: Drug may increase effects of these drugs, causing coronary insufficiency or arrhythmias. Use together cautiously.

Adverse reactions

CNS: nervousness, insomnia, tremor, headache.
CV: *tachycardia,* ***arrhythmias,*** angina pectoris, ***cardiac decompensation and collapse.***
GI: diarrhea, vomiting.
GU: Menstrual irregularities.
Metabolic: weight loss.
Musculoskeletal: accelerated bone maturation in infants and children.
Skin: diaphoresis, allergic skin reactions.
Other: heat intolerance.

Overdose and treatment

Evidence of overdose includes signs and symptoms of hyperthyroidism, including weight loss, increased appetite, palpitations, nervousness, diarrhea, abdominal cramps, sweating, tachycardia, increased pulse rate and blood pressure, angina, arrhythmias, tremor, headache, insomnia, heat intolerance, fever, and menstrual irregularities.

Treatment requires reduction of GI absorption and efforts to counteract central and peripheral effects, primarily sympathetic activity. Use gastric lavage or induce emesis, then follow with activated charcoal if less than 4 hours since ingestion. If patient is comatose or having seizures, inflate the cuff on an endotracheal tube to prevent aspiration. Treatment may include oxygen and artificial ventilation as needed to maintain respiration. It also should include appropriate measures to treat heart failure and control fever, hypoglycemia, and fluid loss. Propranolol (or atenolol, metoprolol, acebutolol, nadolol, or timolol) may be used to combat many of the effects of increased sympathetic activity. Withdraw thyroid therapy gradually over 2 to 6 days, then resume at a lower dosage.

Special considerations

● T_4 is drug of choice for hypothyroidism. Hepatic conversion of T_4 to T_3 is usually adequate. Excessive exogenous supplementation of T_3 usually leads to toxicity.
● Start with lower dosages in elderly patients; patients with long-standing disease, other endo-

crinopathies, or CV disease; and patients with severe hypothyroidism.

● Protect drug from heat and moisture.
● Liotrix therapy alters radioactive iodine (^{131}I) thyroid uptake, protein-bound iodine levels, and T_3 uptake.

Patient monitoring

● Monitor patient's pulse rate and blood pressure.
● Monitor thyroid studies for clinical response to doses given and for dosage adjustment.

Breast-feeding patients

● Minimal amounts of drug appear in breast milk. Use cautiously in breast-feeding women.

Pediatric patients

● Partial hair loss may occur during first few months of therapy. Reassure child and parents that this is temporary. Infants and children may experience accelerated bone maturation.

Geriatric patients

● Elderly patients are more sensitive to effects of drug and may require a lower dosage.

Patient education

● Tell patient to report headache, diarrhea, nervousness, excessive sweating, heat intolerance, chest pain, increased pulse rate, or palpitations.
● Advise patient not to store liotrix in warm and humid areas, such as the bathroom.
● Encourage patient to take a single daily dose in the morning to avoid insomnia.

lisinopril
Prinivil, Zestril

Pharmacologic classification: ACE inhibitor
Therapeutic classification: antihypertensive
Pregnancy risk category: C (D in second and third trimesters)

Indications and dosages

➤ *Mild to severe hypertension. Adults:* Initially, 5 to 10 mg P.O. daily. Most patients are well controlled on 20 to 40 mg daily as a single dose. Doses up to 80 mg have been used.
➤ *Heart failure. Adults:* Initially, 2.5 to 5 mg P.O. daily. Most patients are well controlled on 5 to 20 mg daily as a single dose.
➤ *Acute MI. Adults:* Initially, 5 mg P.O.; then give 5 mg after 24 hours, 10 mg after 48 hours, and 10 mg daily for 6 weeks.

In patients with acute MI with low systolic blood pressure (less than 120 mm Hg), give 2.5 mg P.O. when treatment is started or during the first 3 days after an infarct. If hypotension occurs, a daily maintenance dosage of 5 mg may be given with temporary reductions to 2.5 mg, if needed.
✦ *Dosage adjustment.* In adults with renal impairment, initially, 5 mg P.O. daily if creatinine clearance is between 10 and 30 ml/minute, and 2.5 mg P.O. daily if it's less than 10 ml/minute. Dosage may be adjusted upward until blood pressure is controlled or to maximum of 40 mg daily. Dosage for patients with heart failure who have a creatinine clearance of less than 30 ml/minute is 2.5 mg P.O. daily. Adults with heart failure, hyponatremia (serum sodium less than 130 mEq/L), or moderate to severe renal impairment (creatinine clearance less than 30 ml/min) should receive an initial dose of 2.5 mg.

How supplied

Available by prescription only
Tablets: 5 mg, 10 mg, 20 mg, 40 mg

Pharmacodynamics

Antihypertensive action: Lisinopril inhibits angiotensin-converting enzyme (ACE), preventing the conversion of angiotensin I to angiotensin II, a potent vasoconstrictor. Reduced formation of angiotensin II decreases peripheral arterial resistance and aldosterone secretion, thereby reducing sodium and water retention and blood pressure.

Pharmacokinetics

Absorption: Variable; about 25% of an oral dose is absorbed.
Distribution: Distributed widely in tissues. Plasma protein binding appears insignificant. Minimal amounts enter the brain. Preclinical studies indicate that it crosses the placenta.
Metabolism: Not metabolized.
Excretion: Excreted unchanged in the urine.

Route	Onset	Peak	Duration
P.O.	1 hr	7 hr	24 hr

Contraindications and precautions

ACE inhibitor therapy shouldn't be initiated in hypotensive patients who are at immediate risk of cardiogenic shock and require I.V. administration of a vasopressor agent.

Contraindicated in patients hypersensitive to ACE inhibitors; in those with a history of angioedema related to previous treatment with ACE inhibitor; and in patients during the second and third trimesters of pregnancy.

Use cautiously in patients at risk for hyperkalemia or in those with impaired renal function.

Interactions

Drug-drug. *Diuretics:* May cause excessive hypotension. Monitor blood pressure closely.
Indomethacin: May attenuate the hypotensive effect of lisinopril. Monitor patient closely.
Lithium: May increase plasma lithium levels. Monitor lithium levels.
Potassium-sparing diuretics, potassium supplements: May lead to hyperkalemia. Avoid concurrent use. Monitor serum potassium levels.
Drug-herb. *Capsaicin:* Increased risk of cough. Discourage use together.

Drug-food. *Potassium-containing salt substitutes:* May lead to hyperkalemia. Discourage use together.

Adverse reactions
CNS: *dizziness, headache, fatigue, paresthesia.*
CV: hypotension, *orthostatic hypotension,* chest pain.
EENT: *nasal congestion.*
GI: *diarrhea,* nausea, dyspepsia.
GU: impotence.
Hematologic: *neutropenia, agranulocytopenia.*
Metabolic: hyperkalemia.
Respiratory: *dry, persistent, tickling, nonproductive cough;* dyspnea.
Skin: rash.
Other: *angioedema, anaphylaxis.*

Overdose and treatment
The most likely sign of overdose is hypotension. Recommended treatment is I.V. infusion of normal saline solution.

Special considerations
Consider the recommendations relevant to all ACE inhibitors as well as the following.
• Drug absorption is unaffected by food.
• Discontinue diuretics 2 to 3 days before lisinopril therapy to reduce the risk of hypotension.
• If drug doesn't adequately control blood pressure, diuretics may be added.
• Lower dosage is necessary in patients with impaired renal function.
• Initiate drug therapy in the hospital for heart failure patients because of the risk of severe hypotension.
• Drug shouldn't be used after acute MI in patients at risk for severe hemodynamic deterioration or cardiogenic shock.
• Beneficial effects of lisinopril may require several weeks of therapy.

Patient monitoring
• Review WBC and differential counts before treatment, every 2 weeks for 3 months, and periodically thereafter.
• Monitor patient's peak and trough blood pressures to assess clinical response.

Breast-feeding patients
• Drug may appear in breast milk, but effect on infant is unknown; use cautiously in breast-feeding women.

Pediatric patients
• Safety and efficacy in children haven't been established; use only if potential benefits outweigh risks.

Geriatric patients
• Geriatric patients may require lower doses because of impaired drug clearance. They also may be more sensitive to hypotensive effects of drug.

Patient education
• Tell patient to report light-headedness, especially in first few days of treatment, so dose can be adjusted; signs of infection, such as sore throat or fever, because drug may decrease WBC count; facial swelling or difficulty breathing, because drug may cause angioedema; and loss of taste, which may necessitate discontinuation of drug.
• Advise patient to avoid sudden postural changes to minimize orthostatic hypotension.
• Warn patient to seek medical approval before taking OTC cold preparations.
• Instruct patient to avoid potassium-containing salt substitutes.
• Warn women of childbearing age of the need to avoid pregnancy during therapy.
• Instruct patient to report any adverse events, including persistent dry cough.

lithium carbonate
Carbolith*, Duralith*, Eskalith, Eskalith CR, Lithane, Lithizine*, Lithobid, Lithonate, Lithotabs

lithium citrate
Cibalith-S

Pharmacologic classification: alkali metal
Therapeutic classification: antimanic, antipsychotic
Pregnancy risk category: D

Indications and dosages
➤ *Prevention or control of mania; prevention of depression in patients with bipolar illness. Adults:* For acute episodes: 1.8 g or 30 ml of lithium citrate P.O. daily in two or three divided doses or 20 to 30 mg/kg daily in two or three divided doses to maintain lithium levels at 1 to 1.5 mEq/L.
✦ *Dosage adjustment.* In geriatric patients, 600 to 900 mg daily.
Adults: For maintenance dosage: 900 mg to 1.2 g or 15 to 20 ml of oral solution P.O. daily in two to four divided doses to maintain serum lithium concentration of 0.6 to 1.2 mEq/L. Usual maintenance dosage doesn't exceed 2.4 g daily.
➤ *Major depression* ◊*, schizoaffective disorder* ◊*, schizophrenic disorder* ◊*, alcohol dependence* ◊*. Adults:* 300 mg lithium carbonate P.O. t.i.d. or q.i.d.
➤ *Apparent mixed bipolar disorder in children* ◊*. Children:* Initially, 15 to 60 mg/kg or 0.5 to 1.5 g/m^2 lithium carbonate P.O. daily in three divided doses. Don't exceed usual adult dosage. Adjust dosage based on patient response and serum lithium levels; usual dosage range is 150 to 300 mg daily in divided doses to maintain lithium levels of 0.5 to 1.2 mEq/L.
➤ *Chemotherapy-induced neutropenia in children and patients with AIDS receiv-*

Reactions may be *common,* uncommon, *life-threatening,* or COMMON AND LIFE-THREATENING.

ing zidovudine ◊. *Adults and children:* 300 to 1,000 mg P.O. daily.

How supplied
Available by prescription only
lithium carbonate
Capsules: 150 mg, 300 mg, 600 mg
Tablets: 300 mg
Tablets (extended-release, film-coated): 300 mg
Tablets (film-coated): 300 mg
Tablets (sustained-release): 300 mg, 450 mg
lithium citrate
Syrup (sugarless): 300 mg/5 ml (with 0.3% alcohol)

Pharmacodynamics
Antimanic action: Lithium is thought to exert its antipsychotic and antimanic effects by competing with other cations for exchange at the sodium-potassium ion pump, thus altering cation exchange at the tissue level. It also inhibits adenyl cyclase, reducing intracellular levels of cAMP and, to a lesser extent, cyclic guanosine monophosphate (cGMP).

Pharmacokinetics
Absorption: Rate and extent of absorption vary with dosage form; absorption is complete within 6 hours of oral administration from conventional tablets and capsules.
Distribution: Distributed widely throughout the body, including breast milk; levels in thyroid gland, bone, and brain tissue exceed serum levels. Steady state serum level achieved in 12 hours. Therapeutic effect begins in 5 to 10 days and is maximal within 3 weeks. Therapeutic and toxic serum levels and therapeutic effects show good correlation. Therapeutic range is 0.6 to 1.2 mEq/L; adverse reactions increase as level reaches 1.5 to 2 mEq/L; such levels may be necessary in acute mania. Toxicity usually occurs at levels above 2 mEq/L.
Metabolism: Not metabolized.
Excretion: Excreted 95% unchanged in urine; about 50% to 80% of a given dose is excreted within 24 hours. Level of renal function determines elimination rate.

Route	Onset	Peak	Duration
P.O.	Unknown	½ to 3 hr	Unknown

Contraindications and precautions
Contraindicated if therapy can't be closely monitored and during pregnancy. Use cautiously in the elderly; in patients with thyroid disease, seizure disorders, renal or CV disease, severe dehydration or debilitation, or sodium depletion; and in those receiving neuroleptics, neuromuscular blockers, and diuretics.

Interactions
Drug-drug. *Antacids and other drugs containing aminophylline, caffeine, calcium, sodi-*um, *or theophylline:* May increase lithium excretion by renal competition for elimination, thus decreasing therapeutic effect of lithium. Monitor patient closely.
Carbamazepine, mazindol, methyldopa, phenytoin, tetracyclines: May increase lithium toxicity. Monitor patient closely.
Chlorpromazine: Decreased effects of chlorpromazine. Avoid administering together.
Fluoxetine: Increases lithium serum levels. Monitor patient closely.
Haloperidol: May result in severe encephalopathy characterized by confusion, tremors, extrapyramidal effects, and weakness. Use this combination cautiously.
Indomethacin, phenylbutazone, piroxicam, other NSAIDs: Decreased renal excretion of lithium. May require a 30% reduction in lithium dosage.
Neuromuscular blockers, such as atracurium, pancuronium, and succinylcholine: Lithium may potentiate the effects of these drugs. Monitor patient closely.
Sympathomimetics, especially norepinephrine: Lithium may interfere with pressor effects of these drugs. Monitor patient closely.
Thiazide diuretics: May decrease renal excretion and enhance lithium toxicity. Diuretic dosage may need to be reduced by 30%.
Drug-herb. *Ispaghula, plantain:* Possible decrease in lithium absorption, reducing effect. Discourage use together.
Parsley: May promote or produce serotonin syndrome. Discourage use together.
Psyllium seed: Inhibited GI absorption. Discourage use together.
Drug-food. *Caffeine:* Decreased lithium levels and possible decrease in effect. Tell patients who ingest large amounts of caffeine to inform prescriber before eliminating caffeine. It may be necessary to adjust lithium dosage.
Dietary sodium: May alter renal elimination of lithium. Increased sodium intake may increase elimination of drug; decreased intake may decrease elimination. Monitor serum lithium levels.

Adverse reactions
CNS: tremors, drowsiness, headache, confusion, restlessness, dizziness, psychomotor retardation, lethargy, *coma*, blackouts, *epileptiform seizures*, EEG changes, worsened organic mental syndrome, impaired speech, ataxia, muscle weakness, incoordination.
CV: reversible ECG changes, *arrhythmias*, hypotension, *bradycardia*.
EENT: tinnitus, blurred vision.
GI: dry mouth, metallic taste, nausea, vomiting, anorexia, diarrhea, *thirst*, abdominal pain, flatulence, indigestion.
GU: *polyuria*, glycosuria, *renal toxicity* with long-term use, decreased creatinine clearance, albuminuria.

Hematologic: *leukocytosis with WBC count of 14,000 to 18,000/mm3* (reversible); elevated neutrophil count.

Metabolic: goiter, transient hyperglycemia, hypothyroidism (lowered T_3, T_4, and protein-bound iodine, but elevated ^{131}I uptake), hyponatremia.

Skin: pruritus, rash, diminished or absent sensation, drying and thinning of hair, psoriasis, acne, alopecia.

Other: ankle and wrist edema.

Overdose and treatment

Vomiting and diarrhea occur within 1 hour of acute ingestion (induce vomiting in noncomatose patients if it's not spontaneous). Death has occurred in patients ingesting 10 to 60 g of lithium; patients have ingested 6 g with minimal toxic effects. Serum lithium levels above 3.4 mEq/L are potentially fatal.

Overdose with long-term lithium ingestion may follow altered pharmacokinetics, drug interactions, or volume or sodium depletion; sedation, confusion, hand tremors, joint pain, ataxia, muscle stiffness, increased deep tendon reflexes, visual changes, and nystagmus may occur. Symptoms may progress to coma, movement abnormalities, tremors, seizures, and CV collapse.

Treatment is symptomatic and supportive; closely monitor vital signs. If emesis isn't feasible, treat with gastric lavage. Monitor fluid and electrolyte balance; correct sodium depletion with normal saline solution. Institute hemodialysis if serum level is above 3 mEq/L, and in severely symptomatic patients unresponsive to fluid and electrolyte correction, or if urine output decreases significantly. Serum rebound of tissue lithium stores (from high volume distribution) commonly occurs after dialysis and may necessitate prolonged or repeated hemodialysis. Peritoneal dialysis may help but is less effective.

Special considerations

● Lithium is used investigationally to increase WBC count in patients undergoing cancer chemotherapy. It also has been used investigationally to treat cluster headaches, aggression, organic brain syndrome, and tardive dyskinesia. Drug has been used to treat SIADH.
● EEG changes include diffuse slowing, widening of frequency spectrum, potentiation, and disorganization of background rhythm.
● Shake syrup formulation before administration.
● Discontinue drug before electroconvulsive therapy (ECT).
● Administer drug with food or milk to reduce GI upset.
● Expect lag of 1 to 3 weeks before beneficial effects of drug are noticed. Other psychotropic medications (such as chlorpromazine) may be necessary during interim period.
● Adjust fluid and salt ingestion to compensate if excessive loss occurs through protracted sweating or diarrhea. Patient should have fluid intake of 2,500 to 3,000 ml daily and a balanced diet with adequate salt intake.
● Lithane tablets contain tartrazine, a dye that may precipitate an allergic reaction in certain individuals, particularly asthmatics sensitive to aspirin.
● Drug causes false-positive test results on thyroid function tests.
● Acute neurotoxicity with delirium has occurred in patients receiving lithium and ECT. Reduce lithium dosage or withdraw before ECT.

Patient monitoring

● Monitor baseline ECG, thyroid and renal studies, and electrolyte levels. Monitor lithium blood levels 8 to 12 hours after first dose, usually before morning dose, two or three times weekly the first month, then weekly to monthly on maintenance therapy.
● Determination of serum drug levels is crucial to safe use of drug. Don't use drug in patients who can't have regular serum drug level checks. Be sure patient or responsible family member can comply with instructions.
● When lithium blood levels are below 1.5 mEq/L, adverse reactions usually remain mild.
● Monitor fluid intake and output, especially when surgery is scheduled.
● Observe patient for signs of edema or sudden weight gain.
● Outpatient follow-up of thyroid and renal functions should occur every 6 to 12 months. Thyroid should be palpated to check for enlargement.
● Check urine for specific gravity below 1.015, which may indicate diabetes insipidus.
● Drug may alter glucose tolerance in diabetic patients. Monitor blood glucose levels closely.
● Monitor serum levels and signs of impending toxicity.
● Monitor drug dosing carefully when patient's initial manic symptoms begin to subside because the ability to tolerate high serum lithium levels decreases as symptoms resolve. Dose must be adjusted based upon lithium level, patient tolerance, and clinical response.

Pregnant patients

● Lithium has been used during pregnancy in life-threatening situations and severe disease when other therapies couldn't be used or were ineffective. Fetal toxicity includes increased risk of cardiovascular abnormalities, Down syndrome, clubfoot, meningomyelocele, transient hypothyroidism with goiter, transient nephrogenic diabetes insipidus, muscular hypotonia, and apnea.

Breast-feeding patients

● Lithium level in breast milk is 33% to 50% that of maternal serum level. Women should avoid breast-feeding during treatment with lithium.

Reactions may be *common*, uncommon, *life-threatening*, or COMMON AND LIFE-THREATENING.

Pediatric patients
• Drug isn't recommended for use in children under age 12.

Geriatric patients
• Elderly patients are more susceptible to overdose and toxic effects, especially dyskinesias. These patients usually respond to a lower dosage.

Patient education
• Explain that lithium has a narrow therapeutic margin of safety. A serum drug level that's even slightly high can be dangerous.
• Warn patient and family to watch for signs of toxicity (diarrhea, vomiting, dehydration, drowsiness, muscle weakness, tremor, fever, and ataxia) and to expect transient nausea, polyuria, thirst, and discomfort during first few days. If toxic symptoms occur, tell patient to withhold one dose and report symptoms promptly.
• Warn patient to avoid activities that require alertness and good psychomotor coordination until CNS response to drug is determined.
• Advise patient to maintain adequate water intake and adequate—but not excessive—salt in diet.
• Explain importance of regular follow-up visits to measure lithium serum levels.
• Tell patient to avoid large amounts of caffeine, which will interfere with effectiveness of drug.
• Advise patient to seek medical approval before beginning a weight-loss program.
• Tell patient not to switch brands of lithium or take other prescription or OTC drugs or herbal remedies without medical approval. Different brands may not provide equivalent effect.
• Tell patient to take drug with food or milk.
• Warn patient against stopping this drug abruptly.
• Tell patient to explain to close friend or family members the signs of lithium overdose in case emergency aid is needed.
• Instruct patient to carry identification and instruction card with toxicity and emergency information.

---

lomefloxacin hydrochloride
Maxaquin

Pharmacologic classification: fluoro-quinolone
Therapeutic classification: broad-spectrum antibiotic
Pregnancy risk category: C

Indications and dosages
➤ *Acute bacterial exacerbations of chronic bronchitis caused by* Haemophilus influenzae *or* Moraxella catarrhalis; *uncomplicated urinary tract infections (cystitis) caused by* Escherichia coli, Klebsiella pneumoniae, Proteus mirabilis, *or* Staphylococcus saprophyticus. *Adults:* 400 mg P.O. daily for 10 days.

➤ *Complicated urinary tract infections caused by* E. coli, K. pneumoniae, P. mirabilis, *or* Pseudomonas aeruginosa; *possibly effective against infections caused by* Citrobacter diversus *or* Enterobacter cloacae. *Adults:* 400 mg P.O. daily for 14 days.
➤ *Prophylaxis of infections after transurethral surgical procedures. Adults:* 400 mg P.O. 2 to 6 hours before surgery as a single dose.
➤ *Uncomplicated gonorrhea.* Adults: 400 mg P.O. as a single dose.
✦ *Dosage adjustment.* In adults with renal impairment and creatinine clearance of 10 to 40 ml/minute, give loading dose of 400 mg P.O. on first day, followed by 200 mg P.O. daily for duration of therapy. Hemodialysis removes negligible amounts of drug.

How supplied
Available by prescription only
Tablets: 400 mg

Pharmacodynamics
Antibiotic action: Lomefloxacin inhibits bacterial DNA gyrase, an enzyme necessary for bacterial replication. Drug is bactericidal.

Pharmacokinetics
Absorption: Rapidly absorbed from the GI tract; absolute bioavailability is 95% to 98%. Food impairs absorption by reducing total amount absorbed and slowing absorption rate.
Distribution: Only 10% is bound to plasma proteins.
Metabolism: About 10% is metabolized in the liver.
Excretion: Mostly excreted unchanged in urine; about 10% is excreted as metabolites. Solubility in urine is pH dependent. About 10% of a dose appears unchanged in the feces. Half-life is 8 hours. Steady state is reached after 2 days of once-daily therapy.

Route	Onset	Peak	Duration
P.O.	Unknown	1½ hr	Unknown

Contraindications and precautions
Contraindicated in patients hypersensitive to drug or other fluoroquinolones. Use cautiously in patients with known or suspected CNS disorders, such as seizures or cerebral arteriosclerosis.

Interactions
Drug-drug. *Antacids, minerals, sucralfate:* These drugs bind with lomefloxacin in the GI tract and impair its absorption. Give antacids and sucralfate at least 4 hours before or 2 hours after lomefloxacin.
Cimetidine: Other quinolones show substantially increased plasma half-lives. Monitor patient for toxicity.

Cyclosporine, warfarin: Other quinolones increase the effects or serum levels of these drugs. Lomefloxacin hasn't been tested for these effects. Monitor patient for toxicity.

Probenecid: Decreases excretion of lomefloxacin. Don't administer together.

Drug-lifestyle. *Sun exposure:* Photosensitivity reactions may occur. Advise patient to take precautions.

Adverse reactions

CNS: *dizziness, headache,* abnormal dreams, fatigue, malaise, asthenia, agitation, anorexia, anxiety, confusion, depersonalization, depression, increased appetite, insomnia, nervousness, somnolence, *seizures, coma,* hyperkinesia, tremor, vertigo, paresthesia, syncope.

CV: flushing, hypotension, hypertension, edema, *arrhythmias,* tachycardia, *bradycardia,* extrasystoles, cyanosis, angina pectoris, *MI, cardiac failure, pulmonary embolism,* cerebrovascular disorder, cardiomyopathy, phlebitis.

EENT: epistaxis, abnormal vision, conjunctivitis, eye pain, earache, tinnitus.

GI: *diarrhea, nausea,* thirst, dry mouth, tongue discoloration, taste perversion, pseudomembranous colitis, abdominal pain, dyspepsia, vomiting, flatulence, constipation, inflammation, dysphagia, bleeding.

GU: dysuria, hematuria, anuria, leukorrhea, epididymitis, orchitis, vaginitis, vaginal moniliasis, intermenstrual bleeding, perineal pain.

Hematologic: thrombocythemia, *thrombocytopenia,* lymphadenopathy, increased fibrinolysis.

Hepatic: elevated liver enzyme levels.

Metabolic: hypoglycemia.

Musculoskeletal: chest or back pain, leg cramps, arthralgia, myalgia.

Respiratory: dyspnea, *bronchospasm,* respiratory disorder or infection, increased sputum, stridor.

Skin: pruritus, skin disorder, skin exfoliation, eczema, increased diaphoresis, rash, urticaria, *photosensitivity.*

Other: *anaphylaxis,* chills, allergic reaction, facial edema, flulike symptoms, decreased heat tolerance, gout.

Overdose and treatment

Treatment of overdose includes emptying the stomach by induced vomiting or gastric lavage, observing patient closely, and providing supportive care. Drug isn't significantly removed by hemodialysis or peritoneal dialysis.

Special considerations

● Drug shouldn't be used for empiric treatment of acute exacerbations of chronic bronchitis when suspected pathogen is *Streptococcus pneumoniae* because this organism demonstrates resistance to drug. Because blood drug levels don't readily exceed the minimum inhibitory concentration against *Pseudomonas aeruginosa,* drug shouldn't be used to treat bacteremia caused by this organism, but it has been used successfully to treat complicated urinary tract *Pseudomonas* infections.

● Achilles and other tendon ruptures have been reported. Discontinue medication if pain, inflammation, or tendon rupture occurs.

Patient monitoring

● Monitor renal and hepatic function tests and CBC in patients with impairments.

Breast-feeding patients

● It isn't known whether drug appears in breast milk. Because of risk of serious adverse effects on the infant, a decision should be made to discontinue the drug or breast-feeding.

Pediatric patients

● Because studies have shown that quinolones can cause arthropathy in immature animals, avoid using these drugs in children under age 18.

Patient education

● Remind patient to take all of drug prescribed, even after he feels better.

● Advise patient to take drug on an empty stomach.

● Tell patient to avoid potentially hazardous tasks that require alertness, such as driving, until adverse CNS effects of drug are known.

● Instruct patient to avoid sunlight or artificial ultraviolet light and to call immediately if signs of photosensitivity occur.

● Caution patient to avoid mineral supplements or vitamins with iron or minerals within 2 hours before or after taking drug.

● Tell patient that sucralfate or antacids containing magnesium or aluminum shouldn't be taken within 4 hours before or 2 hours after taking drug.

● Instruct patient to drink fluids liberally.

lomustine (CCNU)
CeeNU, CeeNU Dose Pack

Pharmacologic classification: alkylating agent, nitrosourea (not specific to cell cycle phase)
Therapeutic classification: antineoplastic
Pregnancy risk category: D

Indications and dosages

Dosages and indications vary. Check current literature for recommended protocol. Wait at least 6 weeks between repeat courses.

➤ **Brain tumors, Hodgkin's disease, lymphomas.** *Adults and children:* 100 to 130 mg/m^2 P.O. as single dose q 6 weeks.

Reactions may be *common,* uncommon, *life-threatening,* or COMMON AND LIFE-THREATENING.

✦ *Dosage adjustment.* Reduce dose according to bone marrow depression using the following guidelines.

Nadir after prior dose		Percentage of prior dose to be given
WBCs/ mm³	Platelets/ mm³	
> 4,000	100,000	100%
3,000-3,999	75,000-99,999	100%
2,000-2,999	25,000-74,999	70%
< 2,000	< 25,000	50%

Repeat doses shouldn't be given until WBC count is more than 4,000/mm³ and platelet count is more than 100,000/mm³. Hematologic toxicity is delayed and cumulative; don't give repeat courses before 6 weeks.

How supplied
Available by prescription only
Capsules: 10 mg, 40 mg, 100 mg
Dose pack: Two capsules lomustine 10 mg, two capsules lomustine 40 mg, two capsules lomustine 100 mg

Pharmacodynamics
Antineoplastic action: Lomustine exerts its cytotoxic activity through alkylation, resulting in the inhibition of DNA and RNA synthesis. As with other nitrosourea compounds, lomustine modifies cellular proteins and alkylate proteins, resulting in an inhibition of protein synthesis. Cross-resistance exists between lomustine and carmustine.

Pharmacokinetics
Absorption: Rapidly and well absorbed across the GI tract after oral administration.
Distribution: Distributed widely into body tissues. Because of its high lipid solubility, drug and its metabolites cross the blood-brain barrier to a significant extent.
Metabolism: Metabolized rapidly and extensively in the liver. Some of the metabolites have cytotoxic activity.
Excretion: Metabolites are excreted primarily in urine, with smaller amounts excreted in feces and through the lungs. Plasma elimination of drug is biphasic, with an initial phase half-life of 6 hours and a terminal phase of 1 to 2 days. Extended half-life of the terminal phase is thought to be caused by enterohepatic circulation and protein-binding.

Route	Onset	Peak	Duration
P.O.	Unknown	Unknown	Unknown

Contraindications and precautions
Contraindicated in patients hypersensitive to drug. Use cautiously in patients with decreased platelet, WBC, or RBC counts and in those receiving other myelosuppressants.

Interactions
None reported.

Adverse reactions
CNS: disorientation, lethargy, ataxia.
GI: *nausea, vomiting,* stomatitis.
GU: *nephrotoxicity,* progressive azotemia, *renal failure.*
Hematologic: *anemia, leukopenia,* delayed up to 6 weeks, lasting 1 to 2 weeks; *thrombocytopenia,* delayed up to 4 weeks, lasting 1 to 2 weeks; *bone marrow suppression,* delayed up to 6 weeks.
Hepatic: *hepatotoxicity.*
Respiratory: pulmonary fibrosis.
Skin: alopecia.
Other: *secondary malignant disease.*

Overdose and treatment
Signs and symptoms of overdose include myelosuppression, nausea, and vomiting. Treatment is usually supportive, including antiemetics and transfusion of blood components.

Special considerations
● Drug has been used investigationally to treat bronchiogenic carcinoma, non-Hodgkin's lymphoma, malignant melanoma, breast cancer, renal cell carcinoma, and GI carcinoma.
● Give drug 2 to 4 hours after meals. Drug is more completely absorbed if taken on an empty stomach. To avoid nausea, give antiemetic before administering.
● Anorexia may persist for 2 to 3 days after a given dose.
● Dosage adjustment may be required in event of decreased platelet, WBC, or RBC count.
● Avoid all I.M. injections when platelet count is below 100,000/mm³.
● Use anticoagulants cautiously. Watch closely for signs of bleeding.
● Because drug crosses the blood-brain barrier, it may be used to treat primary brain tumors.

Patient monitoring
● Monitor CBC weekly. Drug usually isn't administered more than every 6 weeks; bone marrow toxicity is cumulative and delayed.
● Frequently assess renal and hepatic status.

Breast-feeding patients
● Metabolites of lomustine have been found in breast milk. Discontinue breast-feeding because of increased risk of serious adverse reactions, mutagenicity, and carcinogenicity in the infant.

Patient education
● Emphasize importance of continuing medication despite nausea and vomiting.
● Stress importance of taking the exact dose.

• Tell patient to immediately report if vomiting occurs shortly after a dose is taken.
• Advise patient to avoid exposure to people with infections.
• Tell patient to promptly report a sore throat, fever, or unusual bruising or bleeding.
• Advise patient to use effective contraceptive measures during drug therapy.

loperamide hydrochloride
Imodium, Imodium A-D, Kaopectate II, Maalox Anti-Diarrheal, Pepto Diarrhea Control

Pharmacologic classification: piperidine derivative
Therapeutic classification: antidiarrheal
Pregnancy risk category: B

Indications and dosages
➤*Acute, nonspecific diarrhea. Adults and children over age 12:* Initially, 4 mg P.O.; then 2 mg after each unformed stool. Maximum dose is 16 mg daily.
Children ages 9 to 11: 2 mg P.O. t.i.d. on first day.
Children ages 6 to 8: 2 mg P.O. b.i.d. on first day.
Children ages 2 to 5: 1 mg P.O. t.i.d. on first day.
    Maintenance dosage is one-third to one-half the initial dose (0.1 mg/kg only after each unformed stool) not to exceed dose recommended on the first day. Discontinue if no improvement after 48 hours.
➤*Chronic diarrhea. Adults:* Initially, 4 mg P.O.; then 2 mg after each unformed stool until diarrhea subsides. Adjust dose to individual response. Discontinue if 16 mg is used for at least 10 days.
Children ◇: 0.08 to 0.24 mg/kg daily in two to three divided doses.
Directions for patient self-medication
Adults: 4 teaspoons or 2 tablets P.O. after the first loose bowel movement, followed by 2 teaspoons or 1 tablet after each subsequent loose bowel movement. Don't exceed 8 mg daily.
Children ages 9 to 11 or who weigh 27 to 43 kg (60 to 95 lb): 2 teaspoons or 1 tablet P.O. after first loose bowel movement, followed by 1 teaspoon or ½ tablet after each subsequent loose bowel movement. Don't exceed 6 mg daily.
Children ages 6 to 8 or who weigh 22 to 27 kg (48 to 59 lb): 2 teaspoons or 1 tablet P.O. after first loose bowel movement, followed by 1 teaspoon or ½ tablet after each subsequent loose bowel movement. Don't exceed 4 mg daily.

How supplied
Available by prescription only
Capsules: 2 mg
Available without a prescription
Solution: 1 mg/5 ml
Tablets: 2 mg

Pharmacodynamics
Antidiarrheal action: Loperamide reduces intestinal motility by acting directly on intestinal mucosal nerve endings; tolerance to antiperistaltic effect doesn't develop. Drug also may inhibit fluid and electrolyte secretion by an unknown mechanism. Although it's chemically related to opiates, it hasn't shown any physical dependence characteristics in humans, and it possesses no analgesic activity.

Pharmacokinetics
Absorption: Absorbed poorly from the GI tract.
Distribution: Distribution isn't well characterized.
Metabolism: Absorbed loperamide is metabolized in the liver.
Excretion: Excreted primarily in feces; less than 2% is excreted in urine.

Route	Onset	Peak	Duration
P.O.	Unknown	2½-5 hr	24 hr

Contraindications and precautions
Contraindicated in children under age 2; in patients hypersensitive to drug; and in patients in whom constipation must be avoided. Also, OTC use is contraindicated in patients with a fever exceeding 101° F (38.3° C) or if blood is present in the stool. Use cautiously in patients with hepatic impairment.

Interactions
Opioid analgesics: May cause severe constipation. Avoid use together.

Adverse reactions
CNS: drowsiness, fatigue, dizziness.
GI: dry mouth; abdominal pain, distention, or discomfort; *constipation;* nausea; vomiting.
Skin: rash, *hypersensitivity reactions.*

Overdose and treatment
Effects of overdose include constipation, GI irritation, and CNS depression. Treatment is with activated charcoal if ingestion was recent. If patient is vomiting, activated charcoal may be given in a slurry when patient can retain fluids. Or, gastric lavage may be performed, followed by administration of activated charcoal slurry. Monitor patient for CNS depression; treat respiratory depression with naloxone.

Special considerations
• After administration via nasogastric tube, flush tube to clear it and ensure passage of drug to stomach.

Patient monitoring
• Patient should be monitored for reduced stools or lack of improvement.
• Monitor fluid and electrolytes if severe diarrhea occurs.

Reactions may be *common,* uncommon, *life-threatening,* or COMMON AND LIFE-THREATENING.

Breast-feeding patients

● It isn't known whether drug appears in breast milk. Use cautiously.

Pediatric patients

● Drug is approved for use in children age 2 and older; however, children may be more susceptible to adverse CNS effects.

Patient education

● Warn patient to take drug only as directed and not to exceed recommended dose.

● Caution patient to avoid driving and other tasks requiring alertness because drug may cause drowsiness and dizziness.

● Instruct patient to call if no improvement occurs in 48 hours or if fever develops.

lopinavir/ritonavir

Kaletra

Pharmacologic classification: protease inhibitor
Therapeutic use: antiviral
Pregnancy risk category: C

Indications and dosages

➤ *Treatment of HIV infection in combination therapy with other antiretroviral agents.* Adults and children over age 12: 400 mg lopinavir/100 mg ritonavir (3 capsules or 5 ml) P.O. b.i.d. with food.

✦ *Dosage adjustment.* In treated adults and children ages 6 months to 12 years who weigh more than 50 kg (110 lb) and who also take efavirenz or nevirapine, consider dose increase to 533 mg lopinavir/133 mg ritonavir (4 capsules or 6.5 ml).

Children ages 6 months to 12 years who weigh more than 40 kg (88 lb): 400 mg lopinavir/100 mg ritonavir (3 capsules or 5 ml) P.O. b.i.d. with food.

✦ *Dosage adjustment.* In treated adults and children ages 6 months to 12 years who weigh more than 40 to 50 kg (88 to 110 lb) and who also take efavirenz or nevirapine, consider dose increase to 11 mg lopinavir/2.75 mg ritonavir/kg (5 ml or 3 capsules).

Children ages 6 months to 12 years who weigh more than 30 to 40 kg (66 to 88 lb): 10 mg lopinavir/2.5 mg ritonavir/kg (3.5 ml) P.O. b.i.d. with food.

✦ *Dosage adjustment.* In treated patients also taking efavirenz or nevirapine, consider dose increase to 11 mg lopinavir/2.75 mg ritonavir/kg (4.5 ml).

Children ages 6 months to 12 years who weigh more than 25 to 30 kg (55 to 66 lb): 10 mg lopinavir/2.5 mg ritonavir/kg (3 ml) P.O. b.i.d. with food.

✦ *Dosage adjustment.* In treated patients also taking efavirenz or nevirapine, consider dose increase to 11 mg lopinavir/2.75 mg ritonavir/kg (4 ml).

Children ages 6 months to 12 years who weigh more than 20 to 25 kg (44 to 55 lb): 10 mg lopinavir/2.5 mg ritonavir/kg (2.5 ml) P.O. b.i.d. with food.

✦ *Dosage adjustment.* In treated patients also taking efavirenz or nevirapine, consider dose increase to 11 mg lopinavir/2.75 mg ritonavir/kg (3.25ml).

Children ages 6 months to 12 years who weigh more than 15 to 20 kg (33 to 44 lb): 10 mg lopinavir/2.5 mg ritonavir/kg (2.25 ml) P.O. b.i.d. with food.

✦ *Dosage adjustment.* In treated patients also taking efavirenz or nevirapine, consider dose increase to 11 mg lopinavir/2.75 mg ritonavir/kg (2.5 ml).

Children ages 6 months to 12 years who weigh 10 to 15 kg (22 to 33 lb): 12 mg lopinavir/3 mg ritonavir/kg (1.75 ml) P.O. b.i.d. with food.

✦ *Dosage adjustment.* In treated patients also taking efavirenz or nevirapine, consider dose increase to 13 mg lopinavir/3.25 mg ritonavir/kg (2 ml).

Children ages 6 months to 12 years who weigh 7 to 10 kg (15 to 22 lb): 12 mg lopinavir/3 mg ritonavir/kg (1.25 ml) P.O. b.i.d. with food.

✦ *Dosage adjustment.* In treated patients also taking efavirenz or nevirapine, consider dose increase to 13 mg lopinavir/3.25 mg ritonavir/kg (1.5 ml).

How supplied

Capsules: lopinavir 133.3 mg/ritonavir 33.3 mg.
Solution: lopinavir 400 mg/ritonavir 100 mg per 5 ml (80 mg/20 mg per ml)

Pharmacodynamics

Lopinavir inhibits the HIV protease, thus preventing the cleavage of the Gag-Pol polyprotein, resulting in the production of immature, noninfectious viral particles. Ritonavir inhibits the metabolism of lopinavir, thereby increasing plasma levels of lopinavir.

Pharmacokinetics

Absorption: Peak levels are achieved in 4 hours. Kaletra is better absorbed when taken with food.
Distribution: Lopinavir is highly bound to plasma proteins (98% to 99%).
Metabolism: Lopinavir is extensively metabolized by the CYP3A isoenzyme, which is part of the P-450 pathway. Ritonavir is a potent inhibitor of the CYP3A, which inhibits the metabolism of lopinavir, and therefore increases plasma levels of lopinavir.
Excretion: The drug is excreted in the urine and feces. Less than 3% of the drug is excreted unchanged. The half-life is about 5-6 hours.

Route	Onset	Peak	Duration
P.O.	Unknown	4 hr	5-6 hr

Contraindications and precautions

Contraindicated in patients hypersensitive to any of drug's ingredients. Use cautiously in patients with a history of pancreatitis or with hepatic impairment, hepatitis B or C, marked elevations in liver enzyme levels, or hemophilia. Also use cautiously in elderly patients.

Interactions

Drug-drug. *Amiodarone, bepridil, lidocaine, quinidine:* Increased antiarrhythmic levels. Use cautiously, and monitor drug levels if possible.
Amprenavir, indinavir, saquinavir: Increased levels of these drugs. Avoid use together.
Antiarrhythmics (flecainide, propafenone), pimozide: Increased risk of cardiac arrhythmias. Don't use together.
Atorvastatin, cerivastatin: Increased levels of these drugs. Use lowest possible dose and monitor patient carefully.
Atovaquone, methadone: Decreased levels of these drugs. Consider increased doses of these drugs.
Carbamazepine, dexamethasone, phenobarbital, phenytoin: Decreased lopinavir levels. Use cautiously.
Clarithromycin: Increased clarithromycin levels in patients with renal impairment. Adjust clarithromycin dose.
Cyclosporine, rapamycin, tacrolimus: Increased levels of these drugs. Monitor therapeutic levels.
Delavirdine, ritonavir: Increased lopinavir levels. Avoid use together.
Didanosine: Decreased absorption of didanosine because Kaletra is taken with food. Give didanosine 1 hour before or 2 hours after Kaletra.
Dihydroergotamine, ergonovine, ergotamine, methylergonovine: Increased risk of ergot toxicity characterized by peripheral vasospasm and ischemia. Don't use together.
Disulfiram, metronidazole: Risk of disulfiram-like reaction. Avoid concomitant use.
Efavirenz, nevirapine: Decreased lopinavir levels. Consider increased Kaletra dose.
Felodipine, nicardipine, nifedipine: Increased levels of these drugs. Use cautiously. Monitor patient.
Itraconazole, ketoconazole: Increased levels of these drugs. Don't give more than 200 mg daily of these drugs.
Lovastatin, simvastatin: Increased risk of adverse reactions, such as myopathy and rhabdomyolysis. Avoid concomitant use.
Midazolam, triazolam: Increased risk of prolonged or increased sedation or respiratory depression. Don't use together.
Oral contraceptives (ethinyl estradiol): Decreased effectiveness of contraceptives. Recommend alternative contraception measures.
Rifabutin: Increased rifabutin levels. Decrease rifabutin dose by 75%. Monitor patient for adverse effects.
Rifampin: Decreased effectiveness of Kaletra. Avoid concomitant use.

Sildenafil: Increased sildenafil levels. Reduce sildenafil dose. Use cautiously, and monitor patient for adverse reactions.
Warfarin: Drug may affect warfarin level. Monitor PT and INR.
Drug-herb. *St. John's wort:* Loss of virologic response and possible resistance to drug. Discourage concomitant use.
Drug-food. Increased absorption of drug. Give drug with food.

Adverse reactions

CNS: asthenia, headache, insomnia, malaise, abnormal dreams, agitation, amnesia, anxiety, ataxia, confusion, depression, dizziness, dyskinesia, emotional lability, encephalopathy, hypertonia, nervousness, neuropathy, paresthesia, peripheral neuritis, somnolence, abnormal thinking, tremors.
CV: chest pain, ***deep vein thrombosis,*** hypertension, palpitations, thrombophlebitis, vasculitis, edema.
EENT: sinusitis, abnormal vision, eye disorder, otitis media, tinnitus.
GI: abdominal pain, abnormal stools, *diarrhea, nausea,* vomiting, anorexia, cholecystitis, constipation, dry mouth, dyspepsia, dysphagia, enterocolitis, eructation, esophagitis, fecal incontinence, flatulence, gastritis, gastroenteritis, GI disorder, hemorrhagic colitis, increased appetite, ***pancreatitis,*** sialadenitis, stomatitis, ulcerative stomatitis, elevated amylase level.
GU: abnormal ejaculation, taste perversion, hypogonadism, renal calculus, urine abnormality.
Hematologic: anemia, ***leukopenia, neutropenia; thrombocytopenia*** in children.
Hepatic: elevated liver enzyme levels, hyperbilirubinemia in children.
Metabolic: Cushing's syndrome, hypothyroidism, dehydration, decreased glucose tolerance, lactic acidosis, weight loss, hyperglycemia, hyperuricemia, *hypercholesterolemia, elevated triglycerides,* hyponatremia in children.
Musculoskeletal: back pain, athralgia, arthrosis, myalgia.
Respiratory: bronchitis, dyspnea, lung edema.
Skin: rash, acne, alopecia, dry skin, exfoliative dermatitis, furunculosis, nail disorder, pruritus, benign skin neoplasm, skin discoloration, sweating.
Other: pain, chills, facial edema, fever, flu syndrome, viral infection, lymphadenopathy, peripheral edema, decreased libido, gynecomastia.

Overdose and treatment

Experience of acute overdose is limited. Treatment is supportive and symptomatic. Induce emesis or perform gastric lavage. Activated charcoal may be used to remove unabsorbed drug. Dialysis is unlikely to help with drug removal. There's no known antidote.

Oral solution contains 42% alcohol. Ingestion of the product by a young child may result in alcohol-related toxicity.

Reactions may be *common*, uncommon, ***life-threatening***, or COMMON AND LIFE-THREATENING.

Special considerations
• To monitor maternal-fetal outcomes of pregnant women exposed to Kaletra, an antiretroviral registry has been established. Health care providers are encouraged to enroll patients by calling 1-800-258-4263.
⚠ ALERT Many drug interactions are possible. Review current medications that patient is taking.
• Give drug with food.
• Refrigerated drug remains stable until expiration date on package. If stored at room temperature, drug should be used within 2 months.

Patient monitoring
• Monitor patient for signs of fat redistribution, including central obesity, buffalo hump, peripheral wasting, breast enlargement, and cushingoid appearance.
• Monitor total cholesterol and triglycerides before starting therapy and periodically thereafter.
• Monitor patient for signs of pancreatitis: nausea, vomiting, abdominal pain, increased lipase and amylase values.
• Monitor patient for signs of bleeding.

Breast-feeding patients
• The CDC recommends that HIV-infected mothers not breast-feed their infants to avoid HIV transmission. It's not known whether the drug appears in breast milk.

Pediatric patients
• Safety and efficacy in children less than age 6 months haven't been established.

Patient education
• Tell patient to take drug with food.
• Tell patient also taking didanosine to take it 1 hour before or 2 hours after Kaletra.
• Advise patient to report side effects to prescriber.
• Tell patient to immediately report severe nausea, vomiting, or abdominal pain.
• Warn patient to tell prescriber about any other prescription or nonprescription medicine that he's taking, including herbal supplements.
• Tell patient that drug isn't a cure for HIV.

---

loracarbef
Lorabid

Pharmacologic classification: synthetic beta-lactam antibiotic of carbacephem class
Therapeutic classification: antibiotic
Pregnancy risk category: B

Indications and dosages
➤ **Secondary bacterial infections of acute bronchitis.** *Adults and adolescents age 13 and older:* 200 to 400 mg P.O. q 12 hours for 7 days.
➤ **Acute bacterial exacerbations of chronic bronchitis.** *Adults and adolescents age 13 and older:* 400 mg P.O. q 12 hours for 7 days.

➤ **Pneumonia.** *Adults and adolescents age 13 and older:* 400 mg P.O. q 12 hours for 14 days.
➤ **Pharyngitis or tonsillitis.** *Adults and adolescents age 13 and older:* 200 mg P.O. q 12 hours for 10 days.
Children ages 6 months to 12 years: 15 mg/kg P.O. daily in divided doses q 12 hours for 10 days.
➤ **Sinusitis.** *Adults and adolescents age 13 and older:* 400 mg P.O. q 12 hours for 10 days.
Children ages 6 months to 12 years: 15 mg/kg P.O. q 12 hours for 10 days.
➤ **Acute otitis media.** *Children ages 6 months to 12 years:* 30 mg/kg (oral suspension) P.O. daily in divided doses q 12 hours for 10 days.
➤ **Uncomplicated skin and skin-structure infections.** *Adults and adolescents age 13 and older:* 200 mg P.O. q 12 hours for 7 days.
➤ **Impetigo.** *Children:* 15 mg/kg P.O. daily in divided doses q 12 hours for 7 days.
➤ **Uncomplicated cystitis.** *Adults and adolescents age 13 and older:* 200 mg P.O. daily for 7 days.
➤ **Uncomplicated pyelonephritis.** *Adults and adolescents age 13 and older:* 400 mg P.O. q 12 hours for 14 days.
✦ *Dosage adjustment.* Adults and children with renal impairment and creatinine clearance of 50 ml/minute or more don't require dose and interval changes. In patients with creatinine clearance of 10 to 49 ml/minute, half usual dose at same interval or normal recommended dose at twice the usual dosage interval; in those with creatinine clearance below 10 ml/minute, usual dose q 3 to 5 days. Hemodialysis patients should be given another dose after dialysis.

How supplied
Available by prescription only
Powder for oral suspension: 100 mg/5 ml, 200 mg/5 ml
Pulvules: 200 mg, 400 mg

Pharmacodynamics
Antibiotic action: Loracarbef exerts its bactericidal action by binding to essential target proteins of the bacterial cell wall, leading to inhibition of cell-wall synthesis. Loracarbef is active against gram-positive aerobes, such as *Staphylococcus aureus, S. saprophyticus, Streptococcus pneumoniae,* and *S. pyogenes,* and gram-negative aerobes, such as *Escherichia coli, Haemophilus influenzae,* and *Moraxella catarrhalis.*

Pharmacokinetics
Absorption: After oral administration, drug is about 90% absorbed from the GI tract. When pulvules are taken with food, peak plasma levels are 50% to 60% of those achieved on an empty stomach. (Effect of food on rate and extent of absorption of suspension form hasn't been studied.) Absorption of suspension form is greater than that of pulvule.
Distribution: About 25% of circulating drug is bound to plasma proteins.

Metabolism: Doesn't appear to be metabolized.
Excretion: Eliminated primarily in urine. Elimination half-life in patients with normal renal function averages 1 hour.

Route	Onset	Peak	Duration
P.O.	Unknown	½-1 hr	Unknown

Contraindications and precautions
Contraindicated in patients hypersensitive to drug or other cephalosporins and in patients with diarrhea caused by pseudomembranous colitis. Use cautiously in pregnant and breast-feeding women.

Interactions
Drug-drug. *Probenecid:* Decreased excretion of loracarbef, causing increased plasma levels. Monitor patient for toxicity.

Adverse reactions
CNS: headache, somnolence, nervousness, insomnia, dizziness.
CV: vasodilation.
GI: diarrhea, nausea, vomiting, abdominal pain, anorexia, pseudomembranous colitis.
GU: vaginal candidiasis, transient increases in BUN and creatinine levels.
Hematologic: *transient thrombocytopenia, leukopenia,* eosinophilia.
Hepatic: transient elevations in AST, ALT, and alkaline phosphatase levels.
Skin: rash, urticaria, pruritus, *erythema multiforme.*
Other: *hypersensitivity reactions,* including *anaphylaxis.*

Overdose and treatment
Toxic symptoms after overdose of beta-lactams such as loracarbef may include nausea, vomiting, epigastric distress, and diarrhea.

Forced diuresis, peritoneal dialysis, hemodialysis, or hemoperfusion hasn't been established as beneficial for an overdose of loracarbef. Hemodialysis is effective in hastening the elimination of loracarbef from plasma in patients with chronic renal failure.

Special considerations
● Consider the increased rate of absorption if oral suspension is to be substituted for pulvule. Pulvules shouldn't be substituted for oral suspension when treating otitis media.
● Pseudomembranous colitis has been reported with nearly all antibacterial agents and may range from mild to life-threatening. Therefore, diagnosis must be considered in patients with diarrhea subsequent to drug administration.
● To reconstitute powder for oral suspension, add 30 ml of water in two portions to the 50-ml bottle or 60 ml of water in two portions to the 100-ml bottle; shake after each addition.
● After reconstitution, oral suspension is stable for 14 days at 59° to 86° F (15° to 30° C).
● Drug can cause positive direct Coombs' test.

Patient monitoring
● Culture and sensitivity tests should be done before giving first dose. Therapy may begin pending test results.
● Drug may cause overgrowth of nonsusceptible bacteria or fungi. Patient needs to be monitored for signs and symptoms of superinfection.

Breast-feeding patients
● It isn't known whether drug appears in breast milk. Use caution when administering drug to breast-feeding women.

Pediatric patients
● Safety and efficacy in infants under age 6 months haven't been established.

Patient education
● Instruct patient to take drug at least 1 hour before or at least 2 hours after eating.
● Tell patient to take drug exactly as prescribed, even after he feels better.
● Inform patient that oral suspension can be stored at room temperature for 14 days. Instruct patient to discard unused portion after 14 days.

loratadine
Claritin

Pharmacologic classification: tricyclic antihistamine
Therapeutic classification: antihistaminic
Pregnancy risk category: B

Indications and dosages
➤ *Symptomatic treatment of seasonal allergic rhinitis and indicated for treatment of idiopathic chronic urticaria.*
Adults and children age 6 and older: 10 mg P.O. daily.
Children ages 2 to 5: 5 mg P.O. daily.
✦ *Dosage adjustment.* In adults and children age 6 and older with liver impairment or glomerular filtration rate below 30 ml/minute, adjust dose to 10 mg every other day. In children ages 2 to 5 with liver or renal impairment, adjust dose to 5 mg every other day.
➤ *Perennial allergic rhinitis◇. Adults:* 10 mg P.O. daily.

How supplied
Available by prescription only
Syrup: 1 mg/ml
Tablets: 10 mg
Tablets (rapidly distintegrating): 10 mg

Pharmacodynamics
Antihistaminic action: Loratadine is a long-acting tricyclic antihistamine with selective peripheral H_1-receptor antagonistic activity.

Pharmacokinetics

Absorption: Readily absorbed. Because loratadine's peak plasma level may be delayed by 1 hour with a meal, administer drug on an empty stomach.
Distribution: About 97% is bound to plasma protein. Drug doesn't readily cross the blood-brain barrier.
Metabolism: Extensively metabolized to an active metabolite (descarboethoxyloratadine), primarily by cytochrome P-450 3A4 and, to a lesser extent, by cytochrome P-450 2D6.
Excretion: About 80% of dose is equally excreted via urine and feces. Mean elimination half-life is 8¼ hours for loratadine. Drug isn't eliminated by hemodialysis; it's unknown whether drug is eliminated by peritoneal dialysis.

Route	Onset	Peak	Duration
P.O.	1-3 hr	8-10 hr	24 hr

Contraindications and precautions
Contraindicated in patients hypersensitive to drug. Use cautiously in patients with hepatic impairment and in breast-feeding women.

Interactions
Drug-drug. *Drugs known to inhibit hepatic metabolism:* Should be coadministered cautiously until definitive interaction studies can be completed.
Drug-herb. *Licorice:* May prolong the QT interval and be potentially additive. Discourage concomitant use.

Adverse reactions
CNS: headache, somnolence, fatigue.
GI: dry mouth.

Overdose and treatment
Somnolence, tachycardia, and headache have been reported with overdoses of 40 to 180 mg. If overdose occurs, institute symptomatic and supportive measures promptly and maintain for as long as necessary.
 Treatment consists of emesis with ipecac syrup, except in patients with impaired consciousness, followed by administration of activated charcoal to adsorb any remaining drug. If vomiting is unsuccessful or contraindicated, perform gastric lavage with normal saline solution. Saline cathartics also may be of value for rapid dilution of bowel contents.

Special considerations
● No information exists to indicate that drug abuse or dependency occurs.
● Store drug in a cool, dry place away from heat and direct sunlight.

Patient monitoring
● Monitor renal and hepatic function in patients with preexisting conditions.

Breast-feeding patients
● Loratadine appears in breast milk. Antihistamine therapy is contraindicated in breast-feeding women.

Pediatric patients
● Safety and efficacy in children under age 2 haven't been established.

Patient education
● Instruct patient to take drug on an empty stomach at least 2 hours after a meal and to avoid eating for at least 1 hour after taking drug.
● Tell patient to take drug only once daily. Tell him to call if symptoms persist or worsen.
● Warn patient to stop taking drug 4 days before allergy skin tests to preserve accuracy of tests.

lorazepam
Apo-Lorazepam*, Ativan, Novo-Lorazem*

Pharmacologic classification: benzodiazepine
Therapeutic classification: antianxiety, sedative-hypnotic
Controlled substance schedule: IV
Pregnancy risk category: D

Indications and dosages
➤ *Anxiety, tension, agitation, irritability, especially in anxiety neuroses or organic (especially GI or CV) disorders.*
Adults: Initially, 2 to 3 mg P.O. daily in two to three divided doses. Usual range is 2 to 6 mg P.O. daily in divided doses; maximum dose is 10 mg daily.
➤ *Insomnia. Adults:* 2 to 4 mg P.O. h.s.
➤ *Preoperatively. Adults:* 0.05 mg/kg I.M. 2 hours before surgery (maximum, 4 mg). Or, 0.044 mg/kg (maximum total dose is 2 mg) I.V. 15 to 20 minutes before surgery; in adults under age 50, dosage may be increased to 0.05 mg/kg (maximum, 4 mg) I.V. when decreased recall of preoperative events is desired.
➤ *Management of nausea and vomiting caused by emetogenic chemotherapy ◇.*
Adults: 2.5 mg P.O. the evening before chemotherapy and repeat just after the initiation of chemotherapy. Or, 1.5 mg/m² (maximum 3 mg) I.V. over 5 minutes 45 minutes before chemotherapy.
✦ *Dosage adjustment.* Geriatric patients should initially receive 1 to 2 mg P.O. daily in divided doses. Then dosage is divided p.r.n.
➤ *Status epilepticus ◇. Adults and children:* 0.05 to 0.1 mg/kg I.V. Doses may be repeated at 10- to 15-minute intervals as necessary for seizure control. Or, adults may be given 4 to 8 mg I.V.

How supplied
Available by prescription only
Injection: 2 mg/ml, 4 mg/ml
Solution: 2 mg/ml

Tablets: 0.5 mg, 1 mg, 2 mg
Tablets (S.L.)*: 1 mg, 2 mg

Pharmacodynamics
Anxiolytic and sedative actions: Lorazepam depresses the CNS at the limbic and subcortical levels of the brain. It produces an antianxiety effect by influencing the effect of the neurotransmitter gamma-aminobutyric acid on its receptor in the ascending reticular activating system, which increases inhibition and blocks both cortical and limbic arousal after stimulation of the reticular formation.

Pharmacokinetics
Absorption: When administered orally, is well absorbed through the GI tract.
Distribution: Distributed widely throughout the body. Drug is about 85% protein-bound.
Metabolism: Metabolized in the liver to inactive metabolites.
Excretion: Metabolites are excreted in urine as glucuronide conjugates.

Route	Onset	Peak	Duration
P.O.	1 hr	2 hr	12-24 hr
I.V.	5 min	1-1½ hr	6-8 hr
I.M.	15-30 min	1-1½ hr	6-8 hr

Contraindications and precautions
Contraindicated in patients with acute angle-closure glaucoma or hypersensitivity to drug, other benzodiazepines, or its vehicle (used in parenteral dosage form).

Use cautiously in patients with pulmonary, renal, or hepatic impairment and in elderly, acutely ill, or debilitated patients. Don't use in pregnant women, especially during the first trimester of pregnancy.

Interactions
Drug-drug. *Antidepressants, antihistamines, barbiturates, general anesthetics, MAO inhibitors, narcotics, phenothiazines:* Lorazepam potentiates CNS depressant effects of these drugs. Use together cautiously.
Cimetidine and possibly disulfiram: Diminished hepatic metabolism of lorazepam, which increases its plasma level. Avoid use together.
Scopolamine: Combined use of parenteral lorazepam and scopolamine may cause an increased risk of hallucinations, irrational behavior, and increased sedation. Use together cautiously.
Drug-herb. *Calendula, catnip, hops, kava, lady's slipper, passionflower, valerian:* May increase sedative effect of the drug. Discourage use together.
Drug-lifestyle. *Alcohol use:* Lorazepam potentiates the CNS depressant effects of alcohol. Advise patient not to consume alcohol during drug therapy.
Heavy smoking: Accelerated lorazepam metabolism, thus lowering clinical effectiveness. Discourage smoking.

Adverse reactions
CNS: *drowsiness,* amnesia, insomnia, agitation, *sedation,* dizziness, weakness, unsteadiness, disorientation, depression, headache.
EENT: visual disturbances.
GI: abdominal discomfort, nausea, change in appetite.
Other: *acute withdrawal syndrome* (after sudden discontinuation in physically dependent patients).

Overdose and treatment
Signs and symptoms of overdose include somnolence, confusion, coma, hypoactive reflexes, dyspnea, labored breathing, hypotension, bradycardia, slurred speech, and unsteady gait or impaired coordination.

Treatment requires support of blood pressure and respiration until drug effects subside; monitor vital signs. Mechanical ventilatory assistance via endotracheal tube may be required to maintain a patent airway and support adequate oxygenation. Flumazenil, a specific benzodiazepine antagonist, may be useful. Use I.V. fluids and vasopressors such as dopamine and phenylephrine to treat hypotension, if necessary. If patient is conscious, induce emesis. Use gastric lavage if ingestion was recent, but only if an endotracheal tube is present to prevent aspiration. After emesis or lavage, administer activated charcoal with a cathartic as a single dose. Dialysis is of limited value.

Special considerations
● Lorazepam is one of the preferred benzodiazepines for patients with hepatic disease.
● Use lowest possible effective dose to avoid oversedation.
● Parenteral lorazepam appears to possess potent amnesic effects.
● For the oral concentrated solution, add dose to 30 ml or more of water, juice, or soda, or to semisolid foods.
● Oral drug is given in divided doses, with the largest dose given before bedtime.
⚠ ALERT Arteriospasm may result from intra-arterial injection of lorazepam. Don't administer by this route.
● For I.V. administration, dilute lorazepam with an equal volume of a compatible diluent, such as D₅W, sterile water for injection, or normal saline solution.
● Drug may be injected directly into a vein or into the tubing of a compatible I.V. infusion, such as normal saline solution or D₅W solution. The rate of lorazepam I.V. injection shouldn't exceed 2 mg/minute. Emergency resuscitative equipment should be available when administering I.V.
● Diluted lorazepam solutions must be given immediately.
● Don't use drug solutions if they're discolored or contain a precipitate.
● I.M. doses of lorazepam are given undiluted, deep into a large muscle mass.

Reactions may be *common,* uncommon, *life-threatening,* or COMMON AND LIFE-THREATENING.

Patient monitoring

● Monitor hepatic function studies to prevent cumulative effects and to ensure adequate drug metabolism.

● Monitor renal function tests.

Breast-feeding patients

● Drug may appear in breast milk. Don't administer to breast-feeding women.

Pediatric patients

● Safety of oral lorazepam in children under age 12 hasn't been established. Safety of sublingual or parenteral lorazepam in children under age 18 hasn't been established. Neonates haven't been closely observed for withdrawal symptoms when mother took lorazepam for a prolonged period during pregnancy.

Geriatric patients

● These patients are more sensitive to CNS depressant effects of lorazepam. They may need assistance with walking and daily activities when therapy starts or dosage increases.

● Lower doses usually are effective in elderly patients because of decreased elimination.

● Parenteral administration of drug is more likely to cause apnea, hypotension, bradycardia, and cardiac arrest in elderly patients.

Patient education

● Caution patient not to change drug regimen without specific instructions.

● Teach safety measures, as appropriate, to protect from injury, such as gradual position changes and supervised walking.

● Advise patient of possible retrograde amnesia after I.V. or I.M. use.

● Tell patient to avoid large amounts of caffeine-containing products, which may interfere with effectiveness of drug.

● Advise patient about risk of physical and psychological dependence with long-term use.

● Tell patient to stop drug slowly (over 8 to 12 weeks) after long-term therapy.

losartan potassium
Cozaar

Pharmacologic classification: angiotensin II receptor antagonist
Therapeutic classification: antihypertensive
Pregnancy risk category: C (D in second and third trimesters)

Indications and dosages

➤ *Hypertension. Adults:* Initially, 25 to 50 mg P.O. daily. Maintenance dosage is 25 to 100 mg P.O. once daily or b.i.d.

How supplied

Available by prescription only
Tablets: 25 mg, 50 mg

Pharmacodynamics

Antihypertensive action: Losartan is an angiotensin II receptor antagonist; it blocks the vasoconstrictor and aldosterone-secreting effects of angiotensin II by selectively blocking the binding of angiotensin II to its receptor sites found in many tissues, including vascular smooth muscle.

Pharmacokinetics

Absorption: Well absorbed and undergoes substantial first-pass metabolism; systemic bioavailability is about 33%.
Distribution: Both losartan and its active metabolite are highly bound to plasma proteins, primarily albumin.
Metabolism: Cytochrome P-450 2C9 and 3A4 are involved in the biotransformation of drug to its metabolites.
Excretion: Drug and its metabolites are primarily excreted in feces with a small amount excreted in urine.

Route	Onset	Peak	Duration
P.O.	Unknown	1 hr	Unknown

Contraindications and precautions

Contraindicated in patients hypersensitive to drug. Use cautiously in patients with impaired renal or hepatic function.

Interactions

None significant.

Adverse reactions

CNS: dizziness, insomnia.
EENT: nasal congestion, sinus disorder, sinusitis.
GI: diarrhea, dyspepsia.
Musculoskeletal: muscle cramps, myalgia, back or leg pain.
Respiratory: cough, upper respiratory tract infection.

Overdose and treatment

The most likely signs of overdose are hypotension and tachycardia; bradycardia could occur from parasympathetic stimulation. If symptomatic hypotension occurs, initiate supportive treatment. Neither losartan nor its active metabolite can be removed by hemodialysis.

Special considerations

● Use the lowest dose (25 mg) initially in patients with impaired hepatic function and in those who are intravascularly volume-depleted (receiving diuretic therapy).

● Drug can be used alone or with other antihypertensives.

● If antihypertensive effect measured at trough (using once-daily dosing) is inadequate, a twice-daily regimen at the same total daily dose or an increased dose may give a more satisfactory response.

● Patients with severe heart failure whose renal function depends on the angiotensin-aldosterone system have experienced acute renal failure during therapy with ACE inhibitors. Manufacturer of losartan states that drug would be expected to do the same. Closely monitor patient, especially during first few weeks of therapy.

Patient monitoring
• Monitor patient taking diuretics for hypertension for symptomatic hypotension.
• Monitor patient's renal function (serum creatinine and BUN levels).

Pregnant patients
• Drugs such as losartan that act directly on the renin-angiotensin system can cause fetal and neonatal morbidity and death when administered to pregnant women; these problems haven't been detected when exposure has been limited to the first trimester. If pregnancy is suspected, discontinue drug.

Breast-feeding patients
• It isn't known whether drug appears in breast milk. Because of the potential for adverse effects on the breast-fed infant, a decision should be made to discontinue the drug or breast-feeding, taking into account the importance of drug to the woman.

Pediatric patients
• Safety and efficacy in children haven't been established.

Patient education
• Instruct patient not to discontinue drug abruptly.
• Tell patient to avoid sodium substitutes; these products may contain potassium, which can cause hyperkalemia in patients taking losartan.
• Inform woman of childbearing age about the consequences of second- and third-trimester exposure to losartan; instruct her to call immediately if pregnancy is suspected.

lovastatin
Mevacor

Pharmacologic classification: lactone, 3-hydroxy-3-methylglutaryl-coenzyme A (HMG-CoA) reductase inhibitor
Therapeutic classification: cholesterol-lowering agent
Pregnancy risk category: X

Indications and dosages
➤ *Reduction of low-density lipoprotein and total cholesterol levels in patients with primary hypercholesterolemia (types IIa and IIb), atherosclerosis.* Adults: Initially, 20 mg P.O. once daily with evening meal. For patients with severely elevated cholesterol levels (over 300 mg/dl), initial dose should be 40 mg. Recommended range is 20 to 80 mg in single or divided doses.

✦ *Dosage adjustment.* For patients also taking immunosuppressive drugs, 10 mg P.O. daily, not to exceed 20 mg daily.

How supplied
Available by prescription only
Tablets: 10 mg, 20 mg, 40 mg

Pharmacodynamics
Antilipemic action: Lovastatin, an inactive lactone, is hydrolyzed to the beta-hydroxy acid, which specifically inhibits HMG-CoA reductase. This enzyme is an early (and rate-limiting) step in the synthetic pathway of cholesterol. At therapeutic doses, the enzyme isn't blocked, and biologically necessary amounts of cholesterol can still be synthesized.

Pharmacokinetics
Absorption: About 30% of an oral dose is absorbed in animals. Administration of drug with food improves plasma levels of total inhibitors by about 30%. Onset of action is about 3 days, with maximal therapeutic effects seen in 4 to 6 weeks.
Distribution: Less than 5% of an oral dose reaches the systemic circulation because of extensive first-pass hepatic extraction; the liver is the principal site of action for the drug. Both the parent compound and its principal metabolite are highly bound (more than 95%) to plasma proteins. Lovastatin crosses the placenta and the blood-brain barrier.
Metabolism: Converted to the active B hydroxy acid form in the liver. Other metabolites include the 6' hydroxy derivative and two unidentified compounds.
Excretion: About 80% is excreted primarily in feces, about 10% in urine.

Route	Onset	Peak	Duration
P.O.	Unknown	2 hr	Unknown

Contraindications and precautions
Contraindicated in patients hypersensitive to drug, in those with active liver disease or conditions of unexplained persistent elevations of serum transaminase levels, in pregnant and breast-feeding women, and in women of childbearing age unless there's no risk of pregnancy.

Use cautiously in patients who consume excessive amounts of alcohol or have history of liver disease.

Interactions
Drug-drug. *Cholestyramine, colestipol:* May enhance lipid-reducing effects but may decrease bioavailability of lovastatin. Patient requires close monitoring.
Cyclosporine, erythromycin, gemfibrozil, niacin: May increase risk of severe myopathy or rhabdomyolysis. Use together cautiously.

Reactions may be *common*, uncommon, *life-threatening*, or COMMON AND LIFE-THREATENING.

Isradipine: May increase clearance of lovastatin and its metabolites. Patient requires careful monitoring.

Itraconazole: Coadministration with lovastatin increases HMG-CoA reductase inhibitor levels. Therapy with lovastatin should be temporarily interrupted if systemic azole antifungal treatment is required.

Warfarin: Increased anticoagulant effect. Monitor PT and INR.

Drug-herb. *Pectin:* Decreased lovastatin effect. Tell patient to avoid use together.

Drug-food. *Grapefruit juice:* Elevated drug levels and increased risk of adverse effects. Tell patient to take with liquids other than grapefruit juice.

Drug-lifestyle. *Alcohol use:* May increase hepatic effects. Advise patient to avoid alcohol use. *Sun exposure:* Photosensitivity reaction. Advise patient to take precautions.

Adverse reactions

CNS: headache, dizziness, peripheral neuropathy, insomnia.
CV: chest pain.
EENT: blurred vision.
GI: constipation, diarrhea, dyspepsia, flatulence, abdominal pain or cramps, heartburn, nausea, vomiting.
Hepatic: elevated serum transaminase levels, abnormal liver test results.
Musculoskeletal: muscle cramps, myalgia, myositis, ***rhabdomyolysis.***
Skin: rash, pruritus, alopecia, photosensitivity.

Overdose and treatment
No information available.

Special considerations

● Initiate drug therapy only after diet and other nonpharmacologic therapies have proved ineffective. Patient should be on a standard cholesterol-lowering diet and continue on this diet during therapy.
● Administer drug with evening meal; absorption is enhanced and cholesterol biosynthesis is greater in the evening.
● Therapeutic response occurs in about 2 weeks, with maximum effects in 4 to 6 weeks.
● Store tablets at room temperature in a light-resistant container.
● Don't exceed 20 mg daily if patient is receiving immunosuppressive drugs.

Patient monitoring

● Patient must be monitored for signs of myositis; have patient report muscle aches and pains.
● Liver function tests are needed frequently during initiation of therapy and periodically thereafter.
● Monitor serum lipoprotein, triglycerides, and serum cholesterol periodically during therapy.

Breast-feeding patients
● Breast feeding isn't recommended during therapy with lovastatin.

Pediatric patients
● Safety and efficacy in children haven't been established.

Patient education
● Stress importance of lowering cholesterol.
● Advise patient to restrict alcohol intake.
● Instruct patient to take drug with evening meal.
● Tell patient to report adverse reactions, particularly muscle aches and pains, and to take precautions with exposure to sun and other ultraviolet light until tolerance is determined.

loxapine hydrochloride
Loxitane C, Loxitane IM

loxapine succinate
Loxapac*, Loxitane

Pharmacologic classification: dibenzoxazepine
Therapeutic classification: antipsychotic
Pregnancy risk category: NR

Indications and dosages

➤ *Psychotic disorders. Adults:* Initially, 10 mg P.O. b.i.d. (in severe schizophrenia, 50 mg P.O. daily); usual therapeutic and maintenance dosage is 60 to 100 mg P.O. daily b.i.d. to q.i.d. (dose varies from patient to patient) or 12.5 to 50 mg I.M. q 4 to 6 hours or longer. Maximum daily dose is 250 mg. After desired symptom control, change to oral therapy. Don't administer drug I.V.

How supplied
Available by prescription only
Capsules: 5 mg, 10 mg, 25 mg, 50 mg
Injection: 50 mg/ml
Oral concentrate: 25 mg/ml

Pharmacodynamics
Antipsychotic action: Loxapine is the only tricyclic antipsychotic; it's structurally similar to amoxapine. Loxapine is thought to exert its antipsychotic effects by postsynaptic blockade of CNS dopamine receptors, thus inhibiting dopamine-mediated effects. Loxapine has many other central and peripheral effects; its most prominent adverse reactions are extrapyramidal.

Pharmacokinetics
Absorption: Absorbed rapidly and completely from the GI tract. First-pass metabolism results in lower systemic availability.
Distribution: Distributed widely throughout the body, including breast milk. Steady state serum level is achieved within 3 to 4 days. Drug is 91% to 99% protein-bound.

Metabolism: Metabolized extensively by the liver, forming a few active metabolites; duration of action is 12 hours.
Excretion: Mostly excreted as metabolites in urine; some is excreted in feces by way of the biliary tract. About 50% is excreted in urine and feces within 24 hours.

Route	Onset	Peak	Duration
P.O., I.M.	½ hr	1½-3 hr	12 hr

Contraindications and precautions

Contraindicated in patients hypersensitive to dibenzoxazepines and in patients experiencing coma, severe CNS depression, or drug-induced depressed states. Use cautiously in patients with seizure or CV disorders, glaucoma, or history of urine retention.

Interactions

Drug-drug. *Aluminum- and magnesium-containing antacids and antidiarrheals:* Decreased loxapine absorption and therapeutic effects. Separate administration times.
Antiarrhythmics, disopyramide, quinidine, procainamide: Increased risk of arrhythmias and conduction defects. Use together cautiously.
Anticholinergics, including antidepressants, antihistamines, antiparkinsonians, atropine, MAO inhibitors, meperidine, phenothiazines: Oversedation, paralytic ileus, visual changes, and severe constipation. Avoid use together.
Beta blockers: May inhibit loxapine metabolism, increasing plasma levels and toxicity. Use together cautiously.
Bromocriptine: Loxapine may antagonize therapeutic effect of bromocriptine on prolactin secretion. Monitor patient for effect.
Centrally acting antihypertensive drugs, such as clonidine, guanabenz, guanadrel, guanethidine, methyldopa, and reserpine: Loxapine may inhibit blood pressure response. Use together cautiously.
CNS depressants, including analgesics, anesthetics (general, spinal, and epidural), barbiturates, narcotics, tranquilizers, and parenteral magnesium sulfate: Additive effects are likely. Use together cautiously.
Dopamine: Decreased vasoconstricting effects of high-dose dopamine. Avoid use together.
Levodopa: Decreased effectiveness and increased toxicity of levodopa (by dopamine blockade). Avoid use together.
Lithium: May result in severe neurologic toxicity with an encephalitis-like syndrome and a decreased therapeutic response to loxapine. Avoid use together.
Nitrates: May cause hypotension. Use together cautiously.
Sympathomimetics, including ephedrine, epinephrine, and phenylephrine (often found in nasal sprays), appetite suppressants: Decreased stimulatory and pressor effects. Loxapine may cause epinephrine reversal, an inhibition of the vasopressor effect of epinephrine. Use together cautiously.
Drug-lifestyle. *Alcohol use:* Additive effects are likely. Tell patient to avoid use together.

Adverse reactions

CNS: *extrapyramidal reactions, sedation, drowsiness, **seizures,** numbness, confusion, syncope, tardive dyskinesia, **neuroleptic malignant syndrome,** pseudoparkinsonism, EEG changes, dizziness.
CV: *orthostatic hypotension, tachycardia,* ECG changes, hypertension.
EENT: *blurred vision,* nasal congestion.
GI: *dry mouth, constipation,* nausea, vomiting, paralytic ileus.
GU: *urine retention,* menstrual irregularities.
Hematologic: *leukopenia, agranulocytosis, thrombocytopenia.*
Hepatic: jaundice.
Metabolic: weight gain.
Skin: *mild photosensitivity,* allergic reactions, rash, pruritus.
Other: gynecomastia.

Overdose and treatment

CNS depression is characterized by deep, unarousable sleep and possible coma, hypotension or hypertension, extrapyramidal symptoms, abnormal involuntary muscle movements, agitation, seizures, arrhythmias, ECG changes, hypothermia or hyperthermia, and autonomic nervous system dysfunction. Treatment is symptomatic and supportive, including maintaining vital signs, airway, stable body temperature, and fluid and electrolyte balance.

Don't induce vomiting: drug inhibits cough reflex, and aspiration may occur. Use gastric lavage, then activated charcoal and saline cathartics; hemodialysis may be helpful. Regulate body temperature as needed. Treat hypotension with I.V. fluids; don't give epinephrine. Treat seizures with parenteral diazepam or barbiturates; arrhythmias with parenteral phenytoin (1 mg/kg with rate adjusted to blood pressure); and extrapyramidal reactions with benztropine 1 to 2 mg or parenteral diphenhydramine 10 to 50 mg.

Special considerations

● Tardive dyskinesia may occur, usually after prolonged use. It may not appear until months or years after treatment and may disappear spontaneously or persist for life.
● Avoid combining drug with alcohol or other depressants.
● Dilute liquid concentrate with orange or grapefruit juice just before giving.
● Dose of 10 mg is therapeutic equivalent of 100 mg chlorpromazine.
● Photosensitivity may occur with loxapine.
● Drug causes false-positive test results for urinary porphyrins, urobilinogen, amylase, and 5-hydroxyindoleacetic acid because of darkening of urine by metabolites; it also causes false-

positive urine pregnancy test results using human chorionic gonadotropin.

Patient monitoring
• Patient needs to be assessed periodically for abnormal body movement.
• Obtain baseline blood pressure measurements before starting therapy and monitor regularly.
• Periodic ophthalmic testing should be performed.

Pediatric patients
• Drug isn't recommended for children under age 16.

Geriatric patients
• Elderly patients are highly sensitive to antimuscarinic, hypotensive, and sedative effects of drug and have a higher risk of extrapyramidal adverse reactions, such as parkinsonism and tardive dyskinesia.
• Higher plasma levels develop in these patients and, therefore, they require lower initial dosage and more gradual dosage adjustment.

Patient education
• Warn patient against activities that require alertness and good psychomotor coordination until CNS response to drug is determined. Drowsiness and dizziness usually subside after first few weeks.
• Recommend sugarless gum or candy, mouthwash, ice chips, or artificial saliva to alleviate dry mouth.
• Advise patient to get up slowly to avoid orthostatic hypotension.

Lyme disease vaccine (recombinant OspA)
LYMErix

Pharmacologic classification: vaccine, bacterial-recombinant
Therapeutic classification: biological
Pregnancy risk category: C

Indications and dosages
➤ *Active immunization against Lyme disease. Children and adults ages 15 to 70:* 30 mcg I.M. in deltoid region; repeat dose at 1 and 12 months after first dose. Safety and efficacy of this vaccine are based on administration of second and third doses several weeks before the onset of the disease transmission season.

How supplied
Available by prescription only
Single-dose vials and prefilled syringes: 30 mcg/0.5 ml

Pharmacodynamics
Lyme disease prophylaxis: The vaccine stimulates specific antibodies directed against *Borrelia burgdorferi* (a bacterial spirochete that causes Lyme disease). The vaccine contains lipoprotein OspA, an outer surface protein of *B. burgdorferi.*

Pharmacokinetics
No information available.

Route	Onset	Peak	Duration
I.M.	Unknown	Unknown	Unknown

Contraindications and precautions
Contraindicated in patients hypersensitive to vaccine or its components. Don't administer vaccine to patients with treatment-resistant Lyme arthritis (antibiotic refractory) or moderate or severe febrile illness. Lyme disease vaccine shouldn't be given to patients receiving anticoagulants unless potential benefit outweighs risk.

Use cautiously in immunosuppressed patients or in those receiving immunosuppressive therapy because the expected immune response may not occur. For patients receiving immunosuppressive therapy, consider deferring vaccination for 3 months after therapy.

Also use cautiously in persons who may have allergic reactions to packaging for the LYMErix syringe, which contains dry natural rubber. The vial packaging doesn't contain rubber.

Interactions
None reported.

Adverse reactions
CNS: *headache, fatigue,* dizziness, depression, hypoesthesia, paresthesia.
GI: diarrhea, nausea.
EENT: pharyngitis, rhinitis, sinusitis.
Musculoskeletal: *arthralgia,* back pain, myalgia, arthritis, arthrosis, stiffness, tendinitis.
Respiratory: bronchitis, cough, upper respiratory tract infection.
Skin: *rash, injection site pain, redness, soreness, swelling,* injection site reaction, contact dermatitis.
Other: chills or rigors, fever, viral infection, flulike symptoms.

Overdose and treatment
No information available.

Special considerations
• Before immunization, review the patient's history for possible vaccine sensitivity, allergies, previous vaccination-related adverse reactions, and occurrence of any adverse event–related symptoms or signs. Epinephrine injection (1:1,000) and other appropriate agents used for control of immediate allergic reactions must be immediately available.
• Shake well before withdrawal and use. Inspect visually for particulate matter or discoloration before administration. With thorough agitation, LYMErix is a turbid white suspension. Discard if it appears otherwise. Use vaccine as supplied; no

dilution or reconstitution is necessary. Discard any vaccine remaining in a single-dose vial.

• Packaging for vaccine prefilled syringe contains dry natural rubber, which may cause allergic reactions; packaging for the vial doesn't contain natural rubber.

• A separate sterile syringe and needle or a sterile disposable unit must be used for each patient to prevent transmission of infectious agents. Dispose of needles properly; don't recap.

• Administer vaccine by I.M. injection in the deltoid region. Don't inject I.V., I.D., or S.C.

• No data are available on the immune response to vaccine when administered with other vaccines. When concomitant administration of other vaccines is required, they should be given with different syringes and at different injection sites.

• It's recommended that vaccine not be administered to antibiotic-resistant Lyme arthritis patients.

• As with other I.M. injections, vaccine shouldn't be given to individuals on anticoagulant therapy or with clotting disorders, unless the potential benefit clearly outweighs the risk.

• Store between 36° and 46° F (2° and 8° C). Don't freeze; discard if product has been frozen.

• LYMErix vaccination may result in a positive IgG enzyme-linked immunosorbent assay in the absence of infection.

Patient monitoring

• Monitor patient for adverse reactions and report any such reactions to 1-800-822-7967.

Pregnant patients

• Prescribers are encouraged to register pregnant women who received the vaccine by calling 1-800-366-8900.

Breast-feeding patients

• It isn't known whether vaccine appears in breast milk; use cautiously in breast-feeding women.

Pediatric patients

• Safety and efficacy in children under age 15 haven't been evaluated. Avoid giving to this age group.

Geriatric patients

• Vaccine isn't indicated for patients over age 70.

Patient education

• Inform patient that this vaccine is specific for preventing, not treating, Lyme disease.

• Inform patients, parents, or guardians of the benefits and risks of immunization with the vaccine, and of the importance of completing the immunization series.

• Ask patient about the occurrence of any symptoms or signs after a previous dose of the same vaccine and advise him to report any adverse events.

• Instruct patient to tell health care provider administering vaccine if he's taking anticoagulant

drugs (warfarin, heparin) or other blood-thinning drugs such as aspirin.

• Advise patient of ways to prevent other tick-borne diseases (wearing long-sleeved shirts, long pants, tucking pants into socks, and treating clothing with tick repellents). In addition, tell patient to carefully check himself for the presence of ticks when returning from endemic areas.

• Instruct patient on the appropriate way to remove ticks (use fine-pointed tweezers to avoid squashing the tick during removal from skin).

lymphocyte immune globulin (antithymocyte globulin [equine], ATG)
Atgam

Pharmacologic classification: immuno-globulin
Therapeutic classification: immuno-suppressive
Pregnancy risk category: C

Indications and dosages

➤ *Prevention of acute renal allograft rejection. Adults and children:* 15 mg/kg I.V. daily for 14 days; then same dosage every other day for next 14 days (to a total of 21 doses in 28 days). Administer the first dose of ATG within 24 hours before or after transplantation.

➤ *Treatment of acute renal allograft rejection. Adults and children:* 10 to 15 mg/kg I.V. daily for 14 days; if necessary, same dosage may be given every other day for another 14 days (to a total of 21 doses in 28 days). Begin ATG therapy at the first sign of acute rejection.

➤ *Aplastic anemia. Adults and children:* 10 to 20 mg/kg I.V. daily for 8 to 14 days, followed by alternate-day therapy for an additional 14 days (total of 21 doses in 28 days).

➤ *Skin allotransplantation◇. Adults:* 10 mg/kg I.V. 24 hours before allograft; then 10 to 15 mg/kg every other day. Maintenance dosage varies and can range from 5 to 40 mg/ kg daily, based on clinical response and clinical indicators of immunosuppressive activity. Therapy usually continues until allografts cover less than 20% of total body surface area; often, this requires 40 to 60 days of treatment.

➤ *Bone marrow allotransplantation◇; graft-versus-host disease after bone marrow transplantation◇. Adults:* 7 to 10 mg/kg I.V. every other day for six doses.

How supplied

Available by prescription only
Injection: 50 mg of equine IgG per ml, in 5-ml ampules

Pharmacodynamics

Immunosuppressive action: The exact mechanism hasn't been fully defined but may involve elimination of antigen reactive T cells (T lymphocytes) in peripheral blood or alteration of T-cell function. The effects of antilymphocyte preparations, including ATG, on T cells are variable and complex. Whether the effects of ATG are mediated through a specific subset of T cells hasn't been determined.

Pharmacokinetics
Absorption: Peak plasma levels of equine IgG after I.V. administration of ATG vary, depending on patient's ability to catabolize foreign IgG.
Distribution: Distribution of ATG into body fluids and tissues hasn't been fully described. Because antilymphocyte serum reportedly is poorly distributed into lymphoid tissues (such as spleen, lymph nodes), it's likely that ATG is also poorly distributed into these tissues.

No information is available on transplacental distribution of ATG. However, such distribution is likely because other immunoglobulins cross the placenta. Virtually all transplacental passage of immunoglobulins occurs during the last 4 weeks of pregnancy.
Metabolism: No information available.
Excretion: Plasma half-life of equine IgG averages about 6 days (range is 1.5 to 13 days). About 1% of a dose of ATG is excreted in urine, principally as unchanged equine IgG. In one report, mean urinary level of equine IgG was about 4 mcg/ml after about 21 doses of ATG over 28 days.

Route	Onset	Peak	Duration
I.V.	Immediate	5 days	Unknown

Contraindications and precautions
Contraindicated in patients hypersensitive to drug. An intradermal skin test is recommended at least 1 hour before first dose. Marked local swelling or erythema larger than 10 mm indicates an increased potential for severe systemic reaction, such as anaphylaxis. Severe reactions to skin test, such as hypotension, tachycardia, dyspnea, generalized rash, or anaphylaxis, usually preclude further administration of drug.

Use cautiously in patients receiving other immunosuppressive medications, such as corticosteroids or azathioprine.

Interactions
Drug-drug. *Other immunosuppressive therapy (azathioprine, corticosteroids, graft irradiation):* May intensify immunosuppression, an effect that can be used to therapeutic advantage; however, such therapy may increase vulnerability to infection and possibly the risk of lymphoma or lymphoproliferative disorders. Patient requires close monitoring.

Adverse reactions
CNS: malaise, *seizures, headache.*
CV: *hypotension,* chest pain, thrombophlebitis, tachycardia, edema, iliac vein obstruction, renal artery stenosis.

EENT: *laryngospasm.*
GI: *nausea, vomiting, diarrhea,* epigastric pain, abdominal distention, stomatitis.
Hematologic: LEUKOPENIA, THROMBOCYTOPENIA, *hemolysis, aplastic anemia.*
Hepatic: elevated liver enzyme levels.
Metabolic: hyperglycemia.
Musculoskeletal: *myalgia, arthralgia.*
Respiratory: hiccups, *dyspnea, pulmonary edema.*
Skin: *rash, pruritus, urticaria.*
Other: *febrile reactions,* serum sickness, *anaphylaxis, infections,* night sweats, lymphadenopathy, *chills.*

Overdose and treatment
No information available.

Special considerations
● Drug has been used to treat aplastic anemia, lymphoma, agranulocytosis, and as an adjunct in bone marrow, cardiac allotransplantation, and skin allotransplantation.
● To minimize risks of leukopenia and infection, some clinicians recommend that azathioprine and corticosteroid dosages be reduced by 50% when ATG is used with these drugs for the prevention or treatment of renal allograft rejection.
● Some clinicians elect to administer prophylactic platelet transfusion in patients receiving drug for aplastic anemia because of high risk of thrombocytopenia.
● Dilute drug concentrate for injection before I.V. infusion. Dilute required dose of ATG in normal saline solution or half-normal saline solution (usually 250 to 1,000 ml); final concentration preferably shouldn't exceed 1 mg of equine IgG per ml. Infuse over at least 4 hours.
● Infusion in dextrose or highly acidic solutions isn't recommended.
● Invert I.V. infusion solution container into which ATG concentrate is added to prevent contact of undiluted ATG with air inside the container. Refrigerate diluted solutions of ATG at 36° to 46° F (2° to 8° C) if administration is delayed. Reconstituted solutions shouldn't be used after 12 hours (including infusion time), even if stored at 36° to 46° F.
● Because of risk of severe systemic reaction (anaphylaxis), manufacturer recommends an intradermal skin test before administration of ATG. The skin test procedure consists of intradermal injection of 0.1 ml of a 1:1,000 dilution of ATG concentrate for injection in normal saline solution injection (5 mcg of equine IgG). Administer a control test using normal saline solution injection in the other arm to facilitate interpretation of the results. If a wheal or area of erythema exceeding 10 mm in diameter (with or without pseudopod formation) and itching or marked local swelling develops, infusion of ATG requires extreme caution; severe and potentially fatal systemic reactions can occur in patients with a positive skin test. A systemic reaction to the skin test

such as generalized rash, tachycardia, dyspnea, hypotension, or anaphylaxis rules out further administration of ATG. The predictive value of the ATG skin test hasn't been clearly established, and an allergic reaction may occur despite a negative skin test.

• The manufacturer hasn't yet determined the total number of ATG doses (10 to 20 mg/kg per dose) that can be safely administered. Some renal allograft recipients have received up to 50 doses in 4 months; others, up to four 28-day courses of 21 doses each without an increased risk of adverse effects.

Patient monitoring

• Anaphylaxis may occur at any time during drug therapy and may be indicated by hypotension, respiratory distress, or pain in the chest, flank, or back. Monitor patient closely.

• Observe patient receiving drug for signs of leukopenia, thrombocytopenia, and concurrent infection.

• Monitor peripheral blood levels of rosette-forming cells (RFCs) in order to guide therapy in allograft recipient (maintain RFCs at 10% of treatment level).

• Monitor patient for signs of infection during ATG therapy.

Breast-feeding patients

• Although it isn't known whether drug appears in breast milk, other immunoglobulins do. Breast-feeding women should consider an alternative feeding method.

Pediatric patients

• Safety and efficacy in children haven't been established. Drug has had limited use in children ages 3 months to 19 years.

Patient education

• Warn patient that a febrile reaction is likely.

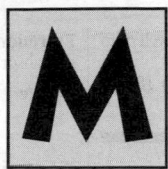

magaldrate (aluminum magnesium hydroxide)
Iosopan, Lowsium, Magaldrate, Riopan

Pharmacologic classification: aluminum-magnesium salt
Therapeutic classification: antacid
Pregnancy risk category: C

Indications and dosages
➤ *Indigestion or hyperacidity caused by peptic ulcer, gastritis, peptic esophagitis, hiatal hernia. Adults:* 5 to 10 ml (suspension) P.O. between meals and h.s. with water.

How supplied
Available without a prescription
Suspension: 540 mg/5 ml

Pharmacodynamics
Antacid action: Magaldrate neutralizes gastric acid, reducing the direct acid irritant effect. This increases gastric pH, which inactivates pepsin. Magaldrate also enhances mucosal barrier integrity and improves gastroesophageal sphincter tone.

Pharmacokinetics
Absorption: Aluminum may be absorbed systemically. Magnesium also may be absorbed, posing a risk to patients with renal failure. Absorption is unrelated to mechanism of action.
Distribution: Distribution is primarily local.
Metabolism: None.
Excretion: Excreted in feces; some aluminum and magnesium may appear in breast milk. Duration of action is prolonged.

Route	Onset	Peak	Duration
P.O.	20 min	Unknown	20-180 min

Contraindications and precautions
Contraindicated in patients with severe renal disease. Use cautiously in patients with mild renal impairment.

Interactions
Drug-drug. *Anticoagulants, antimuscarinics, chenodiol, chlordiazepoxide, coumadin, diazepam, digoxin, isoniazid, phenothiazines (especially chlorpromazine), phosphates, quinolones, tetracycline, and vitamin A:* Decreased absorption of these drugs, thus lessening their effectiveness. Separate administration times.
Enteric-coated drugs: Magaldrate may cause premature release of these drugs. Separate doses of magaldrate and all oral drugs by 1 to 2 hours.
Levodopa: Concurrent administration may increase levodopa absorption, increasing risk of toxicity. Separate administration times.
Drug-herb. *Melatonin:* Additive inhibitory effects on the *N*-methyl-*D*-aspartate receptor. Discourage use together.

Adverse reactions
GI: mild constipation, diarrhea.
GU: increased urine pH levels.
Metabolic: decreased serum potassium levels, increased serum gastrin levels.

Overdose and treatment
No information available.

Special considerations
● Shake suspension well; give with small amounts of water or fruit juice.
● After administration through nasogastric tube, flush tube with water to clear it and ensure passage of drug to stomach.
● Give drug at least 1 hour apart from enterically coated medications.
● Suspension contains saccharin and sorbitol.
● Most formulations contain less than 0.5 mg of sodium per tablet (or 5 ml of liquid).

Patient monitoring
● Monitor renal function and serum phosphate, potassium, and magnesium levels in patients with renal disease.

Breast-feeding patients
● Some aluminum and magnesium may appear in breast milk. However, no problems have been linked to use in breast-feeding women.

Pediatric patients
● Use of drug as an antacid in children under age 6 requires a well-established diagnosis because children typically give vague descriptions of symptoms.

Patient education
● Caution patient to take drug only as directed and 1 or 2 hours apart from other oral medications.

• Remind patient to shake suspension well or to chew tablets thoroughly.
• Warn patient not to take more than 18 teaspoonfuls in a 24-hour period.

magnesium hydroxide
Milk of Magnesia, Phillips' Milk of Magnesia, Concentrated Phillips' Milk of Magnesia

Pharmacologic classification: magnesium salt
Therapeutic classification: antacid, antiulcer agent, laxative
Pregnancy risk category: NR

Indications and dosages
➤ **Constipation, bowel evacuation before surgery.** *Adults and children over age 6:* 10 to 20 ml concentrated Milk of Magnesia P.O.; 15 to 60 ml Milk of Magnesia P.O.
➤ **Laxative effects.** *Adults:* 30 to 60 ml P.O., usually h.s.
Children ages 6 to 11: 15 to 30 ml P.O.
Children ages 2 to 5: 5 to 15 ml P.O.
➤ **Antacid effects.** *Adults:* 5 to 15 ml (liquid) P.O., p.r.n., up to q.i.d.; 2.5 to 7.5 ml (liquid concentrate) P.O., p.r.n., up to q.i.d.; 2 to 4 tablets P.O., p.r.n., up to q.i.d.
Children: 2.5 to 5 ml P.O., p.r.n.

How supplied
Available without a prescription
Liquid: 400 mg/5 ml, 800 mg/5 ml
Suspension: 77.5 mg/g
Suspension (concentrated): 10 ml (equivalent to 30 ml of milk of magnesia)
Tablets: 300 mg, 600 mg
Tablets (chewable): 311 mg

Pharmacodynamics
Antiulcer action: Magnesium hydroxide neutralizes gastric acid, decreasing the direct acid irritant effect. This increases pH, which, in turn, leads to pepsin inactivation. Magnesium hydroxide also enhances mucosal barrier integrity and improves gastric and esophageal sphincter tone.
Antacid action: Drug reacts rapidly with hydrochloric acid in the stomach to form magnesium chloride and water.
Laxative action: Magnesium hydroxide produces its laxative effect by increasing the osmotic gradient in the gut and drawing in water, causing distention that stimulates peristalsis and bowel evacuation.

Pharmacokinetics
Absorption: About 15% to 30% may be absorbed systemically (posing a potential risk to patients with renal failure).
Distribution: None.
Metabolism: None.

Excretion: Unabsorbed drug is excreted in feces; absorbed drug is excreted rapidly in urine.

Route	Onset	Peak	Duration
P.O.	½-3 hr	Variable	Variable

Contraindications and precautions
Contraindicated in patients with abdominal pain, nausea, vomiting, or other symptoms of appendicitis or acute surgical abdomen and in those with myocardial damage, heart block, fecal impaction, rectal fissures, intestinal obstruction or perforation, or renal disease. Also contraindicated in patients about to deliver.
Use cautiously in patients with rectal bleeding.

Interactions
Drug-drug. *Chlordiazepoxide, chlorpromazine, dicumarol, digoxin, iron salts, isoniazid:* Use of magnesium hydroxide with aluminum hydroxide may decrease the absorption rate of these drugs. Separate administration times.
Enteric-coated tablets: Premature release of enteric-coated drugs. Separate administration times.
Quinolones, tetracyclines: Decreased absorption of these drugs. Separate administration times.

Adverse reactions
GI: *abdominal cramping, nausea, diarrhea,* laxative dependence (with long-term or excessive use).
Metabolic: fluid and electrolyte disturbances (with daily use).

Overdose and treatment
No information available.

Special considerations
• Give drug at least 1 hour apart from enteric-coated drugs; shake suspension well.
• After giving drug through nasogastric tube, flush tube with water to clear it.

Patient monitoring
• Monitor patient for signs and symptoms of hypermagnesemia, especially if patient has impaired renal function.

Breast-feeding patients
• Some magnesium may appear in breast milk, but no problems have been reported with use by breast-feeding women.

Pediatric patients
• Use as an antacid in children under age 6 requires a well-established diagnosis because children tend to give vague descriptions of symptoms.

Patient education
• Caution patient to avoid overuse to prevent laxative dependence.
• Instruct patient to shake suspension well or to chew tablets well.

Reactions may be *common*, uncommon, *life-threatening*, or COMMON AND LIFE-THREATENING.

• Encourage patient using drug as a laxative to maintain adequate fluid intake, diet, and exercise.

magnesium salicylate
Extra Strength Doan's, Magan, Mobidin

Pharmacologic classification: salicylate
Therapeutic classification: nonnarcotic analgesic, anti-inflammatory, antipyretic
Pregnancy risk category: C

Indications and dosages
➤**Arthritis.** *Adults:* 545 mg to 1.2 g t.i.d. or q.i.d.
➤**Analgesia, antipyresis.** *Adults and children over age 11:* 300 to 600 mg P.O. q 4 hours, p.r.n.
➤**Analgesia (self-medicated).** *Adults and children over age 11:* 500 mg to 1 g P.O. initially, then 500 mg q 4 hours, p.r.n., not to exceed 3.5 g in 24 hours. Absorption of buffered or enteric-coated aspirin is increased by simultaneous administration. Use cautiously in children; may receive the following doses q 4 hours, p.r.n., not to exceed five doses in 24 hours.
Children age 11: 450 mg P.O.
Children ages 9 to 10: 375 mg P.O.
Children ages 6 to 8: 300 mg P.O.
Children ages 4 to 5: 225 mg P.O.
Children ages 2 to 3: 150 mg P.O.
Children under age 2: Dose must be individualized.

How supplied
Available by prescription only
Tablets: 545 mg, 600 mg
Available without a prescription
Tablets: 325 mg, 500 mg

Pharmacodynamics
Analgesic action: Produces analgesia by an ill-defined effect on the hypothalamus (central action) and by blocking generation of pain impulses (peripheral action). The peripheral action may involve inhibition of prostaglandin synthesis.
Anti-inflammatory action: Thought to exert anti-inflammatory effect by inhibiting prostaglandin synthesis; may also inhibit the synthesis or action of other mediators of inflammation.
Antipyretic action: Relieves fever by acting on the hypothalamic heat-regulating center to produce peripheral vasodilation. This increases peripheral blood supply and promotes sweating, which leads to loss of heat and to cooling by evaporation.

Pharmacokinetics
Absorption: Magnesium salicylate is absorbed rapidly and completely from GI tract.
Distribution: Highly protein-bound.
Metabolism: Hydrolyzed in liver.

Excretion: Metabolites excreted in urine.

Route	Onset	Peak	Duration
P.O.	Rapid	20 min	Unknown

Contraindications and precautions
Contraindicated in patients hypersensitive to drug, salicylates, or NSAIDs and in those with severe chronic renal insufficiency because of risk of magnesium toxicity. Also contraindicated in patients with bleeding disorders. Use cautiously in patients with hypoprothrombinemia or vitamin K deficiency.

Interactions
Drug-drug. *Ammonium chloride, other urine acidifiers:* Increased magnesium salicylate blood levels. Monitor patient for magnesium salicylate toxicity.
Antacids, other urine alkalizers: Decreased magnesium salicylate blood levels. Monitor patient for decreased salicylate effect.
Anticoagulants, thrombolytics: Potentiated platelet-inhibiting effects of magnesium salicylate. Monitor patient for bruising or bleeding.
Corticosteroids: Enhanced magnesium salicylate elimination. Monitor patient for decreased salicylate effect.
Drugs that are highly protein-bound (such as phenytoin, sulfonylureas, warfarin): May cause displacement of either drug; possible adverse effects. Monitor patient.
Other GI-irritant drugs (antibiotics, corticosteroids, other NSAIDs): May potentiate adverse GI effects of magnesium salicylate. Use together cautiously.
Drug-lifestyle. *Alcohol use:* Increased risk of GI bleeding. Discourage concurrent use.

Adverse reactions
EENT: *tinnitus, hearing loss.*
GI: *nausea, vomiting, GI distress.*
Hepatic: abnormal liver function test results; increased serum levels of AST, ALT, alkaline phosphatase, and bilirubin; *hepatitis.*
Skin: rash, bruising.
Other: *hypersensitivity reactions (anaphylaxis,* asthma), *Reye's syndrome.*

Overdose and treatment
Signs and symptoms of overdose include metabolic acidosis with respiratory alkalosis.

To treat, empty stomach immediately by inducing emesis with ipecac syrup if patient is conscious, or by gastric lavage. Give activated charcoal via nasogastric tube.

Special considerations
• Drug has been linked to a lower frequency of GI disturbances.
• Drug has a less profound inhibiting effect on platelet aggregation than other salicylates.
• High doses of drug may cause false-positive urine glucose test results using copper sulfate

method. Drug may cause false-negative urine glucose test results using glucose enzymatic method.
● Stop drug if patient develops dizziness, tinnitus, or hearing impairment.

Patient monitoring
● Obtain hemoglobin and PT tests periodically.
● Monitor serum magnesium levels to prevent magnesium toxicity, especially in patients with renal insufficiency.

Breast-feeding patients
● Salicylates appear in breast milk; avoid use of magnesium salicylate in breast-feeding women.

Pediatric patients
● Safety of long-term magnesium salicylate use in children hasn't been established.
● Because of drug's link to Reye's syndrome, the Centers for Disease Control and Prevention recommends that children with chickenpox or flu-like symptoms not be given salicylates.
● Febrile, dehydrated children can develop toxicity rapidly.

Geriatric patients
● Patients over age 60 may be more susceptible to the toxic effects of magnesium salicylate. Use it cautiously.
● The effects of salicylates on renal prostaglandins may cause fluid retention and edema, a significant drawback for elderly patients and those with heart failure.

Patient education
● Instruct patient to follow prescribed regimen and to report problems.
● Advise patient not to take drug longer than 10 days without medical supervision.
● Caution patient to keep drug out of children's reach.

magnesium sulfate

Pharmacologic classification: mineral/electrolyte
Therapeutic classification: anticonvulsant
Pregnancy risk category: A

Indications and dosages
➤ **Hypomagnesemic seizures.** *Adults:* 1 g I.V. or I.M. Or, 1 to 2 g (as 10% solution) I.V. over 15 minutes; then 1 g I.M. q 4 to 6 hours, based on patient's response and magnesium blood levels.
➤ **Seizures secondary to hypomagnesemia in acute nephritis.** *Children:* 0.2 ml/kg of 50% solution I.M. q 4 to 6 hours, p.r.n., or 100 to 200 mg/kg as a 1% to 3% solution I.V. given slowly over 1 hour with the first half of dose in the first 15 to 20 minutes. Also, 0.1 to 0.2 ml/kg of 20% solution (20 to 40 mg/kg) I.M. Adjust dosage according to magnesium blood levels and seizure response.

➤ **Life-threatening arrhythmias.** *Adults:* For patient with sustained ventricular tachycardia or torsades de pointes, give 1 to 6 g I.V. over several minutes followed by 3 to 20 mg/minute I.V. infusion for 5 to 48 hours depending on patient response and serum magnesium levels. For patient with paroxysmal atrial tachycardia, give 3 to 4 g I.V. over 30 seconds.
➤ **Prevention or control of seizures in preeclampsia or eclampsia.** *Adults:* Initially, 4 g I.V. in 250 ml D₅W and 4 to 5 g deep I.M. into each buttock (using undiluted 50% magnesium sulfate injection); then 4 to 5 g deep I.M. into alternate buttock q 4 hours, p.r.n. Or, 4 g I.V. as a loading dose followed by 1 to 3 g hourly as an I.V. infusion. Maximum daily dose, 30 to 40 g. Or, 8 to 15 g depending on weight of patient (8 g for 45-kg [100-lb] patient and 15 g for 90-kg [198-lb] patient); 4 g of magnesium sulfate (as magnesium sulfate injection or magnesium sulfate in D₅W) is given I.V. and the remaining dose is given I.M. using undiluted 50% magnesium sulfate injection. Dosage over next 24 hours based on serum level and urinary excretion of magnesium following initial dose. Later doses should be sufficient to replace magnesium excreted in urine, about 65% of the initial dose given I.M. q 6 hours.
✦ **Dosage adjustment.** In severe renal insufficiency, maximum dose is 20 g in 48 hours.
➤ **Barium poisoning, asthma.** *Adults:* 1 to 2 g I.V.
➤ **Management of preterm labor◇.** *Adults:* 4 to 6 g I.V. over 20 minutes as a loading dose, followed by maintenance infusions of 2 to 4 g/hour for 12 to 24 hours as tolerated after contractions subside.
➤ **Mild hypomagnesemia.** *Adults:* 1 to 3 g I.M. q 6 hours for 4 doses. Or, 5 g in 1 L of D₅W or dextrose 5% in normal saline solution I.V. over 3 hours.
➤ **Reduction of CV morbidity and mortality caused by acute MI.** *Adults:* 2 g I.V. over 5 to 15 minutes, followed by infusion of 18 g over 24 hours (12.5 mg/min). Start therapy as soon as possible, and no longer than 6 hours after MI.

How supplied
Available by prescription only
Injection for I.V. use: 4% (4, 20, and 40 g); 8% (4g)
Parenteral injection: 10%, 12.5%, 50%
Parenteral injection for I.V. use: 1% (1 and 10 g) in D₅W; 2% (10 and 20 g) in D₅W

Pharmacodynamics
Anticonvulsant action: Magnesium sulfate has CNS and respiratory depressant effects. It acts peripherally, causing vasodilation; moderate doses cause flushing and sweating, whereas high doses cause hypotension. It prevents or controls seizures by blocking neuromuscular transmission.

Drug is sometimes used in pregnant women to prevent or control preeclamptic or eclamptic seizures; it also is used to treat hypomagnesemic seizures in adults, and in children with acute nephritis.

Pharmacokinetics

Absorption: Effective anticonvulsant serum levels are 2.5 to 7.5 mEq/L.
Distribution: Magnesium sulfate is distributed widely throughout the body.
Metabolism: None.
Excretion: Excreted unchanged in urine; some appears in breast milk.

Route	Onset	Peak	Duration
I.V.	1-2 min	Rapid	½ hr
I.M.	1 hr	Unknown	3-4 hr

Contraindications and precautions

Parenteral administration of drug contraindicated in patients with heart block or myocardial damage. Use cautiously in patients with impaired renal function and in women in labor. Don't give to patients with toxemia of pregnancy during the 2 hours preceding delivery.

Interactions

Drug-drug. *Antidepressants, antipsychotics, anxiolytics, barbiturates, general anesthetics, hypnotics, narcotics:* May increase CNS depressant effects. Reduced dosages may be required.
Cardiac glycosides: Changes in cardiac conduction in digitalized patients may lead to heart block if I.V. calcium is administered. Avoid use together, if possible.
Succinylcholine, tubocurarine: Potentiated and prolonged neuromuscular blocking action of these drugs. Use cautiously.
Drug-lifestyle. *Alcohol use:* Increased CNS depressant effects. Tell patient to avoid use together.

Adverse reactions

CNS: drowsiness, *depressed reflexes,* flaccid paralysis.
CV: *hypotension, flushing, circulatory collapse,* depressed cardiac function.
Metabolic: hypocalcemia.
Respiratory: *respiratory paralysis.*
Skin: diaphoresis.
Other: hypothermia.

Overdose and treatment

Signs and symptoms of overdose with magnesium sulfate include a sharp decrease in blood pressure, respiratory paralysis, ECG changes (increased PR, QRS, and QT intervals), heart block, and asystole.

Treatment requires artificial ventilation and I.V. calcium salt to reverse respiratory depression and heart block. Usual dose is 5 to 10 mEq of calcium (10 to 20 ml of a 10% calcium gluconate solution).

Special considerations

⚠ ALERT Read label closely to ensure proper dosage and concentration.
● Inject I.V. bolus slowly to avoid respiratory or cardiac arrest.
● Administer by constant infusion pump if possible; maximum infusion rate is 150 mg/minute. Rapid drip causes feeling of heat.
● Discontinue drug as soon as needed effect is achieved.
● Level of magnesium sulfate for I.V. administration shouldn't exceed 20% and rate shouldn't exceed 150 mg/minute (1.5 ml of a 10% concentration or equivalent). For I.M. administration in adults, levels of 25% or 50% are generally used; in infants and children, levels shouldn't exceed 20% (200 mg/ml).
● Respiratory rate must be 16 breaths per minute or more before each dose. Keep I.V. calcium gluconate 20% on hand.
● To calculate grams of magnesium in a percentage of solution: $X\% = X$ g/100 ml (for example, $25\% = 25$ g/100 ml = 250 mg/ml).

Patient monitoring

● Monitor serum magnesium level and clinical status to avoid overdose.
● When giving repeated doses, test knee jerk reflex before each dose; if absent, discontinue magnesium. Use of drug beyond this point risks respiratory center failure.
● When using drug as a tocolytic agent, monitor patient for magnesium toxicity and monitor I.V. infusion to avoid circulatory overload.
● After use in toxemic women within 24 hours before delivery, newborn requires observation for signs of magnesium toxicity, including neuromuscular and respiratory depression.

Breast-feeding patients

● Drug appears in breast milk; in patients with normal renal function, all magnesium sulfate is excreted within 24 hours of discontinuing drug. Alternative feeding method is recommended during therapy.

Pediatric patients

● Drug isn't indicated for pediatric use.

Patient education

● Inform patient about short-term need for drug, and address any questions or concerns.

mannitol
Osmitrol, Resectisol

Pharmacologic classification: osmotic diuretic
Therapeutic classification: diuretic
Pregnancy risk category: C

Indications and dosages
➤ *Test dose for marked oliguria or suspected inadequate renal function.* Adults

and children over age 12: 200 mg/kg or 12.5 g as a 15% or 20% solution I.V. over 3 to 5 minutes. Response is adequate if 30 to 50 ml urine/hour is excreted over 2 to 3 hours. May repeat test dose one time if response is inadequate the first time.

Children age 12 and under ◊: 0.2 g/kg or 6 g/m² I.V. over 3 to 5 minutes.

➤ *Treatment of oliguria. Adults and children over age 12:* 50 to 100 g as a 15% to 20% solution I.V. over 90 minutes to several hours.

Children age 12 and under: 2 g/kg or 60 g/m² I.V.

➤ *Prevention of oliguria or acute renal failure. Adults and children over age 12:* 50 to 100 g followed by a 5% to 10% solution I.V. Exact level is determined by fluid requirements.

➤ *Treatment of edema and ascites. Adults and children over age 12:* 100 g as a 10% to 20% solution I.V. over 2 to 6 hours.

Children age 12 and under ◊: 2 g/kg or 60 g/m² I.V. as a 15% to 20% solution over 2 to 6 hours.

➤ *To reduce intraocular pressure or intracranial pressure. Adults and children over age 12:* 1.5 to 2 g/kg as a 15% to 25% solution I.V. over 30 to 60 minutes (60 to 90 minutes before surgery if used preoperatively).

Children age 12 and under ◊: 2 g/kg or 60 g/m² I.V. as a 15% to 20% solution over 30 to 60 minutes.

➤ *To promote diuresis in drug intoxication. Adults and children over age 12:* 25 g loading dose followed by an infusion maintaining 100 to 500 ml urine output/hour and positive fluid balance (of 1 to 2 L). For patients with barbiturate poisoning, give 0.5 g/kg followed by a 5% to 10% solution. Or, 1 L of 10% solution during first hour. Subsequent dosing based on urine output, urine pH, and fluid balance.

Children age 12 and under ◊: 2 g/kg or 60 g/m² of 5% to 10% solution as needed.

➤ *Urologic irrigation. Adults:* 2.5% to 5% irrigating solution via indwelling urethral catheter.

How supplied
Available by prescription only
Injection: 5%, 10%, 15%, 20%, 25%
Urogenital solution: 5 g/100 ml distilled water

Pharmacodynamics
Diuretic action: Mannitol increases the osmotic pressure of glomerular filtrate, inhibiting tubular reabsorption of water and electrolytes, thus promoting diuresis. This action also promotes urinary elimination of certain drugs. This effect is useful for prevention and management of acute renal failure or oliguria. This action is also useful for reduction of intracranial or intraocular pressure because mannitol elevates plasma osmolality, enhancing flow of water into extracellular fluid.

Pharmacokinetics
Absorption: Not absorbed from the GI tract. I.V. mannitol lowers intracranial pressure in 15 minutes and intraocular pressure in 30 to 60 minutes; it produces diuresis in 1 to 3 hours.
Distribution: Remains in the extracellular compartment. It doesn't cross the blood-brain barrier.
Metabolism: Metabolized minimally to glycogen in the liver.
Excretion: Filtered by the glomeruli; half-life in adults with normal renal function is about 100 minutes.

Route	Onset	Peak	Duration
I.V.	¼-1 hr	1-3 hr	3-8 hr

Contraindications and precautions
Contraindicated in patients hypersensitive to drug and in those with anuria, severe pulmonary congestion, frank pulmonary edema, severe heart failure, severe dehydration, metabolic edema, progressive renal disease or dysfunction, or active intracranial bleeding except during craniotomy. Use cautiously in pregnant patients.

Interactions
Drug-drug. *Cardiac glycosides:* May enhance the possibility of digitalis toxicity. Monitor serum digoxin levels.
Diuretics, including carbonic anhydrase inhibitors: Increased effects of these drugs. Monitor patient closely.
Lithium: Enhanced renal excretion of lithium and lower serum lithium levels. Monitor lithium levels.

Adverse reactions
CNS: *seizures,* dizziness, headache.
CV: edema, thrombophlebitis, hypotension, hypertension, *heart failure,* tachycardia, angina-like chest pain.
EENT: blurred vision, rhinitis.
GI: thirst, dry mouth, nausea, vomiting, *diarrhea.*
GU: urine retention.
Metabolic: fluid and electrolyte imbalance, dehydration.
Skin: urticaria.
Other: local pain, fever, chills.

Overdose and treatment
Signs and symptoms of overdose include polyuria, cellular dehydration, hypotension, and CV collapse.

Discontinue infusion and institute supportive measures. Hemodialysis removes mannitol and decreases serum osmolality.

Special considerations
● For maximum pressure reduction during surgery, give drug 1 to 1½ hours preoperatively.
● Give drug I.V. via an in-line filter with great care to avoid extravasation.

Reactions may be *common*, uncommon, *life-threatening*, or COMMON AND LIFE-THREATENING.

• Don't give with whole blood; agglutination will occur.

• Mannitol solutions commonly crystallize at low temperatures; place crystallized solutions in a hot water bath, shake vigorously to dissolve crystals, and cool to body temperature before use. Don't use solutions with undissolved crystals.

• Don't give more than 1 liter of fluids in excess of urine output daily.

• Store drug at 59° to 86° F (15° to 30° C) and protect from freezing.

Patient monitoring

• Use with extreme caution in patients with compromised renal function; monitor vital signs (including CVP) hourly. Monitor input and output, weight, renal function, fluid balance, and serum and urine sodium and potassium levels daily.

Breast-feeding patients

• Safety of drug in breast-feeding women hasn't been established.

Pediatric patients

• Dosage for children under age 12 hasn't been established.

Geriatric patients

• Geriatric or debilitated patients need close observation and possibly lower dosages. Excessive diuresis promotes rapid dehydration, leading to hypovolemia, hypokalemia, and hyponatremia.

Patient education

• Tell patient that he may feel thirsty or have a dry mouth; emphasize importance of drinking only the amount of fluids provided.

• With initial doses, warn patient to change positions slowly, especially when rising from lying or sitting position, to prevent dizziness from orthostatic hypotension.

• Instruct patient to immediately report shortness of breath, apnea, or pain in the chest, back, or legs.

---

measles, mumps, and rubella virus vaccine, live
M-M-R II

Pharmacologic classification: vaccine
Therapeutic classification: viral vaccine
Pregnancy risk category: C

Indications and dosages

➤ *Measles, mumps, and rubella immunization. Adults (born after 1957):* Two doses of 0.5 ml S.C. in outer aspect of upper arm, given at least 1 month apart.

Children: Initially, 0.5 ml S.C. in outer aspect of upper arm at age 12 to 15 months; second dose at age 4 to 6 years. Second dose may be given earlier if at least 4 weeks have elapsed since first dose and both doses are given beginning at or after age 12 months.

How supplied

Available by prescription only
Injection: Single-dose vial containing not less than 1,000 TCID$_{50}$ (tissue culture infective doses) of attenuated measles virus derived from Enders' attenuated Edmonston strain (grown in chick embryo culture); 20,000 TCID$_{50}$ of the Jeryl Lynn (B level) mumps strain (grown in chick embryo culture); and 1,000 TCID$_{50}$ of the Wistar RA 27/3 strain of rubella virus (propagated in human diploid cell culture)

Pharmacodynamics

Measles, mumps, and rubella prophylaxis: This vaccine promotes active immunity to measles (rubeola), mumps, and German measles (rubella) by inducing production of antibodies.

Pharmacokinetics

Absorption: Antibodies are usually evident 2 to 3 weeks after injection. Vaccine-induced immunity is expected to be lifelong.
Distribution: No information available.
Metabolism: No information available.
Excretion: No information available.

Route	Onset	Peak	Duration
S.C.	Unknown	Unknown	< 11 yr

Contraindications and precautions

Contraindicated in immunosuppressed patients; in those with cancer, blood dyscrasias, gamma globulin disorders, fever, active untreated tuberculosis, or anaphylactic reactions to neomycin or eggs; in those receiving corticosteroid or radiation therapy; and in pregnant women. Use cautiously in patients with history of cerebral injury, individual or family history of seizures, or any other condition in which stress resulting from fever should be avoided.

Interactions

Drug-drug. *Immune serum globulin or transfusions of blood or blood products:* May interfere with the immune response to the vaccine. Whenever possible, defer vaccination for 3 months in these situations.
Immunosuppressive drugs: May interfere with the response to vaccine. Avoid use together if possible.

Adverse reactions

CNS: syncope, malaise, headache.
CV: vasculitis.
EENT: otitis media, conjunctivitis, sore throat.
GI: diarrhea, vomiting.
Respiratory: cough.
Skin: urticaria, rash.
Other: fever, regional lymphadenopathy, *anaphylaxis,* erythema at injection site.

Overdose and treatment
No information available.

Special considerations
• Drug can be given to patient with HIV infection who doesn't have severe immunosuppression.
• Obtain a thorough history of allergies, especially to antibiotics, eggs, chicken, or chicken feathers, and of reactions to immunizations.
• Perform a skin test to assess vaccine sensitivity (against a control of normal saline solution in the opposing limb) in patients with history of anaphylactoid reactions to egg ingestion. Administer a prick (intracutaneous) or scratch test with a 1:10 dilution. Read results after 5 to 30 minutes. A positive reaction is a wheal with or without pseudopodia and surrounding erythema.
• Epinephrine solution 1:1,000 should be available to treat allergic reactions.
• Most adults born before 1957 are believed to have been infected with naturally occurring disease, and vaccination isn't necessary; however, vaccination should be offered if they are considered susceptible.
• Use only the diluent supplied. Discard reconstituted solution after 8 hours.
• Drug shouldn't be given I.V. Use a 25G, ⅝-inch needle and inject S.C., preferably into the outer aspect of the upper arm. Use a sterile syringe free of preservatives, antiseptics, and detergents for each injection, because these substances may inactivate the live virus vaccine.
• Solution may be used if red, pink, or yellow, but it must be clear.
• Vaccine shouldn't be given less than 1 month before or after immunization with other live virus vaccines—except for monovalent or trivalent live oral poliovirus vaccine or poliovirus vaccine, inactivated, which may be given simultaneously at separate sites using separate syringes.
• Vaccine may not offer any protection when given within a few days after exposure to natural measles, mumps, or rubella.
• Give passive immunization with immune serum globulin, if necessary, when immediate protection against measles is required in patients who cannot receive the measles vaccine component. Don't give any live virus vaccine component simultaneously with immune serum globulin.
• Revaccination is unnecessary if the child received two doses of vaccine at least 1 month apart, beginning after the first birthday.
• Store vaccine at 36° to 46° F (2° to 8° C) and protect from light.
• Measles, mumps, and rubella vaccine may temporarily decrease the response to tuberculin skin testing. If a tuberculin skin test is necessary, administer it either before or simultaneously with this vaccine.

Patient monitoring
• Patient should be observed for allergic reactions.

Breast-feeding patients
• It isn't known whether measles or mumps virus components appear in breast milk. Rubella virus or virus antigen transfers into breast milk in about 68% of women. Few adverse effects have been linked to breast-feeding after immunization with rubella-containing vaccines. The risk-benefit ratio suggests that breast-feeding women may be immunized with the rubella component, if necessary.

Pediatric patients
• Children under age 15 months may not respond to one, two, or all three of vaccine components, because retained maternal antibodies may interfere with immune response. However, vaccination at age 12 months is recommended if child lives in a high-risk area, because the benefits outweigh the risk of a slightly lower efficacy of vaccine.

Patient education
• Tell patient to expect tingling sensations in the limbs or joint aches and pains that may resemble arthritis, beginning several days to several weeks after vaccination. These symptoms usually resolve within 1 week. Other effects include pain and inflammation at the injection site and a low-grade fever, a rash, or difficulty breathing. Recommend acetaminophen to alleviate adverse reactions, such as fever.
• Tell patient to report distressing adverse reactions.
• Advise women of childbearing age not to become pregnant for 3 months after receiving vaccine.

measles and rubella virus vaccine, live, attenuated
M-R-Vax II

Pharmacologic classification: vaccine
Therapeutic classification: viral vaccine
Pregnancy risk category: C

Indications and dosages
➤ *Measles and rubella immunization.*
Adults and children age 15 months and older: 0.5 ml in outer aspect of the upper arm. For adequate protection against measles, a two-dose schedule is recommended (at least 1 month between doses).

How supplied
Available by prescription only
Injection: Single-dose vial containing not less than 1,000 TCID$_{50}$ (tissue culture infective doses) each of attenuated measles virus derived from Enders' attenuated Edmonston strain (grown in chick embryo culture) and the Wistar RA 27/3 strain of rubella virus (propagated in human diploid cell culture)
    Note: 10-dose and 50-dose vials are available to government agencies and institutions.

Pharmacodynamics
Measles and rubella prophylaxis: Vaccine promotes active immunity to measles (rubeola) and German measles (rubella) virus by inducing production of antibodies.

Pharmacokinetics
Absorption: Antibodies are usually detectable 2 to 3 weeks after injection. Duration of vaccine-induced immunity is expected to be lifelong.
Distribution: No information available.
Metabolism: No information available.
Excretion: No information available.

Route	Onset	Peak	Duration
S.C.	Unknown	Unknown	< 11 yr

Contraindications and precautions
Contraindicated in immunosuppressed patients; in those with cancer, blood dyscrasias, gamma globulin disorders, fever, active untreated tuberculosis, or anaphylactic reactions to eggs or neomycin; in those receiving corticosteroid or radiation therapy; and in pregnant women. Use cautiously in patients with history of cerebral injury, individual or family history of seizures, or any other condition in which stress resulting from fever should be avoided.

Interactions
Drug-drug. *Immune serum globulin or transfusions of blood or blood products:* May interfere with the immune response to the vaccine. Whenever possible, defer vaccination for 3 months in these situations.
Immunosuppressants: May interfere with response to vaccine. Avoid use together if possible.

Adverse reactions
CNS: syncope, malaise, headache.
CV: vasculitis.
EENT: sore throat.
GI: vomiting, diarrhea.
Respiratory: cough.
Skin: rash.
Other: fever, lymphadenopathy, erythema, burning, or stinging at injection site, *anaphylaxis*.

Overdose and treatment
No information available.

Special considerations
● Drug can be given to patient with HIV infection who doesn't have severe immunosuppression.
● Obtain a thorough history of allergies, especially to antibiotics, eggs, chicken, or chicken feathers, and of reactions to immunizations.
● Skin testing is necessary to assess vaccine sensitivity (against a control of normal saline solution in the opposing limb) in patients with history of anaphylactoid reactions to eggs. Administer a prick (intracutaneous) or scratch test with a 1:10 dilution. Read results after 5 to 30 minutes.

A positive reaction is a wheal with or without pseudopodia and surrounding erythema.
● Epinephrine solution 1:1,000 should be available to treat allergic reactions.
● Drug shouldn't be given I.V. Use a 25G, ⅝-inch needle and inject S.C., preferably into the outer aspect of the upper arm.
● Use a sterile syringe free of preservatives, antiseptics, and detergents for each injection because these substances may inactivate the live virus vaccine.
● Use only diluent supplied. Discard reconstituted solution after 8 hours.
● Solution may be used if red, pink, or yellow, but it must be clear.
● Vaccine shouldn't be given less than 1 month before or after immunization with other live-virus vaccines, except for mumps virus vaccine and monovalent or trivalent live oral poliovirus vaccine, and poliovirus vaccine, inactivated, which may be given simultaneously.
● Vaccine may not offer protection when given within a few days' exposure to natural measles or rubella.
● According to Centers for Disease Control and Prevention recommendations, measles, mumps and rubella (MMR) is the preferred vaccine.
● Passive immunization is given with immune serum globulin when immediate protection against measles is required in patients who can't receive the measles vaccine component. Don't give either vaccine component simultaneously with immune serum globulin.
● Store vaccine at 36° to 46° F (2° to 8° C) and protect from light.
● Revaccination is usually given between 4 to 6 years of age. Measles virus vaccine, live, MMR II, or MR-VAX II may be used.
● Measles and rubella vaccine may temporarily decrease response to tuberculin skin testing. If a tuberculin skin test is necessary, give it either before or simultaneously with measles and rubella vaccine.

Patient monitoring
● Patient should be monitored for adverse allergic reaction.

Breast-feeding patients
● No data are available regarding distribution of measles and rubella virus components in breast milk. Rubella virus or virus antigen may appear in breast milk in about 68% of patients. Few adverse effects have been linked to breast-feeding after immunization with rubella-containing vaccines. The risk-benefit ratio suggests that breast-feeding women may be immunized with the rubella component, if necessary.

Pediatric patients
● Children under age 15 months may not respond to one or both of the vaccine components because retained maternal antibodies may interfere

with the immune response; revaccination is recommended after age 15 months.

Patient education
● Tell patient to expect tingling sensations in the limbs or joint aches and pains that may resemble arthritis, beginning several days to several weeks after vaccination. These symptoms usually resolve within 1 week. Other effects include pain and inflammation at the injection site and a low-grade fever, rash, or difficulty breathing. Recommend acetaminophen for relief of fever.
● Encourage patient to report distressing adverse reactions.
● Advise women of childbearing age not to become pregnant for 3 months after receiving the vaccine.

measles virus vaccine, live, attenuated
Attenuvax

Pharmacologic classification: vaccine
Therapeutic classification: viral vaccine
Pregnancy risk category: C

Indications and dosages
➤ *Immunization. Adults and children age 15 months and older:* 0.5 ml (1,000 units) S.C. in outer aspect of the upper arm. Give two doses at least 1 month apart. For children, usual schedule is the first dose at age 15 months and a second dose at the entry of school (age 4 to 6 years).

How supplied
Available by prescription only
Injection: Single-dose vial containing not less than 1,000 TCID$_{50}$ (tissue culture infective doses) per 0.5 ml of attenuated measles virus derived from Enders' attenuated Edmonston strain grown in chick embryo culture.
Note: 10-dose and 50-dose vials are available to government agencies and institutions.

Pharmacodynamics
Measles prophylaxis: Measles virus vaccine promotes active immunity to measles virus by inducing production of antibodies.

Pharmacokinetics
Absorption: Antibodies are usually evident 2 to 3 weeks after injection. Duration of vaccine-induced immunity is at least 13 to 16 years and probably lifelong in most immunized persons.
Distribution: No information available.
Metabolism: No information available.
Excretion: No information available.

Route	Onset	Peak	Duration
S.C.	Few days	Unknown	13 yr

Contraindications and precautions
Contraindicated in immunosuppressed patients; in those with cancer, blood dyscrasias, gamma globulin disorders, fever, active untreated tuberculosis, or anaphylaxis or anaphylactoid reactions to neomycin or eggs; in those receiving corticosteroid or radiation therapy; and in pregnant patients. Use cautiously in patients with history of cerebral injury, individual or family history of seizures, or any other condition where stress resulting from fever should be avoided.

Interactions
Drug-drug. *Immune serum globulin or transfusions of blood or blood products:* May interfere with the immune response to the vaccine. Whenever possible, defer vaccination for 3 months in these situations.
Immunosuppressants: May interfere with the response to vaccine. Avoid use together if possible.
Meningococcal vaccine: Administration of meningococcal vaccine with measles virus vaccine can result in a reduced seroconversion rate to meningococci. Avoid administration together.

Adverse reactions
CNS: *febrile seizures.*
GI: anorexia.
Hematologic: *leukopenia.*
Skin: rash, erythema, swelling, tenderness at injection site.
Other: fever, lymphadenopathy, *anaphylaxis.*

Overdose and treatment
No information available.

Special considerations
● Obtain a thorough history of allergies, especially to immunizations, antibiotics, eggs, chicken, or chicken feathers.
● Measles vaccine shouldn't be given less than 1 month before or after immunization with other live-virus vaccines, except for mumps virus vaccine, rubella virus vaccine, or monovalent or trivalent live oral poliovirus vaccine or poliovirus vaccine, inactivated, which may be given simultaneously.
● Vaccine may offer some protection when given within a few days after exposure to natural measles and substantial protection when given a few days before exposure.
● According to Centers for Disease Control and Prevention recommendations, measles, mumps, and rubella is the preferred vaccine.
● Passive immunization is given with immune serum globulin if immediate protection against measles is required in patients who can't receive the measles vaccine.
● Patients with a history of anaphylactoid reactions to eggs should first have a skin test to assess vaccine sensitivity (using a control of normal saline solution in the other arm). Administer a prick (intracutaneous) or scratch test with a

1:10 dilution. Read results after 5 to 30 minutes. A positive reaction is a wheal with or without pseudopodia and surrounding erythema.

• Patients who received measles vaccine live when under age 1 year should be considered susceptible to measles, and therefore should be revaccinated.

• Epinephrine solution 1:1,000 should be available to treat allergic reactions.

• Drug shouldn't be given I.V. Use a 25G, ⅝-inch needle and inject S.C., preferably into the outer aspect of the upper arm. Use a sterile syringe free of preservatives, antiseptics, and detergents for each injection, because these substances may inactivate the live-virus vaccine.

• Use diluent supplied. Discard reconstituted solution after 8 hours.

• Store vaccine at 35° to 46° F (2° to 8° C), and protect from light. Solution may be used if red, pink, or yellow, but it must be clear.

• Measles vaccine temporarily may decrease the response to tuberculin skin testing. If a tuberculin skin test is necessary, administer it either before or simultaneously with the measles vaccine.

Patient monitoring

• Patient should be monitored for adverse allergic reaction.

Breast-feeding patients

• It isn't known if vaccine appears in breast milk. Use cautiously in breast-feeding women.

Pediatric patients

• Children under age 15 months may not respond to the vaccine, because retained maternal antibodies may interfere with the immune response; revaccination is recommended after age 15 months.

Patient education

• Tell patient to expect pain and inflammation at the injection site, fever, rash, general malaise, or difficulty breathing. Recommend acetaminophen for relief of fever.

• Encourage patient to report distressing adverse reactions.

• Advise women of childbearing age not to become pregnant for 3 months after receiving the vaccine.

---

mebendazole

Vermox

Pharmacologic classification: benzimidazole
Therapeutic classification: anthelmintic
Pregnancy risk category: C

Indications and dosages

➤ **Pinworm infestations.** *Adults and children over age 2:* 100 mg P.O. as a single dose. If infection persists 2 weeks later, repeat treatment.

➤ *Other roundworm, whipworm, and hookworm infestations◇; trichostrongylosis◇.* *Adults and children over age 2:* 100 mg P.O. b.i.d. for 3 days. If infection persists 3 weeks later, repeat treatment. Or, for treatment of hookworm, whipworm, or roundworm, 500 mg P.O. as a single dose.

➤ *Trichinosis◇.* *Adults:* 200 to 400 mg P.O. t.i.d. for 3 days; then 400 to 500 mg t.i.d. for 10 days.

➤ *Capillariasis◇.* *Adults:* 200 mg P.O. b.i.d. for 20 days.

➤ *Toxocariasis◇.* *Adults and children:* 200 to 400 mg P.O. daily divided into two doses for 5 days.

➤ *Dracunculiasis◇.* *Adults:* 400 to 800 mg P.O. daily for 6 days.

➤ *Mansonella perstans infestations◇.* *Adults:* 100 mg P.O. b.i.d. for 30 days.

➤ *Angiostrongylus cantonensis infestations◇.* *Adults and children:* 100 mg P.O. b.i.d. for 5 days.

➤ *Onchocerciasis◇.* *Adults:* 1 g P.O. b.i.d. for 28 days.

➤ *Treatment of hydatid disease (echinococcosis)◇.* *Adults:* 40 mg/kg P.O. for 1 to 6 months. Or, sequential 2-week courses of 50 mg/kg daily, 200 mg/kg daily, and 50 mg/kg daily for 21 to 30 days.

➤ *Angiostrongylus costaricensis◇.* *Adults and children:* 600 to 1,200 mg P.O. daily divided t.i.d. for 10 days.

How supplied

Available by prescription only
Tablets (chewable): 100 mg

Pharmacodynamics

Anthelmintic action: Mebendazole inhibits uptake of glucose and other low-molecular-weight nutrients in susceptible helminths, depleting the glycogen stores they need for survival and reproduction. It has a broad spectrum and may be useful in mixed infections. It's considered a drug of choice in the treatment of ascariasis, capillariasis, enterobiasis, trichuriasis, and uncinariasis; it has been used investigationally to treat echinococciasis, onchocerciasis, and trichinosis.

Pharmacokinetics

Absorption: About 5% to 10% is absorbed. Absorption varies widely among patients.
Distribution: Highly bound to plasma proteins; it crosses the placenta.
Metabolism: Metabolized to inactive 2-amino-5(6)-benzimidazolyl phenylketone.
Excretion: Most of a dose is excreted in feces; 2% to 10% is excreted in urine in 48 hours as either unchanged drug or the 2-amine metabolite. Half-life is 3 to 9 hours. It isn't known if drug appears in breast milk.

Route	Onset	Peak	Duration
P.O.	Unknown	2-4 hr	Variable

Contraindications and precautions
Contraindicated in patients hypersensitive to drug.

Interactions
Drug-drug. *Anticonvulsants, including carbamazepine and phenytoin:* May enhance mebendazole metabolism and decrease its efficacy. Monitor patient for clinical effect.
Cimetidine: Inhibits mebendazole metabolism and may increase its plasma level. Use together cautiously.

Adverse reactions
GI: occasional, transient abdominal pain and diarrhea in massive infection and expulsion of worms.
Other: fever.

Overdose and treatment
Signs and symptoms of overdose may include GI disturbances and altered mental status.
No specific recommendations exist; treatment is supportive. After recent ingestion (within 4 hours), empty stomach by induced emesis or gastric lavage. Follow with activated charcoal to decrease absorption.

Special considerations
● Tablets may be chewed, swallowed whole, or crushed and mixed with food.
● Laxatives, enemas, or dietary restrictions are unnecessary.
● Collect stool specimens in a clean, dry container and transfer to a properly labeled container to send to laboratory; ova may be destroyed by toilet bowl water, urine, and some drugs.
● Store drug at 59° to 77° F (15° to 25° C) in well-closed container; product expires 3 years from date of manufacture.

Patient monitoring
● High-dose treatment of hydatid disease and trichinosis is investigational. Frequently monitor WBC counts to detect drug toxicity, especially during initial therapy.

Breast-feeding patients
● Safety in breast-feeding women hasn't been established.

Pediatric patients
● Give drug to children under age 2 only when potential benefits justify risks.

Patient education
● Teach patient and family members personal hygiene measures to prevent reinfection, including washing perianal area and changing undergarments and bedclothes daily; washing hands and cleaning fingernails before meals and after defecation; and sanitary disposal of feces.
● Advise patient to bathe often, by showering, if possible.

● Advise patient to keep hands away from mouth, to keep fingernails short, and to wear shoes to avoid hookworm. Explain that ova are easily transmitted directly and indirectly by hands, food, or contaminated articles. Washing clothes in household washing machine will destroy ova.
● Instruct patient to handle bedding carefully because shaking will send ova into the air, and to disinfect toilet facilities and vacuum or damp-mop floors daily to reduce number of ova.
● Encourage patient's family and contacts to be checked for infestation and treated, if necessary

mechlorethamine hydrochloride (nitrogen mustard)
Mustargen

Pharmacologic classification: alkylating agent (not specific to cell cycle phase)
Therapeutic classification: antineoplastic
Pregnancy risk category: D

Indications and dosages
Dosage and indications may vary. Check current literature for recommended protocols.
➤ *Hodgkin's disease, bronchogenic carcinoma, chronic lymphocytic leukemia, chronic myelocytic leukemia, lymphosarcoma, polycythemia vera.* *Adults:* 0.4 mg/kg I.V. per course of therapy as a single dose or 0.1 to 0.2 mg/kg on 2 to 4 successive days q 3 to 6 weeks. Give through running I.V. infusion. Dose reduced in prior radiation therapy or chemotherapy to 0.2 to 0.4 mg/kg. Dose based on ideal or actual body weight, whichever is less.
➤ *Intracavitary doses for neoplastic effusions.* *Adults:* 0.2 to 0.4 mg/kg.
➤ *Treatment of advanced Hodgkin's disease (MOPP regimen).* *Adults:* 6 mg/m^2 given I.V. on days 1 and 8 of 28-day cycle. In subsequent cycles, dose is based on leukocyte count.

How supplied
Available by prescription only
Injection: 10-mg vials

Pharmacodynamics
Antineoplastic action: Mechlorethamine exerts its cytotoxic activity through the basic processes of alkylation. Drug causes cross-linking of DNA strands, single-strand breakage of DNA, abnormal base pairing, and interruption of other intracellular processes, resulting in cell death.

Pharmacokinetics
Absorption: Well absorbed after oral administration; however, because drug is very irritating to tissue, it must be given I.V. After intracavitary administration, mechlorethamine is absorbed in-

---

Reactions may be *common*, uncommon, *life-threatening*, or COMMON AND LIFE-THREATENING.

completely, probably from deactivation by body fluids in the cavity.

Distribution: Doesn't cross the blood-brain barrier.

Metabolism: Undergoes rapid chemical transformation and reacts quickly with various cellular components before being deactivated.

Excretion: Metabolites are excreted in urine. Less than 0.01% of an I.V. dose is excreted unchanged in urine.

Route	Onset	Peak	Duration
I.V., intracavitary	Few seconds, few minutes	Unknown	Unknown

Contraindications and precautions

Contraindicated in patients hypersensitive to drug and in those with infectious diseases. Use cautiously in patients with severe anemia or depressed neutrophil or platelet count and in those who have recently undergone chemotherapy or radiation therapy.

Interactions

None reported.

Adverse reactions

CNS: weakness, vertigo.
CV: *thrombophlebitis.*
EENT: tinnitus, deafness.
GI: *nausea, vomiting, anorexia.*
GU: menstrual irregularities, impaired spermatogenesis.
Hematologic: *thrombocytopenia, lymphocytopenia, agranulocytosis,* nadir of myelosuppression occurring by days 4 to 10 and lasting 10 to 21 days; mild anemia begins in 2 to 3 weeks.
Hepatic: jaundice.
Metabolic: hyperuricemia.
Skin: *alopecia,* rash, sloughing, severe irritation (if drug extravasates or touches skin).
Other: precipitation of herpes zoster, *anaphylaxis,* amyloidosis.

Overdose and treatment

Signs and symptoms of overdose include severe leukopenia, anemia, thrombocytopenia, and a hemorrhagic diathesis with subsequent delayed bleeding. Death may follow.

Treatment is usually supportive and includes transfusion of blood components and antibiotic treatment of complicating infections.

Special considerations

• Avoid contact with skin or mucous membranes. Wear gloves when preparing solution and during administration to prevent accidental skin contact. If contact occurs, wash with copious amounts of water.
• To prevent hyperuricemia with resulting uric acid nephropathy, allopurinol may be given; keep patient well hydrated.

• Drug has been used topically to treat mycosis fungoides.
• To reconstitute powder, use 10 ml of sterile water for injection or normal saline solution to give a concentration of 1 mg/ml.
• When reconstituted, drug is a clear colorless solution. Don't use if solution is discolored or if droplets of water are visible within vial before reconstitution.
• Solution is very unstable. Prepare immediately before infusion and use within 15 minutes. Discard unused solution.
• Dilution of drug into a large volume of I.V. solution isn't recommended, because it may react with the diluent and isn't stable for a prolonged period.
• Drug may be given I.V. push over a few minutes into the tubing of a freely flowing I.V. infusion. Following administration, flush vein for 2.5 minutes with running I.V. solution or inject 5 to 10 ml of solution into sidearm.
• Treatment of extravasation includes local injections of a 1/6 M sodium thiosulfate solution. Prepare solution by mixing 4 ml of sodium thiosulfate 10% with 6 ml of sterile water for injection. Also, apply ice packs for 6 to 12 hours to minimize local reactions.
• During intracavitary administration, patient should be turned from side to side every 15 minutes for 1 hour to distribute drug.
• Avoid all I.M. injections when platelet count is low.

Patient monitoring

• Monitor uric acid levels, CBC, and liver function tests.
• Use anticoagulants cautiously. Watch closely for signs of bleeding.

Breast-feeding patients

• It isn't known if drug appears in breast milk. However, because of the potential for serious adverse reactions, mutagenicity, and carcinogenicity in the infant, breast-feeding isn't recommended.

Patient education

• Tell patient to avoid exposure to people with infections.
• Advise patient that adequate fluid intake is very important to facilitate excretion of uric acid.
• Reassure patient that hair should grow back after treatment has ended.
• Tell patient to promptly report signs or symptoms of bleeding or infection.
• Advise patient to use contraception while using drug.

meclizine hydrochloride
Antivert, Antivert/25, Antrizine,
Bonine, Dizmiss, Meclizine, Meni-D,
Ru-Vert M

Pharmacologic classification: piperazine-
derivative antihistamine
Therapeutic classification: antiemetic, antivertigo
Pregnancy risk category: B

Indications and dosages
➤ *Dizziness.* Adults and children age 12 or
older: 25 to 100 mg P.O. daily in divided doses.
Dosage varies with patient response.
➤ *Motion sickness.* Adults and children age
12 or older: 25 to 50 mg P.O. 1 hour before travel; may repeat dose daily for duration of journey.

How supplied
Available with or without a prescription
Capsules: 25 mg
Tablets: 12.5 mg, 25 mg, 50 mg
Tablets (chewable): 25 mg

Pharmacodynamics
Antiemetic action: Meclizine probably inhibits
nausea and vomiting by centrally decreasing sensitivity of labyrinth apparatus that relays stimuli
to the chemoreceptor trigger zone and stimulates
the vomiting center in the brain.
Antivertigo action: Drug decreases labyrinth
excitability and conduction in vestibular-cerebellar
pathways.

Pharmacokinetics
Absorption: Well absorbed.
Distribution: Well distributed throughout the
body and crosses the placenta.
Metabolism: Probably metabolized in the liver.
Excretion: Half-life is about 6 hours. Drug is ex-
creted unchanged in feces; metabolites are found
in urine.

Route	Onset	Peak	Duration
P.O.	1 hr	Unknown	8-24 hr

Contraindications and precautions
Contraindicated in patients hypersensitive to drug.
Use cautiously in patients with asthma, glauco-
ma, or prostatic hyperplasia.

Interactions
Drug-drug. *CNS depressants, such as antianxiety drugs, barbiturates, sleeping aids,
and tranquilizers:* Increased sedative effects.
Use together cautiously.
*Other ototoxic drugs, such as aminoglycosides,
cisplatin, loop diuretics, salicylates, and vancomycin:* Meclizine may mask signs of ototoxicity. Avoid use together.

Drug-lifestyle. *Alcohol use:* Additive sedative
and CNS depressant effects. Advise patient to avoid
alcohol use.

Adverse reactions
CNS: *drowsiness,* restlessness, excitation, ner-
vousness, auditory and visual hallucinations.
CV: hypotension, palpitations, tachycardia.
EENT: blurred vision, diplopia, tinnitus, dry nose
and throat.
GI: dry mouth, constipation, anorexia, nausea,
vomiting, diarrhea.
GU: urine retention, urinary frequency.
Skin: urticaria, rash.

Overdose and treatment
Signs and symptoms of moderate overdose may
include hyperexcitability alternating with drowsiness. Seizures, hallucinations, and respiratory
paralysis may occur in profound overdose. Anticholinergic symptoms, such as dry mouth, flushed
skin, fixed and dilated pupils, and GI symptoms,
are common, especially in children.

Treat overdose by using gastric lavage to empty stomach contents; emesis with ipecac syrup
may be ineffective. Treat hypotension with vasopressors, and control seizures with diazepam or
phenytoin. Don't give stimulants.

Special considerations
• Tablets may be placed in mouth and allowed to
dissolve without water, or they may be chewed
or swallowed whole.
• Abrupt withdrawal of drug after long-term use
may cause paradoxical reactions or sudden reversal of improved state.
• Discontinue meclizine 4 days before diagnostic skin tests to avoid preventing, reducing, or
masking test response.

Patient monitoring
• Monitor patient for excessive CNS effects.

Breast-feeding patients
• Safety in breast-feeding women hasn't been
established.

Pediatric patients
• Safety and efficacy for use in children haven't
been established. Don't use in children under
age 12; infants and children under age 6 may experience paradoxical hyperexcitability.

Geriatric patients
• Geriatric patients are usually more sensitive to
adverse effects of antihistamines and are especially likely to experience a greater degree of
dizziness, sedation, hyperexcitability, dry mouth,
and urine retention than younger patients.

Patient education
• Instruct patient to avoid activities that require
mental alertness and physical coordination, such
as driving and operating dangerous machinery.

Reactions may be *common*, uncommon, *life-threatening*, or COMMON AND LIFE-THREATENING.

medroxyprogesterone acetate

Amen, Curretab, Cycrin, Depo-Provera, Provera

Pharmacologic classification: progestin
Therapeutic classification: antineoplastic
Pregnancy risk category: X

Indications and dosages

➤ *Abnormal uterine bleeding from hormonal imbalance. Adults:* 5 to 10 mg P.O. daily for 5 to 10 days beginning on day 16 to 21 of menstrual cycle. If patient has received estrogen, then 10 mg P.O. daily for 10 days beginning on day 16 of cycle. If bleeding is controlled satisfactorily, give two subsequent cycles of combination therapy.

➤ *Secondary amenorrhea. Adults:* 5 to 10 mg P.O. daily for 5 to 10 days, preferably beginning on day 16 to 21 of menstrual cycle. If patient has received estrogen, then 10 mg P.O. daily for 10 days.

➤ *Endometrial or renal carcinoma (adjunct). Adults:* 400 to 1,000 mg I.M. weekly. If disease improves or stabilizes in a few weeks or months, 400 mg/month.

➤ *Paraphilia in men ◊. Adults:* Initially, 200 mg I.M. b.i.d. or t.i.d. or 500 mg I.M. weekly. Adjust dosage based on response.

➤ *Contraception in women. Adults:* 150 mg I.M. q 3 months; give first injection on first 5 days of menstrual cycle.

How supplied

Available by prescription only
Injection: 150 mg/ml, 400 mg/ml
Tablets: 2.5 mg, 5 mg, 10 mg

Pharmacodynamics

Progestational action: Parenteral medroxyprogesterone suppresses ovulation, causes thickening of cervical mucus, and induces sloughing of the endometrium.
Antineoplastic action: Drug may inhibit growth progression of progestin-sensitive endometrial or renal cancer tissue by an unknown mechanism.

Pharmacokinetics

Absorption: Absorption is slow after I.M. administration.
Distribution: Not well characterized.
Metabolism: Primarily hepatic; not well characterized.
Excretion: Primarily renal; not well characterized.

Route	Onset	Peak	Duration
P.O., I.M.	Unknown	Unknown	Unknown

Contraindications and precautions

Contraindicated in pregnant patients, patients hypersensitive to drug, and patients with active or previous thromboembolic disorders, cerebral vascular disease, apoplexy, breast cancer, undiagnosed abnormal vaginal bleeding, missed abortion, or hepatic dysfunction. Tablets are also contraindicated in patients with liver dysfunction or known or suspected malignant disease of the genital organs.

Use cautiously in patients with diabetes mellitus, seizures, migraines, cardiac or renal disease, asthma, or depression.

Interactions

Drug-drug. *Aminoglutethimide:* May increase the hepatic metabolism of medroxyprogesterone, possibly decreasing its therapeutic effect. Avoid use together.

Adverse reactions

CNS: depression.
CV: thrombophlebitis, *pulmonary embolism*, edema, *thromboembolism, CVA.*
EENT: exophthalmos, diplopia.
GU: breakthrough bleeding, dysmenorrhea, amenorrhea, cervical erosion, abnormal secretions.
Hepatic: cholestatic jaundice.
Metabolic: changes in weight.
Skin: rash, pain, induration, sterile abscesses, acne, pruritus, melasma, alopecia, hirsutism.
Other: breast tenderness, enlargement, or secretion.

Overdose and treatment

No information available.

Special considerations

• Use parenteral form only for I.M. administration. Inject deep into large muscle mass, preferably the gluteal muscle. Monitor patient for development of sterile abscesses.
• Shake suspension vigorously just before use to ensure complete suspension of drug.
• Drug has been used to treat obstructive sleep apnea and to manage paraphilia.
• When used as a long-acting contraceptive, rule out pregnancy before starting therapy.
• Store drug between 59° and 86° F (15° and 30° C); avoid freezing.

Patient monitoring

• Monitor serum glucose in diabetic patient.

Breast-feeding patients

• Drug has been detected in breast milk. Infants exposed to drug via breast milk have shown no adverse developmental or behavioral effects through puberty.

Patient education

• Tell patient not to take drug if she becomes pregnant.
• Advise patient to report chest pain, difficulty breathing, or leg pain.
• Warn patient about signs of CVA.

medroxyprogesterone acetate and estradiol cypionate
Lunelle

Pharmacologic classification: estrogen/progestin
Therapeutic classification: combined hormonal contraceptive
Pregnancy risk category: X

Indications and dosages
➤ *Prevention of pregnancy.* Women over age 16 who have achieved menarche: 0.5 ml I.M. into deltoid, gluteus maximus, or anterior thigh. Give first injection within first 5 days of onset of a normal menstrual period, within 5 days of a complete first trimester abortion, or at least 4 weeks postpartum if not breast-feeding (at least 6 weeks postpartum if breast-feeding). Give second and subsequent injections monthly (28 to 30 days, not to exceed 33 days) after previous injection.

How supplied
Available by prescription only
Injection: 25 mg medroxyprogesterone acetate and 5 mg estradiol cypionate per 0.5 ml

Pharmacodynamics
Medroxyprogesterone acetate and estradiol cypionate inhibit secretion of gonadotropins, which prevents follicular maturation and ovulation. Other possible actions include thickening of cervical mucus, reduction of the volume of cervical mucus, and thinning of the endometrium.

Pharmacokinetics
Absorption: Maximum plasma level typically occurs within 1 to 10 days postinjection for medroxyprogesterone and 1 to 7 days postinjection for estradiol cypionate.
Distribution: Medroxyprogesterone acetate binds primarily to serum albumin. Estradiol is primarily bound to SHBG and albumin. About 3% of estradiol remains unbound. Unbound estrogens are known to modulate pharmacologic response.
Metabolism: Medroxyprogesterone acetate is metabolized to numerous derivatives. Estradiol cypionate is metabolized to a parent active compound.
Excretion: Most medroxyprogesterone is excreted in the urine as glucuronide conjugates with only small amounts as sulfates. Estrogen metabolites are primarily excreted in the urine as glucorunides and sulfates.

Route	Onset	Peak	Duration
I.M.	1 day	7-10 days	28-30 days

Contraindications and precautions
Contraindicated in patients with known or suspected pregnancy, thrombophlebitis or thromboembolic disorders, a history of deep vein thrombophlebitis or thromboembolic disorders, and cerebral vascular or coronary artery disease. Also contraindicated in patients with undiagnosed abnormal genital bleeding and in patients with liver dysfunction or disease (such as history of hepatic adenoma or carcinoma), or history of cholestatic jaundice of pregnancy or jaundice with prior hormonal contraceptive use, including severe pruritus of pregnancy. Contraindicated in patients with carcinoma of the endometrium, breast, or other known or suspected estrogen-dependent neoplasia. Also contraindicated in patients hypersensitive to any of the ingredients, patients who smoke heavily (15 or more cigarettes per day) and are over age 35, and patients with severe hypertension, diabetes with vascular involvement, headaches with focal neurologic symptoms, and valvular heart disease with complications.

Use cautiously in patients with hypertension, hyperlipidemias, obesity, diabetes, and liver dysfunction. Also use cautiously in patients who smoke and in patients with a history of depression.

Interactions
Drug-drug. *Acetaminophen:* Decreased plasma levels. Monitor patient.
Aminoglutethimide: May decrease medroxyprogesterone acetate levels. Recommend additional birth control.
Antibiotics (ampicillin, griseofulvin, tetracycline): Decreased contraceptive effectiveness. Recommend additional birth control.
Anticonvulsants (carbamazepine, phenobarbital, phenytoin): Increased metabolism of some synthetic estrogens and progestins, which could result in reduced contraceptive effectiveness. Recommend additional birth control.
Cyclosporine, prednisolone, theophylline: Increased levels of these drugs. Monitor serum levels, and adjust as needed.
Phenylbutazone: May decrease contraceptive effectiveness and increase menstrual irregularities. Recommend additional birth control.
Rifampin: Increased metabolism of some synthetic estrogens and progestins, resulting in decreased contraceptive effectiveness and more irregular bleeding. Recommend additional birth control.
Drug-herb. *St John's wort:* May induce hepatic enzymes (cytochrome P-450) and transporter proteins, reduce the effectiveness of contraceptives, and result in breakthrough bleeding. Discourage use or advise the use of a second method of contraception.
Drug-lifestyle. *Smoking:* Increased risk of thromboembolic disorders. Discourage smoking.

Reactions may be *common*, uncommon, *life-threatening*, or COMMON AND LIFE-THREATENING.

Adverse reactions

CNS: emotional lability, depression, headache, nervousness, dizziness, asthenia.
GI: abdominal pain, nausea, enlarged abdomen.
GU: amenorrhea, dysmenorrhea, menorrhagia, metrorrhagia, vaginal candidiasis, vulvovaginal disorder.
Metabolic: weight gain.
Skin: acne, alopecia.
Other: breast tenderness, decreased libido.

Overdose and treatment

Overdose may cause nausea, vomiting, vaginal bleeding, or other menstrual irregularities. Supportive measures are recommended.

Special considerations

● The use of oral contraceptives is linked to increased risk of MI, CVA, hepatic neoplasia, and gallbladder disease.
● Monthly injection is effective for contraception during the first cycle of use when administered as recommended.
● If more than 33 days have elapsed since last injection, pregnancy should be considered and another injection shouldn't be given until pregnancy is ruled out.
● Shortening the injection interval could lead to a change in menstrual pattern.
● Don't use bleeding episodes to guide the injection schedule.
● Shake the aqueous suspension vigorously just before use to ensure a uniform suspension.
● Provide yearly physical examinations. Monitor breast exam closely in women with breast nodules or family history of breast cancer.
● When switching patients from other methods of birth control, drug should be given in a manner that ensures continuous contraceptive coverage based on the mechanism of action from both methods. For example, patients switching from oral contraceptives should have their first injection within 7 days after taking their last active pill.
● Discontinue use at least 4 weeks before and for 2 weeks after elective surgery that may be linked to increased risk of thromboembolism.
● Don't use during periods of prolonged immobilization or within 4 weeks after childbirth.
● Injection should be stored at 59° to 86° F (15° to 30° C).

Breast-feeding patients

● Effects of drug in nursing mothers haven't been evaluated and are unknown. However, estrogen administration to nursing mothers has resulted in a decrease in the quantity and quality of breast milk.
● Small amounts of combined hormonal contraceptives have been identified in milk with no deleterious effects to the child. However, breast-feeding women shouldn't begin a combined hormonal contraceptive until 6 weeks postpartum.

Pediatric patients

● Use of this product before menarche isn't indicated.
● Safety and efficacy are expected to be the same in adolescents under 16 years of age.

Geriatric patients

● Not indicated in postmenopausal women.

Patient education

⚠ **ALERT** Teach patient that this product is intended to prevent pregnancy and won't protect against sexually transmitted diseases such as HIV (AIDS), genital warts, genital herpes, chlamydia, gonorrhea, hepatitis B, and syphillis.
● Advise patient that injection must be given every 28 to 30 days. If more than 33 days have passed since an injection, pregnancy must be ruled out before another injection can be given.
● Tell patient that menstrual bleeding patterns may be disrupted while receiving drug. Advise patient to report excessive or prolonged bleeding.
● Tell patient that weight gain may occur while taking drug.
● Advise patient who wears contact lenses to have an eye examination if visual changes or changes in lens tolerance develop while taking drug.

megestrol acetate
Megace

Pharmacologic classification: progestin
Therapeutic classification: antineoplastic
Pregnancy risk category: X

Indications and dosages

Dosage and indications may vary. Check current literature for recommended protocol.
➤ *Palliative treatment of breast carcinoma. Adults:* 40 mg (tablets) P.O. q.i.d.
➤ *Palliative treatment of endometrial carcinoma. Adults:* 10 to 80 mg (tablets) P.O. q.i.d.
➤ *Anorexia, cachexia, or weight loss in patients with AIDS. Adults:* 800 mg (suspension) P.O. daily; 100 to 400 mg for AIDS-related cachexia.
➤ *Anorexia or cachexia in patients with neoplastic disease* ◇. *Adults:* 480 to 600 mg P.O. daily.

How supplied

Available by prescription only
Suspension: 200 mg/5 ml
Tablets: 20 mg, 40 mg

Pharmacodynamics

Antineoplastic action: Megestrol inhibits growth and causes regression of progestin-sensitive breast and endometrial cancer tissue by an unknown mechanism.

Weight-raising action: Mechanism for weight gain is unknown. Drug may stimulate appetite by interfering with the production of mediators such as cachectin.

Pharmacokinetics

Absorption: Well absorbed across the GI tract after oral administration.
Distribution: Appears to be stored in fatty tissue and is highly bound to plasma proteins.
Metabolism: Completely metabolized in the liver.
Excretion: Metabolites are eliminated primarily through the kidneys.

Route	Onset	Peak	Duration
P.O.	Unknown	Unknown	Unknown

Contraindications and precautions

Contraindicated in patients hypersensitive to drug and in pregnant patients (especially during first 4 months). Use cautiously in patients with history of thrombophlebitis.

Interactions

None reported.

Adverse reactions

CV: thrombophlebitis, hypertension, edema, chest pain.
EENT: pharyngitis.
GI: increased appetite, nausea, vomiting, diarrhea, flatulence.
GU: breakthrough menstrual bleeding, impotence.
Hepatic: hepatomegaly.
Metabolic: weight gain, hyperglycemia.
Musculoskeletal: carpal tunnel syndrome.
Respiratory: *pulmonary embolism,* dyspnea, pneumonia, cough.
Skin: alopecia, rash, pruritus, candidiasis.
Other: decreased libido.

Overdose and treatment

No information available.

Special considerations

• Investigational uses include prevention of contraception, treatment of prostatic hypertrophy, endometriosis, and endometrial hyperplasias.
• Store tablets at 59° to 86° F (15° to 30° C) and oral suspension at 77° F (25° C) or less.
• Blood glucose levels may increase in diabetic patients.
• Drug is relatively nontoxic with a low risk of adverse effects.
• In patients with cancer, 2 months is an adequate trial period.

Patient monitoring

• Monitor hemapoietic function and liver function.

Patient education

• Inform patient that therapeutic response isn't immediate.

meloxicam

Mobic

Pharmacologic classification: enolic acid NSAID
Therapeutic classification: anti-inflammatory, analgesic
Pregnancy risk category: C

Indications and dosages

➤ *Relief of the signs and symptoms of osteoarthritis.* Adults: 7.5 mg P.O. once daily. May increase as needed to maximum dose of 15 mg daily.

How supplied

Available by prescription only
Tablets: 7.5 mg.

Pharmacodynamics

The mechanism of action of meloxicam may be related to prostaglandin (cyclooxygenase) synthetase inhibition.

Pharmacokinetics

Absorption: The bioavailability after oral administration is 89% and doesn't appear to be affected by either food or antacids. Steady state conditions are reached after 5 days of daily administration.
Distribution: Meloxicam is 99.4% bound to human plasma proteins (primarily albumin).
Metabolism: Meloxicam is almost completely metabolized to pharmacologically inactive metabolites.
Excretion: Meloxicam is excreted in both the urine and the feces primarily as metabolites. The elimination half-life ranges from 15 to 20 hours.

Route	Onset	Peak	Duration
P.O.	Unknown	Unknown	Unknown

Contraindications and precautions

Contraindicated in patients hypersensitive to meloxicam and in patients who have experienced asthma, urticaria, or allergic-type reactions after taking aspirin or other NSAIDs. Avoid use in late pregnancy.

Use with extreme caution in patients with a history of ulcers or GI bleeding. Use cautiously in patients with dehydration, anemia, hepatic disease, renal disease, hypertension, fluid retention, heart failure, and asthma. Also use cautiously in elderly and debilitated patients because of increased risk of fatal GI bleeding.

Interactions
Drug-drug. *ACE Inhibitors:* Diminished anti-hypertensive effects. Monitor patient's blood pressure.
Aspirin: Increased risk of adverse effects. Avoid concurrent use.
Furosemide, thiazide diuretics: Reduced sodium excretion, leading to sodium retention. Monitor patient for edema and increased blood pressure.
Lithium: Increased lithium levels. Monitor plasma lithium levels closely during treatment.
Warfarin: May increase PT or INR and increase risk of bleeding complications. Monitor PT and INR, and monitor patient for bleeding.
Drug-lifestyle. *Alcoholism, smoking:* Increased risk of GI irritation and bleeding. Monitor patient for bleeding.

Adverse reactions
CNS: dizziness, headache, insomnia, fatigue, *seizures*, paresthesia, tremor, vertigo, anxiety, confusion, depression, nervousness, somnolence, malaise, syncope.
CV: *arrhythmias*, palpitations, tachycardia, angina, **heart failure**, hypertension, hypotension, *MI*, edema.
EENT: pharyngitis, abnormal vision, conjunctivitis, tinnitus.
GI: abdominal pain, diarrhea, dyspepsia, flatulence, nausea, constipation, colitis, dry mouth, duodenal ulcer, esophagitis, gastric ulcer, gastritis, gastroesophageal reflux, *hemorrhage*, *pancreatitis*, vomiting, increased appetite, taste perversion.
GU: albuminuria, elevated BUN and creatinine levels, hematuria, urinary frequency, *renal failure*, urinary tract infection.
Hematologic: anemia, *leukopenia*, purpura, *thrombocytopenia*.
Hepatic: elevated liver function test results, bilirubinemia, *hepatitis*.
Metabolic: dehydration, weight increase or decrease.
Musculoskeletal: arthralgia, back pain.
Respiratory: upper respiratory tract infection, asthma, *bronchospasm*, dyspnea, coughing.
Skin: rash, pruritus, alopecia, bullous eruption, photosensitivity, sweating, urticaria.
Other: accidental injury, allergic reaction, fever, *angioedema*, flulike symptoms.

Overdose and treatment
Signs and symptoms of acute NSAID overdose include lethargy, drowsiness, nausea, vomiting, epigastric pain, and GI bleeding. Severe poisoning may result in acute renal failure, hepatic dysfunction, respiratory depression, coma, seizures, CV collapse, and cardiac arrest. Anaphylactoid reactions may also occur.

There is no antidote and patients should be managed with symptomatic and supportive care. Within 1 hour of the overdose, induce vomiting or perform gastric lavage. Activated charcoal is recommended for patients seen 1 to 2 hours after overdose. Activated charcoal may be given repeatedly for substantial overdose or severely symptomatic patient. Cholestyramine may be useful following an overdose. Forced diuresis, alkalinization of urine, hemodialysis, or hemoperfusion may not be useful because of high protein-binding.

Special considerations
⚠ ALERT Drug may produce allergic-type reactions in patients hypersensitive to aspirin and other NSAIDs.
● Patients with a history of ulcers or GI bleeding have a higher risk of GI bleeding while taking NSAIDs such as meloxicam. Other risk factors for GI bleeding include treatment with corticosteroids or anticoagulants, longer duration of NSAID treatment, smoking, alcoholism, older age, and poor overall health.
● Rehydrate patients who are dehydrated before starting treatment with meloxicam.
● Periodically monitor CBC and chemistry profile for patients on long-term treatment.

Patient monitoring
● Monitor patient for signs and symptoms of overt and occult bleeding.
● NSAIDs such as meloxicam can cause fluid retention; closely monitor patients who have hypertension, edema, or heart failure.
● Meloxicam may be hepatotoxic and elevations of ALT or AST levels have been reported and should be monitored if they occur. If clinical signs and symptoms consistent with liver disease develop, or if systemic manifestations such as eosinophilia or rash occur, the drug should be discontinued.

Breast-feeding patients
● It is unknown whether meloxicam appears in breast milk. However, because it may enter milk and it has the potential for serious adverse reactions in nursing infants, a decision should be made whether to discontinue nursing or to discontinue the drug, taking into account the importance of the drug to the mother.

Pediatric patients
● Safety and effectiveness in children under age 18 haven't been established.

Geriatric patients
● As with any NSAID, use cautiously when treating elderly patients.

Patient education
● Tell patient to report any history of allergic reactions to aspirin or other NSAIDs before starting therapy.
● Teach patient to report signs and symptoms of GI ulcerations and bleeding (vomiting blood, blood in stool, and black, tarry stools) and to seek medical advice when observing any indicative signs.

• Instruct patient to report any skin rash, weight gain, or edema.

• Advise patient to report warning signs of hepatotoxicity (nausea, fatigue, lethargy, pruritus, jaundice, right upper quadrant tenderness and "flulike" symptoms).

• Warn patient with a prior history of asthma that the asthma may reoccur while taking meloxicam and to stop taking the drug and notify prescriber.

• Tell woman to notify prescriber if she becomes pregnant or is planning to become pregnant while taking this drug.

• Inform patient that it may take several days before consistent pain relief is achieved.

melphalan (phenylalanine mustard)
Alkeran

Pharmacologic classification: alkylating agent (not specific to cell cycle phase)
Therapeutic classification: antineoplastic
Pregnancy risk category: D

Indications and dosages
Dosage and indications may vary. Check current literature for recommended protocol.
➤*Multiple myeloma. Adults:* 6 mg P.O. daily for 2 to 3 weeks; then stop therapy for 4 weeks. When WBC and platelet count begin to increase, start maintenance dosage of 2 mg P.O. daily. Or, give 0.15 mg/kg daily P.O. for 7 days or 0.25 mg/kg daily P.O. for 4 days at 4- to 6-week intervals, usually with prednisone; monitor patient's blood counts. Other dosing methods: 10 mg P.O. for 7 to 10 days. When platelet and leukocyte counts exceed 100,000/µL and 4000/µL, respectively, start maintenance therapy at 2 mg P.O. daily. Dose adjusted by 1 to 3 mg based on hematologic response.

For I.V. use, give 16 mg/m² over 15 to 20 minutes once at 2-week intervals for four doses. Monitor patient's blood counts and reduce dose as necessary. After satisfactory recovery, repeat dose at 4-week intervals.
➤*Epithelial ovarian cancer. Adults:* 200 mcg/kg daily P.O. for 5 days, repeated q 4 to 5 weeks if blood counts return to normal.
✦*Dosage adjustment.* I.V. melphalan dose is reduced by 50% in patients with renal impairment to reduce severe leukopenia and drug-related death.

How supplied
Available by prescription only
Powder for injection: 50 mg
Tablets (scored): 2 mg

Pharmacodynamics
Antineoplastic action: Melphalan exerts its cytotoxic activity by forming cross-links of strands of DNA and RNA and inhibiting protein synthesis.

Pharmacokinetics
Absorption: Absorption from GI tract is incomplete and variable. One study found that absorption ranged from 25% to 89% after an oral dose of 0.6 mg/kg.
Distribution: Distributes rapidly and widely into total body water. Drug is initially 50% to 60% bound to plasma proteins and eventually increases to 80% to 90% over time.
Metabolism: Extensively deactivated by the process of hydrolysis.
Excretion: Elimination has been described as biphasic, with an initial half-life of 8 minutes and a terminal half-life of 2 hours. Melphalan and its metabolites are excreted primarily in urine, with 10% of an oral dose excreted as unchanged drug.

Route	Onset	Peak	Duration
P.O., I.V.	Unknown	Unknown	Unknown

Contraindications and precautions
Contraindicated in patients hypersensitive to drug and in those whose disease is known to be resistant to drug. Patients hypersensitive to chlorambucil may have cross-sensitivity to melphalan.

Use cautiously in patients with impaired renal function, severe leukopenia, thrombocytopenia, anemia, or chronic lymphocytic leukemia.

Interactions
Drug-drug. *Cimetidine:* Inhibits GI absorption. Avoid administration together.
Cisplatin, cyclosporine: May increase nephrotoxicity. Monitor renal function closely in patients receiving melphalan and cyclosporine together or melphalan and cisplatin together.
Interferon alpha: May decrease melphalan levels. Monitor patient carefully.
Drug-food. *Food:* Reduces bioavailability of melphalan. Advise patient to take drug on an empty stomach.

Adverse reactions
CNS: transient paralysis, peripheral neuritis.
CV: hypotension, tachycardia, edema, thrombosis, phlebitis, *pulmonary embolism.*
GI: nausea, vomiting, diarrhea, oral ulceration.
Hematologic: *thrombocytopenia, leukopenia, bone marrow suppression,* hemolytic anemia.
Hepatic: *hepatotoxicity.*
Respiratory: *pneumonitis, pulmonary fibrosis,* dyspnea, *bronchospasm.*
Skin: pruritus, alopecia, urticaria, vesiculation and tissue necrosis.
Other: *anaphylaxis, hypersensitivity, secondary malignancy.*

Overdose and treatment
Signs and symptoms of overdose include myelosuppression, hypocalcemia, severe nausea, vomiting, ulceration of the mouth, decreased con-

---

Reactions may be *common*, uncommon, *life-threatening*, or COMMON AND LIFE-THREATENING.

sciousness, seizures, muscular paralysis, and cholinomimetic effects.

Treatment is usually supportive and includes transfusion of blood components.

Special considerations
• Fever may enhance elimination of the drug.
• Use anticoagulants, aspirin, and aspirin-containing products cautiously.
• Oral dose may be taken all at one time.
• Give drug on an empty stomach because absorption is decreased by food.
• Discontinue therapy temporarily or reduce dosage if WBC count goes below 3,000/mm³ or platelet count goes below 100,000/mm³.
• Avoid I.M. injections when platelet count is less than 100,000/mm³.
• Consider dosage reduction in patients with renal failure receiving I.V. melphalan.
• Increased bone marrow suppression was observed in patients with BUN levels of 30 mg/dl or more.
• Follow procedure for proper handling and disposal of antineoplastic drugs.
• Reconstitute powder for injection by adding 10 ml of provided diluent to 50-mg vial using a 20G or larger needle; produces a concentration of 5 mg/ml. Add diluent rapidly and shake vial until solution is clear. Don't refrigerate because a precipitate may form. Immediately, dilute further in normal saline solution for injection to provide a solution not exceeding 0.45 mg/ml. Give over 15 to 20 minutes; infuse solution within 60 minutes from time of reconstitution.

Patient monitoring
• Frequent hematologic monitoring, including CBC, is necessary for accurate dosage adjustments and prevention of toxicity.
• Monitor renal function, especially if BUN is greater than 30 mg/dL.

Breast-feeding patients
• It isn't known if melphalan appears in breast milk. However, because of risk of serious adverse reactions, mutagenicity, and carcinogenicity in the infant, breast-feeding isn't recommended.

Patient education
• Instruct patient to continue taking drug despite nausea and vomiting.
• Tell patient to call immediately if vomiting occurs shortly after taking a dose.
• Explain that adequate fluid intake is important to facilitate excretion of uric acid.
• Instruct patient to avoid exposure to people with infections.
• Reassure patient that hair should grow back after treatment has ended.
• Tell patient to promptly report signs and symptoms of infection or bleeding.
• Advise women of childbearing age to avoid becoming pregnant while receiving drug therapy.

meningococcal polysaccharide vaccine
Menomune-A/C/Y/W-135

Pharmacologic classification: vaccine
Therapeutic classification: bacterial vaccine
Pregnancy risk category: C

Indications and dosages
➤ *Meningococcal meningitis prophylaxis.* *Adults and children over age 2:* 0.5 ml S.C. *Children ages 3 to 18 months ◊:* 0.5 ml S.C. for two doses 3 months apart.

How supplied
Available by prescription only
Injection: A killed bacterial vaccine in single-dose, 10-dose, and 50-dose vials with vial of diluent

Pharmacodynamics
Meningitis prophylaxis action: Vaccine promotes active immunity to meningitis caused by *Neisseria meningitidis.*

Pharmacokinetics
No information available.

Route	Onset	Peak	Duration
S.C.	Unknown	Unknown	3 yr

Contraindications and precautions
Contraindicated in immunosuppressed patients hypersensitive to thimerosal. Defer vaccination in patients with acute illness. Avoid use during pregnancy unless clearly needed.

Interactions
Drug-drug. *Vaccines containing whole-cell pertussis or whole-cell typhoid antigens:* Combined endotoxin effect. Don't use together.

Adverse reactions
CNS: headache, malaise.
GU: nephropathy.
Musculoskeletal: muscle cramps.
Other: *pain, tenderness, erythema, induration* (at injection site); *anaphylaxis;* chills; fever.

Overdose and treatment
No information available.

Special considerations
• Obtain a thorough history of patient's allergies and reactions to immunizations.
• Don't give meningitis vaccine I.D., I.M., or I.V.; safety and efficacy haven't been established.
• Keep epinephrine solution 1:1,000 available to treat allergic reactions.
• Booster responses to second doses of vaccine are poor and unpredictable.

• Older children and adults in high-risk exposure areas should consider revaccination every 3 to 5 years.

• The 50-dose vial of vaccine is intended for jet injector administration only and generally shouldn't be given using syringes and needles. Discard any unused vaccine.

• Reconstitute vaccine with diluent provided. Shake until dissolved. Discard reconstituted solution after 5 days.

• Store vaccine between 36° and 46° F (2° and 8° C).

• Protective antibody levels may be achieved within 10 to 14 days after vaccination.

Patient monitoring
• Monitor patient for adverse allergic reactions.

Breast-feeding patients
• It isn't known if vaccine appears in breast milk. Use cautiously in breast-feeding women.

Pediatric patients
• Vaccine isn't recommended for children under age 2, but has been used investigationally in children ages 3 to 24 months.

• In a child age 3 to 6 months, vaccine may provide short-term protection against serotype A meningococcal disease.

• In a child as young as 6 months, vaccine may provide short-term protection against serotype C meningococcal disease.

• Children under age 4 vaccinated in high-risk exposure areas should be revaccinated 2 to 3 years after primary immunization.

Patient education
• Tell patient that pain and inflammation may occur at injection site. Recommend acetaminophen to alleviate adverse reactions, such as fever.

• Encourage patient to report distressing adverse reactions.

• Advise patient on use of contraceptives, if necessary.

• Explain that vaccine will provide immunity only to meningitis caused by one type of bacteria.

menotropins
Humegon, Pergonal

Pharmacologic classification: gonadotropin
Therapeutic classification: ovulation stimulant, spermatogenesis stimulant
Pregnancy risk category: X

Indications and dosages
➤ **Production of follicular maturation.**
Adults: 75 IU each of follicle-stimulating hormone (FSH) and luteinizing hormone (LH) I.M. daily for 9 to 12 days, followed by 10,000 USP units chorionic gonadotropin (CG) I.M. 1 day after last dose of menotropins; may repeat for two more menstrual cycles if evidence of ovulation,

but pregnancy doesn't occur. Then, if ovulation or follicular development doesn't occur, increase to 150 IU each of FSH and LH I.M. daily for 9 to 12 days, followed by 10,000 USP units CG I.M. 1 day after last dose of menotropins; may repeat for two menstrual cycles if evidence of ovulation, but pregnancy doesn't occur.

Note: If the ovaries are abnormally enlarged or if total urinary estrogen excretion is more than 100 mcg daily, or if urinary estriol excretion is more than 50 mcg daily, hold CG dose because hyperstimulation syndrome is more likely to occur.

➤ **Stimulation of spermatogenesis.** *Adults:* After 5,000 USP units of CG I.M. 3 times weekly for 4 to 6 months of treatment; 1 ampule (75 IU FSH/LH) I.M. three times weekly (given with 2,000 USP units CG twice weekly) for at least 4 months. If no improvement occurs after 4 months, treatment may continue with 75 IU FSH/LH three times weekly or 150 IU FSH/LH three times weekly. Dosage of CG doesn't change.

How supplied
Available by prescription only
Injection: 75 IU of LH and 75 IU of FSH activity per ampule; 150 IU of LH and 150 IU of FSH activity per ampule

Pharmacodynamics
Ovulation stimulant action: Drug causes growth and maturation of the ovarian follicle in women who don't have primary ovarian failure by mimicking the action of endogenous LH and FSH. Additional treatment with CG is usually required to achieve ovulation.

Spermatogenesis stimulant action: Drug causes spermatogenesis when coadministered with CG in men with primary or secondary pituitary hypofunction.

Pharmacokinetics
Absorption: Administered parenterally.
Distribution: Unknown.
Metabolism: Unknown.
Excretion: Excreted in urine.

Route	Onset	Peak	Duration
I.M.	9-12 days	Unknown	Unknown

Contraindications and precautions
Contraindicated in patients hypersensitive to drug; in women with primary ovarian failure, uncontrolled thyroid or adrenal dysfunction, pituitary tumor, abnormal uterine bleeding, uterine fibromas, or ovarian cysts or enlargement; in pregnant women; and in men with normal pituitary function, primary testicular failure, or infertility disorders other than hypogonadotropic hypogonadism.

Interactions
None reported.

Adverse reactions
CNS: *CVA,* headache, malaise, dizziness.
CV: tachycardia.
GI: nausea, vomiting, diarrhea, abdominal cramps, bloating.
GU: *ovarian enlargement with pain and abdominal distention, ovarian hyperstimulation syndrome* (sudden severe abdominal pain, distention, nausea, vomiting, weight gain, and dyspnea followed by hypovolemia, hemoconcentration, electrolyte imbalance, pleural effusion, ascites, and hemoperitoneum), ovarian cysts, ectopic pregnancy.
Musculoskeletal: musculoskeletal aches, joint pains.
Respiratory: *atelectasis, acute respiratory distress syndrome, pulmonary embolism, pulmonary infarction, arterial occlusion,* dyspnea, tachypnea.
Skin: rash.
Other: fever, multiple births, *hypersensitivity reactions, anaphylaxis,* gynecomastia, chills.

Overdose and treatment
The most common dose-related adverse effect appears to be ovarian hyperstimulation syndrome.
Drug should be discontinued. Symptomatic and supportive care measures include bed rest, fluid and electrolyte replacement, and analgesics.

Special considerations
• Drug is given only by I.M. route.
• Reconstitute drug with 1 to 2 ml of sterile saline injection. Use immediately and discard any unused portion.
• Pregnancies that follow ovulation induced with menotropins show a relatively high frequency of multiple births.
• Store drug at 37° to 86° F (3° to 30° C).

Patient monitoring
• Monitor patient at least every other day for enlarged ovaries or hyperstimulation syndrome during and for 2 weeks after therapy.

Breast-feeding patients
• Drug isn't indicated for use in breast-feeding women.

Patient education
• Teach patient signs and tests that indicate time of ovulation, such as increase in basal body temperature and increased cervical mucus.
• Warn patient to immediately report symptoms of ovarian hyperstimulation syndrome, such as abdominal distention and pain, dyspnea, and vaginal bleeding.
• Warn patient that multiple births are possible. Ectopic pregnancy and congenital malformations have been reported in pregnancies following treatment.
• Encourage daily intercourse from day before CG is given until ovulation occurs.

• Advise patient that she should be examined at least every other day for signs of excessive ovarian stimulation during therapy and for 2 weeks after treatment is discontinued.

meperidine hydrochloride (pethidine hydrochloride)
Demerol

Pharmacologic classification: opioid
Therapeutic classification: analgesic, adjunct to anesthesia
Controlled substance schedule: II
Pregnancy risk category: C

Indications and dosages
➤ *Moderate to severe pain.* *Adults:* 50 to 150 mg P.O., I.M., or S.C. q 3 to 4 hours; or continuous infusion of 15 to 35 mg/hour.
Children: 1.1 to 1.8 mg/kg P.O., I.M., or S.C. q 3 to 4 hours or 175 mg/m² daily in six divided doses. Maximum single dose for children shouldn't exceed 100 mg.
➤ *Preoperatively.* *Adults:* 50 to 100 mg I.M. or S.C. 30 to 90 minutes before surgery.
Children: 1 to 2 mg/kg I.M. or S.C. 30 to 90 minutes before surgery. Don't exceed adult dose.
➤ *Support of anesthesia.* *Adults:* Repeated slow I.V. injections of fractional doses (10 mg/ml) or continuous I.V. infusion of 1 mg/ml. Titrate dose to meet patient's needs.
➤ *Obstetric analgesia.* *Adults:* 50 to 100 mg I.M. or S.C. when pain becomes regular; may repeat at 1- to 3-hour intervals.

How supplied
Available by prescription only
Injection: 10 mg/ml, 25 mg/ml, 50 mg/ml, 75 mg/ml, 100 mg/ml
Liquid: 50 mg/5 ml
Tablets: 50 mg, 100 mg

Pharmacodynamics
Analgesic action: Meperidine is a narcotic agonist with actions and potency similar to those of morphine, with principal actions at the opiate receptors. It's recommended for the relief of moderate to severe pain.

Pharmacokinetics
Absorption: Given orally, drug is only half as effective as when given parenterally.
Distribution: Distributed widely throughout the body and is 60% to 80% bound to plasma proteins.
Metabolism: Metabolized primarily by hydrolysis in the liver to an active metabolite, normeperidine.
Excretion: About 30% is excreted in urine as the *N*-demethylated derivative; about 5% is excreted unchanged. Excretion is enhanced by acidifying the urine. Half-life of parent compound is

3 to 5 hours and the half-life of metabolite is 8 to 21 hours.

Route	Onset	Peak	Duration
P.O.	15 min	1-1½ hr	2-4 hr
I.V.	1 min	5-7 min	2-4 hr
I.M.	10-15 min	30-50 min	2-4 hr
S.C.	10-15 min	40-60 min	2-4 hr

Contraindications and precautions

Contraindicated in patients hypersensitive to drug and in those who have received MAO inhibitors within the past 14 days.

Use cautiously in geriatric or debilitated patients and in those with increased intracranial pressure, head injury, asthma, other respiratory conditions, supraventricular tachycardia, seizures, acute abdominal conditions, renal or hepatic disease, hypothyroidism, Addison's disease, urethral stricture, or prostatic hyperplasia.

Interactions

Drug-drug. *Anticholinergics:* May cause paralytic ileus. Monitor patient closely.
Cimetidine: May increase respiratory and CNS depression, causing confusion, disorientation, apnea, or seizures. Reduce meperidine dosage.
CNS depressants, such as antihistamines, barbiturates, benzodiazepines, general anesthetics, muscle relaxants, narcotic analgesics, phenothiazines, sedative-hypnotics, and tricyclic antidepressants. Potentiate respiratory and CNS depression, sedation, and hypotensive effects of drugs. Use together cautiously.
General anesthetics: Severe CV depression may result from use together. Use together cautiously.
Isoniazid: Meperidine can potentiate adverse effects of isoniazid. Avoid use together.
MAO inhibitors: May precipitate unpredictable and occasionally fatal reactions, even in patients who may receive MAO inhibitors within 14 days of receiving meperidine. Avoid use together.
Narcotic antagonist: Patients who become physically dependent on drug may experience acute withdrawal syndrome if given a narcotic antagonist. Avoid use together.
Drug-herb. *Parsley:* May promote or produce serotonin syndrome. Discourage use together.
Drug-lifestyle. *Alcohol use:* Potentiates respiratory and CNS depression, sedation, and hypotensive effects of drug. Discourage use together.

Adverse reactions

CNS: *sedation, somnolence, clouded sensorium, euphoria, dizziness,* paradoxical excitement, tremor, **seizures** (with large doses), headache, hallucinations, syncope, *light-headedness.*
CV: *hypotension,* **bradycardia,** tachycardia, **cardiac arrest, shock.**
GI: *constipation,* ileus, dry mouth, *nausea, vomiting,* biliary tract spasms.
GU: *urine retention.*

Respiratory: *respiratory depression, respiratory arrest.*
Skin: pruritus, urticaria, *diaphoresis.*
Other: physical dependence, muscle twitching, phlebitis (after I.V. delivery); pain (at injection site); local tissue irritation, induration (after S.C. injection).

Overdose and treatment

The most common signs and symptoms of meperidine overdose are CNS depression, respiratory depression, skeletal muscle flaccidity, cold and clammy skin, mydriasis, bradycardia, and hypotension. Other acute toxic effects include hypothermia, shock, apnea, cardiopulmonary arrest, circulatory collapse, pulmonary edema, and seizures.

To treat acute overdose, first establish adequate respiratory exchange via a patent airway and ventilation as needed; give a narcotic antagonist (naloxone) to reverse respiratory depression. (Because the duration of action of meperidine is longer than that of naloxone, repeated dosing is necessary.) Naloxone shouldn't be given unless the patient has clinically significant respiratory or CV depression. Monitor vital signs.

If within 2 hours of ingestion of an oral overdose, empty the patient's stomach immediately by inducing emesis (ipecac syrup) or using gastric lavage. Use cautiously to avoid risk of aspiration. Give activated charcoal via nasogastric tube for further removal of meperidine, and acidify urine to help remove drug.

Provide symptomatic and supportive treatment (continued respiratory support, correction of fluid or electrolyte imbalance). Monitor laboratory values, vital signs, and neurologic status closely.

Special considerations

● Drug may be given to patients allergic to morphine.
● Commercial preparations contain sodium metabisulfite, which may cause allergic reactions in susceptible individuals.
● Question patient carefully regarding possible use of MAO inhibitors within the past 14 days.
● Concentration of 10 mg/ml should only be used with compatible infusion device and doesn't require further dilution.
● Because drug toxicity commonly appears after several days of treatment, this drug isn't recommended for treatment of chronic pain.
● Meperidine may be given slowly through an I.V. line, preferably as a diluted solution. S.C. injection is very painful. During I.V. administration, tachycardia may occur, possibly as a result of atropine-like effects of the drug.
● Oral dose is less than half as effective as parenteral dose. Give I.M. if possible. When changing from parenteral to oral route, increase dosage.
● Syrup has local anesthetic effect. Give with water.
● Alternating meperidine with a peripherally active non-opioid analgesic, such as aspirin, acetaminophen, or an NSAID, may improve pain control while allowing lower opioid dosages.

Reactions may be *common*, uncommon, *life-threatening*, or COMMON AND LIFE-THREATENING.

• Injectable meperidine is compatible with saline and D_5W solutions and their combinations, and with lactated Ringer's and sodium lactate solutions.
• Drug increases plasma amylase or lipase levels through increased biliary tract pressure; levels may be unreliable for 24 hours after meperidine administration.

Patient monitoring
• Meperidine and its active metabolite normeperidine accumulate. Monitor patient for neurotoxic effects, especially in burn patients and those with poor renal function, sickle cell anemia, or cancer.

Breast-feeding patients
• Drug appears in breast milk; use cautiously in breast-feeding women.

Pediatric patients
• Drug shouldn't be given to infants under age 6 months.

Geriatric patients
• Lower doses are usually indicated for geriatric patients because they may be more sensitive to therapeutic and adverse effects of drug.

Patient education
• Caution patient about CNS drug effects. Warn patient to avoid driving and other potentially hazardous activities that require mental alertness until CNS effects of drug are known.
• Advise patient to avoid alcohol.
• Tell patient to take drug before pain becomes intense.

mephenytoin
Mesantoin

Pharmacologic classification: hydantoin derivative
Therapeutic classification: anticonvulsant
Pregnancy risk category: NR

Indications and dosages
➤ **Generalized tonic-clonic or complex-partial seizures.** *Adults:* 50 to 100 mg P.O. daily; may increase by 50 to 100 mg at weekly intervals. Usual maintenance dosage is 200 to 600 mg daily in three equally divided doses. Doses up to 800 mg daily may be required.
Children: Initial dose is 50 to 100 mg P.O. daily. May increase slowly by 50 to 100 mg at weekly intervals. Dosage must be adjusted individually. Usual maintenance dosage is 100 to 400 mg daily (or 3 to 15 mg/kg daily or 100 to 450 mg/m²/day) in three equally divided doses.

How supplied
Available by prescription only
Tablets: 100 mg

Pharmacodynamics
Anticonvulsant action: Like other hydantoin derivatives, mephenytoin stabilizes the neuronal membranes and limits seizure activity either by increasing efflux or by decreasing influx of sodium ions across cell membranes in the motor cortex during generation of nerve impulses. Like phenytoin, mephenytoin appears to have antiarrhythmic effects.

Mephenytoin is used for prophylaxis of tonic-clonic (grand mal), psychomotor, focal, and jacksonian-type partial seizures in patients refractory to less toxic agents. It's usually combined with phenytoin, phenobarbital, or primidone; phenytoin is preferred because it causes less sedation than barbiturates. Mephenytoin also is used with succinimides to control combined absence and tonic-clonic disorders; combined use with oxazolidinediones, paramethadione, or trimethadione isn't recommended because of the increased hazard of blood dyscrasias.

Pharmacokinetics
Absorption: Absorbed from the GI tract.
Distribution: Distributed widely throughout the body; good seizure control without toxicity occurs when serum levels of drug and major metabolite reach 25 to 40 mcg/ml.
Metabolism: Metabolized by the liver.
Excretion: Excreted in urine.

Route	Onset	Peak	Duration
P.O.	30 min	Unknown	24-48 hr

Contraindications and precautions
Contraindicated in patients with hydantoin hypersensitivity.

Interactions
Drug-drug. *Antihistamines, chloramphenicol, cimetidine, diazepam, diazoxide, disulfiram, isoniazid, phenylbutazone, oral anticoagulants, salicylates, sulfamethizole, valproate:* Therapeutic effects and toxicity of mephenytoin may be increased. Monitor patient closely.
Folic acid: Therapeutic effects of mephenytoin may be decreased. Use together cautiously.
Oral contraceptives: Decreased contraceptive effect. Recommend alternative means of contraception.
Drug-lifestyle. *Alcohol use:* May reduce therapeutic effects of drug. Discourage use together.

Adverse reactions
CNS: ataxia, *drowsiness,* fatigue, irritability, choreiform movements, depression, tremor, insomnia, dizziness.
EENT: conjunctivitis, diplopia, nystagmus, gingival hyperplasia.
GI: nausea and vomiting.
Hematologic: *leukopenia, neutropenia, agranulocytosis, thrombocytopenia,* eosinophilia, leukocytosis.
Hepatic: elevated liver function test results.

Musculoskeletal: polyarthropathy.
Respiratory: *pulmonary fibrosis.*
Skin: rash, exfoliative dermatitis, *Stevens-Johnson syndrome, fatal dermatitides.*
Other: edema, lymphadenopathy.

Overdose and treatment

Signs and symptoms of acute mephenytoin toxicity may include restlessness, dizziness, drowsiness, nausea, vomiting, nystagmus, ataxia, dysarthria, tremor, and slurred speech. Hypotension, respiratory depression, and coma may follow. Death may result from respiratory and circulatory depression.

Treat overdose with gastric lavage or emesis and follow up with supportive treatment. Carefully monitor vital signs and fluid and electrolyte balance. Forced diuresis is of little or no value. Hemodialysis or peritoneal dialysis may be helpful.

Special considerations

● Decreased alertness and coordination are most pronounced at start of treatment. Patient may need help with walking and other activities for first few days.
● Drug shouldn't be discontinued abruptly. Transition from mephenytoin to other anticonvulsant drug should progress over 6 weeks.
● When patient is receiving phenobarbital, continue phenobarbital until the transition to the other anticonvulsant is completed. Then attempt a gradual withdrawal of phenobarbital.
● Safe use of mephenytoin during pregnancy hasn't been established. Use drug during pregnancy only when clearly needed.

Patient monitoring

● CBC and platelet counts should be performed before therapy, after 2 weeks of initial therapy, and after 2 weeks on maintenance dosage; they should be repeated every month for 1 year and, subsequently, at 3-month intervals. If neutrophil count declines to 1,600 to 2,500/mm³, obtain CBC every 2 weeks.
● Discontinue drug if neutrophil count is less than 1,600/mm³.

Breast-feeding patients

● Safe use during breast-feeding hasn't been established. Alternative feeding method is recommended.

Pediatric patients

● Children usually require from 100 to 400 mg/day.

Patient education

● Tell patient never to discontinue drug or change dosage except as prescribed and to avoid alcohol, which decreases effectiveness of drug and increases sedative effects.
● Explain that follow-up laboratory tests are essential for safe use.

● Instruct patient to report unusual changes immediately (cutaneous reaction, sore throat, glandular swelling, fever, mucous membrane swelling).

meprobamate
Apo-Meprobamate*, Equanil, Meprospan-200, Meprospan-400, Miltown, Neuramate

Pharmacologic classification: carbamate
Therapeutic classification: antianxiety
Controlled substance schedule: IV
Pregnancy risk category: D

Indications and dosages

➤**Anxiety and tension.** *Adults:* 1.2 to 1.6 g P.O. daily in three or four equally divided doses. Maximum dose, 2.4 g daily (sustained-release capsules, 400 to 800 mg b.i.d.).
Children ages 6 to 12: 100 to 200 mg P.O. b.i.d. or t.i.d. Or, 25 mg/kg daily or 700 mg/m² daily in two or three divided doses. Sustained-release capsules, 200 mg b.i.d.
➤**Preoperative sedation and relief of anxiety.** *Adults:* 400 mg P.O.
Children: 200 mg P.O.

How supplied

Available by prescription only
Capsules (sustained-release): 200 mg, 400 mg
Tablets: 200 mg, 400 mg, 600 mg

Pharmacodynamics

Anxiolytic action: Cellular mechanism is unknown, but drug causes nonselective CNS depression similar to that of barbiturates. Meprobamate acts at multiple sites in the CNS, including the thalamus, hypothalamus, limbic system, and spinal cord, but not the medulla or reticular activating system.

Pharmacokinetics

Absorption: Well absorbed after oral administration. Sedation usually occurs within 1 hour.
Distribution: Distributed throughout the body; 20% is protein-bound. Drug appears in breast milk at two to four times the serum level; meprobamate crosses the placenta.
Metabolism: Metabolized rapidly in the liver to inactive glucuronide conjugates. Half-life of drug is 6 to 17 hours.
Excretion: Metabolites of drug and 10% to 20% of a single dose as unchanged drug are excreted in urine.

Route	Onset	Peak	Duration
P.O.	Unknown	Unknown	Unknown

Contraindications and precautions

Contraindicated in patients with porphyria and in those hypersensitive to meprobamate or related compounds, such as carbromal, carisoprodol, mebutamate, and tybamate. Avoid use of drug in pregnant women (during first trimester) and breast-feeding women.

Use cautiously in geriatric or debilitated patients and in those with impaired renal or hepatic function, seizure disorders, or suicidal tendencies.

Interactions
Drug-drug. *Antihistamines, barbiturates, narcotics, tranquilizers, or other CNS depressants:* Potentiated effects. Use together cautiously.
Drug-lifestyle. *Alcohol use:* Potentiated effects. Advise patient to use caution.

Adverse reactions
CNS: *drowsiness,* ataxia, dizziness, slurred speech, headache, syncope, vertigo, *seizures.*
CV: palpitations, tachycardia, hypotension, *arrhythmias.*
GI: nausea, vomiting, diarrhea.
Hematologic: *aplastic anemia, thrombocytopenia, agranulocytosis.*
Skin: pruritus, urticaria, erythematous maculopapular rash, *hypersensitivity reactions.*

Overdose and treatment
Signs and symptoms of overdose include drowsiness, lethargy, ataxia, coma, hypotension, shock, and respiratory depression.

Treatment of overdose is supportive and symptomatic, including maintaining adequate ventilation and a patent airway, with mechanical ventilation, if needed.

Treat hypotension with fluids and vasopressors as needed. Empty gastric contents by emesis or lavage if ingestion was recent, followed by activated charcoal and a cathartic. Treat seizures with parenteral diazepam. Peritoneal dialysis and hemodialysis may effectively remove drug. Serum levels of more than 100 mcg/ml may be fatal.

Special considerations
• Safety precautions are needed; such as raised bed rails, especially for geriatric patients, when starting treatment or increasing the dose. Patient may need assistance when walking.
• Drug abuse and addiction may occur.
• Withdraw drug gradually; otherwise, withdrawal symptoms may occur if patient has been taking drug for a long time. After abrupt withdrawal of long-term therapy, patient may experience severe generalized tonic-clonic seizures.
• Store drug at 59° to 86° F (15° to 30° C); it expires 2 to 5 years from date of manufacture.
• Drug may falsely elevate urinary 17-ketosteroids, 17-ketogenic steroids (as determined by the Zimmerman reaction), and 17-hydroxycorticosteroid levels (as determined by the Glenn-Nelson technique).

Patient monitoring
• Assess level of consciousness and vital signs frequently.

• Evaluate CBC periodically during long-term therapy.
• Monitor hepatic and renal function.

Breast-feeding patients
• Drug is found in breast milk at two to four times the serum level. Don't use in breast-feeding women.

Pediatric patients
• Safety hasn't been established in children under age 6.

Geriatric patients
• Geriatric patients may have more pronounced CNS effects. Use lowest dose possible.

Patient education
• Tell patient to avoid alcohol and other CNS depressants, such as antihistamines, narcotics, and tranquilizers, while taking drug, unless prescribed.
• Advise patient not to increase dose or frequency and not to abruptly discontinue or decrease dose unless prescribed.
• Tell patient to avoid tasks that require mental alertness or physical coordination until CNS effects of drug are known.
• Recommend sugarless candy or gum or ice chips to relieve dry mouth.
• Advise patient to report sore throat, fever, or unusual bleeding or bruising.
• Inform patient of potential for physical or psychological dependence with long-term use.

mercaptopurine (6-MP)
Purinethol

Pharmacologic classification: antimetabolite (specific to S phase of cell cycle)
Therapeutic classification: antineoplastic
Pregnancy risk category: D

Indications and dosages
Dosage and indications may vary. Check current literature for recommended protocols.
➤*Acute lymphoblastic leukemia (in children), chronic myelocytic leukemia.*
Adults: 2.5 mg/kg P.O. daily as a single dose, increased to 5 mg/kg daily (only if, after 4 weeks, there's no clinical improvement or signs of toxicity). Or, 80 to 100 mg/m² daily. Maintenance dosage is 1.5 to 2.5 mg/kg daily.
Children: 2.5 mg/kg P.O. daily. Or, 70 mg/m² daily. Maintenance dosage is 1.5 to 2.5 mg/kg daily.
➤*Acute myeloblastic leukemia. Adults:* 500 mg/m² daily P.O. in combination with other therapies.

How supplied
Available by prescription only
Tablets (scored): 50 mg

Pharmacodynamics

Antineoplastic action: Mercaptopurine is converted intracellularly to its active form, which exerts its cytotoxic antimetabolic effects by competing for an enzyme required for purine synthesis. This results in inhibition of DNA and RNA synthesis. Cross-resistance exists between mercaptopurine and thioguanine.

Pharmacokinetics

Absorption: Absorption after an oral dose is incomplete and variable; about 50% of a dose is absorbed. Serum levels peak in 2 hours.
Distribution: Distributes widely into total body water. Drug crosses the blood-brain barrier, but the CSF level is too low for treatment of meningeal leukemias.
Metabolism: Extensively metabolized in the liver. It appears to undergo extensive first-pass metabolism, contributing to its low bioavailability.
Excretion: Excreted in urine.

Route	Onset	Peak	Duration
P.O.	Unknown	2 hr	Unknown

Contraindications and precautions

Contraindicated in patients whose disease has shown resistance to drug. Use cautiously in pregnant patients, patients with depressed neutrophil or platelet counts after chemotherapy or radiation therapy, and patients with impaired renal or hepatic function.

Interactions

Drug-drug. *Allopurinol at doses of 300 to 600 mg daily:* Increased toxic effects of mercaptopurine, especially myelosuppression. Reduce dosage by 25% to 30% when giving with allopurinol.
Co-trimoxazole: Enhanced marrow suppression. Use together cautiously.
Hepatotoxic drugs: Increased potential for hepatotoxicity. Use together cautiously.
Warfarin: Decreased anticoagulant activity of warfarin with use together. Monitor PT and INR.

Adverse reactions

GI: *nausea, vomiting, anorexia, painful oral ulcers, diarrhea, **pancreatitis**, GI ulceration.*
Hematologic: *leukopenia, thrombocytopenia,* anemia.
Hepatic: *jaundice, **hepatotoxicity**.*
Metabolic: hyperuricemia.
Skin: rash, hyperpigmentation.

Overdose and treatment

Signs and symptoms of overdose include myelosuppression, nausea, vomiting, and hepatic necrosis.

Treatment is usually supportive and includes transfusion of blood components and antiemetics. Hemodialysis is thought to be of marginal use because of the rapid intracellular incorporation

of mercaptopurine into active metabolites with long persistence.

Special considerations

● Investigational uses include prevention of rejection of homografts, treatment of various autoimmune diseases, treatment of Crohn's disease, and treatment of chronic active hepatitis.
● Drug is sometimes called 6-mercaptopurine or 6-MP.
● Dose modifications may be required following chemotherapy or radiation therapy or if patient has depressed neutrophil or platelet counts or impaired hepatic or renal function.
● Hepatic dysfunction is reversible when drug is stopped. Watch for jaundice, clay-colored stools, and frothy dark urine, and stop drug if hepatic tenderness occurs. Monitor hepatic function during start of therapy.
● Avoid all I.M. injections when platelet count is less than 100,000/mm³.
● Store tablets at room temperature and protect from light.
● Drug may also cause falsely elevated serum glucose and uric acid values when sequential multiple analyzer is used.

Patient monitoring

● Monitor weekly blood counts; watch for precipitous decline. Hematologic adverse effects may persist for several days after the drug is discontinued.
● Monitor intake and output. Push fluids (3 L/day).
● Monitor hepatic function and hematologic values weekly during therapy.
● Monitor serum uric acid levels. If allopurinol is necessary, use very cautiously.
● Observe patient for signs of bleeding and infection.

Breast-feeding patients

● It isn't known if drug appears in breast milk. However, because of the potential for serious adverse reactions, mutagenicity, and carcinogenicity in the infant, breast-feeding isn't recommended.

Pediatric patients

● Adverse GI reactions are less common in children than in adults.

Patient education

● Warn patient that improvement may take 2 to 4 weeks or longer.
● Tell patient to continue medication despite nausea and vomiting.
● Instruct patient to immediately report vomiting that occurs shortly after taking a dose.
● Warn patient to avoid alcoholic beverages while taking drug.
● Urge patient to ensure adequate fluid intake to increase urine output and facilitate the excretion of uric acid.

Reactions may be *common*, uncommon, *life-threatening*, or COMMON AND LIFE-THREATENING.

• Advise patient to avoid exposure to people with infections. Tell patient to immediately report signs of unusual bleeding or infection.
• Advise women of childbearing age not to become pregnant while taking drug.

meropenem
Merrem IV

Pharmacologic classification: carbapenem derivative
Therapeutic classification: antibiotic
Pregnancy risk category: B

Indications and dosages
➤ *Complicated appendicitis and peritonitis caused by viridans group streptococci,* Escherichia coli, Klebsiella pneumoniae, Pseudomonas aeruginosa, Bacteroides fragilis, B. thetaiotaomicron, *and* Peptostreptococcus *sp.; bacterial meningitis caused by* Streptococcus pneumoniae, Haemophilus influenzae, *and* Neisseria meningitidis. Recommended concentration not to exceed 50 mg/ml. *Adults:* Give 1 g I.V. q 8 hours over 15 to 30 minutes as I.V. infusion or over about 3 to 5 minutes as I.V. bolus injection (5 to 20 ml).
Children age 3 months and older who weigh 50 kg (110 lb) or less: 20 mg/kg (intra-abdominal infection) or 40 mg/kg (bacterial meningitis) q 8 hours over 15 to 30 minutes as I.V. infusion or over about 3 to 5 minutes as I.V. bolus injection (5 to 20 ml). For children who weigh more than 50 kg, give 1 g q 8 hours for treating intra-abdominal infections and 2 g q 8 hours for treating meningitis.
✦ *Dosage adjustment.* In adults with renal impairment, give 1 g q 12 hours if creatinine clearance is 26 to 50 ml/minute, 500 mg q 12 hours if it's 10 to 25 ml/minute, and 500 mg q 24 hours if it's less than 10 ml/minute. There's no clinical experience in children with renal impairment.

How supplied
Available by prescription only
Powder for injection: 500 mg/15 ml, 500 mg/20 ml, 500 mg/100 ml, 1 g/15 ml, 1 g/30 ml, 1 g/100 ml

Pharmacodynamics
Antibiotic action: Meropenem inhibits cell wall synthesis in bacteria. It readily penetrates the cell wall of most gram-positive and gram-negative bacteria to reach penicillin-binding protein targets.

Pharmacokinetics
Absorption: Administered I.V.
Distribution: Distributed into most body fluids and tissues, including CSF. It's only about 2% bound to plasma protein.

Metabolism: Thought to undergo minimal metabolism. One inactive metabolite has been identified.
Excretion: Excreted unchanged primarily in urine. Elimination half-life of drug in adults with normal renal function and children age 2 and older is about 1 hour and 1½ hours in children age 3 months to 2 years.

Route	Onset	Peak	Duration
I.V.	Unknown	1 hr	Unknown

Contraindications and precautions
Contraindicated in patients hypersensitive to any component of drug or other drugs in the same class and in those who have demonstrated anaphylactoid reactions to beta-lactams. Use cautiously in patients with history of seizure disorders or impaired renal function.

Interactions
Drug-drug. *Probenecid:* Competes with meropenem for active tubular secretion and thus inhibits the renal excretion of meropenem. Avoid use together.

Adverse reactions
CNS: headache, syncope, insomnia, agitation, delirium, confusion, dizziness, *seizures,* nervousness, paresthesia, hallucinations, somnolence, anxiety, depression.
CV: *heart failure, cardiac arrest, MI, pulmonary embolism,* tachycardia, chest pain, hypertension, *bradycardia,* hypotension.
GI: diarrhea, nausea, vomiting, constipation, abdominal pain or enlargement, oral candidiasis, anorexia.
GU: dysuria, *kidney failure,* increased creatinine clearance or BUN levels, RBCs in urine.
Hematologic: bleeding events; anemia; increased or decreased platelet count; increased eosinophil count; prolonged or shortened PT, INR, or partial thromboplastin time; decreased hemoglobin or hematocrit; decreased WBC count.
Hepatic: *hepatic failure;* cholestatic jaundice; jaundice; flatulence; ileus; increased levels of ALT, AST, alkaline phosphatase, LD, and bilirubin.
Musculoskeletal: back pain.
Respiratory: *apnea, hypoxia,* respiratory disorder, dyspnea.
Skin: rash, pruritus, urticaria, sweating.
Other: *hypersensitivity reactions; anaphylaxis;* inflammation, pain, edema, phlebitis, or thrombophlebitis at injection site; pain; *sepsis; shock;* fever; peripheral edema.

Overdose and treatment
Signs and symptoms of overdose are unknown.
If overdose occurs, discontinue drug and give general supportive treatment until renal elimination occurs. Meropenem and its metabolite are readily removed by hemodialysis.

Special considerations

● Don't use drug to treat methicillin-resistant staphylococci.

● Obtain specimen for culture and sensitivity tests before giving first dose. Therapy may begin pending test results.

● Serious and occasionally fatal hypersensitivity (anaphylactoid) reactions have been reported in patients receiving therapy with beta-lactams. Before therapy starts, ascertain whether previous hypersensitivity reactions to penicillins, cephalosporins, other beta-lactams, and other allergens have occurred.

● Discontinue drug immediately if an allergic reaction occurs. Serious anaphylactoid reactions require immediate emergency treatment with epinephrine, oxygen, I.V. corticosteroids, and airway management. Other therapy may also be required as indicated by the patient's condition.

● Seizures and other CNS adverse reactions caused by meropenem therapy commonly occur in patients with CNS disorders, bacterial meningitis, and compromised renal function.

● If seizures occur during meropenem therapy, decrease dosage or discontinue meropenem.

● For I.V. bolus, add 10 ml of sterile water for injection to 500 mg/20 ml vial size or 20 ml to 1 g/30 ml vial size to provide 50 mg/ml. Shake to dissolve and let stand until clear.

● For I.V. infusion, infusion vials (500 mg/100 ml and 1 g/100 ml) may be directly reconstituted with a compatible infusion fluid to provide 2.5 to 50 mg/ml. Or, an injection vial may be reconstituted and the resulting solution added to an I.V. container and further diluted with an appropriate infusion fluid. ADD-Vantage vials shouldn't be used.

● For ADD-Vantage vials, reconstitute only with half-normal saline solution injection, normal saline solution injection, or D_5W injection in 50-, 100-, or 250-ml Abbott ADD-Vantage flexible diluent containers. Follow manufacturer guidelines closely when using ADD-Vantage vials.

● Don't mix with or physically add meropenem to solutions containing other drugs. Infuse drug over 15 to 30 minutes.

● Use freshly prepared solutions of meropenem immediately whenever possible. Stability of drug varies with type of drug used (injection vial, infusion vial, or ADD-Vantage container). Consult manufacturer's literature for details.

Patient monitoring

● Drug may cause overgrowth of nonsusceptible bacteria or fungi. Monitor patient for signs and symptoms of superinfection.

● Periodic assessment of organ system functions, including renal, hepatic, and hematopoietic, is recommended during prolonged therapy.

Breast-feeding patients

● It isn't known if drug appears in breast milk; use cautiously in breast-feeding women.

Pediatric patients

● Safety and efficacy haven't been established in children under age 3 months.

Geriatric patients

● Use cautiously in geriatric patients because of decreased renal function. Dosage adjustment is recommended in patients of advanced age whose creatinine clearance levels are less than 50 ml/minute.

Patient education

● Tell patient to report pain, inflammation, or swelling at I.V. site.

● Advise breast-feeding patient of risk of transmitting drug to infant through breast milk.

● Instruct patient to report adverse reactions or symptoms of superinfection.

mesalamine (5-aminosalicylic acid)

Asacol, Pentasa, Rowasa

Pharmacologic classification: salicylate
Therapeutic classification: anti-inflammatory
Pregnancy risk category: B

Indications and dosages

➤ *Active mild to moderate distal ulcerative colitis, proctosigmoiditis, proctitis.* Adults: 800 mg (delayed-release tablets) P.O. t.i.d. for 6 weeks or 1 g (controlled-release capsules) q.i.d. for up to 8 weeks.

Or, use 1 rectal suppository b.i.d. for 3 to 6 weeks. For maximum benefit, the suppository should be retained for 1 to 3 hours or longer. Usual dosage of mesalamine suspension enema in 60-ml units is one rectal instillation (4 g) once daily, preferably h.s., retained for about 8 hours.

Lower doses of suspension enemas of 4 g q 2 to 3 nights or 1 g daily have been effective ◇.

➤ *Maintenance of remission of ulcerative colitis* ◇. Adults: 1.6 g P.O. daily in divided doses for 6 months. Or, 60 ml (4 g) rectal suspension q 2 to 3 nights or 1 to 3 g rectal suspension daily.

How supplied

Available by prescription only
Capsules (controlled-release): 250 mg
Rectal suspension: 4 g/60 ml, in units of 7 disposable bottles
Suppositories: 500 mg
Tablets (delayed-release): 400 mg

Pharmacodynamics

Anti-inflammatory action: Unknown, but action appears to be topical rather than systemic. Mucosal production of arachidonic acid metabolites, both through cyclooxygenase pathways (such as prostaglandins) and lipoxygenase pathways (such as leukotrienes and hydroxyeicosatetraenoic acids) is increased in patients with chronic inflammatory bowel disease; possibly, mesalamine may diminish inflammation by blocking cyclooxygenase and inhibiting prostaglandin production in the colon.

Pharmacokinetics

Absorption: Drug given by rectal suppository or suspension enema is poorly absorbed from the colon. Extent of absorption depends on retention time, with considerable individual variation. Oral tablets are coated with an acrylic resin that delays the release of drug until tablet is beyond the terminal ileum. About 72% of a dose reaches the colon; 28% of a dose is absorbed. Absorption isn't affected by food. Capsules are formulated to release therapeutic levels throughout the GI tract. About 20% to 30% is absorbed.
Distribution: Maximum plasma levels of oral mesalamine and N-acetyl 5-aminosalicylic acid are about twice as high as those seen with sulfasalazine therapy. At steady state, about 10% to 30% of daily 4-g rectal dose can be recovered in cumulative 24-hour urine collections.
Metabolism: Undergoes acetylation, but site is unknown. Most absorbed drug is excreted in urine as the N-acetyl-5-aminosalicylic acid metabolite. Elimination half-life of drug is ½ to 1½ hours; half-life of acetylated metabolite is 5 to 10 hours. Steady-state plasma levels show no accumulation of either free or metabolized drug during repeated daily administrations.
Excretion: After rectal administration, drug is mostly excreted in feces as parent drug and metabolite. After oral administration, drug is mostly excreted in urine as metabolite.

Route	Onset	Peak	Duration
P.O., P.R.	Unknown	3-12 hr	Unknown

Contraindications and precautions

Contraindicated in patients hypersensitive to drug, its components (sulfite in rectal preparation), or salicylates. Use cautiously in patients with impaired renal function.

Interactions

None reported.

Adverse reactions

CNS: headache, dizziness, fatigue, malaise, asthenia, chills, anxiety, depression, hyperesthesia, paresthesia, tremor.
CV: chest pain.
GI: abdominal pain, cramps, discomfort, flatulence, diarrhea, rectal pain, bloating, nausea, *pancolitis, **pancreatitis,** vomiting, constipation, eructation.
GU: dysuria, hematuria, urinary urgency.
Musculoskeletal: arthralgia, myalgia, back pain.
Respiratory: wheezing.
Skin: itching, rash, urticaria, hair loss.
Other: fever, hypertonia.

Overdose and treatment

No information available.

Special considerations

● Drug has been used to treat Crohn's disease.
● Rectal suspension contains potassium metabisulfite, which may produce an allergic reaction in susceptible people.
● Although effects of drug may be evident in 3 to 21 days, usual course of therapy is 3 to 6 weeks depending on symptoms and sigmoidoscopic findings. Clinical studies haven't determined whether suspension enema will modify relapse rates after the 6-week, short-term treatment.

Patient monitoring

● Monitor renal function studies during therapy.

Breast-feeding patients

● It isn't known if drug or its metabolites appear in breast milk. Avoid breast-feeding during therapy.

Pediatric patients

● Safety and efficacy for use in children haven't been established.

Patient education

● Tell patient to swallow tablets whole and not to crush or chew them.
● Tell patient to retain suppository as long as possible (at least 1 to 3 hours) for maximum effectiveness.
● Instruct patient in correct use of rectal suspension:
– Shake bottle well to make sure the suspension is homogeneous.
– Remove the protective sheath from the applicator tip. Holding the bottle at the neck won't cause medication to be discharged.
– Lie on the left side (to facilitate migration into the sigmoid colon) with the lower leg extended and the upper right leg flexed forward for balance; or use the knee-chest position.
– Gently insert the applicator tip in the rectum, pointing toward the umbilicus.
– Steadily squeeze the bottle to discharge the preparation into the colon.
● Patient instructions are included with every 7 units.

mesna
Mesnex

Pharmacologic classification: thiol derivative
Therapeutic classification: uroprotectant
Pregnancy risk category: B

Indications and dosages

➤ *Prevention of ifosfamide-induced hemorrhagic cystitis. Adults:* Calculate daily dose as 60% of the ifosfamide dose. Administer in three equally divided bolus doses: Give first dose at time of ifosfamide injection. Subsequent doses are given at 4 and 8 hours following ifosfamide. Or, administer in four divided doses just before ifosfamide dose and then at 4, 8, and 12 hours after ifosfamide. Or, administer at time of ifosfamide dose and then at 3, 6, and 9 hours after ifosfamide dose.

Protocols that use 1.2 g/m² ifosfamide would employ 240 mg/m² mesna at 0, 4, and 8 hours after ifosfamide.

Continuous mesna I.V. infusion is given at 100% ifosfamide dosage and may be mixed in the same I.V. solution. Continue regimen as long as ifosfamide is given; it may have to continue for additional 8 to 24 hours as a result of shorter mesna half-life.

➤ *Prophylaxis in bone marrow recipients receiving cyclophosphamides*◇.
Adults: 60% to 160% of the cyclophosphamide daily dose given in three to five divided doses or by continuous infusion. Or, in patients receiving cyclophosphamide, 50 to 60 mg/kg I.V. daily for 2 to 4 days; give 10 mg/kg I.V. loading dose of mesna followed by 60 mg/kg by way of continuous I.V. infusion over 24 hours. Give mesna regimen with each cyclophosphamide dose and continue for an additional 24 hours.

How supplied
Available by prescription only
Injection: 100 mg/ml in 2- and 10-ml ampules

Pharmacodynamics
Uroprotectant action: Mesna disulfide is reduced to mesna in the kidney and reacts with the urotoxic metabolites of ifosfamide to detoxify the drug and protect the urinary system.

Pharmacokinetics
Absorption: Administered I.V.
Distribution: Remains in the vascular compartment; doesn't distribute through tissues.
Metabolism: Rapidly metabolized to mesna disulfide, its only metabolite.
Excretion: In the kidneys, 33% of the dose is eliminated in the urine in 24 hours; half-life of mesna and mesna disulfide are ½ and 1¼ hours, respectively.

Route	Onset	Peak	Duration
I.V.	Unknown	Unknown	Unknown

Contraindications and precautions
Contraindicated in patients hypersensitive to mesna or thiol-containing compounds.

Interactions
None reported.

Adverse reactions
Because mesna is used with ifosfamide and other chemotherapeutic drugs, it's difficult to determine adverse reactions attributable solely to mesna.
CNS: headache, fatigue.

CV: hypotension.
GI: soft stools, nausea, vomiting, diarrhea, dysgeusia.
Musculoskeletal: limb pain.
Other: *allergy.*

Overdose and treatment
No information available. There's no known antidote.

Special considerations
● The parent form of the drug has been administered orally by preparing extemporaneous oral solutions by mixing injection with flavored syrup to produce a concentration of 20 to 50 mg/ml. Solutions are stable for 7 days at 75° F (24° C). If carbonated beverage, apple juice, or orange juice is used, solution is stable for at least 24 hours at 41° F (5° C).
● Patients receiving mesna for ifosfamide-induced hemorrhagic cystitis should be adequately hydrated (2 L of oral or I.V. fluid before and during ifosfamide therapy).
● Multidose vials may be stored and used for up to 8 days.
● Discard unused mesna from open ampules. It will form an inactive oxidation product (dimesna) upon exposure to oxygen.
● Dilute appropriate dose in D₅W injection, normal saline solution injection, or lactated Ringer's injection to a level of 20 mg/ml. Once diluted, solution is stable for 24 hours at room temperature. However, the manufacturer recommends refrigerating the solution and using within 6 hours (contains no preservatives).
● Infuse I.V. solution over 15 to 30 minutes.
● Mesna is physically incompatible with cisplatin and carboplatin. Don't add mesna to cisplatin infusions.
● Store drug at 59° to 86° F (15° to 30° C); expires 5 years from date of manufacture.
● Drug may also cause falsely elevated serum glucose and uric acid values when sequential multiple analyzer is used.

Patient monitoring
● Monitor morning urine specimen for erythrocytes, which may precede hemorrhagic cystitis.

Breast-feeding patients
● It isn't known if mesna appears in breast milk.

Pediatric patients
● Safety in children hasn't been established. However, drug has been used for prophylaxis of ifosfamide-induced hemorrhagic cystitis in infants and children ages 4 to 16 and for prophylaxis of cyclophosphamide-induced hemorrhagic cystitis in children age 5 months and older.
● Multidose vials contain benzyl alcohol.

Patient education
● Instruct patient to report hematuria or allergy immediately.

Reactions may be *common*, uncommon, *life-threatening*, or COMMON AND LIFE-THREATENING.

mesoridazine besylate
Serentil

Pharmacologic classification: phenothiazine (piperidine derivative)
Therapeutic classification: antipsychotic
Pregnancy risk category: NR

Indications and dosages
➤**Schizophrenia in patients unresponsive to treatment with other antipsychotics.** *Adults:* 50 mg P.O. t.i.d. Adjust dose as needed. Total daily dose range is 100 to 400 mg P.O. daily. Or, 25 mg I.M., repeated in 30 to 60 minutes, p.r.n. Total range is 25 to 200 mg I.M. daily.
➤**Psychoneurotic effects (anxiety).** *Adults and children over age 12:* 25 mg P.O. t.i.d. Maximum, 150 mg daily.
➤**Alcoholism.** *Adults and children over age 12:* 25 mg P.O. b.i.d. Maximum, 200 mg daily.
➤**Behavioral problems from chronic brain syndrome.** *Adults and children over age 12:* 25 mg P.O. t.i.d. Maximum, 300 mg daily.

How supplied
Available by prescription only
Injection: 25 mg/ml
Oral concentrate: 25 mg/ml (0.6% alcohol)
Tablets: 10 mg, 25 mg, 50 mg, 100 mg

Pharmacodynamics
Antipsychotic action: A metabolite of thioridazine, mesoridazine is thought to exert antipsychotic effects by postsynaptic blockade of CNS dopamine receptors, thereby inhibiting dopamine-mediated effects. Drug has many other central and peripheral effects; it produces both alpha and ganglionic blockade and counteracts histamine- and serotonin-mediated activity. Its most prominent adverse reactions are antimuscarinic and sedative; it causes fewer extrapyramidal effects than other antipsychotics.

Pharmacokinetics
Absorption: Appears to be well absorbed from the GI tract following oral administration. I.M. dosage form is absorbed rapidly.
Distribution: Distributed widely into the body, including breast milk. Steady state serum level is achieved within 4 to 7 days. Drug is 91% to 99% protein-bound.
Metabolism: Metabolized extensively by the liver; no active metabolites are formed.
Excretion: Mostly excreted as metabolites in urine; some excreted in feces via biliary tract.

Route	Onset	Peak	Duration
P.O., I.M.	Unknown	2-4 hr	4-6 hr

Contraindications and precautions
Contraindicated in patients hypersensitive to drug and in those experiencing severe CNS depression or coma. Also contraindicated in patients with a history of arrhythmias or those who are predisposed to prolonged QTc interval. Contraindicated in combination with other drugs that are known to prolong the QTc interval.

Interactions
Drug-drug. *Aluminum- and magnesium-containing antacids and antidiarrheals:* Decreased absorption. Separate administration times.
Antiarrhythmics, disopyramide, procainamide, quinidine, other drugs known to prolong the QTc interval: Increased risk of arrhythmias and conduction defects. Avoid use together.
Anticholinergics, including antidepressants, antihistamines, antiparkinsonians, atropine, MAO inhibitors, meperidine, phenothiazines: Oversedation, paralytic ileus, visual changes, and severe constipation. Use together cautiously.
Beta blockers: May inhibit mesoridazine metabolism, increasing plasma levels and toxicity. Monitor patient for signs of toxicity.
Bromocriptine: Mesoridazine may antagonize therapeutic effect of bromocriptine on prolactin secretion. Use together cautiously.
Centrally acting antihypertensives, such as clonidine, guanabenz, guanadrel, guanethidine, methyldopa, reserpine: Mesoridazine may inhibit blood pressure response to these drugs. Monitor blood pressure frequently.
CNS depressants, including analgesics, anesthetics (general, spinal, epidural), barbiturates, opioids, parenteral magnesium sulfate, tranquilizers: Oversedation, respiratory depression, and hypotension. Avoid use together.
High dose dopamine: Decreased vasoconstricting effects. Monitor patient for clinical effects.
Levodopa: Decreased effectiveness and increased toxicity of levodopa. Use together cautiously.
Lithium: May result in severe neurologic toxicity with an encephalitis-like syndrome and a decreased therapeutic response to mesoridazine. Avoid use together.
Metrizamide: Increased risk of seizures. Use together cautiously.
Nitrates: Hypotension. Monitor blood pressure.
Phenobarbital: Enhanced renal excretion of mesoridazine. Monitor patient for clinical effects.
Phenytoin: Mesoridazine may inhibit metabolism and increase toxicity of phenytoin. Decrease phenytoin dosage if necessary.
Propylthiouracil: Increased risk of agranulocytosis. Monitor hemapoeitic studies.
Sympathomimetics, including ephedrine, epinephrine, and phenylephrine (often found in nasal sprays), or appetite suppressants: May decrease their stimulatory and pressor effects. Use together cautiously.
Drug-food. *Caffeine:* Increased metabolism of drug. Tell patient to use together cautiously.
Drug-lifestyle. *Alcohol use:* Additive effects. Advise patient to avoid alcohol.
Heavy smoking: Increased metabolism. Advise patient to avoid smoking.

Sun exposure: Increased risk of photosensitivity reactions. Recommend that patient use sunscreen or limit sun exposure.

Adverse reactions

CNS: extrapyramidal reactions, *tardive dyskinesia, sedation, drowsiness, tremor, rigidity, weakness, EEG changes, dizziness,* **neuroleptic malignant syndrome.**
CV: *hypotension, tachycardia, ECG changes.*
EENT: *ocular changes, blurred vision, retinitis pigmentosa, nasal congestion.*
GI: *dry mouth, constipation, nausea, vomiting.*
GU: *urine retention, menstrual irregularities, inhibited ejaculation.*
Hematologic: leukopenia, agranulocytosis, aplastic anemia, eosinophilia, **thrombocytopenia.**
Hepatic: jaundice, abnormal liver function test results.
Metabolic: weight gain, elevated test results for protein-bound iodine.
Skin: *mild photosensitivity, allergic reactions, pain at I.M. injection site, sterile abscess, rash.*
Other: *gynecomastia.*

Overdose and treatment

CNS depression is characterized by deep, unarousable sleep and possible coma, hypotension or hypertension, extrapyramidal symptoms, abnormal involuntary muscle movements, agitation, seizures, arrhythmias, ECG changes, hypothermia or hyperthermia, and autonomic nervous system dysfunction.

Treatment is symptomatic and supportive, including maintaining vital signs, airway, stable body temperature, and fluid and electrolyte balance.

Patients who have overdosed should receive immediate CV monitoring, including ECG to detect arrhythmias. Drugs such as disopyramide, procainamide, and quinidine that may produce additive QT prolongation should also be avoided in patients being treated for overdose.

Don't induce vomiting; drug inhibits cough reflex, and aspiration may occur. Use gastric lavage, then activated charcoal and saline cathartics; dialysis doesn't help. Regulate body temperature as needed. Treat hypotension with I.V. fluids; don't give epinephrine. Treat seizures with parenteral diazepam or barbiturates; arrhythmias, with parenteral phenytoin (15 mg to 18 mg/kg not exceeding 50 mg/min, with rate titrated to blood pressure); treat extrapyramidal reactions with benztropine at 1 to 2 mg or parenteral diphenhydramine at 10 to 50 mg.

Special considerations

● Protect drug from light. Slight yellowing of injection or concentrate is common and doesn't affect potency. Discard markedly discolored solutions.
● Oral liquid and parenteral forms may cause contact dermatitis. Wear gloves when preparing solutions, and avoid contact with skin and clothing.

● I.M. form is irritating. Give by deep I.M. injection, only in upper outer quadrant of buttocks. Massage slowly afterward to prevent sterile abscess. Injection may sting.
🄽 **ALERT** Watch for evidence of neuroleptic malignant syndrome (extrapyramidal effects, hyperthermia, autonomic disturbance), which is rare but commonly fatal. It isn't necessarily related to length of drug use or type of neuroleptic; however, more than 60% of affected patients are men.
● Withhold dose if jaundice, symptoms of blood dyscrasia (fever, sore throat, infection, cellulitis, weakness), or persistent extrapyramidal reactions (longer than a few hours) develop, especially in children or pregnant women.
● Don't withdraw drug abruptly unless severe adverse reactions make it necessary.
● After abrupt withdrawal of long-term therapy, gastritis, nausea, vomiting, dizziness, tremor, feeling of warmth or cold, diaphoresis, tachycardia, headache, or insomnia may occur.
🄽 **ALERT** Don't confuse Serentil with Serevent or Aventyl.
● Mesoridazine causes false-positive test results for urinary porphyrins, urobilinogen, amylase, and 5-hydroxyindoleacetic acid, because of darkening of urine by metabolites; it also causes false-positive urine pregnancy test results using human chorionic gonadotropin.

Patient monitoring

● Monitor vital signs, especially during parenteral therapy.
● Monitor hematopoietic and liver function studies.
● Obtain baseline ECG and serum potassium levels before starting treatment.
● Serum potassium level should be normalized before treatment.
● Patients with a QTc interval greater than 450 msec shouldn't receive Serentil.
● Obtain periodic ECG and serum potassium level. Discontinue drug if patient has a QTc interval greater than 500 msec.
● Monitor patient for tardive dyskinesia, which may occur after prolonged use. It may not appear until months or years later and may disappear spontaneously or persist for life, despite ending drug.

Pediatric patients

● Drug isn't recommended for children under age 12.

Patient education

● Warn patient to avoid activities that require alertness and good psychomotor coordination until CNS effects of drug are known. Tell patient that drowsiness and dizziness usually subside after a few weeks.
● Advise patient to change position slowly.
● Warn patient to avoid alcohol while taking this drug.

Reactions may be *common*, uncommon, *life-threatening*, or COMMON AND LIFE-THREATENING.

● Instruct patient to relieve dry mouth with sugarless gum or hard candy.
● Advise patient to use sunblock and to wear protective clothing to avoid photosensitivity reactions.

---

metaproterenol sulfate
Alupent, Metaprel

Pharmacologic classification: adrenergic
Therapeutic classification: bronchodilator
Pregnancy risk category: C

Indications and dosages
➤ **Bronchial asthma and reversible bronchospasm. Oral form.** *Adults and children over age 9 or who weigh more than 27 kg (60 lb):* 20 mg P.O. t.i.d. or q.i.d.
Children ages 6 to 9 or who weigh less than 27 kg: 10 mg P.O. t.i.d. or q.i.d.
Children under age 6: 1.3 to 2.6 mg/kg P.O. daily in divided doses.
Inhaled form
Adults and children age 12 and older: Administered by metered aerosol, two or three inhalations q 3 to 4 hours with at least 2 minutes between inhalations; no more than 12 inhalations in 24 hours. Administered by hand bulb nebulizer, 10 inhalations of an undiluted 5% solution or, administered by intermittent positive pressure breathing, 0.3 ml (range, 0.2 to 0.3 ml of a 5% solution diluted in about 2.5 ml of a normal saline solution or 2.5 ml of a commercially available 0.4% or 0.6% solution for nebulization).
Children ages 6 to 11: 0.1 ml (range 0.1 to 0.2 ml) of 5% solution diluted with normal saline solution to final volume of 3 ml. Administer by nebulizer.
    Note: To relieve acute bronchospasm, usually don't need to repeat more than q 4 hours. If part of bronchospastic pulmonary disease treatment regimen, administer three to four times daily.

How supplied
Available by prescription only
Aerosol inhaler: 0.65 mg/metered spray
Nebulizer inhaler: 0.4%, 0.6%, 5% solution
Syrup: 10 mg/5 ml
Tablets: 10 mg, 20 mg

Pharmacodynamics
Bronchodilator action: Metaproterenol relaxes bronchial smooth muscle and peripheral vasculature by stimulating $beta_2$-adrenergic receptors, thus decreasing airway resistance by way of bronchodilation. It has lesser effect on $beta_1$ receptors and has little or no effect on alpha-adrenergic receptors. In high doses, it may cause CNS and cardiac stimulation, resulting in tachycardia, hypertension, or tremors.

Pharmacokinetics
Absorption: Well-absorbed from the GI tract.
Distribution: Widely distributed throughout the body.
Metabolism: Extensively metabolized on first pass through the liver.
Excretion: Excreted in urine, mainly as glucuronic acid conjugates.

Route	Onset	Peak	Duration
P.O.	15 min	1 hr	1-4 hr
Inhalation	1 min	1 hr	1-2½ hr
Nebulizer	5-30 min	1 hr	1-2½ hr

Contraindications and precautions
Contraindicated in patients hypersensitive to drug or its ingredients and in those with tachycardia, arrhythmias related to tachycardia, peripheral or mesenteric vascular thrombosis, profound hypoxia, or hypercapnia. Also contraindicated during anesthesia with cyclopropane or halogenated hydrocarbon general anesthetics.
    Use cautiously in patients with hypertension, hyperthyroidism, heart disease, diabetes, or cirrhosis and in those receiving cardiac glycosides.

Interactions
Drug-drug. *Beta blockers, especially propranolol:* Antagonized bronchodilating effects of metaproterenol. Avoid use together.
Cardiac glycosides, general anesthetics (especially chloroform, cyclopropane, halothane, and trichloroethylene), levodopa, theophylline derivatives, thyroid hormones: May increase the potential for cardiac effects, including severe ventricular tachycardia, arrhythmias, and coronary insufficiency. Use together cautiously.
MAO inhibitors, tricyclic antidepressants: May potentiate their CV actions. Use together cautiously.
Sympathomimetics: May produce additive effects and toxicity. Use together cautiously.
Xanthines, other sympathomimetics, other CNS-stimulating drugs: Increased CNS stimulation. Monitor patient closely.

Adverse reactions
CNS: *nervousness, weakness, drowsiness, tremor, vertigo, headache.*
CV: *tachycardia, hypertension, palpitations, cardiac arrest.*
GI: *vomiting, nausea, heartburn, dry mouth.*
Respiratory: *paradoxical bronchiolar constriction with excessive use,* cough, dry and irritated throat.
Skin: rash, *hypersensitivity reactions.*

Overdose and treatment
Signs and symptoms of overdose include exaggeration of common adverse reactions, particularly nausea and vomiting, arrhythmias, angina, hypertension, and seizures.
    Treatment includes supportive and symptomatic measures. Monitor vital signs closely.

Support CV status. Use cardioselective beta₁-adrenergic blockers (acebutolol, atenolol, metoprolol) to treat symptoms with extreme caution; they may induce severe bronchospasm or asthmatic attack.

Special considerations

● Adverse reactions are dose-related and characteristic of sympathomimetics, and may persist a long time because of the long duration of action of metaproterenol.
● Excessive or prolonged use may lead to decreased effectiveness.
● Avoid simultaneous administration of adrenocorticoid inhalation aerosol. Allow at least 5 minutes to lapse between using the two aerosols.
● Aerosol treatments may be used with oral tablet dosing.
● Store tablets and oral solution at 59° to 86° F (15° to 30° C) in tight, light-resistant containers. Store oral inhalation and nebulizer solution at 59° to 86° F (15° to 30° C).
● Drug may reduce sensitivity of spirometry in diagnosis of asthma.

Patient monitoring

● Monitor patient for signs and symptoms of toxic effects, such as nausea and vomiting, tremors, and arrhythmias.

Pediatric patients

● Oral inhalation in children under age 12 isn't recommended because safety and efficacy haven't been established. Safety and efficacy of oral preparations in children under age 6 haven't been established.

Geriatric patients

● Geriatric patients may be more sensitive to the therapeutic and adverse effects of drug.

Patient education

● Instruct patient to use only as directed and to take no more than two inhalations at one time with 1- to 2-minute intervals between. Remind patient to save applicator; refills may be available.
● Tell patient to take missed dose if remembered within 1 hour. After 1 hour, patient should skip dose and resume regular schedule. The patient shouldn't double the dose.
● Tell patient to store drug away from heat and light, and safely out of reach of children.
● Tell patient to immediately notify prescriber if condition worsens or no relief occurs.
● Warn patient to avoid simultaneous use of adrenocorticoid aerosol and to allow at least 5 minutes to elapse between using the two aerosols.
● Tell patient that he may experience an unpleasant taste after using oral inhaler.
● Instruct patient to shake container, exhale through nose as completely as possible, administer aerosol while inhaling deeply through mouth, and hold breath for 10 seconds before exhaling

slowly. Patient should wait 1 to 2 minutes before repeating inhalations.
● Tell patient that drug may have shorter duration of action after prolonged use. Advise patient to report failure to respond to usual dose.
● Warn patient not to increase dose or frequency unless prescribed; serious adverse reactions are possible.

metaraminol bitartrate
Aramine

Pharmacologic classification: adrenergic
Therapeutic classification: vasopressor
Pregnancy risk category: C

Indications and dosages

➤ *Prevention of hypotension. Adults:* 2 to 10 mg I.M. or S.C. At least 10 minutes should elapse prior to repeat dosing.
Children: 0.1 mg/kg or 3 mg/m² S.C. or I.M.
➤ *Hypotension in severe shock. Adults:* 0.5 to 5 mg direct I.V. followed by I.V. infusion. If necessary, mix 15 to 100 mg (up to 500 mg has been used) in 500 ml normal saline solution or D₅W; titrate infusion based on blood pressure response.
Children: 0.01 mg/kg or 0.3 mg/m² direct I.V. followed by I.V. infusion (dilution of 1 mg in 25 ml of diluent) if necessary, of 0.4 mg/kg or 12 mg/m² diluted and titrated to maintain desired blood pressure.
➤ *Priapism ◊ . Adults:* 1 to 2 mg injected into corpus cavernosum of the penis.

How supplied

Available by prescription only
Injection: 10 mg/ml parenteral

Pharmacodynamics

Vasopressor action: Drug acts predominantly by direct stimulation of alpha-adrenergic receptors, which constrict both capacitance and resistance blood vessels, resulting in increased total peripheral resistance; increased systolic and diastolic blood pressure; decreased blood flow to vital organs, skin, and skeletal muscle; and constriction of renal blood vessels, which reduces renal blood flow. It also has a direct stimulating effect on beta₁ receptors of the heart, producing a positive inotropic response, and an indirect effect, releasing norepinephrine from its storage sites, which, with repeated use, may result in tachyphylaxis. Metaraminol also acts as a weak or false neurotransmitter by replacing norepinephrine in sympathetic nerve endings. Its main effects are vasoconstriction and cardiac stimulation. It doesn't usually cause CNS stimulation but may cause contraction of pregnant uterus and uterine blood vessels because of its alpha-adrenergic effects.

Pharmacokinetics
Absorption: Pressor effects may persist 20 to 90 minutes, depending on route of administration and patient variability.
Distribution: Not completely known.
Metabolism: In vitro tests suggest that drug isn't metabolized. Effects appear to be terminated by uptake of drug into tissues and by urinary excretion.
Excretion: Excreted in urine; may be accelerated by acidifying urine.

Route	Onset	Peak	Duration
I.V.	1-2 min	Unknown	20 min
I.M.	10 min	Unknown	< 90 min
S.C.	5-20 min	Unknown	< 90 min

Contraindications and precautions
Contraindicated in patients hypersensitive to drug and in those receiving anesthesia with cyclopropane and halogenated hydrocarbon anesthetics.

Use cautiously in patients with cardiac or thyroid disease, hypertension, peripheral vascular disease, cirrhosis, history of malaria, or sulfite sensitivity; in those receiving cardiac glycosides; and in pregnant patients.

Interactions
Drug-drug. *Alpha blockers:* Pressor effects may be decreased, but not completely blocked. Use together cautiously.
Atropine: Blocks the reflex bradycardia caused by metaraminol and enhances its pressor response. Use together cautiously.
Beta blockers: Mutual inhibition of therapeutic effects with increased potential for hypertension, and excessive bradycardia with possible heart block. Avoid use together.
Cardiac glycosides, general anesthetics, levodopa, maprotiline, other sympathomimetics, thyroid hormones: Increased cardiac effects may result. Use together cautiously.
Diuretics used as antihypertensives, guanadrel, guanethidine, rauwolfia alkaloids: Decreased hypotensive effects. Monitor blood pressure frequently.
Doxapram, ergot alkaloids, mazindol, methylphenidate, or trimethaphan: Pressor effects may be increased. Use together cautiously.
MAO inhibitors: May prolong and intensify cardiac stimulant and vasopressor effects. Don't administer metaraminol until 14 days after MAO inhibitors have been discontinued.

Adverse reactions
CNS: apprehension, dizziness, headache, tremor.
CV: hypertension; hypotension; palpitations; **arrhythmias,** including sinus or **ventricular tachycardia; cardiac arrest;** flushing.
GI: nausea.
Skin: diaphoresis.
Other: abscess, necrosis, sloughing with extravasation.

Overdose and treatment
Signs and symptoms of overdose include severe hypertension, arrhythmias, seizures, cerebral hemorrhage, acute pulmonary edema, and cardiac arrest.

Treatment requires discontinuation of drug followed by supportive and symptomatic measures. Monitor vital signs closely. Use atropine for reflex bradycardia and propranolol for tachyarrhythmias. Use a sympatholytic agent to relieve hypertension.

Special considerations
● Commercial preparations contain sodium bisulfite, which may cause allergic reactions in susceptible people.
● Correct blood volume depletion before administration. Metaraminol isn't a substitute for blood, plasma, fluids, or electrolyte replacement.
● Drug must be diluted before I.V. use. Preferred solutions for dilution are normal saline solution or D_5W injection. Select injection site carefully. I.V. route is preferred, using large veins. Avoid extravasation. Monitor infusion rate; use of infusion-controlling device preferred. Withdraw drug gradually; recurrent hypotension may follow abrupt withdrawal.
● When administering I.M. or S.C., allow at least 10 minutes to elapse before administering additional doses because maximum effect isn't immediately apparent.
● To treat extravasation, infiltrate site promptly with 10 to 15 ml normal saline solution containing 5 to 10 mg phentolamine, using fine needle.
● Cumulative effect possible after prolonged use. Excessive vasopressor response may persist after drug is withdrawn.
● Keep emergency drugs on hand to reverse effect of metaraminol: atropine for reflex bradycardia, phentolamine for extravasation, and propranolol for tachyarrhythmias.
● Don't mix in bag or syringe with other medications.

Patient monitoring
● Blood pressure and heart rate and rhythm should be checked during and after metaraminol administration until patient is stable.
● Monitor diabetic patients closely. Insulin adjustments may be needed.
● Fluid and electrolyte status must be monitored carefully.

Breast-feeding patients
● It isn't known if drug appears in breast milk. Use cautiously in breast-feeding women.

Pediatric patients
● Because safety hasn't been fully established, use cautiously.

Geriatric patients
● Geriatric patients may be more sensitive to effects of drug.

Patient education
- Ask patient about sulfite allergy before giving drug; vials contain sodium bisulfite.
- Inform patient that he'll need frequent assessment of vital signs.
- Advise patient to report adverse reactions.

---

metformin hydrochloride
Glucophage, Glucophage XR

Pharmacologic classification: biguanide
Therapeutic classification: antidiabetic
Pregnancy risk category: B

Indications and dosages
➤ *Adjunct to diet and exercise to lower blood glucose level in patients with non-insulin-dependent diabetes mellitus.*
Adults: If using regular-release form, initially, give 500 mg P.O. b.i.d. with morning and evening meals or 850 mg P.O. once daily with morning meal. When 500-mg dose is used, increase dose by 500 mg weekly to maximum dose of 2,500 mg daily, p.r.n. Or, 500 mg P.O. b.i.d. May be increased to 850 mg P.O. b.i.d. after 2 weeks. When 850-mg dose is used, increase dose 850 mg every other week to maximum daily dose of 2,550 mg, p.r.n. If patient needs more than 2 g daily, administer in three divided doses.

If using extended-release form, start therapy at 500 mg P.O. q.d. with the evening meal. May increase dose in weekly increments of 500 mg up to a maximum dose of 2,000 mg once daily. If higher doses are required, consider using the regular-release form up to its maximum dose.

How supplied
Available by prescription only
Tablets: 500 mg, 850 mg, 1,000 mg
Tablets (extended-release): 500 mg

Pharmacodynamics
Antidiabetic action: Drug decreases hepatic glucose production and intestinal absorption of glucose and improves insulin sensitivity (increases peripheral glucose uptake and utilization).

Pharmacokinetics
Absorption: Absorbed from GI tract with absolute bioavailability being about 50% to 60%. Food decreases the extent and slightly delays absorption.
Distribution: Negligibly bound to plasma proteins. It partitions into erythrocytes, most likely as a function of time.
Metabolism: Not metabolized.
Excretion: 90% is excreted in urine. Elimination half-life in plasma is about 6¼ hours and 17½ hours in blood.

Route	Onset	Peak	Duration
P.O.	Unknown	Unknown	Unknown

Contraindications and precautions
Contraindicated in patients hypersensitive to drug and in those with heart failure, renal disease, or metabolic acidosis. Drug should be temporarily withheld in patients undergoing radiologic studies involving parenteral administration of iodinated contrast materials because use of such products may result in acute renal dysfunction. Discontinue drug if a hypoxic state develops. Avoid use in patients with hepatic disease.

Use cautiously in geriatric, debilitated, or malnourished patients and in those with adrenal or pituitary insufficiency because of increased susceptibility to developing hypoglycemia.

Interactions
Drug-drug. *Calcium channel blockers, corticosteroids, estrogens, isoniazid, nicotinic acid, oral contraceptives, phenothiazines, phenytoin, sympathomimetics, thiazides or other diuretics, thyroid agents:* May produce hyperglycemia. Monitor patient's glycemic control. Metformin dosage may need to be increased.
Cationic drugs such as amiloride, cimetidine, digoxin, morphine, procainamide, quinidine, quinine, ranitidine, triamterene, trimethoprim, and vancomycin: Potential to compete for common renal tubular transport systems, which may increase metformin plasma levels. Monitor patient's blood glucose level.
Nifedipine: Increased metformin plasma levels. Monitor patient closely. Metformin dosage may need to be decreased.
Drug-herb. *Guar gum:* Decreased hypoglycemic effect. Monitor blood glucose levels.

Adverse reactions
GI: unpleasant or metallic taste, diarrhea, nausea, vomiting, abdominal bloating, flatulence, anorexia.
Hematologic: *megaloblastic anemia.*
Metabolic: *lactic acidosis.*
Skin: rash, dermatitis.

Overdose and treatment
Hypoglycemia hasn't been observed with ingestion of up to 85 g of metformin, although lactic acidosis has occurred. Hemodialysis may be useful for removing accumulated drug from patients in whom metformin overdose is suspected.

Special considerations
- Give drug with meals; give once-daily dose with breakfast, twice-daily dose with breakfast and dinner. For extended-release form, give daily dose with dinner.
- When transferring patients from standard oral hypoglycemic agents other than chlorpropamide to metformin, no transition period is necessary. When transferring patients from chlorpropamide, use care during the first 2 weeks because of prolonged retention of chlorpropamide in the body, increasing risk of hypoglycemia during this time.

• If patient doesn't respond to 4 weeks of maximum dose of metformin, add an oral sulfonylurea while continuing metformin at the maximum dose. If patient still doesn't respond after several months of concomitant therapy at maximum doses, discontinue both agents and start insulin therapy.
• Risk of drug-induced lactic acidosis is very low. Reported cases have occurred primarily in diabetic patients with significant renal insufficiency, multiple concomitant medical or surgical problems, and multiple concomitant medications. Risk of lactic acidosis increases with advanced age and degree of renal impairment.
• Discontinue drug immediately if patient develops conditions caused by hypoxemia or dehydration because of risk of lactic acidosis linked to these conditions.
• Suspend therapy temporarily for surgical procedures (except minor procedures not associated with restricted intake of food and fluids) or radiologic procedures involving parenteral administration of iodinated contrast, and don't restart until patient's oral intake has resumed and renal function is normal.

Patient monitoring
• Assess patient's renal function before beginning therapy and then annually thereafter. If renal impairment is detected, another antidiabetic agent should be prescribed.
• Monitor patient's blood glucose level regularly to evaluate effectiveness.
• Patient needs close monitoring during times of increased stress, such as infection, fever, surgery, or trauma. Insulin therapy may be required in these situations.
• Monitor patient's hematologic status for megaloblastic anemia. Patients with inadequate vitamin B_{12} or calcium intake or absorption appear to be predisposed to developing subnormal vitamin B_{12} levels. These patients should have serum vitamin B_{12} levels checked routinely at 2- to 3-year intervals.
• Check glycosylated hemoglobin every 3 months to monitor continued response.

Breast-feeding patients
• It isn't known if metformin appears in breast milk. Because of the potential for serious adverse effects in nursing infants, drug shouldn't be administered to breast-feeding women.

Pediatric patients
• Safety and efficacy in children haven't been established. Studies in maturity-onset diabetes of the young haven't been conducted.

Geriatric patients
• Administer cautiously to geriatric patients because they may have decreased renal function.

Patient education
• Instruct patient to discontinue drug immediately and report unexplained hyperventilation, myalgia, malaise, unusual somnolence, or other nonspecific symptoms of early lactic acidosis.
• Warn patient not to consume excessive amounts of alcohol while taking metformin.
• Instruct patient about nature of diabetes and importance of following therapeutic regimen; adhering to specific diet, weight reduction, exercise and personal hygiene programs; and avoiding infection. Explain how and when to monitor blood glucose level, and teach recognition of hypoglycemia and hyperglycemia.
• Tell patient not to change drug dosage without medical approval. Encourage him to report abnormal blood glucose levels.
• Advise patient not to take other medications, including OTC drugs, without medical approval.
• Instruct patient to carry medical identification regarding diabetic status.

methadone hydrochloride
Dolophine, Methadose, Physeptone*

Pharmacologic classification: opioid
Therapeutic classification: analgesic, narcotic detoxification adjunct
Controlled substance schedule: II
Pregnancy risk category: C

Indications and dosages
➤ **Severe pain.** *Adults:* 2.5 to 10 mg P.O., I.M., or S.C. q 3 to 4 hours, p.r.n., or around-the-clock. *Children* ◊: 0.7 mg/kg P.O. q 4 to 6 hours
➤ **Relief of severe, chronic pain.** *Adults:* 5 to 20 mg P.O. q 6 to 8 hours.
➤ **Narcotic abstinence syndrome.** *Adults:* 15 to 20 mg P.O. daily (highly individualized).
   Maintenance dosage is 20 to 120 mg P.O. daily. Adjust dose, p.r.n. Daily doses above 120 mg require special state and federal approval. If patient feels nauseated, give one-fourth of total P.O. dose in two injections, S.C. or I.M. Treatment is 30 (short-term) to 180 (long-term) days.

How supplied
Available by prescription only
Injection: 10 mg/ml
Oral solution: 5 mg/5 ml, 10 mg/5 ml, 10 mg/ml (concentrate)
Tablets: 5 mg, 10 mg, 40 mg for oral solution (for narcotic abstinence syndrome)

Pharmacodynamics
Analgesic action: Methadone is an opiate agonist that has analgesic activity via an affinity for the opiate receptors similar to that of morphine. It's recommended for severe, chronic pain and is also used in detoxification and maintenance of patients with opiate abstinence syndrome.

Pharmacokinetics
Absorption: Well absorbed from the GI tract. Oral administration delays onset and prolongs duration of action as compared to parenteral administration.
Distribution: Highly bound to tissue protein, which may explain its cumulative effects and slow elimination.
Metabolism: Metabolized primarily in the liver by N-demethylation.
Excretion: Half-life is prolonged (7 to 11 hours) in patients with hepatic dysfunction. Urinary excretion, the major route, is dose-dependent. Methadone metabolites are also excreted in the feces via the bile.

Route	Onset	Peak	Duration
P.O.	½-1 hr	½-2 hr	4-6 hr
I.M.	10-20 min	1-2 hr	4-5 hr

Contraindications and precautions
Contraindicated in patients hypersensitive to drug. Use cautiously in geriatric or debilitated patients and in those with severe renal or hepatic impairment, acute abdominal conditions, hypothyroidism, Addison's disease, prostatic hyperplasia, urethral stricture, head injury, increased intracranial pressure, asthma, or other respiratory disorders.

Interactions
Drug-drug. *CNS depressants, such as antidepressants, antihistamines, barbiturates, benzodiazepines, general anesthetics, muscle relaxants, narcotic analgesics, phenothiazines, and sedative-hypnotics:* Potentiated respiratory and CNS depression, sedation, and hypotensive effects. Use together cautiously.
Cimetidine: Increased respiratory and CNS depression, causing confusion, disorientation, apnea, or seizures. Such use usually requires reduced dosage of methadone.
Opioid antagonists: Patients who become physically dependent on methadone may experience acute withdrawal syndrome if given these drugs. Use cautiously, and monitor patient closely.
Rifampin: May reduce blood level of methadone. Monitor patient.
Drug-lifestyle. *Alcohol use:* Potentiated respiratory and CNS depression, sedation, and hypotensive effects. Discourage use together.

Adverse reactions
CNS: *sedation, somnolence, clouded sensorium, euphoria, dizziness, choreic movements, seizures,* headache, insomnia, agitation, *lightheadedness,* syncope.
CV: *hypotension,* **bradycardia, shock, cardiac arrest,** palpitations, edema.
EENT: visual disturbances.
GI: *nausea, vomiting, constipation, ileus, dry mouth, anorexia, biliary tract spasm,* increased plasma amylase levels.
GU: *urine retention.*

Respiratory: *respiratory depression, respiratory arrest.*
Skin: *diaphoresis,* pruritus, urticaria.
Other: physical dependence, pain at injection site, tissue irritation and induration after S.C. injection, *decreased libido.*

Overdose and treatment
The most common signs and symptoms of overdose are CNS depression, respiratory depression, and miosis (pinpoint pupils). Others include hypotension, bradycardia, hypothermia, shock, apnea, cardiopulmonary arrest, circulatory collapse, pulmonary edema, and seizures. Toxicity may result from accumulation of drug over several weeks.

To treat acute overdose, first establish adequate respiratory exchange by way of a patent airway and ventilation as needed; administer an opioid antagonist (naloxone) to reverse respiratory depression. Because the duration of action of methadone is longer than that of naloxone, repeated naloxone dosing is necessary. The antagonist naloxone shouldn't be given unless the patient has clinically significant respiratory or CV depression. Monitor vital signs closely.

If patient is seen within 2 hours of ingestion of an oral overdose, empty the stomach immediately by inducing emesis (ipecac syrup) or using gastric lavage. Use cautiously to avoid risk of aspiration. Administer activated charcoal through nasogastric tube for further removal of drug in an oral overdose.

Provide symptomatic and supportive treatment (continued respiratory support, correction of fluid or electrolyte imbalance). Monitor laboratory values, vital signs, and neurologic status closely.

Special considerations
Consider the recommendations relevant to all opioids as well as the following.
• Verify that patient is in a methadone maintenance program for management of narcotic addiction and, if so, at what dosage, and continue that program appropriately.
• Dispersible tablets may be dissolved in 4 oz (120 ml) of water or fruit juice; oral concentrate must be diluted to at least 30 ml, but when used for detoxification, must be diluted with at least 3 oz (90 ml) of water before use.
⚑ ALERT Diluents used for diluting methadone and levomethadyl acetate should differ in color and taste to avoid confusion.
• Oral liquid form (not tablet form) is legally required and is the only form available in drug maintenance programs.
• Regimented scheduling (around-the-clock) is beneficial in severe, chronic pain. Tolerance may develop with long-term use, requiring a higher dose to achieve the same degree of analgesia.
• Patient treated for narcotic abstinence syndrome usually requires an additional analgesic if pain control is necessary.

Reactions may be *common*, uncommon, ***life-threatening***, or COMMON AND LIFE-THREATENING.

• Physical and psychological tolerance or dependence may occur. Be aware of potential for abuse.

Patient monitoring
• Patient requires observation for increased sedation, respiratory depression, stabilization of symptoms of withdrawal, and pain relief.

Breast-feeding patients
• Methadone appears in breast milk; it may cause physical dependence in breast-feeding infants of women on methadone maintenance therapy.

Pediatric patients
• Drug isn't recommended for use in children. Safe use as maintenance drug in adolescent addicts hasn't been established.

Geriatric patients
• Lower doses are usually indicated for geriatric patients because they may be more sensitive to the therapeutic and adverse effects of drug.

Patient education
• If appropriate, tell patient that constipation is often severe during maintenance with methadone. Instruct him to take a stool softener or other laxative.

• Caution patient to avoid activities that require full alertness, such as driving and operating machinery, because of potential for drowsiness.

methamphetamine hydrochloride
Desoxyn, Desoxyn Gradumets

Pharmacologic classification: amphetamine
Therapeutic classification: CNS stimulant, short-term adjunctive anorexigenic agent, sympathomimetic amine
Controlled substance schedule: II
Pregnancy risk category: C

Indications and dosages
➤ *Attention deficit hyperactivity disorder.* Children age 6 and older: Initially, 5 mg P.O. once daily or b.i.d., with 5-mg increments weekly, p.r.n. Usual effective dose is 20 to 25 mg daily.
➤ *Short-term adjunct in exogenous obesity.* Adults: 2.5 to 5 mg P.O. b.i.d. to t.i.d. 30 minutes before meals or 10 to 15 mg daily (extended-release) P.O. in morning. Don't use for more than a few weeks.

How supplied
Available by prescription only
Tablets: 5 mg
Tablets (extended-release): 5 mg, 10 mg, 15 mg

Pharmacodynamics
CNS stimulant action: Amphetamines are sympathomimetic amines with CNS stimulant activi-ty; in hyperactive children, they have a paradoxical calming effect.
Anorexigenic action: Anorexigenic effects are thought to occur in the hypothalamus, where decreased smell and taste acuity decreases appetite; they may involve other systemic and metabolic effects. They may be tried for short-term control of refractory obesity, with calorie restriction and behavior modification.

The cerebral cortex and reticular activating system appear to be the primary sites of activity; amphetamines release nerve terminal stores of norepinephrine, promoting nerve impulse transmission. At high dosages, effects are mediated by dopamine.

Amphetamines are used to treat narcolepsy and as adjuncts to psychosocial measures in attention deficit hyperactivity disorder in children. The precise mechanisms of action in these conditions are unknown.

Pharmacokinetics
Absorption: Rapidly absorbed from the GI tract after oral administration.
Distribution: Widely distributed throughout the body. Drug crosses the placenta and enters breast milk.
Metabolism: Metabolized in the liver to at least seven metabolites.
Excretion: Excreted in urine.

Route	Onset	Peak	Duration
P.O.	Unknown	Unknown	24 hr

Contraindications and precautions
Contraindicated in patients hypersensitive to sympathomimetic amines, patients with idiosyncratic reactions to them, agitated patients, patients who have taken an MAO inhibitor within 14 days, patients with a history of drug abuse, and patients with moderate to severe hypertension, hyperthyroidism, symptomatic CV disease, advanced arteriosclerosis, or glaucoma.

Use cautiously in geriatric, debilitated, asthenic, or psychopathic patients and in those with history of suicidal or homicidal tendencies.

Interactions
Drug-drug. Acetazolamide, antacids, sodium bicarbonate: Enhanced reabsorption of methamphetamine and prolonged duration of action. Monitor patient closely.
Antihypertensives: Possible antagonized antihypertensive effects. Monitor patient closely.
Ascorbic acid: Enhanced methamphetamine excretion and shortened duration of action. May need to increase methamphetamine dose.
Barbiturates: Antagonized methamphetamine by CNS depression. Avoid use together.
CNS stimulants: Additive effects. Avoid use together.
General anesthesia: Increased risk of arrhythmias. Monitor patient closely.

Haloperidol, phenothiazines: Decreased methamphetamine effects. Monitor patient closely.
Insulin: Drug may alter insulin requirements. Monitor serum glucose.
MAO inhibitors (or drugs with MAO-inhibiting activity, such as furazolidone) or within 14 days of such therapy: May cause hypertensive crisis. Avoid use together.
Drug-herb. *Melatonin:* Enhanced monoaminergic effects of methamphetamine and possible worsened insomnia. Discourage use together.
Drug-food. *Caffeine:* Additive effects. Discourage use together.

Adverse reactions
CNS: *nervousness, insomnia, irritability,* talkativeness, dizziness, headache, hyperexcitability, tremor, euphoria.
CV: hypertension, *tachycardia, palpitations, arrhythmias.*
EENT: blurred vision, mydriasis.
GI: dry mouth, metallic taste, diarrhea, constipation, anorexia.
GU: impotence.
Metabolic: elevated plasma corticosteroid levels.
Skin: urticaria.
Other: altered libido.

Overdose and treatment
Signs and symptoms of overdose include increasing restlessness, tremor, hyperreflexia, tachypnea, confusion, aggressiveness, hallucinations, and panic. Fatigue and depression usually follow the excitement stage. Other symptoms may include arrhythmias, shock, alterations in blood pressure, nausea, vomiting, diarrhea, and abdominal cramps. Death is usually preceded by seizures and coma.

Treat overdose symptomatically and supportively. If ingestion was recent (within 4 hours), use gastric lavage or emesis and sedate with barbiturate; monitor vital signs and fluid and electrolyte balance. I.V. phentolamine is suggested for treatment of severe acute hypertension. Chlorpromazine is useful in decreasing CNS stimulation and sympathomimetic effects. Urine acidification may enhance excretion. Saline catharsis (magnesium citrate) may hasten GI evacuation of unabsorbed long-acting forms. Hemodialysis or peritoneal dialysis may be effective in severe cases.

Special considerations
● Drug isn't recommended for first-line treatment of obesity.
● Don't crush long-acting forms.
● Rapid withdrawal after prolonged use may lead to depression, somnolence, and increased appetite.

Patient monitoring
● When treating behavioral disorders in children, consider a periodic discontinuation of the drug to evaluate effectiveness and the need for continued therapy.

Breast-feeding patients
● Amphetamines appear in breast milk. An alternative method of feeding should be used.

Pediatric patients
● Drug isn't recommended for weight reduction in children under age 12.

Geriatric patients
● Geriatric or debilitated patients may be especially sensitive to effects of methamphetamine. Use drug cautiously.

Patient education
● Warn patient that potential for abuse is high. Discourage use to combat fatigue.
● Advise patient to avoid caffeine-containing drinks and alcohol, to take drug 1 hour before next meal, and to take last daily dose at least 6 hours before bedtime to prevent insomnia. Sustained-release (long-acting) forms should be taken at the start of the day.
● Warn patient not to increase dosage unless prescribed.
● Inform patient that methamphetamine may impair ability to engage in potentially hazardous activities, such as operating machinery or driving a motor vehicle.

methimazole
Tapazole

Pharmacologic classification: thyroid hormone antagonist
Therapeutic classification: antihyperthyroid
Pregnancy risk category: D

Indications and dosages
➤ **Hyperthyroidism, preparation for thyroidectomy, thyrotoxic crisis.** *Adults:* 15 mg P.O. daily if mild; 30 to 40 mg P.O. daily if moderately severe; 60 mg P.O. daily if severe. All are given in three equally divided doses q 8 hours. Continue until patient is euthyroid; then start maintenance dosage of 5 to 15 mg daily. Continue initial dosage for 2 months.
Children: 0.4 mg/kg daily P.O. divided q 8 hours. Continue until patient is euthyroid; then start maintenance dosage of 0.2 mg/kg daily divided q 8 hours.

How supplied
Available by prescription only
Tablets: 5 mg, 10 mg

Pharmacodynamics
Antithyroid action: In treating hyperthyroidism, methimazole inhibits synthesis of thyroid hormone by interfering with the incorporation of iodide into tyrosyl. Methimazole also inhibits the

formation of iodothyronine. As preparation for thyroidectomy, methimazole inhibits synthesis of the thyroid hormone and causes a euthyroid state, reducing surgical problems during thyroidectomy; as a result, the mortality for a single-stage thyroidectomy is low. Iodide reduces the vascularity of the gland, making it less friable. For treating thyrotoxic crisis (thyrotoxicosis), propylthiouracil theoretically is preferred over methimazole because it inhibits peripheral deiodination of thyroxine to triiodothyronine.

Pharmacokinetics
Absorption: Absorbed rapidly from the GI tract (80% to 95% bioavailable).
Distribution: Readily crosses the placenta and is distributed into breast milk. Drug is concentrated in the thyroid, and isn't protein-bound.
Metabolism: Undergoes hepatic metabolism.
Excretion: About 80% of drug and its metabolites are excreted renally; 7% is excreted unchanged. Half-life is between 5 and 13 hours.

Route	Onset	Peak	Duration
P.O.	Rapid	½-1 hr	Unknown

Contraindications and precautions
Contraindicated in patients hypersensitive to drug and in breast-feeding women. Use cautiously in pregnant women.

Interactions
Drug-drug. *Adrenocorticoids, corticotropin, propylthiouracil:* May require a dosage adjustment of the steroid when thyroid status changes. Monitor patient carefully.
Anticoagulants: Antivitamin K action of methimazole potentiates the action of anticoagulants. Monitor PT and INR.
Bone marrow depressants: Increased risk of agranulocytosis. Monitor CBC.
Hepatotoxic drugs: Increased risk of hepatotoxicity. Monitor liver function tests. Use together cautiously.
Iodinated glycerol, lithium, potassium iodide: May potentiate hypothyroid and goitrogenic effects. Use together cautiously.

Adverse reactions
CNS: headache, drowsiness, vertigo, paresthesia, neuritis, neuropathies, CNS stimulation, depression.
GI: diarrhea, nausea, vomiting (may be dose-related), salivary gland enlargement, loss of taste, epigastric distress.
GU: nephritis.
Hematologic: *agranulocytosis, leukopenia, thrombocytopenia, aplastic anemia.*
Hepatic: jaundice, hepatic dysfunction, ***hepatitis.***
Metabolic: hypothyroidism.
Musculoskeletal: arthralgia, myalgia.

Skin: rash, urticaria, discoloration, pruritus, erythema nodosum, exfoliative dermatitis, lupus-like syndrome.
Other: fever, lymphadenopathy.

Overdose and treatment
Signs and symptoms of overdose include nausea, vomiting, epigastric distress, fever, headache, arthralgia, pruritus, edema, and pancytopenia.

Treatment is supportive; perform gastric lavage or induce emesis, if possible. If bone marrow depression develops, fresh whole blood, corticosteroids, and anti-infectives may be required.

Special considerations
● Best response occurs if dosage is administered around-the-clock and given at the same time each day with respect to meals.
● Doses of more than 40 mg daily increase the risk of agranulocytosis.
● A beta blocker, most often propranolol, is given to manage the peripheral signs of hyperthyroidism, primarily tachycardia.
● Euthyroid state may take several months to develop.
● Sulfonamide-type adverse reactions can occur.

Patient monitoring
● Monitor CBC in patients with signs and symptoms of illness.
● Monitor liver function tests, especially if hepatic dysfunction is suspected.

Pregnant patients
● Drug can induce goiter and hypothyroidism in developing fetus. Manufacturer states that drug may be used judiciously to treat hyperthyroidism during pregnancy.

Breast-feeding patients
● Patient should discontinue breast-feeding before beginning therapy because drug appears in breast milk. However, if breast-feeding is necessary, propylthiouracil is the preferred antithyroid agent.

Patient education
● Tell patient to take drug at regular intervals around-the-clock and to take it at the same time each day in relation to meals.
● If GI upset occurs, advise patient to take drug with meals.
● Tell patient to promptly report fever, sore throat, malaise, unusual bleeding, yellowing of eyes, nausea, or vomiting.
● Advise patient not to store drug in bathroom; heat and humidity cause it to deteriorate.
● Tell patient to inform other health care providers of drug use.
● Teach patient how to recognize the signs of hyperthyroidism and hypothyroidism and what to do if they occur.

methocarbamol
Robaxin

Pharmacologic classification: carbamate derivative of guaifenesin
Therapeutic classification: skeletal muscle relaxant
Pregnancy risk category: C

Indications and dosages

➤*Adjunct in acute, painful musculoskeletal conditions. Adults:* 1.5 g P.O. q.i.d. for 2 to 3 days. Maintenance dosage, 4 to 4.5 g P.O. daily in three to six divided doses. Or, 1 g I.M. or I.V. For severe conditions, I.M. or I.V. doses may be administered at 8-hour intervals. Maximum dosage, 3 g daily I.M. or I.V. for 3 consecutive days. Patient may resume I.M. or I.V. use after drug-free interval of 2 days.

➤*Supportive therapy in tetanus management. Adults:* 1 to 2 g I.V. push (300 mg/minute) and an additional 1 to 2 g may be added to I.V. solution. Total initial I.V. dosage, 3 g. Repeat I.V. infusion of 1 to 2 g q 6 hours until nasogastric tube can be inserted. Total adult P.O. dose may be up to 24 g daily to manage tetanus. *Children:* 15 mg/kg or 500 mg/m² I.V. Don't inject faster than 180 mg/m²/minute. May be repeated q 6 hours, if necessary, to total dosage of 1.8 g/m² daily for 3 consecutive days.

How supplied
Available by prescription only
Injection: 100 mg/ml parenteral in 10 ml vial
Tablets: 500 mg, 750 mg
Tablets (film-coated): 500 mg, 750 mg

Pharmacodynamics
Skeletal muscle relaxant action: Drug doesn't relax skeletal muscle directly. Its effects appear to be related to its sedative action; however, the exact mechanism of action is unknown.

Pharmacokinetics
Absorption: Rapidly and completely absorbed from the GI tract.
Distribution: Widely distributed throughout the body.
Metabolism: Extensively metabolized in liver by way of dealkylation and hydroxylation. Half-life of drug is between 1 and 2 hours.
Excretion: Rapidly and almost completely excreted in urine, mainly as its glucuronide and sulfate metabolites (40% to 50%), as unchanged drug (10% to 15%), and the rest as unidentified metabolites.

Route	Onset	Peak	Duration
P.O.	30 min	2 hr	Unknown
I.V.	Immediate	Immediate	Unknown
I.M.	Unknown	Unknown	Unknown

Contraindications and precautions
Contraindicated in patients hypersensitive to drug and in those with impaired renal function (injectable form) or seizure disorder (injectable form). Safe use of methocarbamol in regard to fetal development hasn't been established. Therefore, drug shouldn't be used in women who are or may become pregnant, especially during early pregnancy, unless the benefits outweigh the possible hazards.

Interactions
Drug-drug. *Anticholinesterase drugs:* In patients with myasthenia gravis, severe weakness may result if given methocarbamol. Avoid use together.
CNS depressants, including anxiolytics, narcotics, psychotics, and tricyclic antidepressants: May cause additive CNS depression. Use together cautiously.
Drug-lifestyle. *Alcohol use:* May cause additive CNS depression. Discourage use together.

Adverse reactions
CNS: drowsiness, dizziness, light-headedness, headache, syncope, mild muscular incoordination with I.M. or I.V. use, *seizures* with I.V. use, vertigo.
CV: flushing, hypotension, *bradycardia* with I.M. or I.V. use.
EENT: blurred vision, conjunctivitis, nystagmus, diplopia.
GI: nausea, GI upset, metallic taste.
GU: hematuria with I.V. use, discoloration of urine.
Skin: urticaria, pruritus, rash.
Other: thrombophlebitis, extravasation with I.V. use, fever, *anaphylaxis* with I.M. or I.V. use.

Overdose and treatment
Signs and symptoms of overdose include extreme drowsiness, nausea, vomiting, and arrhythmias.

Treatment includes symptomatic and supportive measures. If ingestion was recent, empty stomach by emesis or gastric lavage (may reduce absorption). Maintain adequate airway. Monitor urine output and vital signs, and administer I.V. fluids, if needed.

Special considerations
• Don't administer S.C. Give I.V. undiluted at no more than 300 mg per minute. May also be given by I.V. infusion after diluting in D₅W or normal saline solution.
• For I.V. administration, dilute 1 g of drug with up to 250 ml of D₅W or normal saline solution injection. Don't refrigerate I.V. solution because precipitate and haze may occur.
• Methocarbamol solutions containing 4 mg/ml in sterile water for injection, 5% dextrose, or normal saline solution injection are stable for 6 days at room temperature.
• Inspect all solutions before administration for particles and haze.
• Patient should be supine during and for at least 10 to 15 minutes after I.V. injection.

- To give via nasogastric tube, crush tablets and suspend in water or normal saline solution.
- When used in tetanus, follow manufacturer's instructions.
- Patient's urine may turn black, blue, brown, or green if left standing.
- Patient will need assistance with walking after parenteral administration.
- Extravasation of I.V. solution may cause thrombophlebitis and sloughing from hypertonic solution.
- Oral administration should replace parenteral use as soon as feasible.
- Adverse reactions after oral administration are usually mild and transient and subside with dosage reduction.
- For I.M. administration, don't give more than 500 mg in each gluteal region.
- Store at 59° to 86° F (15° to 30° C). Avoid freezing injection.
- Methocarbamol therapy alters results of laboratory tests for urine 5-hydroxyindoleacetic acid using quantitative method of Udenfriend (false-positive) and for urine vanillylmandelic acid (false-positive when Gitlow screening test used; no problem when quantitative method of Sunderman used).

Patient monitoring
- Monitor vital signs during I.V. or I.M. administration.

Breast-feeding patients
- Drug appears in breast milk in small amounts. Patient shouldn't breast-feed during treatment.

Pediatric patients
- For children under age 12, use only as recommended for tetanus.

Geriatric patients
- Lower doses are indicated, because geriatric patients are more sensitive to effects of drug.

Patient education
- Tell patient urine may turn black, blue, green, or brown.
- Warn patient that drug may cause drowsiness. Patient should avoid hazardous activities that require alertness until degree of CNS depression can be determined.
- Advise patient to change positions slowly, particularly from recumbent to upright, and to dangle legs before standing.
- Advise patient to avoid alcoholic beverages and use OTC cold or cough preparations carefully because some contain alcohol.
- Tell patient to store drug away from heat and light (not in bathroom medicine cabinet) and safely out of reach of children.
- Tell patient to take missed dose if remembered within 1 hour. After 1 hour, patient should skip that dose and resume regular schedule. He shouldn't double the dose.

methotrexate, methotrexate sodium
Folex, Mexate, Mexate-AQ, Rheumatrex Dose Pack

Pharmacologic classification: antimetabolite (specific to S phase of cell cycle)
Therapeutic classification: antineoplastic
Pregnancy risk category: X

Indications and dosages
Dosage and indications may vary. Check current literature for recommended protocols.
➤ *Trophoblastic tumors (choriocarcinoma, hydatidiform mole).* *Adults:* 15 to 30 mg P.O. or I.M. daily for 5 days. Repeat after 1 or more weeks, according to response or toxicity.
Adults◇: 10 to 15 mg via the hypogastric artery until toxicity or therapeutic response occurs; 3 to 5 courses are usually needed.
➤ *Acute lymphoblastic leukemia.* *Adults and children:* 3.3 mg/m² P.O. daily for 4 to 6 weeks or until remission occurs; then 20 to 30 mg/m² P.O. or I.M. twice weekly or 2.5 mg/kg I.V. q 14 days. (Used with prednisone.)
➤ *Prophylaxis against meningeal leukemia.* 12 mg/m² or 15 mg intrathecally. Consult specific references for intervals and dosing.
➤ *Meningeal leukemia.* *Adults and children:* 12 mg/m² intrathecally to a maximum dose of 15 mg q 2 to 5 days until CSF is normal. Or, 12 mg/m² once weekly for 2 weeks; then once monthly. Use only vials of powder with no preservatives; dilute using normal saline solution injection without preservatives. Use only new vials of drug and diluent. Use immediately after reconstitution.
➤ *Burkitt's lymphoma (stage I or II).* *Adults:* 10 to 25 mg P.O. daily for 4 to 8 days with 7- to 10-day rest intervals.
➤ *Lymphosarcoma (stage III; malignant lymphoma).* *Adults:* 0.625 to 2.5 mg/kg daily P.O., I.M., or I.V.
➤ *Mycosis fungoides (advanced).* *Adults:* 2.5 to 10 mg P.O. daily or 50 mg I.M. weekly; or 25 mg I.M. twice weekly for several weeks to months.
➤ *Psoriasis (severe).* *Adults:* Initially, a 5- to 10-mg test dose should be given 1 week before therapy. Then, 2.5 to 5 mg P.O. at 12-hour intervals for three doses each week or at 8-hour intervals for four doses each week. May increase by 2.5 mg/week, not to exceed 25 to 30 mg/week. Or, 10 to 25 mg P.O., I.M., or I.V. as single weekly dose. May increase by 2.5 to 5 mg/week, not to exceed 50 mg/week. Or, 2.5 mg P.O. daily for 5 days followed by a 2-day rest period. Dosage shouldn't exceed 6.25 mg/day. Improvement within 4 weeks should be noted with optimum results in 2 to 3 months.
➤ *Rheumatoid arthritis (severe, refractory).* *Adults:* 7.5 to 20 mg weekly P.O. in single or divided doses.
Adults◇: 7.5 to 15 mg I.M. once weekly.

◇ Unlabeled clinical use

➤*Adjunct treatment in osteosarcoma.*
Adults: Give 12 g/m² as a 4-hour I.V. infusion.
➤*Head and neck carcinoma* ◊. *Adults:* 40 to 60 mg/m² I.V. once weekly. Response limited to 4 months.

How supplied
Available by prescription only
Injection: 20-mg, 25-mg, 50-mg, 100-mg, 250-mg, 1-g vials, lyophilized powder, preservative-free; 25-mg/ml vials, preservative-free solution; 2.5-mg/ml, 25-mg/ml vials, lyophilized powder, preserved
Tablets (scored): 2.5 mg

Pharmacodynamics
Antineoplastic action: Methotrexate exerts its cytotoxic activity by tightly binding with dihydrofolic acid reductase, an enzyme crucial to purine metabolism, resulting in an inhibition of DNA, RNA, and protein synthesis.

Pharmacokinetics
Absorption: Absorption across the GI tract appears to be dose-related. Lower doses are essentially completely absorbed, while absorption of larger doses is incomplete and variable. I.M. doses are absorbed completely.
Distribution: Distributed widely throughout the body, with the highest levels found in the kidneys, gallbladder, spleen, liver, and skin. Drug crosses the blood-brain barrier but doesn't achieve therapeutic levels in the CSF. About 50% of the drug is bound to plasma protein.
Metabolism: Metabolized slightly in the liver.
Excretion: Excreted primarily into urine as unchanged drug. Elimination has been described as biphasic, with a first phase half-life averaging 1½ to 3½ hours and a terminal phase half-life of 8 to 15 hours.

Route	Onset	Peak	Duration
P.O.	Unknown	1-2 hr	Unknown
I.V.	Unknown	Immediate	Unknown
I.M.	Unknown	½-1 hr	Unknown
Intra-thecal	Unknown	Unknown	Unknown

Contraindications and precautions
Contraindicated in patients hypersensitive to drug and patients who are pregnant or breast-feeding. Also contraindicated in patients with psoriasis or rheumatoid arthritis who also have alcoholism, alcoholic liver, chronic liver disease, immunodeficiency syndromes, or blood dyscrasias.

Use cautiously in very young, geriatric, or debilitated patients and in those with impaired renal or hepatic function, bone marrow suppression, aplasia, leukopenia, thrombocytopenia, anemia, folate deficiency, infection, peptic ulcer, or ulcerative colitis. Drug exits slowly from third space compartments resulting in a prolonged terminal plasma half-life and risk of toxicity.

Interactions
Drug-drug. *Folic acid:* May decrease methotrexate effectiveness. Use together cautiously.
Hepatotoxic drugs, such as azathioprine, retinoids, and sulfasalazine: Increased risk of hepatotoxicity. Monitor patient closely.
Immunizations: May not be effective when given during methotrexate therapy. Vaccines shouldn't be given during methotrexate therapy.
NSAIDs, salicylates, sulfonamides, sulfonylureas: May increase the therapeutic and toxic effects of methotrexate by displacing methotrexate from plasma proteins, increasing the levels of free methotrexate. Avoid use together if possible.
Oral antibiotics, such as chloramphenicol, nonabsorbable broad-spectrum antibiotics, and tetracycline: May decrease absorption of the drug. Use together cautiously.
Phenytoin: Increased risk of seizures. Patient requires careful monitoring.
Probenecid: Increases the therapeutic and toxic effects of methotrexate. Combined use requires a lower methotrexate dosage.
Pyrimethamine: Similar pharmacologic action. Avoid use together.
Drug-lifestyle. *Sun exposure:* Increased risk of photosensitivity reactions. Advise patient to take precautions.

Adverse reactions
CNS: *arachnoiditis* (within hours of intrathecal use), subacute *neurotoxicity* (may begin a few weeks later), *necrotizing demyelinating leukoencephalopathy* (may occur a few years later), malaise, fatigue, dizziness, headache, drowsiness, *seizures.*
CV: *sudden death.*
EENT: pharyngitis, gingivitis, blurred vision.
GI: stomatitis, diarrhea, abdominal distress, anorexia, GI ulceration and bleeding, enteritis, *nausea, vomiting.*
GU: nephropathy, *tubular necrosis, renal failure,* hematuria, menstrual dysfunction, defective spermatogenesis, cystitis.
Hematologic: WBC and platelet count nadirs occurring on day 7; anemia, ecchymoses, *leukopenia, thrombocytopenia* (all dose-related).
Hepatic: acute toxicity (elevated transaminase level), *chronic toxicity (cirrhosis, hepatic fibrosis).*
Metabolic: diabetes, hyperuricemia.
Musculoskeletal: arthralgia, myalgia, osteoporosis (in children, with long-term use).
Respiratory: *pulmonary fibrosis; pulmonary interstitial infiltrates; pneumonitis;* dry, nonproductive cough.
Skin: alopecia, *urticaria, pruritus, hyperpigmentation, erythematous rash, psoriatic lesions (aggravated by exposure to sun), rash, photosensitivity.*
Other: fever, chills, reduced resistance to infection, soft tissue necrosis, osteonecrosis, *septicemia.*

Reactions may be common, uncommon, *life-threatening*, or COMMON AND LIFE-THREATENING.

Overdose and treatment

Signs and symptoms of overdose include myelosuppression, anemia, nausea, vomiting, dermatitis, alopecia, and melena.

The antidote for hematopoietic toxicity of methotrexate (diagnosed or anticipated) is calcium leucovorin, started as soon as possible and within 1 hour after methotrexate administration. The dosage of leucovorin should produce plasma levels higher than those of methotrexate. Since leucovorin blunts therapeutic response of methotrexate, consult specific disease protocol for details.

Special considerations

● Methotrexate has been used to treat breast cancer, bladder carcinoma, and various solid tumors. In addition, it has been used investigationally for its immunosuppressive and anti-inflammatory effects in various conditions.
● Methotrexate may be given undiluted by I.V. push.
● Drug can be diluted to a larger volume with normal saline solution for I.V. infusion.
● Use reconstituted solutions of preservative-free drug within 24 hours after mixing.
● For intrathecal delivery, use only preservative-free forms. Dilute with unpreserved normal saline solution.
● Dose modification may be required in impaired hepatic or renal function, bone marrow depression, aplasia, leukopenia, thrombocytopenia, or anemia. Use cautiously in patients with infection, peptic ulcer, or ulcerative colitis and in very young, old, or debilitated patients.
● GI adverse reactions may require drug discontinuation.
● ◼ ALERT Rash, redness, or ulcerations in mouth or pulmonary adverse reactions may signal serious complications.
● Alkalinize urine by giving sodium bicarbonate tablets to prevent precipitation of drug, especially with high doses. Maintain urine pH at more than 6.5. Reduce dose if BUN level is 20 to 30 mg/dl or serum creatinine level is 1.2 to 2 mg/dl. Stop drug if BUN level is more than 30 mg/dl or serum creatinine level is more than 2 mg/dl.
● Avoid all I.M. injections in patients with thrombocytopenia.
● Leucovorin rescue is necessary with high-dose protocols (doses greater than 100 mg).
● Methotrexate may alter results of the laboratory assay for folate by inhibiting the organism used in the assay, thus interfering with the detection of folic acid deficiency.

Patient monitoring

● Monitor uric acid levels.
● Monitor intake and output daily. Force fluids (2 to 3 L daily).
● Watch for increases in AST, ALT, and alkaline phosphatase levels, which may signal hepatic dysfunction. Methotrexate shouldn't be used when the potential for "third spacing" exists.

● Monitor patient for bleeding (especially GI) and infection.
● Monitor temperature daily, and watch for cough, dyspnea, and cyanosis.

Breast-feeding patients

● Drug appears in breast milk. To avoid risk of serious adverse reactions, mutagenicity, and carcinogenicity in the infant, discontinue breast-feeding during therapy.

Patient education

● Emphasize importance of continuing drug despite nausea and vomiting. Advise patient to call immediately if vomiting occurs shortly after taking a dose.
● Encourage patient to maintain adequate fluid intake to increase urine output, to prevent nephrotoxicity, and to facilitate excretion of uric acid.
● Instruct patients also taking leucovorin to take exactly as prescribed to avoid potentially serious adverse effects.
● Warn patient to avoid alcoholic beverages during therapy.
● Caution patient to avoid conception during and immediately after therapy because of possible abortion or congenital anomalies.
● Tell patient to avoid prolonged exposure to sunlight and to use a highly protective sunscreen when exposed to sunlight.
● Teach patient good mouth care to prevent superinfection of oral cavity.
● Advise patient that hair should grow back after treatment has ended.
● Recommend salicylate-free analgesics for pain relief or fever reduction.
● Tell patient to avoid exposure to people with infections and to report signs of infection immediately.
● Advise patient to report unusual bruising or bleeding promptly.

methyldopa
Aldomet, Apo-Methyldopa*,
Dopamet*, Novomedopa*

Pharmacologic classification: centrally acting antiadrenergic
Therapeutic classification: antihypertensive
Pregnancy risk category: B (oral); C (I.V.)

Indications and dosages

➤ *Moderate to severe hypertension.* Adults: Initially, 250 mg P.O. b.i.d. or t.i.d. in first 48 hours; then increased or decreased, p.r.n., q 2 days. Or, 250 to 500 mg I.V. q 6 hours (maximum dose, 1 g q 6 hours). Adjust dosage if other antihypertensive drugs are added to or deleted from therapy.

Maintenance dosage is 500 mg to 2 g P.O. daily in two to four divided doses. Maximum recommended daily dose is 3 g. I.V. infusion dose is

250 to 500 mg given over 30 to 60 minutes q 6 hours. Maximum I.V. dose, 1 g q 6 hours.
Children: Initially, 10 mg/kg P.O. daily or 300 mg/m² P.O. daily in two to four divided doses. Or, 20 to 40 mg/kg I.V. daily or 0.6 to 1.2 g/m² I.V. daily in four divided doses. Increase dosage at least q 2 days until desired response occurs. Maximum daily dose is 65 mg/kg, 2 g/m², or 3 g, whichever is least.

How supplied
Available by prescription only
Tablets: 125 mg, 250 mg, 500 mg
Injection (as methyldopate hydrochloride): 250 mg/5 ml in 5-ml vials

Pharmacodynamics
Antihypertensive action: Exact mechanism of antihypertensive effect is unknown; it's thought to be caused by a metabolite of methyldopa, alpha-methylnorepinephrine, which stimulates central inhibitory alpha-adrenergic receptors, decreasing total peripheral resistance. Drug may act as a false neurotransmitter. Drug may also reduce plasma renin activity.

Pharmacokinetics
Absorption: Absorbed partially from the GI tract. Absorption varies, but usually about 50% of an oral dose is absorbed. No correlation exists between plasma level and antihypertensive effect. After I.V. administration, blood pressure usually begins to decrease in 4 to 6 hours.
Distribution: Distributed throughout the body and is bound weakly to plasma proteins.
Metabolism: Metabolized extensively in the liver and intestinal cells.
Excretion: Drug and its metabolites are excreted in urine; unabsorbed drug is excreted unchanged in feces. Elimination half-life is about 2 hours.

Route	Onset	Peak	Duration
P.O.	Unknown	4-6 hr	12-48 hr
I.V.	Unknown	4-6 hr	10-16 hr

Contraindications and precautions
Contraindicated in patients hypersensitive to drug and in those with active hepatic disease (such as acute hepatitis) and active cirrhosis. Also contraindicated if previous methyldopa therapy has been linked to liver disorders. Use cautiously in patients with impaired hepatic function, in those receiving MAO inhibitors, and in breast-feeding women.

Interactions
Drug-drug. *Anesthetics:* Increased effects. Patients undergoing surgery may require reduced dosages of anesthetics.
Antihypertensives: Potentiated antihypertensive effects. Use together cautiously.
Diuretics: May increase hypotensive effect of methyldopa. Use together cautiously.
Haloperidol: May produce dementia and sedation. Use together cautiously.

Lithium: May increase risk of lithium toxicity. Monitor lithium levels.
Oral iron therapy: May decrease hypotensive effects and increase serum levels of levodopa. Use together cautiously.
Phenothiazines, tricyclic antidepressants: May cause a reduction in antihypertensive effects. Monitor patient's blood pressure.
Phenoxybenzamine: May cause reversible urinary incontinence. Avoid use together.
Sympathomimetic amines such as phenylpropanolamine: Potentiated pressor effects. Use together cautiously.
Tolbutamide: Methyldopa may impair tolbutamide metabolism. Monitor serum glucose levels.
Drug-herb. *Capsicum:* May reduce antihypertensive effects. Discourage use together.

Adverse reactions
CNS: *sedation, headache, weakness, dizziness,* decreased mental acuity, paresthesia, parkinsonism, involuntary choreoathetoid movements, psychic disturbances, depression, nightmares.
CV: *bradycardia,* orthostatic hypotension, aggravated angina, ***myocarditis,*** edema.
EENT: *nasal congestion.*
GI: nausea, vomiting, diarrhea, ***pancreatitis,*** dry mouth, constipation.
GU: amenorrhea, impotence, altered serum creatinine, altered urine uric acid.
Hematologic: *hemolytic anemia, thrombocytopenia, leukopenia, bone marrow depression.*
Hepatic: *hepatic necrosis,* abnormal liver function tests, ***hepatitis.***
Skin: rash.
Other: gynecomastia, galactorrhea, drug-induced fever, decreased libido.

Overdose and treatment
Evidence of overdose includes sedation, hypotension, impaired AV conduction, and coma.
   After recent (within 4 hours) ingestion, empty stomach by induced emesis or gastric lavage. Give activated charcoal to reduce absorption; then treat symptomatically and supportively. In severe cases, hemodialysis may be considered.

Special considerations
● Patients with impaired renal function may require smaller maintenance dosage.
● Multiple dosing may decrease patient compliance, but b.i.d. dosing may provide adequate control with decreased cost.
● Methyldopate hydrochloride is administered I.V. Administration by I.M. or S.C. route isn't recommended because of unpredictable absorption.
● Patients receiving methyldopa may become hypertensive after dialysis because drug is dialyzable.
● Sedation and drowsiness usually disappear with continued therapy; bedtime dosage will minimize this effect. Orthostatic hypotension may indicate a need for dosage reduction. Some patients tolerate entire daily dose in the evening or h.s.

Reactions may be *common*, uncommon, *life-threatening*, or COMMON AND LIFE-THREATENING.

- Tolerance may develop after 2 to 3 weeks.
- Signs of hepatotoxicity may occur 2 to 4 weeks after therapy begins.
- For I.V. use, add required dose of drug to 100 ml of 5% dextrose injection. Or, a concentration of 100 mg/ml may be used. ADD-Vantage vials contain 50 mg/ml and should be reconstituted per manufacturer direction. Administer I.V. infusion over 30 to 60 minutes.
- Methyldopa may cause falsely high levels of urine catecholamines, interfering with the diagnosis of pheochromocytoma. A positive direct antiglobulin (Coombs') test may also occur.

Patient monitoring

- At the start of therapy and periodically throughout, monitor hemoglobin, hematocrit, and RBC count for hemolytic anemia; also monitor liver function tests.
- Take blood pressure in supine, sitting, and standing positions during dosage adjustment; take blood pressure at least every 30 minutes during I.V. infusion until patient is stable.
- Monitor intake, output, and daily weights to detect sodium and water retention; voided urine exposed to air may darken because of the breakdown of methyldopa or its metabolites.
- Monitor patient for signs and symptoms of drug-induced depression.

Pregnant patients

- Methyldopa is the most extensively used hypotensive agent in pregnant women.

Breast-feeding patients

- Drug appears in breast milk; the American Academy of Pediatrics considers methyldopa to be compatible with breast-feeding.

Pediatric patients

- Safety and efficacy in children haven't been established; use only if potential benefits outweigh risks.

Geriatric patients

- Dosage reductions may be necessary in geriatric patients because they're more sensitive to sedation and hypotension.

Patient education

- Teach patient signs and symptoms of adverse effects, such as jerky movements, and about the need to report them; he should also report excessive weight gain (5 lb weekly), signs of infection, or fever.
- Teach patient to minimize adverse effects by taking drug at bedtime until tolerance develops to sedation, drowsiness, and other CNS effects; by avoiding sudden position changes to minimize orthostatic hypotension; and by using ice chips, hard candy, or gum to relieve dry mouth.
- Warn patient to avoid hazardous activities that require mental alertness until sedative effects subside.

- Instruct patient to call for instructions before taking OTC cold preparations.

methylergonovine maleate
Methergine

Pharmacologic classification: ergot alkaloid
Therapeutic classification: oxytocic
Pregnancy risk category: C

Indications and dosages

➤ *Prevention and treatment of postpartum hemorrhage from uterine atony or subinvolution. Adults:* 0.2 mg I.M. or I.V. q 2 to 4 hours for maximum five doses. Following initial I.M. or I.V. dose, may give 0.2 to 0.4 mg P.O. q 6 to 12 hours for maximum 7 days. Decrease dose if severe cramping occurs.
➤ *Diagnosis of coronary artery spasm◊. Adults:* 0.1 to 0.4 mg I.V.

How supplied

Available by prescription only
Injection: 0.2 mg/ml ampule
Tablets: 0.2 mg

Pharmacodynamics

Oxytocic action: Drug stimulates contractions of uterine and vascular smooth muscle. The intense uterine contractions are followed by periods of relaxation. Drug produces vasoconstriction primarily of capacitance blood vessels, causing increased central venous pressure and elevated blood pressure. Drug increases the amplitude and frequency of uterine contractions and tone, which therefore impedes uterine blood flow.

Pharmacokinetics

Absorption: Absorption is rapid, with 60% of an oral dose appearing in the bloodstream.
Distribution: Distribution appears to be rapidly distributed into tissues.
Metabolism: Extensive first-pass metabolism precedes hepatic metabolism.
Excretion: Excreted primarily in feces, with a small amount in urine.

Route	Onset	Peak	Duration
P.O.	5-10 min	30 min	3 hr
I.V.	Immediate	Unknown	45 min
I.M.	2-5 min	Unknown	3 hr

Contraindications and precautions

Contraindicated in pregnant women and patients with hypertension, toxemia, or sensitivity to ergot preparations. Use cautiously during first stage of labor and in patients with renal or hepatic disease, sepsis, or obliterative vascular disease.

Interactions

Drug-drug. *Ergot alkaloids, sympathomimetic amines:* Enhanced vasoconstrictor potential. Use together cautiously.

Local anesthetics with vasoconstrictors (lidocaine with epinephrine): Enhanced vasoconstriction. Use together cautiously.
Drug-lifestyle. *Smoking (nicotine):* Enhanced vasoconstriction. Advise patient to stop smoking.

Adverse reactions
CNS: dizziness, headache, *seizures, CVA* (with I.V. use), hallucinations.
CV: hypertension, transient chest pain, palpitations, hypotension.
EENT: tinnitus, nasal congestion.
GI: *nausea, vomiting, diarrhea,* foul taste.
GU: hematuria.
Musculoskeletal: leg cramps.
Respiratory: dyspnea.
Skin: diaphoresis.
Other: thrombophlebitis.

Overdose and treatment
Signs and symptoms of overdose include seizures, gangrene, nausea, vomiting, diarrhea, dizziness, changing blood pressure, weak pulse, chest pain, tingling, and numbness and coldness in limbs.

Treatment of oral overdose requires that the patient drink tap water, milk, or vegetable oil to delay absorption. Follow with gastric lavage or emesis and then activated charcoal and cathartics. Treat seizures with anticonvulsants and hypercoagulability with heparin; use vasodilators to improve blood flow as required. Gangrene may require surgical amputation.

Special considerations
● Contractions begin 5 to 15 minutes after P.O. administration, 2 to 5 minutes after I.M. injection, and immediately following I.V. injection. They continue 3 hours or more after P.O. or I.M. administration, 45 minutes after I.V. delivery.
● Don't administer I.V. routinely because of the possibility of inducing sudden hypertensive and CV accidents.
● If I.V. administration is considered essential as a life-saving measure, dilute the desired dose with normal saline solution injection to a volume of 5 ml and give slowly over at least 60 seconds.
● Store tablets in tightly closed, light-resistant containers. Discard if discolored.
● Store I.V. solutions below 77° F (25° C). Administer only if solution is clear and colorless.

Patient monitoring
● Monitor patient's blood pressure, pulse rate, and uterine response.
● Watch for sudden change in vital signs or frequent periods of uterine relaxation.
● Assess vaginal bleeding.

Breast-feeding patients
● Ergot alkaloids inhibit lactation.
● Drug appears in breast milk, and ergotism has been reported in breast-fed infants.

Patient education
● Advise patient to stop smoking during therapy.
● Warn patient of adverse reactions.

methylphenidate hydrochloride
Concerta, Methylin, Methylin ER, Ritalin, Ritalin-SR

Pharmacologic classification: piperidine CNS stimulant
Therapeutic classification: CNS stimulant (analeptic)
Controlled substance schedule: II
Pregnancy risk category: NR (C for Concerta)

Indications and dosages
➤ *Attention deficit hyperactivity disorder (ADHD).* Ritalin, Methylin. *Children age 6 and older:* Initially 5 mg P.O. daily before breakfast and lunch, increased in 5- to 10-mg increments weekly, p.r.n., until an optimum daily dose of 2 mg/kg is reached, not to exceed 60 mg daily.
➤ *ADHD.* Concerta. *Children age 6 and older not currently taking methylphenidate or patients taking stimulants other than methylphenidate:* 18 mg P.O. (extended-release) once daily in the morning. Adjust dosage by 18 mg at weekly intervals to a maximum of 54 mg daily taken once daily in the morning.
Children age 6 and older currently taking methylphenidate: If the previous methylphenidate daily dose is 5 mg b.i.d. or t.i.d. or 20 mg sustained release, the recommended dose of Concerta is 18 mg P.O. every morning. If the previous methylphenidate daily dose is 10 mg b.i.d. or t.i.d. or 40 mg sustained release, the recommended dose of Concerta is 36 mg P.O. every morning. If the previous methylphenidate daily dose is 15 mg b.i.d. or t.i.d. or 60 mg sustained release, the recommended dose of Concerta is 54 mg P.O. every morning. Maximum daily dose is 54 mg
➤ *Narcolepsy.* Ritalin, Methylin. *Adults:* 10 mg P.O. b.i.d. or t.i.d. 30 to 45 minutes before meals. Dosage varies with patient needs; average dose is 40 to 60 mg daily.

When using sustained-release tablets, calculate regular dose in q-8-hour intervals and administer as such.

How supplied
Available by prescription only
Tablets: 5 mg, 10 mg, 20 mg
Tablets (extended-release): 10 mg, 18 mg, 20 mg, 36 mg, 54 mg
Tablets (sustained-release): 20 mg

Pharmacodynamics
Analeptic action: The cerebral cortex and reticular activating system appear to be the primary sites of activity; methylphenidate releases nerve terminal stores of norepinephrine, promoting

nerve impulse transmission. At high doses, effects are mediated by dopamine.

Drug is used to treat narcolepsy and as an adjunct to psychosocial measures in ADHD. Like amphetamines, it has a paradoxical calming effect in hyperactive children.

Pharmacokinetics
Absorption: Absorbed rapidly and completely after oral administration.
Distribution: Unknown.
Metabolism: Metabolized by the liver.
Excretion: Excreted in urine.

Route	Onset	Peak	Duration
P.O.	Unknown	2-5 hr	Unknown

Contraindications and precautions
Contraindicated in patients hypersensitive to drug and in those with glaucoma, motor tics, family history of or diagnosis of Tourette syndrome, or history of marked anxiety, tension, or agitation. Don't use Concerta in patients with severe GI narrowing (pathologic or iatrogenic), such as small bowel inflammatory disease, short gut syndrome from adhesions or decreased transit time, history of peritonitis, cystic fibrosis, chronic intestinal pseudoobstruction, or Meckel's diverticulum.

Use cautiously in patients with history of seizures, drug abuse, hypertension, or EEG abnormalities. Also use cautiously in patients with a history of drug dependence or alcoholism. Use Concerta cautiously in patients with hypertension and in patients whose underlying medical condition could be compromised by increased blood pressure or heart rate, such as those with hypertension, heart failure, recent MI, or hyperthyroidism.

Interactions
Drug-drug. *Anticonvulsants (phenobarbital, phenytoin, primidone), coumarin anticoagulants, phenylbutazone, tricyclic antidepressants:* Methylphenidate may inhibit metabolism and increase serum levels of these drugs. Patient may need dosage adjustment if concomitant therapy is necessary.
Bretylium, guanethidine: Decreased hypotensive effects. Monitor patient for clinical effect.
MAO inhibitors (or drugs with MAO-inhibiting activity) or within 14 days of such therapy: May cause severe hypertension. Avoid use together.
Drug-lifestyle. *Caffeine:* May enhance CNS stimulant effects of methylphenidate and decrease effectiveness of drug in ADHD. Discourage use together.

Adverse reactions
CNS: *nervousness, insomnia, Tourette syndrome, dizziness, headache, akathisia, dyskinesia,* **seizures,** drowsiness.
CV: *palpitations, angina, tachycardia, changes in blood pressure and pulse rate,* **arrhythmias.**
EENT: pharyngitis, sinusitis

GI: nausea, abdominal pain, anorexia, vomiting.
Hematologic: *thrombocytopenia, thrombocytopenic purpura, leukopenia,* anemia.
Metabolic: weight loss.
Respiratory: cough, upper respiratory tract infection.
Skin: rash, urticaria, *exfoliative dermatitis, erythema multiforme.*

Overdose and treatment
Evidence of overdose may include euphoria, confusion, delirium, coma, toxic psychosis, agitation, headache, vomiting, dry mouth, mydriasis, self-injury, fever, diaphoresis, tremors, hyperreflexia, hyperpyrexia, muscle twitching, seizures, flushing, hypertension, tachycardia, palpitations, and arrhythmias.

Treat overdose symptomatically and supportively. Use gastric lavage or emesis in patients with intact gag reflex. Maintain airway and circulation. Closely monitor vital signs and fluid and electrolyte balance. Maintain patient in cool room, monitor temperature, minimize external stimulation, and protect him against self-injury. External cooling blankets may be needed.

Special considerations
• Methylphenidate is the drug of choice for ADHD. Therapy is usually discontinued after puberty.
• If paradoxical aggravation of symptoms occurs during therapy, reduce dosage or discontinue drug.
• If improvement fails to occur after appropriate dosage adjustment over a one-month period, discontinue drug.
• Drug isn't intended to treat severe depression or normal fatigue.
• Drug may decrease seizure threshold in seizure disorders. If seizures occur, discontinue drug.
• Intermittent drug-free periods when stress is least evident (weekends, school holidays) may help prevent development of tolerance and permit decreased dosage when drug is resumed. Sustained-release form allows convenience of single, at-home dosing for school children.
• Drug has abuse potential; discourage use to combat fatigue. Some abusers dissolve tablets and inject drug.
• After high-dose and long-term use, abrupt withdrawal may unmask severe depression. Lower dosage gradually to prevent acute rebound depression.
• Drug impairs ability to perform tasks requiring mental alertness.
• Be sure patient obtains adequate rest; fatigue may result as drug wears off.
• Discourage methylphenidate use for analeptic effect; CNS stimulation superimposed on CNS depression may cause neuronal instability and seizures.
• Don't administer drug to women of childbearing age unless potential benefits outweigh the possible risks.
• Store drug in tight, light-resistant containers.

Patient monitoring

• Monitor start of therapy closely; drug may precipitate Tourette syndrome.

• Check vital signs regularly for increased blood pressure or other signs of excessive stimulation; avoid late-day or evening dosing, especially of long-acting dosage forms, to minimize insomnia.

• Monitor CBC, differential, and platelet counts when patient is taking drug long-term.

• Monitor height and weight; drug has been linked to growth suppression.

Pediatric patients

• Drug isn't recommended for ADHD in children under age 6. It has been linked to growth suppression; all patients should be monitored.

Patient education

• Explain rationale for therapy and the risks and benefits that may be anticipated.

• Tell patient to avoid drinks containing caffeine to prevent added CNS stimulation.

• Tell patient not to alter dosage unless prescribed.

• Advise narcoleptic patient to take first dose on awakening; advise ADHD patient to take last dose several hours before bedtime to avoid insomnia.

• Tell patient not to chew or crush sustained-release forms.

• Tell patient taking Concerta that the tablet shell may appear in stool.

• Warn patient to avoid using drug to mask fatigue, to obtain adequate rest, and to call if excessive CNS stimulation occurs.

• Advise patient to avoid hazardous activities that require mental alertness until degree of sedative effect is determined.

methylprednisolone (systemic)
Medrol

methylprednisolone acetate
depMedalone 40, depMedalone 80, Depoject-40, Depoject-80, Depo-Medrol, Depopred-40, Depopred-80, Duralone-40, Duralone-80, Medralone, Rep-Pred 40, Rep-Pred 80

methylprednisolone sodium succinate
A-methapred, Solu-Medrol

Pharmacologic classification: glucocorticoid
Therapeutic classification: anti-inflammatory, immunosuppressant
Pregnancy risk category: C

Indications and dosages
➤ *Multiple sclerosis.* methylprednisolone (systemic). *Adults:* 200 mg P.O. daily for 1 week, followed by 80 mg every other day for 1 month.

➤ *Inflammation.* methylprednisolone. *Adults:* 2 to 60 mg P.O. daily in four divided doses, depending on disease being treated.
Children: 0.117 to 1.66 mg/kg daily or 3.3 to 50 mg/m² P.O. daily in three to four divided doses.
methylprednisolone acetate
Adults: 10 to 80 mg I.M. daily; or 4 to 80 mg into joints and soft tissue, p.r.n., q 1 to 5 weeks; or 20 to 60 mg intralesionally.
methylprednisolone sodium succinate
Adults: 10 to 250 mg I.M. or I.V. q 4 hours.
Children: 0.03 to 0.2 mg/kg or 1 to 6.25 mg m² I.M. or I.V. daily in 1 or 2 divided doses.

➤ *Shock.* methylprednisolone sodium succinate. *Adults:* 100 to 250 mg I.V. at 2- to 6-hour intervals or 30 mg/kg I.V. initially and repeat q 4 to 6 hours, p.r.n. Or, after original I.V. push dose, 30 mg/kg I.V. infusion q 12 hours for 24 to 48 hours.

➤ *Severe lupus nephritis* ◇. *Adults:* 1 g I.V. over 1 hour for 3 days. Therapy is then continued orally at 0.5 mg/kg daily.
Children: 30 mg/kg I.V. every other day for six doses.

➤ *Treatment or minimization of motor and sensory defects caused by acute spinal cord injury* ◇. *Adults:* Initially, 30 mg/kg I.V. over 15 minutes followed in 45 minutes by I.V. infusion of 5.4 mg/kg/hour for 23 hours.

➤ *Adjunct to moderate-severe* **Pneumocystis carinii** *pneumonia* ◇. *Adults and children over age 13:* 30 mg I.V. b.i.d. for 5 days; 30 mg I.V. daily for 5 days; 15 mg I.V. daily for 11 days (or until completion of anti-infective regimen).

How supplied
Available by prescription only
methylprednisolone
Tablets: 2 mg, 4 mg, 8 mg, 16 mg, 24 mg, 32 mg
methylprednisolone acetate
Injection: 20 mg/ml, 40 mg/ml, 80 mg/ml suspension
methylprednisolone sodium succinate
Injection: 40 mg, 125 mg, 500 mg, 1,000 mg, 2,000 mg/vial

Pharmacodynamics
Anti-inflammatory action: Methylprednisolone stimulates the synthesis of enzymes needed to decrease the inflammatory response. It suppresses the immune system by reducing activity and volume of the lymphatic system, thus producing lymphocytopenia (primarily of T lymphocytes), decreasing immunoglobulin and complement levels, decreasing passage of immune complexes through basement membranes, and possibly by depressing reactivity of tissue to antigen-antibody interactions.

Drug is an intermediate-acting glucocorticoid. It has essentially no mineralocorticoid activity but is a potent glucocorticoid, with five times the potency of an equal weight of hydrocortisone. It's used primarily as an anti-inflammatory agent and immunosuppressant.

Pharmacokinetics
Absorption: Absorbed readily after oral administration.
Distribution: Distributed rapidly to muscle, liver, skin, intestines, and kidneys. Adrenocorticoids are distributed into breast milk and through the placenta.
Metabolism: Metabolized in the liver to inactive glucuronide and sulfate metabolites.
Excretion: Inactive metabolites and small amounts of unmetabolized drug are excreted by the kidneys. Insignificant quantities of drug are excreted in feces. Biological half-life of methylprednisolone is 18 to 36 hours.

Route	Onset	Peak	Duration
P.O.	Rapid	2-3 hr	30-36 hr
I.V.	Rapid	Immediate	7 days
I.M.	6-48 hr	4-8 days	1-4 wk
Intra-articular	Rapid	7 days	1-5 wk

Contraindications and precautions
Contraindicated in patients allergic to any component of the formulation, in those with systemic fungal infections, and in premature infants (acetate and succinate).

Use cautiously in patients with renal disease, GI ulceration, hypertension, osteoporosis, diabetes mellitus, hypothyroidism, cirrhosis, diverticulitis, nonspecific ulcerative colitis, recent intestinal anastomoses, thromboembolic disorders, seizures, myasthenia gravis, heart failure, tuberculosis, emotional instability, ocular herpes simplex, and psychotic tendencies.

Interactions
Drug-drug. *Amphotericin B, diuretic therapy:* May enhance hypokalemia. Monitor serum potassium level.
Antacids, cholestyramine, colestipol: Decreased corticosteroid effect. Separate administration times.
Anticholinesterase: Profound weakness. Use together cautiously.
Barbiturates, phenytoin, rifampin: May cause decreased corticosteroid effects because of increased hepatic metabolism. Monitor patient for potential dosage adjustment.
Cyclosporine: Levels of cyclosporine may increase. Use together cautiously.
Estrogens: Reduced metabolism of corticosteroids. Patient may need dosage adjustment.
Insulin, oral antidiabetics: Increased risk of hyperglycemia. Dosage adjustment may be needed.
Isoniazid, salicylates: Increased metabolism. May require dosage adjustment of isoniazid or salicylates.

Oral anticoagulants: Decreased effectiveness. Monitor PT and INR.
Ulcerogenic drugs such as NSAIDs: Increased risk of GI ulceration. Use together cautiously.
Vaccines: Decreased effectiveness of vaccines. Vaccine shouldn't be administered during corticosteroid therapy.

Adverse reactions
Most adverse reactions to corticosteroids are dose- or duration-dependent.
CNS: *euphoria, insomnia,* psychotic behavior, pseudotumor cerebri, vertigo, headache, paresthesia, *seizures.*
CV: *heart failure,* hypertension, edema, *arrhythmias,* thrombophlebitis, *thromboembolism, fatal arrest or circulatory collapse* (following rapid administration of large I.V. doses).
EENT: cataracts, glaucoma.
GI: *peptic ulceration,* GI irritation, increased appetite, *pancreatitis,* nausea, vomiting.
GU: menstrual irregularities, increased urine glucose and calcium levels.
Metabolic: hypokalemia, hyperglycemia, hypocalcemia, decreased serum thyroxine and triiodothyronine levels, carbohydrate intolerance, growth suppression in children, cushingoid state (moonface, buffalo hump, central obesity).
Musculoskeletal: muscle weakness, osteoporosis.
Skin: delayed wound healing, acne, various skin eruptions.
Other: hirsutism, susceptibility to infections, *acute adrenal insufficiency that may occur with increased stress (infection, surgery, or trauma) or abrupt withdrawal after long-term therapy.*

Overdose and treatment
Acute ingestion, even in massive doses, is rarely a clinical problem. Toxic signs and symptoms rarely occur if drug is used for less than 3 weeks, even at large doses. However, chronic use causes adverse physiologic effects, including suppression of the hypothalamus-pituitary-adrenal axis, cushingoid appearance, muscle weakness, and osteoporosis.

Special considerations
• Methylprednisolone may be administered orally. Methylprednisolone sodium succinate may be administered by I.M. or I.V. injection or by I.V. infusion, usually at 4- to 6-hour intervals.
• Methylprednisolone acetate suspension may be administered by intra-articular, intrasynovial, intrabursal, intralesional, or soft tissue injection. It has a slow onset but a long duration of action. Injectable forms are usually used only when the oral forms can't be used.
• Determine whether patient is sensitive to other corticosteroids.
• Drug may be used for alternate-day therapy.

• Most adverse reactions to corticosteroids are dose- or duration-dependent.

• For better results and less toxicity, give a once-daily dose in the morning.

• Give oral dose with food when possible. Critically ill patients may need concomitant antacid or H_2-receptor antagonist therapy.

• Salt forms aren't interchangeable.

⚠ ALERT Don't give Solu-Medrol intrathecally because severe adverse reactions have been reported.

• Give I.M. injection deep into gluteal muscle. Avoid S.C. injection because atrophy and sterile abscesses may occur.

• Dermal atrophy may occur with large doses of acetate salt. Use several small injections rather than a single large dose, and rotate injection sites.

• Don't use acetate if immediate onset of action is needed.

• Discard reconstituted solution after 48 hours.

• Always adjust to lowest effective dose.

• Gradually reduce dosage after long-term therapy.

• Unless contraindicated, give low-sodium diet that's high in potassium and protein. Administer potassium supplements as needed.

⚠ ALERT Don't confuse Solu-Medrol with Solu-Cortef (hydrocortisone sodium succinate) or methylprednisolone with medroxyprogesterone.

• Use only methylprednisolone sodium succinate for I.V. route; never use acetate form. Reconstitute according to manufacturer's directions using supplied diluent, or use bacteriostatic water for injection with benzyl alcohol.

• When administering as direct injection, inject diluted drug into vein or free-flowing compatible I.V. solution over at least 1 minute. For shock, give massive doses over at least 10 minutes to prevent arrhythmias and circulatory collapse. When administering as an intermittent or continuous infusion, dilute solution according to manufacturer's instructions, and give over prescribed duration. If used for continuous infusion, change solution every 24 hours.

Patient monitoring

• Monitor patient's weight, blood pressure, serum electrolyte levels, and sleep patterns. Euphoria may initially interfere with sleep, but patients typically adjust to therapy in 1 to 3 weeks.

• Monitor patient for cushingoid effects, including moonface, buffalo hump, central obesity, thinning hair, hypertension, and increased susceptibility to infection.

• Drug may mask or worsen infections, including latent amebiasis.

• Watch for depression or psychotic episodes, especially in high-dose therapy.

• Diabetic patient may need increased insulin; monitor blood glucose levels.

• Watch for an enhanced response to drug in patients with hypothyroidism or cirrhosis.

• Watch for allergic reaction to tartrazine in patients with sensitivity to aspirin.

Pediatric patients

• Long-term use of adrenocorticoids in children and adolescents may delay growth and maturation.

Geriatric patients

• Compare the risks and benefits of corticosteroid use; lower doses are recommended. Elderly patients may be more susceptible to osteoporosis with prolonged use.

• Monitor blood pressure, blood glucose, and electrolyte levels at least every 6 months.

Patient education

• Tell patient not to stop drug abruptly or without medical consent.

• Instruct patient to take oral form of drug with food.

• Teach patient early signs of adrenal insufficiency: fatigue, muscle weakness, joint pain, fever, anorexia, nausea, dyspnea, dizziness, and fainting.

• Tell patient to carry a card identifying need for supplemental systemic steroids during stress. Medication, dose, and name of prescriber should appear on card.

• Teach patient on long-term therapy to notify prescriber of sudden weight gain or swelling.

• Tell patient on long-term therapy to consult with prescriber about the need for vitamin D or calcium supplement, or a physical exercise program.

• Warn patient to avoid exposure to infections (such as chicken pox or measles) and to report if such exposure occurs.

methysergide maleate
Sansert

Pharmacologic classification: ergot alkaloid
Therapeutic classification: vasoconstrictor
Pregnancy risk category: X

Indications and dosages

➤ *Prevention of vascular headaches, including migraine and cluster headaches.* Adults: 4 to 8 mg P.O. daily in divided doses with meals.

➤ *To control diarrhea in patients with carcinoid disease* ◇. Adults: 2 mg P.O. t.i.d. Adjust dosage as needed and tolerated. Usual dosage range is 4 to 16 mg P.O. t.i.d.

How supplied

Available by prescription only
Tablets: 2 mg

Pharmacodynamics

Vasoconstrictor action: Competitively blocks serotonin peripherally and may act as a serotonin agonist in the CNS (brain stem). Drug's antiserotonin effects result in inhibition of peripheral vasoconstrictor and pressor effects of serotonin, inflammation induced by serotonin, and a reduction in the increased rate of platelet aggregation caused by serotonin.

Reactions may be *common*, uncommon, *life-threatening*, or COMMON AND LIFE-THREATENING.

Mechanism involved in prophylaxis of vascular headaches unknown. However, drug's effectiveness may result from humoral factors affecting the pain threshold and from its central serotonin-agonist effect.

Pharmacokinetics
Absorption: Rapidly absorbed from GI tract.
Distribution: Widely distributed in body tissues.
Metabolism: Metabolized in liver to methylergonovine and glucuronide metabolites.
Excretion: 56% of dose excreted in urine as unchanged drug and metabolites. Plasma elimination half-life is 10 hours.

Route	Onset	Peak	Duration
P.O.	Rapid	Unknown	Unknown

Contraindications and precautions
Contraindicated in debilitated patients, pregnant patients, and patients with severe hypertension or arteriosclerosis, peripheral vascular insufficiency, renal or hepatic disease, coronary artery disease, phlebitis or cellulitis of legs, collagen diseases, fibrotic processes, or valvular heart disease.

Use cautiously in patients with peptic ulcer or suspected coronary artery disease and in those with aspirin or tartrazine allergies.

Interactions
Drug-drug. *Beta blockers:* Possible peripheral ischemia, evidenced by cold limbs with possible peripheral gangrene. Monitor patient closely.
Narcotic analgesics: Drug may reverse analgesic activity. Use cautiously.
Drug-lifestyle. *Alcohol use:* May worsen headaches. Discourage use.
Smoking: Increased adverse effects of drug. Discourage use.

Adverse reactions
CNS: insomnia, drowsiness, *euphoria, vertigo, ataxia,* light-headedness, hyperesthesia, weakness, hallucinations or feelings of dissociation, rapid speech, lethargy.
CV: *fibrotic thickening of cardiac valves and aorta, inferior vena cava, and common iliac branches (retroperitoneal fibrosis);* vasoconstriction, causing chest pain, abdominal pain, vascular insufficiency of lower limbs; cold, numb, painful limbs with or without paresthesia and diminished or absent pulses; flushing; orthostatic hypotension; tachycardia; peripheral edema; murmurs; bruits.
GI: nausea, vomiting, diarrhea, constipation, heartburn.
Hematologic: *neutropenia,* eosinophilia.
Musculoskeletal: arthralgia, myalgia.
Respiratory: *pulmonary fibrosis* (causing dyspnea, tightness and pain in chest, pleural friction rubs, and effusion).
Skin: hair loss, rash.

Overdose and treatment
Signs and symptoms of overdose include hyperactivity, euphoria, dizziness, peripheral vasospasm with diminished or absent pulses, and coldness, mottling, and cyanosis of limbs.

If patient is conscious and ingestion recent, induce emesis; if unconscious, insert cuffed endotracheal tube and perform gastric lavage. Apply warmth (not direct heat) to ischemic limbs if vasospasm occurs.

Special considerations
Consider the recommendations relevant to all ergot alkaloids as well as the following.
● Intervals of 3 to 4 weeks must separate each 6-month course of therapy.
● Adverse reactions occur in up to 50% of patients.
● Drug may contain tartrazine, which can cause an allergic reaction.
● GI effects may be reduced by introducing drug gradually and by giving with food or milk.
● Don't use drug to treat acute episodes of migraine, vascular headache, or muscle contraction headache.
● Dosage should be reduced gradually for 2 to 3 weeks before stopping drug.
● If drug is given for cluster headaches, it's usually administered only during the cluster.
● Drug has also been used to control diarrhea in patients with carcinoid disease.
● Protective effect develops in 1 to 2 days and persists for 1 to 2 days after drug is stopped.

Patient monitoring
● Monitor patient for adverse effects.
● Check WBC count as indicated, vital signs, and ECG.

Breast-feeding patients
● Drug may appear in breast milk. Advise against breast-feeding during therapy.

Pediatric patients
● Drug isn't recommended for use in children because of risk of fibrosis.

Geriatric patients
● Use cautiously in elderly patients.

Patient education
● Tell patient to immediately report signs of numbness or tingling in hands or feet, red or violet blisters on hands and feet, flank or chest pain, shortness of breath, leg cramps when walking, or other signs or symptoms of impaired circulation.
● Tell patient to report illness or infection, which may increase sensitivity to drug effects.
● Advise patient to avoid prolonged exposure to very cold temperatures; cold may increase adverse effects of drug.
● Explain that, after stopping drug, patient's body may need time to adjust depending on amount of drug used and duration of time involved.

● Tell patient to take drug with food.
● Inform patient that drug may cause drowsiness; urge caution when patient is driving or performing other tasks requiring alertness.
● Caution patient to avoid excessive weight gain.

metipranolol hydrochloride
OptiPranolol

Pharmacologic classification: beta blocker
Therapeutic classification: antiglaucoma drug
Pregnancy risk category: C

Indications and dosages
➤ *Ocular conditions in which lowering of intraocular pressure (IOP) would be beneficial (ocular hypertension, chronic open-angle glaucoma). Adults:* Instill 1 drop into affected eye(s) b.i.d. Larger dose or more frequent administration isn't known to be of benefit. If IOP isn't satisfactory, concomitant therapy to lower IOP may be instituted.

How supplied
Available by prescription only
Ophthalmic solution: 0.3% in 5- or 10-ml dropper bottles with 0.004% benzalkonium chloride and ethylenediaminetetraacetic acid

Pharmacodynamics
Antiglaucoma action: Exact mechanism unknown. Appears to be a reduction of aqueous humor production. A slight increase in outflow facility has been demonstrated with metipranolol. Like other noncardioselective beta blockers, metipranolol doesn't have significant local anesthetic (membrane-stabilizing) actions or intrinsic sympathomimetic activity. It does reduce elevated and normal IOP with or without glaucoma with little or no effect on pupil size or accommodation. In patients with IOP above 24 mm Hg, pressure is reduced an average of 20% to 26%.

Pharmacokinetics
Absorption: Intended to act locally, but some systemic absorption may occur. Onset of action occurs in less than 30 minutes.
Distribution: Local distribution.
Metabolism: No information available.
Excretion: No information available; maximum effect occurs in about 2 hours; duration of effect is 12 to 24 hours.

Route	Onset	Peak	Duration
Oph-thalmic	< 30 min	Unknown	12-24 hr

Contraindications and precautions
Contraindicated in patients hypersensitive to drug or its components and in those with bronchial asthma, history of bronchial asthma or severe COPD, sinus bradycardia, second- or third-degree AV block, cardiac failure, and cardiogenic shock.

Use cautiously in patients with nonallergic bronchospasm, chronic bronchitis, emphysema, diabetes mellitus, hyperthyroidism, or cerebrovascular insufficiency.

Interactions
Drug-drug. *Antithyroid drugs, calcium channel blockers, catecholamine-depleting drugs, cimetidine, clonidine, digoxin, haloperidol, hydralazine, insulin, lidocaine, morphine, nondepolarizing neuromuscular blockers, NSAIDs, oral contraceptives, phenobarbital, phenothiazines, prazosin, rifampin, salicylates, sympathomimetics, theophylline, thyroid hormones:* May interfere with drug action. Use together cautiously.
Systemic beta blockers: Potential for additive effects. Use together cautiously.
Drug-lifestyle. *Smoking:* May interfere with drug's effect. Discourage smoking.

Adverse reactions
CNS: headache, anxiety, dizziness, depression, somnolence, nervousness, asthenia, brow ache.
CV: hypertension, *MI,* atrial fibrillation, angina, palpitations, *bradycardia.*
EENT: transient local eye discomfort, tearing, conjunctivitis, eyelid dermatitis, blurred vision, blepharitis, abnormal vision, photophobia, eye edema, rhinitis, epistaxis.
GI: nausea.
Musculoskeletal: myalgia.
Respiratory: dyspnea, bronchitis, cough.
Skin: rash.
Other: *hypersensitivity reactions.*

Overdose and treatment
If ocular overdose occurs, flush eye with copious amounts of water or normal saline solution.

Systemic overdose, after accidental ingestion, may cause bradycardia, hypotension, bronchospasm, or acute cardiac failure. Stop therapy, institute supportive and symptomatic measures, and decrease further absorption (as with gastric lavage)

Special considerations
● Pilocarpine and other miotics, dipivefrin, or systemic carbonic anhydrase inhibitors may be administered concomitantly if IOP isn't adequately controlled.
● Proper administration is essential for optimal therapeutic response; instruct patient in correct techniques.
● The normal eye can retain only about 10 mcl (microliters) of fluid; the average dropper delivers 25 to 50 mcl/drop. Thus, the value of more than 1 drop is questionable. If multiple-drop therapy is indicated, the best interval between drops is 5 minutes.

Reactions may be *common,* uncommon, *life-threatening*, or COMMON AND LIFE-THREATENING.

Patient monitoring
● Monitor patient's response to drug therapy; watch for adverse effects.
● Monitor cardiac status carefully.

Pediatric patients
● Safety and efficacy in children haven't been established.

Breast-feeding patients
● It's unknown if drug appears in breast milk, but systemic beta blockers appear in breast milk. Use cautiously in breast-feeding women.

Patient education
● Tell patient to wash hands thoroughly before administration and then to follow these directions:
– Tilt head back or lie down and gaze upward.
– Gently grasp lower eyelid below eyelashes and pull eyelid away from eye to form a pouch.
– Place dropper directly over eye, avoiding contact of dropper with eye or any surface.
– Look up just before applying drop; look down for several seconds after applying drop. Slowly release eyelid.
   Close eyes gently for 1 to 2 minutes. Closing eyes tightly after instillation may expel drug from pouch.
– Apply gentle pressure to inside corner of eye at bridge of nose to retard drainage of solution out of eye.
● Tell patient to avoid rubbing eye and to minimize blinking.
● Tell patient not to rinse dropper after use.
● Advise patient to check expiration date on bottle before use and not to use eyedrops that have changed color.
● Tell patient who must use more than one drug to wait at least 5 minutes between instillations.

---

metoclopramide hydrochloride
Apo-Metoclop*, Clopra, Maxeran*, Maxolon, Octamide PFS, Reclomide, Reglan

Pharmacologic classification: para-aminobenzoic acid (PABA) derivative
Therapeutic classification: antiemetic, GI stimulant
Pregnancy risk category: B

Indications and dosages
➤ *Prevention or reduction of nausea and vomiting induced by highly emetogenic chemotherapy.* *Adults:* 2 mg/kg I.V. given initially 30 minutes prior to highly emetogenic chemotherapy, followed by two additional doses of 2 mg/kg I.V. given q 2 hours. If emesis isn't controlled, administer doses of 2 mg/kg I.V. may be repeated every 3 hours for three additional doses. If emesis is suppressed following the initial three

doses, reduce dose to 1 mg/kg I.V. for three additional doses given at 3-hour intervals. Some clinicians have used up to 2.75 mg/kg by I.V. infusion to control nausea and vomiting. Diphenhydramine 50 mg I.M. may be necessary to control extrapyramidal symptoms at this dose. Less emetogenic chemotherapy requires initial doses of 1 mg/kg I.V. every 2 hours for three doses then 1 mg/kg every 3 hours for three additional doses.
➤ *Facilitation of small-bowel intubation and to aid in radiologic examinations.* *Adults:* 10 mg I.V. as a single dose over 1 to 2 minutes.
Children ages 6 to 14: 2.5 to 5 mg I.V. over 1 to 2 minutes.
Children under age 6: 0.1 mg/kg I.V. over 1 to 2 minutes
➤ *Delayed gastric emptying secondary to diabetic gastroparesis.* *Adults:* 10 mg P.O. 30 minutes before meals and h.s. for 2 to 8 weeks, depending on response. Or, 10 mg I.M. or I.V. over 2 minutes. Therapy should be reinstituted at the earliest recurrence of symptoms.
➤ *Gastroesophageal reflux.* *Adults:* 10 to 15 mg P.O. q.i.d., taken 30 minutes before meals and h.s. for up to 12 weeks. Geriatric patients may need only 5 mg per dose.
➤ *Postoperative nausea and vomiting.* *Adults:* 10 to 20 mg I.M. near end of surgical procedure, repeated q 4 to 6 hours, p.r.n.
✦ *Dosage adjustment.* If creatinine clearance is less than 40 ml/minute, initial doses should be 50% of usual recommended doses and adjusted as tolerated.

How supplied
Available by prescription only
Injection: 5 mg/ml
Solution: 5 mg/5 ml, 10 mg/ml
Tablets: 5 mg, 10 mg

Pharmacodynamics
Antiemetic action: Metoclopramide inhibits dopamine receptors in the chemoreceptor trigger zone of the brain to inhibit or reduce nausea and vomiting.
GI stimulant action: Drug relieves esophageal reflux by increasing lower esophageal sphincter tone and reduces gastric stasis by stimulating motility of the upper GI tract, thus reducing gastric emptying time.

Pharmacokinetics
Absorption: After oral administration, drug is absorbed rapidly and thoroughly from the GI tract. After I.M. administration, about 74% to 96% of drug is bioavailable.
Distribution: Distributed to most body tissues and fluids, including the brain. Drug crosses the placenta and is distributed in breast milk.
Metabolism: Not metabolized extensively; a small amount is metabolized in the liver via conjugation.

Excretion: Mostly excreted in urine and feces. Hemodialysis and renal dialysis remove minimal amounts.

Route	Onset	Peak	Duration
P.O.	½-1 hr	1-2 hr	1-2 hr
I.V.	1-3 min	Unknown	1-2 hr
I.M.	10-15 min	Unknown	1-2 hr

Contraindications and precautions
Contraindicated in patients in whom stimulation of GI motility might be dangerous (such as those with hemorrhage, mechanical obstruction, or perforation), in patients hypersensitive to drug, and in those with pheochromocytoma or seizure disorders. Use cautiously in patients with history of depression, Parkinson's disease, or hypertension.

Interactions
Drug-drug. *Acetaminophen, aspirin, diazepam, levodopa, lithium, tetracycline:* Increased absorption of these drugs. Patient requires careful monitoring.
Anticholinergics, opiates: May antagonize effect of metoclopramide on GI motility. Avoid use together if possible.
Antihypertensives, CNS depressants (such as sedatives and tricyclic antidepressants): May lead to increased CNS depression. Patient requires careful monitoring.
Butyrophenone antipsychotics, phenothiazine: May potentiate extrapyramidal reactions. Avoid use together if possible.
Cyclosporine: Increased absorption, possibly increasing its immunosuppressive and toxic effects. Patient requires careful monitoring.
Digoxin: Decreased absorption. Monitor serum digoxin levels.
MAO inhibitors: Increased blood pressure. Use together cautiously.
Drug-lifestyle. *Alcohol use:* May lead to increased CNS depression. Discourage use together.

Adverse reactions
CNS: *restlessness, anxiety, drowsiness, fatigue, lassitude, depression, akathisia, insomnia, confusion,* **suicidal ideation, seizures,** hallucinations, headache, dizziness, extrapyramidal symptoms, tardive dyskinesia, dystonic reactions.
CV: transient hypertension, hypotension, supraventricular tachycardia, **bradycardia.**
GI: nausea, bowel disturbances, diarrhea.
GU: urinary frequency, incontinence, prolactin secretion.
Respiratory: *bronchospasm.*
Skin: rash, urticaria.
Other: fever, porphyria, loss of libido.

Overdose and treatment
Effects of overdose include drowsiness, disorientation, dystonia, seizures, and extrapyramidal effects.

Treatment includes symptomatic and supportive care, administration of antimuscarinics, antiparkinsonians, or antihistamines with antimuscarinic activity (such as 50 mg diphenhydramine, given I.M.).

Special considerations
● Drug has been used investigationally to promote postpartum lactation and treat anorexia nervosa, dizziness, migraine, and intractable hiccups. Oral form is being used investigationally to treat nausea and vomiting.
● Don't use drug for more than 12 weeks.
● Metoclopramide is photosensitive and will degrade when exposed to light. Protect all forms from light. Store at 59° to 86° F (15° to 30° C).
● Drug may be used to facilitate nasoduodenal tube placement.
● When oral concentrate is used, dilute with water, juice, or carbonated beverage or mix with semisolid food.
● Diphenhydramine may be used to counteract extrapyramidal effects of high-dose metoclopramide.
● For I.V. push, use undiluted and inject over a 1- to 2-minute period. For I.V. infusion, dilute with 50 ml of D_5W, dextrose 5% in half-normal saline injection, Ringer's injection, or lactated Ringer's injection, and infuse over at least 15 minutes. Solution is stable for 48 hours when stored at 39° to 86° F (4° to 30° C) and protected from light or for 24 hours when exposed to normal light. Drug may be added to total or partial parenteral nutrition.
● Drug is incompatible with cisplatin, methotrexate, cephalosporins, chloramphenicol, and sodium bicarbonate. Consult specific references for compatibility information.
● Administer by I.V. infusion 30 minutes before chemotherapy.

Patient monitoring
● Monitor renal and hepatic studies.

Breast-feeding patients
● Because drug appears in breast milk, use cautiously when administering to breast-feeding women.

Pediatric patients
● Children have an increased risk of adverse CNS effects.

Geriatric patients
● Use drug cautiously, especially if patient has impaired renal function; dosage may need to be decreased.
● Geriatric patients are more likely to experience extrapyramidal symptoms and tardive dyskinesia.

Patient education
● Warn patient to avoid driving for 2 hours after each dose because drug may cause drowsiness.

Reactions may be *common*, uncommon, *life-threatening*, or COMMON AND LIFE-THREATENING.

• Until extent of CNS effect is known, advise patient not to consume alcohol.
• Tell patient to report twitching or involuntary movement.
• Instruct patient to take medication 30 minutes before each meal.

metolazone
Mykrox, Zaroxolyn

Pharmacologic classification: quinazoline derivative (thiazide-like) diuretic
Therapeutic classification: diuretic, antihypertensive
Pregnancy risk category: B

Indications and dosages
➤ **Edema (heart failure).** **Tablets.** *Adults:* 5 to 10 mg P.O. daily. Maintenance dosage may be lower.
➤ **Edema (renal disease).** **Tablets.** *Adults:* 5 to 20 mg P.O. daily. Maintenance dosage may be lower.
➤ **Hypertension.** **Tablets.** *Adults:* 2.5 to 10 mg P.O. daily; maintenance dosage based on patient's blood pressure. If using stepped-care approach, initial dose is 1.25 to 2.5 mg.
Rapid-acting tablets
Adults: 0.5 mg P.O. once daily; may be increased to maximum of 1 mg daily.

How supplied
Available by prescription only
Tablets: 2.5 mg, 5 mg, 10 mg
Tablets (rapid-acting): 0.5 mg (Mykrox)

Pharmacodynamics
Diuretic action: Metolazone increases urinary excretion of sodium and water by inhibiting sodium reabsorption in the cortical diluting tubule of the nephron, thus relieving edema. Metolazone may be more effective in edema caused by impaired renal function than thiazide or thiazide-like diuretics.
Antihypertensive action: Exact mechanism of antihypertensive effect of metolazone is unknown; it may result from direct arteriolar vasodilatation. Metolazone also reduces total body sodium levels and total peripheral resistance.

Pharmacokinetics
Absorption: About 65% of a given dose of metolazone is absorbed after oral administration in healthy subjects; in cardiac patients, absorption falls to 40%. However, rate and extent of absorption vary among preparations.
Distribution: Metolazone is 50% to 70% erythrocyte-bound and about 33% protein-bound. Drug crosses the placenta and is distributed into breast milk.
Metabolism: Insignificant.
Excretion: About 70% to 95% of metolazone is excreted unchanged in urine. Half-life is about

14 hours in healthy subjects; it may be prolonged in patients with decreased creatinine clearance.

Route	Onset	Peak	Duration
P.O.			
Regular	1 hr	8 hr	12-24 hr
Rapid	1 hr	2-4 hr	12-24 hr

Contraindications and precautions
Contraindicated in patients with anuria, hepatic coma or precoma, or hypersensitivity to thiazides or other sulfonamide-derived drugs. Use cautiously in patients with severely impaired renal or hepatic function.

Interactions
Drug-drug. *Amphetamine, quinidine:* Decreased urinary excretion. Monitor patient closely.
Antihypertensives: Potentiated effects. This may be used to therapeutic advantage.
Cholestyramine, colestipol: May bind metolazone, preventing its absorption. Give drugs 1 hour apart.
Diazoxide: Metolazone may potentiate hyperglycemic, hypotensive, and hyperuricemic effects of diazoxide. Use together cautiously.
Digoxin: Increased risk of digoxin toxicity. Monitor electrolytes.
Furosemide: Excessive volume and electrolyte depletion. Monitor fluid and electrolytes.
Insulin, sulfonylurea: Increased requirements in diabetic patients. Monitor patient closely.
Lithium: Elevated serum lithium levels. May necessitate a 50% reduction in lithium dosage.
Methenamine mandelate: Decreased therapeutic effect. Monitor patient closely.
Drug-lifestyle. *Sun exposure:* Increased risk of photosensitivity reactions. Recommend that patient use adequate protection or avoid excessive sun exposure.

Adverse reactions
CNS: *dizziness, headache, fatigue, vertigo, paresthesia, weakness, restlessness, drowsiness, anxiety, depression, nervousness, blurred vision.*
CV: volume depletion and dehydration, orthostatic hypotension, palpitations, vasculitis, chest pain.
GI: anorexia, nausea, *pancreatitis,* epigastric distress, vomiting, abdominal pain, diarrhea, constipation, dry mouth, abdominal bloating.
GU: nocturia, polyuria, frequent urination, impotence.
Hematologic: *aplastic anemia, agranulocytosis, leukopenia.*
Hepatic: jaundice, *hepatitis.*
Metabolic: hyperglycemia and glucose tolerance impairment; fluid and electrolyte imbalances, including hypokalemia, dilutional hyponatremia and hypochloremia, metabolic alkalosis, hypercalcemia.
Musculoskeletal: muscle cramps.
Skin: dermatitis, photosensitivity, rash, purpura, pruritus, urticaria.

Overdose and treatment
Signs and symptoms of overdose include ortho-static hypotension, dizziness, electrolyte abnormalities, GI irritation and hypermotility, diuresis, and lethargy, which may progress to coma.

Treatment is mainly supportive; monitor patient and assist respiratory, CV, and renal function as indicated. Monitor fluid and electrolyte balance. Induce vomiting with ipecac in conscious patient; otherwise, use gastric lavage to avoid aspiration. Don't give cathartics; these promote additional loss of fluids and electrolytes.

Special considerations
● Drug is effective in patients with decreased renal function. If progressive impairment is evident, consider discontinuing or interrupting treatment.
● Metolazone is used as an adjunct in furosemide-resistant edema.
● Drug has been used with furosemide to induce diuresis in patients who didn't respond to either diuretic alone.
● Rapid-acting form (Mykrox) isn't interchangeable with other forms of metolazone. Dosage and uses vary.
● Store at room temperature in tight, light-resistant containers.
● Drug therapy may interfere with tests for parathyroid function and should be discontinued before such tests.

Patient monitoring
● Monitor renal and hepatic function, electrolytes (potassium, sodium, chloride, calcium), and serum glucose levels.

Breast-feeding patients
● Drug appears in breast milk. Safety and efficacy in breast-feeding women haven't been established.

Pediatric patients
● Safety and efficacy in children haven't been established.

Geriatric patients
● Geriatric and debilitated patients need close observation and may need reduced dosages. They're more sensitive to excess diuresis because of age-related changes in CV and renal function. Excess diuresis promotes orthostatic hypotension, dehydration, hypovolemia, hyponatremia, hypomagnesemia, and hypokalemia.

Patient education
● Tell patient to take drug in the morning to prevent nocturia.
● Advise patient to avoid sudden posture changes and to rise slowly to avoid orthostatic hypotension.
● Instruct patient to use a sunblock to prevent photosensitivity reactions.

metoprolol succinate
Toprol XL

metoprolol tartrate
Lopressor

Pharmacologic classification: beta blocker
Therapeutic classification: antihypertensive, adjunctive treatment of acute MI
Pregnancy risk category: C

Indications and dosages
➤ *Mild to severe hypertension. Adults:* Initially, 50 to 100 mg P.O. daily in single or divided doses; usual maintenance dosage is 100 to 450 mg daily. Or, 50 to 100 mg P.O. extended-release tablets daily (maximum dose, 400 mg daily). Dosages may be increased weekly or longer as needed to desired effect.
➤ *Early intervention in acute MI. Adults:* 2.5 to 5 mg I.V. bolus at 2- to 5-minute intervals up to a total of 15 mg over 10 to 15 minutes. Then give 50 mg P.O. 15 minutes after the last I.V. dose, and continue 50 mg P.O. every 6 hours for 48 hours. Maintenance dosage, 100 mg, b.i.d., P.O. or 200 mg of sustained release form PO daily.
➤ *Atrial tachyarrhythmias following acute MI ◊ . Adults:* 2.5 to 5 mg I.V. q 2 to 5 minutes to control rate up to 15 mg over 10 to 15 minutes. Discontinue when therapeutic efficacy is achieved or if systolic blood pressure is less than 100 mm Hg or heart rate is less than 50 bpm.
➤ *Angina. Adults:* 100 mg P.O. daily in two divided doses. Maintenance dosage, 100 to 400 mg daily. Or, 100 mg P.O. extended-release tablets daily (maximum dose, 400 mg daily). Dosages may be increased gradually at weekly intervals p.r.n.
➤ *Stable, symptomatic heart failure of ischemic, hypertensive, or cardiomyopathic origin. Adults:* Using extended-release form, 25 mg P.O. once daily for 2 weeks in patients with New York Heart Association class II heart failure, and 12.5 mg P.O. once daily in patients with more severe heart failure. Double the dose every 2 weeks to the highest tolerable dose, up to 200 mg.

How supplied
Available by prescription only
Injection: 1 mg/ml in 5-ml ampules or prefilled syringes
Tablets: 50 mg, 100 mg
Tablets (extended-release): 25 mg (scored), 50 mg, 100 mg, 200 mg

Pharmacodynamics
Antihypertensive action: Metoprolol is classified as a cardioselective beta$_1$ antagonist; exact mechanism of antihypertensive effect is unknown. Drug may reduce blood pressure by blocking adrenergic receptors, thus decreasing cardiac

---

output; by decreasing sympathetic outflow from the CNS; or by suppressing renin release.

Action after acute MI: The exact mechanism by which metoprolol decreases mortality after MI is unknown. In patients with MI, it reduces heart rate, systolic blood pressure, and cardiac output. Drug also appears to decrease the occurrence of ventricular fibrillation in these patients.

Pharmacokinetics

Absorption: Orally administered metoprolol is absorbed rapidly and almost completely from GI tract; food enhances absorption.

Distribution: Distributed widely throughout the body; about 12% is protein-bound.

Metabolism: Metabolized in the liver to inactive metabolites.

Excretion: About 95% of a given dose of metoprolol is excreted in urine within 72 hours, largely as metabolites.

Route	Onset	Peak	Duration
P.O.			
Regular	15 min	1 hr	6-12 hr
Extended	15 min	6-12 hr	24 hr
I.V.	5 min	20 min	5-8 hr

Contraindications and precautions

Contraindicated in patients hypersensitive to drug or other beta blockers. Also contraindicated in patients with sinus bradycardia, heart block greater than first-degree, cardiogenic shock, or overt cardiac failure when used to treat hypertension or angina. When used to treat MI, drug also is contraindicated in patients with heart rate less than 45 beats/minute, second- or third-degree heart block, PR interval of 0.24 second or longer with first-degree heart block, systolic blood pressure less than 100 mm Hg, or moderate to severe cardiac failure.

Use cautiously in patients with diabetes mellitus, impaired hepatic or respiratory function, diabetes, or heart failure.

Interactions

Drug-drug. *Cardiac glycosides:* Enhanced bradycardia. Monitor patient closely.

Antihypertensives, diuretics: Potentiated antihypertensive effects. Monitor patient carefully.

Sympathomimetics: Antagonized beta-adrenergic effects of sympathomimetic agents. Monitor patient for drug effect.

Verapamil: May increase bioavailability of metoprolol when given together. Avoid use together if possible. If used together, monitor patient closely and adjust metoprolol dose.

Adverse reactions

CNS: *fatigue, dizziness,* depression, insomnia, headaches, nightmares.

CV: *bradycardia, hypotension, heart failure,* cold limbs, Raynaud's disease.

GI: nausea, diarrhea, constipation, flatulence.

Respiratory: dyspnea, *bronchospasm.*

Skin: rash.

Other: decreased libido.

Overdose and treatment

Signs and symptoms of overdose include severe hypotension, bradycardia, heart failure, and bronchospasm.

After acute ingestion, empty stomach by induced emesis or gastric lavage, and give activated charcoal to reduce absorption. Subsequent treatment is usually symptomatic and supportive.

Special considerations

● When used for angina, use only if AV block and left ventricular dysfunction aren't present.

● If heart failure worsens, increase diuretic doses and consider lowering dose of Toprol-XL or temporarily discontinuing it. Don't increase dose until symptoms of worsening heart failure are stabilized.

● Decrease dose of Toprol-XL if heart failure patient experiences symptomatic bradycardia.

● Administer drug with meals to enhance absorption.

● Reduce dosage in patients with impaired hepatic function.

● Avoid late-evening doses to minimize insomnia.

● Store drug at 59° to 86° F (15° to 30° C).

Patient monitoring

● Monitor heart rate, blood pressure, and ECG during I.V. administration.

● Check blood pressure during dosage adjustment and every 3 to 6 months during maintenance therapy.

● Assess patient for signs of mental depression.

Breast-feeding patients

● Metoprolol appears in breast milk. Recommend an alternative feeding method during therapy.

Pediatric patients

● Safety and efficacy in children haven't been established. No dosage recommendation exists for children.

Geriatric patients

● Geriatric patients may need lower maintenance dosages of metoprolol because of delayed metabolism; they also may have enhanced adverse effects. Use cautiously.

Patient education

● Instruct patient to take drug exactly as prescribed and to take it with meals.

● Inform patient not to stop drug abruptly and to notify prescriber about adverse reactions. Inform him that drug must be withdrawn gradually over 1 to 2 weeks.

metronidazole
Apo-Metronidazole*, Flagyl, Flagyl ER, Metric 21, Novonidazol*, Protostat

metronidazole hydrochloride
Flagyl IV, Flagyl IV RTU, Metro I.V.

Pharmacologic classification: nitroimidazole
Therapeutic classification: antibacterial, antiprotozoal, amebicide
Pregnancy risk category: B

Indications and dosages
➤ *Amebic hepatic abscess. Adults:* 500 to 750 mg P.O. t.i.d. for 5 to 10 days. Or, 2.4 g P.O. daily for 1 to 2 days or 500 mg I.V. q 6 hours for 10 days.
Children: 30 to 50 mg/kg P.O. daily (in three doses) for 5 to 10 days. Or, 1.3 g/m² P.O. daily in three divided doses for 5 to 10 days.
➤ *Intestinal amebiasis. Adults:* 750 mg P.O. t.i.d. for 5 to 10 days. Centers for Disease Control and Prevention recommends addition of iodoquinol 650 mg P.O. t.i.d. for 20 days. Or, 2.4 g P.O. daily for 1 to 2 days or 500 mg I.V. q 6 hours for 10 days.
Children◊: 30 to 50 mg/kg P.O. daily (in three divided doses) for 5 to 10 days. Follow this therapy with oral iodoquinol. Or, 1.3 g/m² P.O. daily in three divided doses for 5 to 10 days.
➤ *Trichomoniasis. Adults (both men and women concurrently):* 375-mg capsule P.O. b.i.d. for 7 days, or 500-mg tablet P.O. b.i.d. for 7 days, or a single dose of 2 g P.O. or divided into two doses given on same day.
Children◊: 15 mg/kg P.O. daily (in three doses) for 7 to 10 days. Or, 40 mg/kg P.O. as a single dose. Dose shouldn't exceed 2 g.
Infants over age 4 weeks◊: 10 to 30 mg/kg P.O. daily for 5 to 8 days.
➤ *Refractory trichomoniasis. Adult women:* 500 mg P.O. b.i.d. for 7 days. If repeated failure, 2 g P.O. daily for 3 to 5 days. Or (for repeated failure), 2 to 3.5 g P.O. daily for 3 to 21 days depending on in vitro susceptibility testing.
➤ *Bacterial infections caused by anaerobic microorganisms. Adults:* Loading dose is 15 mg/kg I.V. infused over 1 hour (about 1 g for a 70-kg [154-lb] adult). Maintenance dosage is 7.5 mg/kg I.V. or P.O. q 6 hours (about 500 mg for a 70-kg adult). Administer first maintenance dose 6 hours after the loading dose. Maximum dose shouldn't exceed 4 g daily. Continue therapy for 7 days to 3 weeks.
➤ *Giardiasis◊. Adults:* 250 mg P.O. t.i.d. for 5 days, or 2 g once daily for 3 days. If coexistent amebiasis, 750 mg P.O. t.i.d. for 5 to 10 days.
Children: 5 mg/kg P.O. t.i.d. for 5 to 7 days.
➤ *Prevention of postoperative infection in contaminated or potentially contaminated colorectal surgery. Adults:* 15 mg/kg

infused over 30 to 60 minutes and completed about 1 hour before surgery. Then 7.5 mg/kg infused over 30 to 60 minutes at 6 and 12 hours after initial dose. If used with oral neomycin or oral kanamycin, 750 mg P.O. b.i.d. to t.i.d. beginning 2 days before surgery. Or, 500 mg to 1 g I.V. 1 hour before surgery followed by 500 mg I.V. at 8 and 16 hours postoperatively.
➤ *Bacterial vaginosis◊. Adults:* 500 mg P.O. b.i.d. for 7 days. Or, 2 g P.O. as a single dose. Or, 750 mg (extended-release) P.O. daily for 7 days. If during pregnancy, 250 mg P.O. t.i.d. for 7 days or 2 g P.O. as a single dose.
➤ *Pelvic inflammatory disease. Adults:* 500 mg I.V. q 12 hours with I.V. ofloxacin or I.V. ciprofloxacin and I.V. or oral doxycycline.
➤ *Pelvic inflammatory disease (ambulatory patients)◊. Adults:* 500 mg P.O. b.i.d. for 14 days (given with 400 mg b.i.d. of ofloxacin).
➤ *Infection with* Clostridium difficile◊. *Adults:* 750 mg to 2 g P.O. daily, in three to four divided doses for 7 to 14 days. Or, 500 to 750 mg I.V. q 6 to 8 hours when oral dosing isn't feasible.
➤ Helicobacter pylori *related to peptic ulcer disease◊. Adults:* 250 to 500 mg P.O. t.i.d. to q.i.d. (with other drugs). Continue for 7 to 14 days depending on regimen used.
Children: 15 to 20 mg/kg P.O. daily, divided in two doses for 4 weeks (with other drugs).
➤ *Amebiasis caused by* Dientamoeba fragilis◊. *Children:* 250 mg P.O. t.i.d. for 7 days.
➤ Entamoeba polecki *infection◊. Adults:* 750 mg P.O. t.i.d. for 10 days.
Children: 35 to 50 mg/kg P.O. daily in three divided doses for 10 days.
➤ *Dracunculiasis caused by* Dracunculus medinensis *(guinea worm infection)◊. Adults:* 250 mg P.O. t.i.d. for 10 days.
Children: 25 mg/kg daily P.O. in three divided doses (up to 750 mg daily) for 10 days.
➤ *Balantidiasis caused by* Balantidium coli◊. *Adults:* 750 mg P.O. t.i.d. for 5 days.
Children: 35 to 50 mg/kg P.O. daily in three divided doses for 5 days.
➤ *Symptomatic* Blastocystis hominis *infection◊. Adults:* 750 mg P.O. t.i.d. for 10 days.
➤ *Active Crohn's disease◊. Adults:* 400 mg P.O. b.i.d. For refractory perineal disease, 20 mg/kg (1 to 1.5 g) in three to five divided doses daily.
➤ *Prophylaxis in sexual assault victims◊. Adults:* 2 g P.O. with other drugs.

How supplied
Available by prescription only
Capsules: 375 mg
Injection: 500 mg/dl ready to use
Powder for injection: 500-mg single-dose vials
Tablets: 250 mg, 500 mg
Tablet (extended-release, film-coated): 750 mg
Tablets (film-coated): 250 mg, 500 mg

Reactions may be *common*, uncommon, *life-threatening*, or COMMON AND LIFE-THREATENING.

Pharmacodynamics

Bactericidal, amebicidal, and trichomonacidal actions: The nitro group of metronidazole is reduced inside the infecting organism; this reduction product disrupts DNA and inhibits nucleic acid synthesis. Drug is active in intestinal and extraintestinal sites. It's active against most anaerobic bacteria and protozoa, including *Bacteroides fragilis, B. melaninogenicus, Fusobacterium, Veillonella, Clostridium, Peptococcus, Peptostreptococcus, Entamoeba histolytica, Trichomonas vaginalis, Giardia lamblia,* and *B. coli.*

Pharmacokinetics

Absorption: About 80% of an oral dose is absorbed; food delays the rate but not the extent of absorption.
Distribution: Distributed into most body tissues and fluids, including CSF, bone, bile, saliva, pleural and peritoneal fluids, vaginal secretions, seminal fluids, middle ear fluid, and hepatic and cerebral abscesses. CSF levels approach serum levels in patients with inflamed meninges; they reach about 50% of serum levels in patients with uninflamed meninges. Less than 20% of metronidazole is bound to plasma proteins. It readily crosses the placenta.
Metabolism: Metabolized to an active 2-hydroxymethyl metabolite and also to other metabolites.
Excretion: About 60% to 80% of dose is excreted as parent compound or its metabolites. About 20% of a metronidazole dose is excreted unchanged in urine; about 6% to 15% is excreted in feces. Half-life of drug is 6 to 8 hours in adults with normal renal function; its half-life may be prolonged in patients with impaired hepatic function.

Route	Onset	Peak	Duration
P.O.	Unknown	2 hr	Unknown
I.V.	Immediate	1 hr	Unknown

Contraindications and precautions

Contraindicated in patients hypersensitive to drug or other nitroimidazole derivatives. Use cautiously in patients with history of blood dyscrasia or alcoholism, hepatic disease, retinal or visual field changes, or CNS disorders and in those receiving hepatotoxic drugs.

Interactions

Drug-drug. *Barbiturates, phenytoin:* Reduced antimicrobial effectiveness of metronidazole. Patient may need higher metronidazole dosage.
Cimetidine: Decreased metronidazole clearance. Monitor patient for adverse effects.
Disulfiram: May precipitate psychosis and confusion. Avoid use together.
Lithium: May increase lithium levels. Monitor serum lithium levels.

Oral anticoagulants: Prolonged PT and INR. Monitor patient for increased bruising or bleeding.
Drug-lifestyle. *Alcohol use:* May cause disulfiram-like reaction (nausea, vomiting, headache, abdominal cramps, and flushing). Discourage use together.

Adverse reactions

CNS: vertigo, headache, ataxia, dizziness, syncope, uncoordination, confusion, irritability, depression, weakness, insomnia, *seizures,* peripheral neuropathy.
CV: ECG change (flattened T wave), edema (with I.V. ready-to-use preparation), flushing.
GI: abdominal cramping, stomatitis, metallic taste, epigastric distress, nausea, vomiting, anorexia, diarrhea, constipation, proctitis, dry mouth.
GU: darkened urine, polyuria, dysuria, cystitis, dyspareunia, dryness of vagina and vulva, vaginal candidiasis.
Hematologic: *transient leukopenia, neutropenia, thrombocytopenia.*
Musculoskeletal: fleeting joint pain.
Skin: rash.
Other: overgrowth of nonsusceptible organisms, especially *Candida* (glossitis, furry tongue); fever; thrombophlebitis (after I.V. infusion); decreased libido.

Overdose and treatment

Signs and symptoms of overdose include nausea, vomiting, ataxia, seizures, and peripheral neuropathy.

There's no known antidote for metronidazole; treatment is supportive. If patient doesn't vomit spontaneously, induced emesis or gastric lavage is indicated for an oral overdose; activated charcoal and a cathartic may be used. Diazepam or phenytoin may be used to control seizures.

Special considerations

● Injection contains 28 mEq of sodium per gram of metronidazole.
● Trichomoniasis should be confirmed by wet smear and amebiasis by culture before giving metronidazole.
● When preparing powder for injection, follow manufacturer's instructions carefully; use solution prepared from powder within 24 hours. I.V. solutions must be prepared in three steps: reconstitution with 4.4 ml of normal saline solution injection (with or without bacteriostatic water); dilution with lactated Ringer's injection, D₅W, or normal saline solution; and neutralization with sodium bicarbonate, 5 mEq per 500 mg metronidazole. Final concentration should be 8 mg/ml or less.
● Administer I.V. form by slow infusion only; if used with a primary I.V. fluid system, discontinue the primary fluid during the infusion; don't give by I.V. push.
⚠ ALERT Infuse drug over 30 minutes to 1 hour. Don't give I.V. push.

• Drug may interfere with the chemical analyses of aminotransferases and triglyceride, leading to falsely decreased values.

Patient monitoring
• Monitor patient for candidiasis during I.V. therapy.
• When treating amebiasis, monitor number and character of stools. Send fecal specimens to the laboratory promptly; infestation is detectable only in warm specimens. Repeat fecal studies at 3-month intervals to ensure elimination of organisms.

Pregnant patients
• If indicated during pregnancy for trichomoniasis, the 7-day regimen is preferred over the single-dose regimen. Avoid treatment with metronidazole during the first trimester.

Breast-feeding patients
• Patient should discontinue breast-feeding while taking drug.

Pediatric patients
• Neonates may eliminate drug more slowly than older infants and children.

Patient education
• Inform patient that drug may cause metallic taste and discolored (red-brown) urine.
• Tell patient to take tablets with meals to minimize GI distress and that tablets may be crushed to facilitate swallowing.
• Counsel patient on need for medical follow-up after discharge.
• Advise patient to report adverse effects.
• Tell patient to avoid alcohol and alcohol-containing drugs during therapy and for at least 48 hours after the last dose to prevent disulfiram-like reaction.
• Explain to patient with amebiasis that follow-up examinations of stool specimens are necessary for 3 months after treatment is discontinued, to ensure elimination of amebae.
• To help prevent reinfection of amebiasis, instruct patient and family members in proper hygiene, including disposal of feces and washing of hands after defecation and before handling, preparing, or eating food. Explain the risks of eating raw food and the need to control contamination by flies.
• Encourage other household members and suspected contacts to be tested for amebiasis and, if necessary, treated.
• For patient with trichomoniasis, teach correct personal hygiene, including perineal care.
• Explain that asymptomatic sexual partners of patients being treated for trichomoniasis should be treated simultaneously to prevent reinfection; patient should refrain from intercourse during therapy or have partner use condom.

metronidazole (topical)
MetroCream, MetroGel, MetroGel-Vaginal, Noritate

Pharmacologic classification: nitroimidazole
Therapeutic classification: antiprotozoal, antibacterial
Pregnancy risk category: B

Indications and dosages
➤ *Topical treatment of acne rosacea, pressure ulcer, inflammatory papules or pustules.* Adults: Apply a thin film b.i.d. to affected area during the morning and evening (once daily for Noritate 1% topical gel). Significant results should be seen within 3 weeks and continue for first 9 weeks of therapy.
➤ *Topical treatment of bacterial vaginosis.* Adults: One applicator once daily or b.i.d., vaginally, for 5 days or once at bedtime (nonpregnant women). In low-risk pregnant women, one applicator vaginally b.i.d. for 5 days.
➤ *Treatment of pressure ulcer◇.* Adults: Prepare a 1% aqueous solution or suspension from crushed metronidazole tablets (sterilized); apply t.i.d.

How supplied
Available by prescription only
Topical cream: 0.75%
Topical gel: 0.75%, 1%
Vaginal gel: 0.75%

Pharmacodynamics
Anti-inflammatory action: Although its exact mechanism of action is unknown, topical metronidazole probably exerts an anti-inflammatory effect through its antibacterial and antiprotozoal actions.

Pharmacokinetics
Absorption: Under normal conditions, serum levels of metronidazole after topical administration are negligible.
Distribution: Less than 20% bound to plasma proteins.
Metabolism: Unknown.
Excretion: Unknown after topical or intravaginal application.

Route	Onset	Peak	Duration
Topical	Unknown	Unknown	Unknown
Intra-vaginal	Unknown	8-12 hr	Unknown

Contraindications and precautions
Contraindicated in patients hypersensitive to drug, its ingredients (such as parabens), or other nitroimidazole derivatives. Use cautiously in patients with history of blood dyscrasia. Use vaginal form cautiously in patients with history of CNS disease because risk of seizures or peripheral neuropathy exists.

Reactions may be *common*, uncommon, **life-threatening**, or COMMON AND LIFE-THREATENING.

Interactions

Drug-drug. *Oral anticoagulants:* May potentiate anticoagulant effect. Monitor patient closely for adverse effects.

Drug-lifestyle. *Alcohol use:* May cause disulfiram-like reaction. Discourage use with vaginal form.

Adverse reactions

CNS: dizziness, light-headedness, headache (with vaginal form).

EENT: lacrimation (if topical gel is applied around the eyes).

GI: decreased appetite, cramps, pain, nausea, diarrhea, constipation, metallic or unpleasant taste sensation (with vaginal form).

GU: *cervicitis, vaginitis,* urinary frequency (with vaginal form).

Skin: rash, transient redness, dryness, mild burning, stinging (with vaginal form).

Other: overgrowth of nonsusceptible organisms (with vaginal form).

Overdose and treatment

No information available. Overdose after topical application is unlikely.

Special considerations

• Topical metronidazole therapy hasn't been linked to the adverse reactions observed with parenteral or oral metronidazole therapy. However, some of the drug can be absorbed following topical use. Limited clinical experience hasn't shown any of these adverse effects.

• Vaginal metronidazole has limited reports of systemic-type reactions.

Patient monitoring

• Monitor patient for clinical effect.

Breast-feeding patients

• Drug appears in breast milk. A decision should be made whether to discontinue drug or breast-feeding, after assessing the importance of drug to the woman.

Pediatric patients

• Safety hasn't been established in children.

Patient education

• Advise patient to clean area thoroughly before applying the drug. Patient may use cosmetics after applying the drug.

• Instruct patient to avoid use of drug on eyelids and to apply it cautiously if drug must be used around the eyes.

• If local reactions occur, advise patient to apply drug less frequently or to discontinue use and call for specific instructions.

mexiletine hydrochloride
Mexitil

Pharmacologic classification: lidocaine analogue, sodium channel antagonist
Therapeutic classification: ventricular anti-arrhythmic
Pregnancy risk category: C

Indications and dosages

➤ *Life-threatening documented ventricular arrhythmias, including ventricular tachycardia. Adults:* 200 mg P.O. q 8 hours. May increase or decrease dose in increments of 50 to 100 mg q 8 hours every 2 to 3 days if satisfactory control isn't obtained. Or, give a loading dose of 400 mg with maintenance dosage of 200 mg P.O. q 8 hours. Some patients may respond well to 450 mg q 12 hours. Maximum daily dose shouldn't exceed 1,200 mg.

➤ *Diabetic neuropathy* ◊. *Adults:* 150 mg P.O. daily for 3 days; then, 300 mg P.O. daily for 3 days followed by 10 mg/kg daily.

How supplied

Available by prescription only
Capsules: 150 mg, 200 mg, 250 mg

Pharmacodynamics

Antiarrhythmic action: Mexiletine is structurally similar to lidocaine and exerts similar electrophysiologic and hemodynamic effects. A class IB antiarrhythmic, it suppresses automaticity and shortens the effective refractory period and action potential duration of His-Purkinje fibers and suppresses spontaneous ventricular depolarization during diastole. At therapeutic serum levels, the drug doesn't affect conductive atrial tissue or AV conduction.

Unlike quinidine and procainamide, mexiletine doesn't significantly alter hemodynamics when given in usual doses. Its effects on the conduction system inhibit reentry mechanisms and halt ventricular arrhythmias. Drug doesn't have a significant negative inotropic effect.

Pharmacokinetics

Absorption: About 90% is absorbed from the GI tract. Absorption rate decreases with conditions that speed gastric emptying.

Distribution: Widely distributed throughout the body. About 50% to 60% of circulating drug is bound to plasma proteins. Usual therapeutic drug level is 0.5 to 2 mcg/ml. Although toxicity may occur within this range, levels above 2 mcg/ml are considered toxic and are linked to an increased frequency of adverse CNS effects, warranting dosage reduction.

Metabolism: Metabolized in the liver to relatively inactive metabolites. Less than 10% of a parenteral dose escapes metabolism and reaches the kidneys unchanged. Metabolism is affected by hepatic blood flow, which may be reduced in patients who are recovering from MI and in those with heart failure. Liver disease also limits metabolism.

Excretion: In healthy patients, half-life of drug is 10 to 12 hours. Elimination half-life may be prolonged in patients with heart failure or liver disease. Urinary excretion increases with urine acidification and slows with urine alkalinization.

Route	Onset	Peak	Duration
P.O.	½-2 hr	2-3 hr	Unknown

Contraindications and precautions

Contraindicated in patients with cardiogenic shock or second- or third-degree AV block in the absence of an artificial pacemaker. Use cautiously in patients with hypotension, heart failure, first-degree heart block, ventricular pacemaker, sinus node dysfunction, or seizure disorders.

Interactions

Drug-drug. *Ammonium chloride:* Enhanced mexiletine excretion. Monitor patient carefully.
Antacids that contain aluminum or magnesium hydroxide, atropine, narcotics: May delay mexiletine absorption. Separate administration times.
Carbonic anhydrase inhibitors, high-dose antacids, sodium bicarbonate: Decreased mexiletine excretion. Monitor patient carefully.
Cimetidine: May increase or decrease mexiletine metabolism, resulting in altered drug levels. Monitor patient carefully.
Metoclopramide: May increase metoclopramide absorption. Monitor patient carefully.
Phenobarbital, phenytoin, rifampin: May induce hepatic metabolism of mexiletine and thus reduce serum drug levels. Patient requires careful monitoring.
Theophylline: Increased serum theophylline levels. Monitor serum theophylline levels.
Drug-food. *Caffeine:* decreased caffeine metabolism by 50%. Encourage patient to reduce caffeine intake.

Adverse reactions

CNS: *tremor, dizziness, blurred vision, diplopia, confusion,* light-headedness, incoordination, changes in sleep habits, paresthesia, weakness, fatigue, speech difficulties, tinnitus, depression, *nervousness, headache.*
CV: *new or worsened arrhythmias,* palpitations, chest pain, nonspecific edema, angina.
GI: *nausea, vomiting, upper GI distress, heartburn, diarrhea, constipation, dry mouth, changes in appetite, abdominal pain.*
Hepatic: *altered liver function test results.*
Skin: rash.

Overdose and treatment

Effects of overdose are primarily extensions of adverse CNS effects. Seizures are the most serious effect.

Treatment usually involves symptomatic and supportive measures. In acute overdose, emesis induction or gastric lavage should be performed. Urine acidification may accelerate drug elimination. If patient has bradycardia and hypotension, atropine may be given.

Special considerations

● Administer dosage with meals, if possible.
● Because of proarrhythmic effects, drug is generally not recommended for non-life-threatening arrhythmias.
● When changing from lidocaine to mexiletine, stop infusion when first mexiletine dose is given. Keep infusion line open, however, until arrhythmia appears to be satisfactorily controlled.
● When transferring patient from another Class I oral antiarrhythmic, initial dose of 200 mg should be started 6 to 12 hours after last dose of quinidine; 3 to 6 hours after last dose of procainamide; 6 to 12 hours after last dose of disopyramide; and 8 to 12 hours after last dose of tocainide.
● Patient whose condition isn't controlled by dosing every 8 hours may respond to dosing every 6 hours.
● Many patients who respond well to mexiletine (300 mg or less every 8 hours) can be maintained on an every-12-hour schedule. The same total daily dose is divided into twice-daily doses, which improves patient compliance.
● Tremor (usually a fine hand tremor) is commonly evident in patients taking higher doses of mexiletine.

Patient monitoring

● Monitor blood pressure and heart rate and rhythm for significant change.
● Monitor hepatic function tests.

Breast-feeding patients

● Drug appears in breast milk. Alternative feeding method should be used during therapy.

Geriatric patients

● Most geriatric patients require reduced dosages because of reduced hepatic blood flow and consequent decreased metabolism.
● Geriatric patients also may be more susceptible to CNS adverse effects.

Patient education

● Tell patient to take drug with food to reduce risk of nausea.
● Instruct patient to report if the following occur: unusual bleeding or bruising; signs of infection, such as fever, sore throat, stomatitis, or chills; or fatigue.

Reactions may be *common*, uncommon, *life-threatening*, or COMMON AND LIFE-THREATENING.

mezlocillin sodium
Mezlin

Pharmacologic classification: extended-spectrum penicillin, acylaminopenicillin
Therapeutic classification: antibiotic
Pregnancy risk category: B

Indications and dosages
➤ *Infections caused by susceptible organisms.* Adults: 200 to 300 mg/kg I.V. or I.M. daily given in four to six divided doses. Usual dosage is 3 g q 4 hours or 4 g q 6 hours. For serious infections, up to 24 g daily may be administered. Therapy is usually 10 to 14 days.
Children under age 12: For mild to moderate infection, 50 to 100 mg/kg daily in four divided doses. For more severe infections, 200 to 300 mg/kg per day I.M. or I.V. in divided doses q 4 to 6 hours.
Neonates age 7 days and under ◊ : 75 mg/kg q 12 hours I.V. or I.M.
Neonates age 8 days and older: 75 mg/kg q 8 hours (if weight less than 2 kg [4.4 lb]) or q 6 hours (if weight over 2 kg) I.V. or I.M.
➤ *Uncomplicated urinary tract infections.* Adults: 100 to 125 mg/kg daily I.M. or I.V. in divided doses q 6 hours or 1.5 to 2 g q 6 hours.
➤ *Complicated urinary tract infections.* Adults: 150 to 200 mg/kg I.V. daily divided into q 6 hour doses or 3 g q 6 hours.
➤ *Uncomplicated gonococcal urethritis caused by* Neisseria gonorrhoeae. Adults: 1 to 2 g I.M. or I.V. with 1 g of oral probenecid.
➤ *Surgical prophylaxis.* Adults: 4 g I.V. 30 minutes to 1.5 hours before surgery and repeat I.V. 6 and 12 hours later.
✦ *Dosage adjustment.* In adult patients with renal impairment and creatinine clearance of 10 to 30 ml/minute, give 3 g q 6 to 8 hours for life-threatening or serious infection. For urinary tract infection (UTI), give 1.5 g q 6 to 8 hours. If creatinine clearance is less than 10 ml/minute, give 2 g q 6 to 8 hours for life-threatening or serious infection. For UTI, give 1.5 g q 8 hours.
Patients on hemodialysis should be given 3 to 4 g after each dialysis session, then q 12 hours. Patients on peritoneal dialysis may receive 3 g q 12 hours. In patients with severe hepatic impairment, reduce dose by 50% or double the dosing interval.

How supplied
Available by prescription only
Infusion: 2 g, 3 g, 4 g
Injection: 1 g, 2 g, 3 g, 4 g

Pharmacodynamics
Antibiotic action: Mezlocillin is bactericidal; it adheres to bacterial penicillin-binding proteins, thereby inhibiting bacterial cell wall synthesis.

Extended-spectrum penicillins are more resistant to inactivation by certain beta-lactamases, especially those produced by gram-negative organisms, but are still liable to inactivation by certain others.

Spectrum of activity of drug includes many gram-negative aerobic and anaerobic bacilli, many gram-positive and gram-negative aerobic cocci, and some gram-positive aerobic and anaerobic bacilli, but a large number of these organisms are resistant to mezlocillin. Mezlocillin may be effective against some strains of carbenicillin-resistant and ticarcillin-resistant gram-negative bacilli. Mezlocillin shouldn't be used as sole therapy because of the rapid development of resistance. Some clinicians believe that there's no evidence that it has any advantages over ticarcillin or carbenicillin, at least with respect to cure rates. Drug is less active against *Pseudomonas aeruginosa* than other members of this class, such as piperacillin.

Pharmacokinetics
Absorption: Not absorbed from GI tract.
Distribution: Distributed widely. It penetrates minimally into CSF with uninflamed meninges, crosses the placenta, and is 16% to 42% protein-bound.
Metabolism: Partially metabolized; about 15% of a dose is metabolized to inactive metabolites.
Excretion: Excreted primarily (39% to 72%) in urine by glomerular filtration and renal tubular secretion; up to 30% of a dose is excreted in bile, and some appears in breast milk. Elimination half-life in adults is ¾ to 1½ hours; in extensive renal impairment, half-life is extended to 2 to 14 hours. Mezlocillin is removed by hemodialysis but not by peritoneal dialysis.

Route	Onset	Peak	Duration
I.V.	Immediate	Immediate	Unknown
I.M.	Unknown	45-90 min	Unknown

Contraindications and precautions
Contraindicated in patients hypersensitive to drug or other penicillins. Use cautiously in patients with bleeding tendencies, uremia, hypokalemia, or allergy to cephalosporins.

Interactions
Drug-drug. *Aminoglycoside antibiotics:* Synergistic bactericidal effect against *P. aeruginosa, Escherichia coli, Klebsiella, Citrobacter, Enterobacter, Serratia,* and *Proteus mirabilis.* This is a therapeutic advantage.
Clavulanic acid: Synergistic bactericidal effect against certain beta–lactamase-producing bacteria. This is a therapeutic advantage.
Methotrexate: Delayed elimination and elevated serum levels of methotrexate. Monitor patient closely.
Probenecid: Blocks tubular secretion of penicillins, raising their serum levels. Monitor patient carefully.

Vecuronium bromide: Prolonged neuromuscular blockade. Monitor patient closely.

Adverse reactions
CNS: neuromuscular irritability, *seizures.*
GI: nausea, diarrhea, vomiting, abnormal taste sensation, pseudomembranous colitis, flatulence.
GU: interstitial nephritis.
Hematologic: *bleeding* (with high doses), *neutropenia, thrombocytopenia,* eosinophilia, *leukopenia, hemolytic anemia.*
Metabolic: *hypokalemia.*
Other: *hypersensitivity reactions (anaphylaxis,* edema, fever, chills, rash, pruritus, urticaria), overgrowth of nonsusceptible organisms, *pain at injection site, vein irritation, phlebitis.*

Overdose and treatment
Overdose may cause neuromuscular sensitivity or seizures. A 4- to 6-hour hemodialysis session will remove 20% to 30% of mezlocillin.

Special considerations
● Mezlocillin may be more suitable than carbenicillin or ticarcillin for patients on salt-free diets; mezlocillin contains only 1.85 mEq of sodium per gram.
● Drug is almost always used with another antibiotic such as an aminoglycoside in life-threatening infections.
● For I.M. reconstitution, for each gram, add 3 to 4 ml of sterile water for injection or 1% lidocaine without epinephrine and dissolve.
● Inject I.M. dose slowly over 12 to 15 seconds to minimize pain. Don't exceed 2 g per site.
● For direct I.V. injection, add 9 to 10 ml of sterile water for injection, 5% dextrose injection, normal saline solution injection to each gram of mezlocillin. Shake vigorously and inject desired dose over 3 to 5 minutes. Don't exceed 100 mg/ml. For I.V. infusion, further dilute in 50 to 100 ml of a compatible I.V. solution (such as normal saline solution or 5% dextrose) and infuse over 30 minutes. Reconstitute ADD-Vantage vial according to manufacturer instructions.
● Mezlocillin is incompatible with aminoglycosides and shouldn't be infused in the same I.V. line or solution.
● Solutions are stable for 24 hours to 7 days depending on solution used and storage temperature.
● If precipitate forms during refrigerated storage, warm to 98.6° F (37° C) in warm water bath and shake well. Solution should be clear.
● Because drug is partially dialyzable, dosage may need adjustment in patients undergoing hemodialysis.
● Drug alters tests for urinary or serum proteins; it interferes with turbidimetric methods that use sulfosalicylic acid, trichloroacetic acetic acid, or nitric acid. Positive Coombs' tests have been reported in patients taking mexlocillin.

Patient monitoring
● Monitor serum potassium level and liver function studies.
● Monitor patient with high serum levels for seizures.

Breast-feeding patients
● Drug appears in breast milk; safe use in breast-feeding women hasn't been established. Alternative feeding method is recommended during therapy.

Geriatric patients
● Half-life may be prolonged in geriatric patients because of impaired renal function.

Patient education
● Instruct patient to report adverse reactions promptly.
● Tell patient to alert prescriber if discomfort occurs.
● Caution patient to limit salt intake during mezlocillin therapy because of high sodium content of drug.

miconazole nitrate
Femizol-M, Micatin, Monistat 3, Monistat 7, Monistat-Derm

Pharmacologic classification: imidazole derivative
Therapeutic classification: antifungal
Pregnancy risk category: B

Indications and dosages
➤ *Cutaneous or mucocutaneous fungal infections caused by susceptible organisms.* **Topical use.** *Adults and children:* Apply to affected areas b.i.d. for 2 to 4 weeks.
➤ *Treatment of pityriasis (tinea versicolor).* **Topical use.** *Adults and children over age 2:* Apply cream to affected area once daily.
Vaginal use
Adults: Insert 200-mg suppository h.s. for 3 days, or 100-mg suppository or one applicatorful of vaginal cream h.s. for 7 days.

How supplied
Available by prescription only
Cream: 2%
Vaginal cream: 2%
Vaginal suppositories: 200 mg
Available without a prescription
Cream: 2%
Powder: 2%
Spray: 2%
Vaginal cream: 2%
Vaginal suppositories: 100 mg, 200 mg

Pharmacodynamics
Antifungal action: Miconazole is fungistatic and fungicidal, depending on drug concentration, in *Aspergillus flavus, Candida albicans,*

C. parapsilosis, C. tropicalis, Coccidioides im-mitis, Cryptococcus neoformans, Curvularia, Histoplasma capsulatum, Microsporum canis, Paracoccidioides brasiliensis, Pseudallescheria boydii, Sporothrix schenckii, dermatophytes, and some gram-positive bacteria. Miconazole causes thickening of the fungal cell wall, altering membrane permeability; it also may kill the cell by interference with peroxisomal enzymes, causing accumulation of peroxide within the cell wall. It attacks virtually all pathogenic fungi.

Pharmacokinetics
Absorption: A small amount of drug is systemically absorbed after vaginal administration.
Distribution: Penetrates well into inflamed joints, vitreous humor, and the peritoneal cavity. Distribution into sputum and saliva is poor, and CSF penetration is unpredictable. Over 90% is bound to plasma proteins.
Metabolism: Metabolized in the liver, predominantly to inactive metabolites.
Excretion: Elimination is triphasic; terminal half-life is about 24 hours. Between 10% and 14% of an oral dose is excreted in urine; 50%, in feces. Up to 1% of a vaginal dose is excreted in urine; 14% to 22% of an I.V. dose is excreted in urine. It isn't known if drug appears in breast milk.

Route	Onset	Peak	Duration
Topical, intra-vaginal	Unknown	Unknown	Unknown

Contraindications and precautions
Topical form contraindicated in patients hypersensitive to drug. Use cautiously in patients with hepatic insufficiency.

Interactions
Drug-drug. *Amphotericin B:* May antagonize the effects of amphotericin B. Monitor patient carefully.
Phenytoin: Increased phenytoin levels. Monitor phenytoin levels.
Warfarin: Increased anticoagulant effect. Monitor PT and INR.

Adverse reactions
CNS: headache.
GU: vulvovaginal burning, pruritus, or irritation with vaginal cream; pelvic cramps.
Skin: irritation, burning, maceration, allergic contact dermatitis.

Overdose and treatment
No information available.

Special considerations
• Clean affected area before applying cream. After application, massage area gently until cream disappears.
• Continue topical therapy for at least 1 month; improvement should begin in 1 to 2 weeks. If no

improvement occurs by 4 weeks, reevaluate diagnosis.
• Insert vaginal applicator high into vagina, except in pregnancy.

Patient monitoring
• Monitor patient for clinical effects.

Pregnant patients
• The 7-day vaginal treatment is preferred in pregnant women.

Breast-feeding patients
• Safety hasn't been established in breast-feeding women.

Pediatric patients
• Safety in children under age 1 hasn't been established.

Patient education
• Teach patient the symptoms of fungal infection, and explain treatment rationale.
• Encourage patient to adhere to prescribed regimen and follow-up visits and to report adverse effects.
• Teach patient correct procedure for intravaginal or topical applications.
• To prevent vaginal reinfection, teach correct perineal hygiene and recommend that patient abstain from sexual intercourse during therapy.

midazolam hydrochloride
Versed

Pharmacologic classification: benzodiazepine
Therapeutic classification: preoperative sedative, agent for conscious sedation, adjunct for induction of general anesthesia, amnesic agent
Controlled substance schedule: IV
Pregnancy risk category: D

Indications and dosages
➤*Preoperative sedation (to induce sleepiness or drowsiness and relieve apprehension).* Adults under age 60: 0.07 to 0.08 mg/kg I.M. about ½ to 1 hour before surgery. May be administered with atropine or scopolamine and reduced doses of narcotics.
✦ *Dosage adjustment.* Reduce dosage in patients over age 60, those with COPD, those considered to be high-risk surgical patients, and those who have received concomitant narcotics or other depressants.
➤*Conscious sedation.* Adults under age 60: Initially, 1 to 2.5 mg I.V. administered over at least 2 minutes; repeat in 2 minutes, if needed, in small increments of initial dose over at least 2 minutes to achieve desired effect. Total dose up to 5 mg may be used. Additional doses to maintain desired level of sedation may be given by slow titra-

tion in increments of 25% of dose used to reach the sedation endpoint.

Adults age 60 and older: 1.5 mg or less over at least 2 minutes. If additional titration is needed, give at a rate not exceeding 1 mg over 2 minutes. Total doses exceeding 3.5 mg aren't usually necessary.

➤*Induction of general anesthesia.* *Unpremedicated adults under age 55:* 0.3 to 0.35 mg/kg I.V. over 20 to 30 seconds if patient hasn't received preanesthesia medication, or 0.15 to 0.35 mg/kg (usually 0.25 mg/kg) I.V. over 20 to 30 seconds if patient has received preanesthesia medication. Additional increments of 25% of the initial dose may be needed to complete induction.

Unpremedicated adults age 55 and older: Initially, 0.3 mg/kg. For debilitated patients, initial dose is 0.2 to 0.25 mg/kg. For premedicated patients, 0.15 mg/kg may be sufficient.

➤*Continuous infusion for sedation of intubated and mechanically ventilated patients as a component of anesthesia or during treatment in a critical care setting.* *Adults:* If a loading dose is necessary to rapidly start sedation, give 0.01 to 0.05 mg/kg slowly or infused over several minutes, with dose repeated at 10- to 15-minute intervals until adequate sedation is achieved. For maintenance of sedation, usual infusion rate is 0.02 to 0.10 mg/kg/hour (1 to 7 mg/hour). Titrate infusion rate to the desired amount of sedation. Drug can be titrated up or down by 25% to 50% of the initial infusion rate to achieve optimal sedation without oversedation.

Children: After a loading dose of 0.05 to 0.2 mg/kg over 2 to 3 minutes in intubated patients, an infusion may be started at 0.06 to 0.12 mg/kg/hour (1 to 2 mcg/kg/minute). Dose may be titrated up or down by 25% of initial or subsequent infusion rate to obtain optimal sedation. *Neonates:* Use only on intubated neonates. No loading dose is used. Neonates under 32 weeks' gestation receive infusion rates of 0.03 mg/kg/hour (0.5 mcg/kg/minute). In neonates over 32 weeks' gestation, infusion rates are 0.06 mg/kg/hour (1 mcg/kg/minute). Infusion may be run more rapidly in the first few hours to obtain a therapeutic blood level. Rate of infusion should be frequently and carefully reassessed to administer the lowest possible amount of drug.

➤*Sedation, anxiolysis, and amnesia before diagnostic, therapeutic, or endoscopic procedures or before induction of anesthesia.* *Children ages 6 months to 16 years:* 250 to 500 mcg/kg P.O. up to 20 mg or up to 1 mg/kg. Lower doses may provide adequate therapeutic effect for children age 6 months to 16 years or cooperative patients. Or, 100 to 150 mcg/kg I.M. (up to 500 mcg/kg may be necessary) not to exceed 10 mg.

Children ages 6 months to 5 years: Initially 50 to 100 mcg/kg I.V. up to 600 mcg/kg (usual dose doesn't exceed 6 mg).

Children ages 6 to 12: 25 to 50 mcg/kg I.V. up to 400 mcg/kg (usual dose doesn't exceed 10 mg).

Children ages 13 to 16: 0.07 to 0.08 mg/kg I.M. ½ to 1 hour before surgery; for conscious sedation, 1 to 2.5 mg I.V. over at least 2 minutes.

How supplied

Available by prescription only

Injection: 1 mg/ml in 2-ml, 5-ml, and 10-ml vials; 5 mg/ml in 1-ml, 2-ml, 5-ml, and 10-ml vials; 5 mg/ml in 2-ml disposable syringe
Syrup: 2 mg/ml in 118 ml bottle

Pharmacodynamics

Sedative and anesthetic actions: Although exact mechanism is unknown, midazolam, like other benzodiazepines, is thought to facilitate the action of gamma-aminobutyric acid to provide a short-acting CNS depressant action.

Amnesic action: Mechanism of action by which midazolam causes amnesia isn't known.

Pharmacokinetics

Absorption: Absorption after I.M. administration appears to be 80% to 100% and after oral administration 40 to 50%.

Distribution: Drug has a large volume of distribution and is about 97% protein-bound. Drug crosses the placenta and enters fetal circulation.
Metabolism: Metabolized in the liver.
Excretion: Metabolites are excreted in urine. Half-life of drug is 1¼ to 12⅓ hours.

Route	Onset	Peak	Duration
P.O.	10-20 min	1-2 hr	2-6 hr
I.V.	1½-2½ min	Rapid	2-6 hr
I.M.	15 min	15-60 min	2-6 hr

Contraindications and precautions

Contraindicated in patients hypersensitive to drug, in those with acute angle-closure glaucoma, and in those experiencing shock, coma, or acute alcohol intoxication. Use cautiously in patients with uncompensated acute illnesses and in geriatric or debilitated patients.

Interactions

Drug-drug. *Antidepressants, antihistamines, barbiturates, narcotics, tranquilizers, and other CNS and respiratory depressants:* Potentiated effects. Use together cautiously.

Droperidol, fentanyl, narcotics: Potentiated hypnotic effect of midazolam. Monitor patient carefully.

Erythromycin: May decrease plasma clearance of midazolam. Monitor patient closely.

Inhaled anesthetics: Midazolam may decrease the needed dose of inhaled anesthetics by depressing respiratory drive. Anesthesia dosage may require adjustment.

Isoniazid: May decrease the metabolism of midazolam. Monitor patient closely.

Reactions may be *common*, uncommon, *life-threatening*, or COMMON AND LIFE-THREATENING.

Rifampin: Decreased midazolam levels. Monitor patient for effect.

Drug-herb. *Catnip, kava, lady's slipper, lemon balm, passionflower, sassafras, skullcap, valerian:* Sedative effects may be enhanced. Discourage concurrent use.

Drug-food. *Grapefruit juice:* Increased bioavailability of oral syrup form of drug. Discourage use together.

Drug-lifestyle. *Alcohol use:* Potentiated effects of alcohol. Advise patient to avoid alcohol.

Adverse reactions
CNS: headache, oversedation, drowsiness, amnesia.
CV: hypotension, irregular pulse, *cardiac arrest.*
GI: *nausea,* vomiting.
Respiratory: *hiccups, decreased respiratory rate, apnea, respiratory arrest.*
Other: *pain, tenderness at injection site.*

Overdose and treatment
Signs and symptoms of overdose include confusion, stupor, coma, respiratory depression, and hypotension.

Treatment is supportive. Maintain patent airway, and ensure adequate ventilation with mechanical support, if necessary. Monitor vital signs. Use I.V. fluids or ephedrine to treat hypotension. Flumazenil, a specific benzodiazepine-receptor antagonist, is indicated for complete or partial reversal of the sedative effects.

Special considerations
• Individualized dosages are advised, using the smallest effective dose possible. Use with extreme caution and reduced dosage in geriatric and debilitated patients.
• Medical personnel who administer midazolam should be familiar with airway management. Close monitoring of cardiopulmonary function is required. Continuously monitor patients who have received midazolam to detect potentially life-threatening respiratory depression.
• Laryngospasm and bronchospasm may occur rarely; countermeasures should be available.
• Midazolam can be mixed in the same syringe with morphine, meperidine, atropine, and scopolamine.
• Syrup form must be given only to patients visually monitored by health care professionals.
• Solutions compatible with midazolam include D₅W, normal saline solution, and lactated Ringer's solution.
• Before I.V. administration, ensure the immediate availability of oxygen and resuscitation equipment. Apnea and death have been reported with rapid I.V. administration. Avoid intra-arterial injection because the hazards of this route are unknown. Avoid extravasation. Administer I.V. dose slowly to prevent respiratory depression.
• Benzyl alcohol creates an increased risk of adverse effects, such as hypotension, metabolic acidosis, and kernicterus, in neonates. Take into account the amount of benzyl alcohol when giving high doses of midazolam or other drugs that contain this preservative.
• Give I.M. dose deep into a large muscle mass to prevent tissue injury.
• Don't use solution that's discolored or that contains a precipitate.

Patient monitoring
• Hypotension is more likely in patients premedicated with narcotics. Monitor vital signs.

Breast-feeding patients
• It isn't known if drug appears in breast milk; use cautiously in breast-feeding women.

Pediatric patients
• The safety and efficacy of oral solution in children under age 6 months haven't been established. Monitor the amount of benzyl alcohol when used in neonates.

Geriatric patients
• Geriatric or debilitated patients, especially those with COPD, are at significantly increased risk for respiratory depression and hypotension. Lower doses are indicated. Use cautiously.
• Oral forms aren't recommended.

Patient education
• Advise patient to postpone tasks that require mental alertness or physical coordination until the effects of the drug have worn off.
• Instruct patient as necessary in safety measures, such as supervised walking and gradual position changes, to prevent injury.
• Advise patient to contact prescriber before taking OTC drugs.

mifepristone
Mifeprex

Pharmacologic classification: synthetic steroid
Therapeutic classification: anti-progestational
Pregnancy risk category: NR

Indications & dosages
➤ *Termination of intrauterine pregnancy through 49ᵗʰ day of pregnancy.* Adults: On day 1, give 600 mg (three 200-mg tablets) P.O. as a single dose. On day 3, unless abortion is confirmed by clinical examination or ultrasonographic scan, give misoprostol 400 mcg P.O.

How supplied
Tablets: 200 mg

Pharmacodynamics
Drug is a synthetic steroid with antiprogestational effects. It competitively interacts with progesterone at progesterone-receptor sites, inhibiting

the activity of endogenous and exogenous progesterone, causing termination of pregnancy.

Pharmacokinetics

Absorption: Mifepristone is rapidly absorbed; levels peak in about 90 minutes.
Distribution: Mifepristone is 98% bound to plasma proteins, albumin and α_1-acid glycoprotein.
Metabolism: Mifepristone is metabolized by N-demethylation and terminal hydroxylation to three major metabolites. In vitro studies have shown that CYP-450 3A4 is primarily responsible for the metabolism.
Excretion: Excreted in the feces and urine.

Route	Onset	Peak	Duration
P.O.	Rapid	90 min	11 days

Contraindications and precautions

Contraindicated in patients with confirmed or suspected ectopic pregnancy or undiagnosed adnexal mass, or in patients with an intrauterine device in place. Also contraindicated in patients with chronic adrenal failure, patients on concurrent long-term corticosteroid therapy, and patients with history of allergy to mifepristone, misoprostol, or other prostaglandins. Contraindicated in patients with inherited porphyrias, hemorrhagic disorders, or anticoagulant therapy.

The treatment procedure is contraindicated in patients without access to a medical facility equipped to provide emergency treatment of incomplete abortion, blood transfusions, and emergency resuscitation during the period from the first visit until discharged by the prescriber.

Don't administer to any patient who may be unable to understand the effects of the treatment procedure or to comply with its regimen.

Use cautiously in heavy smokers and patients who have CV disease; hypertension; respiratory, renal, or hepatic disease; insulin-dependent diabetes mellitus; or severe anemia. Also use cautiously in women who are more than 35 years old and who also smoke 10 or more cigarettes per day because such patients were excluded from clinical trials of mifepristone.

Interactions

Drug-drug: *Carbamazepine, dexamethasone, phenobarbital, phenytoin, rifampin:* May induce metabolism and reduce serum mifepristone levels. Use together cautiously.
Drugs that are CYP 3A4 substrates and have narrow therapeutic ranges (general anesthetics): Increased serum levels and prolonged elimination of these drugs. Use together cautiously.
Erythromycin, itraconazole, ketoconazole: May inhibit metabolism and increased serum mifepristone levels. Use together cautiously.
Drug-herb: *St. John's wort:* May induce metabolism and decrease mifepristone levels. Tell patient to use together cautiously.

Drug-food: *Grapefruit juice:* May inhibit metabolism and increase mifepristone levels. Tell patient to use together cautiously.

Adverse reactions

CNS: *headache, dizziness, fatigue,* insomnia, asthenia, anxiety, syncope, fainting.
EENT: sinusitis.
GI: *abdominal cramping, nausea, vomiting, diarrhea,* dyspepsia.
GU: vaginitis, *uterine cramping,* pelvic pain, uterine hemorrhage.
Hematologic: anemia, leukorrhea, decrease in hemoglobin of more than 2 g/dl.
Musculoskeletal: back pain, leg pain.
Other: fever, rigors, viral infections.

Overdose and treatment

No serious adverse reactions were seen with three times the recommended dose of mifepristone. If a patient ingests a massive overdose, she should be observed closely for signs of adrenal failure.

Special considerations

● Drug is supplied only to licensed physicians who sign and return a prescriber's agreement. It isn't available through pharmacies.
● For purposes of this treatment, pregnancy is dated from the first day of the last menstrual period in a presumed 28-day cycle with ovulation occurring at mid-cycle. The duration of pregnancy may be determined from menstrual history and clinical examination. Ultrasonographic scan should be used if the duration of pregnancy is uncertain, or if ectopic pregnancy is suspected.
● Patient must read the medication guide and sign the patient agreement before drug is given.
● Any intrauterine device must be removed before treatment begins.
● Mifepristone and misoprostol treatment for the termination of pregnancy requires three office visits by the patient to the prescriber for proper administration. This treatment may be administered only in a clinic, medical office, or hospital, by or under the supervision of a physician able to assess gestational age and to diagnose ectopic pregnancies. Physician must also be able to provide surgical intervention in cases of incomplete abortion or severe bleeding, or have made plans to provide such care through others, and be able to assure patient access to medical facilities equipped to provide blood transfusions and resuscitation, if necessary.
● During the period following administration of misoprostol, the patient may need medication for cramps or GI symptoms.
● Mifeprex should be stored at controlled room temperature.

Patient monitoring

● Patient must return for a follow up visit about 14 days after administration of Mifeprex to determine by clinical examination or ultrasound

---

Reactions may be *common*, uncommon, **life-threatening**, or COMMON AND LIFE-THREATENING.

that a complete termination of pregnancy has occurred and to assess the degree of bleeding. Patients who have an ongoing pregnancy at this visit have a risk of fetal malformation resulting from the treatment. Surgical termination is recommended.

• Vaginal bleeding and uterine or abdominal cramping are expected effects of the drug. Vaginal bleeding or spotting occurs for an average of 9 to 16 days. Excessive bleeding may require treatment with vasoconstrictors, curettage, saline infusions, and blood transfusions. Persistence of heavy or moderate bleeding at the 14-day follow-up visit may indicate incomplete abortion.

Breast-feeding

• It isn't known whether mifepristone appears in human milk. Breast-feeding women should consult with their prescriber to decide if they should discard their breast milk for a few days following administration.

Patient education

• Give patient a copy of the medication guide and the patient agreement. Review them with patient and discuss any questions the patient has.

• Inform patient of the importance of completing the treatment schedule, and stress the need for a follow-up visit about 14 days after taking Mifeprex.

• Tell the patient to expect vaginal bleeding that may be heavy at times along with uterine cramping.

• Inform patient that vaginal bleeding isn't proof of a complete abortion and that she must return for follow-up to confirm the abortion.

• Inform patient that if treatment fails, surgical intervention may be necessary.

• Supply patient with a name and telephone number to contact in case of emergency.

• Inform patient that she may become pregnant again as soon as termination of pregnancy is complete and before normal menses has returned.

• Teach the patient about forms of contraception.

miglitol
Glyset

Pharmacologic classification: alpha-glucosidase inhibitor
Therapeutic classification: antidiabetic
Pregnancy risk category: B

Indications and dosages

➤ *Monotherapy adjunct to diet to improve glycemic control in patients with type 2 (non-insulin-dependent) diabetes mellitus whose hyperglycemia can't be managed with diet alone, or with a sulfonylurea when diet plus either miglitol or sulfonylurea alone don't result in adequate glycemic control. Adults:* 25 mg P.O.

t.i.d. at the start (with the first bite) of each main meal; dose may be increased after 4 to 8 weeks to 50 mg P.O. t.i.d. The dose may then be further increased after 3 months, based on the glycosylated hemoglobin level, to a maximum of 100 mg P.O. t.i.d.

How supplied

Avaialable by prescription only
Tablets: 25 mg, 50 mg, 100 mg

Pharmacodynamics

Antidiabetic action: Miglitol lowers blood glucose through reversible inhibition of the enzymes alpha-glucosidases in the brush border of the small intestine. Alpha-glucosidases are responsible for the conversion of oligosaccharides and disaccharides to glucose. Inhibition of these enzymes results in delayed glucose absorption and a lowering of postprandial blood glucose. In contrast to sulfonylureas, miglitol has no effect on insulin secretion.

Pharmacokinetics

Absorption: Demonstrates saturable absorption at high doses. A 25-mg dose is completely absorbed, whereas a dose of 100 mg is only 50% to 70% absorbed.
Distribution: Distributes primarily into the extracellular fluid. Protein-binding is negligible (less than 4%).
Metabolism: Not metabolized.
Excretion: Eliminated primarily by renal excretion. More than 95% of a given dose is recovered in the urine as unchanged drug. The elimination half-life is about 2 hours.

Route	Onset	Peak	Duration
P.O.	Unknown	2-3 hr	Unknown

Contraindications and precautions

Miglitol is contraindicated in patients hypersensitive to the drug or any of its components. Also contraindicated in patients with diabetic ketoacidosis, inflammatory bowel disease, colonic ulceration, or partial intestinal obstruction, and in patients predisposed to intestinal obstruction or those with chronic intestinal diseases related to marked disorders of digestion or absorption, or with conditions that may deteriorate as a result of increased gas formation in the intestine.

Drug isn't recommended in patients with significant renal dysfunction (serum creatinine level above 2 mg/dl). Use cautiously in patients also receiving insulin or oral sulfonylureas.

Interactions

Drug-drug. *Digoxin, propranolol, ranitidine:* May decrease the bioavailability of these drugs. Monitor patient for loss of drug efficacy; dose adjustment may be needed.
Intestinal absorbents, such as charcoal, and digestive enzyme preparations, such as amy-

lase and pancreatin: May reduce the effectiveness of miglitol. Avoid use together.

Adverse reactions
GI: *abdominal pain, diarrhea, flatulence.*
Metabolic: decreased serum iron level.
Skin: rash.

Overdose and treatment
Overdose may result in transient increases in adverse GI reactions. No serious systemic reactions are expected.

Special considerations
● An increased risk of hypoglycemia can occur when drug is used with insulin or sulfonylureas; dosage adjustments of these drugs may be needed.
● The management of type 2 diabetes should also include diet control, an exercise program, and regular testing of urine and blood glucose level.
● Give miglitol with the first bite of each main meal.
● Mild to moderate hypoglycemia may be treated with a form of dextrose such as glucose tablets or gel. Severe hypoglycemia may require I.V. glucose or glucagon administration.

Patient monitoring
● When therapy starts or dosage is adjusted, one-hour postprandial plasma glucose may be used to determine therapeutic response.
● Monitor patient for an increased frequency of hypoglycemia.
● Monitor blood glucose levels regularly, especially during increased stress, such as infection, fever, surgery, and trauma.
● Besides having glucose levels checked regularly, monitor glycosylated hemoglobin level every 3 months to evaluate long-term glycemic control.

Breast-feeding patients
● Although the amount of miglitol that appears in breast milk is low, it's recommended that miglitol not be administered to breast-feeding women.

Pediatric patients
● Safety and efficacy of miglitol in children haven't been established.

Geriatric patients
● No significant differences in the safety and effectiveness of miglitol have been observed in placebo-controlled clinical trials between older and younger patients.

Patient education
● Instruct patient about the importance of adhering to diet, weight reduction, and exercise instructions and of having blood glucose and glycosylated hemoglobin levels tested regularly.
● Inform patient that treatment with miglitol relieves symptoms but doesn't cure diabetes.

● Teach patient to recognize signs and symptoms of hyperglycemia and hypoglycemia.
● Instruct patient to treat hypoglycemia with glucose tablets and to have a source of glucose readily available to treat symptoms of hypoglycemia when miglitol is taken with a sulfonylurea or insulin.
● Advise patient to seek medical advice promptly during periods of stress such as fever, trauma, infection, or surgery because medication requirements may change.
● Instruct patient to take miglitol three times a day with the first bite of each main meal.
● Show patient how and when to perform self-monitoring of glucose levels.
● Advise patient that adverse GI effects are most common during the first few weeks of therapy and should improve over time.
● Urge patient to wear or carry medical identification at all times.

milrinone lactate
Primacor

Pharmacologic classification: bipyridine phosphodiesterase inhibitor
Therapeutic classification: inotropic vasodilator
Pregnancy risk category: C

Indications and dosages
➤ *Short-term I.V. therapy for heart failure.* *Adults:* Initial loading dose of 50 mcg/kg I.V. over 10 minutes, followed by continuous infusion/maintenance dosage of 0.375 to 0.75 mcg/kg/minute. Adjust infusion dose based on hemodynamic and clinical response.
✦ *Dosage adjustment.* For patients with renal impairment, refer to the following table.

Creatinine clearance (ml/min)	Infusion rate (mcg/kg/min)
50	0.43
40	0.38
30	0.33
20	0.28
10	0.23
5	0.20

How supplied
Available by prescription only
Cartridge: 5 ml (1mg/ml)
Injection, premixed: 200 mcg/ml
Solution: 1 mg/ml in 10-ml and 20-ml vials

Pharmacodynamics
Inotropic and vasodilator actions: Milrinone is a selective inhibitor of peak III cAMP phosphodiesterase isozyme in cardiac and vascular muscle. This inhibitory action is consistent with

cAMP-mediated increases in intracellular ionized calcium and contractile force in cardiac muscle, as well as with cAMP-dependent contractile protein phosphorylation and relaxation in vascular muscle. In addition to increasing myocardial contractility, milrinone improves diastolic function, shown by improvements in left ventricular diastolic relaxation.

Pharmacokinetics

Absorption: Administered I.V.
Distribution: About 70% is bound to human plasma protein.
Metabolism: About 12% is metabolized to a glucuronide metabolite.
Excretion: After I.V. administration, about 90% is excreted unchanged in urine within 8 hours.

Route	Onset	Peak	Duration
I.V.	5-15 min	1-2 hr	3-6 hr

Contraindications and precautions

Contraindicated in patients hypersensitive to drug, patients with severe aortic or pulmonic valvular disease in place of surgical correction, and patients in the acute phase of an MI. Use cautiously in patients with atrial fibrillation or flutter.

Interactions

None reported.

Adverse reactions

CNS: headache, tremors.
CV: ventricular arrhythmias, ventricular ectopic activity, nonsustained ventricular tachycardia, *sustained ventricular tachycardia, ventricular fibrillation,* hypotension, angina.
Hematologic: *thrombocytopenia.*
Metabolic: hypokalemia.

Overdose and treatment

Hypotension may occur with milrinone overdose because of its vasodilator effect. No specific antidote is known, but general measures for circulatory support should be taken.

Special considerations

● Drug isn't recommended for patients in acute phase of post-MI; clinical studies in this population are lacking.
● Duration of therapy depends on patient responsiveness. Patients have been maintained on infusions of milrinone for up to 5 days.
● If hypotension occurs, administration of milrinone should be reduced or temporarily discontinued until patient's condition stabilizes.
● Milrinone must be further diluted before I.V. administration. Acceptable diluents include half-normal saline solution, normal saline solution, and D₅W. Prepare 100 mcg/ml, 150 mcg/ml, or 200 mcg/ml solutions by adding 180 ml, 113 ml, or 80 ml to the 20-mg (20-ml) vial. Add one-half of the diluent amounts to the 10-ml vial to achieve same concentration.

● When furosemide is injected into an I.V. line containing milrinone, a precipitate forms. Therefore, furosemide shouldn't be administered in an I.V. line that contains milrinone.

Patient monitoring

● Monitor renal function and fluid and electrolyte changes during milrinone therapy. Correct hypokalemia with potassium supplements before or during use of milrinone.

Breast-feeding patients

● It isn't known if drug appears in breast milk. Use cautiously in breast-feeding women.

Pediatric patients

● Safety and efficacy in children haven't been established.

Patient education

● Instruct patient to report adverse reactions, especially angina, promptly.
● Tell patient to report discomfort at the I.V. insertion site.

mineral oil
Fleet Enema Mineral Oil, Kondremul*, Kondremul Plain, Lansoÿl*, Milkinol, Neo-Cultol, Nujol*, Petrogalar Plain

Pharmacologic classification: lubricant oil
Therapeutic classification: laxative
Pregnancy risk category: C

Indications and dosages

➤ *Constipation, preparation for bowel studies or surgery. Adults and children age 12 and older:* 15 to 45 ml P.O. as a single dose or in divided doses, or 120-ml enema.
Children ages 6 to 12: 5 to 15 ml P.O. as a single dose or in divided doses, or 30- to 60-ml enema.
Children ages 2 to 6: 30- to 60-ml enema.

How supplied

Available without a prescription
Emulsion: 2.5 ml/5 ml, 1.4 g/5 ml
Jelly: 180 ml
Rectal oil enema: 120 ml
Suspension: 2.75 ml/5 ml, 4.75 ml/5 ml

Pharmacodynamics

Laxative action: Mineral oil acts mainly in the colon, lubricating the intestine and retarding colonic fluid absorption.

Pharmacokinetics

Absorption: Absorbed minimally; with emulsified drug form, significant absorption occurs.
Distribution: Distributed locally, primarily in the colon.
Metabolism: None.

Excretion: Excreted in feces.

Route	Onset	Peak	Duration
P.O.	6-8 hr	Variable	Variable
P.R.	2-15 min	Unknown	Unknown

Contraindications and precautions
Contraindicated in patients with abdominal pain, nausea, vomiting, or other symptoms of appendicitis or acute surgical abdomen and in those with fecal impaction or intestinal obstruction or perforation. Contraindicated in patients with colostomy, ileostomy, ulcerative colitis, and diverticulitis. Use cautiously in geriatric, debilitated, and young patients.

Interactions
Drug-drug. *Anticoagulants, cardiac glycosides, fat-soluble vitamins (A, D, E, and K), oral contraceptives, sulfonamides:* Impaired absorption of these drugs and vitamins, thus lessening their therapeutic effects. Avoid administration together, and monitor patient for vitamin deficiency.
Stool softeners such as docusate: Increased mineral oil absorption to potentially toxic levels. Avoid use together.

Adverse reactions
GI: *nausea; vomiting; diarrhea* (with excessive use); abdominal cramps, especially in severe constipation; decreased absorption of nutrients and fat-soluble vitamins, resulting in deficiency; slowed healing after hemorrhoidectomy.
Respiratory: *lipid pneumonia.*
Skin: anal pruritus, anal irritation, hemorrhoids, perianal discomfort.
Other: laxative dependence (with long-term or excessive use).

Overdose and treatment
No information available.

Special considerations
● Avoid administering drug to patients lying flat because if drug is aspirated into the lungs, pneumonitis may result.
● Drug shouldn't be given with food because this may delay gastric emptying, resulting in delayed drug action and increased aspiration risk. Separate administration by at least 2 hours.
● To improve taste, give emulsion and suspension with fruit juice or carbonated beverages.
● Prescribe cleansing enema 30 minutes to 1 hour after retention enema.
● Reduce or divide dose or use emulsified drug form to avoid leakage through anal sphincter.
● Mineral oil may impair absorption of fat-soluble vitamins (A, D, E, and K).

Patient monitoring
● Monitor patient for clinical effect.

Pediatric patients
● Mineral oil isn't recommended for children under age 6 because of risk of aspiration. Enema form is contraindicated in children under age 2.

Geriatric patients
● Because of increased aspiration risk, use cautiously in geriatric patients.

Patient education
● Instruct patient not to take mineral oil with stool softeners.
● Warn patient that mineral oil may leak through anal sphincter, especially with repeated use or with enema form. Undergarment protection may be desired.

minocycline hydrochloride
Dynacin, Minocin, Vectrin

Pharmacologic classification: tetracycline
Therapeutic classification: antibiotic
Pregnancy risk category: NR

Indications and dosages
➤ *Infections caused by sensitive organisms.* *Adults:* Initially, 200 mg P.O., I.V.; then 100 mg q 12 hours or 50 mg P.O. q 6 hours.
Children over age 8: Initially, 4 mg/kg P.O., I.V.; then 4 mg/kg P.O. daily, divided q 12 hours. Give I.V. in 500 to 1,000 ml solution without calcium, over 6 hours.
➤ *Gonorrhea in patients sensitive to penicillin.* *Adults:* Initially, 200 mg P.O., then 100 mg q 12 hours for 4 days.
➤ *Syphilis in patients sensitive to penicillin.* *Adults:* Initially, 200 mg P.O.; then 100 mg q 12 hours for 10 to 15 days.
➤ *Meningococcal carrier state.* *Adults:* Initially, 200 mg P.O., then 100 mg P.O. q 12 hours for 5 days.
➤ *Uncomplicated urethral, endocervical, or rectal infection caused by* Chlamydia trachomatis *or* Ureaplasma urealyticum.
Adults: 100 mg P.O. q 12 hours for at least 7 days.
➤ *Uncomplicated gonococcal urethritis in men.* *Adults:* 100 mg P.O. q 12 hours for 5 days.
➤ *Infection with* Mycobacterium marinum.
Adults: 100 mg P.O. q 12 hours for 6 to 8 weeks.
➤ *Cholera.* *Adults:* Initially, 200 mg P.O.; then 100 mg P.O. q 12 hours for 72 hours.
➤ *Acne.* *Adults:* 50 mg P.O. daily to t.i.d.
➤ *Treatment of multibacillary leprosy◇.*
Adults: 100 mg P.O. daily with clofazimine and ofloxacin for 6 months, followed by 100 mg P.O. daily for another 18 months with clofazimine.
➤ *Nocardiosis ◇. Adults:* Usual dose for 12 to 18 months.
➤ *Sclerosis agent for pleural effusions ◇.*
Adults: 300 mg mixed in 40 to 50 ml sodium chloride injection, given via thoracostomy tube.
➤ *Nongonococcal urethritis caused by* C. trachomatis *or* mycoplasma ◇. *Adults:*

100 mg P.O. daily in one or two divided doses for 1 to 3 weeks.

How supplied
Available by prescription only
Capsules: 50 mg, 100 mg
Injection: 100 mg/vial
Suspension: 50 mg/5 ml
Tablets: 50 mg, 100 mg

Pharmacodynamics
Antibacterial action: Minocycline is bacteriostatic; it binds reversibly to ribosomal units, thus inhibiting bacterial protein synthesis.

Minocycline is active against many gram-negative and gram-positive organisms, *Mycoplasma, Rickettsia, Chlamydia,* and spirochetes; it may be more active against staphylococci than other tetracyclines.

The potential vestibular toxicity and cost of minocycline limit its usefulness. It may be more active than other tetracyclines against *Nocardia asteroides;* it's also effective against *M. marinum* infections. It has been used for meningococcal meningitis prophylaxis because of its activity against *Neisseria meningitidis.*

Pharmacokinetics
Absorption: About 90% to 100% is absorbed after oral administration.
Distribution: Widely distributed into body tissues and fluids, including synovial, pleural, prostatic, and seminal fluids; bronchial secretions; saliva; and aqueous humor. CSF penetration is poor. Drug crosses the placenta, and is 70% to 80% protein-bound.
Metabolism: Metabolized partially.
Excretion: Excreted primarily unchanged in urine by glomerular filtration. Plasma half-life is 11 to 22 hours in adults with normal renal function. Some drug appears in breast milk.

Route	Onset	Peak	Duration
P.O.	Unknown	1-4 hr	Unknown
I.V.	Immediate	Immediate	Unknown

Contraindications and precautions
Contraindicated in patients hypersensitive to drug or other tetracyclines. Use cautiously in patients with impaired renal or hepatic function, children under age 8, and patients in last half of pregnancy.

Interactions
Drug-drug. *Antacids containing aluminum, calcium, or magnesium or with laxatives containing magnesium, oral iron products, or sodium bicarbonate:* Decreased oral absorption of minocycline because of chelation. Administer drugs at separate times.
Cimetidine: May decrease absorption of minocycline. Monitor patient.
Digoxin: Increased bioavailability. Decreased digoxin dose may be necessary.

Oral anticoagulants: Increased effects. Decreased anticoagulant dose may be necessary.
Oral contraceptives: May be less effective when administered with minocycline. Advise patient to use alternative birth control.
Penicillins: Tetracyclines may antagonize bactericidal effects of penicillin. Give penicillin 2 to 3 hours before minocycline.
Drug-food. *Dairy products, food:* May decrease minocycline absorption. Discourage use together.
Drug-lifestyle. *Sun exposure:* Increased risk of photosensitivity reactions. Advise patient to use sunscreen and limit sun exposure.

Adverse reactions
CNS: headache, *intracranial hypertension (pseudotumor cerebri),* light-headedness, dizziness, vertigo.
CV: pericarditis.
EENT: dysphagia, glossitis, blurred vision.
GI: *anorexia, epigastric distress, oral candidiasis, nausea, vomiting, diarrhea,* enterocolitis, inflammatory lesions in anogenital region, esophageal ulcerations.
GU: increased BUN level.
Hematologic: *neutropenia,* eosinophilia, *thrombocytopenia,* hemolytic anemia.
Hepatic: elevated liver enzyme levels.
Skin: *maculopapular and erythematous rashes, photosensitivity, increased pigmentation, urticaria, Stevens-Johnsons syndrome.*
Other: *hypersensitivity reactions (anaphylaxis);* permanent discoloration of teeth, enamel defects, and bone growth retardation if used in children under age 8; superinfection; *thrombophlebitis.*

Overdose and treatment
Signs and symptoms of overdose are usually limited to GI tract; give antacids or empty stomach by gastric lavage if ingestion occurred within the preceding 4 hours.

Special considerations
⚠ ALERT Don't confuse Minocin with niacin or Mithracin.
⚠ ALERT Check expiration date. Outdated or deteriorated tetracyclines are highly nephrotoxic and have produced a Fanconi-like syndrome.
● Reconstitute 100 mg powder with 5 ml sterile water for injection, with further dilution of 500 to 1,000 ml for I.V. infusion of 100 to 200 mcg/ml. Infuse over 6 hours.
● Reconstituted solution is stable for 24 hours at room temperature. Use final diluted solution immediately.
● Avoid mixing with solutions containing calcium because a precipitate may form (Ringer's injection and lactated Ringer's injection are compatible).
● Drug causes false-negative results in urine glucose tests using glucose oxidase reagent (Clinistix or glucose enzymatic test strip). Minocycline causes false elevations in fluorometric test results for urinary catecholamines.

Patient monitoring
● Monitor renal and hepatic function in prolonged therapy.

Breast-feeding patients
● Avoid use in breast-feeding women.

Pediatric patients
● Drug isn't recommended for use in children under age 8.

Patient education
● Tell patient to take entire amount of drug prescribed, even after he feels better.
● Instruct patient to take oral form of drug with a full glass of water. Drug may be taken with food. Tell patient not to take within 1 hour of bedtime to avoid esophageal irritation or ulceration.
● Warn patient to avoid driving or other hazardous tasks because of possible adverse CNS effects.
● Caution patient to avoid direct sunlight and ultraviolet light, to wear protective clothing, and to use sunscreen. Photosensitivity reactions may occur within a few minutes to several hours after exposure. Photosensitivity persists for some time after discontinuation of therapy.

minoxidil
Loniten

Pharmacologic classification: peripheral vasodilator
Therapeutic classification: antihypertensive
Pregnancy risk category: C

Indications and dosages
➤ *Severe hypertension. Adults and children over age 12:* Initially, 2.5 to 5 mg P.O. as a single daily dose. Dose may be increased at 3-day intervals (minimum) to 10 mg, 20 mg, and then 40 mg. If rapid control is necessary, dose may be adjusted q 6 hours. Effective dosage range is usually 10 to 40 mg daily in one to two divided doses. Maximum dose is 100 mg/day.
Children under age 12: 0.2 mg/kg (maximum 5 mg) as an initial single daily dose. Effective dosage range is usually 0.25 to 1 mg/kg daily in one or two doses. If necessary, dose is increased after at least 3-day intervals in increments of 50% to 100% until optimal response is attained. If rapid control is necessary, dose may be adjusted q 6 hours. Maximum dose is 50 mg/day.

How supplied
Available by prescription only
Tablets: 2.5 mg, 10 mg

Pharmacodynamics
Antihypertensive action: Drug produces its antihypertensive effect by a direct vasodilating effect on vascular smooth muscle; the effect on resistance vessels (arterioles and arteries) is greater

than that on capacitance vessels (venules and veins).

Pharmacokinetics
Absorption: Absorbed rapidly and almost completely from the GI tract.
Distribution: Distributed widely into body tissues; it isn't bound to plasma proteins.
Metabolism: About 90% of a given dose is metabolized.
Excretion: Excreted primarily in urine. Average plasma half-life is 4¼ hours.

Route	Onset	Peak	Duration
P.O.	½ hr	2-3 hr	2-5 days

Contraindications and precautions
Contraindicated in patients hypersensitive to drug and in those with pheochromocytoma. Use cautiously in patients with impaired renal function or after acute MI.

Interactions
Drug-drug. *Diuretics, hypotensive agents:* increased hypotensive effects. May be used to therapeutic advantage.
Guanethidine: May cause profound orthostatic hypotension. Discontinue guanethidine 1 to 3 days before starting minoxidil.

Adverse reactions
CV: *edema, tachycardia, pericardial effusion and tamponade, **heart failure**, ECG changes,* rebound hypertension.
GI: *nausea, vomiting.*
Metabolic: *weight gain.*
Respiratory: pulmonary edema.
Skin: rash, ***Stevens-Johnson syndrome.***
Other: *hypertrichosis,* gynecomastia, *breast tenderness.*

Overdose and treatment
Evidence of overdose includes hypotension, tachycardia, headache, and skin flushing.

After acute ingestion, empty stomach by induced emesis or gastric lavage, and give activated charcoal to reduce absorption. Further treatment is usually symptomatic and supportive. Administer normal saline solution I.V. to maintain blood pressure. Avoid sympathomimetic drugs, such as epinephrine and norepinephrine, because of their excessive cardiac stimulating action.

Special considerations
● Drug usually is given with other antihypertensives, such as diuretics, beta blockers, or sympathetic nervous system suppressants.
● Patients with renal impairment or a need for dialysis may need smaller maintenance dosages. Because minoxidil is removed by dialysis, it's recommended that, on the day of dialysis, the drug be given immediately after dialysis if dialysis is at

---

Reactions may be *common*, uncommon, *life-threatening*, or COMMON AND LIFE-THREATENING.

9 a.m.; if dialysis is after 3 p.m., the daily dose is given at 7 a.m. (8 hours before dialysis).
• After blood pressure is stabilized, patient should be reevaluated every 3 to 6 months.

Patient monitoring
• Monitor blood pressure and pulse after administration.
• Assess intake, output, and body weight for sodium and water retention.
• Monitor patient for heart failure, pericardial effusion, and cardiac tamponade; have phenylephrine, dopamine, and vasopressin on hand to treat hypotension.

Breast-feeding patients
• Drug appears in breast milk. An alternative feeding method is recommended during therapy.

Pediatric patients
• Because of limited experience in children, use drug and adjust dosage cautiously.

Geriatric patients
• These patients may be sensitive to antihypertensive effects of drug. Dosage adjustment may be necessary because of altered drug clearance. Monitor orthostatic blood pressure in geriatric patients.

Patient education
• Explain that drug is usually taken with other antihypertensives; emphasize importance of taking drug as prescribed.
• Caution patient to report these cardiac symptoms promptly: increased heart rate (more than 20 beats/minute over normal), rapid weight gain, shortness of breath, chest pain, severe indigestion, dizziness, light-headedness, or fainting.
• Tell patient to call prescriber for instructions before taking OTC cold preparations.
• Advise patient that hypertrichosis will disappear 1 to 6 months after stopping drug.

minoxidil (topical)
Minoxidil for Men, Rogaine

Pharmacologic classification: direct-acting vasodilator
Therapeutic classification: hair-growth stimulant
Pregnancy risk category: C

Indications and dosages
➤ *Male-pattern baldness (alopecia androgenetica); diffuse hair loss or thinning in women; adjunct to hair transplantation* ◇. *Adults:* Apply 1 ml to affected area b.i.d. for 4 months or longer.
➤ *Alopecia areata* ◇. *Adults:* 1 ml of 1%, 3%, or 5% solution applied to scalp b.i.d.

How supplied
Available without a prescription
Topical solution: 2% in 60-ml bottle

Pharmacodynamics
Hair-growth stimulation: Exact mechanism by which drug promotes hair growth is unknown. It may alter androgen metabolism in the scalp, or it may exert a local vasodilatation and enhance the microcirculation around the hair follicle. It may also directly stimulate the hair follicle.

Pharmacokinetics
Absorption: Poorly absorbed through intact skin. About 0.3% to 4.5% of a topically applied dose reaches the systemic circulation. Application to skin with decreased integrity may increase systemic absorption.
Distribution: Serum levels are generally negligible.
Metabolism: Metabolism isn't fully described.
Excretion: Eliminated primarily by the kidneys. About 95% of a topically applied dose is eliminated after 4 days.

Route	Onset	Peak	Duration
Topical	Unknown	Unknown	Unknown

Contraindications and precautions
Contraindicated in patients hypersensitive to drug or any component of the solution, or during pregnancy. Use cautiously in patients with renal, cardiac, or hepatic disease; those over age 50; and breast-feeding women.

Interactions
None reported.

Adverse reactions
CNS: headache, dizziness, faintness, light-headedness.
CV: edema, chest pain, hypertension, hypotension, palpitations, increased or decreased pulse rate, *heart failure.*
EENT: sinusitis.
GI: diarrhea, nausea, vomiting.
GU: urinary tract infection, renal calculi, urethritis.
Metabolic: weight gain.
Musculoskeletal: back pain, tendinitis.
Respiratory: bronchitis, upper respiratory infection.
Skin: irritant dermatitis, allergic contact dermatitis, eczema, hypertrichosis, local erythema, pruritus, dry skin or scalp, flaking, alopecia, exacerbation of hair loss.

Overdose and treatment
None reported. However, if topical use produces systemic adverse effects, wash application site thoroughly with soap and water and treat symptoms, as appropriate. Signs and symptoms of oral overdose include hypotension, tachycardia, headache, and skin flushing.

After acute ingestion, empty stomach by induced emesis or gastric lavage, and give activated charcoal to reduce absorption. Further treatment is usually symptomatic and supportive.

Special considerations

• Before treatment with topical minoxidil, patient should have a history and physical examination and should be advised of potential risks; a risk-benefit decision should be made. Patients with cardiac disease should realize that adverse effects may be especially serious. Alert patient to possibility of tachycardia and fluid retention, and monitor patient for increased heart rate, weight gain, or other systemic effects.

• Don't use with other topical agents such as corticosteroids, retinoids, and petrolatum or agents that enhance percutaneous absorption. Rogaine is for topical use only; each milliliter contains 20 or 50 mg minoxidil and accidental ingestion could cause adverse systemic effects.

• Alcohol base will burn and irritate sensitive surfaces (eye, abraded skin, and mucous membranes). If topical minoxidil contacts sensitive areas, flush with copious cool water.

• The 5% topical solution shouldn't be used by women.

• Self-medication should cease and a clinician should be consulted if no hair grows in 8 months for women and 12 months for men using the 2% solution and in 4 months in men using the 5% solution.

Patient monitoring

• Before starting treatment, check that patient has a normal, healthy scalp. Local abrasion or dermatitis may increase absorption and the risk of adverse effects.

• Monitor patient 1 month after starting topical drug therapy and at least every 6 months afterward. Discontinue topical minoxidil if systemic effects occur.

Breast-feeding patients

• Topical minoxidil shouldn't be administered to breast-feeding women.

Pediatric patients

• Safety and efficacy haven't been established for patients under age 18.

Patient education

• Tell patient to avoid inhaling the spray.

• Teach patient to apply topical minoxidil as follows: Dry hair and scalp. Apply 1 ml to the total affected areas twice daily. Total daily dose shouldn't exceed 2 ml. If fingertips are used to apply the drug, wash hands afterward.

• Encourage patient to carefully review patient information leaflet, which is included with each package and in the full product information.

• Inform patient that 4 months of use may be required before results become apparent.

mirtazapine
Remeron

Pharmacologic classification: piperazinoazepine
Therapeutic classification: tetracyclic antidepressant
Pregnancy risk category: C

Indications and dosages

➤ *Depression.* Adults: Initially, 15 mg P.O. h.s. Maintenance dosage ranges from 15 mg to 45 mg daily. Dosage adjustments should be made at intervals no less than 1 to 2 weeks apart.

How supplied

Available by prescription only
Tablets: 15 mg, 30 mg, 45 mg

Pharmacodynamics

Antidepressant action: Unknown.

Pharmacokinetics

Absorption: Rapidly and completely absorbed from the GI tract. Absolute bioavailability of drug is about 50%.
Distribution: About 85% is bound to plasma protein.
Metabolism: Extensively metabolized in the liver.
Excretion: Predominantly eliminated in urine (75%) with 15% excreted in feces. Half-life is between 20 and 40 hours.

Route	Onset	Peak	Duration
P.O.	Unknown	2 hr	Unknown

Contraindications and precautions

Contraindicated in patients hypersensitive to drug. Coadministration with MAO inhibitors is contraindicated.

Use cautiously in patients with CV or cerebrovascular disease, seizure disorders, suicidal ideation, impaired hepatic and renal function, or history of mania or hypomania. Also, use cautiously in pregnant patients and those with conditions that predispose them to hypotension, such as dehydration, hypovolemia, or antihypertensive treatment. Use cautiously in patients with increased intraocular pressure, history of urine retention, or history of angle-closure glaucoma because of anticholinergic properties.

Interactions

Drug-drug. *Diazepam and other CNS depressants:* May cause additive CNS effects. Avoid use together.
MAO inhibitors or within 14 days of starting or stopping an MAO inhibitor: Potential for serious, and sometimes fatal, reactions. Avoid use together.
Drug-lifestyle. *Alcohol use:* Additive CNS effects. Discourage use together.

Adverse reactions
CNS: *somnolence,* dizziness, asthenia, abnormal dreams, abnormal thinking, tremor, confusion.
CV: edema, hypertension.
GI: nausea, *increased appetite, dry mouth, constipation,* vomiting.
GU: urinary frequency.
Metabolic: *weight gain.*
Musculoskeletal: back pain, myalgia.
Respiratory: dyspnea.
Skin: pruritus, rash.
Other: flu syndrome, peripheral edema.

Overdose and treatment
Overdose may result in disorientation, drowsiness, impaired memory, and tachycardia.

Treat as for any antidepressant overdose. If patient is unconscious, establish an airway and provide adequate oxygenation. Consider gastric lavage, induced emesis, or both; also consider activated charcoal. Monitor cardiac and vital signs and provide general symptomatic and supportive measures.

Special considerations
• There should be a drug-free interval of at least 2 weeks when switching from MAO-inhibitor therapy to mirtazapine or from mirtazapine to an MAO inhibitor.

Patient monitoring
• Although risk of agranulocytosis is rare, discontinue drug and monitor patient closely if he develops a sore throat, fever, stomatitis, or other signs of infection with a low WBC count.
• Patient requires close observation because it isn't known if mirtazapine causes physical or psychological dependence.

Breast-feeding patients
• It isn't known if drug appears in breast milk; use cautiously in breast-feeding women.

Pediatric patients
• Safety and efficacy in children haven't been established.

Geriatric patients
• Weight gain occurs predominantly in elderly patients. May be used as therapeutic advantage in patients who need appetite stimulation.
• Administer mirtazapine cautiously to geriatric patients because pharmacokinetic studies reveal decreased clearance in elderly people.

Patient education
• Caution patient not to perform hazardous activities if somnolence occurs.
• Instruct patient not to use alcohol or other CNS depressants while taking drug because of additive effect.
• Tell patient to report signs and symptoms of infection such as fever, chills, sore throat, mucous membrane ulceration, or other possible signs of infection including any flulike complaints.
• Stress importance of compliance with mirtazapine therapy.
• Instruct patient not to take any other medication without medical approval.
• Tell women of childbearing age to report suspected pregnancy immediately.

misoprostol
Cytotec

Pharmacologic classification: prostaglandin E₁ analogue
Therapeutic classification: antiulcer, gastric mucosal protectant
Pregnancy risk category: X

Indications and dosages
➤ *Prevention of gastric ulcer induced by NSAIDs. Adults:* 200 mcg P.O. q.i.d with meals and h.s. Reduce dosage to 100 mcg P.O. q.i.d. in patients who cannot tolerate this dosage.
➤ *Duodenal or gastric ulcer* ◊ *. Adults:* 100 to 200 mcg P.O. q.i.d. with meals and h.s. for 4 to 8 weeks.

How supplied
Available by prescription only
Tablets: 100 mcg, 200 mcg

Pharmacodynamics
Antiulcer action: Misoprostol enhances the production of gastric mucus and bicarbonate and decreases basal, nocturnal, and stimulated gastric acid secretion.

Pharmacokinetics
Absorption: Rapidly absorbed after oral use.
Distribution: Less than 90% bound to plasma proteins.
Metabolism: Rapidly de-esterified to misoprostol acid, the biologically active metabolite. The de-esterified metabolite undergoes further oxidation in several body tissues.
Excretion: About 15% of an oral dose appears in the feces; the balance is excreted in urine. Terminal half-life is 20 to 40 minutes.

Route	Onset	Peak	Duration
P.O.	Unknown	14-20 min	3 hr

Contraindications and precautions
Contraindicated in pregnant and breast-feeding women and in patients allergic to prostaglandins. Uterine rupture may occur if drug used intravaginally in pregnant women to induce labor or induce abortion beyond the first trimester of pregnancy. Uterine perforation may occur if combined vaginal and oral therapy is used to induce abortion in pregnant women.

Interactions
None significant.

Adverse reactions
CNS: headache.
GI: *diarrhea, abdominal pain, nausea, flatulence, dyspepsia, vomiting, constipation.*
GU: hypermenorrhea, dysmenorrhea, spotting, cramps, menstrual disorders, postmenopausal bleeding.

Overdose and treatment
There has been little clinical experience with overdose. Cumulative daily doses of 1,600 mcg have been administered with only minor GI discomfort noted. Treatment should be supportive.

Special considerations
● Drug has been used for treatment and prophylaxis of reflux esophagitis, alcohol-induced gastritis, hemorrhagic gastritis, fat malabsorption in cystic fibrosis, and NSAID-induced nephropathy.
● Misoprostol shouldn't be prescribed for a woman of childbearing age unless she needs NSAID therapy and is at high risk for development of gastric ulcers; is capable of complying with effective contraception practices; has received oral and written warnings about the hazards of therapy, the risk of possible contraception failure, and the hazards this drug would pose to other women of childbearing age who might take it by mistake; and has had a negative serum pregnancy test within 2 weeks before beginning therapy and she'll begin therapy on the second or third day of her next normal menstrual period.
● Diarrhea is usually dose-related and develops within the first 2 weeks of therapy. It can be minimized by administering the drug after meals and at bedtime, and by avoiding magnesium-containing antacids.

Patient monitoring
● Monitor patient for GI distress, especially diarrhea.

Pregnant patients
● Drug shouldn't be used routinely in women of child-bearing age unless they're at high risk for development of ulcers or complications from NSAID-induced ulcers.

Breast-feeding patients
● Breast-feeding isn't recommended because of potential for drug-induced diarrhea in infant.

Pediatric patients
● Safety hasn't been established in children under age 18.

Patient education
● Explain importance of not giving drug to anyone else.

● Make sure patient understands that a miscarriage could result if drug is taken by a pregnant woman.
● Advise patient to take drug as prescribed for duration of therapy.

mitomycin (mitomycin-C; MTC)
Mutamycin

Pharmacologic classification: antineoplastic antibiotic (not specific to cell cycle phase)
Therapeutic classification: antineoplastic
Pregnancy risk category: NR

Indications and dosages
Dosage and indications may vary. Check current literature for recommended protocol. Not indicated as a single-agent primary therapy.
➤ *Stomach and pancreatic adenocarcinoma (with other chemotherapy drugs); cancer of breast◇, colon◇, rectum◇, head◇, neck◇, lung◇, cervix◇. Adults:* 20 mg/m² as a single dose. Repeat cycle q 6 to 8 weeks, adjusting dose, if needed, according to the following table.

Nadir after prior dose		Percentage of prior dose to be given
WBCs/ mm³	Platelets/ mm³	
≥ 3,000	≥ 75,000	100%
2,000-2,999	25,000-74,999	70%
< 2,000	< 25,000	50%

➤ *Bladder cancer◇. Adults:* 20 to 60 mg intravesically once per week for 8 weeks.

How supplied
Available by prescription only
Injection: 5-mg, 20-mg, 40-mg vials

Pharmacodynamics
Antineoplastic action: Mitomycin exerts its cytotoxic activity by a mechanism similar to that of the alkylating agents. The drug is converted to an active compound that forms cross-links between strands of DNA, inhibiting DNA synthesis. Mitomycin also inhibits RNA and protein synthesis to a lesser extent.

Pharmacokinetics
Absorption: Because of its vesicant nature, drug must be administered I.V.
Distribution: Distributes widely into body tissues; animal studies show that the highest levels are found in the kidneys followed by the muscle, eyes, lungs, intestines, and stomach. Drug doesn't cross the blood-brain barrier.

Metabolism: Metabolized by hepatic microsomal enzymes; deactivated in the kidneys, spleen, brain, and heart.

Excretion: Excreted in urine, 10% as unchanged drug. A small portion is eliminated in bile and feces.

Route	Onset	Peak	Duration
I.V.	Unknown	Unknown	Unknown

Contraindications and precautions

Contraindicated in patients hypersensitive to drug and those with thrombocytopenia, coagulation disorders, or an increase in bleeding tendency from other causes. Contraindicated as primary therapy as a single agent to replace surgery or radiotherapy.

Interactions

Drug-drug. *Vinca alkaloids:* Acute shortness of breath and severe bronchospasm have occurred following use of vinca alkaloids in patients who had previously or simultaneously received mitomycin. Patient requires careful monitoring.

Adverse reactions

CNS: headache, neurologic abnormalities, confusion, drowsiness, fatigue, syncope.
EENT: blurred vision.
GI: *nausea, vomiting, anorexia, diarrhea,* hematemesis.
Hematologic: *thrombocytopenia, leukopenia* (may be delayed up to 8 weeks and may be cumulative with successive doses), *microangiopathic hemolytic anemia, characterized by thrombocytopenia, renal failure,* and hypertension.
Respiratory: *interstitial pneumonitis,* pulmonary edema, dyspnea, nonproductive cough, adult respiratory distress syndrome.
Skin: reversible alopecia.
Other: desquamation, induration, pruritus, and pain at injection site; *septicemia;* cellulitis, ulceration, and sloughing with extravasation; fever; pain.

Overdose and treatment

Signs and symptoms of overdose include myelosuppression, nausea, vomiting, and alopecia.

Treatment is usually supportive and includes transfusion of blood components, antiemetics, and antibiotics for infections that may develop.

Special considerations

⚠ ALERT Stop drug if WBC count is less than 4,000/mm³ or platelet count is less than 150,000/mm³. Give no repeat dose until blood counts go above these levels. If disease progresses after two courses of therapy, discontinue use.
● Don't confuse this drug with mitoxantrone. Question any unfamiliar color of the drug.
● To reconstitute 5-mg vial, use 10 ml of sterile water for injection; to reconstitute 20-mg vial, use 40 ml of sterile water for injection; to re-constitute a 40-mg vial, use 80 ml sterile water for injection, to yield 0.5 mg/ml. Let stand at room temperature until complete dissolution occurs.
● Drug may be administered by I.V. push injection slowly over 5 to 10 minutes into the tubing of a freely flowing I.V. infusion.
● Drug can be further diluted to 100 to 150 ml with normal saline solution or D₅W for I.V. infusion (over 30 to 60 minutes or longer).
● Reconstituted solution remains stable for 1 week at room temperature and for 2 weeks if refrigerated.
● Mitomycin has been used intra-arterially to treat certain tumors, for example, into hepatic artery for colon cancer. It has also been given as a continuous daily infusion.
● Ulcers caused by extravasation develop late and dorsal to the extravasation site. Apply cold compresses for at least 12 hours.

Patient monitoring

● Observe patient for evidence of renal toxicity. Don't give drug to patient with a serum creatinine level over 1.7 mg/dl.
● Continue CBC and blood studies at least 7 weeks after therapy is stopped. Monitor patient for signs of bleeding.

Breast-feeding patients

● It isn't known if drug appears in breast milk. To avoid risk of serious adverse reactions, mutagenicity, and carcinogenicity in the infant, breast-feeding isn't recommended.

Patient education

● Tell patient to avoid exposure to people with infections.
● Warn patient not to receive immunizations during therapy and for several weeks afterward. Members of the same household shouldn't receive immunizations during the same period.
● Reassure patient that hair should grow back after treatment has been discontinued.
● Tell patient to call promptly if he develops a sore throat or fever or notices unusual bruising or bleeding.

mitoxantrone hydrochloride
Novantrone

Pharmacologic classification: antibiotic antineoplastic
Therapeutic classification: antineoplastic
Pregnancy risk category: D

Indications and dosages

➤ *Initial treatment for acute nonlymphocytic leukemia with other approved drugs.* Adults: For induction (in combination chemotherapy), 12 mg/m² daily by I.V. infusion on days 1 to 3, and 100 mg/m² of cytosine arabinoside by continuous I.V. infusion (over 24 hours) on days 1 to 7 for 7 days.

Most complete remissions follow initial course of induction therapy. A second course may be given if antileukemic response is incomplete: Give mitoxantrone for 2 days and cytosine for 5 days using the same daily dosage levels. If severe or life-threatening nonhematologic toxicity occurs, withhold second course of therapy until toxicity clears.

➤ *Combined initial therapy for pain related to advanced hormone-refractory prostate cancer. Adults:* 12 to 14 mg/m² I.V. infusion over 15 to 30 minutes q 21 days.

➤ *Worsening relapsing-remitting, secondary progressive, and progressive-relapsing multiple sclerosis. Adults:* 12 mg/m² I.V. once every 3 months.

How supplied
Available by prescription only
Injection: 2 mg mitoxantrone base/ml in 10-ml, 12.5-ml, 15-ml vials

Pharmacodynamics
Antineoplastic action: Mechanism of action isn't fully understood. Drug is a DNA-reactive agent that has cytocidal effects on proliferating and nonproliferating cells, suggestive of lack of cell-phase specificity. It also interferes with RNA and inhibits topoisomerase II.

Pharmacokinetics
Absorption: Administered by I.V. infusion.
Distribution: 78% plasma protein-bound.
Metabolism: Metabolized by the liver.
Excretion: Excretion is via renal and hepatobiliary systems; 6% to 11% of dose is excreted in urine within 5 days: 65% is unchanged drug; 35% is two inactive metabolites. Within 5 days, 25% of dose is excreted in feces.

Route	Onset	Peak	Duration
I.V.	Unknown	Unknown	Unknown

Contraindications and precautions
Contraindicated in patients hypersensitive to mitoxantrone. Use cautiously in patients with prior exposure to anthracyclines or other cardiotoxic drugs. Contraindicated in pregnancy unless potential benefits outweigh hazards to fetus.

Interactions
None reported.

Adverse reactions
CNS: *seizures,* headache.
EENT: conjunctivitis, temporary blue color to sclera, sinusitis.
CV: *heart failure, arrhythmias,* tachycardia.
GI: *bleeding, abdominal pain, diarrhea, nausea, mucositis, vomiting,* stomatitis.
GU: *renal failure,* urinary tract infection, menstrual disorder, amenorrhea.
Hematologic: *myelosuppression.*
Hepatic: jaundice.

Metabolic: hyperuricemia.
Respiratory: *dyspnea, cough,* upper respiratory infection.
Skin: *alopecia, petechiae, ecchymoses.*
Other: *sepsis, fungal infections, fever.*

Overdose and treatment
Accidental overdoses have occurred and have caused severe leukopenia with infection.

Monitor hematologic parameters and treat symptomatically. Antimicrobial therapy may be necessary.

Special considerations
⚕ **ALERT** Don't confuse this drug with mitomycin. Question any unfamiliar color of the drug.
● Safety of administration by routes other than I.V. hasn't been established. Don't use intrathecally.
● To prepare, dilute solutions to at least 50 ml with either normal saline solution or D₅W. Inject slowly into tubing of a freely running I.V. solution of normal saline solution or D₅W over not less than 3 minutes. Discard unused infusion solutions appropriately. Don't mix for infusion with heparin; a precipitate may form. Specific compatibility data aren't available.
● For I.V. infusion over 15 to 30 minutes, further dilute solution.
● After penetration of container, undiluted mitoxantrone concentration may be stored no longer than 7 days at room temperature or 14 days if refrigerated.
● If extravasation occurs, discontinue I.V. and restart in another vein. Mitoxantrone is a nonvesicant and the possibility of severe local reactions is minimal.
● Urine may appear blue-green for 24 hours after administration.
● Bluish discoloration of sclera may occur; this may be a sign of myelosuppression.

Patient monitoring
● Close and frequent monitoring of hematologic and chemical laboratory parameters, including serial CBC and liver function tests, with frequent patient observation is recommended.
● Hyperuricemia may result from rapid lysis of tumor cells. Monitor serum uric acid levels. Start hypouricemic therapy before antileukemic therapy.
● Transient increased AST and ALT levels have occurred 4 to 24 days after mitoxantrone therapy.

Breast-feeding patients
● It isn't known if drug appears in breast milk. Because of potential for serious adverse reactions in infants, discontinue breast-feeding before therapy.

Pediatric patients
● Safety and efficacy in children haven't been established.

Reactions may be *common,* uncommon, *life-threatening,* or COMMON AND LIFE-THREATENING.

Patient education

• Tell patient urine may appear blue-green for 24 hours after administration and sclera may appear bluish.
• Advise patient to call promptly if signs and symptoms of myelosuppression develop, such as fever, sore throat, easy bruising, or excessive bleeding.
• Advise patient to use contraception; tell patient to report suspected pregnancy.
• Tell patient to drink fluids to minimize uric acid nephropathy.

mivacurium chloride
Mivacron

Pharmacologic classification: nondepolarizing neuromuscular blocker
Therapeutic classification: skeletal muscle relaxant
Pregnancy risk category: C

Indications and dosages

➤ *Adjunct to general anesthesia, to facilitate endotracheal intubation, and to provide skeletal muscle relaxation during surgery or mechanical ventilation.*
Dosage is highly individualized. All times of onset and duration of neuromuscular blockade are averages and considerable individual variation is normal.
Adults: Usually, 0.15 mg/kg I.V. push over 5 to 15 seconds provides adequate muscle relaxation within 2 to 3 minutes for endotracheal intubation. Clinically sufficient neuromuscular blockade usually lasts about 15 to 20 minutes. Or, 0.2 mg/kg over 30 seconds or 0.25 mg/kg in doses of 0.15 mg/kg and 0.1 mg/kg 30 seconds later. Spontaneous recovery usually occurs in 25 to 35 minutes. Supplemental doses of 0.1 mg/kg I.V. q 15 to 25 minutes usually maintain muscle relaxation. Or, maintain neuromuscular blockade with a continuous infusion of 4 mcg/kg/minute started simultaneously with initial dose, or 9 to 10 mcg/kg/minute started after evidence of spontaneous recovery of initial dose. When used with isoflurane or enflurane anesthesia, dosage is usually reduced about 35% to 40%.
✦ *Dosage adjustment.* Infusion rate needs to be reduced by 50% in end-stage renal and liver patients.
Children ages 2 to 12: 0.20 mg/kg I.V. push administered over 5 to 15 seconds.
Neuromuscular blockade is usually evident in less than 2 minutes. Although supplemental doses of 0.1 mg/kg I.V. q 15 minutes usually maintain muscle relaxation in adults, maintenance dosages are usually required more frequently in children. Or, maintain neuromuscular blockade with a continuous infusion titrated to effect. Most children respond to 5 to 31 mcg/kg/minute (average, 14 mcg/kg/minute).

How supplied
Available by prescription only
Injection: 2 mg/ml in 5-ml and 10-ml vials
Infusion: 0.5 mg/ml, in 50 ml D$_5$W

Pharmacodynamics
Neuromuscular blocking action: Mivacurium competes with acetylcholine for receptor sites at the motor end-plate. Because this action may be antagonized by cholinesterase inhibitors, mivacurium is considered a competitive antagonist. Drug is a mixture of three stereoisomers, each possessing neuromuscular blocking activity: the cis-trans isomer (36% of the total) and the trans-trans isomer (57% of the total) are about 10 times as potent as the cis-cis isomer (only 6% of the total). The isomers don't interconvert in vivo.

Pharmacokinetics
Absorption: Absorption is rapid.
Distribution: Volume of distribution is small, indicating that drug isn't extensively distributed to tissues.
Metabolism: Rapidly hydrolyzed by plasma pseudocholinesterase to inactive components.
Excretion: Metabolites are excreted in bile and urine. Of the highly active isomers, the cis-trans and trans-trans isomers each have an elimination half-life of less than 2.3 minutes. The less active cis-cis isomer, which is only a small portion of the total drug, has an elimination half-life of 55 minutes.

Route	Onset	Peak	Duration
I.V.	1-2 min	2-5 min	20-35 min

Contraindications and precautions
Contraindicated in patients hypersensitive to drug. Use cautiously in patients with significant CV disease, metastatic cancer, severe electrolyte disturbances, or neuromuscular disease; in those who may be adversely affected by the release of histamine; and in those in whom neuromuscular blockade reversibility is difficult, such as patients with myasthenia gravis or myasthenic syndrome. Use with extreme caution in patients with reduced plasma cholinesterase activity; drug may cause prolonged neuromuscular blockade.

Interactions
Drug-drug. *Aminoglycosides (gentamicin, kanamycin, neomycin, streptomycin), bacitracin, colistimethate, colistin, magnesium salts, polymyxin B, tetracyclines:* May increase muscle weakness. Monitor patient closely.
Carbamazepine, phenytoin: May prolong the time to maximal block or shorten the duration of blockade with neuromuscular blockers. Monitor patient closely.
Glucocorticoids, MAO inhibitors, oral contraceptives: Plasma cholinesterase activity may be diminished by long-term use. Monitor patient closely.

Inhaled anesthetics (especially enflurane, isoflurane), quinidine: May enhance activity or prolong action. Patient requires close monitoring.

Adverse reactions

CNS: dizziness.
CV: *flushing, tachycardia,* **bradycardia, arrhythmias,** *hypotension.*
Musculoskeletal: prolonged muscle weakness, muscle spasms.
Respiratory: **bronchospasm,** wheezing, *respiratory insufficiency or apnea.*
Skin: rash, urticaria, erythema.
Other: phlebitis.

Overdose and treatment

Overdose may result in prolonged neuromuscular blockade. Maintain a patent airway and control respirations until patient recovers neuromuscular function. Antagonists shouldn't be administered until there's some evidence of spontaneous recovery. In clinical trials, administration of 0.03 to 0.064 mg/kg neostigmine methylsulfate or 0.5 mg/kg edrophonium chloride to patients with spontaneous recovery of muscle function resulted in increased muscle strength of about 10% recovery to about 95% recovery within 10 minutes.

Special considerations

• When mivacurium is given I.V. push to adults receiving anesthetic combinations of nitrous oxide and opiates, neuromuscular blockade usually lasts 15 to 20 minutes; most patients recover 95% of muscle strength in 25 to 30 minutes.
• Duration of drug effect is increased about 150% in patients with end-stage renal disease and 300% in patients with hepatic dysfunction.
• Adjust dosage to ideal body weight in obese patients (patients 30% or more above their ideal weight) because of reported prolonged neuromuscular blockade.
• A nerve stimulator and train-of-four monitoring are recommended to document antagonism of neuromuscular blockade and recovery of muscle strength. Before attempting pharmacologic reversal with neostigmine methylsulfate or edrophonium chloride, some evidence of spontaneous recovery should be evident.
• Experimental evidence suggests that acid-base and electrolyte balance may influence actions of and response to nondepolarizing neuromuscular blockers. Alkalosis may counteract paralysis; acidosis may enhance it.
• Mivacurium, like other neuromuscular blockers, doesn't have an effect on consciousness or pain threshold. To avoid patient distress, don't give drug until patient's consciousness is obtunded by general anesthetic.
• Drug is compatible with D₅W, normal saline solution injection, dextrose 5% in normal saline solution injection, lactated Ringer's injection, and dextrose 5% in lactated Ringer's injection. Diluted solutions are stable for 24 hours at room temperature.
• When diluted as directed, mivacurium is compatible with alfentanil, fentanyl, sufentanil, droperidol, and midazolam. Alkaline solutions, such as barbiturate solutions, may form a precipitate. Drug shouldn't be administered through the same I.V. line with alkaline solutions.
• Drug is available as premixed infusion in D₅W. After removing the protective outer wrap, check container for minor leaks by squeezing the bag before administering. Don't add other drugs to the container, and don't use the container in series connections.

Patient monitoring

• Monitor vital signs and respirations until patient is fully recovered from neuromuscular blockade (as evidenced by hand grip, head lift, and ability to cough).

Breast-feeding patients

• It isn't known if drug appears in breast milk. Use cautiously in breast-feeding women.

Pediatric patients

• As with other neuromuscular blockers, dosage requirements for children are higher on a mg/kg basis as compared with adults. Onset and recovery of neuromuscular blockade occur more rapidly in children.

Patient education

• Explain purpose of drug.
• Assure patient that he'll be monitored continuously.

modafinil
Provigil

Pharmacologic classification: nonamphetamine CNS stimulant
Therapeutic classification: analeptic
Controlled substance schedule: IV
Pregnancy risk category: C

Indications and dosages

➤ *Improvement of wakefulness in patients with excessive daytime sleepiness related to narcolepsy.* *Adults:* 200 mg P.O. daily, given as a single dose in the morning.
✦ *Dosage adjustment.* In patients with severe hepatic impairment, 100 mg P.O. daily, given as a single dose in the morning.

How supplied

Available by prescription only
Tablets: 100 mg, 200 mg

Pharmacodynamics

CNS stimulant action: The exact mechanism of action in which modafinil promotes wakefulness is unknown. Modafinil has wake-promoting actions like sympathomimetic agents including amphetamines, but modafinil is structurally distinct from amphetamines and doesn't appear to alter the release of either dopamine or norepinephrine to produce CNS stimulation.

Pharmacokinetics
Absorption: Absorption is rapid.
Distribution: Well distributed in body tissue and moderately bound to plasma protein (about 60%), primarily albumin.
Metabolism: Primarily metabolized (about 90%) in the liver, with subsequent renal elimination of the metabolites.
Excretion: Less than 10% is renally excreted as unchanged drug.

Route	Onset	Peak	Duration
P.O.	Unknown	2-4 hr	Unknown

Contraindications and precautions
Contraindicated in patients hypersensitive to drug. Don't use in patients with history of left ventricular hypertrophy or ischemic ECG changes, chest pain, arrhythmias, or other clinically significant manifestations of mitral valve prolapse in association with CNS stimulant use.

Use cautiously in patients with recent history of MI or unstable angina and in those with history of psychosis. Use cautiously, and in reduced dosages, in patients with severe hepatic impairment, with or without cirrhosis. Also use cautiously in patients concurrently treated with MAO inhibitors and those with a history of psychosis.

Interactions
Drug-drug. *CYP3A4 inducers, such as carbamazepine, phenobarbital, rifampin; CYP3A4 inhibitors, such as itraconazole and ketoconazole:* Altered modafinil levels. Monitor patient closely.
Cyclosporine, theophylline: Reduced serum levels. Use together cautiously.
Diazepam, phenytoin, propranolol, or other agents metabolized by CYP2C19: Increased serum levels of drugs metabolized by this enzyme. Use together cautiously. Dosage adjustment may be necessary.
Hormonal contraceptives: Reduced contraceptive effectiveness. Recommend alternative or additional contraception during modafinil therapy and for 1 month after drug is discontinued.
Methylphenidate: May delay absorption of modafinil by about 1 hour when administered together. Separate administration times.
Phenytoin, warfarin: Increased serum levels of these drugs. Monitor patient closely for toxicity.
Tricyclic antidepressants, such as clomipramine and desipramine: Levels are increased by modafinil. Dosage reduction of these agents may be necessary.

Adverse reactions
CNS: *headache,* nervousness, dizziness, syncope, depression, anxiety, cataplexy, insomnia, paresthesia, dyskinesia, hypertonia, confusion, amnesia, emotional lability, ataxia, tremor.
CV: hypotension, hypertension, vasodilation, *arrhythmias,* chest pain.
EENT: *rhinitis,* pharyngitis, epistaxis, amblyopia, abnormal vision, gingivitis, thirst.
GI: *nausea,* diarrhea, mouth ulcer, dry mouth, anorexia, vomiting.
GU: abnormal urine, urine retention, abnormal ejaculation, albuminuria.
Hematologic: eosinophilia.
Hepatic: abnormal liver function test results.
Metabolic: hyperglycemia.
Musculoskeletal: joint disorder, neck pain, rigid neck.
Respiratory: lung disorder, dyspnea, asthma.
Skin: dry skin.
Other: herpes simplex, chills, fever.

Overdose and treatment
No specific antidote to a modafinil overdose exists.
Start supportive care as appropriate, including CV monitoring. If there are no contraindications, consider induced emesis or gastric lavage.

Special considerations
• Safety and efficacy of dosage in patients with severe renal impairment haven't been determined.
• Although dosages of 400 mg daily as a single dose have been well tolerated, there's no consistent evidence that this dosage confers additional benefit beyond the 200-mg dose.
• Even though food has no effect on overall bioavailability, the absorption of modafinil may be delayed by about 1 hour if given with food.

Patient monitoring
• Monitor patient for misuse or abuse.
• Monitor liver function tests before and during drug therapy.

Breast-feeding patients
• It isn't known if modafinil appears in breast milk. Because many drugs do, give modafinil cautiously to a breast-feeding woman.

Pediatric patients
• Safety and efficacy in patients under age 16 haven't been established.

Geriatric patients
• Safety and efficacy in patients over age 65 haven't been established. In geriatric patients, a lower dosage may be considered because elimination of drug and its metabolites may be reduced.

Patient education
• Advise woman to notify prescriber if she becomes pregnant or intends to become pregnant during therapy.

• Caution patient about increased risk of pregnancy when using steroidal contraceptives (including depot or implantable contraceptives) with modafinil tablets. Recommend alternative or additional contraception during therapy and for 1 month after drug is discontinued.

• Advise woman to notify prescriber if she's breast-feeding an infant.

• Instruct patient to avoid taking any prescription or OTC drugs before consulting with prescriber because of risk of interactions between modafinil and other drugs.

• Urge patient to avoid alcohol during therapy.

• Tell patient to notify prescriber about rash, hives, or a related allergic reaction.

• Modafinil may impair judgment. Advise patient to be cautious while driving and during other activities requiring alertness until effects are known.

moexipril hydrochloride
Univasc

Pharmacologic classification: angiotensin-converting enzyme (ACE) inhibitor
Therapeutic classification: antihypertensive
Pregnancy risk category: C (D second and third trimesters)

Indications and dosages
➤**Hypertension.** *Adults:* Initially, 7.5 mg P.O. once daily one hour before meals for patients not receiving diuretics. If control isn't adequate, dose can be increased or divided dosing may be attempted. Recommended dosage range is 7.5 to 30 mg daily, administered in one or two divided doses 1 hour before meals. For patients receiving diuretics, give 3.75 mg P.O. once daily before meals. Make subsequent dosage adjustments according to blood pressure response.

✦ *Dosage adjustment.* If creatinine clearance is 40 ml/minute or less, start at 3.75 mg P.O. daily, and adjust to a maximum of 15 mg daily. If concomitant diuretic therapy is needed, a loop diuretic is preferred.

How supplied
Available by prescription only
Tablets: 7.5 mg, 15 mg

Pharmacodynamics
Antihypertensive action: Exact mechanism is unknown. Action is thought to result primarily from suppression of the renin-angiotensin-aldosterone system. A metabolite of moexipril, moexiprilat, inhibits ACE and thereby inhibits production of angiotensin II (a potent vasoconstrictor and stimulator of aldosterone secretion). Other mechanisms may also be involved.

Pharmacokinetics
Absorption: Incompletely absorbed from the GI tract with a bioavailability of about 13%. Food significantly decreases bioavailability of drug.

Distribution: Metabolite is about 50% protein-bound.

Metabolism: Metabolized extensively to the active metabolite, moexiprilat.

Excretion: Excreted primarily in feces with a small amount excreted in urine. Half-life of drug is over 2 to 9 hours.

Route	Onset	Peak	Duration
P.O.	½ hr	1½ hr	24 hr

Contraindications and precautions
Contraindicated in patients hypersensitive to drug, pregnant patients, and patients with a history of angioedema related to previous ACE inhibitor therapy. Use cautiously in breast-feeding women and patients with impaired renal function, heart failure, or renal artery stenosis.

Interactions
Drug-drug. *Diuretics:* Increased risk of excessive hypotension. Lower dose of diuretic or moexipril may be necessary.
Lithium: Lithium toxicity. Avoid use together.
Potassium-sparing diuretics, potassium supplements: Increased risk of hyperkalemia. Monitor serum potassium closely.
Drug-food. *Sodium substitutes containing potassium:* Increased risk of hyperkalemia. Discourage use together.

Adverse reactions
CNS: *dizziness,* headache, fatigue.
CV: peripheral edema, hypotension, orthostatic hypotension, chest pain, flushing.
EENT: pharyngitis, rhinitis, sinusitis.
GI: diarrhea, dyspepsia, nausea.
GU: urinary frequency.
Hematologic: *neutropenia.*
Metabolic: hyperkalemia.
Musculoskeletal: myalgia.
Respiratory: *dry, persistent, tickling, nonproductive cough;* upper respiratory tract infection.
Skin: rash.
Other: *anaphylactoid reactions, angioedema,* flu syndrome, pain.

Overdose and treatment
Although no information is available on overdose of moexipril, it's believed that signs and symptoms would be similar to those of other ACE inhibitors with hypotension being the principal adverse reaction.

Because the hypotensive effect of moexipril is achieved through vasodilation and effective hypovolemia, it's reasonable to treat moexipril overdose by infusion of normal saline solution. In addition, renal function and serum potassium should be monitored.

Special considerations
• Because angioedema that involves the tongue, glottis, or larynx may cause a fatal airway

obstruction, keep appropriate therapy, such as S.C. epinephrine 1:1,000 (0.3 to 0.5 ml) available, as well as equipment to ensure a patent airway.

• In patients undergoing major surgery or anesthesia with agents that produce hypotension, moexipril may block the compensatory renin release. Hypotension can be treated with volume expansion.

Patient monitoring

• Monitor patient for hypotension. Excessive hypotension can occur when drug is given with diuretics. Diuretic therapy may be discontinued 2 to 3 days before starting moexipril to decrease potential for excessive hypotensive response. If drug doesn't adequately control blood pressure, diuretic therapy may be restarted cautiously.

• Measure blood pressure at trough (just before a dose) to verify adequate blood pressure control. Drug is less effective in reducing trough blood pressures in blacks than in nonblacks.

• Assess renal function before and periodically throughout therapy. Monitor serum potassium levels.

• Other ACE inhibitors have been linked to agranulocytosis and neutropenia. Monitor CBC with differential counts before therapy, especially in patients who have collagen vascular disease with impaired renal function.

Breast-feeding patients

• It isn't known if drug appears in breast milk; use cautiously in breast-feeding women.

Pediatric patients

• Safety and efficacy in children haven't been established.

Patient education

• Instruct patient to take drug on an empty stomach; meals, particularly those high in fat, can impair absorption.

• Tell patient to avoid sodium substitutes; these products may contain potassium, which can cause hyperkalemia in patients taking this drug.

• Inform patient that light-headedness can occur, especially during the first few days of therapy. Tell him to rise slowly to minimize this effect and to report symptoms. If fainting occurs, tell patient to stop drug and call immediately.

• Instruct patient to use caution in hot weather and during exercise. Inadequate fluid intake, vomiting, diarrhea, and excessive perspiration can lead to light-headedness and syncope.

• Advise patient to report signs of infection, such as fever and sore throat. Also tell patient to report the following signs or symptoms: easy bruising or bleeding; swelling of tongue, lips, face, eyes, mucous membranes, or limbs; difficulty swallowing or breathing; and hoarseness.

• Tell woman to report suspected pregnancy immediately. Drug will need to be discontinued.

molindone hydrochloride
Moban

Pharmacologic classification: dihydroindolone
Therapeutic classification: antipsychotic
Pregnancy risk category: NR

Indications and dosages

➤ *Psychotic disorders. Adults:* 50 to 75 mg P.O. daily in 3 to 4 divided doses, increased 100 mg daily in 3 to 4 days to a maximum of 225 mg daily. Maintenance dosage for mild disease is 5 to 15 mg t.i.d. or q.i.d., moderate disease is 10 to 25 mg t.i.d. or q.i.d., and severe disease is up to 225 mg daily.

➤ *Behavioral complications related to mental retardation, mentally retarded schizophrenic child◇. Children age 3 to 5:* 1 to 2.5 mg P.O. daily as a single dose.

How supplied

Available by prescription only
Oral concentrate: 20 mg/ml
Tablets: 5 mg, 10 mg, 25 mg, 50 mg, 100 mg

Pharmacodynamics

Antipsychotic action: Molindone is unrelated to all other antipsychotics; it's thought to exert its antipsychotic effects by postsynaptic blockade of CNS dopamine receptors, thereby inhibiting dopamine-mediated effects.

Molindone has many other central and peripheral effects; it also produces alpha and ganglionic blockade. Its most prominent adverse reactions are extrapyramidal.

Pharmacokinetics

Absorption: Data are limited, but absorption appears rapid.
Distribution: Distributed widely into the body. Drug is 90% to 95% protein-bound.
Metabolism: Metabolized extensively in the liver.
Excretion: Most of drug is excreted as metabolites in urine; some is excreted in feces by way of the biliary tract. Overall, 90% of a given dose is excreted within 24 hours.

Route	Onset	Peak	Duration
P.O.	Unknown	1½ hr	24-36 hr

Contraindications and precautions

Contraindicated in patients hypersensitive to drug and in those experiencing coma or severe CNS depression. Use cautiously in patients at risk for seizures or when high physical activity is harmful to patient.

Interactions

Drug-drug. *Antiarrhythmics, disopyramide, procainamide, quinidine:* Increased risk of arrhythmias and conduction defects. Avoid use together.

Anticholinergics, including antidepressants, antihistamines, antiparkinsonians, atropine, MAO inhibitors, meperidine, and phenothiazines: Oversedation, paralytic ileus, visual changes, and severe constipation. Use together cautiously.

Beta blockers: May inhibit molindone metabolism, increasing plasma levels and toxicity. Monitor patient for toxicity.

Bromocriptine: Molindone may antagonize therapeutic effect of bromocriptine on prolactin secretion. Use together cautiously.

Centrally acting antihypertensive drugs, such as clonidine, guanabenz, guanadrel, guanethidine, methyldopa, and reserpine: May inhibit blood pressure response to these drugs. Monitor blood pressure carefully.

CNS depressants, including analgesics, anesthetics (general, spinal, or epidural), barbiturates, opioids, parenteral magnesium sulfate, tranquilizers: Oversedation, respiratory depression, and hypotension. Avoid use together.

High-dose dopamine: Decreased vasoconstricting effects. Monitor patient for effects.

Levodopa: Decreased effectiveness and increased toxicity of levodopa. Use together cautiously.

Metrizamide: Increased risk of seizures. Use together cautiously.

Nitrates: Hypotension. Monitor blood pressure.

Phenytoin, tetracycline: Molindone may inhibit absorption. Monitor patient carefully.

Propylthiouracil: Increased risk of agranulocytosis. Monitor hematopoietic studies.

Sympathomimetics, including epinephrine, ephedrine (often found in nasal sprays), phenylephrine, or appetite suppressants: May decrease their stimulatory and pressor effects. Use together cautiously.

Drug-lifestyle. *Alcohol use:* Additive effects. Discourage use together.

Sun exposure: Increased risk of photosensitivity reactions. Recommend that patient use sunscreen and avoid excessive exposure to the sun.

Adverse reactions

CNS: *extrapyramidal reactions, tardive dyskinesia, sedation, drowsiness, depression, euphoria, pseudoparkinsonism, EEG changes, dizziness.*

CV: *orthostatic hypotension, tachycardia, ECG changes.*

EENT: *blurred vision.*

GI: *dry mouth, constipation, nausea.*

GU: *urine retention, menstrual irregularities, inhibited ejaculation.*

Hematologic: ***leukopenia,*** leukocytosis.

Hepatic: jaundice, abnormal liver function test results.

Skin: *mild photosensitivity,* ***allergic reactions.***

Other: *gynecomastia.*

Overdose and treatment

CNS depression is characterized by deep, unarousable sleep and possible coma, hypotension or hypertension, extrapyramidal symptoms, abnormal involuntary muscle movements, agitation, seizures, arrhythmias, ECG changes, hypothermia or hyperthermia, and autonomic nervous system dysfunction.

Treatment is symptomatic and supportive, including maintaining vital signs, airway, stable body temperature, and fluid-electrolyte balance.

Don't induce vomiting; drug inhibits cough reflex, and aspiration may occur. Use gastric lavage, then activated charcoal and saline cathartics; dialysis doesn't help. Regulate body temperature as needed. Treat hypotension with I.V. fluids; don't give epinephrine. Treat seizures with parenteral diazepam or barbiturates; arrhythmias, with parenteral phenytoin; extrapyramidal reactions, with benztropine at 1 to 2 mg or parenteral diphenhydramine at 10 to 50 mg.

Special considerations

● Liquid concentrate contains sodium metabisulfite, which may cause severe allergic reaction in susceptible individuals.

● Drug may cause GI distress and should be administered with food or fluids.

● Dilute concentrate in 2 to 4 oz of liquid, preferably soup, water, juice, carbonated drinks, milk, or puddings.

● Drug may cause pink to brown discoloration of urine.

● Protect liquid form from light and store at 59° to 86° F (15° to 30° C).

● Drug causes false-positive results in urine pregnancy tests using human chorionic gonadotropin and has additive potential for causing seizures with metrizamide myelography.

Patient monitoring

● Monitor patient for CNS adverse effects, especially drowsiness and extrapyramidal symptoms.

● Monitor CBC and liver function tests in long-term therapy.

Pediatric patients

● Drug isn't recommended for children under age 12.

Geriatric patients

● Lower doses are recommended; 30% to 50% of usual dose may be effective. Geriatric patients are at greater risk for tardive dyskinesia and other extrapyramidal effects.

Patient education

● Explain risks of dystonic reaction and tardive dyskinesia to patient and advise him to report abnormal body movements.

● Warn patient to avoid spilling liquid preparation on the skin; rash and irritation may result.

● Advise patient to avoid temperature extremes (hot or cold baths, sunlamps, or tanning beds)

Reactions may be *common,* uncommon, ***life-threatening,*** or COMMON AND LIFE-THREATENING.

because drug may cause thermoregulatory changes.

● Suggest sugarless gum or candy, ice chips, or artificial saliva to relieve dry mouth.

● Warn patient not to take drug with antacids or antidiarrheals; not to drink alcoholic beverages or take other drugs that cause sedation; not to stop taking drug or take any other drug except as instructed; and to take drug exactly as prescribed, without doubling after missing a dose.

● Warn patient about sedative effect. Tell him to report difficult urination, sore throat, dizziness, or fainting.

● Advise patient to get up slowly from a recumbent or seated position to minimize effects of light-headedness.

● Tell patient that liquid concentrate contains sodium metabisulfite, which can cause an allergic reaction to those with a sulfite allergy.

---

montelukast sodium
Singulair

Pharmacologic classification: leukotriene receptor antagonist
Therapeutic classification: antiasthmatic
Pregnancy risk category: B

Indications and dosages
➤ *For prophylaxis and long-term treatment of asthma. Adults and adolescents:* 10 mg P.O. once daily in the evening.
Children ages 6 to 14: 5 mg (chewable tablet) P.O. once daily in the evening.
Children ages 2 to 5: 4 mg (chewable tablet) P.O. once daily in the evening.

How supplied
Available by prescription only
Tablets: 10 mg
Tablets (chewable): 4 mg, 5 mg

Pharmacodynamics
Antiasthmatic action: Montelukast causes inhibition of airway cysteinyl leukotriene receptors. Drug binds with high affinity and selectivity to the $cysLT_1$ receptor, and inhibits the physiologic action of the cysteinyl leukotriene LTD_4. This receptor inhibition reduces early- and late-phase bronchoconstriction resulting from antigen challenge.

Pharmacokinetics
Absorption: Rapidly absorbed after oral administration with mean oral bioavailability of 64%. Food doesn't affect absorption of drug. For chewable tablet, mean oral bioavailability is 73%.
Distribution: Minimally distributed to the tissues with a steady state volume of distribution of 8 to 11 L. Over 99% is bound to plasma proteins.
Metabolism: Extensively metabolized, but plasma levels of metabolites at therapeutic doses are undetectable. In vitro studies with human liver microsomes demonstrate metabolism involvement by cytochromes P-450 3A4 and 2C9.
Excretion: About 86% of an oral dose is metabolized and excreted in the feces, indicating drug and its metabolites are excreted almost exclusively in the bile. Half-life is 2¾ to 5½ hours.

Route	Onset	Peak	Duration
P.O.			
Chewable	Unknown	2-2½ hr	Unknown
Film-coated	Unknown	3-4 hr	Unknown

Contraindications and precautions
Contraindicated in patients hypersensitive to drug or its components. Also contraindicated in patients with acute asthmatic attacks or status asthmaticus. Although airway function is improved in patients with known aspirin hypersensitivity, these patients should avoid aspirin and NSAIDs.

Interactions
Drug-drug. *Phenobarbital, rifampin:* Increased metabolism of drug. Monitor patient closely.

Adverse reactions
CNS: *headache, dizziness,* fatigue, asthenia.
EENT: nasal congestion, dental pain.
GI: dyspepsia, infectious gastroenteritis, abdominal pain.
Respiratory: cough, influenza.
Skin: rash.
Other: fever, trauma.

Overdose and treatment
No information is available on treatment of drug overdose. Provide supportive measures for overdose such as removal of unabsorbed material from the GI tract and clinical monitoring.

Special considerations
● Although dose of inhaled corticosteroids may be reduced gradually, montelukast shouldn't be abruptly substituted for inhaled or oral corticosteroids.
● Drug shouldn't be used as monotherapy for management of exercise-induced bronchospasm.
● No added benefit is achieved with doses above 10 mg daily.

Patient monitoring
● Monitor patient for worsening asthmatic symptoms.

Breast-feeding patients
● It isn't known if drug appears in breast milk. Use cautiously in breast-feeding women.

Pediatric patients
● Safety and efficacy in children under age 6 haven't been established.

Geriatric patients
● No change in safety and effectiveness has been reported in geriatric patients.

Patient education
● Advise patient to take drug daily, even if asymptomatic, and to contact prescriber if asthma isn't well controlled.
● Warn patient that drug isn't beneficial in acute asthma attacks or exercise-induced bronchospasm, and advise him to keep appropriate rescue medications available.
● Advise patient with known aspirin sensitivity not to take aspirin and NSAIDs.
● Warn patient with phenylketonuria that chewable tablet contains phenylalanine, a component of aspartame.
● Advise patients to seek medical attention if short-acting bronchodilators are needed more often than usual or prescribed.

moricizine hydrochloride
Ethmozine

Pharmacologic classification: sodium channel blocker
Therapeutic classification: antiarrhythmic
Pregnancy risk category: B

Indications and dosages
➤*Treatment of documented, life-threatening ventricular arrhythmias when benefit of treatment outweighs risks. Adults:* Dosage must be individualized. Usual range is 600 to 900 mg P.O. daily, given q 8 hours in equally divided doses. Dosage may be adjusted within this range in increments of 150 mg daily at 3-day intervals until desired effect is obtained. Hospitalization is recommended for start of therapy because patient will be at high risk. Patients whose arrhythmias are well controlled during q-8-hour dosing may receive the same dose daily, divided q 12 hours to increase compliance.
✦ *Dosage adjustment.* For patients with hepatic impairment and significant renal dysfunction, give 600 mg or less daily. Monitor ECG before increasing dose.

How supplied
Available by prescription only
Tablets: 200 mg, 250 mg, 300 mg

Pharmacodynamics
Antiarrhythmic action: Although moricizine is chemically related to the neuroleptic phenothiazines, it has no demonstrated dopaminergic activities. It does have potent local anesthetic activity and myocardial membrane-stabilizing effects. A Class I antiarrhythmic agent, it reduces the fast inward current carried by sodium ions. In patients with ventricular tachycardia, moricizine prolongs AV conduction but has no significant effect on ventricular repolarization. Intra-atrial conduction or atrial effective refractory periods aren't consistently affected and moricizine has minimal effect on sinus cycle length and sinus node recovery time. This may be significant in patients with sinus node dysfunction.

In patients with impaired left ventricular function, moricizine has minimal effects on measurements of cardiac performance: cardiac index, stroke volume, pulmonary artery wedge pressure, systemic or pulmonary vascular resistance, and ejection fraction either at rest or during exercise. A small but consistent increase in resting blood pressure and heart rate are seen. Moricizine has no effect on exercise tolerance in patients with ventricular arrhythmias, heart failure, or angina pectoris.

Moricizine has antiarrhythmic activity similar to that of disopyramide, propranolol, and quinidine. Arrhythmia "rebound" isn't noted after discontinuation of therapy.

Pharmacokinetics
Absorption: Administration within 30 minutes of mealtime delays absorption and lowers peak plasma levels but has no effect on extent of absorption.
Distribution: 95% plasma protein-bound.
Metabolism: Undergoes significant first-pass metabolism resulting in an absolute bioavailability of about 38%. At least 26 metabolites have been identified with no single one representing at least 1% of the administered dose. It has been shown to induce its own metabolism.
Excretion: About 56% is excreted in feces, 39% in urine; some is also recycled through enterohepatic circulation.

Route	Onset	Peak	Duration
P.O.	1 hr	½-2 hr	10-24 hr

Contraindications and precautions
Contraindicated in patients with cardiogenic shock, those hypersensitive to drug, and those with second- or third-degree AV block or right bundle branch block when associated with left hemiblock (bifascicular block), unless an artificial pacemaker is present. Stop breast-feeding or drug because drug appears in breast milk.

Use cautiously in patients with renal or hepatic impairment, sick sinus syndrome, coronary artery disease, or left ventricular function.

Interactions
Drug-drug. *Cimetidine:* Decreased moricizine clearance by 49% when used together; no significant changes in efficacy or tolerance have been observed. Patients should receive decreased doses of cimetidine (not more than 600 mg daily).
Digoxin: Prolonged PR interval. Monitor patient carefully.
Propranolol: May produce a small additive increase in the PR interval. Monitor patient carefully.

Theophylline: Theophylline clearance increases and plasma half-life decreases. Monitor theophylline levels.

Adverse reactions

CNS: *dizziness, headache, fatigue,* hyperesthesia, anxiety, asthenia, nervousness, paresthesia, sleep disorders.

CV: *proarrhythmic events (ventricular tachycardia, premature ventricular contractions, supraventricular arrhythmias),* ECG abnormalities (including *conduction defects, sinus pause, junctional rhythm,* or *AV block*), *heart failure,* palpitations, chest pain, *cardiac death,* hypotension, hypertension, vasodilation, cerebrovascular events.

EENT: blurred vision.

GI: *nausea, vomiting, abdominal pain, dyspepsia, diarrhea, dry mouth.*

GU: urine retention, urinary frequency, dysuria.

Musculoskeletal: musculoskeletal pain.

Respiratory: dyspnea.

Skin: diaphoresis, rash.

Other: drug-induced fever, thrombophlebitis.

Overdose and treatment

Signs and symptoms of overdose include emesis, lethargy, coma, syncope, hypotension, conduction disturbances, exacerbation of heart failure, MI, sinus arrest, arrhythmias, and respiratory failure. No specific antidote has been identified.

Treatment should be supportive and include careful monitoring of cardiac, respiratory, and CNS changes. Gastric evacuation with care to avoid aspiration may be used as well.

Special considerations

● When switching from another antiarrhythmic to moricizine, withdraw previous therapy one to two half-lives before starting moricizine. Start moricizine 6 to 12 hours after last dose of quinidine and disopyramide; 3 to 6 hours after last dose of procainamide; 8 to 12 after encainide, propaferone, tocainide, or mexiletine; and 12 to 24 hours after flecainide.

Patient monitoring

● Electrolyte imbalances should be corrected before starting therapy; hypokalemia, hyperkalemia, or hypomagnesemia may alter effects of drug.
● Monitor patient for increased dizziness and nausea with 12-hour dosing.

Breast-feeding patients

● Appears in breast milk. Because of the potential for adverse reactions in the breast-fed infant, a decision whether to continue therapy must be made.

Pediatric patients

● Safety and efficacy haven't been established.

Patient teaching

● Instruct patient to take drug as prescribed to maintain adequate arrhythmia control.

morphine hydrochloride*
Morphitec*, M.O.S.*

morphine sulfate
Astramorph PF, Duramorph, Epimorph*, Infumorph, Kadian, MS Contin, MSIR, MS/L, MS/S, OMS Concentrate, Oramorph SR, RMS Uniserts, Roxanol, Statex*

Pharmacologic classification: opioid
Therapeutic classification: narcotic analgesic
Controlled substance schedule: II
Pregnancy risk category: C

Indications and dosages

➤ *Severe pain. Adults:* 10 mg q 4 hours S.C. or I.M., or 10 to 30 mg P.O., or 10 to 20 mg P.R. q 4 hours, p.r.n., or around the clock. May be injected slow I.V. (over 4 to 5 minutes) 2.5 to 15 mg diluted in 4 to 5 ml water for injection. May also give controlled-release tablets 15 to 30 mg q 12 hours. As an intermittent epidural injection, 5 mg via an epidural catheter q 24 hours. For continuous epidural infusion (device not implanted surgically), initial dose is 2.4 mg per 24 hours. May increase 1 to 2 mg daily, as needed. For a surgically implanted device, 3.5 to 7.5 mg daily or 4.5 to 10 mg daily if opiate tolerant. Intrathecal dose is one-tenth epidural dose; 0.2 to 1 mg may provide adequate relief in patients not tolerant to opiates.

Children: 0.1 to 0.2 mg/kg S.C. or I.M. q 4 hours. Maximum dose is 15 mg. May also give 0.05 to 0.1 mg/kg I.V. very slowly. In some situations, morphine may be administered by continuous I.V. infusion or by intraspinal and intrathecal injection.

➤ *Severe chronic pain related to cancer. Adults:* Initial loading dose of 15 mg followed by 0.8 to 10 mg /hour continuous I.V. or S.C. infusion. Adjust to effect.

Children: 0.025 to 2.6 mg/kg/hour by I.V. infusion or 0.025 to 1.79 mg/kg/hour by S.C. infusion.

➤ *Preoperative sedation and adjunct to anesthesia. Adults:* 8 to 10 mg I.M., S.C., or I.V.

➤ *Postoperative analgesia. Children:* 0.01 to 0.04 mg/kg/hour by continuous I.V. infusion. *Neonates:* 0.015 to 0.02 mg/kg/hour by continuous I.V. infusion.

➤ *Control of pain caused by acute MI. Adults:* Initially, 2 to 15 mg I.M., S.C., or I.V. Additional doses of 1 to 4 mg I.V. may be given q 5 minutes, p.r.n.

➤ *Control of angina pain. Adults:* 2 to 5 mg I.V. q 5 to 30 minutes, p.r.n., in pain unrelieved by three doses of S.L. nitroglycerin.

➤*Adjunctive treatment of acute pulmonary edema. Adults:* 10 to 15 mg I.V. at a rate not exceeding 2 mg/minute.
➤*Analgesia during labor. Adults*: 10 mg I.M. or S.C.

How supplied
Available by prescription only
*morphine hydrochloride**
Suppositories: 20 mg, 30 mg
Syrup: 1 mg/ml, 5 mg/ml, 10 mg/ml, 20 mg/ml, 50 mg/ml
Tablets: 10 mg, 20 mg, 40 mg, 60 mg
morphine sulfate
Capsules: 15 mg, 30 mg
Capsules (sustained-release): 20 mg, 50 mg, 100 mg
Injection (with preservative): 1 mg/ml, 2 mg/ml, 3 mg/ml, 4 mg/ml, 5 mg/ml, 8 mg/ml, 10 mg/ml, 15 mg/ml, 25 mg/ml, 50 mg/ml
Injection (without preservative): 500 mcg/ml, 1 mg/ml, 10 mg/ml, 15 mg/ml, 25 mg/ml
Oral solution: 10 mg/5 ml, 20 mg/5 ml, 20 mg/5 ml, 100 mg/5 ml
Suppositories: 5 mg, 10 mg, 20 mg, 30 mg
Tablets: 15 mg, 30 mg
Tablets (extended-release): 15 mg, 30 mg, 60 mg, 100 mg
Tablets (soluble): 10 mg, 15 mg, 30 mg

Pharmacodynamics
Analgesic action: Morphine is the principal opium alkaloid, the standard for opiate agonist analgesic activity. Mechanism of action is thought to be via the opiate receptors, altering patient's perception of pain. Morphine is particularly useful in severe, acute pain or severe, chronic pain. Morphine also has a central depressant effect on respiration and on the cough reflex center.

Pharmacokinetics
Absorption: Absorption is variable from the GI tract.
Distribution: Distributed widely through the body.
Metabolism: Metabolized primarily in the liver. One metabolite, morphine 6-glucuromide, is active.
Excretion: Excreted in the urine and bile. Morphine 6-glucuromide may accumulate after continuous dosing in patients with renal failure, leading to enhanced and prolonged opiate activity.

Route	Onset	Peak	Duration
P.O.	1 hr	1-2 hr	4-12 hr
I.V.	5 min	20 min	4-5 hr
I.M.	10-30 min	30-60 min	4-5 hr
S.C.	10-30 min	50-90 min	4-5 hr
P.R.	20-30 min	20-60 min	4-5 hr
Epidural	15-60 min	15-60 min	24 hr
Intrathecal	15-60 min	30-60 min	24 hr

Contraindications and precautions
Contraindicated in patients hypersensitive to drug and patients with conditions that would preclude administration of opioids by I.V. route (acute bronchial asthma or upper airway obstruction).

Use cautiously in geriatric or debilitated patients and in those with head injury, increased intracranial pressure, seizures, pulmonary disease, prostatic hyperplasia, hepatic or renal disease, acute abdominal conditions, hypothyroidism, Addison's disease, or urethral strictures.

Interactions
Drug-drug. *Anticholinergics:* May cause paralytic ileus. Monitor patient carefully.
Cimetidine: Increased respiratory and CNS depression. Reduced dosage of morphine is usually necessary.
CNS depressants, such as antihistamines, barbiturates, benzodiazepines, general anesthetics, narcotic analgesics, MAO inhibitors, muscle relaxants, phenothiazines, sedative-hypnotics, tricyclic antidepressants: Potentiated respiratory and CNS depression, sedation, and hypotensive effects of drug. Use together cautiously.
General anesthetics: Severe CV depression may result. Use together cautiously.
Narcotic antagonist: Patients who become physically dependent on this drug may experience acute withdrawal syndrome if given a narcotic antagonist. Avoid use together.
Drug-lifestyle. *Alcohol use:* Potentiated effects of drug. Discourage use together.

Adverse reactions
CNS: sedation, somnolence, clouded sensorium, euphoria, **seizures** (with large doses), dizziness, nightmares (with long-acting oral forms), light-headedness, hallucinations, nervousness, depression, syncope.
CV: *hypotension,* **bradycardia, shock, cardiac arrest,** tachycardia, hypertension.
GI: *nausea, vomiting, constipation, ileus, dry mouth, biliary tract spasms, anorexia,* increased plasma amylase levels.
GU: *urine retention.*
Hematologic: *thrombocytopenia.*
Respiratory: *respiratory depression, apnea, respiratory arrest.*
Skin: pruritus, skin flushing (with epidural administration); *diaphoresis; edema.*
Other: *physical dependence, decreased libido.*

Overdose and treatment
Rapid I.V. administration may result in overdose because of the delay in maximum CNS effect (30 minutes). The most common effects of morphine overdose are respiratory depression, with or without CNS depression, and miosis (pinpoint pupils). Other acute toxic effects include hypotension, bradycardia, hypothermia, shock, apnea, cardiopulmonary arrest, circulatory collapse, pulmonary edema, and seizures.

Reactions may be *common*, uncommon, *life-threatening*, or COMMON AND LIFE-THREATENING.

To treat acute overdose, first establish adequate respiratory exchange by way of a patent airway and ventilation, as needed; administer a narcotic antagonist (naloxone) to reverse respiratory depression. (Because duration of action of morphine is longer than that of naloxone, repeated naloxone dosing is necessary.) Naloxone shouldn't be given in the absence of clinically significant respiratory or CV depression. Monitor vital signs closely.

If patient is seen within 2 hours of ingestion of an oral overdose, empty the stomach immediately by inducing emesis (ipecac syrup) or using gastric lavage. Use cautiously to avoid risk of aspiration. Administer activated charcoal via nasogastric tube for further removal of drug in an oral overdose.

Provide symptomatic and supportive treatment (continued respiratory support, correction of fluid or electrolyte imbalance). Monitor laboratory parameters, vital signs, and neurologic status closely.

Special considerations
⚑ ALERT Don't confuse morphine with hydromorphone.
● Morphine is the drug of choice in relieving pain of MI; it may cause transient decrease in blood pressure.
● Regimented (around-the-clock) scheduling is beneficial in severe, chronic pain.
● Oral solutions of various levels are available, as well as a new intensified oral solution.
● There's a greater fluctuation in pain control with extended-release preparations.
● Note the disparity between oral and parenteral doses.
⚑ ALERT For continuous epidural or intrathecal infusion, morphine is administered via a controlled-infusion device. Take care when refilling the reservoir of such devices to ensure that medication is instilled into the proper port. A technical error could result in life-threatening respiratory depression.
● Morphine sulfate 10 or 25 mg/ml injections are intended for use with continuous, controlled microinfusion devices.
● For I.V. use, morphine 25 mg/ml is diluted to 0.1 to 1 mg/ml in D_5W. A higher concentration may be used for patients with fluid restriction.
● Long-term therapy in patients with advanced renal disease may lead to toxicity as a result of accumulation of the active metabolite.
● Some morphine injections contain sulfites which may cause allergic-type reactions.
● For S.L. administration, measure oral solution with tuberculin syringe, and administer dose a few drops at a time to allow maximal S.L. absorption and to minimize swallowing.
● Refrigeration of rectal suppositories isn't necessary. In some patients, rectal and oral absorption may not be equivalent.

● Preservative-free preparations are available for epidural and intrathecal administration. The use of the epidural route is increasing.
● Morphine may worsen or mask gallbladder pain.

Patient monitoring
● Epidural morphine has proven to be an excellent analgesic for patients with postoperative pain. After epidural administration, monitor patient closely for respiratory depression up to 24 hours after the injection. Check respiratory rate and depth according to protocol (such as every 15 minutes for 2 hours, then hourly for 18 hours). Some clinicians advocate a dilute naloxone infusion of 5 to 10 mcg/kg/hour during the first 12 hours to minimize respiratory depression without altering pain relief.
● Careful monitoring of patient's vital signs during morphine administration is needed.

Breast-feeding patients
● Morphine appears in breast milk. A woman should wait 2 to 3 hours after last dose before breast-feeding to avoid sedating the infant.

Pediatric patients
● Safety and efficacy of epidural and intrathecal dosing in children haven't been established. Safety and efficacy of morphine in neonates haven't been established. Children may be more sensitive to opiates on a body-weight basis.

Geriatric patients
● Lower doses are usually indicated for geriatric patients, who may be more sensitive to the therapeutic and adverse effects of drug.

Patient education
● Tell patient that oral liquid form of morphine may be mixed with a glass of fruit juice immediately before it's taken, if desired, to improve the taste.
● Tell patient taking long-acting morphine tablets to swallow them whole. Tablets shouldn't be broken, crushed, or chewed before swallowing.

moxifloxacin hydrochloride
Avelox

Pharmacologic classification: fluoroquinolone
Therapeutic classification: antibiotic
Pregnancy risk category: C

Indications and dosages
➤*Acute bacterial sinusitis caused by* **Haemophilus influenzae, Moraxella catarrhalis** *or* **Streptococcus pneumoniae.**
Adults: 400 mg P.O. once daily for 10 days.
➤*Acute bacterial exacerbation of chronic bronchitis caused by* **H. influenzae, H. parainfluenzae, Klebsiella pneumoniae, M.**

catarrhalis, Staphylococcus aureus, *or* **S. pneumoniae.** *Adults:* 400 mg P.O. once daily for 5 days.

➤ *Mild to moderate community-acquired pneumonia caused by* **Chlamydia pneumoniae, H. influenzae, M. catarrhalis, M. pneumoniae,** *or* **S. pneumoniae.** *Adults:* 400 mg P.O. once daily for 10 days.

➤ *Uncomplicated skin and skin structure infections caused by* **Staphylococcus aureus** *or* **S. pyogenes.** *Adults:* 400 mg P.O. once daily for 7 days.

How supplied
Available by prescription only
Tablets (film-coated): 400 mg

Pharmacodynamics
Antibactericidal action: Inhibits the activity of topoisomerase I (DNA gyrase) and topoisomerase IV in susceptible bacteria. These enzymes are necessary for bacterial DNA replication, transcription, repair, and recombination.

Pharmacokinetics
Absorption: Well absorbed after oral administration; absolute bioavailability of about 90%. Plasma levels peak within 1 to 3 hours; steady state reached after 3 days on a 400-mg, once-daily dose.
Distribution: Widely distributed; volume of 1.7 to 2.7 L/kg. Plasma protein–binding about 50%. Penetrates well into nasal and bronchial secretions, sinus mucosa, and saliva.
Metabolism: Metabolized to inactive glucuronide and sulfate conjugates. About 14% of dose converted to glucuronide metabolite. Sulfate metabolite accounts for about 38% of dose.
Excretion: About 45% excreted unchanged; about 20% in urine and 25% in feces. Sulfate metabolite eliminated primarily in feces; glucuronide metabolite renally excreted. Mean elimination half-life about 12 hours.

Route	Onset	Peak	Duration
P.O.	Unknown	1-3 hr	Unknown

Contraindications and precautions
Contraindicated in patients hypersensitive to drug, its components, or fluoroquinolone antimicrobials. Safety and efficacy haven't been documented in children, adolescents under age 18, and pregnant or lactating women.

Use cautiously in patients with prolonged QT interval and uncorrected hypokalemia. Use cautiously in patients with known or suspected CNS disorders or in the presence of other risk factors that may predispose patients to seizures or lower seizure threshold.

Interactions
Drug-drug. *Antacids; didanosine; metal cations, such as aluminum, magnesium, iron, zinc; multivitamins; sucralfate:* Metal cations chelate with moxifloxacin, resulting in decreased absorption and lower serum levels. Administer drug at least 4 hours before or 8 hours after drugs containing metal cations.

Antipsychotics, erythromycin, tricyclic antidepressants: May have additive effect when used with these drugs. Monitor patient and ECG closely; use drug cautiously.

Class IA (such as procainamide, quinidine) or Class III (such as amiodarone, sotalol) antiarrhythmics: Lack of clinical experience. Avoid concurrent use.

NSAIDs: Increased risk of CNS stimulation and seizures. Don't use together.

Drug-lifestyle. *Sun exposure:* Although photosensitivity hasn't occurred with moxifloxacin, it has been reported with other fluoroquinolones. Tell patient to take precautions.

Adverse reactions
CNS: dizziness, headache.
CV: prolongation of QT interval.
EENT: taste perversion.
GI: abdominal pain; diarrhea; dyspepsia; nausea; vomiting; hyperlipidemia; increased amylase, GGT, and LD levels.
Hematologic: thrombocythemia, *thrombocytopenia*, eosinophilia, *leukopenia*, increase or decrease in PT.
Hepatic: abnormal liver function test results.
Metabolic: hyperglycemia.

Overdose and treatment
In acute overdose, immediately empty the stomach. Monitor ECG closely because of the risk of QT interval prolongation. Provide adequate hydration and supportive care.

Special considerations
● Drug may be administered without regard to meals. Give at same time each day to provide consistent absorption. Provide liberal fluid intake.
● Urge patient to complete the course of therapy.
● Administer moxifloxacin 4 hours before or 8 hours after antacids, sucralfate, and products containing iron or zinc.
● Store drug at controlled room temperature.
● NSAIDs may increase risk of CNS stimulation and seizures when used with fluoroquinolones such as moxifloxacin.
● Rupture of Achilles and other tendons has been linked to fluoroquinolones. If pain, inflammation, or rupture of a tendon occurs, stop drug.
● Drug hasn't been studied and isn't recommended in patients with moderate to severe hepatotoxicity (Child Pugh Classes B and C).
● The most common adverse reactions are nausea, vomiting, stomach pain, diarrhea, dizziness, and headache.
● CNS reactions caused by fluoroquinolones include dizziness, confusion, tremors, hallucinations, depression, and, rarely, suicidal thoughts or acts. These reactions may occur after initial

dose. Stop drug and institute appropriate therapy if any of these reactions occur.
• Serious hypersensitivity reactions, including anaphylaxis, have occurred in patients receiving fluoroquinolones. Stop drug and institute supportive measures as indicated
• Pseudomembranous colitis may occur with moxifloxacin as with other antimicrobials. Consider this diagnosis if diarrhea develops.

Patient monitoring
• Watch for hypersensitivity reactions, CNS toxicities (including seizures), QT interval prolongation, pseudomembranous colitis, phototoxicity, and tendon rupture.
• Monitor patient for response to drug therapy.

Breast-feeding patients
• Drug may appear in breast milk. Benefits must be weighed against risks to breast-feeding infant.

Pediatric patients
• Safety and efficacy haven't been established in children under age 18.

Geriatric patients
• Drug is safe and effective in elderly patients.

Patient education
• Tell patient to take drug once daily, at same time each day.
• Advise patient to finish entire course of therapy, even if condition has improved.
• Tell patient to drink plenty of fluids and to take drug 4 hours before or 8 hours after antacids, sucralfate, or products containing iron or zinc.
• Most common adverse reactions include nausea, vomiting, stomach pain, diarrhea, dizziness, and headache. Tell patient to avoid hazardous activities until effects of drug are known.
• Advise patient to call if he experiences allergic reaction, heart palpitations, fainting, persistent diarrhea, severe sunburn, injury to a muscle tendon, or seizures.

mumps skin test antigen
MSTA

Pharmacologic classification: viral antigen
Therapeutic classification: skin test antigen
Pregnancy risk category: C

Indications and dosages
➤ *Assessment of cell-mediated immunity.* *Adults and children:* 0.1 ml I.D. into inner surface of forearm.

How supplied
Available by prescription only
Injection: 40 complement-fixing units/ml suspension; 10 tests/1-ml vial

Pharmacodynamics
Antigenic action: Isn't indicated for the immunization, diagnosis, or treatment of mumps virus infection. The status of cell-mediated immunity can be determined from use of mumps with other antigens. In vitro tests (such as lymphocyte stimulation and assays for T and B cells) are necessary to diagnose a specific disorder.

Pharmacokinetics
Absorption: After I.D. injection, examine test site in 48 to 72 hours.
Distribution: Must be given I.D.; S.C. injection invalidates test.
Metabolism: Not applicable.
Excretion: Not applicable.

Route	Onset	Peak	Duration
Intra-dermal	Unknown	Unknown	Unknown

Contraindications and precautions
Contraindicated in persons sensitive to avian protein (chicken, eggs, or feathers) and in those hypersensitive to thimerosal. Use cautiously in elderly and immunosuppressed patients.

Interactions
Drug-drug. *Cimetidine:* May increase delayed-sensitivity responses. Use cautiously.
Immunosuppressants, viral vaccines: Responses may be suppressed. Monitor patient closely.

Adverse reactions
CNS: headache, drowsiness.
GI: nausea, anorexia.
Other: tenderness, pruritus, and rash at injection site. Occasionally, *severe delayed-hypersensitivity reaction* will produce vesiculation, local tissue necrosis, abscess, and scar formation, *anaphylaxis,* Arthus reaction, urticaria, *angioedema,* shortness of breath, excessive perspiration.

Overdose and treatment
None reported.

Special considerations
• Obtain history of allergies and reactions to skin tests. In patients hypersensitive to feathers, eggs, or chicken, a severe reaction may follow administration of mumps skin test antigen.
• After injection, observe patient for 15 minutes for possible immediate-type systemic allergic reaction. Keep epinephrine 1:1,000 available.
• Accurate dosage (0.1 ml) and administration are essential.
• Pseudopositive reactions may occur in patients with egg protein sensitivity.
• Examine injection site within 48 to 72 hours, interpreting as follows:
Positive reaction—Induration of 5 mm or more, with or without erythema, indicates sensitivity.

Negative reaction—Induration less than 5 mm means the individual hasn't been sensitized to mumps or is anergic.

● Reactivity to test may be depressed or suppressed for as long as 6 weeks in individuals who have received concurrent virus vaccines, in those who are receiving a corticosteroid or other immunosuppressants, in those who have had viral infections, and in malnourished patients.

● Mumps skin test antigen isn't used to assess exposure to mumps; it's used in assessing T-cell function for immunocompetence because most normal individuals will exhibit a positive reaction.

● Cold packs or topical corticosteroids may provide relief of pain, pruritus, and discomfort if a local reaction occurs.

● Store vial in refrigerator.

Patient monitoring
● Watch for sensitivity or allergic reaction.
● Monitor patient receiving immunosuppressant drugs for response to therapy.

Breast-feeding patients
● Although appearance of drug in breast milk is unlikely, benefit to breast-feeding patient should be weighed against possible risk to infant.

Geriatric patients
● Elderly patients who don't react to test are considered anergic.

Patient education
● Tell patient to report unusual adverse effects.
● Explain that induration will disappear in a few days.

mumps virus vaccine, live
Mumpsvax

Pharmacologic classification: vaccine
Therapeutic classification: viral vaccine
Pregnancy risk category: C

Indications and dosages
➤ **Immunization.** *Adults and children over age 1:* 1 vial (0.5 ml) S.C. in outer aspect of the upper arm.

How supplied
Available by prescription only
Injection: single-dose vial containing not less than 20,000 TCID$_{50}$ (tissue culture infective doses) of attenuated mumps virus derived from Jeryl Lynn mumps strain (grown in chick embryo culture) and vial of diluent

Pharmacodynamics
Mumps prophylactic action: Vaccine promotes active immunity to mumps.

Pharmacokinetics
Absorption: Antibodies usually are evident 2 to 3 weeks after injection. Duration of vaccine-induced immunity is at least 20 years and probably lifelong.
Distribution: No information available.
Metabolism: No information available.
Excretion: No information available.

Route	Onset	Peak	Duration
S.C.	Unknown	Unknown	> 15 yr

Contraindications and precautions
Contraindicated in immunosuppressed patients; in those with cancer, blood dyscrasias, gamma globulin disorders, fever, untreated active tuberculosis, or anaphylaxis or anaphylactoid reactions to neomycin or eggs; in those receiving corticosteroid or radiation therapy; and in pregnant women.

Interactions
Drug-drug. *Immune serum globulin or transfusions of blood or blood products:* May interfere with immune response to vaccine. If possible, defer vaccination for 3 months in these situations.
Immunosuppressant drugs: May interfere with response to vaccine. Avoid use together.

Adverse reactions
CNS: *malaise.*
GI: *diarrhea.*
Skin: *rash.*
Other: *slight fever, mild allergic reactions, mild lymphadenopathy, injection-site reaction.*

Overdose and treatment
No information available.

Special considerations
● Mumps vaccine shouldn't be used in delayed hypersensitivity (anergy) skin testing.
● Obtain a thorough history of patient's allergies, especially to antibiotics, eggs, chicken, or chicken feathers, and of reactions to immunizations.
● Skin testing is done to assess vaccine sensitivity (against a control of normal saline solution in the opposite arm) in patients with history of anaphylactoid reactions to egg ingestion. Administer an I.D. or scratch test with a 1:10 dilution. Read results after 5 to 30 minutes. A positive reaction is a wheal with or without pseudopodia and surrounding erythema. If sensitivity test is positive, consider desensitization.
● The FDA requires documentation of manufacturer, lot number, date of administration, and name, address, and title of person giving vaccine.
● Vaccine can be used in HIV-infected patients who don't have severe immunosuppression.
● Have epinephrine solution 1:1,000 available to treat allergic reactions.

• Don't administer vaccine I.V. Use a 25G, ⅝-inch needle and inject S.C., preferably into the outer aspect of the upper arm.
• Use only diluent supplied. Discard reconstituted solution after 8 hours.
• Refrigerate and protect from light. Solution may be red, pink, or yellow, but it must be clear.
• Don't give vaccine less than 1 month before or after immunization with other live virus vaccines—except for live, attenuated measles virus vaccine, live rubella virus vaccine, or monovalent or trivalent live oral poliovirus vaccine or poliovirus vaccine, inactivated, which may be administered simultaneously.
• Vaccine doesn't offer protection when given after exposure to natural mumps.
• Revaccination is recommended at age 4 to 6.
• Vaccine temporarily may decrease the response to tuberculin skin testing. If a tuberculin skin test is necessary, administer it either before or simultaneously with mumps vaccine.

Patient monitoring
• Monitor patient for allergic response.

Breast-feeding patients
• It isn't known if vaccine appears in breast milk. No problems have been reported. Use vaccine cautiously in breast-feeding women.

Pediatric patients
• Vaccine isn't recommended for children under age 1 because retained maternal mumps antibodies may interfere with immune response.

Patient education
• Tell patient that he may experience pain and inflammation at the injection site and a low-grade fever, rash, or general malaise.
• Encourage patient to report distressing adverse reactions.
• Recommend acetaminophen to alleviate adverse reactions, such as fever.
• Tell women of childbearing age to avoid pregnancy for 3 months after vaccination. Provide contraceptive information, if necessary.

---

mupirocin (pseudomonic acid A)
Bactroban

mupirocin calcium
Bactroban Nasal

Pharmacologic classification: antibiotic
Therapeutic classification: topical antibacterial
Pregnancy risk category: B

Indications and dosages
➤ *Topical treatment of impetigo caused by* Staphylococcus aureus, *beta-hemolytic* Streptococcus, *and* Streptococcus pyogenes.
Adults and children: Apply a small amount to affected area t.i.d. for 1 to 2 weeks. Treated area may be covered with a gauze dressing, if desired.
➤ *Eradication of nasal colonization of methicillin-resistant* S. aureus. *Adults:* Apply one-half of a single-use tube to each nostril b.i.d. for 5 days. Press and release the sides of the nose repeatedly for 1 minute to disperse the medication through the nares.

How supplied
Available by prescription only
Cream: 2%
Ointment: 2% (1-g single-use tubes, 15 g, 30 g)
Ointment for intranasal use: 2%

Pharmacodynamics
Antibacterial action: Mupirocin is structurally unrelated to other agents and is produced by fermentation of the organism *Pseudomonas fluorescens.* Mupirocin inhibits bacterial protein synthesis by reversibly and specifically binding to bacterial isoleucyl transfer-RNA synthetase. Mupirocin shows no cross-resistance with chloramphenicol, erythromycin, gentamicin, lincomycin, methicillin, neomycin, novobiocin, penicillin, streptomycin, or tetracycline.

Pharmacokinetics
Absorption: No absorption 24 hours after application under occlusive dressing.
Distribution: Highly protein-bound (about 95%). A substantial decrease in activity can be expected in the presence of serum (as in exudative wounds).
Metabolism: Slightly metabolized locally in the skin to monic acid.
Excretion: Eliminated locally by desquamation of the skin.

Route	Onset	Peak	Duration
Topical	Unknown	Unknown	Unknown

Contraindications and precautions
Contraindicated in patients hypersensitive to drug. Use cautiously in patients with burns or impaired renal function.

Interactions
None reported.

Adverse reactions
CNS: headache with nasal use.
EENT: rhinitis, pharyngitis, and burning with nasal use.
GI: taste perversion with nasal use.
Respiratory: upper respiratory congestion and cough with nasal use.
Skin: burning, pruritus, stinging, rash, pain, and erythema with topical use.

Overdose and treatment
No information available.

Special considerations
• If sensitivity or chemical irritation occurs, stop drug and start appropriate alternative therapy.
• When used on burns or extensive open wounds, absorption of polyethylene glycol vehicle is possible and may result in serious renal toxicity.

Patient monitoring
• Patients not showing a clinical response within 3 to 5 days should be re-evaluated.
• Monitor patient for superinfection. Use of antibiotics (prolonged or repeated) may result in bacterial or fungal overgrowth of nonsusceptible organisms.

Breast-feeding patients
• It isn't known if drug appears in breast milk. Use cautiously.

Patient education
• Tell patient to wash and dry affected areas thoroughly and apply thin film, rubbing in gently.
• Tell patient to use single-use tube for nasal application for one application and to discard tube. Tell him to apply one-half of the ointment from the tube into one nostril and the remaining into the other nostril, in the morning and evening.
• Warn patient to avoid contact with eyes and mucous membranes.

---

muromonab-CD3
Orthoclone OKT3

Pharmacologic classification: monoclonal antibody
Therapeutic classification: immunosuppressant
Pregnancy risk category: C

Indications and dosages
➤ *Acute allograft rejection in renal, cardiac, and hepatic transplant patients.*
Adults: 5 mg/day I.V. bolus for 10 to 14 days. Begin once acute renal rejection is diagnosed.

How supplied
Injection: 5 mg/5 ml in 5-ml ampules

Pharmacodynamics
Immunosuppressive action: Reverses graft rejection, probably by interfering with T-cell function that promotes acute renal rejection. Interacts with and prevents the function of the T-cell antigen receptor complex in the cellular membrane, which influences antigen recognition and is essential for signal transduction. Reacts with most peripheral T cells in blood and in body tissues, and blocks all known T-cell functions.

Pharmacokinetics
Absorption: Administered I.V.
Distribution: No information available.
Metabolism: No information available.
Excretion: No information available.

Route	Onset	Peak	Duration
I.V.	Immediate	Unknown	Unknown

Contraindications and precautions
Contraindicated in patients hypersensitive to drug or to other products of murine (mouse) origin and in those with antimurine antibody titers of 1:1,000 or more. Also contraindicated in patients with fluid overload (as evidenced by chest X-ray or a weight gain greater than 3% within week before treatment) or a history of seizures or predisposition to seizures. Also contraindicated in pregnant and breast-feeding women.

Interactions
Drug-drug. *Immunosuppressants (azathioprine, cyclosporine):* May potentiate immunosuppressive effects of these drugs. Monitor patient closely.
Live-virus vaccines: May potentiate replication and increase effects of vaccine. Defer immunization if possible. If given, monitor response.

Adverse reactions
CNS: *tremor, headache, **seizures, asthenia,** fatigue, lethargy, malaise, dizziness, meningitis, confusion, depression, nervousness, somnolence.
CV: chest pain, *tachycardia, hypertension,* vasodilation, **arrhythmias, bradycardia,** *hypotension,* vascular occlusion, *edema.*
EENT: photophobia, tinnitus.
GI: *nausea, vomiting, diarrhea,* anorexia, abdominal pain.
GU: *renal dysfunction.*
Hematologic: *leukopenia, **thrombocytopenia,** leukocytosis, anemia.
Respiratory: pulmonary edema, *dyspnea,* wheezing, *abnormal chest sounds,* hyperventilation, hypoxia, pneumonia, respiratory congestion.
Skin: diaphoresis, pruritus, *rash.*
Other: *fever, chills,* infection, **anaphylaxis,** cytokine release syndrome (from flulike symptoms to shock), **aseptic meningitis, risk of neoplasia.**

Overdose and treatment
Overdose may cause hyperthermia, severe chills, myalgia, vomiting, diarrhea, edema, oliguria, pulmonary edema, and acute renal failure. Hemolytic-uremic syndrome may also occur. Treatment is symptomatic and supportive.

Special considerations
• A reaction is common within ½ to 6 hours after the first dose, consisting of significant fever, chills, dyspnea, and malaise. Pulmonary edema

---

Reactions may be *common*, uncommon, *life-threatening*, or COMMON AND LIFE-THREATENING.

may occur if patient isn't pretreated with a corticosteroid.

• To prepare solution, draw into a syringe through a low protein-binding 0.2 or 0.22 micrometer filter. Discard filter and attach needle for I.V. bolus injection.

• Because drug is a protein solution, it may develop a few fine translucent particles, which don't affect its potency.

• Give I.V. bolus in less than 1 minute. Don't give by I.V. infusion or with other drug solutions.

• Manufacturer recommends that, if patient's temperature exceeds 100° F (37.8° C), you should lower it with antipyretics before giving drug.

• Immunosuppressive therapy increases susceptibility to infection and to lymphoproliferative disorders. Lymphomas may follow immunosuppressive therapy; their occurrence seems related to the intensity and duration of immunosuppression rather than specific drugs because most patients receive a combination of treatments.

• Reduce concomitant immunosuppressive therapy to daily dose of prednisone 0.5 mg/kg and azathioprine 25 mg. Reduce or stop cyclosporine. Maintenance immunosuppression can resume 3 days before stopping muromonab-CD3.

• Refrigerate drug at 36° to 46° F (2° to 8° C). Don't freeze or shake.

Patient monitoring

• Chest X-ray taken within 24 hours before treatment must be clear of fluid; monitor WBC counts and differentials at intervals during treatment.

• Monitor patient for drug's effect on circulating T cells using flow cytometry or by expressing the CD3 antigen by in vitro assay.

Breast-feeding patients

• Safety in breast-feeding women hasn't been established. It's unknown if drug appears in breast milk.

Pediatric patients

• Safety and efficacy in children haven't been established. Patients as young as age 2 have had no unexpected adverse effects.

Patient education

• Tell patient to expect fever, chills, dyspnea, chest pain, nausea, and vomiting with first dose.

---

mycophenolate mofetil
CellCept

Pharmacologic classification: mycophenolic acid derivative
Therapeutic classification: immunosuppressive
Pregnancy risk category: C

Indications and dosages

➤ *Prophylaxis of organ rejection in patients receiving allogeneic renal trans-*plants. *Adults:* 1 g P.O. or I.V. b.i.d. Use with corticosteroids and cyclosporine.

➤ *Prophylaxis of organ rejection in patients receiving cardiac transplants.* *Adults:* 1.5 g P.O. or I.V. over no less than 2 hours b.i.d. Use with corticosteroids and cyclosporine.

➤ *Prophylaxis of organ rejection in patients receiving allogeneic hepatic transplants. Adults:* 1.5 g P.O. b.i.d. or 1 g I.V. over at least 2 hours b.i.d. Use with corticosteroids and cyclosporine.

How supplied

Available by prescription only
Capsules: 250 mg
Oral suspension: 200 mg/ml (after reconstitution)
Powder for injection: 500 mg
Tablets: 500 mg

Pharmacodynamics

Immunosuppressive action: Inhibits proliferative responses of T- and B-lymphocytes, suppresses antibody formation by B-lymphocytes, and may inhibit recruitment of leukocytes into sites of inflammation and graft rejection.

Pharmacokinetics

Absorption: Absorbed from the GI tract. Absolute bioavailability of drug and active metabolite is 94%.
Distribution: About 97% is bound to plasma protein.
Metabolism: Undergoes complete presystemic metabolism to mycophenolic acid.
Excretion: Mainly excreted in urine with a small amount in feces. Half-life is about 18 hours.

Route	Onset	Peak	Duration
P.O.	Unknown	½-1¼ hr	7½-18 hr
I.V.	Unknown	Unknown	10-17 hr

Contraindication and precautions

Contraindicated in patients hypersensitive to drug, mycophenolic acid, or any component of drug product. Drug shouldn't be used during pregnancy unless the benefits outweigh the risks. Use cautiously in patients with GI disorders.

Interactions

Drug-drug. *Acyclovir, ganciclovir:* Increased risk of toxicity for both drugs. Monitor patient closely.
Antacids with magnesium and aluminum hydroxides: Decreased absorption of mycophenolate mofetil. Administer drugs separately.
Cholestyramine: May interfere with enterohepatic recirculation, decreasing mycophenolate bioavailability. Don't give together.
Oral contraceptives: Mycophenolate may affect efficacy of oral contraceptives. Advise patient to use alternative contraceptives measures.

Adverse reactions

CNS: *asthenia, tremor,* insomnia, dizziness, *headache.*

CV: chest pain, hypertension, edema.

EENT: pharyngitis.

GI: *diarrhea, constipation, nausea, dyspepsia, vomiting, oral candidiasis, abdominal pain.*

GU: *urinary tract infection, hematuria,* kidney tubular necrosis.

Hematologic: *anemia,* **leukopenia,** THROMBOCYTOPENIA, hypochromic anemia, leukocytosis.

Metabolic: *hypercholesterolemia, hypophosphatemia, hypokalemia,* hyperkalemia, hyperglycemia.

Musculoskeletal: *back pain.*

Respiratory: *dyspnea, cough,* bronchitis, pneumonia.

Skin: *acne,* rash.

Other: *pain, fever, sepsis, possible immunosuppression-induced infection or lymphoma.*

Overdose and treatment

Although there's no reported experience of overdose, doses of 4 to 5 g daily compared with 3 g daily cause an increase in nausea, vomiting, or diarrhea and occasional hematologic abnormalities in some patients. Treatment includes use of bile acid sequestrants to increase excretion of drug.

Special considerations

● Avoid doses exceeding 1 g b.i.d. in patients with severe chronic renal impairment (glomerular filtration rate below 25 ml/minute) outside the immediate post-transplant period.

● Because of potential teratogenic effects, don't open capsules and don't crush tablets. Also, avoid inhaling powder in capsules or allowing direct contact with skin or mucous membranes. If such contact occurs, wash thoroughly with soap and water; rinse eyes with plain water.

● Immunosuppression-induced infection or lymphoma may occur.

● Don't give I.V. solution by rapid or bolus method; it must be given over 2 hours or more.

● Reconstitute by injecting 14 ml D_5W into a 500-mg vial; shake and inspect for particles or discoloration (solution is slightly yellow). Discard if particles or discoloration is present. To prepare a 1-g dose, further dilute two reconstituted vials in 140 ml of D_5W injection. To prepare a 1.5-g dose, further dilute three reconstituted vials in 210 ml of D_5W injection. The final concentration of both preparations is 6 mg/ml. Drug is incompatible with other I.V. infusion solutions and must be given at an exclusive site.

● Use solution within 4 hours of reconstitution and dilution. Store at 77° F (25° C).

● Oral solution should be reconstituted by a pharmacist prior to dispensing.

● Don't mix oral solution with other drugs.

Patient monitoring

● Monitor patient's CBC regularly. If neutropenia develops, interrupt therapy, reduce dose, perform appropriate diagnostic tests, or give additional treatment.

Breast-feeding patients

● It isn't known if drug appears in breast milk. Use in breast-feeding women isn't recommended.

Pediatric patients

● Safety and efficacy in children haven't been established.

Patient education

● Warn patient not to open capsules or crush tablets; instruct him to swallow them whole on an empty stomach.

● Instruct patient about need for repeated appropriate laboratory tests during drug therapy.

● Give patient complete dosage instructions and inform him of increased risk of lymphoproliferative diseases and other malignancies.

● Explain that drug is used with other drug therapies. Stress importance of not interrupting or stopping these drugs without medical approval.

● Inform women that a pregnancy test should be done within 1 week before beginning therapy and that effective contraception must be used before, during, and for 6 weeks after therapy is completed, even when there's history of infertility (unless the result of hysterectomy). Also, two forms of contraception must be used simultaneously unless abstinence is chosen. If pregnancy occurs despite these measures, she must contact her prescriber immediately.

Reactions may be *common*, uncommon, *life-threatening*, or COMMON AND LIFE-THREATENING.

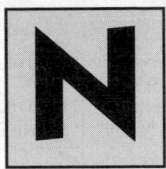

nabumetone
Relafen

Pharmacologic classification: NSAID
Therapeutic classification: antiarthritic
Pregnancy risk category: C

Indications and dosages
➤ *Acute and long-term treatment of rheumatoid arthritis or osteoarthritis.*
Adults: Initially, 1,000 mg P.O. daily as a single dose or in divided doses b.i.d. Adjust dosage based on patient response. Maximum recommended daily dose, 2,000 mg.

How supplied
Available by prescription only
Tablets: 500 mg, 750 mg

Pharmacodynamics
Anti-inflammatory action: Nabumetone probably acts by inhibiting the synthesis of prostaglandins. Drug also has analgesic and antipyretic action.

Pharmacokinetics
Absorption: Well absorbed from the GI tract. After absorption, about 35% is rapidly transformed to 6-methoxy-2-naphthylacetic acid (6MNA), the principal active metabolite; the balance is transformed to unidentified metabolites. Administration with food increases the absorption rate and peak levels of 6MNA but doesn't change total drug absorbed.
Distribution: 6MNA is more than 99% bound to plasma proteins.
Metabolism: 6MNA is metabolized to inactive metabolites in the liver.
Excretion: Metabolites are excreted primarily in urine. About 9% appears in the feces. Elimination half-life is about 24 hours. Half-life is increased in patients with renal failure.

Route	Onset	Peak	Duration
P.O.	Unknown	2-4 hr	Unknown

Contraindications and precautions
Contraindicated in patients with hypersensitivity reactions, history of aspirin- or NSAID-induced asthma, urticaria, or other allergic-type reactions. Also contraindicated during third trimester of pregnancy.

Use cautiously in patients with impaired renal or hepatic function, heart failure, hypertension, conditions that predispose to fluid retention, and history of peptic ulcer disease.

Interactions
Drug-drug. *Drugs that are highly bound to plasma proteins, such as warfarin:* Nabumetone may displace drug. Use together cautiously.

Adverse reactions
CNS: *dizziness, headache,* fatigue, insomnia, nervousness, somnolence.
CV: vasculitis, edema.
EENT: *tinnitus.*
GI: *diarrhea, dyspepsia, abdominal pain, constipation, flatulence, nausea,* dry mouth, gastritis, stomatitis, anorexia, vomiting, *bleeding,* ulceration.
Respiratory: dyspnea, pneumonitis.
Skin: *pruritus, rash,* increased diaphoresis.

Overdose and treatment
After an accidental overdose, empty the stomach by induced emesis or lavage. Activated charcoal may limit the amount of drug absorbed.

Special considerations
● Because NSAIDs impair the synthesis of renal prostaglandins, they can decrease renal blood flow and lead to reversible renal function impairment, especially in patients with renal failure, liver dysfunction, or heart failure; geriatric patients; and patients who take diuretics. Monitor these patients closely during therapy.

Patient monitoring
● During long-term therapy, periodically monitor renal and liver function, CBC, and hematocrit.
● Monitor patient carefully for signs and symptoms of GI bleeding.

Breast-feeding patients
● Because of risk of serious toxicity to the infant, use in breast-feeding women isn't recommended.

Pediatric patients
● Safety and efficacy in children haven't been established.

Geriatric patients
● No differences in safety or efficacy have been noted in geriatric patients.

Patient education
● Tell patient to take drug with food, milk, or antacids to enhance drug absorption.

• Stress importance of follow-up examinations to detect adverse GI effects.
• Teach patient signs and symptoms of GI bleeding, and tell him to report them immediately.
• Advise patient to limit alcohol intake because of risk of additive GI toxicity.

nadolol
Corgard

Pharmacologic classification: beta blocker
Therapeutic classification: antihypertensive, antianginal
Pregnancy risk category: C

Indications and dosages
➤ *Hypertension. Adults:* Initially, 20 to 40 mg P.O. once daily. Dosage may be increased in 40- to 80-mg increments daily at 2- to 14-day intervals until optimum response occurs. Usual maintenance dosage is 40 or 80 mg once daily. Doses of up to 240 or 320 mg daily may be necessary. Rarely, up to 640 mg daily.
➤ *Long-term prophylactic management of chronic stable angina pectoris. Adults:* Initially, 40 mg P.O. once daily. Dosage may be increased in 40- to 80-mg increments daily at 3- to 7-day intervals until optimum response occurs. Usual maintenance dosage is 40 or 80 mg once daily. Doses of up to 160 or 240 mg daily may be needed.
➤ *Arrhythmias* ◇. *Adults:* 60 to 160 mg P.O. daily.
➤ *Prophylaxis of vascular headache* ◇. *Adults:* 20 to 40 mg P.O. once daily; may gradually increase to 120 mg daily, if necessary.
✦ *Dosage adjustment.* For renally impaired patients, refer to the following table.

Creatinine clearance (ml/min)	Dosing interval
> 50	q 24 hr
31-50	q 24-36 hr
10-30	q 24-48 hr
< 10	q 40-60 hr

How supplied
Available by prescription only
Tablets: 20 mg, 40 mg, 80 mg, 120 mg, 160 mg

Pharmacodynamics
Antihypertensive action: Mechanism of antihypertensive effect is unknown. Drug may reduce blood pressure by blocking adrenergic receptors, thus decreasing cardiac output; by decreasing sympathetic outflow from the CNS; or by suppressing renin release.
Antianginal action: Nadolol decreases myocardial oxygen consumption, thus relieving angina, by blocking catecholamine-induced increas-

es in heart rate, myocardial contraction, and blood pressure.

Pharmacokinetics
Absorption: 30% to 40% of a dose of nadolol is absorbed from the GI tract. Absorption isn't affected by food.
Distribution: Distributed throughout the body; drug is about 30% protein-bound.
Metabolism: Not metabolized.
Excretion: Most of a given dose is excreted unchanged in urine; the remainder is excreted in feces. Plasma half-life is about 20 hours. Antihypertensive and antianginal effects persist for about 24 hours.

Route	Onset	Peak	Duration
P.O.	Unknown	2-4 hr	Unknown

Contraindications and precautions
Contraindicated in patients with bronchial asthma, sinus bradycardia, greater than first-degree heart block, and cardiogenic shock. Use cautiously in patients with hyperthyroidism, heart failure, diabetes, chronic bronchitis, emphysema, and impaired renal or hepatic function. Also use cautiously in those receiving general anesthesia before undergoing surgery.

Interactions
Drug-drug. *Antiarrhythmics:* Possible additive or antagonistic cardiac effects and additive toxic effects. Use together cautiously.
Antihypertensives, diuretics, and, at high doses, the neuromuscular blocking effect of tubocurarine and related drugs: Potentiated antihypertensive effects. Use together cautiously
Antimuscarinics, such as atropine: May antagonize nadolol-induced bradycardia. Use together cautiously.
Sympathomimetics, such as epinephrine and isoproterenol: Antagonized effects of these drugs. Use together cautiously.
Drug-lifestyle. *Cocaine use:* Inhibited therapeutic effects of nadolol. Inform patient of this interaction.

Adverse reactions
CNS: fatigue, dizziness.
CV: *bradycardia, hypotension, heart failure,* peripheral vascular disease, rhythm and conduction disturbances.
GI: nausea, vomiting, diarrhea, abdominal pain, constipation, anorexia.
Respiratory: *increased airway resistance.*
Skin: rash.
Other: fever.

Overdose and treatment
Evidence of overdose includes severe hypotension, bradycardia, heart failure, and bronchospasm.
    After acute ingestion, empty patient's stomach by induced emesis or gastric lavage and give ac-

---

Reactions may be *common*, uncommon, *life-threatening*, or COMMON AND LIFE-THREATENING.

tivated charcoal to reduce absorption. Magnesium sulfate may be given orally as a cathartic. Subsequent treatment is usually symptomatic and supportive.

Special considerations
● Dosage adjustments may be necessary in patients with renal impairment.
● Nadolol has been used as an antiarrhythmic and as prophylaxis for migraine headaches.
● If long-term therapy is used, gradually decrease dose over 1 to 2 weeks before discontinuing drug. Abrupt withdrawal can exacerbate angina and cause an MI.

Patient monitoring
● Monitor blood pressure closely at start of therapy and during dosage adjustments; once condition is stabilized, monitor patient at 3- to 6-month intervals.
● Monitor patient for reflex bradycardia, which may be treated with atropine.
● Monitor patients with hyperthyroidism and diabetes carefully; symptoms may be masked by drug therapy.

Breast-feeding patients
● Drug appears in breast milk; an alternative feeding method is recommended during therapy.

Pediatric patients
● Safety and efficacy in children haven't been established; use only if potential benefit outweighs risk.

Geriatric patients
● These patients may need lower maintenance dosages of nadolol because of increased bioavailability or delayed metabolism; they also may experience enhanced adverse effects.

Patient education
● Tell patient not to stop nadolol abruptly. Drug should be tapered.

---

nafcillin sodium
Nafcil, Nallpen, Unipen

Pharmacologic classification: penicillinase-resistant penicillin
Therapeutic classification: antibiotic
Pregnancy risk category: B

Indications and dosages
➤ *Systemic infections caused by susceptible organisms (methicillin-sensitive* **Staphylococcus aureus***).* *Adults:* 250 to 500 mg P.O. q 4 to 6 hours for mild to moderate infections and 1 g q 4 to 6 hours for more severe infections. Or, 500 mg I.M. q 4 hours or 500 to 1,000 mg I.V. q 4 hours depending on severity of the infection.

Children over age 1 month: 50 to 100 mg/kg P.O. daily, in divided doses q 6 hours. Or, 50 to 200 mg/kg daily I.M. or I.V. in divided doses q 4 to 6 hours depending on the severity of the infection.
Neonates: 30 to 40 mg/kg daily P.O. divided equally into three to four doses. Or, 20 mg/kg daily I.M. in two equally divided doses. Or, 40 mg/kg daily I.M. in two equally divided doses q 12 hours if neonate is less than 7 days old and 60 to 200 mg/kg daily in equally divided doses q 8 hours if neonate is 7 to 28 days old. For mild to moderate infection, may give 50 to 100 mg/kg daily I.V. in divided doses q 6 hours. For more severe infections, 100 to 200 mg/kg daily I.V. divided q 4 to 6 hours. Or, 25 mg/kg I.V. q 12 hours (if less than 7 days old and under 2 kg [4.4 lb]) or q 8 hours (if less than 7 days old and over 2 kg or over 7 days old and less than 2 kg) or q 6 hours (if over 7 days old and over 2 kg).
➤ *Meningitis. Neonates under age 7 days who weigh less than 2 kg:* 50 mg/kg I.V. q 12 hours.
Neonates under age 7 days who weigh more than 2 kg: 50 mg/kg I.V. q 8 hours.
Neonates over age 7 days who weigh less than 2 kg: 50 mg/kg I.V. q 8 hours.
Neonates over age 7 days who weigh more than 2 kg: 50 mg/kg I.V. q 6 hours.
➤ *Acute or chronic osteomyelitis caused by susceptible organism. Adults:* 1 to 2 g I.V. q 4 hours for 4 to 8 weeks.
➤ *Meningitis caused by susceptible organisms. Adults:* 100 to 200 mg/kg daily I.V. in divided doses q 4 to 6 hours.
➤ *Native valve endocarditis caused by susceptible organisms. Adults:* 2 g I.V. q 4 hours for 4 to 6 weeks in combination with gentamicin.

How supplied
Available by prescription only
Capsules: 250 mg
Injection: 500 mg, 1 g, 2 g
I.V. infusion piggyback: 1 g, 2 g
Tablets: 500 mg

Pharmacodynamics
Antibiotic action: Nafcillin is bactericidal; it adheres to bacterial penicillin-binding proteins, thus inhibiting bacterial cell wall synthesis. Nafcillin resists the effects of penicillinases—enzymes that inactivate penicillin—and is active against many strains of penicillinase-producing bacteria; this activity is most important against penicillinase-producing staphylococci; some strains may remain resistant. Nafcillin is also active against a few gram-positive aerobic and anaerobic bacilli but has no significant effect on gram-negative bacilli.

Pharmacokinetics
Absorption: Absorbed erratically and poorly from the GI tract; Food decreases absorption.

Distribution: Distributed widely; CSF penetration is poor but enhanced by meningeal inflammation. Drug crosses the placenta and is 70% to 90% protein-bound.

Metabolism: Metabolized primarily in the liver; it undergoes enterohepatic circulation. Dosage adjustment isn't necessary for patients in renal failure.

Excretion: Excreted primarily in bile; about 25% to 30% is excreted in urine unchanged. It may also appear in breast milk. Elimination half-life in adults is ½ to 1½ hours.

Route	Onset	Peak	Duration
P.O.	Unknown	½-2 hr	Unknown
I.V.	Immediate	Immediate	Unknown
I.M.	Unknown	½-1 hr	Unknown

Contraindications and precautions

Contraindicated in patients hypersensitive to drug or other penicillins. Use cautiously in patients with GI distress or sensitivity to cephalosporins.

Interactions

Drug-drug. *Aminoglycosides:* Synergistic bactericidal effects against *S. aureus.* However, the drugs are physically and chemically incompatible and are inactivated when mixed or given together. Don't mix in same solution.
Cyclosporines: Subtherapeutic cyclosporine levels. Monitor cyclosporine levels.
Hepatotoxic drugs: May increase the risk of hepatotoxicity. Monitor patient carefully.
Drug-food. *Fruit juice or carbonated beverages:* Acidity may inactivate drug. Don't give together.

Adverse reactions

CV: vein irritation, thrombophlebitis.
GI: *nausea,* vomiting, diarrhea, pseudomembranous colitis.
Hematologic: *transient leukopenia, neutropenia, granulocytopenia, thrombocytopenia* with high doses.
Other: *hypersensitivity reactions* (chills, fever, rash, pruritus, urticaria, *anaphylaxis*).

Overdose and treatment

Signs and symptoms of overdose include neuromuscular irritability or seizures.

There are no specific recommendations. Treatment is supportive. After recent ingestion (4 hours or less), empty stomach by induced emesis or gastric lavage; follow with activated charcoal to reduce absorption. Nafcillin isn't appreciably removed by hemodialysis.

Special considerations

● I.V. administration is the preferred route.
● Give drug with water; acid in fruit juice or carbonated beverage may inactivate it.
● Give dose on empty stomach; food decreases absorption.
● Drug is incompatible with aminoglycosides.

● Infuse I.V. nafcillin for short time periods (24 to 48 hours) if possible to reduce risk of thrombophlebitis.
● If used to treat infections caused by group A beta-hemolytic streptococci, continue therapy for at least 10 days to decrease risk of rheumatic fever or glomerulonephritis.

Patient monitoring

● Renal, hepatic, and hematologic systems should be evaluated periodically during prolonged nafcillin therapy.

Breast-feeding patients

● Nafcillin appears in breast milk; use drug cautiously in breast-feeding women.

Pediatric patients

● Nafcillin that's been reconstituted with bacteriostatic water for injection with benzyl alcohol shouldn't be used in neonates because of toxicity.

Geriatric patients

● Half-life may be prolonged because of impaired hepatic and renal function.

Patient education

● Tell patient to report severe diarrhea or allergic reactions promptly.

nalbuphine hydrochloride
Nubain

Pharmacologic classification: narcotic agonist-antagonist, opioid partial agonist
Therapeutic classification: analgesic, adjunct to anesthesia
Pregnancy risk category: NR

Indications and dosages

➤ *Moderate to severe pain.* *Adults:* 10 to 20 mg S.C., I.M., or I.V. q 3 to 6 hours, p.r.n., or around the clock. Maximum dose, 160 mg daily.
➤ *Supplement to anesthesia.* *Adults:* 0.3 mg/kg to 3 mg/kg I.V. over 10 to 15 minutes. Maintenance dosage, 0.25 to 0.5 mg/kg I.V.

How supplied

Available by prescription only
Injection: 1.5 mg/ml, 10 mg/ml, 20 mg/ml

Pharmacodynamics

Analgesic action: Analgesia is believed to result from action of drug at opiate receptor sites in the CNS, relieving moderate to severe pain. The narcotic antagonist effect may result from competitive inhibition at opiate receptors. Like other opioids, nalbuphine causes respiratory depression, sedation, and miosis. In patients with coronary artery disease or MI, it appears to produce no substantial changes in heart rate, pulmonary artery or wedge pressure, left ventricular end-diastolic pressure, pulmonary vascular resistance, or cardiac index.

Pharmacokinetics
Absorption: When administered orally, drug is about one-fifth as effective as an analgesic as it is when given I.M., apparently because of first-pass metabolism in the GI tract and liver.
Distribution: Not appreciably bound to plasma proteins.
Metabolism: Metabolized in the liver.
Excretion: Excreted in urine and to some degree in bile.

Route	Onset	Peak	Duration
I.V.	2-3 min	30 min	3-6 hr
I.M.	15 min	1 hr	3-6 hr
S.C.	15 min	Unknown	3-6 hr

Contraindications and precautions
Contraindicated in patients hypersensitive to drug. Use cautiously in patients with history of drug abuse, emotional instability, head injury, increased intracranial pressure, impaired ventilation, MI accompanied by nausea and vomiting, upcoming biliary surgery, and hepatic or renal disease.

Interactions
Drug-drug. *Barbiturate anesthetics, such as thiopental:* Additive CNS and respiratory depressant effects and, possibly, apnea. Use together very cautiously.
Cimetidine: May increase narcotic nalbuphine toxicity. A narcotic antagonist may be needed if toxicity occurs.
CNS depressants (antihistamines, barbiturates, benzodiazepines, muscle relaxants, narcotic analgesics, phenothiazines, sedative-hypnotics, tricyclic antidepressants): Potentiated respiratory and CNS depression, sedation, and hypotensive effects. Reduced doses of nalbuphine are usually necessary.
Digitoxin, phenytoin, rifampin: Drug accumulation and enhanced effects may result. Monitor patient carefully for toxicity.
General anesthetics: May cause severe CV depression. Avoid use together.
Narcotic antagonist: Patients who become physically dependent on drug may experience acute withdrawal syndrome if given high doses of a narcotic antagonist. Use cautiously, and monitor patient closely.

Adverse reactions
CNS: *headache, sedation, dizziness, vertigo,* nervousness, depression, restlessness, crying, euphoria, hostility, unusual dreams, confusion, hallucinations, speech difficulty, delusions.
CV: hypertension, hypotension, tachycardia, *bradycardia.*
EENT: blurred vision, *dry mouth.*
GI: cramps, dyspepsia, bitter taste, *nausea, vomiting,* constipation, biliary tract spasms.
GU: urinary urgency.

Respiratory: *respiratory depression,* dyspnea, asthma, *pulmonary edema.*
Skin: pruritus, burning, urticaria, *clamminess.*

Overdose and treatment
The most common signs and symptoms of nalbuphine overdose are CNS depression, respiratory depression, and miosis. Other acute toxic effects include hypotension, bradycardia, hypothermia, shock, apnea, cardiopulmonary arrest, circulatory collapse, pulmonary edema, and seizures.

To treat acute overdose, first establish adequate respiratory exchange via a patent airway and ventilation as needed; administer a narcotic antagonist (naloxone) to reverse respiratory depression. Because the duration of action of nalbuphine is longer than that of naloxone, repeated naloxone dosing is necessary. Naloxone shouldn't be given in the absence of clinically significant respiratory or CV depression. Monitor vital signs closely.

Provide symptomatic and supportive treatment, such as continued respiratory support and correction of fluid or electrolyte imbalance. Monitor laboratory values, vital signs, and neurologic status closely.

Special considerations
● Some commercial preparations contain sodium metabisulfite which may cause allergic reactions in susceptible people.
● Drug is incompatible with diazepam and pentobarbital.
● Nalbuphine may obscure the signs and symptoms of an acute abdominal condition or worsen gallbladder pain.
● Drug may cause orthostatic hypotension in ambulatory patients.
● Before administration, inspect all parenteral products to rule out particulates and discoloration.
● Parenteral administration of drug provides better analgesia than oral administration. Give I.V. doses by slow I.V. injection, preferably in diluted solution. Rapid I.V. injection increases the risk of adverse effects.
● Drug causes respiratory depression, which at 10 mg is equal to the respiratory depression produced by 10 mg of morphine.
● Drug may interfere with enzymatic tests for detection of opioids.
● Store at 59° to 86° F (15° to 30° C) and protect from light.

Patient monitoring
● When drug is used during labor and delivery, neonate must be assessed for signs of respiratory depression.
● Drug also acts as a narcotic antagonist; it may precipitate abstinence syndrome in narcotic-dependent patients. Give 25% of usual dose in these patients and monitor patient for signs and symptoms of withdrawal.

Breast-feeding patients
● It isn't known if drug appears in breast milk. Use cautiously in breast-feeding women.

Pediatric patients
● Safety in children under age 18 hasn't been established.

Geriatric patients
● Lower doses are usually indicated for geriatric patients, who may be more sensitive to therapeutic and adverse effects of drug.

Patient education
● Instruct patient to avoid driving or operating machinery because drug may cause dizziness and fatigue.

nalidixic acid
NegGram

Pharmacologic classification: quinolone antibiotic
Therapeutic classification: urinary tract anti-infective
Pregnancy risk category: B

Indications and dosages
➤ *Acute and chronic urinary tract infections caused by susceptible gram-negative organisms.* Adults: 1 g P.O. q.i.d. for 7 to 14 days; 2 g P.O. daily for long-term use. Up to 6 g daily have been used for severe urinary tract infection.
Children over age 3 months: 55 mg/kg P.O. daily divided q.i.d. for 7 to 14 days; 33 mg/kg P.O. daily divided q.i.d. for long-term use.

How supplied
Available by prescription only
Suspension: 250 mg/5 ml
Tablets: 250 mg, 500 mg, 1 g

Pharmacodynamics
Antimicrobial action: Bactericidal. Inhibits microbial synthesis of DNA. Spectrum of action includes most gram-negative organisms except *Pseudomonas.* (About 2% to 14% of patients develop nalidixic acid-resistant organisms during therapy.)

Pharmacokinetics
Absorption: Well absorbed from GI tract; levels peak in 1 to 2 hours.
Distribution: Concentrates in renal tissue and seminal fluid. Doesn't penetrate prostatic tissue. Only minimal amounts appear in CSF and placenta. Drug is highly protein-bound.
Metabolism: Metabolized to more active hydroxynalidixic acid and inactive conjugates in liver.
Excretion: 13% of drug metabolites and 2% to 3% of unchanged drug excreted via kidneys. In

patients with normal renal function, plasma half-life is 1 to 2½ hours. In anuric patients, half-life is prolonged up to 21 hours.

Route	Onset	Peak	Duration
P.O.	Unknown	1-3 hr	Unknown

Contraindications and precautions
Contraindicated in patients hypersensitive to drug, in those with seizure disorders, and in infants under age 3 months. Use cautiously in prepubertal children and patients with impaired renal or hepatic function, pulmonary disease, or severe cerebral arteriosclerosis.

Interactions
Drug-drug. *Antacids:* Decreased absorption of nalidixic acid. Don't give together.
Dicumarol, warfarin: Excessive anticoagulation. Monitor patient closely.
Photosensitizing drugs: Possible additive effects. Inform patient about increased sensitivity to sun exposure, and recommend precautions.
Drug-lifestyle. *Sun exposure:* Photosensitivity reactions. Tell patient to take precautions.

Adverse reactions
CNS: drowsiness, weakness, headache, dizziness, vertigo, *seizures,* malaise, confusion, hallucinations, psychosis, *increased intracranial pressure and bulging fontanelles in infants and children.*
EENT: sensitivity to light, change in color perception, diplopia, blurred vision.
GI: *abdominal pain, nausea, vomiting,* diarrhea.
Hematologic: eosinophilia, *leukopenia, thrombocytopenia,* hemolytic anemia.
Musculoskeletal: arthralgia, joint stiffness.
Skin: pruritus, photosensitivity, urticaria, rash.
Other: *angioedema, anaphylactoid reaction.*

Overdose and treatment
Toxicity may cause psychosis, seizures, increased intracranial pressure, metabolic acidosis, lethargy, nausea, and vomiting. However, because nalidixic acid is rapidly excreted, such reactions usually resolve in 2 to 3 hours.

Special considerations
● Drug is ineffective against *Pseudomonas* infection or infection outside the urinary tract.
● Resistant bacteria may emerge after first 48 hours of therapy (especially if inadequate doses are given).
● Although CNS toxicity is rare, brief seizures, increased intracranial pressure, and toxic psychosis may occur in infants, children, and elderly patients.
● False-positive reactions may occur in urine glucose tests using cupric sulfate reagents (such as Benedict's test, Fehling's solution, and Clinitest), from reaction between glucuronic acid (liberat-

---

Reactions may be *common,* uncommon, *life-threatening,* or COMMON AND LIFE-THREATENING.

ed by urinary metabolites of nalidixic acid) and cupric sulfate. Urine 17-ketosteroid and urine 17-ketogenic steroid levels may be falsely elevated because nalidixic acid interacts with *m*-dinitrobenzene, used to measure these urine metabolites. Urinary vanillylmandelic acid levels may also be falsely elevated.

Patient monitoring
• Obtain culture and sensitivity tests before starting therapy and repeat as needed.
• Obtain CBC and renal and liver function studies periodically during long-term therapy.

Pregnant patients
• Drug can be used during second and third trimesters of pregnancy; however, safety hasn't been established for use in first trimester.

Breast-feeding patients
• Low levels of drug appear in breast milk. In one case, hemolytic anemia occurred in infant of uremic mother taking 1 g q.i.d. Lower drug excretion and elevated serum level resulted in higher level in milk. Use cautiously in breast-feeding women.

Pediatric patients
• Don't give drug to infants under 3 months old because safety hasn't been established.
• Don't give drug to prepubertal children because it can erode cartilage in weight-bearing joints.

Patient education
• Instruct patient to report visual disturbances; they usually disappear with dosage reduction.
• Warn patient about possible photosensitivity. Explain that photosensitivity reactions usually resolve 2 to 8 weeks after therapy ends, but that bullae may continue after exposure to sunlight or mild skin trauma for up to 3 months after therapy ends.
• Advise patient to take drug with food or milk to avoid GI upset.
• Warn patient to drive cautiously because drug may cause drowsiness or blurred vision.

naloxone hydrochloride
Narcan

Pharmacologic classification: narcotic (opioid) antagonist
Therapeutic classification: narcotic antagonist
Pregnancy risk category: B

Indications and dosages
➤ *Known or suspected narcotic-induced respiratory depression, including that caused by natural and synthetic narcotics, methadone, nalbuphine, pentazocine, and propoxyphene.* Adults: 0.4 to 2 mg I.V., S.C., or I.M., repeated q 2 to 3 minutes, p.r.n. If

no response occurs after 10 mg have been given, question diagnosis of narcotic-induced toxicity. Or, 0.4 mg I.V. loading dose followed by 0.4 mg/hour infusion.
Children: 0.01 mg/kg I.V.; give a subsequent dose of 0.1 mg/kg if needed. Dosage for continuous infusion is 0.024 to 0.16 mg/kg/hour. If I.V. route isn't available, dose may be given I.M. or S.C. in divided doses. Or, 0.1 mg/kg I.V. q. 2 to 3 minutes, p.r.n., in neonates and children up to age 5 and 2 mg I.V. q 2 to 3 minutes, p.r.n., in children age 6 and older.
➤ *Postoperative narcotic depression.*
Adults: 0.1 to 0.2 mg I.V. q 2 to 3 minutes, p.r.n., until desired response is obtained. Or, 0.005 mg/kg I.V. and repeat in 15 minutes, p.r.n., or administer 0.01 mg/kg I.M. for the second dose. May give continuous infusion at 0.0037 mg/kg/hour.
Children: 0.005 to 0.01 mg/kg dose I.M., I.V., or S.C., repeated q 2 to 3 minutes, p.r.n., until desired degree of reversal is obtained.
Neonates (asphyxia neonatorum): 0.01 mg/kg I.V. into umbilical vein repeated q 2 to 3 minutes, p.r.n.
Concentration for use in neonates and children is 0.02 mg/ml.
➤ *Naloxone challenge for diagnosing opiate dependence* ◊. *Adults:* 0.16 mg I.M. naloxone; if no signs of withdrawal after 20 to 30 minutes, give second dose of 0.24 mg I.V.

How supplied
Available by prescription only
Injection: 0.4 mg/ml, 1 mg/ml with preservatives, and 0.02 mg/ml, 0.4 mg/ml paraben-free

Pharmacodynamics
Narcotic (opioid) antagonism: Naloxone is essentially a pure antagonist. In patients who have received an opioid agonist or other analgesic with narcotic-like effects, naloxone antagonizes most of the opioid effects, especially respiratory depression, sedation, and hypotension. Because the duration of action of naloxone in most cases is shorter than that of the opioid, opiate effects may return as those of naloxone dissipate. Naloxone doesn't produce tolerance or physical or psychological dependence. The precise mechanism of action is unknown, but is thought to involve competitive antagonism of more than one opiate receptor in the CNS.

Pharmacokinetics
Absorption: Rapidly inactivated after oral administration; therefore, it's given parenterally. The duration of action is longer after I.M. use and higher doses, when compared with I.V. use and lower doses.
Distribution: Rapidly distributed into body tissues and fluids.
Metabolism: Rapidly metabolized in the liver, primarily by conjugation.

Excretion: Excreted in urine. Plasma half-life has been reported to be from 60 to 90 minutes in adults and 3 hours in neonates.

Route	Onset	Peak	Duration
I.V.	1-2 min	5-15 min	Variable
I.M., S.C.	2-5 min	5-15 min	Variable

Contraindications and precautions
Contraindicated in patients hypersensitive to drug. Use cautiously in patients with cardiac irritability and opiate addiction. When given to a narcotic addict, naloxone may produce an acute abstinence syndrome. Use cautiously, and monitor patient closely.

Interactions
Drug-drug. *Cardiotoxic drugs:* May cause serious CV effects. Use together cautiously.

Adverse reactions
CNS: *tremors, seizures.*
CV: tachycardia, hypertension, hypotension, *ventricular fibrillation, cardiac arrest.*
GI: nausea, vomiting.
Respiratory: *pulmonary edema.*
Skin: diaphoresis.
Other: withdrawal symptoms (in narcotic-dependent patients with higher-than-recommended doses).

Overdose and treatment
No serious adverse reactions to naloxone overdose are known except those of acute abstinence syndrome in narcotic-dependent persons.

Special considerations
● Before administration, inspect all parenteral products to rule out particulates and discoloration.
● Take a careful drug history to rule out possible narcotic addiction, to avoid inducing withdrawal symptoms (apply cautions also to the neonate of an addicted mother).
● Because naloxone has a shorter duration of action than most narcotics, vigilance and repeated doses are usually necessary to manage acute narcotic overdose in a nonaddicted patient.
● Naloxone isn't effective in treating respiratory depression caused by nonopioid drugs.
● Naloxone can be diluted in D₅W or normal saline solution. Use within 24 hours after mixing.
● Naloxone is the safest drug to use when the cause of respiratory depression is uncertain.
● Naloxone may be given by continuous I.V. infusion, which is necessary in many cases to control the adverse effects of epidurally administered morphine. Usual dose is 2 mg in 500 ml of D₅W or normal saline solution.
● Don't mix drug with preparations containing bisulfite, metabisulfite, long-chain anions, high molecular weight anions, or any solution having an alkaline pH.

● Injections are stable at pH of 2.5 to 5.

Patient monitoring
● Avoid depending on drug too much; carefully monitor airway, breathing, and circulation. Maintain adequate respiratory and CV status at all times.
● Because respiratory overshoot may occur, monitor patient for a respiratory rate that's higher than it was before the respiratory depression. Respiratory rate increases in 1 to 2 minutes, and the effect lasts 1 to 4 hours.

Breast-feeding patients
● It isn't known if drug appears in breast milk.

Geriatric patients
● Lower doses are usually indicated for geriatric patients because they may be more sensitive to therapeutic and adverse effects of drug.

Patient education
● Inform family about need for and administration of drug.
● Reassure family that patient will be monitored closely until narcotic effects resolve.

---

naltrexone hydrochloride
Depade, ReVia

Pharmacologic classification: narcotic (opioid) antagonist
Therapeutic classification: narcotic detoxification adjunct
Pregnancy risk category: C

Indications and dosages
➤ *Adjunct for maintenance of opioid-free state in detoxified patients. Adults:* Don't attempt treatment until naloxone challenge is negative and patient has been opioid-free for 7 to 10 days, verified by analyzing urine for opioids. Initially, 25 mg P.O. If no withdrawal signs occur within 1 hour, give another 25 mg. Or, 10- to 12.5-mg initial dose followed by 10- to 12.5-mg incremental increases daily to 50 mg. Or, 5 mg initially with incremental 10-mg increases hourly to 50 mg. Once patient has been started on 50 mg q 24 hours, flexible maintenance schedule may be used. From 50 to 150 mg may be given daily, depending on the schedule prescribed, but the average daily dose is 50 mg.
➤ *Alcoholism (short-term therapy). Adults:* 50 mg P.O. daily.

How supplied
Available by prescription only
Tablets: 50 mg

Pharmacodynamics
Opioid antagonism: Naltrexone is essentially a pure opiate (narcotic) antagonist. Like naloxone, it has little or no agonist activity. Its precise

mechanism of action is unknown, but it may competitively antagonize more than one opiate receptor in the CNS. When given to patients who haven't recently received opiates, it has little or no pharmacologic effect. At oral doses of 30 to 50 mg daily, it produces minimal analgesia, only slight drowsiness, and no respiratory depression. However, pharmacologic effects, including psychotomimetic effects, increased systolic or diastolic blood pressure, respiratory depression, and decreased oral temperature, which suggest opiate agonist activity, have reportedly occurred in a few patients. In patients who have received single or repeated large doses of opiates, naltrexone attenuates or produces a complete but reversible block of the pharmacologic effects of the narcotic. Naltrexone doesn't produce physical or psychological dependence, and tolerance to its antagonist activity reportedly doesn't develop.

Pharmacokinetics

Absorption: Well absorbed after oral administration. It undergoes extensive first-pass hepatic metabolism. (Only 5% to 40% of an oral dose reaches the systemic circulation unchanged.)
Distribution: About 21% to 28% protein-bound. Extent and duration of antagonist activity appear directly related to plasma and tissue drug levels. It's widely distributed throughout the body, but varies considerably among people.
Metabolism: Oral naltrexone undergoes extensive first-pass hepatic metabolism. Its major metabolite is believed to be a pure antagonist and may contribute to its efficacy. Drug and hepatic metabolites may undergo enterohepatic recirculation.
Excretion: Excreted mainly by the kidneys. Elimination half-life is about 4 hours; that of its major active metabolite is about 13 hours.

Route	Onset	Peak	Duration
P.O.	15-30 min	1 hr	24 hr

Contraindications and precautions

Contraindicated in patients receiving opioid analgesics. Also contraindicated in opioid-dependent patients, patients in acute opioid withdrawal, patients with positive urine screen for opioids, and patients with acute hepatitis or liver failure. Also contraindicated in patients hypersensitive to drug.

Use cautiously in patients with mild hepatic disease or history of hepatic impairment.

Interactions

Drug-drug. *Drugs that alter hepatic metabolism:* May increase or decrease serum naltrexone levels. Monitor patient for this effect.
Opioid-containing drugs, such as cough and cold preparations, antidiarrheals, and opioid analgesics: Attenuated opioid activity. Avoid use together.
Thioridazine: Lethargy and somnolence may occur. Use together cautiously.

Adverse reactions

CNS: *insomnia, anxiety, nervousness, headache,* depression, dizziness, fatigue, somnolence, *suicidal ideation.*
GI: *nausea, vomiting,* anorexia, *abdominal pain,* constipation, increased thirst.
GU: delayed ejaculation, decreased potency.
Hematologic: lymphocytosis.
Hepatic: *hepatotoxicity.*
Musculoskeletal: *muscle and joint pain.*
Skin: rash.
Other: chills.

Overdose and treatment

Overdose hasn't been documented. Test subjects have received 800 mg daily (16 tablets) for up to 1 week and shown no evidence of toxicity.

In case of overdose, provide symptomatic and supportive treatment in a closely supervised environment. Contact a local or regional poison control center for further information.

Special considerations

● For naloxone challenge test, which should be negative before patient receives naltrexone, give 0.2 mg I.V. If no signs of withdrawal occur after 30 seconds, give another 0.6 mg I.V. Or, give 0.8 mg S.C. and observe patient for 20 minutes for signs of withdrawal. If acute abstinence signs and symptoms are present, don't administer naltrexone. If inconclusive results, may repeat challenge with 1.6 mg I.V.
● Naltrexone has been used investigationally for the treatment of methadone dependence.
● Before administration, take a careful drug history to rule out possible narcotic use. Don't attempt treatment until the patient has been opiate-free for 7 to 10 days. Verify self-reporting of abstinence from narcotics by urinalysis. No withdrawal signs or symptoms should be reported by patient or be evident.
● Because naltrexone can precipitate potentially severe opiate withdrawal, it shouldn't be used in patients receiving opiates or in nondetoxified patients physically dependent on opiates.
● Drug can cause hepatocellular injury if given at higher-than-recommended doses. Naltrexone can cause or exacerbate signs and symptoms of abstinence in anyone not completely opioid-free.

Patient monitoring

● Obtain liver function tests before giving naltrexone and every month for 6 months to establish a baseline and evaluate possible drug-induced hepatotoxicity.
● In an emergency that demands analgesia obtainable only with opiates, a patient who has been receiving naltrexone may need a higher narcotic dose than usual, which may cause deeper and more prolonged respiratory depression.

Breast-feeding patients
● It isn't known if drug appears in breast milk. Use drug cautiously in breast-feeding women, especially because of its known hepatotoxicity.

Pediatric patients
● Safety of naltrexone in children under age 18 hasn't been established.

Geriatric patients
● Use in elderly patients isn't documented, but dosage probably should be reduced.

Patient education
● Inform patient that opioid drugs, including cough and cold preparations, antidiarrheal products, and narcotic analgesics may not be effective during naltrexone use; recommend a non-narcotic alternative if available.
● Warn patient not to take narcotics while taking naltrexone because serious injury, coma, or death may result.
● Explain that drug causes no tolerance or dependence.
● Tell patient to report withdrawal signs and symptoms (tremors, vomiting, bone or muscle pains, sweating, abdominal cramps).
● Tell patient to wear or carry medical identification that alerts medical personnel to naltrexone use. Also, tell him to inform new health care providers that he's receiving drug.

nandrolone decanoate
Androlone-D, Deca-Durabolin, Hybolin Decanoate, Neo-Durabolic

Pharmacologic classification: anabolic steroid
Therapeutic classification: erythropoietic, anabolic
Controlled substance schedule: III
Pregnancy risk category: X

Indications and dosages
➤ **Anemia caused by renal insufficiency.**
Adults: 100 to 200 mg I.M. weekly in men; 50 to 100 mg/week I.M. in women.
Children ages 2 to 13: 25 to 50 mg I.M. q 3 to 4 weeks.

How supplied
Available by prescription only
Injection: 50 mg/ml, 100 mg/ml, 200 mg/ml (in oil)

Pharmacodynamics
Androgenic action: Nandrolone exerts inhibitory effects on hormone-responsive breast tumors and metastases.
Erythropoietic action: Nandrolone stimulates kidney production of erythropoietin, leading to increases in red blood cell mass and volume.

Anabolic action: Nandrolone may reverse corticosteroid-induced catabolism and promote tissue development in severely debilitated patients.

Pharmacokinetics
Absorption: Well absorbed.
Distribution: Slowly released from I.M. depot following injection and is hydrolyzed to free nandrolone by plasma esterase.
Metabolism: Metabolized in the liver.
Excretion: Both the unchanged drug and its metabolites are excreted in the urine. The elimination half-life of nandrolone is 6 to 8 days.

Route	Onset	Peak	Duration
I.M.	Unknown	3-6 days	Unknown

Contraindications and precautions
Contraindicated in pregnant women, breast-feeding women, patients hypersensitive to anabolic steroids, men with breast cancer or prostate cancer, patients with nephrosis, patients experiencing the nephrotic phase of nephritis, and women with breast cancer and hypercalcemia.

Use cautiously in patients with renal, cardiac, or hepatic disease; diabetes; epilepsy; migraine; or other conditions that may be aggravated by fluid retention.

Interactions
Drug-drug. *Adrenocorticosteroids or adrenocorticotropic hormone:* Increased risk of fluid and electrolyte retention. Monitor patient for this effect.
Insulin, oral antidiabetics: Decreased blood glucose levels; may require adjustment of antidiabetic or insulin.
Warfarin-type anticoagulants: Increased PT and INR. Monitor PT and INR.

Adverse reactions
CNS: excitation, insomnia, habituation, depression.
CV: edema.
GI: nausea, vomiting, diarrhea.
GU: bladder irritability, *hypoestrogenic effects in women (flushing; diaphoresis; vaginitis, including itching, dryness, and burning; vaginal bleeding; nervousness; emotional lability; menstrual irregularities).*
Hematologic: elevated serum lipid levels, suppression of clotting factors.
Hepatic: reversible jaundice, *peliosis hepatitis,* elevated liver enzyme levels, *liver cell tumors.*
Metabolic: increased serum sodium, potassium, calcium and phosphate; abnormal results of fasting plasma glucose, glucose tolerance, and metyrapone tests; decreased thyroid function test results and 17-ketosteroid levels.
Skin: pain and induration at injection site.

Reactions may be *common*, uncommon, *life-threatening*, or COMMON AND LIFE-THREATENING.

Other: *excessive hormonal effects in men (prepubertal-premature epiphyseal closure,* acne, priapism, *growth of body and facial hair,* phallic enlargement; postpubertal-testicular atrophy, oligospermia, decreased ejaculatory volume, impotence, gynecomastia, epididymitis), androgenic effects in women (acne, edema, *weight gain, hirsutism,* hoarseness, clitoral enlargement, *decreased breast size,* changes in libido, male-pattern baldness, *oily skin or hair*).

Overdose and treatment
No information available.

Special considerations
● Administer nandrolone injections I.M. deep into the gluteal muscle.
● An adequate iron intake is necessary for maximum response when patient is receiving nandrolone decanoate injections.
● Therapy should be intermittent, if possible.
● Duration of therapy depends on patient response and the occurrence of adverse reactions.

Patient monitoring
● Monitor liver function test results, urine and serum calcium levels (in women with breast cancer), serum lipid and cholesterol levels, and CBC periodically.
● Prepubertal patients should have X-ray studies every 6 months to evaluate bone age.

Breast-feeding patients
● It isn't known if anabolic steroids appear in breast milk. Because of the risk of serious adverse reactions in breast-fed infants, a decision should be made to discontinue breast-feeding or drug.

Pediatric patients
● The adverse effects of giving androgens to young children aren't fully understood, but the risk of serious disturbances (premature epiphyseal closure, masculinization of females, or precocious development in males) exists. Weigh the benefits and risks before starting therapy in young children.

Geriatric patients
● Assess elderly men for the development of prostatic hypertrophy and prostatic carcinoma.

Patient education
● Instruct diabetic patient to monitor glucose levels closely because glucose tolerance may be altered.
● Tell women to report menstrual irregularities, acne, deepening of voice, male-pattern baldness, or hirsutism.
● Tell patient to notify prescriber about persistent GI upset, nausea, vomiting, changes in skin color, or ankle swelling.

naphazoline hydrochloride
AK-Con, Albalon Liquifilm, Allerest, Clear Eyes, Clear Eyes ACR, Comfort Eye Drops, Degest 2, Nafazair, Naphcon, Naphcon Forte, Privine, VasoClear, Vasocon

Pharmacologic classification: sympathomimetic
Therapeutic classification: decongestant, vasoconstrictor
Pregnancy risk category: C

Indications and dosages
➤ *Ocular congestion, irritation, itching.*
Adults: Instill 1 to 3 drops (0.1% solution) q 3 to 4 hours or 1 to 2 drops (0.012% to 0.03% solution) in eye daily to q.i.d for 3 to 4 days.
➤ *Nasal congestion. Adults and children over age 12:* 1 or 2 drops or sprays (0.05% solution), p.r.n. May repeat doses q 6 hours. Treatment not to exceed 3 to 5 days.
Children ages 6 to 12: 1 to 2 drops or sprays (0.025% solution), p.r.n. May repeat doses q 6 hours.

How supplied
Available by prescription only
Ophthalmic solution: 0.1%
Available without a prescription
Nasal drops or sprays: 0.05% (solution)
Ophthalmic solution: 0.012%, 0.02%, 0.025% (generic), 0.03%

Pharmacodynamics
Decongestant action: Naphazoline produces vasoconstriction by local and alpha-adrenergic action on blood vessels of the conjunctiva or nasal mucosa; therefore, it reduces blood flow and nasal congestion.

Pharmacokinetics
Absorption: Well absorbed intranasally.
Distribution: Unknown.
Metabolism: Unknown.
Excretion: Unknown.

Route	Onset	Peak	Duration
Oph-thalmic	10 min	Unknown	2-6 hr
Nasal	10 min	Unknown	2-6 hr

Contraindications and precautions
Contraindicated in patients hypersensitive to ingredients of drug and in those with acute angle-closure glaucoma. Use of 0.1% solution is contraindicated in children. Use cautiously in patients with hyperthyroidism, cardiac disease, hypertension, or diabetes mellitus.

Interactions
Drug-drug. *MAO inhibitors:* May result in an increased adrenergic response and hypertensive crisis. Avoid use together.

Adverse reactions
CNS: headache, dizziness, nervousness, weakness (with ophthalmic form); marked sedation (with nasal form).
CV: hypertension, *cardiac irregularities.*
EENT: transient eye stinging, pupillary dilation, eye irritation, photophobia, blurred vision, increased intraocular pressure, keratitis, lacrimation (with ophthalmic form); rebound nasal congestion (with excessive or long-term use), sneezing, stinging, dryness of mucosa (with nasal form).
GI: nausea (with ophthalmic form).
Skin: diaphoresis (with ophthalmic form)
Other: systemic effects in children after excessive or long-term use.

Overdose and treatment
Signs and symptoms of overdose include CNS depression, sweating, decreased body temperature, bradycardia, shocklike hypotension, decreased respiration, CV collapse, and coma.

Activated charcoal or gastric lavage may be used initially to treat accidental ingestion; administer early before sedation occurs. Monitor vital signs and ECG, as ordered. Treat seizures with I.V. diazepam.

Special considerations
• Naphazoline is the most widely used ocular decongestant.
• Don't shake container.
• Use drug cautiously in diabetic patients prone to diabetic ketoacidosis.

Patient monitoring
• Monitor patient for blurred vision, pain, or lid edema.

Pediatric patients
• Use in infants and children may result in CNS depression, leading to coma and marked reduction in body temperature. Although drug is available without a prescription, parents shouldn't use nasal solution containing 0.025% naphazoline hydrochloride in children under age 6, and 0.05% naphazoline hydrochloride in children under age 12.
• Use drug cautiously in children with severe cardiac disease or poorly controlled hypertension.

Patient education
• Teach patient how to instill ophthalmic or nasal drug; tell him not to share it with others.
• Advise patient to report blurred vision, eye pain, or lid swelling when using ophthalmic drug.
• Inform patient using ophthalmic solution that photophobia may follow pupil dilation; tell patient to report this effect promptly.

• Warn patient not to exceed recommended dosage. Rebound nasal congestion and conjunctivitis may occur with frequent or prolonged use.
• Tell patient to report nasal congestion that persists after 5 days of using nasal solution.

naproxen
Naprosyn, EC-Naprosyn

naproxen sodium
Aleve, Anaprox, Anaprox DS, Naprelan

Pharmacologic classification: NSAID
Therapeutic classification: nonnarcotic analgesic, antipyretic, anti-inflammatory
Pregnancy risk category: B

Indications and dosages
➤ *Mild to moderately severe musculoskeletal or soft tissue irritation.* **naproxen.** *Adults:* 250 to 500 mg P.O. b.i.d. Or, 250 mg in the morning and 500 mg in the evening. Or, 375 to 500 mg P.O. b.i.d. delayed release.
naproxen sodium
Adults: 275 to 550 mg P.O. b.i.d. Or, 275 mg in the morning and 550 mg in the evening. Or, 750 to 1,000 mg P.O. once daily (controlled-release).
➤ *Mild to moderate pain, primary dysmenorrhea.* **naproxen.** *Adults:* 500 mg P.O. to start, followed by 250 mg P.O. q 6 to 8 hours, p.r.n. Maximum, 1.25 g naproxen daily.
naproxen sodium
Adults: 550 mg P.O. to start, followed by 275 mg P.O. q 6 to 8 hours, p.r.n. Maximum, 1.375 g naproxen sodium daily. For self-medication, 220 mg q 8 to 12 hours. Maximum, 660 mg for adults under age 65 or 440 mg daily for adults age 65 and older. Tell patient not to self-medicate for more than 10 days.
➤ *Acute gout.* **naproxen.** *Adults:* 750 mg P.O. initially; then 250 mg q 8 hours until episode subsides.
naproxen sodium
Adults: 825 mg P.O. initially; then 275 mg q 8 hours until attack has subsided. Or, 1,000 mg P.O. to 1,500 mg (controlled-release tablets) P.O. daily on the first day; then 1,000 mg P.O. daily until attack subsides.
➤ *Juvenile rheumatoid arthritis.* **naproxen.** *Children:* 10 mg/kg daily P.O. in two divided doses.

How supplied
Available by prescription only
naproxen
Oral suspension: 125 mg/5 ml
Tablets: 250 mg, 375 mg, 500 mg
Tablets (delayed-release): 375 mg, 500 mg
naproxen sodium
Tablets: 220 mg

Reactions may be *common*, uncommon, *life-threatening*, or COMMON AND LIFE-THREATENING.

Tablets (controlled-release): 375 mg, 500 mg
Tablets (film-coated): 275 mg, 550 mg
Available without a prescription
naproxen sodium
Capsules, gelcaps, tablets: 220 mg

Pharmacodynamics

Analgesic, antipyretic, and anti-inflammatory actions: Mechanisms of action are unknown; naproxen is thought to inhibit prostaglandin synthesis.

Pharmacokinetics

Absorption: Absorbed rapidly and completely from the GI tract.
Distribution: Highly protein-bound. It crosses the placenta and appears in milk.
Metabolism: Metabolized in the liver.
Excretion: Excreted in urine. Half life is 10 to 20 hours.

Route	Onset	Peak	Duration
P.O.	1 hr	2-4 hr	7 hr

Contraindications and precautions

Contraindicated in patients hypersensitive to drug and in those with asthma, rhinitis, or nasal polyps. Use cautiously in elderly patients and those with a history of peptic ulcer disease or renal, CV, GI, or hepatic disease.

Interactions

Drug-drug. *Acetaminophen, anti-inflammatory drugs, gold compounds:* Increased nephrotoxicity. Monitor renal function test results.
Anticoagulants and thrombolytics, such as coumadin derivatives, heparin, streptokinase, and urokinase: May potentiate anticoagulant effects. Monitor PT and INR.
Antihypertensives, diuretics: Decreased effects of these drugs. Using together may increase risk of nephrotoxicity. Avoid use together.
Anti-inflammatory drugs, corticosteroids, corticotropin, salicylates: May cause increased GI adverse reactions, including ulceration and hemorrhage. Use together very cautiously.
Aspirin, cefamandole, cefoperazone, dextran, dipyridamole, mezlocillin, parenteral carbenicillin, piperacillin, plicamycin, salicylates, sulfinpyrazone, ticarcillin, valproic acid, and other anti-inflammatory drugs: Increased risk of bleeding problems. Use together very cautiously.
Aspirin: May decrease the bioavailability of naproxen. Monitor patient for lack of effectiveness.
Coumadin derivatives, nifedipine, phenytoin, verapamil: Increased risk of toxicity. Monitor patient closely.
Insulin, oral antidiabetics: May potentiate hypoglycemic effects. Monitor serum glucose levels.
Lithium, methotrexate: Increased nephrotoxicity may occur. Monitor renal function test results.

Adverse reactions

CNS: *headache, drowsiness, dizziness,* vertigo.
CV: *edema,* palpitations.
EENT: visual disturbances, *tinnitus,* auditory disturbances.
GI: *epigastric distress, occult blood loss, nausea, peptic ulceration,* constipation, dyspepsia, heartburn, diarrhea, stomatitis, thirst.
GU: nephrotoxicity.
Hematologic: *thrombocytopenia,* eosinophilia, *agranulocytosis, neutropenia,* hemolysis, ecchymoses.
Hepatic: elevated liver enzyme levels.
Respiratory: dyspnea.
Skin: *pruritus, rash,* urticaria, ecchymosis, diaphoresis, purpura.

Overdose and treatment

Signs and symptoms of overdose include drowsiness, heartburn, indigestion, nausea, and vomiting.

To treat naproxen overdose, empty patient's stomach immediately by inducing emesis with ipecac syrup or by performing gastric lavage. Administer activated charcoal via nasogastric tube. Provide symptomatic and supportive measures, including respiratory support and correction of fluid and electrolyte imbalances. Monitor laboratory parameters and vital signs closely. Hemodialysis is ineffective in removing naproxen.

Special considerations

● Keep in mind that 220 mg, 275 mg, and 550 mg of naproxen sodium equals 200 mg, 250 mg, and 500 mg of naproxen, respectively.
● Naproxen and its metabolites may interfere with urinary 5-hydroxyindoleacetic acid and 17-hydroxy-corticosteroid determinations.
● Use lowest possible effective dose; 250 mg of naproxen is equivalent to 275 mg of naproxen sodium.
● Relief usually begins within 2 weeks after beginning therapy with naproxen.
● Institute safety measures to prevent injury resulting from possible CNS effects.

Patient monitoring

● Monitor fluid balance. Watch for signs and symptoms of fluid retention, especially significant weight gain.
● Monitor liver function test results, renal function test results, CBC, and bleeding times during long-term therapy.

Breast-feeding patients

● Because they appear in breast milk, avoid using naproxen and naproxen sodium during breast-feeding.

Pediatric patients

● Safety of naproxen in children under age 2 hasn't been established.
● Safety of naproxen sodium in children hasn't been established.
● No age-related problems have been reported.

Geriatric patients
● Patients over age 60 are more sensitive to adverse effects (especially GI toxicity).
● The effect of naproxen on renal prostaglandins may cause fluid retention and edema. This may be significant in elderly patients, especially those with heart failure.

Patient education
● Caution patient to avoid taking naproxen with OTC drugs.
● Teach patient signs and symptoms of possible adverse reactions and tell him to report them promptly.
● Instruct patient to check his weight every 2 to 3 days and to report any gain of 3 lb (1.4 kg) or more within 1 week.
● Instruct patient in safety measures; advise him to avoid activities that require alertness until CNS effects are known.
● Warn patient against combining naproxen with naproxen sodium because both drugs circulate in the blood as naproxen anion.
● Teach patient not to break or crush controlled- or delayed-release tablets.

naratriptan hydrochloride
Amerge

Pharmacologic classification: selective 5-hydroxytryptamine$_1$ (5-HT$_1$) receptor subtype agonist
Therapeutic classification: antimigraine
Pregnancy risk category: C

Indications and dosages
➤ *Treatment of acute migraine headache attacks with or without aura. Adults:* 1 or 2.5 mg P.O. as a single dose. Dose should be individualized, depending on the possible benefit of the 2.5-mg dose and the greater risk of adverse events. If headache returns or if only partial response occurs, may repeat dose after 4 hours, for maximum dose of 5 mg within 24 hours.
✦ *Dosage adjustment.* In patients with mild to moderate renal or hepatic impairment, consider a lower initial dose; don't exceed maximum dose of 2.5 mg over a 24-hour period. Don't use in patients with severe renal or hepatic impairment.

How supplied
Available by prescription only
Tablets: 1 mg, 2.5 mg

Pharmacodynamics
Antimigraine action: Naratriptan binds with high affinity to 5-HT$_{1D}$ and 5-HT$_{1B}$ receptors. One theory suggests that activation of 5-HT$_{1D/1B}$ receptors located on intracranial blood vessels leads to vasoconstriction, which is linked to the migraine relief. Another hypothesis suggests that activation of 5-HT$_{1D/1B}$ receptors on sensory nerve endings in the trigeminal system results in the inhibition of proinflammatory neuropeptide release.

Pharmacokinetics
Absorption: Well absorbed with about 70% oral bioavailability.
Distribution: Steady state volume of distribution is 170 L/kg. Plasma protein–binding is 28% to 31%.
Metabolism: In vitro, naratriptan is metabolized by many P-450 cytochrome isoenzymes to inactive metabolites.
Excretion: Predominantly eliminated in urine, with 50% of dose recovered unchanged and 30% as metabolites. Mean elimination half-life is 6 hours.

Route	Onset	Peak	Duration
P.O.	Unknown	2-3 hr	Unknown

Contraindications and precautions
Contraindicated in patients hypersensitive to drug or its components and in those with history or evidence of ischemic cardiac disease, cerebrovascular disease (such as CVA or transient ischemic attack), or peripheral vascular disease (such as ischemic bowel disease). Also contraindicated in patients with significant underlying CV diseases, including angina pectoris, MI, and silent myocardial ischemia. Drug shouldn't be given to patients with uncontrolled hypertension because of potential increase in blood pressure. Contraindicated in patients with severe renal impairment (creatinine clearance less than 15 ml/minute) or hepatic impairment (Child-Pugh grade C) and in those with hemiplegic or basilar migraine.

Drug or other 5-HT$_1$ agonists are also contraindicated in patients with risk factors for coronary artery disease, such as hypertension, hypercholesterolemia, obesity, diabetes, strong family history of coronary artery disease, women with surgical or physiologic menopause, men over age 40, or smokers.

Interactions
Drug-drug. *Ergot-containing or ergot-type drugs or other 5-HT$_1$ agonists:* Prolonged vasospastic reactions. Use of these drugs within 24 hours of naratriptan is contraindicated.
Oral contraceptives: Increased naratriptan levels. Monitor patient closely.
Selective serotonin reuptake inhibitors, such as fluoxetine, fluvoxamine, paroxetine, and sertraline: Weakness, hyperreflexia, and incoordination when given with 5-HT$_1$ agonists. Use together cautiously.
Drug-lifestyle. *Smoking:* Increased clearance of naratriptan by 30%. Advise patient to avoid smoking.

Adverse reactions
CNS: paresthesia, dizziness, drowsiness, malaise, fatigue, vertigo, syncope.

Reactions may be *common*, uncommon, *life-threatening*, or COMMON AND LIFE-THREATENING.

CV: palpitations, increased blood pressure, tachyarrhythmias, *ECG changes (PR or QT prolongation, ST/T wave abnormalities) PVCs, atrial flutter, atrial fibrillation.*
EENT: ear, nose, and throat infections; photophobia.
GI: nausea, hyposalivation, vomiting.
Other: warm or cold temperature sensations; pressure, tightness, or heaviness sensations.

Overdose and treatment
Blood pressure may increase significantly 30 minutes to 6 hours after ingestion of an overdose; it may return to normal within 8 hours without pharmacologic intervention, or patient may need antihypertensive treatment.

No specific antidote exists. Perform ECG monitoring for evidence of ischemia. Monitor patient for at least 24 hours after an overdose or while symptoms persist. The effect of hemodialysis or peritoneal dialysis on drug is unknown.

Special considerations
● Use drug only when a clear diagnosis of migraine has been established. It's not intended for preventing migraines or for managing hemiplegic or basilar migraine.
● Safety and effectiveness haven't been established for cluster headaches.

Patient monitoring
● If patient has risk factors for coronary artery disease but a satisfactory CV evaluation, first dose should be given in a medically equipped facility. Consider ECG monitoring.
● Periodically reevaluate cardiac status in patients who have or develop risk factors for coronary artery disease.

Pregnant patients
● To monitor fetal outcomes of patients exposed to naratriptan during pregnancy, call 1-800-722-9292.

Breast-feeding patients
● Use cautiously in breast-feeding women.

Pediatric patients
● Safety and efficacy in children under age 18 haven't been established.

Geriatric patients
● Don't give drug to elderly patients.

Patient education
● Tell patient that drug is intended to relieve, not prevent, migraine headaches.
● Instruct patient not to use drug if pregnancy is suspected or confirmed.
● Tell patient to notify prescriber about risk factors for coronary artery disease.
● Instruct patient to take a dose soon after headache starts. If there's no response to the first

tablet, tell patient to seek medical approval before taking second tablet.
● Tell patient that if more relief is needed after the first tablet, such as when a partial response occurs or if the headache returns, he may take a second tablet but not sooner than 4 hours after the first tablet. Caution him not to exceed two tablets in 24 hours.

nateglinide
Starlix

Pharmacologic classification: amino acid derivative
Therapeutic classification: antidiabetic
Pregnancy risk category: C

Indications and dosages
➤*Alone or with metformin, to lower blood glucose levels in patients with type 2 diabetes whose hyperglycemia isn't adequately controlled by diet and exercise and who haven't received long-term treatment with other antidiabetics.* *Adults:* 120 mg P.O. t.i.d., taken 1 to 30 minutes before meals. If patient's glycosylated hemoglobin (HbA1c) is near goal when treatment starts, he may receive 60 mg P.O. t.i.d.

How supplied
Available by prescription only
Tablets: 60 mg, 120 mg

Pharmacodynamics
Blood glucose–lowering action: Nateglinide lowers blood glucose levels by stimulating insulin secretion from the pancreas. This action is dependent on the presence of functioning beta cells in the pancreas. The extent of insulin release is relative to blood glucose levels.

Pharmacokinetics
Absorption: Drug is rapidly absorbed when taken immediately before a meal. Levels peak within 1 hour. The rate of absorption is slower when nateglinide is taken with or after a meal, but the extent of absorption is unaffected.
Distribution: Drug is extensively bound (98%) to plasma proteins, primarily albumin.
Metabolism: Drug is metabolized in the liver by hydroxylation followed by glucuronide conjugation. It's mainly metabolized by the cytochrome P-450 isoenzymes CYP2C9 (70%) and CYP3A4 (30%).
Excretion: Nateglinide and its metabolites are rapidly and completely eliminated in urine and feces after oral use. Average elimination half-life in healthy people and those with type 2 diabetes is about 1.5 hours.

Route	Onset	Peak	Duration
P.O.	20 min	1 hr	4 hr

Contraindications and precautions

Contraindicated in patients hypersensitive to the drug and in patients with type 1 diabetes or diabetic ketoacidosis.

Use cautiously in elderly patients, malnourished patients, and patients with moderate to severe liver dysfunction or adrenal or pituitary insufficiency.

Interactions

Drug-drug: *MAO inhibitors, nonselective beta blockers, NSAIDs, salicylates:* May potentiate the hypoglycemic action of nateglinide. Monitor patient for hypoglycemia, and monitor blood glucose levels closely.
Corticosteroids, sympathomimetics, thiazides, thyroid products: May reduce the hypoglycemic action of nateglinide. Monitor patient for hyperglycemia, and monitor blood glucose levels closely.

Adverse reactions

CNS: dizziness.
GI: diarrhea.
Metabolic: hypoglycemia.
Musculoskeletal: back pain, arthropathy.
Respiratory: *upper respiratory tract infection,* bronchitis, coughing.
Other: flu symptoms, accidental trauma.

Overdose and treatment

No adverse events were noted at a dosage of 720 mg daily for 7 days. However, an overdose may result in hypoglycemia.

Hypoglycemic symptoms without loss of consciousness should be treated with oral glucose and adjustments in dosage, meal patterns, or both. Severe hypoglycemic reactions with coma, seizures, or other neurologic symptoms should be treated with I.V. glucose. Dialysis isn't effective in removing nateglinide.

Special considerations

● Don't use with or instead of glyburide or other oral antidiabetics. Drug may be used with metformin.
● Give drug 1 to 30 minutes before a meal. If a patient misses a meal, skip the scheduled dose.
● Risk of hypoglycemia rises with strenuous exercise, alcohol ingestion, insufficient caloric intake, and use with other oral antidiabetics.
● Symptoms of hypoglycemia may be masked in patients with autonomic neuropathy or those who use beta blockers.
● Insulin may be needed for glycemic control in patients with fever, infection, trauma, or impending surgery.
● Effectiveness may decline over time.

Patient monitoring

● Monitor blood glucose levels regularly to evaluate drug effectiveness.
● Observe patient for evidence of hypoglycemia, including sweating, rapid pulse, trembling, confusion, headache, irritability, and nausea. To minimize the risk of hypoglycemia, the dose of nateglinide should be followed immediately by a meal. If hypoglycemia occurs and the patient remains conscious, give an oral form of glucose. If unconscious, give I.V. glucose.
● Monitor blood glucose levels closely when other drugs are started or stopped to detect possible drug interactions.
● Periodically monitor HbA1c levels.

Breast-feeding patients

● It isn't known if nateglinide appears in breast milk. Use by nursing mothers should be avoided.

Pediatric patients

● The safety and efficacy of nateglinide in children hasn't been determined.

Geriatric patients

● No special dosage adjustments are usually necessary. However, some people may have greater sensitivity to the glucose-lowering effects than others.

Patient education

● Tell patient to take nateglinide1 to 30 minutes before a meal.
● To reduce the risk of hypoglycemia, advise patient to skip the scheduled dose if he skips a meal.
● Educate patient about the risk of hypoglycemia and its signs and symptoms (sweating, rapid pulse, trembling, confusion, headache, irritability, and nausea). Advise the patient to treat these symptoms by eating or drinking something containing sugar.
● Teach patient how to monitor and log blood sugar levels to evaluate diabetes control.
● Instruct patient to adhere to the prescribed diet and exercise regimen.
● Explain the possible long-term complications of diabetes and the importance of regular preventive therapy.
● Encourage patient to wear or carry medical identification that shows he has diabetes.

nedocromil sodium
Tilade

Pharmacologic classification: pyranoquinoline
Therapeutic classification: anti-inflammatory respiratory inhalant
Pregnancy risk category: B

Indications and dosages

➤ *Maintenance therapy in mild to moderate bronchial asthma. Adults and children age 6 and older:* 2 inhalations q.i.d., preferably at regular intervals; may gradually decrease dosing interval to b.i.d.

Reactions may be *common*, uncommon, ***life-threatening***, or COMMON AND LIFE-THREATENING.

How supplied
Available by prescription only
Inhalation aerosol: 1.75 mg per actuation in 16.2-g canister (U.S.); 2 mg per actuation in 16.2-g canister (Canada)

Pharmacodynamics
Anti-inflammatory and antiallergic action: Drug inhibits activation and release of inflammatory mediators from various cell types in the lumen and mucosa of the bronchial tree. These mediators, which include the leukotrienes, histamine, and prostaglandins, are preformed or derived from arachidonic acid metabolism. A range of human cells linked to asthma may be involved. As a result, nedocromil exhibits specific anti-inflammatory properties when administered topically to the bronchial mucosa. It has demonstrated a significant inhibitory effect on allergen-induced early and late asthmatic reactions and on bronchial hyperresponsiveness. Nedocromil also may affect sensory nerves in the lung. The result is inhibition of bradykinin-induced bronchoconstriction.

Pharmacokinetics
Absorption: 2% to 3% of amount swallowed after nedocromil inhalation is absorbed. From 6% to 9% of nedocromil deposited in the lungs is completely absorbed.
Distribution: Distributed to plasma only. About 89% is reversibly bound to plasma proteins when plasma levels range between 0.5 and 50 mcg/ml.
Metabolism: Not metabolized.
Excretion: Rapidly excreted unchanged in the bile and urine. Half-life is about 1½ to 3⅓ hours.

Route	Onset	Peak	Duration
Inhalation	Unknown	30 min	3½ hr

Contraindications and precautions
Contraindicated in patients hypersensitive to the formulation or in patients experiencing an acute asthmatic attack or acute bronchospasm.

Interactions
None reported.

Adverse reactions
CV: chest pain.
CNS: headache, dysphonia, fatigue.
EENT: rhinitis, pharyngitis.
GI: nausea, vomiting, dyspepsia, abdominal pain, dry mouth, *unpleasant taste*.
Respiratory: upper respiratory tract infection, cough, increased sputum, bronchitis, dyspnea, *bronchospasm*.

Overdose and treatment
Because nedocromil doesn't pass the blood-brain barrier, symptoms of overdose probably require nothing more than observing patient and stopping drug when appropriate.

Special considerations
● Dosage may be reduced to two inhalations three times daily and then twice daily after several weeks, when patient's asthma is under control.
● In maintenance therapy, drug must be used regularly, even during symptom-free periods, to achieve benefit.
● Reduced severity of clinical symptoms or need for accessory therapy is a sign of improvement that usually occurs in the first 2 weeks if patient responds to therapy.
● When nedocromil is added to an existing regimen of bronchodilators or given with inhaled or oral corticosteroids, the steroid or bronchodilator dosage may be reduced in some patients. However, reduction should be gradual and under close medical supervision to avoid worsening asthma.
● Don't exceed 14 mg within 24 hours.
● In some patients, bronchospasm may be prevented by a single dose of nedocromil before activities that precipitate asthma, such as exercise or exposure to cold air, pollutants, or allergens.

Patient monitoring
● Monitor patient for response to therapy.

Breast-feeding patients
● It isn't known if drug appears in breast milk. Use cautiously when administering drug to breast-feeding women.

Pediatric patients
● Safety and efficacy haven't been established for children under age 6.

Patient education
● Warn patient that drug has no direct bronchodilating action and can't replace bronchodilators during an acute asthmatic attack.
● Tell patient that drug is an adjunct to the regular bronchodilator regimen and may reduce the need for corticosteroids or bronchodilators.
● Emphasize that drug should be taken regularly for best results. Most patients report benefits after 1 week of use; some require longer treatment before improvement occurs.
● Teach patient how to use the inhaler. Instruct him to shake canister immediately before use and to invert it just before actuation. Prime inhaler with 3 actuations before first use or if unused for more than 7 days.
● Advise patient to clean inhaler at least twice weekly and to remove canister before rinsing inhaler in hot running water. Allow inhaler to air dry overnight.

nefazodone hydrochloride
Serzone

Pharmacologic classification: phenylpiperazine
Therapeutic classification: antidepressant
Pregnancy risk category: C

Indications and dosages
➤ *Depression. Adults:* Initially, 200 mg daily P.O. divided into two doses. Dosage increased in 100- to 200-mg increments daily at intervals of no less than 1 week, p.r.n. Usual dosage range, 300 to 600 mg daily.
✦ *Dosage adjustment.* In adults age 65 and older, initial dosage is 50 mg P.O. b.i.d. Increase slowly as needed. Usual dosage is 200 to 400 mg daily.

How supplied
Available by prescription only
Tablets: 50 mg, 100 mg, 150 mg, 200 mg, 250 mg

Pharmacodynamics
Antidepressive action: Action of drug isn't precisely defined. It inhibits neuronal uptake of serotonin and norepinephrine. It also occupies central 5-hydroxytryptamine$_1$ (serotonin) and alpha$_1$-adrenergic receptors.

Pharmacokinetics
Absorption: Rapidly and completely absorbed but, because of extensive metabolism, its absolute bioavailability is only about 20%. Food delays absorption and reduces bioavailability.
Distribution: More than 99% is bound to plasma proteins.
Metabolism: Extensively metabolized by n-dealkylation and aliphatic and aromatic hydroxylation.
Excretion: Excreted in urine. Half-life of drug is 2 to 4 hours.

Route	Onset	Peak	Duration
P.O.	Unknown	1 hr	Unknown

Contraindications and precautions
Contraindicated in patients hypersensitive to drug or other phenylpiperazine antidepressants. Don't use within 14 days of MAO inhibitor therapy or with pimozide.

Use cautiously in patients with CV or cerebrovascular disease that could be worsened by hypotension (such as history of MI, angina, or CVA) or conditions that would predispose patient to hypotension (such as dehydration, hypovolemia, or antihypertensive treatment). Use cautiously in patients with a history of mania.

Interactions
Drug-drug. *Alprazolam, triazolam:* Potentiated effects of these drugs. Avoid use together. If necessary, dosages of alprazolam and triazolam may need to be reduced greatly.
CNS active drugs: May alter CNS activity. Use together cautiously.
Digoxin: Increased digoxin levels. Use together cautiously, and monitor digoxin levels.
Highly plasma protein–bound drugs: May increase risk and severity of adverse reactions. Monitor patient closely.
Pimozide: May cause decreased pimozide metabolism, leading to increased levels and cardiotoxicity. Avoid use together.
MAO inhibitors: May cause severe excitation, hyperpyrexia, seizures, delirium, or coma. Avoid use together.
Drug-herb. *St. John's wort:* Increased sedative and hypnotic effects. Discourage use together.

Adverse reactions
CNS: *headache, somnolence, dizziness, asthenia,* insomnia, *light-headedness, confusion,* memory impairment, paresthesia, abnormal dreams, decreased concentration, ataxia, incoordination, psychomotor retardation, tremor, hypertonia.
CV: orthostatic hypotension, vasodilation, hypotension, peripheral edema.
EENT: *blurred vision, abnormal vision,* pharyngitis, tinnitus, visual field defect.
GI: *dry mouth, nausea, constipation,* dyspepsia, diarrhea, increased appetite, vomiting, thirst, taste perversion.
GU: urinary frequency, urinary tract infection, urine retention, vaginitis, breast pain.
Musculoskeletal: neck rigidity, arthralgia.
Respiratory: cough.
Skin: pruritus, rash.
Other: infection, flu syndrome, chills, fever.

Overdose and treatment
Overdose may cause nausea, vomiting, and somnolence. Other drug-related adverse reactions may occur.

Provide symptomatic and supportive treatment for hypotension or excessive sedation. Use gastric lavage if needed.

Special considerations
● Allow at least 1 week after stopping drug before giving patient an MAO inhibitor. Also, allow at least 14 days after stopping an MAO inhibitor before starting nefazodone.
● Drug therapy may precipitate mania or hypomania in patients with bipolar or other affective disorders.

Patient monitoring
● Monitor patient for suicidal tendencies. Give a minimum supply of drug.
● Monitor liver function test results in patients with hepatic dysfunction.

Breast-feeding patients
● It isn't known if nefazodone appears in breast milk; use cautiously in breast-feeding women.

Reactions may be *common*, uncommon, *life-threatening*, or COMMON AND LIFE-THREATENING.

Pediatric patients

• Safety and efficacy in children under age 18 haven't been established.

Geriatric patients

• Because of increased systemic exposure to nefazodone, begin treatment at half the usual dose, but increase dose over the same dosage range as in younger patients.

• Observe usual precautions in elderly patients who have ongoing medical illnesses or are receiving other drugs.

Patient education

• Warn patient not to engage in potentially hazardous activities until CNS effects are known.

• Instruct men to stop drug immediately and seek medical attention if they have prolonged or inappropriate erections.

• Instruct women to report planned, suspected, or known pregnancy during therapy.

• Instruct patient not to drink alcoholic beverages during therapy.

• Tell patient to report rash, hives, or other related allergic reactions.

• Inform patient that several weeks of therapy may be needed to obtain the full antidepressant effect. Once improvement occurs, advise patient not to discontinue drug until directed.

---

nelfinavir mesylate
Viracept

Pharmacologic classification: HIV protease inhibitor
Therapeutic classification: antiviral
Pregnancy risk category: B

Indications and dosages

➤ *Treatment of HIV infection when antiretroviral therapy is warranted. Adults:* 750 mg P.O. t.i.d with meal or light snack.
Children ages 2 to 13: 20 to 30 mg/kg/dose P.O. t.i.d. with meal or light snack. Maximum, 750 mg t.i.d. Recommended pediatric dosage given t.i.d. is shown in the following table.

Body weight (kg)	No. of level 1-g scoops	No. of level teaspoons	No. of tablets
7-8.4	4	1	-
8.5-10.4	5	1.25	-
10.5-11.9	6	1.5	-
12-13.9	7	1.75	-
14-15.9	8	2	-
16-17.9	9	2.25	-
18-22.9	10	2.5	2
≥ 23	15	3.75	3

Children ages 2 to 13 who weigh 23 to 53 kg (50 to 116 lb) ◊: 25 to 30 mg/kg P.O. t.i.d. up to 1,250 or 1,500 mg per dose.
➤ *Post-exposure prophylaxis following occupational exposure to HIV* ◊. *Adults:* 750 mg P.O. t.i.d. with oral zidovudine and lamivudine for 4 weeks.

How supplied

Available by prescription only
Powder: 50 mg/g of powder
Tablets: 250 mg

Pharmacodynamics

Antiviral action: Inhibition of the protease enzyme prevents cleavage of the viral polyprotein, resulting in production of an immature, noninfectious virus.

Pharmacokinetics

Absorption: Absolute bioavailability isn't determined. Food increases absorption of drug.
Distribution: Apparent volume of drug distribution is 2 to 7 L/kg. More than 98% of drug is bound to plasma protein.
Metabolism: Metabolized in the liver by multiple cytochrome P-450 isoforms, including CYP3A.
Excretion: Terminal half-life is 3½ to 5 hours. Drug is primarily excreted in the feces.

Route	Onset	Peak	Duration
P.O.	Unknown	2-4 hr	Unknown

Contraindications and precautions

Contraindicated in patients hypersensitive to any component of drug. Use cautiously in patients with hepatic dysfunction or hemophilia types A and B.

Interactions

Drug-drug. *Amiodarone, ergot derivatives, midazolam, quinidine, triazolam:* Increased levels of these drugs, which may increase risk for serious or life-threatening adverse events. Avoid use together.
Anti-HIV protease inhibitors, such as indinavir or saquinavir: May increase levels of both drugs. Use together cautiously.
Carbamazepine, phenobarbital, phenytoin: May reduce the effectiveness of nelfinavir by decreasing nelfinavir levels. Use together cautiously.
Drugs primarily metabolized by CYP3A, such as dihydropyridine or calcium channel blockers: May increase levels of these drugs and decrease nelfinavir levels. Use together cautiously.
HMG-CoA inhibitors such as lovastatin, simvastatin: May increase levels of antilipemic drugs. Avoid using together.
Oral contraceptives: Nelfinavir may decrease contraceptive levels. Advise patient to use appropriate contraceptive during therapy.
Rifabutin: Increased rifabutin levels. Reduce rifabutin dosage to half the usual amount.

Rifampin: Decreased nelfinavir levels. Don't use together.

Ritonavir: May increase nelfinavir levels. Use together cautiously.

Sildenafil: May increase adverse effects of sildenafil. Use together cautiously.

Drug-herb. *St. John's wort:* Decreased nelfinavir levels. Discourage concurrent use.

Adverse reactions
CNS: anxiety, depression, dizziness, emotional lability, hyperkinesia, insomnia, malaise, migraine headache, paresthesia, *seizures*, sleep disorders, somnolence, *suicidal ideation*, asthenia.
EENT: iritis, eye disorders, pharyngitis, rhinitis, sinusitis.
GI: abdominal pain, nausea, *diarrhea*, flatulence, anorexia, dyspepsia, epigastric pain, GI bleeding, *pancreatitis*, mouth ulceration, vomiting.
GU: sexual dysfunction, kidney calculus, urine abnormality.
Hematologic: anemia, *leukopenia, thrombocytopenia*.
Hepatic: *hepatitis*.
Metabolic: dehydration, diabetes mellitus, hyperlipidemia, hyperuricemia, hypoglycemia.
Musculoskeletal: back pain, arthralgia, arthritis, cramps, myalgia, myasthenia, myopathy.
Respiratory: dyspnea.
Skin: rash, dermatitis, folliculitis, fungal dermatitis, pruritus, sweating, urticaria.
Other: fever, redistribution or accumulation of body fat.

Overdose and treatment
Information is limited. Unabsorbed drug may be removed by emesis or gastric lavage; activated charcoal may also be used. Dialysis isn't beneficial.

Special considerations
● Decision to use drug is based on surrogate marker changes in patients who received drug in combination with nucleoside analogues or alone for up to 24 weeks. There are no results from controlled trials evaluating the effect on survival or risk of opportunistic fungal infections.
● Drug dosage is same whether used alone or in combination with other antiretroviral agents.
● Antiretroviral activity may be increased when used in combination with approved reverse transcriptase inhibitors.
● Administer oral powder in children unable to take tablets; may mix oral powder with water, milk, formula, soy formula, soy milk, or dietary supplements. Acidic foods or juice aren't recommended due to bitter taste.
● Don't reconstitute with water in its original container.
● Use reconstituted powder within 6 hours.

Patient monitoring
● Monitor CBC with differential (especially neutrophils) and chemistries, although patient has a low risk of laboratory abnormalities.
● Alkaline phosphatase, amylase, CK, LD, AST, ALT, and GGT levels may increase; monitor patient closely.
● Monitor patient for toxicity and disease progression.

Pregnant patients
● Use only when clearly needed. To monitor maternal and fetal outcomes, register patient by calling 1-800-258-4263.

Breast-feeding patients
● It isn't known if drug appears in breast milk. Although safety hasn't been established, advise HIV-infected women not to breast-feed in order to avoid HIV transmission to the infant.

Pediatric patients
● Safety and efficacy haven't been established in children under age 2.

Patient education
● Advise patient to take drug with food.
● Inform patient that drug isn't a cure for HIV infection.
● Tell patient that long-term effects of drug are currently unknown and that there's evidence that drug reduces risk of HIV transmission to others.
● Advise patient to take drug daily as prescribed and not to alter dose or discontinue drug without medical approval.
● If patient misses a dose, tell him to take the dose as soon as possible and return to his normal schedule. Advise against doubling the dose.
● Tell patient that diarrhea is the most common adverse effect and that it can be controlled with loperamide, if necessary.
● Explain to patient that body fat may accumulate or redistribute during therapy.
● Instruct patient taking oral contraceptives to use alternate or additional contraceptive measures.
● Advise patient to report use of other prescribed or OTC drugs.

neomycin sulfate
Mycifradin, Myciguent, Neo-fradin, Neo-Tabs

Pharmacologic classification: aminoglycoside
Therapeutic classification: antibiotic
Pregnancy risk category: D

Indications and dosages
➤ *Infectious diarrhea caused by enteropathogenic* **Escherichia coli.** *Adults:* 50 mg/kg P.O. daily in four divided doses for 2 to 3 days. *Children:* 50 to 100 mg/kg P.O. daily divided q 4 to 6 hours for 2 to 3 days.

➤ *Suppression of intestinal bacteria preoperatively.* Adults: 1 g P.O. q 1 hour for four doses; then 1 g q 4 hours for rest of 24 hours. A saline cathartic should precede therapy.
Children: 40 to 100 mg/kg P.O. daily divided q 4 to 6 hours. First dose should be preceded by saline cathartic.

2- to 3-day regimen
Adults and children: 88 mg/kg P.O. in six equally divided doses at 4-hour intervals. Or, for 8 a.m. surgery, 1 g of neomycin and 1 g of erythromycin base P.O. at 1 p.m., 2 p.m., and 11 p.m. on the day preceding surgery.

➤ *Adjunctive treatment in hepatic coma.* Adults: 1 to 3 g P.O. q.i.d. for 5 to 6 days; 200 ml of 1% or 100 ml of 2% solution as enema retained for 20 to 60 minutes q 6 hours.
Children: 50 to 100 mg/kg P.O. daily in divided doses for 5 to 6 days.

➤ *Treatment of hypercholesterolemia* ◇. Adults: 500 mg to 2 g P.O. daily in two or three divided doses.

➤ *External ear canal infection.* Adults and children: 2 to 5 drops into ear canal t.i.d. or q.i.d. for 7 to 10 days.

➤ *Topical bacterial infections, burns, wounds, skin grafts, following surgical procedure, lesions, pruritus, trophic ulcerations, and edema.* Adults and children: Rub in small amount gently b.i.d., t.i.d., or as directed.

✦ *Dosage adjustment.* Use reduced dosage in adults and children with renal failure. Specific recommendations aren't available.

How supplied
Available by prescription only
Oral solution: 125 mg/5 ml
Otic suspension: 5 mg/ml (with polymyxin B sulfate 10,000 units/ml and hydrocortisone 1%)
Tablets: 500 mg
Available without a prescription
Cream: 0.5%
Ointment: 0.5%

Pharmacodynamics
Antibiotic action: Neomycin is bactericidal; it binds directly to the 30S ribosomal subunit, thus inhibiting bacterial protein synthesis. Its spectrum of action includes many aerobic gram-negative organisms and some aerobic gram-positive organisms. Drug is far less active against many gram-negative organisms than are amikacin, gentamicin, netilmicin, and tobramycin. Given orally or as retention enema, neomycin inhibits ammonia-forming bacteria in the GI tract, reducing ammonia and improving neurologic status of patients with hepatic encephalopathy. It's rarely given systemically because of its high potential for ototoxicity and nephrotoxicity.

Pharmacokinetics
Absorption: Absorbed poorly (about 3%) after oral use, although absorption is enhanced in pa-

tients with impaired GI motility or mucosal intestinal ulcerations. Neomycin isn't absorbed through intact skin; it may be absorbed from wounds, burns, or skin ulcers.
Distribution: Crosses the placenta. Oral administration restricts distribution to the GI tract.
Metabolism: Not metabolized.
Excretion: Excreted primarily in urine by glomerular filtration. Elimination half-life in adults is 2 to 3 hours; in severe renal damage, half-life may extend to 24 hours. After oral administration, neomycin is excreted primarily unchanged in feces.

Route	Onset	Peak	Duration
P.O.	Unknown	1-4 hr	8 hr
Topical	Unknown	Unknown	Unknown

Contraindications and precautions
Contraindicated in patients hypersensitive to drug. Oral form contraindicated in patients sensitive to other aminoglycosides and in those with intestinal obstruction. Don't give drug parenterally.

Use oral form cautiously in elderly patients and patients with impaired renal function, neuromuscular disorders, or ulcerative bowel lesions. Use topical form cautiously in patients with extensive skin conditions.

Interactions
Drug-drug. *Oral anticoagulants*: Potentiated effects of anticoagulant. Dosage adjustment of anticoagulants may be necessary.

Adverse reactions
EENT: *ototoxicity* with oral use.
GI: nausea, vomiting, diarrhea, malabsorption syndrome, and *Clostridium difficile*–related colitis with oral use.
GU: *nephrotoxicity* with oral use.
Skin: *rash, contact dermatitis,* and urticaria with topical use.
Other: *neuromuscular blockade* with topical use.

Overdose and treatment
Overdose may cause ototoxicity, nephrotoxicity, and neuromuscular toxicity.

After recent ingestion (4 hours or less), empty patient's stomach by induced emesis or gastric lavage; follow with activated charcoal to reduce absorption. Remove drug by hemodialysis or peritoneal dialysis; treatment with calcium salts or anticholinesterases reverses neuromuscular blockade.

Special considerations
● Monitor renal function: output, specific gravity, urinalysis, BUN and creatinine levels, and creatinine clearance during therapy.
● Evaluate patient's hearing before and during prolonged therapy. Onset of deafness may occur several weeks after drug is stopped.

• Watch for superinfection, such as fever or other evidence of new infection.

• In adjunctive treatment of hepatic coma, decrease patient's dietary protein and assess neurologic status frequently during therapy.

• For preoperative disinfection, provide a low-residue diet and a cathartic immediately before oral administration of neomycin, as ordered.

• The ototoxic and nephrotoxic properties of neomycin limit its usefulness.

• Neomycin is nonabsorbable at recommended dosage. However, more than 4 g daily may be systemically absorbed and lead to nephrotoxicity.

• Drug is available with polymyxin B as a bladder irrigant.

• In hepatic coma, decrease dietary protein and reassess neurologic status frequently.

Preoperative bowel contamination

• Provide low-residue diet and cathartic immediately before administration of oral neomycin; follow-up enemas may be necessary to completely empty bowel.

Topical therapy

• Don't apply to more than 20% of body surface.

• Don't apply to any body surface of patient with decreased renal function without considering risk/benefit ratio.

Otic therapy

• Reculture persistent drainage.

• Drug is best used in combination with other antibiotics.

• Avoid touching ear with dropper.

Patient monitoring

• Monitor patient for hypersensitivity or contact dermatitis.

• Monitor renal function during drug therapy.

• Patient's hearing should be evaluated before and during prolonged drug therapy.

• Monitor patient for superinfection.

Patient education

• Instruct patient to report adverse reactions promptly.

• Encourage adequate fluid intake.

neostigmine bromide
neostigmine methylsulfate
Prostigmin

Pharmacologic classification: cholinesterase inhibitor
Therapeutic classification: muscle stimulant
Pregnancy risk category: C

Indications and dosages

➤*Antidote for nondepolarizing neuromuscular blocking agents. Adults:* 0.5 to 2 mg slow I.V. Repeat, p.r.n. Maximum total dose, 5 mg. Give 0.6 to 1.2 mg atropine sulfate I.V. before antidote dose if patient is bradycardic.

Neonates, infants, and children: 0.04 mg/kg/dose I.V. with atropine sulfate (0.02 mg/kg atropine) with each dose of neostigmine.

➤*Prevention of postoperative abdominal distention and bladder atony. Adults:* 0.25 mg I.M. or S.C. q 4 to 6 hours for 2 to 3 days.

➤*Treatment of postoperative abdominal distention and bladder atony. Adults:* 0.5 to 1 mg S.C. or I.M. If given for urine retention and there's no response in 1 hour, catheterize patient and repeat dose q 3 hours for five doses after bladder is emptied.

➤*Diagnosis of myasthenia gravis*◇. *Adults:* 0.022 mg/kg I.M. Give atropine 0.011 mg/kg I.V. with dose or I.M. 30 minutes before dose. If cholinergic reaction occurs, stop test and give atropine sulfate 0.4 to 0.6 mg I.V. If the results are inconclusive, retest on another day using 0.031 mg/kg I.M. of neostigmine preceded by atropine 0.01 mg/kg.

Children: 0.025 to 0.04 mg/kg I.M. preceded by 0.011 mg/kg S.C. of atropine sulfate.

➤*Symptomatic control of myasthenia gravis. Adults:* 0.5 to 2.5 mg S.C., I.V., or I.M. Oral dose can range from 15 to 375 mg daily (average 150 mg in 24 hours). Subsequent dosages must be individualized, based on response and tolerance of adverse effects. Therapy may be required day and night.

Children: 7.5 to 15 mg P.O. t.i.d. or q.i.d. Or, 0.333 mg/kg or 10 mg/m² P.O. 6 times daily.

Neonates: 0.1 to 0.2 S.C. or 0.03 mg/kg I.M. q 2 to 4 hours or 1 to 4 mg P.O. q 2 to 3 hours. Gradual dose reduction as symptoms improve.

➤*Supraventricular tachycardia from tricyclic antidepressant overdose*◇. *Children:* 0.5 to 1 mg I.V. followed by 0.25 to 0.5 mg q 1 to 3 hours, p.r.n.

➤*Decrease small bowel transit time during radiography*◇. *Adults:* 0.5 to 0.75 mg S.C.

How supplied

Available by prescription only
Injection: 0.5 mg/ml, 1 mg/ml, 2 mg/ml
Tablets: 15 mg

Pharmacodynamics

Muscle stimulant action: Neostigmine blocks hydrolysis of acetylcholine by cholinesterase, resulting in acetylcholine accumulation at cholinergic synapses, which leads to increased cholinergic receptor stimulation at the myoneural junction.

Pharmacokinetics

Absorption: Poorly absorbed (1% to 2%) from GI tract after oral administration.
Distribution: About 15% to 25% of dose binds to plasma proteins.
Metabolism: Hydrolyzed by cholinesterases and metabolized by microsomal liver enzymes. Duration of effect varies considerably, depending on patient's physical and emotional status and on disease severity.

Reactions may be *common,* uncommon, *life-threatening,* or COMMON AND LIFE-THREATENING.

Excretion: About 80% of dose is excreted in urine as unchanged drug and metabolites in the first 24 hours after administration.

Route	Onset	Peak	Duration
P.O.	45-75 min	1-2 hr	2-4 hr
I.V.	4-8 min	1-2 hr	2-4 hr
I.M., S.C.	20-30 min	1-2 hr	2-4 hr

Contraindications and precautions
Contraindicated in patients hypersensitive to cholinergics or to bromide and in those with peritonitis or mechanical obstruction of the intestine or urinary tract. Use cautiously in patients with bronchial asthma, bradycardia, seizure disorders, recent coronary occlusion, vagotonia, hyperthyroidism, arrhythmias, and peptic ulcer.

Interactions
Drug-drug. *Atropine, corticosteroids, magnesium, procainamide, quinidine:* May reverse cholinergic effect of neostigmine on muscle. Observe patient for drug effect.
Cholinergic drugs: May cause additive toxicity. Avoid use together.
Succinylcholine: May prolong respiratory depression. Monitor patient carefully.

Adverse reactions
CNS: dizziness, seizures, headache, muscle weakness, loss of consciousness, drowsiness, syncope.
CV: *bradycardia,* hypotension, tachycardia, AV block, *cardiac arrest,* flushing.
EENT: blurred vision, lacrimation, miosis.
GI: *nausea, vomiting, diarrhea, abdominal cramps,* excessive salivation, flatulence, increased peristalsis.
GU: urinary frequency.
Musculoskeletal: *muscle cramps,* muscle fasciculations, arthralgia.
Respiratory: *bronchospasm,* dyspnea, *respiratory depression, respiratory arrest,* increased secretions.
Skin: rash, urticaria, diaphoresis.
Other: *hypersensitivity reactions (anaphylaxis).*

Overdose and treatment
Signs and symptoms of overdose include headache, nausea, vomiting, diarrhea, blurred vision, miosis, excessive tearing, bronchospasm, increased bronchial secretions, hypotension, incoordination, excessive sweating, muscle weakness, cramps, fasciculations, paralysis, bradycardia or tachycardia, excessive salivation, and restlessness or agitation.

Discontinue drug immediately. Support respiration; bronchial suctioning may be performed. Atropine may be given to block muscarinic effects of neostigmine, but it won't counter paralytic effects of drug on skeletal muscle. Avoid atropine overdose because it may lead to bronchial plug formation.

Special considerations
● If muscle weakness is severe, determine if it stems from drug toxicity or from worsening of myasthenia gravis. A test dose of edrophonium I.V. will aggravate drug-induced weakness but will temporarily relieve disease-related weakness.
● Hospitalized patients may be able to manage a bedside supply of tablets to take themselves.
● Give drug with food or milk to reduce the chance for GI adverse effects.
● To diagnose myasthenia gravis, discontinue all anticholinergics for at least 8 hours before neostigmine administration.
● When giving drug to patient with myasthenia gravis, schedule largest dose before anticipated periods of fatigue. If patient has dysphagia, schedule this dose 30 minutes before each meal.
● Stop all other cholinergic drugs during neostigmine therapy because of risk of additive toxicity.
● When giving neostigmine to prevent abdominal distention and GI distress, inserting a rectal tube may help passage of gas.
● Administering atropine with neostigmine can relieve or eliminate adverse reactions; these symptoms may indicate neostigmine overdose and will be masked by atropine.
● Patients may develop resistance to drug.

Patient monitoring
● Monitor patient's vital signs, particularly pulse.

Breast-feeding patients
● Neostigmine may appear in breast milk, possibly resulting in infant toxicity. Evaluate patient's clinical status to see if breast-feeding or drug should be discontinued.

Pediatric patients
● Safety and efficacy in children haven't been fully established.

Geriatric patients
● These patients may be more sensitive to effects of neostigmine. Use cautiously.

Patient education
● Instruct patient to observe and record changes in muscle strength.

nevirapine
Viramune

Pharmacologic classification: nonnucleoside reverse transcriptase inhibitor
Therapeutic classification: antiviral
Pregnancy risk category: C

Indications and dosages
➤ *Treatment of patients with HIV-1 infection (with other antiretrovirals). Adults and adolescents:* 200 mg P.O. daily for first 14 days, followed by 200 mg P.O. q 12 hours.

Children ages 2 months to 8 years: 4 mg/kg P.O. once daily for first 14 days, followed by 7 mg/kg P.O. q 12 hours thereafter. Maximum, 400 mg daily.

Children age 8 and older: 4 mg/kg P.O. once daily for first 14 days, followed by 4 mg/kg P.O. q 12 hours thereafter. Maximum, 400 mg daily. Or, children may receive 120 mg/m² P.O. daily for first 14 days, followed by 120 to 200 mg/m² q 12 hours.

Neonates◊: 5 mg/kg P.O. daily for first 14 days followed by 120 mg/m² q 12 hours for next 14 days; then 200 mg/m² q 12 hours.

How supplied
Available by prescription only
Oral suspension: 50 mg/5 ml
Tablets: 200 mg

Pharmacodynamics
Antiviral action: Nevirapine binds directly to reverse transcriptase and blocks RNA-dependent and DNA-dependent DNA polymerase activities by disrupting the catalytic site of the enzyme.

Pharmacokinetics
Absorption: Readily absorbed.
Distribution: Widely distributed, crosses the placenta, and appears in breast milk. It's about 60% bound to plasma proteins.
Metabolism: Extensively metabolized in the liver.
Excretion: Metabolites are primarily excreted in urine; a small amount of drug is excreted in feces.

Route	Onset	Peak	Duration
P.O.	Unknown	4 hr	Unknown

Contraindications and precautions
Contraindicated in patients hypersensitive to drug. Use cautiously in patients with impaired renal or hepatic function because the pharmacokinetics of nevirapine haven't been evaluated in these patients.

Interactions
Drug-drug. *Drugs extensively metabolized by P-450 CYP3A:* Nevirapine may lower levels of these drugs. Adjust dosages of these drugs if needed.
Ketoconazole: Decreased ketoconazole levels. Avoid using together.
Oral contraceptives, protease inhibitors: Decreased plasma levels of these drugs. Don't administer together.
Drug-herb. *St. John's wort:* Decreased nevirapine levels. Discourage concurrent use.

Adverse reactions
CNS: headache, peripheral neuropathy, paresthesia.
GI: nausea, diarrhea, abdominal pain, ulcerative stomatitis.
Hematologic: *decreased neutrophil count,* eosinophilia.

Hepatic: *hepatitis,* abnormal liver function test results, *hepatotoxicity.*
Musculoskeletal: myalgia.
Skin: *rash, Stevens-Johnson syndrome,* facial edema, epidermic necrolysis.
Other: fever.

Overdose and treatment
No information available.

Special considerations
● Nevirapine is usually used in three-drug regimens.
● Resistant virus emerges rapidly when drug is given alone. Always administer with at least one other antiretroviral.
● Using a 200-mg lead-in dose may decrease rash.
● Discontinue drug if patient develops a severe rash or a rash accompanied by fever, blistering, oral lesions, conjunctivitis, swelling, muscle or joint aches, or general malaise. If rash occurs during the initial 14 days, don't increase dosage until it has resolved. Most rashes occur during the first 6 weeks of therapy.
● Severe, life-threatening cases of hepatotoxicity, including hepatitis, hepatic necrosis and hepatic failure have been reported.
● If therapy is interrupted for more than 7 days, restart it as though giving drug for the first time.
● If disease progresses during therapy, consider alternative antiretroviral therapy.

Patient monitoring
● Monitor clinical chemistry tests, including liver function tests, before starting and regularly throughout therapy.
● Drug must be stopped temporarily in patients with moderate or severe liver function test abnormalities (excluding GGT) until values have returned to baseline. May restart drug at half the previous dose level. If moderate or severe liver function test abnormalities recur, discontinue drug therapy. Monitor LFTs closely.
● Patient should be monitored for development of rash.

Breast-feeding patients
● Drug appears in breast milk. HIV-infected women shouldn't breast-feed.

Pediatric patients
● Safety and efficacy in children haven't been established.

Patient education
● Inform patient that drug doesn't cure HIV infection and that illnesses linked to advanced HIV-1 infection may still occur. Also, tell patient that drug doesn't reduce risk of transmission of HIV-1 to others through sexual contact or blood contamination.
● Instruct patient to report rash immediately. Therapy may need to be stopped temporarily.

Reactions may be *common*, uncommon, *life-threatening*, or COMMON AND LIFE-THREATENING.

- Stress the importance of taking drug exactly as prescribed. Tell patient to take a missed dose as soon as possible but not to double the next dose if he skips one.
- Tell patient not to take other medications without medical approval.
- Advise women of childbearing age to avoid oral contraceptives and other hormonal methods of birth control during therapy.

niacin (vitamin B₃, nicotinic acid)
Niacor, Niaspan, Nico-400, Nicobid, Nicotinex, Slo-Niacin

niacinamide (nicotinamide)
Pharmacologic classification: B-complex vitamin
Therapeutic classification: vitamin B₃, antilipemic, peripheral vasodilator
Pregnancy risk category: A (C if greater than RDA)

Indications and dosages
▶ *Pellagra. Adults:* 300 to 500 mg in divided doses P.O., depending on severity of niacin deficiency. Maximum recommended dose is 500 mg daily divided into 10 50-mg doses.
Children: Up to 300 mg P.O. daily, depending on severity of niacin deficiency.
▶ *Peripheral vascular disease and circulatory disorders. Adults:* 100 to 150 mg P.O. three to five times daily. Or, 1,000 to 2,000 g once daily at bedtime.
▶ *Adjunctive treatment of hyperlipidemias, especially those related to hypercholesterolemia. Adults:* 1.5 to 6 g P.O. daily in two to four divided doses with or after meals. Maximum, 9 g daily. Or, initial dose of 100 mg P.O. t.i.d., increasing by 300 mg daily at 4- to 7-day intervals. Or, 500 mg P.O. t.i.d. with gradual increase to desired effect.
▶ *Hartnup disease. Adults:* 50 to 200 mg P.O. daily in divided doses.
▶ *Dietary supplement. Adults:* 10 to 20 mg P.O. daily.

How supplied
Available by prescription only
Capsules: 500 mg
Tablets (extended-release): 500 mg, 750 mg, 1,000 mg; 21-day starter pack containing seven each of 375-mg, 500-mg, and 750-mg strength.
Available without a prescription
Capsules (timed-release): 125 mg, 250 mg, 300 mg, 400 mg, 500 mg, 750 mg
Elixir: 50 mg/5 ml
Tablets: 25 mg, 50 mg, 100 mg, 125 mg, 250 mg, 400 mg, 500 mg
Tablets (timed-release): 250 mg, 500 mg, 750 mg

Pharmacodynamics
Vitamin replacement action: As a vitamin, niacin functions as a coenzyme essential to tissue respiration, lipid metabolism, and glycogenolysis. Niacin deficiency causes pellagra, which causes dermatitis, diarrhea, and dementia; administration of niacin cures pellagra. Niacin lowers cholesterol and triglyceride levels by an unknown mechanism.
Vasodilating action: Niacin acts directly on peripheral vessels, dilating cutaneous vessels and increasing blood flow, predominantly in the face, neck, and chest.
Antilipemic action: Mechanism of action is unknown. Nicotinic acid inhibits lipolysis in adipose tissues, decreases hepatic esterification of triglyceride, and increases lipoprotein lipase activity. It reduces serum cholesterol and triglyceride levels.

Pharmacokinetics
Absorption: Absorbed rapidly from the GI tract. Cholesterol and triglyceride levels decrease after several days.
Distribution: Coenzymes are distributed widely in body tissues; niacin appears in breast milk.
Metabolism: Metabolized by the liver to active metabolites.
Excretion: Excreted in urine.

Route	Onset	Peak	Duration
P.O.	Unknown	45 min	Unknown

Contraindications and precautions
Contraindicated in patients with hepatic dysfunction, active peptic ulcer, severe hypotension, arterial hemorrhage, or hypersensitivity to drug. Use cautiously in patients with history of liver disease, peptic ulcer, allergy, gout, gallbladder disease, diabetes mellitus, or coronary artery disease.

Interactions
Drug-drug. *Aspirin:* May decrease the metabolic clearance of nicotinic acid. Use together cautiously.
Sympathetic blocking agents: May cause added vasodilation and hypotension. Use together cautiously.

Adverse reactions
Most reactions are dose-dependent.
CV: *excessive peripheral vasodilation,* hypotension, atrial fibrillation, ***arrhythmias,*** *flushing.*
EENT: toxic amblyopia.
GI: *nausea, vomiting, diarrhea,* possible activation of peptic ulceration, epigastric or substernal pain.
Hepatic: *hepatic dysfunction.*
Metabolic: hyperglycemia, hyperuricemia.
Skin: pruritus, dryness, tingling.

Overdose and treatment
Niacin is a water-soluble vitamin and seldom causes toxicity in patients with normal renal function.

Special considerations
• The Recommended Daily Allowance of niacin is 19 mg in men, 15 mg in women, and 5 to 20 mg in children.
• Megadoses of niacin usually aren't recommended.
• Premedication with aspirin, use of the slow-release formulation, and gradual dose adjustments may reduce flushing response.
• Niacin therapy alters fluorometric test results for urine catecholamines and results for urine glucose tests using cupric sulfate (Benedict's reagent).

Patient monitoring
• Monitor hepatic function and blood glucose levels early in therapy.

Breast-feeding patients
• There have been no reports of problems in breast-feeding women taking normal daily doses as dietary requirement.

Patient education
• Explain disease process and rationale for therapy. Stress that use of niacin to treat hyperlipidemia or to dilate peripheral vessels isn't simply taking a vitamin but taking a serious medicine. Emphasize the importance of complying with therapy.
• Instruct patient not to substitute sustained-release (timed) tablets for intermediate-release tablets in equivalent doses. Severe hepatic toxicity, including necrosis, has occurred.
• Explain that cutaneous flushing and warmth commonly occur in the first 2 hours; this will cease with continued therapy.
• To minimize the effects of orthostatic hypotension, advise against making sudden postural changes.
• To reduce flushing response, instruct patient to avoid hot liquids early in therapy.
• Advise patient to take drug with meals to minimize GI irritation.
• To prevent recurrence of pellagra after symptoms subside, advise adequate nutrition and adequate supplements to meet RDAs.

nicardipine hydrochloride
Cardene, Cardene I.V., Cardene SR

Pharmacologic classification: calcium channel blocker
Therapeutic classification: antianginal, antihypertensive
Pregnancy risk category: C

Indications and dosages
➤ *Hypertension; management of chronic stable angina. Adults:* Initially, 20 mg P.O.

t.i.d. Adjust dosage based on patient response. Usual dosage range, 20 to 40 mg t.i.d. For extended-release capsules (hypertension only), start at 30 mg b.i.d. Usual dose, 30 to 60 mg b.i.d.
➤ *Short-term management of hypertension when oral therapy isn't feasible or possible. Adults:* Initially, 5 mg/hour by I.V. infusion; increase by 2.5 mg/hour q 5 to 15 minutes to a maximum of 15 mg/hour, p.r.n. Maintenance infusion is 3 mg/hour. When transferring to oral therapy, give conventional capsule 1 hour before stopping infusion.
   Note: If patient is already taking nicardipine and needs short-term I.V. management of hypertension, give 0.5 mg/hour if dose is 20 mg q 8 hours, 1.2 mg/hour if dose is 30 mg q 8 hours, or 2.2 mg/hour if dose is 40 mg q 8 hours.
✦ *Dosage adjustment.* In patients with hepatic dysfunction, therapy should begin at 20 mg P.O. twice daily; carefully adjust subsequent dosage based on patient response.

How supplied
Available by prescription only
Capsules: 20 mg, 30 mg
Capsules (extended-release): 30 mg, 45 mg, 60 mg
Injection: 2.5 mg/ml in 10-ml ampules

Pharmacodynamics
Antihypertensive and antianginal actions: Nicardipine inhibits the flux of calcium ions into cardiac and smooth muscle cells. Drug appears to act specifically on vascular muscle. It may cause a smaller decrease in cardiac output than other calcium channel blockers because of its vasodilatory effect.

Pharmacokinetics
Absorption: Completely absorbed after oral administration. Absorption may be decreased if drug is taken with food. Therapeutic blood levels are 28 to 50 ng/ml.
Distribution: Extensively (more than 95%) bound to plasma proteins.
Metabolism: A substantial first-pass effect reduces absolute bioavailability to about 35%. Drug is extensively metabolized in the liver, and the process is saturable. Increasing dosage yields nonlinear increases in blood levels.
Excretion: Elimination half-life of drug is about 8½ hours after steady state levels are reached.

Route	Onset	Peak	Duration
P.O.			
Immediate	½-1½ min	1-2 hr	Unknown
Sustained	20 min	1-4 hr	12 hr
I.V.	Immediate	Immediate	Unknown

Contraindications and precautions
Contraindicated in patients hypersensitive to drug and in those with advanced aortic stenosis. Use cautiously in patients with impaired renal or he-

patic function, cardiac conduction disturbances, hypotension, or heart failure.

Interactions

Drug-drug. *Cimetidine:* Increased nicardipine levels. Monitor patient for increased effects.
Cyclosporine: Increased cyclosporine levels. Monitor patient carefully.
Fentanyl anesthesia: Severe hypotension. Monitoring blood pressure frequently.
Drug-food. *Grapefruit juice:* Increased bioavailability of drug. Advise patient to avoid taking drug with grapefruit juice.
High fat meal: Decreased bioavailability of nicardipine by 20% to 30%. Tell patient to take drug between meals if possible.

Adverse reactions

CNS: dizziness, light-headedness, headache, paresthesia, asthenia.
CV: *peripheral edema, palpitations,* angina, tachycardia, *flushing.*
GI: nausea, abdominal discomfort, dry mouth.
Skin: rash.

Overdose and treatment

Overdose may produce hypotension, bradycardia, drowsiness, confusion, and slurred speech. Treatment is supportive, with vasopressors given as needed. Calcium gluconate given I.V. may be useful to counteract the effects of drug.

Special considerations

• Allow at least 3 days between oral dosage changes to ensure steady state plasma levels.
• When treating patients who have chronic stable angina, S.L. nitroglycerin, prophylactic nitrate therapy, and beta blockers may be continued.
• Dilute solution in ampule before I.V. infusion. Recommended dilution is 0.1 mg/ml in dextrose or saline solution.
• When using I.V. route, change I.V. site every 12 hours to minimize vein irritation.

Patient monitoring

• When treating hypertension, measure blood pressure at trough level (about 8 hours after dose or just before next dose). Because prominent effects may occur during peak levels, measure blood pressure 1 to 2 hours after conventional dose and 2 to 4 hours after extended-release dose. Base dosage adjustment on blood pressure 2 to 4 hours after oral dose.
• Monitor blood pressure during I.V. administration because nicardipine I.V. decreases peripheral resistance.

Breast-feeding patients

• Substantial levels of drug have been found in the milk of animals given nicardipine. Breast-feeding isn't recommended.

Pediatric patients

• Safety in children under age 18 hasn't been established.

Patient education

• Tell patient to take oral form of drug exactly as prescribed.
• Advise patient to report chest pain immediately. Some patients may experience increased frequency, severity, or duration of chest pain at the beginning of therapy or during dosage adjustments.

nicotine
Habitrol, Nicoderm, Nicotrol, Nicotrol Inhaler, Nicotrol NS, ProStep

Pharmacologic classification: nicotinic cholinergic agonist
Therapeutic classification: smoking cessation aid
Pregnancy risk category: D

Indications and dosages

➤ *Relief of nicotine withdrawal symptoms in patients trying to stop smoking.*
Adults: One transdermal system applied to a nonhairy part of the upper trunk or upper outer arm. Dosage varies slightly with product selected.
Habitrol, Nicoderm
Initially, one 21-mg daily system applied daily for 6 weeks. After 24 hours, system removed and a new system applied to a different site. Then, dosage tapered to 14 mg daily for 2 to 4 weeks. Finally, dosage tapered to 7 mg daily if necessary. Nicotine substitution and gradual withdrawal should take 8 to 12 weeks.
✦ *Dosage adjustment.* Patients who weigh less than 45 kg (100 lb), have CV disease, or smoke less than half a pack of cigarettes daily should start therapy with the 14-mg daily system.
Nicotrol
Adults: One 15-mg system applied daily for 6 weeks. System applied upon waking and removed h.s. because patch provides systemic delivery over 16 hours.
Nicotrol NS
Adults: Initially, 1 or 2 doses/hour (1 dose = 2 sprays, one in each nostril). Encourage patient to use at least the recommended minimum of 8 doses daily. Maximum recommended dose is 40 mg or 80 sprays daily. Treatment shouldn't exceed 3 months, with dosage reduced gradually during those 3 months.
ProStep
Adults: Initially, one 22-mg system applied daily for 4 to 8 weeks. After 24 hours, system removed and a new system applied to a different site. Those who successfully stop smoking during the 4- to 8-week period may discontinue drug. Or, treatment may continue for another 2 to 4 weeks at lower dosage (11 mg daily). Nicotine substitu-

tion and gradual withdrawal should take 6 to 12 weeks.

✦ *Dosage adjustment.* Patients who weigh less than 45 kg should start therapy with the 11-mg daily system.

Nicotrol inhaler

Adults: Initial dose is 6 to 16 cartridges daily. Best effect is achieved with continuous puffing. Recommended treatment is up to 3 months and, if needed, gradual reduction over the next 6 to 12 weeks.

How supplied

Available with and without a prescription

Transdermal system: Designed to release nicotine at a fixed rate

Habitrol—21 mg daily, 14 mg daily, and 7 mg daily

Nicoderm—21 mg daily, 14 mg daily, 7 mg daily

Nicotrol—15 mg daily

ProStep—22 mg daily, 11 mg daily

Nasal spray: metered spray pump

Nicotrol NS—10 mg/ml

Available by prescription only

Nicotrol inhaler—10 mg cartridge, supplying 4 mg of nicotine

Pharmacodynamics

Nicotinic cholinergic action: Nicotine transdermal system and nasal spray provide nicotine, the chief stimulant alkaloid found in tobacco products, which stimulates nicotinic acetylcholine receptors in the CNS, neuromuscular junction, autonomic ganglia, and adrenal medulla.

Pharmacokinetics

Absorption: Rapidly absorbed.

Distribution: Plasma protein–binding of drug is below 5%.

Metabolism: Metabolized by the liver, kidney, and lungs. Over 20 metabolites have been identified. Primary metabolites are cotinine (15%) and trans-3-hydroxycotinine (45%).

Excretion: Excreted primarily in urine as metabolites; about 10% is excreted unchanged. With high urine flow rates or acidified urine, up to 30% can be excreted unchanged.

Route	Onset	Peak	Duration
Trans-dermal	Unknown	3-9 hr	Unknown
Intranasal	Unknown	4-15 min	Unknown
Inhalation	Unknown	15 min	Unknown

Contraindications and precautions

Contraindicated in patients hypersensitive to nicotine or any components. Also contraindicated in nonsmokers and in patients with recent MI, life-threatening arrhythmias, and severe or worsening angina pectoris.

Use cautiously in patients with hyperthyroidism, pheochromocytoma, insulin-dependent diabetes, or peptic ulcer disease.

Interactions

Drug-drug. *Acetaminophen, caffeine, imipramine, oxazepam, pentazocine, propranolol, theophylline:* Cessation of smoking may decrease induction of hepatic enzymes responsible for metabolizing certain drugs. Dosage reduction of these drugs may be necessary.

Adrenergic agonists, such as isoproterenol and phenylephrine; adrenergic antagonists, such as labetalol and prazosin: Cessation of smoking may decrease levels of circulating catecholamines. Dosage adjustment of these drugs may be necessary.

Insulin: Cessation of smoking may increase the amount of S.C. insulin absorbed. Adjust insulin dosage.

Propoxyphene: Cessation of smoking may increase first-pass metabolism of propoxyphene. Dose adjustments may be necessary.

Drug-herb. *Blue cohosh:* Increased nicotine effects. Tell patient not to use together.

Adverse reactions

CNS: somnolence, dizziness, *headache, insomnia,* paresthesia, abnormal dreams, nervousness.

CV: hypertension.

EENT: pharyngitis, sinusitis.

GI: abdominal pain, constipation, dyspepsia, nausea, diarrhea, vomiting, dry mouth.

GU: dysmenorrhea.

Musculoskeletal: back pain, myalgia.

Respiratory: increased cough.

Skin: *local or systemic erythema, pruritus, burning at application site,* cutaneous hypersensitivity, rash, diaphoresis.

Overdose and treatment

Overdose could produce symptoms caused by acute nicotine poisoning, including nausea, vomiting, diarrhea, weakness, respiratory failure, hypotension, and seizures.

Treat symptomatically. Barbiturates or benzodiazepines may be used to treat seizures, and atropine may attenuate excessive salivation or diarrhea. Administer fluids for hypotension; increase urine flow to enhance elimination of drug.

Special considerations

● Transdermal nicotine has been used investigationally to manage ulcerative colitis.

● Discourage use of transdermal system for more than 3 months. Chronic nicotine consumption by any route can be dangerous and habit-forming.

● Patients who can't stop cigarette smoking during the first 4 weeks of therapy probably will not benefit from continued use of drug. They may benefit from counseling to identify factors that helped to prevent cessation. Encourage patient to minimize or eliminate factors that contributed to treatment failure and to try again, possibly after some interval.

● Health care workers' exposure to the nicotine in the transdermal systems should be minimal;

however, avoid unnecessary contact with the system. After contact, wash hands with water alone because soap can enhance absorption.
• Nicotrol NS isn't recommended for patients with chronic nasal disorders or severe reactive airway disease.
• Increased cough is a common occurrence in patients using the inhaler.
• Although use of nicotine replacement therapy isn't recommended in patients with recent MI, it may be preferable to cigarette smoking in patients experiencing withdrawal.

Patient monitoring
• Monitor patient for correct use of system to prevent overdose or failure of program.

Breast-feeding patients
• Nicotine passes freely into breast milk and is readily absorbed after oral use. Weigh the infant's risk of exposure to nicotine against the risk of exposure from continued smoking by the mother.

Pediatric patients
• Safety and efficacy in children haven't been established.
• The amount of nicotine in a patch could prove fatal to a child if ingested; even used patches contain a substantial amount of residual nicotine.

Patient education
• Tell patient to remove patch and to immediately report a generalized rash or persistent or severe local skin reactions, such as pruritus, edema, or erythema.
• Make sure patient understands that nicotine can evaporate from the transdermal system once it's removed from its protective packaging. Explain that patch should be applied promptly after removing protective packaging.
• Caution patient not to alter the patch (by folding or cutting, for example) before applying it.
• Tell patient not to store patch at temperatures above 86° F (30° C).
• Teach patient how to dispose of transdermal system by removing it and folding it in half by bringing the adhesive sides together. If the system comes in a protective pouch, tell patient to dispose of used patch in the pouch that contained the new system. Stress that careful disposal is necessary to prevent accidental poisoning of children or pets.
• Make sure patient reads and understands the information dispensed with drug.
• Urge patient not to smoke while using the system because increased nicotine levels could cause adverse effects.
• Explain that patient is likely to experience nasal irritation, which may become less bothersome with continued use of Nicotrol NS.

• Warn patient to keep used and unused transdermal systems and metered spray bottles safely out of the reach of children and pets.

nicotine polacrilex (nicotine resin complex)
Nicorette, Nicorette DS

Pharmacologic classification: nicotinic agonist
Therapeutic classification: smoking cessation aid
Pregnancy risk category: X

Indications and dosages
➤ *Aid in managing nicotine dependence.*
Serves as a temporary aid to smokers seeking to give up smoking while participating in a behavior modification program under medical supervision. Generally, a smoker with the physical type of nicotine dependence is most likely to benefit from use of nicotine chewing gum. *Adults:* One piece of gum chewed slowly and intermittently for 30 minutes whenever the urge to smoke occurs. Most patients need about 9 to 12 pieces of gum daily during first month. Patients using the 2-mg strength shouldn't exceed 24 pieces of gum daily if unsupervised or 30 pieces if supervised; those using the 4-mg strength shouldn't exceed 24 pieces of gum daily.

How supplied
Available with and without a prescription
Chewing gum: 2 mg or 4 mg nicotine resin complex per square

Pharmacodynamics
Nicotine replacement action: Nicotine is an agonist at the nicotinic receptors in the peripheral nervous system and CNS and produces both behavioral stimulation and depression. It acts on the adrenal medulla to aid in overcoming physical dependence on nicotine during withdrawal from habitual smoking.

Pharmacokinetics
Absorption: Bound to ion-exchange resin and released only during chewing. Blood level depends on the vigor with which gum is chewed.
Distribution: Distribution into tissues hasn't been fully characterized. It crosses the placenta and appears in breast milk.
Metabolism: Metabolized mainly by the liver, less so by the kidneys and lungs. Main metabolites are cotinine and nicotine-19-N-oxide.
Excretion: Both nicotine and its metabolites are excreted in urine, with about 10% to 20% excreted unchanged. Excretion of nicotine is increased in acid urine and by high urine output.

Route	Onset	Peak	Duration
P.O.	Unknown	15-30 min	Unknown

Contraindications and precautions

Contraindicated in nonsmokers, pregnant patients, and patients with recent MI, life-threatening arrhythmias, severe or worsening angina pectoris, or active temporomandibular joint disease.

Use cautiously in patients with hyperthyroidism, pheochromocytoma, insulin-dependent diabetes, peptic ulcer disease, a history of esophagitis, oral or pharyngeal inflammation, or dental conditions that might be aggravated by chewing gum.

Interactions

Drug-drug. *Adrenergic agonists, adrenergic blockers:* Nicorette gum and smoking can increase cortisol and catecholamine levels. Dose adjustments may be necessary.
Imipramine, pentazocine, theophylline: Smoking cessation with or without nicotine substitutes may reverse the increased metabolism caused by smoking. Dosage adjustments may be necessary.
Insulin: Smoking cessation may increase insulin absorption. Adjust insulin dosage.
Propoxyphene: Smoking cessation may reduce the first-pass metabolism of propoxyphene. Dose adjustments may be necessary.
Drug-herb. *Blue cohosh:* May increase nicotine effects. Tell patient not to use together.
Drug-food. *Caffeine:* Smoking may increase caffeine metabolism. Monitor patient for effect.
Food and beverages: Inhibited absorption. Advise patient to avoid eating and drinking 15 minutes before and during gum chewing.

Adverse reactions

CNS: dizziness, light-headedness, irritability, insomnia, headache, paresthesia.
CV: atrial fibrillation.
EENT: throat soreness, jaw muscle ache (from chewing).
GI: nausea, vomiting, indigestion, eructation, anorexia, excessive salivation.
Other: hiccups, sweating.

Overdose and treatment

The risk of overdose is minimized by early nausea and vomiting that result from excessive nicotine intake. Poisoning causes nausea, vomiting, salivation, abdominal pain, diarrhea, cold sweats, headache, dizziness, disturbed hearing and vision, mental confusion, and weakness.

Treatment includes emesis—give ipecac syrup if it hasn't occurred. A saline cathartic will speed the passage of gum through the GI tract. Give gastric lavage followed by activated charcoal if patient is unconscious. Provide supportive treatment of respiratory paralysis and CV collapse as needed.

Special considerations

● Patients most likely to benefit from Nicorette gum are smokers with a high physical dependence. Typically, they smoke more than 15 cigarettes daily, prefer high-nicotine brands of cigarettes, usually inhale the smoke, smoke the first cigarette within 30 minutes of arising, and find the first morning cigarette the hardest to give up.
● Patient may reduce dosage by making pieces of gum smaller or by altering the time chewed.
● Smoking cessation typically takes 2 to 3 months with gradual dose reduction.
● Although nicotine replacement therapy isn't recommended in patients with recent MI, it may be considered preferable to cigarette smoking in patients experiencing nicotine withdrawal.
● CV effects of nicotine are usually dependent on dose. Nonsmokers have experienced CNS-mediated symptoms of hiccuping, nausea, and vomiting, even with a small dose. A smoker chewing a 2-mg piece of gum every hour usually doesn't experience CV adverse effects.

Patient monitoring

● Reevaluate patient at least monthly to determine response to therapy.

Breast-feeding patients

● Nicotine appears in breast milk and is readily absorbed after oral use. Weigh infant's risk of exposure to nicotine from transdermal patch against risk of exposure from continued smoking.

Patient education

● Instruct patient to chew gum slowly and intermittently for about 30 minutes to promote slow and even buccal absorption of nicotine. Fast chewing causes faster absorption and produces more adverse reactions. After about 15 chews, advise the patient to park the gum between the cheek and gum for a few minutes.
● Instruct patient to chew one piece of gum instead of having a cigarette whenever the urge to smoke occurs. Most patients need about 10 pieces of gum daily during the first month of treatment.
● Tell patient who has successfully abstained to gradually withdraw gum use after 3 months; caution against using it for more than 6 months.
● Inform patient that gum is sugar-free and usually doesn't stick to dentures.

nifedipine
Adalat, Adalat CC, Procardia, Procardia XL

Pharmacologic classification: calcium channel blocker
Therapeutic classification: antianginal
Pregnancy risk category: C

Indications and dosages

➤ *Management of Prinzmetal's (variant) angina or chronic stable angina.* **Adults:** Starting dose is 10 mg P.O. t.i.d. Usual effective dosage range is 10 to 20 mg t.i.d. Some patients may need up to 30 mg q.i.d. Or, 30 to 60 mg (extended-release) P.O. daily. Gradually increased at 7- to 14-day intervals or more frequently, if neccssary. Maximum, 180 mg daily for capsules, 120 mg for extended-release tablets.

➤ **Hypertension.** *Adults:* Initially, 30 to 60 mg P.O. once daily (extended-release). Adjust dosage at 7- to 14-day intervals based on patient tolerance and response. Maximum, 120 mg daily.

➤ **Quick reduction of blood pressure** ◇. *Adults:* 10 to 20 mg q 20 to 30 minutes; capsule should be bitten and then swallowed.

How supplied
Available by prescription only
Capsules: 10 mg, 20 mg
Tablets (extended-release): 30 mg, 60 mg, 90 mg

Pharmacodynamics
Antianginal action: Nifedipine dilates systemic arteries, resulting in decreased total peripheral resistance and modestly decreased systemic blood pressure with a slightly increased heart rate, decreased afterload, and increased cardiac index. Reduced afterload and the subsequent decrease in myocardial oxygen consumption probably account for the value of nifedipine in treating chronic stable angina. In Prinzmetal's angina, nifedipine inhibits coronary artery spasm, increasing myocardial oxygen delivery.

Pharmacokinetics
Absorption: About 90% of a dose is absorbed rapidly from the GI tract after oral administration; however, only about 65% to 70% of drug reaches the systemic circulation because of a significant first-pass effect in the liver. Therapeutic serum levels are 25 to 100 ng/ml.
Distribution: About 92% to 98% of circulating nifedipine is bound to plasma proteins.
Metabolism: Metabolized in the liver.
Excretion: Excreted in urine and feces as inactive metabolites. Elimination half-life is 2 to 5 hours.

Route	Onset	Peak	Duration
P.O.			
Regular	20 min	½-1 hr	4-8 hr
Extended	20 min	6 hr	24 hr

Contraindications and precautions
Contraindicated in patients hypersensitive to drug. Use cautiously in elderly patients and patients with heart failure or hypotension.

Use cautiously in patients with unstable angina who aren't currently taking a beta blocker because a higher risk of MI has been reported. Use extended-release form cautiously in patients with GI narrowing.

Interactions
Drug-drug. *Beta blockers:* May worsen angina, heart failure, and hypotension. Use together cautiously.
Cimetidine: May decrease nifedipine metabolism. Use together cautiously.

Digoxin: May increase serum digoxin levels. Monitor serum digoxin level.
Fentanyl: May cause excessive hypotension. Use together cautiously.
Hypotensive drugs: May precipitate excessive hypotension. Use together cautiously.
Phenytoin: May increase phenytoin levels. Monitor phenytoin levels.
Drug-herb. *Melatonin:* Interferes with antihypertensive effect of nifedipine. Discourage use together.
Drug-food. *Grapefruit juice:* Increased bioavailability of drug. Advise patient to avoid taking drug with grapefruit juice.

Adverse reactions
CNS: *dizziness, light-headedness, headache, weakness,* syncope, nervousness.
CV: *peripheral edema,* hypotension, palpitations, *heart failure, MI, flushing.*
EENT: nasal congestion.
GI: *nausea,* diarrhea, constipation, abdominal discomfort.
Hepatic: increased alkaline phosphate, LD, AST, and ALT levels.
Metabolic: hypokalemia.
Musculoskeletal: muscle cramps.
Respiratory: dyspnea, cough, *pulmonary edema.*
Skin: rash, pruritus.
Other: fever.

Overdose and treatment
Effects of overdose are extensions of pharmacologic effects, primarily peripheral vasodilation and hypotension.

Treatment includes such basic support measures as hemodynamic and respiratory monitoring. If patient needs blood pressure support with a vasoconstrictor, norepinephrine may be given. Elevate limbs and correct any fluid deficit.

Special considerations
• Nifedipine has been used investigationally to treat Raynaud's phenomenon and preterm labor.
⚡ **ALERT** Warn patient not to switch brands. Procardia XL and Adalat CC aren't therapeutically equivalent because of major differences in their pharmacokinetics.
• Initial doses and increased dosage may worsen angina briefly. Reassure patient that this effect is temporary.
• Nifedipine isn't available in S.L. form. No advantage has been found in S.L. or intrabuccal use.
• Although rebound effect hasn't been observed when drug is stopped, reduce dosage slowly.

Patient monitoring
• Monitor blood pressure regularly, especially if patient is also taking beta blockers or antihypertensives.

Geriatric patients
● Use drug cautiously in geriatric patients because they may be more sensitive to effects of drug and duration of effect may be prolonged. Orthostatic blood pressures should be monitored.

Patient education
● Instruct patient to swallow capsules whole without breaking, crushing, or chewing them unless instructed otherwise.
● Tell patient that he may experience annoying hypotensive effects early in therapy and during dosage adjustment; urge compliance with therapy.

nimodipine
Nimotop

Pharmacologic classification: calcium channel blocker
Therapeutic classification: cerebral vasodilator
Pregnancy risk category: C

Indications and dosages
➤ *Improvement of neurologic deficits after subarachnoid hemorrhage from ruptured congenital aneurysms. Adults:* 60 mg P.O. q 4 hours for 21 days. Therapy should begin within 96 hours of subarachnoid hemorrhage.
✦ *Dosage adjustment.* In adults with hepatic impairment, 30 mg P.O. q 4 hours.
➤ *Migraine headache◇. Adults:* 120 mg P.O. daily in divided doses, 1 hour before or at least 2 hours after meals.

How supplied
Available by prescription only
Capsules: 30 mg

Pharmacodynamics
Neuronal-sparing action: Inhibits calcium ion influx across cardiac and smooth muscle cells, thus decreasing myocardial contractility and oxygen demand, and dilates coronary arteries and arterioles. Although exact mechanism unknown, it's believed that dilation of the small cerebral resistance vessels with increased collateral circulation is possible.

Pharmacokinetics
Absorption: Well absorbed after oral administration. However, because of extensive first-pass metabolism, bioavailability is only about 3% to 30%.
Distribution: More than 95% protein-bound.
Metabolism: Extensively metabolized in liver. Drug and metabolites undergo enterohepatic recycling.

Excretion: Less than 1% excreted as parent drug. Elimination half-life is 1 to 9 hours.

Route	Onset	Peak	Duration
P.O.	Unknown	1 hr	Unknown

Contraindications and precautions
No known contraindications. Use cautiously in patients with hepatic failure.

Interactions
Drug-drug. *Antihypertensives:* Enhanced hypotensive effect. Monitor patient's blood pressure. *Calcium channel blockers:* May enhance CV effects of these drugs. Monitor patient closely. *Phenytoin:* Increased phenytoin levels. Monitor serum phenytoin levels.
Drug-food. *Food:* Decreased absorption. Give drug 1 hour before or 2 hours after meals.

Adverse reactions
CNS: headache, psychic disturbances.
CV: decreased blood pressure, flushing, edema, tachycardia.
GI: nausea, diarrhea, abdominal discomfort.
Musculoskeletal: muscle cramps.
Respiratory: dyspnea.
Skin: dermatitis, rash.

Overdose and treatment
Overdose may cause nausea, weakness, drowsiness, confusion, bradycardia, and decreased cardiac output. Calcium gluconate I.V. has been used to treat calcium channel blocker overdose.

Special considerations
● Unlike other calcium channel blockers, nimodipine isn't used for angina pectoris or hypertension.
● Use lower doses in patients with hepatic failure. Start therapy at 30 mg P.O. every 4 hours, and closely monitor blood pressure and heart rate.
● If patient can't swallow capsules, puncture ends of liquid-filled capsule with an 18G needle and draw the contents into syringe. Instill dose into patient's nasogastric tube and rinse tube with 30 ml of normal saline solution.

Patient monitoring
● Monitor blood pressure and heart rate in all patients, especially at start of therapy.
● Monitor patient for therapeutic effect.

Pediatric patients
● Safety and efficacy in children haven't been established.

Breast-feeding patients
● Substantial amounts of drug may appear in breast milk. Advise against breast-feeding during therapy.

Reactions may be *common*, uncommon, *life-threatening*, or COMMON AND LIFE-THREATENING.

Patient education
● Advise patient to rise from supine position slowly to avoid dizziness and hypotension, especially at start of therapy.
● Food decreases absorption. Advise patient to take drug 1 hour before or 2 hours after meals.

nisoldipine
Sular

Pharmacologic classification: calcium channel blocker
Therapeutic classification: antihypertensive
Pregnancy risk category: C

Indications and dosages
➤ *Hypertension. Adults:* Initially, 20 mg P.O. once daily; then increased by 10 mg/week or at longer intervals, p.r.n. Usual maintenance dosage, 20 to 40 mg once daily. Don't exceed 60 mg daily.
✦ *Dosage adjustment.* In patients over age 65 and those with hepatic dysfunction, give starting dose of 10 mg P.O. once daily. Monitor blood pressure closely during dosage adjustment.

How supplied
Available by prescription only
Tablets (extended-release): 10 mg, 20 mg, 30 mg, 40 mg

Pharmacodynamics
Antihypertensive action: Nisoldipine prevents the entry of calcium ions into vascular smooth muscle cells, causing dilation of the arterioles, which in turn decreases peripheral vascular resistance.

Pharmacokinetics
Absorption: Relatively well absorbed from GI tract. High-fat foods significantly affect release of drug from the coat-core formulation.
Distribution: About 99% is bound to plasma protein.
Metabolism: Extensively metabolized with five major metabolites identified.
Excretion: Excreted in urine; half-life ranges from 7 to 12 hours.

Route	Onset	Peak	Duration
P.O.	Unknown	6-12 hr	24 hr

Contraindications and precautions
Contraindicated in patients hypersensitive to dihydropyridine calcium channel blockers. Use cautiously in patients receiving beta blockers or in those who have compromised ventricular or hepatic function and heart failure.

Interactions
Drug-drug. *Cimetidine:* Increased bioavailability and peak level of nisoldipine. Use together cautiously.

Quinidine: Decreased bioavailability but not peak level of nisoldipine. Monitor blood pressure.
Drug-food. *High-fat meals:* May decrease drug absorption. Advise patient not to take drug with these foods.
Grapefruit juice: Increased levels and pharmacologic effect of nisoldipine. Avoid use together.

Adverse reactions
CNS: *headache,* dizziness.
CV: vasodilation, palpitations, chest pain, *peripheral edema.*
EENT: pharyngitis, sinusitis.
GI: nausea.
Skin: rash.

Overdose and treatment
Overdose with similar drugs leads to pronounced hypotension. Treatment should focus on CV support, including monitoring of CV and respiratory function, elevation of limbs, and judicious use of calcium infusion, pressor agents, and fluids.

Special considerations
● Extended-release form of drug makes it unsuitable for use in hypertensive emergency.

Patient monitoring
● Monitor patient carefully. Some patients, especially those with severe obstructive coronary artery disease, have increased frequency, duration, or severity of angina or even acute MI after calcium channel blocker therapy starts or dosage increases.
● Monitor blood pressure regularly, especially early in therapy and during dosage adjustment.

Breast-feeding patients
● It isn't known if drug appears in breast milk. Use of drug in breast-feeding women isn't recommended.

Pediatric patients
● Safety and efficacy in children haven't been established.

Geriatric patients
● Elderly patients may have two- to three-fold higher plasma levels than younger patients, requiring cautious dosing.

Patient education
● Tell patient to take drug exactly as prescribed, even if he feels better.
● Advise patient to swallow tablet whole and not to chew, divide, or crush tablets unless instructed otherwise.
● Tell patient not to take drug with a high-fat meal or with grapefruit products.
● Advise patient to rise slowly from supine position to avoid dizziness and hypotension, especially at beginning of therapy.

nitrofurantoin macrocrystals
Macrobid, Macrodantin

nitrofurantoin microcrystals
Furadantin

Pharmacologic classification: nitrofuran
Therapeutic classification: urinary tract anti-infective
Pregnancy risk category: B

Indications and dosages
➤ *Initial or recurrent urinary tract infections caused by susceptible organisms.*
Adults and children over age 12: 50 to 100 mg P.O. q.i.d. or 100 mg dual-release capsules q 12 hours for 7 days.
Children ages 1 month to 12 years: 5 to 7 mg/kg/24 hours P.O. daily, divided q.i.d.
➤ *Long-term suppression therapy. Adults:* 50 to 100 mg P.O. daily h.s. as a single dose.
Children: As low as 1 mg/kg daily P.O. in a single dose or two divided doses.

How supplied
Available by prescription only
macrocrystals
Capsules: 25 mg, 50 mg, 100 mg
Capsules (dual-release): 100 mg
microcrystals
Suspension: 25 mg/5 ml

Pharmacodynamics
Antibacterial action: Nitrofurantoin has bacteriostatic action at low levels and possible bactericidal action at high levels. Although its exact mechanism of action is unknown, it may inhibit bacterial enzyme systems, interfering with bacterial carbohydrate metabolism. Drug is most active at an acidic pH.

Spectrum of activity includes many common gram-positive and gram-negative urinary pathogens, including *Escherichia coli, Staphylococcus aureus,* enterococci, and certain strains of *Klebsiella,* and *Enterobacter.* Organisms that usually resist nitrofurantoin include *Acinetobacter, Proteus, Providencia, Pseudomonas,* and *Serratia.*

Pharmacokinetics
Absorption: When administered orally, drug is well absorbed (mainly by the small intestine) from GI tract. Presence of food aids dissolution of drug and speeds absorption. The macrocrystal form exhibits slower dissolution and absorption; it causes less GI distress.
Distribution: Crosses into bile and placenta. 60% binds to plasma proteins. Plasma half-life is about 20 minutes. Urine levels peak in about 30 minutes when drug is given as microcrystals, somewhat later when given as macrocrystals.
Metabolism: Metabolized partially in the liver.

Excretion: About 30% to 50% of dose is eliminated by glomerular filtration and tubular secretion into urine as unchanged drug within 24 hours. Some drug may appear in breast milk.

Route	Onset	Peak	Duration
P.O.	Unknown	Unknown	Unknown

Contraindications and precautions
Contraindicated in pregnant women at term (38 to 42 weeks' gestation). Also contraindicated during labor and delivery and when the onset of labor is imminent. Contraindicated in children age 1 month and under and in patients with moderate to severe renal impairment, anuria, oliguria, or creatinine clearance under 60 ml/minute.

Use cautiously in patients with impaired renal function, anemia, diabetes mellitus, electrolyte abnormalities, vitamin B deficiency, debilitating disease, or G6PD deficiency.

Interactions
Drug-drug. *Magnesium trisilicate antacids:* May decrease nitrofurantoin absorption. Separate administration times.
Probenecid, sulfinpyrazone: Reduced renal excretion of nitrofurantoin. Monitor patient for increased toxicity and decreased clinical effect.
Quinolone derivatives, such as cinoxacin, ciprofloxacin, nalidixic acid, and norfloxacin: May antagonize anti-infective effects. Monitor patient for decreased clinical effect.
Drug-food. *Food:* Enhances bioavailability of nitrofurantoin. Give drug with food.

Adverse reactions
CNS: *peripheral neuropathy,* headache, dizziness, drowsiness, *ascending polyneuropathy* (with high doses or renal impairment).
GI: *anorexia, nausea, vomiting,* abdominal pain, *diarrhea.*
GU: overgrowth of nonsusceptible organisms in the urinary tract.
Hematologic: *hemolysis in patients with G6PD deficiency* (reversed after stopping drug), *agranulocytosis, thrombocytopenia.*
Hepatic: *hepatitis, hepatic necrosis,* elevated bilirubin and alkaline phosphatase.
Metabolic: decreased serum glucose.
Respiratory: *pulmonary sensitivity reactions* (cough, chest pain, fever, chills, dyspnea, pulmonary infiltration with consolidation or pleural effusion), *asthmatic attacks in patients with history of asthma.*
Skin: maculopapular, erythematous, or eczematous eruption; pruritus; urticaria; *exfoliative dermatitis; Stevens-Johnson syndrome,* transient alopecia.
Other: *hypersensitivity reactions (anaphylaxis),* drug fever.

Overdose and treatment
Acute overdose may result in nausea and vomiting. Treat symptomatically. No specific antidote

is known. Increase fluid intake to promote urinary excretion of drug. Nitrofurantoin is dialyzable.

Special considerations
• Obtain culture and sensitivity tests before starting therapy, and repeat as needed.
• Oral suspension may be mixed with water, milk, fruit juice, and formulas.
• Drug may turn urine brown or rust-yellow.
• Continue treatment for at least 3 days after sterile urine specimens have been obtained.
• Long-term therapy may cause overgrowth of nonsusceptible organisms, especially *Pseudomonas*.
• Nitrofurantoin may cause false-positive results in urine glucose tests using cupric sulfate reagents (such as Benedict's test, Fehling's solution, or Clinitest) because it reacts with these reagents.

Patient monitoring
• Monitor CBC regularly.
• Monitor fluid intake and output and pulmonary status.

Breast-feeding patients
• Safety hasn't been established. Although drug appears in low levels in breast milk, no adverse reactions have been reported except in infants with G6PD deficiency, in whom hemolytic anemia may develop.

Pediatric patients
• Contraindicated in infants under age 1 month because their immature enzyme systems increase the risk of hemolytic anemia.

Patient education
• Instruct patient to take drug with food or milk to minimize GI distress. Have patient report any unpleasant side effects.
• Caution patient that drug may cause false-positive results in urine glucose tests using cupric sulfate reduction method (Clinitest) but not in glucose oxidase test (glucose enzymatic test strip, Diastix, or Chemstrip uG).
• Emphasize that bedtime dose is important because drug will remain in bladder longer.
• Warn patient that drug may turn urine brown or rust-yellow.

nitrofurazone
Furacin

Pharmacologic classification: synthetic antibacterial nitrofuran derivative
Therapeutic classification: topical antibacterial
Pregnancy risk category: C

Indications and dosages
➤ *Adjunct for major burns (especially when resistance to other anti-infectives occurs); prevention of skin graft infection before or after surgery.* Adults and children: Apply directly to lesion or to dressings used to cover affected area daily or as indicated, depending on severity of burn. Apply once daily or every few days, depending on dressing technique.

How supplied
Available by prescription only
Cream: 0.2%
Ointment: 0.2% soluble dressing
Topical solution: 0.2%

Pharmacodynamics
Antibacterial action: Exact mechanism of action is unknown. However, it appears that drug inhibits bacterial enzymes involved in carbohydrate metabolism. Nitrofurazone has a broad spectrum of activity against gram-positive and gram-negative organisms.

Pharmacokinetics
Absorption: Limited drug absorption with topical use.
Distribution: None.
Metabolism: None.
Excretion: None.

Route	Onset	Peak	Duration
Topical	Unknown	Unknown	Unknown

Contraindications and precautions
Contraindicated in patients hypersensitive to drug. Use cautiously in patients with known or suspected renal impairment.

Interactions
None reported.

Adverse reactions
Skin: *erythema, pruritus,* burning, edema, severe reactions (vesiculation, denudation, ulceration), *allergic contact dermatitis.*

Overdose and treatment
Discontinue use and cleanse area with mild soap and water.

Special considerations
• Investigationally, drug has been administered orally for the treatment of refractory African trypanosomiasis, acute bacillary dysentry, and testicular tumors. Diluted nitrofurazone solution with 6 to 10 parts of sterile water has been used for bladder irrigation.
• Avoid contact with eyes and mucous membranes.
• If undiluted solution is cloudy, warm to 122° to 140° F (50° to 60° C).
• Prepare solutions for wet dressings by diluting nitrofurazone solution with distilled water (equal parts of each).

• Use diluted solutions within 24 hours after preparation; discard diluted solution that becomes cloudy.

Patient monitoring
• Monitor patient for overgrowth of nonsusceptible organisms, including fungi and *Pseudomonas*.

Breast-feeding patients
• Safety in breast-feeding women hasn't been established. Potential benefits to woman must be weighed against risks to infant.

Patient education
• Teach patient proper application of drug and to apply directly on lesion or place on gauze.
• Tell patient to avoid exposure of drug to direct sunlight, excessive heat, strong fluorescent lighting, and alkaline materials.

---

nitroglycerin (glyceryl trinitrate)

Oral, extended-release
Nitro-Bid, Nitroglyn, Nitrong

Sublingual
NitroQuick, Nitrostat

Translingual
Nitrolingual

I.V.
Nitro-Bid IV, Tridil

Topical
Nitro-Bid, Nitrol

Transdermal
Deponit, Minitran, Nitro-Derm, Nitrodisc, Nitro-Dur, Transderm-Nitro

Transmucosal
Nitrogard

Pharmacologic classification: nitrate
Therapeutic classification: antianginal, vasodilator
Pregnancy risk category: C

Indications and dosages
➤ **Prophylaxis against chronic anginal attacks.** *Adults:* 2.5 to 9 mg P.O. q 8 to 12 hours. Or, ½ inch of 2% ointment, increasing in ½-inch increments until desired effect is achieved. Range of dosage with ointment is 0.5 to 4 inches q 4 to 6 hours. Usual dose is 1 to 2 inches. Or, transdermal disc or pad may be applied to hairless site once daily. However, to prevent tolerance, topical forms shouldn't be worn overnight.

➤ **Relief of acute angina pectoris, prophylaxis to prevent or minimize anginal attacks when taken immediately before stressful events.** *Adults:* One S.L. tablet dissolved under the tongue or in the buccal pouch immediately after onset of anginal attack. May repeat q 5 minutes for 15 to 30 minutes for a maximum of three doses. Or, using Nitrolingual spray, spray one or two doses into mouth, preferably onto or under the tongue. May repeat q 3 to 5 minutes to a maximum of three doses within a 15-minute period. Or, transmucosally, 1 to 3 mg q 3 to 5 hours during waking hours.

➤ **Hypertension, heart failure, angina.** Nitroglycerin is indicated to control hypertension related to surgery, to treat heart failure caused by MI, to relieve angina pectoris in acute situations, and to produce controlled hypotension during surgery (by I.V. infusion). *Adults:* Initial infusion rate is 5 mcg/minute. May be increased by 5 mcg/minute q 3 to 5 minutes until a response is noted. If a 20-mcg/minute rate does not produce desired response, dosage may be increased by as much as 10 to 20 mcg/minute q 3 to 5 minutes.

➤ **Acute MI.** *Adults:* Initially, 12.5 to 25 mcg I.V. followed by an infusion at 10 to 20 mcg/minute; increase 5 to 10 mcg/minute q 5 to 10 minutes as needed. Maximum dose is 200 mcg/minute. Decrease or discontinue if mean arterial pressure is under 80 mm Hg or systolic blood pressure under 90 mm Hg.

➤ **Hypertensive crisis◇.** *Adults:* Infuse at 5 to 100 mcg/minute I.V.

How supplied
Available by prescription only
Aerosol (lingual): 0.4 mg/metered spray
Capsules (sustained-release): 2.5 mg, 6.5 mg, 9 mg, 13 mg
I.V.: 0.5 mg/ml, 0.8 mg/ml, 5 mg/ml
I.V. premixed solutions in dextrose: 100 mcg/ml, 200 mcg/ml, 400 mcg/ml
Tablets (buccal, controlled-release): 1 mg, 2 mg, 3 mg
Tablets (S.L.): 0.15 mg, 0.3 mg, 0.4 mg, 0.6 mg
Topical: 2% ointment
Transdermal: 0.1-mg, 0.2-mg, 0.3-mg, 0.4-mg, 0.6-mg/hour systems, 0.8-mg/hour systems

Pharmacodynamics
Antianginal action: Nitroglycerin relaxes vascular smooth muscle of both the venous and arterial beds, resulting in a net decrease in myocardial oxygen consumption. It also dilates coronary vessels, leading to redistribution of blood flow to ischemic tissue. Systemic and coronary vascular effects of drug, which may vary slightly with the various nitroglycerin forms, probably account for its value in treating angina.
Vasodilating action: Nitroglycerin dilates peripheral vessels, making it useful (in I.V. form) in producing controlled hypotension during surgical procedures and in controlling blood pres-

---

sure in perioperative hypertension. Because peripheral vasodilation decreases venous return to the heart (preload), nitroglycerin also helps to treat pulmonary edema and heart failure. Arterial vasodilation decreases arterial impedance (afterload), thereby decreasing left ventricular work and aiding the failing heart. These combined effects may prove valuable in treating some patients with acute MI.

Pharmacokinetics

Absorption: Well-absorbed from the GI tract. However, because it undergoes first-pass metabolism in the liver, it's incompletely absorbed into the systemic circulation. Onset of action for oral preparations is slow (except for S.L. tablets). After S.L. administration, absorption from the oral mucosa is relatively complete. Nitroglycerin also is well absorbed after topical administration as an ointment or transdermal system.

Distribution: Distributed widely throughout the body. About 60% of circulating drug is bound to plasma proteins.

Metabolism: Metabolized in the liver and serum to 1,3 glyceryl dinitrate; 1,2 glyceryl dinitrate; and glyceryl mononitrate. Dinitrate metabolites have a slight vasodilatory effect.

Excretion: Metabolites are excreted in urine; elimination half-life is about 1 to 4 minutes.

Route	Onset	Peak	Duration
P.O.	20-45 min	Unknown	3-8 hr
Buccal	3 min	Unknown	3-5 hr
S.L.	1-3 min	Unknown	½-1 hr
I.V.	Immediate	Immediate	3-5 min
Translingual	2-4 min	Unknown	½-1 hr
Topical	30 min	Unknown	2-12 hr
Transdermal	30 min	Unknown	24 hr

Contraindications and precautions

Contraindicated in patients hypersensitive to nitrates and in those with early MI (S.L. form), severe anemia, increased intracranial pressure, angle-closure glaucoma, orthostatic hypotension, and allergy to adhesives (transdermal form). I.V. form is contraindicated in patients hypersensitive to I.V. form, cardiac tamponade, restrictive cardiomyopathy, or constrictive pericarditis. Extended-release preparations shouldn't be used in patients with organic or functional GI hypermotility or malabsorption syndrome.

Use cautiously in patients with hypotension or volume depletion.

Interactions

Drug-drug. *Antihypertensives, phenothiazines:* May cause additive hypotensive effects. Use together cautiously.

Ergot alkaloids: May precipitate angina. Avoid use together.

Sildenafil: Potentiates hypotensive effects of nitrates. Don't use together.

Drug-lifestyle. *Alcohol use:* May cause additive hypotensive effects. Discourage use together.

Adverse reactions

CNS: *headache, sometimes with throbbing; dizziness;* weakness.

CV: *orthostatic hypotension, tachycardia, flushing, palpitations,* fainting.

GI: nausea, vomiting, sublingual burning.

Skin: cutaneous vasodilation, contact dermatitis (patch), rash.

Other: *hypersensitivity reactions.*

Overdose and treatment

Effects of overdose result primarily from vasodilation and methemoglobinemia and include hypotension, persistent throbbing headache, palpitations, visual disturbances, flushing of the skin, sweating (with skin later becoming cold and cyanotic), nausea and vomiting, colic, bloody diarrhea, orthostasis, initial hyperpnea, dyspnea, slow respiratory rate, bradycardia, heart block, increased intracranial pressure with confusion, fever, paralysis, tissue hypoxia (from methemoglobinemia) leading to cyanosis, and metabolic acidosis, coma, clonic seizures, and circulatory collapse. Death may result from circulatory collapse or asphyxia.

Treatment includes gastric lavage followed by administration of activated charcoal to remove remaining gastric contents. Monitor blood gas measurements and methemoglobin levels, as indicated. Supportive care includes respiratory support and oxygen administration, passive movement of the limbs to aid venous return, and recumbent positioning.

Special considerations

⚠ ALERT Don't confuse Nitro-Bid with Nicobid or nitroglycerin with nitroprusside.

● Ask all patients about the use of sildenafil (Viagra) before using nitrates.

● Use only S.L. and translingual forms to relieve acute anginal attack.

● S.L. dose may be taken before anticipated stress or at bedtime if angina is nocturnal.

● To apply ointment, spread in uniform thin layer to hairless part of skin except distal parts of arms or legs, because absorption won't be maximal at these sites. Don't rub in. Cover with plastic film to aid absorption and to protect clothing. If using Tape-Surrounded Appli-Ruler (TSAR) system, keep TSAR on skin to protect patient's clothing and ensure that ointment remains in place. If serious adverse effects develop in patients using ointment or transdermal system, remove product at once or wipe ointment from skin. Be sure to avoid contact with ointment.

● Remove transdermal patch before defibrillation. Aluminum backing may cause patch to explode when exposed to electric current.

• When terminating transdermal nitroglycerin treatment for angina, gradually reduce dosage and frequency of application over 4 to 6 weeks.
• Administration as I.V. infusion requires special nonabsorbent tubing supplied by manufacturer; regular plastic tubing may absorb up to 80% of drug. Prepare infusion in a glass bottle or container.
• If drug causes headache, which is especially likely with early doses, aspirin or acetaminophen may be indicated. Dosage may need to be reduced temporarily.
• Drug may cause orthostatic hypotension. To minimize it, patient should change to upright position slowly, move up and down stairs carefully, and lie down at the first sign of dizziness.
• To prevent withdrawal symptoms, reduce dosage gradually after long-term use of oral or topical preparations.
• Nitrate tolerance may develop.
• Nitroglycerin may interfere with serum cholesterol determination tests using the Zlatkis-Zak color reaction, resulting in falsely decreased values.

Patient monitoring
• When administering drug to patients during initial days after acute MI, monitor hemodynamic and clinical status carefully.
• Monitor blood pressure and intensity and duration of patient's response to drug.

Pediatric patients
• Methemoglobinemia may occur in infants receiving large doses of nitroglycerin.

Patient education
• Instruct patient to take drug regularly, if prescribed, and to keep S.L. form accessible at all times. Drug is physiologically necessary but not addictive.
• Teach patient to take oral tablet on empty stomach, either 30 minutes before or 1 to 2 hours after meals, to swallow oral tablets whole, and to chew chewable tablets thoroughly before swallowing.
• Instruct patient to take S.L. tablet at first sign of anginal attack. Tell him to wet tablet with saliva, place it under the tongue until completely absorbed, and sit down and rest. If no relief occurs after three tablets, he should call for help or go to a hospital emergency room. If he complains of tingling sensation with S.L. form, he may try holding tablet in buccal pouch.
• Advise patient to store S.L. tablets in original container or other container specifically approved for this use away from heat and light. Tell him to keep cap to bottle tightly closed.
• Instruct patient to place transmucosal tablet under upper lip or in buccal pouch, to let it dissolve slowly over a 3- to 5-hour period, and not to chew or swallow tablet. Advise him that dissolution rate may increase if he touches tablet with tongue or drinks hot liquids.

• If patient is receiving nitroglycerin lingual aerosol (Nitrolingual), instruct him how to use this device correctly. Remind him not to inhale spray but to release it onto or under the tongue. Also tell him not to swallow immediately after administering the spray but to wait about 10 seconds before swallowing.
• Caution patient to use care when wearing transdermal patch near a microwave oven because leaking radiation may heat metallic backing of patch and cause burns.
• Warn patient that headache may follow initial doses but that this symptom may respond to usual headache remedies or dosage reduction (dosage should be reduced only with medical approval). Assure patient that headache usually subsides gradually with continued treatment.
• Instruct patient to avoid alcohol while taking drug because severe hypotension and CV collapse may occur.
• Warn patient that drug may cause dizziness or flushing and that he should move to an upright position slowly.
• Tell patient to report blurred vision, dry mouth, or persistent headache.

---

nitroprusside sodium
Nipride*, Nitropress

Pharmacologic classification: vasodilator
Therapeutic classification: antihypertensive
Pregnancy risk category: C

Indications and dosages
➤ *Hypertensive emergencies. Adults and children:* Initial dose is 0.25 to 3 mcg/kg/minute by I.V. infusion titrated to blood pressure, with a range of 0.3 to 10 mcg/kg/minute. Maximum infusion rate is 10 mcg/kg/minute for 10 minutes. If an adequate blood pressure response isn't achieved at this rate, discontinue infusion.
➤ *Acute heart failure. Adults and children:* I.V. infusion titrated to cardiac output and systemic blood pressure. Same dosage range as for hypertensive emergencies.

How supplied
Available by prescription only
Injection: 50 mg/2-ml, 50 mg/5-ml vials

Pharmacodynamics
Antihypertensive action: Nitroprusside acts directly on vascular smooth muscle, causing peripheral vasodilation.

Pharmacokinetics
Absorption: Administered by I.V. route. I.V. infusion of nitroprusside reduces blood pressure almost immediately.
Distribution: Unknown.
Metabolism: Metabolized rapidly in erythrocytes and tissues to a cyanide radical and then converted to thiocyanate in the liver.

Excretion: Excreted primarily as metabolites in urine. Blood pressure returns to pretreatment level 1 to 10 minutes after completion of infusion.

Route	Onset	Peak	Duration
I.V.	Immediate	Unknown	10 min

Contraindications and precautions

Contraindicated in patients hypersensitive to drug and in those with compensatory hypertension (as in arteriovenous shunt or coarctation of the aorta), inadequate cerebral circulation, congenital optic atrophy, or tobacco-induced amblyopia.

Use cautiously in patients with renal or hepatic disease, increased intracranial pressure, hypothyroidism, hyponatremia, or low vitamin B_{12} levels.

Interactions

Drug-drug. *Antihypertensives:* May potentiate antihypertensive effects of nitroprusside. Use together cautiously.

General anesthetics, particularly enflurane and halothane: Potentiated hypotensive effects. Patient requires careful blood pressure monitoring.

Pressor agents such as epinephrine: May cause an increase in blood pressure during nitroprusside therapy. Monitor blood pressure carefully.

Sildenafil: Potentiates hypotensive effects of nitrates. Don't use together.

Adverse reactions

CNS: *headache, dizziness, loss of consciousness, apprehension, increased intracranial pressure, restlessness.*

CV: *bradycardia, hypotension, tachycardia, palpitations, ECG changes,* flushing.

GI: *nausea, abdominal pain, ileus.*

GU: *increased serum creatinine.*

Metabolic: *acidosis, methemoglobinemia, hypothyroidism.*

Musculoskeletal: *muscle twitching.*

Skin: pink color, rash, diaphoresis.

Other: *thiocyanate toxicity, cyanide toxicity, venous streaking, irritation at infusion site.*

Overdose and treatment

Signs and symptoms of overdose include the adverse reactions listed above and increased tolerance to the antihypertensive effects of drug.

Treat overdose by giving nitrites to induce methemoglobin formation. Discontinue drug and give amyl nitrite inhalations for 15 to 30 seconds each minute until a 3% sodium nitrite solution can be prepared. Give amyl nitrite cautiously to minimize risk of additional hypotension secondary to vasodilation. Then give the sodium nitrite solution by I.V. infusion at no more than 2.5 to 5 ml/minute up to a total dose of 10 to 15 ml. Follow with I.V. sodium thiosulfate infusion (12.5 g in 50 ml of D_5W solution) over 10 minutes. If necessary, repeat infusions of sodium nitrite and sodium thiosulfate at half the initial doses. Further treatment involves symptomatic and supportive care.

Special considerations

- Ask all patients about the use of sildenafil (Viagra) before giving nitrates.
- Drug may be used to produce controlled hypotension during anesthesia, to reduce bleeding from surgical procedure.
- Hypertensive patients are more sensitive to nitroprusside than normotensive patients. Also, patients taking other antihypertensive drugs are extremely sensitive to nitroprusside. Nitroprusside has been used in patients with acute MI, refractory heart failure, and severe mitral regurgitation.
- The goal of therapy is to reduce the mean arterial pressure by 25% within minutes to 2 hours.
- Prepare solution using D_5W solution; don't use bacteriostatic water for injection or sterile saline solution for reconstitution; because of light sensitivity, foil-wrap I.V. solution (but not tubing). Fresh solutions have faint brownish tint; discard after 24 hours.
- The concentrated solution is further diluted in 250, 500, or 1,000 ml 5% dextrose injection to produce 200, 100, or 50 mcg/ml, respectively.
- Infuse drug with infusion pump.
- Drug is best run piggyback through a peripheral line with no other medications; don't adjust rate of main I.V. line while drug is running because even small boluses can cause severe hypotension.

Patient monitoring

- Monitor blood pressure at least every 5 minutes at start of infusion and every 15 minutes thereafter during infusion.
- Nitroprusside can cause cyanide toxicity; therefore, check serum thiocyanate levels every 72 hours. Levels above 100 mcg/ml are linked to cyanide toxicity, which can produce profound hypotension, metabolic acidosis, dyspnea, ataxia, and vomiting. If such symptoms occur, discontinue infusion and reevaluate therapy. Keep cyanide antidote available.

Breast-feeding patients

- It isn't known if drug appears in breast milk; administer cautiously to breast-feeding women.

Geriatric patients

- These patients may be more sensitive to antihypertensive effects of drug.

Patient education

- Advise patient to report CNS symptoms, such as headache or dizziness, promptly.

nizatidine
Axid, Axid AR

Pharmacologic classification: H₂-receptor
antagonist
Therapeutic classification: antiulcer
Pregnancy risk category: B

Indications and dosages
➤ *Treatment of active duodenal ulcer,
gastric ulcer.* Adults: 300 mg P.O. once daily
h.s. Or, 150 mg P.O. b.i.d. for up to 8 weeks.
➤ *Maintenance therapy for duodenal ulcer patients.* Adults: 150 mg P.O. once daily
h.s. for up to 1 year.
➤ *Gastroesophageal reflux disease.* Adults:
150 mg P.O. b.i.d. up to 12 weeks.
➤ *Heartburn (self-medication).* Adults and
children age 12 and older: One 75-mg capsule
P.O. 30 to 60 minutes before meals; use up to
b.i.d. not to exceed continuous therapy for 2
weeks.
✦ *Dosage adjustment.* In adults with renal impairment, refer to this table.

Creatinine clearance (ml/min)	Active duodenal ulcer	Maintenance
20-50	150 mg/day	150 mg q other day
< 20	150 mg q other day	150 mg q 3 days

How supplied
Available by prescription only
Capsules: 150 mg, 300 mg
Available without a prescription
Capsules: 75 mg

Pharmacodynamics
Antiulcer action: Nizatidine is a competitive,
reversible inhibitor of H₂ receptors, particularly those in gastric parietal cells.

Pharmacokinetics
Absorption: Well absorbed (more than 90%)
after oral administration. Absorption may be
slightly enhanced by food, and slightly impaired
by antacids.
Distribution: About 35% is bound to plasma
protein.
Metabolism: Probably undergoes hepatic metabolism. About 40% of excreted drug is metabolized; the remainder is excreted unchanged.
Excretion: More than 90% of an oral dose is excreted in urine within 12 hours. Renal clearance
is about 500 ml/minute, which indicates excretion by active tubular secretion. Less than 6% of
an administered dose is eliminated in the feces.
Elimination half-life is 1 to 2 hours. Moderate to
severe renal impairment significantly prolongs

half-life and decreases clearance of nizatidine.
In anephric persons, half-life is 3½ to 11 hours;
plasma clearance is 7 to 14 L/hour.

Route	Onset	Peak	Duration
P.O.	½ hr	½-3 hr	12 hr

Contraindications and precautions
Contraindicated in patients hypersensitive to H₂-
receptor antagonists. Use cautiously in patients
with impaired renal function.

Interactions
Drug-drug. *High doses of aspirin (3,900 mg
daily) with nizatidine (150 mg twice daily):*
Increased serum salicylate levels. Monitor salicylate levels.
Drug-food. *Tomato-based mixed-vegetable
juices:* May decrease potency of drug when used
together. Advise patient not to use together.

Adverse reactions
CNS: somnolence.
CV: *arrhythmias.*
Hematologic: eosinophilia.
Hepatic: hepatocellular injury, elevated liver
function test results.
Metabolic: hyperuricemia.
Skin: *diaphoresis,* rash, urticaria.
Other: fever.

Overdose and treatment
Expected effects of overdose are cholinergic, including lacrimation, salivation, emesis, miosis,
and diarrhea. Treatment may include use of activated charcoal, emesis, or lavage, with clinical
monitoring and supportive therapy.

Special considerations
● Because drug is excreted primarily by the kidneys, reduce dosage in patients with moderate to
severe renal insufficiency.
● Nizatidine is partially metabolized in the liver.
In patients with normal renal function and uncomplicated hepatic dysfunction, the disposition
of nizatidine is similar to that in patients with normal hepatic function.
● For patients on maintenance therapy, consider
that effects of continuous drug therapy for over
1 year aren't known.
● False-positive tests for urobilinogen may occur
during nizatidine therapy.

Patient monitoring
● Monitor liver function test results in prolonged
therapy.
● Monitor BUN and creatinine levels in patients
with renal impairment.

Breast-feeding patients
● Use cautiously in breast-feeding women. Nizatidine is secreted and concentrated in the milk
of lactating rats.

Reactions may be *common*, uncommon, *life-threatening*, or COMMON AND LIFE-THREATENING.

Pediatric patients
● Safety and efficacy in children haven't been established.

Geriatric patients
● Safety and efficacy appear similar to those in younger patients, but elderly patients tend to have reduced renal function.

Patient education
● Tell patient not to mix drug with tomato-based mixed-vegetable juices.
● Urge patient to avoid cigarette smoking, which can increase gastric acid secretion and worsen disease.
● Advise patient to report abdominal pain and blood in stools or emesis immediately.

---

norepinephrine bitartrate (formerly levarterenol bitartrate)
Levophed

Pharmacologic classification: adrenergic (direct-acting)
Therapeutic classification: vasopressor
Pregnancy risk category: C

Indications and dosages
➤ **To maintain blood pressure in acute hypotensive states.** *Adults:* Initially, 8 to 12 mcg/minute I.V. infusion, adjusted to maintain desired blood pressure. Maintenance dosage, 2 to 4 mcg/minute.
Children: Initially, 2 mcg/minute or 2 mcg/m^2/minute by I.V. infusion, adjusted to maintain desired blood pressure. For advanced cardiac life support, initial infusion rate is 0.1 mcg/kg/minute adjusted to maximum of 2 mcg/kg/min.
➤ **GI bleeding** ◊. *Adults:* 8 mg in 250 ml normal saline solution given intraperitoneally. Or, 8 mg in 100 ml of normal saline solution given via a nasogastric tube q hour for 6 to 8 hours and then q 2 hours for 4 to 6 hours.

How supplied
Available by prescription only
Injection: 1 mg/ml parenteral

Pharmacodynamics
Vasopressor action: Norepinephrine acts mainly by direct stimulation of alpha-adrenergic receptors, constricting both capacitance and resistance blood vessels. This results in increased total peripheral resistance; increased systolic and diastolic blood pressure; decreased blood flow to vital organs, skin, and skeletal muscle; and constriction of renal blood vessels, which reduces renal blood flow. It also has a direct stimulating effect on beta$_1$ receptors of the heart, producing a positive inotropic response. Its main therapeutic effects are vasoconstriction and cardiac stimulation.

Pharmacokinetics
Absorption: Pressor effect occurs rapidly after infusion, is of short duration, and stops within 1 to 2 minutes after infusion is stopped.
Distribution: Localizes in sympathetic nerve tissues. It crosses the placenta but not the blood-brain barrier.
Metabolism: Metabolized in the liver and other tissues to inactive compounds.
Excretion: Excreted in urine primarily as sulfate and glucuronide conjugates. Small amounts are excreted unchanged in urine.

Route	Onset	Peak	Duration
I.V.	Immediate	Immediate	1-2 min after infusion ends

Contraindications and precautions
Contraindicated in patients with mesenteric or peripheral vascular thrombosis, profound hypoxia, hypercapnia, or hypotension resulting from blood volume deficit and during cyclopropane and halothane anesthesia.

Use cautiously in patients with sulfite allergies or in those receiving MAO inhibitors or triptyline- or imipramine-type antidepressants.

Interactions
Drug-drug. *Antihistamines (some), ergot alkaloids (parenteral), guanethidine, MAO inhibitors, methyldopa, oxytocic drugs, tricyclic antidepressants:* Severe, prolonged hypertension. Avoid use together.
Atropine: Blocks the reflex bradycardia caused by norepinephrine and enhances its pressor effects. Use together cautiously.
Beta blockers: Increased risk of hypertension. Propranolol may be used to treat arrhythmias occurring during norepinephrine administration. Use together cautiously.
Furosemide and other diuretics: May decrease arterial responsiveness. Monitor blood pressure for effect.
General anesthetics: Norepinephrine may cause increased arrhythmias. Use together cautiously.

Adverse reactions
CNS: anxiety, weakness, dizziness, tremor, restlessness, insomnia.
CV: *bradycardia, severe hypertension, arrhythmias.*
Respiratory: respiratory difficulties, *asthmatic episodes.*
Other: *anaphylaxis,* irritation or necrosis with extravasation.

Overdose and treatment
Signs and symptoms of overdose include severe hypertension, photophobia, retrosternal or pharyngeal pain, intense sweating, vomiting, cere-

---

bral hemorrhage, seizures, and arrhythmias. Monitor vital signs closely.

Treatment includes supportive and symptomatic measures. Use atropine for reflex bradycardia, phentolamine for extravasation, and propranolol for tachyarrhythmias.

Special considerations
• Correct blood volume depletion before administration. Norepinephrine isn't a substitute for blood, plasma, fluid, or electrolyte replacement.
• Select injection site carefully. Administration by I.V. infusion requires an infusion pump or other device to control flow rate. If possible, infuse into antecubital vein of the arm or the femoral vein. Change injection sites for prolonged therapy. Must be diluted before use with 5% dextrose or with saline (dilution with saline alone isn't recommended). Monitor infusion rate. Withdraw drug gradually; recurrent hypotension may follow abrupt withdrawal.
• Prepare infusion solution by adding 4 mg norepinephrine to 1 L of 5% dextrose. The resulting solution contains 4 mcg/ml.
• To treat extravasation, infiltrate site promptly with 10 to 15 ml saline solution containing 5 to 10 mg phentolamine, using a fine needle.
• Some clinicians add phentolamine (5 to 10 mg) to each liter of infusion solution as a preventive against sloughing, should extravasation occur.
• In patients with previously normal blood pressure, adjust flow rate to maintain blood pressure at low normal (usually 80 to 100 mm Hg systolic); in hypertensive patients, maintain systolic no more than 40 mm Hg below preexisting pressure level.
• Avoid contact of drug with iron salts, alkalies, or oxidizing agents.
• Protect solution from light. Discard solution that's discolored or contains a precipitate.

Patient monitoring
• Observe patient constantly during norepinephrine administration. Obtain baseline blood pressure and pulse before therapy, and repeat every 2 minutes until stabilization. Repeat every 5 minutes during administration.
• In addition to vital signs, monitor patient's mental state, skin temperature of limbs, and skin color (especially earlobes, lips, and nail beds).
• Monitor intake and output. Norepinephrine reduces renal blood flow, which may cause decreased urine output initially.

Pediatric patients
• Use cautiously in children.

Geriatric patients
• Drug hasn't been evaluated systematically in patients age 65 or older. Start with low dose and adjust based on response.

Patient education
• Inform patient of need for frequent monitoring of vital signs.
• Advise patient to report adverse reactions.

---

norethindrone
Micronor, Nor-Q.D.

norethindrone acetate
Aygestin, Norlutate*

Pharmacologic classification: progestin
Therapeutic classification: contraceptive
Pregnancy risk category: X

Indications and dosages
➤ *Amenorrhea, abnormal uterine bleeding, endometriosis. Adults:* 2.5 to 10 mg norethindrone acetate P.O. daily on days 5 to 10 of second half of menstrual cycle.
➤ *Endometriosis. Adults:* 5 mg norethindrone acetate P.O. daily for 14 days; then increase by 2.5 mg/day q 2 weeks up to 15 mg/day. Daily therapy may be continued consecutively for 6 to 9 months; if breakthrough bleeding occurs, temporarily discontinue therapy.
➤ *Contraception. Adults:* 0.35 mg norethindrone P.O. daily, beginning day 1 of menstrual cycle and continuing uninterrupted thereafter.

How supplied
Available by prescription only
norethindrone
Tablets: 0.35 mg
norethindrone acetate
Tablets: 5 mg

Pharmacodynamics
Contraceptive action: Norethindrone suppresses ovulation, causes thickening of cervical mucus, and induces sloughing of the endometrium.

Pharmacokinetics
Absorption: Well absorbed after oral administration.
Distribution: Distributed into bile and breast milk and is about 80% protein-bound.
Metabolism: Primarily metabolized in the liver, where it undergoes extensive first-pass metabolism.
Excretion: Excreted primarily in feces. Elimination half-life is 5 to 14 hours.

Route	Onset	Peak	Duration
P.O.	Unknown	Unknown	Unknown

Contraindications and precautions
Contraindicated in pregnant patients, patients hypersensitive to drug, and patients with thromboembolic disorders, cerebral apoplexy, or history of these conditions; breast cancer;

---

undiagnosed abnormal vaginal bleeding; severe hepatic disease; or missed abortion.

Use cautiously in patients with diabetes mellitus, seizures, migraine, cardiac or renal disease, asthma, or mental depression.

Interactions
Drug-drug. *Bromocriptine:* Amenorrhea or galactorrhea, which interferes with the action of bromocriptine. Don't use together.

Adverse reactions
CNS: depression.
CV: thrombophlebitis, edema, ***thromboembolism, CVA.***
EENT: exophthalmos, diplopia, retinal thrombosis.
GU: breakthrough bleeding, dysmenorrhea, amenorrhea, cervical erosion, abnormal secretions.
Hepatic: cholestatic jaundice.
Metabolic: changes in weight, decreased pregnanediol excretion, increased serum alkaline phosphatase and amino acid levels, decreased glucose tolerance.
Respiratory: ***pulmonary embolism.***
Skin: melasma, rash, acne, pruritus.
Other: breast tenderness, enlargement, or secretion.

Overdose and treatment
No information available.

Special considerations
⚠ ALERT Don't confuse Micronor with Micro K or Micronase.
⚠ ALERT Norethindrone acetate is twice as potent as norethindrone. Norethindrone acetate shouldn't be used for contraception.
• Use as a test for pregnancy isn't appropriate; drug may cause birth defects and masculinization of female fetus.
• Preliminary estrogen treatment is usually needed in menstrual disorders.

Patient monitoring
• Monitor liver function test results in patients with hepatic impairment.
• Observe patient for signs of edema.
• Monitor blood pressure.

Patient education
• Explain possible adverse effects of progestins before patient takes first dose. Also, urge patient to carefully read package insert before taking drug.
• Tell patient to take drug at same time every day when used as a contraceptive.
⚠ ALERT Tell patient to report unusual symptoms immediately and to stop drug and notify prescriber about visual disturbances or migraine.
• Teach woman how to perform routine breast self-examination.
• Tell patient to report suspected pregnancy.

• Tell patient with visual disturbances or migraine to stop drug and notify prescriber immediately.
• If using as a method of contraception, tell patient that risk of pregnancy increases with each tablet missed. If she misses one tablet, tell her to take it as soon as she remembers and then take the next tablet at the regular time. If she misses two tablets, tell her to take one as soon as she remembers, take the next regular dose at the usual time, and use a nonhormonal method of contraception in addition to norgestrel until 14 tablets have been taken. If she misses three or more tablets, tell her to discontinue drug and use a nonhormonal method of contraception until after her menstrual period. Instruct patient to perform a pregnancy test if her menstrual period doesn't occur within 45 days.

---

norfloxacin (ophthalmic)
Chibroxin

Pharmacologic classification: fluoroquinolone
Therapeutic classification: broad-spectrum antibiotic
Pregnancy risk category: C

Indications and dosages
➤ ***Conjunctivitis caused by susceptible strains of bacteria.*** *Adults and children age 1 and older:* 1 or 2 drops in the affected eye q.i.d. for up to 7 days. If condition warrants, 1 to 2 drops may be applied q 2 hours during the waking hours of first 1 to 2 days of treatment.

How supplied
Available by prescription only
Ophthalmic solution: 0.3% in 5-ml containers

Pharmacodynamics
Antibiotic action: Ophthalmic norfloxacin inhibits bacterial DNA gyrase, an enzyme needed for bacterial replication. Drug is bacteriostatic or bactericidal, depending on level.

Pharmacokinetics
Absorption: Systemic absorption of ophthalmic norfloxacin is limited.
Distribution: No information available.
Metabolism: No information available.
Excretion: No information available.

Route	Onset	Peak	Duration
Ophthalmic	Unknown	Unknown	Unknown

Contraindications and precautions
Contraindicated in patients hypersensitive to norfloxacin or other fluoroquinolone antibiotics. Don't inject drug into eye.

Interactions
Drug-food. *Caffeine.* Systemically administered drug interferes with caffeine metabolism. Use cautiously in patients receiving these drugs.

Adverse reactions
EENT: local burning or discomfort, itching, chemosis, photophobia, conjunctival hyperemia, white crystalline precipitates, lid margin crusting, *hypersensitivity reactions.*
GI: nausea, bad or bitter taste.

Overdose and treatment
A topical overdose may be flushed from the eye with warm tap water.

Special considerations
● Drug is indicated for treatment of conjunctivitis when caused by susceptible bacteria. Known susceptible strains include *Acinetobacter calcoaceticus, Aeromonas hydrophila, Haemophilus influenzae, Proteus mirabilis, Serratia marcescens, Staphylococcus aureus, S. epidermidis, S. warnerii, Streptococcus pneumoniae,* and *Pseudomonas aeruginosa.*

Patient monitoring
● Monitor patient for overgrowth of nonsusceptible organisms, including fungi.

Breast-feeding patients
● It isn't known if drug appears in breast milk. Use cautiously in breast-feeding women.

Patient education
● Advise patient to wash hands before and after instilling solution.
● Teach patient how to instill drug correctly. Remind him not to touch the tip of the bottle with his hands or to touch it to the eye or surrounding tissue.
● Instruct patient not to share washcloths or towels with other family members to avoid spreading infection. Tell him not to share drug with others.
● Tell patient to store drug at room temperature and to protect it from light.
● Advise patient not to wear contact lenses during therapy.

norfloxacin (systemic)
Noroxin

Pharmacologic classification: fluoroquinolone
Therapeutic classification: broad-spectrum antibiotic
Pregnancy risk category: C

Indications and dosages
➤ *Complicated and uncomplicated urinary tract infections caused by certain gram-negative and gram-positive bacteria. Adults:* For complicated infection, 400 mg P.O. b.i.d. for 10 to 21 days. For uncomplicated infection, 400 mg P.O. b.i.d. for 3 to 10 days. Don't exceed 800 mg daily.
✦ *Dosage adjustment.* Patients with creatinine clearance less than 30 ml/minute should receive 400 mg/day for appropriate duration of therapy.
➤ *Uncomplicated gonorrhea. Adults:* 800 mg P.O. as a single dose.
➤ *Prostatitis. Adults:* 400 mg P.O. q 12 hours for 28 days.
➤ *Gastroenteritis* ◇. *Adults:* 400 mg P.O. b.i.d. for 5 days.
➤ *Traveler's diarrhea* ◇. *Adults:* 400 mg P.O. b.i.d. for up to 3 days.

How supplied
Available by prescription only
Tablets: 400 mg

Pharmacodynamics
Antibacterial action: Norfloxacin is generally bactericidal. It inhibits DNA gyrase, blocking DNA synthesis. Spectrum of activity includes most aerobic gram-positive and gram-negative urinary pathogens, including *Pseudomonas aeruginosa.*

Pharmacokinetics
Absorption: About 30% to 40% of dose is absorbed from the GI tract; as dose increases, percentage of absorbed drug decreases. Food may reduce absorption.
Distribution: Distributed into renal tissue, liver, gallbladder, prostatic fluid, testicles, seminal fluid, bile, and sputum. From 10% to 15% binds to plasma proteins.
Metabolism: Unknown.
Excretion: Most of systemically absorbed drug is excreted by the kidneys, with about 30% appearing in feces. In patients with normal renal function, plasma half-life is 3 to 4 hours; up to 8 hours in severe renal impairment.

Route	Onset	Peak	Duration
P.O.	Unknown	½-2 hr	Unknown

Contraindications and precautions
Contraindicated in patients hypersensitive to fluoroquinolones. Use cautiously in patients with renal impairment or conditions predisposing them to seizure disorders, such as cerebral arteriosclerosis.

Interactions
Drug-drug. *Antacids:* Decreased absorption. Administer drugs at separate times.
Multivitamins containing divalent or trivalent cations: May interfere with norfloxacin absorption. Separate administration times.
Nitrofurantoin: Antagonizes antibacterial activity of norfloxacin. Monitor patient for clinical effect.

Probenecid: May increase norfloxacin levels. Monitor patient for toxicity.

Warfarin: Prolonged PT. Monitor PT and INR. Monitor patient for increased bruising and bleeding.

Xanthine derivatives, such as aminophylline and theophylline: May increase theophylline level. Monitor patient for xanthine-related toxicities.

Drug-food. *Food:* Interferes with norfloxacin absorption. Give drug 1 hour before or 2 hours after meals.

Drug-lifestyle. *Sun exposure:* May cause photosensitivity reaction. Advise patient to take precautions.

Adverse reactions

CNS: fatigue, somnolence, headache, dizziness, *seizures,* depression, insomnia.
GI: nausea, constipation, flatulence, heartburn, dry mouth, abdominal pain, diarrhea, vomiting, anorexia.
GU: increased serum creatinine and BUN levels, crystalluria.
Hematologic: eosinophilia, *neutropenia,* decreased hematocrit.
Hepatic: transient elevations of AST, ALT, and alkaline phosphatase levels.
Musculoskeletal: back pain, tendinitis.
Skin: photosensitivity.
Other: *hypersensitivity reactions* (rash, *anaphylactoid reaction*), fever, hyperhidrosis.

Overdose and treatment
No information available.

Special considerations
● Obtain culture and sensitivity tests before starting therapy; repeat as needed throughout therapy.
● Patient should be well hydrated before and during therapy to avoid crystalluria.

Patient monitoring
● Monitor baseline and follow-up BUN levels, creatinine clearance, CBC, and liver function tests.
● Observe patient for signs and symptoms of resistant infection or reinfection.

Breast-feeding patients
● Safety in breast-feeding women hasn't been established; alternative feeding method is recommended during treatment with norfloxacin.

Pediatric patients
● Contraindicated in children because animal studies suggest a risk of arthropathy.

Patient education
● Instruct patient to continue taking drug as directed, even if he feels better.
● Advise patient to take drug 1 hour before or 2 hours after meals and antacids.

● Warn patient that drug may cause dizziness that impairs his ability to perform tasks that require alertness and coordination.
● Instruct patient to avoid excessive exposure to sunlight.

norgestrel
Ovrette

Pharmacologic classification: progestin
Therapeutic classification: contraceptive
Pregnancy risk category: X

Indications and dosages
➤ **Contraception.** *Adults:* 1 tablet P.O. daily, beginning on first day of menstruation.

How supplied
Available by prescription only
Tablets: 0.075 mg

Pharmacodynamics
Contraceptive action: Norgestrel suppresses ovulation and causes thickening of cervical mucus.

Pharmacokinetics
Absorption: Well absorbed after oral administration.
Distribution: No information available.
Metabolism: No information available.
Excretion: No information available.

Route	Onset	Peak	Duration
P.O.	Unknown	Unknown	Unknown

Contraindications and precautions
Contraindicated in pregnant patients, patients hypersensitive to drug, and patients with thromboembolic disorders, cerebral apoplexy, or history of these conditions; breast cancer; undiagnosed abnormal vaginal bleeding; severe hepatic disease; or missed abortion.

Use cautiously in patients with renal or cardiac disease, diabetes mellitus, migraine, seizures, asthma, or mental depression.

Interactions
Drug-drug. *Bromocriptine:* May cause amenorrhea or galactorrhea, which interferes with the action of bromocriptine. Don't administer together.

Adverse reactions
CNS: *cerebral thrombosis or hemorrhage,* migraine, depression.
CV: thrombophlebitis, *pulmonary embolism,* edema, *thromboembolism, CVA.*
EENT: exophthalmos, diplopia.
GU: *breakthrough bleeding, change in menstrual flow,* dysmenorrhea, spotting, amenorrhea, cervical erosion.

◇ Unlabeled clinical use

Hepatic: cholestatic jaundice, increased serum alkaline phosphatase.
Metabolic: increased amino acid levels, altered weight, decreased pregnanediol excretion, decreased glucose tolerance.
Skin: melasma, rash, acne, pruritus.
Other: breast tenderness, enlargement, or secretion.

Overdose and treatment
No information available.

Special considerations
● Norgestrel is also known as the minipill.
● Failure rate of the progestin-only contraceptive is about three times higher than that of combination contraceptives.
● Ovrette tablets contain tartrazine. Use cautiously in patients with tartrazine or aspirin sensitivity.

Patient monitoring
● Monitor liver function test results in patients with hepatic impairment and patients receiving prolonged therapy.

Breast-feeding patients
● If possible, advise breast-feeding women not to use oral contraceptives until infant is completely weaned because drug may interfere with lactation by decreasing the quantity and quality of breast milk. Recommend other means of contraception.

Patient education
● Tell patient to take drug at the same time every day, even during menstruation.
● Advise patient of increased risk of serious CV adverse reactions linked to heavy smoking, especially while taking oral contraceptives.
● Tell patient that risk of pregnancy increases with each tablet missed. If she misses one tablet, tell her to take it as soon as she remembers and then take the next tablet at the regular time. If she misses two tablets, tell her to take one as soon as she remembers, take the next regular dose at the usual time, and use a nonhormonal method of contraception in addition to norgestrel until 14 tablets have been taken. If she misses three or more tablets, tell her to discontinue drug and use a nonhormonal method of contraception until after her menstrual period. Instruct patient to perform a pregnancy test if her menstrual period doesn't occur within 45 days.
● Advise patient to report excessive bleeding or bleeding between menstrual cycles immediately.
● Instruct patient to use a second method of birth control for the first cycle on norgestrel, or for 3 weeks after starting the hormonal contraceptive, to ensure full protection.
● Advise patient who wishes to become pregnant to wait at least 3 months after discontinuing norgestrel, to prevent birth defects.

nortriptyline hydrochloride
Aventyl, Pamelor

Pharmacologic classification: tricyclic antidepressant
Therapeutic classification: antidepressant
Pregnancy risk category: NR

Indications and dosages
➤*Depression; panic disorder◇. Adults:* 25 mg P.O. t.i.d. or q.i.d., gradually increasing to a maximum of 150 mg daily. Or, entire dosage may be given h.s.
Elderly patients or adolescents: 30 to 50 mg P.O. daily or in divided doses.

How supplied
Available by prescription only
Capsules: 10 mg, 25 mg, 50 mg, 75 mg
Solution: 10 mg/5 ml (4% alcohol)

Pharmacodynamics
Antidepressant action: Drug is thought to exert antidepressant effects by inhibiting reuptake of norepinephrine and serotonin in CNS nerve terminals (presynaptic neurons), which results in increased levels and enhanced activity of these neurotransmitters in the synaptic cleft. Nortriptyline inhibits reuptake of serotonin more actively than norepinephrine; it's less likely than other tricyclic antidepressants to cause orthostatic hypotension.

Pharmacokinetics
Absorption: Absorbed rapidly from the GI tract after oral administration.
Distribution: Distributed widely into the body, including the CNS and breast milk, and is 95% protein-bound. Steady state serum levels occur in 2 to 4 weeks. Therapeutic serum level ranges from 50 to 150 ng/ml.
Metabolism: Metabolized by the liver; a significant first-pass effect may account for variability of serum levels in different patients taking the same dosage.
Excretion: Mostly excreted in urine; some in feces, via the biliary tract.

Route	Onset	Peak	Duration
P.O.	Unknown	7-8½ hr	Unknown

Contraindications and precautions
Contraindicated in patients hypersensitive to drug, patients in acute recovery phase of MI, and patients who have taken an MAO inhibitor within 14 days. Use cautiously in patients receiving thyroid medication and those with glaucoma, suicidal tendencies, CV disease, hyperthyroidism, or a history of urine retention or seizures.

Interactions
Drug-drug. *Antiarrhythmics (such as disopyramide, procainamide, and quinidine),*

pimozide, thyroid medications: May increase risk of arrhythmias and conduction defects. Use together cautiously.

Anticholinergics, including antihistamines, antiparkinsonians, atropine, meperidine, and phenothiazines: Oversedation, paralytic ileus, visual changes, and severe constipation. Use together cautiously.

Barbiturates: Induced nortriptyline metabolism and decreased therapeutic efficacy. Monitor patient closely.

Beta blockers, cimetidine, methylphenidate, oral contraceptives, propoxyphene: May inhibit nortriptyline metabolism, increasing plasma levels. Monitor patient for toxicity.

Centrally acting antihypertensives, such as clonidine, guanabenz, guanadrel, guanethidine, methyldopa, and reserpine: Decreased hypotensive effects. Monitor blood pressure.

CNS depressants, including analgesics, anesthetics, barbiturates, narcotics, and tranquilizers: Additive effects (oversedation). Use together cautiously.

Disulfiram, ethchlorvynol: May cause delirium and tachycardia. Avoid use together.

Haloperidol, phenothiazines: Decreased nortriptyline metabolism. Monitor patient closely.

Metrizamide: Increased risk of seizures. Avoid use together, if possible.

Sympathomimetics, including epinephrine, phenylephrine, and ephedrine (often found in nasal sprays): May increase blood pressure. Use together cautiously.

Warfarin: May increase PT and cause bleeding. Monitor PT and INR. Monitor patient for increased bruising and bleeding.

Drug-herb. *Evening primrose oil:* Possible additive or synergistic effect resulting in decreased seizure threshold and increased risk of seizures. Discourage use together.

Drug-lifestyle. *Alcohol use:* Additive effects. Advise patient to avoid alcohol.

Heavy smoking: Induced nortriptyline metabolism and decreased therapeutic efficacy. Advise patient to avoid smoking.

Adverse reactions
CNS: *drowsiness, dizziness, seizures,* tremor, weakness, confusion, headache, nervousness, EEG changes, extrapyramidal reactions, *CVA,* insomnia, nightmares, hallucinations, paresthesia, ataxia, agitation.

CV: *tachycardia,* hypertension, hypotension, *MI,* heart block, prolonged conduction time (elongation of QT and PR intervals, flattened T waves on ECG).

EENT: *blurred vision,* tinnitus, mydriasis.

GI: dry mouth, *constipation,* nausea, vomiting, anorexia, paralytic ileus.

GU: *urine retention,* elevated liver function test results.

Hematologic: *bone marrow depression, agranulocytosis,* eosinophilia, ***thrombocytopenia.***

Metabolic: increased serum glucose levels.

Skin: rash, urticaria, photosensitivity, *diaphoresis.*

Other: *hypersensitivity reaction.*

After abrupt withdrawal of long-term therapy: nausea, headache, malaise (doesn't indicate addiction).

Overdose and treatment
The first 12 hours after acute ingestion are a stimulatory phase characterized by excessive anticholinergic activity, including agitation, irritation, confusion, hallucinations, hyperthermia, parkinsonian symptoms, seizures, urine retention, dry mucous membranes, pupillary dilation, constipation, and ileus. This is followed by CNS depressant effects, including hypothermia; decreased or absent reflexes; sedation; hypotension; cyanosis; and cardiac irregularities, including tachycardia, conduction disturbances, and quinidine-like effects on the ECG.

Severity of overdose is best indicated by prolonging QRS complex beyond 100 ms, which usually indicates a serum level above 1,000 ng/ml. Metabolic acidosis may follow hypotension, hypoventilation, and seizures.

Treatment is symptomatic and supportive, including maintaining a patent airway, stable body temperature, and fluid and electrolyte balance. Induce emesis with ipecac syrup if patient is conscious; follow with gastric lavage and activated charcoal to prevent further absorption. Dialysis is usually ineffective. Consider use of cardiac glycosides or physostigmine if serious CV abnormalities or cardiac failure occurs. Treat seizures with parenteral diazepam or phenytoin; arrhythmias with parenteral phenytoin or lidocaine; and acidosis with sodium bicarbonate. Don't use quinidine, procainamide or disopyramide to treat arrhythmias, since these agents can further depress myocardial conduction and contractility. Don't give barbiturates; these may enhance CNS and respiratory depressant effects.

Special considerations
Consider recommendations relevant to all tricyclic antidepressants as well as the following.
• Drug may be given at bedtime to reduce daytime sedation. Tolerance to sedative effects usually develops in early weeks of therapy.
• Withdraw drug gradually over a few weeks and at least 48 hours before surgical procedures.
• Drug is available in liquid form.
• In patients with bipolar disorders, drug may cause symptoms of the manic phase to emerge.

Patient monitoring
• Monitor nortriptyline level if dose is over 100 mg daily.

Breast-feeding patients
• Nortriptyline appears in breast milk in low levels; potential benefit to woman should outweigh potential harm to infant.

Pediatric patients
● Drug isn't recommended for children. Lower dosages may be indicated for adolescents.

Geriatric patients
● Lower dosages may be indicated. These patients have an increased risk for adverse cardiac effects. Nortriptyline is less likely to cause hypotension than other tricyclic antidepressants.

Patient education
● Explain that patient may not see full effects of drug therapy for up to 4 weeks after start of therapy.
● Warn patient about sedative effects.
● Recommend taking full daily dose at bedtime to prevent daytime sedation.
● Instruct patient to avoid drinking alcoholic beverages, doubling doses after missing one, or discontinuing drug abruptly, unless instructed.
● Caution about possible dizziness. Tell patient to lie down for about 30 minutes after each dose at start of therapy and to avoid sudden position changes, to prevent dizziness. Orthostatic hypotension is usually less severe than with amitriptyline.
● Urge patient to report unusual reactions promptly, such as confusion, movement disorders, fainting, rapid heartbeat, or difficulty urinating.
● Tell patient to store drug away from children.
● Suggest relieving dry mouth with sugarless chewing gum or candy.
● Advise patient to avoid activities that require physical and mental alertness, such as driving a car or operating machinery.

nystatin
Mycostatin, Nilstat

Pharmacologic classification: polyene macrolide
Therapeutic classification: antifungal
Pregnancy risk category: B

Indications and dosages
➤ *GI infections. Adults:* 500,000 to 1 million units as oral tablets, t.i.d.
➤ *Oropharyngeal candidiasis. Adults and children:* 400,000 to 600,000 units of oral suspension q.i.d. Or, 200,000 to 400,000 units (lozenges) four to five times daily for up to 14 days; allow to dissolve in mouth.
Infants: 200,000 units of oral suspension q.i.d.
Neonates and premature infants: 100,000 units of oral suspension q.i.d.
➤ *Oropharyngeal candidiasis in HIV-infected patients. Adults:* 500,000 to 1,000,000 units 3 to 5 times daily as oral suspension or tablets (dissolved in mouth). Or, oral lozenges may be used.
➤ *Cutaneous or mucocutaneous candidal infections. Topical use:* Apply to affected

areas b.i.d. or t.i.d. until healing is complete (about 2 weeks).
Vaginal use: 100,000 units, as vaginal tablets, inserted high into vagina daily or b.i.d. for 14 days.
For prevention of thrush in the neonate, 100,000- to 200,000-unit vaginal tablets daily for 3 to 6 weeks before delivery.
➤ *Candidal diaper dermatitis. Infants:* 100,000 units of oral suspension P.O. q.i.d. as an adjunct to topical nystatin therapy.

How supplied
Available by prescription only
Cream: 100,000 units/g
Lozenges: 200,000 units
Ointment: 100,000 units/g
Powder: 100,000 units/g
Powder for suspension: 50-, 150-, 500-million units; 1-, 2-, 5-billion units
Suspension: 100,000 units/ml
Tablets: 500,000 units
Vaginal suppositories: 100,000 units

Pharmacodynamics
Antifungal action: Nystatin is both fungistatic and fungicidal. It binds to sterols in the fungal cell membrane, altering its permeability and allowing leakage of intracellular components. It acts against various yeasts and fungi, including *Candida albicans.*

Pharmacokinetics
Absorption: Not absorbed from GI tract or through intact skin or mucous membranes.
Distribution: No detectable amount is available for tissue distribution.
Metabolism: No detectable amount is systemically available for metabolism.
Excretion: Oral nystatin is excreted almost entirely unchanged in feces.

Route	Onset	Peak	Duration
P.O., topical, intra-vaginal	Unknown	Unknown	Unknown

Contraindications and precautions
Contraindicated in patients hypersensitive to drug.

Interactions
None reported.

Adverse reactions
GI: transient nausea, diarrhea (usually with large oral dosage), vomiting (with oral administration or vaginal tablets).
Skin: occasional contact dermatitis from preservatives in some forms (with topical administration or vaginal tablets).

Overdose and treatment
Overdose may result in nausea, vomiting, and diarrhea. Treatment is unnecessary because toxicity is negligible.

Special considerations
• Avoid contact between drug and hands; hypersensitivity is rare but can occur.
• For treatment of oral candidiasis, patient should have a clean mouth and should hold suspension in mouth for several minutes before swallowing. For infant thrush, medication should be swabbed on oral mucosa.
• May give immunosuppressed patient vaginal tablets (100,000 units) orally to provide prolonged drug contact with oral mucosa; or, use clotrimazole troche.
• For candidiasis of the feet, patient should dust powder on shoes and stockings as well as feet for maximal contact and effectiveness.
• Avoid occlusive dressings or ointment on moist covered body areas that favor yeast growth.
• To prevent maceration, use cream on intertriginous areas and powder on moist lesions.
• Clean affected skin gently before topical application; cool, moist compresses applied for 15 minutes between applications help soothe dry skin.
• Douches may be used by nonpregnant women for aesthetic reasons; they should use preparations that don't contain antibacterials, which may alter flora and promote reinfection.
• Protect drug from light, air, and heat.
• Drug is ineffective in systemic fungal infection.

Patient monitoring
• Monitor patient for proper use of medication and for clinical effect.

Breast-feeding patients
• Safety in breast-feeding women hasn't been established.

Patient education
• Teach patient signs and symptoms of candidal infection. Inform patient about predisposing factors, such as use of antibiotics, oral contraceptives, and corticosteroids; diabetes; infected sexual partners; and tight-fitting pantyhose and undergarments.
• Teach good oral hygiene. Explain that overuse of mouthwash and poorly fitting dentures, especially in elderly patients, may alter flora and promote infection.
• Tell patient to continue using vaginal cream through menstruation; emphasize importance of washing applicator thoroughly after each use.
• Advise patient to change stockings and undergarments daily; teach good skin care.
• Teach patient how to administer the dosage form prescribed.
• Tell patient to continue drug for at least 48 hours after symptoms clear to prevent reinfection.

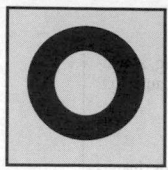

octreotide acetate
Sandostatin, Sandostatin LAR Depot

Pharmacologic classification: synthetic octapeptide
Therapeutic classification: somatotropic hormone
Pregnancy risk category: B

Indications and dosages
➤ *Flushing and diarrhea caused by carcinoid tumors.* *Adults:* Initially, 100 to 600 mcg daily S.C. in two to four divided doses for first 2 weeks of therapy (usual daily dose, 300 mcg). Subsequent dosage based on individual response. Or, 50 to 500 mcg I.V., repeated p.r.n.; prolonged I.V. infusion (for example, 50 mcg/hour) infused over 8 to 24 hours also may be used. Or, 20 mg I.M. of suspension q 4 weeks for 2 months (after using injection for at least 2 weeks). Continue S.C. injection of immediate release for at least first 2 weeks of therapy with long-acting formulation. After 2 months, increase dose to 30 mg or decrease to 10 mg I.M. q 4 weeks, p.r.n.
➤ *Prevention of carcinoid crisis from surgery.* *Adults:* 250 to 500 mcg S.C. 1 to 2 hours before induction of anesthesia.
➤ *Symptomatic treatment of watery diarrhea caused by vasoactive intestinal peptide-secreting tumors (VIPomas).* *Adults:* Initially, 200 to 300 mcg daily S.C. in two to four divided doses for first 2 weeks of therapy. Subsequent dosage based on individual response, but usually won't exceed 450 mcg daily. Also, 10 to 30 mg I.M. of suspension based on growth hormone concentration, insulin-like growth factor 1 (IGF-1), and symptom control q 4 weeks for 2 months (after using injection for at least 2 weeks). Continue S.C. injection of immediate release for at least first 2 weeks of therapy with long-acting formulation. After 2 months, increase dose to 30 mg or decrease to 10 mg I.M. q 4 weeks as needed.
➤ *Acromegaly.* *Adults:* Initially, 50 mcg t.i.d. S.C. Subsequent dosage based on individual response. Usual dosage is 100 to 200 mcg S.C. t.i.d. but some patients may need up to 500 mcg t.i.d. for maximum effectiveness. Patients currently receiving S.C. Sandostatin may be switched directly to Sandostatin LAR in a dose of 20 mg I.M. of suspension q 4 weeks for 3 months (after using S.C. injection for at least 2 weeks). After 3 months of receiving Sandostatin LAR, dosage adjustment is based on growth hormone concentration, IGF-

1, and symptom control. Dose ranges from 10 to 40 mg I.M. q 4 weeks.

How supplied
Available by prescription only
Injection: 0.05 mg/ml, 0.1 mg/ml, and 0.5 mg/ml in 1-ml ampules; 0.2 mg/ml and 1 mg/ml in 5-ml multidose vials
Injection suspension, extended-release: 10 mg/5 ml, 20 mg/5 ml, 30 mg/5 ml

Pharmacodynamics
Antidiarrheal action: Octreotide mimics the action of naturally occurring somatostatin and decreases the secretion of gastroenterohepatic peptides that may contribute to adverse effects in patients with metastatic carcinoid tumors and VIPomas. It isn't known if drug affects the tumor directly.

Pharmacokinetics
Absorption: Absorbed rapidly and completely after injection.
Distribution: Distributed to the plasma, where it binds to serum lipoprotein and albumin.
Metabolism: Eliminated from the plasma at a slower rate than the naturally occurring hormone. Apparent half-life is about 1½ hours, with a duration of effect of up to 12 hours.
Excretion: About 35% appears unchanged in urine.

Route	Onset	Peak	Duration
S.C.	½ hr	½ hr	< 12 hr

Contraindications and precautions
Contraindicated in patients hypersensitive to drug or its components.

Interactions
Drug-drug. *Cyclosporine*: Decreased cyclosporine levels. Monitor patient closely.

Adverse reactions
CNS: dizziness, light-headedness, fatigue, headache.
CV: *bradycardia,* conduction abnormalities, *arrhythmias.*
EENT: blurred vision.
GI: *nausea, diarrhea, abdominal pain or discomfort, loose stools,* vomiting, fat malabsorption, gallstones or biliary sludge, flatulence, constipation.
GU: urinary frequency, urinary tract infection.

Reactions may be *common*, uncommon, *life-threatening*, or COMMON AND LIFE-THREATENING.

Metabolic: hyperglycemia, hypoglycemia, hypothyroidism, suppressed secretion of growth hormone and gastroenterohepatic peptides (gastrin, glucagon, insulin, motilin, pancreatic polypeptide, secretin, and VIP).
Musculoskeletal: backache, joint pain.
Skin: flushing, edema, wheals, erythema or pain at injection site, alopecia, pain or burning at S.C. injection site.
Other: flulike symptoms.

Overdose and treatment

Doses of 1,000 mcg have been administered as an I.V. bolus in volunteers without adverse effects. Drug may produce metabolic changes in certain patients.

Special considerations

● Fluid and electrolyte balance may be altered after start of octreotide therapy.
● Half-life may be altered in patients with end-stage renal failure who are undergoing dialysis. Dosage adjustment may be necessary.
● Octreotide suspension must be given under clinical supervision. Suspension is for I.M. use only into the gluteal muscle and should be stored refrigerated at $36°$ to $46°$ F ($2°$ to $8°$ C) and protected from light. Warm to room temperature for 30 to 60 minutes before mixing.
● I.V. injection may be given undiluted for carcinoid crisis. For I.V. infusion, dilute drug in 50 to 200 ml of normal saline solution or D_5W injection. Infuse over 15 to 30 minutes. Drug remains stable for 24 hours. Store ampules in the refrigerator. Drug may be stored at room temperature for 14 days. Injection is incompatible with total parenteral nutrition solution.

Patient monitoring

● Monitor baseline and periodic tests of thyroid function because long-term effects of drug on hypothalamic-pituitary function aren't known.
● Monitor laboratory values during therapy, such as urinary 5-hydroxyindoleacetic acid, plasma serotonin, plasma substance P for carcinoid tumors, and plasma VIP for VIPomas.
● Mild, transient hypoglycemia or hyperglycemia may occur during therapy. Monitor patient for signs of glucose imbalance.
● Drug may alter fat absorption and aggravate fat malabsorption. Periodically monitor 72-hour fecal fat and serum carotene.
● Drug may decrease vitamin B_{12} levels during chronic treatment. Monitor patient's vitamin B_{12} levels.
● Patients with acromegaly are more likely to experience adverse GI effects and bradycardia. Monitor patient closely.

Breast-feeding patients

● It isn't known if drug appears in breast milk.

Pediatric patients

● Doses of 1 to 10 mcg/kg appear to be well tolerated in children.

Patient education

● Because drug may cause gallstones, tell patient to report abdominal discomfort promptly.

---

olanzapine
Zyprexa, Zyprexa Zydis

Pharmacologic classification: thienobenzodiazepine derivative
Therapeutic classification: antipsychotic
Pregnancy risk category: C

Indications and dosages

➤*Acute manic episodes in bipolar disorder, schizophrenia. Adults:* Initially, 5 to 10 mg P.O. once daily. Adjust dosage in 5-mg increments daily at intervals of at least 1 week. Most patients respond to 10 mg daily; don't exceed 20 mg daily.

How supplied

Available by prescription only
Tablets: 2.5 mg, 5 mg, 7.5 mg, 10 mg
Tablets, orally disintegrating: 5 mg, 10 mg, 15 mg, 20 mg

Pharmacodynamics

Unknown. Drug acts as an antagonist at dopamine (D_{1-4}) and serotonin (5-HT$_{2A/2C}$) receptors; it also may exhibit antagonist-binding at adrenergic, cholinergic, and histaminergic receptors.

Pharmacokinetics

Absorption: Food doesn't affect rate or extent of absorption. About 40% of dose is eliminated by first pass metabolism.
Distribution: Distributes extensively throughout the body, with a volume of distribution of about 1,000 L. Drug is 93% protein-bound, primarily to albumin and alpha$_1$-acid glycoprotein.
Metabolism: Metabolized by direct glucuronidation and cytochrome P-450-mediated oxidation.
Excretion: About 57% appears in urine and 30% in feces as metabolites. Only 7% of dose is recovered in urine unchanged. Elimination half-life ranges from 21 to 54 hours.

Route	Onset	Peak	Duration
P.O.	Unknown	6 hr	Unknown

Contraindications and precautions

Contraindicated in patients hypersensitive to drug. Use cautiously in patients with heart disease, cerebrovascular disease, conditions that predispose to hypotension (gradual dosage adjustment minimizes the risk), history of seizures or conditions that could lower the seizure threshold, and hepatic impairment. Also, use cautiously in elderly patients, patients at risk for aspiration pneumonia, and patients with a history of paralytic ileus, significant prostatic hypertrophy, or angle-closure glaucoma.

Interactions
Drug-drug. *Antihypertensives, diazepam:* May potentiate hypotensive effects. Monitor blood pressure closely.
Carbamazepine, omeprazole, rifampin: May increase olanzapine clearance. Monitor patient for drug effect.
Dopamine agonists, levodopa: May antagonize effects of these drugs. Use together cautiously.
Fluvoxamine: May inhibit olanzapine elimination. Monitor patient for toxicity.
Drug-herb. *Nutmeg:* May reduce symptom control in patients taking olanzapine or interfere with existing therapy for psychiatric illnesses. Discourage use together.
Drug-lifestyle. *Alcohol use:* May potentiate hypotensive effects. Advise patient to avoid alcohol.

Adverse reactions
CNS: *somnolence, agitation, insomnia, headache, nervousness, hostility, parkinsonism, dizziness,* anxiety, personality disorder, *akathisia,* hypertonia, tremor, amnesia, articulation impairment, euphoria, stuttering, dystonic or dyskinetic events, tardive dyskinesia, *neuroleptic malignant syndrome, suicide attempt.*
CV: orthostatic hypotension, tachycardia, chest pain, hypotension, edema.
EENT: amblyopia, blepharitis, corneal lesion, *rhinitis,* pharyngitis.
GI: constipation, dry mouth, abdominal pain, increased appetite, increased salivation, nausea, vomiting, thirst.
GU: premenstrual syndrome, hematuria, metrorrhagia, urinary incontinence, urinary tract infection.
Hematologic: increased eosinophil count.
Hepatic: increased ALT, AST, and GGT levels.
Metabolic: weight gain or loss, increased CK and serum prolactin levels.
Musculoskeletal: joint pain, limb pain, back pain, neck rigidity, twitching.
Respiratory: increased cough, dyspnea.
Skin: vesiculobullous rash.
Other: fever, intentional injury, flu syndrome.

Overdose and treatment
Signs and symptoms of overdose may include drowsiness and slurred speech. There's no specific antidote to olanzapine; treatment should be symptomatic. Monitor patient for hypotension, circulatory collapse, obtundation, seizures, or dystonic reactions. Gastric lavage with activated charcoal and sorbitol may be effective. Drug isn't removed by dialysis. Avoid epinephrine, dopamine, or other sympathomimetics with beta-agonist activity.

Special considerations
⚠ ALERT Don't confuse Zyprexa, which is an antipsychotic, with Zyrtec, which is an antihistamine. The two drugs look alike, sound alike, and have similar dosing. Store separately.
● Therapy may start at 5 mg in patients who are debilitated, predisposed to hypotension, or pharmacologically sensitive to drug. It also may start at 5 mg in patients who have an altered metabolism because of smoking status, gender, or age.

Patient monitoring
● Monitor patient for signs of neuroleptic malignant syndrome (hyperpyrexia, muscle rigidity, altered mental status, autonomic instability), a rare but frequently fatal adverse reaction that can occur with antipsychotic drug therapy. Drug should be stopped immediately and patient monitored and treated.
● Monitor baseline and periodic liver function test results.

Breast-feeding patients
● Drug appears in breast milk. Advise breast-feeding women to use alternative feeding methods during therapy.

Pediatric patients
● Safety and efficacy in children under age 18 haven't been established.

Geriatric patients
● Drug may be started at lower dose because clearance may be decreased in elderly patients. Half-life is 1½ times greater in this population.

Patient education
● Warn patient to avoid hazardous tasks until adverse CNS effects of drug are known.
● Caution patient against exposure to extreme heat; drug may impair ability of the body to reduce core temperature.
● Advise patient to avoid alcohol.
● Tell patient to rise slowly to avoid orthostatic hypotension.
● Advise patient to use ice chips or sugarless candy or gum to relieve dry mouth.
● Inform patient not to take prescription or OTC drugs without medical approval because of potential drug interactions.

olsalazine sodium
Dipentum

Pharmacologic classification: salicylate
Therapeutic classification: anti-inflammatory
Pregnancy risk category: C

Indications and dosages
➤ *Maintenance of remission of ulcerative colitis in patients intolerant of sulfasalazine. Adults:* 1 g P.O. daily in two divided doses.

How supplied
Available by prescription only
Capsules: 250 mg

Pharmacodynamics
Anti-inflammatory action: Mechanism of action is unknown but appears to be topical rather than systemic. Drug is converted to mesalamine (5-aminosalicylic acid; 5-ASA) in the colon. Presumably, mesalamine diminishes inflammation by blocking cyclooxygenase and inhibiting prostaglandin production in the colon.

Pharmacokinetics
Absorption: After oral administration, about 2.4% of a single dose is absorbed.
Distribution: Once metabolized to 5-ASA, drug is absorbed slowly from the colon, resulting in very high local levels.
Metabolism: 0.1% is metabolized in the liver; remainder will reach the colon, where it's rapidly converted to 5-ASA by colonic bacteria.
Excretion: Less than 1% is recovered in urine.

Route	Onset	Peak	Duration
P.O.	Unknown	1 hr	Unknown

Contraindications and precautions
Contraindicated in patients hypersensitive to salicylates. Use cautiously in patients with renal disease.

Interactions
Drug-drug. *Warfarin:* Increased PT. Monitor PT and INR.

Adverse reactions
CNS: headache, depression, vertigo, dizziness, fatigue.
GI: *diarrhea,* nausea, *abdominal pain,* dyspepsia, bloating, anorexia, stomatitis.
Musculoskeletal: arthralgia.
Skin: rash, itching.

Overdose and treatment
Decreased motor activity and diarrhea can occur. Treat overdose symptomatically and supportively.

Special considerations
● Diarrhea from drug therapy is difficult to distinguish from underlying condition.

Patient monitoring
● Monitor CBC with differential and liver function tests periodically.

Breast-feeding patients
● It isn't known if drug appears in breast milk. Use cautiously in breast-feeding women.

Pediatric patients
● Safety and efficacy in children haven't been established.

Patient education
● Advise patient to take drug with food and in evenly divided doses.
● Urge patient to call prescriber if diarrhea develops or worsens.

---

omeprazole
Prilosec

Pharmacologic classification: substituted benzimidazole
Therapeutic classification: gastric acid suppressant
Pregnancy risk category: C

Indications and dosages
➤ *Active duodenal ulcer. Adults:* 20 mg P.O. daily for 4 to 8 weeks.
➤ *Helicobacter pylori eradication to reduce risk of duodenal ulcer recurrence.* **Triple therapy.** *Adults:* 20 mg P.O. b.i.d. plus 500 mg clarithromycin P.O. b.i.d. plus 1,000 mg amoxicillin P.O. b.i.d. for 10 days. In patients with an ulcer present at the time that therapy starts, an additional 18 days of omeprazole 20 mg once daily is recommended alone for ulcer healing and symptom relief. (Also see entries for clarithromycin and amoxicillin.)
Dual therapy
Adults: 40 mg P.O. q morning plus 500 mg clarithromycin P.O. t.i.d. for 14 days followed by 14 days of omeprazole 20 mg daily. (Also see entry for clarithromycin.)
➤ *Severe erosive esophagitis; symptomatic, poorly responsive gastroesophageal reflux disease (GERD). Adults:* 20 mg P.O. daily for 4 to 12 weeks. Patients with GERD should have failed initial therapy with an H_2 antagonist. May continue with maintenance dosage of 20 mg daily for up to 1 year.
➤ *Pathological hypersecretory conditions (such as Zollinger-Ellison syndrome). Adults:* Initial dosage is 60 mg P.O. daily; adjust dosage based on patient response. Administer daily doses exceeding 80 mg in divided doses. Doses up to 120 mg t.i.d. have been administered. Continue therapy as long as clinically indicated.
➤ *Gastric ulcer. Adults:* 40 mg P.O. daily for 4 to 8 weeks.
✦ *Dosage adjustment.* Dosage adjustments may be needed in patients with hepatic impairment. Dosage adjustments may be needed in Asian patients because of increased bioavailability of drug in this population.

How supplied
Available by prescription only
Capsules (delayed-release): 10 mg, 20 mg, 40 mg

Pharmacodynamics
Antisecretory action: Omeprazole inhibits the activity of the acid (proton) pump, H^+/K^+ adeno-

sine triphosphatase (ATPase), located at the secretory surface of the gastric parietal cell. This blocks the formation of gastric acid.

Pharmacokinetics
Absorption: Omeprazole is acid-labile, and the formulation contains enteric-coated granules that permit absorption after drug leaves the stomach. Absorption is rapid. Bioavailability is about 40% because of instability in gastric acid as well as a substantial first-pass effect. Bioavailability increases slightly with repeated dosing, possibly because of drug's effect on gastric acidity.
Distribution: About 95% protein-bound.
Metabolism: Primarily metabolized in the liver.
Excretion: Primarily excreted by the kidneys. Plasma half-life is ½ to 1 hour, but drug effects may persist for days.

Route	Onset	Peak	Duration
P.O.	1 hr	2 hr	< 3 days

Contraindications and precautions
Contraindicated in patients hypersensitive to drug or its components.

Interactions
Drug-drug. *Ampicillin esters, iron derivatives, itraconazole, ketoconazole:* Poor bioavailability because optimal absorption of these drugs requires a low gastric pH. Avoid use together.
Diazepam, phenytoin, propranolol, theophylline, warfarin: Effects may be impaired by omeprazole. Patient needs close monitoring for decreased effect or toxicity.
Drug-herb. *Male fern:* Inactivated in alkaline environments. Advise patient concerning this effect.
Pennyroyal: May change the rate at which toxic metabolites of pennyroyal form. Discourage use together.

Adverse reactions
CNS: headache, dizziness, asthenia.
GI: diarrhea, abdominal pain, nausea, vomiting, constipation, flatulence.
Musculoskeletal: back pain.
Respiratory: cough, upper respiratory tract infection.
Skin: rash.

Overdose and treatment
Reports of overdose are rare. Symptoms include confusion, drowsiness, blurred vision, tachycardia, nausea, vomiting, diaphoresis, dry mouth, and headache. Doses up to 360 mg daily have been well tolerated.

Treatment should be symptomatic and supportive. Dialysis is of little value because of the extent of binding to plasma proteins.

Special considerations
● Drug increases its own bioavailability with repeated administration. It's labile in gastric acid;

less of it is lost to hydrolysis because drug elevates gastric pH.
● Capsules shouldn't be crushed.
● If administered through a feeding tube, an acidic fluid such as orange juice may decrease risk of clogging tube.
● Serum gastrin levels rise in most patients during first 2 weeks of therapy.

Patient monitoring
● Monitor patient for effects of therapy.
● Monitor liver function tests in patients with hepatic impairment.

Breast-feeding patients
● It isn't known if drug appears in breast milk. Patient should avoid breast-feeding during therapy.

Pediatric patients
● Safety in children hasn't been established.

Patient education
● Explain importance of taking drug exactly as prescribed.
● Tell patient to take 30 minutes before meals and not to crush capsules.

ondansetron hydrochloride
Zofran, Zofran ODT

Pharmacologic classification: serotonin (5-HT$_3$) receptor antagonist
Therapeutic classification: antiemetic
Pregnancy risk category: B

Indications and dosages
➤ *Prevention of nausea and vomiting caused by initial and repeat courses of emetogenic chemotherapy, including high-dose cisplatin. Adults and children age 4 and older:* Three I.V. doses of 0.15 mg/kg with first dose infused over 15 minutes beginning 30 minutes before start of chemotherapy, with subsequent doses of 0.15 mg/kg administered 4 and 8 hours after first dose. In adults, may also administer as a single dose of 32 mg, infused over 15 minutes, 30 minutes before start of chemotherapy. *Adults and children over age 12:* Initially, 8 mg P.O. starting 30 minutes before start of chemotherapy, with a repeat dose after the first dose; then q 12 hours for 1 to 2 days after completion of chemotherapy.
Children ages 4 to 11: Initially, 4 mg given P.O. 30 minutes before start of chemotherapy with subsequent doses 4 and 8 hours after initial dose. Then 4 mg given P.O. q 8 hours for 1 to 2 days after completion of chemotherapy.
➤ *Prevention of radiation-induced nausea and vomiting. Adults:* 8 mg P.O. t.i.d. First dose should be 1 to 2 hours before radiation treatment. Patients receiving single, high-dose radiation to abdomen should continue q-8-hour dosing for 1 to 2 days.

Reactions may be *common*, uncommon, *life-threatening*, or COMMON AND LIFE-THREATENING.

➤ **Prevention of postoperative nausea and vomiting.** *Adults:* 16 mg P.O. 1 hour before anesthesia or 4 mg I.V. immediately before anesthesia or soon after operation. Or, 4 mg I.M. undiluted as a single injection.

Children ages 2 to 12 who weigh more than 40 kg (88 lb): 4 mg I.V. as a single dose.

Children ages 2 to 12 who weigh 40 kg or less: 0.1 mg/kg I.V. as a single dose.

✦ **Dosage adjustment.** In patients with severe hepatic impairment, total daily dose shouldn't exceed 8 mg.

How supplied

Available by prescription only
Injection: 2 mg/ml in 20-ml multidose vials, 2-ml single-dose vials
Injection, premixed: 32 mg/50 ml in D_5W single-dose vial
Oral solution: 4 mg/5 ml
Orally disintegrating tablets: 4 mg, 8 mg
Tablets: 4 mg, 8 mg, 24 mg

Pharmacodynamics

Antiemetic action: Not well known. Ondansetron isn't a dopamine-receptor antagonist. Because serotonin receptors of the $5\text{-}HT_3$ type occur peripherally on vagal nerve terminals and centrally in the chemoreceptor trigger zone, it's uncertain if antiemetic action is mediated centrally, peripherally, or both.

Pharmacokinetics

Absorption: Absorption is variable with oral administration; bioavailability is 50% to 60%.
Distribution: 70% to 76% protein-bound.
Metabolism: Extensively metabolized by hydroxylation on the indole ring, followed by glucuronide or sulfate conjugation.
Excretion: 5% recovered in urine as parent compound. Half-life in adults is 3½ to 6 hours.

Route	Onset	Peak	Duration
P.O.	Unknown	2 hr	Unknown
I.V.	Unknown	Unknown	Unknown

Contraindications and precautions

Contraindicated in patients hypersensitive to drug. Use cautiously in patients with hepatic failure. Orally disintegrating tablet contains aspartame; use cautiously in patients with phenylketonuria.

Interactions

Drug-herb. *Horehound:* May enhance serotonergic effects. Discourage use together.

Adverse reactions

CNS: *headache, malaise, fatigue, dizziness, sedation,* anxiety, agitation, oculogyric crisis.
CV: chest pain, hypotension.
GI: *diarrhea, constipation,* abdominal pain, xerostomia.
GU: urine retention, gynecologic disorders.
Hepatic: transient elevation of AST and ALT levels.

Musculoskeletal: *musculoskeletal pain.*
Respiratory: *hypoxia.*
Skin: rash, injection-site reaction.
Other: chills, fever, *anaphylaxis.*

Overdose and treatment

Doses more than 10 times recommended dose have been given without incident. If overdose is suspected, manage with supportive therapy.

Special considerations

● Drug may be administered I.V. undiluted over 2 to 5 minutes.
● For infusion, dilute drug in 50 ml of compatible solution and infuse over 15 minutes.
● Ondansetron is stable at room temperature for 48 hours after dilution with normal saline solution, D_5W, 5% dextrose and normal saline solution, 5% dextrose and half-normal saline, or 3% saline.

Patient monitoring

● Monitor liver function tests if giving repeated doses.
● For patients undergoing abdominal surgery, watch for ileus, gastric distension, or both.

Breast-feeding patients

● It isn't known if drug appears in breast milk. Use cautiously in breast-feeding women.

Pediatric patients

● Little information is available for use in children age 3 and under for preventing chemotherapy-induced nausea and vomiting, and in children under age 2 for preventing postoperative nausea and vomiting.

Geriatric patients

● No age-related problems have been reported.

Patient education

● Advise patient to alert prescriber if adverse effects occur.

opium tincture, deodorized (laudanum)

opium tincture, camphorated (paregoric)

Pharmacologic classification: opiate
Therapeutic classification: antidiarrheal
Controlled substance schedule: II (deodorized), III (camphorated)
Pregnancy risk category: B (D for high doses or long term)

Indications and dosages

Note: Don't confuse opium tincture with camphorated opium tincture.

➤ **Acute, nonspecific diarrhea.** *Adults:* 0.6 ml opium tincture (range, 0.3 to 1 ml) P.O. q.i.d.

(maximum dose, 6 ml daily). Or, 5 to 10 ml camphorated opium tincture daily, b.i.d., t.i.d., or q.i.d. until diarrhea subsides.
Children: 0.25 to 0.5 ml/kg camphorated opium tincture daily, b.i.d., t.i.d., or q.i.d. until diarrhea subsides.
➤ *Severe opiate withdrawal symptoms in neonates. Neonates*: Camphorated opium tincture or a 1:25 dilution of opium tincture in water, given as 0.2 ml P.O. q 3 hours. Adjust dosage to control withdrawal symptoms. Increase by 0.05 ml q 3 hours until symptoms are controlled. Once symptoms are stabilized for 3 to 5 days, gradually decrease dosage over a 2-to 4-week period.

How supplied
Available by prescription only
opium tincture
Alcoholic solution: Equivalent to morphine 10 mg/ml
opium tincture, camphorated
Alcoholic solution: Each 5 ml contains morphine, 2 mg; anise oil, 0.2 ml; benzoic acid, 20 mg; camphor, 20 mg; glycerin, 0.2 ml; and ethanol to make 5 ml

Pharmacodynamics
Antidiarrheal action: Opium contains several ingredients. The most active, morphine, increases GI smooth-muscle tone, inhibits motility and propulsion, and diminishes secretions. By inhibiting peristalsis, the drug delays passage of intestinal contents, increasing water resorption and relieving diarrhea.

Pharmacokinetics
Absorption: Absorbed variably from the gut.
Distribution: Although opium alkaloids are distributed widely in the body, the low doses used to treat diarrhea act primarily in the GI tract. Camphor crosses the placenta.
Metabolism: Metabolized rapidly in the liver.
Excretion: Opium is excreted in urine; opium alkaloids (especially morphine) enter breast milk.

Route	Onset	Peak	Duration
P.O.	Unknown	Unknown	4-5 hr

Contraindications and precautions
Contraindicated in patients with acute diarrhea caused by poisoning until toxic material is removed from GI tract or in those with diarrhea caused by organisms that penetrate intestinal mucosa. Use cautiously in patients with asthma, prostatic hyperplasia, hepatic disease, or history of opium dependence.

Interactions
Drug-drug. *Other CNS depressants:* Additive effect. Use together cautiously.
Metoclopramide: May antagonize the effects of metoclopramide. Avoid use together.

Adverse reactions
CNS: dizziness, light-headedness.
GI: nausea, vomiting, increased serum amylase and lipase levels.
Other: physical dependence (after long-term use).

Overdose and treatment
Signs and symptoms of overdose include drowsiness, hypotension, seizures, and apnea. Empty stomach by induced emesis or gastric lavage; maintain patent airway. Use naloxone to treat respiratory depression. Monitor patient for signs and symptoms of CNS or respiratory depression.

Special considerations
● Mix drug with sufficient water to ensure passage to stomach.
⚠ ALERT Deodorized opium tincture (laudanum) is 25 times more potent than camphorated form (paregoric); take care not to confuse these drugs. Camphorated form is more dilute, and teaspoon doses are easier to measure than dropper quantities of opium tincture.
● When camphorated opium tincture is added to water, a milky fluid forms.
● Risk of physical dependence on drug increases with long-term use.
● Don't refrigerate drug.
● Opium tincture and camphorated tincture may prevent delivery of technetium-99m disofenin to the small intestine during hepatobiliary imaging tests; delay test until 24 hours after last dose.

Patient monitoring
● Monitor vital signs and bowel function.

Breast-feeding patients
● Because opium alkaloids, especially morphine, appear in breast milk, risks must be weighed against benefits.

Pediatric patients
● Opium tincture has been used to treat withdrawal symptoms in infants whose mothers are narcotic addicts.

Patient education
● Warn patient that physical dependence may result from long-term use.
● Advise patient to use caution when performing hazardous tasks because drug may cause drowsiness, dizziness, and blurred vision.
● Instruct patient to report diarrhea that persists longer than 48 hours because drug is indicated only for short-term use.
● Advise patient to take drug with food if it causes nausea, vomiting, or constipation.
● Instruct patient to call prescriber immediately if he has difficulty breathing or shortness of breath.
● Instruct patient to drink adequate fluids while diarrhea persists.

---

oprelvekin
Neumega

Pharmacologic classification: recombinant human interleukin eleven (rhIL-11)
Therapeutic classification: human thrombopoietic growth factor
Pregnancy risk category: C

Indications and dosages
➤ *Prevention of severe thrombocytopenia and reduction of need for platelet transfusions after myelosuppressive chemotherapy in patients with non-myeloid malignancies at high risk for severe thrombocytopenia.* Adults: 50 mcg/kg S.C. once daily. Begin dosing 6 to 24 hours after completion of chemotherapy and stop at least 2 days before starting the next cycle of chemotherapy. Continue dosing until the postnadir platelet count is 50,000 cells/microliter or more.

How supplied
Available by prescription only
Injection: 5-mg, single-dose vial with diluent

Pharmacodynamics
Thrombopoietic growth factor action: Main activity is stimulation of megakaryocytopoiesis and thrombopoiesis. Thrombopoietic growth factor directly stimulates proliferation of hematopoietic stem cells and megakaryocyte progenitor cells. Platelets produced in response to oprelvekin possess a normal life-span and are functionally normal. Bone-forming and bone-resorbing cells are potential targets for oprelvekin. In some instances, platelet counts began to increase relative to baseline between 5 and 9 days after the start of oprelvekin therapy. After treatment stops, platelet counts continue to increase for up to 7 days and return to baseline within 14 days.

Pharmacokinetics
Absorption: When administered S.C., absolute bioavailability is over 80%.
Distribution: Plasma levels peak 3 to 5 hours after S.C. dose.
Metabolism: Mostly metabolized before excretion; routes of metabolism unknown.
Excretion: Excreted primarily by kidneys; terminal half-life is about 7 hours.

Route	Onset	Peak	Duration
S.C.	Unknown	3-5 hr	Unknown

Contraindications and precautions
Contraindicated in patients hypersensitive to drug or its components. Use cautiously in patients with heart failure, a risk for heart failure, or a history of heart failure that is currently well controlled. Also use cautiously in patients with a history of papilledema, atrial arrhythmias, or CNS tumors. Use cautiously in patients receiving cardiac drugs, patients who previously received doxorubicin, and elderly patients.

Interactions
Drug-drug. *Diuretics, ifosfamide:* Severe, possibly fatal, hypokalemia. Use together with extreme caution.

Adverse reactions
CNS: *asthenia, headache, insomnia, dizziness,* paresthesia, *syncope.*
CV: *tachycardia, vasodilation, palpitations, atrial flutter or fibrillation, edema.*
EENT: blurred vision, *conjunctival injection, pharyngitis, rhinitis,* eye hemorrhage.
GI: *oral candidiasis, nausea, vomiting, diarrhea, mucositis.*
Hematologic: *neutropenic fever,* decreased hemoglobin level, increased plasma fibrinogen level, increased level of von Willebrand factor.
Metabolic: dehydration; decreased serum albumin, protein (transferrin and gamma globulins), and calcium levels.
Respiratory: *dyspnea, cough, pleural effusions.*
Skin: *rash,* skin discoloration, exfoliative dermatitis, transient rash at injection site.
Other: *fever.*

Overdose and treatment
If overdose occurs, stop drug and observe patient for signs of cardiac toxicity.

Special considerations
● Administer by S.C. route in abdomen, thigh, hip, or upper arm.
● Store drug and diluent in refrigerator until ready for reconstitution.
● Reconstitute single-dose vial with 1 ml of supplied diluent. Avoid excessive or vigorous agitation. Discard unused drug.
● Use reconstituted drug within 3 hours.
● Some patients may develop antibodies to drug.

Patient monitoring
● Closely monitor fluid and electrolyte status (especially potassium levels) in patients receiving long-term diuretic therapy.
● Obtain CBC before chemotherapy and at regular intervals during drug therapy. Drug isn't indicated following myeloablative chemotherapy.

Breast-feeding patients
● It isn't known if drug appears in breast milk. Depending on importance of drug to mother, stop either breast-feeding or drug.

Patient education
● Provide patient with information leaflet available from manufacturer. A copy can also be obtained from drug package insert.
● If patient will self-administer, show him how to prepare and administer drug.

• Advise patient to give each dose at about the same time each day.
• Tell patient to refrigerate drug before reconstitution and not to reconstitute until ready to use. Also, inform patient that reconstituted drug is stable at room temperature or in refrigerator for up to 3 hours.
• Tell patient not to reuse vial that has been reconstituted and entered by a syringe, and to discard remaining solution after giving dose.
• Instruct patient to call immediately if swelling, chest pain, irregular heart beat, blurred vision, difficulty breathing, or fatigue occurs.

---

orlistat
Xenical

Pharmacologic classification: lipase inhibitor
Therapeutic classification: antiobesity drug
Pregnancy risk category: B

Indications and dosages
➤ *Management of obesity, including weight loss and weight maintenance with a reduced-calorie diet; reduction of risk of weight regain after weight loss.* Adults: 120 mg P.O. t.i.d. with each main meal that contains fat (during or up to 1 hour after the meal).

How supplied
Available by prescription only
Capsules: 120 mg

Pharmacodynamics
Antiobesity action: As a reversible inhibitor of lipases, orlistat forms a bond with the active site of gastric and pancreatic lipases. These inactivated enzymes are unavailable to hydrolyze dietary fat, in the form of triglycerides, into absorbable free fatty acids and monoglycerides. Because the undigested triglycerides aren't absorbed, the resulting caloric deficit may have a positive effect on weight control. The recommended dose of 120 mg t.i.d. inhibits dietary fat absorption by about 30%.

Pharmacokinetics
Absorption: Systemic exposure to orlistat is minimal because only a small amount of the drug is absorbed.
Distribution: More than 99% binds to plasma proteins; lipoproteins and albumin are major binding proteins.
Metabolism: Primarily metabolized within the GI wall.
Excretion: Most of unabsorbed drug is excreted in feces.

Route	Onset	Peak	Duration
P.O.	Unknown	8 hr	Unknown

Contraindications and precautions
Contraindicated in patients hypersensitive to orlistat or its components and in patients with chronic malabsorption syndrome or cholestasis. Also, exclude organic causes of obesity such as hypothyroidism before starting orlistat therapy.
Use cautiously in patients with a risk of anorexia nervosa or bulimia or a history of hyperoxaluria or calcium oxalate nephrolithiasis. Use cautiously in patients receiving cyclosporine because of potential changes in cyclosporine absorption related to variations in dietary intake.

Interactions
Drug-drug. *Fat-soluble vitamins such as vitamin E and beta-carotene:* Absorption may be decreased by drug. Separate administration times by 2 hours.
Pravastatin: Increased pravastatin levels and additive lipid-lowering effect. Monitor patient.
Warfarin: May alter coagulation parameters. Monitor PT and INR.

Adverse reactions
CNS: *headache,* dizziness, fatigue, sleep disorder, anxiety, depression.
CV: pedal edema.
EENT: otitis.
GI: *oily spotting, flatus with discharge, fecal urgency, fatty or oily stool, oily evacuation, increased defecation, abdominal pain,* fecal incontinence, nausea, infectious diarrhea, rectal pain, vomiting.
GU: menstrual irregularity, vaginitis, urinary tract infection.
Musculoskeletal: *back pain,* pain in legs, arthritis, myalgia, joint disorder, tendonitis.
Respiratory: *influenza, upper respiratory tract infection,* lower respiratory tract infection.
Skin: rash, dry skin.
Other: tooth and gingival disorders.

Overdose and treatment
If an overdose occurs, stop drug and observe patient for 24 hours. Systemic effects attributable to lipase inhibitiion should reverse rapidly.

Special considerations
• Drug is recommended for patients with an initial body mass index of 30 kg/m² or more, or 27 kg/m² or more if patient has other risk factors, such as hypertension, diabetes, or dyslipidemia.
• Advise patient to adhere to dietary guidelines. GI effects may increase when patient takes orlistat with high-fat foods—specifically, when more than 30% of total daily calories come from fat.
• Orlistat reduces absorption of some fat-soluble vitamins and beta-carotene. Patient may need a multivitamin supplement that contains fat-soluble vitamins during orlistat therapy.
• It's unknown if orlistat is safe and effective when therapy lasts more than 2 years.

Reactions may be *common*, uncommon, *life-threatening*, or COMMON AND LIFE-THREATENING.

• As with any weight loss agent, the risk of mis-use exists in certain patient populations, such as patients with anorexia nervosa or bulimia.

Patient monitoring
• In diabetic patients, improved metabolic control may accompany weight loss, so the dosage of oral antidiabetic or insulin may need to be reduced. Monitor serum glucose.

Pregnant patients
• Not recommended for use in pregnant women; effects on fetus aren't known.

Breast-feeding patients
• It isn't known if orlistat appears in breast milk; breast-feeding women shouldn't take the drug.

Pediatric patients
• Safety and efficacy haven't been established.

Geriatric patients
• It isn't known if elderly patients respond differently to the drug than younger patients.

Patient education
• Advise patient to follow a nutritionally balanced, reduced-calorie diet that derives only 30% of its calories from fat. The daily intake of fat, carbohydrate, and protein should be distributed over three main meals. If a meal is occasionally missed or contains no fat, patient can omit a dose.
• To ensure adequate nutrition, advise patient to take a daily multivitamin supplement that contains fat-soluble vitamins at least 2 hours before or after orlistat, such as at bedtime.
• Tell patient with diabetes that weight loss may improve glycemic control, so oral antidiabetic (such as a sulfonylurea or metformin) or insulin dosage may be reduced during orlistat therapy.
• Tell women to inform prescriber if pregnancy or breast-feeding is planned.

orphenadrine citrate
Banflex, Flexoject, Flexon, Myolin, Myotrol, Norflex

orphenadrine hydrochloride
Disipal*

Pharmacologic classification: diphenhydramine analogue
Therapeutic classification: skeletal muscle relaxant
Pregnancy risk category C

Indications and dosages
➤*Adjunct in painful, acute musculoskeletal conditions. Adults:* 100 mg P.O. b.i.d. Or, 60 mg I.V. or I.M. q 12 hours. If given with acetylsalicylic acid and caffeine, 25 to 50 mg P.O. t.i.d. to q.i.d.

➤*Leg cramps* ◊. *Adults:* 100 mg P.O. h.s.

How supplied
Available by prescription only
Injection: 30 mg/ml parenteral
Tablets: 50 mg, 100 mg
Tablets (extended-release): 100 mg

Pharmacodynamics
Skeletal muscle relaxant action: Orphenadrine doesn't relax skeletal muscle directly. Atropine-like central action on cerebral motor centers or on the medulla may be the mechanism by which it reduces skeletal muscle spasm. Its reported analgesic effect may add to its skeletal muscle relaxant properties.

Pharmacokinetics
Absorption: Rapidly absorbed from the GI tract.
Distribution: Widely distributed.
Metabolism: Pathway unknown, but drug is almost completely metabolized to at least eight metabolites.
Excretion: Excreted in urine, mainly as its metabolites. Small amounts are excreted unchanged. Half-life is about 14 hours.

Route	Onset	Peak	Duration
P.O.	1 hr	2 hr	4-6 hr
I.V., I.M.	Unknown	Unknown	Unknown

Contraindications and precautions
Contraindicated in patients hypersensitive to drug and patients with glaucoma; prostatic hyperplasia; pyloric, duodenal, or bladder neck obstruction; myasthenia gravis; and peptic ulceration.
Use cautiously in elderly or debilitated patients and in those with tachycardia, cardiac disease, arrhythmias, or sulfite allergy.

Interactions
Drug-drug. *Anticholinergics:* May increase anticholinergic effects. Use together cautiously.
CNS depressants (such as antipsychotics, anxiolytics, and tricyclic antidepressants), propoxyphene: May produce additive CNS effects. Concurrent use requires reduction of both drugs.
MAO inhibitors: May increase CNS adverse effects. Use together cautiously.
Drug-lifestyle. *Alcohol use:* Additive CNS effects. Advise patient to avoid combined use.

Adverse reactions
CNS: weakness, *drowsiness,* light-headedness, confusion, agitation, tremor, headache, dizziness, hallucinations, syncope.
CV: palpitations, tachycardia.
EENT: dilated pupils, blurred vision, difficulty swallowing, increased intraocular pressure.
GI: constipation, *dry mouth,* nausea, vomiting, epigastric distress.
GU: urinary hesitancy, urine retention.
Hematologic: *aplastic anemia.*

◊ Unlabeled clinical use

Skin: urticaria, pruritus.
Other: *anaphylaxis.*

Overdose and treatment

Overdose may cause dry mouth, blurred vision, urine retention, tachycardia, confusion, paralytic ileus, deep coma, seizures, shock, respiratory arrest, arrhythmias, and death.

Treatment is symptomatic and supportive. If ingestion is recent, induce emesis or gastric lavage followed by activated charcoal. Monitor vital signs and fluid and electrolyte balance.

Special considerations

● When giving drug I.V., inject slowly over 5 minutes. Keep patient supine during and 5 to 10 minutes after injection. Paradoxical initial bradycardia may occur; it usually stops in 2 minutes.
● Some orphenadrine citrate injections may contain sodium bisulfite, which can cause allergic-type reactions, including anaphylaxis.

Patient monitoring

● Monitor blood, urine, and liver function tests periodically during prolonged therapy.
● Monitor vital signs, especially intake and output, noting urine retention.

Pediatric patients

● Safety and efficacy in children under age 12 haven't been established.

Geriatric patients

● These patients may be more sensitive to effects of drug.

Patient education

● Suggest ice chips, sugarless gum, hard candy, or saliva substitutes to relieve dry mouth.
● Tell patient to avoid hazardous activities until CNS depressant effects can be determined.
● Warn patient to avoid alcohol.
● Tell patient to store drug away from heat and light (not in bathroom medicine cabinet) and safely out of reach of children.
● Instruct patient to take missed dose if remembered within 1 hour. If beyond 1 hour, patient should skip that dose and return to regular schedule. Warn against doubling the dose.

oseltamivir phosphate
Tamiflu

Pharmacologic classification: influenza virus neuraminidase inhibitor
Therapeutic classification: antiviral
Pregnancy risk category: C

Indications and dosages

➤ *Treatment of uncomplicated, acute influenza A and B infection in adults symptomatic for 2 days or less.* Adults: 75 mg P.O. twice daily for 5 days, beginning within 2 days of symptom onset.
Children age 1 and older who weigh more than 40 kg (88 lb), adults unable to swallow capsule: 75 mg (6.2 ml) P.O. twice daily for 5 days, beginning within 2 days of symptom onset.
Children age 1 and older who weigh 23 to 39 kg (51 to 87 lb): 60 mg (5 ml) P.O. twice daily for 5 days, beginning within 2 days of symptom onset.
Children age 1 and older who weigh 15 to 39 kg (33 to 86 lb): 45 mg (3.8ml) P.O. twice daily for 5 days, beginning within 2 days of symptom onset.
Children age 1 and older who weigh 15 kg or less: 30 mg (2.5 ml) P.O. twice daily for 5 days, beginning within 2 days of symptom onset.
✦ *Dosage adjustment.* For adults with renal impairment (creatinine clearance less than 30 ml/minute), 75 mg P.O. once daily for 5 days, beginning within 2 days of symptom onset.
➤ *Prophylaxis of influenza following close contact with an infected person.* Adults and adolescents age 13 and older: 75 mg P.O. once daily for at least 7 days, beginning within 2 days of exposure. During a community outbreak, 75 mg P.O. once daily for up to 6 weeks.
✦ *Dosage adjustment.* For patients with renal impairment (creatinine clearance less than 30 ml/minute), 75 mg P.O. every other day for 5 days, beginning within 2 days of exposure.

How supplied

Available by prescription only.
Capsules: 75 mg
Suspension: 12 mg/ml

Pharmacodynamics

Antiviral action: Oseltamivir is hydrolyzed in the liver to its active form, oseltamivir carboxylase. Oseltamivir carboxylase inhibits the enzyme neuraminidase in influenza virus particles. This action is thought to inhibit viral replication, possibly by interfering with viral particle aggregation and release from the host cell.

Pharmacokinetics

Absorption: Well absorbed after oral administration. More than 75% of dose reaches the systemic circulation as oseltamivir carboxylase. Peak level of oseltamivir is 65.2 ng/ml whereas that of oseltamivir carboxylase is 348 ng/ml.
Distribution: Serum protein–binding is low for both oseltamivir (42%) and oseltamivir carboxylase (3%). Volume of distribution of oseltamivir carboxylase is 23 to 26 L.
Metabolism: Oseltamivir is extensively metabolized by hepatic esterases to its active component, oseltamivir carboxylase. Oseltamivir is neither a substrate nor an inhibitor of cytochrome P-450 oxidases.
Excretion: Oseltamivir carboxylase is almost entirely eliminated in urine via glomerular fil-

tration and tubular secretion. Less than 20% of oral dose is eliminated in feces.

Route	Onset	Peak	Duration
P.O.	Unknown	Unknown	Unknown

Contraindications and precautions

Contraindicated in patients hypersensitive to any component of the formulation. Use cautiously in patients with chronic cardiac disease, chronic respiratory disease, or any acute medical illness requiring hospitalization. Efficacy of oseltamivir hasn't been established in these settings.

Interactions

None reported.

Adverse reactions

CNS: dizziness, insomnia, headache, vertigo, fatigue.
GI: abdominal pain, diarrhea, nausea, vomiting.
Respiratory: bronchitis, cough.

Overdose and treatment

Single doses as high as 1,000 mg have been linked to only nausea and vomiting. The entire 5-day course of therapy provides a total dose of 750 mg.

Special considerations

● Oseltamivir doesn't appear to interfere with normal humoral antibody response to influenza.
● Efficacy of oseltamivir against influenza virus type A and B has been demonstrated in clinical trials. There's no evidence supporting the use of oseltamivir in the treatment of other viral infections.
● Administration of oseltamivir with meals may alleviate adverse GI effects.
● Nausea and vomiting are the most frequent adverse effects.
● Store drug at 59° to 86° F (15° to 30° C).

Patient monitoring

● Monitor patient for adverse GI effects and for response to drug.

Breast-feeding patients

● It isn't known if drug appears in breast milk. The potential benefits and risks of oseltamivir therapy on the breast-fed infant must be considered.

Pediatric patients

● Safety and efficacy in children haven't been established.

Geriatric patients

● Dosage reduction isn't required for elderly patients unless creatinine clearance is less than 30 ml/minute.

Patient education

● Advise patient to contact prescriber as soon as possible to begin treatment within 2 days of symptom onset.
● Tell patient to complete the full 5 days of treatment, even if he feels better.
● Inform patient that oseltamivir may be taken with or without meals. Nausea or vomiting may be relieved by taking drug with food or milk.
● Advise patient to take a missed dose as soon as possible unless the nest dose is due within 2 hors. In that case, tell him to skip the dose.
● Tell patient that drug doesn't replace the influenza virus vaccine. If patient is at risk for influenza, he should continue to receive the vaccine each fall.

oxacillin sodium
Bactocill

Pharmacologic classification: penicillinase-resistant penicillin
Therapeutic classification: antibiotic
Pregnancy risk category: B

Indications and dosages

➤ *Systemic infections caused by* Staphylococcus aureus. *Adults and children who weigh more than 40 kg (88 lb):* 500 mg P.O. q 4 to 6 hours for mild to moderate infections. Dose is 1 g P.O. q 4 to 6 hours when changing from I.V. to P.O. therapy. Or, 250 to 500 mg I.M. or I.V. q 4 to 6 hours. For more severe infections, 1 g or more I.V. or I.M. q 4 to 6 hours. Serious infections are treated for 1 to 2 weeks.
Children over age 1 month who weigh less than 40 kg: 50 to 100 mg/kg P.O. daily, divided into doses given q 4 to 6 hours. Or, 50 to 200 mg/kg I.M. or I.V. daily, divided into doses given q 4 to 6 hours. Doses vary based on severity of infection.

➤ *Acute or chronic osteomyelitis caused by susceptible organisms. Adults:* 1.5 to 2 g I.V. q 4 hours for 4 to 8 weeks or I.V. dose for 5 to 28 days followed by P.O. dose for 3 to 6 weeks for a total of 6 weeks of therapy.

➤ *Treatment of native valve endocarditis caused by methicillin-susceptible staphylococci. Adults:* 2 g I.V. q 4 hours for 4 to 6 weeks with gentamicin for the first 3 to 5 days.

➤ *Treatment of prosthetic valve endocarditis caused by methicillin-susceptible staphylococci. Adults:* 2 g I.V. q 4 hours for 6 weeks or longer with gentamicin and rifampin.
✦ *Dosage adjustment.* In adults with creatinine clearance below 10 ml/minute, 1 g I.M. or I.V. q 4 to 6 hours.

How supplied

Available by prescription only
Capsules: 250 mg, 500 mg

Injection: 250 mg, 500 mg, 1 g, 2 g, 4 g
I.V. infusion: 1 g, 2 g, 4 g
Oral solution: 250 mg/5 ml (after reconstitution)

Pharmacodynamics

Antibiotic action: Oxacillin is bactericidal; it adheres to bacterial penicillin-binding proteins, thus inhibiting bacterial cell wall synthesis. Oxacillin resists the effects of penicillinases—enzymes that inactivate penicillin—and is thus active against many strains of penicillinase-producing bacteria; this activity is most important against penicillinase-producing staphylococci; some strains may remain resistant. Oxacillin is also active against a few gram-positive aerobic and anaerobic bacilli but has no significant effect on gram-negative bacilli.

Pharmacokinetics

Absorption: Absorbed rapidly but incompletely from the GI tract; it's stable in an acid environment. Food decreases absorption.
Distribution: Distributed widely. CSF penetration is poor but enhanced by meningeal inflammation. Oxacillin crosses the placenta, and is 89% to 94% protein-bound.
Metabolism: Metabolized partially.
Excretion: Excreted primarily in urine by renal tubular secretion and glomerular filtration; it also appears in breast milk and in small amounts in bile. Elimination half-life in adults is ½ to 1 hour, extended to 2 hours in severe renal impairment. Dosage adjustments aren't required in patients with creatinine clearance less than 10 ml/minute.

Route	Onset	Peak	Duration
P.O.	Unknown	½-2 hr	Unknown
I.V.	Immediate	Immediate	Unknown
I.M.	Unknown	½ hr	Unknown

Contraindications and precautions

Contraindicated in patients hypersensitive to drug or other penicillins. Use cautiously in neonates, infants, and patients with other drug allergies, especially to cephalosporins.

Interactions

Drug-drug. *Aminoglycosides:* Produces synergistic bactericidal effects against *S. aureus*. This is a therapeutic effect.
Probenecid: Blocks renal tubular secretion of penicillins, increasing their serum levels. Use together cautiously.
Drug-food. *Food:* Decreases absorption. Tell patient that drug should be taken on an empty stomach.
Fruit juice and carbonated beverages: Interference with absorption. Tell patient that drug should be taken with water.

Adverse reactions

CNS: neuropathy, neuromuscular irritability, *seizures*, lethargy, hallucinations, anxiety, confusion, agitation, depression, dizziness, fatigue.
GI: oral lesions, nausea, vomiting, diarrhea, enterocolitis, *pseudomembranous colitis*.
GU: interstitial nephritis, nephropathy.
Hematologic: *thrombocytopenia*, eosinophilia, *hemolytic anemia, neutropenia,* anemia, *agranulocytosis.*
Hepatic: elevated liver enzyme levels.
Other: *hypersensitivity reactions* (fever, chills, rash, urticaria, *anaphylaxis,* overgrowth of nonsusceptible organisms, *thrombophlebitis*).

Overdose and treatment

Overdose may cause neuromuscular sensitivity or seizures. There are no specific recommendations. Treatment is supportive. After recent ingestion (within 4 hours), empty the stomach by induced emesis or gastric lavage; follow with activated charcoal to reduce absorption. Oxacillin isn't appreciably removed by peritoneal dialysis or hemodialysis.

Special considerations

● Prosthetic valve endocarditis caused by coagulase-negative staphylococci is usually methicillin-resistant.
● When drug is given for group A beta-hemolytic streptococci, continue therapy for at least 10 days to decrease risk of glomerulonephritis and rheumatic fever.
● Give oral drug with water; acid in fruit juice or carbonated beverage may inactivate drug.
● Give oral dose on empty stomach; food decreases absorption.
● Except in osteomyelitis, don't give by I.M. or I.V. route unless patient can't take oral dose.
● For oral preparation, add amount of water specified on bottle to yield 250 mg/5 ml. Add water in 2 parts and shake vigorously.
● For I.M. preparation, add 1.4, 2.8, 5.7, 11.4, or 21.8 ml of sterile water for injection or half-normal or normal saline solution injection to vial containing 250 mg, 500 mg, 1 g, 2 g, or 4 g, respectively. Final solution is 250 mg/1.5 ml.
● For intermittent I.V. injection, use sterile water for injection or normal saline solution injection; add 5 ml to 250-mg vial to equal 50 mg/ml. Add 5 ml, 10 ml, 20 ml, or 40 ml to vials containing 500 mg, 1 g, 2 g, or 4 g, respectively, and 93 ml to 10-g pharmacy bulk package to produce 100 mg/ml. Inject slowly over 10 minutes. For continuous I.V. infusion, further dilute with compatible solution to 0.5 to 40 mg/ml. Infuse over 30 to 60 minutes. Drug loses 10% of potency within 6 hours of dilution.
● Thaw commercial solutions at room temperature or in refrigerator.
● Oxacillin is incompatible with aminoglycosides in the same I.V. infusion.
● Oxacillin alters tests for urinary and serum proteins; turbidimetric urine and serum proteins are

often falsely positive or elevated in tests using sulfosalicylic acid or trichloroacetic acid.
• Oxacillin may falsely decrease serum aminoglycoside levels.

Patient monitoring
• Monitor renal and hepatic function and hematologic function; watch for elevated AST and ALT levels.

Breast-feeding patients
• Oxacillin appears in breast milk. Use drug cautiously in breast-feeding women.

Pediatric patients
• Elimination of oxacillin is reduced in neonates. Transient hematuria, azotemia, and albuminuria have occurred in some neonates receiving oxacillin. Monitor renal function closely.

Geriatric patients
• Half-life of drug may be prolonged in elderly patients because of impaired renal function.
• These patients have an increased risk of thrombophlebitis during I.V. infusion.

Patient education
• Explain need to take oral preparations without food and to follow with water only, not fruit juice or carbonated beverages.
• Tell patient to report allergic reactions or severe diarrhea promptly.
• Emphasize importance of completing the full course of therapy.

---

oxaprozin
Daypro

Pharmacologic classification: NSAID
Therapeutic classification: nonnarcotic analgesic, antipyretic, anti-inflammatory
Pregnancy risk category: C

Indications and dosages
➤ *Management of acute or chronic osteoarthritis or rheumatoid arthritis. Adults:* Initially, 1,200 mg P.O. daily. Individualize to smallest effective dosage to minimize adverse reactions. Smaller patients or those with mild symptoms may need only 600 mg daily. Maximum daily dose is 1,800 mg or 26 mg/kg, whichever is lower, in divided doses.
✦ *Dosage adjustment.* For patients with renal impairment or those undergoing hemodialysis, initial dose is 600 mg P.O. daily.

How supplied
Available by prescription only
Caplets: 600 mg

Pharmacodynamics
Analgesic, antipyretic, and anti-inflammatory actions: Exact mechanism of action isn't clearly

defined. Drug inhibits several steps along the arachidonic acid pathway of prostaglandin synthesis. One of the modes of action is presumed to be a result of the inhibition of cyclooxygenase activity and prostaglandin synthesis at the site of inflammation.

Pharmacokinetics
Absorption: Demonstrates high oral bioavailability (95%). Food may reduce the rate of absorption, but extent of absorption is unchanged.
Distribution: About 99.9% bound to albumin in plasma.
Metabolism: Primarily metabolized in the liver by microsomal oxidation (65%) and glucuronic acid conjugation (35%).
Excretion: Glucuronide metabolites are excreted in urine (65%) and feces (35%). Elimination half-life in adults is 42 to 50 hours.

Route	Onset	Peak	Duration
P.O.	Unknown	3-5 hr	Unknown

Contraindications and precautions
Contraindicated in patients hypersensitive to drug or with the syndrome of nasal polyps, angioedema, and bronchospastic reaction to aspirin or other NSAIDs.
Use cautiously in patients with renal or hepatic dysfunction, history of peptic ulcer, hypertension, CV disease, or conditions predisposing to fluid retention.

Interactions
Drug-drug. *Aspirin:* Oxaprozin displaces salicylates from plasma protein binding, increasing the risk of salicylate toxicity. Avoid use together.
Beta blockers such as metoprolol: May cause a transient increase in blood pressure after 14 days of therapy. Monitor blood pressure.
Oral anticoagulants: May increase the risk of bleeding. Monitor PT and INR. Monitor patient for increased bruising or bleeding.
Drug-lifestyle. *Sun exposure:* May cause photosensitivity reactions. Advise patient to take precautions.

Adverse reactions
CNS: depression, sedation, somnolence, confusion, sleep disturbances.
EENT: tinnitus, blurred vision.
GI: *nausea, dyspepsia, diarrhea, constipation,* abdominal pain or distress, anorexia, flatulence, vomiting, *hemorrhage,* stomatitis, ulcer.
GU: dysuria, urinary frequency.
Hematologic: prolonged bleeding time.
Hepatic: elevated liver function test results (with long-term use).
Skin: *rash,* photosensitivity.

Overdose and treatment
No information specific to oxaprozin overdose is available. Common symptoms of acute overdose with other NSAIDs, including lethargy, drowsi-

ness, nausea, vomiting, and epigastric pain, are generally reversible with supportive care. GI bleeding and coma have occurred after NSAID overdose. Hypertension, acute renal failure, and respiratory depression are rare.

Gut decontamination may be indicated in symptomatic patients seen within 4 hours of ingestion or after a large overdose (5 to 10 times the usual dose). This is accomplished by emesis or activated charcoal with an osmotic cathartic.

Special considerations
• Serious GI toxicity, including peptic ulceration and bleeding, can occur in patients taking NSAIDs despite the absence of GI symptoms. Patients at risk for peptic ulceration and bleeding are those with history of serious GI events, alcoholism, smoking, or other factors linked to peptic ulcer disease.
• Dosages exceeding 1,200 mg daily should be used for patients who weigh more than 50 kg (110 lb), who have normal renal and hepatic function, who are at low risk of peptic ulceration, and whose severity of disease justifies maximal therapy.
• Most patients tolerate once-daily dosing. Divided doses may be tried in patients unable to tolerate single doses.

Patient monitoring
• Periodically monitor liver function tests in patients receiving long-term therapy, and closely monitor patients with abnormal results. Elevated liver function test results can occur after long-term use. These findings may persist, worsen, or resolve with continued therapy. Rarely, patients may progress to severe hepatic dysfunction.
• Anemia may occur in patients receiving oxaprozin. Monitor hemoglobin level or hematocrit in patients receiving prolonged therapy at intervals appropriate for their clinical situation.

Breast-feeding patients
• Studies of oxaprozin appearing in breast milk haven't been conducted. Use cautiously in breast-feeding women.

Pediatric patients
• Safety and efficacy in children haven't been established.

Geriatric patients
• Elderly patients may need a reduced dose because of low body weight or disorders caused by aging.
• These patients are less likely than younger patients to tolerate adverse reactions linked to oxaprozin.

Patient education
• Warn patient to immediately report signs and symptoms of GI bleeding or visual or auditory adverse reactions.

• Tell patient to take drug with milk or meals if adverse GI reactions occur.
• Because photosensitivity reactions may occur, advise patient to use a sunblock, wear protective clothing, and avoid prolonged exposure to sunlight.

oxazepam
Apo-Oxazepam*, Novoxapam*, Ox-pam*, Serax

Pharmacologic classification: benzodiazepine
Therapeutic classification: antianxiety agent, sedative-hypnotic
Controlled substance schedule: IV
Pregnancy risk category: D

Indications and dosages
➤ *Alcohol withdrawal, severe anxiety.*
Adults: 15 to 30 mg P.O. t.i.d. or q.i.d.
➤ *Tension, mild to moderate anxiety.*
Adults: 10 to 15 mg P.O. t.i.d. or q.i.d.
✦ *Dosage adjustment.* In older adults, give 10 mg P.O. t.i.d.; then increase to 15 mg t.i.d. or q.i.d., p.r.n.

How supplied
Available by prescription only
Capsules: 10 mg, 15 mg, 30 mg
Tablets: 15 mg

Pharmacodynamics
Anxiolytic and sedative-hypnotic actions: Oxazepam depresses the CNS at the limbic and subcortical levels of the brain. It produces an antianxiety effect by enhancing the effect of the neurotransmitter gamma-aminobutyric acid on its receptor in the ascending reticular activating system, which increases inhibition and blocks both cortical and limbic arousal.

Pharmacokinetics
Absorption: When administered orally, oxazepam is well absorbed through the GI tract.
Distribution: Distributed widely throughout the body; 85% to 95% protein-bound.
Metabolism: Metabolized in the liver to inactive metabolites.
Excretion: Metabolites are excreted in urine as glucuronide conjugates. Half-life of drug is 5¾ to 20 hours.

Route	Onset	Peak	Duration
P.O.	Unknown	2-4 hr	Unknown

Contraindications and precautions
Contraindicated in patients hypersensitive to drug and patients with psychosis. Use cautiously in elderly or debilitated patients; in those with history of drug abuse; and in those in whom decreased blood pressure is linked to cardiac problems.

Reactions may be *common*, uncommon, *life-threatening*, or COMMON AND LIFE-THREATENING.

Interactions

Drug-drug. *Antacids:* May decrease rate but not extent of oxazepam absorption. Separate administration times of these drugs.

Antidepressants, antihistamines, barbiturates, general anesthetics, MAO inhibitors, narcotics, phenothiazines: Potentiated CNS depressant effects of these drugs. Avoid use together, if possible.

Cimetidine, disulfiram: Risk of decreased hepatic metabolism and increase plasma levels of oxazepam. Monitor patient carefully.

Levodopa: Inhibited therapeutic effects of levodopa. Monitor patient closely.

Theophylline: May antagonize the effects of benzodiazepines. Monitor patient for effect.

Drug-herb. *Catnip, kava, lady's slipper, lemon balm, passionflower, sassafras, skullcap, valerian:* Sedative effects may be enhanced. Discourage use together.

Drug-lifestyle. *Alcohol use:* Potentiated CNS depressant effects. Tell patient to avoid use together. *Caffeine:* May antagonize effects of benzodiazepines. Monitor patient for effect.

Heavy smoking: Accelerated oxazepam metabolism and reduced effectiveness. Advise patient to avoid use together.

Adverse reactions

CNS: *drowsiness, lethargy,* dizziness, vertigo, headache, syncope, tremor, slurred speech, changes in EEG patterns.
CV: edema.
GI: nausea.
Hepatic: *hepatic dysfunction.*
Skin: rash.
Other: altered libido.

Overdose and treatment

Signs and symptoms of overdose include somnolence, confusion, coma, hypoactive reflexes, dyspnea, labored breathing, hypotension, bradycardia, slurred speech, and unsteady gait or impaired coordination.

Support blood pressure and respiration until drug effects have subsided; monitor vital signs. Mechanical ventilatory assistance via endotracheal tube may be needed to maintain a patent airway and support oxygenation. Flumazenil, a specific benzodiazepine antagonist, may be useful and should be kept readily available. As needed, give I.V. fluids and vasopressors, such as dopamine and phenylephrine, to treat hypotension. If the patient is conscious, induce emesis. Use gastric lavage if ingestion was recent, but only if an endotracheal tube is present to prevent aspiration. After emesis or lavage, administer activated charcoal with a cathartic as a single dose. Dialysis is of limited value.

Special considerations

● Oxazepam tablets contain tartrazine dye; check patient's history for allergy to this substance.
● Store drug in a cool, dry place away from light.

● Use of drug for greater than 4 months hasn't been established.
● Gradually reduce dosage (over 8 to 12 weeks) after long-term use.

Patient monitoring
● Monitor hepatic and renal function studies to ensure normal function.

Breast-feeding patients
● The breast-fed infant of a woman who uses oxazepam may become sedated, have feeding difficulties, or lose weight. Avoid use in breast-feeding women.

Pediatric patients
● Safety in children under age 6 hasn't been established. Closely observe neonate for withdrawal symptoms if mother took oxazepam for a prolonged period during pregnancy.

Geriatric patients
● These patients are more susceptible to CNS depressant effects of oxazepam. Some may need assistance with walking and activities of daily living when therapy starts or dosage increases.
● Reduced dosages are usually effective in elderly patients because of their decreased elimination.

Patient education
● Advise patient not to change part of drug regimen without medical approval.
● Instruct patient in safety measures, such as gradual position changes and assisted ambulation, to prevent injury.
● Because sleepiness may not occur for up to 2 hours after taking oxazepam, tell patient to wait before taking an additional dose.
● Advise patient of risk for physical and psychological dependence with long-term use of oxazepam.
● Tell patient not to stop drug suddenly if he has been taking it for a long time.

oxcarbazepine
Trileptal

Pharmacologic classification: carboxamide derivative
Therapeutic classification: antiepileptic
Pregnancy risk category: C

Indications and dosages
➤ *Adjunctive therapy for partial seizures in patients with epilepsy. Adults:* Initially, 300 mg P.O. b.i.d. Increase by a maximum of 600 mg daily (300 mg P.O b.i.d.) at weekly intervals. Recommended daily dose is 1,200 mg P.O. divided b.i.d.
Children ages 4 to 16: Initially 8 to 10 mg/kg daily P.O. divided b.i.d., not to exceed 600 mg daily. The target maintenance dose depends on

patient weight and should be divided b.i.d. If patient weighs 20 to 29 kg (44 to 64 lb), then the target maintenance dose is 900 mg daily. If patient weighs 29.1 to 39 kg (65 to 86 lb), target maintenance dose is 1,200 mg daily. If patient weighs more than 39 kg, target maintenance dose is 1,800 mg daily. Target doses should be achieved over 2 weeks.

➤ *Conversion to monotherapy for partial seizures in patients with epilepsy.* *Adults:* Initially, 300 mg P.O. b.i.d., with simultaneous reduction in antiepileptic dosage. Increase oxcarbazepine by a maximum of 600 mg daily at weekly intervals over 2 to 4 weeks. Recommended daily dose is 2,400 mg P.O. divided b.i.d. Concomitant antiepileptics should be withdrawn over 3 to 6 weeks.

➤ *Monotherapy for partial seizures in patients with epilepsy.* *Adults:* Initially, 300 mg P.O. b.i.d. Increase dosage by 300 mg daily every third day to a daily dose of 1,200 mg divided b.i.d.

✦ *Dosage adjustment.* For adults with creatinine clearance less than 30 ml/minute, start with 150 mg P.O. b.i.d. (half the usual starting dose) and increase slowly to achieve the desired response.

How supplied

Available by prescription only
Tablets (film-coated): 150 mg, 300 mg, 600 mg

Pharmacodynamics

Anticonvulsant action: Unknown. Antiseizure activity is thought to occur through the blockade of voltage-sensitive sodium channels which ultimately may prevent seizure spread in the brain. Increased potassium conductance and modulation of high-voltage activated calcium channels may also contribute to anticonvulsant effects.

Pharmacokinetics

Absorption: Oxcarbazepine is completely absorbed following oral administration.
Distribution: About 40% of 10-monohydroxy (MHD) metabolite is bound to serum proteins, mostly to albumin.
Metabolism: Oxcarbazepine is rapidly metabolized in the liver to MHD, which is mainly responsible for drug effects. Minor amounts (4% of dose) are oxidized to the pharmacologically inactive 10,11-dihydroxy metabolite.
Excretion: Oxcarbazepine and its metabolites are primarily excreted by the kidneys. More than 95% appears in urine, with less than 1% as unchanged oxcarbazepine. Fecal excretion accounts for less than 4%. Half-life of parent compound is about 2 hours, and half-life of MHD is about 9 hours. Children under age 8 have about 30% to 40% increased clearance of drug.

Route	Onset	Peak	Duration
P.O.	Unknown	Variable	Unknown

Contraindications and precautions

Contraindicated in patients hypersensitive to oxcarbazepine or its components. Use cautiously in patients who have had hypersensitivity reactions to carbamazepine.

Interactions

Drug-drug. *Carbamazepine, valproic acid, verapamil:* Decreased levels of the active metabolite of oxcarbazepine. Monitor patient and serum levels closely.
Felodipine: Decreased felodipine level. Monitor patient closely.
Hormonal contraceptives: Decreased plasma levels of ethinylestradiol and levonorgestrel, rendering oral contraceptives less effective. Women of childbearing age should use alternative forms of contraception.
Phenobarbital: Decreased serum levels of the active metabolite of oxcarbazepine and increased phenobarbital level. Monitor patient closely.
Phenytoin: Decreased serum levels of the active metabolite of oxcarbazepine. May increase phenytoin level in adults receiving high doses of oxcarbazepine. Monitor phenytoin levels closely when starting therapy in these patients.
Drug-lifestyle. *Alcohol:* Increased CNS depression. Avoid concomitant use.

Adverse reactions

CNS: *fatigue,* asthenia, feeling abnormal, *headache, dizziness, somnolence, ataxia, abnormal gait,* insomnia, *tremor,* nervousness, agitation, abnormal coordination, speech disorder, confusion, anxiety, amnesia, *aggravated seizures,* hypoesthesia, emotional lability, impaired concentration, *vertigo.*
CV: hypotension, edema, chest pain.
EENT: *nystagmus, diplopia, abnormal vision,* abnormal accommodation, rhinitis, sinusitis, pharyngitis, epistaxis, toothache, ear ache.
GI: *nausea, vomiting, abdominal pain,* diarrhea, dyspepsia, constipation, gastritis, anorexia, dry mouth, rectal hemorrhage, taste perversion, thirst.
GU: urinary tract infection, urinary frequency, vaginitis.
Metabolic: hyponatremia, weight increase, decreased thyroxine level.
Musculoskeletal: muscle weakness, back pain.
Respiratory: *upper respiratory tract infection,* coughing, bronchitis, chest infection.
Skin: acne, hot flushes, purpura, rash, bruising, increased sweating.
Other: fever, allergy, lymphadenopathy, infection.

Overdose and treatment

Give symptomatic and supportive treatment as appropriate. There is no specific antidote. Consider removing drug by gastric lavage, inactivating it with activated charcoal, or both.

Reactions may be *common*, uncommon, *life-threatening*, or COMMON AND LIFE-THREATENING.

Special considerations

ALERT Question patient about history of hypersensitivity to carbamazepine because 25% to 30% of these patients may develop hypersensitivity to oxcarbazepine. Stop drug immediately if signs or symptoms of hypersensitivity occur.

• Oxcarbazepine has been linked to several nervous system–related adverse events including psychomotor slowing, difficulty with concentration, speech or language problems, somnolence, fatigue, and coordination abnormalities, including ataxia and gait disturbances.

ALERT Withdraw drug gradually to minimize risk of increased seizure frequency.

Patient monitoring

• Monitor patient for signs and symptoms of hyponatremia, including nausea, malaise, headache, lethargy, confusion, or decreased sensation.

• Monitor serum sodium levels in patients receiving oxcarbazepine for maintenance treatment, especially those who receive other therapies that may decrease serum sodium levels.

Breast-feeding patients

• The drug and its active metabolite appear in breast milk. Because of the risk of serious adverse reactions in infants, a decision must be made to stop either drug or breast-feeding.

Pediatric patients

• Oxcarbazepine is indicated only for adjunctive therapy in children ages 4 to 16.

Geriatric patients

• Doses may need to be adjusted in elderly patients to compensate for age-related decreases in creatinine clearance.

Patient education

• Medication may be taken with or without food.
• Advise patient not to interrupt or stop drug without medical advice.
• Urge patient to report signs and symptoms of hyponatremia, such as nausea, malaise, headache, lethargy or confusion.
• Caution patient to avoid hazardous activities until drug effects are known.
• Advise women using oral contraceptives for birth control to use another form of birth control during therapy.
• Tell patient to avoid alcohol while taking drug.
• Advise patient to tell prescriber about any previous hypersensitivity reactions to carbamazepine.

oxtriphylline

Apo-Oxtriphylline*, Choledyl, Choledyl SA

Pharmacologic classification: xanthine derivative
Therapeutic classification: bronchodilator
Pregnancy risk category: C

Indications and dosages

➤ *To relieve acute bronchial asthma and reversible bronchospasm caused by chronic bronchitis and emphysema.* Adults (nonsmokers): 4.7 mg/kg P.O. q 8 hours.
Adults (smokers) and children ages 9 to 16: 4.7 mg/kg q 6 hours.
Children ages 1 to 9: 6.2 mg/kg P.O. q 6 hours.

For all patients, if total daily maintenance dosage is established at about 800 to 1,200 mg, one sustained-action tablet q 12 hours may be substituted.

How supplied

Available by prescription only
Elixir: 100 mg/5 ml*
Syrup: 50 mg/5 ml*
Tablets (delayed release): 100 mg, 200 mg
Tablets (sustained release): 400 mg, 600 mg

Pharmacodynamics

Bronchodilating action: Oxtriphylline exerts bronchodilating action after it is converted to theophylline. (Oxtriphylline is 64% anhydrous theophylline.) Theophylline antagonizes adenosine receptors in the bronchi and may inhibit phosphodiesterase and increase levels of cyclic adenosine monophosphate, thus relaxing smooth muscle of the respiratory tract.

Pharmacokinetics

Absorption: Drug is well absorbed; rate of absorption and onset of action depend on dosage form.
Distribution: Drug is distributed rapidly throughout body fluids and tissues.
Metabolism: Oxtriphylline, the choline salt of theophylline, is converted to theophylline, then metabolized to inactive compounds.
Excretion: Drug is excreted in the urine as theophylline (10%) and theophyllic metabolites.

Route	Onset	Peak	Duration
P.O.	Variable	Unknown	Unknown

Contraindications and precautions

Contraindicated in patients hypersensitive to xanthines (caffeine, theobromine) and in those with arrhythmias, especially tachyarrhythmias.

Use cautiously in young and elderly patients and those with impaired renal or hepatic function, peptic ulcer, COPD, cardiac failure, cor pulmonale, glaucoma, severe hypoxemia, hypertension, compromised cardiac or circulatory function, angina, acute MI, sulfite sensitivity, hyperthyroidism, or diabetes mellitus.

Interactions
Drug-drug. *Allopurinol (high dose), cimetidine, macrolides (erythromycin, troleandomycin), propranolol, quinolones:* May increase oxtriphylline level by decreasing hepatic clearance. Monitor oxtriphylline level.
Adenosine: Decreased antiarrhythmic effect. Larger doses of adenosine may be needed or adenosine may be ineffective.
Aminoglutethimide, barbiturates: Decreased oxtriphylline effects via enhanced metabolism. Monitor patient for effect.
Lithium: Increased lithium excretion. Monitor patient for effect.
Drug-lifestyle. *Marijuana, nicotine use:* Decreased oxtriphylline effects via enhanced metabolism. Discourage marijuana and nicotine use.

Adverse reactions
CNS: restlessness, dizziness, headache, insomnia, irritability, *seizures*, muscle twitching.
CV: palpitations, sinus tachycardia, extrasystoles, flushing, marked hypotension, *arrhythmias*.
GI: nausea, vomiting, epigastric pain, diarrhea.
Respiratory: tachypnea, *respiratory arrest*.
Skin: rash.

Overdose and treatment
Signs and symptoms of overdose include nausea, vomiting, insomnia, irritability, tachycardia, extrasystoles, tachypnea, and tonic-clonic seizures. The onset of toxicity may be sudden and severe, with arrhythmias and seizures as the first signs.

Induce emesis except in convulsing patients; follow with activated charcoal and cathartics. Treat arrhythmias with lidocaine and seizures with I.V. benzodiazepine; support CV and respiratory systems.

Special considerations
● Don't crush sustained-release tablets.
● Store drug at 59° to 86° F (15° to 30° C) and away from heat and light.
● Oxtriphylline may falsely elevate serum uric acid levels measured by colorimetric methods.
● Theophylline levels may be falsely elevated in patients taking furosemide, phenylbutazone, probenecid, some cephalosporins, sulfa drugs, theobromine, caffeine, tea, chocolate, cola beverages, or acetaminophen, depending on assay method used.

Patient monitoring
● Monitor vital signs and intake and output. Watch for CNS stimulation and CV adverse reactions.

Breast-feeding patients
● Drug appears in breast milk and may cause irritability, insomnia, or fretfulness in the breast-fed infant.

Pediatric patients
● Use cautiously in neonates.

Geriatric patients
● Decrease dosage in elderly patients, and monitor them closely.

Patient education
● Instruct patient about drug and dosage schedule; if a dose is missed, tell him to take it as soon as possible. Warn against doubling the dose.
● Advise patient about adverse effects and signs of possible toxicity. Urge patient to report signs of excessive CNS stimulation (nervousness, tremors, akathisia).
● Warn patient to avoid consuming large quantities of xanthine-containing foods and beverages.

oxybutynin chloride
Ditropan, Ditropan XL

Pharmacologic classification: synthetic tertiary amine
Therapeutic classification: antispasmodic
Pregnancy risk category: B

Indications and dosages
➤ *For relief of symptoms of bladder instability caused by voiding in patients with uninhibited and reflex neurogenic bladder.* Adults: 5 mg P.O. b.i.d. to t.i.d. to maximum of 5 mg q.i.d.
Children over age 5: 5 mg P.O. b.i.d. to maximum of 5 mg t.i.d.

How supplied
Available by prescription only
Syrup: 5 mg/5 ml
Tablets: 5 mg
Tablets (extended release): 5 mg, 10 mg, 15 mg

Pharmacodynamics
Antispasmodic action: Oxybutynin reduces the urge to void, increases bladder capacity, and reduces the frequency of detrusor muscle contractions. Drug exerts a direct spasmolytic action and an antimuscarinic action on smooth muscle.

Pharmacokinetics
Absorption: Absorbed rapidly.
Distribution: No data available.
Metabolism: Metabolized by the liver.
Excretion: Excreted principally in urine.

Route	Onset	Peak	Duration
P.O.	½-1 hr	3-4 hr	6-10 hr

Contraindications and precautions
Contraindicated in patients hypersensitive to drug and patients with myasthenia gravis, GI obstruction, glaucoma, adynamic ileus, megacolon, severe colitis, ulcerative colitis when megacolon is

present, or obstructive uropathy. Also contraindicated in geriatric or debilitated patients with intestinal atony and in hemorrhaging patients with unstable CV status.

Use cautiously in elderly patients and patients with impaired renal or hepatic function, autonomic neuropathy, or reflux esophagitis.

Interactions

Drug-drug. *Acetaminophen:* Delayed absorption of acetaminophen because of oxybutynin effect on smooth muscle. Monitor patient.
Atenolol: Increased atenolol absorption. Monitor patient.
CNS depressants: Additive sedative effects. Use together cautiously.
Digoxin: May increase digoxin levels. Monitor serum digoxin levels.
Haloperidol: Worsening of schizophrenia, decreased serum levels of haloperidol, and development of tardive dyskinesia. Use together cautiously, if at all.
Levodopa: Decreased effects of levodopa. Monitor patient for effect.
Phenothiazine: Increased risk of anticholinergic adverse effects. Monitor patient closely.

Adverse reactions

CNS: dizziness, insomnia, restlessness, hallucinations, asthenia.
CV: *palpitations, tachycardia,* vasodilation.
EENT: mydriasis, cycloplegia, decreased lacrimation, amblyopia.
GI: nausea, vomiting, *constipation, dry mouth,* decreased GI motility.
GU: *urinary hesitancy, urine retention.*
Skin: rash.
Other: decreased diaphoresis, fever, suppressed lactation.

Overdose and treatment

Signs and symptoms of overdose include restlessness, excitement, psychotic behavior, flushing, hypotension, circulatory failure, and fever. In severe cases, paralysis, respiratory failure, and coma may occur.

Treatment requires gastric lavage. Activated charcoal may be given, and a cathartic. Physostigmine may reverse symptoms of anticholinergic intoxication. Treat hyperpyrexia symptomatically with ice bags or other cold applications and alcohol sponges. Maintain artificial respiration if respiratory muscles are paralyzed.

Special considerations

• Stop drug periodically to determine whether patient still needs it.
• Store drug in tight, light-resistant container at 59° to 86° F (15° to 30° C); drug expires 4 years from date of manufacture.

Patient monitoring

• Monitor patient with hepatic and renal disease.

Breast-feeding patients

• It isn't known if drug appears in breast milk. Use cautiously in breast-feeding women.

Pediatric patients

• Dosage guidelines haven't been established for children under age 5.

Geriatric patients

• These patients may be more sensitive to antimuscarinic effects. Drug is contraindicated in elderly and debilitated patients with intestinal atony.

Patient education

• Instruct patient regarding drug and dosage schedule; tell him to take a missed dose as soon as possible and not to double the dose.
• Tell patient not to crush or chew extended-release tablets. They may be taken without regard to food.
• Explain that extended-release tablets don't disintegrate and are eliminated in feces.
• Warn patient about possible decreased mental alertness or visual changes.
• Remind patient to use drug cautiously in warm climate to minimize risk of heatstroke that may occur because of decreased sweating.

oxycodone hydrochloride

Endocodone, M-oxy, Oxycontin, OxyFAST, OxyIR, Percolone, Roxicodone, Supeudol*

Pharmacologic classification: opioid
Therapeutic classification: analgesic
Controlled substance schedule: II
Pregnancy risk category: C

Indications and dosages

➤ *Moderate to severe pain. Adults:* 5 mg P.O. q 6 hours.
➤ *Chronic pain. Adults:* Initially, 10-mg sustained-release tablet P.O. q 12 hours; may increase dose q 1 to 2 days. Dosing frequency shouldn't be increased.

How supplied

Available by prescription only
Capsules: 5 mg
Oral solution: 5 mg/ml, 20 mg/ml
Tablets: 5 mg, 15 mg, 30 mg
Tablets (sustained-release): 10 mg, 20 mg, 40 mg, 80 mg, 160 mg

Pharmacodynamics

Analgesic action: Oxycodone acts on opiate receptors, providing analgesia for moderate to moderately severe pain. Acute pain, rather than chronic pain, appears to be more responsive.

Pharmacokinetics

Absorption: After oral administration.
Distribution: Rapidly distributed.

Metabolism: Metabolized in the liver.
Excretion: Excreted principally by the kidneys.

Route	Onset	Peak	Duration
P.O.			
Immediate	10-15 min	1 hr	3-12 hr
Sustained	Unknown	Unknown	Unknown

Contraindications and precautions
Contraindicated in patients hypersensitive to drug. Use cautiously in elderly or debilitated patients and in those with head injury, increased intracranial pressure, seizures, asthma, COPD, prostatic hyperplasia, severe hepatic or renal disease, acute abdominal conditions, urethral stricture, hypothyroidism, Addison's disease, or arrhythmias.

Interactions
Drug-drug. *Anticholinergics:* May cause paralytic ileus. Use together cautiously.
Anticoagulants: Oxycodone products that contain aspirin may increase anticoagulant effects. Monitor clotting times, and use together cautiously.
Cimetidine: May increase respiratory and CNS depression, causing confusion, disorientation, apnea, or seizures. Avoid use together.
CNS depressants, such as antihistamines, barbiturates, benzodiazepines, general anesthetics, muscle relaxants, narcotic analgesics, phenothiazines, sedative-hypnotics, and tricyclic antidepressants: Potentiated respiratory and CNS depression, sedation, and hypotensive effects of drug. Use together with extreme caution.
Digitoxin, phenytoin, rifampin: Drug accumulation and enhanced effects may result from use with other drugs that are extensively metabolized in the liver. Monitor patient closely.
General anesthetics: Severe CV depression. Use together with extreme caution.
Opioid agonist-antagonist or a single dose of an antagonist: Patients who become physically dependent on oxycodone may experience acute withdrawal syndrome. Avoid use together in this situation.
Drug-lifestyle. *Alcohol use:* Potentiated respiratory and CNS depression, sedation, and hypotensive effects of drug. Advise patient to avoid combined use.

Adverse reactions
CNS: *sedation, somnolence, clouded sensorium, euphoria, dizziness, light-headedness, seizures.*
CV: *hypotension, bradycardia.*
GI: *nausea, vomiting, constipation,* ileus, increased plasma amylase and lipase levels.
GU: *urine retention.*
Hepatic: increased liver enzyme levels.
Respiratory: *respiratory depression.*
Skin: *diaphoresis,* pruritus, rash.
Other: physical dependence.

Overdose and treatment
The most common signs and symptoms of a severe overdose are CNS depression, respiratory depression, and miosis. Other acute toxic effects include hypotension, bradycardia, hypothermia, shock, apnea, cardiopulmonary arrest, circulatory collapse, pulmonary edema, and seizures.

To treat acute overdose, first establish adequate respiratory exchange via a patent airway and ventilation as needed; give a narcotic antagonist (naloxone) to reverse respiratory depression. Because the duration of action of oxycodone is longer than that of naloxone, repeated naloxone dosing is necessary. Don't give naloxone unless patient has clinically significant respiratory or CV depression. Monitor vital signs closely.

If within 2 hours of ingestion of an oral overdose, empty the stomach immediately via induced emesis (ipecac syrup) or gastric lavage. Use caution to avoid risk of aspiration. Administer activated charcoal via nasogastric tube for further removal of drug. Provide symptomatic and supportive treatment, including continued respiratory support and correction of fluid or electrolyte imbalance. Monitor laboratory values, vital signs, and neurologic status closely. Dialysis may be helpful if aspirin-containing products are involved.

Special considerations
• Some commercial preparations contain sodium metabisulfite, which may cause an allergic reaction in susceptible people.
• Single-agent oxycodone solution or tablets are ideal for patients who can't take aspirin or acetaminophen.
• The sustained-release preparation isn't intended for preoperative or immediate postoperative pain in patients not already taking the drug. Drug is only indicated for postoperative use if patient was receiving it before surgery or if pain is expected to persist for a long time. It also isn't intended for p.r.n. use.
• Oxycodone has high abuse potential.
• Drug may obscure signs and symptoms of an acute abdominal condition and it may worsen gallbladder pain.
• Consider prescribing a stool softener for patients receiving long-term therapy.
• The 80 mg sustained-release tablets are for opioid-tolerant patients.
• Patients being transferred from 5- to 25-mg daily conventional dose should receive 10 to 20 mg q 12 hours of the sustained-release preparation. If conventional dose is 30 to 45 mg or 50 to 60 mg daily, the sustained-release dose is 20 to 30 mg q 12 hours or 30 to 40 mg q 12 hours, respectively.
• Chewing, crushing, snorting, or injecting the sustained-release preparation can lead to overdose and death.

Patient monitoring
• Monitor patient for relief of pain and development of tolerance to drug effects.

Reactions may be *common*, uncommon, *life-threatening*, or COMMON AND LIFE-THREATENING.

Breast-feeding patients
• It isn't known if drug appears in breast milk. Use cautiously in breast-feeding women.

Pediatric patients
• Dosage may be individualized for children; however, safety and effectiveness in children haven't been established.

Geriatric patients
• Lower doses are usually indicated for elderly patients, who may be more sensitive to therapeutic and adverse effects of drug.

Patient education
• For full analgesic effect, teach patient to take drug before onset of intense pain.
• Warn patient about possibility of decreased alertness or visual changes.

oxymetazoline hydrochloride
Afrin, Allerest 12 Hour Nasal Spray, Chlorphed-LA, Dristan Long Lasting, Duramist Plus, Duration, 4-Way Long Lasting Spray, Neo-Synephrine 12 Hour Nasal Spray, Nostrilla Long Acting Nasal Decongestant, NTZ Long Acting Decongestant Nasal Spray, OcuClear, Sinarest 12 Hour Nasal Spray, Vicks Sinex Long-Acting, Visine L.R.

Pharmacologic classification: sympathomimetic
Therapeutic classification: decongestant, vasoconstrictor
Pregnancy risk category: C

Indications and dosages
➤ *Nasal congestion. Adults and children over age 6:* 2 to 3 drops or sprays of 0.05% solution in each nostril q 10 to 12 hours for no more than 3 to 5 days. Dosage for younger children hasn't been established.
➤ *Relief of minor eye redness. Adults and children over age 6:* 1 to 2 drops in the conjunctival sac up to q.i.d. (spaced at least 6 hours apart).

How supplied
Available without a prescription
Nasal drops or spray: 0.05%
Nasal solution: 0.025% (drops) for children
Ophthalmic solution: 0.025%

Pharmacodynamics
Decongestant action: Oxymetazoline produces local vasoconstriction of arterioles through alpha receptors to reduce blood flow and nasal congestion.

Pharmacokinetics
Absorption: Occasional systemic absorption may occur.
Distribution: Unknown.
Metabolism: Unknown.
Excretion: Unknown.

Route	Onset	Peak	Duration
Ophthalmic	5 min	Unknown	6 hr
Nasal	5-10 min	6 hr	< 12 hr

Contraindications and precautions
Contraindicated in patients hypersensitive to drug. Ophthalmic form contraindicated in patients with angle-closure glaucoma.

Use cautiously in patients with hyperthyroidism, cardiac disease, or hypertension and in those receiving MAO inhibitors. Use nasal solution cautiously in patients with diabetes mellitus. Use ophthalmic form cautiously in those with eye disease, infection, or injury.

Interactions
Drug-drug. *Beta blockers:* May increase systemic adverse effects. Monitor patient carefully.
Local anesthetics: May increase absorption of ophthalmic form. Monitor patient closely.
Tricyclic antidepressants: May potentiate the pressor effects from significant systemic absorption of the decongestant. Monitor patient carefully.

Adverse reactions
CNS: headache; insomnia; drowsiness, dizziness, and possible sedation from nasal form; lightheadedness and nervousness from ophthalmic form.
CV: palpitations; *CV collapse* and hypertension with nasal form; tachycardia, *bradycardia*, and irregular heartbeat with ophthalmic form.
EENT: rebound nasal congestion or irritation with excessive or long-term use, dryness of nose and throat, increased nasal discharge, stinging, sneezing (with nasal form); *transient stinging upon instillation,* blurred vision, reactive hyperemia, keratitis, lacrimation, increased intraocular pressure (with ophthalmic form).
Other: systemic effects in children (with excessive or long-term use of nasal form); trembling (with ophthalmic form).

Overdose and treatment
Signs and symptoms of overdose include somnolence, sedation, sweating, CNS depression with hypertension, bradycardia, decreased cardiac output, rebound hypertension, CV collapse, depressed respirations, and coma.

If drug is ingested, emesis isn't recommended (unless given early) because of rapid onset of sedation. Activated charcoal or gastric lavage may be used initially. Monitor vital signs and ECG. Treat seizures with I.V. diazepam.

Special considerations
● Excessive dosing may irritate nasal mucosa and cause rebound congestion (nasal) or rebound hyperemia (ophthalmic).

Patient monitoring
● Watch for adverse reactions in patients with CV disease, diabetes mellitus, or prostatic hypertrophy because systemic absorption can occur.

Pediatric patients
● Children may exhibit increased adverse effects from systemic absorption; 0.05% nasal solution is contraindicated in children under age 6; 0.025% nasal solution should be used in children under age 2 only under medical direction and supervision.

Geriatric patients
● Use drug cautiously in elderly patients with cardiac disease, poorly controlled hypertension, or diabetes mellitus.

Patient education
● Emphasize that only one person should use dropper bottle or nasal spray.
● Advise patient not to exceed recommended dosage and to use drug only when needed.
● Tell patient to stop drug and report symptoms that persist after 3 days of self-medication.
● Tell patient that nasal mucosa may sting, burn, or become dry.
● Warn patient that excessive use may cause bradycardia, hypotension, dizziness, and weakness.
● Show patient how to apply drug. Have him bend head forward and sniff spray briskly or apply light pressure on lacrimal sac after instillation of eyedrop.

---

oxymorphone hydrochloride
Numorphan

Pharmacologic classification: opioid
Therapeutic classification: analgesic
Controlled substance schedule: II
Pregnancy risk category: C

Indications and dosages
➤ *Moderate to severe pain. Adults:* 1 to 1.5 mg I.M. or S.C. q 4 to 6 hours, p.r.n. or around the clock. Or, 0.5 mg I.V. q 4 to 6 hours, p.r.n. or around the clock. Or, 1 suppository P.R. q 4 to 6 hours, p.r.n. or around the clock.

How supplied
Available by prescription only
Injection: 1 mg/ml, 1.5 mg/ml
Suppository: 5 mg

Pharmacodynamics
Analgesic action: Oxymorphone relieves moderate to severe pain via agonist activity at the opiate receptors. It has little or no antitussive effect.

Pharmacokinetics
Absorption: Well absorbed after P.R., S.C., I.M., or I.V. administration.
Distribution: Widely distributed.
Metabolism: Primarily metabolized in the liver.
Excretion: Excreted primarily in the urine as oxymorphone conjugates.

Route	Onset	Peak	Duration
I.V.	5-10 min	15-30 min	3-4 hr
I.M.	10-15 min	½-1½ hr	3-6 hr
S.C.	10-20 min	1-1½ hr	3-6 hr
P.R.	15-30 min	2 hr	3-6 hr

Contraindications and precautions
Contraindicated in patients hypersensitive to drug. Use cautiously in elderly or debilitated patients and in those with head injury, increased intracranial pressure, seizures, asthma, COPD, acute abdomen conditions, prostatic hyperplasia, severe renal or kidney disease, urethral stricture, respiratory depression, Addison's disease, arrhythmias, or hypothyroidism.

Interactions
Drug-drug. *Anticholinergics:* May cause paralytic ileus. Use together cautiously.
Cimetidine: May increase respiratory and CNS depression, causing confusion, disorientation, apnea, or seizures. Avoid use together.
CNS depressants, such as antihistamines, barbiturates, benzodiazepines, general anesthetics, muscle relaxants, opiates, phenothiazines, sedative-hypnotics, and tricyclic antidepressants: Potentiated respiratory and CNS depression, sedation, and hypotensive effects of drug. Use together with extreme caution.
Digitoxin, phenytoin, rifampin: Drug accumulation and enhanced effects may result from use with other drugs that are extensively metabolized in the liver. Monitor patient closely.
General anesthetics: Severe CV depression. Use together with extreme caution.
Opioid agonist-antagonist or a single dose of an antagonist: Patients who become physically dependent on oxycodone may experience acute withdrawal syndrome. Avoid use together in this situation.
Drug-lifestyle. *Alcohol use:* Potentiated respiratory and CNS depression, sedation, and hypotensive effects of drug. Advise patient to avoid combined use.

Adverse reactions
CNS: *sedation, somnolence, clouded sensorium, euphoria,* dizziness, **seizures** (with large doses), light-headedness, headache.
CV: *hypotension,* **bradycardia.**
GI: *nausea, vomiting, constipation,* ileus, increased plasma amylase levels.
GU: *urine retention.*
Respiratory: ***respiratory depression.***
Skin: pruritus.

Reactions may be *common,* uncommon, ***life-threatening***, or COMMON AND LIFE-THREATENING.

Other: physical dependence.

Overdose and treatment
The most common signs and symptoms of oxymorphone overdose are CNS depression, including extreme somnolence progressing to stupor and coma; respiratory depression; and miosis. Other acute toxic effects include hypotension, bradycardia, hypothermia, shock, apnea, cardiopulmonary arrest, circulatory collapse, pulmonary edema, and seizures.

To treat acute overdose, first establish adequate respiratory exchange via a patent airway and ventilation, as needed; give a narcotic antagonist (naloxone) to reverse respiratory depression. Because duration of action of drug is longer than that of naloxone, repeated naloxone dosing is necessary. Don't give naloxone unless patient has significant respiratory or CV depression. Monitor vital signs closely.

Provide symptomatic and supportive treatment, including continued respiratory support and correction of fluid or electrolyte imbalance. Monitor laboratory values, vital signs, and neurologic status closely.

Special considerations
• Parenteral administration of drug is also indicated for preoperative medication, support of anesthesia, obstetric analgesia, and relief of anxiety in dyspnea caused by acute left-sided heart failure and pulmonary edema.
• Keep an opiate antagonist and oxygen available after I.V. administration.
• Refrigerate oxymorphone suppositories.
• Drug is well absorbed P.R. and is an alternative to opioids with more limited dosage forms.
• Drug may worsen gallbladder pain.

Patient monitoring
• Monitor vital signs and respiratory status.

Breast-feeding patients
• It isn't known if drug appears in breast milk. Use cautiously in breast-feeding women.

Pediatric patients
• Don't use in children under age 12.

Geriatric patients
• Lower doses are usually indicated for elderly patients, who may be more sensitive to therapeutic and adverse effects of drug.

Patient education
• Tell patient to ask for drug before pain is intense.
• Caution ambulatory patient about getting out of bed and walking. Patient should avoid driving or other potentially hazardous activities until CNS effects are known.
• Instruct patient to store suppositories in the refrigerator.
• Advise patient to avoid alcohol.

oxytocin
Pitocin, Syntocinon

Pharmacologic classification: exogenous hormone
Therapeutic classification: oxytocic, lactation stimulant
Pregnancy risk category: C

Indications and dosages
➤ *Induction of labor.* *Adults:* Initially, no more than 0.5 to 1 milliunits/minute I.V. infusion. Rate of infusion may be increased slowly (1 to 2 milliunits/minute at 30- to 60-minute intervals until response occurs). Decrease rate when labor is firmly established.
➤ *Augmentation of labor.* *Adults:* Initially, 2 milliunits/minute I.V. infusion. Rate of infusion may be increased slowly to maximum of 20 milliunits/minute.
➤ *Reduction of postpartum bleeding after expulsion of placenta.* *Adults:* 20 to 40 milliunits/minute by I.V. infusion to total of 10 units (or 10 units I.M.) after delivery of the placenta.
➤ *To induce abortion.* *Adults:* 10 units mixed in 500 ml D₅W or normal saline solution I.V. at 10 to 100 milliunits/minute (not to exceed 30 units in 12 hours)
➤ *Oxytocin challenge test to assess fetal distress in high-risk pregnancies of greater than 31 weeks' gestation* ◇. *Adults:* Prepare solution by adding 5 to 10 units oxytocin to 1 L of 5% dextrose injection, yielding 5 to 10 milliunits/ml. Infuse 0.5 milliunits/minute, gradually increasing at 15-minute intervals to maximum of 20 milliunits/minute. Stop infusion when three moderate uterine contractions occur in a 10-minute interval. Response of fetal heart rate to test may be used to evaluate prognosis.

How supplied
Available by prescription only
Injection: 10-units/ml ampules, vials, and closed injection system

Pharmacodynamics
Oxytocic action: Oxytocin increases the sodium permeability of uterine myofibrils, indirectly stimulating the contraction of uterine smooth muscle. The threshold for response is lowered when estrogen levels are high. Uterine response increases with the length of the pregnancy and increases further during active labor. Response mimics labor contractions.

Pharmacokinetics
Absorption: Destroyed in the GI tract.
Distribution: Distributed throughout the extracellular fluid; small amounts may enter the fetal circulation.
Metabolism: Metabolized rapidly in the kidneys and liver. In early pregnancy, a circulating enzyme, oxytocinase, can inactivate the drug.

Excretion: Only small amounts are excreted in the urine as oxytocin. Half-life is 3 to 5 minutes.

Route	Onset	Peak	Duration
I.V.	Immediate	Unknown	1 hr
I.M.	3-5 min	Unknown	2-3 hr

Contraindications and precautions
Contraindicated in patients hypersensitive to drug and in those with severe toxemia, hypertonic uterine patterns, total placenta previa, and vasoprevia. Also contraindicated when cephalopelvic disproportion is present; when delivery requires conversion, as in transverse lie; in fetal distress when delivery isn't imminent; and in prematurity and other obstetric emergencies.

Use cautiously during first and second stages of labor and in patients with history of cervical or uterine surgery (including cesarean section), grand multiparity, uterine sepsis, traumatic delivery, overdistended uterus, or invasive cervical cancer.

Interactions
Drug-drug. *Cyclopropane anesthesia:* May modify CV effects of oxytocin. Use together cautiously.
Sympathomimetics: May increase pressor effects, possibly resulting in postpartum hypertension. Avoid use together.
Thiopental anesthesia: Delays the induction of anesthesia. Use together cautiously.

Adverse reactions
Maternal
CNS: *subarachnoid hemorrhage* (from hypertension), *seizures or coma* (from water intoxication).
CV: *hypertension;* increased heart rate, systemic venous return, and cardiac output; *arrhythmias.*
GI: nausea, vomiting.
GU: tetanic uterine contractions, *abruptio placentae, impaired uterine blood flow,* pelvic hematoma, *increased uterine motility, uterine rupture, postpartum hemorrhage.*
Hematologic: *afibrinogenemia* (may be related to postpartum bleeding).
Other: *hypersensitivity reactions (anaphylaxis), water retention.*
Fetal
CNS: *infant brain damage.*
EENT: retinal hemorrhage.
CV: *bradycardia,* PVCs, arrhythmias.
Hepatic: *jaundice.*
Respiratory: *anoxia, asphyxia.*
Other: *low Apgar scores.*

Overdose and treatment
Signs and symptoms of overdose include hyperstimulation of the uterus, causing tetanic contractions and possible uterine rupture, cervical laceration, abruptio placentae, impaired uterine blood flow, amniotic fluid embolism, and fetal trauma. Drug has a very short half-life; halt therapy and start supportive care.

Special considerations
● Drug must be given by I.V. infusion, not I.V. bolus injection. Use an infusion device.
● Have magnesium sulfate (20% solution) available for relaxation of the myometrium.
● Drug isn't recommended for routine I.M. use. However, 10 units may be given I.M. after delivery of the placenta to control postpartum uterine bleeding.
● I.V. infusion rates up to 6 milliunits/minute produce maternal plasma levels similar to spontaneous labor. Rates exceeding 9 to 10 milliunits/minute are rarely needed.
● Solution containing 10 milliunits/ml may be prepared by adding 10 units of oxytocin to 1 L of normal saline solution or D_5W. Solution containing 20 milliunits/ml may be prepared by adding 10 units of oxytocin to 500 ml of normal saline solution or D_5W.
● Oxytocin injection is incompatible with fibrinolysin, norepinephrine bitartrate, prochlorperazine edisylate, and warfarin sodium.
● Discontinue drug if uterine contractions are prolonged (more than 90 seconds), intrauterine pressure rises, or uterine motility interferes with fetal heart rate.

Patient monitoring
● When giving the oxytocin challenge test, monitor fetal heart rate and uterine contractions immediately before and during infusion. If fetal heart rate doesn't change during test, repeat in 1 week. If late deceleration in fetal heart rate is noted, consider terminating pregnancy.
● During long infusions, watch for signs of water intoxication.
● Record uterine contractions, heart rate, blood pressure, intrauterine pressure, fetal heart rate, and character of blood loss every 15 minutes.
● Drug may produce an antidiuretic effect; monitor fluid intake and output.

Breast-feeding patients
● Minimal amounts of drug enter breast milk. Risks must be evaluated.

Patient education
● Explain possible adverse effects of drug.

Reactions may be *common,* uncommon, *life-threatening,* or COMMON AND LIFE-THREATENING.

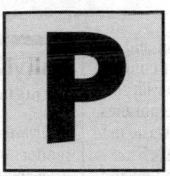

paclitaxel
Taxol

Pharmacologic classification: novel anti-microtubule
Therapeutic classification: antineoplastic
Pregnancy risk category: D

Indications and dosages
➤*First-line and subsequent therapy for advanced carcinoma of the ovary. Adults (previously untreated):* 175 mg/m² over 3 hours every 3 weeks followed by cisplatin 75 mg/m². Or, 135 mg/m² over 24 hours with cisplatin 75 mg/m² every 3 weeks. Subsequent courses shouldn't be repeated until neutrophil count is at least 1,500 cells/mm³ and platelet count is at least 100,000 cells/mm³.
Adults (previously treated): 135 or 175 mg/m² I.V. over 3 hours q 3 weeks. Subsequent courses shouldn't be repeated until neutrophil count is at least 1,500 cells/mm³ and platelet count is at least 100,000 cells/mm³.
➤*Breast cancer after failure of combination chemotherapy for metastatic disease or relapse within 6 months of adjuvant chemotherapy (prior therapy should have included an anthracycline unless clinically contraindicated). Adults:* 175 mg/m² I.V. over 3 hours q 3 weeks.
➤*AIDS-related Kaposi's sarcoma. Adults:* 135 mg/m² I.V. over 3 hours q 3 weeks, or 100 mg/m² I.V. over 3 hours q 2 weeks.

How supplied
Available by prescription only
Injection: 30 mg/5 ml

Pharmacodynamics
Antineoplastic action: Prevents depolymerization of cellular microtubules, thus inhibiting the normal reorganization of the microtubule network necessary for mitosis and other vital cellular functions.

Pharmacokinetics
Absorption: No information available.
Distribution: About 89% to 98% bound to serum proteins.
Metabolism: Possibly metabolized in liver.
Excretion: Not fully understood.

Route	Onset	Peak	Duration
I.V.	Unknown	Unkown	Unknown

Contraindications and precautions
Contraindicated in patients hypersensitive to drug or polyoxyethylated castor oil, a vehicle used in drug solution. Also contraindicated in patients with baseline neutrophil counts below 1,500/mm³. Use cautiously in patients who have received radiation therapy.

Interactions
Drug-drug. *Cisplatin:* Myelosuppression may be greater when cisplatin is given before rather than after paclitaxel. Consider this effect before therapy.
Cyclosporine, dexamethasone, diazepam, etoposide, ketoconazole, quinidine, teniposide, verapamil, vincristine: Inhibited paclitaxel metabolism. Use together cautiously.

Adverse reactions
CNS: *peripheral neuropathy.*
CV: ***bradycardia,*** *hypotension, abnormal ECG.*
GI: *nausea, vomiting, diarrhea, mucositis.*
Hematologic: ***neutropenia, leukopenia, thrombocytopenia,*** *anemia, bleeding.*
Hepatic: *elevated liver enzyme levels.*
Musculoskeletal: *myalgia, arthralgia.*
Skin: *alopecia.*
Other: *hypersensitivity reactions (****anaphylaxis****), phlebitis, cellulitis at injection site, infections.*

Overdose and treatment
Primary complications of overdose include bone marrow suppression, peripheral neurotoxicity, and mucositis. No specific antidote for overdose is known.

Special considerations
● Severe hypersensitivity reactions characterized by dyspnea, hypotension, angioedema, and generalized urticaria have occurred in 2% of patients receiving paclitaxel. To reduce risk or severity of these reactions, pretreat patients with corticosteroids (such as dexamethasone), antihistamines (such as diphenhydramine), and H₂-receptor antagonists (such as cimetidine or ranitidine).
● Don't rechallenge patients who experience severe hypersensitivity reactions to drug.
● In patients who experience severe neutropenia (neutrophil count below 500 cells/mm³ for 1 week or longer) or severe peripheral neuropathy during drug therapy, reduce dosage by 20% for subsequent courses. Risk and severity of neurotoxicity and hematologic toxicity increase with dose, especially above 190 mg/m².

• Use caution during drug preparation and administration; wear gloves. If solution contacts skin, wash immediately and thoroughly with soap and water. If drug contacts mucous membranes, flush thoroughly with water. Mark all waste materials with CHEMOTHERAPY HAZARD labels.

• Concentrate must be diluted before infusion. Compatible solutions include normal saline solution injection, D_5W, dextrose 5% in normal saline solution injection, and 5% dextrose in lactated Ringer's injection. Dilute to a final concentration of 0.3 to 1.2 mg/ml. Diluted solutions are stable for 27 hours at room temperature.

• Prepare and store infusion solutions in glass containers. Undiluted concentrate shouldn't contact polyvinyl chloride I.V. bags or tubing. Store diluted solution in glass or polypropylene bottles, or use polypropylene or polyolefin bags. Administer through polyethylene-lined administration sets, and use an in-line filter with a microporous membrane not exceeding 0.22 microns.

Patient monitoring
• Bone marrow toxicity is the most frequent and dose-limiting toxicity. Frequent blood count monitoring is necessary during therapy. Packed RBC or platelet transfusions may be necessary in severe cases. Take bleeding precautions as appropriate.

• If patient develops significant conduction abnormalities during drug administration, provide appropriate therapy and monitor cardiac function continuously during subsequent drug therapy.

• Continuously monitor patient for 30 minutes after starting infusion. Closely monitor patient throughout infusion.

Breast-feeding patients
• It isn't known if drug appears in breast milk. Because of potential for serious adverse reactions in breast-fed infants, breast-feeding should be stopped during therapy.

Pediatric patients
• Safety and effectiveness in children haven't been established.

Patient education
• Advise woman of childbearing age to avoid becoming pregnant during therapy because of potential harm to fetus.

• Warn patient that alopecia occurs in almost all patients.

• Teach patient to recognize and immediately report signs and symptoms of peripheral neuropathy, such as tingling, burning, and numbness in limbs. Although mild symptoms are common, severe symptoms occur infrequently. Dosage reduction may be necessary.

palivizumab
Synagis

Pharmacologic classification: recombinant monoclonal antibody $IgG1_K$
Therapeutic classification: respiratory syncytial virus (RSV) prophylaxis
Pregnancy risk category: C

Indications and dosages
➤ *Prevention of serious lower respiratory tract disease caused by RSV in children at high risk. Children:* 15 mg/kg I.M. monthly throughout RSV season. Give first dose before RSV season.

How supplied
Available by prescription only
Injection: 100 mg single-use vial

Pharmacodynamics
RSV prophylaxis drug action: Exhibits neutralizing and fusion-inhibitory activity against RSV, which inhibits RSV replication.

Pharmacokinetics
Absorption: Not reported.
Distribution: Not reported.
Metabolism: Not reported.
Excretion: Half-life is about 18 days.

Route	Onset	Peak	Duration
I.M.	Unknown	Unknown	Unknown

Contraindications and precautions
Contraindicated in children with history of severe reaction to drug or its components. Use cautiously in patients with thrombocytopenia or any coagulation disorder.

Interactions
None reported.

Adverse reactions
CNS: nervousness.
EENT: *otitis media, rhinitis,* pharyngitis, sinusitis, conjunctivitis, oral candidiasis.
GI: diarrhea, vomiting, gastroenteritis.
Hematologic: anemia.
Hepatic: liver function abnormality (increased ALT, AST levels).
Respiratory: *upper respiratory tract infection,* cough, wheeze, bronchiolitis, *apnea,* pneumonia, bronchitis, asthma, croup, dyspnea.
Skin: *rash,* fungal dermatitis, eczema, seborrhea.
Other: pain, hernia, failure to thrive, injection site reaction, viral infection, flu syndrome.

Overdose and treatment
No information available.

Special considerations
● Drug is intended for prophylaxis and not for treatment of RSV infection.
● Patient should receive monthly doses throughout RSV season, even if patient develops RSV infection. In northern hemisphere, RSV season typically lasts from November to April.
● To reconstitute, slowly add 1 ml of sterile water for injection into a 100-mg vial. Gently swirl vial for 30 seconds to avoid foaming. Don't shake vial. Let reconstituted solution stand at room temperature for 20 minutes.
● Vial doesn't contain preservative; use within 6 hours of reconstitution.
● Give drug in anterolateral aspect of thigh. Don't use gluteal muscle routinely as injection site because of risk of damaging sciatic nerve. Injection volumes over 1 ml should be given as a divided dose. Don't administer I.V.
● Anaphylactoid reactions after drug administration haven't been observed but can occur after administration of proteins. If anaphylaxis or severe allergic reaction occurs, give epinephrine (1:1,000) and provide supportive care as needed.

Patient monitoring
● Monitor patient for adverse effects.
● Monitor hepatic enzymes.

Patient education
● Explain to parent or caregiver that drug is used to prevent RSV, not to treat it.
● Advise parent that monthly injections are recommended throughout RSV season (November to April in northern hemisphere).
● Advise parent to report adverse reactions immediately.

pamidronate disodium
Aredia

Pharmacologic classification: bisphosphonate, pyrophosphate analogue
Therapeutic classification: antihypercalcemic
Pregnancy risk category: C

Indications and dosages
➤ *Moderate to severe hypercalcemia related to malignancy (with or without metastases). Adults:* Dosage depends on severity of hypercalcemia. Serum calcium levels should be corrected for serum albumin. Corrected serum calcium (CCa) is calculated using the following formula:

$$\begin{matrix} \text{CCa} \\ \text{(mg/dl)} \end{matrix} = \begin{matrix} \text{serum Ca} \\ \text{(mg/dl)} \end{matrix} + \begin{matrix} 0.8 \ (4 - \text{serum albumin}) \\ \text{(g/dl)} \end{matrix}$$

Repeat doses shouldn't be given sooner than 7 days to allow for full response to initial dose.
✦ *Dosage adjustment.* Patients with moderate hypercalcemia (CCa levels of 12 to 13.5 mg/dl) may receive 60 to 90 mg I.V. infusion as a single dose over 2 to 24 hours. Patients with severe hypercalcemia (CCa levels over 13.5 mg/dl) may receive 90 mg I.V. infusion as a single dose over 2 to 24 hours.
➤ *Paget's disease. Adults:* 30 mg I.V. daily over 4 hours for 3 consecutive days for total dose of 90 mg.
➤ *Osteolytic bone lesions of multiple myeloma. Adults:* 90 mg I.V. daily over 4 hours once monthly.
➤ *Osteolytic bone lesions of breast cancer. Adults:* 90 mg I.V. daily over 2 hours q 3 to 4 weeks.

How supplied
Available by prescription only
Injection: 30 mg/vial, 60 mg/vial, 90 mg/vial

Pharmacodynamics
Antihypercalcemic action: Inhibits bone resorption. Adsorbs to hydroxyapatite crystals in bone and may directly block dissolution of calcium phosphate. Apparently doesn't inhibit bone formation or mineralization.

Pharmacokinetics
Absorption: Rapid onset; duration of action up to 6 months in bone.
Distribution: After I.V. administration, about 50% to 60% of dose rapidly absorbed by bone; drug also taken up by kidneys, liver, spleen, teeth, and tracheal cartilage.
Metabolism: None.
Excretion: Excreted by kidneys; average of 51% of dose excreted in urine within 72 hours of administration.

Route	Onset	Peak	Duration
I.V.	Unknown	Unknown	Unknown

Contraindications and precautions
Contraindicated in patients hypersensitive to drug or other bisphosphonates, such as etidronate. Use with extreme caution in patients with impaired renal function.

Interactions
Drug-drug. *Calcium-containing solutions:* Drug may form precipitate when mixed with solutions containing calcium. Don't mix together.

Adverse reactions
CNS: *seizures,* fatigue, headache, somnolence.
CV: atrial fibrillation, syncope, tachycardia, *hypertension.*
GI: *abdominal pain, anorexia, constipation, nausea, vomiting,* GI hemorrhage.
Hematologic: *leukopenia, thrombocytopenia,* anemia.
Metabolic: *hypophosphatemia, hypokalemia, hypomagnesemia, hypocalcemia.*
Musculoskeletal: *bone pain.*

Other: *fever, infusion-site reaction, generalized pain.*

Overdose and treatment
Symptomatic hypocalcemia could result from overdose; treat with I.V. calcium.

Special considerations
● Reconstitute vial with 10 ml sterile water for injection. Once drug is completely dissolved, add to 250-ml (2-hour infusion), 500-ml (4-hour infusion), or 1,000-ml (up to 24-hour infusion) bag of half-normal or normal saline solution injection or D₅W. Don't mix with infusion solutions that contain calcium, such as Ringer's injection or lactated Ringer's injection. Administer in single I.V. solution, in separate line from all other drugs. Inspect to rule out precipitates before administering.
● Injection solution is stable for 24 hours when refrigerated. Give only by I.V. infusion. Nephropathy may occur when drug is given as a bolus.
● Infusions longer than 2 hours may reduce the risk of renal toxicity, especially in patients with preexisting renal insufficiency.

Patient monitoring
● Because drug can cause electrolyte disturbances, careful monitoring of serum electrolytes (especially calcium, phosphate, and magnesium) is essential. Short-term administration of calcium may be necessary in patients with severe hypocalcemia. Also monitor hemoglobin and creatinine levels, CBC, differential, and hematocrit.
● Carefully monitor patients with anemia, leukopenia, or thrombocytopenia during first 2 weeks after therapy.
● Monitor patient's temperature; 27% of patients have a slightly elevated temperature for 24 to 48 hours after therapy.

Breast-feeding patients
● It isn't known if drug appears in breast milk. Use cautiously in breast-feeding women.

Pediatric patients
● Safety and efficacy in children haven't been established.

Patient education
● Explain use and administration of drug to patient and family.
● Instruct patient to report adverse reactions promptly.

pancreatin
Donnazyme, Hi-Vegi-Lip, 4X Pancreatin, 8X Pancreatin, Pancrezyme 4X

Pharmacologic classification: pancreatic enzyme
Therapeutic classification: digestant
Pregnancy risk category: C

Indications and dosages
➤ **Exocrine pancreatic secretion insufficiency, digestive aid in cystic fibrosis, steatorrhea, and other disorders of fat metabolism secondary to insufficient pancreatic enzymes.** *Adults and children:* 1 to 2 tablets P.O. with each meal.

How supplied
Available without a prescription
Hi-Vegi-Lip
Tablets (enteric-coated): 2,400 mg pancreatin; 4,800 units lipase; 60,000 units protease; 60,000 units amylase
4X Pancreatin, Pancrezyme 4X
Tablets (enteric-coated): 2,400 mg pancreatin; 12,000 units lipase; 60,000 units protease; 60,000 units amylase
8X Pancreatin
Tablets (enteric-coated): 7,200 mg pancreatin; 22,500 units lipase; 180,000 units protease; 180,000 units amylase
Available by prescription only
Donnazyme
Tablets: 500 mg pancreatin; 1,000 units lipase; 12,500 units protease; 12,500 units amylase

Pharmacodynamics
Digestive action: Proteolytic, amylolytic, and lipolytic enzymes enhance the digestion of proteins, starches, and fats. Drug is sensitive to acids and is more active in neutral or slightly alkaline environments.

Pharmacokinetics
Absorption: Not absorbed; acts locally in GI tract.
Distribution: None.
Metabolism: None.
Excretion: Excreted in feces.

Route	Onset	Peak	Duration
P.O.	Unknown	Unknown	1-2 hr

Contraindications and precautions
Contraindicated in patients hypersensitive to drug or pork protein or enzymes. Also contraindicated in those with acute pancreatitis or acute exacerbations of chronic pancreatitis. Use cautiously in pregnant or breast-feeding women.

Interactions
Drug-drug. *Antacids that contain calcium or magnesium:* Pancreatin activity may be reduced. Don't administer together.
Products that contain iron: Decreased absorption of these drugs. Monitor patient for decreased effectiveness.

Adverse reactions
GI: perianal irritation, nausea, diarrhea (with high doses).
Metabolic: increased serum uric acid.
Skin: rash.
Other: *allergic reactions.*

Overdose and treatment
Toxicity may cause hyperuricuria, hyperuricemia, diarrhea, abdominal cramps, and transient intestinal upset. If necessary, provide symptomatic treatment.

Special considerations
● For maximal effect, give dose just before or during a meal.
● Tablets may not be crushed or chewed; follow with a glass of water to ensure complete swallowing.
● Diet should balance fat, protein, and starch intake properly to avoid indigestion. Dosage varies according to degree of maldigestion and malabsorption, amount of fat in diet, and enzyme activity of individual preparations.
● Adequate replacement decreases number of bowel movements and improves stool consistency.
● Use only after confirmed diagnosis of exocrine pancreatic insufficiency. Not effective in GI disorders unrelated to pancreatic enzyme deficiency.
● Enteric coating may reduce availability of enzyme in upper portion of jejunum and shouldn't be chewed. Swallow promptly to avoid mucosal irritation.

Patient monitoring
● Monitor dietary intake.
● Monitor therapeutic effect.

Patient education
● Explain use of drug, and advise storage away from heat and light.
● Make sure patient or family understands special dietary instructions for the patient's disease. Advise against changing brands without medical approval.

pancrelipase
Cotazym, Cotazym-S, Creon 5, Creon 10, Creon 20, Ilozyme, Ku-Zyme HP, Pancrease, Pancrease MT-4, Pancrease MT-10, Pancrease MT-16, Pancrease MT-20, Ultrase, Ultrase MT-12, Ultrase MT-18, Ultrase MT-20, Viokase, Zymase

Pharmacologic classification: pancreatic enzyme
Therapeutic classification: digestant
Pregnancy risk category: C

Indications and dosages
➤ *Exocrine pancreatic secretion insufficiency, cystic fibrosis in adults and children, steatorrhea, other disorders of fat metabolism secondary to insufficient pancreatic enzymes. Adults:* 4,000 to 20,000 units (or more) lipase with meals and snacks. Dose must be adjusted to patient's response.
Children ages 7 to 12: 4,000 to 12,000 units lipase with meals and snacks. Dose must be adjusted to patient's response.
Children ages 1 to 6: 4,000 to 8,000 units lipase with meals and 4,000 units with snacks. Dose must be adjusted to patient's response.
Children ages 6 to 12 months: 2,000 units lipase with meals and snacks. Dose must be adjusted to patient's response.
➤ *Patients with pancreatectomy or obstructive pancreatic duct. Adults:* 8,000 to 16,000 units lipase at 2-hour intervals; may increase dose to 64,000 to 88,000 units in severe cases.

How supplied
Available by prescription only
Cotazym
Capsules: 8,000 units lipase; 30,000 units protease; 30,000 units amylase
Cotazym-S
Capsules: 5,000 units lipase; 20,000 units protease; 20,000 units amylase
Creon 5
Capsules (enteric-coated microspheres): 5,000 units lipase; 16,600 units protease; 18,750 units amylase
Creon 10
Capsules (delayed-release): 10,000 units lipase; 37,500 units protease; 33,200 units amylase
Creon 20
Capsules (delayed-release): 20,000 units lipase; 75,000 units protease; 66,400 units amylase
Ilozyme
Tablets: 11,000 units lipase; 30,000 units protease; 30,000 units amylase
Ku-Zyme HP
Capsules: 8,000 units lipase; 30,000 units protease; 30,000 units amylase

Pancrease
Capsules: 4,000 units lipase; 25,000 units protease; 20,000 units amylase
Pancrease MT-4
Capsules (enteric-coated microtablets): 4,000 units lipase; 12,000 units protease; 12,000 units amylase
Pancrease MT-10
Capsules (enteric-coated microtablets): 10,000 units lipase; 30,000 units protease; 30,000 units amylase
Pancrease MT-16
Capsules (enteric-coated microtablets): 16,000 units lipase; 48,000 units protease; 48,000 units amylase
Pancrease MT-20
Capsules (enteric-coated microtablets): 20,000 units lipase; 44,000 units protease; 56,000 units amylase
Ultrase
Capsules (enteric-coated microspheres): 4,500 units lipase; 25,000 units protease; 20,000 units amylase
Ultrase MT-12
Capsules (enteric-coated microtablets): 12,000 units lipase; 39,000 units protease; 39,000 units amylase
Ultrase MT-18
Enteric-coated minitablets: 18,000 units lipase; 58,500 units protease; 58,500 units amylase
Ultrase MT-20
Capsules (enteric-coated microtablets): 20,000 units lipase; 65,000 units protease; 65,000 units amylase
Viokase
Powder: 16,800 units lipase; 70,000 units protease; 70,000 units amylase
Tablets: 8,000 units lipase; 30,000 units protease; 30,000 units amylase
Zymase
Capsules: 12,000 units lipase; 24,000 units protease; 24,000 units amylase

Pharmacodynamics
Digestive action: Proteolytic, amylolytic, and lipolytic enzymes enhance the digestion of proteins, starches, and fats. Drug is sensitive to acids and is more active in neutral or slightly alkaline environments.

Pharmacokinetics
Absorption: Not absorbed; acts locally in GI tract.
Distribution: None.
Metabolism: None.
Excretion: Excreted in feces.

Route	Onset	Peak	Duration
P.O.	Variable	Variable	Variable

Contraindications and precautions
Contraindicated in patients with severe hypersensitivity to pork and in those with acute pancreatitis or acute exacerbations of chronic pancreatic diseases. Use cautiously in pregnant or breast-feeding women.

Interactions
Drug-drug. *Antacids that contain calcium or magnesium:* Pancrelipase activity may be reduced by these drugs. Don't give together.
Products that contain iron: Decreased absorption of these drugs. Monitor patient for decreased effectiveness.

Adverse reactions
GI: *nausea,* cramping, diarrhea (high doses).
Metabolic: increased serum uric acid.
Other: *allergic reaction.*

Overdose and treatment
Toxicity may cause hyperuricuria, hyperuricemia, diarrhea, and transient GI upset.

Special considerations
● For maximal effect, administer dose just before or during a meal. Patient should drink a glass of water or juice to ensure complete swallowing.
● Preparations may not be crushed or chewed.
● Use only after confirmed diagnosis of exocrine pancreatic insufficiency. Not effective in GI disorders unrelated to enzyme deficiency.
● Dosage varies with degree of maldigestion and malabsorption, amount of fat in diet, and enzyme activity of individual preparations.
● Adequate replacement decreases number of bowel movements and improves stool consistency.
● Enteric coating on some products may reduce availability of enzyme in upper portion of jejunum.

Patient monitoring
● Monitor patient for effectiveness of therapy.
● Monitor patient for adverse effects.

Pediatric patients
● For young children, mix powders with applesauce and give at mealtime. Avoid allowing patient to inhale powder. Older children may swallow capsules with food.
● Capsules may be opened to facilitate swallowing. Contents may be sprinkled on food, but a pH of 5.5 or greater is necessary to ensure stability.
● Dosage for children under age 6 months hasn't been established.

Patient education
● Teach patient or family proper use of drug, and advise storage away from heat and light.
● Make sure patient or family understands special dietary instructions for the patient's disease.
● Advise against changing brands without medical approval.

---

pancuronium bromide
Pavulon

Pharmacologic classification: nondepolarizing neuromuscular blocker
Therapeutic classification: skeletal muscle relaxant
Pregnancy risk category: C

Indications and dosages
➤ *Adjunct to anesthesia to induce skeletal muscle relaxation, facilitate intubation and ventilation, and weaken muscle contractions in induced seizures.* Dose depends on anesthetic used, individual needs, and response. Doses are representative and must be adjusted. *Adults and children over age 1 month:* Initially, 0.04 to 0.1 mg/kg I.V.; then 0.01 mg/kg q 25 to 60 minutes if needed.

How supplied
Available by prescription only
Injection: 1 mg/ml, 2 mg/ml parenteral

Pharmacodynamics
Skeletal muscle relaxant action: Prevents acetylcholine (ACh) from binding to receptors on the motor end-plate, thus blocking depolarization. May increase heart rate through direct blocking effect on ACh receptors of the heart; increase is dose-related. Causes little or no histamine release and no ganglionic blockade.

Pharmacokinetics
Absorption: Onset and duration are dose-related. After 0.06 mg/kg dose, effects begin to subside in 35 to 45 minutes. Repeated doses may increase magnitude and duration of action.
Distribution: 87% bound to plasma proteins.
Metabolism: No information available; small amounts may be metabolized by liver.
Excretion: Mainly excreted unchanged in urine; some through biliary excretion.

Route	Onset	Peak	Duration
I.V.	30-45 sec	3-4½ min	35-65 min

Contraindications and precautions
Contraindicated in patients hypersensitive to bromides, in those with tachycardia, and in those for whom even a minor increase in heart rate is undesirable.

Use cautiously in elderly or debilitated patients and in those with respiratory depression, myasthenia gravis, myasthenic syndrome of lung, bronchogenic cancer, dehydration, thyroid disorders, collagen diseases, porphyria, electrolyte disturbances, hyperthermia, toxemic states, or impaired renal, pulmonary, or hepatic function. Also, use large doses cautiously in patients undergoing cesarean section.

Interactions
Drug-drug. *Aminoglycoside antibiotics, beta blockers, clindamycin, depolarizing neuromuscular blocking drugs, furosemide, general anesthetics, lincomycin, lithium, parenteral magnesium salts, polymyxin antibiotics, potassium-depleting drugs, quinidine, quinine, thiazide diuretics, other nondepolarizing neuromuscular blocking drugs:* Potentiated pancuronium effects. Monitor patient closely.
Opioid analgesics: Increased respiratory depression. Monitor vital signs, especially respiratory rate.
Succinylcholine: Enhanced and prolonged neuromuscular blocking effects of pancuronium. Monitor patient closely.

Adverse reactions
CV: tachycardia, increased blood pressure.
Musculoskeletal: residual muscle weakness.
Respiratory: *prolonged, dose-related respiratory insufficiency or apnea.*
Skin: transient rashes.
Other: excessive salivation, *allergic or idiosyncratic hypersensitivity reactions.*

Overdose and treatment
Toxicity may cause respiratory depression, apnea, and CV collapse. Use a peripheral nerve stimulator to monitor response and to evaluate neuromuscular blockade. Maintain an adequate airway and manual or mechanical ventilation until patient can maintain adequate ventilation unassisted. Neostigmine, edrophonium, or pyridostigmine may be used to reverse effects.

Special considerations
● Administration requires direct medical supervision, with emergency respiratory support available.
● If using succinylcholine, allow its effects to subside before giving pancuronium.
● Store drug in refrigerator and not in plastic container or syringes. Plastic syringes may be used to administer dose.
● Don't mix in same syringe or give through same needle with barbiturates or other alkaline solutions.
● Reduce dosage when ether or other inhalation anesthetics that enhance neuromuscular blockade are used.
● Large doses may increase frequency and severity of tachycardia.
● Drug doesn't relieve pain or alter consciousness; assess patient's need for analgesic or sedative.

Patient monitoring
● Monitor baseline electrolyte levels, intake and output, and vital signs, especially heart rate and respiration.
● Monitor patient for cardiac function, oxygen saturation, and blood pressure.

Breast-feeding patients
• It isn't known if drug appears in breast milk. Use cautiously in breast-feeding women.

Pediatric patients
• Dosage for neonates under age 1 month must be carefully individualized. For infants over age 1 month and children, see adult dosage.

Geriatric patients
• The usual adult dose must be individualized depending on response.

Patient education
• Explain all events and procedures to patient because he can still hear.

---

pantoprazole
Prontonix

Pharmacologic classification: substituted benzimidazole
Therapeutic classification: proton pump inhibitor that suppresses gastric acid production.
Pregnancy risk category: B

Indications and dosages
➤ *Erosive esophagitis caused by gastro-esophageal reflux disease (GERD).* *Adults:* 40 mg P.O. once daily for up to 8 weeks. For patients who haven't healed after 8 weeks, another 8-week course may be considered.

How supplied
Available by prescription only
Tablets (delayed-release): 40 mg

Pharmacodynamics
Proton pump–inhibiting action: Pantoprazole inhibits the activity of the proton pump by binding to hydrogen-potassium adenosine triphosphatase, located at secretory surface of the gastric parietal cells, to suppress gastric acid secretion.

Pharmacokinetics
Absorption: Well absorbed with an absolute bioavailability of 77%. Serum levels peak at 2½ hours. Food may delay its absorption up to 2 hours; however, the extent of absorption is not affected.
Distribution: Distributes mainly in the extracellular fluid. Protein-binding is about 98%, mainly to albumin.
Metabolism: Extensively metabolized in the liver through the cytochrome P-450 (CYP) system. The main metabolic pathway is demethylation by CYP2C19 with subsequent sulfation. Other pathways include oxidation by CYP3A4. No evidence suggests that any metabolites have significant pharmacologic activity.

Excretion: About 71% is excreted in urine and 18% excreted in feces by biliary excretion. There is no renal excretion of unchanged drug.

Route	Onset	Peak	Duration
P.O.	Unknown	2½ hr	Unknown

Contraindications and precautions
Contraindicated in patients hypersensitive to any component of the formulation.

Interactions
Drug-drug. *Ampicillin esters, iron salts, ketoconazole:* May decrease absorption of these drugs. Monitor patient closely.
Drug-food. *Food:* Delayed absorption of pantoprazole for up to 2 hours; however, extent of absorption isn't affected. Can be given without regard to meals.

Adverse reactions
CNS: headache, insomnia, asthenia, migraine, anxiety, dizziness.
CV: chest pain.
EENT: pharyngitis, rhinitis, sinusitis.
GI: diarrhea, flatulence, abdominal pain, eructation, constipation, dyspepsia, gastroenteritis, gastrointestinal disorder, nausea, vomiting.
GU: rectal disorder, urinary frequency, urinary tract infection.
Hepatic: abnormal liver function test results.
Metabolic: hyperglycemia, hyperlipemia.
Musculoskeletal: back pain, neck pain, arthralgia, hypertonia.
Respiratory: bronchitis, increased cough, dyspnea, upper respiratory tract infection.
Skin: rash.
Other: flu syndrome, infection, pain.

Overdose and treatment
Overdosage with 400 to 600 mg has caused no adverse effects. Pantoprazole isn't removed by hemodialysis.

Special considerations
• Can be given without regards to meals.
• Drug shouldn't be used for maintenance therapy beyond 16 weeks.
• Symptomatic response to therapy doesn't preclude the presence of gastric malignancy.

Breast-feeding patients
• It isn't known if pantoprazole appears in breast milk. Use cautiously in nursing women.

Pediatric patients
• Safety and effectiveness haven't been established.

Patient education
• Instruct patient to take exactly as prescribed and at about the same time every day.
• Advise patient that drug can be taken without regard to meals.

Reactions may be *common*, uncommon, *life-threatening*, or COMMON AND LIFE-THREATENING.

• Urge patient to swallow tablet whole and not to crush, split, or chew it.
• Tell patient that antacids don't affect pantoprazole absorption.

papaverine hydrochloride
Pavabid, Pavabid Plateau Caps

Pharmacologic classification: benzylisoquinoline derivative, opiate alkaloid
Therapeutic classification: peripheral vasodilator
Pregnancy risk category: C

Indications and dosages
➤ *Relief of cerebral and peripheral ischemia caused by arterial spasm and myocardial ischemia; treatment of coronary occlusion and certain cerebral angiospastic states. Adults.* 75 to 300 mg P.O. three to five times daily. Or, 150 to 300 mg sustained-release form q 8 to 12 hours. Or, 30 to 120 mg I.M. or I.V. q 3 hours, as indicated. In treatment of extrasystoles, give two doses 10 minutes apart. *Children:* 6 mg/kg I.M. or I.V. q.i.d.
➤ *Impotence* ◊. *Adults:* 2.5 to 37.5 mg by intracavernous injection.

How supplied
Available by prescription only
Capsules (sustained-release): 150 mg
Injection: 30 mg/ml in 2- and 10-ml ampules

Pharmacodynamics
Vasodilating action: Relaxes smooth muscle directly by inhibiting phosphodiesterase, thus increasing the level of cyclic adenosine monophosphate. There is considerable controversy over effectiveness of drug. Some clinicians find little evidence of clinical value.

Pharmacokinetics
Absorption: 54% of orally administered drug is bioavailable. Plasma levels peak 1 to 2 hours after oral dose; half-life varies from 12 to 24 hours, but levels can be maintained by giving drug at 6-hour intervals. Sustained-release forms sometimes absorbed poorly and erratically.
Distribution: Tends to localize in adipose tissue and liver; remainder distributed throughout body. About 90% protein-bound.
Metabolism: Metabolized by liver.
Excretion: Excreted in urine as metabolites.

Route	Onset	Peak	Duration
P.O.	Unknown	1-2 hr	Unknown
I.V., I.M.	Unknown	Unknown	Unknown

Contraindications and precautions
I.V. use is contraindicated in patients with Parkinson's disease or complete AV block. Use cautiously in patients with glaucoma or hepatic dysfunction.

Interactions
Drug-drug. *CNS depressants:* Papaverine's effects may be potentiated. Monitor patient closely. *Levodopa:* Decreased antiparkinsonian effects; exacerbation of such symptoms as rigidity and tremors. Monitor patient for effect.
Morphine: Synergic response. Monitor patient closely.
Drug-lifestyle. *Heavy smoking:* May interfere with therapeutic effect of papaverine because nicotine constricts blood vessels. Discourage smoking.

Adverse reactions
CNS: *headache,* vertigo, drowsiness, sedation, malaise.
CV: *increased heart rate, increased blood pressure* (with parenteral use), depressed AV and intraventricular conduction, **arrhythmias.**
GI: constipation, *nausea,* anorexia, abdominal pain, diarrhea.
Hepatic: *hepatitis, cirrhosis.*
Respiratory: increased depth and rate of respiration.
Skin: *diaphoresis, flushing,* rash.

Overdose and treatment
Signs and symptoms of overdose include drowsiness, weakness, nystagmus, diplopia, incoordination, and lassitude, progressing to coma with cyanosis and respiratory depression.

To slow drug absorption, give activated charcoal, water, or milk; then evacuate stomach contents by gastric lavage or emesis and then catharsis. Hemodialysis may be helpful.

Special considerations
• Papaverine is an opiate; however, it has strikingly different pharmacologic properties than other drugs in this group.
• Drug may be given orally, I.M., or, when immediate effect is needed, by slow I.V. injection. Inject I.V. slowly over 1 to 2 minutes; arrhythmias and fatal apnea may follow rapid injection.
• Papaverine injection is incompatible with lactated Ringer's injection; a precipitate will form.

Patient monitoring
• Monitor vital signs and cardiac rhythm during and after I.V. administration.
• Monitor hepatic enzyme levels.

Breast-feeding patients
• It isn't known if drug appears in breast milk. Safety in breast-feeding women hasn't been established.

Pediatric patients
• Children's doses are administered parenterally.

Geriatric patients
• Elderly patients are at greater risk for papaverine-induced hypothermia.

Patient education

- Advise patient to avoid sudden postural changes to minimize possible orthostatic hypotension.
- Instruct patient to report nausea, abdominal distress, anorexia, constipation, diarrhea, jaundice, rash, sweating, tiredness, or headache.

paricalcitol
Zemplar

Pharmacologic classification: vitamin D analogue
Therapeutic classification: hyperparathyroidism drug
Pregnancy risk category: C

Indications and dosages
➤ *Prevention and treatment of secondary hyperparathyroidism caused by chronic renal failure.* *Adults:* 0.04 to 0.1 mcg/kg (2.8 to 7 mcg) by I.V. bolus no more than every other day during dialysis. Doses as high as 0.24 mcg/kg (16.8 mcg) have been safely administered. If satisfactory response isn't observed, dose may be increased by 2 to 4 mcg at 2- to 4-week intervals.

How supplied
Available by prescription only
Injection: 5 mcg/ml, 1-ml and 2-ml vials

Pharmacodynamics
Antihyperparathyroid action: Synthetic vitamin D analogue shown to reduce parathyroid hormone (PTH) levels.

Pharmacokinetics
Absorption: Administered I.V.
Distribution: No information available.
Metabolism: No information available.
Excretion: Eliminated primarily by hepatobiliary excretion; 74% in feces and 16% in urine. Half-life is about 15 hours.

Route	Onset	Peak	Duration
I.V.	Immediate	Unknown	15 hr

Contraindications and precautions
Contraindicated in patients hypersensitive to drug or its components and in those with evidence of vitamin D toxicity or hypercalcemia. Use cautiously in patients taking digitalis compounds. Patients taking digoxin are at greater risk for digitalis toxicity during therapy because of possible hypercalcemia.

Interactions
None reported.

Adverse reactions
CNS: light-headedness, malaise.
CV: palpitations.
GI: dry mouth, GI bleeding, *nausea,* vomiting.

Hepatic: reduced serum total alkaline phosphatase level.
Respiratory: pneumonia.
Other: chills, edema, fever, flu syndrome, *sepsis.*

Overdose and treatment
Overdose may cause hypercalcemia. Symptoms include weakness, headache, nausea, vomiting, constipation, anorexia, pancreatitis, ectopic calcification, cardiac arrhythmias, and death.

Treatment should include correcting electrolyte abnormalities, assessing cardiac abnormalities, and hemodialysis or peritoneal dialysis against a calcium-free dialysate.

Special considerations
- In patients with chronic renal failure, appropriate types of phosphate-binding compounds may be needed to control serum phosphorus levels, but excessive use of compounds containing aluminum should be avoided.
- Drug is given only as an I.V. bolus. Discard unused portion.
- Inspect drug for particulate matter and discoloration before use.
- Store drug at 59° to 86° F (15° to 30° C).
- As PTH level decreases, paricalcitol dose may need to be decreased.

Patient monitoring
- Watch for ECG abnormalities.
- Monitor patient for symptoms of hypercalcemia.
- Monitor serum calcium and phosphorus levels twice weekly when dose is being adjusted; then monitor levels monthly. Measure PTH level every 3 months during therapy.

Breast-feeding patients
- It isn't known if drug appears in breast milk. Use cautiously in breast-feeding women.

Pediatric patients
- Safety and efficacy in children haven't been established.

Geriatric patients
- No significant difference in safety and efficacy was reported in patients over age 65.

Patient education
- Stress importance of adhering to a dietary regimen of calcium supplementation and phosphorus restriction during therapy.
- Caution against use of phosphate or vitamin D–related compounds during therapy.
- Explain need for frequent laboratory tests.
- Instruct patient with chronic renal failure to take phosphate-binding compounds as prescribed but to avoid excessive use of compounds containing aluminum.
- Alert patient to early symptoms of hypercalcemia and vitamin D intoxication, such as weakness, headache, somnolence, nausea, vomiting,

dry mouth, constipation, muscle pain, bone pain, and metallic taste.
• Instruct patient to promptly report adverse reactions.
• Remind patient taking digoxin to watch for signs of digitalis toxicity.

paroxetine hydrochloride
Paxil

Pharmacologic classification: selective serotonin reuptake inhibitor (SSRI)
Therapeutic classification: antidepressant
Pregnancy risk category: C

Indications and dosages
➤ *Depression. Adults:* Initially, 20 mg P.O. daily, preferably in the morning. Increased by 10 mg daily at 1-week intervals to maximum of 50 mg daily, if necessary.
➤ *Obsessive-compulsive disorder. Adults:* Initially, 20 mg P.O. daily, preferably in the morning. Increased by 10 mg daily at 1-week intervals to target dose of 40 mg daily. Maximum, 60 mg daily.
➤ *Panic disorder. Adults:* Initially, 10 mg P.O. daily, preferably in the morning. Increased by 10 mg daily at 1-week intervals to target dose of 40 mg daily. Maximum, 60 mg daily.
➤ *Social anxiety disorder. Adults:* 20 mg P.O. daily.
✦ *Dosage adjustment.* For elderly or debilitated patients or patients with severe hepatic or renal disease, 10 mg P.O. daily, preferably in the morning. Increased by 10 mg daily at 1-week intervals, p.r.n., to maximum of 40 mg daily.
➤ *Diabetic neuropathy* ◊. *Adults:* 10 to 60 mg P.O. daily.
➤ *Headaches* ◊. *Adults:* 10 to 50 mg P.O. daily.
➤ *Premature ejaculation* ◊. *Adults:* 20 mg P.O. daily.

How supplied
Available by prescription only
Suspension: 10 mg/5ml
Tablets: 10 mg, 20 mg, 30 mg, 40 mg

Pharmacodynamics
Antidepressant action: Exact mechanism unknown. Presumed to be linked to potentiation of serotonergic activity in the CNS, from inhibition of neuronal reuptake of serotonin.

Pharmacokinetics
Absorption: Completely absorbed after oral dosing.
Distribution: Distributed throughout body, including CNS, with only 1% remaining in plasma. About 93% to 95% bound to plasma protein.
Metabolism: About 36% metabolized in liver. Principal metabolites are polar and conjugated products of oxidation and methylation; readily cleared.

Excretion: About 64% excreted in urine (2% as parent compound, 62% as metabolite).

Route	Onset	Peak	Duration
P.O.	Unknown	2-8 hr	Unknown

Contraindications and precautions
Contraindicated in patients hypersensitive to drug and in those taking MAO inhibitors or within 14 days of discontinuing an MAO inhibitor. Use cautiously in those with a history of seizures or mania; those with severe, concurrent systemic illness; and those at risk for volume depletion.

Interactions
Drug-drug. *Cimetidine:* Decreased hepatic metabolism of paroxetine; risk of toxicity. Dosage adjustments may be needed.
Digoxin: Decreased digoxin levels. Monitor patient closely.
MAO inhibitors: Increased risk of serious, sometimes fatal, adverse reactions. Avoid concomitant use and don't use paroxetine within 14 days of discontinuing MAO inhibitors.
Phenobarbital: Induced paroxetine metabolism and reduced plasma levels. Adjust dosage as needed.
Phenytoin: Altered pharmacokinetics of phenytoin. Adjust dosage as needed.
Procyclidine: Increased procyclidine levels. Monitor patient for excessive anticholinergic effects.
Sumatriptan: Weakness, hyperreflexia and incoordination. Monitor patient closely.
Theophylline: Increased theophylline levels. Monitor patient closely.
Tryptophan: Increased adverse reactions, such as diaphoresis, headache, nausea, and dizziness. Avoid concomitant use.
Warfarin: Increased risk of bleeding. Monitor INR.
Drug-herb. *St. John's wort:* Serotonin levels may rise too high, causing serotonin syndrome. Discourage concomitant use.
Drug-lifestyle. *Alcohol use:* Increased risk of adverse CNS effects. Discourage use.

Adverse reactions
CNS: *somnolence, dizziness, insomnia, tremor, nervousness,* anxiety, paresthesia, confusion, *headache,* agitation, *asthenia,* abnormal dreams.
CV: palpitations, vasodilation, orthostatic hypotension, chest pain.
EENT: lump or tightness in throat, dysgeusia, visual disturbances, double vision.
GI: *dry mouth, nausea, constipation, diarrhea,* flatulence, vomiting, dyspepsia, increased or decreased appetite, abdominal pain.
GU: ejaculatory disturbances, decreased libido, male genital disorders (including anorgasmia, erectile difficulties, delayed ejaculation or orgasm, impotence, and sexual dysfunction), urinary frequency, other urinary disorders, female genital disorders (including anorgasmia, difficulty with orgasm).

---

* Canada only   ◊ Unlabeled clinical use

Musculoskeletal: myopathy, myalgia, myasthenia.
Skin: *diaphoresis,* rash, pruritus.
Other: yawning.

Overdose and treatment
Toxicity may cause nausea, vomiting, dizziness, sweating, facial flushing, drowsiness, sinus tachycardia, and dilated pupils. Perform gastric evacuation by emesis, lavage, or both. In most cases, 20 to 30 g of activated charcoal may then be used every 4 to 6 hours during the first 24 to 48 hours after ingestion.

Special caution must be taken with a patient who receives or recently received paroxetine if the patient ingests an excessive quantity of a tricyclic antidepressant; accumulation of the parent tricyclic and its active metabolite may increase the possibility of clinically significant sequelae and extend the time needed for close medical observation.

Special considerations
● At least 14 days should elapse between stopping an MAO inhibitor and starting drug therapy. Similarly, at least 14 days should elapse between stopping paroxetine and starting MAO inhibitor.

Patient monitoring
● Hyponatremia may occur with paroxetine use, especially in elderly patients, those taking diuretics, and those who are otherwise volume depleted. Monitor serum sodium levels.
● If signs of psychosis occur or increase, reduce dosage. Monitor patients for suicidal tendencies and allow them only a minimum supply of drug.

Breast-feeding patients
● Drug appears in breast milk. Use cautiously in breast-feeding women.

Pediatric patients
● Safety and effectiveness in children haven't been established.

Geriatric patients
● Use cautiously and in lower dosages in elderly patients.

Patient education
● Caution patient not to operate hazardous machinery, including automobiles, until reasonably certain that drug doesn't affect ability to engage in such activity.
● Tell patient that he may notice improvement in 1 to 4 weeks but that he must continue with prescribed regimen to obtain continued benefits.
● Instruct patient to call before taking other drugs, including OTC preparations and herbal remedies, while taking paroxetine.
● Tell patient to abstain from alcohol while taking drug.

pegaspargase
(PEG-L-asparaginase)
Oncaspar

Pharmacologic classification: modified version of the enzyme L-asparaginase
Therapeutic classification: antineoplastic
Pregnancy risk category: C

Indications and dosages
➤ *Acute lymphoblastic leukemia (ALL) in patients who need L-asparaginase but have developed hypersensitivity to its native forms.* Adults and children with body surface area (BSA) of at least 0.6 m²: 2,500 IU/m² I.M. or I.V. q 14 days.
Children with BSA less than 0.6 m²: 82.5 IU/kg I.M. or I.V. q 14 days.

Note: Moderate to life-threatening hypersensitivity reactions require stopping L-asparaginase treatment.

How supplied
Available by prescription only
Injection: 750 IU/ml in single-use vial

Pharmacodynamics
Antineoplastic action: Modified version of the enzyme L-asparaginase that exerts cytotoxic activity by inactivating the amino acid asparagine. Because leukemic cells can't synthesize their own asparagine, protein synthesis and eventually synthesis of DNA and RNA are inhibited.

Pharmacokinetics
No information available.

Route	Onset	Peak	Duration
I.M., I.V.	Unknown	Unknown	Unknown

Contraindications and precautions
Contraindicated in patients with pancreatitis or a history of it; those who have had significant hemorrhagic events linked to prior L-asparaginase therapy; and those with previous serious allergic reactions, such as generalized urticaria, bronchospasm, laryngeal edema, hypotension, or other unacceptable adverse reactions to pegaspargase.

Use cautiously in pregnant patients and those with hepatic dysfunction.

Interactions
Drug-drug. *Aspirin, dipyridamole, heparin, NSAIDs, warfarin:* Imbalances in coagulation factors; possible bleeding or thrombosis. Monitor patient for increased bleeding; monitor PT and INR.
Methotrexate: May interfere with action of drugs such as methotrexate that require cell replication for lethal effects. Watch for decreased effect.
Other protein-bound drugs: Increased toxicity of these drugs. Pegaspargase may also interfere with enzymatic detoxification of other drugs, particularly in liver. Monitor patient closely.

Adverse reactions

CNS: seizures, headache, malaise, paresthesia, *status epilepticus,* somnolence, *coma,* mental status changes, dizziness, emotional lability, mood changes, parkinsonism, confusion, disorientation, fatigue.

CV: hypotension, tachycardia, chest pain, subacute bacterial endocarditis, hypertension, peripheral edema.

EENT: mouth tenderness, epistaxis.

GI: nausea, vomiting, abdominal pain, anorexia, diarrhea, constipation, indigestion, flatulence, GI pain, mucositis, *pancreatitis* (sometimes fulminant and fatal), increased serum amylase and lipase levels, severe colitis.

GU: increased BUN level, increased creatinine level, increased urinary frequency, hematuria, severe hemorrhagic cystitis, renal dysfunction, *renal failure.*

Hematologic: *thrombosis;* prolonged PT, prolonged partial thromboplastin time, decreased antithrombin III, *disseminated intravascular coagulation,* decreased fibrinogen, hemolytic anemia, *leukopenia, pancytopenia, agranulocytosis, thrombocytopenia,* increased thromboplastin, easy bruising, ecchymoses, *hemorrhage* (may be fatal).

Hepatic: jaundice, abnormal liver function test results, bilirubinemia, increased ALT and AST levels, ascites, hypoalbuminemia, fatty changes in liver, *liver failure.*

Metabolic: hyperuricemia, hyponatremia, uric acid nephropathy, hypoproteinemia, proteinuria, weight loss, metabolic acidosis, increased blood ammonia level, hyperglycemia, hypoglycemia.

Musculoskeletal: arthralgia, myalgia, musculoskeletal pain, joint stiffness, cramps, pain in limbs.

Respiratory: cough, *severe bronchospasm,* upper respiratory tract infection.

Skin: itching, alopecia, fever blister, purpura, hand whiteness, fungal changes, nail whiteness and ridging, erythema simplex, petechial rash, injection pain or reaction, localized edema.

Other: hypersensitivity reactions, including *anaphylaxis,* rash, erythema, edema, pain, fever, chills, urticaria, dyspnea, and *bronchospasm;* night sweats; infection; *sepsis; septic shock.*

Overdose and treatment

Only three cases of overdose (10,000 IU/m^2 as an I.V. infusion) have been reported. One patient had a slight increase in liver enzymes, another developed a rash, and the third had no adverse effects. No other information is available.

Special considerations

• I.M. is preferred route because it causes a lower risk of hepatotoxicity, coagulopathy, and GI and renal disorders than I.V. route.

• Drug shouldn't be given if it has ever been frozen. Although its appearance may not change, its activity is destroyed after freezing.

• Avoid excessive agitation; don't shake. Keep refrigerated at 36° to 46° F (2° to 8° C). Don't use

if cloudy, precipitated, or stored at room temperature for more than 48 hours. Don't freeze. Discard unused portions. Use only one dose per vial; don't reenter vial. Don't save unused drug for later administration.

• When administering I.M., limit volume at a single injection site to 2 ml. If volume to be administered is greater than 2 ml, use multiple injection sites.

• When administered I.V., give over 1 to 2 hours in 100 ml of normal saline solution or 5% dextrose injection through an infusion that is already running.

• Pegaspargase should be the sole induction drug only when a combined regimen using other chemotherapeutic drugs is inappropriate because of toxicity or other specific patient-related factors or because patient is refractory to other therapy.

• Because drug may be a contact irritant, handle and administer solution with care; wear gloves. Avoid inhalation of vapors and contact with skin or mucous membranes, especially eyes. In case of contact, wash with copious amounts of water for at least 15 minutes.

Patient monitoring

• Hypersensitivity reactions to drug, including life-threatening anaphylaxis, may occur during therapy, especially in patients hypersensitive to other forms of L-asparaginase. Observe patient for 1 hour and keep resuscitation equipment and other emergency products on hand.

• Circulating lymphoblasts commonly decline after therapy starts. Patient may have a marked rise in serum uric acid as well. As a guide to the effects of therapy, monitor patient's peripheral blood count and bone marrow. Obtain frequent serum amylase determinations to detect early evidence of pancreatitis. Monitor blood glucose level during therapy because hyperglycemia may occur. When using pegaspargase with hepatotoxic chemotherapy, monitor patient for liver dysfunction. Pegaspargase may affect some plasma proteins; therefore, monitoring of fibrinogen, PT, and partial thromboplastin time may be indicated.

Breast-feeding patients

• It isn't known if drug appears in breast milk. Because of potential for serious adverse reactions in breast-fed infants, stop either breast-feeding or drug, taking into account importance of drug to mother.

Pediatric patients

• Safety and efficacy in infants under age 1 haven't been established.

Patient education

• Tell patient to report hypersensitivity reactions immediately.

• Instruct patient not to take other drugs, including OTC preparations, without medical approval; pegaspargase increases the risk of bleed-

ing when given with certain drugs, such as aspirin, and may increase toxicity of other drugs.
• Instruct patient to report signs and symptoms of infection (fever, chills, malaise); drug may have immunosuppressive activity.

peginterferon alfa-2b
PEG-Intron

Pharmacologic classification: biological response modifier
Therapeutic classification: antiviral
Pregnancy risk category: C

Indications and dosages
➤ **Chronic hepatitis C in patients not previously treated with interferon alpha.**
Adults: Give S.C. once weekly for 48 weeks on same day each week, initial dose based on weight as follows.
Adults who weigh 37 to 45 kg (81 to 99 lb): 40 mcg (0.4 ml) of 100-mcg/ml strength
Adults who weigh 46 to 56 kg (100 to 123 lb): 50 mcg (0.5 ml) of 100-mcg/ml strength
Adults who weigh 57 to 72 kg (124 to 158 lb): 64 mcg (0.4 ml) of 160-mcg/ml strength
Adults who weigh 73 to 88 kg (159 to 194 lb): 80 mcg (0.5 ml) of 160-mcg/ml strength
Adults who weigh 89 to 106 kg (195 to 233 lb): 96 mcg (0.4 ml) of 240-mcg/ml strength
Adults who weigh 107 to 136 kg (234 to 299 lb): 120 mcg (0.5 ml) of 240-mcg/ml strength
Adults who weigh 137 to 160 kg (300 to 352 lb): 150 mcg (0.5 ml) of 300-mcg/ml strength
✦ **Dosage adjustment.** For patient who develops a serious adverse reaction, stop drug or decrease dose to one-half starting dose. If neutrophil count is below 0.75×10^9/L, reduce dose. If below 0.50×10^9/L, discontinue drug. If platelet count is below 80×10^9/L, reduce dose. If below 50×10^9/L, discontinue drug.

How supplied
Available by prescription only
Injection: 100 mcg/ml, 160 mcg/ml, 240 mcg/ml, 300 mcg/ml

Pharmacodynamics
Antiviral action: Interferon alfa-2b binds to specific membrane receptors on the cell surface, initiating induction of certain enzymes, suppression of cell proliferation, immunomodulation activities, and inhibition of viral replication in infected cells. PEG-Intron increases levels of effector proteins, increases body temperature, and decreases leukocyte and platelet counts.

Pharmacokinetics
Absorption: Serum levels peak 15 to 44 hours after a dose and effects last for 48 to 72 hours.
Distribution: Unknown.
Metabolism: Mean elimination half-life is about 40 hours.

Excretion: About 30% is excreted by the kidneys.

Route	Onset	Peak	Duration
S.C.	Unknown	15-44 hr	Unknown

Contraindications and precautions
Contraindicated in patients hypersensitive to peginterferon alfa-2b or any of its components. Also contraindicated in patients with autoimmune hepatitis or decompensated liver disease.

Use cautiously in patients with psychiatric disorders, diabetes mellitus, CV disease, renal failure (creatinine clearance below 50 ml/minute), pulmonary infiltrates, and pulmonary function impairment. Also use cautiously in patients with autoimmune, ischemic, and infectious disorders.

Interactions
None reported.

Adverse reactions
CNS: dizziness, hypertonia, depression, insomnia, anxiety, emotional lability, irritability, headache, fatigue, malaise, **suicidal behavior.**
CV: flushing.
EENT: pharyngitis, sinusitis.
GI: nausea, anorexia, diarrhea, abdominal pain, vomiting, dyspepsia, right upper quadrant pain.
Hematologic: *neutropenia, thrombocytopenia.*
Hepatic: hepatomegaly, elevated ALT levels.
Metabolic: hypothyroidism, hyperthyroidism, weight decrease.
Musculoskeletal: musculoskeletal pain.
Respiratory: cough.
Skin: alopecia, pruritus, dry skin, rash, injection site inflammation or reaction, increased sweating, injection site pain.
Other: viral infection, fever, flulike symptoms, rigors.

Overdose and treatment
In a clinical study, 13 patients received a dose greater than that prescribed. The maximum dose received was 3.45 mcg/kg weekly for about 12 weeks. No serious reactions resulted from overdose.

Special considerations
• Don't use drug in patients with diabetes or thyroid disorders that can't be controlled with medication. Drug may cause or aggravate hypothyroidism, hyperthyroidism, or diabetes.
• Don't use in patients who have failed other alpha-interferon treatment, patients who have received liver or other organ transplants, or patients with HIV or HBV.
• Initiate treatment in patient that is well-hydrated.

Patient monitoring
• Perform ECG on patient with cardiac history before starting drug.
• Perform eye exam in patients with diabetes or hypertension before starting drug. Retinal he-

morrhages, cotton wool spots, and retinal artery or vein obstruction may occur.
• Monitor patient with history of MI or arrhythmias closely for hypotension, arrhythmias, tachycardia, cardiomyopathy, and MI.
• Monitor patient for depression and other psychiatric illness. If symptoms are severe, discontinue drug and refer for psychiatric care.
• Monitor patient for signs and symptoms of colitis, such as abdominal pain, bloody diarrhea, and fever. Discontinue drug if colitis occurs. Symptoms should resolve 1 to 3 weeks after stopping drug.
• Monitor patient for evidence of pancreatitis or hypersensitivity reactions, and discontinue drug if these occur.
• Monitor patient with pulmonary disease for dyspnea, pulmonary infiltrates, pneumonitis, and pneumonia.
• Monitor patient with renal disease for signs and symptoms of toxicity.
• Monitor CBC, platelet, AST, ALT, bilirubin, and TSH levels before starting drug and periodically during treatment.
• Discontinue use in patients with severe neutropenia or thrombocytopenia.

Breast-feeding patients
• It isn't known whether peginterferon alfa-2b appears in breast milk. Because of the risk of adverse reactions in nursing infants, a decision must be made whether to discontinue nursing or the drug.

Pediatric patients
• Safety and effectiveness in children under age 18 haven't been established.

Geriatric patients
• No differences in pharmacokinetics have been seen in elderly patients.

Patient education
• Advise patient on the appropriate use of drug and the benefits and risks linked to treatment. Tell patient that adverse reactions may continue for several months after treatment is stopped.
• Advise patient to immediately report symptoms of depression or suicidal ideation.
• Instruct patient on the importance of proper disposal of needles and syringes, and caution against reuse of needles and syringes.
• Tell patient that drug isn't known to prevent transmission of hepatitis C virus to others. It also isn't known whether drug will cure hepatitis C or prevent cirrhosis, liver failure, or liver cancer that may result from hepatitis C infection.
• Advise patient that lab tests are required before starting therapy and periodically thereafter.
• Tell patient to take drug at bedtime and to use antipyretics to decrease the effects of flulike symptoms.

pemoline
Cylert

Pharmacologic classification: oxazolidinedione derivative, CNS stimulant
Therapeutic classification: analeptic
Controlled substance schedule: IV
Pregnancy risk category: B

Indications and dosages
➤ *Attention deficit hyperactivity disorder (ADHD). Children age 6 and older:* Initially, 37.5 mg P.O. in the morning. Daily dosage can be increased by 18.75 mg weekly. Effective dosage range is 56.25 to 75 mg daily. Maximum, 112.5 mg daily.
Note: Because of its association with life-threatening hepatic failure, pemoline shouldn't be considered first-line therapy for ADHD.
➤ *Narcolepsy* ◇ *. Adults:* 50 to 200 mg daily, in divided doses after breakfast and lunch.

How supplied
Available by prescription only
Tablets: 18.75 mg, 37.5 mg, 75 mg
Tablets (chewable and povidone-containing): 37.5 mg

Pharmacodynamics
Analeptic action: Differs structurally from methylphenidate and amphetamines; however, like those drugs, pemoline has a paradoxical calming effect in children with ADHD. Mechanism of action is unknown. May be mediated through dopaminergic mechanisms. CNS stimulant effect has been studied in narcolepsy in adults, in fatigue, in depressed and schizophrenic states, and in elderly patients.

Pharmacokinetics
Absorption: Well absorbed after oral administration. Therapeutic effects peak within 4 hours and last for about 8 hours.
Distribution: No information available. Drug is 50% protein-bound.
Metabolism: Metabolized by liver to active and inactive metabolites.
Excretion: Drug and metabolites excreted in urine; 75% of oral dose excreted within 24 hours.

Route	Onset	Peak	Duration
P.O.	Unknown	2-4 hr	Unknown

Contraindications and precautions
Contraindicated in patients hypersensitive to drugs, patients with idiosyncratic reactions to drug, and patients with hepatic dysfunction. Use cautiously in patients with impaired renal function.

Interactions
Drug-drug. *Anticonvulsants:* Decreased seizure threshold. Monitor patient closely.

Drug-food. *Caffeine:* Decreased efficacy of pemoline in ADHD. Discourage use.

Adverse reactions

CNS: *insomnia,* dyskinetic movements, irritability, fatigue, mild depression, dizziness, headache, drowsiness, hallucinations, **seizures,** *Tourette syndrome,* abnormal oculomotor function.
GI: anorexia, abdominal pain, nausea.
Hematologic: *aplastic anemia.*
Hepatic: elevated liver enzyme levels, *hepatic failure.*
Skin: rash.

Overdose and treatment

Toxicity may cause irregular respiration, hyperreflexia, restlessness, tachycardia, hallucinations, excitement, and agitation.

Treat overdose symptomatically and supportively. Use gastric lavage if symptoms aren't severe. Monitor vital signs and fluid and electrolyte balance. Maintain patient in a cool room, monitor temperature, and minimize external stimulation; protect patient from self-injury. Chlorpromazine or haloperidol usually can reverse CNS stimulation. Hemodialysis may help.

Special considerations

• Give drug in a single morning dose for maximum daytime benefit and to minimize insomnia.
• Explain that therapeutic effects may not appear for 3 to 4 weeks and that intermittent drug-free periods when stress is least evident (weekends, school holidays) may help assess patient's condition, prevent development of tolerance, and permit decreased dosage when drug is resumed.
• Abrupt withdrawal after high-dose long-term use may unmask severe depression. Lower dosage gradually to prevent acute rebound depression.
• Drug impairs ability to perform tasks requiring mental alertness.
• Make sure patient obtains adequate rest; fatigue may result as drug wears off.
• Discourage pemoline use for analeptic effect because drug has abuse potential; CNS stimulation superimposed on CNS depression may cause neuronal instability and seizures.
• Carefully follow manufacturer's directions for reconstitution, storage, and administration of all preparations. Pemoline has been used to treat narcolepsy in adults (50 to 200 mg divided twice daily) as well as depression and schizophrenia, but these uses are controversial.

Patient monitoring

• Monitor start of therapy closely; drug may precipitate Tourette syndrome.
• Check vital signs regularly for increased blood pressure or other signs of excessive stimulation.
• Monitor blood and urine glucose levels in diabetic patients; drug may alter insulin requirements.
• Monitor CBC, differential, and platelet counts while patient receives long-term therapy.

• Determine baseline and periodically assess liver function tests. If abnormalities occur, stop drug.
• Monitor height and weight; drug may cause growth suppression.

Pediatric patients

• Drug isn't recommended for ADHD in children under age 6.

Patient education

• Explain rationale for therapy and anticipated risks and benefits; teach signs and symptoms of adverse reactions and need to report these.
• Tell patient to avoid drinks containing caffeine to prevent added CNS stimulation.
• Urge patient or parent not to alter dosage without medical approval.
• Warn against using drug to mask fatigue. Tell patient to obtain adequate rest and report excessive CNS stimulation.
• Advise diabetic patient to monitor blood glucose levels because drug may alter insulin needs.
• Advise patient to avoid tasks that require mental alertness until degree of sedative effect is determined.

---

penbutolol sulfate
Levatol

Pharmacologic classification: beta blocker
Therapeutic classification: antihypertensive
Pregnancy risk category: C

Indications and dosages

➤ *Mild to moderate hypertension. Adults:* 20 mg P.O. once daily. Usually given with other antihypertensives, such as thiazide diuretics. Doses as high as 40 to 80 mg daily and as low as 10 mg daily have been effective.

How supplied

Available by prescription only
Tablets: 20 mg

Pharmacodynamics

Antihypertensive action: Blocks both beta$_1$- and beta$_2$-adrenergic receptors. Antihypertensive effects may be related to peripheral antiadrenergic effects that lead to decreased cardiac output, a central effect that leads to decreased sympathetic tone, or decreased renin secretion by the kidneys.

Pharmacokinetics

Absorption: Almost completely absorbed after oral administration. Plasma levels peak in 2 to 3 hours.
Distribution: 80% to 98% bound to plasma proteins.
Metabolism: Metabolized by liver. Several metabolites identified; some retain partial pharmacologic activity.

Reactions may be *common,* uncommon, *life-threatening,* or COMMON AND LIFE-THREATENING.

Excretion: Average elimination half-life of parent drug is 5 hours; some metabolites persist for 20 hours or more. Most metabolites excreted in urine.

Route	Onset	Peak	Duration
P.O.	1 hr	1½-3 hr	24 hr

Contraindications and precautions

Contraindicated in patients hypersensitive to drug or other beta blockers and in those with sinus bradycardia, cardiogenic shock, overt cardiac failure, greater than first-degree heart block, bronchial asthma, bronchospastic disease, or chronic bronchitis.

Use cautiously in patients with heart failure controlled by drug therapy, diabetes, or history of bronchospastic disease.

Interactions

Drug-drug. *Clonidine:* Paradoxical hypertension when combined with beta blockers; enhanced rebound hypertension when clonidine is withdrawn. Use together cautiously.

Doxazosin, prazosin, terazosin: Enhanced first dose orthostatic hypotension with these drugs. Use together cautiously.

Insulin, oral antidiabetics: Altered hypoglycemic response. Monitor patient closely.

Lidocaine: Increased volume of lidocaine distribution; may increase loading dose requirements in some patients. Adjust dosage as needed.

Oral calcium antagonists: Enhanced hypotensive effects of beta blockers; predispose patient to bradycardia and arrhythmias. Monitor patient closely.

Reserpine, other catecholamine-depleting drugs: Additive effects. Avoid using together.

Adverse reactions

CNS: *dizziness,* headache, fatigue, insomnia, asthenia.
CV: chest pain, ***bradycardia, heart failure.***
GI: nausea, diarrhea, dyspepsia.
GU: impotence.
Metabolic: interference with glucose or insulin tolerance tests.
Respiratory: cough, dyspnea.
Skin: excessive diaphoresis.

Overdose and treatment

Toxicity may cause bradycardia, bronchospasm, heart failure, and severe hypotension.

After emptying the stomach by lavage (for acute oral ingestion), administer symptomatic and supportive care. Bradycardia may be treated with atropine or cautious use of isoproterenol. Cardiac glycosides, glucagon hydrochloride, dobutamine, and diuretics may be useful in treating heart failure, and vasopressors, such as epinephrine or alpha-adrenergic agonists, may be used to counter severe hypotension. In refractory cases of hypotension, administration of glucagon

hydrochloride may be useful. Treat bronchospasm with aminophylline or isoproterenol.

Special considerations

● Like other beta blockers, penbutolol may cause patients to exhibit hypersensitivity to catecholamines upon withdrawal.
● Full effect of a 20-mg or 40-mg dose is seen in 2 weeks. When 10 mg is used, it may take 4 to 6 weeks to see full effect.
● To discontinue drug, slowly taper dosage over 1 to 2 weeks, especially in patients with ischemic heart disease. If symptoms of angina develop, immediately resume therapy, at least temporarily, and take steps to control the patient's unstable angina.

Patient monitoring

● Monitor blood pressure to determine effectiveness of therapy.
● Perform periodic ECG. Monitor patient for early signs of heart failure.

Breast-feeding patients

● It isn't known if drug appears in breast milk. Use cautiously in breast-feeding women.

Pediatric patients

● Safety and effectiveness in children haven't been established.

Geriatric patients

● Pharmacokinetic studies indicate no difference in plasma half-life in healthy elderly patients compared with patients on renal dialysis.

Patient education

● Advise patient not to stop drug abruptly because sudden withdrawal of other beta blockers has precipitated angina and MI.
● Tell patient to report adverse effects immediately, particularly slow heart rate, chest congestion, cough, wheezing, or shortness of breath from mild exertion.
● Teach patient about disease and therapy. Explain why it's important to continue taking drug, even when feeling well.
● Advise patient to report unpleasant adverse effects promptly.
● Tell patient to call before taking OTC products.

---

penicillamine
Cuprimine, Depen

Pharmacologic classification: chelating drug
Therapeutic classification: heavy metal antagonist, antirheumatic
Pregnancy risk category: NR

Indications and dosages

➤ **Wilson's disease.** *Adults:* 250 mg P.O. q.i.d. ½ to 1 hour before meals and at least 2 hours after evening meal. Adjust dose to achieve urinary copper excretion of 0.5 to 1 mg daily. Doses over 2 g are seldom necessary.

➤ *Cystinuria. Adults:* 250 mg P.O. daily in four divided doses; then gradually increase dosage. Usual dose is 2 g daily (range, 1 to 4 g daily). Adjust dose to achieve urinary cystine excretion of less than 100 mg daily when renal calculi are present, or 100 to 200 mg daily when no calculi are present.

➤ *Rheumatoid arthritis, Felty's syndrome. Adults:* Initially, 125 to 250 mg P.O. daily, with increases of 125 to 250 mg daily at 1- to 3-month intervals if necessary. Maximum, 1.5 g daily.

➤ *Adjunctive treatment of heavy metal poisoning* ◇. *Adults:* 500 to 1,500 mg P.O. daily for 1 to 2 months.

➤ *Primary biliary cirrhosis* ◇. *Adults:* Initially, 250 mg P.O. daily, with increases of 250 mg q 2 weeks. Maximum, 1 g daily in divided doses.

How supplied
Available by prescription only
Capsules: 125 mg, 250 mg
Tablets: 250 mg

Pharmacodynamics
Antirheumatic action: Mechanism unknown; depresses circulating IgM rheumatoid factor (but not total circulating immunoglobulin levels) and depresses T-cell but not B-cell activity. Also depolymerizes some macroglobulins (for example, rheumatoid factor).

Chelating action: Forms stable, soluble complexes with copper, iron, mercury, lead, and other heavy metals that are excreted in urine; particularly useful in chelating copper in patients with Wilson's disease. Also combines with cystine to form a complex more soluble than cystine alone, thereby reducing free cystine below the level of urinary stone formation.

Pharmacokinetics
Absorption: Well absorbed after oral administration; serum levels peak at 3 hours.
Distribution: Limited data available.
Metabolism: Metabolized by liver to inactive compounds.
Excretion: Only small amounts excreted unchanged; after 24 hours, about 50% of drug excreted in urine and about 50% in feces.

Route	Onset	Peak	Duration
P.O.	Unknown	3 hr	Unknown

Contraindications and precautions
Contraindicated in patients hypersensitive to drug, pregnant women, patients with a history of penicillamine-related aplastic anemia or agranulocytosis, patients with significant renal or hepatic insufficiency, and patients receiving gold salts, immunosuppressants, antimalarials, or phenylbutazone because of the increased risk of serious hematologic effects.

Use cautiously in patients allergic to penicillin (cross reaction is rare); in those who receive a second course of therapy and who may have become sensitized and are more likely to have allergic reactions; and in patients who develop proteinuria not linked to Goodpasture's syndrome.

Interactions
Drug-drug. *Antacids, iron salts:* Decreased penicillamine absorption. Separate administration times.
Antimalarials, cytotoxic drugs, gold therapy, oxyphenbutazone, phenylbutazone: Serious hematologic and renal effects. Don't administer together.
Digoxin: Increased serum digoxin levels. Monitor serum levels.

Adverse reactions
EENT: oral ulcerations, glossitis, cheilosis, tinnitus, optic neuritis.
GI: anorexia, nausea, vomiting, dyspepsia, alteration in taste, metallic taste, diarrhea, dysgeusia, *hypogeusia.*
GU: *proteinuria.*
Hematologic: eosinophilia, *leukopenia, thrombocytopenia, aplastic anemia, agranulocytosis,* thrombotic thrombocytopenia purpura, hemolytic anemia or iron deficiency anemia, lupus-like syndrome, *bone marrow suppression.*
Hepatic: cholestatic jaundice, *pancreatitis,* hepatic dysfunction.
Metabolic: thyroiditis.
Musculoskeletal: arthralgia, myasthenia gravis.
Respiratory: pneumonitis, Goodpasture's syndrome.
Skin: *pruritus; erythematous rash;* intensely pruritic rash with scaly, macular lesions on trunk; pemphigoid reactions; urticaria; alopecia; *exfoliative dermatitis;* increased skin friability; purpuric or vesicular ecchymoses; wrinkling.
Other: lymphadenopathy, drug fever.

Overdose and treatment
There are no reports of significant drug overdose. Induce emesis unless unconscious or gag reflex is absent; otherwise empty stomach by gastric lavage and then administer activated charcoal and sorbitol. Thereafter, treat supportively. Treat seizures with diazepam (or pyridoxine if previously successful). Hemodialysis will remove penicillamine.

Special considerations
● Stop drug if patient has signs of hypersensitivity or drug fever, usually with other allergic signs and symptoms (if Wilson's disease, may rechallenge), or if the following occur: rash developing 6 months or more after start of therapy, pemphigoid reaction, hematuria or proteinuria with hemoptysis or pulmonary infiltrates, gross or persistent microscopic hematuria or proteinuria greater than 2 g daily in patients with rheuma-

toid arthritis, platelet count below 100,000/mm³ or leukocyte count below 3,500/mm³, or if either shows three consecutive decreases (even within normal range).

⚠ **ALERT** Don't confuse penicillamine with polycillin and the various types of penicillin.

• Patients with Wilson's disease or cystinuria may need daily pyridoxine (vitamin B₆) supplementation.

• Prescribe drug to be taken 1 hour before or 2 hours after meals or other drugs to facilitate absorption.

• For initial treatment of Wilson's disease, 10 to 40 mg of sulfurated potash should be administered with each meal during penicillamine therapy for 6 months to 1 year, and then discontinued.

• Drug therapy may cause positive test results for antinuclear antibody with or without clinical systemic lupus erythematosus-like syndrome.

• Hemodialysis will remove penicillamine.

Patient monitoring
• Perform urinalyses and CBC (including differential blood count) every 2 weeks for 6 months, then monthly. Perform kidney and liver functions studies, usually every 6 months. Watch for fever or allergic reactions (rash, joint pain, easy bruising). Check routinely for proteinuria, and handle patient carefully to avoid skin damage.

• About one-third of patients receiving drug experience an allergic reaction. Monitor patient for signs and symptoms of allergic reaction.

Breast-feeding patients
• It isn't known if drug appears in breast milk. Safety hasn't been established in breast-feeding women; an alternative to breast-feeding is recommended during therapy.

Pediatric patients
• Check for possible iron deficiency resulting from long-term use. Safety and efficacy for juvenile rheumatoid arthritis haven't been established in children.

Geriatric patients
• Lower doses may be indicated. Monitor renal and hepatic function closely. Toxicity may be more common in elderly patients.

Patient education
• Provide health education for patients with Wilson's disease, rheumatoid arthritis, or cystinuria; explain disease process and rationale for therapy and explain that results may not be evident for 3 months.

• Encourage compliance with therapy and follow-up visits.

• Stress importance of reporting immediately any fever, chills, sore throat, bruising, bleeding, or allergic reaction.

• Tell patient to take drug on an empty stomach 30 minutes to 1 hour before meals or 2 hours after ingesting food, antacids, mineral supplements, vitamins, or other drugs. Tell patient to drink large amounts of water, especially at night.

• Advise patient receiving drug for rheumatoid arthritis that an exacerbation of disease may occur during therapy. This usually can be controlled by concurrent use of NSAIDs.

• Advise patient taking drug for Wilson's disease to maintain a low-copper (less than 2 mg daily) diet by excluding foods with high copper content, such as chocolate, nuts, liver, and broccoli. Also, sulfurated potash may be administered with meals to minimize copper absorption.

penicillin G benzathine
Bicillin L-A, Permapen

penicillin G benzathine and procaine
Bicillin C-R

penicillin G potassium
Pfizerpen

penicillin G procaine
Ayercillin*, Bicillin C-R, Wycillin

penicillin G sodium

Pharmacologic classification: natural penicillin
Therapeutic classification: antibiotic
Pregnancy risk category: B

Indications and dosages
➤ **Congenital syphilis.** penicillin G benzathine. *Children under age 2:* 50,000 units/kg I.M. as a single injection.

➤ **Group A streptococcal upper respiratory infections, diphtheria, yaws, pinta, and bejel.** penicillin G benzathine. *Adults:* 1.2 million units I.M. as a single injection.
Children who weigh 27 kg (60 lb) or more: 900,000 units I.M. in a single injection.
Children who weigh less than 27 kg: 300,000 to 600,000 units I.M. in a single injection.

➤ **Prophylaxis of poststreptococcal rheumatic fever.** penicillin G benzathine. *Adults and children:* 1.2 million units I.M. once monthly.

➤ **Syphilis of less than 1 year's duration.** penicillin G benzathine. *Adults:* 2.4 million units I.M. in a single dose.

➤ **Syphilis of more than 1 year's duration.** penicillin G benzathine. *Adults:* 2.4 million units I.M. weekly for 3 successive weeks.

➤ **Moderate to severe systemic infections.** penicillin G potassium, sodium. *Adults:* 12 to 24 million units I.M. or I.V. daily, given in divided doses q 4 hours.
Children: 25,000 to 300,000 units/kg I.M. or I.V. daily, given in divided doses q 4 hours.

➤ *Moderate to severe systemic infections, pneumococcal pneumonia.* penicillin G procaine. *Adults:* 600,000 to 1.2 million units I.M. daily as a single dose or q 6 to 12 hours. *Children:* 300,000 units I.M. daily as a single dose.

➤ *Uncomplicated gonorrhea.* penicillin G procaine. *Adults and children over age 12:* 1 g probenecid P.O; then, 30 minutes later, 4.8 million units of penicillin G procaine I.M., divided into two injection sites.

✦ *Dosage adjustment.* For patients with renal impairment, refer to the table.

Creatinine clearance (ml/min)	Dosage (after full loading dose)
10-50	50% of usual dose q 4 to 5 hr; or, give usual dose q 8 to 12 hr
< 10	50% of usual dose q 8 to 12 hr; or, give usual dose q 12 to 18 hr

How supplied
Available by prescription only
penicillin G benzathine
Injection: 300,000 units/ml; 600,000 units/ml; 1.2 million units/2 ml; 2.4 million units/4 ml
Suspension: 250,000 units/5 ml*; 500,000 units/ml*
penicillin G benzathine and procaine
Injection: 300,000 units/ml; 600,000 units/ml
penicillin G potassium
Injection (premixed, frozen): 1 million units/50 ml, 2 million units/50 ml, 3 million units/50 ml
Powder for injection: 1 million units, 5 million units, 10 million units, 20 million units
penicillin G procaine
Injection: 600,000 units/ml
penicillin G sodium
Powder for injection: 1 million units*, 5 million units, 10 million units*

Pharmacodynamics
Antibiotic action: Bactericidal. Adheres to penicillin-binding proteins, thus inhibiting bacterial cell wall synthesis. Spectrum of activity includes most non–penicillinase-producing strains of gram-positive and gram-negative aerobic cocci, spirochetes, and some gram-positive aerobic and anaerobic bacilli.

Pharmacokinetics
Penicillin G is available as four salts, each having the same bactericidal action, but designed to offer greater oral stability (potassium salt) or to prolong duration of action by slowing absorption after I.M. injection (benzathine and procaine salts).
Absorption: Sodium and potassium salts of penicillin G absorbed rapidly after I.M. injection; peak

serum levels within 15 to 30 minutes. Slower absorption of other salts. Serum levels of penicillin G procaine peak in 1 to 4 hours, with drug detectable in serum for 1 to 2 days; serum levels of penicillin G benzathine peak in 13 to 24 hours, with serum levels detectable for 1 to 4 weeks.
Distribution: Penicillin G distributed widely into synovial, pleural, pericardial, ascitic fluids; bile, liver, skin, lungs, kidneys, muscle, intestines, tonsils, maxillary sinuses, saliva, and erythrocytes. Poor CSF penetration but enhanced in patients with inflamed meninges. Penicillin G crosses placenta; is 45% to 68% protein-bound.
Metabolism: Between 16% and 30% of I.M. dose metabolized to inactive compounds.
Excretion: Excreted primarily in urine by tubular secretion; 20% to 60% of dose recovered in 6 hours. Some drug appears in breast milk. Elimination half-life in adults is about ½ to 1 hour. Severe renal impairment prolongs half-life; penicillin G is removed by hemodialysis and is only minimally removed by peritoneal dialysis.

Route	Onset	Peak	Duration
I.M., I.V.	Varies	Varies	Varies

Contraindications and precautions
Contraindicated in patients hypersensitive to drug or other penicillins. Use cautiously in patients with drug allergies (especially to cephalosporins or imipenem). Penicillin G potassium is contraindicated in patients with renal failure.

Interactions
Drug-drug. *Aminoglycosides:* Synergistic therapeutic effects, chiefly against enterococci; this combination is most effective in enterococcal bacterial endocarditis. However, drugs are physically and chemically incompatible; inactivated when mixed or given together. Administer separately.
Clavulanate: Enhanced effect of penicillin G against certain beta–lactamase-producing bacteria. Clavulanate may be used for this purpose.
Heparin, oral anticoagulants: Increased risk of bleeding. Monitor PTT, PT, and INR.
Methotrexate: Large doses of penicillin may interfere with renal tubular secretion of methotrexate; delayed elimination and elevated serum levels of methotrexate. Monitor patient for toxicity.
NSAIDs, sulfinpyrazone: Prolonged penicillin half-life. Monitor patient for effectiveness.
Oral contraceptives: Decreased effectiveness. Suggest using alternative forms of contraception.
Potassium-sparing diuretics: Possible hyperkalemia when used with parenteral penicillin G potassium. Monitor serum potassium.
Probenecid: Blocked tubular secretion of penicillin, raising its serum levels. Probenecid may be used for this purpose.

Adverse reactions
CNS: neuropathy, *seizures,* lethargy, hallucinations, anxiety, confusion, agitation, depression, dizziness, fatigue.

Reactions may be *common,* uncommon, *life-threatening,* or COMMON AND LIFE-THREATENING.

CV: thrombophlebitis (with penicillin G potassium only).
GI: nausea, vomiting, enterocolitis, pseudomembranous colitis.
GU: interstitial nephritis, nephropathy.
Hematologic: eosinophilia, hemolytic anemia, *thrombocytopenia, leukopenia*, anemia, *agranulocytosis*.
Metabolic: possible severe potassium poisoning with high doses (hyperreflexia, *seizures, coma*).
Other: hypersensitivity reactions (maculopapular and *exfoliative dermatitis*, chills, fever, edema, *anaphylaxis*); pain and sterile abscess at injection site; overgrowth of nonsusceptible organisms (with penicillin G potassium and procaine).

Overdose and treatment

Signs and symptoms of overdose include neuromuscular irritability and seizures. Drug can be removed by hemodialysis.

Special considerations

⚡ **ALERT** Don't confuse the various types of penicillin, polycillin, and penicillamine.
● Keep emergency equipment on hand to manage possible anaphylaxis.
● Because penicillins are dialyzable, patients undergoing hemodialysis may need dosage adjustments.
● Administer by deep I.M. injection in upper outer quadrant of buttock. In infants and small children, use midlateral aspect of thigh.
⚡ **ALERT** Never give penicillin G benzathine or penicillin G procaine by I.V. route. Inadvertent I.V. administration has caused cardiac arrest and death.
● Drug can be given as a continuous infusion for meningitis.
● Penicillin G alters test results for urine and serum protein levels and interferes with turbidimetric methods using sulfosalicylic acid, trichloracetic acid, acetic acid, and nitric acid. It doesn't interfere with tests using bromophenol blue (Albustix, Albutest, Multistix), but alters urine glucose testing using cupric sulfate (Benedict's reagent); use Diastix, Chemstrip uG, or glucose enzymatic test strip instead. Penicillin G may cause falsely elevated results of urine specific gravity tests in patients with low urine output and dehydration, and falsely elevated Norymberski and Zimmermann test results for 17-ketogenic steroids; causes false-positive CSF protein test results (Folin-Ciocalteau method) and may cause positive Coombs' test results.
● Penicillin G may falsely decrease serum aminoglycoside levels. Adding beta-lactamase to sample inactivates penicillin, rendering assay more accurate. Or sample can be spun down and frozen immediately after collection.

Patient monitoring

● Monitor patient closely for possible hypernatremia (with sodium) or hyperkalemia (with potassium).
● Patients with poor renal function are predisposed to high blood levels, which may cause seizures. Monitor renal function.

Breast-feeding patients

● Drug appears in breast milk; use in breast-feeding women may sensitize infant to penicillin.

Geriatric patients

● Half-life is prolonged in elderly patients because of impaired renal function.

Patient education

● Tell patient that drug must be injected deep into a large muscle mass.
● Instruct patient to report allergic symptoms and any adverse reactions.

---

penicillin V potassium

Betapen-VK, Ledercillin VK, Nadopen-V*, Pen Vee K, PVF K*, V-Cillin K, Veetids

Pharmacologic classification: natural penicillin
Therapeutic classification: antibiotic
Pregnancy risk category: B

Indications and dosages

➤ *Mild to moderate susceptible infections. Adults and children ages 12 and over:* 125 to 500 mg (200,000 to 800,000 units) P.O. q 6 hours.
Children ages 1 month to 12 years: 15 to 62.5 mg/kg P.O. daily, divided into doses given q 6 to 8 hours.
➤ *Necrotizing ulcerative gingivitis. Adults:* 250 to 500 mg P.O. q 6 to 8 hours.
➤ *Lyme disease ◇. Adults:* 250 to 500 mg P.O. q.i.d. for 10 to 20 days.
➤ *Prophylaxis for pneumococcal infection ◇. Adults:* 250 mg P.O. b.i.d.
Children over age 5: 125 mg P.O. b.i.d.

How supplied

Available by prescription only
Solution: 125 mg/5 ml, 250 mg/5 ml (after reconstitution)
Tablets: 250 mg, 500 mg
Tablets (film-coated): 250 mg, 500 mg

Pharmacodynamics

Antibiotic action: Bactericidal. Adheres to penicillin-binding proteins, thus inhibiting bacterial cell wall synthesis. Spectrum of activity includes most non–penicillinase-producing strains of gram-positive and gram-negative aerobic cocci, spirochetes, and some gram-positive aerobic and anaerobic bacilli.

Pharmacokinetics

Absorption: Penicillin V has greater acid stability and is absorbed more completely than penicillin G after oral administration. About 60% to 75% of oral dose of penicillin V absorbed. Serum levels peak at 60 minutes in fasting subjects; food has no significant effect.

Distribution: Distributed widely into synovial, pleural, pericardial, and ascitic fluids and into bile, liver, skin, lungs, kidneys, muscle, intestines, tonsils, maxillary sinuses, saliva, and erythrocytes. CSF penetration is poor but enhanced in patients with inflamed meninges. Penicillin V crosses placenta and is 75% to 89% protein-bound.

Metabolism: Between 35% and 70% is metabolized to inactive compounds.

Excretion: Excreted primarily in urine by tubular secretion; 26% to 65% of dose recovered in 6 hours. Some drug appears in breast milk. Elimination half-life in adults is ½ hour; severe renal impairment prolongs half-life.

Route	Onset	Peak	Duration
P.O.	Unknown	½-1 hr	Unknown

Contraindications and precautions

Contraindicated in patients hypersensitive to drug or other penicillins. Use cautiously in patients with drug allergies (especially to cephalosporins or imipenem).

Interactions

Drug-drug. *Aminoglycosides:* Synergistic therapeutic effects, chiefly against enterococci. However, drugs are physically and chemically incompatible; inactivated when given together. Don't administer together.

Anticoagulants, heparin: Increased risk of bleeding. Monitor PTT, PT, and INR.

Oral contraceptives that contain estrogen: Decreased efficacy; possible breakthrough bleeding. Suggest alternative method of contraception.

Probenecid: Blocked tubular secretion of penicillin; higher serum levels of drug. Probenecid may be used for this purpose.

Sulfinpyrazone: Prolonged penicillin V half-life. Watch for clinical effectiveness.

Adverse reactions

CNS: neuropathy.

GI: *epigastric distress,* vomiting, diarrhea, *nausea,* black "hairy" tongue.

GU: nephropathy.

Hematologic: eosinophilia, hemolytic anemia, *leukopenia, thrombocytopenia.*

Other: hypersensitivity reactions (rash, urticaria, fever, laryngeal edema, *anaphylaxis*), overgrowth of nonsusceptible organisms.

Overdose and treatment

Signs and symptoms of overdose include neuromuscular sensitivity and seizures. No specific recommendations are available. Treatment is supportive. After recent ingestion (within 4 hours), empty stomach by induced emesis or gastric lavage; follow with activated charcoal to reduce absorption.

Special considerations

⚠ **ALERT** Don't confuse the various types of penicillin, polycillin, and penicillamine.

● Give oral dose 1 hour before or 2 hours after meals for maximum absorption.

● After reconstitution, oral solution is stable for 14 days if refrigerated.

● Penicillin V alters test results for urine and serum protein levels and interferes with turbidimetric methods using sulfosalicylic acid, trichloracetic acid, acetic acid, and nitric acid. Penicillin V doesn't interfere with tests using bromophenol blue (Albustix, Albutest, Multistix) and may falsely decrease serum aminoglycoside levels.

Patient monitoring

● Monitor patient for overgrowth of nonsusceptible organisms.

● Monitor therapeutic effect.

Breast-feeding patients

● Drug appears in breast milk; use in breast-feeding women may sensitize infant to penicillins.

Geriatric patients

● Half-life may be prolonged in elderly patients because of impaired renal function.

Patient education

● Tell patient to take drug on an empty stomach for maximum absorption.

● Instruct patient to swallow drug only with water because acid in fruit juices and carbonated beverages impairs absorption.

---

pentamidine isethionate
NebuPent, Pentacarinat, Pentam 300

Pharmacologic classification: diamidine derivative
Therapeutic classification: antiprotozoal
Pregnancy risk category: C

Indications and dosages

➤ *Pneumonia caused by* **Pneumocystis carinii.** *Adults and children:* 4 mg/kg I.V. or I.M. once daily for 14 to 21 days. As alternative dose in children, 150 mg/m² daily for 5 days; then 100 mg/m² for duration of therapy.

➤ *Prophylaxis against* P. carinii *pneumonia (PCP) in persons at high risk for the disease◇. Adults:* 300 mg by inhalation once q 4 weeks. Aerosol form of drug should be given with Respirgard II jet nebulizer.

➤ *Infection with* Trypanosoma gambiense ◇. *Adults:* 3-4 mg/kg I.V. or I.M. once daily or every other day to up to a total of 7 to 10 doses.

Reactions may be *common,* uncommon, *life-threatening,* or COMMON AND LIFE-THREATENING.

➤ **Leishmaniasis** ◊. *Adults:* 2 to 4 mg/kg I.V. or I.M. daily or every other day up to 15 doses.

How supplied
Available by prescription only
Injection: 300-mg vials
Solution for inhalation: 300 mg

Pharmacodynamics
Antiprotozoal action: Mechanism unknown. May inhibit synthesis of RNA, DNA, proteins, or phospholipids. May also interfere with several metabolic processes, particularly certain energy-yielding reactions and reactions involving folic acid. Spectrum of activity includes *P. carinii* and *Trypanosoma* organisms.

Pharmacokinetics
Absorption: Daily I.M. doses (4 mg/kg) produce surprisingly few plasma level fluctuations. Plasma levels usually increase slightly 1 hour after I.M. injection. Little information on pharmacokinetics with I.V. administration. Limited absorption after aerosol administration.
Distribution: Extensively tissue-bound. Poor CNS penetration. Extent of plasma protein-binding unknown.
Metabolism: No information available.
Excretion: Mostly excreted unchanged in urine. Extensive tissue-binding may account for appearance in urine 6 to 8 weeks after therapy ends.

Route	Onset	Peak	Duration
I.V.	Unknown	1 hr	Unknown
I.M., Inhalation	Unknown	½ hr	Unknown

Contraindications and precautions
Contraindicated in patients hypersensitive to drug. Use cautiously in patients with hepatic or renal dysfunction, hypertension, hypotension, hypoglycemia, hypocalcemia, leukopenia, thrombocytopenia, or anemia.

Interactions
Drug-drug. *Aminoglycosides, amphotericin B, capreomycin, cisplatin, colistin, methoxyflurane, polymyxin B, vancomycin:* Additive nephrotoxic effects. Use together cautiously.

Adverse reactions
CNS: confusion, hallucinations, *fatigue, dizziness,* headache.
CV: *hypotension, ventricular tachycardia,* chest pain, edema.
EENT: pharyngitis.
GI: nausea, metallic taste, decreased appetite, vomiting, diarrhea, abdominal pain, anorexia, bad taste in mouth.
GU: *elevated serum creatinine level, acute renal failure.*
Hematologic: *leukopenia, thrombocytopenia,* anemia.
Hepatic: elevated liver function test results.

Metabolic: hyperkalemia, hypocalcemia, *hypoglycemia,* hyperglycemia.
Musculoskeletal: myalgia.
Respiratory: *congestion, cough, bronchospasm, shortness of breath,* pneumothorax.
Skin: *rash, Stevens-Johnson syndrome.*
Other: *night sweats, chills, sterile abscess, pain or induration at injection site.*

Overdose and treatment
No information available.

Special considerations
● Make sure patient is adequately hydrated before giving drug; dehydration may lead to hypotension and renal toxicity.
● I.V. infusion avoids risk of local reactions and is as safe as I.M. injection when given slowly, over at least 60 minutes. To prepare drug for I.V. infusion, add 3 to 5 ml of sterile water for injection or D_5W to 300-mg vial to yield 100 mg/ml or 60 mg/ml, respectively. Withdraw desired dose and dilute further into 50 to 250 ml of D_5W; infuse over at least 60 minutes. Diluted solution remains stable for 48 hours.
● To prepare drug for I.M. injection, add 3 ml of sterile water for injection to 300-mg vial to yield 100 mg/ml. Withdraw desired dose and inject deep I.M.
● Keep emergency drugs and equipment (including emergency airway, vasopressors, and I.V. fluids) on hand.
● When inhalation solution is used for prophylaxis against PCP, high-risk individuals include persons infected with HIV with a history of PCP; patients who have never had an episode of PCP but whose CD4+ T cells are below 20% of total lymphocytes, or whose CD4+ T-cell count is below 200/mm².
● To administer by inhalation, dilute dose in 6 ml of sterile water and deliver at 6 L/minute from a 50-p.s.i. compressed air source until reservoir is dry. Alternative delivery systems (other than the Respirgard II) are under investigation but currently aren't recommended.
● Patients who develop wheezing or cough during pentamidine aerosol therapy may benefit by pretreatment (at least 5 minutes before pentamidine administration) with a bronchodilator.

Patient monitoring
● To minimize risk of hypotension, patient should be supine during I.V. administration. Because sudden, severe hypotension may develop after I.M. injection or during I.V. infusion, closely monitor blood pressure during infusion and several times thereafter until patient is stable.
● Monitor daily blood glucose, BUN, and serum creatinine levels.
● Periodically monitor electrolyte levels, CBC, platelet count, and liver function tests.
● Observe patient for signs and symptoms of hypoglycemia.

Patient education
● Instruct patient to use aerosol device until chamber is empty, which may take up to 45 minutes.
● Warn patient that I.M. injection is painful.
● Instruct patient to complete full course of therapy, even if feeling better.

---

pentazocine hydrochloride
Talwin*, Talwin Nx (with naloxone hydrochloride)

pentazocine lactate
Talwin

Pharmacologic classification: narcotic agonist-antagonist, opioid partial agonist
Therapeutic classification: analgesic, adjunct to anesthesia
Controlled substance schedule: IV
Pregnancy risk category: NR (C for Talwin-Nx)

Indications and dosages
➤*Moderate to severe pain. Adults:* 50 to 100 mg P.O. q 3 to 4 hours, p.r.n., or around the clock. Maximum oral dose is 600 mg daily. Or 30 mg I.M., I.V., or S.C. q 3 to 4 hours, p.r.n., or around the clock. Maximum parenteral dose is 360 mg daily. Doses above 30 mg I.V. or 60 mg I.M. or S.C. not recommended.

For patients in labor, give 30 mg I.M. or 20 mg I.V. in 2- to 3-hour intervals.

How supplied
Available by prescription only
Injection: 30 mg/ml
Tablets: 50 mg

Pharmacodynamics
Analgesic action: Exact mechanism unknown. Believed to be a competitive antagonist at some receptors and an agonist at others, resulting in relief of moderate pain.

Can produce respiratory depression, sedation, miosis, and antitussive effects. Also may cause psychotomimetic and dysphoric effects. In patients with coronary artery disease, drug elevates mean aortic pressure, left ventricular end-diastolic pressure, and mean pulmonary artery pressure. In patients with acute MI, I.V. drug increases systemic and pulmonary arterial pressures and systemic vascular resistance.

Pharmacokinetics
Absorption: Well absorbed after oral or parenteral administration. However, orally administered drug undergoes first-pass metabolism in liver; less than 20% of dose reaches systemic circulation unchanged. Increased bioavailability in patients with hepatic dysfunction; patients with cirrhosis absorb 60% to 70% of drug. Onset of analgesia in 15 to 30 minutes; peak effect at 15 to 60 minutes.

Distribution: Widely distributed in body.
Metabolism: Metabolized in liver, mainly by oxidation and secondarily by glucuronidation. Metabolism may be prolonged in patients with impaired hepatic function.
Excretion: Duration of effect is 3 hours. Considerable variability among patients in its urinary excretion. Small amounts excreted in feces after oral or parenteral administration.

Route	Onset	Peak	Duration
P.O.	15-30 min	1-3 hr	2-3 hr
I.V.	2-3 min	15-30 min	2-3 hr
I.M., S.C.	10-20 min	30-60 min	2-3 hr

Contraindications and precautions
Contraindicated in patients hypersensitive to drug or its components and in children under age 12. Use cautiously in patients with impaired renal or hepatic function, acute MI, head injury, increased intracranial pressure, or respiratory depression.

Interactions
Drug-drug. *Barbiturates (such as thiopental):* If administered within a few hours of these drugs, pentazocine may produce additive CNS and respiratory depressant effects; possible apnea. Separate administration times if used together.
Cimetidine: Increased pentazocine toxicity; disorientation, respiratory depression, apnea, and seizures. Monitor patient; be prepared to give naloxone if toxicity occurs.
CNS depressants (antihistamines, barbiturates, benzodiazepines, muscle relaxants, narcotic analgesics, phenothiazines, sedative-hypnotics, tricyclic antidepressants): Potentiated respiratory and CNS depression, sedation, and hypotensive effects. Reduced doses of pentazocine usually are needed.
Drugs extensively metabolized in liver (digitoxin, phenytoin, rifampin): Drug accumulation and enhanced effects. Monitor patient for toxicity.
General anesthetics: Possibly severe CV depression. Avoid concomitant use.
Narcotic agonist-antagonist, single dose of an antagonist: Patients who become physically dependent on pentazocine may experience acute withdrawal syndrome. Use cautiously; monitor patient closely.
Drug-lifestyle. *Alcohol use:* Potentiated respiratory and CNS depression, sedation, and hypotensive effects. Discourage concurrent use.

Adverse reactions
CNS: *sedation,* visual disturbances, hallucinations, drowsiness, *dizziness, light-headedness,* confusion, *euphoria,* headache, syncope, psychotomimetic effects.
CV: circulatory depression, *shock,* hypertension, hypotension.
EENT: blurred vision, nystagmus.

Reactions may be *common,* uncommon, *life-threatening,* or COMMON AND LIFE-THREATENING.

GI: dry mouth, *nausea, vomiting,* constipation, taste alteration.
GU: urine retention.
Hematologic: WBC depression.
Respiratory: *respiratory depression,* dyspnea, *apnea.*
Skin: induration, nodules, sloughing, and sclerosis of injection site; diaphoresis; pruritus.
Other: hypersensitivity reactions (*anaphylaxis*), physical and psychological dependence.

Overdose and treatment
The signs and symptoms of overdose haven't been defined because of lack of clinical experience with overdose.

If overdose occurs, use supportive measures (including oxygen, I.V. fluids, vasopressors) as necessary. Consider mechanical ventilation. Parenteral naloxone is an effective antagonist for respiratory depression because of pentazocine.

Special considerations
• Tablets aren't well absorbed.
• Don't mix in same syringe with soluble barbiturates.
• Pentazocine may obscure signs and symptoms of an acute abdominal condition or worsen gallbladder pain.
• Drug possesses narcotic antagonist properties. May precipitate abstinence syndrome in narcotic-dependent patients.
• Talwin-Nx, the available oral pentazocine, contains the narcotic antagonist naloxone, which prevents illicit I.V. use.
• Use S.C. route only when necessary. Severe tissue damage is possible at injection site.

Patient monitoring
• Drug may cause orthostatic hypotension in ambulatory patients. Have patient sit down to relieve symptoms.
• Monitor blood pressure as needed.

Breast-feeding patients
• It isn't known if drug appears in breast milk; use cautiously in breast-feeding women.

Pediatric patients
• Drug isn't recommended for children under age 12.

Geriatric patients
• Lower doses are usually indicated for elderly patients, who may be more sensitive to therapeutic and adverse effects of drug.

Patient education
• Tell patient to report rash, confusion, disorientation, or other serious adverse effects.
• Warn patient that Talwin-Nx is for oral use only. Severe reactions may result if tablets are crushed, dissolved, and injected.
• Tell patient to avoid use of alcohol and other CNS depressants.

pentobarbital sodium
Nembutal

Pharmacologic classification: barbiturate
Therapeutic classification: anticonvulsant, sedative-hypnotic
Controlled substance schedule: II (suppositories, schedule III)
Pregnancy risk category: D

Indications and dosages
➤ *Sedation.* *Adults:* 20 to 40 mg P.O. b.i.d., t.i.d., or q.i.d.
Children: 2 to 6 mg/kg P.O. daily in divided doses, to maximum of 100 mg/dose.
➤ *Insomnia.* *Adults:* 100 mg P.O. h.s. or 150 to 200 mg deep I.M.; 120 to 200 mg P.R.
Children: 2 to 6 mg/kg I.M., up to maximum of 100 mg/dose. Or 30 mg P.R. (ages 2 months to 1 year), 30 to 60 mg P.R. (ages 1 to 4), 60 mg P.R. (ages 5 to 12), 60 to 120 mg P.R. (ages 12 to 14).
➤ *Preanesthetic action.* *Adults:* 150 to 200 mg I.M. or P.O. in two divided doses.
➤ *Anticonvulsant action.* *Adults:* Initially, 100 mg I.V.; after 1 minute additional doses may be given. Maximum dose is 500 mg.
Children: 50 mg initially; after 1 minute additional small doses may be given until desired effect is obtained.

How supplied
Available by prescription only
Capsules: 50 mg, 100 mg
Elixir: 18.2 mg/5 ml
Injection: 50 mg/ml, 1-ml and 2-ml disposable syringes; 2-ml, 20-ml, and 50-ml vials
Suppositories: 30 mg, 60 mg, 120 mg, 200 mg

Pharmacodynamics
Sedative-hypnotic action: Exact cellular site and mechanism of action unknown. Acts throughout the CNS as a nonselective depressant with a fast onset of action and short duration of action. Particularly sensitive to this drug is the reticular activating system, which controls CNS arousal. Pentobarbital decreases both presynaptic and postsynaptic membrane excitability by facilitating the action of gamma-aminobutyric acid (GABA).
Anticonvulsant action: Suppresses spread of seizure activity produced by epileptogenic foci in the cortex, thalamus, and limbic systems by enhancing the effect of GABA. Both presynaptic and postsynaptic excitability are decreased, and the seizure threshold is raised.

Pharmacokinetics
Absorption: Absorbed rapidly after oral or rectal administration; onset of action in 10 to 15 minutes. Serum levels peak 30 to 60 minutes after oral use. After I.M. injection, onset of action is within 10 to 15 minutes. After I.V. administra-

◊ Unlabeled clinical use

tion, onset of action is immediate. Serum levels needed for sedation and hypnosis are 1 to 5 mcg/ml and 5 to 15 mcg/ml, respectively. After oral or rectal administration, duration of hypnosis is 1 to 4 hours.

Distribution: Distributed widely throughout body. About 35% to 45% protein-bound. Accumulates in fat with long-term use.

Metabolism: Metabolized in liver.

Excretion: 99% eliminated as glucuronide conjugates and other metabolites in urine. Terminal half-life ranges from 35 to 50 hours; duration of action 3 to 4 hours.

Route	Onset	Peak	Duration
P.O.	20 min	½-1 hr	1-4 hr
I.V.	Immediate	Immediate	15 min
I.M.	10-25 min	Unknown	Unknown
P.R.	20 min	Unknown	1-4 hr

Contraindications and precautions

Contraindicated in patients hypersensitive to barbiturates and in those with porphyria or severe respiratory disease when dyspnea or obstruction is evident. Use cautiously in elderly or debilitated patients and in those with acute or chronic pain, mental depression, suicidal tendencies, history of drug abuse, or impaired hepatic function.

Interactions

Drug-drug. *Antidepressants, antihistamines, narcotics, sedative-hypnotics, tranquilizers:* Potentiated or added CNS and respiratory depressant effects. Monitor patient closely.

Corticosteroids, digitoxin, doxycycline, oral contraceptives (and other estrogens), theophylline (and other xanthines): Enhanced hepatic metabolism. Monitor patient for clinical effectiveness.

Disulfiram, MAO inhibitors, valproic acid: Decreased metabolism of pentobarbital. Monitor patient for toxicity.

Griseofulvin: Impaired effectiveness of this drug; decreased absorption from GI tract. Separate administration times.

Rifampin: Decreased pentobarbital levels; increases hepatic metabolism. Adjust dosage as needed.

Warfarin, other oral anticoagulants: Enhanced enzymatic degradation of these drugs. Increased doses of anticoagulants may be needed.

Drug-lifestyle. *Alcohol use:* Potentiated or added CNS and respiratory depressant effects. Discourage use.

Adverse reactions

CNS: *drowsiness, lethargy, hangover,* paradoxical excitement in elderly patients, somnolence, syncope, hallucinations, change in EEG patterns.

CV: *bradycardia,* hypotension.

GI: nausea, vomiting.

Hematologic: exacerbation of porphyria.

Respiratory: *respiratory depression.*

Skin: rash, urticaria, STEVENS-JOHNSON SYNDROME.

Other: *angioedema,* physical and psychological dependence.

Overdose and treatment

Toxicity may cause unsteady gait, slurred speech, sustained nystagmus, somnolence, confusion, respiratory depression, pulmonary edema, areflexia, and coma. Typical shock syndrome with tachycardia and hypotension may occur. Jaundice, hypothermia, then fever and oliguria also may occur. Serum levels greater than 10 mcg/ml may produce profound coma; levels greater than 30 mcg/ml may be fatal.

To treat, maintain and suport ventilation and pulmonary function as necessary; support cardiac function and circulation with vasopressors and I.V. fluids, as needed. If patient is conscious and gag reflex is intact, induce emesis (if ingestion was recent) by administering ipecac syrup. If emesis is contraindicated, perform gastric lavage while a cuffed endotracheal tube is in place to prevent aspiration. Follow with administration of activated charcoal or soduim chloride cathartic. Measure intake or output, vital sighs, and laboratory parameters. Maintain body temperature.

Alkalinization of urine may be helpful in removing drug from body. Hemodialysis may be useful in severe overdose.

Special considerations

● Reserve I.V. injection for emergency treatment. Be prepared for emergency resuscitative measures.

● Avoid I.V. administration at a rate exceeding 50 mg/minute to prevent hypotension and respiratory depression.

● High-dose therapy for elevated intracranial pressure may require mechanically assisted ventilation.

● Administer I.M. dose deep into large muscle mass. Don't administer more than 5 ml into any one site.

● Discard solution that is discolored or contains precipitate.

● Administration of full loading doses over short periods of time to treat status epilepticus will require ventilatory support in adults.

● To assure accuracy of dosage, don't divide suppositories.

● Drug has no analgesic effect and may cause restlessness or delirium in patients with pain.

● Nembutal tablets contain tartrazine dye, which may cause allergic reactions in susceptible persons.

● To prevent rebound of rapid-eye-movement sleep after prolonged therapy, discontinue gradually over 5 to 6 days.

● Pentobarbital may cause a false-positive phentolamine test. Drug's physiologic effects may impair the absorption of cyanocobalamin Co 57; it may decrease serum bilirubin levels in neonates, epileptic patients, and patients with congenital nonhemolytic unconjugated hyperbilirubinemia.

Reactions may be *common,* uncommon, *life-threatening,* or COMMON AND LIFE-THREATENING.

Patient monitoring
• Monitor vital signs, especially respirations.
• Monitor patient for changes in neurologic status.

Breast-feeding patients
• Drug appears in breast milk. Don't administer to breast-feeding women.

Pediatric patients
• Barbiturates may cause paradoxical excitement in children. Use cautiously.

Geriatric patients
• Elderly patients usually need lower doses because of increased susceptibility to CNS depressant effects of pentobarbital. Confusion, disorientation, and excitability may occur in elderly patients. Use cautiously.

Patient education
• Advise pregnant patient of potential hazard to fetus or neonate when taking drug late in pregnancy. Withdrawal symptoms can occur.
• Tell patient not to take drug continuously for longer than 2 weeks.
• Emphasize the dangers of combining drug with alcohol. An excessive depressant effect is possible even if drug is taken the evening before ingestion of alcohol.

pentoxifylline
Trental

Pharmacologic classification: xanthine derivative
Therapeutic classification: hemorrheologic agent
Pregnancy risk category: C

Indications and dosages
➤ **Intermittent claudication from chronic occlusive vascular disease.** *Adults:* 400 mg P.O. t.i.d. with meals.

How supplied
Available by prescription only
Tablets (extended-release): 400 mg

Pharmacodynamics
Hemorrheologic action: Improves capillary blood flow by increasing erythrocyte flexibility and reducing blood viscosity.

Pharmacokinetics
Absorption: Absorbed almost completely from GI tract but undergoes first-pass hepatic metabolism. Absorption slowed by food. Levels peak in 2 to 4 hours; clinical effect requires 2 to 4 weeks of continued therapy.
Distribution: No information available; bound to erythrocyte membrane.
Metabolism: Metabolized extensively by erythrocytes and liver.

Excretion: Metabolites excreted principally in urine; less than 4% of drug excreted in feces. Half-life of unchanged drug is about ½ to ¾ hour; half-life of metabolites is about 1 to 1½ hours.

Route	Onset	Peak	Duration
P.O.	Unknown	1 hr	Unknown

Contraindications and precautions
Contraindicated in patients who are intolerant to pentoxifylline or methylxanthines (such as caffeine, theophylline, and theobromine) and in patients with recent cerebral or retinal hemorrhage. Use cautiously in elderly patients.

Interactions
Drug-drug. *Antihypertensives:* Increased hypotensive response. Monitor blood pressure.
Drugs that inhibit platelet aggregation, oral anticoagulants (such as warfarin): Bleeding abnormalities. Monitor PT and INR.
Theophylline: Increased theophylline levels. Monitor patient closely.

Adverse reactions
CNS: headache, dizziness.
CV: angina, chest pain.
GI: dyspepsia, nausea, vomiting, flatus, bloating.

Overdose and treatment
Signs and symptoms of overdose include flushing, hypotension, seizures, somnolence, loss of consciousness, fever, and agitation. There's no known antidote. Empty stomach by gastric lavage and use activated charcoal; treat symptoms and support respiration and blood pressure.

Special considerations
• If GI and CNS adverse effects occur, decrease dosage to twice daily. If adverse effects persist, stop drug.
• Drug is useful in patients who aren't good candidates for surgery.
• Don't crush or break timed-release tablets; make sure patient swallows them whole.

Patient monitoring
• Monitor blood pressure regularly, especially in patients taking antihypertensives.
• Monitor INR, especially in patients taking anticoagulants such as warfarin.

Breast-feeding patients
• Drug appears in breast milk. An alternative to breast-feeding is recommended during therapy.

Pediatric patients
• Safety and efficacy haven't been established for patients under age 18.

Geriatric patients
• Elderly patients may have increased bioavailability and decreased excretion of drug and, thus,

are at higher risk for toxicity; adverse reactions may be more common in elderly patients.

Patient education
• Explain need for continuing therapy for at least 8 weeks; warn patient not to stop drug during this period without approval.
• Advise taking drug with meals to minimize GI distress.
• Tell patient to report GI or CNS adverse reactions; dosage reduction may be needed.

pergolide mesylate
Permax

Pharmacologic classification: dopaminergic agonist
Therapeutic classification: antiparkinsonian
Pregnancy risk category: B

Indications and dosages
➤ *Adjunct to levodopa-carbidopa in the management of Parkinson's disease.*
Adults: Initially, 0.05 mg P.O. daily for first 2 days. Gradually increase dosage by 0.1 to 0.15 mg q third day over next 12 days of therapy. Subsequent dosage can be increased by 0.25 mg q third day until optimum response occurs. Mean therapeutic daily dose is 3 mg.
   Drug is usually administered in divided doses t.i.d. Gradual reductions in levodopa-carbidopa dosage may be made during dosage adjustment.

How supplied
Available by prescription only
Tablets: 0.05 mg, 0.25 mg, 1 mg

Pharmacodynamics
Antiparkinsonian action: Stimulates dopamine receptors at both D_1 and D_2 sites. Acts by directly stimulating postsynaptic receptors in the nigrostriatal system.

Pharmacokinetics
Absorption: Well absorbed after oral administration. Half-life is about 24 hours.
Distribution: About 90% bound to plasma proteins.
Metabolism: Metabolized to at least 10 different compounds; some retain some pharmacologic activity.
Excretion: Excreted primarily by kidneys.

Route	Onset	Peak	Duration
P.O.	Unknown	Unknown	Unknown

Contraindications and precautions
Contraindicated in patients hypersensitive to drug or to ergot alkaloids. Use cautiously in patients prone to arrhythmias and underlying psychiatric disorders.

Interactions
Drug-drug. *Dopamine antagonists (such as butyrophenones, metoclopramide, phenothiazines, thioxanthenes):* Antagonized effects of pergolide. Use together cautiously.
Other drugs known to affect protein-binding: Pergolide is extensively protein-bound. Use cautiously if pergolide is administered with these drugs.

Adverse reactions
CNS: headache, asthenia, *dyskinesia, dizziness, hallucinations, dystonia, confusion, somnolence,* insomnia, anxiety, depression, tremor, abnormal dreams, personality disorder, psychosis, abnormal gait, akathisia, extrapyramidal syndrome, incoordination, akinesia, hypertonia, neuralgia, speech disorder, twitching, paresthesia.
CV: *orthostatic hypotension,* vasodilation, palpitations, hypotension, syncope, hypertension, *arrhythmias, MI.*
EENT: *rhinitis,* epistaxis, abnormal vision, diplopia, eye disorder.
GI: dry mouth, taste perversion, abdominal pain, *nausea, constipation,* diarrhea, dyspepsia, anorexia, vomiting.
GU: urinary frequency, urinary tract infection, hematuria.
Hematologic: anemia.
Metabolic: weight gain.
Musculoskeletal: chest, neck, and back pain; arthralgia; bursitis; myalgia.
Respiratory: dyspnea.
Skin: rash, diaphoresis.
Other: flu syndrome; chills; infection; facial, peripheral, or generalized edema.

Overdose and treatment
Toxicity may cause hypotension, vomiting, hallucinations, involuntary movements, palpitations, and arrhythmias. Provide supportive treatment. Monitor cardiac function and protect the patient's airway. Antiarrhythmics and sympathomimetics may be necessary to support CV function. Adverse CNS effects may be treated with dopaminergic antagonists such as phenothiazines. If indicated, gastric lavage or induced emesis may be used to empty the stomach of its contents. Orally administered activated charcoal may be useful in attenuating absorption.

Special considerations
• Adverse effects (primarily hallucinations and confusion) have occurred in some patients taking pergolide.

Patient monitoring
• Monitor blood pressure.
• Monitor patient for adverse effects.

Breast-feeding patients
• It isn't known if drug appears in breast milk. Safety in breast-feeding women hasn't been established.

Reactions may be *common,* uncommon, *life-threatening,* or COMMON AND LIFE-THREATENING.

Pediatric patients
● Safety in children hasn't been established.

Patient education
● Inform patient of potential for adverse effects. Warn patient to avoid activities that could expose him to injury secondary to orthostatic hypotension and syncope.
● Caution patient to rise slowly to avoid orthostatic hypotension, particularly at start of therapy.

perindopril erbumine
Aceon

Pharmacologic classification: angiotensin converting enzyme (ACE) inhibitor
Therapeutic classification: antihypertensive
Pregnancy risk category: C (first trimester), D (second and third trimesters)

Indications and dosages
➤ **Essential hypertension.** *Adults:* Initially, 4 mg P.O. once daily. Increase dosage until blood pressure is controlled or to a maximum of 16 mg/day; usual maintenance dose is 4 to 8 mg once daily; may be given in two divided doses.
Elderly patients: Initially, 4 mg P.O. daily as one dose or in two divided doses. Dosage increases exceeding 8 mg/day should occur only under close medical supervision.
✦ **Dosage adjustment.** For renally impaired patients, initially, 2 mg P.O. daily with a maximum maintenance dose of 8 mg daily. Don't use in patients with creatinine clearance less than 30 ml/minute. For patients taking diuretics: initially, 2 to 4 mg P.O. daily as one dose or in two divided doses with close medical supervision for several hours and until blood pressure has stabilized. Adjust dosage based on patient's blood pressure response.

How supplied
Available by prescription only
Tablets: 2 mg, 4 mg, 8 mg

Pharmacodynamics
Antihypertensive action: A prodrug that is converted by the liver to the active metabolite perindoprilat. Perindoprilat is thought to lower blood pressure through inhibition of ACE activity, thereby preventing the conversion of angiotensin I to angiotensin II, a potent vasoconstrictor. Inhibition of ACE results in decreased vasoconstriction and decreased aldosterone, thus reducing sodium and water retention and lowering blood pressure.

Pharmacokinetics
Absorption: Rapidly absorbed after oral administration; levels peak in about 1 hour. Absolute oral bioavailability around 75%. Plasma level of perindopril and perindoprilat increased about twofold in elderly patients.

Distribution: Perindopril and perindoprilat about 60% and 10% to 20% bound to plasma proteins, respectively. Drug interaction resulting from effects on protein-binding aren't anticipated.
Metabolism: Perindopril extensively metabolized by liver to perindoprilat.
Excretion: About 4% to 12% of dose excreted in urine as unchanged drug. Reduced drug clearance in elderly patients and in those with heart failure or renal insufficiency.

Route	Onset	Peak	Duration
P.O.	Unknown	1 hr	Unknown

Contraindications and precautions
Contraindicated in patients hypersensitive to perindopril or other ACE inhibitors and in those with history of angioedema secondary to ACE inhibitors. Also contraindicated in pregnant women.

Use cautiously in patients with history of angioedema unrelated to ACE inhibitor therapy. Also use cautiously in patients with impaired renal function, heart failure, ischemic heart disease, cerebrovascular disease or renal artery stenosis, and in patients with collagen vascular disease, such as systemic lupus erythematosus or scleroderma.

Interactions
Drug-drug. *Diuretics:* Additive hypotensive effect. Monitor patient closely.
Lithium: Increased serum lithium level; possible symptoms of lithium toxicity. Use of a diuretic may further increase risk of lithium toxicity. Use together cautiously; monitor serum lithium level.
Potassium-sparing diuretics (amiloride, spironolactone, triamterene), potassium supplements, other drugs capable of increasing serum potassium (cyclosporine, heparin, indomethacin): Additive hyperkalemic effect. Use together cautiously; monitor serum potassium level frequently.
Drug-herb. *Capsaicin:* Increased risk of cough. Discourage concomitant use.
Drug-food. *Salt substitutes that contain potassium:* Increased risk of hyperkalemia. Tell patient to use together cautiously.

Adverse reactions
CNS: dizziness, asthenia, sleep disorder, paresthesia, depression, somnolence, nervousness, *headache.*
CV: palpitations, edema, chest pain, abnormal ECG.
EENT: rhinitis, sinusitis, ear infection, pharyngitis, tinnitus.
GI: dyspepsia, diarrhea, abdominal pain, nausea, vomiting, flatulence.
GU: proteinuria, urinary tract infection, male sexual dysfunction, menstrual disorder.
Hepatic: increased ALT level.
Metabolic: increased triglyceride level.

Musculoskeletal: back pain, hypertonia, neck pain, joint pain, myalgia, arthritis, low or upper extremity pain.
Respiratory: *cough,* upper respiratory tract infection.
Skin: rash.
Other: viral infection, fever, injury, seasonal allergy.

Overdose and treatment
Hypotension would be the most likely result of perindopril overdose. Treatment should be symptomatic and supportive. Discontinue perindopril and observe patient closely. Treat dehydration, electrolyte imbalances, and hypotension using established protocols.

Special considerations
● Angioedema involving face, limbs, lips, tongue, glottis, and larynx has been reported in patients treated with perindopril. Stop drug and observe patient until swelling disappears. If swelling is confined to face and lips, it probably will resolve without treatment, but antihistamines may be useful in relieving symptoms. Angioedema involving with tongue, glottis, or larynx may be fatal because of airway obstruction. Appropriate therapy, such as S.C. epinephrine solution, should be promptly administered.
● Patients with history of angioedema unrelated to ACE inhibitor therapy may be at increased risk for angioedema while receiving an ACE inhibitor.
● Excessive hypotension can occur when drug is given with diuretics. If possible, diuretic therapy should be stopped 2 to 3 days before starting perindopril to decrease potential for excessive hypotensive response. If it isn't possible to stop diuretic, consider starting with a lower dose of perindopril or decreasing diuretic dose.
● Hypotension can occur when initiating therapy or adjusting doses in patients who have been volume- or salt-depleted as a result of prolonged diuretic therapy, dietary salt restriction, dialysis, diarrhea, or vomiting. Volume and salt depletion should be corrected before starting drug.
● ACE inhibitors have rarely been linked to a syndrome of cholestatic jaundice, fulminant hepatic necrosis, and death. Stop drug in patients who develop jaundice or marked elevations of hepatic enzyme levels during therapy.

Patient monitoring
● Other ACE inhibitors have been linked to agranulocytosis and neutropenia. Monitor CBC with differential before therapy, especially in renally impaired patients with systemic lupus erythematosus or scleroderma.
● Monitor patients at risk for hypotension closely during start of therapy and for the first 2 weeks of treatment, and whenever perindopril dosage or concomitant diuretic is increased. If severe hypotension occurs, place patient in supine position and treat symptomatically.

● Monitor renal function before and periodically throughout therapy. Drug shouldn't be used in patients with creatinine clearance less than 30 ml/minute.
● Monitor serum potassium levels closely.

Breast-feeding patients
● It isn't known if drug appears in breast milk. Because many drugs do, use cautiously in breast-feeding women.

Pediatric patients
● Safety and effectiveness of drug in children haven't been established.

Geriatric patients
● Plasma levels of perindopril and perindoprilat in patients over age 70 are about twice those observed in younger patients. With the exception of dizziness and possibly rash, adverse effects don't appear to increase in elderly patients. Doses above 8 mg/day should be administered cautiously and under close medical supervision.

Patient education
● Inform patient that angioedema, including laryngeal edema, can occur during therapy, especially with first dose. Advise patient to stop taking drug and immediately report any signs or symptoms of angioedema (swelling of face, limbs, eyes, lips, or tongue; hoarseness; or difficulty in swallowing or breathing).
● Advise patient to report promptly any sign of infection (such as sore throat, fever) or jaundice (yellowing of eyes or skin).
● Advise patient to avoid salt substitutes containing potassium unless instructed otherwise.
● Caution patient that light-headedness may occur, especially during first few days of therapy. Advise patient to report light-headedness and, if fainting occurs, to stop drug and call promptly.
● Caution patient that inadequate fluid intake or excessive perspiration, diarrhea, or vomiting can lead to an excessive drop in blood pressure.
● Advise woman of childbearing age of consequences of second and third trimester exposure to drug. Advise her to call immediately if pregnancy is suspected.

permethrin
Acticin, Elimite, Nix

Pharmacologic classification: synthetic pyrethroid
Therapeutic classification: scabicide, pediculicide
Pregnancy risk category: B

Indications and dosages
➤ *Pediculosis. Adults and children:* Apply sufficient volume to saturate the hair and scalp. Leave on hair for 10 minutes before rinsing.

Reactions may be *common*, uncommon, *life-threatening*, or COMMON AND LIFE-THREATENING.

➤ **Scabies.** *Adults and children:* Thoroughly massage into skin from head to soles of feet. Treat infants on hairline, neck, scalp, temple, and forehead. Remove cream by washing after 8 to 14 hours. One application is curative.

How supplied
Available by prescription only
Acticin, Elimite
Cream: 5%
Available without a prescription
Nix
Cream Rinse: 1%

Pharmacodynamics
Scabicide action: Acts on the parasites' nerve cell membranes to disrupt the sodium channel current, thereby paralyzing parasites.

Pharmacokinetics
Absorption: Not fully investigated; probably less than 2% of amount applied.
Distribution: No information available.
Metabolism: Rapidly metabolized by ester hydrolysis to inactive metabolites.
Excretion: Metabolites excreted in urine. Residue on hair detectable for up to 10 days.

Route	Onset	Peak	Duration
Topical	10-15 min	Unknown	10 days

Contraindications and precautions
Contraindicated in patients hypersensitive to pyrethrins or chrysanthemums.

Interactions
None reported.

Adverse reactions
Skin: pruritus, *burning, stinging,* edema, tingling, numbness or scalp discomfort, mild erythema, scalp rash.

Overdose and treatment
For accidental ingestion, perform gastric lavage and use general supportive measures.

Special considerations
• A single treatment is usually effective. Although combing of nits isn't needed for effectiveness, drug package supplies a fine-tooth comb.
• A second application may be needed if lice are seen 7 days after initial application.
• Permethrin has been shown to be at least as effective as lindane (Kwell) in treating head lice.

Patient monitoring
• Monitor patient for therapeutic effect.

Breast-feeding patients
• It isn't known if drug appears in breast milk. Either discontinue breast-feeding temporarily or stop drug.

Pediatric patients
• Safety and efficacy in children under age 2 haven't been established.

Patient education
• Tell patient or caregiver to wash hair with shampoo, rinse it thoroughly, and then towel dry.
• Tell patient or caregiver to apply sufficient amount to saturate hair and scalp.
• Instruct patient to report itching, redness, or swelling of scalp.
• Advise patient that drug is for external use only and to avoid contact with mucous membranes.

perphenazine
Apo-Perphenazine*, Trilafon

Pharmacologic classification: phenothiazine (piperazine derivative)
Therapeutic classification: antipsychotic, antiemetic
Pregnancy risk category: NR

Indications and dosages
➤ **Psychosis.** *Adults:* Initially, 8 to 16 mg P.O. b.i.d., t.i.d., or q.i.d., increasing to 64 mg daily. Or administer 5 to 10 mg I.M.; change to P.O. as soon as possible.
➤ **Mental disturbances, acute alcoholism, nausea, vomiting, hiccups.** *Adults:* 5 to 10 mg I.M., p.r.n. Maximum dose is 15 mg daily in ambulatory patients; 30 mg daily in hospitalized patients; or 8 to 16 mg P.O. daily in divided doses.

Perphenazine may be given slowly by I.V. drip at 1 mg/2 minutes with continuous blood pressure monitoring (rarely used). A maximum of 5 mg I.V. diluted to 0.5 mg/ml with normal saline solution may be given for severe hiccups or vomiting. Extended-release form may be given 8 to 16 mg P.O. b.i.d. for outpatients; 8 to 32 mg P.O. b.i.d. for inpatients.

How supplied
Available by prescription only
Injection: 5 mg/ml
Oral concentrate: 16 mg/5 ml
Tablets: 2 mg, 4 mg, 8 mg, 16 mg

Pharmacodynamics
Antipsychotic action: Thought to exert antipsychotic effects by postsynaptic blockade of CNS dopamine receptors, thus inhibiting dopamine-mediated effects; antiemetic effects are attributed to dopamine receptor blockade in the medullary chemoreceptor trigger zone. Has many other central and peripheral effects: produces both alpha and ganglionic blockade and counteracts histamine- and serotonin-mediated activity. Most serious adverse reactions are extrapyramidal.

Pharmacokinetics

Absorption: Rate and extent of absorption vary with administration route. Oral tablet absorption erratic and variable, with onset of action ranging from ½ to 1 hour; oral concentrate absorption much more predictable. I.M. drug absorbed rapidly.

Distribution: Distributed widely into body, including breast milk. 91% to 99% protein-bound. After oral tablet administration, peak effect at 2 to 4 hours; steady state serum levels achieved within 4 to 7 days.

Metabolism: Metabolized extensively by liver; no active metabolites formed.

Excretion: Mostly excreted in urine via kidneys; some in feces via biliary tract.

Route	Onset	Peak	Duration
P.O., I.M., I.V.	½- 1 hr	2-4 hr	Unknown

Contraindications and precautions

Contraindicated in patients hypersensitive to drug; in patients experiencing coma; in those with CNS depression, blood dyscrasia, bone marrow depression, liver damage, or subcortical damage; and in those receiving large doses of CNS depressants.

Use cautiously in elderly or debilitated patients; in those with alcohol withdrawal, psychic depression, suicidal tendencies, adverse reaction to other phenothiazines, impaired renal function, or respiratory disorders; and in patients receiving other CNS depressants or anticholinergics.

Interactions

Drug-drug. *Antacids that contain aluminum and magnesium, antidiarrheals:* Inhibited absorption. Separate administration times by at least 2 hours.

Antiarrhythmics, disopyramide, procainamide, quinidine: Increased risk of arrhythmias and conduction defects. Monitor patient closely.

Appetite suppressants, sympathomimetics (such as ephedrine [commonly found in nasal sprays], epinephrine, phenylephrine, phenylpropanolamine): Decreased stimulatory and pressor effects. Monitor patient closely.

Atropine, other anticholinergics (such as antidepressants, antihistamines, antiparkinsonians, MAO inhibitors, meperidine, phenothiazines): Oversedation, paralytic ileus, visual changes, and severe constipation. Monitor patient closely.

Beta blockers: Inhibited perphenazine metabolism; increased plasma levels. Watch for toxicity.

Bromocriptine: Antagonized prolactin secretion. Monitor patient closely.

Centrally acting antihypertensives (such as clonidine, guanabenz, guanadrel, guanethidine, methyldopa, reserpine): Inhibited blood pressure response. Monitor blood pressure.

CNS depressants (such as analgesics; barbiturates; epidural, general, spinal anesthetics; narcotics; tranquilizers), parenteral magnesium sulfate: Oversedation, respiratory depression, and hypotension. Monitor patient closely.

Epinephrine: Phenothiazines can cause epinephrine reversal and hypotensive response when epinephrine is used for pressor effects. Avoid concomitant use.

High-dose dopamine: Decreased vasoconstricting effects. Monitor patient closely.

Levodopa: Decreased effectiveness; increased risk of levodopa toxicity. Use together cautiously.

Lithium: Severe neurologic toxicity with encephalitis-like syndrome; decreased therapeutic response to perphenazine. Avoid using together.

Metrizamide: Increased risk of seizures. Monitor patient closely.

Nitrates: Hypotension. Monitor blood pressure.

Phenobarbital: Enhanced renal excretion of perphenazine. Adjust dosage as needed.

Phenytoin: Inhibited metabolism and increased risk of phenytoin toxicity. Monitor patient closely.

Propylthiouracil: Increased risk of agranulocytosis. Monitor hematologic studies.

Drug-food. *Caffeine:* Decreased therapeutic response to perphenazine. Discourage use.

Drug-lifestyle. *Alcohol use:* Additive effects. Discourage use.

Heavy smoking: Decreased therapeutic response to perphenazine. Discourage smoking.

Sun exposure: Possible photosensitivity reactions. Tell patient to take precautions.

Adverse reactions

CNS: *neuroleptic malignant syndrome, extrapyramidal reactions, tardive dyskinesia,* sedation, pseudoparkinsonism, EEG changes, dizziness, adverse behavioral effects, *seizures,* drowsiness.

CV: *orthostatic hypotension,* tachycardia, ECG changes, *cardiac arrest.*

EENT: ocular changes, *blurred vision,* nasal congestion.

GI: *dry mouth, constipation,* nausea, vomiting, diarrhea, ileus.

GU: *urine retention,* dark urine, menstrual irregularities, inhibited ejaculation.

Hematologic: *leukopenia,* galactorrhea, *agranulocytosis,* eosinophilia, *hemolytic anemia, thrombocytopenia.*

Hepatic: jaundice, abnormal liver function test results.

Metabolic: hyperglycemia, hypoglycemia, weight gain.

Skin: *mild photosensitivity, allergic reactions,* pain at I.M. injection site, sterile abscess.

Other: gynecomastia, SIADH.

Overdose and treatment

CNS depression is characterized by deep, unarousable sleep and possible coma, hypotension or hypertension, extrapyramidal symptoms, dystonia, abnormal involuntary muscle movements, agitation, seizures, arrhythmias, ECG changes, hy-

---

Reactions may be *common*, uncommon, *life-threatening*, or COMMON AND LIFE-THREATENING.

pothermia or hyperthermia, and autonomic nervous system dysfunction.

Treatment is symptomatic and supportive, including maintaining vital signs, airway, stable body temperature, and fluid and electrolyte balance.

Induce vomiting in a conscious patient with ipecac syrup even if spontaneous vomiting has occurred. Don't induce vomiting in patients with impaired consciousness. Use gastric lavage, then activated charcoal and soduim chloride cathartics; dialysis is usually ineffective. Regulate body temperature as needed. Treat hypotension with I.V. fluids. Don't give epinephrine. Treat seizures with parenteral diazepam or barbiturates; arrhythmias with parenteral phenytoin (1 mg/kg with rate titrated to blood pressure); and extrapyramidal reactions with benztropine at 1 to 2 mg or parenteral diphenhydramine at 10 to 50 mg.

Special considerations
• Oral formulations may cause stomach upset; administer with food or fluid.
• Dilute the concentrate in 2 to 4 oz (60 to 120 ml) of liquid (water, caffeine-free carbonated drinks, fruit juice, tomato juice, milk, or puddings). Dilute every 5 ml of concentrate with 60 ml of suitable fluid. Shake oral concentrate before administration.
• Liquid formulation may cause rash upon contact with skin.
• I.M. injection may cause skin necrosis; avoid extravasation.
• Administer I.M. injection deep into upper outer quadrant of buttocks. Massaging injection site may prevent formation of abscesses.
• Don't administer drug for injection if it's excessively discolored or contains precipitate.
• After abrupt withdrawal of long-term therapy, patient may experience gastritis, nausea, vomiting, dizziness, tremor, feeling of warmth or cold, diaphoresis, tachycardia, headache, and insomnia.
• Perphenazine causes false-positive test results for urinary porphyrins, urobilinogen, amylase, and 5-hydroxyindoleacetic acid because of darkening of urine by metabolites; also causes false-positive urine pregnancy test results using human chorionic gonadotropin.

Patient monitoring
• Monitor blood pressure before and after parenteral administration.
• Monitor serum glucose level, CBC, and liver function tests.

Breast-feeding patients
• Drug appears widely in breast milk; use cautiously. Potential benefits to mother should outweigh potential harm to infant.

Pediatric patients
• Drug isn't recommended for children under age 12.

Geriatric patients
• Use lower doses in elderly patients, and adjust to effect; 30% to 50% of the usual dose may be effective. Elderly patients have an increased risk of adverse effects, especially tardive dyskinesia and other extrapyramidal effects.

Patient education
• Explain risks of dystonic reactions and tardive dyskinesia, and tell patient to report abnormal body movements.
• Instruct patient to avoid sun exposure and to wear sunscreen when going outdoors to prevent photosensitivity reactions and to avoid using sun lamps and tanning beds, which may cause burning of the skin or skin discoloration.
• Tell patient to avoid spilling liquid; contact with skin may cause rash and irritation.
• Warn patient not to take extremely hot or cold baths and to avoid exposure to temperature extremes; drug may cause thermoregulatory changes.
• Advise patient to take drug exactly as prescribed and not to double missed doses.
• Inform patient that interactions with many other drugs are possible. Advise patient to seek medical approval before taking herbal or OTC products.
• Instruct patient not to stop taking drug suddenly; any adverse reactions may be alleviated by a dosage reduction. Patient should promptly report difficulty urinating, sore throat, dizziness, or fainting.
• Tell patient to avoid hazardous activities that require alertness until drug's effect is known. Reassure patient that sedative effects of drug should become tolerable within a few weeks.
• Tell patient not to drink alcohol or take other drugs that may cause excessive sedation.
• Explain which fluids are appropriate for diluting the concentrate (not apple juice or drinks containing caffeine); explain dropper technique of measuring dose.
• Recommend sugarless hard candy or chewing gum, ice chips, or artificial saliva to relieve dry mouth.
• Tell patient not to crush or chew sustained-release form.

phenazopyridine hydrochloride
Azo-Standard, Baridium, Geridium, Phenazo*, Prodium, Pyridiate, Pyridium, Urogesic

Pharmacologic classification: azo dye
Therapeutic classification: urinary analgesic
Pregnancy risk category: B

Indications and dosages
➤ **Pain with urinary tract irritation or infection.** *Adults:* 200 mg P.O. t.i.d. Give drug after meals.

◊ Unlabeled clinical use

How supplied
Available by prescription only
Tablets: 100 mg, 200 mg
Available without prescription
Tablets: 95 mg

Pharmacodynamics
Analgesic action: Mechanism unknown. Has a local anesthetic effect on urinary tract mucosa.

Pharmacokinetics
Absorption: No information available.
Distribution: Traces thought to enter CSF and cross placenta.
Metabolism: Metabolized in liver.
Excretion: Excreted by kidneys; 65% excreted unchanged in urine. Totally excreted on average in 20.4 hours.

Route	Onset	Peak	Duration
P.O.	Unknown	Unknown	Unknown

Contraindications and precautions
Contraindicated in patients hypersensitive to drug and in those with glomerulonephritis, severe hepatitis, uremia, pyelonephritis during pregnancy, or renal insufficiency.

Interactions
None reported.

Adverse reactions
CNS: headache.
GI: nausea, GI disturbances.
Hematologic: hemolytic anemia, methemoglobinemia.
Skin: rash, pruritus.
Other: *anaphylactoid reactions.*

Overdose and treatment
Toxicity may cause methemoglobinemia (most obvious as cyanosis), along with renal and hepatic impairment and failure.

To treat overdose, empty stomach immediately by inducing emesis with ipecac syrup or by gastric lavage. Administer methylene blue, 1 to 2 mg/kg I.V., or 100 to 200 mg ascorbic acid P.O. to reverse methemoglobinemia. Provide symptomatic and supportive measures (respiratory support and correction of fluid and electrolyte imbalances). Monitor laboratory parameters and vital signs closely. Contact local or regional poison information center for specific instructions.

Special considerations
• Drug colors urine red or orange; may stain fabrics.
• Use only as an analgesic.
• May be used with an antibiotic to treat urinary tract infections.
• Discontinue drug in 2 days with concurrent antibiotic use.
• Drug may alter results of Diastix, Chemstrip uG, glucose enzymatic test strip, Acetest, and Ketostix.

Clinitest should be used to obtain accurate urine glucose test results. Drug may also interfere with Ehrlich's test for urine urobilinogen; phenolsulfonphthalein excretion tests of kidney function; sulfobromophthalein excretion tests of liver function; and urine tests for protein, corticosteroids, or bilirubin.
• Administer with food or fluids to reduce GI upset.

Patient monitoring
• Monitor patient for decrease in pain caused by urinary tract infection.
• Watch for continued symptoms of urinary tract infection.
• Repeat urinalysis as indicated.
• Evaluate response to therapy; assess urinary function, such as output, complaints of burning, pain, and frequency. Monitor vital signs, especially temperature. Encourage patient to force fluids (if not contraindicated). Monitor intake and output.

Breast-feeding patients
• It isn't known if drug appears in breast milk. Safe use in breast-feeding women hasn't been established.

Geriatric patients
• Use cautiously in elderly patients because of possible decreased renal function.

Patient education
• Instruct patient in measures to prevent urinary tract infection.
• Caution patient that drug colors urine red or orange and may stain clothing.
• Tell patient that stains on clothing may be removed with a 0.25% solution of sodium dithionite or hydrosulfite.
• Advise patient to take missed dose as soon as possible but not to double doses.
• Instruct patient to report symptoms that worsen or don't resolve.

phenelzine sulfate
Nardil

Pharmacologic classification: MAO inhibitor
Therapeutic classification: antidepressant
Pregnancy risk category: C

Indications and dosages
➤ *Severe depression. Adults:* 15 mg P.O. t.i.d. Increase rapidly to 60 mg daily; maximum daily dose is 90 mg. Onset of maximum therapeutic effect is 2 to 6 weeks. Some clinicians reduce dosage after response occurs; maintenance dose may be as low as 15 mg daily or every other day.

How supplied
Available by prescription only
Tablets: 15 mg

Reactions may be *common*, uncommon, *life-threatening*, or COMMON AND LIFE-THREATENING.

Pharmacodynamics

Antidepressant action: Depression is thought to result from low CNS levels of neurotransmitters, including norepinephrine and serotonin. Phenelzine inhibits MAO, an enzyme that normally inactivates amine-containing substances, thus increasing the level and activity of these substances.

Pharmacokinetics

Absorption: Absorbed rapidly and completely from GI tract.
Distribution: No information available.
Metabolism: Metabolized in liver.
Excretion: Excreted primarily in urine within 24 hours; some drug excreted in feces via biliary tract. Relatively short half-life, but enzyme inhibition is prolonged and unrelated to half-life.

Route	Onset	Peak	Duration
P.O.	Unknown	2-4 hr	≤ 10 days

Contraindications and precautions

Contraindicated in patients hypersensitive to drug and in those with heart failure, pheochromocytoma, hypertension, liver disease, or CV disease. Also contraindicated during therapy with other MAO inhibitors (isocarboxazid, tranylcypromine); within 14 days of such therapy or within 14 days of elective surgery requiring general anesthesia; with cocaine use; or with local anesthesia containing sympathomimetic vasoconstrictors. Contraindicated within 2 weeks of selective serotonin reuptake inhibitor antidepressant use. Contraindicated by some manufacturers in patients over age 60 because of possibility of existing cerebrosclerosis with damaged vessels.

Use cautiously in patients at risk for diabetes, suicide, or seizure disorders and in those receiving thiazide diuretics or spinal anesthetics.

Interactions

Drug-drug. *Amphetamines, ephedrine, phenylephrine, other related drugs:* Enhanced pressor effects. Avoid concomitant use.
Barbiturates, dextromethorphan, narcotics, tricyclic antidepressants, other sedatives: Increased adverse reactions. Use cautiously and reduce dosage of phenelzine.
Disulfiram: Possible tachycardia, flushing, or palpitations. Monitor patient closely.
General, spinal anesthetics: Severe hypotension and excessive CNS depression. Avoid concomitant use.
Local anesthetics (lidocaine, procaine): Decreased effectiveness of these drugs; poor nerve block. Stop phenelzine for at least 1 week before giving these drugs.
OTC cold, hay fever, weight-reduction products: Serious CV toxicity. Avoid concomitant use.
Serotonergic drugs (fluoxetine, fluvoxamine, paroxetine, sertraline), tricyclic antidepressants: Serious adverse effects. At least a 2-week waiting period between drug use is recommended.

Drug-herb. *Cacao:* Potentiated vasopressor effects. Discourage use.
Ephedra: Possible severe reactions, including hypertensive crisis. Discourage concurrent use.
Ginseng: Possible adverse reactions, including headache, tremors, mania, insomnia, irritability, visual hallucinations. Discourage use.
Drug-food. *Foods high in caffeine, tryptophan, tyramine:* May precipitate hypertensive crisis. Discourage use.
Drug-lifestyle. *Alcohol use:* Increased adverse reactions. Discourage alcohol use or reduce dosage.

Adverse reactions

CNS: *dizziness,* vertigo, headache, hyperreflexia, tremor, muscle twitching, *insomnia,* drowsiness, weakness, fatigue.
CV: orthostatic hypotension, edema.
GI: dry mouth, *anorexia,* nausea, constipation.
GU: elevated urinary catecholamine levels, sexual disturbances.
Hematologic: elevated WBC count.
Hepatic: elevated liver function test results.
Metabolic: weight gain.
Skin: diaphoresis.

Overdose and treatment

Signs and symptoms of toxicity become apparent slowly (within 24 to 48 hours) and may last for up to 2 weeks. Agitation, flushing, tachycardia, hypotension, hypertension, palpitations, increased motor activity, twitching, increased deep tendon reflexes, seizures, hyperpyrexia, cardiorespiratory arrest, and coma may occur. Doses of 375 mg to 1.5 g have been ingested with fatal and nonfatal results.

Give 5 to 10 mg phentolamine I.V. push for hypertensive crisis; treat seizures, agitation, or tremors with I.V. diazepam; tachycardia with beta blockers; and fever with cooling blankets. Monitor vital signs and fluid and electrolyte balance. Use of sympathomimetics (such as norepinephrine or phenylephrine) is contraindicated in hypotension caused by MAO inhibitors.

Special considerations

● Exercise precautions for use of MAO inhibitors, given alone or with other drugs, for 14 days after stopping drug.
● Consider inherent risk of suicide until significant improvement of depressive state occurs. High-risk patients should have close supervision during initial therapy. To reduce risk of suicidal overdose, prescribe smallest quantity of tablets consistent with good management.
● At start of therapy, patient should lie down for 1 hour after taking phenelzine; to prevent dizziness from orthostatic blood pressure changes, sudden changes to standing position should be avoided.
● Unlike therapy with other MAO inhibitors, therapy with phenelzine and tricyclic antidepressants is generally well tolerated.

Patient monitoring
- Monitor blood pressure closely at start of therapy.
- Monitor patient for adverse effects.

Pediatric patients
- Drug isn't recommended for children under age 16.

Geriatric patients
- Drug isn't recommended for patients over age 60.

Patient education
- Warn patient not to take alcohol, other CNS depressants, or OTC products (such as cold, hay fever, or diet preparations) without medical approval.
- Explain that many foods and beverages (such as wine, beer, cheeses, preserved fruits, meats, and vegetables) may interact with drug. A list of foods to avoid can usually be obtained from the dietary department or pharmacy at most hospitals.
- Tell patient to avoid hazardous activities that require alertness until drug's full CNS effects are known. Suggest taking drug at bedtime to minimize daytime sedation.
- Instruct patient to take drug exactly as prescribed and not to double the dose if one is missed.
- Tell patient not to stop drug abruptly and to report any problems; dosage reduction can relieve most adverse reactions.

phenobarbital
Barbita, Solfoton

phenobarbital sodium
Luminal

Pharmacologic classification: barbiturate
Therapeutic classification: anticonvulsant, sedative-hypnotic
Controlled substance schedule: IV
Pregnancy risk category: D

Indications and dosages
➤ *All forms of epilepsy except absence seizures, febrile seizures in children.*
Adults: 60 to 100 mg P.O. daily, divided t.i.d. or given as single dose h.s. Or, give 200 to 300 mg I.M. or I.V. and repeat q 6 hours, p.r.n.
Children: 1 to 6 mg/kg P.O. daily, usually divided q 12 hours. It can, however, be administered once daily. Or give 4 to 6 mg/kg I.V. or I.M. daily and monitor patient's blood levels.
➤ *Status epilepticus. Adults and children:* 10 to 20 mg/kg I.V. over 10 to 15 minutes (don't exceed 60 mg/min). Repeat if necessary.

➤ *Sedation. Adults:* 30 to 120 mg P.O., I.M., or I.V. daily in two or three divided doses. Maximum dose is 400 mg/24 hours.
Children: 8 to 32 mg P.O. daily.
➤ *Insomnia. Adults:* 100 to 200 mg P.O. or 100 to 320 mg I.M.
➤ *Preoperative sedation. Adults:* 100 to 200 mg I.M. 60 to 90 minutes before surgery.
Children: 1 to 3 mg/kg I.V. or I.M. 60 to 90 minutes before surgery.

How supplied
Available by prescription only
Capsules: 16 mg
Elixir: 15 mg/5 ml; 20 mg/5 ml
Injection: 30 mg/ml, 60 mg/ml, 65 mg/ml, 130 mg/ml
Tablets: 15 mg, 16 mg, 30 mg, 60 mg, 100 mg

Pharmacodynamics
Anticonvulsant action: Exact cellular site and mechanism of action unknown. Suppresses spread of seizure activity produced by epileptogenic foci in the cortex, thalamus, and limbic systems by enhancing the effect of GABA. Both presynaptic and postsynaptic excitability are decreased; also raises the seizure threshold.
Sedative-hypnotic action: Acts throughout the CNS as a nonselective depressant with a slow onset of action and a long duration of action. Particularly sensitive to this drug is the reticular activating system, which controls CNS arousal. Phenobarbital decreases both presynaptic and postsynaptic membrane excitability by facilitating the action of GABA.

Pharmacokinetics
Absorption: Well absorbed after oral administration, with 70% to 90% reaching bloodstream. 100% absorption after I.M. administration. After oral administration, serum levels peak in 1 to 2 hours; levels in CNS peak at 1 to 3 hours. Onset of action occurs 20 to 60 minutes or longer after oral dosing; onset after I.V. administration is about 5 minutes. Serum level of 10 mcg/ml needed to produce sedation; 40 mcg/ml usually produces sleep. Levels of 20 to 40 mcg/ml considered therapeutic for anticonvulsant therapy.
Distribution: Distributed widely throughout body. About 25% to 30% protein-bound.
Metabolism: Metabolized by hepatic microsomal enzyme system.
Excretion: 25% to 50% of dose eliminated unchanged in urine; remainder excreted as metabolites of glucuronic acid. Drug's half-life is 5 to 7 days.

Route	Onset	Peak	Duration
P.O.	1 hr	8-12	10-12 hr
I.V.	5 min	½ hr	4-10 hr
I.M.	> 5 min	> ½ hr	4-10 hr

Reactions may be *common*, uncommon, *life-threatening*, or COMMON AND LIFE-THREATENING.

Contraindications and precautions

Contraindicated in patients with barbiturate hypersensitivity or history of manifest or latent porphyria, hepatic dysfunction, respiratory disease with dyspnea or obstruction, or nephritis.

Use cautiously in elderly or debilitated patients and in those with acute or chronic pain, depression, suicidal tendencies, history of drug abuse, blood pressure alterations, CV disease, shock, or uremia.

Interactions

Drug-drug. *Antidepressants, antihistamines, narcotics, phenothiazines, tranquilizers, other sedative-hypnotics:* Potentiated CNS and respiratory depressant effects. Monitor patient closely.

Corticosteroids, digitoxin, doxycycline, oral contraceptives (and other estrogens), theophylline (and other xanthines): Enhanced hepatic metabolism of these drugs. Monitor patient for clinical effectiveness; adjust dosage as needed.

Disulfiram, MAO inhibitors, valproic acid: Decreased metabolism of phenobarbital and increased toxicity. Monitor serum levels.

Griseofulvin. Decreased absorption from GI tract. Separate administration times by at least 2 hours.

Rifampin: Decreased phenobarbital levels due to increased hepatic metabolism. Monitor serum levels; adjust dosage as needed.

Warfarin, other oral anticoagulants: Enhanced enzymatic degradation of these drugs. Increased dosages of anticoagulant may be needed.

Drug-herb. *Evening primrose oil:* Possible increase in anticonvulsant requirement. Discourage concurrent use.

Drug-lifestyle. *Alcohol use:* Potentiated CNS and respiratory depressant effects. Discourage use.

Adverse reactions

CNS: *drowsiness, lethargy, hangover,* paradoxical excitement in elderly patients, somnolence, change in EEG patterns.

CV: *bradycardia,* hypotension.

GI: nausea, vomiting.

Hematologic: exacerbation of porphyria.

Respiratory: *respiratory depression, apnea.*

Skin: rash, *erythema multiforme, Stevens-Johnson syndrome,* urticaria, pain, swelling, thrombophlebitis, necrosis, nerve injury at injection site.

Other: *angioedema,* physical and psychological dependence.

Overdose and treatment

Toxicity may cause unsteady gait, slurred speech, sustained nystagmus, somnolence, confusion, respiratory depression, pulmonary edema, areflexia, and coma. Typical shock syndrome with tachycardia and hypotension along with jaundice, oliguria, and chills followed by fever may occur.

Treatment aims to maintain and support ventilation and pulmonary function as necessary; and to support cardiac function and circulation with vasopressors and IV fluids as needed. If patient is conscious and gag reflex is intact, induce emesis (if ingestion was recent) by administering ipecac syrup. If emesis is contraindicated, perform gastric lavage while a cuffed endotracheal tube is in place to prevent aspiration. Follow with administration of activated charcoal or sodium chloride cathartic. Measure intake and output, vital signs and laboratory parameters. Maintain body temperature.

Alkalinization of urine may be helpful in removing drug from body; hemodialysis may be useful in severe overdose. Oral activated charcoal may enhance drug elimination regardless of its route of administration.

Special considerations

- Oral solution may be mixed with water or juice to improve taste.
- Don't crush or break extended-release form; this will impair drug action.
- Reconstitute powder for injection with 2.5 to 5 ml sterile water for injection. Roll vial in hands; don't shake.
- Use a larger vein for I.V. administration to prevent extravasation.
- Avoid I.V. administration at more than 60 mg/minute to prevent hypotension and respiratory depression. It may take up to 30 minutes after I.V. administration to achieve maximum effect.
- Administer parenteral dose within 30 minutes of reconstitution because drug hydrolyzes in solution and on exposure to air.
- Keep emergency resuscitation equipment on hand when administering phenobarbital I.V.
- Administer I.M. dose deep into large muscle mass to prevent tissue injury.
- Don't use injectable solution if it contains a precipitate.
- Administration of full loading doses over short periods of time to treat status epilepticus will require ventilatory support in adults.
- Full therapeutic effects aren't seen for 2 to 3 weeks, except when loading dose is used.
- Drug may cause a false-positive phentolamine test. Physiologic drug effect may impair absorption of cyanocobalamin Co 57; it may decrease serum bilirubin levels in neonates, epileptics, and patients with congenital nonhemolytic unconjugated hyperbilirubinemia. Barbiturates may increase sulfobromophthalein retention.

Patient monitoring

- Monitor vital signs when giving via I.V. route.
- Monitor phenobarbital levels as needed.

Breast-feeding patients

- Drug appears in breast milk; avoid use in breast-feeding women.

Pediatric patients
• Paradoxical hyperexcitability may occur in children. Use cautiously.
• Use of phenobarbital extended-release capsules isn't recommended in children under age 12.

Geriatric patients
• Elderly patients are more sensitive to drug's effects and usually need lower doses. Confusion, disorientation, and excitability may occur in elderly patients.

Patient education
• Advise patient of potential for physical and psychological dependence with prolonged use.
• Warn patient to avoid alcohol and other CNS depressants while taking drug. An excessive depressant effect is possible even if drug is taken the evening before alcohol ingestion.
• Caution patient not to stop taking drug suddenly because this could cause a withdrawal reaction.
• Advise patient to avoid driving and other hazardous activities that require alertness until adverse CNS effects of drug are known.

---

phentermine hydrochloride
Adipex-P, Fastin, Ionamin, Obe-Nix, Phentride, Teramine

Pharmacologic classification: amphetamine congener
Therapeutic classification: short-term adjunctive anorexigenic, indirect-acting sympathomimetic amine
Controlled substance schedule: IV
Pregnancy risk category: X

Indications and dosages
➤ *Short-term adjunct in exogenous obesity. Adults:* 8 mg P.O. t.i.d. ½ hour before meals. Or, 15 to 37.5 mg daily before breakfast. Or, 15 to 30 mg daily before breakfast (resin complex).

How supplied
Available by prescription only
Capsules and tablets: 8 mg, 15 mg, 18.75 mg, 30 mg, 37.5 mg
Capsules (resin complex, sustained-release): 15 mg, 30 mg, 37.5 mg

Pharmacodynamics
Anorexigenic action: Indirect-acting sympathomimetic amine; causes fewer and less severe adverse reactions from CNS stimulation than do amphetamines, and potential for addiction is lower. Anorexigenic effects are thought to follow direct stimulation of the hypothalamus; they may involve other CNS and metabolic effects.

Pharmacokinetics
Absorption: Absorbed readily after oral administration; therapeutic effects last 4 to 6 hours.

Distribution: Distributed widely throughout body.
Metabolism: No information available.
Excretion: Excreted in urine.

Route	Onset	Peak	Duration
P.O.	Unknown	Unknown	12-14 hr

Contraindications and precautions
Contraindicated in patients hypersensitive to sympathomimetic amines, patients with idiosyncratic reactions to them, agitated patients, and patients with hyperthyroidism, moderate to severe hypertension, advanced arteriosclerosis, symptomatic CV disease, or glaucoma. Also contraindicated within 14 days of MAO inhibitor therapy. Use cautiously in patients with mild hypertension.

Interactions
Drug-drug. *Acetazolamide, antacids, sodium bicarbonate:* Increased renal reabsorption of phentermine and prolonged duration of action. Monitor patient closely.
General anesthetics: Arrhythmias. Monitor patient closely.
Guanethidine, other antihypertensives: Decreased hypotensive effects. Monitor blood pressure.
Haloperidol, phenothiazines: Decreased phentermine effects. Monitor patient for clinical effect.
Insulin: Altered insulin requirements in diabetic patient. Monitor blood glucose levels.
MAO inhibitors (drugs with MAO-inhibiting effects): Concomitant use or use within 14 days may cause hypertensive crisis. Avoid concomitant use.
Drug-food. *Caffeine:* Additive CNS stimulation. Discourage excessive use.

Adverse reactions
CNS: overstimulation, headache, euphoria, dysphoria, dizziness, *insomnia.*
CV: *palpitations, tachycardia,* increased blood pressure.
GI: dry mouth, dysgeusia, constipation, diarrhea, other GI disturbances.
GU: impotence, dysuria, polyuria, urinary frequency.
Skin: urticaria.
Other: altered libido.

Overdose and treatment
Toxicity may cause restlessness, tremor, hyperreflexia, fever, tachypnea, dizziness, confusion, aggressive behavior, hallucinations, blood pressure changes, arrhythmias, nausea, vomiting, diarrhea, and cramps. Fatigue and depression usually follow CNS stimulation; then possible seizures, coma, and death. Chlorpromazine may antagonize CNS stimulation. Acidification of urine may hasten excretion.

Reactions may be *common*, uncommon, *life-threatening*, or COMMON AND LIFE-THREATENING.

Special considerations

• Intermittent courses of treatment (6 weeks on, 4 weeks off) are as effective as continuous use.
• Greatest weight loss occurs in first weeks of therapy and loss diminishes in succeeding weeks. When such tolerance develops, drug should be discontinued instead of increasing dosage.
• Don't crush sustained-release forms.
• Give morning dose 2 hours after breakfast.

Patient monitoring

• Monitor patient's weight loss.
• Monitor patient for adverse effects.

Pediatric patients

• Drug isn't recommended for children under age 12.

Patient education

• Advise patient to take morning dose 2 hours after breakfast, not to crush or chew sustained-release products, and to avoid caffeine.
• Tell patient to take last daily dose at least 6 hours before bedtime to prevent insomnia.
• Warn patient not to take drug more frequently than prescribed.
• Advise patient that drug may produce dizziness, fatigue, or drowsiness.
• Tell patient to call if palpitations occur.
• Tell diabetic patients to closely monitor blood glucose level. Adjustment in eating habits, body weight, and activity and change in dosage of antidiabetic may be needed.

phentolamine mesylate
Regitine

Pharmacologic classification: alpha-adrenergic blocker
Therapeutic classification: antihypertensive for pheochromocytoma; cutaneous vasodilator
Pregnancy risk category: C

Indications and dosages

➤ *Aid for diagnosis of pheochromocytoma.* Adults: 5 mg I.V. or I.M.
Children: 1 mg I.V., or 3 mg I.M
➤ *Control or prevention of paroxysmal hypertension immediately before or during pheochromocytomectomy.* Adults: 5 mg I.M. or I.V. 1 to 2 hours preoperatively, repeated as necessary; 5 mg I.V. during surgery if indicated.
Children: 1 mg I.M. or I.V. 1 to 2 hours preoperatively, repeated as necessary; 1 mg I.V. during surgery if indicated.
➤ *Prevention or treatment of dermal necrosis and sloughing of extravasation after I.V. administration of norepinephrine (or dopamine* ◊ *). Adults and children:* Inject 5 to 10 mg in 10 ml of normal saline solution into affected area, or add 10 mg to each liter of I.V. fluids containing norepinephrine.

➤ *Adjunctive treatment of left-sided heart failure secondary to acute MI* ◊ . *Adults:* 170 to 400 mcg/minute by I.V. infusion.
➤ *Treatment adjunct for men with impotence (neurogenic or vascular)* ◊ . *Adults:* 0.5 to 1 mg by intracavernosal injection. Usually administered with 30 mg papaverine injection.
➤ *Hypertensive crisis from sympathomimetic amines* ◊ . *Adults:* 5 to 15 mg I.V.

How supplied

Available by prescription only
Injection: 5 mg/ml in 1-ml vials

Pharmacodynamics

Antihypertensive action: Competitively antagonizes endogenous and exogenous amines at presynaptic and postsynaptic alpha-adrenergic receptors, decreasing both preload and afterload.
Cutaneous vasodilation action: Blocks epinephrine- and norepinephrine-induced vasoconstriction.

Pharmacokinetics

Absorption: Administered I.V.
Distribution: No information available.
Metabolism: No information available.
Excretion: About 10% of dose excreted unchanged in urine; excretion of remainder unknown. Short duration of action; plasma half-life is 19 minutes after I.V. administration.

Route	Onset	Peak	Duration
I.V.	Immediate	Unknown	Unknown
I.M.	Unknown	Unknown	Unknown

Contraindications and precautions

Contraindicated in patients hypersensitive to drug and in those with angina, coronary artery disease, or MI or history of MI. Use cautiously in patients with peptic ulcer or gastritis.

Interactions

Drug-drug. *Ephedrine, epinephrine:* Antagonized vasoconstrictor and hypertensive effects of these drugs. Avoid using together.

Adverse reactions

CNS: *dizziness, weakness, flushing, **cerebrovascular occlusion,** cerebrovascular spasm.*
CV: *hypotension, **shock, arrhythmias,** tachycardia, **MI.***
EENT: *nasal congestion.*
GI: *diarrhea, nausea, vomiting.*

Overdose and treatment

Toxicity may cause hypotension, dizziness, fainting, tachycardia, vomiting, lethargy, and shock.

Use norepinephrine if necessary to increase blood pressure. Don't use epinephrine; it stimulates alpha and beta receptors and causes vasodilation and further drop in blood pressure.

Special considerations
• Usual doses of phentolamine have little effect on blood pressure of normal individuals or patients with essential hypertension.
• Before test for pheochromocytoma, have patient rest in supine position until blood pressure is stabilized. When drug is administered I.V., inject dose rapidly after effects of venipuncture on blood pressure have passed. A marked decrease in blood pressure will be seen immediately, with maximum effect seen within 2 minutes.
• When possible, sedatives, analgesics, and all other drugs should be withdrawn at least 24 hours (preferably 48 to 72 hours) before phentolamine test; antihypertensives should be withdrawn and test shouldn't be performed until blood pressure returns to pretreatment levels; rauwolfia drugs should be withdrawn at least 4 weeks before test.
• Drug has been used to treat hypertension resulting from clonidine withdrawal and to treat reaction to sympathetic amines or other drugs or foods in patients taking MAO inhibitors.
• Drug has been used in patients with MI with left-sided heart failure in an attempt to reduce infarct size and decrease left ventricular ejection impedance. Drug has also been used to treat supraventricular premature contractions.

Patient monitoring
• When testing for pheochromocytoma, record blood pressure immediately after injection, at 30-second intervals for first 3 minutes, and at 1-minute intervals for next 7 minutes. When drug is given I.M., maximum effect occurs within 20 minutes. Record blood pressure every 5 minutes for 30 to 45 minutes after injection.
• Watch for test response. A positive test response occurs when patient's blood pressure decreases at least 35 mm Hg systolic and 25 mm Hg diastolic; a negative test response occurs when patient's blood pressure remains unchanged, is elevated, or decreases less than 35 mm Hg systolic and 25 mm Hg diastolic.

Breast-feeding patients
• It isn't known if drug appears in breast milk; because of possible adverse reactions in infant, stop either breast-feeding or drug based on importance of drug to mother.

Pediatric patients
• Infants and children may be more susceptible to drug effects.

Geriatric patients
• Administer cautiously because elderly patients may be more sensitive to adverse effects.

Patient education
• Teach patient about phentolamine test, if indicated.
• Tell patient to report adverse effects at once.
• Tell patient not to take sedatives or narcotics for at least 24 hours before test.

phenylephrine hydrochloride
Nasal products
Alconefrin 12, Alconefrin 25, Neo-Synephrine, Nostril, Rhinall, Sinex

Parenteral
Neo-Synephrine

Ophthalmic
AK-Dilate, AK-Nefrin, Isopto Frin, Mydfrin, Neo-Synephrine, Prefrin Liquifilm

Pharmacologic classification: adrenergic
Therapeutic classification: vasoconstrictor
Pregnancy risk category: C

Indications and dosages
➤ *Hypotensive emergencies during spinal anesthesia.* Adults: Initially, 0.1 to 0.2 mg I.V.; subsequent doses should also be low (0.1 mg).
➤ *Prevention of hypotension during spinal or inhalation anesthesia.* Adults: 2 to 3 mg S.C. or I.M. 3 to 4 minutes before anesthesia.
➤ *Mild to moderate hypotension.* Adults: 1 to 10 mg S.C. or I.M. (initial dose shouldn't exceed 5 mg). Additional doses may be given in 1 to 2 hours if needed. Or 0.1 to 0.5 mg slow I.V. injection (initial dose shouldn't exceed 0.5 mg). Additional doses may be given q 10 to 15 minutes. *Children:* 0.1 mg/kg or 3 mg/m^2 I.M. or S.C.
➤ *Paroxysmal supraventricular tachycardia.* Adults: Initially, 0.5 mg rapid I.V.; subsequent doses may be increased in increments of 0.1 to 0.2 mg. Maximum dose shouldn't exceed 1 mg.
➤ *Prolongation of spinal anesthesia.* Adults: 2 to 5 mg added to anesthetic solution.
➤ *Adjunct in the treatment of severe hypotension or shock.* Adults: 0.1 to 0.18 mg/minute I.V. infusion. After blood pressure stabilizes, maintain at 0.04 to 0.06 mg/minute, adjusted to patient response.
➤ *Vasoconstrictor for regional anesthesia.* Adults: 1 mg phenylephrine added to 20 ml local anesthetic.
➤ *Mydriasis (without cycloplegia).* Adults: Instill 1 or 2 drops 2.5% or 10% solution in eye before procedure. May be repeated in 10 to 60 minutes if needed.
➤ *Posterior synechia (adhesion of iris).* Adults: Instill 1 drop of 10% solution in eye 3 or more times daily with atropine sulfate.
➤ *Diagnosis of Horner's or Raeder's syndrome.* Adults: Instill a 1% or 10% solution in both eyes.
➤ *Initial treatment of postoperative malignant glaucoma.* Adults: Instill 1 drop of a 10% solution with 1 drop of a 1% to 4% atropine sulfate solution 3 or more times daily.

Reactions may be *common*, uncommon, *life-threatening*, or COMMON AND LIFE-THREATENING.

➤ *Nasal, eustachian tube, or sinus* ◇ *congestion. Adults and children over age 12:* Apply 2 to 3 drops or 1 to 2 sprays of 0.25% to 1% solution instilled in each nostril; or a small quantity of 0.5% nasal jelly applied into each nostril. Apply jelly or spray to nasal mucosa.
Children ages 6 to 12: Apply 2 to 3 drops or 1 to 2 sprays in each nostril.
Children under age 6: Apply 2 to 3 drops or sprays of 0.125% or 0.16% solution in each nostril.

Drops, spray, or jelly can be given q 4 hours, p.r.n.
➤ *Conjunctival congestion. Adults:* 1 to 2 drops of 0.08% to 0.25% solution applied to conjunctiva q 3 to 4 hours, p.r.n.

How supplied
Available by prescription only
Injection: 10 mg/ml parenteral
Ophthalmic solution: 0.12%, 2.5%, 10%
Available without a prescription
Nasal solution: 0.125%, 0.16%, 0.25%, 0.5%, 1%
Nasal spray: 0.25%, 0.5%, 1%

Pharmacodynamics
Vasopressor action: Acts predominantly by direct stimulation of alpha-adrenergic receptors, which constrict resistance and capacitance blood vessels, resulting in increased total peripheral resistance; increased systolic and diastolic blood pressure; decreased blood flow to vital organs, skin, and skeletal muscle; and constriction of renal blood vessels, reducing renal blood flow. Main therapeutic effect is vasoconstriction.

Also may act indirectly by releasing norepinephrine from its storage sites. Doesn't stimulate beta receptors except in large doses (activates beta$_1$ receptors). Tachyphylaxis (tolerance) may follow repeated injections.

Other alpha-adrenergic effects include action on the dilator muscle of the pupil (producing contraction) and local decongestant action in the arterioles of the conjunctiva (producing constriction).

Acts directly on alpha-adrenergic receptors in the arterioles of conjunctiva nasal mucosa, producing constriction. Vasoconstricting action on skin, mucous membranes, and viscera slows the vascular absorption rate of local anesthetics, which prolongs their action, localizes anesthesia, and decreases the risk of toxicity.

May cause contraction of pregnant uterus and constriction of uterine blood vessels.

Pharmacokinetics
Absorption: Pressor effects almost immediately after I.V. injection; last 15 to 20 minutes. After I.M. injection, onset is within 10 to 15 minutes; lasts ½ to 2 hours. After S.C. injection, onset is within 10 to 15 minutes; lasts 50 to 60 minutes. Nasal or conjunctival decongestant effects last 30 minutes to 4 hours. Peak effects for mydriasis 15

to 60 minutes for 2.5% solution; 10 to 90 minutes for 10% solution. Mydriasis recovery time is 3 hours for 2.5% solution; 3 to 7 hours for 10% solution.
Distribution: No information available.
Metabolism: Metabolized in liver and intestine by MAO.
Excretion: No information available.

Route	Onset	Peak	Duration
I.V.	Immediate	Unknown	15-20 min
I.M.	10-15 min	Unknown	½-2 hr
S.C.	10-15 min	Unknown	50-60 min
Ophthalmic	Rapid	10-90 min	3-7 hr
Nasal	Rapid	Unknown	½-4 hr

Contraindications and precautions
All forms are contraindicated in patients hypersensitive to drug. Injected form is also contraindicated in those with severe hypertension or ventricular tachycardia. Ophthalmic form is also contraindicated in patients with angle-closure glaucoma and in those who wear soft contact lenses.

Use all forms cautiously in elderly patients and in patients with hyperthyroidism or cardiac disease. Use nasal and ophthalmic forms cautiously in patients with type 1 diabetes mellitus, hypertension, or advanced arteriosclerotic changes and in children who have low body weight. Use injectable form cautiously in patients with severe atherosclerosis, bradycardia, partial heart block, myocardial disease, or allergy to sulfites.

Interactions
Drug-drug. *Alpha blockers, antihypertensives, diuretics used as antihypertensives, guanadrel, guanethidine, nitrates, rauwolfia alkaloids:* Decreased pressor response (hypotension). Monitor patient closely.
Cardiac glycosides, epinephrine, general anesthetics (cyclopropane, halothane), guanadrel, guanethidine, levodopa, MAO inhibitors, tricyclic antidepressants, other sympathomimetics: Increased risk of arrhythmias, including tachycardia. Monitor patient closely; don't use with MAO inhibitors.
Cycloplegic antimuscarinics (such as atropine): Increased mydriatic response to phenylephrine. Use together cautiously.
Doxapram, ergot alkaloids, MAO inhibitors, mazindol, methyldopa, oxytocics: Potentiated pressor effects. Monitor patient closely; don't use with MAO inhibitors.
Levodopa: Decreased mydriatic response to phenylephrine. Use together cautiously.
Nitrates: Reduced antianginal effects. Evaluate response to therapy.
Thyroid hormones: Increased effects of either drug. Monitor patient closely.

Adverse reactions

CNS: *headache;* excitability (with injected form); brow ache (with ophthalmic form); tremor, dizziness, nervousness (with nasal form).

CV: *bradycardia, arrhythmias,* hypertension (with injected form); *hypertension* (with 10% solution), tachycardia, palpitations, *PVCs, MI* (with ophthalmic form); *palpitations, tachycardia, PVCs,* hypertension.

EENT: transient eye burning or stinging on instillation, blurred vision, increased intraocular pressure, keratitis, lacrimation, reactive hyperemia of eye, allergic conjunctivitis, rebound miosis (with ophthalmic form); transient burning or stinging, dryness of nasal mucosa, rebound nasal congestion with continued use (with nasal form).

GI: nausea (with nasal form).

Respiratory: *asthmatic episodes.*

Skin: pallor (with nasal form), dermatitis (with ophthalmic form), tissue sloughing with extravasation (with injected form), diaphoresis (with ophthalmic form).

Other: tachyphylaxis (may occur with continued use), *anaphylaxis, decreased organ perfusion* (with prolonged use), trembling.

Overdose and treatment

Toxicity may cause exaggeration of common adverse reactions, palpitations, paresthesia, vomiting, arrhythmias, and hypertension.

Use atropine sulfate to block reflex bradycardia; phentolamine to treat excessive hypertension; and propranolol to treat cardiac arrhythmias, or levodopa to reduce excessive mydriatic effect of ophthalmic preparation as necessary.

Special considerations

● Give I.V. through large veins, and monitor flow rate. To treat extravasation ischemia, infiltrate site promptly and liberally with 10 to 15 ml of saline solution containing 5 to 10 mg of phentolamine through fine needle. Topical nitroglycerin has also been used.

● Hypovolemic states should be corrected before administration of drug; phenylephrine shouldn't be used in place of fluid, blood, plasma, and electrolyte replacement.

● Drug is chemically incompatible with butacaine, sulfate, alkalies, ferric salts, and oxidizing drugs and metals.

Ophthalmic form

● Apply digital pressure to lacrimal sac during and for 1 to 2 minutes after instillation to prevent systemic absorption.

● Prolonged exposure to air or strong light may cause oxidation and discoloration. Don't use if solution is brown or contains precipitate.

● To prevent contamination, don't touch applicator tip to any surface. Instruct patient in proper technique.

● Drug may cause false-normal tonometry readings.

Nasal form

● Prolonged or long-term use may result in rebound congestion and chronic swelling of nasal mucosa.

● To reduce risk of rebound congestion, use weakest effective dose.

● After use, rinse tip of spray bottle or dropper with hot water and dry with clean tissue. Wipe tip of nasal jelly container with clean, damp tissues.

Patient monitoring

● During I.V. administration, monitor pulse, blood pressure, and CVP every 2 to 5 minutes. Control flow rate and dosage to prevent excessive increases. I.V. overdoses can induce ventricular arrhythmias.

● Monitor patient for adverse effects.

Breast-feeding patients

● It isn't known if drug appears in breast milk; use cautiously in breast-feeding women.

Pediatric patients

● Infants and children may be more susceptible than adults to drug's effects. Because of risk of precipitating severe hypertension, only ophthalmic solutions containing 0.5% or less should be used in infants under age 1. The 10% ophthalmic solution is contraindicated in infants. Most manufacturers recommend that the 0.5% nasal solution not be used in children under age 12 except under medical supervision, and the 0.25% nasal solution shouldn't be used in children under age 6 except under medical supervision.

Geriatric patients

● Effects may be exaggerated in elderly patients. In patients over age 50, phenylephrine (ophthalmic solution) appears to alter the response of the dilator muscle of the pupil so that rebound miosis may occur the day after drug is given.

Patient education

● Tell patient to store away from heat, light, and humidity (not in bathroom medicine cabinet) and out of children's reach.

● Warn patient to use only as directed. If using OTC product, patient should follow directions on label and not use more often or in larger doses than prescribed or recommended.

● Caution patient not to exceed recommended dosage regardless of formulation; patient shouldn't double, decrease, or omit doses nor change dosage intervals unless so instructed.

● Tell patient to call if drug provides no relief in 2 days after using ophthalmic solution or 3 days after using nasal solution.

● Explain that systemic absorption from nasal and conjunctival membranes can occur. Patient should report systemic reactions, such as dizziness and chest pain, and stop drug.

Ophthalmic form

● Instruct patient not to use if solution is brown or contains a precipitate.

Reactions may be *common*, uncommon, *life-threatening*, or COMMON AND LIFE-THREATENING.

• Tell patient to wash hands before applying and to use finger to apply pressure to lacrimal sac during and for 1 to 2 minutes after instillation to decrease systemic absorption.

• Warn patient to avoid touching tip to any surface to prevent contamination.

• Inform patient that after applying drops, pupils will become unusually large. Patient should use sunglasses to protect eyes from sunlight and other bright lights, and call if effects persist 12 hours or more.

Nasal form

• After use, tell patient to rinse tip of spray bottle or dropper with hot water and dry with clean tissue or wipe tip of nasal jelly container with clean, damp tissues.

• Instruct patient to blow nose gently (with both nostrils open) to clear nasal passages before using drug.

• Teach patient appropriate method:
– Drops: Tilt head back while sitting or standing up, or lie on bed and hang head over side. Stay in position a few minutes to permit drug to spread through nose.
– Spray: With head upright, squeeze bottle quickly and firmly to produce 1 or 2 sprays into each nostril; wait 3 to 5 minutes, blow nose and repeat dose.
– Jelly: Place in each nostril and sniff well back into nose.

• Tell patient that increased fluid intake helps keep secretions liquid.

• Warn patient to avoid using OTC drugs with phenylephrine to prevent possible hazardous interactions.

---

phenytoin, phenytoin sodium, phenytoin sodium (extended)
Dilantin, Dilantin Infatab, Dilantin Kapseals, Dilantin-125

phenytoin sodium (prompt)
Pharmacologic classification: hydantoin derivative
Therapeutic classification: anticonvulsant
Pregnancy risk category: D

Indications and dosages
➤ **Generalized tonic-clonic seizures, status epilepticus, nonepileptic seizures (post–head trauma, Reye's syndrome).** *Adults:* Loading dose is 10 to 15 mg/kg I.V. slowly, not to exceed 50 mg/minute; oral loading dose is 1 g divided into three doses (400 mg, 300 mg, 300 mg) given at 2-hour intervals. Once controlled, maintenance dose is 300 mg P.O. daily (extended only); initially use a dose divided t.i.d. (extended or prompt).
Children: Loading dose is 15 to 20 mg/kg I.V. at 50 mg/minute, or P.O. divided q 8 to 12 hours;

then start maintenance dose of 4 to 8 mg/kg P.O. or I.V. daily, divided q 12 hours.

➤ **Neuritic pain (migraine, trigeminal neuralgia, and Bell's palsy).** *Adults:* 200 to 600 mg P.O. daily in divided doses.

➤ **Skeletal muscle relaxant.** *Adults:* 200 to 600 mg P.O. daily, p.r.n.

➤ **Ventricular arrhythmias unresponsive to lidocaine or procainamide, and arrhythmias induced by cardiac glycosides ◊.** *Adults:* 50 to 100 mg q 10 to 15 minutes, p.r.n., not to exceed 15 mg/kg. Infusion rate shouldn't exceed 50 mg/minute (slow I.V. push). *Alternative method:* 100 mg I.V. q 15 minutes until adverse effects develop, arrhythmias are controlled, or 1 g has been given. Also may administer entire loading dose of 1 g I.V. slowly at 25 mg/minute. Can be diluted in normal saline solution. I.M. route isn't recommended because of pain and erratic absorption.

➤ **Prophylactic control of seizures during neurosurgery.** *Adults:* 100 to 200 mg I.V. at intervals of about 4 hours during perioperative and postoperative periods.

How supplied
Available by prescription only
phenytoin
Oral suspension: 30 mg/5 ml*, 125 mg/5 ml
Tablets (chewable): 50 mg
phenytoin sodium
Injection: 50 mg/ml
phenytoin sodium (extended)
Capsules: 30 mg, 100 mg
phenytoin sodium (prompt)
Capsules: 100 mg

Pharmacodynamics
Anticonvulsant action: Like other hydantoin derivatives, phenytoin stabilizes neuronal membranes and limits seizure activity by either increasing efflux or decreasing influx of sodium ions across cell membranes in the motor cortex during generation of nerve impulses. Phenytoin exerts its antiarrhythmic effects by normalizing sodium influx to Purkinje's fibers in patients with cardiac glycoside–induced arrhythmias. It's indicated for generalized tonic-clonic (grand mal) and partial seizures.
Other actions: Inhibits excessive collagenase activity in patients with epidermolysis bullosa.

Pharmacokinetics
Absorption: Absorbed slowly from small intestine; absorption is form-dependent and bioavailability may differ among products. For extended-release capsules, serum levels peak at 4 to 12 hours; for prompt-release products, levels peak at 1½ to 3 hours. I.M. doses absorbed erratically; about 50% to 75% of I.M. dose absorbed in 24 hours.
Distribution: Widely distributed throughout body; therapeutic plasma levels 10 to 20 mcg/ml; 5 to 10 mcg/ml in some patients. Lateral nystag-

mus may occur at levels above 20 mcg/ml; ataxia usually at levels above 30 mcg/ml; significantly decreased mental capacity at 40 mcg/ml. About
90% protein-bound; less so in uremic patients.
Metabolism: Metabolized by liver to inactive
metabolites.
Excretion: Excreted in urine; exhibits dose-
dependent (zero-order) elimination kinetics.
Above a certain dosage level, small increases in
dosage disproportionately increase serum levels.

Route	Onset	Peak	Duration
P.O.	Unknown	1½- 12 hr	Unknown
I.V.	Immediate	1-2 hrs	Unknown
I.M.	Unknown	Unknown	Unknown

Contraindications and precautions
Contraindicated in patients with hydantoin hypersensitivity, sinus bradycardia, SA block, sec-
ond- or third-degree AV block, or Adams-Stokes
syndrome.

Use cautiously in elderly or debilitated patients; in those with hepatic dysfunction, hypotension, myocardial insufficiency, diabetes, or
respiratory depression; and in those receiving
hydantoin derivatives.

Interactions
Drug-drug. Phenytoin interacts with many drugs.
Diminished therapeutic effects and toxic reactions commonly are the result of recent changes
in drug therapy.
*Allopurinol, amiodarone, benzodiazepines,
chloramphenicol, chlorpheniramine, cimetidine, diazepam, disulfiram, fluconazole, ibuprofen, imipramine, isoniazid, metronidazole,
miconazole, omeprazole, phenacemide, phenylbutazone, salicylates, succinimides, trimethoprim, valproic acid:* Increased therapeutic effects of phenytoin. Monitor patient.
*Amiodarone, APAP, carbamazepine, cortico-
steroids, cyclosporine, dicumarol, digitoxin,
disopyramide, dopamine, doxycycline, estrogens, furosemide, haloperidol, levodopa,
mebendazole, meperidine, methadone, metyrapone, oral contraceptives, phenothiazines,
quinidine, sulfonylureas:* Decreased effects of
these drugs via increased hepatic metabolism.
Adjust dosages as needed.
*Antacids, antineoplastics, barbiturates, calci-
um, calcium gluconate, carbamazepine, charcoal, diazoxide, folic acid, loxapine, nitrofurantoin, pyridoxine, rifampin, sucralfate,
theophylline:* Decreased therapeutic effects of
phenytoin. Monitor patient.
Antipsychotic drugs: Lowered seizure threshold. Use together cautiously.
Drug-lifestyle. *Alcohol use:* Decreased therapeutic effects. Discourage use.

Adverse reactions
CNS: *ataxia, slurred speech,* dizziness, insomnia, nervousness, twitching, headache, *mental
confusion, decreased coordination.*

CV: periarteritis nodosa, hypotension.
EENT: *nystagmus, diplopia,* blurred vision, *gin-
gival hyperplasia* (especially in children).
GI: *nausea, vomiting,* constipation.
Hematologic: *thrombocytopenia, leukopenia, agranulocytosis, pancytopenia,*
macrocythemia, megaloblastic anemia.
Hepatic: *toxic hepatitis.*
Metabolic: hyperglycemia, decreased protein-
bound iodine.
Musculoskeletal: osteomalacia.
Skin: scarlatiniform or morbilliform rash; bullous, *exfoliative,* or purpuric dermatitis;
Stevens-Johnson syndrome; lupus erythematosus; *hirsutism; toxic epidermal necrolysis;* photosensitivity; pain, necrosis, and inflammation at injection site; discoloration of skin
(purple glove syndrome) if given by I.V. push in
back of hand.
Other: lymphadenopathy, hypertrichosis.

Overdose and treatment
Early toxicity may cause drowsiness, nausea, vomiting, nystagmus, ataxia, dysarthria, tremor, and
slurred speech; then hypotension, arrhythmias,
respiratory depression, and coma. Death is caused
by respiratory and circulatory depression. Estimated lethal dose in adults is 2 to 5 g.

Treat overdose with gastric lavage or emesis
and follow with suportive treatment. Carefully
monitor vital signs and fluid and electrolye balance. Forced diuresis is of little or no value. Hemodialysis or peritoneal dialysis may be helpful.

Special considerations
● Only extended-release capsules are approved
for once-daily dosing; all other forms are given
in divided doses every 8 to 12 hours.
● Oral or nasogastric feeding may interfere with
absorption of oral suspension; separate dosing
and feeding times as much as possible, but by no
less than 1 hour. During continuous tube feeding, tube should be flushed before and after dose.
● If suspension is used, shake well.
● I.M. administration should be avoided; it's
painful and drug absorption is erratic.
● Mix I.V. doses in normal saline solution and
use within 30 minutes; mixtures with D_5W will
precipitate. Don't refrigerate solution; don't mix
with other drugs. In-line filter is recommended.
● If using I.V. bolus, use slow (50 mg/minute)
I.V. push or constant infusion; too-rapid I.V. injection may cause hypotension and circulatory
collapse. Don't use I.V. push in veins on back of
hand; larger veins are needed to prevent discoloration caused by purple glove syndrome.
● Abrupt withdrawal may precipitate status epilepticus.
● Phenytoin commonly is abbreviated as DPH
(diphenylhydantoin), an older drug name.
● Drug may interfere with the 1-mg dexamethasone suppression test.

Reactions may be *common,* uncommon, *life-threatening,* or COMMON AND LIFE-THREATENING.

Patient monitoring
• Monitoring of serum levels is essential because of dose-dependent excretion.
• When giving I.V., monitor ECG, blood pressure, and respiratory status continuously.

Breast-feeding patients
• Drug appears in breast milk; an alternative to breast-feeding is recommended during therapy.

Pediatric patients
• Special pediatric-strength suspension (30 mg/5 ml) is available in Canada only. Take extreme care to use correct strength. Don't confuse with adult strength (125 mg/5 ml).

Geriatric patients
• Elderly patients metabolize and excrete drug slowly; they may require lower dosages.

Patient education
• Tell patient to use same brand of phenytoin consistently. Changing brands may change effect.
• Instruct patient to take drug with food or milk to minimize GI distress.
• Warn patient not to stop drug, except with medical supervision; to avoid hazardous activities that require alertness until CNS effect is determined; and to avoid alcoholic beverages, which can decrease effectiveness of drug and increase adverse reactions.
• Encourage patient to wear a medical identification bracelet or necklace.
• Stress good oral hygiene to minimize overgrowth and sensitivity of gums.

---

physostigmine salicylate
Antilirium

physostigmine sulfate
Eserine

Pharmacologic classification: cholinesterase inhibitor
Therapeutic classification: antimuscarinic antidote, antiglaucoma
Pregnancy risk category: C
Ophthalmic ointment: 0.25%

Indications and dosages
➤ *Tricyclic antidepressant and anticholinergic poisoning. Adults:* 0.5 to 2 mg I.M. or I.V. given slowly (not to exceed 1 mg/minute I.V.). Dosage individualized and repeated, p.r.n., q 10 minutes.
Children: Reserve for life-threatening situations only. Initial pediatric I.V. or I.M. dose of physostigmine salicylate is 0.02 mg/kg. Dose may be repeated at 5- to 10-minute intervals to maximum of 2 mg if no adverse cholinergic signs are present.

➤ *Postanesthesia care. Adults:* 0.5 to 1 mg I.M. or I.V. given slowly (not to exceed 1 mg/minute I.V.). Dosage individualized and repeated, p.r.n., q 10 to 30 minutes.
➤ *Open-angle glaucoma. Adults:* Apply ointment to lower fornix up to t.i.d.

How supplied
Available by prescription only
Injection: 1 mg/ml

Pharmacodynamics
Antimuscarinic action: Competitively blocks acetylcholine hydrolysis by cholinesterase, resulting in acetylcholine accumulation at cholinergic synapses; that antagonizes the muscarinic effects of overdose with antidepressants and anticholinergics. With ophthalmic use, miosis and ciliary muscle contraction increase aqueous humor outflow and decrease intraocular pressure.

Pharmacokinetics
Absorption: Well absorbed from GI tract, mucous membranes, and subcutaneous tissues when given I.M. or I.V.; effects peak within 5 minutes. After ophthalmic use, may be absorbed orally after passage through nasolacrimal duct.
Distribution: Distributed widely; crosses blood-brain barrier.
Metabolism: Cholinesterase hydrolyzes drug relatively quickly. Duration of effect is 1 to 2 hours after I.V. administration, 12 to 48 hours after ophthalmic use.
Excretion: Only small amount excreted in urine. Exact mode of excretion unknown.

Route	Onset	Peak	Duration
I.V.	3-5 min	5 min	½-5 hr
I.M.	3-5 min	20-30 min	½-5 hr
Oph-thalmic	10-30 min	Unknown	12-48 hr

Contraindications and precautions
Injected form contraindicated in patients with mechanical obstruction of the intestine or urogenital tract, asthma, gangrene, diabetes, CV disease, or vagotonia and in those receiving choline esters or depolarizing neuromuscular blockers.

Ophthalmic form is contraindicated in patients with intolerance to physostigmine and in those with active uveitis or corneal injury. Use injectable form cautiously during pregnancy.

Interactions
Drug-drug. *Succinylcholine:* Prolonged respiratory depression. Monitor patient closely.
Systemic cholinergic drugs: Additive toxicity. Monitor patient for toxicity.
Drug-herb. *Jaborandi tree, pill-bearing spurge:* Additive effects. Discourage use together.

Adverse reactions
CNS: weakness; headache (ophthalmic form); *seizures, restlessness, excitability* (injected form).
CV: slow or irregular heartbeat (ophthalmic form); *bradycardia,* hypotension (injected form).
EENT: blurred vision, eye pain, burning, redness, stinging, eye irritation, twitching of eyelids, watering of eyes (ophthalmic form); miosis (injected form).
GI: nausea, vomiting, diarrhea; epigastric pain, *excessive salivation* (injected form).
GU: loss of bladder control (ophthalmic form); urinary urgency (injected form).
Respiratory: *bronchospasm,* bronchial constriction, shortness of breath, dyspnea (injected form).
Skin: diaphoresis.

Overdose and treatment
Toxicity may cause headache, nausea, vomiting, diarrhea, blurred vision, miosis, myopia, excessive tearing, bronchospasm, increased bronchial secretions, hypotension, incoordination, excessive sweating, muscle weakness, bradycardia, excessive salivation, restlessness or agitation, and confusion.

Suppport respiration; bronchial suctioning may be performed. Discontinue drug immediately. Atropine may be given to block muscarinic effects. Avoid atropine overdose because it may cause bronchial plug formation.

Special considerations
ALERT Watch closely for adverse reactions, particularly CNS disturbances. Raise side rails if patient becomes restless or hallucinates. Adverse reactions may indicate drug toxicity.
Injectable form
● Effectiveness is typically immediate and dramatic but it may be transient.
● Give I.V. at controlled rate; use direct injection at no more than 1 mg/minute in adults or 0.5 mg/minute in children.
● Observe solution for discoloration. Don't use if darkened, which may indicate loss of potency.
● Atropine sulfate injection should always be available as an antagonist and antidote for most of physostigmine's effects.
● The commercially available formulation of physostigmine salicylate injection contains sodium bisulfite, a sulfite that can cause allergic-type reactions, including anaphylaxis and life-threatening or less severe asthmatic episodes in susceptible individuals.
Ophthalmic form
● After applying ointment, have patient close eyelids and roll eyes.

Patient monitoring
● Monitor patient's vital signs.
● Monitor patient for adverse effects.

Breast-feeding patients
● It isn't known if drug appears in breast milk. Safety and efficacy in breast-feeding women haven't been established.

Geriatric patients
● Use cautiously when administering to elderly patients because they may be more sensitive to drug's effects.

Patient education
● Teach patient how to administer ophthalmic ointment.
● Instruct patient not to close his eyes tightly or blink unnecessarily after instilling ointment.
● Warn patient that he may experience blurred vision and difficulty seeing after initial instillation.
● Instruct patient to report abdominal cramps, diarrhea, or excessive salivation.
● Remind patient to wait 10 minutes after instillation before using another eye preparation.

pilocarpine hydrochloride
Adsorbocarpine, Akarpine, Isopto Carpine, Miocarpine*, Ocusert Pilo, Pilocar, Pilopine HS

pilocarpine nitrate
Minims Pilocarpine*, Pilagan

Pharmacologic classification: cholinergic agonist
Therapeutic classification: miotic
Pregnancy risk category: C

Indications and dosages
➤ *Chronic open-angle glaucoma; before or instead of emergency surgery in acute narrow-angle glaucoma. Adults and children:* Instill 1 or 2 drops of a 1% to 4% solution in the lower conjunctival sac q 4 to 12 hours (dosage should be based on periodic tonometric readings) or apply ½-inch ribbon of 4% gel (Pilopine HS) h.s.
Or apply one Ocusert Pilo System (20 or 40 mcg/hour) q 7 days.
➤ *Emergency treatment of acute narrow-angle glaucoma. Adults and children:* 1 drop of 2% solution q 5 minutes for three to six doses; then 1 drop q 1 to 3 hours until pressure is controlled.
➤ *To counteract mydriatic effects of sympathomimetics. Adults:* 1 drop of 1% solution in affected eye.

How supplied
Available by prescription only
pilocarpine hydrochloride
Solution: 0.25%, 0.5%, 1%, 2%, 3%, 4%, 5%, 6%, 8%, 10%
Gel: 4%

Reactions may be *common*, uncommon, *life-threatening*, or COMMON AND LIFE-THREATENING.

Releasing-system insert: 20 mcg/hour, 40 mcg/hour
pilocarpine nitrate
Solution: 1%, 2%, 4%

Pharmacodynamics

Miotic action: Stimulates cholinergic receptors of the sphincter muscles of the iris, resulting in miosis. Also produces ciliary muscle contraction, resulting in accommodation with deepening of the anterior chamber, and vasodilation of conjunctival vessels of the outflow tract.

Pharmacokinetics

Absorption: Drops act within 10 to 30 minutes; peak effect at 2 to 4 hours. With Ocusert Pilo System, 0.3 to 7 mg of drug are released during initial 6-hour period; during remainder of 1-week insertion period, release rate is within 20% of rated value. Effect seen in 1½ to 2 hours; maintained for the 1-week life of insertion.
Distribution: No information available.
Metabolism: No information available.
Excretion: Duration of effect of drops is 4 to 6 hours.

Route	Onset	Peak	Duration
Oph-thalmic	10-30 min	30-85 min	4-8 hr

Contraindications and precautions

Contraindicated in patients hypersensitive to drug or when cholinergic effects such as constriction are undesirable (for example, in acute iritis, some forms of secondary glaucoma, pupillary block glaucoma, acute inflammatory disease of the anterior chamber).

Use cautiously in patients with acute cardiac failure, bronchial asthma, peptic ulcer, hyperthyroidism, GI spasm, urinary obstruction, and Parkinson's disease.

Interactions

Drug-drug. *Demecarium, echothiophate, isoflurophate:* Decreased pilocarpine effects. Monitor patient closely.
Epinephrine derivatives, timolol: Enhanced reductions in intraocular pressure. Monitor patient closely.

Adverse reactions

CV: hypertension, tachycardia.
EENT: periorbital or supraorbital headache, *myopia,* ciliary spasm, *blurred vision,* conjunctival irritation, transient stinging and burning, keratitis, lens opacity, retinal detachment, lacrimation, changes in visual field, *brow pain.*
GI: nausea, vomiting, diarrhea, salivation.
Respiratory: *bronchoconstriction, pulmonary edema.*
Skin: diaphoresis.
Other: *hypersensitivity reactions.*

Overdose and treatment

Toxicity may cause flushing, vomiting, bradycardia, bronchospasm, increased bronchial secretion, sweating, tearing, involuntary urination, hypotension, and tremors. Vomiting is usually spontaneous with accidental ingestion; if not, induce emesis and then use activated charcoal or cathartic. Treat dermal exposure by washing areas twice with water. Use epinephrine to treat CV responses. Atropine sulfate is antidote of choice. Flush eye with water or sodium chloride to treat local overdose. Doses up to 20 mg are generally considered nontoxic.

Special considerations

• Drug may be used alone or with mannitol, urea, glycerol, or acetazolamide. May be used to counteract effects of mydriatic and cycloplegic products after surgery or ophthalmoscopic examination and may be used alternately with atropine to break adhesions.

Patient monitoring

• Monitor tonometric readings.
• Monitor patient for adverse effects.

Patient education

• Warn patient that vision will be temporarily blurred, that miotic pupil may make surroundings appear dim and that transient brow ache and myopia are common at first; assure patient that adverse effects subside 10 to 14 days after therapy begins.
• Instruct patient to check for presence of pilocarpine ocular system at bedtime and upon arising.
• Tell patient that if systems in both eyes are lost, they should be replaced as soon as possible. If one system is lost, it may be replaced with a fresh system or the system remaining in other eye may be removed and both replaced with fresh systems so that both systems will subsequently be replaced on same schedule.
• Instruct patient that if Ocusert System falls out of eye during sleep, he should wash hands, then rinse Ocusert in cool tap water and reposition it in eye. Don't use insert if deformed.
• Inform patient that systems should be replaced every 7 days.
• Provide patient with a copy of manufacturer's instructions for pilocarpine ocular system.
• Tell patient to use caution in night driving and other activities in poor illumination because miotic pupil diminishes side vision and illumination.
• Stress importance of complying with prescribed medical regimen.
• Reassure patient that adverse effects will subside.
• Teach patient correct way to instill drops and to apply light finger pressure on lacrimal sac for 1 minute after administration to minimize systemic absorption.

• Instruct patient to apply gel at bedtime because it will cause blurred vision.

pilocarpine hydrochloride
Salagen

Pharmacologic classification: cholinergic agonist
Therapeutic classification: antixerostomia
Pregnancy risk category: C

Indications and dosages
➤ *Treatment of symptoms of xerostomia from salivary gland hypofunction caused by radiotherapy for cancer of the head and neck. Adults:* 5 mg P.O. t.i.d. Dosage may be increased to 10 mg P.O. t.i.d., p.r.n.

How supplied
Available by prescription only
Tablets: 5 mg

Pharmacodynamics
Antixerostomia action: Increases secretion of the salivary glands, which eliminates dryness.

Pharmacokinetics
Absorption: Absorbed in GI tract. High-fat meal may decrease absorption rate.
Distribution: No information available.
Metabolism: Inactivation thought to occur at neuronal synapses and probably in plasma.
Excretion: Drug and minimally active or inactive degradation products excreted in urine.

Route	Onset	Peak	Duration
P.O.	20 min	1 hr	3-5 hr

Contraindications and precautions
Contraindicated in patients hypersensitive to pilocarpine, in those with uncontrolled asthma, and when miosis is undesirable, such as in acute iritis and angle-closure glaucoma.
    Use cautiously in patients with CV disease, controlled asthma, chronic bronchitis, COPD, cholelithiasis, biliary tract disease, nephrolithiasis, and cognitive or psychiatric disturbances.

Interactions
Drug-drug. *Beta-adrenergic antagonists:* Increased risk of conduction disturbances. Use together cautiously.
Drugs with anticholinergic effects: Antagonized anticholinergic effects of oral pilocarpine. Use together cautiously.
Drugs with parasympathomimetic effects: Additive pharmacologic effects. Monitor patient closely.

Adverse reactions
CNS: *dizziness, headache,* tremor.
CV: hypertension, tachycardia, edema.

EENT: *rhinitis,* lacrimation, amblyopia, pharyngitis, voice alteration, conjunctivitis, epistaxis, sinusitis, abnormal vision.
GI: *nausea,* dyspepsia, diarrhea, abdominal pain, vomiting, dysphagia, taste perversion.
GU: *urinary frequency.*
Musculoskeletal: *asthenia,* myalgia.
Skin: *flushing,* rash, pruritus.
Other: *sweating, chills.*

Overdose and treatment
Taking 100 mg of oral pilocarpine is considered potentially fatal. Treat with atropine titration (0.5 mg to 1 mg S.C. or I.V.) and supportive measures to maintain respiration and circulation. Epinephrine (0.3 mg to 1 mg S.C. or I.M.) may also be useful during severe CV depression or bronchoconstriction. It isn't known if pilocarpine is dialyzable.

Special considerations
• Patient should undergo careful examination of fundus before therapy begins; retinal detachment has been reported with pilocarpine use in patients with preexisting retinal disease.

Patient monitoring
• Monitor patient for signs and symptoms of pilocarpine toxicity characterized by exaggeration of its parasympathomimetic effects, including headache, visual disturbance, lacrimation, sweating, respiratory distress, GI spasm, nausea, vomiting, diarrhea, AV block, tachycardia, bradycardia, hypotension, hypertension, shock, mental confusion, cardiac arrhythmia, and tremors.

Breast-feeding patients
• It isn't known if drug appears in breast milk. Because of potential for serious adverse reactions in breast-feeding infants, stop either breast-feeding or drug, taking into account importance of drug to mother.

Pediatric patients
• Safety and effectiveness in children haven't been established.

Patient education
• Warn patient that drug may cause visual disturbances (especially at night) that could impair the ability to drive safely.
• Tell patient to drink plenty of fluids to prevent dehydration if drug causes excessive sweating. If adequate fluid intake can't be maintained, tell patient to call.

---

pimozide
Orap

Pharmacologic classification: diphenyl-butylpiperidine
Therapeutic classification: antipsychotic
Pregnancy risk category: C

Indications and dosages
➤ **Suppression of severe motor and phonic tics in patients with Tourette syndrome.**
Adults and children over age 12: Initially, 1 to 2 mg daily in divided doses. Then, increase dosage, p.r.n., every other day. Maintenance dosage, from 7 to 16 mg daily. Maximum, 20 mg daily.
Children under age 12: 0.05 mg/kg h.s.; increase at 3-day intervals to maximum of 0.2 mg/kg. Maximum, 10 mg daily.

How supplied
Available by prescription only
Tablets: 2 mg

Pharmacodynamics
Antipsychotic action: Mechanism unknown. Thought to exert effects by postsynaptic or presynaptic blockade of CNS dopamine receptors, thus inhibiting dopamine-mediated effects. Also has anticholinergic, antiemetic, and anxiolytic effects and produces mild alpha blockade.

Pharmacokinetics
Absorption: Absorbed slowly and incompletely from GI tract; bioavailability about 50%. Plasma levels peak in 4 to 12 hours (usually in 6 to 8 hours).
Distribution: Distributed widely into body.
Metabolism: Metabolized by liver; a significant first-pass effect exists.
Excretion: About 40% of dose excreted in urine as parent drug and metabolites in 3 to 4 days; about 15% excreted in feces via biliary tract within 3 to 6 days.

Route	Onset	Peak	Duration
P.O.	Unknown	4-12 hr	Unknown

Contraindications and precautions
Contraindicated in patients hypersensitive to drug, in treatment of simple tics or tics other than those linked to Tourette syndrome, with drug therapy known to cause motor and phonic tics, and in congenital long QT interval syndrome or history of arrhythmias. Also contraindicated in patients with severe toxic CNS depression and in those experiencing coma.

Use cautiously in patients with impaired renal or hepatic function, glaucoma, prostatic hyperplasia, seizure disorders, or EEG abnormalities.

Interactions
Drug-drug. *Amphetamines, methylphenidate, pemoline:* Tourette-like tic; exacerbation of existing tics. Monitor patient closely.
Anticonvulsants (carbamazepine, phenobarbital, phenytoin): Seizures. An anticonvulsant dosage increase may be needed.
Antidepressants, disopyramide, phenothiazines, procainamide, quinidine, other antiarrhythmics, other antipsychotics: Further depress cardiac conduction and prolong QT interval, resulting in serious arrhythmias. Monitor patient closely if concomitant use is necessary.
CNS depressants (such as analgesics; anxiolytics; barbiturates; epidural, general, spinal anesthetics; narcotics; parenteral magnesium sulfate; tranquilizers): Oversedation and respiratory depression due to additive CNS depressant effects. Avoid concomitant use.
Drug-lifestyle. *Alcohol use:* Oversedation and respiratory depression due to additive CNS depressant effects. Discourage use.

Adverse reactions
CNS: *parkinsonian-like symptoms,* drowsiness, headache, insomnia, **neuroleptic malignant syndrome,** other extrapyramidal signs and symptoms (dystonia, akathisia, hyperreflexia, opisthotonos, oculogyric crisis), *tardive dyskinesia, sedation, adverse behavioral effects.*
CV: *ECG changes (prolonged QT interval),* hypotension, hypertension, tachycardia.
EENT: visual disturbances.
GI: *dry mouth, constipation.*
GU: impotence, urinary frequency.
Musculoskeletal: muscle rigidity.
Skin: rash, diaphoresis.

Overdose and treatment
Signs and symptoms of overdose include severe extrapyramidal reactions, hypotension, respiratory depression, coma, and ECG abnormalities, including prolongation of QT interval, inversion or flattening of T waves, and new appearance of U waves. Treat with gastric lavage to remove unabsorbed drug. Maintain blood pressure with I.V. fluids, plasma expanders, or norepinephrine. Don't use epinephrine. Treat extrapyramidal symptoms with parenteral diphenhydramine. Monitor patient for adverse effects for at least 4 days because of drug's prolonged half-life (55 hours).

Special considerations
● Extrapyramidal reactions develop in about 10% to 15% of patients at normal doses. Reactions are especially likely to occur during early days of therapy.
● If excessive restlessness and agitation occur, therapy with a beta blocker, such as propranolol or metoprolol, may be helpful.

Patient monitoring
● Obtain baseline ECG before therapy and then periodically to monitor CV effects.

• Maintain patient's serum potassium level within normal range; decreased potassium levels increase risk of arrhythmias. Monitor potassium level in patients with diarrhea and in those who are taking diuretics.
• Assess patient periodically for abnormal body movement.

Pediatric patients
• Use and efficacy in children under age 12 are limited. Dosage should be kept at lowest possible level. Use of drug in children for any disorder other than Tourette syndrome isn't recommended.

Geriatric patients
• Elderly patients are more likely to develop cardiac toxicity and tardive dyskinesia even at normal doses.

Patient education
• Inform patient of risks and signs and symptoms of dystonic reactions and tardive dyskinesia.
• Advise patient to take drug exactly as prescribed, not to double missed doses, not to share drug with others, and not to stop taking it suddenly.
• Explain that drug's therapeutic effect may not be seen for several weeks.
• Urge patient to report unusual effects promptly.
• Tell patient not to take drug with alcohol, sleeping medications, or other drugs that may cause drowsiness without medical approval.
• Recommend use of sugarless hard candy or chewing gum, ice chips, or artificial saliva to relieve dry mouth.
• To prevent dizziness at start of therapy, tell patient to lie down for 30 minutes after taking each dose and to avoid sudden changes in posture, especially when rising to upright position.
• To minimize daytime sedation, suggest taking entire daily dose at bedtime.
• Warn patient to avoid hazardous activities that require alertness until drug's effects are known.

pindolol
Visken

Pharmacologic classification: beta blocker
Therapeutic classification: antihypertensive
Pregnancy risk category: B

Indications and dosages
➤ *Hypertension.* *Adults:* Initially, 5 mg P.O. b.i.d. increased by 10 mg daily q 3 to 4 weeks up to maximum of 60 mg/day. Usual dosage is 10 to 30 mg daily, given in two or three divided doses. In some patients, once-daily dosing may be possible.
➤ *Angina* ◊. *Adults:* 15 to 40 mg daily P.O. in three or four divided doses.

How supplied
Available by prescription only
Tablets: 5 mg, 10 mg

Pharmacodynamics
Antihypertensive action: Exact mechanism unknown. Doesn't consistently affect cardiac output or renin release, and other mechanisms such as decreased peripheral resistance probably contribute to hypotensive effect. Because pindolol has some intrinsic sympathomimetic activity—that is, beta-agonist sympathomimetic activity—it may be useful in patients who develop bradycardia with other beta-blockers. It's a nonselective beta-blocker, inhibiting both $beta_1$ and $beta_2$ receptors.

Pharmacokinetics
Absorption: After oral administration, absorbed rapidly from GI tract; peak plasma levels in 1 to 2 hours. Effect on heart rate usually occurs in 3 hours. Food doesn't reduce bioavailability but may increase rate of GI absorption.
Distribution: Distributed widely throughout body; 40% to 60% protein-bound.
Metabolism: About 60% to 65% of dose metabolized by liver.
Excretion: In adults with normal renal function, 35% to 50% of dose excreted unchanged in urine; half-life about 3 to 4 hours. Antihypertensive effect usually lasts 24 hours.

Route	Onset	Peak	Duration
P.O.	Unknown	1-2 hr	24 hr

Contraindications and precautions
Contraindicated in patients hypersensitive to drug and in those with bronchial asthma, severe bradycardia, heart block greater than first degree, cardiogenic shock, or overt cardiac failure.
    Use cautiously in patients with heart failure, nonallergic bronchospastic disease, diabetes, hyperthyroidism, or impaired renal or hepatic function.

Interactions
Drug-drug. *Other antihypertensives:* Potentiated antihypertensive effects. Monitor blood pressure.

Adverse reactions
CNS: *insomnia, fatigue, dizziness, nervousness,* vivid dreams, weakness, paresthesia.
CV: *edema,* **bradycardia, heart failure,** chest pain.
GI: *nausea,* abdominal discomfort.
Hepatic: elevated serum transaminase, alkaline phosphatase, LD, and uric acid levels.
Musculoskeletal: *muscle pain, joint pain.*
Respiratory: *increased airway resistance,* dyspnea.
Skin: rash, pruritus.

Reactions may be *common,* uncommon, *life-threatening,* or COMMON AND LIFE-THREATENING.

Overdose and treatment

Toxicity may cause severe hypotension, brady-cardia, heart failure, and bronchospasm.

Special considerations

• Always check patient's apical pulse rate before giving drug. If extremes in pulse rate are detect-ed, withhold drug and reevaluate drug therapy.
• Maximum therapeutic response may not be seen for 2 weeks or more.
• Withdraw drug over 1 to 2 weeks after long-term therapy.
• Beta blockers may mask tachycardia caused by hyperthyroidism. In patients with suspected thy-rotoxicosis, withdraw beta blocker gradually, to avoid thyroid storm.
ALERT Don't confuse pindolol with Parlodel, Panadol, or Plendil.

Patient monitoring

• Monitor blood pressure frequently. A vasopressor may be needed in the event of hypotension.
• Monitor blood glucose levels in diabetic pa-tients closely because drug masks certain signs and symptoms of hypoglycemia.
• Monitor hepatic studies.

Breast feeding patients

• Drug appears in breast milk; an alternative to breast-feeding is recommended during therapy.

Pediatric patients

• Safety and efficacy in children haven't been es-tablished; use only if potential benefit outweighs risk.

Geriatric patients

• Elderly patients may need lower maintenance drug doses because of increased bioavailability or delayed metabolism; they also may experience enhanced adverse effects. Half-life of drug may be increased in elderly patients.

Patient education

• Tell patient to take drug exactly as prescribed.
• Tell patient to report adverse reactions imme-diately.

---

pioglitazone hydrochloride
Actos

Pharmacologic classification: thiazolidine-dione
Therapeutic classification: antidiabetic
Pregnancy risk category: C

Indications and dosages

➤ *Monotherapy adjunct to diet and ex-ercise to improve glycemic control in pa-tients with type 2 diabetes mellitus; com-bination therapy with a sulfonylurea, metformin, or insulin when diet and ex-ercise plus single drug doesn't result in* *adequate glycemic control. Adults:* Initial-ly, 15 or 30 mg P.O. once daily. For patients who respond inadequately to initial dose, dose may be increased in increments. Maximum, 45 mg daily. If used in combination therapy, maximum is 30 mg daily.

How supplied

Available by prescription only
Tablets: 15 mg, 30 mg, 45 mg

Pharmacodynamics

Antidiabetic action: Lowers blood glucose lev-els by decreasing insulin resistance in the pe-riphery and in the liver, resulting in increased insulin-dependent glucose disposal and decreased glucose output by the liver. Potent and highly se-lective agonist for receptors found in insulin-sensitive tissues, such as adipose tissue, skele-tal muscle, and liver. Activation of these receptors modulates the transcription of a number of insulin-responsive genes involved in control of glucose and lipid metabolism.

Pharmacokinetics

Absorption: When taken on empty stomach, rapidly absorbed and measurable in serum within 30 minutes; levels peak within 2 hours. Food delays time to peak serum levels slightly (to 3 to 4 hours), but doesn't affect overall extent of absorption.
Distribution: Drug and metabolites more than 98% protein-bound, primarily to serum albumin.
Metabolism: Extensively metabolized by liver. Three pharmacologically active metabolites: M-II, M-III, and M-IV.
Excretion: About 15% to 30% of dose recov-ered in urine, primarily as metabolites and their conjugates. Majority of oral dose excreted into bile and eliminated in feces. Half-life ranges from 3 to 7 hours.

Route	Onset	Peak	Duration
P.O.	Unknown	Within 2 hr	Unknown

Contraindications and precautions

Contraindicated in patients hypersensitive to drug or its components. Drug shouldn't be used in pa-tients with type 1 diabetes mellitus or for the treat-ment of diabetic ketoacidosis, in patients with clinical evidence of active liver disease or serum ALT level greater than two and one-half times up-per limit of normal, or in those who experienced jaundice while taking troglitazone. Don't use in patients with New York Heart Association Class III or IV heart failure. Use cautiously in patients with edema or heart failure.

Interactions

Drug-drug. *Ketoconazole:* May inhibit metab-olism of pioglitazone. Monitor patient's blood glucose levels more frequently.
Oral contraceptives: Decreased effectiveness of contraceptives. Advise patient to consider addi-tional birth control measures.

Adverse reactions
CNS: headache.
CV: *edema* (with insulin).
EENT: sinusitis, pharyngitis.
Hematologic: anemia.
Metabolic: *hypoglycemia* (with combination therapy), aggravated diabetes mellitus, weight gain, decreased triglyceride levels, increased high-density lipoprotein cholesterol.
Musculoskeletal: myalgia.
Respiratory: *upper respiratory tract infection.*
Other: tooth disorder

Overdose and treatment
Limited data available. Supportive treatment should be initiated depending on patient's clinical presentation.

Special considerations
● Because ovulation may resume in premenopausal, anovulatory women with insulin resistance, contraceptive measures may need to be considered.
● Drug should be used in pregnancy only if benefit justifies risk to fetus. Insulin is the preferred antidiabetic for use during pregnancy.
● Management of type 2 diabetes should include diet control. Because caloric restrictions, weight loss, and exercise help improve insulin sensitivity and help make drug therapy effective, these measures are essential for proper diabetes management.

Patient monitoring
● Liver enzyme levels should be measured at start of therapy, every 2 months for first year, and then periodically. Liver function tests also should be performed in patients who develop signs and symptoms of liver dysfunction, such as nausea, vomiting, abdominal pain, fatigue, anorexia, or dark urine. Stop drug if patient develops jaundice or if results of liver functions tests show ALT elevations greater than three times upper limit of normal.
● Patients with heart failure should be observed for increased edema during therapy.
● While patient is receiving drug, hemoglobin levels and hematocrit may decrease, usually during the first 4 to 12 weeks of therapy. Monitor patient.
● Watch for hypoglycemia in patients receiving drug with insulin or a sulfonylurea and adjust dosage of these products as needed.
● Besides having blood glucose levels checked regularly, patients should also have glycosylated hemoglobin checked periodically to evaluate therapeutic response to drug.

Breast-feeding patients
● It isn't known if drug appears in breast milk. Because many drugs appear in breast milk, pioglitazone shouldn't be administered to breast-feeding women.

Pediatric patients
● Safety and effectiveness in children haven't been evaluated.

Geriatric patients
● No significant differences in drug safety and effectiveness have been observed between patients ages 65 and older and younger patients.

Patient education
● Instruct patient to adhere to dietary instructions and to have blood glucose levels and glycosylated hemoglobin tested regularly.
● Teach patient taking pioglitazone with insulin or oral antidiabetics the signs and symptoms of hypoglycemia.
● Advise patient to call during periods of stress, such as fever, trauma, infection, or surgery, because drug requirements may change.
● Notify patient that blood tests for liver function will be performed before therapy, every 2 months for the first year, and then periodically.
● Tell patient to report unexplained nausea, vomiting, abdominal pain, fatigue, anorexia, or dark urine immediately because these may indicate potential liver problems.
● Inform patient that drug can be taken with or without meals.
● Tell patient that, if a dose is missed, he shouldn't double the dose the next day.
● Advise anovulatory, premenopausal women with insulin resistance that drug may cause resumption of ovulation and contraceptive measures may need to be considered.

piperacillin sodium
Pipracil

Pharmacologic classification: extended-spectrum penicillin, acylaminopenicillin
Therapeutic classification: antibiotic
Pregnancy risk category: B

Indications and dosages
➤ *Infections caused by susceptible organisms.* Adults and children over age 12: Serious infection: 12 to 18 g daily I.V. in divided doses q 4 to 6 hours. Uncomplicated urinary tract infection (UTI) and community-acquired pneumonia: 6 to 8 g/day I.V. in divided doses q 6 to 12 hours. Complicated UTI: 8 to 16 g daily I.V. in divided doses q 6 to 8 hours. Uncomplicated gonorrhea: 2 g I.M. as a single dose. Maximum daily dose is 24 g.
Children ages 1 month to 12 years: 50 mg/kg I.V. over 30 minutes q 4 hours.
➤ *Prophylaxis of surgical infections.* *Adults:* Intra-abdominal surgery: 2 g I.V. before surgery, 2 g during surgery, and 2 g q 6 hours after surgery for no more than 24 hours. Vaginal hysterectomy: 2 g I.V. before surgery, 2 g 6 hours after first dose then 2 g 12 hours after second dose. Cesarean section: 2 g I.V. after cord is

clamped; then 2 g q 4 hours for two doses. Abdominal hysterectomy: 2 g I.V. before surgery, 2 g in postanesthesia care unit, and 2 g after 6 hours.

✦ *Dosage adjustment.* For adults with renal impairment, refer to the table.

Creatinine clearance (ml/min)	Urinary tract infection		Serious systemic infection
	Uncomplicated	Complicated	
20-40	*	3 g q 8 hr	4 g q 8 hr
< 20	3 g q 12 hr	3 g q 12 hr	4 g q 12 hr

*No dosage adjustment necessary

How supplied
Available by prescription only
Bulk vial: 40 g
Infusion: 2 g, 3 g, 4 g
Injection: 2 g, 3 g, 4 g

Pharmacodynamics
Antibiotic action: Bactericidal. Adheres to bacterial penicillin-binding proteins, thus inhibiting bacterial cell wall synthesis. Extended-spectrum penicillins are more resistant to inactivation by certain beta-lactamases, especially those produced by gram-negative organisms, but are still liable to inactivation by certain others. Because of the potential for rapid development of bacterial resistance, drug shouldn't be used as a sole drug in the treatment of an infection.

Piperacillin's spectrum of activity includes many gram-negative aerobic and anaerobic bacilli, many gram-positive and gram-negative aerobic cocci, and some gram-positive aerobic and anaerobic bacilli. Piperacillin may be effective against some strains of carbenicillin-resistant and ticarcillin-resistant gram-negative bacilli. Piperacillin is more active against *Pseudomonas aeruginosa* than are other extended-spectrum penicillins.

Pharmacokinetics
Absorption: Plasma levels peak 30 to 50 minutes after I.M. dose.
Distribution: Distributed widely after parenteral administration; penetrates minimally into uninflamed meninges and slightly into bone and sputum. 16% to 22% protein bound; crosses placenta.
Metabolism: None significant.
Excretion: 42% to 90% excreted in urine by renal tubular secretion and glomerular filtration; also excreted in bile and breast milk. Elimination half-life in adults is about ½ to 1½ hours; in extensive renal impairment, half-life extended to about 2 to 6 hours; in combined hepatorenal

dysfunction, half-life may extend from 11 to 32 hours. Drug is removed by hemodialysis but not by peritoneal dialysis.

Route	Onset	Peak	Duration
I.V.	Immediate	Immediate	Unknown
I.M.	Unknown	30-50 min	Unknown

Contraindications and precautions
Contraindicated in patients hypersensitive to drug or other penicillins. Use cautiously in patients with other drug allergies (especially to cephalosporins), bleeding tendencies, uremia, or hypokalemia.

Interactions
Drug-drug. *Aminoglycoside antibiotics:* Synergistic bactericidal effects against *Pseudomonas aeruginosa, Escherichia coli, Klebsiella, Citrobacter, Enterobacter, Serratia,* and *Proteus mirabilis.* However, drugs are physically and chemically incompatible; inactivated when mixed or given together. Don't give together.
Clavulanic acid, sulbactam, tazobactam: Synergistic bactericidal effects against certain beta-lactamase-producing bacteria. May be used together for this effect.
Methotrexate: Large doses of penicillins may interfere with renal tubular secretion of methotrexate; delayed elimination and elevated serum levels of methotrexate. Monitor patient for toxicity.
Oral contraceptives: Decreased efficacy. Suggest other means of contraception.
Probenecid: Blocked tubular secretion of piperacillin, raising serum levels of drug. Probenecid may be used for this purpose.
Vecuronium: Prolonged neuromuscular blockade. Monitor patient closely.

Adverse reactions
CNS: *seizures,* headache, dizziness, fatigue.
GI: nausea, diarrhea, vomiting, pseudomembranous colitis.
GU: interstitial nephritis.
Hematologic: *bleeding* (with high doses), *neutropenia,* eosinophilia, *leukopenia, thrombocytopenia.*
Hepatic: elevations in liver function test results.
Metabolic: *hypokalemia,* hypernatremia.
Musculoskeletal: prolonged muscle relaxation.
Other: hypersensitivity reactions (edema, fever, chills, rash, pruritus, urticaria, *anaphylaxis*), overgrowth of nonsusceptible organisms, pain at injection site, vein irritation, phlebitis.

Overdose and treatment
Overdose may cause neuromuscular hypersensitivity and seizures resulting from CNS irritation by high drug levels. A 4- to 6-hour hemodialysis will remove 10% to 50% of drug.

Special considerations
● Piperacillin is usually given with another antibiotic such as an aminoglycoside in life-threatening situations.
● Drug may be more suitable than carbenicillin or ticarcillin for patients on salt-free diets; piperacillin contains only 1.85 mEq of sodium per gram.
● Drug may be administered by direct I.V. injection, given slowly over at least 5 minutes; chest discomfort occurs if injection is given too rapidly.
● Patients with cystic fibrosis are most susceptible to fever or rash from piperacillin.
● Use reduced dosage in patients with creatinine clearance below 40 ml/minute.
● Because drug is dialyzable, patients undergoing hemodialysis may need dosage adjustments.
● Drug may falsely decrease serum aminoglycoside levels; drug may cause positive Coombs' tests.

Patient monitoring
● Monitor serum electrolytes, especially potassium.
● Monitor neurologic status. High serum levels of this drug may cause seizures.
● Monitor CBC, differential, and platelets. Drug may cause thrombocytopenia. Observe patient carefully for signs of occult bleeding.

Breast-feeding patients
● Drug appears in breast milk; use cautiously in breast-feeding women.

Pediatric patients
● Safe use in children under age 12 hasn't been established.

Geriatric patients
● Half-life may be prolonged in elderly patients because of impaired renal function.

Patient education
● Tell patient to report adverse reactions promptly.
● Advise patient to limit salt intake during therapy because drug contains 1.85 mEq of sodium/g.

piperacillin sodium and tazobactam sodium
Zosyn

Pharmacologic classification: extended-spectrum penicillin/beta-lactamase inhibitor
Therapeutic classification: antibiotic
Pregnancy risk category: B

Indications and dosages
➤ *Moderate to severe infections caused by piperacillin-resistant, piperacillin/tazobactam-susceptible, beta-lactamase–producing strains of microorganisms in the following conditions: appendicitis (complicated by rupture or abscess) and peritonitis caused by* Escherichia coli, Bacteroides fragilis, B. ovatus, B. thetaio-

taomicron, B. vulgatus; *skin and skin-structure infections caused by* Staphylococcus aureus; *postpartum endometritis or pelvic inflammatory disease caused by* E. coli; *moderately severe community-acquired pneumonia caused by* Haemophilus influenzae. *Adults:* 3.375 g (3 g piperacillin/0.375 g tazobactam) q 6 hours as a 30-minute I.V. infusion.
✦ *Dosage adjustment.* For adult or child over age 12 with creatinine clearance of 20 to 40 ml/minute, give 2.25 g (2 g piperacillin/0.25 g tazobactam) q 6 hours. If creatinine clearance is less than 20 ml/minute, give same dose q 8 hours. In hemodialysis patients, give same dose q 8 hours with a supplemental dose of 0.75 g (0.67 g piperacillin/0.08 g tazobactam) after each dialysis period.

Creatinine clearance (ml/min)	Recommended dosage
> 40	12 g/1.5 g/day in divided doses of 3.375 g q 6 hr
20-40	8 g/1 g/day in divided doses of 2.25 g q 6 hr
< 20	6 g/0.75 g/day in divided doses of 2.25 g q 8 hr

Note: Stop therapy if hypersensitivity reactions or signs and symptoms of bleeding occur.

How supplied
Available by prescription only
Powder for injection (equivalent to piperacillin/tazobactam in a ratio of 8 to 1): 2.25 g, 3.375 g, 4.5 g

Pharmacodynamics
Antibiotic action: Piperacillin is an extended-spectrum penicillin that inhibits cell-wall synthesis during microorganism multiplication; tazobactam increases piperacillin effectiveness by inactivating beta-lactamases, which destroy penicillins.

Pharmacokinetics
Absorption: No information available.
Distribution: Both piperacillin and tazobactam are about 30% bound to plasma proteins.
Metabolism: Piperacillin metabolized to minor microbiologically active desethyl metabolite; tazobactam metabolized to single metabolite that lacks pharmacologic and antibacterial activities.
Excretion: Both piperacillin and tazobactam eliminated via kidneys by glomerular filtration and tubular secretion. Piperacillin excreted rapidly as unchanged drug (68% of dose); tazobactam excreted as unchanged drug (80%) in urine.

Piperacillin, tazobactam, and desethyl piperacillin also secreted into bile.

Route	Onset	Peak	Duration
I.V.	Immediate	Immediate	Unknown

Contraindications and precautions

Contraindicated in patients hypersensitive to drug or other penicillins. Use cautiously in patients with drug allergies (especially to cephalosporins), bleeding tendencies, uremia, or hypokalemia.

Interactions

Drug-drug. *Aminoglycosides:* Substantial inactivation of aminoglycoside. Don't mix in same I.V. container.
Heparin, oral anticoagulants, other drugs affecting blood coagulation system or thrombocyte function: Prolonged effectiveness. Monitor coagulation parameters more frequently.
Probenecid: Increased blood levels of piperacillin/tazobactam. Probenecid may be used for this purpose.
Vecuronium: Prolonged neuromuscular blockade of vecuronium. Monitor patient closely.

Adverse reactions

CNS: *headache, insomnia,* agitation, dizziness, anxiety.
CV: hypertension, tachycardia, chest pain, edema.
EENT: rhinitis.
GI: *diarrhea, nausea, constipation,* vomiting, dyspepsia, stool changes, abdominal pain.
GU: interstitial nephritis.
Hematologic: *leukopenia,* anemia, eosinophilia, *thrombocytopenia.*
Respiratory: dyspnea.
Skin: rash (including maculopapular, bullous, urticarial, and eczematoid), pruritus.
Other: fever, pain, candidiasis, inflammation and phlebitis at I.V. site, *anaphylaxis.*

Overdose and treatment

No information available.

Special considerations

● Pseudomembranous colitis has been reported with nearly all antibacterial drugs, including piperacillin/tazobactam, and may range in severity from mild to life-threatening. Therefore, consider this diagnosis in patients with diarrhea after piperacillin/tazobactam administration.
● Bacterial and fungal superinfection may occur and warrants appropriate measures.
● Use piperacillin/tazobactam with an aminoglycoside to treat infections caused by *Pseudomonas aeruginosa.*
● Piperacillin/tazobactam contains 2.35 mEq (54 mg) of sodium per g of piperacillin in combination product. Consider this when treating patients requiring restricted sodium intake.
● As with other semisynthetic penicillins, piperacillin has been linked to increased risk of fever and rash in patients with cystic fibrosis.

● Reconstitute piperacillin/tazobactam with 5 ml of diluent per 1 g of piperacillin. Appropriate diluents include sterile or bacteriostatic water for injection, normal saline solution injection, bacteriostatic normal saline solution injection, D_5W, dextrose 5% in normal saline solution injection, or dextran 6% in normal saline solution injection. Don't use lactated Ringer's injection. Shake until dissolved. Further dilution can be made to a final desired volume.
● Infuse over at least 30 minutes. Stop primary infusion during administration if possible. Don't mix with other drugs.
● Use single-dose vials immediately after reconstitution. Discard unused drug after 24 hours if held at room temperature; 48 hours if refrigerated. Once diluted, drug is stable in I.V. bags for 24 hours at room temperature or 1 week if refrigerated.
● As with other penicillins, piperacillin/tazobactam may result in false-positive reaction for urine glucose using a copper-reduction method such as Clinitest. Glucose tests based on enzymatic glucose oxidase reactions (such as Diastix or glucose enzymatic test strip) are recommended.

Patient monitoring

● Obtain specimen for culture and sensitivity tests before giving first dose. Therapy may begin pending results.
● Perform periodic electrolyte determinations in patients with low potassium reserves; hypokalemia can occur when patient with potentially low potassium reserves receives cytotoxic therapy or diuretics.

Breast-feeding patients

● Low levels of piperacillin appear in breast milk (no information on tazobactam levels). Use piperacillin/tazobactam cautiously in breast-feeding women.

Pediatric patients

● Safety and effectiveness in children under age 12 haven't been established.

Patient education

● Tell patient to report adverse reactions promptly.

pirbuterol acetate
Maxair

Pharmacologic classification: beta-adrenergic agonist
Therapeutic classification: bronchodilator
Pregnancy risk category: C

Indications and dosages

➤ *Prevention and reversal of bronchospasm; asthma. Adults and children age 12 and over:* 1 or 2 inhalations (0.2 to 0.4 mg) repeated q 4 to 6 hours. Not to exceed 12 inhalations daily.

How supplied
Available by prescription only
Inhaler: 0.2 mg per inhalation

Pharmacodynamics
Bronchodilating action: Stimulates beta$_2$-adrenergic receptors and increases the activity of intracellular adenylate cyclase, an enzyme that catalyzes the conversion of adenosine triphosphate to cyclic adenosine monophosphate (cAMP). Elevated cellular cAMP is related to bronchodilation and inhibition of the cellular release of mediators of immediate hypersensitivity.

Pharmacokinetics
Absorption: Serum levels achieved after inhalation of usual dose.
Distribution: Drug acts locally.
Metabolism: Metabolized in liver.
Excretion: About 50% of inhaled dose recovered in urine as parent drug and metabolites.

Route	Onset	Peak	Duration
Inhalation	5 min	½-1 hr	5 hr

Contraindications and precautions
Contraindicated in patients hypersensitive to drug. Use cautiously in patients with CV disorders, hyperthyroidism, diabetes, or seizure disorders and in those who are sensitive to sympathomimetic amines.

Interactions
Drug-drug. *MAO inhibitors, tricyclic antidepressants:* Enhanced vascular effects of beta-adrenergic agonists. Use together cautiously.
Propranolol, other beta blockers: Decreased bronchodilating effects of beta agonists. Avoid using together.

Adverse reactions
CNS: tremor, nervousness, dizziness, insomnia, headache, vertigo.
CV: tachycardia, palpitations, chest tightness.
EENT: dry or irritated throat.
GI: dry mouth, nausea, vomiting, diarrhea.
Respiratory: cough.

Overdose and treatment
Anginal pain, hypertension, and tachycardia may result from overdose. Sedatives or barbiturates may be necessary to counteract any adverse CNS effects; cautious use of beta blockers may be useful to counteract cardiac effects.

Special considerations
● Don't administer to patients who are receiving other beta-adrenergic bronchodilators.

Patient monitoring
● Monitor patients for worsening symptoms of asthma.
● Watch for increased inhaler use.

Breast-feeding patients
● It isn't known if drug appears in breast milk. Use cautiously in breast-feeding women.

Pediatric patients
● Use in children under age 12 isn't recommended.

Patient education
● Warn patient not to exceed recommended maximum dose of 12 inhalations daily. He should call if a previously effective dosage doesn't control symptoms because this may signify a worsening of disease.
● Tell patient to call promptly if he experiences increased bronchospasm after using drug.
● Teach patient how to use metered dose inhaler correctly. Have him shake container, exhale through the nose, administer aerosol while inhaling deeply on mouthpiece of inhaler, hold breath for a few seconds, then exhale slowly. Tell him to allow at least 2 minutes between inhalations, and to wait at least 5 minutes before using his corticosteroid inhalant (if he's also taking inhalational corticosteroids).

piroxicam
Apo-Piroxicam*, Feldene, Novo-Pirocam*

Pharmacologic classification: NSAID
Therapeutic classification: nonnarcotic analgesic, antipyretic, anti-inflammatory
Pregnancy risk category: B (D in third trimester or near delivery)

Indications and dosages
➤ *Osteoarthritis, rheumatoid arthritis.*
Adults: 20 mg P.O. once daily. If desired, the dose may be divided.
➤ *Juvenile rheumatoid arthritis◇. Children who weigh 15 to 30 kg (33 to 67 lb):* 5 mg P.O.
Children who weigh 31 to 45 kg (68 to 100 lb): 10 mg P.O.
Children who weigh 46 to 55 kg (101 to 121 lb): 15 mg P.O.

How supplied
Available by prescription only
Capsules: 10 mg, 20 mg

Pharmacodynamics
Analgesic, antipyretic, and anti-inflammatory actions: Exact mechanisms unknown. Thought to inhibit prostaglandin synthesis.

Pharmacokinetics
Absorption: Absorbed rapidly from GI tract. Peak effect seen 3 to 5 hours after dosing. Food delays absorption.
Distribution: Highly protein-bound.
Metabolism: Metabolized in liver.

Excretion: Excreted in urine. Long half-life (about 50 hours) allows for once-daily dosing.

Route	Onset	Peak	Duration
P.O.	1 hr	3-5 hr	48-72 hr

Contraindications and precautions

Contraindicated in patients hypersensitive to drug, in those with bronchospasm or angioedema precipitated by aspirin or NSAIDs, during pregnancy, or while breast-feeding.

Use cautiously in elderly patients and in patients with GI disorders, hypertension, conditions predisposing to fluid retention, or history of renal, peptic ulcer, or cardiac disease.

Interactions

Drug-drug. *Acetaminophen, gold compounds, other anti-inflammatories:* Increased nephrotoxicity. Monitor patient for toxicity.

Anticoagulants, thrombolytics (coumarin derivatives, heparin, other highly protein-bound drugs): May potentiate anticoagulant effects. Monitor PTT, PT, and INR.

Antihypertensives, diuretics: Decreased effectiveness of these drugs; using piroxicam with diuretics may increase risk of nephrotoxicity. Monitor patient.

Anti-inflammatories, corticotropin, salicylates, corticosteroids: GI adverse effects, including ulceration and hemorrhage. Use together cautiously.

Aspirin: Decreased bioavailability of piroxicam. Don't administer together.

Coumarin derivatives, nifedipine, phenytoin, verapamil: Piroxicam may displace highly protein-bound drugs. Monitor patient for toxicity.

Drugs that inhibit platelet aggregation (such as aspirin, cefamandole, cefoperazone, dextran, dipyridamole, mezlocillin, piperacillin, plicamycin, salicylates, sulfinpyrazone, ticarcillin, valproic acid, other anti-inflammatories): Possible bleeding problems. Monitor patient.

Insulin, oral antidiabetics: Potentiated hypoglycemic effects. Monitor serum glucose level.

Lithium, methotrexate: Decreased renal clearance of these drugs. Monitor plasma levels.

Drug-herb. *Dong quai, feverfew, garlic, ginger, horse chestnut, red clover:* Possible increased risk of bleeding. Discourage use together.

St. John's wort, dong quai: Increased risk of photosensitivity. Advise patient to avoid unprotected exposure to sunlight.

Drug-lifestyle. *Alcohol use:* Increased GI adverse effects, including ulceration and hemorrhage. Discourage alcohol use.

Sun exposure: Photosensitivity reaction. Tell patient to take precautions.

Adverse reactions

CNS: headache, drowsiness, dizziness, somnolence, vertigo.
CV: peripheral edema.
EENT: auditory disturbances.

GI: *epigastric distress, nausea, occult blood loss,* **peptic ulceration, severe GI bleeding,** diarrhea, constipation, abdominal pain, dyspepsia, flatulence, anorexia, stomatitis.
GU: *nephrotoxicity,* elevated BUN level.
Hematologic: prolonged bleeding time, anemia, *leukopenia, aplastic anemia, agranulocytosis,* eosinophilia, *thrombocytopenia.*
Hepatic: elevated liver enzyme levels.
Skin: pruritus, rash, urticaria, *photosensitivity.*

Overdose and treatment

To treat piroxicam overdose, empty stomach immediately by inducing emesis with ipecac syrup or by gastric lavage. Administer activated charcoal via nasogastric tube. Provide symptomatic and supportive measures, such as respiratory support and correction of fluid and electrolyte imbalances. Monitor laboratory parameters and vital signs closely.

Special considerations

• Drug is usually administered as a single dose.
• Adverse skin reactions are more common with piroxicam than with other NSAIDs; photosensitivity reactions are the most common.
• Drug hasn't been proven safe for fetus.

Patient monitoring

• Effectiveness isn't usually seen for at least 2 weeks after therapy begins. Evaluate response to drug as evidenced by reduced symptoms.
• Monitor renal and hepatic function and CBC periodically during therapy.

Breast-feeding patients

• Drug may inhibit lactation. Drug appears in breast milk at 1% of maternal serum levels; avoid use in breast-feeding women.

Pediatric patients

• Safe use of long-term piroxicam in children hasn't been established.

Geriatric patients

• Patients over age 60 are more sensitive to drug's adverse effects. Use cautiously. Because of its effect on renal prostaglandins, drug may cause fluid retention and edema. This may be significant in elderly patients and in those with heart failure.

Patient education

• Advise patient to call before taking OTC or herbal products.
• Caution patient to avoid hazardous activities until CNS effects are known. Instruct patient in safety measures to prevent injury.
• Review adverse effects. Tell patient to report them immediately.
• Encourage patient to comply with recommended medical follow-up.
• Tell patient to avoid aspirin and alcohol.

plasma protein fraction
Plasmanate, Plasma-Plex, Plasmatein, Protenate

Pharmacologic classification: blood derivative
Therapeutic classification: plasma volume expander
Pregnancy risk category: C

Indications and dosages
➤ **Shock.** *Adults:* Varies with patient's condition and response, but usually 250 to 500 ml (12.5 to 25 g protein) I.V., not to exceed 10 ml/minute.
Children: 22 to 33 ml/kg I.V. infused at rate of 5 to 10 ml/minute.
Small children and infants: 15 ml/2.2 kg (1 lb) I.V. infused at rate of 5 to 10 ml/minute (Plasma-Plex).
➤ **Hypoproteinemia.** *Adults:* 1,000 to 1,500 ml I.V. daily. Maximum infusion rate is 8 ml/minute (500 ml infused in 30 to 45 minutes).

How supplied
Available by prescription only
Injection: 5% solution in 50-ml, 250-ml, 500-ml vials

Pharmacodynamics
Plasma-expanding action: Supplies colloid to the blood and expands plasma volume. Causes fluid to shift from interstitial spaces into the circulation and slightly increases the plasma protein level. Comprised mostly of albumin, but may contain up to 17% alpha and beta globulins and not more than 1% gamma globulin.

Pharmacokinetics
The pharmacokinetics of plasma protein fraction (PPF) are similar to its chief constituent, albumin (about 83% to 90%).
Absorption: Albumin isn't adequately absorbed from GI tract.
Distribution: Albumin accounts for about 50% of plasma proteins. Distributed into intravascular space and extravascular sites, including skin, muscle, and lungs. In patients with reduced circulating blood volumes, hemodilution secondary to albumin administration lasts for many hours; in patients with normal blood volume, excess fluid and protein are lost from intravascular space within a few hours.
Metabolism: Albumin synthesized in liver, but liver isn't involved in clearance of albumin from plasma in healthy individuals.
Excretion: Little is known about albumin excretion in healthy individuals. Administration of albumin decreases hepatic albumin synthesis and increases albumin clearance if plasma oncotic pressure is high. In certain pathologic states, liv-

er, kidneys, or intestines may provide elimination mechanisms.

Route	Onset	Peak	Duration
I.V.	Immediate	Immediate	Unknown

Contraindications and precautions
Contraindicated in patients with severe anemia or heart failure and in those undergoing cardiac bypass. Use cautiously in patients with impaired renal or hepatic function, low cardiac reserve, or restricted salt intake.

Interactions
None reported.

Adverse reactions
CNS: headache.
CV: hypotension (after rapid infusion or intra-arterial administration), *vascular overload*, tachycardia.
GI: nausea, vomiting, hypersalivation.
Metabolic: increased plasma protein levels.
Musculoskeletal: back pain.
Respiratory: dyspnea, *pulmonary edema*.
Skin: rash.
Other: flushing, chills, fever.

Overdose and treatment
Rapid infusion can cause circulatory overload and pulmonary edema. Watch patient for signs of hypervolemia; monitor blood pressure and central venous pressure. Treatment is symptomatic.

Special considerations
● Don't use solution if cloudy, contains sediment, or has been frozen. Store at room temperature; freezing may break bottle and allow bacterial contamination.
● Use opened solution promptly, discarding unused portion after 4 hours; solution contains no preservatives and becomes unstable.
● One unit is usually considered to be 250 ml of the 5% concentration.
⚠ ALERT Avoid rapid I.V. infusion. Rate is individualized according to patient's age, condition, and diagnosis. Maximum dose is 250 g/48 hours; don't give faster than 10 ml/minute. Decrease infusion rate to 5 to 8 ml/minute as plasma volume approaches normal.
● PPF is also used in treatment of burns; dosage depends on extent and severity of burn.
● No cross-matching is needed. PPF shouldn't be administered with same administration set of solutions containing protein hydrolysates, amino acid solutions, or alcohol.
● If patient is dehydrated, give additional fluids either P.O. or I.V.
● Each liter contains 130 to 160 mEq of sodium before dilution with any additional I.V. fluids; a 250-ml container of the 5% concentration contains about 33 to 40 mEq sodium.

Reactions may be *common*, uncommon, *life-threatening*, or COMMON AND LIFE-THREATENING.

Patient monitoring
• Monitor blood pressure frequently; slow or stop infusion if hypotension suddenly occurs. Vital signs should return to normal gradually.
• Observe patient for signs of vascular overload (heart failure, pulmonary edema, widening pulse pressure indicating increased cardiac output) and signs of hemorrhage or shock (after surgery or trauma); be alert for bleeding sites not evident at lower blood pressure.
• Monitor intake and output (watch especially for decreased output), hemoglobin and serum protein and electrolyte levels, and hematocrit to help determine ongoing dosage.

Breast-feeding patients
• Drug may inhibit lactation. Drug appears in breast milk at 1% of maternal serum levels; avoid use in breast-feeding women.

Pediatric patients
• Safe use of long-term piroxicam in children hasn't been established.

Geriatric patients
• Patients over age 60 are more sensitive to drug's adverse effects. Use cautiously. Because of its effect on renal prostaglandins, drug may cause fluid retention and edema. This may be significant in elderly patients and in those with heart failure.

Patient education
• Explain use and administration of drug to patient and family.
• Tell patient to report adverse reactions promptly.

plicamycin
Mithracin

Pharmacologic classification: antibiotic antineoplastic (not specific to cell cycle phase)
Therapeutic classification: antineoplastic, hypocalcemic
Pregnancy risk category: X

Indications and dosages
Dosage and indications may vary. Check current literature for recommended protocol.
➤ *Hypercalcemia. Adults:* 25 mcg/kg I.V. daily over 4 to 6 hours for 3 to 4 days. Repeat at intervals of 1 week, p.r.n.
➤ *Testicular cancer. Adults:* 25 to 30 mcg/kg I.V. daily over 4 to 6 hours for up to 10 days (based on ideal body weight or actual weight, whichever is less).
➤ *Paget's disease ◇. Adults:* 15 mcg/kg I.V. daily over 4 to 6 hours for up to 10 days.

How supplied
Available by prescription only
Injection: 2,500-mcg vials

Pharmacodynamics
Antineoplastic action: Exerts cytotoxic activity by intercalating between DNA base pairs and also binding to the outside of the DNA molecule. The result is inhibition of DNA-dependent RNA synthesis.
Hypocalcemic action: Exact mechanism unknown. May block the hypercalcemic effect of vitamin D or may inhibit the effect of parathyroid hormone upon osteoclasts, preventing osteolysis. Both mechanisms reduce serum calcium levels.

Pharmacokinetics
Absorption: Not administered orally.
Distribution: Distributed mainly into Kupffer's cells of liver, into renal tubular cells, and along formed bone surfaces. Crosses blood-brain barrier; achieves appreciable levels in CSF.
Metabolism: Poorly understood.
Excretion: Eliminated primarily through kidneys.

Route	Onset	Peak	Duration
I.V.	1-2 days	3 days	7-10 days

Contraindications and precautions
Contraindicated in patients with thrombocytopenia, bone marrow suppression, or coagulation and bleeding disorders and in women who are or who may become pregnant. Use cautiously in patients with impaired renal or hepatic function.

Interactions
None reported.

Adverse reactions
CNS: drowsiness, weakness, lethargy, headache, malaise.
GI: *nausea, vomiting,* anorexia, diarrhea, stomatitis.
GU: increased BUN and serum creatinine levels.
Hematologic: *leukopenia, thrombocytopenia, bleeding syndrome*.
Hepatic: *elevated liver enzyme levels, hepatotoxicity*.
Metabolic: decreased *serum calcium,* potassium, and phosphorus levels.
Skin: facial flushing, rash.
Other: fever, cellulitis with extravasation, phlebitis.

Overdose and treatment
Toxicity may cause myelosuppression, electrolyte imbalance, and coagulation disorders. Treatment includes transfusion of blood components. Patient's renal and hepatic status should be closely monitored.

Special considerations
• To reconstitute drug, use 4.9 ml of sterile water to give a concentration of 500 mcg/ml. Reconstitute drug immediately before administration, and discard unused solution.
• Drug may be further diluted with normal saline solution or D_5W to a volume of 1,000 ml and administered as an I.V. infusion over 4 to 6 hours.

• To reduce nausea, give antiemetics before administering drug.

• Although drug may be administered by I.V. push injection, this method is discouraged because of the higher risk and greater severity of GI toxicity. Nausea and vomiting are greatly diminished as infusion rate is decreased.

• Infusions of plicamycin in 1,000 ml D₅W are stable for up to 24 hours.

• If I.V. infiltrates, infusion should be stopped immediately and ice packs applied before restarting an I.V. in other arm.

• Therapeutic effect in hypercalcemia may not be seen for 24 to 48 hours; may last 3 to 15 days.

• Avoid drug contact with skin or mucous membranes.

• Store lyophilized powder in refrigerator.

Patient monitoring

• Monitor LDH, AST, ALT, alkaline phosphatase, BUN, creatinine, potassium, calcium, and phosphorus levels.

• Monitor platelet count and PT before and during therapy.

• Check serum calcium levels. Monitor patient for tetany, carpopedal spasm, Chvostek's sign, and muscle cramps because a sharp drop in calcium levels is possible.

• Watch for signs of bleeding. Facial flushing may be an early indicator.

Breast-feeding patients

• It isn't known if drug appears in breast milk. Because of potential for serious adverse reactions, mutagenicity, and carcinogenicity in infant, breast-feeding isn't recommended.

Patient education

• Tell patient to use salicylate-free drugs for pain relief or fever reduction.

• Instruct patient to avoid exposure to people with infections and to call immediately if signs of infection or unusual bleeding occur.

• Inform patient that he and household members shouldn't receive immunizations during therapy and for several weeks after therapy.

• Advise patient to use contraceptive measures during therapy.

pneumococcal vaccine, polyvalent

Pneumovax 23, Pnu-Imune 23

Pharmacologic classification: vaccine
Therapeutic classification: bacterial vaccine
Pregnancy risk category: C

Indications and dosages

➤ *Pneumococcal immunization. Adults and children over age 2:* 0.5 ml I.M. or S.C. as a one-time dose.

How supplied

Available by prescription only
Injection: 25 mcg each of 23 polysaccharide isolates of *Streptococcus pneumoniae* per 0.5-ml dose, in 1-ml and 5-ml vials and disposable syringes.

Pharmacodynamics

Pneumonia prophylaxis: Promotes active immunity against the 23 most prevalent pneumococcal types.

Pharmacokinetics

Absorption: Protective antibodies produced within 3 weeks after injection. Duration of vaccine-induced immunity at least 5 years in adults.
Distribution: No information available.
Metabolism: No information available.
Excretion: No information available.

Route	Onset	Peak	Duration
I.M., S.C.	2-3 wk	Unknown	5 yr

Contraindications and precautions

Contraindicated in patients hypersensitive to drug or its components (phenol). Also contraindicated in patients with Hodgkin's disease who have received extensive chemotherapy or nodal irradiation.

Interactions

Drug-drug. *Corticosteroids, other immunosuppressants:* Impaired immune response to vaccine; vaccination should be avoided.

Adverse reactions

CNS: headache.
GI: nausea, vomiting.
Musculoskeletal: myalgia, arthralgia.
Skin: rash.
Other: adenitis, ***anaphylaxis***, serum sickness, *slight fever, soreness at injection site,* severe local reaction caused by revaccination within 3 years.

Overdose and treatment

No information available.

Special considerations

• Obtain thorough history of allergies and reactions to immunizations.

• Persons with asplenia who received the 14-valent vaccine should be revaccinated with the 23-valent vaccine.

• Have epinephrine solution 1:1,000 available to treat allergic reactions.

• Use deltoid or midlateral thigh. Don't inject I.V. Avoid intradermal administration because this may cause severe local reactions.

• Polyvalent pneumococcal vaccine also may be administered to children to prevent pneumococcal otitis media.

• Candidates for pneumococcal vaccine include persons ages 65 and older; adults and children ages 2 and older with chronic illness, asplenia,

or splenic dysfunction; and those with sickle-cell anemia and HIV infection.
● Vaccine also is recommended for patients awaiting organ transplants, those receiving radiation therapy or cancer chemotherapy, persons in nursing homes and orphanages, and bedridden individuals.
● If different sites and separate syringes are used, pneumococcal vaccine may be administered simultaneously with influenza, DTP, poliovirus, or *Haemophilus* b polysaccharide vaccines.
● Store vaccine at 36° to 46° F (2° to 8° C). Reconstitution or dilution is unnecessary.

Patient monitoring
● Monitor patient for adverse effects.

Breast-feeding patients
● It isn't known if vaccine appears in breast milk. Use cautiously in breast-feeding women.

Pediatric patients
● Children under age 2 don't respond satisfactorily to pneumococcal vaccine. Safety and efficacy of vaccine haven't been established.

Patient education
● Tell patient to expect redness, soreness, swelling, and pain at injection site after vaccination. Patient may also develop fever, joint or muscle aches and pains, rash, itching, general weakness, or difficulty breathing.
● Encourage patient to report distressing adverse reactions promptly.
● Advise patient to use acetaminophen to relieve adverse reactions promptly.

poliovirus vaccine, inactivated (IPV)
IPOL

poliovirus vaccine, live, oral, trivalent (Sabin vaccine, TOPV)
Orimune

Pharmacologic classification: vaccine
Therapeutic classification: viral vaccine
Pregnancy risk category: C

Indications and dosages
➤ *Poliovirus immunization (primary series).* *Adolescents and older children:* Two 0.5-ml doses administered 8 weeks apart. Give third 0.5-ml dose 6 to 12 months after second dose.
Infants: 0.5 ml at ages 2 months, 4 months, and 18 months. Optional dose may be given at 6 months when substantial risk of exposure exists.
Supplementary: All children entering elementary school (ages 4 to 6) who have completed the primary series should receive a single follow-up dose of TOPV. Booster vaccination beyond elementary school isn't routinely recommended.

Adults age 18 and over: TOPV shouldn't be given to persons age 18 and over who haven't received at least one prior dose of TOPV. Enhanced potency inactivated polio vaccine (eIPV) should be used if polio vaccination is indicated.
If less than 4 weeks are available before protection is needed, a single dose of TOPV is recommended, then IPV later if the person remains at increased risk.
Persons traveling to countries with endemic or epidemic polio who previously completed a primary series should receive a single follow-up dose of TOPV. Don't administer vaccine to neonates under age 6 weeks.
➤ *Poliovirus immunization (IPV).* *Infants and children (primary series):* 0.5 ml S.C. or I.M. at 2 months, 4 months, 6 to 18 months, and at 4 to 6 years. Minimum interval between doses is 4 weeks. Or use sequential IPV/oral poliovirus vaccine (OPV) regimen: IPV given at 2 and 4 months of age, then OPV at 12 to 18 months and 4 to 6 years.
Adults: Three doses: Two doses 0.5 ml S.C. or I.M., 4 to 8 weeks apart, and third dose given 6 to 12 weeks after second dose.

How supplied
Available by prescription only
poliovirus vaccine, inactivated (IPV)
Injectable suspension: 40 D antigen units of type 1 (Mahoney), 8 D antigen units of type 2 (MEF-1), and 32 D antigen units of type 3 (Saukett) per 0.5 ml
poliovirus vaccine, live, oral, trivalent
Oral vaccine: mixture of three viruses (types 1, 2, and 3), grown in monkey kidney tissue culture, in 0.5-ml single-dose Dispettes

Pharmacodynamics
Polio prophylaxis: TOPV and IPV promote immunity to poliomyelitis by inducing humoral and secretory antibodies and antibodies in the lymphatic tissue of the GI tract.

Pharmacokinetics
Absorption: Antibody response to vaccine occurs within 7 to 10 days after ingestion; peaks around 21 days. Duration of immunity thought to be lifelong.
Distribution: No information available.
Metabolism: No information available.
Excretion: No information available.

Route	Onset	Peak	Duration
P.O.	7-10 days	21 days	Years
I.M., S.C.	Unknown	Unknown	Years

Contraindications and precautions
Oral vaccine is contraindicated in immunosuppressed patients, in those with cancer or immunoglobulin abnormalities, and in those receiving radiation, antimetabolite, alkylating drug, or corticosteroid therapy. These patients should receive IPV. Injectable vaccine is contraindicat-

ed in patients hypersensitive to neomycin, streptomycin, or polymyxin B.

Use cautiously in siblings of children with known immunodeficiency syndrome.

Interactions
Drug-drug. *Corticosteroids, other immunosuppressants:* Impaired immune response to vaccine. Defer vaccination with TOPV until immunosuppressant is stopped; or inactivated poliovirus vaccine may be used.
Immune serum globulin, transfusions of blood or blood products: Interference with immune response to vaccine. Defer vaccination for 3 months in these situations.

Adverse reactions
CNS: sleepiness.
GI: decreased appetite.
Skin: induration, erythema.
Other: crying, *fever, hypersensitivity reactions, poliomyelitis, pain* (at injection site).

Overdose and treatment
No information available.

Special considerations
● Obtain thorough history of allergies, especially to antibiotics, and of reactions to immunizations.
● Vaccine isn't effective in modifying or preventing existing or incubating poliomyelitis.
● Adults and immunocompromised persons who haven't been vaccinated should receive IPV (Salk) in three doses, given 1 month apart, before other household contacts are immunized with TOPV.
● TOPV isn't for parenteral use. Dose may be administered directly or mixed with distilled water, chlorine-free tap water, simple syrup USP, or milk. It also may be placed on bread, cake, or a sugar cube.
● Keep TOPV frozen until used. It may be refrigerated up to 30 days once thawed, if unopened. Opened vials may be refrigerated up to 7 days. IPV should be refrigerated; don't freeze.
● Color change from pink to yellow has no effect on efficacy of TOPV as long as vaccine remains clear. Yellow color results from storage at low temperatures.
● Vaccine may temporarily decrease response to tuberculin skin testing. If a tuberculin test is necessary, administer either before, simultaneously with, or at least 8 weeks after TOPV.

Patient monitoring
● Check parents' immunization history when they bring in child for vaccine; this is an excellent time for parents to receive booster immunizations.
● Monitor patient for adverse effects.

Breast-feeding patients
● It isn't known if drug appears in breast milk. Breast-feeding doesn't interfere with successful immunization; no interruption in feeding schedule is necessary.

Pediatric patients
● Poliovirus vaccine shouldn't be administered to neonates under age 6 weeks.

Patient education
● Inform patient that risk of vaccine-associated paralysis is extremely small for vaccines, susceptible family members, and other close contacts (about 1 case per 2.6 million patients receiving the vaccines).
● Encourage patient to report distressing adverse reactions promptly.

polyethylene glycol-electrolyte solution (PEG-ES)
Colovage, CoLyte, GoLYTELY, NuLytely, OCL

Pharmacologic classification: polyethylene glycol 3350 nonabsorbable solution
Therapeutic classification: laxative and bowel evacuant
Pregnancy risk category: C

Indications and dosages
➤ *Bowel preparation before GI examination. Adults:* 240 ml P.O. q 10 minutes until 4 L are consumed or rectal effluent is clear. Typically, administer 4 hours before examination, allowing 3 hours for drinking and 1 hour for bowel evacuation.
➤ *Management of acute iron overdose* ◊.
Children under age 3: 0.5 L/hour.

Note: If a patient experiences severe bloating, distention, or abdominal pain, slow or temporarily stop administration until symptoms abate.

How supplied
Available by prescription only
Powder for oral solution: polyethylene glycol (PEG) 3350 (6 g), anhydrous sodium sulfate (568 mg), sodium chloride (146 mg), potassium chloride (74.5 mg/100 ml) (Colovage); PEG 3350 (120 g), sodium sulfate (3.36 g), sodium chloride (2.92 g), potassium chloride (1.49 g/2 L) (CoLyte); PEG 3350 (236 g), sodium sulfate (22.74 g), sodium bicarbonate (6.74 g), sodium chloride (5.86 g), potassium chloride (2.97 g/4.8 L) (GoLYTELY); PEG 3350 (420 g), sodium bicarbonate (5.72 g), sodium chloride (11.2 g), potassium chloride (1.48 g/4 L) (NuLytely); PEG 3350 (6 g), sodium sulfate decahydrate (1.29 g), sodium chloride (146 mg), potassium chloride (75 mg), polysorbate-80 (30 mg/100 ml) (OCL)

Pharmacodynamics
Laxative and bowel evacuant action: Acts as an osmotic product. With sodium sulfate as the major sodium source, active sodium absorption is markedly reduced. Diarrhea results, which rapidly cleans the bowel, usually within 4 hours.

Reactions may be *common*, uncommon, **life-threatening**, or COMMON AND LIFE-THREATENING.

Pharmacokinetics
Absorption: Nonabsorbable solution. Onset of action within 30 to 60 minutes.
Distribution: Not applicable; not absorbed.
Metabolism: Not applicable; not absorbed.
Excretion: Excreted via GI tract.

Route	Onset	Peak	Duration
P.O.	1 hr	Variable	Variable

Contraindications and precautions
Contraindicated in patients with GI obstruction or perforation, gastric retention, toxic colitis, ileus, or megacolon.

Interactions
Drug-drug. *Oral drugs:* Drug given within 1 hour before start of therapy may be flushed from GI tract and not absorbed. Avoid oral drug within this time frame.

Adverse reactions
EENT: rhinorrhea.
GI: *nausea, bloating, cramps, vomiting, abdominal fullness,* anal irritation.
Skin: urticaria, dermatitis.
Other: *anaphylaxis.*

Overdose and treatment
No information available.

Special considerations
● Drug may be given via nasogastric tube (at 20 to 30 ml/minute, or 1.2 to 1.8 L/hour) to patients unwilling or unable to drink preparation. First bowel movement should occur within 1 hour.
● Tap water may be used to reconstitute solution. Shake container vigorously several times to ensure powder is completely dissolved. After reconstitution to 4 L with water, the solution contains PEG 3350 17.6 mmol/L, sodium 125 mmol/L, sulfate 40 mmol/L (CoLyte 80 mmol/L), chloride 35 mmol/L, bicarbonate 20 mmol/L, and potassium 10 mmol/L (1 mmol/L = 1 mEq/L).
● Store reconstituted solution in refrigerator (chilling before administration improves palatability); use within 48 hours.
● Don't add flavorings or additional ingredients to solution before use.
● No major shifts in fluid or electrolyte balance have been reported.
● Patient preparation for barium enema may be less satisfactory with this solution because it may interfere with barium coating of colonic mucosa using the double-contrast technique.

Patient monitoring
● Monitor patient for adverse GI reactions.

Patient education
● Instruct patient to fast about 3 to 4 hours before ingesting solution.
● Tell patient not to take solid foods less than 2 hours before solution is administered. Also inform him that no foods except clear liquids are permitted after administration of solution until examination is completed.

---

polysaccharide iron complex
Hytinic, Niferex, Niferex-150, Nu-Iron, Nu-Iron 150

Pharmacologic classification: oral iron supplement
Therapeutic classification: hematinic
Pregnancy risk category: NR

Indications and dosages
➤ *Uncomplicated iron-deficiency anemia.*
Adults and children age 12 and older: 150 to 300 mg P.O. daily as capsules or tablets or 1 to 2 teaspoonfuls of elixir P.O. daily.
Children ages 6 to 12: 150 mg to 300 mg P.O. daily as tablets or 1 teaspoonful of elixir P.O. daily.
Children ages 2 to 6: ½ teaspoonful of elixir P.O. daily.

How supplied
Available without a prescription
Capsules: 150 mg
Solution: 100 mg/5 ml
Tablets (film-coated): 50 mg

Pharmacodynamics
Hematinic action: Provides elemental iron, an essential component in the formation of hemoglobin.

Pharmacokinetics
Absorption: Although iron is absorbed from entire length of GI tract, duodenum and proximal jejunum are primary absorption sites. Up to 10% of iron absorbed by healthy individuals; patients with iron-deficiency anemia may absorb up to 60%. Enteric coating and some extended-release formulas have decreased absorption; designed to release iron past points in GI tract of highest absorption. Food may decrease absorption by 33% to 50%.
Distribution: Iron is transported through GI mucosal cells directly into blood; immediately bound to a carrier protein, transferrin, and transported to bone marrow for incorporation into hemoglobin. Iron is highly protein-bound.
Metabolism: Iron is liberated by hemoglobin destruction but is conserved and reused by body.
Excretion: Healthy individuals lose only small amounts of iron each day. Men and postmenopausal women lose about 1 mg/day; premenopausal women about 1.5 mg/day. Loss usually occurs in nails, hair, feces, and urine; trace amounts lost in bile and sweat.

Route	Onset	Peak	Duration
P.O.	Few days	2-10 days	2 mo

Contraindications and precautions
Contraindicated in patients hypersensitive to drug or its components and in those with hemochromatosis and hemosiderosis.

Interactions
Drug-drug. *Antacids, cholestyramine resin, cimetidine, tetracycline, vitamin E:* Decreased iron absorption. Separate administration times by 2 to 4 hours.
Chloramphenicol: Delayed response to iron therapy. Monitor patient closely.
Fluoroquinolones, levodopa, methyldopa, penicillamine: Decreased absorption of these drugs, possibly resulting in decreased serum levels or efficacy. Monitor patient.
Vitamin C: Increased iron absorption. Give together.
Drug-food. *Coffee, dairy products, eggs, tea, whole-grain breads and cereals:* Decreased iron absorption. Separate use by 2 to 4 hours.
Foods high in vitamin C: Increased iron absorption. Give with these foods.

Adverse reactions
GI: nausea, constipation, black stools, epigastric pain. (Linked to iron therapy; however, few, if any, occur with polysaccharide-iron complex. Iron-containing liquids may cause temporary staining of teeth.)

Overdose and treatment
The lethal dose of iron is between 200 and 250 mg/kg; fatalities have occurred with lower doses. Symptoms may follow ingestion of 20 to 60 mg/kg. Signs and symptoms of acute overdose may occur as follows. Between 30 minutes and 8 hours after ingestion, patient may experience lethargy, nausea and vomiting, green then tarry stools, weak and rapid pulse, hypotension, dehydration, acidosis, and coma. If death isn't immediate, symptoms may clear for about 24 hours. At 12 to 48 hours, symptoms may return, accompanied by diffuse vascular congestion, pulmonary edema, shock, seizures, anuria, hyperthermia, then possibly death.

Treatment requires immediate support of airway, respiration, and circulation. Induce emesis with ipecac in conscious patients with intact gag reflex; for unconscious patients, empty stomach by gastric lavage.

Follow emesis with lavage, using 1% sodium bicarbonate solution to convert iron to less irritating, poorly absorbed form. (Phosphate solutions have been used, but carry risk of other adverse effects.) Perform radiographic evaluation of abdomen to determine continued presence of excess iron; if serum iron levels exceed 350 mg/dl, deferoxamine may be used for systemic chelation. Survivors are likely to sustain organ damage, including pyloric or antral stenosis, hepatic cirrhosis, CNS damage, and intestinal obstruction.

Special considerations
● Administer iron with juice (preferably orange juice) or water, but not with milk or antacids.
● Polysaccharide iron complex is nontoxic and there are relatively few, if any, GI adverse effects linked to other iron preparations.
● Oral iron may turn stools black. This unabsorbed iron is harmless; however, it could mask melena.
● Polysaccharide iron complex may blacken feces and may interfere with test for occult blood in stool; guaiac and orthotoluidine tests may yield false-positive results. Benzidine test usually isn't affected. Iron overload may decrease uptake of technetium 99m and interfere with skeletal imaging.

Patient monitoring
● Monitor hemoglobin level and hematocrit and reticulocyte counts during therapy.

Breast-feeding patients
● Iron supplements are often recommended for breast-feeding women; no adverse effects documented.

Pediatric patients
● Iron overdose may be fatal in children; treat patient immediately.

Geriatric patients
● Because iron-induced constipation is common in elderly patients, stress proper diet to minimize this adverse effect. Elderly patients may need higher doses of iron because as reduced gastric secretions and achlorhydria may lower capacity for iron absorption.

Patient education
● Inform parents that as few as three or four tablets can cause serious iron poisoning in children.
● If patient misses a dose, tell him to take it as soon as he remembers but not to double the dose.
● Advise patient to avoid certain foods that may impair oral iron absorption, including yogurt, cheese, eggs, milk, whole-grain breads and cereals, tea, and coffee.
● Teach patient dietary measures to follow for preventing constipation.

potassium iodide (KI, SSKI)
Pima, Thyro-Block

Pharmacologic classification: electrolyte
Therapeutic classification: antihyperthyroid, expectorant
Pregnancy risk category: D

Indications and dosages
➤ *Expectorant. Adults:* 300 to 600 mg t.i.d. or q.i.d.
Children: 60 to 250 mg q.i.d.
➤ *Preoperative thyroidectomy. Adults and children:* 50 to 250 mg (or 1 to 5 drops) SSKI

t.i.d.; or 0.1 to 0.3 ml (or 3 to 5 drops) Lugol's solution t.i.d.; give drug for 10 to 14 days before surgery.

▶ **Nuclear radiation protection.** *Adults and children:* 0.13 ml P.O. of SSKI (130 mg) immediately before or after initial exposure will block 90% of radioactive iodine. Same dosage given 3 to 4 hours after exposure will provide 50% block. Drug should be administered for up to 10 days under medical supervision.

Infants under age 1: Half the adult dosage.

▶ **To replenish iodine** ◊. *Adults:* 5 to 10 mg/day.

Children: 1 mg/day.

▶ **Management of thyrotoxic crisis.** *Adults:* 500 mg P.O. q 4 hours (about 10 drops of a potassium iodide solution containing 1 g/ml). Or 1 ml of strong iodine solution P.O. t.i.d.

▶ **Cutaneous sporotrichosis** ◊. *Adults:* 65 to 325 mg P.O. t.i.d.

How supplied
Available by prescription only
Saturated solution (SSKI): 1 g/ml
Strong iodine solution (Lugol's solution): iodine 50 mg/ml and potassium iodide 100 mg/ml
Syrup: 325 mg/5 ml
Tablets: 130 mg

Pharmacodynamics
Expectorant action: Exact mechanism unknown. Thought to reduce viscosity of mucus by increasing respiratory tract secretions.
Antihyperthyroid action: Acts directly on the thyroid gland to inhibit synthesis and release of thyroid hormone.

Pharmacokinetics
Absorption: Absorption similar to iodinated amino acids.
Distribution: Distributed extracellularly.
Metabolism: No information available.
Excretion: Excreted by kidneys.

Route	Onset	Peak	Duration
P.O.	< 24 hours	10-15 days	Unknown

Contraindications and precautions
Contraindicated in patients with tuberculosis, acute bronchitis, iodide hypersensitivity, or hyperkalemia. Some formulations contain sulfites, which may precipitate allergic reactions in hypersensitive individuals.

Use cautiously in patients with hypocomplementemic vasculitis, goiter, or autoimmune thyroid disease.

Interactions
Drug-drug. *Drugs that contain potassium, potassium-sparing diuretics:* Possible hyperkalemia and subsequent arrhythmia or cardiac arrest. Avoid concomitant use.

Lithium: Potentiated hypothyroid and goitrogenic effects of potassium iodide. Use together cautiously.

Adverse reactions
EENT: inflammation of salivary glands, periorbital edema.
GI: nausea, vomiting, stomach pain, diarrhea, burning mouth and throat, sore teeth and gums, *metallic taste.*
Metabolic: altered thyroid function tests.
Skin: acneiform rash.
Other: fever, *hypersensitivity reactions.*

Overdose and treatment
Acute overdose is rare; angioedema, laryngeal edema, and cutaneous hemorrhages may occur. Treat hyperkalemia immediately; salt and fluid intake help eliminate iodide. Iodism (chronic iodine poisoning) may follow prolonged use; symptoms include metallic taste, sore mouth, swollen eyelids, sneezing, skin eruptions, nausea, vomiting, epigastric pain, and diarrhea.

Special considerations
● Dilute with 6 oz (180 ml) of water, fruit juice, or broth to reduce GI distress and disguise strong, salty metallic taste; advise patient to use a straw to avoid tooth discoloration.
● Store in light-resistant container because exposure to light liberates traces of free iodine; if crystals develop in solution, dissolve them by placing container in warm water and carefully agitating it.
● Drug may cause flare-up of adolescent acne or other rash.
⚠ **ALERT** Sudden withdrawal may precipitate thyroid storm.
● Maintain fluid intake when using drug as an expectorant; adequate hydration encourages optimal expectorant action.

Patient monitoring
● Monitor serum potassium levels before and during therapy; patients taking any diuretic, especially potassium-sparing diuretics, are at risk for hyperkalemia.
● Monitor patient for adverse effects.

Breast-feeding patients
● Drug appears in breast milk. Avoid use breast-feeding women; it may cause rash and thyroid suppression in infant.

Pediatric patients
● Strong iodine solution is used for treating Graves' disease in neonates (1 drop every 8 hours).

Geriatric patients
● Serum potassium determinations may be needed in elderly patients with renal dysfunction.

Patient education

• Enteric-coated tablets are seldom used because of reports of small-bowel lesions with possible obstruction, perforation, and hemorrhage; when prescribed, give tablet with small amount of water, and tell patient to swallow tablet whole (don't crush or chew) and follow with 8 oz (240 ml) of water or juice.

• Advise patient to drink all of solution prepared and to use a straw to avoid discoloring teeth.

• Review signs and symptoms of iodism with patient, and instruct patient to report such symptoms, especially abdominal pain, distention, nausea, vomiting, or GI bleeding.

• Caution patient not to use OTC drugs without approval; many preparations contain iodides and could potentiate drug. For the same reason, patient should report ingestion of iodized salt and shellfish.

---

potassium salts, oral

potassium acetate

potassium bicarbonate
K+ Care ET, K-Electrolyte, K-Ide, Klor-Con/EF, K•Lyte, K-Vescent

potassium chloride
Apo-K*, Cena-K, Gen-K, K+8, K-10*, Kalium Durules*, Kaochlor S-F, Kaon-Cl, Kaon Cl-10, Kato, Kay Ciel, K+ Care, KCL*, K-Dur, K-Ide, K-Lease, K-Long*, K-Lor, Klor-Con, Klorvess, Klotrix, K-Lyte/Cl Powder, K-Med 900*, K-Norm, K-Sol, K-Tab, Micro-K Extencaps, Micro-K 10 Extencaps, Potasalan, Rum-K, Slow-K, Ten-K

potassium gluconate
Glu-K, Kaon

Pharmacologic classification: potassium supplement
Therapeutic classification: therapeutic drug for electrolyte balance
Pregnancy risk category: C

Indications and dosages

➤ *Hypokalemia. Adults and children:* 40- to 100-mEq tablets divided into two to four doses daily. Use I.V. potassium chloride when oral replacement isn't feasible or when hypokalemia is life-threatening. Dosage up to 20 mEq/hour at 60 mEq/L or less. Further dose based on serum potassium determinations. Don't exceed 150 mEq daily (3 mEq/kg in children).

Further doses are based on serum potassium levels and blood pH. I.V. potassium replacement should be carried out only with ECG monitoring and frequent serum potassium determinations.

➤ *Prevention of hypokalemia. Adults and children:* Initially, 20 mEq of potassium supplement P.O. daily, in divided doses. Adjust dosage, p.r.n., based on serum potassium levels.

➤ *Potassium replacement. Adults and children:* Potassium chloride should be diluted in a suitable I.V. solution (not more than 40 mEq/L) and administered at no more than 20 mEq/hour. Don't exceed 400 mEq daily (3 mEq/kg/day or 40 mEq/m²/day for children). I.V. potassium replacement should be carried out only with ECG monitoring and frequent serum potassium determinations.

➤ *Acute MI ◇. Adults:* High dose—80 mEq/L at 1.5 ml/kg/hour for 24 hours with an I.V. infusion of 25% dextrose and 50 units/L regular insulin. Low dose—40 mEq/L at 1 ml/kg/hour for 24 hours, with an I.V. infusion of 10% dextrose and 20 units/L regular insulin.

How supplied
Available by prescription only
Liquid: 15 mEq/15 ml, 20 mEq/15 ml, 30 mEq/15 ml, 40 mEq/15 ml
Tablets (effervescent): 20 mEq, 25 mEq, 50 mEq
potassium acetate
Vials: 2 mEq/ml, 4 mEq/ml in 20-ml vials
potassium chloride
Powder: 15 mEq/package, 20 mEq/package, and 25 mEq/package
Tablets (sustained-release): 6.7 mEq, 8 mEq, 10 mEq, 20 mEq
potassium gluconate
Liquid: 20 mEq/15 ml
Tablets: 2 mEq

Pharmacodynamics
Potassium replacement action: Potassium, the main cation in body tissue, is necessary for physiologic processes such as maintaining intracellular tonicity, maintaining a balance with sodium across cell membranes, transmitting nerve impulses, maintaining cellular metabolism, contracting cardiac and skeletal muscle, maintaining acid-base balance, and maintaining normal renal function.

Pharmacokinetics
Absorption: Well absorbed from GI tract. Should be taken with meals and sipped slowly over a 5- to 10-minute period to decrease irritation. Potassium bicarbonate doesn't correct hypochloremic alkalosis.
Distribution: Normal serum levels of potassium range from 3.8 to 5 mEq/L. Plasma potassium levels up to 7.7 mEq/L may be normal in neonates. Up to 60 mEq/L of potassium may be found in gastric secretions and diarrhea fluid.
Metabolism: None significant.
Excretion: Excreted largely by kidneys. Small amounts may be excreted via skin and intestinal tract, but intestinal potassium usually is reab-

---

sorbed. A healthy patient on a potassium-free diet will excrete 40 to 50 mEq of potassium daily.

Route	Onset	Peak	Duration
I.V., P.O.	Varies	Varies	Varies

Contraindications and precautions
Contraindicated in patients with severe renal impairment with oliguria, anuria, or azotemia; in those with untreated Addison's disease; and in those with acute dehydration, heat cramps, hyperkalemia, hyperkalemic form of familial periodic paralysis, or conditions caused by extensive tissue breakdown.

Use cautiously in patients with cardiac or renal disease.

Interactions
Drug-drug. *ACE inhibitors (captopril), potassium-sparing diuretics:* Severe hyperkalemia. Use cautiously.

Anticholinergics that slow GI motility: Increased chance of GI irritation and ulceration. Use together cautiously.

Digoxin: Potential for arrhythmias. Potassium isn't recommended in digitalized patients with severe or complete heart block.

Products that contain potassium: Hyperkalemia within 1 to 2 days. Monitor patient closely.

Drug-food. *Salt substitutes that contain potassium salts:* Severe hyperkalemia. Avoid concurrent use.

Adverse reactions
CNS: paresthesia of the limbs, listlessness, mental confusion, weakness or heaviness of legs, flaccid paralysis.

CV: hypotension, *arrhythmias, cardiac arrest, heart block,* ECG changes.

GI: nausea, vomiting, abdominal pain, diarrhea.

Metabolic: hyperkalemia.

Respiratory: *respiratory paralysis.*

Other: pain and redness at infusion site, fever.

Overdose and treatment
Toxicity is evidenced by increased serum potassium level and characteristic ECG changes, including tall peaked T waves, depression of ST segment, disappearance of P wave, prolonged QT interval, and widening and slurring of the QRS complex. Late signs of toxicity include weakness, paralysis of voluntary muscles, respiratory distress, and dysphagia. These may precede severe or fatal cardiac toxicity. Hyperkalemia produces symptoms paradoxically similar to those of hypokalemia.

In patients with a potassium level greater than 6.5 mEq/L, supportive therapy may include the following interventions (with continuous ECG monitoring): Infuse 40 to 160 mEq sodium bicarbonate I.V. over a 5-minute interval; repeat in 10 to 15 minutes if ECG abnormalities persist. Infuse 300 to 500 ml of dextrose 10% to 25% over 1 hour. Insulin (5 to 10 units per 20 g of dextrose) should be added to the infusion or, ideally, administered as a separate injection.

Patients with absent P waves or broad QRS complex who aren't receiving cardiotonic glycosides should immediately be given 0.5 g to 1 g of calcium gluconate or another calcium salt I.V. over a 2-minute period (with continuous ECG monitoring) to antagonize cardiotoxic effect of potassium. May be repeated in 1 to 2 minutes if ECG abnormalities persist.

To remove potassium from body, use sodium polystyrene sulfonate resin, hemodialysis, or peritoneal dialysis. Administer potassium-free I.V. fluids when hyperkalemia is linked to water loss.

Special considerations
● In patients receiving cardiac glycosides, removing potassium too rapidly may result in digitalis toxicity.

● Don't give potassium during immediate postoperative period until urine flow is established.

● Give parenteral potassium by slow infusion only, never by I.V. push or I.M. Dilute I.V. potassium preparations with large volume of parenteral solutions.

● Give oral potassium supplements with extreme caution because its many forms deliver varying amounts of potassium. Patient may tolerate one product better than another.

● Potassium gluconate doesn't correct hypokalemic hypochloremic alkalosis.

● Enteric-coated tablets aren't recommended because of potential for GI bleeding and small-bowel ulcerations.

● Tablets in wax matrix sometimes lodge in esophagus and cause ulceration in cardiac patients who have esophageal compression due to enlarged left atrium. In such patients and in those with esophageal or GI stasis or obstruction, use liquid form.

● Drug is often used orally with diuretics that cause potassium excretion. Potassium chloride is most useful because diuretics waste chloride ions. Hypokalemic alkalosis is treated best with potassium chloride.

● Don't crush sustained-released potassium products.

Patient monitoring
● Monitor serum potassium, BUN, and serum creatinine levels before starting therapy.

● Monitor ECG, pH, serum potassium levels, and other electrolytes during therapy.

Breast-feeding patients
● Potassium supplements appear in breast milk. Safety in breast-feeding women hasn't been established; use potassium only when benefits to mother outweigh risks to infant.

Pediatric patients
● Use cautiously in children.

Patient education
• Tell patient potassium is available only with a prescription because the wrong amount may cause severe reactions.
• Suggest diluting liquid potassium product in at least 4 to 8 oz (120 to 240 ml) of water; to take it after meals; and to sip liquid potassium slowly to minimize GI irritation.
• Tell patient to dissolve powder, soluble tablets, or granules completely in at least 4 oz (120 ml) of water or juice, and to allow fizzing to finish before drinking.
• Instruct patient not to crush or chew sustained-release capsules; contents of capsule can be opened and sprinkled onto applesauce or other soft food.
• Tell patient to stop taking drug and report immediately if the following reactions occur: confusion; irregular heartbeat; numbness of feet, fingers, or lips; shortness of breath; anxiety; excessive tiredness or weakness of legs; unexplained diarrhea; nausea and vomiting; stomach pain; or bloody or black stools. Such reactions are rare.
• Tell patient that expelling a whole tablet (sustained-release tablet) in stool is normal. The body eliminates the shell after absorbing the potassium.
• Warn patient to avoid salt substitutes except when prescribed.

pralidoxime chloride (2-PAM chloride, 2-pyridine aldoxime methochloride)
Protopam

Pharmacologic classification: quaternary ammonium oxime
Therapeutic classification: antidote
Pregnancy risk category: C

Indications and dosages
➤ *Organophosphate pesticide poisoning.*
Adults: 1 to 2 g I.V. in 100 ml of normal saline solution over 15 to 30 minutes. May repeat in 1 hour if muscle weakness continues. For subconjunctival injection, give 0.1 to 0.2 ml of a 5% solution.
Children: 20 to 40 mg/kg I.V. in 100 ml of normal saline solution over 15 to 30 minutes. May repeat in 1 hour if muscle weakness continues.
   Drug is most effective when given within 24 hours of exposure. It should be given with atropine.
➤ *Anticholinesterase overdose.* *Adults:* 1 to 2 g I.V.; then increments of 250 mg q 5 minutes.

How supplied
Available by prescription only
Injection: 1 g/20 ml vial (without diluent or syringe); 1 g/20 ml vial with diluent, syringe, needle, alcohol swab (emergency kit); 600 mg/2 ml auto-injector, parenteral

Pharmacodynamics
Antidote action: Reactivates cholinesterase that has been inactivated by phosphorylation due to exposure to an organophosphate pesticide or related compound. One of the few drugs that correct a biochemical lesion, pralidoxime acts by removing the phosphoryl group from the active site of the inhibited enzyme, freezing and reactivating acetylcholinesterase. It also directly reacts with and detoxifies the organophosphorus molecule and may also react with cholinesterase to protect it from inhibition.
   Cholinesterase reactivation occurs primarily at the neuromuscular junction where pralidoxime exerts its most critical effect—reversal of respiratory paralysis or paralysis of other skeletal muscles. Reactivation also occurs at autonomic effector sites and, to a lesser degree, within the CNS. Pralidoxime is effective against nicotinic signs and symptoms but it doesn't substantially influence muscarinic effects. Therefore, it's used in conjunction with atropine, which ameliorates muscarinic symptoms and directly blocks the effects of accumulation of excess acetylcholine at various sites, including the respiratory center.

Pharmacokinetics
Absorption: After I.V. administration, plasma levels peak in 5 to 15 minutes; after I.M., in 10 to 20 minutes.
Distribution: Distributed throughout extracellular water; not appreciably bound to plasma protein. Doesn't readily pass into CNS. Distribution into breast milk is unknown. Therapeutic levels achieved in eye after subconjunctival injection.
Metabolism: Exact mechanism unknown; likely hepatic metabolism.
Excretion: Excreted rapidly in urine as unchanged drug and metabolite; 80% to 90% of I.V. or I.M. dose excreted unchanged within 12 hours.

Route	Onset	Peak	Duration
I.V.	Unknown	5-15 min	Unknown
I.M.	Unknown	10-20 min	Unknown
S.C.	Unknown	Unknown	Unknown

Contraindications and precautions
Contraindicated in patients hypersensitive to drug or its components. Use cautiously in patients with myasthenia gravis.

Interactions
Drug-drug. *Barbiturates:* Potentiated by anticholinesterase. Use cautiously.
CNS depressants, drugs that lower seizure threshold (aminophylline, morphine, phenothiazines, reserpine, succinylcholine, theophylline, other respiratory depressants), skeletal muscle relaxants: Possible potentiation or decreased effect of these drugs. Avoid use in patients with anticholinesterase poisoning.

Adverse reactions
CNS: dizziness, headache, drowsiness.

Reactions may be *common*, uncommon, *life-threatening*, or COMMON AND LIFE-THREATENING.

CV: tachycardia, hypertension.
EENT: blurred vision, diplopia, impaired accommodation.
GI: nausea.
Hepatic: transient elevation of AST, ALT, CK, and liver enzyme levels.
Musculoskeletal: muscle weakness.
Respiratory: hyperventilation.
Other: mild to moderate pain at injection site.

Overdose and treatment
Toxicity may cause dizziness, headache, blurred vision, diplopia, impaired accommodation, nausea, and tachycardia. However, these effects may also result from organophosphate toxicity or the use of atropine. Treatment is supportive.

Special considerations
● Reconstitute drug with 20 ml of sterile water for injection to provide a solution containing 50 mg/ml. For I.V. infusion, dilute calculated dose to a volume of 100 ml with normal saline solution injection. Use within a few hours.
● Drug usually is administered by I.V. infusion over 15 to 30 minutes. Rapid administration has produced tachycardia, laryngospasm, muscle rigidity, and transient neuromuscular blockade. Hypertension may also occur, related to dose and rate of infusion; it may be treated by stopping infusion or slowing rate of infusion. Phentolamine 5 mg I.V. quickly reverses pralidoxime-induced hypertension.
● In patients with pulmonary edema, or when I.V. infusion isn't practical, or a more rapid effect is needed, drug may be given by slow I.V. injection over at least 5 minutes. It may also be given I.M. or S.C.
● Institute treatment of organophosphate poisoning without waiting for laboratory test results. Begin pralidoxime and atropine therapy simultaneously. Give 2 to 6 mg of atropine I.V. (I.M. if patient is cyanotic) every 5 to 60 minutes in adults until muscarinic effects (dyspnea, cough, salivation, bronchospasm) subside. Repeat dosage if signs reappear. Maintain some degree of atropinism for at least 48 hours.
● Use reduced dosage in renally impaired patients.
● Treatment is most effective when started within first 24 hours, preferably within a few hours after poisoning. Even severe poisoning may be reversed if drug is given within 48 hours. Monitor effect of therapy by ECG because of possible heart block due to the anticholinesterase. Continued absorption of the anticholinesterase from the lower bowel constitutes new toxic exposure that may require additional doses of pralidoxime every 3 to 8 hours, or over several days
● After dermal exposure, patient's clothing should be removed and hair and skin should be washed with sodium bicarbonate, soap, water, or alcohol as soon as possible. While cleaning patient, caregiver should wear gloves and protective clothing to avoid contamination. Patient may need a second washing.

● Drug isn't effective in treating toxic exposure to phosphorus, inorganic phosphates, or organophosphates that don't have anticholinesterase activity.
● Give I.V. sodium thiopental or diazepam if seizures interfere with respiration.
● Subconjunctival injection is currently an unapproved method of administration but has been used to reverse adverse ocular effects resulting from systemic overdose or splashing of an organophosphate into eye.

Patient monitoring
● Assess vital signs and insert I.V. line. Drug administration requires close medical supervision and close observation of patient for at least 24 hours.
● Draw blood for RBC and cholinesterase levels before giving pralidoxime.
● Closely monitor blood pressure during infusion.

Breast-feeding patients
● It isn't known if drug appears in breast milk. Use caution when administering drug to breast-feeding women.

Pediatric patients
● Safety hasn't been established.

Patient education
● Warn patient that mild to moderate pain may occur 20 to 40 minutes after I.M. injection.

---

pramipexole hydrochloride
Mirapex

Pharmacologic classification: nonergot dopamine agonist
Therapeutic classification: antiparkinsonian
Pregnancy risk category: C

Indications and dosages
➤ *Idiopathic Parkinson's disease. Adults:* Initially, 0.375 mg P.O. daily given in three divided doses; don't increase more than q 5 to 7 days. Increase dose by 0.75 mg in divided doses weekly until maximum dose of 1.5 mg t.i.d. is reached after 7 weeks of therapy. Maintenance dose ranges from 1.5 to 4.5 mg daily administered in three divided doses.
✦ *Dosage adjustment.* For patients with impaired renal function and creatinine clearance of 35 to 59 ml/minute, initial dose is 0.125 mg P.O. b.i.d. and maintenance maximum dose is 1.5 mg b.i.d. For patients with creatinine clearance of 15 to 34 ml/minute, initial dose is 0.125 mg P.O. daily and maintenance maximum dose is 1.5 mg daily.

How supplied
Available by prescription only
Tablets: 0.125 mg, 0.25 mg, 0.5 mg, 1 mg, 1.5 mg

Pharmacodynamics

Antiparkinsonian action: Thought to stimulate dopamine (D_2 and D_3) receptors in striatum; pramipexole influences striatal neuronal firing rates via activation of dopamine receptors in the striatum and the substantia nigra, the site of neurons that send projections to the striatum.

Pharmacokinetics

Absorption: Rapidly absorbed; levels peak in about 2 hours. Absolute bioavailability over 90%, suggesting it's well absorbed and undergoes little presystemic metabolism. Food doesn't affect extent of absorption, but increases time of maximum plasma level by about 1 hour.

Distribution: Extensively distributed; volume of distribution of about 500 L. About 15% bound to plasma proteins; also distributed into RBCs. Terminal half-life 8 to 12 hours; steady state reached within 2 days of dosing.

Metabolism: 90% of dose excreted unchanged in urine.

Excretion: Excreted mainly in urine. Nonrenal routes may contribute a small extent to elimination; no metabolites identified in plasma or urine. Drug secreted by renal tubules, probably by organic transport system.

Route	Onset	Peak	Duration
P.O.	Rapid	2 hr	8-12 hr

Contraindications and precautions

Contraindicated in patients hypersensitive to drug or its components. Use cautiously in those who have renal impairment, such as elderly patients, because dosing may need to be adjusted.

Interactions

Drug-drug. *Cimetidine, diltiazem, quinidine, quinine, ranitidine, triamterene, verapamil:* Decreased clearance of pramipexole. Adjust pramipexole dose if used together.
Dopamine antagonists (butyrophenones, metoclopramide, phenothiazines, thiothixenes): Diminished effectiveness of pramipexole. Monitor patient closely.
Levodopa: Increased levodopa maximum plasma levels. Adjust levodopa dosage as needed.

Adverse reactions

CNS: *dizziness,* somnolence, malaise, *insomnia,* hallucinations, *confusion,* amnesia, hypoesthesia, dystonia, akathisia, thought abnormalities, myoclonus, *asthenia, dyskinesia, extrapyramidal syndrome, dream abnormalities,* gait abnormalities, hypertonia, paranoid reaction, delusions, sleep disorders.
CV: chest pain, peripheral edema, *orthostatic hypotension,* general edema.
EENT: accommodation abnormalities, diplopia, rhinitis, vision abnormalities.
GI: dry mouth, anorexia, *constipation,* dysphagia, nausea.

GU: impotence, urinary frequency, urinary tract infection, urinary incontinence.
Musculoskeletal: arthritis, twitching, bursitis, myasthenia.
Respiratory: dyspnea, pneumonia.
Skin: skin disorders.
Other: decreased libido, fever, unevaluable reaction, *accidental injury.*

Overdose and treatment

No known antidote; if signs of CNS stimulation occur, a phenothiazine or other butyrophenone neuroleptic agent may be given. Management of overdose may require general supportive measures with gastric lavage, IV fluids and ECG monitoring.

Special considerations

● If drug needs to be discontinued, do so over a 1-week period.
◳ **ALERT** Neuroleptic malignant syndrome (elevated temperature, muscular rigidity, altered consciousness, and autonomic instability) without obvious cause has occurred with rapid dose reduction or withdrawal of or changes in antiparkinsonian therapy.
● Adjust dosage gradually. Increase dosage to achieve maximum therapeutic effect, balanced against the main adverse effects of dyskinesia, hallucinations, somnolence, and dry mouth.

Patient monitoring

● Drug may cause orthostatic hypotension, especially during dose escalation; monitor patient carefully.
● Monitor patient for adverse effects.

Breast-feeding patients

● It isn't known if drug appears in breast milk. Use cautiously in breast-feeding women.

Pediatric patients

● Safety and efficacy in children haven't been established.

Geriatric patients

● Drug clearance decreases with age because half-life and clearance are about 40% longer and 30% lower, respectively, in patients ages 65 and older.

Patient education

● Tell patient to take drug only as prescribed.
● Instruct patient not to rise rapidly after sitting or lying down because of risk of orthostatic hypotension.
● Caution patient not to drive or operate complex machinery until response to drug is known.
● Tell patient to use caution before taking drug with other CNS depressants.
● Advise patient to take drug with food if nausea develops.
● Caution patient to not stop drug abruptly.

Reactions may be *common*, uncommon, **life-threatening**, or COMMON AND LIFE-THREATENING.

pravastatin sodium
Pravachol

Pharmacologic classification: HMG-CoA
reductase inhibitor
Therapeutic classification: antilipemic
Pregnancy risk category: X

Indications and dosages
➤*Reduction of low-density lipoprotein
and total cholesterol levels, apolipoprotein b, triglycerides and increase high-
density lipoprotein in patients with primary hypercholesterolemia and mixed
dyslipidemia (types IIa and IIb), primary prevention of coronary events. Adults:*
Initially, 10 to 20 mg daily h.s. Adjust dosage q
4 weeks based on patient tolerance and response;
maximum daily dose is 40 mg. Most elderly
patients respond to a daily dose of 20 mg or less.

How supplied
Available by prescription only
Tablets: 10 mg, 20 mg, 40 mg

Pharmacodynamics
Antilipemic action: Inhibits the enzyme 3-
hydroxy-3-methylglutaryl-coenzyme A (HMG-CoA)
reductase. This hepatic enzyme is an early (and
rate limiting) step in the synthetic pathway of cholesterol.

Pharmacokinetics
Absorption: Rapidly absorbed; plasma levels
peak in 1 to 1½ hours. Average oral absorption
is 34%; absolute bioavailability of 17%. Food reduces bioavailability, but same drug effects if drug
is taken with or 1 hour before meals.
Distribution: Plasma levels proportional to dose,
but don't necessarily correlate perfectly with lipid-
lowering effects. About 50% bound to plasma
proteins. Undergoes extensive first-pass extraction, possibly because of active transport system
into hepatocytes.
Metabolism: Metabolized by liver. At least six
metabolites identified; some active.
Excretion: Excreted by liver and kidneys.

Route	Onset	Peak	Duration
P.O.	Unknown	1-1½ hr	Unknown

Contraindications and precautions
Contraindicated in patients hypersensitive to
drug; in those with active liver disease or conditions that cause unexplained, persistent elevations of serum transaminase levels; in pregnant and breast-feeding women; and in women
of childbearing age unless there is no risk of
pregnancy.
    Use cautiously in patients who consume large
quantities of alcohol or have history of liver disease.

Interactions
Drug-drug. *Cholestyramine, colestipol:* Decreased plasma levels of pravastatin. Administer
pravastatin 1 hour before or 4 hours after these
drugs.
Cimetidine, ketoconazole, spironolactone: Increased risk of endocrine dysfunction. No intervention appears necessary; take complete drug
history in patients who develop endocrine dysfunction.
*Erythromycin, fibric acid derivatives (clofi-
brate, gemfibrozil), high doses of niacin (1 g
or more nicotinic acid daily), immunosuppressants (such as cyclosporine):* Increased
risk of rhabdomyolysis. Monitor patient closely
if drugs must be given together.
Gemfibrozil: Decreased protein-binding and urinary clearance of pravastatin. Avoid concomitant
use.
Hepatotoxic drugs: Increased risk of hepatotoxicity. Use together cautiously.
Drug-herb. *Red yeast rice:* Contains components similar to those of statin drugs, increasing
the risk of adverse events or toxicity. Discourage
concomitant use.
Drug-lifestyle. *Chronic alcohol abuse:* Increased risk of hepatotoxicity. Monitor patient
closely.
Sun exposure: Photosensitivity reaction. Tell patient to take precautions.

Adverse reactions
CNS: headache, dizziness, fatigue.
CV: chest pain.
EENT: rhinitis.
GI: vomiting, diarrhea, heartburn, abdominal
pain, constipation, flatulence, nausea.
GU: *renal failure* secondary to myoglobinuria,
urinary abnormality.
Hepatic: increased AST, ALT, CK, alkaline phos-
phatase, and bilirubin levels.
Metabolic: abnormal thyroid function test re-
sults.
Musculoskeletal: myositis, myopathy, *localized
muscle pain,* myalgia, **rhabdomyolysis.**
Respiratory: cough.
Skin: rash.
Other: flulike symptoms, photosensitivity, in-
fluenza, common cold.

Overdose and treatment
No information available. Treat symptomatically.

Special considerations
● Stop drug temporarily in patients with an acute
condition that suggests a developing myopathy
or in patients with risk factors that may predispose them to development of renal failure secondary to rhabdomyolysis (including severe acute
infection; severe endocrine, metabolic, or electrolyte disorders; hypotension; major surgery; or
uncontrolled seizures).
● Initiate drug therapy only after diet and other
nonpharmacologic therapies have proved inef-

fective. Patients should continue a cholesterol-lowering diet during therapy.
• Give drug in evening, preferably at bedtime. Drug may be given without regard to meals.
• Dosage adjustments should be made about every 4 weeks. May reduce dosage if cholesterol levels fall below target range.

Patient monitoring
• Watch for signs of myositis. Rarely, myopathy and marked elevations of CK level, possibly leading to rhabdomyolysis and renal failure secondary to myoglobinuria, have occurred.
• Monitor therapeutic effect.

Breast-feeding patients
• Drug appears in breast milk. Women shouldn't breast-feed while taking drug.

Pediatric patients
• Safety and efficacy in children under age 18 haven't been established.

Geriatric patients
• Maximum effectiveness is usually evident with daily doses of 20 mg or less.

Patient education
• Teach patient appropriate dietary management (restricting total fat and cholesterol intake), weight control, and exercise. Explain importance of these interventions in controlling serum lipids.
• Because of drug's possible impact on liver function, advise patient to restrict alcohol intake.
• Tell patient to call if he experiences adverse reactions, particularly muscle aches and pains.
• Inform patient to take drug at bedtime.

---

prazosin hydrochloride
Minipress

Pharmacologic classification: alpha-adrenergic blocker
Therapeutic classification: antihypertensive
Pregnancy risk category: C

Indications and dosages
➤ **Hypertension.** *Adults:* Initially, 1 mg P.O. b.i.d. or t.i.d.; gradually increased to maximum of 20 mg daily. Usual maintenance dose is 6 to 15 mg daily in divided doses. If other antihypertensives or diuretics are added to prazosin therapy, reduce dose of prazosin to 1 or 2 mg t.i.d. and then gradually increase as necessary.
➤ **Benign prostatic hyperplasia** ◇. *Adults:* Initially, 2 mg P.O. b.i.d. Dose may range from 1 to 9 mg/day.

How supplied
Available by prescription only
Capsules: 1 mg, 2 mg, 5 mg

Pharmacodynamics
Antihypertensive action: Selectively and competitively inhibits alpha-adrenergic receptors, causing arterial and venous dilation, reducing peripheral vascular resistance and blood pressure.
Hypertrophic action: Alpha blockade in nonvascular smooth muscle causes relaxation, notably in prostatic tissue, thereby reducing urinary symptoms in men with benign prostatic hyperplasia.

Pharmacokinetics
Absorption: Variable absorption from GI tract. Antihypertensive effect begins in about 2 hours; peaks in 2 to 4 hours. Full antihypertensive effect may not occur for 4 to 6 weeks.
Distribution: Distributed throughout body; about 97% protein-bound.
Metabolism: Metabolized extensively in liver.
Excretion: Over 90% of dose excreted in feces via bile; remainder excreted in urine. Plasma half-life is 2 to 4 hours. Antihypertensive effect lasts less than 24 hours.

Route	Onset	Peak	Duration
P.O.	½-1½ hr	2-4 hr	7-10 hr

Contraindications and precautions
No known contraindications. Use cautiously in patients receiving antihypertensives and in those with chronic renal failure.

Interactions
Drug-drug. *Diuretics, other antihypertensives:* Increased hypotensive effects. Monitor blood pressure regularly.
Other highly protein-bound drugs: Prazosin is highly bound to plasma proteins and may interact with these drugs. Monitor patient closely.
Drug-herb. *Butcher's broom:* Reduced effects of drug. Discourage use.

Adverse reactions
CNS: *dizziness,* headache, drowsiness, nervousness, paresthesia, weakness, *first-dose syncope,* depression.
CV: edema, orthostatic hypotension, *palpitations.*
EENT: blurred vision, tinnitus, conjunctivitis, nasal congestion, epistaxis.
GI: vomiting, diarrhea, abdominal cramps, constipation, *nausea.*
GU: increased BUN levels, priapism, impotence, urinary frequency, incontinence.
Hematologic: transient fall in leukocyte count.
Hepatic: liver function test abnormalities.
Metabolic: increased serum uric acid levels.
Musculoskeletal: arthralgia, myalgia.
Respiratory: dyspnea.
Skin: pruritus.
Other: fever.

Reactions may be *common,* uncommon, **life-threatening**, or COMMON AND LIFE-THREATENING.

Overdose and treatment
Toxicity may cause hypotension and drowsiness. After acute ingestion, empty stomach by induced emesis or gastric lavage, and give activated charcoal to reduce absorption. Further treatment is usually symptomatic and supportive. Prazosin isn't dialyzable.

Special considerations
● First-dose syncope (dizziness, light-headedness, and syncope) may occur ½ to 1 hour after initial dose; it may be severe, with loss of consciousness, if initial dose exceeds 2 mg. Effect is transient and may be diminished by giving drug at bedtime, by limiting initial dose of prazosin to 1 mg, by subsequently increasing dosage gradually, and by introducing other antihypertensives into patient's regimen cautiously; it's more common during febrile illness and more severe if patient has hyponatremia. Always increase dosage gradually and have patient sit or lie down if he experiences dizziness.
● Prazosin's effect is most pronounced on diastolic blood pressure.
● Drug has been used to treat vasospasm caused by Raynaud's syndrome. It also has been used with diuretics and cardiac glycosides to treat severe heart failure, to manage the signs and symptoms of pheochromocytoma preoperatively, and to treat ergotamine-induced peripheral ischemia.
● Drug alters results of screening tests for pheochromocytoma and causes increases in levels of the urinary metabolite of norepinephrine and vanillylmandelic acid.

Patient monitoring
● Monitor blood pressure, especially at start of therapy and with changes in dosing.
● Monitor patient for adverse effects.

Breast-feeding patients
● Small amounts of drug appear in breast milk; an alternative to breast-feeding is recommended during therapy.

Pediatric patients
● Safety and efficacy in children haven't been established; use only when potential benefit outweighs risk.

Geriatric patients
● Elderly patients may be more sensitive to hypotensive effects and may need lower doses because of altered drug metabolism.

Patient education
● Teach patient about his disease and therapy, and explain that he must take drug exactly as prescribed, even when feeling well; advise him never to stop drug suddenly because severe rebound hypertension may occur, and to promptly report malaise or unusual adverse effects.
● Tell patient to avoid hazardous activities that require mental alertness until tolerance develops to sedation, drowsiness, and other CNS effects; to avoid sudden position changes to minimize orthostatic hypotension; and to use ice chips, candy, or gum to relieve dry mouth.
● Warn patient to seek medical approval before taking OTC cold preparations.

prednisolone (systemic)
Delta-Cortef, Prelone

prednisolone acetate
Cotolone, Key-Pred 25, Predalone 50, Predcor-50

prednisolone sodium phosphate
Hydeltrasol, Key-Pred-SP, Pediapred, Orapred

prednisolone tebutate
Nor-Pred T.B.A., Predate TBA, Predcor-TBA, Prednisol TBA

Pharmacologic classification: glucocorticoid, mineralocorticoid
Therapeutic classification: anti-inflammatory, immunosuppressant
Pregnancy risk category: C

Indications and dosages
➤ *Severe inflammation, modification of body's immune response to disease.* Adults: 2.5 to 15 mg P.O. b.i.d., t.i.d., or q.i.d. *Children:* 0.14 to 2 mg/kg or 4 to 60 mg/m² daily in divided doses.
prednisolone acetate
Adults: 2 to 30 mg I.M. q 12 hours.
prednisolone sodium phosphate
Adults: 2 to 30 mg I.M. or I.V. q 12 hours, or into joints, lesions, and soft tissue, p.r.n.
prednisolone tebutate
Adults: 4 to 40 mg into joints and lesions, p.r.n.

How supplied
Available by prescription only
prednisolone
Syrup: 5 mg/ml, 15 mg/5 ml
Tablets: 5 mg
prednisolone acetate
Injection: 25 mg/ml, 50 mg/ml suspension
prednisolone sodium phosphate
Injection: 20 mg/ml solution
Oral liquid: 6.7 mg (5 mg base)/5 ml; Orapred: 20.2 mg (15 mg base)/5ml
prednisolone tebutate
Injection: 20 mg/ml suspension

Pharmacodynamics
Anti-inflammatory action: Prednisolone stimulates the synthesis of enzymes needed to decrease the inflammatory response. It suppresses

the immune system by reducing activity and volume of the lymphatic system, thus producing lymphocytopenia (primarily of T-lymphocytes), decreasing immunoglobulin and complement levels, decreasing passage of immune complexes through basement membranes, and possibly by depressing reactivity of tissue to antigen-antibody interactions.

The mineralocorticoids regulate electrolyte homeostasis by acting renally at the distal tubules to enhance the reabsorption of sodium ions (and thus water) from the tubular fluid into the plasma and enhance the excretion of both potassium and hydrogen ions.

Prednisolone is an adrenocorticoid with both glucocorticoid and mineralocorticoid properties. It's a weak mineralocorticoid with only half the potency of hydrocortisone but is a more potent glucocorticoid, having four times the potency of equal weight of hydrocortisone. It's used primarily as an anti-inflammatory drug and an immunosuppressant. It's not used for mineralocorticoid replacement therapy because of the availability of more specific and potent drugs.

Prednisolone may be administered orally. Prednisolone sodium phosphate is highly soluble, has a rapid onset and a short duration of action, and may be given I.M. or I.V. Prednisolone acetate and tebutate are suspensions that may be administered by intra-articular, intrasynovial, intrabursal, intralesional, or soft-tissue injection. They have a slow onset but a long duration of action.

Pharmacokinetics
Absorption: Absorbed readily after oral administration. After oral and I.V. administration, effects peak in about 1 to 2 hours. Acetate and tebutate suspensions for injection have a variable absorption rate over 24 to 48 hours, depending on whether injected into intra-articular space or muscle, and on blood supply to that muscle. Slow systemic absorption after intra-articular injection.
Distribution: Removed rapidly from blood and distributed to muscle, liver, skin, intestines, and kidneys. Extensively bound to plasma proteins (transcortin and albumin); only unbound portion is active. Adrenocorticoids distributed into breast milk and through placenta.
Metabolism: Metabolized in liver to inactive glucuronide and sulfate metabolites.
Excretion: Inactive metabolites, and small amounts of unmetabolized drug, excreted in urine. Insignificant drug quantities excreted in feces. Biological half-life 18 to 36 hours.

Route	Onset	Peak	Duration
P.O.	Rapid	1-2 hr	3-36 hr
I.V.	Rapid	1 hr	Unknown
I.M.	Rapid	1 hr	4 wk

Contraindications and precautions
Contraindicated in patients hypersensitive to drug or its components and in those with systemic fungal infections.

Use cautiously in patients with a recent MI, GI ulcer, renal disease, hypertension, osteoporosis, diabetes mellitus, hypothyroidism, cirrhosis, diverticulitis, nonspecific ulcerative colitis, recent intestinal anastomoses, thromboembolic disorders, seizures, myasthenia gravis, heart failure, tuberculosis, ocular herpes simplex, emotional instability, or psychotic tendencies.

Interactions
Drug-drug. *Amphotericin B, diuretics:* Enhanced hypokalemia. Monitor serum potassium level.
Antacids, cholestyramine, colestipol: Decreased prednisolone absorption. Separate administration times.
Barbiturates, phenytoin, rifampin: Decreased corticosteroid effects because of increased hepatic metabolism. Monitor patient.
Cardiac glycosides: Possible hypokalemia may increase risk of toxicity in patients receiving these drugs. Monitor serum potassium level.
Estrogens: Reduced metabolism of prednisolone via increased level of transcortin; half-life of corticosteroid prolonged because of increased protein-binding. Adjust dosage as needed.
Insulin, oral antidiabetics: Hyperglycemia. Adjust dosages of these drugs as needed.
Isoniazid, salicylates: Increased metabolism of these drugs. Monitor patient closely.
Oral anticoagulants: Decreased effects. Monitor PT and INR.
Ulcerogenic drugs (such as NSAIDs): Increased risk of GI ulceration. Use together cautiously.

Adverse reactions
CNS: *euphoria, insomnia,* psychotic behavior, pseudotumor cerebri, vertigo, headache, paresthesia, **seizures.**
CV: *heart failure, thromboembolism,* hypertension, edema, ***arrhythmias,*** thrombophlebitis.
EENT: cataracts, glaucoma.
GI: *peptic ulceration,* GI irritation, increased appetite, **pancreatitis,** nausea, vomiting.
GU: menstrual irregularities.
Metabolic: hypokalemia, hyperglycemia, carbohydrate intolerance.
Musculoskeletal: muscle weakness, osteoporosis, growth suppression in children.
Skin: delayed wound healing, acne, various skin eruptions, hirsutism.
Other: susceptibility to infections; ***acute adrenal insufficiency (with increased stress from infection, surgery, or trauma);*** cushingoid state (moonface, buffalo hump, central obesity).

Overdose and treatment
Acute ingestion, even in massive doses, is rarely a clinical problem. Toxic signs and symptoms

rarely occur if drug is used for less than 3 weeks, even at large dosage ranges. However, chronic use causes adverse physiologic effects, including suppression of the hypothalamic-pituitary-adrenal axis, cushingoid appearance, muscle weakness, and osteoporosis.

Special considerations

• Determine whether patient is sensitive to other corticosteroids.
• Always adjust to lowest effective dose.
• Prednisolone salts (sodium phosphate and tebutate) are used parenterally less often than other corticosteroids that have more potent anti-inflammatory action.
• Drug may be used for alternate-day therapy.
• Most adverse reactions to corticosteroids are dose- or duration-dependent.
• Give oral dose with food when possible to reduce GI irritation. Patient may need medication to prevent GI irritation.
• Give I.M. injection deeply into gluteal muscle. Rotate injection sites to prevent muscle atrophy. Avoid S.C. injection because atrophy and sterile abscesses may occur.
• Prednisolone acetate isn't for I.V. use.
• Unless contraindicated, give low-sodium diet that's high in potassium and protein. Administer potassium supplements as needed.
• Drug may mask or worsen infections, including latent amebiasis.
• Gradually reduce dosage after long-term therapy.
ALERT After abrupt withdrawal patient may experience rebound inflammation, fatigue, weakness, arthralgia, fever, dizziness, lethargy, depression, fainting, orthostatic hypotension, dyspnea, anorexia, hypoglycemia. After prolonged use, sudden withdrawal may cause acute adrenal insufficiency and death.
ALERT Don't confuse prednisolone with prednisone.
• Use only prednisolone sodium phosphate for I.V. administration. When administering as direct injection, inject undiluted over at least 1 minute. When administering as intermittent or continuous infusion, dilute solution according to manufacturer's instructions. Use D_5W or normal saline solution as diluent for I.V. infusion.
• Prednisolone suppresses reactions to skin tests; causes false-negative results in the nitroblue tetrazolium test for systemic bacterial infections.

Patient monitoring

• Monitor patient's weight, blood pressure, and serum electrolyte levels.
• Monitor patient for cushingoid effects, including moonface, buffalo hump, central obesity, thinning hair, hypertension, and increased susceptibility to infection.
• Watch for depression or psychotic episodes, especially during high-dose therapy.

• Diabetic patient may need increased insulin; monitor blood glucose levels.

Pediatric patients

• Prolonged use of adrenocorticoids or corticotropin may suppress growth and maturation in children and adolescents.

Geriatric patients

• Elderly patients may be more susceptible to osteoporosis with long-term use.

Patient education

• Tell patient not to stop drug abruptly or without prescriber's consent.
• Instruct patient to take oral form of drug with food or milk.
• Tell patient symptoms of early adrenal insufficiency: fatigue, muscle weakness, joint pain, fever, anorexia, nausea, dyspnea, dizziness, and fainting.
• Instruct patient to carry or wear medical identification indicating his need for supplemental systemic glucocorticoids during stress. It should include prescriber's name, name of drug, and dosage taken.
• Warn patient on long-term therapy about cushingoid effects (moonface, buffalo hump) and the need to notify prescriber about sudden weight gain or swelling.
• Tell patient to report slow healing.
• Advise patient receiving long-term therapy to consider exercise or physical therapy. Advise him about vitamin D or calcium supplement.
• Instruct patient to avoid exposure to infections and to notify prescriber if exposure occurs.
• Tell patient to avoid immunizations while taking drug.
• Advise patient to be aware of signs of infection; some of these signs may be masked during drug use.

prednisolone acetate (ophthalmic)
Econopred, Pred Forte, Pred Mild

prednisolone sodium phosphate
AK-Pred, Inflamase Forte, Inflamase Mild, I-Pred, Ocu-Pred

Pharmacologic classification: corticosteroid
Therapeutic classification: ophthalmic anti-inflammatory
Pregnancy risk category: C

Indications and dosages

➤ *Inflammation of palpebral and bulbar conjunctiva, cornea, and anterior segment of globe; corneal injury; graft rejection. Adults and children:* Instill 1 or 2 drops in eye. In severe conditions, may be used hourly, tapering to discontinuation as inflammation subsides. In mild conditions, may be used four to six times daily.

How supplied
Available by prescription only
prednisolone acetate
Suspension: 0.12%, 0.125%, 1%
prednisolone sodium phosphate
Solution: 0.125%, 1%

Pharmacodynamics
Anti-inflammatory action: Corticosteroids stimulate the synthesis of enzymes needed to decrease the inflammatory response. Prednisolone, a synthetic corticosteroid, has about four times the anti-inflammatory potency of an equal weight of hydrocortisone. Prednisolone acetate is poorly soluble and therefore has a slower onset of action, but a longer duration of action, when applied in a liquid suspension. The sodium phosphate salt is highly soluble and has a rapid onset but short duration of action.

Pharmacokinetics
Absorption: After ophthalmic use, absorbed through aqueous humor. Systemic absorption rarely occurs.
Distribution: After ophthalmic use, distributed throughout local tissue layers. Any drug absorbed into circulation is rapidly removed from blood and distributed into muscle, liver, skin, intestines, and kidneys.
Metabolism: After ophthalmic use, corticosteroids primarily metabolized locally. Small amount absorbed into systemic circulation is metabolized primarily in liver to inactive compounds.
Excretion: Inactive metabolites excreted by kidneys, primarily as glucuronides and sulfates, but also as unconjugated products. Small amounts of metabolites excreted in feces.

Route	Onset	Peak	Duration
Oph-thalmic	Unknown	Unknown	Unknown

Contraindications and precautions
Contraindicated in patients with acute, untreated, purulent ocular infections; acute superficial herpes simplex (dendritic keratitis); vaccinia, varicella, or other viral or fungal eye diseases; or ocular tuberculosis. Use cautiously in patients with corneal abrasions that may be contaminated (especially with herpes).

Interactions
None reported.

Adverse reactions
EENT: increased intraocular pressure; thinning of cornea, interference with corneal wound healing, increased susceptibility to viral or fungal corneal infection, corneal ulceration; with excessive or long-term use: discharge, discomfort, foreign body sensation, glaucoma exacerbation, cataracts, visual acuity and visual field defects, optic nerve damage.
Other: systemic effects and adrenal suppression with excessive or long-term use.

Overdose and treatment
No information available.

Special considerations
● Shake suspension and check dosage before administering. Store in tightly covered container.

Patient monitoring
● Monitor tonometric readings in patients on long-term therapy.
● Monitor therapeutic effect.

Patient education
● Teach patient how to apply eyedrops.
● Tell patient not to share drug, washcloths, or towels with family members.
● Tell patient to call if improvement doesn't occur within several days or if pain, itching, or swelling of eye occurs.

---

prednisone
Apo-Prednisone*, Deltasone, Meticorten, Orasone, Prednicen-M, Sterapred, Winpred*

Pharmacologic classification: adrenocorticoid
Therapeutic classification: anti-inflammatory, immunosuppressant
Pregnancy risk category: C

Indications and dosages
➤ *Severe inflammation, modification of body's immune response to disease. Adults:* 5 to 60 mg P.O. daily in single dose or divided doses. Maximum daily dose is 250 mg. Maintenance dose given once daily or every other day. Dosage must be individualized.
Children: 0.14 to 2 mg/kg or 4 to 60 mg/m^2 P.O. daily in divided doses; or may use the following dosage schedule:
Children ages 11 to 18: 20 mg P.O. q.i.d.
Children ages 5 to 10: 15 mg P.O. q.i.d.
Children ages 18 months to 4 years: 7.5 to 10 mg P.O. q.i.d.
➤ *Adjunct to anti-infective therapy in treatment of moderate to severe* Pneumocystis carinii *pneumonia* ◇. *Adults or children over age 13 with AIDS:* 40 mg P.O. b.i.d. for 5 days; then 40 mg. P.O. once daily for 5 days; then 20 mg P.O. once daily for 11 days (or until completion of the concurrent anti-infective regimen).

How supplied
Available by prescription only
Oral solution: 5 mg/ml, 5 mg/5 ml
Syrup: 5 mg/5 ml

Reactions may be *common*, uncommon, **life-threatening**, or COMMON AND LIFE-THREATENING.

Tablets: 1 mg, 2.5 mg, 5 mg, 10 mg, 20 mg, 50 mg

Pharmacodynamics

Immunosuppressant action: Stimulates the synthesis of enzymes needed to decrease the inflammatory response. Suppresses the immune system by reducing activity and volume of the lymphatic system, thus producing lymphocytopenia (primarily of T-lymphocytes), decreasing immunoglobulin and complement levels, decreasing passage of immune complexes through basement membranes, and possibly by depressing reactivity of tissue to antigen-antibody interactions.

Anti-inflammatory action: One of the intermediate-acting glucocorticoids, with greater glucocorticoid activity than cortisone and hydrocortisone but less anti-inflammatory activity than betamethasone, dexamethasone, and paramethasone. About four to five times more potent as an anti-inflammatory than hydrocortisone, but has only half the mineralocorticoid activity of an equal weight of hydrocortisone. The oral glucocorticoid of choice for anti-inflammatory or immunosuppressive effects.

Pharmacokinetics

Absorption: Absorbed readily after oral administration; effects peak in about 1 to 2 hours.
Distribution: Distributed rapidly to muscle, liver, skin, intestines, and kidneys. Extensively bound to plasma proteins (transcortin and albumin); only unbound portion is active. Distributed into breast milk and through placenta.
Metabolism: Metabolized in liver to active metabolite prednisolone, which is then metabolized to inactive glucuronide and sulfate metabolites.
Excretion: Inactive metabolites and small amounts of unmetabolized drug excreted by kidneys. Insignificant drug quantities also excreted in feces. Biological half-life of prednisone is 18 to 36 hours.

Route	Onset	Peak	Duration
P.O.	Variable	1-2 hr	Variable

Contraindications and precautions

Contraindicated in patients hypersensitive to drug and in those with systemic fungal infections.

Use cautiously in patients with GI ulcer, renal disease, hypertension, osteoporosis, diabetes mellitus, hypothyroidism, cirrhosis, diverticulitis, nonspecific ulcerative colitis, recent intestinal anastomoses, thromboembolic disorders, seizures, myasthenia gravis, heart failure, tuberculosis, ocular herpes simplex, emotional instability, and psychotic tendencies.

Interactions

Drug-drug. *Amphotericin B, diuretics:* Enhanced hypokalemia. Monitor serum potassium level.

Antacids, cholestyramine, colestipol: Decreased prednisone absorption. Separate administration times.
Barbiturates, phenytoin, rifampin: Decreased corticosteroid effects because of increased hepatic metabolism. Monitor patient.
Cardiac glycosides: Possible hypokalemia may increase risk of toxicity in patients receiving these drugs. Monitor serum potassium level.
Estrogens: Reduced metabolism of prednisone via increased level of transcortin; half-life of corticosteroid prolonged because of increased protein-binding. Adjust dosage as needed.
Insulin, oral antidiabetics: Hyperglycemia. Adjust dosages of these drugs as needed.
Isoniazid, salicylates: Increased metabolism of these drugs. Monitor patient closely.
Oral anticoagulants: Decreased effects. Monitor PT and INR.
Ulcerogenic drugs (such as NSAIDs): Increased risk of GI ulceration. Use together cautiously.
Drug-herb. *Alfalfa sprouts, astragulus, echinacea, licorice:* Possible interference with immunosuppressive effect of drug. Discourage concomitant use.

Adverse reactions

Most adverse reactions to corticosteroids are dose- or duration-dependent.
CNS: *euphoria, insomnia,* psychotic behavior, pseudotumor cerebri, vertigo, headache, paresthesia, *seizures.*
CV: hypertension, edema, *arrhythmias,* thrombophlebitis, *thromboembolism, heart failure.*
EENT: cataracts, glaucoma.
GI: *peptic ulceration,* GI irritation, increased appetite, *pancreatitis,* nausea, vomiting.
GU: menstrual irregularities.
Metabolic: hypokalemia, hyperglycemia, carbohydrate intolerance.
Musculoskeletal: muscle weakness, osteoporosis, growth suppression in children.
Skin: delayed wound healing, acne, various skin eruptions, hirsutism.
Other: susceptibility to infections; *acute adrenal insufficiency (with increased stress from infection, surgery, or trauma);* cushingoid state (moonface, buffalo hump, central obesity).

Overdose and treatment

Acute ingestion, even in massive doses, is rarely a clinical problem. Toxic signs and symptoms rarely occur if drug is used for less than 3 weeks, even at large dosage ranges. However, chronic use causes adverse physiologic effects, including suppression of the hypothalamic-pituitary-adrenal axis, cushingoid appearance, muscle weakness, and osteoporosis.

Special considerations

● Determine whether patient is sensitive to other corticosteroids.
● Drug may be used for alternate-day therapy.

◇ Unlabeled clinical use

• Always adjust to lowest effective dose.
• Most adverse reactions to corticosteroids are dose- or duration-dependent.
• For better results and less toxicity, give a once-daily dose in the morning.
• Unless contraindicated, give oral dose with food when possible to reduce GI irritation. Patient may need medication to prevent GI irritation.
• The oral solution may be diluted in juice or other flavored diluent or semi-solid food (such as applesauce) before administration.
• Drug may mask or worsen infections, including latent amebiasis.
• Unless contraindicated, give low-sodium diet that's high in potassium and protein. Administer potassium supplements as needed.

⚠ ALERT Gradually reduce dosage after long-term therapy. After abrupt withdrawal: rebound inflammation, fatigue, weakness, arthralgia, fever, dizziness, lethargy, depression, fainting, orthostatic hypotension, dyspnea, anorexia, hypoglycemia. After prolonged use, sudden withdrawal may cause acute adrenal insufficiency and death.

⚠ ALERT Don't confuse prednisone with prednisolone.

• For patients who can't swallow tablets, liquid forms are available. The oral concentrate (5 mg/ml) may be diluted in juice or another flavored diluent or mixed in semisolid food (such as applesauce) before administration.
• Prednisone suppresses reactions to skin tests; causes false-negative results in the nitroblue tetrazolium test for systemic bacterial infections.

Patient monitoring
• Monitor patient's weight, blood pressure, and serum electrolyte levels.
• Monitor patient for cushingoid effects, including moonface, buffalo hump, central obesity, thinning hair, hypertension, and increased susceptibility to infection.
• Watch for depression or psychotic episodes, especially during high-dose therapy.
• Diabetic patient may need increased insulin; monitor blood glucose levels.

Beast-feeding patients
• Prednisone is distributed into breast milk; breast-feeding during use is not recommended.

Pediatric patients
• Prolonged use of prednisone in children or adolescents may delay growth and maturation.

Geriatric patients
• Elderly patients may be more susceptible to osteoporosis with long-term use.

Patient education
• Tell patient not to stop drug abruptly or without prescriber's consent.
• Instruct patient to take drug with food or milk.
• Teach patient evidence of early adrenal insufficiency: fatigue, muscle weakness, joint pain, fever, anorexia, nausea, dyspnea, dizziness, and fainting.
• Instruct patient to carry or wear medical identification indicating his need for supplemental systemic glucocorticoids during stress. It should include prescriber's name, name of drug, and dosage taken.
• Warn patient on long-term therapy about cushingoid effects (moonface, buffalo hump) and the need to notify prescriber about sudden weight gain or swelling.
• Advise patient receiving long-term therapy to consider exercise or physical therapy. Also, advise patient about vitamin D or calcium supplement.
• Tell patient to report slow healing.
• Advise patient receiving long-term therapy to have periodic ophthalmic examinations.
• Instruct patient to avoid exposure to infections and to contact prescriber if exposure occurs.
• Tell patient to report fluid retention if it occurs.
• Instruct patient to not become immunized during drug therapy.
• Advise patient to be aware of signs of infection; some of these signs may be masked during drug use.

primaquine phosphate

Pharmacologic classification: 8-aminoquinoline
Therapeutic classification: antimalarial
Pregnancy risk category: C

Indications and dosages
➤ **Radical cure of relapsing vivax malaria, eliminating symptoms and infection completely, and prevention of relapse.**
Adults: 15 mg (base) P.O. daily for 14 days (26.3-mg tablet equals 15 mg of base), or 79 mg (45-mg base) once weekly for 8 weeks.
Children: 0.3 mg (base)/kg daily for 14 days, or 0.9 mg (base)/kg daily once weekly for 8 weeks.
➤ **Pneumocystis carinii** *pneumonia* ◇.
Adults: 15 to 30 mg (base) P.O. daily.

How supplied
Available by prescription only
Tablets: 26.3 mg (15-mg base)

Pharmacodynamics
Antimalarial action: Disrupts the parasitic mitochondria, thereby interrupting metabolic processes requiring energy. Spectrum of activity includes preerythrocytic and exoerythrocytic forms of *Plasmodium falciparum, P. malariae, P. ovale,* and *P. vivax.* Nifurtimox (Lampit), an investigational drug available from the Centers for Disease Control and Prevention, is preferred for intracellular parasites.

Pharmacokinetics
Absorption: Well absorbed from GI tract; levels peak in 2 to 6 hours.
Distribution: Distributed widely into liver, lungs, heart, brain, skeletal muscle, and other tissues.
Metabolism: Carboxylated rapidly in liver.
Excretion: Only small amount of drug excreted unchanged in urine. Plasma half-life is 4 to 10 hours.

Route	Onset	Peak	Duration
P.O.	Unknown	1-3 hr	Unknown

Contraindications and precautions
Contraindicated in patients with systemic diseases in which granulocytopenia may develop (such as lupus erythematosus or rheumatoid arthritis) and in those taking bone marrow suppressants and potentially hemolytic drugs.

Use cautiously in patients with previous idiosyncratic reaction (manifested by hemolytic anemia, methemoglobinemia, or leukopenia) and in those with family or personal history of favism, erythrocytic G6PD deficiency, or nicotinamide adenine dinucleotide (NADH) methemoglobin reductase deficiency.

Interactions
Drug-drug. *Aluminum salts, magnesium:* Decreased GI absorption. Separate administration times.
Quinacrine: Potentiated toxic effects of primaquine. Use together cautiously.

Adverse reactions
GI: nausea, vomiting, epigastric distress, abdominal cramps.
Hematologic: *leukopenia, hemolytic anemia in G6PD deficiency,* methemoglobinemia in NADH methemoglobin reductase deficiency.

Overdose and treatment
Toxicity may cause abdominal distress, vomiting, CNS and CV disturbances, cyanosis, methemoglobinemia, leukocytosis, leukopenia, and anemia.

Special considerations
● Primaquine is often used with a fast-acting antimalarial such as chloroquine.
⚠ **ALERT** Light-skinned patients taking more than 30 mg daily, dark-skinned patients taking more than 15 mg daily, and patients with severe anemia or suspected sensitivity should have frequent blood studies and urine examinations. A sudden fall in hemoglobin levels or erythrocyte or leukocyte counts, or a marked darkening of urine suggests impending hemolytic reaction.

Patient monitoring
● Before starting therapy, screen patients for possible G6PD deficiency.

● Perform periodic blood studies and urinalyses to monitor patient for impending hemolytic reactions.

Breast-feeding patients
● It isn't known if drug appears in breast milk. Safety in breast-feeding women hasn't been established.

Patient education
● Teach patient signs and symptoms of adverse reactions and to report them if they occur.
● Advise patient to check urine color at each voiding and to report if urine darkens, becomes tinged with red, or decreases in volume.
● Tell patient to take drug with meals to minimize gastric irritation. Don't take with antacids, which may decrease absorption.
● Advise patient to complete entire course of therapy.

primidone
Mysoline

Pharmacologic classification: barbiturate analogue
Therapeutic classification: anticonvulsant
Pregnancy risk category: NR

Indications and dosages
➤ *Generalized tonic-clonic seizures, focal seizures, complex-partial (psychomotor) seizures.* *Adults and children ages 8 and over:* 100 to 125 mg P.O. h.s. on days 1 to 3; 100 to 125 mg P.O. b.i.d. on days 4 to 6; 100 to 125 mg P.O. t.i.d. on days 7 to 9; and maintenance dose of 250 mg P.O. t.i.d. on day 10. May need up to 2 g daily.
Children under age 8: 50 mg P.O. h.s. on days 1 to 3; 50 mg P.O. b.i.d. on days 4 to 6; 100 mg P.O. t.i.d. on days 7 to 9; and maintenance dose of 125 to 250 mg P.O. t.i.d. on day 10.
➤ *Benign familial tremor (essential tremor).* *Adults:* 750 mg P.O. daily.

How supplied
Available by prescription only
Suspension: 250 mg/5 ml
Tablets: 50 mg, 250 mg

Pharmacodynamics
Anticonvulsant action: Mechanism unknown. Acts as a nonspecific CNS depressant used alone or with other anticonvulsants to control refractory tonic-clonic seizures and to treat psychomotor or focal seizures. Some activity may be from phenobarbital, an active metabolite.

Pharmacokinetics
Absorption: Drug absorbed readily from GI tract; serum levels peak at about 3 hours. Phenobarbital appears in plasma after several days of continuous therapy; most laboratory assays detect

both phenobarbital and primidone. Therapeutic levels 5 to 12 mcg/ml for primidone; 10 to 30 mcg/ml for phenobarbital.

Distribution: Primidone distributed widely throughout body.

Metabolism: Primidone metabolized slowly by liver to phenylethylmalonamide (PEMA) and phenobarbital; PEMA is major metabolite.

Excretion: Primidone excreted in urine; substantial amounts appear in breast milk.

Route	Onset	Peak	Duration
P.O.	Unknown	3-4 hr	Unknown

Contraindications and precautions

Contraindicated in patients with phenobarbital hypersensitivity or porphyria.

Interactions

Drug-drug. *Acetazolamide, succinimides:* Decreased primidone levels. Monitor patient closely.
Carbamazepine, phenytoin: Possible decreased effects of primidone; increased conversion to phenobarbital. Monitor serum levels to prevent toxicity.
CNS depressants (such as narcotic analgesics): Excessive depression in patients taking primidone. Avoid using together.
Oral contraceptives: Barbiturates may render oral contraceptives ineffective. Advise patient to consider a different birth control method.
Drug-lifestyle. *Alcohol use:* Excessive depression in patients taking primidone. Discourage use.

Adverse reactions

CNS: *drowsiness, ataxia,* emotional disturbances, vertigo, hyperirritability, fatigue, paranoia.
EENT: *diplopia,* nystagmus.
GI: anorexia, nausea, vomiting.
GU: impotence, polyuria.
Hematologic: megaloblastic anemia, ***thrombocytopenia.***
Hepatic: abnormalities in liver function test results.
Skin: morbilliform rash.

Overdose and treatment

Signs and symptoms of toxicity resemble those of barbiturate intoxication, including CNS and respiratory depression, areflexia, oliguria, tachycardia, hypotension, hypothermia, and coma. Shock may occur. Treat overdose supportively: in conscious patient with intact gag reflex, induce emesis with ipecac; follow in 30 minutes with repeated doses of activated charcoal. Use lavage if emesis isn't feasible. Alkalinization of urine and forced diuresis may hasten excretion. Hemodialysis may be necessary. Monitor vital signs and fluid and electrolyte balance.

Special considerations

• Abrupt withdrawal of drug may cause status epilepticus; dosage should be reduced gradually.

• Barbiturates impair ability to perform tasks requiring mental alertness such as driving.

Patient monitoring

• Perform a CBC and liver function tests every 6 months.
• Monitor patient for adverse effects.

Breast-feeding patients

• Considerable amounts of drug appear in breast milk. Use an alternative to breast-feeding during therapy.

Pediatric patients

• Drug may cause hyperexcitability in children under age 6.

Geriatric patients

• Reduce dosage in elderly patients; many have decreased renal function.

Patient education

• Explain rationale for therapy and potential risks and benefits.
• Teach patient signs and symptoms of adverse reactions.
• Tell patient to avoid alcohol and other sedatives to prevent added CNS depression.
• Instruct patient not to stop drug or to alter dosage without medical approval.
• Advise patient to avoid hazardous tasks that require mental alertness until degree of sedative effect is determined. Tell patient that dizziness and incoordination are common at first but will disappear.
• Recommend that patient wear a medical identification bracelet or necklace identifying him as having a seizure disorder and listing drug.
• Tell patient to shake oral suspension well before use.

probenecid
Benemid

Pharmacologic classification: sulfonamide-derivative
Therapeutic classification: uricosuric
Pregnancy risk category: NR

Indications and dosages

➤ **Adjunct to penicillin therapy.** *Adults and children over age 14 or weighing over 50 kg (110 lb):* 500 mg P.O. q.i.d.
Children ages 2 to 14 or weighing under 50 kg: Initially, 25 mg/kg or 700 mg/m² daily; then 40 mg/kg or 1.2 g/m² divided q.i.d.
➤ **Single-dose penicillin treatment of gonorrhea.** *Adults:* 1 g P.O. given together with penicillin treatment, or 1 g P.O. 30 minutes before I.M. dose of penicillin.
➤ **Hyperuricemia related to gout.** *Adults:* 250 mg P.O. b.i.d. for first week, then 500 mg b.i.d., to maximum of 2 to 3 g daily.

Reactions may be *common*, uncommon, ***life-threatening***, or COMMON AND LIFE-THREATENING.

➤ *To diagnose parkinsonian syndrome or mental depression* ◇. *Adults:* 500 mg P.O. q 12 hours for five doses.

How supplied
Available by prescription only
Tablets: 500 mg

Pharmacodynamics
Uricosuric action: Competitively inhibits the active reabsorption of uric acid at the proximal convoluted tubule, thereby increasing urinary excretion of uric acid.
Adjunctive action in antibiotic therapy: Competitively inhibits secretion of weak organic acids, such as penicillins, cephalosporins, and other beta-lactam antibiotics, thereby increasing serum levels of these drugs.

Pharmacokinetics
Absorption: Completely absorbed after oral administration; serum levels peak in 2 to 4 hours.
Distribution: Distributed throughout body; about 75% protein-bound. CSF levels about 2% of serum levels.
Metabolism: Metabolized in liver to active metabolites, with some uricosuric effect.
Excretion: Drug and metabolites excreted in urine; drug (but not metabolites) actively reabsorbed.

Route	Onset	Peak	Duration
P.O.	Unknown	2-4 hr	Unknown

Contraindications and precautions
Contraindicated in patients hypersensitive to drug, in those with uric acid kidney stones or blood dyscrasias; in acute gout attack; and in children under age 2. Use cautiously in patients with impaired renal function or peptic ulcer.

Interactions
Drug-drug. *Aminosalicylic acid, dapsone, methotrexate, nitrofurantoin:* Increased serum levels; increased risk of toxicity of these drugs. Monitor patient for toxicity.
Bumetanide, ethacrynic acid, furosemide: Impaired natriuretic effects of these drugs. Adjust dosages as needed.
Cephalosporins, ketamine (possibly), penicillins, sulfonamides, thiopental (possibly), other beta-lactam antibiotics: Significant increased or prolonged effects of these drugs. Monitor patient closely.
Chlorpropamide, other oral sulfonylureas: Enhanced hypoglycemic effects. Adjust dosages as needed.
Diuretics, pyrazinamide: Increased uric acid levels. Increased doses of probenecid may be needed.
Indomethacin, naproxen: Decreased excretion of these drugs. Use lower dosages.
Salicylates: Inhibited uricosuric effect of probenecid only in doses that achieve levels of

50 mcg/ml or more; occasional use of low-dose aspirin doesn't interfere.
Weak organic acids: Inhibited urinary excretion of these drugs. Monitor patient.
Zidovudine: Increased bioavailability of zidovudine; cutaneous eruptions accompanied by systemic symptoms (including malaise, myalgia, or fever) possible. Monitor patient for toxicity.
Drug-lifestyle. *Alcohol use:* Decreased uric acid levels of probenecid. Increased doses of probenecid may be needed with alcohol use.

Adverse reactions
CNS: *headache,* dizziness.
GI: anorexia, nausea, vomiting, sore gums.
GU: urinary frequency, renal colic, nephrotic syndrome.
Hematologic: *hemolytic anemia, aplastic anemia, anemia.*
Hepatic: *hepatic necrosis.*
Skin: dermatitis, pruritus.
Other: flushing, fever, exacerbation of gout, hypersensitivity reactions (including *anaphylaxis*).

Overdose and treatment
Toxicity may cause nausea, copious vomiting, stupor, coma, and tonic-clonic seizures. Treat supportively, using mechanical ventilation, if needed; induce emesis or use gastric lavage, as apopropriate. Control seizures with I.V. phenobarbital and phenytoin.

Special considerations
● When used for hyperuricemia related to gout, probenecid has no analgesic or anti-inflammatory actions and no effect on acute attacks; start therapy after attack subsides. Because drug may increase frequency of acute attacks during first 6 to 12 months of therapy, prophylactic doses of colchicine or an NSAID should be given during first 3 to 6 months of probenecid therapy.
● Give with food, milk, or prescribed antacids to lessen GI upset.
● Maintain adequate hydration with high fluid intake to prevent formation of uric acid stones. Also maintain alkalinization of urine.
● Drug has been used in the diagnosis of parkinsonian syndrome and mental depression.
● Probenecid causes false-positive test results for urinary glucose with tests using cupric sulfate reagent (Benedict's reagent, Clinitest, and Fehling's test); perform tests with glucose oxidase reagent (Diastix, Chemstrip uG, or glucose enzymatic test strip) instead.

Patient monitoring
● Monitor BUN and serum creatinine levels closely; drug is ineffective in severe renal insufficiency.
● Monitor uric acid levels and adjust dosage to lowest dose that maintains normal uric acid levels.

Breast-feeding patients
● It isn't known if drug appears in breast milk. An alternative to breast-feeding is recommended during therapy.

Pediatric patients
● Drug is contraindicated in infants under age 2.

Geriatric patients
● Lower dosages are indicated in elderly patients.

Patient education
● Instruct patient not to stop drug without medical approval.
● Warn patient not to use drug for pain or inflammation and not to increase dose during gouty attack.
● Tell patient to drink 8 to 10 glasses of fluid daily and to take drug with food to minimize GI upset.
● Warn patient to avoid aspirin and other salicylates, which may antagonize probenecid's uricosuric effect.
● Caution diabetic patients to use glucose enzymatic test strip, Diastix, or Chemstrip uG for urine glucose testing.

procainamide hydrochloride
Procanbid, Pronestyl, Pronestyl-SR

Pharmacologic classification: procaine derivative
Therapeutic classification: ventricular antiarrhythmic, supraventricular antiarrhythmic
Pregnancy risk category: C

Indications and dosages
➤ *Symptomatic PVCs; life-threatening ventricular tachycardia, atrial fibrillation and flutter unresponsive to quinidine* ◇*; paroxysmal atrial tachycardia* ◇.
Adults: 50 to 100 mg q 5 minutes by slow I.V. push, no faster than 25 to 50 mg/minute, until arrhythmias disappear, adverse effects develop, or 500 mg has been given. When arrhythmias disappear, give continuous infusion of 1 to 6 mg/minute. Usual effective loading dose is 500 to 600 mg. If arrhythmias recur, repeat bolus as above and increase infusion rate. For I.M. administration, give 50 mg/kg divided q 3 to 6 hours; during surgery, 100 to 500 mg I.M. For oral therapy, initiate dosage at 50 mg/kg P.O. in divided doses q 3 hours until therapeutic levels are reached. Once patient is stable, may substitute sustained-release form q 6 hours or extended-release form at dose of 50 mg/kg in two divided doses q 12 hours.
➤ *Loading dose to prevent atrial fibrillation or paroxysmal atrial tachycardia* ◇. *Adults:* 1 to 1.25 g P.O. If arrhythmias persist after 1 hour, give additional 750 mg. If no change occurs, give 500 mg to 1 g q 2 hours until arrhythmias disappear or adverse effects occur.
➤ *Loading dose to prevent ventricular tachycardia. Adults:* 1 g P.O. Maintenance dose is 50 mg/kg daily given at 3-hour intervals; average is 250 to 500 mg q 4 hours but 1 to 1.5 g q 4 to 6 hours may be needed.
➤ *Malignant hyperthermia* ◇. *Adults:* 200 to 900 mg I.V.; then an infusion.

How supplied
Available by prescription only
Capsules: 250 mg, 375 mg, 500 mg
Injection: 100 mg/ml, 500 mg/ml
Tablets: 250 mg, 375 mg, 500 mg
Tablets (extended-release): 500 mg, 1 g
Tablets (sustained-release): 250 mg, 500 mg, 750 mg

Pharmacodynamics
Antiarrhythmic action: A class IA antiarrhythmic that depresses phase 0 of the action potential. Considered a myocardial depressant because it decreases myocardial excitability and conduction velocity and may depress myocardial contractility. Also possesses anticholinergic activity, which may modify direct myocardial effects. In therapeutic doses, drug reduces conduction velocity in the atria, ventricles, and His-Purkinje system. Its effectiveness in controlling atrial tachyarrhythmias stems from its ability to prolong the effective refractory period (ERP) and increase the action potential duration in the atria, ventricles, and His-Purkinje system. Because ERP prolongation exceeds action potential duration, tissue remains refractory even after returning to resting membrane potential (membrane-stabilizing effect).

Procainamide shortens the effective refractory period of the AV node. Drug's anticholinergic action also may increase AV node conductivity. Suppression of automaticity in the His-Purkinje system and ectopic pacemakers accounts for drug's effectiveness in treating ventricular premature beats. At therapeutic doses, procainamide prolongs the PR and QT intervals. (This effect may be used as an index of drug effectiveness and toxicity.) The QRS complex usually isn't prolonged beyond normal range; the QT interval isn't prolonged to the extent achieved with quinidine.

Procainamide exerts a peripheral vasodilatory effect; with I.V. administration, it may cause hypotension, which limits the administration rate and amount of drug deliverable.

Pharmacokinetics
Absorption: Rate and extent of absorption from intestines vary; usually, 75% to 95% of oral dose absorbed. With tablets and capsules, plasma levels peak in about 1 hour. Extended-release tablets formulated to provide sustained and relatively constant rate of release and absorption throughout small intestine. After drug's release, extended wax matrix isn't absorbed and may appear in feces after 15 minutes to 1 hour. With I.M. in-

---

jection, onset of action in about 10 to 30 minutes; peak levels in about 1 hour.
Distribution: Distributed widely in most body tissues, including CSF, liver, spleen, kidneys, lungs, muscles, brain, and heart. Only about 15% binds to plasma proteins. Usual therapeutic range of serum procainamide levels is 4 to 8 mcg/ml. Some experts suggest that a range of 10 to 30 mcg/ml for the sum of procainamide and N-acetyl procainamide (NAPA) serum levels is therapeutic.
Metabolism: Drug is acetylated in liver to form NAPA. Acetylation rate determined genetically and affects NAPA formation. (NAPA also exerts antiarrhythmic activity.)
Excretion: Procainamide and NAPA metabolite excreted in urine. Procainamide's half-life is about 2½ to 4¾ hours; NAPA's half-life is about 6 hours. In patients with heart failure or renal dysfunction, half-life increases; in such patients, dosage reduction required to avoid toxicity.

Route	Onset	Peak	Duration
P.O.	1-2 hr	½- 1½ hr	Unknown
I.V.	Immediate	Immediate	Unknown
I.M.	10-30 min	15-60 min	Unknown

Contraindications and precautions
Contraindicated in patients hypersensitive to procaine and related drugs; in those with complete, second-, or third-degree heart block in the absence of an artificial pacemaker; and in patients with myasthenia gravis or systemic lupus erythematosus. Also contraindicated in patients with atypical ventricular tachycardia (torsades de pointes) because procainamide may aggravate this condition

Use cautiously in patients with ventricular tachycardia during coronary occlusion, heart failure or other conduction disturbances (bundle-branch heart block, sinus bradycardia, cardiac glycoside intoxication), impaired renal or hepatic function, preexisting blood dyscrasia, or bone marrow suppression.

Interactions
Drug-drug. *Anticholinergics (atropine, diphenhydramine, tricyclic antidepressants):* Additive anticholinergic effects. Monitor patient closely.
Antihypertensives: Additive hypotensive effects (most common with I.V. procainamide). Monitor blood pressure.
Cholinergics (neostigmine, pyridostigmine, which are used to treat myasthenia gravis): May negate effects of these drugs. Increase dosage.
Cimetidine: Impaired renal clearance of procainamide and NAPA, with elevated serum drug levels. Adjust dose if used together.
Neuromuscular blockers (such as decamethonium bromide, gallium triethiodide, metocurine iodide, pancuronium bromide, succinylcholine chloride, tubocurarine chloride):

Potentiated effects of neuromuscular blockers. Monitor patient closely.
Other antiarrhythmics: Additive or antagonistic cardiac effects; possible additive toxic effects. Monitor patient for toxicity.
Drug-herb. *Jimsonweed:* Possible adverse effect on CV system function. Discourage use.
Licorice: Possible prolonged QT interval; potentially additive. Discourage use together.

Adverse reactions
CNS: hallucinations, confusion, *seizures,* depression, dizziness.
CV: *hypotension, ventricular asystole, bradycardia, AV block, ventricular fibrillation* (after parenteral use).
GI: nausea, vomiting, anorexia, diarrhea, bitter taste.
Hematologic: *thrombocytopenia, neutropenia* (especially with sustained-release forms), *agranulocytosis, hemolytic anemia.*
Hepatic: increased liver function test results.
Skin: *maculopapular rash, urticaria, pruritus, flushing, angioneurotic edema.*
Other: *fever, lupuslike syndrome* (especially after prolonged administration), positive antinuclear antibody (ANA) titers, positive direct antiglobulin (Coombs') tests.

Overdose and treatment
Toxicity may cause severe hypotension, widening QRS complex, junctional tachycardia, intraventricular conduction delay, ventricular fibrillation, oliguria, confusion and lethargy, and nausea and vomiting. Treatment involves general supportive measures, including respiratory and CV support, with hemodynamic and ECG monitoring. Ater recent ingestion of oral form, gastric lavage, emesis, and activated charcoal may be used to decrease absorption. Phenylephrine or norepinephrine may be used to treat hypotension after adequate hydration has been ensured. Hemodialysis may be effective in removing procainamide and NAPA. A 1/6 M solution of sodium lactate may reduce procainamide's cardiotoxic effect.

Special considerations
⚠ **ALERT** In treating atrial fibrillation and flutter, ventricular rate may accelerate because of vagolytic effects on the AV node; to prevent this effect, a cardiac glycoside may be administered before procainamide therapy begins.
● Infusion pump or microdrip system and timer should be used to monitor infusion precisely.
● For initial oral therapy, use conventional capsules and tablets; use extended-release tablets only for maintenance therapy.
● I.V. drug form is more likely to cause adverse cardiac effects, possibly resulting in severe hypotension.
● Procainamide will invalidate bentiromide test results; discontinue at least 3 days before ben-

tiromide test. Procainamide may alter edrophonium test results.

Patient monitoring
• Monitor patient receiving infusions at all times.
• Monitor blood pressure and ECG continuously during I.V. administration. Watch for prolonged QT interval and QRS complex (50% or greater widening), heart block, or increased arrhythmias. When these ECG signs appear, stop drug and monitor patient closely.
• Monitor therapeutic serum levels of procainamide: 3 to 10 mcg/ml (most patients are controlled at 4 to 8 mcg/ml; may exhibit toxicity at levels greater than 16 mcg/ml). Monitor NAPA levels as well; some clinicians feel that procainamide and NAPA levels should be 10 to 30 mcg/ml.
• Baseline and periodic determinations of ANA titers, lupus erythematosus cell preparations, and CBCs may be indicated because procainamide therapy (usually long-term) has been linked to a syndrome resembling systemic lupus erythematosus.
• In prolonged use of oral form, perform ECGs occasionally to determine continued need for drug.

Breast-feeding patients
• Procainamide and NAPA appear in breast milk. An alternative to breast-feeding is recommended for breast-feeding women.

Pediatric patients
• Manufacturer hasn't established dosage guidelines for children. For treating arrhythmias, the suggested dosage is 40 to 60 mg/kg of standard tablets or capsules, P.O. daily, given in four to six divided doses; or 3 to 6 mg/kg I.V. over 5 minutes, then a drip of 0.02 to 0.08 mg/kg/minute.

Geriatric patients
• Elderly patients may need reduced dosage. Because of highly variable metabolism, monitoring of serum levels is recommended.

Patient education
• Stress importance of taking drug exactly as prescribed.
• Instruct patient to report fever, rash, muscle pain, diarrhea, bleeding, bruises, or pleuritic chest pain.
• Tell patient not to crush or break sustained-release tablets.
• Reassure patient who is taking extended-release form that a wax-matrix "ghost" from tablet may be passed in stools. Drug is completely absorbed before this occurs.

procarbazine hydrochloride
Matulane, Natulan*

Pharmacologic classification: antibiotic antineoplastic (specific to S phase of cell cycle)
Therapeutic classification: antineoplastic
Pregnancy risk category: D

Indications and dosages
Dosage and indications may vary. Check current literature for recommended protocol.
➤ *Hodgkin's disease, lymphomas, brain and lung cancer. Adults:* 2 to 4 mg/kg daily P.O. in single or divided doses for the first week; then 4 to 6 mg/kg daily until response or toxicity occurs. Maintenance dose is 1 to 2 mg/kg daily. *Children:* 50 mg/m² daily P.O. for first week; then 100 mg/m² daily until response or toxicity occurs. Maintenance dose is 50 mg/m² P.O. daily after bone marrow recovery.

How supplied
Available by prescription only
Capsules: 50 mg

Pharmacodynamics
Antineoplastic action: Exact mechanism unknown. Appears to have several sites of action, resulting in inhibition of DNA, RNA, and protein synthesis. Has also been reported to damage DNA directly and to inhibit the mitotic S phase of cell division.

Pharmacokinetics
Absorption: Rapidly and completely absorbed after oral administration.
Distribution: Distributed widely into body tissues; highest levels found in liver, kidneys, intestinal wall, and skin. Crosses blood-brain barrier.
Metabolism: Extensively metabolized in liver. Some metabolites have cytotoxic activity.
Excretion: Drug and metabolites excreted primarily in urine.

Route	Onset	Peak	Duration
P.O.	Unknown	Unknown	Unknown

Contraindications and precautions
Contraindicated in patients hypersensitive to drug and in those with inadequate bone marrow reserve as shown by bone marrow aspiration. Use cautiously in patients with impaired renal or hepatic function.

Interactions
Drug-drug. *CNS depressants:* Enhanced CNS depression through additive mechanism. Monitor patient.
Digoxin: Possible decreased serum digoxin levels. Monitor serum digoxin levels.

Reactions may be *common*, uncommon, *life-threatening*, or COMMON AND LIFE-THREATENING.

Levodopa: Flushing and significant rise in blood pressure. Use together cautiously.

MAO inhibitors, selective serotonin reuptake inhibitors, sympathomimetics, tricyclic antidepressants: Inhibition of MAO by procarbazine; hypertensive crisis, tremors, excitation, and cardiac palpitations. Don't use together.

Narcotics: CNS depressant effects causing deep coma and death. Don't use together.

Drug-food. *Foods containing tyramine:* Inhibition of MAO by procarbazine; hypertensive crisis, tremors, excitation, and cardiac palpitations. Discourage use together.

Drug-lifestyle. *Alcohol use:* Disulfiram-like reaction. Discourage alcohol use.

Sun exposure: Photosensitivity reactions. Tell patient to take precautions.

Adverse reactions

CNS: nervousness, depression, headache, dizziness, *coma, seizures,* insomnia, nightmares, paresthesia, neuropathy, *hallucinations,* confusion.

CV: hypotension, tachycardia, syncope.

EENT: retinal hemorrhage, nystagmus, photophobia.

GI: *nausea, vomiting,* anorexia, stomatitis, dry mouth, dysphagia, diarrhea, constipation.

GU: hematuria, urinary frequency, nocturia.

Hematologic: *bleeding tendency, thrombocytopenia, leukopenia, anemia,* hemolytic anemia.

Respiratory: *pleural effusion,* pneumonitis, cough.

Skin: dermatitis, pruritus, rash, reversible alopecia.

Other: *allergic reactions,* gynecomastia.

Overdose and treatment

Toxicity may cause myalgia, arthralgia, fever, weakness, dermatitis, alopecia, paresthesia, hallucinations, tremors, seizures, coma, myelosuppression, nausea, and vomiting.

Treatment is usually supportive and includes transfusion of blood components, antiemetics, antipyretics and appropriate antianxiety agents.

Special considerations

● Nausea and vomiting may be decreased if drug is taken at bedtime and in divided doses.

● Procarbazine inhibits MAO. Use procarbazine cautiously with MAO inhibitors, tricyclic antidepressants and selective serotonin reuptake inhibitors, other drugs that interact with MAO inhibitors, or tyramine-rich foods.

● Use cautiously in patients with inadequate bone marrow reserve, leukopenia, thrombocytopenia, anemia, and impaired hepatic or renal function.

● Store capsules in dry environment.

Patient monitoring

● Watch for signs of bleeding and monitor patient for other adverse effects.

Breast-feeding patients

● It isn't known if drug appears in breast milk. Because of potential for serious adverse reactions, mutagenicity, and carcinogenicity in infant, breast-feeding isn't recommended.

Pediatric patients

● Severe reactions, such as tremors, seizures, and coma, have occurred in children receiving drug.

Patient education

● Emphasize importance of continuing drug despite nausea and vomiting.

● Advise patient to call immediately if vomiting occurs shortly after taking dose.

● Warn patient that drowsiness may occur, so patient should avoid hazardous activities that require alertness until drug's effect is established.

● Warn patient not to drink alcoholic beverages or eat foods containing tyramine while taking drug.

● Instruct patient to stop drug and call immediately if disulfiram-like reaction occurs (chest pains, rapid or irregular heartbeat, severe headache, stiff neck).

● Tell patient to avoid exposure to people with infections.

● Warn patient to avoid prolonged sun exposure because photosensitivity occurs during therapy.

● Tell patient to call if a sore throat or fever or unusual bruising or bleeding occurs.

prochlorperazine
Compazine, Stemetil*

prochlorperazine edisylate
Compazine

prochlorperazine maleate
Compazine, Compazine Spansule, Stemetil*

Pharmacologic classification: phenothiazine (piperazine derivative)
Therapeutic classification: antipsychotic, antiemetic, anxiolytic
Pregnancy risk category: C

Indications and dosages

➤ *Preoperative nausea control. Adults:* 5 to 10 mg I.M. 1 to 2 hours before induction of anesthesia, repeated once in 30 minutes if necessary; or 5 to 10 mg I.V. 15 to 30 minutes before induction of anesthesia, repeated once if necessary; or 20 mg/L D_5W and normal saline solution by I.V. infusion, added to infusion 15 to 30 minutes before induction. Maximum parenteral dosage is 40 mg daily.

➤ *Severe nausea, vomiting. Adults:* 5 to 10 mg P.O. t.i.d. or q.i.d. Or, 15 mg of sustained-release form P.O. on arising. Or, 10 mg of sustained-release form P.O. q 12 hours. Or, 25 mg P.R. b.i.d. Or, 5 to 10 mg I.M. injected deeply into upper outer quadrant of gluteal region. Repeat q 3 to 4 hours, p.r.n. May be given I.V. Maximum parenteral dose is 40 mg daily.

Children weighing 18 to 39 kg (39 to 86 lb): 2.5 mg P.O. or P.R. t.i.d.; or 5 mg P.O. or P.R. b.i.d.; or 0.132 mg/kg deep I.M. injection. (Control usually obtained with one dose.) Maximum, 15 mg daily.

Children weighing 14 to 17 kg (31 to 38 lb): 2.5 mg P.O. or P.R. b.i.d. or t.i.d.; or 0.132 mg/kg deep I.M. injection. (Control usually is obtained with one dose.) Maximum, 10 mg daily.

Children weighing 9 to 14 kg (20 to 30 lb): 2.5 mg P.O. or P.R. daily or b.i.d.; or 0.132 mg/kg deep I.M. injection. (Control usually is obtained with one dose.) Maximum, 7.5 mg daily.

➤ *Anxiety. Adults:* 5 mg P.O. t.i.d. or q.i.d.
➤ *Psychotic disorders. Adults:* 5 to 10 mg P.O. or 10 to 20 mg I.M. t.i.d. or q.i.d.; up to 150 mg daily P.O. for hospitalized patients.

How supplied

Available by prescription only
prochlorperazine maleate
Tablets: 5 mg, 10 mg, 25 mg
prochlorperazine edisylate
Injection: 5 mg/ml
Spansules (sustained-release): 10 mg, 15 mg
Suppositories: 2.5 mg, 5 mg, 25 mg
Syrup: 1 mg/ml

Pharmacodynamics

Antipsychotic action: Thought to exert antipsychotic effects by postsynaptic blockade of CNS dopamine receptors, thus inhibiting dopamine-mediated effects.

Antiemetic action: Effects attributed to dopamine receptor blockade in the medullary chemoreceptor trigger zone.

Has many other central and peripheral effects: Produces alpha and ganglionic blockade and counteracts histamine- and serotonin-mediated activity. Most prevalent adverse reactions are extrapyramidal. Used primarily as an antiemetic; ineffective against motion sickness.

Pharmacokinetics

Absorption: Rate and extent of absorption vary with administration route. Oral tablet absorption is erratic and variable; onset of action ranging from ½ to 1 hour. Oral concentrate absorption more predictable. I.M. drug absorbed rapidly.

Distribution: Distributed widely into body, including breast milk. 91% to 99% protein-bound. Peak effect at 2 to 4 hours; steady state serum levels within 4 to 7 days.

Metabolism: Metabolized extensively by liver; no active metabolites formed. Duration of action about 3 to 4 hours; 10 to 12 hours for extended-release form.

Excretion: Mostly excreted in urine via kidneys; some excreted in feces via biliary tract.

Route	Onset	Peak	Duration
P.O.	30-40 min	Unknown	3-12 hr
I.V.	Unknown	Unknown	Unknown
I.M.	10-20 min	Unknown	3-4 hr
P.R.	1 hr	Unknown	3-4 hr

Contraindications and precautions

Contraindicated in patients hypersensitive to phenothiazines and in those with CNS depression including coma; during pediatric surgery; when using spinal or epidural anesthetic, adrenergic blockers, or ethanol; and in infants under age 2.

Use cautiously in patients with impaired CV function, glaucoma, or seizure disorders; in those who have been exposed to extreme heat; and in children with acute illness.

Interactions

Drug-drug. *Antacids containing aluminum and magnesium; antidiarrheals:* Inhibited absorption. Separate administration times by at least 2 hours.

Antiarrhythmics, disopyramide, procainamide, quinidine: Increased risk of arrhythmias and conduction defects. Avoid using together.

Appetite suppressants, sympathomimetics (such as ephedrine [commonly found in nasal sprays], epinephrine, phenylephrine): Decreased stimulatory and pressor effects; possible epinephrine reversal (hypotensive response to epinephrine). Use together cautiously; don't use with epinephrine.

Atropine, other anticholinergics (such as antidepressants, antihistamines, antiparkinsonians, MAO inhibitors, meperidine, phenothiazines): Oversedation, paralytic ileus, visual changes, and severe constipation. Avoid concomitant use.

Beta blockers: Inhibited prochlorperazine metabolism, increasing plasma levels and toxicity. Adjust dosage as needed.

Bromocriptine: Antagonized prolactin secretion. Monitor patient closely.

Centrally acting antihypertensives (such as clonidine, guanabenz, guanadrel, guanethidine, methyldopa, reserpine): Inhibited blood pressure response. Monitor blood pressure.

CNS depressants (such as anesthetics [epidural, general, spinal], barbiturates, narcotics, parenteral magnesium sulfate, tranquilizers): Oversedation, respiratory depression, and hypotension. Monitor patient closely.

High-dose dopamine: Decreased vasoconstricting effects. Monitor patient closely.

Levodopa: Decreased effectiveness and increased toxicity of levodopa. Monitor patient for drug effect.

Lithium: Severe neurologic toxicity with encephalitis-like syndrome; decreased thera-

---

Reactions may be *common*, uncommon, **_life-threatening_**, or COMMON AND LIFE-THREATENING.

peutic response to prochlorperazine. Avoid using together.

Metrizamide: Increased risk of seizures. Use together cautiously.

Nitrates: Hypotension. Monitor blood pressure.

Phenobarbital: Enhanced renal excretion of perphenazine. Adjust dosage as needed.

Phenytoin: Inhibited metabolism and increased toxicity of phenytoin. Monitor patient closely.

Propylthiouracil: Increased risk of agranulocytosis. Monitor hematologic studies.

Drug-herb. *Kava:* Possible increased risk of dystonic reactions. Discourage use together.

Yohimbe: Phenothiazines may increase the risk of toxicity. Discourage use together.

Drug-food. *Caffeine:* Decreased therapeutic response to prochlorperazine. Discourage use.

Drug-lifestyle. *Alcohol use:* Additive effects. Discourage use.

Heavy smoking: Increased prochlorperazine metabolism. Discourage smoking.

Sun exposure: Photosensitivity reactions. Tell patient to take precautions.

Adverse reactions

CNS: *extrapyramidal reactions,* sedation, pseudoparkinsonism, EEG changes, dizziness.

CV: *orthostatic hypotension,* tachycardia, ECG changes.

EENT: *ocular changes, blurred vision.*

GI: *dry mouth, constipation,* ileus, increased appetite.

GU: *urine retention,* dark urine, menstrual irregularities, inhibited ejaculation, hyperprolactinemia,

Hematologic: *transient leukopenia, agranulocytosis, thrombocytopenia, hemolytic anemia.*

Hepatic: *cholestatic jaundice.*

Metabolic: weight gain, hyperglycemia or hypoglycemia.

Skin: mild photosensitivity, *allergic reactions, exfoliative dermatitis.*

Other: gynecomastia.

Overdose and treatment

Toxicity may cause CNS depression characterized by deep, unarousable sleep and possible coma, hypotension or hypertension, extrapyramidal symptoms, dystonia, abnormal involuntary muscle movements, agitation, seizures, arrhythmias, ECG changes, hypothermia or hyperthermia, and autonomic nervous system dysfunction.

To treat overdose, don't induce vomiting. Drug inhibits cough reflex, and aspiration may occur. Use gastric lavage, then activated charcoal and saline cathartics; dialysis doesn't help. Regulate body temperature as needed. Treat hypotension with I.V. fluids. Don't give epinephrine. Treat seizures with parenteral diazepam or barbiturates; arrhythmias with parenteral phenytoin (1 mg/kg with rate titrated to blood pressure); and extrapyramidal reactions with benztropine or parenteral diphenhydramine 2 mg/kg/minute.

Special considerations

● Liquid and injectable formulations may cause a rash after contact with skin.

● Drug may cause a pink to brown discoloration of urine.

● Drug is linked to a high risk of extrapyramidal effects and, in institutionalized psychiatric patients, photosensitivity reactions; patient should avoid exposure to sunlight or heat lamps.

● Oral formulations may cause stomach upset. Administer with food or fluid.

● Don't give sustained-release form to children.

● Solution for injection may be slightly discolored. Don't use if excessively discolored or if a precipitate is evident. Contact pharmacist.

● Dilute concentrate in 60 to 120 ml (2 to 4 oz) of water. Store suppository form in a cool place.

● Give I.V. dose slowly (5 mg/minute). I.M. injection may cause skin necrosis; take care to prevent extravasation. Don't mix with other drugs in syringe. Don't administer S.C.

● Administer I.M. injection deep into upper outer quadrant of buttock. Massaging area after administration may prevent formation of abscesses.

● Drug is ineffective in treating motion sickness.

● Protect liquid form from light.

● Prochlorperazine causes false-positive test results for urinary porphyrins, urobilinogen, amylase, and 5-hydroxyindoleacetic acid because of darkening of urine by metabolites; also causes false-positive urine pregnancy results in tests using human chorionic gonadotropin as the indicator.

Patient monitoring

● Monitor patient's blood pressure before and after parenteral administration.

● Monitor therapeutic effect.

Breast-feeding patients

● Drug may appear in breast milk; use cautiously. Potential benefits to mother should outweigh potential harm to infant.

Pediatric patients

● Drug isn't recommended for patients under age 2 or weighing less than 20 lb (9 kg).

Geriatric patients

● Elderly patients tend to require lower dosages, adjusted to individual effects. These patients are at greater risk for adverse reactions, especially tardive dyskinesia, other extrapyramidal effects, and hypotension.

Patient education

● Explain risks of dystonic reactions and tardive dyskinesia. Tell patient to promptly report abnormal body movements.

● Tell patient to avoid sun exposure and to wear sunscreen when going outdoors to prevent photosensitivity reactions. (Note that heat lamps and tanning beds also may cause skin burning or skin discoloration.)

- Tell patient to avoid spilling liquid form. Contact with skin may cause rash and irritation.
- Warn patient to avoid extremely hot or cold baths and exposure to temperature extremes, sunlamps, or tanning beds; drug may cause thermoregulatory changes.
- Advise patient to take drug exactly as prescribed, not to double the doses after missing one, and not to share drug with others.
- Warn patient to avoid alcohol or drugs that may cause excessive sedation.
- Tell patient to dilute concentrate in water; explain dropper technique of measuring dose; teach correct use of suppository.
- Tell patient that hard candy, chewing gum, or ice chips can alleviate dry mouth.
- Urge patient to store drug safely away from children.
- Inform patient that interactions are possible with many drugs. Warn him to seek medical approval before taking OTC or herbal products.
- Warn patient not to stop taking drug suddenly and to promptly report difficulty urinating, sore throat, dizziness, or fainting. Reassure patient that most reactions can be relieved by reducing dosage.
- Caution patient to avoid hazardous activities that require alertness until drug's effect is known. Reassure patient that sedative effects subside and become tolerable in several weeks.

progesterone
Crinone

Pharmacologic classification: progestin
Therapeutic classification: progestin, contraceptive
Pregnancy risk category: X

Indications and dosages
➤ *Amenorrhea. Adults:* 5 to 10 mg I.M. daily for 6 to 8 days. Or, for secondary amenorrhea, one application of 4% gel vaginally every other day to a total of six doses. If no response, may use Crinone 8% every other day to a total of six doses.

➤ *Dysfunctional uterine bleeding. Adults:* 5 to 10 mg I.M. daily for 6 days. Or a single 50 to 100 mg I.M. dose.

➤ *Corpus luteum insufficiency. Adults:* 12.5 mg I.M. initiated within several days of ovulation and continuing for 2 weeks. May continue for up to 11th week of gestation. Or, for infertility, one application of 8% gel vaginally, daily or b.i.d. If pregnancy occurs, treatment may be continued until placental autonomy is achieved up to 10 to 12 weeks.

How supplied
Available by prescription only
Gel: 4% (45 mg), 8% (90 mg)
Injection: 50 mg/ml (in oil)

Pharmacodynamics
Contraceptive action: Suppresses ovulation, thickens cervical mucus, and induces endometrial sloughing.

Pharmacokinetics
Absorption: Must be administered parenterally; inactivated by liver after oral administration.
Distribution: Little information available.
Metabolism: Progesterone reduced to pregnanediol in liver, then conjugated with glucuronic acid. Short plasma half-life of progesterone (several minutes).
Excretion: Glucuronide-conjugated pregnanediol excreted in urine.

Route	Onset	Peak	Duration
I.M., P.O., intrauterine, vaginal	Unknown	Unknown	Unknown

Contraindications and precautions
Contraindicated in patients hypersensitive to drug and in those with thromboembolic disorders or cerebral apoplexy (or history of these conditions), breast cancer, undiagnosed abnormal vaginal bleeding, severe hepatic disease, or missed abortion.

Use cautiously in patients with diabetes mellitus, seizures, migraines, cardiac or renal disease, asthma, or mental depression.

Interactions
Drug-drug. *Bromocriptine:* Progesterone may cause amenorrhea or galactorrhea, interfering with bromocriptine's action. Don't use concurrently.
Drug-herb. *Red clover:* May interfere with hormonal therapies. Discourage concurrent use.

Adverse reactions
CNS: depression, somnolence, headache.
CV: thrombophlebitis, ***thromboembolism, CVA, pulmonary embolism,*** edema.
GI: nausea, constipation, diarrhea, vomiting.
GU: breakthrough bleeding, dysmenorrhea, amenorrhea, cervical erosion, abnormal secretions, nocturia, breast tenderness, enlargement, or secretion; decreased pregnanediol excretion.
Hepatic: cholestatic jaundice.
Metabolic: increased serum alkaline phosphatase and amino acid levels.
Skin: melasma, rash, acne, pruritus, pain at injection site.

Overdose and treatment
No information available.

Special considerations
- Parenteral form is for I.M. administration only. Inject deep into large muscle mass, preferably gluteal muscle.

Reactions may be *common*, uncommon, ***life-threatening***, or COMMON AND LIFE-THREATENING.

• Large doses of progesterone may cause a moderate catabolic effect and a transient increase in sodium and chloride excretion.

Patient monitoring
• Check parenteral injection sites for irritation.
• Monitor patient for adverse effects.

Breast-feeding patients
• Because drug appears in breast milk, its use is contraindicated in breast-feeding women.

Patient education
• Advise patient that withdrawal bleeding usually occurs 2 to 3 days after stopping drug.
• Instruct patient to call promptly if she suspects pregnancy during therapy.
• For patient using Crinone gel, advise her not to use gel concurrently with other local intravaginal therapy. If other local intravaginal therapy is used concurrently, there should be at least a 6-hour period before or after gel administration.

---

promethazine hydrochloride
Anergan 25, Anergan 50, Histantil*, Phencen-50, Phenergan, Phenergan Fortis, Phenergan Plain, PhenoJect-50, V-Gan-25, V-Gan-50

Pharmacologic classification: phenothiazine derivative
Therapeutic classification: antiemetic antivertigo, antihistamine (H₁-receptor antagonist), preoperative, postoperative, or obstetric sedative and adjunct to analgesics
Pregnancy risk category: C

Indications and dosages
➤ *Motion sickness. Adults:* 25 mg P.O. b.i.d.
Children: 12.5 to 25 mg P.O., I.M., or P.R. b.i.d.
➤ *Nausea. Adults:* 12.5 to 25 mg P.O., I.M., or P.R. q 4 to 6 hours, p.r.n.
Children: 0.25 to 0.5 mg/kg I.M. or P.R. q 4 to 6 hours, p.r.n.
➤ *Rhinitis, allergy symptoms. Adults:* 12.5 to 25 mg P.O. before meals and h.s., or 25 mg P.O. h.s.
Children: 6.25 to 12.5 mg P.O. t.i.d., or 25 mg P.O. or P.R. h.s.
➤ *Sedation. Adults:* 25 to 50 mg P.O. or I.M. h.s. or p.r.n.
Children: 12.5 to 25 mg P.O., I.M., or P.R. h.s.
➤ *Routine preoperative or postoperative sedation or as an adjunct to analgesics.*
Adults: 25 to 50 mg I.M., I.V., or P.O.
Children: 12.5 to 25 mg I.M., I.V., or P.O.
➤ *Obstetric sedation.* 25 to 50 mg I.M. or I.V. in early stages of labor, and 25 to 75 mg after labor is established; repeat q 2 to 4 hours, p.r.n. Maximum, 100 mg daily.

How supplied
Available by prescription only
Injection: 25 mg/ml, 50 mg/ml
Suppositories: 12.5 mg, 25 mg, 50 mg
Syrup: 6.25 mg/5 ml, 25 mg/5 ml
Tablets: 12.5 mg, 25 mg, 50 mg

Pharmacodynamics
Antiemetic and antivertigo actions: The central antimuscarinic actions of antihistamines probably are responsible for their antivertigo and antiemetic effects; promethazine also is believed to inhibit the medullary chemoreceptor trigger zone.
Antihistamine action: Competes with histamine for the H₁-receptor, thereby suppressing allergic rhinitis and urticaria; drug doesn't prevent the release of histamine.
Sedative action: Mechanism unknown; probably causes sedation by reducing stimuli to the brain-stem reticular system.

Pharmacokinetics
Absorption: Well absorbed from GI tract. Onset begins 20 minutes after P.O., P.R., or I.M. administration; within 3 to 5 minutes after I.V. administration. Effects usually last 4 to 6 hours but may last for 12 hours.
Distribution: Distributed widely throughout body; crosses placenta.
Metabolism: Metabolized in liver.
Excretion: Metabolites excreted in urine and feces.

Route	Onset	Peak	Duration
P.O.	15-60 min	Unknown	< 12 hr
I.V.	3-5 min	Unknown	< 12 hr
I.M., P.R.	20 min	Unknown	< 12 hr

Contraindications and precautions
Contraindicated in patients hypersensitive to drug; in those with intestinal obstruction, prostatic hyperplasia, bladder neck obstruction, seizure disorders, coma, CNS depression, or stenosing peptic ulcerations; in newborns, premature neonates, and breast-feeding patients; and in acutely ill or dehydrated children.

Use cautiously in patients with asthma or cardiac, pulmonary, or hepatic disease.

Interactions
Drug-drug. *Epinephrine:* Partial adrenergic blockade; further hypotension. Monitor blood pressure.
Levodopa: Possible block of levodopa's antiparkinsonian action. Monitor patient.
MAO inhibitors: Interference with detoxification of antihistamines and phenothiazines; prolonged and intensified sedative and anticholinergic effects. Avoid concomitant use.
Other antihistamines or CNS depressants (such as anxiolytics, barbiturates, sleeping aids, tranquilizers): Additive CNS depression. Use together cautiously.

Drug-herb. *Kava*: Increased risk or severity of dystonic reactions. Discourage concomitant use. *Yobimbe:* Increased risk of toxicity. Discourage concomitant use.

Drug-lifestyle. *Alcohol use:* Additive CNS depression. Discourage use.
Sun exposure: Photosensitivity reactions. Tell patient to take precautions.

Adverse reactions
CNS: *sedation,* confusion, sleepiness, dizziness, disorientation, extrapyramidal symptoms, *drowsiness.*
CV: hypotension, hypertension.
EENT: blurred vision.
GI: nausea, vomiting, *dry mouth.*
GU: urine retention.
Hematologic: *leukopenia, agranulocytosis, thrombocytopenia.*
Metabolic: hyperglycemia.
Skin: photosensitivity, rash.

Overdose and treatment
Toxicity may cause CNS depression (sedation, reduced mental alertness, apnea, and CV collapse) or CNS stimulation (insomnia, hallucinations, tremors, or seizures). Atropine-like signs and symptoms, such as dry mouth, flushed skin, fixed and dilated pupils, and GI symptoms, are common, especially in children.

Empty stomach by gastric lavage; don't induce vomiting. Treat hypotension with vasopressors, and control seizures with diazepam or phenytoin; correct acidosis and electrolyte imbalance. Urinary acidification promotes excretion of drug. Don't give stimulants.

Special considerations
● Pronounced sedative effects may limit use in some ambulatory patients.
● The 50 mg/ml concentration is for I.M. use only; inject deep into large muscle mass. Don't administer drug S.C.; this may cause chemical irritation and necrosis. Drug may be administered I.V. in concentrations not to exceed 25 mg/ml and at a rate not to exceed 25 mg/minute. When using I.V. drip, wrap in aluminum foil to protect drug from light.
● Promethazine and meperidine (Demerol) may be mixed in same syringe.
● Stop drug 4 days before diagnostic skin tests to avoid preventing, reducing, or masking test response. Promethazine may cause either false-positive or false-negative pregnancy test results. It also may interfere with blood grouping in the ABO system.

Patient monitoring
● Monitor patient for adverse effects.

Breast-feeding patients
● Antihistamines such as promethazine shouldn't be used during breast-feeding. Many of these drugs appear in breast milk, exposing infants to

risks of unusual excitability, especially premature infants and other neonates, who may experience seizures.

Pediatric patients
● Use cautiously in children with respiratory dysfunction. Safety and efficacy in children younger than age 2 haven't been established; don't give drug to infants under age 3 months.

Geriatric patients
● Elderly patients are usually more sensitive to adverse effects of antihistamines and are especially likely to experience a greater degree of dizziness, sedation, hyperexcitability, dry mouth, and urine retention than younger patients. Symptoms usually respond to a decrease in dosage.

Patient education
● Warn patient about possible photosensitivity and ways to avoid it.
● When treating motion sickness, tell patient to take first dose 30 to 60 minutes before travel; on succeeding days, he should take dose upon arising and with evening meal.

propafenone hydrochloride
Rythmol

Pharmacologic classification: sodium channel antagonist
Therapeutic classification: antiarrhythmic
Pregnancy risk category: C

Indications and dosages
➤ *Suppression of documented life-threatening ventricular arrhythmias.*
Adults: Initially, 150 mg P.O. q 8 hours. Dose may be increased to 225 mg q 8 hours after 3 or 4 days; if necessary, increase dose to 300 mg q 8 hours. Maximum daily dose is 900 mg.
✦ *Dosage adjustment.* Reduce dosage in patients with hepatic failure to 20% to 30% of usual dosage.

How supplied
Available by prescription only
Tablets: 150 mg, 225 mg, 300 mg

Pharmacodynamics
Antiarrhythmic action: Reduces the inward sodium current in myocardial cells and Purkinje fibers; also has weak beta-adrenergic blocking effects. Slows the upstroke velocity of the action potential (phase 0 depolarization) and slows conduction in the AV node, His-Purkinje system, and intraventricular conduction system and prolongs the refractory period in the AV node.

Pharmacokinetics
Absorption: Well absorbed from GI tract; absorption not affected by food. Significant first-pass effect; limited bioavailability. Increases with

dosage. Absolute bioavailability is 3.4% with 150-mg tablet; 10.6% with 300-mg tablet. Plasma levels peak about 3 hours after administration.
Distribution: Rapidly distributed into lung, liver, and heart tissue. The degree of protein-binding is concentration dependent. Drug crosses the placenta and appears in breast milk. Distribution of drug and its metabolites hasn't been fully described.
Metabolism: Metabolized in liver, with a significant first-pass effect. Two active metabolites identified: 5-hydroxypropafenone and N-depropylpropafenone. 10% of all patients and patients receiving quinidine metabolize drug more slowly. Little (if any) 5-hydroxypropafenone present in plasma.
Excretion: Elimination half-life 2 to 10 hours in normal metabolizers (about 90% of patients); can be as long as 10 to 32 hours in slow metabolizers.

Route	Onset	Peak	Duration
P.O.	Unknown	3½ hr	Unknown

Contraindications and precautions
Contraindicated in patients hypersensitive to drug and in those with severe or uncontrolled heart failure; cardiogenic shock; SA, AV, or intraventricular disorders of impulse conduction in the absence of a pacemaker; bradycardia; marked hypotension; bronchospastic disorders; or electrolyte imbalance.

Use cautiously in patients with renal or hepatic failure or heart failure, and in those receiving other cardiac depressant drugs.

Interactions
Drug-drug. *Beta blockers (such as metoprolol, propranolol):* Increased plasma levels of these drugs. Use together cautiously.
Cimetidine: Increased propafenone levels. Monitor patient closely.
Digoxin: Dose-related increase in digoxin levels, ranging from 35% at 450 mg daily to 85% at 900 mg daily. Monitor digoxin levels closely; adjust digoxin dosage as necessary.
Local anesthetics: Increased risk of CNS toxicity. Use together cautiously.
Quinidine: Competitively inhibits one of the metabolic pathways for propafenone, increasing its half-life. Don't give together.
Warfarin: Increased INR. Monitor PT and INR.

Adverse reactions
CNS: anxiety, ataxia, *dizziness,* drowsiness, fatigue, headache, insomnia, syncope, tremor.
CV: atrial fibrillation, *bradycardia,* bundle-branch block, angina, chest pain, edema, first-degree AV block, hypotension, increased QRS complex duration, intraventricular conduction delay, palpitations, *heart failure, proarrhythmic events (ventricular tachycardia, PVCs, ventricular fibrillation).*
EENT: blurred vision.

GI: abdominal pain or cramps, constipation, diarrhea, dyspepsia, anorexia, flatulence, *nausea, vomiting,* dry mouth, unusual taste.
Musculoskeletal: joint pain.
Respiratory: dyspnea.
Skin: diaphoresis, rash.

Overdose and treatment
Toxicity symptoms usually develop within 3 hours of ingestion. Hypotension, somnolence, bradycardia, conduction disturbances, ventricular arrhythmias, and seizures have been reported. Rhythm and blood pressure may be controlled with dopamine and isoproterenol; seizures may respond to I.V. diazepam.

Special considerations
● Propafenone pharmacokinetics are complex; studies have shown that a threefold increase in daily dose (from 300 to 900 mg daily) may produce a tenfold increase in plasma levels. Dosage must be individualized for each patient.

Patient monitoring
● Monitor patient with impaired hepatic function carefully.
● Watch for toxicity, especially if there has been a recent dosage change.

Breast-feeding patients
● It isn't known if drug appears in breast milk. Because of potential for serious toxicity in infant, consider an alternative to breast-feeding during therapy.

Geriatric patients
● In elderly patients and patients with substantial heart disease, increase dosage more gradually during initial phase of treatment.

Patient education
● Instruct patient to report signs and symptoms of infection, such as sore throat, chills, and fever.

propantheline bromide
Pro-Banthine, Propanthel*

Pharmacologic classification: anticholinergic
Therapeutic classification: antimuscarinic, GI antispasmodic
Pregnancy risk category: C

Indications and dosages
➤ *Adjunctive treatment of peptic ulcer, irritable bowel syndrome, and other GI disorders; to reduce duodenal motility during diagnostic radiologic procedures.*
Adults: 15 mg P.O. t.i.d. before meals, and 30 mg h.s. up to 60 mg q.i.d.
Elderly patients: 7.5 mg P.O. t.i.d. before meals.
Children: Antispasmodic dose 2 to 3 mg/kg daily P.O. divided q 4 to 6 hours and h.s. Antisecre-

tory dose 1.5 mg/kg daily P.O. divided q 6 to 8 hours.

How supplied
Available by prescription only
Tablets: 7.5 mg, 15 mg

Pharmacodynamics
Anticholinergic action: Competitively blocks acetylcholine's actions at cholinergic neuroeffector sites, decreasing GI motility and inhibiting gastric acid secretion.

Pharmacokinetics
Absorption: Only about 10% to 25% of drug absorbed (absorption varies among patients).
Distribution: Doesn't cross blood-brain barrier; little else known about distribution.
Metabolism: Appears to undergo considerable metabolism in upper small intestine and liver.
Excretion: Absorbed drug excreted in urine as metabolites and unchanged drug.

Route	Onset	Peak	Duration
P.O.	1½ hr	2-6 hr	6 hr

Contraindications and precautions
Contraindicated in patients hypersensitive to anticholinergics and in those with angle-closure glaucoma, obstructive uropathy, obstructive disease of the GI tract, severe ulcerative colitis, myasthenia gravis, paralytic ileus, intestinal atony, unstable CV status in acute hemorrhage, or toxic megacolon.

Use cautiously in patients with impaired renal or hepatic function, autonomic neuropathy, hyperthyroidism, coronary artery disease, arrhythmias, heart failure, hypertension, hiatal hernia related to gastric reflux, or ulcerative colitis and in those living in a hot or humid environment.

Interactions
Drug-drug. *Antacids:* Decreased oral absorption of anticholinergics. Administer propantheline at least 1 hour before antacids.
Atenolol: Increased absorption; enhanced atenolol effects. Use together cautiously.
Digoxin: Slowly dissolving tablets may yield higher serum digoxin levels when administered with anticholinergics. Monitor serum digoxin levels.
Drugs with anticholinergic effects: Additive toxicity. Use together cautiously.
Ketoconazole, levodopa: Decreased GI absorption. Monitor patient.
Oral potassium supplements (especially wax-matrix formulations): Increased potassium-induced GI ulcerations. Monitor patient closely.

Adverse reactions
CNS: headache, insomnia, drowsiness, dizziness, *confusion or excitement in elderly patients,* nervousness, weakness.
CV: *palpitations,* tachycardia.

EENT: *blurred vision,* mydriasis, increased intraocular pressure, cycloplegia, drying of salivary secretions.
GI: *dry mouth,* constipation, loss of taste, nausea, vomiting, paralytic ileus, bloated feeling.
GU: *urinary hesitancy, urine retention,* impotence.
Skin: urticaria, decreased sweating or possible anhidrosis, other dermal signs and symptoms.
Other: allergic reactions (***anaphylaxis***).

Overdose and treatment
Toxicity may cause curare-like symptoms such as respiratory paralysis and such peripheral effects as headache; dilated, nonreactive pupils; blurred vision; flushed, hot, dry skin; dryness of mucous membranes; dysphagia; decreased or absent bowel sounds; urine retention; hyperthermia; tachycardia; hypertension; and increased respirations. In severe cases, physostigmine may be administered to block propantheline's antimuscarinic effects.

Special considerations
● Drug may be used with histamine$_2$ receptor to treat Zollinger-Ellison syndrome as an unlabeled use.
● Adjust drug until therapeutic effect is obtained or adverse effects become intolerable.

Patient monitoring
● Monitor patient for adverse effects.

Breast-feeding patients
● Drug may appear in breast milk, possibly resulting in infant toxicity. Don't use in breast-feeding women. Drug may decrease milk production.

Geriatric patients
● Administer drug cautiously to elderly patients. Lower dosages are recommended.

Patient education
● Instruct patient to swallow tablets whole rather than chewing or crushing them.

propofol
Diprivan

Pharmacologic classification: phenol derivative
Therapeutic classification: anesthetic
Pregnancy risk category: B

Indications and dosages
➤***Induction and maintenance of sedation in mechanically ventilated intensive care unit patients.*** *Adults:* Initially, 5 mcg/kg/minute I.V. for 5 minutes (0.3 mg/kg/hour). Subsequent increments of 5 to 10 mcg/kg/minute (0.3 to 0.6 mg/kg/hour) over 5 to 10 minutes until desired level of sedation is achieved. Mainte-

nance rates of 5 to 50 mcg/kg/minute (0.3 to 3 mg/kg/hour) or higher may be needed. Minimum amount necessary should be used. Lower dosages are needed for patients over age 55.

➤*Induction of anesthesia. Adults:* Individualize doses based on patient's condition and age. Most patients classified as American Society of Anesthesiologists (ASA) Physical Status category (PS) I or II under age 55 need 2 to 2.5 mg/kg I.V. Drug is usually administered in a 40-mg bolus q 10 seconds until desired response is obtained.

Children age 3 and over: 2.5 to 3.5 mg/kg I.V. over 20 to 30 seconds.

Elderly, debilitated, or hypovolemic patients or patients in ASA PS III or IV: Half of the usual induction dose (20-mg bolus q 10 seconds).

➤*Maintenance of anesthesia. Adults:* May give as a variable rate infusion, titrated to clinical effect. Most patients may be maintained with 0.1 to 0.2 mg/kg/minute (6 to 12 mg/kg/hour).

Elderly, debilitated, or hypovolemic patients or patients in ASA PS III or IV: Half the usual maintenance dose (0.05 to 0.1 mg/kg/minute or 3 to 6 mg/kg/hour).

Children age 3 and over: 125 to 300 mcg/kg/minute I.V.

How supplied
Available by prescription only
Injection: 10 mg/ml in 20-ml ampules and 50-ml and 100-ml infusion vials

Pharmacodynamics
Anesthetic action: Produces a dose-dependent CNS depression similar to benzodiazepines and barbiturates. However, it can be used to maintain anesthesia through careful titration of infusion rate.

Pharmacokinetics
Absorption: Must be administered I.V.
Distribution: Terminal half-life of 1 to 3 days.
Metabolism: Metabolized within liver and tissues; metabolites not fully characterized.
Excretion: Excreted through kidneys. However, termination of drug action is probably caused by redistribution out of CNS as well as metabolism.

Route	Onset	Peak	Duration
I.V.	< 40 sec	Unknown	10-15 min

Contraindications and precautions
Contraindicated in patients hypersensitive to propofol or components of the emulsion, including soybean oil, egg lecithin, and glycerol. Because drug is administered as an emulsion, administer cautiously to patients with a disorder of lipid metabolism (such as pancreatitis, primary hyperlipoproteinemia, and diabetic hyperlipidemia). Use cautiously if patient is receiving lipids as part of a total parenteral nutrition infusion; I.V. lipid dose may need to be reduced. Use

cautiously in elderly or debilitated patients and in those with circulatory disorders.

Don't use drug in obstetric anesthesia because safety of fetus hasn't been established. Also avoid in patients with increased intracranial pressure or impaired cerebral circulation because the reduction in systemic arterial pressure caused by drug may substantially reduce cerebral perfusion pressure.

Don't use drug in children under age 3. Don't use for sedation in children in intensive care units or under monitored anesthesia care sedation.

Drug should be administered under direct medical supervision by persons familiar with airway management and the administration of I.V. anesthetics.

Interactions
Drug-drug. *Inhalational anesthetics (enflurane, halothane, isoflurane), supplemental anesthetics (nitrous oxide, opiates):* Enhanced anesthetic and CV actions of propofol expected. Use together cautiously.

Opiate analgesics or sedatives: Intensified reduction of systolic, diastolic, mean arterial pressure, and cardiac output. Decrease induction dose requirements as needed.

Adverse reactions
CNS: headache, dizziness, twitching, clonicmyoclonic movement.
CV: *hypotension,* **bradycardia,** hypertension.
GI: nausea, vomiting, abdominal cramping.
GU: discolored urine.
Metabolic: hyperlipidemia.
Respiratory: *apnea,* cough, hiccups.
Skin: flushing.
Other: fever, *injection site burning or stinging, pain,* tingling or numbness, coldness.

Overdose and treatment
Specific information not available. However, treatment of overdose may include support of respiration and administration of fluids, pressor agents, and anticholinergics as indicated.

Special considerations
● Although the hemodynamic effects of drug can vary, its major effect in patients maintaining spontaneous ventilation is arterial hypotension (arterial pressure can decrease as much as 30%) with little or no change in heart rate and cardiac output. However, significant depression of cardiac output may occur in patients undergoing assisted or controlled positive pressure ventilation.
● Drug has no vagolytic activity. Premedication with anticholinergics, such as glycopyrrolate or atropine, may help manage potential increases in vagal tone caused by other drugs or surgical manipulations.
⚑ ALERT Don't mix propofol with other drugs or blood products. If it's to be diluted before infusion, use only D_5W and don't dilute to a concentration of less than 2 mg/ml. After dilution,

drug appears to be more stable in glass containers than plastic.
• When administered into a running I.V. catheter, emulsion is compatible with D₅W, lactated Ringer's injection, lactated Ringer's and 5% dextrose injection, 5% dextrose and 0.45% saline injection, and 5% dextrose and 0.2% saline injection.
• Store emulsion above 40° F (4° C) and below 72° F (22° C). Refrigeration isn't recommended.
• If used for sedation of mechanically ventilated patients, wake patient every 24 hours.
• Use strict aseptic technique when administering drug; discard unused drug after 12 hours.

Patient monitoring
• Monitor patients receiving drug for signs of significant hypotension or bradycardia. Treatment may include increased rate of fluid administration, pressor drugs, elevation of lower legs, or atropine.
• Watch for apnea during induction; may persist for longer than 60 seconds. Ventilatory support may be needed.

Breast-feeding patients
• Drug appears in breast milk; don't use in breast-feeding women.

Pediatric patients
• Safety in children hasn't been established.

Geriatric patients
• Drug's pharmacokinetics aren't influenced by chronic hepatic cirrhosis, chronic renal failure, or gender.

Patient education
• Reassure patient that he'll be monitored appropriately during drug administration.

---

propoxyphene hydrochloride
Darvon

propoxyphene napsylate
Darvocet-N 50, Darvocet-N 100, Darvon-N

Pharmacologic classification: opioid
Therapeutic classification: analgesic
Controlled substance schedule: IV
Pregnancy risk category: NR

Indications and dosages
➤ *Mild to moderate pain.* Adults: 65 mg (hydrochloride) P.O. q 4 hours, p.r.n., or 100 mg (napsylate) P.O. q 4 hours, p.r.n.

How supplied
Available by prescription only
propoxyphene hydrochloride
Capsules: 65 mg

propoxyphene napsylate
Suspension: 50 mg/5 ml
Tablets: 100 mg
propoxyphene hydrochloride and acetaminophen
Tablets: 65 mg propoxyphene hydrochloride, 650 mg acetaminophen
propoxyphene napsylate and acetaminophen
Tablets: 50 mg propoxyphene napsylate, 325 mg acetaminophen; 100 mg propoxyphene napsylate, 650 mg acetaminophen

Pharmacodynamics
Analgesic action: Exerts analgesic effect via opiate agonist activity and alters patient's response to painful stimuli, particularly mild to moderate pain.

Pharmacokinetics
Absorption: After oral administration, absorbed primarily in upper small intestine. Equimolar doses of the hydrochloride and napsylate salts provide similar plasma levels. Onset of analgesia in 20 to 60 minutes; analgesic effects peak in 2 to 2½ hours.
Distribution: Enters CSF. Assumed to cross placental barrier; however, placental fluid and fetal blood levels not determined.
Metabolism: Degraded mainly in liver; about one-quarter of dose metabolized to norpropoxyphene, an active metabolite.
Excretion: Excreted in urine. Duration of effect 4 to 6 hours.

Route	Onset	Peak	Duration
P.O.	15-60 min	2-2½ hr	4-6 hr

Contraindications and precautions
Contraindicated in patients hypersensitive to drug. Use cautiously in patients with impaired renal or hepatic function, emotional instability, or history of drug or alcohol abuse.

Interactions
Drug-drug. *Antidepressants such as doxepin:* Propoxyphene may inhibit metabolism of these drugs. Lower dosage of antidepressant as needed.
Carbamazepine: Increased carbamazepine's effects. Monitor serum carbamazepine levels.
Drugs highly metabolized in liver (digitoxin, phenytoin, rifampin): Possible accumulation of either drug. Withdrawal symptoms may result if used together. Avoid using together.
General anesthetics: Possible severe CV depression. Use cautiously and monitor patient closely.
Opiate antagonist: Patients who become physically dependent on propoxyphene may experience acute withdrawal syndrome when given a single dose. Use cautiously and monitor patient closely.
Other CNS depressants (antidepressants, antihistamines, barbiturates, benzodiazepines, gen-

---

Reactions may be *common*, uncommon, *life-threatening*, or COMMON AND LIFE-THREATENING.

eral anesthetics, muscle relaxants, narcotic analgesics, phenothiazines, sedative-hypnotics): Potentiation of adverse effects (respiratory depression, sedation, hypotension). Reduced doses of propoxyphene are usually needed.

Drug-lifestyle. *Alcohol use:* Potentiated CNS depressant effects of propoxyphene. Discourage use.

Adverse reactions

CNS: *dizziness, sedation,* headache, euphoria, light-headedness, weakness, hallucinations.
GI: *nausea, vomiting,* constipation, abdominal pain.
Hepatic: abnormal liver function tests.
Respiratory: *respiratory depression.*
Other: psychological and physical dependence.

Overdose and treatment

Toxicity may cause CNS depression, respiratory depression, and miosis (pinpoint pupils); hypotension, bradycardia, hypothermia, shock, apnea, cardiopulmonary arrest, circulatory collapse, pulmonary edema, and seizures may also occur.

Drug is known to cause ECG changes (prolonged QRS complex) and nephrogenic diabetes insipidus in acute toxic doses. Death from acute overdose is most likely to occur within first hour. Signs and symptoms of overdose with propoxyphene combination products may include salicylism from aspirin or acetaminophen toxicity.

Administer a narcotic antagonist (naloxone) to reverse respiratory depression. Don't give naloxone in the absence of clinically significant respiratory or CV depression.

If patient show symptoms within 2 hours of ingestion of an oral overdose, empty the stomach immediately by inducing emesis or gastric lavage. Use caution to avoid risk of aspiration. Administer activated charcoal via nasogastric tube for further removal of drug in an oral overdose.

Provide symptomatic and supportive treatment. Anticonvulsants may be needed; monitor laboratory parameters, vital signs, and neurologic status closely. Dialysis may be helpful in the treatment of overdose with propoxyphene combination products containing aspirin or acetaminophen.

Special considerations

• Propoxyphene may obscure signs and symptoms of an acute abdominal condition or worsen gallbladder pain.
• Don't prescribe for drug maintenance purposes in narcotic addiction.
• Drug can be considered a mild narcotic analgesic, but pain relief is equivalent to that of aspirin.
• Drug may cause false decrease in test for urinary corticosteroid excretion.

Patient monitoring

• Monitor patient for effectiveness of treatment.

• Watch for signs of dependence.

Breast-feeding patients

• Drug appears in breast milk; use cautiously in breast-feeding women.

Pediatric patients

• Insufficient data exists to establish safety and aqppropriate dosage regimen, therefore it is not recommended for use in pediatric patients.

Geriatric patients

• Lower doses are usually indicated for elderly patients because they may be more sensitive to therapeutic and adverse effects of drug.

Patient education

• Warn patient not to exceed recommended dosage.
• Tell patient to avoid use of alcohol because it will cause additive CNS depressant effects.
• Warn patient of additive depressant effect that can occur if drug is prescribed for medical conditions requiring use of sedatives, tranquilizers, muscle relaxants, antidepressants, or other CNS-depressant drugs.
• Tell patient to take drug with food if GI upset occurs.

propranolol hydrochloride
Inderal, Inderal LA

Pharmacologic classification: beta blocker
Therapeutic classification: antihypertensive, antianginal, antiarrhythmic, adjunctive therapy of migraine, adjunctive therapy of MI
Pregnancy risk category: C

Indications and dosages

➤ *Hypertension. Adults:* Initially, 80 mg P.O. daily in two to four divided doses or sustained-release form once daily. Increase at 3- to 7-day intervals to maximum daily dose of 640 mg. Usual maintenance dose is 160 to 480 mg daily.
Children ◇: 1 mg/kg P.O. daily (maximum daily dose is 16 mg/kg).
➤ *Management of angina pectoris. Adults:* 10 to 20 mg t.i.d. or q.i.d., or one 80-mg sustained-release capsule daily. Dosage may be increased at 7- to 10-day intervals. Average optimum dose is 160 to 240 mg daily.
➤ *Supraventricular, ventricular, and atrial arrhythmias; tachyarrhythmias caused by excessive catecholamine action during anesthesia, hyperthyroidism, and pheochromocytoma. Adults:* 1 to 3 mg I.V. diluted in 50 ml D_5W or normal saline solution infused slowly, not to exceed 1 mg/minute. After 3 mg have been infused, another dose may be given in 2 minutes; subsequent doses no sooner than q 4 hours. Usual maintenance dose is 10 to 30 mg P.O. t.i.d. or q.i.d.

► *Prevention of frequent, severe, un-controllable, or disabling migraine or vascular headache.* *Adults:* Initially, 80 mg daily in divided doses or one sustained-release capsule once daily. Usual maintenance dose is 160 to 240 mg daily, divided t.i.d. or q.i.d.

► *To reduce mortality after MI.* *Adults:* 180 to 240 mg P.O. daily in divided doses. Usually administered in three to four doses daily, beginning 5 to 21 days after infarct.

► *Hypertrophic subaortic stenosis.* *Adults:* 10 to 20 mg P.O. t.i.d. or q.i.d. before meals and h.s.

► *Preoperative pheochromocytoma.* *Adults:* 60 mg P.O. daily.

► *Adjunctive treatment of anxiety* ◇. *Adults:* 10 to 80 mg P.O. 1 hour before anxiety-provoking activity.

► *Essential, familial, or senile movement tremors* ◇. *Adults:* 40 mg P.O. b.i.d., as tolerated and needed.

How supplied
Available by prescription only
Capsules (extended-release): 60 mg, 80 mg, 120 mg, 160 mg
Injection: 1 mg/ml
Solution: 20 mg/5 ml, 40 mg/5 ml, 80 mg/ml (concentrated)
Tablets: 10 mg, 20 mg, 40 mg, 60 mg, 80 mg

Pharmacodynamics
Antihypertensive action: Exact mechanism unknown. May reduce blood pressure by blocking adrenergic receptors (thus decreasing cardiac output), by decreasing sympathetic outflow from the CNS, and by suppressing renin release.
Antianginal action: Decreases myocardial oxygen consumption by blocking catecholamine access to beta-adrenergic receptors, thus relieving angina.
Antiarrhythmic action: Decreases heart rate and prevents exercise-induced increases in heart rate. Also decreases myocardial contractility, cardiac output, and SA and AV nodal conduction velocity.
Migraine prophylactic action: Thought to result from inhibition of vasodilation.
MI prophylactic action: Exact mechanism unknown.

Pharmacokinetics
Absorption: Absorbed almost completely from GI tract; food enhances absorption. Plasma levels peak 60 to 90 minutes after giving regular-release tablets. After I.V. administration, peak levels in about 1 minute, with virtually immediate onset of action.
Distribution: Distributed widely throughout body; more than 90% protein-bound.
Metabolism: Almost total hepatic metabolism; oral dosage form undergoes extensive first-pass metabolism.

Excretion: About 96% to 99% of given dose excreted in urine as metabolites; remainder excreted in feces as unchanged drug and metabolites. Biological half-life about 4 hours.

Route	Onset	Peak	Duration
P.O.	30 min	1-1½ hr	12 hr
I.V.	1 min	Immediate	5 min

Contraindications and precautions
Contraindicated in patients with bronchial asthma, sinus bradycardia and heart block greater than first-degree, cardiogenic shock, and heart failure (unless failure is secondary to a tachyarrhythmia that can be treated with propranolol).

Use cautiously in elderly patients; in patients with impaired renal or hepatic function, nonallergic bronchospastic diseases, diabetes mellitus, or thyrotoxicosis; and in those receiving other antihypertensives.

Interactions
Drug-drug. *Aluminum hydroxide antacid:* Decreased GI absorption. Separate administration times.
Antidiabetics, insulin: Altered dosage requirements in previously stable diabetic patients. Monitor serum glucose level.
Antihypertensives (especially catecholamine-depleting drugs such as reserpine): Potentiated antihypertensive effects. Monitor blood pressure.
Atropine, tricyclic antidepressants, other drugs with anticholinergic effects: Possible antagonized propranolol-induced bradycardia. Monitor patient closely.
Calcium channel blockers (especially I.V. verapamil): Depressed myocardial contractility or AV conduction. Rarely, concurrent I.V. use of a beta blocker and verapamil has resulted in serious adverse reactions, especially in patients with severe cardiomyopathy, heart failure, or recent MI. Use together cautiously.
Cimetidine: Decreased clearance of propranolol via inhibition of hepatic metabolism. Watch for enhanced beta-blocking effects.
Epinephrine: Severe vasoconstriction. Monitor blood pressure and observe patient carefully.
NSAIDs: Possible antagonized hypotensive effects. Monitor patient closely.
Phenytoin, rifampin: Accelerated clearance of propranolol. Adjust dosage as needed.
Sympathomimetics (such as isoproterenol, MAO inhibitors): Antagonized beta-adrenergic stimulating effects. Monitor patient closely.
Tubocurarine and related compounds: High doses of propranolol may potentiate neuromuscular blocking effect. Monitor patient closely.
Drug-herb. *Betel palm:* Reduced temperature-elevating effects and enhanced CNS effects. Discourage use together.
Drug-lifestyle. *Alcohol use:* Slowed rate of absorption. Discourage use.

Reactions may be *common*, uncommon, *life-threatening*, or COMMON AND LIFE-THREATENING.

Adverse reactions

CNS: *fatigue, lethargy,* vivid dreams, hallucinations, mental depression, light-headedness, insomnia.
CV: *bradycardia, hypotension, heart failure,* intermittent claudication, *worsening of AV block.*
GI: nausea, vomiting, diarrhea, abdominal cramping.
GU: increased BUN levels.
Hematologic: *agranulocytosis.*
Hepatic: elevated serum transaminase, alkaline phosphatase, and LD levels.
Respiratory: *bronchospasm.*
Skin: rash.
Other: fever.

Overdose and treatment

Toxicity may cause severe hypotension, bradycardia, heart failure, and bronchospasm. After acute ingestion, induce emesis or empty stomach by gastric lavage; follow with activated charcoal to reduce absorption, and administer symptomatic and supportive care. Treat bradycardia with atropine (0.25 to 1 mg); if no response, administer isoproterenol cautiously. Treat cardiac failure with cardiac glycosides and diuretics and hypotension with glucagon or vasopressors, epinephrine is preferred. Treat bronchospasm with isoproterenol and aminophylline.

Special considerations

● Propranolol also has been used to treat aggression and rage, stage fright, recurrent GI bleeding in cirrhotic patients, and menopausal symptoms.
● Never administer propranolol as an adjunct in treatment of pheochromocytoma unless patient has been pretreated with alpha blockers.

Patient monitoring

● Monitor serum glucose level; drug may mask signs of hypoglycemia.
● Monitor patient for adverse effects.

Breast-feeding patients

● Drug appears in breast milk; an alternative to breast-feeding is recommended during therapy.

Pediatric patients

● Safety and efficacy in children haven't been established; use only if potential benefit outweighs risk.

Geriatric patients

● Elderly patients may need lower maintenance doses because of increased bioavailability or delayed metabolism; they also may experience enhanced adverse effects.

Patient education

● Warn patient not to stop drug abruptly.
● Instruct patient on proper use, dosage, and potential adverse effects of drug.

● Tell patient to call before taking OTC drugs that may interact with propranolol, such as nasal decongestants or cold preparations.

---

propylthiouracil (PTU)
Propyl-Thyracil*

Pharmacologic classification: thyroid hormone antagonist
Therapeutic classification: antihyperthyroid
Pregnancy risk category: D

Indications and dosages

➤ *Hyperthyroidism.* *Adults:* 300 to 450 mg P.O. daily in divided doses. Continue until patient is euthyroid; then start maintenance dose of 100 mg daily to t.i.d.
Neonates and children: 5 to 7 mg/kg P.O. daily in divided doses q 8 hours. Or give according to age.
Children ages 6 to 10: 50 to 150 mg P.O. daily in divided doses q 8 hours.
Children over age 10: 100 mg P.O. t.i.d. Continue until patient is euthyroid; then start maintenance dose of 25 mg t.i.d. to 100 mg b.i.d.

How supplied

Available by prescription only
Tablets: 50 mg

Pharmacodynamics

Antithyroid action: When used to treat hyperthyroidism, PTU inhibits synthesis of thyroid hormone by interfering with the incorporation of iodine into thyroglobulin; it also inhibits the formation of iodothyronine. Besides blocking hormone synthesis, it also inhibits the peripheral deiodination of thyroxine to triiodothyronine (liothyronine). Clinical effects become evident only when the preformed hormone is depleted and circulating hormone levels decline.

As preparation for thyroidectomy, PTU inhibits synthesis of the thyroid hormone and causes a euthyroid state, reducing surgical problems during thyroidectomy; as a result, the mortality for a single-stage thyroidectomy is low. Iodide reduces the vascularity of the gland and makes it less friable.

When used in treating thyrotoxic crisis, PTU inhibits peripheral deiodination of thyroxine to triiodothyronine. Theoretically, it's preferred over methimazole in thyroid storm because of its peripheral action.

Pharmacokinetics

Absorption: About 80% absorbed rapidly and readily from GI tract. Levels peak in 1 to 1½ hours.
Distribution: Appears to be concentrated in thyroid gland. Readily crosses placenta; distributed into breast milk. 75% to 80% protein-bound.
Metabolism: Metabolized rapidly in liver.

Excretion: About 35% of dose excreted in urine. Half-life is 1 to 2 hours in patients with normal renal function; 8½ hours in anuric patients.

Route	Onset	Peak	Duration
P.O.	Unknown	1-1½ hr	Unknown

Contraindications and precautions
Contraindicated in patients hypersensitive to drug and in breast-feeding patients. Use cautiously in pregnant patients.

Interactions
Drug-drug. *Adrenocorticoids, corticotropin:* Altered effects. May require dosage adjustment of the steroid when thyroid status changes.
Bone marrow depressants: Increased risk of agranulocytosis. Monitor hematologic studies.
Hepatotoxic drugs: Increased risk of hepatotoxicity. Monitor patient for toxicity.
Iodinated glycerol, lithium, potassium iodide: Potentiated hypothyroid effects. Monitor patient closely.
Oral anticoagulants: Potentiated by anti–vitamin K activity attributed to PTU. Monitor PT and INR.

Adverse reactions
CNS: headache, drowsiness, vertigo, paresthesia, neuritis, neuropathies, CNS stimulation, depression.
CV: vasculitis.
EENT: visual disturbances.
GI: diarrhea, *nausea, vomiting* (may be dose-related), epigastric distress, salivary gland enlargement, loss of taste.
GU: nephritis.
Hematologic: *agranulocytosis, thrombocytopenia, aplastic anemia, leukopenia,* altered INR.
Hepatic: altered AST, ALT, and LD levels, jaundice, *hepatotoxicity.*
Metabolic: altered selenomethionine levels and liothyronine uptake, dose-related hypothyroidism (mental depression; hypoprothrombinemia and bleeding; cold intolerance; hard, nonpitting edema).
Musculoskeletal: arthralgia, myalgia.
Skin: rash, urticaria, skin discoloration, pruritus, erythema nodosum, exfoliative dermatitis, lupuslike syndrome.
Other: fever, lymphadenopathy.

Overdose and treatment
Toxicity may cause nausea, vomiting, epigastric distress, fever, headache, arthralgia, pruritus, edema, and pancytopenia.

Treatment of toxicity includes withdrawal of drug in the presence of agranulocytosis, pancytopenia, hepatitis, fever, or exfoliative dermatitis. For depression of bone marrow, treatment may require antibiotics and transfusions of fresh whole blood. For hepatitis, treatment includes rest, adequate diet, and symptomatic support, including analgesics, gastric lavage, I.V. fluids, and mild sedation.

Special considerations
● Best response occurs when drug is administered around the clock and given at the same time each day in respect to meals.
● A beta blocker, usually propranolol, commonly is given to manage peripheral signs of hyperthyroidism, which are primarily cardiac-related (tachycardia).
● Stop drug if patient develops severe rash or enlarged cervical lymph nodes.

Patient monitoring
● Watch for signs and symptoms of hypothyroidism (mental depression; cold intolerance; hard, nonpitting edema; hair loss).
● Monitor therapeutic effect.

Breast-feeding patients
● Drug appears in breast milk. Avoid breast-feeding during treatment. However, if breast-feeding is necessary, PTU is the preferred antithyroid drug.

Patient education
● Warn patient to avoid using self-prescribed cough medicines; many contain iodine.
● Suggest taking drug with meals to reduce GI adverse effects.
● Instruct patient to store drug in a light-resistant container and not to store in the bathroom; heat and humidity may cause drug to deteriorate.
● Tell patient to promptly report fever, sore throat, malaise, unusual bleeding, yellowing of eyes, nausea, or vomiting.
● Advise patient to have medical review of thyroid status before undergoing surgery (including dental surgery).
● Teach patient how to recognize signs of hyperthyroidism and hypothyroidism and what to do if they occur.

protamine sulfate

Pharmacologic classification: antidote
Therapeutic classification: heparin antagonist
Pregnancy risk category: C

Indications and dosages
➤ *Heparin overdose. Adults and children:* Dosage based on venous blood coagulation studies, usually 1 mg for each 90 units of heparin derived from lung tissue or 1 mg for each 115 units of heparin derived from intestinal mucosa. Give by slow I.V. injection over 1 to 3 minutes. Maximum dose is 50 mg in any 10-minute period.

How supplied
Available by prescription only
Injection: 10 mg/ml in 5-ml ampule, 25-ml ampule, 5-ml vial, 10-ml vial, 25-ml vial

---

Reactions may be *common*, uncommon, ***life-threatening***, or COMMON AND LIFE-THREATENING.

Pharmacodynamics

Heparin antagonism: Has weak anticoagulant activity; however, when given in the presence of heparin, forms a salt that neutralizes anticoagulant effects of both drugs.

Pharmacokinetics

Absorption: Heparin-neutralizing effect within 30 to 60 seconds.
Distribution: No information available.
Metabolism: Fate of heparin-protamine complex unknown; appears to be partially degraded, with release of some heparin.
Excretion: Binding action lasts about 2 hours.

Route	Onset	Peak	Duration
I.V.	30-60 sec	Unknown	2 hr

Contraindications and precautions

Contraindicated in patients hypersensitive to drug. Use cautiously after cardiac surgery.

Interactions

None reported.

Adverse reactions

CV: fall in blood pressure, *bradycardia, circulatory collapse.*
GI: nausea, vomiting.
Hematologic: shortens heparin-prolonged PTT.
Respiratory: dyspnea, *pulmonary edema, acute pulmonary hypertension.*
Other: transitory flushing, feeling of warmth, *anaphylaxis, anaphylactoid reactions,* lassitude.

Overdose and treatment

Overdose may cause bleeding secondary to interaction with platelets and proteins including fibrinogen. Replace blood loss with blood transfusions or fresh frozen plasma. If hypotension occurs, consider treating with fluids, epinephrine, dobutamine, or dopamine.

Special considerations

● Check for possible fish allergy.
● Dosage is based on blood coagulation studies as well as on route of administration of heparin and time elapsed since heparin was administered.
● Don't mix protamine with any other drug.
● Reconstitute powder by adding 5 ml sterile water to 50-mg vial (25 ml to 250-mg vial); discard unused solution.
● Slow I.V. administration (over 1 to 3 minutes) decreases adverse effects; have antishock equipment available.

Patient monitoring

● Watch for sudden fall in blood pressure. Monitor patient continually, and check vital signs frequently.
● Monitor therapeutic effect.

Breast-feeding patients

● It is not known whether drug appears in breast milk. Use cautiously in breast-feeding women.

Pediatric patients

● Safety and efficacy haven't been established.

Patient education

● Advise patient that he may experience transitory flushing or feel warm after I.V. administration.

pseudoephedrine hydrochloride

pseudoephedrine sulfate

Cenafed, Decofed, Efidac/24, Genaphed, Novafed, PediaCare Infants' Decongestant Drops, Pseudogest, Sudafed, Triaminic AM

Pharmacologic classification: adrenergic
Therapeutic classification: decongestant
Pregnancy risk category: B

Indications and dosages

➤ *Nasal and eustachian tube decongestant. Adults and children age 12 and over:* 60 mg P.O. q 4 to 6 hours. Maximum dose is 240 mg daily, or 120 mg P.O. extended-release tablet q 12 hours.
Children ages 6 to 11: Administer 30 mg P.O. q 4 to 6 hours. Maximum dose is 120 mg daily.
Children ages 2 to 5: 15 mg P.O. q 4 to 6 hours. Maximum dose is 60 mg daily, or 4 mg/kg or 125 mg/m² P.O. divided q.i.d.

How supplied

Available without a prescription
Capsules: 60 mg
Capsules (extended-release): 120 mg
Oral solution: 7.5 mg/0.8 ml, 15 mg/5 ml, 30 mg/5 ml
Tablets: 30 mg, 60 mg
Tablets (extended-release): 120 mg, 240 mg

Pharmacodynamics

Decongestant action: Directly stimulates alpha-adrenergic receptors of respiratory mucosa to produce vasoconstriction; shrinkage of swollen nasal mucous membranes; reduction of tissue hyperemia, edema, and nasal congestion; an increase in airway (nasal) patency and drainage of sinus excretions; and opening of obstructed eustachian ostia. Relaxation of bronchial smooth muscle may result from direct stimulation of beta-adrenergic receptors. Mild CNS stimulation may also occur.

Pharmacokinetics

Absorption: Nasal decongestion within 30 minutes; lasts 4 to 6 hours after oral dose of 60-mg tablet or oral solution. Effects last 8 hours after

60-mg dose; up to 12 hours after 120-mg dose of extended-release form.

Distribution: Widely distributed throughout body.

Metabolism: Incompletely metabolized in liver by N-demethylation to inactive compounds.

Excretion: 55% to 75% of dose excreted unchanged in urine; remainder excreted as unchanged drug and metabolites.

Route	Onset	Peak	Duration
P.O.	½ hr	½-1 hr	4-12 hr

Contraindications and precautions

Contraindicated in patients with severe hypertension or severe coronary artery disease; in those receiving MAO inhibitors; and in breast-feeding women. Extended-release preparations are contraindicated in children under age 12.

Use cautiously in elderly patients and in patients with hypertension, cardiac disease, diabetes, glaucoma, hyperthyroidism, or prostatic hyperplasia.

Interactions

Drug-drug. *Beta blockers:* Increased pressor effects of pseudoephedrine. Monitor patient.
MAO inhibitors: Potentiated pressor effects of pseudoephedrine. Use together cautiously.
Methyldopa, reserpine: Reduced antihypertensive effects. Monitor blood pressure.
Tricyclic antidepressants: Antagonized effects of pseudoephedrine. Monitor patient.
Other sympathomimetics: Additive effects. Monitor patient for toxicity.

Adverse reactions

CNS: *anxiety,* transient stimulation, tremor, dizziness, headache, insomnia, *nervousness.*
CV: *arrhythmias, palpitations,* tachycardia.
GI: anorexia, nausea, vomiting, dry mouth.
GU: difficulty urinating.
Respiratory: respiratory difficulties.
Skin: pallor.

Overdose and treatment

Toxicity may cause exaggeration of common adverse reactions, particularly seizures, arrhythmias, and nausea and vomiting.

Treatment of toxicity may include an emetic and gastric lavage within 4 hours of ingestion. Charcoal is effective only if administered within 1 hour, unless extended-release form was used. Forced diuresis will increase elimination. Don't force diuresis in severe overdose. I.V. propranolol may control cardiac toxicity; I.V. diazepam may be helpful to manage delirium or seizures; dilute potassium chloride solutions (I.V.) may be given for hypokalemia.

Special considerations

● Administer last daily dose several hours before bedtime to minimize insomnia.

● If symptoms persist longer than 5 days or fever is present, reevaluate therapy.

Patient monitoring
● Observe patient for complaints of headache or dizziness.
● Monitor blood pressure.

Breast-feeding patients
● Drug appears in breast milk. Avoid use in breast-feeding women; infant may be susceptible to drug effects.

Pediatric patients
● Don't use extended-release form in children under age 12.

Geriatric patients
● Elderly patients may be sensitive to effects of drug; lower dose may be needed. Overdose may cause hallucinations, CNS depression, seizures, and death in patients over age 60. Use extended-release preparations with caution in elderly patients.

Patient education
● If patient finds swallowing capsules difficult, suggest opening capsules and mixing contents with applesauce, jelly, honey, or syrup. Mixture must be swallowed without chewing.

● Tell patient that dry mouth may occur and suggest using ice chips, sugarless gum, or hard candy for relief.

● Instruct patient to take missed dose if remembered within 1 hour. If beyond 1 hour, patient should skip missed dose and resume regular schedule; he shouldn't double dose.

● Tell patient to store drug away from heat and light (not in bathroom medicine cabinet) and safely out of reach of children.

● Caution patient that many OTC preparations may contain sympathomimetics, which can cause additive, hazardous reactions.

● Advise patient to take last dose at least 2 to 3 hours before bedtime to avoid insomnia.

psyllium
Cillium, Fiberall, Hydrocil Instant, Konsyl, Konsyl-D, Metamucil, Naturacil, Reguloid, Serutan, Syllact, V-Lax

Pharmacologic classification: adsorbent
Therapeutic classification: bulk laxative
Pregnancy risk category: C

Indications and dosages

➤ *Constipation, bowel management, irritable bowel syndrome.* *Adults:* 1 to 2 rounded teaspoons P.O. in full glass of liquid daily, b.i.d., or t.i.d., then second glass of liquid; or 1 packet P.O. dissolved in water daily; or 2 wafers b.i.d. or t.i.d.

Reactions may be *common,* uncommon, *life-threatening,* or COMMON AND LIFE-THREATENING.

Children over age 6: 1 level teaspoon P.O. in ½ glass of liquid h.s.

How supplied
Available without a prescription
Chewable pieces: 1.7 g/piece, 3.4 g/piece
Granules: 2.5 g/teaspoon, 4.03 g/teaspoon
Powder: 3.3 g/teaspoon, 3.4 g/teaspoon, 3.5 g/teaspoon, 4.94 g/teaspoon
Powder (effervescent): 3.4 g/packet, 3.7 g/packet
Wafers: 1.7 g/wafer, 3.4 g/wafer

Pharmacodynamics
Laxative action: Adsorbs water in the gut; also serves as a source of indigestible fiber, increasing stool bulk and moisture, thus stimulating peristaltic activity and bowel evacuation.

Pharmacokinetics
Absorption: None; onset of action varies from 12 hours to 3 days.
Distribution: Distributed locally in gut.
Metabolism: Not metabolized.
Excretion: Excreted in feces.

Route	Onset	Peak	Duration
P.O.	12-24 hr	3 days	Variable

Contraindications and precautions
Contraindicated in patients hypersensitive to drug; in those with abdominal pain, nausea, vomiting, or other symptoms of appendicitis; and in those with intestinal obstruction or ulceration, disabling adhesions, or difficulty swallowing.

Interactions
Drug-drug. *Anticoagulants, cardiac glycosides, salicylates:* Psyllium may adsorb oral drugs. Separate administration times by at least 2 hours.

Adverse reactions
GI: nausea, vomiting, diarrhea (with excessive use); esophageal, gastric, small intestinal, and rectal obstruction when drug is taken in dry form; abdominal cramps, especially in severe constipation.

Overdose and treatment
No cases of overdose have been reported; probable clinical effects include abdominal pain and diarrhea.

Special considerations
• Before administering drug, add at least 8 oz (240 ml) of water or juice and stir for a few seconds (improves drug's taste). Have patient drink mixture immediately to prevent it from congealing; then have him drink another glass of fluid.
• Drug may reduce appetite if administered before meals.
• Psyllium and other bulk laxatives most closely mimic natural bowel function and don't cause laxative dependence; they are especially useful for patients with postpartum constipation or diverticular disease, for debilitated patients, for irritable bowel syndrome, and for chronic laxative users.
• Give diabetic patients a sugar-free and sodium-free psyllium product.

Patient monitoring
• Monitor patient for adverse GI effects.
• Monitor therapeutic effect.

Breast-feeding patients
• Because drug isn't absorbed, it's presumably safe for use in breast-feeding women.

Patient education
• Warn patient not to swallow drug in dry form; he should mix it with at least 8 oz (240 ml) of fluid, stir briefly, drink immediately (to prevent mixture from congealing), and then drink another 8 oz of fluid.
• Explain that drug may reduce appetite if taken before meals; recommend taking drug 2 hours after meals and any other oral drug.
• Advise diabetic patient and patient with restricted sodium or sugar intake to avoid psyllium products containing salt or sugar. Advise patient who must restrict phenylalanine intake to avoid psyllium products containing aspartame.

pyrantel pamoate
Antiminth, Combantrin*, Pin-X, Reese's Pinworm

Pharmacologic classification: pyrimidine derivative
Therapeutic classification: anthelmintic
Pregnancy risk category: C

Indications and dosages
► **Roundworm and pinworm infections.**
Adults and children over age 2: Single dose of 11 mg/kg P.O. Maximum dose is 1 g. For pinworm infection, dose should be repeated in 2 weeks.

How supplied
Available by prescription only
Oral suspension: 50 mg/ml
Tablets: 62.5 mg

Pharmacodynamics
Anthelmintic action: Causes the release of acetylcholine and inhibits cholinesterases, paralyzing the worms. Active against *Ancylostoma duodenale, Ascaris lumbricoides, Enterobius vermicularis, Necator americanus,* and *Trichostrongylus orientalis.*

Pharmacokinetics
Absorption: Absorbed poorly; peak levels in 1 to 3 hours.
Distribution: Little information available.
Metabolism: Small amount of absorbed drug metabolized partially in liver.

Excretion: Over 50% of oral dose excreted unchanged in feces; about 7% excreted in urine as unchanged drug or known metabolites.

Route	Onset	Peak	Duration
P.O.	Variable	1-3 hr	Variable

Contraindications and precautions
Contraindicated in patients hypersensitive to drug and during pregnancy. Use cautiously in patients with hepatic dysfunction or severe malnutrition or anemia.

Interactions
Drug-drug. *Piperazine:* Antagonized effects of piperazine. Avoid using together.

Adverse reactions
CNS: headache, dizziness, drowsiness, insomnia.
GI: anorexia, nausea, vomiting, gastralgia, abdominal cramps, diarrhea, tenesmus.
Hepatic: transient elevation of AST level.
Skin: rash.
Other: fever, weakness.

Overdose and treatment
Treatment of overdose is largely supportive, particularly of CV and respiratory functions. After recent ingestion (within 4 hours), empty stomach by induced emesis or gastric lavage. Follow with activated charcoal to decrease absorption. Osmotic cathartics may be helpful.

Special considerations
• Shake suspension well before measuring to ensure accurate dosage.
• Drug may be given with milk, fruit juice, or food.
• Laxatives, enemas, or dietary restrictions are unnecessary.
• Protect drug from light.
• Treat all family members.

Patient monitoring
• Monitor patient for adverse effects.
• Monitor therapeutic effect.

Breast-feeding patients
• It isn't known if drug appears in breast milk. Safety in breast-feeding women hasn't been established.

Pediatric patients
• Safety and efficacy in children under age 2 haven't been established.

Patient education
• Tell patient to wash perianal area daily and to change undergarments and bedclothes daily.
• To help prevent reinfection, instruct patient and family members in personal hygiene, including sanitary disposal of feces and hand washing and nail cleaning after defecation and before handling, preparing, or eating food.

• Explain routes of transmission and tell patient to encourage other household members and suspected contacts to be tested and, if necessary, treated.

pyrazinamide
PMS-Pyrazinamide*, Tebrazid*

Pharmacologic classification: synthetic pyrazine analogue of nicotinamide
Therapeutic classification: antituberculotic
Pregnancy risk category: C

Indications and dosages
➤ **Adjunctive treatment of tuberculosis (when primary and secondary antituberculotics can't be used or have failed).**
Adults: 15 to 30 mg/kg P.O. daily, in one or more doses. Maximum dose is 3 g daily. Or a twice-weekly dose of 50 to 70 mg/kg (based on lean body weight) has been developed to promote patient compliance. Lower dosage is recommended in patients with decreased renal function.

How supplied
Available by prescription only
Tablets: 500 mg

Pharmacodynamics
Antibiotic action: Mechanism unknown. May be bactericidal or bacteriostatic depending on organism susceptibility and drug level at infection site. Active only against *Mycobacterium tuberculosis.* Considered adjunctive in tuberculosis therapy and is given with other drugs to prevent or delay development of resistance to pyrazinamide by *M. tuberculosis.*

Pharmacokinetics
Absorption: Well absorbed after oral administration; serum levels peak 2 hours after oral dose.
Distribution: Distributed widely into body tissues and fluids, including lungs, liver, and CSF; 50% protein-bound. Not known if drug crosses placenta.
Metabolism: Hydrolyzed in liver; some hydrolysis occurs in stomach.
Excretion: Excreted almost completely in urine by glomerular filtration. Not known if drug appears in breast milk. Elimination half-life in adults is 9 to 10 hours; prolonged half-life in renal and hepatic impairment.

Route	Onset	Peak	Duration
P.O.	Unknown	1-2 hr	Unknown

Contraindications and precautions
Contraindicated in patients hypersensitive to drug and in those with severe hepatic disease or acute gout. Use cautiously in patients with diabetes mellitus, renal failure, or gout.

Reactions may be *common,* uncommon, *life-threatening,* or COMMON AND LIFE-THREATENING.

Interactions

Drug-lifestyle. *Sun exposure:* Possible photosensitivity reactions. Tell patient to take precautions.

Adverse reactions

CNS: malaise.
GI: anorexia, nausea, vomiting.
GU: dysuria, interstitial nephritis.
Hematologic: sideroblastic anemia, ***thrombocytopenia***.
Hepatic: *increased liver enzyme levels, **hepatitis***.
Metabolic: temporarily decreased 17-ketosteroid levels, increased protein-bound iodine and urate levels, hyperuricemia, gout.
Musculoskeletal: *arthralgia, myalgia.*
Skin: rash, urticaria, pruritus, photosensitivity.
Other: fever, porphyria.

Overdose and treatment

No specific recommendations are available. Treatment is supportive. After recent ingestion (4 hours or less), empty stomach by induced emesis or gastric lavage. Follow with activated charcoal to decrease absorption.

Special considerations

● In patients with diabetes mellitus, pyrazinamide therapy may hinder stabilization of serum glucose levels.
● In many cases, drug elevates serum uric acid levels. Although usually asymptomatic, a uricosuric drug, such as probenecid or allopurinol, may be necessary.
● Patients with concomitant HIV infection may need a longer course of treatment.
● Pyrazinamide may interfere with urine ketone determinations.

Patient monitoring

● Monitor liver function, especially enzyme and bilirubin levels, and renal function, especially serum uric acid levels, before therapy and thereafter at 2- to 4-week intervals.
● Observe patient for signs of liver damage or decreased renal function.

Breast-feeding patients

● Drug appears in breast milk. Safety in breast-feeding women hasn't been established. An alternative to breast-feeding is recommended during therapy.

Pediatric patients

● Safe use in children hasn't been definitely established.

Geriatric patients

● Because elderly patients commonly have diminished renal function, which decreases drug excretion, drug should be used cautiously.

Patient education

● Explain disease process and rationale for long-term therapy.
● Teach patient signs and symptoms of hypersensitivity and other adverse reactions, and emphasize need to report them; urge patient to report unusual reactions, especially signs of gout.
● Be sure patient understands how and when to take drugs; urge patient to complete entire prescribed regimen, to comply with instructions for around-the-clock dosage, and to keep follow-up appointments.

pyridostigmine bromide
Mestinon, Regonol

Pharmacologic classification: cholinesterase inhibitor
Therapeutic classification: muscle stimulant
Pregnancy risk category: NR

Indications and dosages

➤ *Reversal of the effects of nondepolarizing drugs, curariform antagonist (postoperatively).* *Adults:* 10 to 20 mg I.V. preceded by atropine sulfate 0.6 to 1.2 mg I.V.
➤ *Myasthenia gravis.* *Adults:* 60 to 180 mg P.O. b.i.d. or q.i.d. Usual dose is 600 mg daily, but higher doses may be needed (up to 1,500 mg daily). Give ⅟₃₀ of oral dose I.M. or I.V. Adjust dosage based on patient response and tolerance of adverse effects. Sustained-release and rapid-release forms are often used together depending on patient's symptoms.
Children: 7 mg/kg/24 hours P.O. divided into five or six doses.
Neonates of myasthenic mothers: 0.05 to 0.15 mg/kg I.M.

How supplied

Available by prescription only
Injection: 5 mg/ml in 2-ml ampule or 5-ml vial
Syrup: 60 mg/5 ml
Tablets: 60 mg
Tablets (sustained-release): 180 mg

Pharmacodynamics

Muscle stimulant action: Blocks acetylcholine's hydrolysis by cholinesterase, resulting in acetylcholine accumulation at cholinergic synapses, increasing stimulation of cholinergic receptors at the myoneural junction.

Pharmacokinetics

Absorption: Poorly absorbed from GI tract. Onset of action usually occurs 30 to 45 minutes after oral administration; 2 to 5 minutes after I.V.; 15 minutes after I.M.
Distribution: Little information available; however, may cross placenta, especially when given in large doses.
Metabolism: Exact metabolic fate unknown. Duration of effect usually 3 to 6 hours after oral dose

and 2 to 3 hours after I.V. dose, depending on patient's physical and emotional status and disease severity. Drug hydrolyzed by cholinesterase.
Excretion: Drug and metabolites excreted in urine.

Route	Onset	Peak	Duration
P.O.			
Regular	20-30 min	1-2 hr	3-6 hr
Extended	30-60 min	1-2 hr	6-12 hr
I.V.	2-5 min	Unknown	2-4 hr
I.M.	15 min	Unknown	2-4 hr

Contraindications and precautions
Contraindicated in patients hypersensitive to anticholinesterases and in those with mechanical obstruction of the intestine or urinary tract. Use cautiously in patients with bronchial asthma, bradycardia, or arrhythmias.

Interactions
Drug-drug. *Aminoglycoside antibiotics:* Mild but definite nondepolarizing blocking action of these drugs may accentuate neuromuscular block. Monitor patient for pyridostigmine effectiveness.
Corticosteroids: Decreased cholinergic effect of drug; when corticosteroids are stopped, this effect may increase, possibly affecting muscle strength. Monitor patient.
Ganglionic blockers: Decreased blood pressure; effect usually preceded by abdominal symptoms. Monitor patient and blood pressure closely.
Magnesium: Antagonized beneficial effects of pyridostigmine. Monitor patient for pyridostigmine effectiveness.
Procainamide, quinidine: Reversal of pyridostigmine's cholinergic effect on muscle. Monitor patient for pyridostigmine effectiveness.
Succinylcholine: Prolonged respiratory depression from plasma esterase inhibition, delaying succinylcholine hydrolysis. Monitor patient closely.

Adverse reactions
CNS: headache (with high doses), weakness.
CV: *bradycardia,* hypotension, thrombophlebitis.
EENT: miosis.
GI: abdominal cramps, nausea, vomiting, diarrhea, excessive salivation, increased peristalsis.
Musculoskeletal: muscle cramps, muscle fasciculations.
Respiratory: *bronchospasm, bronchoconstriction,* increased bronchial secretions.
Skin: rash, diaphoresis.

Overdose and treatment
Toxicity may cause nausea, vomiting, diarrhea, blurred vision, miosis, excessive tearing, bronchospasm, increased bronchial secretions, hypotension, incoordination, excessive sweating, muscle weakness, cramps, fasciculations, paralysis, bradycardia or tachycardia, excessive salivation, and restlessness or agitation.

Support respiration; bronchial suctioning may be performed. Discontinue drug immediately. Atropine may be given to block muscarinic effects; however, it won't counter skeletal muscle paralysis. Avoid atropine overdose because it may lead to bronchial plug formation.

Special considerations
• If muscle weakness is severe, determine if this effect stems from drug toxicity or exacerbation of myasthenia gravis. A test dose of edrophonium I.V. will aggravate drug-induced weakness but will temporarily relieve weakness that results from the disease.
• Avoid giving large doses to patients with decreased GI motility because toxicity may result once motility has been restored.
• Give drug with food or milk to reduce risk of muscarinic adverse effects.
• Atropine sulfate should always be readily available as an antagonist for the muscarinic effects of pyridostigmine.
• Stop all other cholinergics during drug therapy to avoid additive toxicity.

Patient monitoring
• Monitor therapeutic effect.
• Watch for resistance to drug.

Breast-feeding patients
• It isn't known if drug appears in breast milk. Because of potential for serious adverse reactions in breast-fed infant, stop either breast-feeding or drug, taking into account importance of drug to mother.

Pediatric patients
• Safety and efficacy haven't been established.

Patient education
• When drug is used in patient with myasthenia gravis, stress importance of taking drug exactly as ordered, on time, and in evenly spaced doses.
• If patient is taking sustained-release tablets, explain how these work and instruct him to take them at the same time each day; swallow tablets whole rather than crushing them.
• Teach patient how to evaluate muscle strength; instruct him to observe changes in muscle strength and to report muscle cramps, rash, or fatigue.

pyridoxine hydrochloride (vitamin B₆)
Aminoxin, Nestrex

Pharmacologic classification: water-soluble vitamin
Therapeutic classification: nutritional supplement
Pregnancy risk category: A (C if greater than RDA)

Indications and dosages
➤ **RDA.** *Neonates and infants to age 6 months:* 0.3 mg daily.

Infants ages 6 months to 1 year: 0.6 mg daily.
Children ages 1 to 3: 1 mg daily.
Children ages 4 to 6: 1.1 mg daily.
Children ages 7 to 10: 1.4 mg daily.
Women ages 11 to 14: 1.4 mg daily.
Women ages 15 to 18: 1.5 mg daily.
Women age 19 and older: 1.6 mg daily.
Women during pregnancy: 2.2 mg daily.
Breast-feeding women: 2.1 mg daily.
Men ages 11 to 14: 1.7 mg daily.
Men age 15 and over: 2 mg daily.
➤**Dietary vitamin B₆ deficiency.** *Adults:* 2.5 to 10 mg P.O., I.M., or I.V. daily for 3 weeks; then 2 to 5 mg daily as a supplement to a proper diet.
Children: 10 to 100 mg I.M. or I.V. to correct deficiency; then an adequate diet with supplementary RDA doses to prevent recurrence.
➤**Seizures related to vitamin B₆ deficiency or dependency.** *Adults and children:* 100 mg I.M. or I.V. in single dose.
➤**Vitamin B₆–responsive anemias or dependency syndrome (inborn errors of metabolism).** *Adults:* 200 to 600 mg P.O. daily for 1 to 2 months; then 30 to 50 mg P.O. daily.
Children: 100 mg I.M. or I.V.; then 2 to 10 mg I.M. or 10 to 100 mg P.O. daily.
➤**Premenstrual syndrome◇.** *Adults:* 40 to 500 mg P.O., I.M., or I.V. daily.
➤**Hyperoxaluria type I◇.** *Adults:* 25 to 300 mg P.O., I.M., or I.V. daily.
➤**Seizures secondary to isoniazid overdose.** *Adults and children:* A dose of pyridoxine hydrochloride equal to the amount of isoniazid ingested is usually given; generally, 1 to 4 g I.V. initially and then 1 g I.M. every 30 minutes until the entire dose has been given.
➤**Prevention of isoniazid- or penicillamine-induced anemia.** *Adults:* 10 to 50 mg P.O. daily.

How supplied
Available by prescription only
Injection: 10-ml vial (100 mg/ml), 30-ml vial (100 mg/ml), 10-ml vial (100 mg/ml, with 1.5% benzyl alcohol), 30-ml vial (100 mg/ml, with 1.5% benzyl alcohol), 10-ml vial (100 mg/ml, with 0.5% chlorobutanol), 1-ml vial (100 mg/ml)
Available without a prescription
Tablets: 10 mg, 25 mg, 50 mg, 100 mg, 200 mg, 250 mg, 500 mg, 500 mg timed-release

Pharmacodynamics
Metabolic action: Natural vitamin B₆ contained in plant and animal foodstuffs is converted to physiologically active forms of vitamin B₆, pyridoxal phosphate, and pyridoxamine phosphate. Exogenous forms of the vitamin are metabolized. Vitamin B₆ acts as a coenzyme in protein, carbohydrate, and fat metabolism and participates in the decarboxylation of amino acids in protein metabolism. Vitamin B₆ also helps convert tryptophan to niacin as well as facilitate the deamination, transamination, and transulfuration of

amino acids. Finally, vitamin B₆ is responsible for the breakdown of glycogen to glucose-1-phosphate in carbohydrate metabolism. The total adult body store consists of 167 mg of pyridoxine. The need for pyridoxine increases with the amount of protein in the diet.

Pharmacokinetics
Absorption: After oral administration, drug and its substituents absorbed readily from GI tract. GI absorption may be diminished in patients with malabsorption syndromes or after gastric resection. Normal serum levels are 30 to 80 ng/ml.
Distribution: Stored mainly in liver. Total body store about 167 mg. Pyridoxal and pyridoxal phosphate most common forms found in blood; highly protein-bound. Pyridoxal crosses placenta; fetal plasma levels five times greater than maternal plasma levels. After maternal intake of 2.5 to 5 mg daily of pyridoxine, level of vitamin in breast milk is about 240 ng/ml.
Metabolism: Degraded to 4-pyridoxic acid in liver.
Excretion: In erythrocytes, pyridoxine is converted to pyridoxal phosphate; pyridoxamine is converted to pyridoxamine phosphate. Phosphorylated form of pyridoxine is transaminated to pyridoxal and pyridoxamine, which is phosphorylated rapidly. Conversion of pyridoxine phosphate to pyridoxal phosphate requires riboflavin. Biological half-life is 15 to 20 days.

Route	Onset	Peak	Duration
P.O., I.V., I.M.	Unknown	Unknown	Unknown

Contraindications and precautions
Contraindicated in patients hypersensitive to pyridoxine.

Interactions
Drug-drug. *Cycloserine, hydralazine, isoniazid, oral contraceptives, penicillamine:* Increased pyridoxine requirements. Adjust dosages as needed.
Levodopa: Reversed therapeutic effects. Monitor patient closely.
Phenobarbital, phenytoin: Possible 50% decrease in serum levels of these anticonvulsants. Use together cautiously.

Adverse reactions
CNS: paresthesia, unsteady gait, numbness, somnolence.

Overdose and treatment
Toxicity may cause ataxia and severe sensory neuropathy after long-term consumption of high daily doses of pyridoxine (2 to 6 g). These neurologic deficits usually resolve after pyridoxine is discontinued.

Special considerations
• Prepare a dietary history. A single vitamin deficiency is unusual; lack of one vitamin often indicates a deficiency of others.
• A dosage of 25 mg/kg/day is well tolerated. Adults consuming 200 mg daily for 33 days and on a normal dietary intake develop vitamin B6 dependency.
• Don't mix with sodium bicarbonate in the same syringe.
• Patients receiving levodopa shouldn't take pyridoxine in doses above 5 mg daily.
• Store in a tight, light-resistant container.
• Don't use injection solution if it contains precipitate. Slight darkening is acceptable.
• Pyridoxine is sometimes useful for treating nausea and vomiting during pregnancy.
• Pyridoxine therapy alters determinations for urobilinogen in the spot test using Ehrlich's reagent, resulting in a false-positive reaction.

Patient monitoring
• Monitor protein intake; excessive protein intake increases pyridoxine requirements.

Breast-feeding patients
• Drug appears in breast milk. Use caution when administering to breast-feeding women. Pyridoxine may inhibit lactation by suppression of prolactin.

Pediatric patients
• Safety and efficacy in children haven't been established. The use of large doses of pyridoxine during pregnancy has been implicated in pyridoxine-dependency seizures in neonates.

Patient education
• Teach patient about dietary sources of vitamin B6, such as yeast, wheat germ, liver, whole grain cereals, bananas, and legumes.

pyrimethamine
Daraprim

Pharmacologic classification: aminopyrimidine derivative (folic acid antagonist)
Therapeutic classification: antimalarial
Pregnancy risk category: C

Indications and dosages
➤ *Malaria prophylaxis and transmission control.* Adults and children over age 10: 25 mg P.O. weekly.
Children ages 4 to 10: 12.5 mg P.O. weekly.
Children under age 4: 6.25 mg P.O. weekly.
  Dosage should be continued for all age-groups for at least 10 weeks after leaving endemic areas.
➤ *Acute attacks of malaria.* Not recommended alone in nonimmune persons; use with faster-acting antimalarials, such as chloroquine, for 2 days to initiate transmission control and suppressive cure. For chloroquine-resistant strain,

administer with sulfonamides and possibly quinine.
Adults and children over age 15: 50 mg P.O. daily for 2 days followed by 25 mg once weekly for at least 10 weeks.
Children ages 4 to 10: 25 mg once daily for 2 days followed by 12.5 mg once weekly for at least 10 weeks.
➤ *Toxoplasmosis. Adults:* 50 to 75 mg P.O. daily for 3 to 4 weeks, with sulfadiazine 2 to 8 g P.O. daily in three or four divided doses.
Children: 1 mg/kg daily P.O. (maximum daily dose is 25 mg) in divided doses q 12 hours for 3 days; then 1 mg/kg daily P.O. for 4 weeks. Administer with sulfadoxine 100 to 200 mg P.O. daily in divided doses.
➤ *Isosporiasis ◇. Adults:* 50 to 75 mg P.O. daily.

How supplied
Available by prescription only
Tablets: 25 mg of pyrimethamine

Pharmacodynamics
Antimalarial action: Inhibits the reduction of dihydrofolate to tetrahydrofolate, thereby blocking folic acid metabolism needed for survival of susceptible organisms. This mechanism is distinct from sulfonamide-induced folic acid antagonism. Drug is active against the asexual erythrocytic forms of susceptible plasmodia and against *Toxoplasma gondii.*

Pharmacokinetics
Absorption: Well absorbed from intestinal tract; serum levels peak within 2 hours.
Distribution: Distributed to kidneys, liver, spleen, and lungs; about 80% bound to plasma proteins.
Metabolism: Metabolized to several unidentified compounds.
Excretion: Excreted in urine and breast milk; elimination half-life 2 to 6 days. Half-life not changed in end-stage renal disease.

Route	Onset	Peak	Duration
P.O.	Unknown	1½-8 hr	2 wk

Contraindications and precautions
Contraindicated in patients hypersensitive to drug and in those with megaloblastic anemia due to folic acid deficiency. Use cautiously in patients with impaired renal or hepatic function, severe allergy or bronchial asthma, G6PD deficiency, or seizure disorders and in those who have been treated with chloroquine.

Interactions
Drug-drug. *Co-trimoxazole, other sulfonamides:* Additive adverse effects. Pyrimethamine and sulfadoxine combination shouldn't be given with these drugs.
Folic acid, para-aminobenzoic acid: Reduced antitoxoplasmic effects of pyrimethamine. May need dosage adjustment.

Lorazepam: Mild hepatotoxicity. Monitor liver function.
Sulfonamides: Pyrimethamine and sulfonamides act synergistically against some organisms; each inhibits folic acid synthesis at a different level. Monitor patient if used together.

Adverse reactions
GI: anorexia, vomiting, atrophic glossitis.
Hematologic: *aplastic anemia,* megaloblastic anemia, *leukopenia, thrombocytopenia, pancytopenia.*

Overdose and treatment
Toxicity may cause anorexia, vomiting, and CNS stimulation, including seizures. Megaloblastic anemia, thrombocytopenia, leukopenia, glossitis, and crystalluria may also occur. Treatment of overdose consists of gastric lavage, then a cathartic; barbiturates may help to control seizures. Leucovorin (folinic acid) in a dosage of 5 to 15 mg daily P.O., I.M., or I.V. for 3 days or longer is used to restore decreased platelet or leukocyte counts.

Special considerations
● No longer considered a first-line antimalarial. Other antimalarials (mefloquine, chloroquine, sulfadoxine) are generally preferred.
● Give drug with meals to minimize GI distress.
◆ Because severe reactions may occur, pyrimethamine with sulfadoxine should be given only to patient traveling to areas where chloroquine-resistant malaria is prevalent and only if traveler will be in such areas longer than 3 weeks.

Patient monitoring
● Monitor CBC, including platelet counts, twice weekly.
● Monitor patient for signs of folate deficiency or bleeding when platelet count is low; if abnormalities appear, decrease dosage or stop drug. Leucovorin (folinic acid) may be prescribed to raise blood counts while reducing dosage or after drug is stopped.

Breast-feeding patients
● Pyrimethamine is contraindicated in breast-feeding women because of the risk of serious adverse reactions in breast-fed infants.

Pediatric patients
● Use cautiously in children.

Patient education
● Teach patient how to recognize signs and symptoms of adverse blood reactions and tell him to report them immediately. Teach emergency measures to control overt bleeding.
● Teach patient signs and symptoms of folate deficiency.
● Counsel patient about need to report adverse effects and to keep follow-up medical appointments.

● Tell patient to keep drug out of reach of children.

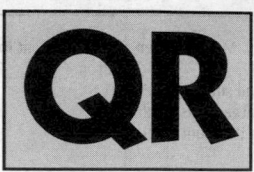

quetiapine fumarate
Seroquel

Pharmacologic classification: dibenzo-
thiazepine derivative
Therapeutic classification: antipsychotic
Pregnancy risk category: C

Indications and dosages
➤ *Management of signs and symptoms
of psychotic disorders. Adults:* Initially, 25 mg
P.O. b.i.d., increased in increments of 25 to 50 mg
b.i.d. or t.i.d. on days 2 and 3, as tolerated, to a
target dosage range of 300 to 400 mg daily by
day 4, divided into two or three doses. Further
dosage adjustments, if indicated, should generally occur at intervals of at least 2 days. Dosages
can be increased or decreased by 25 to 50 mg
b.i.d. Antipsychotic efficacy usually occurs at 150
to 750 mg daily. Safety of doses above 800 mg
daily hasn't been evaluated.
✦ *Dosage adjustment.* In elderly or debilitated patients or those who have hepatic impairment or a predisposition to hypotensive reactions, consider lower doses, slower dosage
adjustment, and careful monitoring during initial dosing period. No specific dosing recommendations are given.

How supplied
Available by prescription only
Tablets: 25 mg, 100 mg, 200 mg

Pharmacodynamics
Antipsychotic action: Exact mechanism of action is unknown. Quetiapine is a dibenzothi-
azepine derivative that is thought to exert antipsychotic activity through antagonism of dopamine
type 2 (D_2) and serotonin type 2 (5-HT_2) receptors. Antagonism at serotonin 5-HT_{1A}, D_1, H_1,
and alpha$_1$- and alpha$_2$-adrenergic receptors may
explain other effects.

Pharmacokinetics
Absorption: Rapidly absorbed after oral administration. Absorption is affected by food, with
maximum level increasing 25% and bioavailability
increasing 15%.
Distribution: Apparent volume of distribution
is 10±4 I/kg. Drug is 83% plasma protein–bound.
Steady state levels are reached within 2 days.
Metabolism: Extensively metabolized by the liver via sulfoxidation and oxidation. Cytochrome
P-450 3A4 is the major isoenzyme involved.

Excretion: Less than 1% of dose is excreted as
unchanged drug. About 73% is recovered in urine
and 20% in feces. Mean terminal half-life is about
6 hours.

Route	Onset	Peak	Duration
P.O.	Unknown	1½ hr	Unknown

Contraindications and precautions
Contraindicated in patients hypersensitive to drug
or its ingredients.
    Use cautiously in patients with CV or cere-
brovascular disease, conditions that predispose
to hypotension, conditions that could contribute
to increased core body temperature, conditions
that could lower the seizure threshold, or a history of seizures. Also use cautiously in patients
at risk for aspiration pneumonia from esophageal
dysmotility and aspiration.

Interactions
Drug-drug. *Antihypertensives:* May potentiate
hypotensive effects. Monitor blood pressure.
Cimetidine: Decreased oral clearance of quetiapine. No dosage adjustment needed.
CNS depressants: Increased CNS effects. Use cautiously together.
Dopamine agonists, levodopa: Quetiapine may
antagonize the effect of these drugs. Monitor patient closely.
*Erythromycin, fluconazole, itraconazole, ke-
toconazole:* Decreased quetiapine clearance. Use
cautiously.
Lorazepam: Reduced lorazepam clearance. Monitor patient.
Phenytoin, thioridazine: Increased oral clearance of quetiapine. Quetiapine dosage may need
adjustment.
Drug-lifestyle. *Alcohol use:* May potentiate cognitive and motor effects. Advise patient to avoid
alcohol during quetiapine therapy.

Adverse reactions
CNS: *dizziness, headache, somnolence,* hyper-
tonia, asthenia, dysarthria.
CV: orthostatic hypotension, tachycardia, palpi-
tations, peripheral edema.
EENT: pharyngitis, rhinitis, ear pain.
GI: dry mouth, dyspepsia, abdominal pain, con-
stipation, anorexia.
Hematologic: *leukopenia.*
Metabolic: *weight gain.*
Musculoskeletal: back pain.
Respiratory: increased cough, dyspnea.
Skin: rash, sweating.

Reactions may be *common*, uncommon, *life-threatening*, or COMMON AND LIFE-THREATENING.

Other: fever, flulike syndrome.

Overdose and treatment
Usually, overdose causes exaggeration of drug effects (drowsiness, sedation, tachycardia, hypotension). Hypokalemia and first-degree heart block also may occur.

For acute overdose, treatment includes establishing and maintaining an airway to ensure adequate oxygenation and ventilation. Consider gastric lavage and administration of activated charcoal or a laxative. Begin CV monitoring, including ECG monitoring, immediately. Avoid use of disopyramide, procainamide, quinidine, and bretylium if antiarrhythmic therapy is indicated. Administer I.V. fluids or sympathomimetic drugs (not epinephrine or dopamine) to treat hypotension and circulatory collapse. For severe extrapyramidal symptoms, give anticholinergic agents.

Special considerations
● Total and free T₄ levels may decrease, although this change usually isn't clinically significant. Although rare, some patients have increased thyroid-stimulating hormone levels and need thyroid replacement.
● Cholesterol and triglyceride levels sometimes increase.
● Asymptomatic, transient, reversible increases in serum transaminase (primarily ALT) levels have been reported. They usually occur during the first 3 weeks of therapy and promptly return to pretreatment levels with continued use.
● Neuroleptic malignant syndrome, a potentially fatal syndrome, has been reported with use of antipsychotic drugs. Signs and symptoms include hyperpyrexia, muscle rigidity, altered mental status, and evidence of autonomic instability. Carefully monitor at-risk patients.
● Use smallest effective dose for shortest duration to minimize risk of tardive dyskinesia.

Patient monitoring
● To detect possible cataract formation, examine the patient's ocular lenses before therapy starts or shortly thereafter and at 6-month intervals during treatment.
● Monitor schizophrenic patient closely during drug therapy because of the inherent risk of suicide.

Pregnant patients
● Instruct women to report planned, suspected, or known pregnancy.

Breast-feeding patients
● Breast-feeding isn't recommended during quetiapine therapy.

Pediatric patients
● Safety and efficacy in children haven't been established.

Geriatric patients
● In general, elderly patients seem to tolerate quetiapine no differently than other adults. However, patients who have problems that could decrease drug clearance, increase response to the drug, decrease tolerance of the drug, or increase the risk of orthostasis may benefit from a reduced starting dosage, slower dosage adjustment, and careful monitoring during the initial treatment period.

Patient education
● Caution patient about the risk of orthostatic hypotension, especially during the first 3 to 5 days of treatment and any time the dosage is adjusted.
● Tell patient to avoid becoming overheated or dehydrated.
● When therapy starts or dosage increases, warn patient to avoid activities that require mental alertness until CNS effects of drug are known.
● Remind patient to have eyes examined at the start therapy and every 6 months during treatment to watch for cataract formation.
● Tell patient to contact prescriber before taking other prescription or OTC drugs.

---

quinapril hydrochloride
Accupril

Pharmacologic classification: angiotensin-converting enzyme (ACE) inhibitor
Therapeutic classification: antihypertensive
Pregnancy risk category: C (D second and third trimesters)

Indications and dosages
➤ **Heart failure.** *Adults:* Initially, 5 mg P.O. b.i.d., when added to conventional therapy including diuretic, cardiac glycoside, or both. Adjust dosage weekly based on response. Usual dosage is 20 to 40 mg P.O. daily divided into two equal doses.
✦ *Dosage adjustment.* Initial dose is 5 mg if creatinine clearance is above 30 ml/minute, 2.5 mg if it's 10 to 30 ml/minute. No recommendation available for creatinine clearance below 10 ml/minute.
➤ **Hypertension in patients not receiving a diuretic.** *Adults:* Initially, 10 or 20 mg P.O. once daily. Adjust dosage at about 2-week intervals based on response. Most patients are controlled at 20, 40, or 80 mg daily, as a single dose or in two divided doses.
➤ **Hypertension in patients receiving a diuretic.** If a patient is currently receiving a diuretic, stop it 2 to 3 days before starting quinapril, if possible, to reduce the risk of hypotension. Initial dosage would then be the same as that listed above. If not possible, give an initial dose of 5 mg P.O. daily. Monitor patient, and adjust dosage as usual.

✦ **Dosage adjustment.** Initial dose is 10 mg P.O. daily if creatinine clearance exceeds 60 ml/minute, 5 mg if it's 30 to 60 ml/minute, and 2.5 mg if it's 10 to 30 ml/minute. No recommendation available for creatinine clearance below 10 ml/minute.

How supplied
Available by prescription only
Tablets: 5 mg, 10 mg, 20 mg, 40 mg

Pharmacodynamics
Antihypertensive action: Quinapril and its active metabolite, quinaprilat, inhibit ACE, preventing conversion of angiotensin I to angiotensin II, a potent vasoconstrictor. Reduced formation of angiotensin II decreases peripheral arterial resistance, decreases aldosterone secretion, reduces sodium and water retention, and lowers blood pressure. Quinapril also has antihypertensive activity in patients with low-renin hypertension.

Pharmacokinetics
Absorption: At least 60% of drug is absorbed. Rate and extent of absorption are decreased 25% to 30% when drug is given during a high-fat meal.
Distribution: About 97% of drug and active metabolite are bound to plasma proteins.
Metabolism: About 38% of an oral dose is de-esterified in the liver to quinaprilat, the active metabolite.
Excretion: Primarily excreted in urine; terminal elimination half-life is about 25 hours.

Route	Onset	Peak	Duration
P.O.	1 hr	2-6 hr	24 hr

Contraindications and precautions
Contraindicated in patients hypersensitive to ACE inhibitors and patients with a history of angioedema from ACE inhibitor treatment. Also contraindicated in patients at immediate risk for cardiogenic shock. Use cautiously in patients with impaired renal function.

Interactions
Drug-drug. *Diuretics, other antihypertensives:* Increased risk of excessive hypotension. Discontinue diuretic or lower dose of quinapril as needed.
Lithium: Increased serum lithium levels and lithium toxicity. Monitor serum lithium levels.
Potassium-sparing diuretics and potassium supplements: May increase risk of hyperkalemia. Don't use together.
Tetracycline: Significantly impaired absorption of tetracycline. Avoid use together.
Drug-herb. *Capsaicin:* Increased risk of cough. Discourage concomitant use.
Licorice: Increased risk of sodium retention and increased blood pressure, which may interfere with effects of ACE inhibitors. Discourage concomitant use.

Drug-food. *Potassium-containing salt substitutes:* May cause hyperkalemia. Tell patient not to use together.

Adverse reactions
CNS: somnolence, vertigo, nervousness, headache, dizziness, fatigue, depression.
CV: palpitations, tachycardia, angina, hypertensive crisis, orthostatic hypotension, chest pain, *rhythm disturbances.*
GI: dry mouth, abdominal pain, constipation, vomiting, nausea, hemorrhage, diarrhea.
Hematologic: *thrombocytopenia, agranulocytosis, neutropenia.*
Hepatic: elevated liver enzyme levels.
Metabolic: hyperkalemia.
Respiratory: *dry, persistent, tickling, nonproductive cough.*
Skin: pruritus, *exfoliative dermatitis, photosensitivity,* diaphoresis.
Other: *angioedema.*

Overdose and treatment
No information is available regarding overdose. The most likely effect is hypotension.

Treat symptomatically. Infusions of normal saline solution have been suggested to treat hypotension. Peritoneal dialysis or hemodialysis isn't beneficial. No data are available to support acidification of urine.

Special considerations
⚕ **ALERT** Because administration with diuretics increases the risk of excessive hypotension, discontinue diuretic therapy 2 to 3 days before start of quinapril, if possible. If quinapril alone doesn't adequately control blood pressure, a diuretic may be carefully added to the regimen.
• Like other ACE inhibitors, drug may cause a dry, persistent, tickling cough; it stops when therapy stops.
• Each quinapril tablet contains magnesium carbonate and magnesium stearate.

Patient monitoring
• Measure blood pressure when drug is at peak levels (2 to 6 hours after dosing) and trough levels (just before a dose) to verify adequate blood pressure control.
• Assess renal and hepatic function before and periodically throughout therapy.
• Monitor CBC and serum potassium levels.

Breast-feeding patients
• Because drug appears in breast milk, use drug cautiously in breast-feeding women.

Pediatric patients
• Safety and efficacy in children haven't been established.

Geriatric patients
• Because elderly patients commonly have decreased renal function, they have an increased

---

risk of higher peak levels and slower elimination of drug.
• No overall differences in safety or efficacy have arisen in elderly patients.

Patient education
• Tell patient to take drug on an empty stomach because meals, particularly high-fat meals, can impair absorption.
• Advise patient to immediately report signs or symptoms of angioedema: difficulty breathing and swelling of face, eyes, lips, or tongue. If these occur, tell patient to stop taking drug and seek medical attention immediately.
• Warn patient that light-headedness may occur, especially during first few days of therapy. Tell him to rise slowly to minimize this effect and to report persistent or severe symptoms. Tell patient to stop taking drug and to immediately call prescriber if he faints.
• Inadequate fluid intake, vomiting, diarrhea, and excessive diaphoresis can lead to light-headedness and syncope. Urge patient to take care in hot weather and during periods of exercise to avoid dehydration and overheating.
• Tell patient to immediately report evidence of infection (sore throat, fever) or easy bruising or bleeding. Other ACE inhibitors have been linked to development of agranulocytosis and neutropenia.

quinidine gluconate
Quinaglute Dura-Tabs, Quinalan

quinidine polygalacturonate
Cardioquin

quinidine sulfate
Apo-Quinidine*, Quinidex Extentabs

Pharmacologic classification: cinchona alkaloid
Therapeutic classification: ventricular antiarrhythmic, supraventricular antiarrhythmic, atrial antitachyarrhythmic
Pregnancy risk category: C

Indications and dosages
➤ *Atrial flutter or fibrillation. Adults:* 200 mg (sulfate or equivalent base) P.O. q 2 to 3 hours for five to eight doses with subsequent daily increases until sinus rhythm is restored or toxic effects develop. Give quinidine only after digitalization to avoid increasing AV conduction. Maximum, 3 to 4 g daily.
   Maintenance dosage, 200 to 400 mg P.O. t.i.d. or q.i.d. Or, 600 mg P.O. q 8 to 12 hours daily (extended-release).
➤ *Paroxysmal supraventricular tachycardia. Adults:* 400 to 600 mg (sulfate) P.O. q 2 to 3 hours until toxic effects develop or arrhythmia subsides.

➤ *Premature atrial contractions, PVCs, paroxysmal AV junctional rhythm or atrial or ventricular tachycardia, maintenance of cardioversion. Adults:* Give test dose of 50 to 200 mg P.O. of sulfate (or 200 mg gluconate I.M.); then monitor vital signs before beginning therapy with 200 to 400 mg P.O. sulfate or equivalent base q 4 to 6 hours. Or, initially, 600 mg of gluconate I.M.; then up to 400 mg q 2 hours, p.r.n. Or, 800 mg I.V. gluconate diluted in 40 ml of D₅W, infused at 16 mg (1 ml)/minute. Or, 300 to 600 mg of sulfate (extended-release) or 324 to 648 mg of gluconate (extended-release) q 8 to 12 hours.
Children: Give test dose of 2 mg/kg; then give 30 mg/kg daily P.O. or 900 mg/m² daily P.O. in five divided doses.
➤ *Malaria (when quinine dihydrochloride is unavailable) ◇. Adults:* Give quinidine gluconate by continuous I.V. infusion. Initial loading dose of 10 mg/kg diluted in 250 ml of normal saline solution injection and infused over 1 to 2 hours, followed by continuous maintenance infusion of 0.02 mg/kg/minute (20 mcg/kg/minute) for 72 hours or until parasitemia is reduced to less than 1% or oral therapy can be started. Or, 10 mg/kg quinidine sulfate P.O. q 8 hours for 5 to 7 days.

How supplied
Available by prescription only
Injection: 80 mg/ml (gluconate)
Tablets: 275 mg (polygalacturonate); 200 mg, 300 mg (sulfate)
Tablets (extended-release): 300 mg (sulfate), 324 mg (gluconate)

Pharmacodynamics
Antiarrhythmic action: A class IA antiarrhythmic, quinidine depresses phase 0 of the action potential. It's considered a myocardial depressant because it decreases myocardial excitability and conduction velocity and may depress myocardial contractility. It also exerts anticholinergic activity, which may modify its direct myocardial effects. In therapeutic doses, quinidine reduces conduction velocity in the atria, ventricles, and His-Purkinje system. It helps control atrial tachyarrhythmias by prolonging the effective refractory period (ERP) and increasing the action potential duration in the atria, ventricles, and His-Purkinje system. Because ERP prolongation exceeds action potential duration, tissue remains refractory even after returning to resting membrane potential (membrane-stabilizing effect).
   Quinidine shortens the effective refractory period of the AV node. Because anticholinergic action of quinidine may increase AV node conductivity, a cardiac glycoside should be administered for atrial tachyarrhythmias before quinidine therapy begins, to prevent ventricular tachyarrhythmias. Quinidine also suppresses automaticity in the His-Purkinje system and ectopic pacemakers, making it useful in treating PVCs. At thera-

peutic doses, quinidine prolongs the QRS complex and QT interval; these ECG effects may be used as an index of drug effectiveness and toxicity.

Pharmacokinetics

Absorption: Although all quinidine salts are well absorbed from the GI tract, individual serum drug levels vary greatly. For extended-release forms, onset of action may be slightly slower but duration of effect is longer because drug delivery system allows longer-than-usual dosing intervals.

Distribution: Drug is well distributed in all tissues except the brain and concentrates in the heart, liver, kidneys, and skeletal muscle. Distribution volume decreases in patients with heart failure, possibly requiring reduction in maintenance dosage. About 80% of drug is bound to plasma proteins; the unbound (active) fraction may increase in patients with hypoalbuminemia from various causes, including hepatic insufficiency. Usual therapeutic serum levels depend on assay method. In specific assay (enzyme multiplied immunoassay technique, high-performance liquid chromatography, fluorescence polarization) levels range from 2 to 5 mcg/ml. In nonspecific assay (fluorometric), they range from 4 to 8 mcg/ml.

Metabolism: About 60% to 80% of drug is metabolized in the liver to two metabolites that may have some pharmacologic activity.

Excretion: About 10% to 30% is excreted in urine within 24 hours as unchanged drug. Urine acidification increases quinidine excretion; alkalinization decreases excretion. Most of drug is eliminated in the urine as metabolites; elimination half-life ranges from 5 to 12 hours (usual half-life is about 6½ hours). Duration of effect ranges from 6 to 8 hours.

Route	Onset	Peak	Duration
P.O.	1-3 hr	1-6 hr	6-8 hr
I.V.	Immediate	Immediate	Unknown
I.M.	½-1½ min	Unknown	Unknown

Contraindications and precautions

Contraindicated in patients hypersensitive to quinidine or related cinchona derivatives, patients with idiosyncratic reactions to them, and patients with intraventricular conduction defects, cardiac glycoside toxicity when AV conduction is grossly impaired, abnormal rhythms caused by escape mechanisms, and a history of drug-induced torsades de pointes or QT syndrome.

Use cautiously in patients with impaired renal or hepatic function, asthma, muscle weakness, or infection accompanied by a fever because hypersensitivity reactions may be masked.

Interactions

Drug-drug. *Antacids, sodium bicarbonate, thiazide diuretics:* Decreased quinidine elimination when urine pH increases. Monitor patient closely.

Anticholinergics: May cause additive anticholinergic effects. Use together cautiously.

Anticonvulsants, such as phenobarbital and phenytoin: Increases rate of quinidine metabolism, decreasing quinidine levels. Monitor drug levels closely.

Cholinergic drugs: May fail to terminate paroxysmal supraventricular tachycardia. Also, anticholinergic effects of quinidine may negate the effects of these drugs when treating myasthenia gravis. Use together cautiously.

Coumarin: May potentiate anticoagulant effect of coumarin, possibly leading to hypoprothrombinemic hemorrhage. Monitor patient closely.

Digitoxin, digoxin: May cause increased (possibly toxic) digoxin levels. Some experts recommend a 50% reduction in digoxin dosage when quinidine therapy starts, with subsequent monitoring of serum levels.

Hypotensive drugs: May cause additive hypotensive effects, mainly when given I.V. Monitor blood pressure closely.

Neuromuscular blockers, such as metocurine iodide, pancuronium bromide, succinylcholine chloride, and tubocurarine chloride: May potentiate anticholinergic effects. Avoid giving quinidine immediately after these drugs; if quinidine must be used, respiratory support may be needed.

Nifedipine: May decrease quinidine levels. Monitor patient closely.

Other antiarrhythmics, such as amiodarone, lidocaine, phenytoin, procainamide, and propranolol: May cause additive or antagonistic cardiac effects and additive toxic effects. Use together cautiously.

Phenothiazines, reserpine: May cause additive cardiac depressant effects. Avoid use together.

Rifampin: May increase quinidine metabolism and decrease serum quinidine levels. Adjust quinidine dosage as needed when rifampin therapy starts or stops.

Verapamil: Possibly significant hypotension in patients with hypertrophic cardiomyopathy. Monitor patient closely.

Drug-herb. *Jimsonweed:* May adversely affect CV function. Discourage use together.

Licorice: May prolong the QT interval and be potentially additive. Tell patient to use cautiously together.

Drug-food. *Grapefruit juice:* Delayed onset of quinidine effect. Tell patient to take with liquid other than grapefruit juice.

Adverse reactions

CNS: *vertigo, headache, light-headedness, fatigue,* confusion, ataxia, depression, dementia.

CV: PVCs, **ventricular tachycardia, atypical ventricular tachycardia (torsades de pointes),** hypotension, **complete AV block,** tachycardia, ECG changes (particularly widening of QRS complex and QT and PR intervals).

EENT: *tinnitus,* excessive salivation, blurred vision, diplopia, photophobia.

Reactions may be *common*, uncommon, ***life-threatening***, or COMMON AND LIFE-THREATENING.

GI: petechial hemorrhage of buccal mucosa, *diarrhea, nausea, vomiting,* anorexia, abdominal pain.

Hematologic: *hemolytic anemia, thrombocytopenia, agranulocytosis.*

Hepatic: *hepatotoxicity.*

Respiratory: *acute asthmatic attack, respiratory arrest.*

Skin: rash, pruritus, urticaria, lupus erythematosus, photosensitivity.

Other: *angioedema,* fever, *cinchonism.*

Overdose and treatment

The most serious effects of overdose include severe hypotension, ventricular arrhythmias (including torsades de pointes), and seizures. QRS complexes and QT and PR intervals may be prolonged, and ataxia, anuria, respiratory distress, irritability, and hallucinations may develop. If ingestion was recent, gastric lavage, emesis, and activated charcoal may be used to decrease absorption. Urine acidification may be used to help increase quinidine elimination.

Treatment involves general supportive measures (including CV and respiratory support) with hemodynamic and ECG monitoring. Metaraminol or norepinephrine may be used to reverse hypotension (after adequate hydration has been ensured). Avoid CNS depressants because CNS depression may occur, possibly with seizures. Cardiac pacing may be necessary. Isoproterenol or ventricular pacing possibly may be used to treat torsades de pointes tachycardia.

I.V. infusion of 1/6 M sodium lactate solution reduces cardiotoxic effect of quinidine. Hemodialysis, although rarely warranted, also may be effective.

Special considerations

⚠ ALERT When changing route of administration or oral salt form, alter dosage to compensate for variations in quinidine base content.

⚠ ALERT Don't confuse quinidine with Quinamm, quinine, or clonidine.

● When drug is used to treat atrial tachyarrhythmias, ventricular rate may be accelerated from anticholinergic effects of drug on AV node. This can be prevented by previous treatment with a digitalis glycoside.

● Because conversion of chronic atrial fibrillation may increase the risk of embolism, give an anticoagulant for several weeks before quinidine therapy begins.

● Use I.V. route only for acute arrhythmias; it's typically avoided because of the risk of severe hypotension.

● Don't use discolored (brownish) quinidine solution.

● For maintenance, give only by oral or I.M. route. Dosage requirements vary. Some patients may need drug q 4 hours, others q 6 hours. Adjust dose by both clinical response and blood levels.

● Decrease dosage in patients with heart failure and hepatic disease.

● Drug may increase toxicity of cardiac glycoside derivatives. Use cautiously in patients receiving cardiac glycosides. Monitor digoxin levels and expect to reduce dosage of cardiac glycoside derivatives. Many clinicians recommend that digoxin dosage be reduced by half when quinidine therapy starts.

● Lidocaine may be effective in treating quinidine-induced arrhythmias because it increases AV conduction.

● Quinidine may cause hemolysis in patients with G6PD deficiency.

● Small amounts of quinidine are removed by hemodialysis; drug isn't removed by peritoneal dialysis.

● Amount of quinidine in the various salt forms varies as follows: *gluconate:* 62% quinidine (324 mg of gluconate, 202 mg sulfate); *polygalacturonate:* 60% quinidine (275 mg polygalacturonate, 166 mg sulfate); *sulfate:* 83% quinidine. The sulfate form is considered the standard dosage preparation.

● Quinidine gluconate is as or more active in vitro as quinine dihydrochloride against *Plasmodium falciparum*. Because the latter drug is only available through the Centers for Disease Control and Prevention, quinidine gluconate may be useful in treating severe malaria when delay of therapy may be life-threatening. The current CDC protocol involves follow-up treatment with either tetracycline or sulfadoxine and pyrimethamine.

Patient monitoring

● Check apical pulse rate, blood pressure, and ECG before starting therapy.

● Monitor ECG, especially when giving large doses. Quinidine-induced cardiotoxicity causes conduction defects (50% widening of the QRS complex), ventricular tachycardia or flutter, frequent PVCs, and complete AV block. When these signs appear, stop drug and monitor patient closely.

● Monitor liver function test results during first 4 to 8 weeks of therapy.

● Adverse GI effects, especially diarrhea, indicate toxicity. Check quinidine blood levels, and suspect toxicity when they exceed 8 mcg/ml. GI symptoms may be minimized by giving drug with meals.

Pregnant patients

● Drug has some oxytocic effects. Safety for use during pregnancy and labor and delivery hasn't been established.

Breast-feeding patients

● Because drug appears in breast milk, an alternative feeding method is recommended during therapy.

Pediatric patients

● Safety and efficacy haven't been established for use in children.

Geriatric patients
● Dosage reduction may be necessary. Because of highly variable metabolism, monitor serum levels.

Patient education
● Instruct patient to report rash, fever, unusual bleeding, bruising, ringing in ears, or visual disturbance.
● Stress importance of taking drug exactly as prescribed.

quinine sulfate

Pharmacologic classification: cinchona alkaloid
Therapeutic classification: antimalarial
Pregnancy risk category: D

Indications and dosages
➤ **Malaria (chloroquine-resistant).** *Adults:* 650 mg P.O. q 8 hours for 10 days, with 25 mg pyrimethamine q 12 hours for 3 days and 500 mg sulfadiazine q.i.d. for 5 days.
Children: 25 mg/kg daily P.O. divided into three doses for 10 days.
➤ **Babesia microti** *infections. Adults:* 650 mg P.O. q 6 to 8 hours for 7 days.
Children: 25 mg/kg daily P.O. divided into three doses for 7 days.
➤ *Nocturnal recumbency leg muscle cramps* ◇ . *Adults:* 200 to 300 mg P.O. h.s. Discontinue if leg cramps subside for several days to determine whether continued therapy is needed.

How supplied
Available by prescription only
Capsules: 260 mg
Tablets: 260 mg, 325 mg

Pharmacodynamics
Antimalarial action: Quinine intercalates into DNA, disrupting the parasite's replication and transcription; it also depresses oxygen uptake and carbohydrate metabolism by parasite. Drug is active against asexual erythrocytic forms of *Plasmodium falciparum, P. malariae, P. ovale,* and *P. vivax* and is used for chloroquine-resistant malaria.
Skeletal muscle relaxant action: Quinine increases refractory period, decreases excitability of the motor end plate, and affects calcium distribution within muscle fibers.

Pharmacokinetics
Absorption: Almost completely absorbed.
Distribution: Distributed widely into the liver, lungs, kidneys, and spleen; CSF levels reach 2% to 5% of serum levels. Quinine is about 70% bound to plasma proteins and readily crosses the placenta.
Metabolism: Metabolized in the liver.

Excretion: Less than 5% is excreted unchanged in urine; small amounts of metabolites appear in feces, gastric juice, bile, saliva, and breast milk. Half-life is 7 to 21 hours in healthy or convalescing persons; it's longer in patients with malaria. Urine acidification hastens elimination.

Route	Onset	Peak	Duration
P.O.	Unknown	1-3 hr	Unknown

Contraindications and precautions
Contraindicated in pregnant patients, patients hypersensitive to drug, and patients with G6PD deficiency, optic neuritis, tinnitus, or history of blackwater fever or thrombocytopenic purpura with previous quinine ingestion.
Use cautiously in patients with arrhythmias and in those taking sodium bicarbonate.

Interactions
Drug-drug. *Acetazolamide, sodium bicarbonate:* May increase quinine levels by decreasing urinary excretion. Monitor patient closely.
Aluminum-containing antacids: May delay or decrease quinine absorption. Avoid use together.
Digitoxin, digoxin: Increased plasma levels of these drugs. Monitor levels closely.
Mefloquine: May cause additive cardiac effects. Don't use together.
Neuromuscular blockers: May potentiate the effects of these drugs. Monitor patient closely.
Warfarin: May potentiate action by depressing synthesis of vitamin K–dependent clotting factors. Monitor PT and INR closely.

Adverse reactions
CNS: severe headache, apprehension, excitement, confusion, delirium, syncope, hypothermia, vertigo, *seizures* (with toxic doses).
CV: hypotension, *CV collapse* (with overdose or rapid I.V. administration), conduction disturbances.
EENT: altered color perception, photophobia, blurred vision, night blindness, amblyopia, scotoma, diplopia, mydriasis, optic atrophy, tinnitus, impaired hearing.
GI: epigastric distress, diarrhea, nausea, vomiting.
GU: renal tubular damage, anuria.
Hematologic: hemolytic anemia, *thrombocytopenia, agranulocytosis,* hypoprothrombinemia, thrombosis at infusion site.
Respiratory: asthma, dyspnea.
Skin: rash, pruritus.
Other: flushing, fever, facial edema, hypoglycemia.

Overdose and treatment
Signs and symptoms of overdose include tinnitus, vertigo, headache, fever, rash, CV effects, GI distress (including vomiting), blindness, apprehension, confusion, and seizures.
Treatment includes gastric lavage followed by supportive measures, which may include fluid and electrolyte replacement, artificial respira-

---

Reactions may be *common*, uncommon, *life-threatening*, or COMMON AND LIFE-THREATENING.

tion, and stabilization of blood pressure and renal function.

Anaphylactoid reactions may require epinephrine, corticosteroids, or antihistamines. Urinary acidification may increase elimination of quinine but will also augment renal obstruction. Hemodialysis or hemoperfusion may be helpful. Vasodilator therapy or stellate blockage may relieve visual disturbances.

Special considerations
• Administer quinine after meals to minimize gastric distress; don't crush tablets because drug irritates gastric mucosa.
• Quinine is no longer used for acute malarial attack by *P. vivax* or for suppression of malaria from resistant organisms.
• Drug falsely elevates urinary catecholamines and may interfere with 17-hydroxycorticosteroid and 17-ketogenic steroid tests.

Patient monitoring
• Discontinue drug if signs of idiosyncrasy or toxicity occur.
• Serum levels of 10 mcg/ml or more may confirm toxicity as the cause of tinnitus or hearing loss.

Breast-feeding patients
• Before giving drug to breast-feeding woman, evaluate infant for possible G6PD deficiency.

Geriatric patients
• Use cautiously in patients with conduction disturbances.

Patient education
• Teach patient about adverse reactions and the need to report them immediately, especially tinnitus and hearing impairment.
• Tell patient to avoid concurrent use of aluminum-containing antacids because they may alter drug absorption.
• Instruct patient to keep drug out of reach of children.

quinupristin-dalfopristin
Synercid

Pharmacologic classification: streptogramin
Therapeutic classification: antibiotic
Pregnancy risk category: B

Indications and dosages
➤ **Serious or life-threatening infections related to vancomycin-resistant** Enterococcus faecium **bacteremia.** *Adults and adolescents age 16 and older:* 7.5 mg/kg by I.V. infusion over 1 hour q 8 hours. Treatment duration should be determined by the site and severity of the infection.
➤ **Complicated skin and skin structure infections caused by** Staphylococcus aureus *(methicillin susceptible) or* Streptococcus pyogenes. *Adults and adolescents age 16 and older:* 7.5 mg/kg by I.V. infusion over 1 hour q 12 hours for at least 7 days.

How supplied
Available by prescription only
Injection: 500 mg/10 ml (150 mg quinupristin and 350 mg dalfopristin)

Pharmacodynamics
Antibiotic action: Quinopristin and dalfopristin work synergistically to inhibit or destroy susceptible bacteria by inhibiting protein synthesis in bacterial cells. Dalfopristin inhibits the early phase of protein synthesis in the bacterial ribosome; quinupristin inhibits the late phase of protein synthesis. Unable to manufacture new proteins, bacterial cells are inactivated or die.

Pharmacokinetics
Absorption: Quinupristin and dalfopristin have differing profiles. Following infusion of multiple 7.5-mg/kg doses every 8 hours, peak quinupristin levels and metabolites are 3.2 mcg/ml; peak dalfopristin levels are 8.0 mcg/ml.
Distribution: Protein-binding is moderate.
Metabolism: Both drugs are converted to several active major metabolites by nonenzymatic reactions.
Excretion: Biliary excretion and fecal elimination accounts for about 75% of both drugs and their metabolites. Urinary excretion accounts for about 15% of quinupristin dose and 19% of dalfopristin dose. Elimination half-lives of quinupristin and dalfopristin are about 0.85 and 0.70 hours, respectively.

Route	Onset	Peak	Duration
I.V.	Unknown	Variable	Unknown

Contraindications and precautions
Contraindicated in patients hypersensitive to drug or other streptogramin antibiotics.

Interactions
Drug-drug: *Calcium channel blockers (such as diltiazem, nifedipine, or verapamil), carbamazepine, diazepam, disopyramide, docetaxel, drugs metabolized by cytochrome P-450 3A4 (including protease inhibitors such as delavirdine, indinavir, lidocaine, nevirapine, and ritonavir), lovastatin, methylprednisolone, midazolam, paclitaxel, tacrolimus, vinblastine:* Increased levels of these drugs and possible increased therapeutic effects and adverse reactions. Use together cautiously.
Cyclosporine: Decreased metabolism and possible increased cyclosporine levels. Monitor cyclosporine levels.
Drugs metabolized by cytochrome P-450 3A4 that increase the QTc interval on the ECG (quinidine and others): Decreased metabolism

of these drugs resulting in prolonged QTc interval. Avoid use together.

Adverse reactions
CNS: headache, pain.
CV: thrombophlebitis.
GI: nausea, diarrhea, vomiting.
Hepatic: *elevated total and conjugated bilirubin,* altered liver function test results.
Musculoskeletal: arthralgia, myalgia.
Skin: rash, pruritus.
Other: *inflammation, pain, edema at infusion site, infusion site reaction.*

Overdose and treatment
Patients who receive an overdose should be observed and given supportive care. Drug isn't removed by peritoneal dialysis or hemodialysis.

Special considerations
⚠ ALERT Quinupristin-dalfopristin isn't active against *Enterococcus faecalis.* Appropriate blood cultures are needed to avoid misidentifying *E. faecalis* as *E. faecium.*
• Drug may cause mild to life-threatening pseudomembranous colitis; consider this diagnosis in patients who develop diarrhea during or after therapy.
• Adverse reactions, such as arthralgia and myalgia, may be reduced by decreasing dosage interval to every 12 hours.
• Reconstitute powder for injection by adding 5 ml of either sterile water for injection or D_5W and gently swirling vial to ensure dissolution; avoid shaking to limit foaming. Reconstituted solutions must be further diluted within 30 minutes.
• The appropriate dose (according to patient's weight) of reconstituted solution should be added to 250 ml of D_5W to make a final concentration of no more than 2 mg/ml. This diluted solution is stable for 5 hours at room temperature or 54 hours if refrigerated.
• Fluid-restricted patient with a central venous catheter may receive dose in 100 ml of D_5W, but this concentration isn't recommended for peripheral venous administration.
• If patient develops moderate to severe peripheral venous irritation, consider increasing infusion volume to 500 or 750 ml, changing injection site, or infusing via central venous catheter.
• Give all doses by I.V. infusion over 1 hour. An infusion pump or device may be used to control rate of infusion.
• Quinupristin-dalfopristin is incompatible with saline and heparin solutions. Don't dilute drug with saline solutions or infuse into lines that contain saline or heparin. Flush line with D_5W before and after each dose.

Patient monitoring
• Monitor I.V. site closely.
• Monitor blood work and vital signs frequently.

• Because nonsusceptible organisms may overgrow, monitor patient closely for signs and symptoms of superinfection.
• Monitor liver function test results during therapy.

Pregnant patients
• Safety hasn't been established for use during pregnancy.

Breast-feeding patients
• It isn't known if drug appears in breast milk. Use cautiously in breast-feeding women.

Pediatric patients
• Safety and efficacy in patients under age 16 haven't been established. In limited clinical trials, children received 7.5 mg every 8 or 12 hours.

Geriatric patients
• No dosage adjustment is needed for elderly patients.

Patient education
• Advise patient to report irritation at I.V. site, pain in joints or muscles, and diarrhea immediately.
• Tell patient about the importance of reporting persistent or worsening symptoms of infection, such as pain or erythema.

rabeprazole sodium
Aciphex

Pharmacologic classification: proton pump inhibitor
Therapeutic classification: antiulcerative
Pregnancy risk category: B

Indications and dosages
➤ *Healing of erosive or ulcerative gastroesophageal reflux disease (GERD).*
Adults: 20 mg P.O. daily for 4 to 8 weeks. Additional 8-week course may be considered, if necessary.
➤ *Maintenance of healing of erosive or ulcerative GERD. Adults:* 20 mg P.O. daily.
➤ *Healing of duodenal ulcers. Adults:* 20 mg P.O. daily after morning meal for up to 4 weeks.
➤ *Treatment of pathologic hypersecretory conditions including Zollinger-Ellison syndrome. Adults:* 60 mg P.O. daily; may be increased, as needed, to 100 mg P.O. daily or 60 mg P.O. twice daily.

How supplied
Available by prescription only
Tablets (delayed-release): 20 mg

Pharmacodynamics
Antiulcerative action: Rabeprazole blocks activity of the acid (proton) pump by inhibiting gastric hydrogen-potassium adenosine triphosphatase

at the secretory surface of the gastric parietal cell, blocking gastric acid secretion.

Pharmacokinetics

Absorption: Drug is acid labile; enteric coating allows it to pass through the stomach relatively intact.
Distribution: 96.3% plasma protein–bound.
Metabolism: Extensively metabolized by the liver to inactive compounds.
Excretion: 90% is eliminated in urine as metabolites. Remaining 10% of metabolites are eliminated in feces. Plasma half-life is 1 to 2 hours.

Route	Onset	Peak	Duration
P.O.	Unknown	2-5 hr	> 24 hr

Contraindications and precautions

Contraindicated in patients hypersensitive to rabeprazole, other benzimidazoles (lansoprazole, omeprazole), or components in these formulations. Use cautiously in patients with severe hepatic impairment.

Interactions

Drug-drug. *Cyclosporine:* May inhibit cyclosporine metabolism. Use together cautiously.
Digoxin, ketoconazole, other gastric pH-dependent drugs: Decreased or increased drug absorption of these drugs at increased pH values. Monitor patient closely.

Adverse reactions

CNS: headache.

Overdose and treatment

Treatment is supportive and symptomatic. There's no specific antidote for rabeprazole overdose, and drug isn't dialyzable because of extensive protein-binding.

Special considerations

● Consider additional courses of therapy when duodenal ulcer or GERD isn't healed after first course.
● Symptomatic response to therapy doesn't preclude presence of GI cancer.

Patient monitoring

● Monitor patient's response to therapy.

Breast-feeding patients

● It isn't known if drug appears in breast milk. Taking into account importance of drug to woman, either stop drug or advise patient to stop breast-feeding.

Pediatric patients

● Safety and efficacy haven't been established.

Geriatric patients

● No differences in safety and efficacy have been observed.

Patient education

● Explain importance of taking drug exactly as prescribed.
● Advise patient to swallow delayed-release tablets whole and not to crush, chew, or split them.
● Advise patient that drug may be taken without regard to meals.

rabies immune globulin, human (RIG)

Hyperab, Imogam Rabies Immune Globulin, BayRab

Pharmacologic classification: immune serum
Therapeutic classification: rabies prophylaxis
Pregnancy risk category: C

Indications and dosages

➤ *Rabies exposure. Adults and children:* 20 IU/kg at time of first dose of rabies vaccine. Use half of dose to infiltrate wound area. Give remainder I.M. (gluteal area preferred). Don't give rabies vaccine and RIG in same syringe or at same site.

How supplied

Available by prescription only
Injection: 150 IU/ml in 2-ml and 10-ml vials

Pharmacodynamics

Postexposure rabies prophylaxis: RIG provides passive immunity to rabies.

Pharmacokinetics

Absorption: After slow I.M. absorption, rabies antibody appears in serum within 24 hours and peaks within 2 to 13 days.
Distribution: Probably crosses the placenta and appears in breast milk.
Metabolism: No information available.
Excretion: Serum half-life for rabies antibody titer is about 24 days.

Route	Onset	Peak	Duration
I.M.	24 hr	Unknown	Unknown

Contraindications and precautions

Don't give repeated doses once vaccine treatment has been started.

Use cautiously in patients hypersensitive to thimerosal, those with immunoglobulin A deficiency, and those with history of systemic allergic reactions following administration of human immunoglobulins.

Interactions

Drug-drug. *Corticosteroids, immunosuppressants:* May interfere with immune response to RIG. Whenever possible, avoid using these drugs during postexposure immunization period. Because antirabies serum may partially suppress antibody response to rabies vaccine, use only the recommended dose of antirabies vaccine.

Live-virus vaccines: RIG may interfere with immune response to live viruses. Don't give live-virus vaccines within 3 months after giving RIG.

Adverse reactions
GU: *nephrotic syndrome.*
Skin: *rash,* pain, redness, and induration at injection site.
Other: slight fever, *anaphylaxis, angioedema.*

Overdose and treatment
No information available.

Special considerations
⚠ ALERT Don't confuse drug with rabies vaccine, which is a suspension of attenuated or killed microorganisms used to confer active immunity. These two drugs are commonly given together prophylactically after exposure to known or suspected rabid animals.
● Obtain a thorough history of the animal bite and the patient's allergies and reactions to immunizations.
● Keep epinephrine solution (1:1,000) available to treat allergic reactions.
● Don't give more than 5 ml I.M. at one injection site; divide I.M. doses exceeding 5 ml between multiple sites.
● Ask patient when he received his last tetanus immunization; a booster may be indicated.
● Patients immunized with a tissue culture–derived rabies vaccine and those who have confirmed adequate rabies antibody titers should receive only the vaccine.
● RIG hasn't been linked to an increased risk of AIDS. The immune globulin is free of HIV, and immune globulin recipients develop no antibodies to HIV.
● Store between 36° and 46° F (2° and 8° C). Don't freeze.

Patient monitoring
● Repeated doses of RIG shouldn't be given after rabies vaccine is started.
● Reactions to antirabies serum may occur up to 12 days after product is given.

Pregnant patients
● Because rabies can be fatal if untreated, use of RIG during pregnancy appears justified. No fetal risk has been reported to date.

Breast-feeding patients
● Safety in breast-feeding women hasn't been established. RIG probably appears in breast milk. An alternative feeding method is recommended.

Pediatric patients
● Safety and efficacy in this population haven't been established.

Patient education
● Explain that the body needs about 1 week to develop immunity to rabies after the vaccine is given. Therefore, patients receive RIG to provide antibodies in their blood for immediate protection against rabies.
● Advise patient to report skin changes, difficulty breathing, or headache.
● Tell patient that local pain, swelling, and tenderness may develop at injection site. Recommend acetaminophen to alleviate these minor effects.

rabies vaccine, adsorbed

Pharmacologic classification: vaccine
Therapeutic classification: viral vaccine
Pregnancy risk category: C

Indications and dosages
➤ **Preexposure prophylaxis rabies immunization for patients in high-risk groups.** *Adults and children:* 1 ml I.M. at 0, 7, and either 21 or 28 days for a total of three injections. Patients at increased risk for rabies should be checked every 6 months and given a booster vaccination, 1 ml I.M., p.r.n., to maintain adequate serum titer.
➤ **Postexposure rabies prophylaxis.** *Adults and children not previously vaccinated against rabies:* 20 IU/kg of human rabies immune globulin (HRIG) I.M. and five 1-ml injections of rabies vaccine, adsorbed, I.M. given one each on days 0, 3, 7, 14, and 28.
Adults and children previously vaccinated against rabies: Two 1-ml injections of rabies vaccine, adsorbed, I.M. given one each on days 0 and 3. HRIG shouldn't be given.

How supplied
Available by prescription only
Injection: 1 ml single-dose vial

Pharmacodynamics
Vaccine action: Promotes active immunity to rabies.

Pharmacokinetics
Absorption: People at high risk should be retested for rabies antibody titer every 6 months.
Distribution: No information available.
Metabolism: No information available.
Excretion: No information available.

Route	Onset	Peak	Duration
I.M.	Unknown	2 wk after 3 doses	Unknown

Contraindications and precautions
Contraindicated in patients who had life-threatening allergic reactions to previous injection of vaccine or its components, including thimerosal. Use cautiously in patients hypersen-

sitive to monkey proteins and patients with a history of non–life-threatening allergic reactions to injected vaccine.

Interactions
Drug-drug. *Antimalarial drugs, corticosteroids, immunosuppressants:* Decreased response to rabies vaccine. Don't use together.

Adverse reactions
CNS: *fatigue, headache, dizziness.*
GI: *abdominal pain, nausea.*
Musculoskeletal: aching of injected muscle, *myalgia.*
Skin: transient pain, erythema, swelling, itching, mild inflammatory reaction at injection site.
Other: *slight fever,* serum sickness–like reactions, *anaphylaxis.*

Overdose and treatment
No information available.

Special considerations
• Keep epinephrine 1:1,000 readily available.
• Administer I.M. into deltoid region in adults and older children; midanterolateral aspect of the thigh is acceptable for younger children. Don't give I.D., close to a peripheral nerve, or into adipose or S.C. tissue.
• Vaccine is normally light pink because of phenol red in the suspension.
• Delay preexposure immunization in acutely ill patient.

Patient monitoring
• If patient has a serious adverse reaction to the vaccine, report it promptly to the manufacturer.

Pregnant patients
• Administration isn't contraindicated because of the potential harm from rabies exposure.

Breast feeding patients
• It isn't known whether vaccine appears in milk or has an effect on nursing infants.

Pediatric patients
• Use cautiously because of limited experience in children.

Patient education
• Tell patient that drug may cause pain, swelling, and itching at injection site; headache; stomach upset; or fever.
• Recommend acetaminophen to alleviate headache, fever, and muscle aches.

rabies vaccine, human diploid cell (HDCV)
Imovax Rabies I.D. Vaccine (inactivated whole virus), Imovax Rabies Vaccine

Pharmacologic classification: vaccine
Therapeutic classification: viral vaccine
Pregnancy risk category: C

Indications and dosages
➤ *Preexposure prophylaxis immunization for persons in high-risk groups. Adults and children:* Three 0.1-ml injections I.D. or three 1-ml injections I.M. Give first dose on day 0 (first day vaccination), second dose on day 7, and third dose on day 21 or 28.
Booster: Persons exposed to rabies virus at their workplace should have antibody titers checked q 6 months. Persons with continued risk of exposure should have antibody titers checked q 2 years. When the titers are inadequate, administer a booster dose.
➤ *Primary postexposure dosage. Adults and children:* Five 1-ml doses I.M. on days 3, 7, 14, and 28 (with rabies immune globulin on day 0). A sixth dose may be given on day 90. For patients who previously received the full HDCV vaccination regimen or who have rabies antibody, give two 1-ml doses I.M. Give first dose on day 0 and second dose 3 days later. Rabies immune globulin (RIG) shouldn't be given.

How supplied
Available by prescription only
I.D. injection: 0.25 IU rabies antigen per dose
I.M. injection: 2.5 IU of rabies antigen/ml in single-dose vial with diluent

Pharmacodynamics
Rabies prophylaxis: Vaccine promotes active immunity to rabies.

Pharmacokinetics
Absorption: After I.D. injection, rabies antibodies appear in the serum within 7 to 10 days.
Distribution: No information available.
Metabolism: No information available.
Excretion: No information available.

Route	Onset	Peak	Duration
I.M., I.D.	1 wk	1-2 mo	> 2 yr

Contraindications and precautions
No contraindications reported after exposure. Acute febrile illness contraindicates use in persons previously exposed. Use cautiously in patients with history of hypersensitivity.

Interactions
Drug-drug. *Corticosteroids, immunosuppressants:* May interfere with development of ac-

tive immunity to rabies vaccine. Avoid use whenever possible.

Adverse reactions
CNS: *headache,* dizziness, *fatigue.*
GI: abdominal pain, diarrhea, *nausea.*
Musculoskeletal: muscle aches.
Other: *anaphylaxis,* *fever, serum sickness, pain, erythema, swelling, itching at injection site.*

Overdose and treatment
No information available.

Special considerations
⚑ ALERT I.D. form is only for preexposure use.
• Obtain a thorough history of allergies, especially to antibiotics, and of reactions to immunizations.
• Keep epinephrine solution (1:1,000) available to treat allergic reactions.
• Reconstitute with diluent provided. Gently shake vial until vaccine is completely dissolved.
• Give I.M. injection in deltoid or upper outer quadrant of gluteus muscle in adults and children. In infants and young children, use midlateral aspect of thigh.
• Store vaccine at 36° to 46° F (2° to 8° C). Don't freeze.

Patient monitoring
• Watch for evidence of serum sickness–like hypersensitivity reactions. Antihistamine treatment may be needed in these patients.

Pregnant patients
• Pregnant women should receive treatment because of possible harm from rabies exposure. Preexposure immunization may also be indicated for a pregnant woman at high risk of exposure.

Breast-feeding patients
• It isn't known if HDCV appears in breast milk or if transmission to breast-feeding infant presents risk. Breast-feeding women should choose an alternative feeding method.

Patient education
• Tell patient that drug may cause pain, swelling, and itching at injection site; headache; stomach upset; or fever.
• Recommend acetaminophen to alleviate headache, fever, and muscle aches.

raloxifene hydrochloride
Evista

Pharmacologic classification: selective estrogen receptor modulator
Therapeutic classification: antiosteoporotic
Pregnancy risk category: X

Indications and dosages
➤ *Prevention and treatment of osteoporosis in postmenopausal women. Adults:*
One 60-mg tablet P.O. once daily.

How supplied
Available by prescription only
Tablets: 60 mg

Pharmacodynamics
Antiosteoporotic action: Decreases bone turnover and reduces bone resorption, evidenced as reduced serum and urine levels of bone turnover markers and increased bone mineral density. Biologic actions of drug are mediated through binding to estrogen receptors resulting in differential expression of multiple estrogen-regulated genes in different tissues.

Pharmacokinetics
Absorption: Rapidly absorbed. Peak levels depend on systemic interconversion and enterohepatic cycling of drug and its metabolites. After oral administration, about 60% of raloxifene is absorbed. Absolute bioavailability is 2%.
Distribution: Apparent volume of distribution is 2,348 I/kg, independent of dose administered. Drug is highly bound to plasma proteins, both albumin and α1-acid glycoprotein, but it doesn't appear to interact with the binding of warfarin, phenytoin, or tamoxifen to plasma proteins.
Metabolism: Undergoes extensive first-pass metabolism to glucuronide conjugates.
Excretion: Primarily excreted in feces, with less than 6% of dose eliminated as glucuronide conjugates in urine. Less than 0.2% of dose is excreted unchanged in urine.

Route	Onset	Peak	Duration
P.O.	Unknown	Unknown	24 hr

Contraindications and precautions
Contraindicated in patients hypersensitive to drug or constituents of tablet. Also contraindicated in pregnant women or those planning pregnancy and in women with history of or currently active venous thromboembolic events, including pulmonary embolism, retinal vein thrombosis, and deep vein thrombosis. Use with hormone replacement therapy or systemic estrogen hasn't been evaluated and isn't recommended. Use cautiously in patients with severe hepatic impairment. Assess risks and benefits in women at high risk for thromboembolic disease secondary to

heart failure, superficial thrombophlebitis, or active malignancy.

Interactions

Drug-drug. *Cholestyramine:* Significant reduction in raloxifene absorption. Don't use together.

Highly protein-bound drugs, such as clofibrate, diazepam, diazoxide, ibuprofen, indomethacin, and naproxen: May interfere with binding sites. Use together cautiously.

Warfarin: Decreased PT. Monitor PT and INR.

Adverse reactions

CNS: depression, insomnia, headache, migraine.
CV: *hot flashes,* chest pain.
EENT: *sinusitis,* pharyngitis, laryngitis.
GI: nausea, dyspepsia, vomiting, flatulence, GI disorder, gastroenteritis, diarrhea, abdominal pain.
GU: vaginitis, urinary tract infection, cystitis, leukorrhea, endometrial disorder, vaginal bleeding.
Metabolic: weight gain.
Musculoskeletal: *arthralgia,* myalgia, arthritis, leg cramps.
Respiratory: increased cough, pneumonia.
Skin: rash, sweating.
Other: breast pain; *infection; flu syndrome;* fever; peripheral edema, increased levels of apolipoprotein A-I; decreased levels of serum total cholesterol, low-density lipoprotein (LDL), fibrinogen, apolipoprotein B, and lipoprotein(a); increased hormone-binding globulin levels.

Overdose and treatment

There have been no reports of overdose. No specific antidote exists for raloxifene overdose. In one study, a dose of 600 mg/day was safely tolerated.

Special considerations

• Discontinue drug at least 72 hours before prolonged immobilization.

• Endometrial proliferation hasn't been linked to drug use. Evaluate unexplained uterine bleeding.

• A decrease in total cholesterol and LDL levels (by 6% and 11% respectively) has been reported. No effect on high-density lipoprotein or triglycerides has been shown.

• There are no data to support drug use in premenopausal women; avoid use in this population.

• Safety and efficacy haven't been evaluated in men.

• Effect on bone mineral density beyond 2 years of therapy isn't known. Safety and efficacy haven't been established beyond 2 years.

Patient monitoring

• The greatest risk for thromboembolic events (deep vein thrombosis, pulmonary embolism, retinal vein thrombosis) occurs during first 4 months of treatment.

• No link has been shown between therapy and breast enlargement, breast pain, or an increased risk of breast cancer. Evaluate breast abnormalities that occur during treatment.

Breast-feeding patients

• It isn't known if drug appears in breast milk. Don't use in breast-feeding women.

Pediatric patients

• Drug hasn't been evaluated in children; don't use in this population.

Geriatric patients

• No age-related differences have been observed in patients ages 42 to 84.

Patient education

• Tell patient to avoid long periods of restricted movement (such as during traveling) because of an increased risk of venous thromboembolic events, such as deep vein thrombosis and pulmonary embolism.

• Inform patient that hot flashes or flushing may occur and will not disappear with continued drug use.

• Tell patient to take supplemental calcium and vitamin D if dietary intake is inadequate.

• Encourage patient to perform weight-bearing exercises. Also, advise her to stop drinking alcohol and smoking.

• Tell patient that drug may be taken without regard for food.

ramipril
Altace

Pharmacologic classification: angiotensin-converting enzyme (ACE) inhibitor
Therapeutic classification: antihypertensive
Pregnancy risk category: C (D second and third trimesters)

Indications and dosages

➤ *Treatment of hypertension, alone or with thiazide diuretics. Adults:* Initially, 2.5 mg P.O. daily in patients not taking a diuretic. Adjust dose based on blood pressure response. Usual maintenance dosage is 2.5 to 20 mg daily as a single dose or in two equal doses.

In patients taking a diuretic, symptomatic hypotension may occur. To minimize it, stop the diuretic, if possible, 2 to 3 days before starting ramipril. If not possible, initial ramipril dose should be 1.25 mg.

✦ *Dosage adjustment.* If creatinine clearance is below 40 ml/minute (serum creatinine above 2.5 mg/dl), recommended initial dose is 1.25 mg daily, adjusted upward to maximum dose of 5 mg based on blood pressure response.

➤ *Heart failure after MI. Adults:* Initially, 2.5 mg P.O. b.i.d. Adjust to target dose of 5 mg P.O. b.i.d.

➤ *To reduce the risk of MI, CVA, and death from CV causes in patients with a history of coronary artery disease, CVA, peripheral vascular disease, or diabetes accompanied by at least one other CV risk factor.* Adults age 55 and older: 2.5 mg daily for 1 week and 5 mg daily for the next 3 weeks; then increased as tolerated to a maintenance dose of 10 mg daily.

How supplied
Available by prescription only
Capsules: 1.25 mg, 2.5 mg, 5 mg, 10 mg

Pharmacodynamics
Antihypertensive action: Ramipril and its active metabolite, ramiprilat, inhibit ACE, preventing conversion of angiotensin I to angiotensin II, a potent vasoconstrictor. Reduced formation of angiotensin II decreases peripheral arterial resistance and, in turn, decreases aldosterone secretion, reduces sodium and water retention, and lowers blood pressure. Ramipril also has antihypertensive activity in patients with low-renin hypertension.

Pharmacokinetics
Absorption: 50% to 60% is absorbed after oral administration.
Distribution: Ramipril is 73% and ramiprilat 56% serum protein–bound.
Metabolism: Ramipril is almost completely metabolized to ramiprilat, which has six times more ACE-inhibiting effects than parent drug.
Excretion: 60% is excreted in urine and 40% in feces. Less than 2% is excreted in urine as unchanged drug.

Route	Onset	Peak	Duration
P.O.	1-2 hr	1-3 hr	24 hr

Contraindications and precautions
Contraindicated in patients hypersensitive to ACE inhibitors and patients with a history of angioedema from ACE inhibitor treatment. Use cautiously in patients with impaired renal function.

Interactions
Drug-drug. *Diuretics:* Excessive hypotension may result if used together. Discontinue diuretic or reduce ramipril dosage as needed.
Lithium: Increased serum lithium levels and lithium toxicity. Monitor levels closely.
Potassium-sparing diuretics, potassium supplements: May result in hyperkalemia. Monitor serum potassium levels.
Drug-herb. *Capsaicin:* Increased risk of cough. Discourage concomitant use.
Drug-food. *Potassium-containing salt substitutes:* May cause hyperkalemia. Urge patient not to use together.
Drug-lifestyle. *Sun exposure:* May cause photosensitivity reaction. Advise patient to take precautions.

Adverse reactions
CNS: asthenia, dizziness, fatigue, headache, *seizures,* vertigo.
CV: orthostatic hypotension, syncope, angina, *arrhythmias, MI,* chest pain.
GI: nausea, vomiting, diarrhea.
Hematologic: *pancytopenia, neutropenia, thrombocytopenia.*
Respiratory: dry, persistent, tickling, nonproductive cough.
Other: *angioedema.*

Overdose and treatment
The most common sign should be hypotension. No cases of overdose have been reported, and specific management of ramipril overdose hasn't been established. Provide supportive care.

Special considerations
● Like other ACE inhibitors, ramipril may cause a dry, persistent, tickling, nonproductive cough that stops when therapy stops.

Patient monitoring
● Monitor blood pressure regularly.
● Monitor CBC and differential counts before and during therapy.
● Assess renal and hepatic function before and periodically throughout therapy.
● Monitor serum potassium levels.

Breast-feeding patients
● Drug shouldn't be given to breast-feeding women.

Pediatric patients
● Safety and efficacy in children haven't been established.

Geriatric patients
● No age-related differences in safety or efficacy have been observed.

Patient education
● Tell patient to report signs or symptoms of angioedema immediately: swelling of face, eyes, lips or tongue or difficulty in breathing. Tell him to stop taking drug and seek medical attention.
● Warn patient that light-headedness can occur, especially during first few days of therapy. Tell him to change positions slowly to reduce hypotensive effect and to report these symptoms. If syncope (fainting) occurs, instruct patient to stop taking drug and call prescriber immediately.
● Warn patient that inadequate fluid intake, vomiting, diarrhea, or excessive perspiration can lead to light-headedness and syncope. Advise caution in excessive heat and during exercise.
● Tell patient to immediately report signs of infection, such as sore throat or fever.

Reactions may be *common,* uncommon, *life-threatening,* or COMMON AND LIFE-THREATENING.

ranitidine
Zantac, Zantac 75, Zantac EFFERdose, Zantac GELdose

Pharmacologic classification: H₂-receptor
antagonist
Therapeutic classification: antiulcer
Pregnancy risk category: B

Indications and dosages
➤ *Duodenal and gastric ulcer (short-term treatment); pathologic hypersecretory conditions such as Zollinger-Ellison syndrome. Adults:* 150 mg P.O. b.i.d. or 300 mg h.s. Doses up to 6 g daily may be given to patients with Zollinger-Ellison syndrome. For parenteral use, 50 mg I.V. or I.M. q 6 to 8 hours.
Children ages 1 month to 16 years: For treatment of duodenal and gastric ulcers, 2 to 4 mg/kg P.O. b.i.d. Maximum, 300 mg daily.
➤ *Maintenance therapy in duodenal or benign gastric ulcer. Adults:* 150 mg P.O. h.s.
Children ages 1 month to 16 years: 2 to 4 mg/kg P.O. once daily. Maximum, 150 mg daily.
➤ *Prevention of stress ulcer. Adults:* Continuous I.V. infusion of 150 mg in 250 ml compatible solution delivered at 6.25 ml/hour using an infusion pump.
➤ *Gastroesophageal reflux disease. Adults:* 150 mg P.O. b.i.d.
➤ *Erosive esophagitis. Adults:* 150 mg or 10 ml (2 teaspoonfuls equivalent to 150 mg of ranitidine) P.O. q.i.d.
➤ *Self-medication for relief of occasional heartburn, acid indigestion, and sour stomach. Adults and adolescents age 12 and older:* 75 mg P.O. once or twice daily; maximum, 150 mg in 24 hours.

How supplied
Available by prescription only
Capsules: 150 mg, 300 mg
Granules (effervescent): 150 mg
Injection: 25 mg/ml
Injection (premixed): 50 mg/50 ml, 50 mg/100 ml
Syrup: 15 mg/ml
Tablets: 150 mg, 300 mg
Tablets (effervescent): 150 mg
Available without a prescription
Tablets: 75 mg

Pharmacodynamics
Antiulcer action: Ranitidine competitively inhibits the action of histamine at H₂-receptors in gastric parietal cells. This reduces basal and nocturnal gastric acid secretion as well as that caused by histamine, food, amino acids, insulin, and pentagastrin.

Pharmacokinetics
Absorption: About 50% to 60% of an oral dose is absorbed; food doesn't significantly affect absorption. After I.M. injection, drug is absorbed rapidly from parenteral sites.
Distribution: Distributed to many body tissues and appears in CSF and breast milk. Drug is about 10% to 19% protein-bound.
Metabolism: Metabolized in the liver.
Excretion: Excreted in urine and feces. Half-life is 2 to 3 hours.

Route	Onset	Peak	Duration
P.O.	1 hr	1-3 hr	13 hr
I.V., I.M.	Unknown	Unknown	Unknown

Contraindications and precautions
Contraindicated in patients hypersensitive to drug and in those with a history of acute porphyria. Use cautiously in patients with impaired renal or hepatic function.

Interactions
Drug-drug. *Antacids:* Decreased ranitidine absorption. Give drugs at least 1 hour apart.
Diazepam: Concurrent use decreases diazepam absorption. Monitor patient closely.
Glipizide: May increase hypoglycemic effect. Adjust glipizide dosage if necessary.
Procainamide: Decreased renal clearance of procainamide. Monitor patient closely for toxicity.
Warfarin: May interfere with warfarin clearance. Monitor patient closely.

Adverse reactions
CNS: malaise, vertigo.
EENT: blurred vision.
Hematologic: *reversible leukopenia, pancytopenia, granulocytopenia, thrombocytopenia.*
Hepatic: elevated liver enzyme levels, jaundice.
Other: burning and itching at injection site, *anaphylaxis,* angioedema, increased serum creatinine levels.

Overdose and treatment
No cases of overdose have been reported. However, treatment would involve emesis or gastric lavage and supportive measures as needed. Drug is removed by hemodialysis.

Special considerations
🔰 **ALERT** Don't confuse Zantac with Zyrtec.
● When giving drug by I.V. push, dilute to a total volume of 20 ml and inject over 5 minutes. No dilution is necessary for I.M. use. Drug also may be given by intermittent I.V. infusion. Dilute 50 mg ranitidine in 100 ml of D₅W and infuse over 15 to 20 minutes.
● Patients with impaired renal function may need dosage adjustment.
● Dialysis removes ranitidine; administer drug after treatment.
● Ranitidine may cause false-positive results in urine protein tests using Multistix.

◇ Unlabeled clinical use

• Debilitated patients may experience reversible confusion, agitation, depression, and hallucinations.

Patient monitoring
• Assess patient for abdominal pain. Note presence of blood in emesis, stool, or gastric aspirate.

Breast-feeding patients
• Drug appears in breast milk; use cautiously in breast-feeding women.

Geriatric patients
• These patients may experience more adverse reactions because of reduced renal clearance.

Patient education
• Instruct patient to take drug as directed, even after pain subsides, to ensure proper healing.
• If patient is taking a single daily dose, advise him to take it at bedtime.
• Instruct patient not to take OTC forms continuously for longer than 2 weeks without medical supervision.
• Tell patient to swallow oral forms whole with water and not to chew tablets.

---

ranitidine bismuth citrate
Tritec

Pharmacologic classification: H_2-receptor antagonist, antimicrobial
Therapeutic classification: antiulcer
Pregnancy risk category: C

Indications and dosages
➤ *Active duodenal ulcer related to* Helicobacter pylori *infection (with clarithromycin).* *Adults:* 400 mg P.O. b.i.d for 28 days with clarithromycin 500 mg P.O. t.i.d. for first 14 days.

How supplied
Available by prescription only
Tablets: 400 mg

Pharmacodynamics
Antiulcer activity: Ranitidine reduces gastric acid secretion by competitively inhibiting histamine at the H_2-receptor of the gastric parietal cells. Bismuth is a topical agent that disrupts the integrity of bacterial cell walls, prevents adhesion of *H. pylori* to gastric epithelium, decreases the development of resistance, and inhibits *H. pylori's* urease, phospholipase, and proteolytic activity.

Pharmacokinetics
Absorption: Dissociates to ranitidine and bismuth following ingestion. Oral bioavailability of bismuth is variable.
Distribution: Volume of distribution of ranitidine is 1.7 L/kg. Ranitidine and bismuth are 15% and 98% protein-bound, respectively.

Metabolism: Metabolized by the liver. It's unknown if bismuth undergoes biotransformation.
Excretion: Primarily eliminated by the kidney. Elimination half-life of ranitidine is about 3 hours. Bismuth is excreted primarily in feces. Bismuth also undergoes minor excretion in the bile and urine. Terminal elimination half-life of bismuth is 11 to 28 days.

Route	Onset	Peak	Duration
P.O.	Unknown	Variable	Variable

Contraindications and precautions
Contraindicated in patients hypersensitive to drug or its components.

Interactions
Drug-drug. *Clarithromycin:* Combination of these drugs shouldn't be used in patients with history of acute porphyria. Also, this combination isn't recommended in patients with creatinine clearance below 25 ml/minute.
Diazepam: Decreased absorption. Separate administration times.
Glipizide: Ranitidine may increase the hypoglycemic effects of glipizide. Monitor glucose levels.
High-dose antacids (170 mEq): May decrease plasma levels of ranitidine and bismuth. Monitor patient closely.
Procainamide: Ranitidine may increase plasma levels of procainamide. Monitor patient closely.
Warfarin: May increase hypoprothrombinemic effects. Monitor PT and INR, and adjust dose as needed.

Adverse reactions
CNS: headache.
GI: constipation, diarrhea.

Overdose and treatment
There has been limited experience with overdose. If overdose occurs, take measures to remove unabsorbed drug from GI tract. Monitor symptoms, and provide supportive care if necessary.

Special considerations
• Drug shouldn't be prescribed alone for treatment of active duodenal ulcers.
• If combination with clarithromycin isn't successful, patient is considered to have clarithromycin-resistant *H. pylori* and shouldn't be retreated with another regimen containing clarithromycin.
• Dialysis removes ranitidine; administer drug after treatment.
• Drug may cause false-positive results in urine protein testing using Multistix; test with sulfosalicylic acid if necessary.

Patient monitoring
• Monitor patient for abdominal pain, and blood in stool or emesis. Drug may cause a temporary and harmless darkening of tongue or stool.

Reactions may be *common*, uncommon, *life-threatening*, or COMMON AND LIFE-THREATENING.

Breast-feeding patients
● Ranitidine appears in breast milk; use cautiously in breast-feeding women.

Pediatric patients
● Safety and efficacy haven't been established in children.

Geriatric patients
● Serum drug levels may be increased in elderly patients.

Patient education
● Inform patient that drug may be taken without regard to food.
● Instruct patient to take drug as directed, even after pain has subsided.
● Stress importance of taking clarithromycin with drug for specified length of time.

---

repaglinide
Prandin

Pharmacologic classification: meglitinide
Therapeutic classification: antidiabetic
Pregnancy risk category: C

Indications and dosages
➤ **Adjunct to diet and exercise in lowering blood glucose levels in patients with type 2 diabetes mellitus whose hyperglycemia can't be controlled by diet and exercise alone.** *Adults:* For patients not previously treated or whose glycosylated hemoglobin (HbA_{1C}) is below 8%, starting dose is 0.5 mg P.O. given 15 minutes before each meal; however, time may vary from immediately before to as long as 30 minutes before meal. For patients previously treated with glucose-lowering drugs and whose HbA_{1c} is 8% or more, initial dose is 1 to 2 mg P.O. with each meal. Recommended dosage range is 0.5 to 4 mg with meals b.i.d., t.i.d., or q.i.d. Maximum, 16 mg daily.

Dosage should be determined by blood glucose response. May double dosage up to 4 mg with each meal until satisfactory blood glucose response is achieved. At least 1 week should elapse between dosage adjustments to assess response to each dose.

Metformin may be added if repaglinide monotherapy is inadequate.

How supplied
Available by prescription only
Tablets: 0.5 mg, 1 mg, 2 mg

Pharmacodynamics
Antidiabetic action: Stimulates the release of insulin from beta cells in the pancreas. Repaglinide closes ATP-dependent potassium channels in the beta cell membrane, which causes depolarization of the B-cell and opening of the calcium channels. The increased calcium influx induces insulin secretion; the overall effect is to lower the blood glucose level.

Pharmacokinetics
Absorption: Rapidly and completely absorbed with oral administration.
Distribution: Mean volume of distribution after I.V. administration during clinical trial was 31 L; protein-binding to albumin exceeded 98%.
Metabolism: Completely metabolized by oxidative biotransformation and conjugation with glucuronic acid. The P-450 isoenzyme system (specifically CYP 3A4) has also been shown to be involved in N-dealkylation of repaglinide. All metabolites are inactive and don't contribute to the blood glucose-lowering effect.
Excretion: About 90% of dose occurs in the feces as metabolites. About 8% of a dose is recovered in the urine as metabolites and less than 0.1% as parent drug. Half-life is about 1 hour.

Route	Onset	Peak	Duration
P.O.	Unknown	1 hr	Unknown

Contraindications and precautions
Contraindicated in patients hypersensitive to drug or its inactive ingredients and in those with insulin-dependent diabetes mellitus or ketoacidosis. Use cautiously in patients with hepatic insufficiency in whom reduced metabolism could lead to elevated blood levels of repaglinide and hypoglycemia.

Interactions
Drug-drug. *Barbiturates, carbamazepine, rifampin:* May increase repaglinide metabolism. Monitor glucose levels.
Beta blockers, chloramphenicol, coumarin, MAO inhibitors, NSAIDs, other highly protein-bound drugs, probenecid, salicylates, sulfonamides: May potentiate hypoglycemic action of repaglinide. Monitor glucose levels.
Calcium channel blockers, corticosteroids, estrogens, isoniazid, nicotinic acid, oral contraceptives, phenothiazines, phenytoin, sympathomimetics, thiazides and other diuretics, thyroid products: May produce hyperglycemia. Monitor glucose levels.
Erythromycin, ketoconazole, miconazole, and similar inhibitors of the P-450 cytochrome system 3A4: Repaglinide metabolism may be inhibited. Monitor glucose levels.
Drug-herb. *Aloe, bitter melon, bilberry leaf, burdock, dandelion, fenugreek, garlic, ginseng:* Possible improved blood glucose control requiring reduced antidiabetic dosage. Explain this effect to patient.

Adverse reactions
CNS: headache.
CV: chest pain, angina.
EENT: rhinitis, sinusitis.
GI: nausea, diarrhea, constipation, vomiting, dyspepsia.

GU: urinary tract infection.
Metabolic: HYPOGLYCEMIA.
Musculoskeletal: arthralgia, back pain.
Respiratory: bronchitis, *upper respiratory tract infection.*
Other: tooth disorder.

Overdose and treatment

Overdose increases the intended effect of lowering blood glucose levels. If patient is conscious and has no loss of neurologic status, treat hypoglycemia aggressively with oral glucose and adjustment to dosage or meal pattern. Monitor patient closely for 24 to 48 hours because hypoglycemia may recur after apparent recovery. If patient has severe hypoglycemia with coma, seizure, or other neurologic impairment, treat immediately with I.V. dextrose 50% solution followed by a continuous infusion of glucose 10% solution. Monitor blood glucose levels carefully.

Special considerations

● Administration of other oral antidiabetics may increase CV mortality compared with diet treatment alone. Although not specifically evaluated for repaglinide, this warning may apply.
● Loss of glycemic control can occur during stress, such as fever, trauma, infection, or surgery. If this occurs, stop drug and give insulin.
● Hypoglycemia may be difficult to recognize in elderly patients and those who take beta blockers.
● Increase dosage cautiously in patients with impaired renal function who need dialysis.

Patient monitoring

● Monitor patient's blood glucose levels periodically to determine minimum effective dose.
● Monitor long-term efficacy by measuring HbA$_{1c}$ levels every 3 months.

Breast-feeding patients

● Although it isn't known if drug appears in breast milk, studies in animals have indicated excretion similar to other glucose-lowering drugs. Because a breast-fed infant has a risk of hypoglycemia, a decision should be made to discontinue drug or breast-feeding.

Pediatric patients

● No studies have been performed in children to determine safety and efficacy.

Geriatric patients

● Elderly patients show no increase in the frequency or severity of hypoglycemia.

Patient education

● Instruct patient on importance of diet and exercise in combination with drug therapy.
● Discuss symptoms of hypoglycemia with patient and family.
● Tell patient to take drug before meals, usually 15 minutes before start of meal; however, time can vary from immediately preceding meal to up to 30 minutes before meal.
● Tell patient to skip a dose if he skips a meal or add an extra dose if he adds a meal.

reteplase, recombinant
Retavase

Pharmacologic classification: tissue-plasminogen activator
Therapeutic classification: thrombolytic enzyme
Pregnancy risk category: C

Indications and dosages

➤ *Management of acute MI. Adults:* Double-bolus injection of 10 + 10 units. Give each bolus I.V. over 2 minutes. If no complications occur after first bolus, such as serious bleeding or anaphylactoid reactions, give second bolus 30 minutes after start of first bolus. Start treatment soon after onset of symptoms of acute MI. There's no experience with repeat courses with reteplase.

How supplied

Available by prescription only
Injection: 10.8 units (18.8 mg)/vial (supplied in kit with components for reconstitution and administration of two single-use vials)

Pharmacodynamics

Thrombolytic action: Drug catalyzes the cleavage of plasminogen to generate plasmin, which leads to fibrinolysis.

Pharmacokinetics

Absorption: Administered I.V.
Distribution: Cleared from plasma at 250 to 450 ml/minute.
Metabolism: Metabolized primarily by the liver and kidney.
Excretion: Plasma half-life of drug is 13 to 16 minutes.

Route	Onset	Peak	Duration
I.V.	Unknown	Unknown	Unknown

Contraindications and precautions

Contraindicated in patients with active internal bleeding, bleeding diathesis, history of CVA, recent intracranial or intraspinal surgery or trauma, severe uncontrolled hypertension, intracranial neoplasm, arteriovenous malformation, or aneurysm.

Use cautiously in pregnant patients, patients age 75 or older, and patients with recent (within 10 days) major surgery, obstetric delivery, organ biopsy, or trauma; previous puncture of noncompressible vessels; cerebrovascular disease; recent GI or GU bleeding; hypertension (systolic pressure 180 mm Hg or more or diastolic pressure 110 mm Hg or more); likelihood of left-sided heart thrombus; subacute bacterial endocarditis; acute pericarditis; hemostatic defects; diabetic hemorrhagic retinopathy; septic thrombophlebitis; and other conditions in which bleeding would be difficult to manage.

Interactions
Drug-drug. *Heparin; oral anticoagulants; platelet inhibitors, such as abciximab, aspirin, and dipyridamole; vitamin K antagonists:* May increase risk of bleeding. Use together cautiously.

Adverse reactions
CNS: *intracranial hemorrhage.*
CV: *arrhythmias, cholesterol embolization.*
GI: *hemorrhage.*
GU: hematuria.
Hematologic: *anemia, bleeding tendency.*
Other: *bleeding* at puncture site.

Overdose and treatment
No information available. Monitor patient for increased bleeding.

Special considerations
● Drug is administered I.V. as a double-bolus injection. If bleeding or anaphylactoid reactions occur after first bolus, second bolus may be withheld.
● Reconstitute drug according to manufacturer's instructions using items provided in the kit.
● Don't give drug with other I.V. drugs through same I.V. line. Heparin and reteplase are incompatible in solution.
● Potency is expressed in units specific to reteplase and not comparable to other thrombolytics.
● Avoid use of noncompressible sites during therapy. If an arterial puncture is needed, use a vessel in the arm. Apply pressure for at least 30 minutes; then apply a pressure dressing. Check site frequently.
● Drug may alter coagulation studies; it remains active in vitro and can lead to degradation of fibrinogen in sample. Collect blood samples in the presence of PPACK (chloromethylketone) at 2-μM concentrations.

Patient monitoring
● Carefully monitor ECG during treatment. Coronary thrombolysis may result in reperfusion arrhythmias. Be prepared to treat bradycardia or ventricular irritability.
● Monitor patient for bleeding. Avoid I.M. injections, invasive procedures, and nonessential handling of patient. Bleeding is the most common adverse reaction and may occur internally or at puncture sites. If local measures don't control serious bleeding, discontinue concurrent anticoagulation therapy. Withhold second bolus of reteplase.

Breast-feeding patients
● It isn't known if drug appears in breast milk. Exercise caution if administered.

Pediatric patients
● Safety and efficacy in children haven't been established.

Geriatric patients
● Use cautiously because risk of intracranial hemorrhage increases with age.

Patient education
● Teach patient and family about use and administration of reteplase.
● Tell patient to report adverse reactions—such as bleeding or allergic reaction—immediately.
● Advise patient about proper dental care to avoid excessive gum trauma.

Rh₀(D) immune globulin, human
Gamulin Rh, HypRho-D, RhoGAM

Rh₀(D) immune globulin, microdose
HypRho-D Mini-Dose, MICRhoGAM, Mini-Gamulin Rh

Pharmacologic classification: immune serum
Therapeutic classification: anti-Rh₀(D)-positive prophylaxis
Pregnancy risk category: C

Indications and dosages
➤**Rh-positive exposure (full-term pregnancy or termination of pregnancy beyond 13 weeks' gestation), threatened abortion.** *Women:* Administer 1 vial I.M. for each 15 ml of estimated fetal packed RBC volume entering patient's blood, as determined by a modified Kleihauer-Betke technique to determine fetal packed RBC volume. Usual (standard) dose after delivery of full-term infant is 1 vial; it must be given within 72 hours after delivery or miscarriage.

If Rh₀(D) immune globulin is indicated before delivery, administer 1 vial (standard dose) at about 28 weeks' gestation and give a second vial within 72 hours of delivery.
➤**Transfusion accidents.** *Premenopausal women:* Consult blood bank or transfusion unit at once. The number of vials (standard dose) to administer is calculated via the following formula:

$$\text{Number of vials} = \frac{\text{volume of whole blood transfused}}{} \times \frac{\text{donor unit hematocrit}}{15}$$

Dose must be given within 72 hours.
➤**Termination of pregnancy (spontaneous or induced abortion or ectopic pregnancy) up to and including 12 weeks' gestation.** *Women:* 1 vial of microdose immune globulin I.M.; ideally, given within 3 hours but

may give up to 72 hours after abortion or miscarriage.

➤ *Amniocentesis or abdominal trauma during pregnancy. Women:* Dosage varies based on extent of estimated fetomaternal hemorrhage.

How supplied
Available by prescription only
Injection: 300 mcg of $Rh_o(D)$ immune globulin/vial (standard dose); 50 mcg of $Rh_o(D)$ immune globulin/vial (microdose)

Pharmacodynamics
Rh reaction prophylaxis: Suppresses the active antibody response and formation of anti-$Rh_o(D)$ in $Rh_o(D)$-negative or D^u-negative individuals exposed to Rh-positive blood. Provides passive immunity to women exposed to Rh-positive fetal blood during pregnancy. Prevents formation of maternal antibodies (active immunity), which prevents hemolytic disease of the Rh-positive newborn in another pregnancy.

Pharmacokinetics
No information available.

Route	Onset	Peak	Duration
I.M.	Unknown	Unknown	Unknown

Contraindications and precautions
Contraindicated in $Rh_o(D)$-positive or D-positive patients and those previously immunized to $Rh_o(D)$ blood factor. Also contraindicated in patients with anaphylactoid or severe systemic reaction to human globulin. Use extreme caution when giving to patients with immunoglobulin A deficiency because of increased risk of anaphylactoid reaction.

Interactions
Drug-drug. *Live-virus vaccines (measles, mumps, rubella):* $Rh_o(D)$ immune globulin may interfere with immune response to vaccine. Don't give live-virus vaccine within 3 months after $Rh_o(D)$ immune globulin. If postpartum women receive both $Rh_o(D)$ immune globulin and rubella virus vaccine within a 3-month period, serologic tests should be performed 6 to 8 weeks after vaccination to confirm seroconversion.

Adverse reactions
Other: discomfort at injection site, slight fever.

Overdose and treatment
No information available.

Special considerations
• Obtain thorough history of allergies and reactions to immunizations.
• Keep epinephrine solution (1:1,000) available to treat allergic reactions.
• For best results, $Rh_o(D)$ immune globulin must be given within 72 hours of Rh-incompatible delivery, spontaneous or induced abortion, or transfusion.
• The microdose formulation is recommended for use after every spontaneous or induced abortion up to and including 12 weeks' gestation unless mother is $Rh_o(D)$-positive or D^u-positive, she has Rh antibodies, or father or fetus is Rh-negative.
• Give I.M. in anterolateral aspect of upper thigh and deltoid muscle. Don't give I.V.
• $Rh_o(D)$ immune globulin hasn't been linked to an increased frequency of AIDS. The immune globulin contains no HIV, and recipients develop no antibodies to HIV.
• Store product between 36° and 46° F (2° and 8° C). Don't freeze.

Patient monitoring
• Immediately after delivery, send a sample of infant's cord blood to laboratory for typing and crossmatching and direct antiglobulin test. Infant must be $Rh_o(D)$-positive or D^u-positive. Confirm that mother is $Rh_o(D)$-negative and D^u-negative.

Breast-feeding patients
• Immune globulins appear in breast milk. Safety in breast-feeding women hasn't been established.

Patient education
• Inform patient that she is receiving this product because her blood has been exposed to the Rh-positive factor. Tell postpartum patient that her body will naturally develop antibodies to destroy this factor, which could threaten future Rh-positive pregnancies.
• Tell patient there is no known risk of HIV infection after receiving product.
• Tell patient that local pain, swelling, and tenderness at injection site may occur after vaccination. Recommend acetaminophen to ease minor discomfort.
• Tell patient to report headache, skin changes, or difficulty breathing.

ribavirin
Virazole

Pharmacologic classification: synthetic nucleoside
Therapeutic classification: antiviral
Pregnancy risk category: X

Indications and dosages
➤ *Treatment of hospitalized infants and young children infected by respiratory syncytial virus (RSV). Infants and young children:* 20-mg/ml solution delivered via the Viratek Small Particle Aerosol Generator (SPAG-2) results in a mist of 190 mcg/L. Treatment continues for 12 to 18 hours daily for at least 3 and no more than 7 days with a flow rate of 12.5 L of mist per minute.

For ventilated patients, use same dose with a pressure- or volume-cycled ventilator and SPAG-2. Patient should be suctioned q 1 to 2 hours and pulmonary pressures checked q 2 to 4 hours.

How supplied
Available by prescription only
Powder to be reconstituted for inhalation: 6 g in 100-ml glass vial

Pharmacodynamics
Antiviral action: Drug action probably involves inhibition of RNA and DNA synthesis, inhibition of RNA polymerase, and interference with completion of viral polypeptide coat.

Pharmacokinetics
Absorption: Some ribavirin is absorbed systemically.
Distribution: Concentrates in bronchial secretions; plasma levels are subtherapeutic for plaque inhibition.
Metabolism: Metabolized to 1,2,4-triazole-3-carboxamide (deribosylated ribavirin).
Excretion: Mostly excreted renally. First phase of drug's plasma half-life is 9½ hours; second phase has extended half-life of 40 hours (from slow drug release from RBC binding sites).

Route	Onset	Peak	Duration
Inhalation	Unknown	Unknown	Unknown

Contraindications and precautions
Contraindicated in patients hypersensitive to drug and women who are or may become pregnant during treatment. Contraindicated in women of childbearing age and their male partners when used with interferon alfa-2b. Women of childbearing age and men must use two forms of contraception during therapy and for 6 months afterward.

Interactions
None reported.

Adverse reactions
CV: *cardiac arrest,* hypotension.
EENT: conjunctivitis, erythema of eyelids.
Hematologic: anemia, reticulocytosis.
Respiratory: worsening respiratory state, *apnea,* bacterial pneumonia, pneumothorax, *bronchospasm.*
Skin: rash.

Overdose and treatment
Unknown in humans; high doses in animals have produced GI symptoms.

Special considerations
• Ribavirin aerosol is indicated for use only for lower respiratory tract infection caused by RSV. Although treatment may begin before test results are available, RSV infection must eventually be confirmed.

• Administer ribavirin aerosol only by SPAG-2. Don't use other aerosol-generating devices.
• Reconstitute solution with USP sterile water for injection or inhalation; then transfer aseptically to sterile 500-ml Erlenmeyer flask. Dilute further with sterile water to 300 ml to yield final level of 20 mg/ml. Solution remains stable for 24 hours at room temperature.
• Don't use bacteriostatic water (or any other water containing antimicrobial agent) to reconstitute drug.
• Discard unused solution in SPAG-2 unit before adding newly reconstituted solution. Change solution at least every 24 hours.
• Drug is most useful for infants with most severe RSV form, typically premature infants and those with underlying disorders such as cardiopulmonary disease. Most other infants and children with RSV infection don't require treatment because disease is self-limiting.
• Drug therapy must be accompanied by appropriate respiratory and fluid therapy.

Patient monitoring
• Monitor ventilator-dependent patients carefully because drug may precipitate in ventilatory apparatus. Change heated wire connective tubing and bacteria filters in series in expiratory limb of the system frequently (such as every 4 hours).

Pregnant patients
• May cause fetal toxicity.

Breast-feeding patients
• It isn't known if drug appears in breast milk. Not recommended for use in breast-feeding women.

Patient education
• Inform parents of need for drug and answer any questions they may have.
• Parents should report any change in child immediately.
• Inform patient that drug may be taken without regard to meals but should be administered in a consistent manner.

riboflavin (vitamin B₂)
Pharmacologic classification: water-soluble vitamin
Therapeutic classification: vitamin B complex vitamin
Pregnancy risk category: A (C if more than the RDA)

Indications and dosages
➤ *Riboflavin deficiency or adjunct to thiamine treatment for polyneuritis or cheilosis secondary to pellagra.* Adults and adolescents age 12 and older: 5 to 30 mg P.O. daily, depending on severity.
Children under age 12: 3 to 10 mg P.O. daily, depending on severity.

➤ *Microcytic anemia related to splenomegaly and glutathione reductase deficiency. Adults:* 10 mg P.O. daily for 10 days.
➤ *Dietary supplementation. Adults:* 1 to
4 mg P.O. daily. For maintenance, increase nutritional intake and supplement with vitamin B
complex.

How supplied
Available without a prescription
Tablets: 25 mg, 50 mg, 100 mg

Pharmacodynamics
Metabolic action: Riboflavin, a coenzyme, functions in the forms of flavin adenine dinucleotide
(FAD) and flavin mononucleotide (FMN) and plays
a vital metabolic role in numerous tissue respiration systems. FAD and FMN act as hydrogen-
carrier molecules for several flavoproteins involved in intermediary metabolism. Riboflavin is
also directly involved in maintaining erythrocyte
integrity.
    Riboflavin deficiency causes a clinical syn-
drome with the following symptoms: cheilosis,
angular stomatitis, glossitis, keratitis, scrotal skin
changes, ocular changes, and seborrheic dermatitis. In severe deficiency, normochromic, normocytic anemia and neuropathy may occur. Clinical signs may become evident after 3 to 8 months
of inadequate riboflavin intake. Administration
of riboflavin reverses signs of deficiency. Riboflavin
deficiency rarely occurs alone and is commonly
related to deficiency of other B vitamins and protein.

Pharmacokinetics
Absorption: Although riboflavin is absorbed
readily from the GI tract, extent of absorption is
limited. Absorption occurs at a specialized segment of the mucosa; drug absorption is limited
by duration of drug's contact with this area. Before being absorbed, riboflavin-5-phosphate is
rapidly dephosphorylated in the GI lumen. GI absorption increases when drug is administered
with food and decreases when hepatitis, cirrhosis, biliary obstruction, or probenecid administration is present.
Distribution: FAD and FMN are distributed widely to body tissues. Free riboflavin is present in the
retina. Riboflavin is stored in limited amounts in
the liver, spleen, kidneys, and heart, mainly in
the form of FAD. FAD and FMN are about 60%
protein-bound in blood. Drug crosses the placenta, and breast milk contains about 400 ng/ml.
Metabolism: Metabolized in the liver.
Excretion: After a single oral dose, biologic half-
life is about 66 to 84 minutes in healthy people.
Drug is metabolized to FMN in erythrocytes, GI
mucosal cells, and the liver; FMN is converted to
FAD in the liver. About 9% of drug is excreted unchanged in urine after normal ingestion. Excretion involves renal tubular secretion and glomerular filtration. Amount renally excreted unchanged
is directly proportional to the dose. Drug removal
by hemodialysis is slower than by natural renal
excretion.

Route	Onset	Peak	Duration
P.O.	Unknown	Unknown	Unknown

Contraindications and precautions
No known contraindications.

Interactions
Drug-drug. *Oral contraceptives:* Decreased riboflavin levels. Riboflavin dosage may need to be
increased.
Propantheline bromide: Delayed absorption rate
of riboflavin but increased total amount absorbed.
Monitor patient closely.
Drug-lifestyle. *Alcohol use:* Impaired intestinal absorption of riboflavin. Advise patient to
avoid alcohol.

Adverse reactions
GU: bright yellow urine with high doses.

Overdose and treatment
No information available.

Special considerations
● RDA of riboflavin is 0.4 to 1.8 mg daily in children, 1.2 to 1.7 mg daily in adults, and 1.6 to 1.8
mg daily in pregnant and breast-feeding women.
● Give oral riboflavin with food to increase absorption.
● Riboflavin therapy alters urinalysis based on
spectrophotometry or color reactions. Riboflavin
produces fluorescent substances in urine and
plasma, which can falsely elevate fluorometric
determinations of catecholamines and urobilinogen.

Patient monitoring
● Obtain patient's dietary history because other
vitamin deficiencies may coexist.

Breast-feeding patients
● Drug crosses the placenta; during pregnancy
and lactation, riboflavin requirements are increased. Increased food intake during this time
usually provides adequate amounts. The National Research Council recommends intake of 1.8
mg daily during first 6 months of breast-feeding.

Patient education
● Teach patient about rich dietary sources of riboflavin, such as whole grain cereals and green
vegetables. Liver, kidney, heart, eggs, and dairy
products are also dietary sources but may not be
appropriate, based on patient's serum cholesterol and triglyceride levels.
● Advise patient to store riboflavin in a tight, light-
resistant container.

Reactions may be *common*, uncommon, *life-threatening*, or COMMON AND LIFE-THREATENING.

rifabutin
Mycobutin

Pharmacologic classification: semisynthetic ansamycin
Therapeutic classification: antibiotic
Pregnancy risk category: B

Indications and dosages
➤ *Primary prevention of disseminated* Mycobacterium avium *complex (MAC) in patients with advanced HIV infection.*
Adults: 300 mg P.O. daily as a single dose or divided b.i.d. with food.

How supplied
Available by prescription only
Capsules: 150 mg

Pharmacodynamics
Antibiotic action: Rifabutin inhibits DNA-dependent RNA polymerase in susceptible strains of *Escherichia coli* and *Bacillus subtilis,* but not in mammal cells. It isn't known whether rifabutin inhibits this enzyme in *M. avium* or in *M. intracellulare,* which compose MAC.

Pharmacokinetics
Absorption: Readily absorbed from the GI tract.
Distribution: Because of its high lipophilicity, rifabutin has a high propensity for distribution and intracellular tissue uptake. About 85% of drug is bound to plasma proteins independent of concentration.
Metabolism: Metabolized in the liver to five metabolites. The 25-0-desacetyl metabolite has an activity equal to parent drug and contributes up to 10% of total antimicrobial activity.
Excretion: Less than 10% is excreted in urine as unchanged drug. About 53% of oral dose is excreted in urine, primarily as metabolites. About 30% is excreted in feces.

Route	Onset	Peak	Duration
P.O.	Unknown	2-4 hr	Unknown

Contraindications and precautions
Contraindicated in patients hypersensitive to drug or other rifamycin derivatives (such as rifampin) and in patients with active tuberculosis because single-agent therapy with rifabutin increases the risk of inducing bacterial resistance to both rifabutin and rifampin.

Use cautiously in patients with neutropenia and thrombocytopenia.

Interactions
Drug-drug. *Drugs metabolized by the liver, zidovudine:* Rifabutin may decrease serum levels of these drugs, although it doesn't affect inhibition of HIV by zidovudine. Dosage adjustments may be necessary.

Oral contraceptives: Decreased contraceptive effectiveness. Instruct patient to use nonhormonal forms of birth control.

Adverse reactions
CNS: headache, insomnia.
GI: dyspepsia, eructation, flatulence, diarrhea, nausea, vomiting, abdominal pain, altered taste, anorexia.
GU: *discolored urine* (brown-orange).
Hematologic: NEUTROPENIA, LEUKOPENIA, *thrombocytopenia,* eosinophilia.
Musculoskeletal: myalgia.
Skin: *rash.*
Other: fever.

Overdose and treatment
Although there's no experience in treating rifabutin overdose, experience with rifamycins suggests that gastric lavage to evacuate gastric contents (within a few hours of overdose), followed by instillation of an activated charcoal slurry into the stomach, may help absorb any remaining drug from the GI tract. Hemodialysis or forced diuresis probably won't enhance systemic elimination of unchanged rifabutin.

Special considerations
Ⓝ ALERT Don't confuse rifabutin with rifampin and rifapentine.
• High-fat meals slow the rate but not extent of drug absorption.

Patient monitoring
• Evaluate patient immediately if complaints develop that are consistent with active tuberculosis during rifabutin prophylaxis, so active disease may be given an effective combination regimen of antituberculotics. Administration of single-agent rifabutin to patients with active tuberculosis increases the risk of tuberculosis that's resistant to rifabutin and rifampin.
• Because rifabutin may lead to neutropenia, and more rarely to thrombocytopenia, consider obtaining hematologic studies periodically in patients receiving rifabutin prophylaxis.

Breast-feeding patients
• It isn't known if drug appears in breast milk. Because of risk for serious adverse effects in breast-fed infants, either breast-feeding or drug should be discontinued, depending on importance of drug to woman.

Pediatric patients
• Although safety and efficacy in children haven't been fully established, several studies indicate that drug may be helpful in children at maximum daily dose of 5 mg/kg.

Geriatric patients
• No specific recommendations have been made for dosage adjustment or monitoring in these patients.

Patient education
● If patient has trouble swallowing, suggest mixing drug with soft foods such as applesauce.
● Advise patient with nausea, vomiting, or other GI upset to take drug with food, in two divided doses.
● Warn patient that urine and other body fluids may become discolored (brown-orange). Caution that clothes and soft contact lenses may become permanently discolored.

---

rifampin
Rifadin, Rimactane

Pharmacologic classification: semisynthetic rifamycin B derivative (macrocyclic antibiotic)
Therapeutic classification: antituberculotic
Pregnancy risk category: C

Indications and dosages
➤**Primary treatment in pulmonary tuberculosis.** *Adults:* 600 mg P.O. or I.V. daily as a single dose. Give P.O. dose 1 hour before or 2 hours after meals.
Children: 10 to 20 mg/kg P.O. or I.V. daily as a single dose. Give P.O. dose 1 hour before or 2 hours after meals. Maximum, 600 mg daily. Concurrent administration of other effective antitubercular drugs is recommended. Treatment usually lasts 6 to 9 months.
➤**Asymptomatic meningococcal carriers.** *Adults:* 600 mg P.O. b.i.d. for 2 days.
Infants and children over age 1 month: 10 mg/kg P.O. b.i.d. for 2 days.
Neonates under age 1 month: 5 mg/kg P.O. b.i.d. for 2 days.
✦ **Dosage adjustment.** Reduce dosage in patients with hepatic dysfunction.
➤**Prevention of infection with Haemophilus influenzae type B.** *Adults and children:* 20 mg/kg (up to 600 mg) once daily for 4 consecutive days.
➤**Leprosy**◊. *Adults:* 600 mg P.O. once monthly, usually with other drugs.

How supplied
Available by prescription only
Capsules: 150 mg, 300 mg
Injection: 600 mg/vial

Pharmacodynamics
Antibiotic action: Rifampin impairs RNA synthesis by inhibiting DNA-dependent RNA polymerase. Rifampin may be bacteriostatic or bactericidal, depending on organism susceptibility and drug level at infection site.

Rifampin acts against *Mycobacterium bovis, M. kansasii, M. marinum, and M. tuberculosis,* some strains of *M. avium, M. avium-intracellulare and M. fortuitum,* and many gram-positive and some gram-negative bacteria. Resistance to rifampin by *M. tuberculosis* can develop rapidly; rifampin is usually given with other antituberculosis drugs to prevent or delay resistance.

Pharmacokinetics
Absorption: Absorbed completely from the GI tract after oral administration. Food delays absorption.
Distribution: Distributed widely into body tissues and fluids, including ascitic, pleural, seminal, and cerebrospinal fluids, tears, and saliva; and into liver, prostate, lungs, and bone. Drug crosses the placenta, and is 84% to 91% protein-bound.
Metabolism: Metabolized extensively in the liver by deacetylation. It undergoes enterohepatic circulation.
Excretion: Undergoes enterohepatic circulation, and drug and metabolite are excreted primarily in bile; drug, but not metabolite, is reabsorbed. From 6% to 30% of rifampin and metabolite appear unchanged in urine in 24 hours; about 60% is excreted in feces. Some drug appears in breast milk. Plasma half-life in adults is 1½ to 5 hours; serum levels rise in obstructive jaundice. Dosage adjustment isn't necessary for patients with renal failure. Rifampin isn't removed by either hemodialysis or peritoneal dialysis.

Route	Onset	Peak	Duration
P.O.	Unknown	2-4 hr	Unknown
I.V.	Unknown	Unknown	Unknown

Contraindications and precautions
Contraindicated in patients hypersensitive to drug. Use cautiously in patients with hepatic disease.

Interactions
Drug-drug. *Anticoagulants, barbiturates, beta blockers, cardiac glycoside derivatives, chloramphenicol, clofibrate, corticosteroids, cyclosporine, dapsone, disopyramide, estrogens, methadone, oral contraceptives, oral sulfonylureas, phenytoin, quinidine, tocainide, verapamil:* Decreased effectiveness of these drugs. Monitor patient closely, and adjust dosage if needed.
Isoniazid: Increased hazard of isoniazid hepatotoxicity. Monitor patient closely.
Oral contraceptives: Rifampin inactivates such drugs and may alter menstrual patterns. Advise oral contraceptive users to substitute other methods.
Para-aminosalicylate: May decrease oral absorption of rifampin, lowering serum levels. Administer drugs 8 to 12 hours apart.
Drug-lifestyle. *Alcohol use:* May increase risk of hepatotoxicity. Advise patient to avoid alcohol during therapy.

Adverse reactions
CNS: headache, fatigue, drowsiness, behavioral changes, dizziness, ataxia, mental confusion, generalized numbness.

Reactions may be *common,* uncommon, **life-threatening**, or COMMON AND LIFE-THREATENING.

EENT: visual disturbances, exudative conjunctivitis.

GI: epigastric distress, anorexia, nausea, vomiting, abdominal pain, diarrhea, flatulence, sore mouth and tongue, pseudomembranous colitis, pancreatitis.

GU: hemoglobinuria, hematuria, menstrual disturbances, *acute renal failure.*

Hematologic: eosinophilia, *thrombocytopenia, transient leukopenia,* hemolytic anemia.

Hepatic: *hepatotoxicity, transient abnormalities in liver function tests.*

Respiratory: shortness of breath, wheezing.

Skin: pruritus, urticaria, rash.

Other: flulike syndrome, discoloration of body fluids, hyperuricemia, *shock,* osteomalacia, porphyria exacerbation.

Overdose and treatment

Signs and symptoms of overdose include lethargy, nausea, and vomiting; hepatotoxicity from massive overdose includes hepatomegaly, jaundice, elevated liver function studies and bilirubin levels, and loss of consciousness. Skin, urine, sweat, saliva, tears, and feces may have red-orange discoloration.

Treat with gastric lavage followed by activated charcoal; if necessary, force diuresis. Perform bile drainage if hepatic dysfunction persists beyond 24 to 48 hours.

Special considerations

⚠ ALERT Don't confuse rifampin with rifabutin or rifapentine.

● Give drug 1 hour before or 2 hours after meals for maximum absorption; capsule contents may be mixed with food or fluid to enhance swallowing.

● Reconstituted solution is stable for 24 hours at room temperature. Use infusion solutions of 100 to 500 ml within 4 hours.

● Increased liver enzyme activity inactivates certain drugs, especially warfarin, corticosteroids, and oral hypoglycemics, requiring dosage adjustments.

● Rifampin alters standard serum folate and vitamin B_{12} assays.

● Rifampin may cause temporary retention of sulfobromophthalein in the liver excretion test; it also may interfere with contrast material in gallbladder studies and urinalysis based on spectrophotometry.

Patient monitoring

● Obtain specimens for culture and sensitivity testing before giving first dose, but don't delay therapy; repeat tests periodically to detect drug resistance.

● Observe patient for adverse reactions, and monitor hematologic studies, renal and liver function studies, and serum electrolyte levels to minimize toxicity. Watch for evidence of hepatic impairment, such as anorexia, fatigue, malaise, jaundice, dark urine, and liver tenderness.

Breast-feeding patients

● Drug may appear in breast milk. Use cautiously in breast-feeding women.

Pediatric patients

● Safety in children under age 5 hasn't been established.

Geriatric patients

● Usual dose in geriatric and debilitated patients is 10 mg/kg once daily. Monitor renal function closely because elderly patients may be more susceptible to toxic effects.

Patient education

● Explain disease process and rationale for long-term therapy.

● Teach signs and symptoms of hypersensitivity and other adverse reactions, and emphasize need to report them if they occur; urge patient to report any unusual reactions.

● Urge patient to comply with prescribed regimen, not to miss doses, and not to discontinue drug without medical approval. Explain importance of follow-up appointments.

● Encourage patient to report promptly any flulike signs or symptoms, weakness, sore throat, loss of appetite, unusual bruising, rash, itching, tea-colored urine, clay-colored stools, or yellow discoloration of eyes or skin.

● Explain that drug turns all body fluids red-orange color; advise patient of possible permanent stains on clothes and soft contact lenses.

rifapentine
Priftin

Pharmacologic classification: cyclopentyl rifamycin
Therapeutic classification: antibiotic
Pregnancy risk category: C

Indications and dosages

➤ *Pulmonary tuberculosis, with at least one other antituberculotic to which the isolate is susceptible. Adults:* During intensive phase of short-course therapy, 600 mg P.O. twice weekly for 2 months, with an interval between doses of at least 72 hours. During continuation phase of short-course therapy, 600 mg P.O. once weekly for 4 months with isoniazid or another drug to which the isolate is susceptible.

How supplied

Available by prescription only
Tablets (film-coated): 150 mg

Pharmacodynamics

Antibiotic action: Rifapentine inhibits DNA-dependent RNA polymerase in susceptible strains of *Mycobacterium tuberculosis*. It has bactericidal activity against the organism both intracellularly and extracellularly. Rifapentine and rifampin share similar antimicrobial action.

Pharmacokinetics
Absorption: Relative bioavailablity after oral absorption is 70%.
Distribution: Bound primarily to albumin.
Metabolism: Unknown.
Excretion: Appears to be excreted through the urine and feces.

Route	Onset	Peak	Duration
P.O.	Unknown	5-6 hr	Unknown

Contraindications and precautions
Contraindicated in patients with history of hypersensitivity to a rifamycin (rifapentine, rifampin, or rifabutin). Use drug cautiously and with frequent monitoring in patients with liver disease.

Interactions
Drug-drug. *Anticonvulsants, antiarrhythmics, antibiotics (including fluoroquinolones), antifungals, barbiturates, benzodiazepines, beta blockers, calcium channel blockers, cardiac glycosides, corticosteroids, clofibrate, haloperidol, HIV protease inhibitors, immunosuppressants, levothyroxine, narcotic analgesics, oral anticoagulants, oral hypoglycemics, oral or other systemic hormonal contraceptives, progestins, quinine, reverse transcriptase inhibitors, sildenafil, theophylline, tricyclic antidepressants:* Rifapentine decreases the activity of these drugs. Dosage adjustments may be needed.

Adverse reactions
CNS: headache, dizziness.
CV: hypertension.
GI: anorexia, nausea, vomiting, dyspepsia, diarrhea.
GU: pyuria, proteinuria, hematuria, urinary casts.
Hematologic: *neutropenia,* lymphopenia, anemia, *leukopenia,* thrombocytosis.
Hepatic: elevated AST and ALT levels.
Metabolic: *hyperuricemia.*
Musculoskeletal: arthralgia.
Respiratory: hemoptysis.
Skin: rash, pruritus, acne, maculopapular rash.
Other: pain.

Overdose and treatment
Overdose hasn't been reported. Gastric lavage followed by activated charcoal may help. Neither hemodialysis nor forced diuresis is suggested. Provide supportive care and close monitoring.

Special considerations
ALERT Don't confuse rifapentine with rifabutin or rifampin.
● Coadministration of pyridoxine (vitamin B_6) is recommended in malnourished patients, patients predisposed to neuropathy (alcoholics, diabetics), and adolescents.
ALERT Drug must be given with appropriate daily companion drugs. Compliance with all medications is crucial for early sputum conversion and protection from relapse of tuberculosis.
● Drug can turn body tissues and fluids red-orange and permanently stain contact lenses.

Patient monitoring
● Rifamycin antibiotics have been linked to hepatotoxicity. Monitor liver function test results before starting therapy.
● Drug therapy may affect liver function test results, CBC, and platelet counts; monitor patient.

Pregnant patients
● Giving drug during the last 2 weeks of pregnancy may lead to postnatal hemorrhage in woman or infant. Monitor clotting parameters closely if drug is given.

Breast-feeding patients
● Because rifapentine may appear in breast milk, it isn't recommended for breast-feeding women.

Pediatric patients
● Safety and efficacy in children under age 12 haven't been established.

Patient education
● Stress importance of strict compliance with drug and daily companion drugs, as well as necessary follow-up visits and laboratory tests.
● Advise patient to use nonhormonal methods of birth control.
● Tell patient to take drug with food if nausea, vomiting, or GI upset occurs.
● Instruct patient to notify prescriber if the following occur: fever, loss of appetite, malaise, nausea, vomiting, darkened urine, yellowish discoloration of the skin and eyes, pain or swelling of the joints, and excessive loose stools or diarrhea.
● Instruct patient to protect pills from heat.

riluzole
Rilutek

Pharmacologic classification: benzothiazole
Therapeutic classification: neuroprotector
Pregnancy risk category: C

Indications and dosages
➤ *Amyotrophic lateral sclerosis (ALS).*
Adults: 50 mg P.O. q 12 hours on an empty stomach.

How supplied
Available by prescription only
Tablets: 50 mg

Pharmacodynamics

Neuroprotector action: It isn't known how riluzole improves signs and symptoms of ALS.

Pharmacokinetics

Absorption: Well absorbed from GI tract (about 90%) with average absolute oral bioavailability of about 60%. A high-fat meal decreases absorption.

Distribution: 96% protein-bound.

Metabolism: Extensively metabolized in the liver to six major and several minor metabolites, not all of which have been identified.

Excretion: Excreted primarily in urine and a small amount in feces. Half-life is 12 hours with repeated doses.

Route	Onset	Peak	Duration
P.O.	Unknown	Unknown	Unknown

Contraindications and precautions

Contraindicated in patients with history of severe hypersensitivity reactions to drug or its components.

Use cautiously in elderly patients and those with hepatic or renal dysfunction. Also use cautiously in women and Japanese patients, who may have a lower metabolic capacity to eliminate drug compared with men and white patients, respectively.

Interactions

Drug-drug. *Allopurinol, methyldopa, sulfasalazine:* Increased risk of hepatotoxicity. Administer together cautiously.

Drug-food. *Any food:* Decreased bioavailability. Give drug 1 hour before or 2 hours after meals. *Charbroiled foods:* May increase riluzole elimination. Advise patient to avoid charbroiled foods.

Drug-lifestyle. *Alcohol use:* May increase risk of hepatotoxicity. Advise patient to avoid alcohol. *Smoking:* May increase riluzole elimination. Advise patient to avoid smoking.

Adverse reactions

CNS: *asthenia*, headache, aggravation reaction, hypertonia, malaise, depression, dizziness, insomnia, somnolence, vertigo, circumoral paresthesia.

CV: phlebitis, hypertension, tachycardia, palpitation, orthostatic hypotension.

EENT: rhinitis, sinusitis.

GI: abdominal pain, *nausea*, vomiting, dyspepsia, anorexia, diarrhea, flatulence, stomatitis, oral candidiasis, dry mouth.

GU: urinary tract infection, dysuria.

Metabolic: weight loss.

Musculoskeletal: back pain, arthralgia.

Respiratory: *decreased lung function*, increased cough.

Skin: pruritus, eczema, alopecia, exfoliative dermatitis.

Other: tooth disorder, peripheral edema.

Overdose and treatment

No information available. In the event of an overdose, stop therapy immediately and give supportive care.

Special considerations

● Use drug cautiously in patients with hepatic or renal dysfunction, in elderly patients, and in women and Japanese patients, who may have a lower metabolic capacity to eliminate drug.

Patient monitoring

● Baseline elevations in liver function studies, especially elevated bilirubin, should preclude riluzole use.

● Perform liver function studies periodically during therapy. In many patients, drug may elevate serum aminotransferase levels; discontinue drug if levels exceed 10 times upper limit of normal range or if clinical jaundice develops.

Breast-feeding patients

● It isn't known if drug appears in breast milk. Because of potential for serious adverse reactions in infants, use of drug in breast-feeding women isn't recommended.

Pediatric patients

● Safety and efficacy haven't been established.

Geriatric patients

● Age-related decreased renal and hepatic function may decrease clearance of riluzole. Administer drug cautiously to elderly patients.

Patient education

● Tell patient or caregiver that drug must be taken regularly and at the same time each day. If a dose is missed, tell patient to take the next tablet as originally planned.

● Instruct patient to report febrile illness; the patient's WBC count should be checked.

● Warn patient to avoid hazardous activities until CNS effects of drug are known.

● Tell patient to store drug at room temperature and protect it from bright light.

● Stress importance of keeping drug out of reach of children.

rimantadine hydrochloride
Flumadine

Pharmacologic classification: adamantine
Therapeutic classification: antiviral
Pregnancy risk category: C

Indications and dosages

➤ *Prophylaxis against influenza A virus.*
Adults and children age 10 and older: 100 mg P.O. b.i.d.; for patients with severe hepatic dysfunction or renal failure (creatinine clearance 10 ml/minute or less) and for elderly patients in

communal settings, a dose reduction to 100 mg
P.O. daily is recommended.
Children under age 10: 5 mg/kg P.O. once daily. Maximum dose, 150 mg.
➤*Treatment of illness caused by various strains of influenza A virus. Adults:*
100 mg P.O. b.i.d. for 7 days from symptom onset; for patients with severe hepatic dysfunction
or renal failure (creatinine clearance 10 ml/
minute or less) and for elderly patients in communal settings, a dose reduction to 100 mg P.O.
daily is recommended.

How supplied
Available by prescription only
Syrup: 50 mg/5 ml
Tablets: 100 mg

Pharmacodynamics
Antiviral action: Mechanism of action isn't fully understood. Drug appears to exert inhibitory
effect early in viral replication cycle, possibly inhibiting uncoating of the virus. Genetic studies
suggest that a virus protein specified by the viri-
on M_2 gene plays an important role in susceptibility of influenza A virus to inhibition by rimantadine.

Pharmacokinetics
Absorption: Tablet and syrup forms are equally absorbed.
Distribution: Plasma protein–binding is about
40%.
Metabolism: Extensively metabolized in the liver.
Excretion: Less than 25% is excreted in urine
as unchanged drug. Elimination half-life of drug
is about 25½ to 32 hours. Hemodialysis doesn't
contribute to drug clearance.

Route	Onset	Peak	Duration
P.O.	Unknown	6 hr	Unknown

Contraindications and precautions
Contraindicated in patients hypersensitive to drug
or to amantadine. Use cautiously in pregnant
patients and patients with impaired renal or hepatic function or seizure disorders (especially
epilepsy).

Interactions
Drug-drug. *Acetaminophen, aspirin:* Reduced
rimantadine levels. Monitor patient for drug effect.
Cimetidine: May decrease total rimantadine clearance by about 16%. Monitor patient for adverse
effects.

Adverse reactions
CNS: insomnia, headache, dizziness, nervousness, fatigue, asthenia.
GI: nausea, vomiting, anorexia, dry mouth, abdominal pain.

Overdose and treatment
Information specific to rimantadine overdose isn't
available. As with any overdose, administer supportive care as indicated. Overdoses of a related
drug, amantadine, have been reported, with reactions ranging from agitation to hallucinations,
cardiac arrhythmia, and death. Administration of
I.V. physostigmine (1 to 2 mg in adults and 0.5 mg
in children; repeated as needed but not to exceed 2 mg/hour) may benefit patients with CNS
effects from overdose of amantadine.

Special considerations
⚠ ALERT Don't confuse rimantadine with amantadine.
● For illnesses related to various strains of influenza A, treatment should begin as soon as possible, preferably within 48 hours after onset of
signs and symptoms, to reduce duration of fever
and systemic symptoms.
● An increased risk of seizures has been observed
in some patients with history of seizures who
weren't taking an anticonvulsant during rimantadine therapy. If seizures develop, discontinue
drug.
● Influenza A–resistant strains can emerge during therapy. Patients taking drug may still be able
to spread the disease.

Patient monitoring
● Because of risk of drug metabolites accumu-
lating during multiple dosing, monitor patient
with any degree of renal insufficiency for adverse
effects, and adjust dosage as necessary.

Breast-feeding patients
● Drug shouldn't be given to breast-feeding
women because of the potential adverse effects
to the infant.

Pediatric patients
● Drug is recommended for prophylaxis of influenza A. Safety and efficacy of drug in treating
symptomatic influenza infection in children haven't
been established.
● Prophylaxis studies with rimantadine haven't
been performed in children under age 1.

Geriatric patients
● Adverse drug reactions occur more often in el-
derly patients than in the general population.
Monitor these patients closely.

Patient education
● Advise patient to take drug several hours before bedtime to prevent insomnia.
● Inform patient that taking drug doesn't prevent
him from spreading the disease and that he should
limit contact with others until fully recovered.
● Warn patient that drug may cause adverse CNS
effects; he shouldn't drive or perform activities
that require mental alertness until these effects
are known.

Reactions may be *common*, uncommon, *life-threatening*, or COMMON AND LIFE-THREATENING.

risperidone
Risperdal

Pharmacologic classification: benzisoxazole derivative
Therapeutic classification: antipsychotic
Pregnancy risk category: C

Indications and dosages
➤ **Psychosis.** *Adults:* Initially, 1 mg P.O. b.i.d. Increase in increments of 1 mg b.i.d. on days 2 and 3 to a target dosage of 3 mg b.i.d. Wait at least 1 week before adjusting dosage further. Doses above 6 mg daily are no more effective than lower doses and may cause more extrapyramidal reactions.

✦ **Dosage adjustment.** Elderly or debilitated patients, hypotensive patients, or patients with severe renal or hepatic impairment should initially receive 0.5 mg P.O. b.i.d. Increase dosage in increments of 0.5 mg b.i.d. on days 2 and 3 to target dosage of 1.5 mg P.O. b.i.d. Wait at least 1 week before increasing dosage further.

How supplied
Available by prescription only
Solution: 1 mg/ml
Tablets: 0.25 mg, 0.5 mg, 1 mg, 2 mg, 3 mg, 4 mg

Pharmacodynamics
Antipsychotic action: Exact mechanism of action is unknown. Antipsychotic activity may be mediated through a combination of dopamine type 2 (D_2) and serotonin type 2 (5-HT_2) antagonism. Antagonism at receptors other than D_2 and 5-HT_2 may explain other effects of drug.

Pharmacokinetics
Absorption: Well absorbed after oral administration. Absolute oral bioavailability is 70%. Food doesn't affect rate or extent of absorption.
Distribution: Plasma protein–binding is about 90% for drug and 77% for its major active metabolite, 9-hydroxyrisperidone.
Metabolism: Extensively metabolized in the liver to 9-hydroxyrisperidone, which is the predominant circulating species and appears about equi-effective with risperidone with respect to receptor binding activity. About 6% to 8% of whites and a low percentage of Asians show little or no receptor binding activity and are called poor metabolizers.
Excretion: Metabolite is excreted by the kidney. Clearance of drug and its metabolite is reduced in patients with renal impairment.

Route	Onset	Peak	Duration
P.O.	Unknown	1 hr	Unknown

Contraindications and precautions
Contraindicated in patients hypersensitive to drug and in breast-feeding women. Use cautiously in patients with prolonged QT interval, CV disease, cerebrovascular disease, dehydration, hypovolemia, history of seizures, or exposure to extreme heat or conditions that could affect metabolism or hemodynamic responses.

Interactions
Drug-drug. *Antihypertensives:* Possible enhanced effects of certain antihypertensives. Monitor blood pressure closely.
Carbamazepine: May increase risperidone clearance, decreasing its effectiveness. Monitor patient closely.
Clozapine: May decrease risperidone clearance, increasing the risk of toxicity. Monitor patient closely.
CNS depressants: May cause additive CNS depression. Give together cautiously.
Dopamine agonists, levodopa: Risperidone may antagonize the effects of these drugs. Avoid use together.
Drug-lifestyle. *Alcohol use:* Additive CNS depression. Tell patient to avoid use together.
Sun exposure: May cause photosensitivity reactions. Advise patient to take precautions.

Adverse reactions
CNS: *neuroleptic malignant syndrome,* somnolence, *extrapyramidal reactions, headache, insomnia, agitation, anxiety,* tardive dyskinesia, aggressiveness, dizziness.
CV: tachycardia, chest pain, orthostatic hypotension, prolonged QT interval.
EENT: *rhinitis,* sinusitis, pharyngitis, abnormal vision.
GI: *constipation, nausea, vomiting, dyspepsia, abdominal pain, anorexia.*
Metabolic: *weight gain.*
Musculoskeletal: arthralgia, back pain.
Respiratory: coughing, upper respiratory infection.
Skin: rash, dry skin, photosensitivity.
Other: fever, increase serum prolactin levels.

Overdose and treatment
Signs and symptoms of overdose reflect exaggeration of risperidone effects, such as drowsiness, sedation, tachycardia, hypotension, and extrapyramidal symptoms. Hyponatremia, hypokalemia, prolonged QT interval, widened QRS complex, and seizures have been reported.

There's no specific antidote to risperidone overdose; institute appropriate supportive measures. Consider gastric lavage (after intubation, if patient is unconscious) and administration of activated charcoal with a laxative. CV monitoring is essential to detect possible arrhythmias. If antiarrhythmic therapy is administered, disopyramide, procainamide, and quinidine carry a theoretical hazard of QT interval–prolonging effects that might be additive to those of risperidone. Similarly, it's reasonable to expect that the alpha-blocking properties of bretylium might be additive to those of risperidone, resulting in problematic hypotension.

Special considerations

● Risperidone and 9-hydroxyrisperidone appear to lengthen the QT interval in some patients, although there's no average increase in treated patients, even at 12 to 16 mg daily (well above recommended dose). Other drugs that prolong the QT interval have been linked to torsades de pointes, a life-threatening arrhythmia. Bradycardia, electrolyte imbalance, use with other drugs that prolong the QT interval, or congenital prolongation of the QT interval can increase risk for occurrence of this arrhythmia.

● Drug has an antiemetic effect in animals; this may occur in humans, masking signs and symptoms of overdose or of such conditions as intestinal obstruction, Reye's syndrome, and brain tumor.

● When restarting drug therapy for patients who have been off drug, follow initial 3-day dose initiation schedule.

● When switching patient from another antipsychotic to risperidone, immediately discontinue other drug at start of risperidone therapy when medically appropriate.

● Tardive dyskinesia may occur after prolonged risperidone therapy. It may not appear until months or years later and may disappear spontaneously or persist for life despite discontinuation of drug.

Patient monitoring

● Neuroleptic malignant syndrome is rare, but in many cases fatal. It isn't necessarily related to length of drug use or type of neuroleptic. Monitor patient closely for symptoms, including hyperpyrexia, muscle rigidity, altered mental status, irregular pulse, alteration in blood pressure, and diaphoresis.

Pregnant patients

● Instruct women to report planned, suspected, or known pregnancy.

Breast-feeding patients

● Patient should stop breast-feeding during therapy.

Pediatric patients

● Safety and efficacy in children haven't been established.

Geriatric patients

● A lower starting dose is recommended for elderly patients because they have decreased pharmacokinetic clearance; a greater risk of hepatic, renal, or cardiac dysfunction; and a greater tendency toward orthostatic hypotension.

Patient education

● Advise patient to rise slowly from a recumbent or seated position to minimize light-headedness.

● Warn patient not to operate hazardous machinery, including driving a car, until effects of drug are known.

● Tell patient to call before taking new drugs, including OTC drugs, because of potential for interactions.

ritonavir
Norvir

Pharmacologic classification: HIV protease inhibitor
Therapeutic classification: antiviral
Pregnancy risk category: B

Indications and dosages

➤ *Treatment of HIV infection when antiretroviral therapy is warranted.* Adults: 600 mg P.O. b.i.d. with meals. If nausea occurs, this schedule may provide some relief: 300 mg b.i.d., increased at 2- to 3-day intervals by 100 mg b.i.d., up to 600 mg b.i.d.
Children age 2 and older: 400 mg/m² P.O. b.i.d. with other antiretrovirals. To minimize nausea, initially 250 mg/m² b.i.d. May increase by 50 mg/m² b.i.d. at 2- to 3-day intervals.

How supplied

Available by prescription only
Capsules: 100 mg
Oral solution: 80 mg/ml

Pharmacodynamics

Antiviral action: Ritonavir is an HIV protease inhibitor. HIV protease is an enzyme required for proteolytic cleavage of viral polyprotein precursors into individual functional proteins found in infectious HIV. Ritonavir binds to the protease active site and inhibits activity of the enzyme. This inhibition prevents cleavage of viral polyproteins, resulting in formation of immature noninfectious viral particles.

Pharmacokinetics

Absorption: Absorbed better when taken with food; absolute bioavailability hasn't been determined.
Distribution: 98% to 99% bound to plasma proteins.
Metabolism: Metabolized in the liver; P-450 3A (CYP3A) is the major isoform involved in ritonavir metabolism.
Excretion: Primarily excreted in feces, although a small amount has been found in urine. Half-life is 3 to 5 hours.

Route	Onset	Peak	Duration
P.O.	Unknown	2-4 hr	Unknown

Contraindications and precautions

Contraindicated in patients hypersensitive to any components of drug. Use cautiously in patients with hepatic insufficiency.

Reactions may be *common*, uncommon, **life-threatening**, or COMMON AND LIFE-THREATENING.

Interactions

Drug-drug. *Alprazolam, clorazepate, diazepam, estazolam, flurazepam, midazolam, triazolam, zolpidem:* Risk of extreme sedation and respiratory depression. Don't use together.

Alprazolam, methadone: Decreased levels of these drugs. Use together cautiously.

Amiodarone, bepridil, bupropion, clozapine, encainide, flecainide, meperidine, piroxicam, propafenone, propoxyphene, quinidine, rifabutin: Significant increases in levels of these drugs, thus increasing risk of arrhythmias, hematologic abnormalities, seizures, or other potentially serious adverse effects. Don't use together.

Clarithromycin: Increased clarithromycin levels. Patients with renal impairment need a 50% reduction in clarithromycin dosage if creatinine clearance is 30 to 60 ml/minute and a 75% reduction if it's below 30 ml/minute.

Desipramine: Increased desipramine levels. Desipramine dosage may need adjustment.

Disopyramide: Increased risk of cardiac and neurologic events. Use together cautiously.

Disulfiram and other drugs that produce disulfiram-like reactions, such as metronidazole: Increased risk of disulfiram-like reactions because ritonavir formulations contain alcohol. Monitor patient.

Drugs that increase CYP3A activity, such as carbamazepine, dexamethasone, phenobarbital, phenytoin, rifabutin, and rifampin: Increased ritonavir clearance and decreased ritonavir levels. Monitor patient closely.

Glucuronosyltransferases, including oral anticoagulants and immunosuppressants: Loss of therapeutic effects from directly glucuronidated agents. They may need dosage adjustment; monitor drug levels and effects. A dosage reduction of more than 50% may be needed for drugs extensively metabolized by CYP3A.

Ketoconazole: Increased levels of both drugs. Use together cautiously, and monitor patient carefully.

Oral contraceptives: Decreased contraceptive levels. Increase contraceptive dosage or recommend a different contraceptive method, as needed.

Sildenafil: Increased risk of sildenafil-related adverse reactions, including hypotension, vision changes, and priapism. Sildenafil dose shouldn't exceed 25 mg in a 48-hour period.

Theophylline: Decreased theophylline levels. Increase theophylline dosage if needed.

Drug-herb. *St. John's wort:* Substantially reduced drug levels and possible loss of therapeutic effects. Discourage concomitant use.

Drug-food. *Any food:* Increased absorption. Tell patient to take drug with food.

Drug-lifestyle. *Smoking:* Decreased ritonavir levels. Discourage alcohol use.

Adverse reactions

CNS: *asthenia,* headache, circumoral paresthesia, dizziness, insomnia, paresthesia, peripheral paresthesia, somnolence, thinking abnormality,

generalized tonic-clonic seizure, depression.

CV: vasodilation.

EENT: pharyngitis.

GI: *taste perversion,* abdominal pain, anorexia, constipation, *diarrhea, nausea, vomiting,* dyspepsia, flatulence.

Hematologic: *thrombocytopenia.*

Hepatic: abnormal liver function test results.

Musculoskeletal: myalgia.

Skin: sweating.

Other: fever.

Overdose and treatment

Information is limited to one patient who reported paresthesia, which resolved after the dose was decreased. Treatment consists of general supportive measures. Emesis or gastric lavage may be used as well as activated charcoal. Dialysis probably isn't helpful.

Special considerations

● Drug may be given alone or with nucleoside analogues.

● GI tolerance may be improved in patients taking ritonavir and nucleosides by starting ritonavir alone and adding nucleosides before completing 2 weeks of ritonavir monotherapy.

Patient monitoring

● Monitor patient's response to drug therapy.

● Measure plasma HIV-1 RNA levels and CD4+ T-cell counts to determine disease progression and detect need to modify therapy.

Breast-feeding patients

● It isn't known if ritonavir appears in breast milk. However, to prevent transmission of infection HIV-positive women shouldn't breast-feed.

Pediatric patients

● Safety and efficacy in children under age 2 haven't been established.

Patient education

● Inform patient that drug doesn't cure HIV infection and that he may continue to develop opportunistic infections and other complications related to HIV infection.

● Explain that drug doesn't reduce the risk of transmitting HIV to others through sexual contact or blood contamination.

● Caution patient not to adjust dosage or stop drug without medical approval.

● Tell patient that he may improve taste of oral solution by mixing with chocolate milk, Ensure, or Advera within 1 hour of dosing.

● Tell patient that if a dose is missed, he should take the next dose as soon as possible. However, if a dose is skipped, he shouldn't double the next dose.

● Advise patient to report use of other drugs, including OTC drugs, because of possible drug interactions.

rituximab
Rituxan

Pharmacologic classification: monoclonal
antibody
Therapeutic classification: antineoplastic
Pregnancy risk factor: C

Indications and dosages
➤*Relapsed or refractory low-grade or
follicular, CD20-positive, B-cell malignant lymphoma. Adults:* 375 mg/m^2 I.V. infusion once weekly for four doses (days 1, 8, 15,
22). Start initial infusion at 50 mg/hour. If no hypersensitivity or infusion-related events, increase
to 50 mg/hour q 30 minutes to maximum of
400 mg/hour. Start subsequent infusions at
100 mg/hour and increase by increments of
100 mg/hour at 30-minute intervals, to maximum
of 400 mg/hour as tolerated.

How supplied
Available by prescription only
Injection: 10 mg/ml; 10 ml, 50 ml single-use
vials

Pharmacodynamics
Antineoplastic action: A murine/human monoclonal antibody directed against CD20 antigen
found on the surface of normal and malignant B-
lymphocytes. CD20 regulates early steps in cell
cycle initiation and differentiation processes. Binding to this antigen mediates the lysis of the B cells.

Pharmacokinetics
No information available.

Route	Onset	Peak	Duration
I.V.	Variable	Variable	6-12 mo

Contraindications and precautions
Contraindicated in patients with type I hypersensitivity or anaphylactoid reactions to murine proteins or to any component of drug.

Interactions
None reported.

Adverse reactions
CNS: dizziness, *asthenia, headache,* fatigue,
paresthesia, malaise, agitation, insomnia, hypoesthesia, hypertonia, nervousness, anxiety.
CV: *hypotension, arrhythmias,* hypertension,
peripheral edema, chest pain, tachycardia, orthostatic hypotension, *bradycardia.*
EENT: sore throat, rhinitis, sinusitis, lacrimation
disorder, conjunctivitis.
GI: *nausea,* vomiting, abdominal pain or enlargement, diarrhea, dyspepsia, anorexia, increased lactate dehydrogenase, taste perversion.
Hematologic: *leukopenia, thrombocytopenia, neutropenia,* anemia.
Metabolic: hyperglycemia, hypocalcemia.

Musculoskeletal: arthralgia, back pain, myalgia.
Respiratory: *bronchospasm,* dyspnea, cough
increase, bronchitis.
Skin: *pruritus, rash,* urticaria, flushing.
Other: *angioedema, fever, chills, rigors,* pain,
pain at injection site, tumor pain.

Special considerations
● Drug must be given as I.V. infusion; don't give
by I.V. push or as a bolus. Drug may be diluted
to 1 to 4 mg/ml in normal saline solution or D$_5$W.
● Consider giving acetaminophen and diphenhydramine before each infusion because hypersensitivity reactions may occur.
● Stop infusion if serious or life-threatening cardiac arrhythmias occur.
● Human anti-murine antibody (HAMA) and human antichimeric antibody (HACA) have been
detected in less than 1% of patients. If HAMA or
HACA titers appear, patient may develop allergic
or hypersensitivity reactions to drug or other
murine or chimeric monoclonal antibody preparations.
● Immunization safety or efficacy during drug
therapy hasn't been studied.
● Because transient hypotension may occur during infusion, consider withholding antihypertensives 12 hours before infusion.
● Hypotension, bronchospasm, and angioedema
have occurred as part of an infusion-related symptom complex. Have such drugs as epinephrine,
diphenhydramine, and corticosteroids available
to immediately treat such a reaction. Monitor patient's blood pressure closely during infusion. If
an infusion-related symptom complex occurs,
stop infusion and restart at a 50% rate reduction
when symptoms resolve. Recommended treatment may include acetaminophen and diphenhydramine; bronchodilators or I.V. saline may be
indicated. In most cases, patients have been able
to proceed with a full course of therapy.

Patient monitoring
● Monitor patient closely for hypersensitivity reactions.
● Patients with cardiac conditions, including arrhythmias and angina, could have recurrences
during drug therapy and should be monitored
throughout infusion period.
● Perform cardiac monitoring during and after
subsequent drug infusions in patients who develop
clinically significant infusion-related symptoms.
● Obtain CBC at regular intervals, more often in
patients who develop cytopenias.

Breast-feeding patients
● It isn't known if drug appears in breast milk.
Because other antibodies can appear, advise patient to stop breast-feeding until drug can't be
detected in circulation.

Pediatric patients
● Safety and effectiveness in children haven't been
established.

Reactions may be *common,* uncommon, *life-threatening,* or COMMON AND LIFE-THREATENING.

Patient education
- Tell patient to report unusual symptoms during and after infusion.
- Advise patient to disclose history of cardiac problems.
- Instruct patient not to receive any vaccinations (especially live viral vaccines) during therapy unless approved.
- Inform patient that frequent CBCs may be necessary.

rivastigmine tartrate
Exelon

Pharmacologic classification: cholinesterase inhibitor
Therapeutic classification: Alzheimer's agent
Pregnancy risk category: B

Indications and dosages
➤ *Symptomatic treatment of patients with mild to moderate Alzheimer's disease. Adults:* Initially, 1.5 mg P.O. b.i.d. with food. If tolerated, may be increased to 3 mg b.i.d after 2 weeks. Further increases to 4.5 mg bid and 6 mg b.i.d may be implemented as tolerated after 2 weeks on the previous dose. Effective dosage range is 6 to 12 mg daily, with maximum recommended dosage of 12 mg daily.

How supplied
Available by prescription only
Capsules: 1.5 mg, 3 mg, 4.5 mg, 6 mg

Pharmacodynamics
Cognitive function action: Drug is thought to increase acetylcholine levels by reversibly inhibiting its hydrolysis by cholinesterase. Acetylcholine is probably the primary neurotransmitter that is depleted in Alzheimer's disease. By increasing acetylcholine activity, cognitive function may improve.

Pharmacokinetics
Absorption: Drug is rapidly absorbed, and serum levels peak in about 1 hour. Although drug should be taken with food, the time to reach peak levels is delayed by about 1.5 hours. Absolute bioavailability is 36%.
Distribution: Widely distributed throughout body; drug crosses the blood-brain barrier. Protein-binding is about 40%.
Metabolism: Rapidly and extensively metabolized.
Excretion: Elimination is primarily through the kidneys. Half-life is about 1½ hours in patients with normal renal function.

Route	Onset	Peak	Duration
P.O.	Unknown	1 hr	12 hr

Contraindications and precautions
Contraindicated in patients hypersensitive to drug, its components, or other carbamate derivatives.
   Use cautiously in patients who take NSAIDs and patients with a history of ulcers or GI bleeding, sick sinus syndrome or other supraventricular cardiac conditions, asthma or obstructive pulmonary disease, or seizures.

Interactions
Drug-drug. *Anticholinergics:* Possible interference with anticholinergic activity. Monitor patient closely.
Bethanechol, succinylcholine, and other neuromuscular blocking agents or cholinergic antagonists: Possible synergistic effect on rivastigmine. Monitor patient closely.
Drug-lifestyle. *Nicotine:* Increased rivastigmine clearance. Monitor patient closely.

Adverse reactions
CNS: syncope, fatigue, asthenia, malaise, *dizziness, headache,* somnolence, tremor, insomnia, confusion, depression, anxiety, hallucination, aggressive reaction, vertigo, agitation, nervousness, delusion, paranoid reaction.
CV: hypertension, chest pain, peripheral edema.
EENT: rhinitis, pharyngitis.
GI: *nausea, vomiting, diarrhea, anorexia, abdominal pain,* dyspepsia, constipation, flatulence, eructation.
GU: urinary tract infection, urinary incontinence.
Metabolic: weight loss.
Musculoskeletal: back pain, arthralgia, bone fracture.
Respiratory: upper respiratory tract infection, cough, bronchitis.
Skin: increased sweating, rash.
Other: *accidental trauma,* flulike symptoms, pain.

Overdose and treatment
Signs and symptoms of overdose are cholinergic in nature and may include severe nausea, vomiting, salivation, sweating, bradycardia, hypotension, muscle weakness, respiratory depression, respiratory collapse, and seizures.
   Withhold additional doses of drug for 24 hours. Consider giving antiemetics if patient has severe nausea and vomiting. Dialysis isn't recommended because of drug's short half-life.

Special considerations
- Expect significant GI adverse effects, such as nausea, vomiting, anorexia, and weight loss. They're less common during maintenance doses.
⚠ ALERT The manufacturer has issued a warning that severe vomiting has occurred among patients who resumed rivastigmine therapy after an interruption. Revised package labeling states that therapy should resume at the recommended starting dosage (1.5 mg b.i.d.) if therapy is interrupted for more than several days. The dosage

should then be adjusted upward to maintenance levels.
● Dramatic memory improvement is unlikely. As disease progresses, the benefits of rivastigmine may decline.

Patient monitoring
● Monitor patient for symptoms of active or occult GI bleeding.
● Monitor patient for severe nausea, vomiting, and diarrhea, which may lead to dehydration and weight loss.
● Carefully monitor patient with a history of GI bleeding, NSAID use, arrhythmias, seizures, or pulmonary conditions for adverse effects.

Breast-feeding patients
● It isn't known if rivastigmine appears in breast milk. There is no indication for use in nursing mothers.

Pediatric patients
● Safety and effectiveness haven't been evaluated.

Patient education
● Advise patient to report any episodes of nausea, vomiting, or diarrhea.
● Inform patient and caregiver that memory improvement may be subtle and that a more likely result of therapy is a slower decline in memory loss.
● Tell patient to take rivastigmine with food in the morning and evening.
● Urge patient to consult prescriber before taking OTC medications.

rizatriptan benzoate
Maxalt, Maxalt-MLT

Pharmacologic classification: selective 5-hydroxytryptamine (5-HT$_{1b/1d}$) receptor agonist
Therapeutic classification: antimigraine
Pregnancy risk category: C

Indications and dosages
➤ **Treatment of acute migraine headaches with or without aura.** *Adults:* Initially, 5 or 10 mg P.O. If first dose is ineffective, another dose can be given at least 2 hours after first dose. Maximum dose is 30 mg within a 24-hour period. For patients receiving propranolol, 5 mg P.O. up to maximum of three doses (15 mg) in 24 hours.

How supplied
Available by prescription only
Tablets: 5 mg, 10 mg
Tablets (orally disintegrating): 5 mg, 10 mg

Pharmacodynamics
Vasoconstricting action: Rizatriptan is believed to exert its effect by acting as an agonist at serotonin receptors on extracerebral intracranial blood vessels, which results in vasoconstriction of affected vessels, inhibition of neuropeptide release, and reduction of pain transmission in the trigeminal pathways.

Pharmacokinetics
Absorption: Bioavailablity after oral administration is 45%.
Distribution: Minimally plasma-bound.
Metabolism: Primary metabolism takes place via oxidative deamination by monoamine oxidase-A to the indoleacetic acid metabolite.
Excretion: 82% excreted in urine, 12% in feces, after oral administration.

Route	Onset	Peak	Duration
P.O.	Unknown	1-1½ hr	Unknown

Contraindications and precautions
Contraindicated in patients with ischemic heart disease (angina pectoris, history of MI, or documented silent ischemia) and in those with symptoms or findings consistent with ischemic heart disease, coronary artery vasospasm (Prinzmetal's variant angina), or other significant underlying CV disease. Also contraindicated in patients with uncontrolled hypertension or within 24 hours of treatment with another 5-HT agonist or an ergotamine-containing or ergot-type drug such as dihydroergotamine or methysergide. Don't give within 2 weeks of stopping an MAO inhibitor. Also contraindicated in patients hypersensitive to drug or its inactive ingredients.

Use cautiously in patients with hepatic or renal impairment. Use cautiously in patients with risk factors for coronary artery disease (such as hypertension, hypercholesterolemia, smoking, obesity, diabetes, strong family history of coronary artery disease, women with surgical or physiologic menopause, or men over age 40) unless a cardiac evaluation provides evidence that patient is free from cardiac disease.

Interactions
Drug-drug. *Ergot-containing or ergot-type drugs, such as dihydroergotamine and methysergide; other 5-HT$_1$ agonists:* May cause prolonged vasospastic reactions. Avoid use within 24 hours of rizatriptan.
MAO inhibitors (moclobemide), nonselective MAO inhibitors (types A and B; isocarboxazid, pargyline, phenelzine, tranylcypromine): May increase rizatriptan levels. Avoid use together, and allow at least 14 days between stopping an MAO inhibitor and giving rizatriptan.
Propranolol: May increase rizatriptan levels. Reduce rizatriptan dosage if needed.
Selective serotonin reuptake inhibitors, such as fluoxetine, fluvoxamine, paroxetine, and sertraline: May cause weakness, hyperreflexia, and incoordination. Monitor patient closely.

Adverse reactions

CNS: dizziness, headache, somnolence, paresthesia, asthenia, fatigue, hypesthesia, decreased mental acuity, euphoria, tremor.
CV: chest pain, pressure or heaviness, palpitations.
EENT: neck, throat and jaw pain, pressure or heaviness.
GI: dry mouth, nausea, diarrhea, vomiting.
Respiratory: dyspnea.
Skin: flushing.
Other: pain, warm or cold sensations, hot flashes.

Special considerations

• Drug should be used only after a definite diagnosis of migraine is established.
• Don't use drug to prevent migraines or treat hemiplegic migraines, basilar migraines, or cluster headaches.
• Safety of treating more than four headaches in a 30-day period, on average, hasn't been established.
ALERT Women of childbearing age should use barrier contraception during therapy because of the risk of fetal toxicity.
• Orally disintegrating tablets contain phenylalanine.

Patient monitoring

• For patient who has coronary risk factors but a satisfactory cardiac evaluation, monitor patient closely after first dose.
• Assess CV status if patient develops coronary risk factors during treatment.

Pregnant patients

• Advise women to notify prescriber about planned, suspected, or known pregnancy.

Breast-feeding patients

• Instruct women not to breast-feed because effects on infants are unknown.

Pediatric patients

• Safety and efficacy in children under age 18 haven't been established.

Patient education

• Inform patient that drug doesn't prevent migraine headaches.
• For Maxalt-MLT, tell patient to remove blister pack from pouch, and then to remove drug from blister pack immediately before use. Advise against popping tablet out of blister pack; instead, explain that pack should be carefully peeled away with dry hands and tablet placed on tongue and allowed to dissolve. Tell patient to swallow tablet with saliva; no water is needed or recommended.
• Tell patient that orally dissolving tablet doesn't provide more rapid headache relief.
• Advise patient that if headache returns after first dose, a second dose may be taken with medical approval at least 2 hours after the first dose. Advise against taking more than 30 mg in a 24-hour period.
• Inform patient that drug may cause somnolence and dizziness, and warn him to avoid hazardous activities until effects are known.
• Tell patient that food may delay onset of drug action.

rofecoxib
Vioxx

Pharmacologic classification: cyclooxygenase-2 (COX-2) inhibitor
Therapeutic classification: nonnarcotic analgesic, anti-inflammatory
Pregnancy risk category: C

Indications and dosages

➤ **Relief of signs and symptoms of osteoarthritis.** *Adults:* Initially, 12.5 mg P.O. once daily, increased as needed to a maximum of 25 mg P.O. once daily.
➤ **Management of acute pain and treatment of primary dysmenorrhea.** *Adults:* 50 mg P.O. once daily as needed for up to 5 days.

How supplied
Available by prescription only
Oral suspension: 12.5 mg/5 ml, 25 mg/5 ml
Tablets: 12.5 mg, 25 mg, 50 mg

Pharmacodynamics
Analgesic and anti-inflammatory actions: Exact mechanism of action is unknown. Anti-inflammatory effects, analgesic effects, and antipyretic activity may come from inhibition of prostaglandin synthesis, which drug does by inhibiting the COX-2 isoenzyme. At therapeutic serum levels, rofecoxib doesn't inhibit the COX-1 isoenzyme.

Pharmacokinetics
Absorption: Well absorbed, with a mean bioavailability of 93%. The median time for serum levels to peak is 2 to 3 hours.
Distribution: About 87% binds to proteins.
Metabolism: The liver metabolizes the drug to inactive metabolites.
Excretion: Eliminated mainly through hepatic metabolism. Less than 1% of the drug is eliminated from the kidneys as unchanged drug. Half-life is about 17 hours.

Route	Onset	Peak	Duration
P.O.	Unknown	2-9 hr	Unknown

Contraindications and precautions
Contraindicated in patients hypersensitive to rofecoxib or any of its components and in patients who have experienced asthma, urticaria, or allergic-type reactions after taking aspirin or other NSAIDs. Avoid use in patients with advanced kidney disease or moderate or severe hepatic in-

sufficiency. Avoid use in pregnant women because drug may cause the ductus arteriosus to close prematurely.

Use cautiously in patients with asthma, renal disease, liver dysfunction, or abnormal liver function tests. Also use cautiously in patients with a history of ulcer disease or GI bleeding. Use cautiously in patients being treated with oral corticosteroids or anticoagulants, in patients with a history of smoking or alcoholism, and in elderly or debilitated patients because of the increased risk of GI bleeding.

Use cautiously in patients with considerable dehydration. Rehydration is recommended before therapy begins. Use cautiously, and initiate therapy at the lowest recommended dose, in patients with fluid retention, hypertension, or heart failure.

Interactions

Drug-drug. *ACE inhibitors:* Decreased antihypertensive effects. Monitor patient closely.
Aspirin: Increased rate of GI ulceration and other complications. Don't use together, if possible. If used together, monitor patient closely for GI bleeding.
Furosemide, thiazide diuretics: Possible reduced efficacy of these drugs. Monitor patient closely.
Lithium: Increased lithium levels and decreased lithium clearance. Monitor patient closely for lithium toxicity.
Methotrexate: Increased methotrexate levels. Monitor patient closely for methotrexate toxicity.
Rifampin: Decreased rofecoxib levels by about 50%. Start therapy with an increased rofecoxib dosage.
Warfarin: Increased warfarin effects. Monitor INR frequently in the first few days after rofecoxib therapy starts or dosage changes.
Drug-herb. *Dong quai:* Increased risk of photosensitivity and bleeding. Discourage use together.
Feverfew, garlic, ginger, horse chestnut, red clover: Increased risk of bleeding. Discourage use together.
St. John's wort: Increased risk of photosensitivity. Advise patient to avoid unprotected exposure to sunlight.
Drug-lifestyle. *Long-term alcohol use, smoking:* Increased risk of GI bleeding. Monitor patient closely.

Adverse reactions

CNS: headache, asthenia, fatigue, dizziness.
CV: hypertension, leg edema.
EENT: sinusitis.
GI: diarrhea, dyspepsia, epigastric discomfort, heartburn, nausea, abdominal pain.
GU: urinary tract infection.
Musculoskeletal: back pain.
Respiratory: bronchitis, upper respiratory tract infection.
Other: flulike syndrome.

Overdose and treatment

In an overdose, remove unabsorbed drug from GI tract, monitor patient, and provide supportive therapy as needed. Hemodialysis doesn't remove drug; it's unknown if peritoneal dialysis removes it.

Special considerations

⚠ ALERT Patient may be allergic to rofecoxib if he's allergic to aspirin or other NSAIDs.
● Rehydrate patients who are dehydrated before starting rofecoxib.
● Fluid retention and edema have occurred in patients taking rofecoxib. Use the lowest recommended dose cautiously in patients with fluid retention, hypertension, or heart failure.
⚠ ALERT Patients taking rofecoxib have more than twice as many MIs, CVAs, and other cardiac events as those taking naproxen.
● NSAIDs may cause serious GI toxicity. Signs and symptoms include bleeding, ulceration, and perforation of the stomach, small intestine, and large intestine. Such toxicity can occur any time, with or without warning. To minimize the risk of an adverse GI event, use the lowest effective dosage of rofecoxib for the shortest possible duration. Monitor patient closely for GI bleeding.

Patient monitoring

● Drug may be hepatotoxic. Monitor patient for signs and symptoms of hepatotoxicity. Discontinue the drug, as ordered, if any signs and symptoms consistent with liver disease develop.
● Patients undergoing long-term treatment should have their hemoglobin level and hematocrit checked if they develop evidence of anemia or blood loss.

Pregnant patients

● Instruct women to report planned, suspected, or known pregnancy.

Breast-feeding patients

● It isn't known if rofecoxib appears in breast milk. However, because breast-fed infants are at risk for serious adverse reactions, women taking this drug shouldn't breast-feed.

Pediatric patients

● The safety and efficacy of rofecoxib in children under age 18 haven't been evaluated.

Geriatric patients

● No substantial differences in safety and effectiveness exist between elderly and younger patients. Although dosage needs no adjustment in elderly patients, drug should be started at lowest recommended dosage.

Patient education

● Tell patient that drug may be taken without regard to food and that taking the drug with food may decrease GI upset.

Reactions may be *common*, uncommon, *life-threatening*, or common and life-threatening.

• Tell patient that the most common minor adverse effects are dyspepsia, epigastric discomfort, heartburn, and nausea. Explain that taking drug with food may help minimize these effects.
• Warn patient about risk of GI bleeding. Explain that signs and symptoms include bloody vomitus, blood in urine and stool, and black, tarry stools. Advise patient to seek medical advice if he has any of these signs or symptoms.
• Advise patient to report rash, unexplained weight gain, or edema.
• Tell patient to avoid aspirin, aspirin-containing products, and OTC anti-inflammatories such as ibuprofen.
• Tell patient that all NSAIDs, including rofecoxib, may adversely affect the liver. Signs and symptoms of liver toxicity include nausea, fatigue, lethargy, itching, jaundice, right upper quadrant tenderness, and flulike symptoms. Advise patient to stop therapy and seek immediate medical advice if he has any of these signs or symptoms.

ropinirole hydrochloride
Requip

Pharmacologic classification: nonergoline dopamine agonist
Therapeutic classification: antiparkinsonian
Pregnancy risk category: C

Indications and dosages
➤ *Treatment of signs and symptoms of idiopathic Parkinson's disease.* *Adults:* Initially, 0.25 mg P.O. t.i.d. Based on patient response, dosage should then be adjusted at weekly intervals: 0.5 mg t.i.d. after week 1, 0.75 mg t.i.d. after week 2, and 1 mg t.i.d. after week 3. After week 4, dosage may be increased by 1.5 mg daily on a weekly basis up to a dose of 9 mg daily and then increased weekly by up to 3 mg daily to maximum dose of 24 mg daily.

How supplied
Available by prescription only
Tablets: 0.25 mg, 0.5 mg, 1 mg, 2 mg, 4mg, 5 mg

Pharmacodynamics
Antiparkinsonian action: Exact mechanism of action is unknown. Ropinirole is a nonergoline dopamine agonist thought to stimulate postsynaptic dopamine D_2 receptors in the caudate-putamen in the brain.

Pharmacokinetics
Absorption: Rapidly absorbed. Absolute bioavailability is 55%.
Distribution: Widely distributed throughout the body, with an apparent volume of distribution of 7.5 L/kg. Up to 40% is bound to plasma proteins.
Metabolism: Extensively metabolized by cytochrome P-450 CYP1A2 isoenzyme to inactive metabolites.

Excretion: Less than 10% is excreted unchanged in urine. Elimination half-life is 6 hours.

Route	Onset	Peak	Duration
P.O.	Unknown	1-2 hr	6 hr

Contraindications and precautions
Contraindicated in patients hypersensitive to drug or its components. Use cautiously in patients with severe renal or hepatic impairment.

Interactions
Drug-drug. *CNS depressants, including antipsychotics and benzodiazepines:* Increased CNS effects. Use together cautiously.
Dopamine antagonists, including butyrophenones, metoclopramide, phenothiazines, and thioxanthenes: May decrease effectiveness of ropinirole. Avoid use together.
Estrogens: Reduced ropinirole clearance. Adjust ropinirole dosage if needed.
Inhibitors or substrates of cytochrome P-450 CYP1A2, such as ciprofloxacin, fluvoxamine, mexiletine, and norfloxacin: Altered ropinirole clearance. Dosage adjustment of ropinirole may be required.
Drug-lifestyle. *Alcohol use:* Increased CNS effects. Discourage concurrent use.
Smoking: May increase ropinirole clearance. Monitor patient closely.

Adverse reactions
Early Parkinson's disease (without levodopa)
CNS: asthenia, hallucinations, *dizziness,* aggravated Parkinson's disease, *somnolence, fatigue,* headache, confusion, hyperkinesia, hypesthesia, vertigo, amnesia, impaired concentration, malaise.
CV: orthostatic hypotension, orthostatic symptoms, hypertension, *syncope,* edema, chest pain, extrasystoles, *atrial fibrillation,* palpitations, tachycardia.
EENT: pharyngitis, dry mouth, abnormal vision, eye abnormality, xerophthalmia, rhinitis, sinusitis.
GI: *nausea, vomiting, dyspepsia,* flatulence, abdominal pain, anorexia.
GU: urinary tract infection, impotence.
Respiratory: bronchitis, dyspnea.
Skin: flushing, increased sweating.
Other: *viral infection,* pain, yawning, peripheral ischemia.
Advanced Parkinson's disease (with levodopa)
CNS: *dizziness,* aggravated parkinsonism, *somnolence, headache,* insomnia, *hallucinations,* abnormal dreaming, confusion, tremor, *dyskinesia,* anxiety, nervousness, amnesia, hypokinesia, paresthesia, paresis.
CV: hypotension, syncope.
EENT: diplopia, dry mouth.
GI: *nausea,* abdominal pain, vomiting, constipation, diarrhea, dysphagia, flatulence, increased saliva.

GU: urinary tract infection, pyuria, urinary incontinence.
Hematologic: anemia.
Metabolic: weight decrease.
Musculoskeletal: arthralgia, arthritis.
Respiratory: upper respiratory tract infection, dyspnea.
Skin: increased sweating.
Other: injury, *falls*, viral infection, increased drug level, pain.

Overdose and treatment
There are reports of 10 patients ingesting more than 24 mg daily. Evidence of overdose includes mild oro-facial dyskinesia, agitation, increased dyskinesia, grogginess, sedation, orthostatic hypotension, chest pain, confusion, vomiting, and nausea.

Treatment involves general supportive measures and removal of unabsorbed drug.

Special considerations
● Dosage adjustment isn't needed in patients with mild to moderate renal impairment.
● Adjust drug cautiously in patients with severe renal or hepatic impairment.
● Although not reported with ropinirole, a symptom complex resembling neuroleptic malignant syndrome (elevated temperature, muscle rigidity, altered consciousness, autonomic instability) has been reported with rapid dose reduction or withdrawal of antiparkinsonians. If this occurs, stop drug gradually over 7 days and reduce frequency of administration to twice daily for 4 days and then once daily over the remaining 3 days.
● Other adverse events reported with dopaminergic therapy may occur with ropinirole, including withdrawal emergent hyperpyrexia and confusion, and fibrotic complications.
● Ropinirole can potentiate the dopaminergic adverse effects of levodopa and may cause or worsen dyskinesia. If this occurs, the levodopa dosage may need to be decreased.

Patient monitoring
● Monitor alkaline phosphatase and BUN levels because drug may increase them.
● Monitor patient carefully for symptomatic orthostatic hypotension, especially during dose escalation, because dopamine agonists impair systemic regulation of blood pressure.
● Syncope, with or without bradycardia, has been reported. Monitor patient carefully, especially for first 4 weeks of therapy and whenever dosage increases.

Breast-feeding patients
● Drug inhibits prolactin secretion and could inhibit lactation.
● It isn't known if drug appears in breast milk. A decision should be made to stop the drug or breast-feeding, taking into account the importance of drug to the woman.

Pediatric patients
● Safety and efficacy in children haven't been established.

Geriatric patients
● Dosage adjustments aren't necessary.
● Elderly patients are at greater risk of hallucinations than younger patients with Parkinson's disease.

Patient education
● Tell patient to take drug with food to reduce nausea.
● Advise patient that hallucinations may occur.
● Instruct patient to rise slowly from sitting or lying because of risk of orthostatic hypotension, particularly early in therapy or when dosage increases.
● Advise patient to use caution when driving or operating machinery until CNS effects of drug are known.

ropivacaine hydrochloride
Naropin

Pharmacologic classification: aminoamide
Therapeutic classification: local anesthetic
Pregnancy risk category: B

Indications and dosages
➤ *Surgical anesthesia. Adults:* For lumbar epidural administration in surgery, 75- to 200-mg doses (duration, 2 to 6 hours). For lumbar epidural administration for cesarean section, 100 to 150 mg (duration, 2 to 4 hours). For thoracic epidural administration, 25- to 75-mg doses to establish block for postoperative pain relief. For major nerve block (for example, brachial plexus block), 175 to 250 mg (duration, 5 to 8 hours). For field block (such as minor nerve blocks and infiltration), 5 to 200 mg (duration, 2 to 6 hours).
➤ *Labor pain management. Adults:* For lumbar epidural administration, initially, 20 to 40 mg (duration, ½ to 1½ hours); then 12 to 28 mg/hour as continuous infusion or 20 to 30 mg/hour as incremental "top-up" injections.
➤ *Postoperative pain management. Adults:* For lumbar epidural administration, 12 to 20 mg/hour as continuous infusion. For thoracic epidural administration, 8 to 16 mg/hour as continuous infusion. For infiltration (minor nerve block), 2 to 200 mg (duration, 2 to 6 hours).

How supplied
Available by prescription only
E-Z off single-dose vials: 7.5 mg/ml and 10 mg/ml in 10-ml vials
Infusion bottles: 2 mg/ml in 100-ml and 200-ml bottles
Single-dose vials: 2 mg/ml, 7.5 mg/ml, and 10 mg/ml in 20-ml vials; 5 mg/ml in 30-ml vials

---

Single-dose ampules: 2 mg/ml, 7.5 mg/ml, and 10 mg/ml in 20 ml ampules; 5 mg/ml in 30-ml ampules
Sterile-pak single-dose vials: 2 mg/ml, 7.5 mg/ml, and 10 mg/ml in 20-ml vials; 5 mg/ml in 30-ml vials

Pharmacodynamics

Anesthetic action: Drug blocks the generation and conduction of nerve impulses, presumably by increasing the threshold for electrical excitation in the nerve by slowing the propagation of the nerve impulse and by reducing the rate of the action potential. Generally, progression of anesthesia is related to the diameter, myelination and conduction velocity of affected nerve fibers. The order of lost nerve function is as follows: pain, temperature, touch, proprioception, and skeletal muscle tone.

Pharmacokinetics

Absorption: Absorption depends on total dose and concentration of administered drug, route of administration, patient's hemodynamic or circulatory condition, and vascularity of administration site. From the epidural space, drug shows complete and biphasic absorption; mean half-lives of two phases are 14 minutes and 4¼ hours, respectively. The slow absorption is a rate-limiting factor in elimination of drug. Terminal half-life is longer after epidural than after I.V. administration.
Distribution: After intravascular infusion, drug has steady state volume of distribution of 41 ± 7 L. Drug is 94% protein-bound, mainly to α1-acid glycoprotein. An increase in total plasma levels during continuous epidural infusion has been observed, secondary to a postoperative increase in α1-acid glycoprotein.
Metabolism: Extensively metabolized in the liver, via cytochrome P-4501A to 3-hydroxy ropivacaine. About 37% of dose is excreted in the urine as free drug and as a conjugated metabolites. Urinary excretion of metabolites accounts for only 3% of dose.
Excretion: Primarily excreted by the kidneys; 86% of the dose appears in urine after I.V. administration, of which only 1% relates to unchanged drug.

Route	Onset	Peak	Duration
Epidural	Unknown	Unknown	Unknown

Contraindications and precautions

Contraindicated in patients hypersensitive to drug or local anesthetics of amide type.

Use cautiously in debilitated, elderly, and acutely ill patients because accumulation may result. Also use cautiously in patients with hypotension, hypovolemia, impaired CV function, or heart block and in those with hepatic disease, especially repeat doses of drug.

Interactions

Drug-drug. *Amide-type anesthetics:* Additive effects. Use together cautiously.
Fluvoxamine, imipramine, theophylline, verapamil: Possible competitive inhibition of ropivacaine. Use together cautiously.

Adverse reactions

CNS: anxiety, dizziness, headache, hypesthesia, pain, paresthesia.
CV: *bradycardia*, chest pain, *hypotension*, hypertension, tachycardia.
GI: *nausea*, neonatal vomiting, vomiting.
GU: oliguria, urine retention.
Hematologic: anemia.
Hepatic: neonatal jaundice.
Respiratory: *neonatal tachypnea, respiratory distress.*
Skin: pruritus.
Other: back pain, FETAL BRADYCARDIA, *fetal tachycardia*, FETAL DISTRESS, fever, neonatal fever, postoperative complications, rigors.

Overdose and treatment

Treatment should be supportive and symptomatic. Discontinue drug. In case of unintentional subarachnoid injection of drug, establish a patent airway and administer 100% oxygen. This may prevent seizures if they haven't already occurred. Give drug to control seizures as appropriate.

Special considerations

⚠ ALERT Don't inject drug rapidly. Keep emergency equipment and personnel immediately available.
● Drug should be used only by personnel familiar with its use.
● Increase doses in incremental steps.
● Don't use in emergencies where a rapid onset of surgical anesthesia is necessary. Insufficient data are available to support use of drug to produce obstetric paracervical block anesthesia, retrobulbar block, or spinal anesthesia (subarachnoid block). I.V. regional anesthesia (Bier block) shouldn't be performed because of lack of clinical experience and risk of toxic ropivacaine levels.
● To reduce risk of serious adverse reactions, attempt to optimize patients who may be at risk, such as those with complete heart block or hepatic or renal impairment.
● Use an adequate test dose (3 to 5 ml of short-acting local anesthetic solution containing epinephrine) before induction of complete block.
● Don't use drug in ophthalmic surgery.

Patient monitoring

● Watch for early evidence of CNS toxicity, including restlessness, anxiety, incoherent speech, light-headedness, numbness and tingling of mouth and lips, metallic taste, tinnitus, dizziness, blurred vision, tremors, twitching, depression, or drowsiness.

Breast-feeding patients
• Appearance of drug in breast milk hasn't been studied; use together cautiously.

Pediatric patients
• Don't give drug to children under age 12.

Patient education
• Tell patient that he may have a temporary loss of sensation and motor activity in the anesthetized body part after proper administration of lumbar epidural anesthesia.
• Explain that adverse reactions that may occur.

rosiglitazone maleate
Avandia

Pharmacologic classification: thiazolidine-dione
Therapeutic classification: antidiabetic
Pregnancy risk category: C

Indications and dosages
➤ *Monotherapy adjunct to diet and exercise to improve glycemic control in patients with type 2 diabetes mellitus or combination therapy with a sulfonylurea or metformin when diet, exercise, and rosiglitazone alone or diet, exercise, and a sulfonylurea or metformin alone don't provide adequate glycemic control in patients with type 2 diabetes mellitus.*
Adults: Initially, 4 mg P.O. daily in the morning or in divided doses b.i.d. in the morning and evening. Dosage may be increased to 8 mg P.O. daily or in divided doses b.i.d. if fasting plasma glucose level doesn't improve after 12 weeks of treatment.

How supplied
Available by prescription only
Tablets: 2 mg, 4 mg, 8 mg

Pharmacodynamics
Antidiabetic action: Rosiglitazone lowers blood glucose levels by improving insulin sensitivity. Drug is a highly selective and potent agonist for receptors found in key areas of insulin action, such as adipose tissue, skeletal muscle, and liver.

Pharmacokinetics
Absorption: Plasma levels peak about 1 hour after dosing. The absolute bioavailability is 99%.
Distribution: About 99.8% binds to plasma proteins, primarily albumin.
Metabolism: Extensively metabolized, with no unchanged drug excreted in urine. Primarily metabolized through *N*-demethylation and hydroxylation.
Excretion: Following oral administration, about 64% and 23% of dose is eliminated in urine and

feces, respectively. The elimination half-life is 3 to 4 hours.

Route	Onset	Peak	Duration
P.O.	Unknown	1 hr	Unknown

Contraindications and precautions
Contraindicated in patients hypersensitive to rosiglitazone or any of its components and in patients with New York Heart Association Class III and IV cardiac status unless expected benefits outweigh risks. Don't use in patients with active liver disease, increased baseline liver enzyme levels (ALT level more than 2.5 times the upper limit of normal), type 1 diabetes, or diabetic ketoacidosis. Contraindicated in patients who experienced jaundice while taking troglitazone. Because metformin is contraindicated in patients with renal impairment, combination therapy with metformin and rosiglitazone is also contraindicated in such patients.
Use cautiously in patients with edema or heart failure.

Interactions
None reported.

Adverse reactions
CNS: headache, fatigue.
CV: edema.
EENT: sinusitis.
GI: diarrhea.
Hematologic: anemia.
Metabolic: hyperglycemia.
Musculoskeletal: back pain.
Respiratory: upper respiratory tract infection.
Other: injury.

Overdose and treatment
In an overdose, provide supportive treatment appropriate to patient's condition.

Special considerations
• Management of type 2 diabetes should include diet control. Because caloric restriction, weight loss, and exercise help improve insulin sensitivity and help make drug therapy effective, these measures are essential to proper diabetes treatment.
• Patients with normal hepatic enzyme levels who are switched from troglitazone to rosiglitazone should undergo a 1-week washout before starting rosiglitazone.
• For patients whose blood glucose levels are inadequately controlled with metformin, rosiglitazone should be added to—not substituted for—metformin.
• Rosiglitazone can be used as monotherapy in patients with renal impairment.

Patient monitoring
• Liver enzyme levels should be checked before therapy starts, every 2 months for the first 12 months of treatment, and periodically afterward.

If ALT level is elevated during treatment, recheck levels as soon as possible. Discontinue drug if levels remain elevated.

● Hemoglobin level and hematocrit may decrease while patient is receiving this drug, usually during the first 4 to 8 weeks of therapy. Increases in total cholesterol, low-density lipoprotein, and high-density lipoprotein levels and decreases in free fatty acid levels may also occur.

Breast-feeding patients

● It isn't known if rosiglitazone appears in breast milk. Rosiglitazone shouldn't be given to breast-feeding women.

Pediatric patients

● Safety and efficacy of rosiglitazone in children haven't been established.

Geriatric patients

● No substantial differences in safety and efficacy exist between patients over age 65 and younger patients. No dosage adjustments are needed for elderly patients.

Patient education

● Advise patient that rosiglitazone can be taken with or without food.
● Tell patient to immediately report unexplained signs and symptoms, such as nausea, vomiting, abdominal pain, fatigue, anorexia, or dark urine, to his prescriber because these may indicate potential liver problems.
● Inform premenopausal, anovulatory women with insulin resistance that ovulation may resume and contraceptive measures may need to be considered.
● Advise patient that management of diabetes should include diet control. Because caloric restriction, weight loss, and exercise help improve insulin sensitivity and help make drug therapy effective, these measures are essential to proper diabetes treatment.

rubella and mumps virus vaccine, live
Biavax II

Pharmacologic classification: vaccine
Therapeutic classification: viral vaccine
Pregnancy risk category: C

Indications and dosages

➤ **Rubella (German measles) and mumps immunization.** *Adults and children over age 1:* 1 vial (0.5 ml) S.C. in outer aspect of the upper arm.

How supplied

Available by prescription only
Injection: Single-dose vial containing not less than 1,000 $TCID_{50}$ (tissue culture infective doses) of the Wistar RA 27/3 rubella virus (propa-

gated in human diploid cell culture) and not less than 20,000 $TCID_{50}$ of the Jeryl Lynn mumps strain (grown in chick embryo cell culture)

Pharmacodynamics

Live rubella and mumps prophylaxis: Vaccine promotes active immunity to rubella and mumps viruses by inducing production of antibodies.

Pharmacokinetics

Absorption: Antibodies are usually detectable within 2 to 6 weeks; duration of vaccine-induced immunity is expected to be lifelong.
Distribution: No information available.
Metabolism: No information available.
Excretion: No information available.

Route	Onset	Peak	Duration
S.C.	Unknown	Unknown	10½ yr

Contraindications and precautions

Contraindicated in pregnant women, immunosuppressed patients, patients receiving corticosteroids (except as replacement therapy) or radiation therapy, and patients with cancer, blood dyscrasias, gamma globulin disorders, fever, active untreated tuberculosis, or history of anaphylaxis or anaphylactoid reactions to neomycin or eggs.

Interactions

Drug-drug. *Immune serum globulin or transfusions of blood and blood products:* May impair immune response to vaccine. Defer vaccination for 3 months.
Immunosuppressants: May interfere with response to vaccine. Monitor patient closely.

Adverse reactions

Musculoskeletal: arthritis, arthralgia.
Other: polyneuritis; rash; thrombocytopenic purpura; urticaria; fever; diarrhea; *anaphylaxis;* lymphadenopathy; pain, erythema, and induration at injection site.

Overdose and treatment

No information available.

Special considerations

● Keep epinephrine solution (1:1,000) available to treat allergic reactions.
● Rubella and mumps vaccine shouldn't be given less than 1 month before or after immunization with other live-virus vaccines, except for monovalent or trivalent live poliovirus vaccine or live, attenuated measles virus vaccine, which may be given simultaneously.
● Use only the diluent supplied. Discard reconstituted vaccine after 8 hours.
● Inject S.C. (not I.M.) into the outer aspect of the upper arm.
● Women who have rubella antibody titers of 1:8 or greater (by hemagglutination inhibition) need

not be vaccinated with the rubella vaccine component.

● Although rubella vaccine administration should be deferred in patients with febrile illness, it may be administered to susceptible children with mild illness such as upper respiratory tract infection.

● According to Centers for Disease Control and Prevention recommendations, measles, mumps, and rubella is the preferred vaccine.

● Women who aren't immune to rubella are at risk for congenital rubella injury to the fetus if exposed to it during pregnancy.

● Store vaccine at 36° to 46° F (2° to 8° C) and protect from light. Solution may be used if red, pink, or yellow, but it must be clear.

● Rubella and mumps vaccine may temporarily decrease the response to tuberculin skin testing. If a tuberculin skin test is needed, administer it either before or simultaneously with rubella and mumps vaccine.

● Revaccination or booster isn't required if patient was previously vaccinated at age 1 or older; however, there's no conclusive evidence of an increased risk of adverse reactions for persons who are already immune when vaccinated.

● Vaccine won't offer protection when given after exposure to natural rubella or mumps, but there's no evidence that it would be harmful.

Patient monitoring

● Obtain a thorough history of allergies (especially to antibiotics, eggs, chicken, or chicken feathers) and of reactions to immunizations.

● Perform skin testing first to assess vaccine sensitivity (against a control of normal saline solution in the opposite arm) in patients with history of anaphylactoid reactions to egg ingestion. Administer I.D. or scratch test with a 1:10 dilution. Read results after 5 to 30 minutes. Positive reaction is a wheal with or without pseudopodia and surrounding erythema.

Pregnant patients

● Tell women of childbearing age to avoid pregnancy for 3 months after immunization. Provide contraceptive information if necessary.

Breast-feeding patients

● Rubella virus or virus antigen appears in breast milk in about 68% of patients. Few adverse effects have been linked to breast-feeding after immunization with rubella-containing vaccines. Give vaccine cautiously to breast-feeding women.

Pediatric patients

● Live rubella and mumps virus vaccine isn't recommended for children under age 1 because retained maternal antibodies may interfere with immune response.

Patient education

● Tell patient that tingling sensations in limbs or arthritis-like aches and pains in joints may occur starting several days to several weeks after vaccination. These symptoms usually resolve within 1 week. Pain and inflammation at injection site and low-grade fever, rash, or breathing difficulties may also occur. Encourage patient to report distressing adverse reactions.

● Recommend acetaminophen to relieve fever or other minor discomfort.

rubella virus vaccine, live
Meruvax II

Pharmacologic classification: vaccine
Therapeutic classification: viral vaccine
Pregnancy risk category: C

Indications and dosages

➤ **Rubella (German measles) immunization.** Adults and children over age 1: 1 vial (0.5 ml) S.C.

How supplied

Available by prescription only
Injection: Single-dose vial containing not less than 1,000 TCID$_{50}$ (tissue culture infective doses) of the Wistar RA 27/3 strain of rubella virus propagated in human diploid cell culture

Pharmacodynamics

Rubella prophylaxis: Vaccine promotes active immunity to rubella by inducing production of antibodies.

Pharmacokinetics

Absorption: Antibodies are usually detectable 2 to 6 weeks after injection; duration of vaccine-induced immunity is expected to be lifelong.
Distribution: No information available.
Metabolism: No information available.
Excretion: No information available.

Route	Onset	Peak	Duration
S.C.	2-6 wk	Unknown	> 10 yr

Contraindications and precautions

Contraindicated in pregnant women, immunosuppressed patients, patients receiving corticosteroids (except as replacement therapy) or radiation therapy, and patients with cancer, blood dyscrasias, gamma globulin disorders, fever, active untreated tuberculosis, or history of hypersensitivity to neomycin.

Interactions

Drug-drug. *Immune serum globulin or transfusions of blood and blood products:* May impair immune response to vaccine. If possible, defer vaccination for 3 months.
Immunosuppressants: May reduce response to vaccine. Monitor patient closely. Defer vaccination until immunosuppressant is discontinued, if possible.

Adverse reactions

CNS: polyneuritis, malaise, headache.
EENT: sore throat.
Musculoskeletal: arthralgia, arthritis.
Skin: rash, *thrombocytopenic purpura*, urticaria.
Other: fever; *anaphylaxis;* lymphadenopathy; pain, erythema, and induration at injection site.

Overdose and treatment

No information available.

Special considerations

● Keep epinephrine solution (1:1,000) available to treat allergic reactions.
● Don't give rubella vaccine less than 1 month before or after immunization with other live virus vaccines, except for monovalent or trivalent live poliovirus vaccine; live, attenuated measles virus vaccine; or live mumps virus vaccine, which may be administered simultaneously.
● Don't inject I.M. Inject S.C. into the outer aspect of the upper arm.
● Use only diluent supplied. Discard 8 hours after reconstituting.
● Store vaccine at 36° to 46° F (2° to 8° C), and protect from light. Solution may be used if red, pink, or yellow, but it must be clear.
● Vaccine won't offer protection when given after exposure to natural rubella, although there's no evidence that it would be harmful.
● Although rubella vaccine administration should be deferred in patients with febrile illness, it may be administered to susceptible children with mild illnesses such as upper respiratory tract infection.
● Rubella vaccine may temporarily decrease response to tuberculin skin testing. If a tuberculin test is necessary, administer it either before, simultaneously with, or at least 8 weeks after rubella vaccine.
● Women who have rubella antibody titers of 1:8 or greater (by hemagglutination inhibition) need not be vaccinated with rubella virus vaccine.
● Revaccination or booster dose is required if patient was previously vaccinated under age 1. The Advisory Committee on Immunization Practices and the American Academy of Pediatrics currently recommend that a second dose be routinely given at ages 4 to 6 or 11 to 12. It may be given at any other time provided at least 1 month has elapsed since the first dose. There's no conclusive evidence of an increased risk of adverse reactions for persons who are already immune when revaccinated.

Patient monitoring

● Obtain a thorough history of allergies, especially to antibiotics, and of reactions to immunizations.

Pregnant patients

● Women who aren't immune to rubella are at risk for congenital rubella injury to the fetus if exposed to rubella during pregnancy. Tell women of childbearing age to avoid pregnancy for 3 months after rubella immunization. Provide contraceptive information if necessary.

Breast-feeding patients

● Rubella virus or virus antigen appears in breast milk in about 68% of patients. Few adverse effects have been linked to breast-feeding after immunization with rubella-containing vaccines. Risk-benefit ratio suggests that breast-feeding women may be immunized, if necessary.

Pediatric patients

● Live, attenuated rubella virus vaccine isn't recommended for children under age 1 because retained maternal antibodies may impair immune response.

Patient education

● Tell patient that tingling sensations in limbs or arthritis-like aches and pains in joints may occur starting several days to several weeks after vaccination. These symptoms usually resolve within 1 week. Pain and inflammation at injection site and low-grade fever, rash, or breathing difficulties may also occur. Encourage patient to report distressing adverse reactions.
● Recommend acetaminophen to relieve fever or other minor discomfort after vaccination.

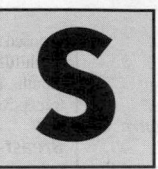

salmeterol xinafoate
Serevent

Pharmacologic classification: selective beta$_2$-adrenergic stimulating agonist
Therapeutic classification: bronchodilator
Pregnancy risk category: C

Indications and dosages
➤ **Long-term maintenance treatment of asthma; prevention of bronchospasm in patients with nocturnal asthma or reversible obstructive airway disease who require regular treatment with short-acting beta agonists.** Aerosol. *Adults and children over age 12:* Two inhalations (42 mcg) b.i.d. in the morning and evening about 12 hours apart.
Powder
Adults and children age 4 and older: One inhalation (50 mcg) twice daily, in the morning and evening about 12 hours apart.
➤ **Prevention of exercise-induced bronchospasm.** Aerosol. *Adults and children over age 12:* Two inhalations (42 mcg) at least 30 to 60 minutes before exercise.
Powder
Adults and children age 4 and older: Two inhalations (50 mcg) at least 30 minutes before exercise.
➤ **COPD or emphysema ◇.** Aerosol. *Adults:* 2 inhalations (42 mcg) twice daily about 12 hours apart, morning and evening.

How supplied
Available by prescription only
Inhalation aerosol: 25 mcg per activation in 6.5-g canister (60 activations), 25 mcg per activation in 13-g canister (120 activations)
Inhalation powder: 50 mcg/blister

Pharmacodynamics
Bronchodilator action: Salmeterol selectively stimulates beta$_2$-adrenergic receptors, resulting in bronchodilation. Drug also blocks the release of histamine from mast cells lining the respiratory tract, which produces vasodilation and increases ciliary motility.

Pharmacokinetics
Absorption: Because of the low therapeutic dose, systemic levels of salmeterol are low or undetectable after inhalation.
Distribution: Highly bound to human plasma proteins (94% to 99%).
Metabolism: Extensively metabolized by hydroxylation.
Excretion: Excreted primarily in feces.

Route	Onset	Peak	Duration
Inhalation	10-20 min	3 hr	12 hr

Contraindications and precautions
Contraindicated in patients hypersensitive to drug or its formulation. Use cautiously in patients with coronary insufficiency, arrhythmias, hypertension, other CV disorders, thyrotoxicosis, or seizure disorders and in those unusually responsive to sympathomimetics.

Interactions
Drug-drug. *Beta-adrenergic agonists, theophylline, or other methylxanthines:* Possible adverse cardiac effects with excessive use of salmeterol. Monitor patient closely.
MAO inhibitors, tricyclic antidepressants: Risk of severe adverse CV effects. Avoid use of salmeterol within 14 days of MAO inhibitor.

Adverse reactions
CNS: *headache,* sinus headache, tremor, nervousness, giddiness.
CV: tachycardia, palpitations, *ventricular arrhythmias.*
EENT: *nasopharyngitis,* nasal cavity or sinus disorder.
GI: nausea, vomiting, diarrhea, heartburn.
Musculoskeletal: joint and back pain, myalgia.
Respiratory: *upper respiratory tract infection,* cough, lower respiratory tract infection, *bronchospasm.*
Other: hypersensitivity reactions (rash, urticaria).

Overdose and treatment
Overdose may result in exaggerated pharmacologic adverse effects of beta-adrenoceptor agonists: tachycardia, arrhythmias, tremor, headache, and muscle cramps. Overdose can lead to clinically significant prolongation of the QT interval, which can produce ventricular arrhythmias. Cardiac arrest and death may be linked to abuse of salmeterol. Other signs of overdose may include hypokalemia and hyperglycemia.

In these cases, stop therapy with salmeterol and all beta-adrenergic–stimulant drugs, provide supportive therapy, and consider judicious use of a beta blocker, bearing in mind the possibility that such agents can produce bronchospasm. Cardiac monitoring is recommended in cases of

---

Reactions may be *common,* uncommon, *life-threatening,* or COMMON AND LIFE-THREATENING.

salmeterol overdose. Dialysis isn't appropriate treatment.

Special considerations
● Don't use drug in patients whose asthma can be managed by occasional use of a short-acting, inhaled beta₂-agonist such as albuterol.

⚠ ALERT Paradoxical bronchospasms (which can be life-threatening) have been reported with salmeterol. If they occur, discontinue salmeterol immediately and start alternative therapy.

● Salmeterol shouldn't be inhaled more than twice daily (morning and evening) at the recommended dose. Provide patient with a short-acting inhaled beta₂-agonist for treatment of symptoms that occur despite regular twice-daily use of salmeterol.
● Salmeterol isn't a substitute for oral or inhaled corticosteroids.

Patient monitoring
● Monitor patient's response to drug therapy.

Breast-feeding patients
● Give drug cautiously to breast-feeding women because it isn't known if drug appears in breast milk.

Pediatric patients
● Safety and efficacy of aerosol in children under age 12 haven't been established.

Geriatric patients
● As with other beta₂-agonists, salmeterol should be used with extreme caution in elderly patients who have CV disease and who could be adversely affected by this class of drugs.

Patient education
● Inform patient that drug isn't meant to relieve acute asthmatic symptoms. Instead, acute symptoms should be treated with an inhaled, short-acting bronchodilator that has been prescribed for symptomatic relief.
● Patients receiving salmeterol twice daily shouldn't use additional doses to prevent exercise-induced bronchospasm.
● Instruct patient on the proper use of the salmeterol inhalation devices, and tell patient to review the illustrated instructions in the package insert.
● Tell patient to shake the aerosol container well before using.
● Remind patient to take drug at 12-hour intervals for optimum effect and to take it even when he's feeling better.
● If patient takes a short-acting inhaled beta₂-agonist daily, tell him to stop taking it daily and to start taking it only as needed if asthma symptoms develop while taking salmeterol.
● If patient takes an inhaled corticosteroid, tell him to continue using it regularly. Warn him not to take other drugs without medical approval.
● Tell patient not to use inhalation powder with a spacer.

● Tell patient to notify prescriber if short-acting agonist no longer provides sufficient relief or if more than four inhalations are being used daily. This may be a sign that asthma symptoms are worsening.
● Caution against washing the mouthpiece or any part of the inhalation powder device. Tell patient to keep it dry.

---

saquinavir
Fortovase

saquinavir mesylate
Invirase

Pharmacologic classification: HIV-1 and HIV-2 proteinase inhibitor
Therapeutic classification: antiviral
Pregnancy risk category: B

Indications and dosages
➤ *Adjunct treatment of advanced HIV infection in selected patients.* Adults: 600 mg (Invirase, three 200-mg capsules) P.O. t.i.d. taken within 2 hours after a full meal and with a nucleoside analogue. Or, 1,200 mg (Fortovase, six 200-mg capsules) t.i.d. within 2 hours after a full meal with a nucleoside analogue.
✦ *Dosage adjustment.* If toxicity develops with saquinavir or saquinavir mesylate, interrupt drug therapy. In combination therapy with nucleoside analogues, base dosage adjustments of the nucleoside analogue on the known toxicity profile of specific drug.

How supplied
Available by prescription only
Saquinavir
Capsules (soft gelatin): 200 mg
Saquinavir mesylate
Capsules (hard gelatin): 200 mg

Pharmacodynamics
Antiviral action: Saquinavir inhibits the activity of HIV protease and prevents the cleavage of HIV polyproteins, which are essential for the maturation of HIV.

Pharmacokinetics
Absorption: Poorly absorbed from the GI tract. Higher saquinavir levels are achieved with Fortovase compared with Invirase. Fortovase has a relative bioavailability of 331% of Invirase.
Distribution: About 98% bound to plasma proteins.
Metabolism: Rapidly metabolized.
Excretion: Excreted mainly in feces.

Route	Onset	Peak	Duration
P.O.	Unknown	Unknown	Unknown

Contraindications and precautions

Contraindicated in patients hypersensitive to drug or components of capsule. Coadministration is contraindicated with ergot alkaloids and derivatives, midazolam, and triazolam.

Interactions

Drug-drug. *Amprenavir:* Decreased amprenavir levels. Use together cautiously.

Delavirdine: Increased saquinavir levels. Use together cautiously, and monitor hepatic enzymes.

Indinavir, nelfinavir, ritonavir: Increased saquinavir levels. Use together cautiously.

Ketoconazole: Increased saquinavir levels. Avoid use together.

Macrolide antibiotics such as clarithromycin: Increased levels of both drugs. Use together cautiously.

Rifabutin, rifampin: Decreased steady state saquinavir levels. Give rifabutin and saquinavir together cautiously. Don't use with rifampin.

Sildenafil: Increased peak plasma levels and increased risk of sildenafil-related adverse reactions, such as hypotension, vision changes, and priapism. Sildenafil dose shouldn't exceed 25 mg in a 48-hour period.

Drug-herb. *St. John's wort:* May substantially reduce drug levels and therapeutic effects. Warn against concomitant use.

Drug-food. *Any food:* Increased drug absorption. Advise patient to take drug with food.

Adverse reactions

CNS: paresthesia, headache.
EENT: pharyngitis, rhinitis, epistaxis.
GI: diarrhea, ulcerated buccal mucosa, abdominal pain, nausea, *pancreatitis.*
Musculoskeletal: asthenia, musculoskeletal pain.
Respiratory: bronchitis, dyspnea, hemoptysis, upper respiratory tract disorder, cough.
Skin: rash.

Overdose and treatment

Limited information available. One patient in clinical studies ingested 8 g as a single dose with no evidence of acute toxicity. Emesis was induced 2 to 4 hours after ingestion.

Special considerations

● If serious or severe toxicity occurs during treatment, discontinue drug until the cause is identified or toxicity resolves. Dose modification isn't needed when drug is resumed.

● Invirase will be phased out and replaced by Fortovase. Be aware of the dosing differences.

Patient monitoring

● Evaluate CBC, platelets, electrolytes, uric acid, liver enzymes, and bilirubin before therapy starts and at appropriate intervals during therapy.

● Monitor plasma HIV-1 RNA levels and CD4+ T-cell counts to determine risk of disease progression and need to modify antiretroviral therapy.

Pregnant patients

● Use drug only when clearly needed. There are no adequate and controlled studies.

Breast-feeding patients

● Although safety of drug hasn't been established in breast-feeding women, to avoid transmitting virus to infant, women with HIV infection shouldn't breast-feed.

Pediatric patients

● Safety and efficacy in children under age 16 haven't been established.

Patient education

● Warn patient of adipogenic effects such as redistribution or accumulation of body fat.

● Inform patient that drug should be taken within 2 hours following a full meal.

● Tell patient to report adverse reactions.

● Inform patient that drug usually is given with other AIDS-related antivirals.

● Tell patient to use Fortovase within 3 months when stored at room temperature or refer to expiration date on the label if capsules are refrigerated.

---

sargramostim (granulocyte-macrophage colony-stimulating factor, GM-CSF)
Leukine

Pharmacologic classification: biologic response modifier
Therapeutic classification: colony-stimulating factor
Pregnancy risk category: C

Indications and dosages

➤ *Acceleration of hematopoietic reconstitution after autologous bone marrow transplantation in patients with malignant lymphoma, acute lymphoblastic leukemia, or Hodgkin's disease. Adults:* 250 mcg/m² daily for 21 consecutive days given as a 2-hour I.V. infusion daily, beginning 2 to 4 hours after the bone marrow transplant. Don't administer within 24 hours of last dose of chemotherapy or within 12 hours after last dose of radiotherapy because of potential sensitivity of rapidly dividing progenitor cells to cytotoxic chemotherapeutic or radiologic therapies.

✦ *Dosage adjustment.* Reduce dosage by half or temporarily discontinue if severe adverse reactions occur. Therapy may be resumed when reaction abates. If blast cells appear or increase to 10% or more of the WBC count or if progression of the underlying disease occurs, discontinue therapy. If absolute neutrophil count is more than 20,000 cells/mm³ or if WBC counts are more than 50,000 cells/mm³, discontinue therapy temporarily or reduce the dose by half.

➤ **Bone marrow transplantation failure or engraftment delay.** *Adults:* 250 mcg/m² daily for 14 days as a 2-hour I.V. infusion. Same course may be repeated after 7 days off therapy if engraftment hasn't occurred. Third course of 500 mcg/m² for 14 days may be given after another 7 days off therapy if engraftment hasn't occurred.

➤ **Acute myelogenous leukemia.** *Adults:* 250 mcg/m² daily by I.V. infusion over 4 hours. Start therapy about day 11 or 4 days following completion of induction therapy. Use only if bone marrow is hypoplastic (fewer than 5% blasts on day 10). Continue until absolute neutrophil count exceeds 1,500/mm³ for 3 consecutive days or for a maximum of 42 days.

➤ **Myelodysplastic syndromes** ◊. *Adults:* 15 to 500 mcg/m² daily by I.V. infusion over 1 to 12 hours.

➤ **Aplastic anemia** ◊. *Adults:* 15 to 480 mcg/m² daily by I.V. infusion over 1 to 12 hours.

How supplied
Available by prescription only
Injection (preservative-free): 250 mcg, 500 mcg (as lyophilized powder) in single-dose vials

Pharmacodynamics
Immunostimulant action: Sargramostim is a 127-amino acid glycoprotein manufactured by recombinant DNA technology in a yeast expression system. It differs from the natural human granulocyte-macrophage colony-stimulating factor by the substitution of leucine for arginine at position 23. The carbohydrate moiety may also be different. Sargramostim induces cellular responses by binding to specific receptors on cell surfaces of target cells. Blood counts return to normal or baseline levels within 2 to 10 days after stopping treatment.

Pharmacokinetics
Absorption: Blood levels detectable within 5 minutes after S.C. administration.
Distribution: Bound to specific receptors on target cells.
Metabolism: Unknown.
Excretion: Unknown.

Route	Onset	Peak	Duration
I.V., S.C.	15 min	2-4 hr	Unknown

Contraindications and precautions
Contraindicated in patients with excessive leukemic myeloid blasts in bone marrow or peripheral blood and in those hypersensitive to drug or its components or to yeast-derived products. Also contraindicated with simultaneous administration of or with 24 hours preceding or following chemotherapy or radiotherapy.

Use cautiously in patients with impaired renal or hepatic function, cardiac disease, fluid retention, hypoxia, pulmonary infiltrates, or heart failure.

Interactions
Drug-drug. *Corticosteroids, lithium:* May potentiate myeloproliferative effects of sargramostim. Use together cautiously.

Adverse reactions
CNS: *malaise, CNS disorders, asthenia.*
CV: *blood dyscrasias, edema,* supraventricular arrhythmia, pericardial effusion, *peripheral edema.*
GI: *nausea, vomiting, diarrhea, anorexia, GI disorders, stomatitis.*
GU: *urinary tract disorder,* abnormal kidney function.
Hematologic: *hemorrhage,* stimulation of hematopoiesis.
Hepatic: *liver damage.*
Musculoskeletal: *bone pain.*
Respiratory: *dyspnea, lung disorders,* pleural effusion.
Skin: *alopecia, rash.*
Other: *fever, mucous membrane disorder,* sepsis.

Overdose and treatment
Doses up to 16 times recommended have been administered with the following reversible adverse reactions: WBC counts up to 200,000/mm³, dyspnea, malaise, nausea, fever, rash, sinus tachycardia, headache, and chills. The maximum dose that can be administered safely has yet to be determined. If overdose is suspected, monitor WBC count increase and respiratory symptoms.

Special considerations
● To prepare, reconstitute with 1 ml sterile water for injection. Don't reenter or reuse the single-dose vial. Discard unused portion. Direct stream of sterile water against side of vial and gently swirl contents to minimize foaming. Avoid excessive or vigorous agitation or shaking. Dilute in normal saline solution. If final concentration is less than 10 mcg/ml, add albumin (human) at a final concentration of 0.1% to the saline before addition of sargramostim to prevent adsorption to components of the delivery system. For a final concentration of 0.1% human albumin, add 1 mg human albumin per milliliter normal saline solution. Administer as soon as possible after admixture, because sargramostim has no preservative, and within 6 hours of reconstitution or dilution. Don't add other medications to infusion solution without compatibility and stability data. Discard unused solution after 6 hours. Don't infuse drug using an in-line membrane filter because absorption of drug could occur.
● Transient rash and local injection site reactions may occur; no serious allergic or anaphylactoid reactions have been reported.
● Drug can act as a growth factor for any tumor type, particularly myeloid malignancies.

• Unlabeled indications include use to increase WBC counts in patients with myelodysplastic syndromes and in patients with AIDS on zidovudine; to decrease nadir of leukopenia secondary to myelosuppressive chemotherapy; to decrease myelosuppression in preleukemic patients; to correct neutropenia in patients with aplastic anemia; and to decrease transplant-associated organ system damage, particularly of the liver and kidneys.

• Drug accelerates myeloid recovery in patients receiving bone marrow purged from monoclonal antibodies.

• Refrigerate sterile powder, reconstituted solution, and diluted solution for injection. Don't freeze or shake. Don't use after expiration date.

Patient monitoring

• Stimulation of marrow precursors may result in rapid elevation of WBC count; biweekly monitoring of CBC count with differential, including examination for blast cells, is recommended.

• The effect of drug may be limited in patients who have received extensive radiotherapy to hematopoietic sites for treatment of primary disease in the abdomen or chest or have been exposed to several agents (alkylating agents, anthracycline antibiotics, antimetabolites) before autologous bone marrow transplant.

Breast-feeding patients

• It isn't known if drug appears in breast milk. Use cautiously in breast-feeding women.

Pediatric patients

• Safety and efficacy in children haven't been established; however, available data suggest no differences in toxicity. The type and frequency of adverse reactions are comparable to those seen in adults.

Patient education

• Review administration schedule with patient and caregivers. Answer any questions and address concerns.

scopolamine hydrobromide

Isopto Hyoscine, Scopace,
Transderm-Scop

Pharmacologic classification: anticholinergic
Therapeutic classification: antimuscarinic, cycloplegic mydriatic
Pregnancy risk category: C

Indications and dosages

➤*Antimuscarinic, adjunct to anesthesia, prevention of nausea and vomiting.*
Adults: 0.3 to 0.6 mg I.M., S.C., or I.V. (after dilution with sterile water for injection) as a single dose. Apply transdermal system the evening before surgery. In cesarean section, apply 1 hour before surgery.

Children: 0.006 mg/kg I.M., S.C., or I.V. (after dilution with sterile water for injection) as a single daily dose. Maximum dose, 0.3 mg.

➤*Prevention of nausea and vomiting caused by motion sickness. Adults:* 1 transdermal patch applied behind the ear 4 hours before anticipated exposure to motion. Or, 0.25 to 0.8 mg P.O. 1 hour before exposure to motion; then t.i.d., as needed.

➤*Cycloplegic refraction. Adults:* 1 to 2 drops 0.25% solution in eye 1 hour before refraction. *Children:* 1 drop 0.25% solution b.i.d. for 2 days before refraction.

➤*Iritis, uveitis. Adults:* 1 to 2 drops of 0.25% solution daily or up to t.i.d.
Children: 1 drop of 0.25% solution up to t.i.d.

How supplied

Available by prescription only
Injection: 0.3 and 1 mg/ml in 1-ml vials; 0.4 mg/ml, 0.86 mg/ml in 0.5-ml ampules
Ophthalmic solution: 0.25%
Tablets (soluble): 0.4 mg
Transdermal system: 1.5 mg

Pharmacodynamics

Antimuscarinic action: Scopolamine inhibits muscarinic action of acetylcholine on autonomic effectors, decreasing secretions and GI motility. It also blocks vagal inhibition of SA node.
Mydriatic action: Scopolamine competitively blocks acetylcholine at cholinergic neuroeffector sites, antagonizing effects of acetylcholine on the sphincter muscle and ciliary body, producing mydriasis and cycloplegia.

Pharmacokinetics

Absorption: Rapidly absorbed when administered I.M. or S.C. Systemic drug absorption may occur from drug passage through the nasolacrimal duct.
Distribution: Distributed widely throughout body tissues. Drug crosses the placenta and probably the blood-brain barrier.
Metabolism: Probably metabolized completely in the liver; however, its exact metabolic fate is unknown. Mydriatic and cycloplegic effects persist for 3 to 7 days.
Excretion: Probably in urine as metabolites.

Route	Onset	Peak	Duration
P.O.	Unknown	1 hr	Unknown
I.M., I.V., S.C.	Varies	Varies	Varies
Ophthalmic	Rapid	15-45 min	< 1 wk
Transdermal	4 hr	24 hr	72 hr

Contraindications and precautions

Scopolamine is contraindicated in patients hypersensitive to the drug, any other belladonna alkaloid, or any ingredient or component in the formulation or administration system.

Reactions may be *common*, uncommon, *life-threatening*, or COMMON AND LIFE-THREATENING.

Systemic form is contraindicated in patients with angle-closure glaucoma, obstructive uropathy, obstructive disease of the GI tract, asthma, chronic pulmonary disease, myasthenia gravis, paralytic ileus, intestinal atony, unstable CV status in acute hemorrhage, or toxic megacolon. Ophthalmic form is contraindicated in patients with shallow anterior chamber and angle-closure glaucoma.

Soluble tablets are contraindicated in patients with prostatic hyperplasia or impaired renal or hepatic function; they should be used cautiously in patients with cardiac disease.

Use systemic form cautiously in patients in hot or humid environments and in patients with autonomic neuropathy, hyperthyroidism, coronary artery disease, arrhythmias, heart failure, hypertension, hiatal hernia with reflux esophagitis, hepatic or renal disease, or ulcerative colitis. Use ophthalmic form cautiously in infants, children, elderly patients, and patients with cardiac disease.

Use transdermal form cautiously in patients with history of seizures or psychosis.

Interactions
Drug-drug. *Anticholinergics, such as ketoconazole and levodopa:* Decreased GI absorption. Separate administration times by 2 to 3 hours.
CNS depressants, including sedative-hypnotics and tranquilizers: May increase CNS depression. Monitor patient closely.
Digoxin: Increased serum digoxin levels. Monitor patient for digitalis toxicity.
Drugs with anticholinergic effects: May cause additive toxicity. Avoid use together.
Oral potassium supplements, especially wax-matrix formulations: Potassium-induced GI ulcerations may be increased. Use together cautiously.
Drug-herb. *Jaborandi, pill-bearing spurge:* Decreased scopolamine effects. Monitor patient closely.
Squaw vine: Tannic acid may decrease metabolic breakdown or scopolamine. Discourage concomitant use.
Drug-lifestyle. *Alcohol use:* Increased risk of CNS depression. Advise patient to avoid alcohol.
Sun exposure: Possible photophobia with ophthalmic form. Urge patient to take precautions.

Adverse reactions
CNS: disorientation, restlessness, irritability, dizziness, drowsiness, headache, confusion, hallucinations, delirium.
CV: tachycardia, palpitations and *paradoxical bradycardia* with systemic form.
EENT: blurred vision; photophobia; increased intraocular pressure; dilated pupils and difficulty swallowing with systemic form; ocular congestion with prolonged use; conjunctivitis, dry eyes, itching eyes, transient stinging and burning, and edema with ophthalmic form.

GI: dry mouth; *constipation, nausea, vomiting, and epigastric distress* with systemic form.
GU: urinary hesitancy and urine retention with systemic form.
Respiratory: bronchial plugging and depressed respirations with systemic form.
Skin: rash and flushing with systemic form, dryness or contact dermatitis with ophthalmic form.
Other: fever with systemic form.

Overdose and treatment
Effects of overdose include excitability, seizures, CNS stimulation followed by depression, and such psychotic symptoms as disorientation, confusion, hallucinations, delusions, anxiety, agitation, delirium, and restlessness. Peripheral effects include dilated, nonreactive pupils; blurred vision; flushed, hot, dry skin; dryness of mucous membranes; dysphagia; decreased or absent bowel sounds; urine retention; hyperthermia; tachycardia; hypertension; and increased respiration.

Treatment is primarily symptomatic and supportive, as needed. Maintain patent airway. Remove transdermal system. If patient is awake and alert, induce emesis (or use gastric lavage) and follow with a sodium chloride cathartic and activated charcoal to prevent further drug absorption. In severe life-threatening cases, physostigmine may be administered to block the antimuscarinic effects of scopolamine. Give fluids, as needed, to treat shock; diazepam to control psychotic symptoms; and pilocarpine (instilled into the eyes) to relieve mydriasis. If urine retention develops, catheterization may be necessary.

Special considerations
● Intermittent and continuous I.V. infusions aren't recommended.
● Some patients, especially elderly patients, may experience transient excitement or disorientation.
Ophthalmic form
● Have patient lie down, tilt head back, or look at ceiling to aid instillation.
● Apply pressure to the lacrimal sac for 1 minute after instillation to reduce the risk of systemic drug absorption.
Transdermal form
● Patch delivers about 1 mg in 72 hours. Remove it when antiemetic effect is no longer required.

Patient monitoring
● Therapeutic doses may produce amnesia, drowsiness, and euphoria (desired effects for use as an adjunct to anesthesia). Monitor patient for these effects, and reorient patient as needed.

Breast-feeding patients
● Scopolamine appears in breast milk. Use cautiously in nursing women.

Pediatric patients
• Safety and efficacy of soluble tablets or transdermal system haven't been established in children. Use ophthalmic form cautiously, if at all, in infants and young children.

Geriatric patients
• Give drug cautiously and in decreased amounts to elderly patients.

Patient education
Ophthalmic form
• Instruct patient to apply pressure to bridge of nose for about 1 minute after instillation.
• Advise patient not to close eyes tightly or blink for about 1 minute after instillation.
Transdermal form
• Tell patient to wash hands after applying the patch.
• Instruct patient to use only one patch at a time.

secobarbital sodium
Seconal

Pharmacologic classification: barbiturate
Therapeutic classification: sedative-hypnotic
Controlled substance schedule: II
Pregnancy risk category: D

Indications and dosages
➤ *Preoperative sedation. Adults:* 200 to 300 mg P.O. 1 to 2 hours before surgery.
Children: 2 to 6 mg/kg P.O. (maximum dose, 100 mg).
➤ *Insomnia. Adults:* 100 mg P.O.

How supplied
Available by prescription only
Capsules: 100 mg

Pharmacodynamics
Sedative-hypnotic action: Secobarbital acts throughout the CNS as a nonselective depressant with a rapid onset and short duration of action. Particularly sensitive to this drug is the reticular activating system, which controls CNS arousal. Secobarbital decreases both presynaptic and postsynaptic membrane excitability by facilitating the action of gamma-aminobutyric acid. The exact cellular site and mechanisms of action are unknown.

Pharmacokinetics
Absorption: After oral administration, 90% is absorbed rapidly. Levels of 1 to 5 mcg/ml are needed to produce sedation; 5 to 15 mcg/ml are needed for hypnosis.
Distribution: Distributed rapidly throughout body tissues and fluids; about 30% to 45% is protein-bound.
Metabolism: Oxidized in the liver to inactive metabolites. Duration of action is 3 to 4 hours.

Excretion: About 95% of a dose is eliminated as glucuronide conjugates and other metabolites in urine. Drug has an elimination half-life of about 30 hours.

Route	Onset	Peak	Duration
P.O.	15 min	15-30 min	1-4 hr

Contraindications and precautions
Contraindicated in patients with respiratory disease involving dyspnea or obstruction and in patients hypersensitive to barbiturates or porphyria.

Use cautiously in patients with acute or chronic pain, depression, suicidal tendencies, history of drug abuse, or impaired hepatic or renal function.

Interactions
Drug-drug. *Antidepressants, antihistamines, narcotics, sedative-hypnotics, tranquilizers:* Secobarbital may add to or potentiate CNS and respiratory depressant effects. Use together cautiously.
Corticosteroids, digitoxin (not digoxin), doxycycline, oral contraceptives and other estrogens, theophylline and other xanthines, warfarin and other oral anticoagulants: Enhanced metabolism of these drugs. Monitor patient for lack of effect.
Disulfiram, MAO inhibitors, valproic acid: Decreased metabolism of secobarbital and increased risk of toxicity. Reduce barbiturate dosage.
Griseofulvin: Secobarbital impairs griseofulvin effectiveness by decreasing absorption from the GI tract. Monitor effectiveness of griseofulvin.
Rifampin: May decrease secobarbital levels by increasing metabolism. Monitor patient for decreased effect.
Drug-lifestyle. *Alcohol use:* May potentiate CNS depressant effects. Advise patient to avoid alcohol.

Adverse reactions
CNS: *drowsiness, lethargy, hangover,* paradoxical excitement in elderly patients, somnolence, altered EEG patterns.
GI: nausea, vomiting.
Hematologic: worsening of porphyria.
Hepatic: decreased serum bilirubin levels.
Respiratory: *respiratory depression.*
Skin: rash, urticaria, *Stevens-Johnson syndrome,* tissue reactions, injection-site pain.
Other: *angioedema,* physical and psychological dependence.

Overdose and treatment
Signs and symptoms of overdose include unsteady gait, slurred speech, sustained nystagmus, somnolence, confusion, respiratory depression, pulmonary edema, areflexia, and coma. Typical shock syndrome with tachycardia and hypotension, jaundice, hypothermia followed by fever, and oliguria may occur.

Maintain and support ventilation and pulmonary function as necessary; support cardiac

---

Reactions may be *common,* uncommon, *life-threatening,* or COMMON AND LIFE-THREATENING.

function and circulation with vasopressors and I.V. fluids as needed. If patient is conscious and gag reflex is intact, induce emesis (if ingestion was recent) by administering ipecac syrup. If emesis is contraindicated, perform gastric lavage while a cuffed endotracheal tube is in place to prevent aspiration. Follow with administration of activated charcoal or sodium chloride cathartic. Measure intake and output, vital signs, and laboratory parameters; maintain body temperature. Roll patient from side to side every 30 minutes to avoid pulmonary congestion.

Alkalinization of urine may help remove drug from the body; hemodialysis may be useful in severe overdose.

Special considerations

● Assess mental status before starting therapy. Elderly patients are more sensitive to adverse CNS effects; watch for paradoxical excitement.

● Take precautions to prevent hoarding or overdosing by patients who are depressed, suicidal, or drug-dependent or who have history of drug abuse.

● Inspect patient's skin. Skin eruptions may precede potentially fatal reactions to barbiturate therapy. Discontinue drug when skin reactions occur. In some patients, high fever, stomatitis, headache, or rhinitis may precede skin reactions.

● Long-term use isn't recommended; drug loses its efficacy in promoting sleep after 14 days of continued use.

● Secobarbital may cause a false-positive phentolamine test. The physiologic effects of the drug may impair absorption of cyanocobalamin C57.

Patient monitoring

● Watch for signs of barbiturate toxicity: coma, pupillary constriction, cyanosis, clammy skin, and hypotension. Overdose can be fatal.

● Monitor hepatic and renal studies frequently to prevent possible toxicity.

Breast-feeding patients

● Because drug appears in breast milk, don't administer to breast-feeding women.

Pediatric patients

● Drug may cause paradoxical excitement in children; use cautiously.

Geriatric patients

● These patients are more susceptible to effects of drug and usually need lower doses. Confusion, disorientation, and excitability may occur.

Patient education

● Inform patient that morning hangover is common after hypnotic dose, which suppresses REM sleep.

● Caution patient not to perform activities that require mental alertness or physical coordination.

selegiline hydrochloride (L-deprenyl hydrochloride)
Carbex, Eldepryl

Pharmacologic classification: MAO inhibitor
Therapeutic classification: antiparkinsonian
Pregnancy risk category: C

Indications and dosages

➤ *Adjunctive treatment to levodopa-carbidopa in the management of symptoms linked to Parkinson's disease. Adults:* 10 mg P.O. daily, taken as 5 mg at breakfast and 5 mg at lunch. After 2 or 3 days of therapy, begin gradual decrease of levodopa-carbidopa dosage.

How supplied

Available by prescription only
Capsules: 5 mg
Tablets: 5 mg

Pharmacodynamics

Antiparkinsonian action: Probably acts by selectively inhibiting MAO type B (found mostly in the brain). At higher-than-recommended doses, it's a nonselective inhibitor of MAO, including MAO type A found in the GI tract. It may also directly increase dopaminergic activity by decreasing the reuptake of dopamine into nerve cells. It has pharmacologically active metabolites (amphetamine and methamphetamine) that may contribute to this effect.

Pharmacokinetics

Absorption: Rapidly absorbed; about 73% of dose is absorbed.
Distribution: After a single dose, plasma levels are below detectable levels (less than 10 ng/ml).
Metabolism: Three metabolites have been detected in the serum and urine: N-desmethyl-deprenyl, amphetamine, and methamphetamine.
Excretion: About 45% appears as a metabolite in urine after 48 hours.

Route	Onset	Peak	Duration
P.O.	Unknown	½-2 hr	Unknown

Contraindications and precautions

Contraindicated in patients hypersensitive to drug and in those receiving meperidine and other opioids.

Interactions

Drug-drug. *Adrenergic drugs:* May increase the pressor response. Use together cautiously.
Fluoxetine: May result in serotonin syndrome. Avoid use together. Allow 5 weeks between stopping fluoxetine and starting selegiline.
Meperidine: Fatal interactions have been reported. Don't use together.
Drug-herb. *Ginseng:* May cause headache, tremors, mania. Discourage use together.

Drug-food. *Cacao:* May cause vasopressor effects. Discourage use together.
Foods high in tyramine: May cause hypertensive crisis. Monitor blood pressure.
Drug-lifestyle. *Alcohol use:* Excessive depressant effect is possible. Advise patient to avoid alcohol.

Adverse reactions
CNS: malaise, *dizziness,* increased tremor, chorea, loss of balance, restlessness, increased bradykinesia, facial grimacing, stiff neck, dyskinesia, involuntary movements, twitching, increased apraxia, behavioral changes, fatigue, headache, confusion, hallucinations, vivid dreams, anxiety, insomnia, lethargy.
CV: orthostatic hypotension, hypertension, hypotension, *arrhythmias,* palpitations, new or increased anginal pain, tachycardia, peripheral edema, syncope.
EENT: blepharospasm.
GI: dry mouth, *nausea,* vomiting, constipation, weight loss, abdominal pain, anorexia or poor appetite, dysphagia, diarrhea, heartburn.
GU: slow urination, transient nocturia, prostatic hyperplasia, urinary hesitancy, urinary frequency, urine retention, sexual dysfunction.
Skin: rash, hair loss, diaphoresis.

Overdose and treatment
Limited experience with overdose suggests that symptoms may include hypotension and psychomotor agitation. Because selegiline becomes a nonselective MAO inhibitor in high doses, consider the possibility of symptoms of MAO inhibitor poisoning: drowsiness, dizziness, hyperactivity, agitation, seizures, coma, hypertension, hypotension, cardiac conduction disturbances, and CV collapse. These symptoms may not develop immediately after ingestion; delays of 12 hours or more are possible.

Provide supportive treatment and closely monitor the patient for worsening of symptoms. Emesis or lavage may be helpful in the early stages of overdose treatment. Avoid phenothiazine derivatives and CNS stimulants; adrenergic agents may provoke an exaggerated response. Diazepam may be useful in treating seizures.

Special considerations
• Some patients who have increased levodopa-related adverse reactions (including dyskinesias) will need a reduction of levodopa-carbidopa dosage. Most need a reduction of 10% to 30%.

Patient monitoring
• Monitor patient's response to drug therapy.

Breast-feeding patients
• It isn't known if drug appears in breast milk. Use cautiously in breast-feeding women.

Patient education
• Advise patient not to take more than 10 mg daily. There's no evidence that higher doses improve efficacy and it may increase adverse reactions.
• Tell patient to move about cautiously at the start of therapy because dizziness may occur, which can cause falls.
• Because drug is an MAO inhibitor, tell patient about the possibility of an interaction with tyramine-containing foods. Tell patient to immediately report signs or symptoms of hypertension, including severe headache. Reportedly, however, this interaction doesn't occur at the recommended dose; at 10 mg daily, drug inhibits only MAO type B. Therefore, dietary restrictions appear unnecessary, provided that patient doesn't exceed the recommended dose.
• Advise patient to take second dose with lunch to avoid nighttime sedation.

---

sertraline hydrochloride
Zoloft

Pharmacologic classification: selective serotonin reuptake inhibitor
Therapeutic classification: antidepressant
Pregnancy risk category: C

Indications and dosages
➤ *Post-traumatic stress disorder (PTSD) or panic disorder.* Adults: Initially, 25 mg P.O. once daily. Increase to 50 mg P.O. daily after 1 week. If no improvement, dose may be increased up to a maximum of 200 mg P.O. daily. Zoloft is safe and effective in preventing relapse of PTSD and in sustaining symptom improvement over 28 weeks (long-term use) in men and women.
➤ *Depression, obsessive-compulsive disorder (OCD).* Adults: Initially, 50 mg P.O. once daily. Adjust dose as needed and tolerated. Dosage adjustments should be made at intervals of no less than 1 week.
Children ages 6 to 12 (OCD only): Initially, 25 mg P.O. once daily. Increase at intervals no less than 1 week. Maximum, 200 mg daily.
Children ages 13 to 17 (OCD only): Initially, 50 mg P.O. once daily. Increase at intervals no less than 1 week. Maximum, 200 mg daily.
➤ *Premenstrual dysphoric disorder◊.* Adults: 50 to 150 mg P.O. daily.
➤ *Premenstrual ejaculation◊.* Adults: 25 to 50 mg P.O. daily or p.r.n.
✦ *Dosage adjustment.* Use lower dose or less frequent delivery in patients with hepatic impairment. Take particular care in patients with renal failure.

How supplied
Available by prescription only
Oral concentrate: 20 mg/ml
Tablets (film-coated): 25 mg, 50 mg, 100 mg

Reactions may be *common*, uncommon, *life-threatening*, or COMMON AND LIFE-THREATENING.

Pharmacodynamics

Antidepressant action: Sertraline probably acts by blocking the reuptake of serotonin (also known as 5-hydroxytryptamine [5-HT]) into presynaptic neurons in the CNS, prolonging the action of 5-HT.

Pharmacokinetics

Absorption: Well absorbed after oral administration; absorption rate and extent are enhanced when taken with food.

Distribution: In vitro studies indicate that drug is highly protein-bound (more than 98%).

Metabolism: Metabolism is probably hepatic; drug undergoes significant first-pass metabolism. N-desmethylsertraline is substantially less active than the parent compound.

Excretion: Excreted mostly as metabolites in the urine and feces. Mean elimination half-life is 26 hours. Steady state levels are reached within 1 week of daily dosing in young, healthy patients.

Route	Onset	Peak	Duration
P.O.	Unknown	4½-8½ hr	Unknown

Contraindications and precautions

Contraindicated in patients receiving MAO inhibitors. Use cautiously in patients at risk for suicide and in those with seizure disorders, major affective disorder, or diseases or conditions that affect metabolism or hemodynamic responses. Avoid using the oral concentrate dropper, which is made of rubber, if patient has a latex allergy.

Interactions

Drug-drug. *Cimetidine:* Increased sertraline bioavailability, peak plasma levels, and half-life. Monitor patient closely.

Diazepam, tolbutamide: Decreased clearance of these drugs. Monitor patient for increased drug effects.

Disulfiram: Oral concentrate contains alcohol that could cause a reaction. Avoid use together.

MAO inhibitors: Serious mental status changes, hyperthermia, autonomic instability, rapid fluctuations of vital signs, delirium, coma, and death. Drug must not be given within 14 days of an MAO inhibitor.

Warfarin, other highly protein-bound drugs: May cause interactions, increasing the plasma levels of sertraline or the other highly bound drug. Monitor patient closely.

Drug-herb. *St. John's wort:* Increased risk of serotonin syndrome. Discourage concomitant use.

Adverse reactions

CNS: *headache, tremor, dizziness, insomnia, somnolence,* paresthesia, hypoesthesia, *fatigue,* nervousness, anxiety, agitation, hypertonia, twitching, confusion.

CV: palpitations, chest pain, hot flashes.

GI: *dry mouth, nausea, diarrhea, loose stools, dyspepsia,* vomiting, constipation, thirst, flatulence, anorexia, abdominal pain, increased appetite.

GU: *male sexual dysfunction,* polyuria, nocturia, dysuria.

Hepatic: elevated liver enzyme levels.

Metabolic: minor increases in serum cholesterol and triglyceride levels, decreased uric acid levels.

Musculoskeletal: myalgia.

Skin: rash, pruritus, *diaphoresis.*

Overdose and treatment

Experience with sertraline overdose is limited. Treatment is supportive. Establish an airway and maintain adequate ventilation. Because recent studies question the value of forced emesis or lavage, consider the use of activated charcoal in sorbitol to bind drug in the GI tract. There's no specific antidote for sertraline. Monitor vital signs closely. Because drug has a large volume of distribution, hemodialysis, peritoneal dialysis, or forced diuresis probably isn't useful.

Special considerations

● Drug may activate mania or hypomania in patients with cyclic disorders.

● Avoid using the oral concentrate dropper, which is made of rubber, in a patient with a latex allergy.

● Mix oral concentrate with 4 oz (½ cup) of water, ginger ale, or lemon/lime soda and give the dose right away.

Patient monitoring

● Patients who respond during the first 8 weeks of therapy will probably continue to respond to drug, although there are limited studies of drug in depressed patients for periods longer than 16 weeks. If patients are continued on drug for prolonged therapy, periodically monitor the effectiveness of drug. It's unknown if periodic dose adjustments are necessary to maintain effectiveness.

● Record mood changes and monitor patient for suicidal tendencies.

Breast-feeding patients

● It isn't known if drug appears in breast milk. Use cautiously in breast-feeding women.

Pediatric patients

● Safety and efficacy in children with depression or panic disorder haven't been established.

Geriatric patients

● Plasma clearance of drug is slower in elderly patients. Studies indicate that it may take 2 to 3 weeks of daily dosing before steady state levels occur.

● Monitor patient closely for dose-related adverse effects. Elderly patients may be more likely than younger patients to develop hyponatremia and transient SIADH.

Patient education
• Tell patient to take drug once daily, either in the morning or evening, with or without food.
• Advise patient to avoid alcohol while taking drug and to call before taking OTC medications.
• Although problems haven't been reported to date, advise patient to use caution when performing hazardous tasks that require alertness, such as driving and operating heavy machinery. Drugs that influence the CNS may impair judgment.
• Advise patient to mix the oral concentrate with 4 oz. (½ cup) of water, ginger ale, lemon/lime soda only, and to take the dose right away.

sevelamer hydrochloride
Renagel

Pharmacologic class: polymeric phosphate binder
Therapeutic class: hypophosphatemic agent
Pregnancy risk category: C

Indications and dosages
➤ *Reduction of serum phosphorus in patients with endstage renal disease.* Adults: initially, 2 to 4 capsules P.O. t.i.d. with meals, depending on severity of hyperphosphatemia. Gradually adjust dosage based on serum phosphorus level with goal of lowering serum phosphorus level to 6 mg/dl or less. If serum phosphorus level is 9 mg/dl or more, give 4 capsules P.O. t.i.d. with meals. If serum phosphorus level is between 7.5 and 9 mg/dl, give 3 capsules P.O. t.i.d. with meals. If serum phosphorus level is between 6 and 7.5 mg/dl, give 2 capsules P.O. t.i.d. with meals.

How supplied
Available by prescription only
Capsules: 403 mg

Pharmacodynamics
Serum phosphorus–reducing action: Drug works locally to inhibit intestinal phosphate absorption. Decreased serum phosphate level decreases ectopic calcification and osteitis fibrosa. Also lowers LDL and total serum cholesterol.

Pharmacokinetics
Absorption: In healthy patients, drug isn't absorbed systemically. No studies have been done in patients with renal disease.
Distribution: Not reported.
Metabolism: Not reported.
Elimination: Not reported.

Route	Onset	Peak	Duration
P.O.	Unknown	Unknown	Unknown

Contraindications and precautions
Contraindicated in patients hypersensitive to drug or its components and in those with hypophos-phatemia or bowel obstruction. Use cautiously in patients with dysphagia, swallowing disorders, severe GI motility disorders, or major GI tract surgery.

Interactions
None significant.

Adverse reactions
CNS: *headache, pain.*
CV: hypertension, *hypotension,* **thrombosis.**
GI: *vomiting,* nausea, constipation, *diarrhea,* flatulence, *dyspepsia.*
Respiratory: increased cough.
Other: *infection.*

Overdose and treatment
No information available. The risk of systemic toxicity is low.

Special considerations
⚠ **ALERT** Although no drug interactions are known, drug may bind to concomitantly administered drugs and decrease their bioavailability. Administer other drugs 1 hour before or 3 hours after sevelamer. Take special precautions when antiarrhythmics or anticonvulsants are taken with sevelamer.
• Don't crush or break capsules, and administer only with meals.

Patient monitoring
• Monitor serum calcium, bicarbonate, and chloride levels, as ordered.
• Watch for thrombosis (numbness or tingling of limbs, chest pain, shortness of breath).

Patient education
• Instruct patient to take drug with meals and adhere to prescribed diet.
• Inform patient that capsules must be taken whole because contents expand in water; caution him not to open or chew capsules.
• Tell patient to take other drugs as directed, either 1 hour before or 3 hours after sevelamer.
• Review adverse reactions and tell patient to report them immediately. Review signs and symptoms of thrombosis (numbness, tingling limbs, chest pain, changes in level of consciousness).

sibutramine hydrochloride monohydrate
Meridia

Pharmacologic classification: norepinephrine, serotonin, and dopamine reuptake inhibitor
Therapeutic classification: antiobesity
Controlled substance schedule: IV
Pregnancy risk category: C

Indications and dosages
➤ *Management of obesity, including weight loss and maintenance of weight*

loss; should be used in conjunction with a reduced-calorie diet. Adults: 10 mg P.O. once daily with or without food. May increase dose to 15 mg daily after 4 weeks if there is inadequate weight loss. Patients who don't tolerate the 10-mg dose may receive 5 mg daily. Doses above 15 mg daily aren't recommended.

How supplied
Available by prescription only
Capsules: 5 mg, 10 mg, 15 mg

Pharmacodynamics
Antiobesity action: Sibutramine produces its therapeutic effects by inhibiting the reuptake of norepinephrine, serotonin, and dopamine.

Pharmacokinetics
Absorption: Rapidly absorbed from the GI tract. On average, at least 77% is absorbed.
Distribution: Distributed extensively into tissues, especially the liver and kidney with relatively low transfer to the fetus. In vitro, sibutramine and the active desmethyl metabolites M_1 and M_2 are extensively bound (97%, 94%, and 94%, respectively) to human plasma proteins.
Metabolism: Undergoes extensive first-pass metabolism by the cytochrome P-450 3A4 Isoenzyme to M_1 and M_2; elimination half-lives of M_1 and M_2 are 14 and 16 hours, respectively.
Excretion: About 77% of a single oral dose is excreted in the urine.

Route	Onset	Peak	Duration
P.O.	Unknown	3-4 hr	Unknown

Contraindications and precautions
Contraindicated in patients taking MAO inhibitors or other centrally acting appetite-suppressant drugs. Also contraindicated in patients hypersensitive to drug or its inactive ingredients and in those with anorexia nervosa. Don't use drug in patients with history of coronary artery disease, heart failure, arrhythmias, CVA, severe renal failure, hepatic dysfunction, or a history of seizures. Use cautiously in patients with angle-closure glaucoma.

Interactions
Drug-drug. *CNS depressants:* May enhance CNS depression. Use together cautiously.
Dextromethorphan, dihydroergotamine, fentanyl, fluoxetine, fluvoxamine, lithium, MAO inhibitors, meperidine, paroxetine, pentazocine, sertraline, sumatriptan, tryptophan, venlafaxine: May cause hyperthermia, tachycardia, and loss of consciousness. Don't use together. At least 2 weeks should elapse between stopping an MAO inhibitor and starting sibutramine, and vice versa.
Drugs that inhibit cytochrome P-450 3A4 metabolism, such as erythromycin and ketoconazole: May inhibit sibutramine metabolism. Sibutramine dosage may need to be reduced.

Ephedrine, pseudoephedrine: May increase blood pressure or heart rate. Monitor patient carefully.
Drug-lifestyle. *Alcohol use:* May enhance CNS depression. Discourage alcohol use.

Adverse reactions
CNS: asthenia, *headache, insomnia,* dizziness, nervousness, anxiety, depression, paresthesia, somnolence, CNS stimulation, emotional lability, migraine.
CV: tachycardia, vasodilation, hypertension, palpitation, chest pain, generalized edema.
EENT: laryngitis, thirst, *dry mouth, rhinitis, pharyngitis,* sinusitis, ear disorder, ear pain.
GI: taste perversion, *anorexia, constipation,* increased appetite, nausea, dyspepsia, gastritis, vomiting, abdominal pain, rectal disorder.
GU: dysmenorrhea, urinary tract infection, vaginal candidiasis, metrorrhagia.
Hepatic: elevated liver enzyme levels.
Musculoskeletal: arthralgia, myalgia, tenosynovitis, joint disorder, neck or back pain.
Respiratory: increased cough.
Skin: rash, sweating, acne.
Other: herpes simplex, flu syndrome, *allergic reaction.*

Overdose and treatment
There's no specific antidote to sibutramine. Treatment should consist of general measures used in the management of overdose: Establish an airway, monitor cardiac and vital signs, and institute general symptomatic and supportive measures. Cautious use of beta blockers may be indicated to control elevated blood pressure or tachycardia. The benefits of forced diuresis and hemodialysis are unknown.

Special considerations
● Drug is recommended for obese patients with an initial body mass index of 30 kg/m² or more or 27 kg/m² or more in the presence of other risk factors, such as hypertension, diabetes, or dyslipidemia.
● Rule out organic causes of obesity before starting therapy.
● Weight loss can precipitate or exacerbate gallstone formation.
● Although not reported with sibutramine, some centrally acting weight-loss agents have been linked to a rare but fatal condition known as primary pulmonary hypertension.

Patient monitoring
● Measure blood pressure and heart rate before starting therapy, with dose changes, and at regular intervals during therapy because drug is known to increase both blood pressure and heart rate.
● If a patient has not lost at least 4 lb in the first 4 weeks of treatment, reevaluate therapy to consider increasing dosage or stopping drug.

Breast-feeding patients
● It isn't known whether drug or its metabolites appear in breast milk. Avoid use of drug in breast-feeding women.

Pediatric patients
● Safety and efficacy in children under age 16 haven't been established.

Geriatric patients
● Select dosage cautiously for elderly patients because they're more likely to have decreased hepatic, renal, or cardiac function; concurrent disease; and other drug therapy.

Patient education
● Advise patient to read the package insert before starting therapy and to review again each time the prescription is renewed.
● Instruct patient to report rash, hives, or other allergic reactions immediately.
● Tell patient to inform prescriber of other prescription or OTC drugs being taken, especially other weight-reducing agents, decongestants, antidepressants, cough suppressants, lithium, dihydroergotamine, sumatriptan, or tryptophan, as there is a potential for drug interactions.
● Emphasize importance of regular follow-up visits with prescriber.
● Advise patient to use drug with a reduced-calorie diet.

sildenafil citrate
Viagra

Pharmacologic classification: selective inhibitor of cyclic guanosine monophosphate-specific phosphodiesterase type 5
Therapeutic classification: therapy for erectile dysfunction
Pregnancy risk category: B

Indications and dosages
➤ *Treatment of erectile dysfunction.*
Adults: 50 mg P.O. as a single dose, p.r.n., 1 hour before sexual activity. However, patient may take drug 30 minutes to 4 hours before sexual activity. Based on effectiveness and tolerance to patient, may increase dose to maximum single dose of 100 mg or decrease dose to 25 mg. A maximum recommended dosing frequency is once daily.
✦ *Dosage adjustment.* For elderly patients with hepatic impairment or severe renal impairment, and for those concurrently taking potent cytochrome P-450 3A4 inhibitors, consider a starting dose of 25 mg.

How supplied
Available by prescription only
Tablets: 25 mg, 50 mg, 100 mg

Pharmacodynamics
Erectile action: Sildenafil has no direct relaxant effect on isolated human corpus cavernosum, but enhances the effect of nitric oxide (NO) by inhibiting phosphodiesterase type 5 (PDE5), which is responsible for degradation of cyclic guanosine monophosphate (cGMP) in the corpus cavernosum. When sexual stimulation causes local release of NO, inhibition of PDE5 by sildenafil causes increased levels of cGMP in the corpus cavernosum, resulting in smooth muscle relaxation and inflow of blood to the corpus cavernosum.

Pharmacokinetics
Absorption: Rapidly absorbed after oral administration. A high-fat meal delays the rate of absorption by about 1 hour and reduces peak levels by one-third. Absolute bioavailability of sildenafil is about 40%.
Distribution: Widely distributed to body tissues with a mean steady state volume of distribution of 105 L. Both drug and its major active metabolite are 96% bound to plasma proteins. Protein-binding is independent of drug levels.
Metabolism: The primary pathway for sildenafil elimination is metabolism by the CYP 3A4 and CYP 2C9 hepatic microsomal isoenzymes. N-desmethylation converts sildenafil into the major circulating metabolite, which accounts for about 20% of the pharmacologic effects of sildenafil.
Excretion: About 80% of an oral dose is metabolized and excreted in the feces, and about 13% is excreted in the urine.

Route	Onset	Peak	Duration
P.O.	Unknown	½-2 hr	4 hr

Contraindications and precautions
Contraindicated in patients using organic nitrates and in those hypersensitive to drug or its components. Use cautiously in patients who have had an MI, CVA, or life-threatening arrhythmias within the past 6 months; those with a history of cardiac failure, coronary artery disease, or uncontrolled high or low blood pressure; those with anatomic deformation of the penis; and those predisposed to priapism (sickle cell anemia, multiple myeloma, leukemia), retinitis pigmentosa, bleeding disorders, or active peptic ulcers.

Interactions
Drug-drug. *Delavirdine, protease inhibitors:* Increased sildenafil levels, which may increase sildenafil-related adverse reactions, including hypotension, vision changes, and priapism. Sildenafil dose shouldn't exceed 25 mg in a 48-hour period.
Inhibitors of cytochrome P-450 isoforms 3A4, such as cimetidine, erythromycin, itraconazole, and ketoconazole: May reduce sildenafil clearance. Avoid use together.

Reactions may be *common*, uncommon, **life-threatening**, or COMMON AND LIFE-THREATENING.

Nitrates: Sildenafil enhances the hypotensive effects of nitrates. Don't use together.
Rifampin: May reduce sildenafil levels. Monitor effect closely.
Drug-food. *High-fat meals:* Can delay absorption of drug and onset of action by 1 hour. Separate administration time from meals.

Adverse reactions
CNS: *headache,* dizziness.
CV: *flushing.*
EENT: nasal congestion, abnormal vision (photophobia, color blindness).
GI: dyspepsia, diarrhea.
GU: urinary tract infection.
Skin: rash.

Overdose and treatment
In healthy volunteers, doses up to 800 mg produced adverse events similar to those seen at lower doses, but at an increased rate. Use standard supportive measures to treat overdose. Renal dialysis isn't expected to increase clearance.

Special considerations
● Because sexual activity may cause cardiac risk, evaluate patient's CV status before starting therapy.

Patient monitoring
● Monitor patient's compliance with drug regimen.

Pregnant patients
● Drug seems to have favorable teratogenic, embryotoxic, and fetotoxic profiles, and it isn't readily distributed into semen; it isn't expected to be harmful to pregnant partners of men receiving therapy.

Breast-feeding patients
● Drug isn't indicated for use in women.

Pediatric patients
● Drug shouldn't be used in children or neonates.

Geriatric patients
● Healthy people age 65 or older have reduced drug clearance, which results in plasma drug levels about 40% higher than those in younger subjects.

Patient education
● Tell patient that drug doesn't protect against sexually transmitted diseases and that he should use protective measures to prevent infection.
● Advise patient that drug is most rapidly absorbed if taken on an empty stomach.
● Tell patient to notify prescriber of visual changes.
● Urge patient to seek medical attention if erection persists for more than 4 hours.
● Advise patient that drug has no effect in the absence of sexual stimulation.

simethicone
Gas-X, Mylicon, Phazyme

Pharmacologic classification: dispersant
Therapeutic classification: antiflatulent
Pregnancy risk category: C

Indications and dosages
➤ *Flatulence, functional gastric bloating.* *Adults and children over age 12:* 40 to 125 mg P.O. after each meal and h.s.
Children ages 2 to 12: 40 mg (drops) P.O. q.i.d.
Children under age 2: 20 mg (drops) P.O. q.i.d., up to 240 mg daily.

How supplied
Available without a prescription
Capsules: 125 mg
Drops: 40 mg/0.6 ml
Tablets (chewable): 40 mg, 80 mg, 125 mg
Tablets (delayed-release, enteric-coated core): 60 mg, 95 mg

Pharmacodynamics
Antiflatulent action: Simethicone acts as a defoaming agent by decreasing the surface tension of gas bubbles, preventing the formation of mucous-coated gas bubbles.

Pharmacokinetics
Absorption: None.
Distribution: None.
Metabolism: None.
Excretion: Excreted in feces.

Route	Onset	Peak	Duration
P.O.	Immediate	Unknown	Unknown

Contraindications and precautions
Contraindicated in patients hypersensitive to drug.

Interactions
Drug-drug. None significant.

Adverse reactions
GI: expulsion of excessive liberated gas as belching, rectal flatus.

Overdose and treatment
No information available.

Special considerations
● Simethicone is found in many combination antacid products.
● This medication doesn't prevent formation of gas.

Patient monitoring
● Monitor patient's response to drug therapy.

Pediatric patients
● Simethicone isn't recommended as treatment for infant colic; it has limited use in children.

Patient education

• Tell patient to chew tablets thoroughly or to shake suspension well before using.
• Encourage patient to change positions frequently and ambulate to aid flatus passage.

---

simvastatin
Zocor

Pharmacologic classification: HMG-CoA reductase inhibitor
Therapeutic classification: antilipemic, cholesterol-lowering agent
Pregnancy risk category: X

Indications and dosages
➤ *Adjunct to diet for reduction of low-density lipoprotein (LDL) and total cholesterol levels in patients with primary hypercholesterolemia (types IIa and IIb) and mixed dyslipidemia and in patients with coronary heart disease and hypercholesterolemia to reduce the risk of coronary death, nonfatal MI, CVA, transient ischemic attack, and myocardial revascularization procedures. Adults:* Initially, 20 mg P.O. daily in the evening. Dosage adjusted q 4 weeks based on patient tolerance and response. Maximum, 80 mg daily.
Elderly patients: Initially, 5 mg P.O. daily in the evening. Maximum, 20 mg daily.
➤ *Reduction of total cholesterol and LDL levels in patients with homozygous familial hypercholesterolemia. Adults:* 40 mg daily in the evening or 80 mg daily given in three divided doses of 20 mg, 20 mg, and 40 mg in the evening.
➤ *To increase high-density lipoprotein levels in patients with primary hypercholesterolemia and mixed dyslipidemia (Frederickson types IIa and IIb); as an adjunct to diet to reduce elevated total cholesterol, LDL, apolipoprotein B, and triglyceride levels in patients with primary hypercholesterolemia and mixed dyslipidemia. Adults:* Initially, 20 mg P.O. daily in the evening. Adjust dosage at intervals of 4 weeks or more according to baseline LDL levels, recommended goal of therapy, and patient response. Range is 5 to 80 mg daily.
➤ *Hypertriglyceridemia (Frederickson type IV hyperlipidemia), primary dysbetalipoproteinemia (Frederickson type III hyperlipidemia). Adults:* Initially, 20 mg P.O. daily in the evening. Adjust dosage every 4 weeks based on patient response and tolerance. Range is 5 to 80 mg daily as single dose in the evening.
Elderly patients: May be adequately treated with 20 mg daily or less.
✦ *Dosage adjustment.* For patients taking cyclosporine, begin with 5 mg P.O. daily; don't exceed 10 mg P.O. daily. In patients taking fibrates or niacin, maximum is 10 mg P.O. daily. In patients with severe renal insufficiency, start with 5 mg P.O. daily.

How supplied
Available by prescription only
Tablets: 5 mg, 10 mg, 20 mg, 40 mg, 80 mg

Pharmacodynamics
Antilipemic action: Simvastatin inhibits the enzyme 3-hydroxy-3-methylglutaryl-coenzyme A (HMG-CoA) reductase. This hepatic enzyme is an early (and rate-limiting) step in the synthetic pathway of cholesterol.

Pharmacokinetics
Absorption: Readily absorbed; however, extensive hepatic extraction limits the plasma availability of active inhibitors to 5% of a dose or less. Individual absorption varies considerably.
Distribution: Parent drug and active metabolites are more than 95% bound to plasma proteins.
Metabolism: Hydrolysis occurs in the plasma; at least three major metabolites have been identified.
Excretion: Excreted primarily in bile.

Route	Onset	Peak	Duration
P.O.	Unknown	1⅓-2½ hr	Unknown

Contraindications and precautions
Contraindicated in patients hypersensitive to drug, in pregnant and breast-feeding women, in women of childbearing age unless there's no risk of pregnancy, and in patients with active hepatic disease or conditions that cause unexplained persistent elevations of serum transaminase levels.

Use cautiously in patients with history of liver disease and patients consume excessive amounts of alcohol.

Interactions
Drug-drug. *Cimetidine, ketoconazole, spironolactone:* May increase the risk of endocrine dysfunction. No intervention appears necessary; obtain complete drug history for patients in whom endocrine dysfunction develops.
Digoxin: Slightly elevated digoxin levels. Closely monitor digoxin levels at start of simvastatin therapy.
Erythromycin, fibric acid derivatives such as clofibrate and gemfibrozil, high doses of niacin (nicotinic acid at 1 g or more daily), immunosuppressants such as cyclosporine: Increased risk of rhabdomyolysis. Monitor patient closely if use together can't be avoided. Limit daily dose of simvastatin to 10 mg if patient must take cyclosporine.
Hepatotoxic drugs: Increased risk for hepatotoxicity. Avoid use together.
Warfarin: Simvastatin may slightly enhance the anticoagulant effect. Monitor PT at the start of therapy and during dose adjustment.

Reactions may be *common*, uncommon, **life-threatening**, or COMMON AND LIFE-THREATENING.

Drug-herb. *Red yeast rice:* Increased risk of adverse events or toxicity because red yeast rice has components similar to those of statins. Discourage concomitant use.

Drug-food. *Grapefruit juice:* Increased drug levels and increased risk of adverse effects. Give with liquids other than grapefruit juice.

Drug-lifestyle. *Alcohol use:* May increase the risk of hepatotoxicity. Advise patient to avoid alcohol.

Adverse reactions

CNS: headache, asthenia.
GI: abdominal pain, constipation, diarrhea, dyspepsia, flatulence, nausea, vomiting.
Hepatic: elevated liver enzyme levels.
Respiratory: upper respiratory tract infection.

Overdose and treatment

A few overdoses have been reported; no patients had any specific symptoms, and all patients recovered without sequelae. The maximum dose taken was 450 mg. Until further experience is obtained, no specific treatment of overdose can be recommended.

Special considerations

● Start simvastatin only after diet and other non-drug therapies have proved ineffective. Patient should continue a cholesterol-lowering diet during therapy.
● Dose adjustments should be made about every 4 weeks. If the cholesterol levels decrease below the target range, dose may be reduced.

Patient monitoring

● Perform liver function tests frequently at the start of therapy and periodically thereafter.

Pregnant patients

● Safety hasn't been established. Patient should immediately report planned, suspected, or known pregnancy.

Breast-feeding patients

● It isn't known if drug appears in breast milk. Because of the risk to infant, patient should avoid breast-feeding during therapy.

Pediatric patients

● Safety and efficacy in children haven't been established.

Geriatric patients

● Most elderly patients respond to daily dose of 20 mg or less.

Patient education

● Tell patient that drug should be taken in the evening and may be taken without regard to meals.
● Tell patient to report adverse reactions, particularly muscle aches and pains.
● Explain importance of controlling serum lipids to CV health. Teach appropriate dietary management (restricting total fat and cholesterol intake), weight control, and exercise.

sirolimus
Rapamune

Pharmacologic classification: macrocyclic lactone
Therapeutic classification: immuno-suppressant
Pregnancy risk category: C

Indications and dosages

➤ *Prophylaxis, with cyclosporine and corticosteroids, of organ rejection in patients receiving renal transplants.* Adults and adolescents age 13 and older who weigh 40 kg (88 lb) or more: Initially, 6 mg P.O. as a one-time loading dose as soon as possible after transplantation; then maintenance dose of 2 mg P.O. once daily.
Adolescents age 13 and older who weigh less than 40 kg: Initially, 3 mg/m² P.O. as a one-time loading dose after transplantation; then maintenance dose of 1 mg/m² P.O. once daily.
✦ *Dosage adjustment.* In patients with mild to moderate hepatic impairment, reduce maintenance dose by about one-third. It isn't necessary to reduce loading dose.

How supplied

Available by prescription only
Oral solution: 1 mg/ml
Tablets: 1 mg

Pharmacodynamics

Immunosuppressant action: Sirolimus is an immunosuppressant that inhibits T-lymphocyte activation and proliferation that occur in response to antigenic and cytokine stimulation. Drug also inhibits antibody formation.

Pharmacokinetics

Absorption: Rapidly absorbed from GI tract, with mean peak levels occurring in about 1 to 3 hours. Oral bioavailability of the solution is about 14%, and even higher with the tablets. Food decreases peak plasma levels and increases time to peak.
Distribution: Extensively partitioned into formed blood elements. Drug is extensively bound to plasma proteins (about 92%).
Metabolism: Extensively metabolized by the mixed function oxidase system, primarily cytochrome P-450 3A4. Seven major metabolites have been identified in whole blood.
Excretion: Excreted in feces (91%) and in urine (2.2%). Half-life is about 62 hours.

Route	Onset	Peak	Duration
P.O.	Unknown	1-3 hr	Unknown

Contraindications and precautions

Contraindicated in patients hypersensitive to active drug or its derivatives or components. Use cautiously in patients with hyperlipidemia or impaired liver or renal function.

Interactions

Drug-drug. *Aminoglycosides, amphotericin, other nephrotoxic drugs*: Increased risk of nephrotoxicity. Use together cautiously.

Bromocriptine, cimetidine, clarithromycin, clotrimazole, danazol, erythromycin, fluconazole, indinavir, itraconazole, metoclopramide, nicardipine, ritonavir, verapamil, other drugs that inhibit CYP3A4: May decrease sirolimus metabolism, thereby increasing sirolimus levels. Monitor patient closely.

Carbamazepine, phenobarbital, phenytoin, rifabutin, rifapentine, other drugs that induce CYP3A4: May increase sirolimus metabolism, thereby decreasing sirolimus levels. Monitor patient closely.

Cyclosporine (oral solution and capsules): Increased sirolimus levels. Administer sirolimus 4 hours after cyclosporine. After long-term use, sirolimus may reduce cyclosporine clearance, leading to need for reduction in cyclosporine dose.

Diltiazem: Increased sirolimus levels. Monitor patient, and reduce dosage of sirolimus as necessary.

Ketoconazole: Increased rate and extent of sirolimus absorption. Avoid use together.

Live-virus vaccines (BCG, measles, mumps, oral polio, rubella, TY21a typhoid, varicella, yellow fever): Reduced effectiveness of vaccines. Avoid concomitant use.

Rifampin: Decreased sirolimus levels. Consider alternatives to rifampin.

Drug-food. *Grapefruit juice*: Decreased sirolimus metabolism. Avoid concomitant use.

Adverse reactions

CNS: *headache, insomnia, tremor, anxiety, depression, asthenia,* malaise, syncope, confusion, dizziness, emotional lability, hypertonia, hypoesthesia, hypotonia, neuropathy, paresthesia, somnolence.

CV: *hypertension, heart failure, atrial fibrillation,* tachycardia, hypotension, *chest pain, edema, hemorrhage,* palpitations, peripheral vascular disorder, thrombophlebitis, thrombosis, vasodilation.

EENT: facial edema, *pharyngitis,* epistaxis, rhinitis, sinusitis, abnormal vision, cataract, conjunctivitis, deafness, ear pain, otitis media, tinnitus.

GI: *diarrhea, nausea, vomiting, constipation, abdominal pain, dyspepsia,* enlarged abdomen, ascites, peritonitis, anorexia, dysphagia, eructation, esophagitis, flatulence, gastritis, gastroenteritis, gingivitis, gum hyperplasia, ileus, mouth ulceration, oral candidiasis, stomatitis.

GU: dysuria, hematuria, albuminuria, *kidney tubular necrosis, increased creatinine level, urinary tract infection,* pelvic pain, glycosuria, increased BUN level, bladder pain, hydronephrosis, impotence, kidney pain, nocturia, oliguria, pyuria, scrotal edema, testis disorder, *toxic nephropathy,* urinary frequency, urinary incontinence, urine retention.

Hematologic: *anemia,* THROMBOCYTOPENIA, *leukopenia,* thrombotic thrombocytopenic purpura, ecchymosis, leukocytosis, polycythemia, lymphadenopathy.

Hepatic: elevation in liver enzyme levels.

Metabolic: *hypercholesteremia, hyperlipidemia, hypokalemia, weight gain, hypophosphatemia, hyperkalemia,* hypervolemia, Cushing's syndrome, diabetes mellitus, acidosis, dehydration, hypercalcemia, hyperglycemia, hyperphosphatemia, hypocalcemia, hypoglycemia, hypomagnesemia, hyponatremia, weight loss.

Musculoskeletal: *back pain, arthralgia,* myalgia, arthrosis, bone necrosis, leg cramps, osteoporosis, tetany.

Respiratory: *dyspnea, cough, atelectasis, upper respiratory tract infection,* asthma, bronchitis, hypoxia, lung edema, pleural effusion, pneumonia.

Skin: *rash, acne,* hirsutism, fungal dermatitis, pruritus, skin hypertrophy, skin ulcer, sweating.

Other: *fever, pain, peripheral edema,* abscess, cellulitis, chills, flulike syndrome, hernia, infection, *sepsis,* lymphadenopathy, abnormal healing.

Overdose and treatment

Experience with overdose is limited. Give general supportive care. Sirolimus probably isn't dialyzable.

Special considerations

• Following transplantation, antimicrobials for prophylaxis of *Pneumocystis carinii* and *Cytomegalovirus* should be administered for 1 year and 3 months, respectively.

• Drug should be used in a regimen with cyclosporine and corticosteroids.

• Only prescribers experienced in immunosuppressive therapy and management of renal transplant patients should prescribe drug.

• Patients taking drug are more susceptible to infection and possible development of lymphoma, which may result from immunosuppression.

• Oral solution must be diluted before administration. After dilution, the product should be used immediately.

• When diluting oral solution, empty correct amount into glass or plastic container that holds at least 2 oz (60 ml) of water or orange juice. Don't use grapefruit juice or any other liquid. Stir vigorously and have patient drink immediately. Refill container with at least 4 oz (120 ml) of water or orange juice, stir again, and have patient drink entire contents.

Reactions may be *common*, uncommon, **life-threatening**, or COMMON AND LIFE-THREATENING.

● Store away from light, and refrigerate at 36° to 46° F (2° to 8° C.) After opening bottle, use contents within 1 month. If necessary, bottles and pouches may be stored at room temperature (up to 77° F [25° C]) for several days. Drug can be kept in oral dosing syringe for 24 hours at room temperature or refrigerated at 36° to 46° F. Store tablets at 68° to 77° F. Protect from light.

● A slight haze may develop during refrigeration, but this doesn't affect quality of drug. If a haze develops, bring drug to room temperature and shake gently until haze disappears.

Patient monitoring

● Monitor renal function tests because drug use with cyclosporine may cause serum creatinine levels to increase. Dosage adjustment if immunosuppressive regimen may be necessary.

● Monitor cholesterol and triglyceride levels during sirolimus therapy. If hyperlipidemia is detected, interventions, such as diet, exercise, and lipid-lowering drugs, should be initiated. If patient is on sirolimus and cyclosporine is started as an HMG-CoA reductase inhibitor, monitor patient for development of rhabdomyolysis.

● Monitor drug levels in children, patients age 13 or older who weigh less than 40 kg, patients with hepatic impairment, patients receiving drugs that induce or inhibit CYP 3A4, and patients for whom cyclosporine dosage is markedly reduced or discontinued.

Breast-feeding patients

● It's not known if drug appears in breast milk. Because of potential for adverse reactions in breast-feeding infants, a decision should be made to stop either breast-feeding or drug.

Pediatric patients

● Safety and efficacy of drug in children under age 13 haven't been established.

Geriatric patients

● Data suggest that dosing adjustments in elderly patients aren't necessary.

Patient education

● Show patient how to properly store, dilute, and administer drug.

● Inform woman of childbearing age of risks during pregnancy. Tell her to use effective contraception before, during, and for 12 weeks after stopping drug.

● Tell patient to take drug consistently with or without food to stabilize drug absorption.

● Advise patient to take drug 4 hours after taking cyclosporine.

● Tell patient to wash area with soap and water if solution touches skin or mucous membranes; rinse eyes with plain water if solution gets in eyes.

sodium bicarbonate
Bell/ans, Neut, Soda Mint

Pharmacologic classification: alkalinizer
Therapeutic classification: systemic and urinary alkalinizer, systemic hydrogen ion buffer, oral antacid
Pregnancy risk category: C

Indications and dosages

➤ *Adjunct to advanced cardiac life support.* Adults and children over age 2: Although no longer routinely recommended, inject either 300 to 500 ml of a 5% solution or 200 to 300 mEq of a 7.5% or 8.4% solution as rapidly as possible. Base further doses on subsequent blood gas values.

Children age 2 or under: 1 mEq/kg I.V. bolus or intraosseous injection of a 4.2% to 8.4% solution. Dose may be repeated q 10 minutes depending on blood gas values. Don't exceed daily dose of 8 mEq/kg.

➤ *Severe metabolic acidosis. Adults and children:* Dose depends on blood carbon dioxide content, pH, and patient's clinical condition. Generally, administer 90 to 180 mEq/L I.V. during first hour; then adjust, p.r.n.

➤ *Less urgent metabolic acidosis. Adults and adolescents:* 2 to 5 mEq/kg as a 4- to 8-hour I.V. infusion.

➤ *Urine alkalization. Adults:* 48 mEq (4 g) P.O. initially; then 12 to 24 mEq (1 to 2 g) q 4 hours. May need doses of 30 to 48 mEq (2.5 to 4 g) q 4 hours, up to 192 mEq (16 g) daily. *Children:* 1 to 10 mEq (84 to 840 mg)/kg daily.

➤ *Antacid. Adults:* 300 mg to 2 g P.O. one to four times daily.

How supplied

Available by prescription only
Injection: 4% (2.4 mEq/5 ml), 4.2% (5 mEq/10 ml), 5% (297.5 mEq/500 ml), 7.5% (8.92 mEq/10 ml and 44.6 mEq/50 ml), 8.4% (10 mEq/10 ml and 50 mEq/50 ml)
Available without a prescription
Tablets: 325 mg, 500 mg, 520 mg, 650 mg

Pharmacodynamics

Alkalizing buffering action: Sodium bicarbonate is an alkalinizing agent that dissociates to provide bicarbonate ion. Bicarbonate in excess of that needed to buffer hydrogen ions causes systemic alkalinization and, when excreted, urine alkalinization as well.

Oral antacid action: Taken orally, sodium bicarbonate neutralizes stomach acid by the above mechanism.

Pharmacokinetics

Absorption: Well absorbed after oral administration as sodium ion and bicarbonate.
Distribution: Occurs naturally and is confined to the systemic circulation.

Metabolism: None.
Excretion: Filtered and reabsorbed by the kidney; less than 1% of filtered bicarbonate is excreted.

Route	Onset	Peak	Duration
P.O.	Unknown	Unknown	Unknown
I.V.	Immediate	Immediate	Unknown

Contraindications and precautions
Contraindicated in patients with metabolic or respiratory alkalosis; in those who are losing chlorides by vomiting or from continuous GI suction; in those receiving diuretics known to produce hypochloremic alkalosis; and in patients with hypocalcemia in which alkalosis may produce tetany, hypertension, seizures, or heart failure. Orally administered sodium bicarbonate is contraindicated in patients with acute ingestion of strong mineral acids.

Use extreme caution when giving drug to patients with heart failure, renal insufficiency, or other edematous or sodium-retaining conditions.

Interactions
Drug-drug. *Amphetamines, ephedrine, flecainide, mecamylamine, pseudoephedrine, quinidine:* If urine alkalinization occurs, sodium bicarbonate increases half-life of these drugs due to urine alkalization decreasing therapeutic effects. Monitor patient closely.
Chlorpropamide, lithium, methotrexate, salicylates, tetracyclines: Increased urinary excretion of these drugs. Monitor patient closely.
Corticosteroids: May increase sodium retention. Monitor patient closely.

Adverse reactions
GI: gastric distention, belching, flatulence.
Metabolic: *metabolic alkalosis,* hypernatremia, increased serum lactate levels, hyperosmolarity (with overdose).
Other: local pain and irritation at injection site.

Overdose and treatment
Overdose may cause depressed consciousness and obtundation from hypernatremia, tetany from hypocalcemia, arrhythmias from hypokalemia, and seizures from alkalosis. Correct fluid, electrolyte, and pH abnormalities. Monitor vital signs and fluid and electrolytes closely.

Special considerations
⚑ **ALERT** Sodium bicarbonate isn't routinely recommended for use in cardiac arrest because it may produce a paradoxical acidosis from carbon dioxide production.
● Avoid extravasation of I.V. solutions. Addition of calcium salts may cause precipitate; bicarbonate may inactivate catecholamines in solution (epinephrine, phenylephrine, and dopamine).
● Discourage use as an oral antacid because of hazardous excessive systemic absorption.

● Drug may be used as an adjunct to treat hyperkalemia (with dextrose and insulin).

Patient monitoring
● Monitor blood pH, partial pressure of arterial oxygen, partial pressure of arterial carbon dioxide and serum electrolytes.
● Assess patient for milk-alkali syndrome if drug use is long-term.
● Monitor vital signs regularly; when drug is used as urine alkalinizer, monitor urine pH.

Pregnant patients
● Safety hasn't been established for use during pregnancy.

Breast-feeding patients
● It isn't known if sodium bicarbonate appears in breast milk. Use cautiously when administering to breast-feeding women.

Pediatric patients
● Avoid rapid infusion (10 ml/minute) of hypertonic solutions in children under age 2.

Geriatric patients
● Elderly patients with heart failure or other fluid-retaining conditions are at greater risk for increased fluid retention; therefore, use drug cautiously.

Patient education
● Advise patient not to take drug with milk. Doing so may cause hypercalcemia, alkalosis, and possibly renal calculi.
● If patient takes an oral dose form, tell patient to take drug 1 hour before or 2 hours after taking enteric-coated drugs because sodium bicarbonate may cause enteric-coated products to dissolve in the stomach.

sodium ferric gluconate complex
Ferrlecit

Pharmacologic classification: macromolecular iron complex
Therapeutic classification: hematinic
Pregnancy risk category: B

Indications and dosages
➤ *Treatment of iron deficiency anemia in patients undergoing chronic hemodialysis who are receiving supplemental erythropoietin therapy.* *Adults:* Before starting therapeutic doses, give a test dose of 2 ml sodium ferric gluconate complex (25 mg elemental iron) diluted in 50 ml normal saline solution and given I.V. over 1 hour. If test dose is tolerated, give therapeutic dose of 10 ml (125 mg elemental iron) diluted in 100 ml normal saline solution and given I.V. over 1 hour. Most patients require a minimum cumulative dose of 1 g ele-

mental iron administered at more than eight sequential dialysis treatments to achieve a favorable hemoglobin or hematocrit response.

How supplied
Available by prescription only
Injection: 62.5 mg elemental iron (12.5 mg/ml) in 5-ml ampules

Pharmacodynamics
Hematinic action: Sodium ferric gluconate complex restores total body iron content, which is critical for normal hemoglobin synthesis and oxygen transport. Iron deficiency in hemodialysis patients can be due to increased iron utilization (such as from erythropoietin therapy), blood loss (such as from fistula, retention in dialyzer, hematologic testing, menses), decreased dietary intake or absorption, surgery, iron sequestration resulting from inflammatory process, and malignancy.

Sodium ferric gluconate complex restores total body iron content, which is critical for normal hemoglobin synthesis and oxygen transport.

Pharmacokinetics
No information available.

Route	Onset	Peak	Duration
I.V.	Unknown	Unknown	Unknown

Contraindications and precautions
Contraindicated in patients hypersensitive to sodium ferric gluconate complex or its components (such as benzyl alcohol). Also contraindicated in patients with anemias not caused by iron deficiency. Don't administer to patients with iron overload. Use cautiously in elderly patients.

Interactions
None reported.

Adverse reactions
CNS: asthenia, headache, fatigue, malaise, dizziness, paresthesia, agitation, insomnia, somnolence.
CV: syncope, hypotension, hypertension, tachycardia, ***bradycardia,*** angina, chest pain, *MI*, edema, flushing.
EENT: conjunctivitis, abnormal vision, rhinitis.
GI: nausea, vomiting, diarrhea, rectal disorder, dyspepsia, eructation, flatulence, melena, abdominal pain.
GU: urinary tract infection.
Hematologic: abnormal erythrocytes, anemia.
Metabolic: hyperkalemia, hypoglycemia, hypokalemia, hypervolemia.
Musculoskeletal: myalgia, arthralgia, back pain, arm pain, cramps.
Respiratory: dyspnea, coughing, upper respiratory tract infections, pneumonia, pulmonary edema.
Skin: pruritus, increased sweating, rash.

Other: injection site reaction, pain, fever, infection, rigors, chills, flulike syndrome, ***sepsis, carcinoma, hypersensitivity reactions,*** lymphadenopathy.

Overdose and treatment
Serum iron levels greater than 300 mcg/dl (with transferrin oversaturation) may indicate iron poisoning. Symptoms include abdominal pain, diarrhea, or vomiting that progresses to pallor or cyanosis; lassitude; drowsiness; hyperventilation resulting from acidosis; and CV collapse.

Treatment consists of supportive measures. Drug isn't dialyzable.

Special considerations
⚡ ALERT Dosage is expressed in milligrams of elemental iron.
● Drug shouldn't be given to patients with iron overload, which generally occurs in hemoglobinopathies and other refractory anemias.
⚡ ALERT Potentially life-threatening hypersensitivity reactions, characterized by CV collapse, cardiac arrest, bronchospasm, oral or pharyngeal edema, dyspnea, angioedema, urticaria, or pruritus sometimes linked to pain and muscle spasm of chest or back, may occur during infusion. Have adequate supportive measures readily available. Monitor patient closely during infusion.
● Some adverse reactions in hemodialysis patients may be related to dialysis itself or to chronic renal failure.
● Dilute test dose of sodium ferric gluconate complex in 50 ml normal saline solution and administer over 1 hour. Dilute therapeutic doses of drug in 100 ml normal saline solution and give over 1 hour.
● Don't mix sodium ferric gluconate complex with other drugs, or add to parenteral nutrition solutions for I.V. infusion. Use immediately after dilution in normal saline solution.
● Profound hypotension associated with flushing, light-headedness, malaise, fatigue, weakness, or severe chest, back, flank, or groin pain has been reported following rapid I.V. administration of iron. These reactions aren't associated with hypersensitivity reactions and may be due to too rapid administration of drug. Don't exceed recommended rate of administration (2.1 mg/min). Monitor patient closely during infusion.

Patient monitoring
● Monitor hematocrit and hemoglobin, serum ferritin, and iron saturation levels during therapy.
● Check with patient about other potential sources of iron, such as nonprescription iron preparations and iron-containing multiple vitamins with minerals.

Breast-feeding patients
● It's unknown if drug appears in breast milk. Administer drug cautiously to breast-feeding women.

Pediatric patients
• Safety and efficacy of drug haven't been established in children.

Geriatric patients
• It's unknown if patients age 65 and older respond differently than younger patients. In general, use drug cautiously in elderly patients because they may be taking other drugs or may have concomitant disease or decreased hepatic, renal, or cardiac function.

Patient education
• Abdominal pain, diarrhea, vomiting, drowsiness, or hyperventilation may indicate iron poisoning. Advise patient to report any of these symptoms immediately.

sodium fluoride
ACT, Fluorigard, Fluorinse, Fluoritab, Flura-Drops, Flura-Loz, Karidium, Karigel, Karigel-N, Listermint with Fluoride, Luride, Luride Lozi-Tabs, Luride-SF Lozi-Tabs, Pediaflor, Phos-Flur, Point-Two, Prevident, Thera-Flur, Thera-Flur-N

Pharmacologic classification: trace mineral
Therapeutic classification: dental caries prophylactic
Pregnancy risk category: C

Indications and dosages
➤ *Aid in the prevention of dental caries.*
Oral form. *Children ages 6 months to 2 years:* 0.25 mg daily.
Children ages 3 to 5: 0.5 mg daily.
Children ages 6 to 16: 1 mg daily.
✦ *Dosage adjustment.* If fluoride in the drinking water is less than 0.3 ppm, use dosage listed; if fluoride content is 0.3 to 0.6 ppm, use one-half of dosage. Oral fluoride supplements are not necessary in children under age 3 where the fluoride ion concentration in drinking water is 0.3 to 0.6 ppm; if fluoride content exceeds 0.6 ppm, don't use.
Topical form
Adults and children over age 12: 10 ml of 0.09% (0.2% fluoride ion) rinse. Use once daily after thoroughly brushing teeth and rinsing mouth. Rinse around and between teeth for 1 minute, then spit out.
Children ages 6 to 12: 5 ml of 0.09% (0.2% fluoride ion) solution.

How supplied
Available by prescription only
Drops: 0.125 mg/drop (30 ml), 0.125 mg/drop (60 ml, sugar-free), 0.25 mg/drop (19 ml), 0.25 mg/drop (24 ml, sugar-free), 0.5 mg/ml (50 ml)
Gel: 0.1% (65 g, 105 g, 122 g), 0.5% (24 g, 30 g, 60 g, 120 g, 130 g, 250 g), 1.23% (480 ml)

Gel drops: 0.5% (24 ml)
Lozenges: 1 mg
Rinse: 0.09% (240 ml, 480 ml), 0.09% (480 ml, sugar-free)
Tablets: 1 mg (sugar-free)
Tablets (chewable): 0.25 mg, 0.5 mg, 1 mg (sugar-free)
Available without a prescription
Rinse: 0.02%; 0.04%; 0.08%; 0.2%
Gel: 0.1%

Pharmacodynamics
Dental caries prophylactic action: Sodium fluoride acts systemically before tooth eruption and topically afterward by increasing tooth resistance to acid dissolution, by promoting remineralization, and by inhibiting the cariogenic microbial process. Acidulation provides greater topical fluoride uptake by dental enamel than neutral solutions. When topical fluoride is applied to hypersensitive exposed dentin, the formation of insoluble materials within the dentinal tubules blocks transmission of painful stimuli.

Pharmacokinetics
Absorption: Absorbed readily and almost completely from the GI tract. A large amount of an oral dose may be absorbed in the stomach; rate of absorption may depend on the gastric pH. Normal total plasma fluoride levels range from 0.14 to 0.19 mcg/ml.
Distribution: Stored in bones and developing teeth after absorption. Skeletal tissue also has a high storage capacity for fluoride ions. Because of the storage-mobilization mechanism in skeletal tissue, a constant fluoride supply may be provided. Fluoride has been found in all organs and tissues with a low accumulation in noncalcified tissues. Fluoride is distributed into sweat, tears, hair, and saliva. Fluoride crosses the placenta and is distributed into breast milk. Fluoride levels in milk range from about 0.05 to 0.13 ppm and remain fairly constant.
Metabolism: Not metabolized.
Excretion: Excreted rapidly, mainly in urine. About 90% of fluoride is filtered by the glomerulus and reabsorbed by the renal tubules.

Route	Onset	Peak	Duration
P.O.	Unknown	Unknown	Unknown

Contraindications and precautions
Contraindicated in patients hypersensitive to fluoride. Also contraindicated when intake from drinking water exceeds 0.6 ppm.

Interactions
Drug-drug. *Aluminum hydroxide or magnesium:* May impair sodium fluoride absorption. Administer drugs at separate times.
Drug-food. *Dairy foods:* Incompatibility may occur because of formation of calcium fluoride, which is poorly absorbed. Discourage use together.

Reactions may be *common*, uncommon, *life-threatening*, or common and life-threatening.

Adverse reactions
CNS: headache, weakness.
GI: gastric distress.
Skin: hypersensitivity reactions (atopic dermatitis, eczema, urticaria).
Other: staining of teeth.

Overdose and treatment
In children, acute ingestion of 10 to 20 mg of sodium fluoride may cause excessive salivation and GI disturbances; 500 mg may be fatal. GI disturbances include salivation, nausea, abdominal pain, vomiting, and diarrhea. CNS disturbances include CNS irritability, paresthesia, tetany, hyperactive reflexes, seizures, and respiratory or cardiac failure (from the calcium-binding effect of fluoride). Hypoglycemia and hypocalcemia and delayed hyperkalemia are frequent laboratory findings.

By using gastric lavage with 1% to 5% calcium chloride solution, the fluoride may be precipitated. Administer glucose I.V. in saline solution; parenteral calcium administration may be indicated for tetany. Maintain adequate urine output.

Special considerations
• Recommended doses are currently under study. Some evidence suggests that considerably less fluoride is needed for adequate supplementation.
• Tablets can be dissolved in the mouth, chewed, swallowed whole, added to drinking water or fruit juice, or added to water in infant formula or other foods.
• Drops may be administered orally undiluted or added to fluids or food.
• Sodium fluoride may be preferred to stannous fluoride to avoid staining tooth surfaces. Neutral sodium fluoride may also be preferred to acidulated fluoride to avoid dulling of porcelain and ceramic restorations.
• Prolonged intake of drinking water containing a fluoride ion concentration of 0.4 to 0.8 ppm may result in increased density of bone mineral and fluoride osteosclerosis.
• An oral sodium fluoride dose of 40 to 65 mg/day has resulted in adverse rheumatic effects.
• Drug is used investigationally to treat osteoporosis.

Patient monitoring
• Fluoride supplementation must be continuous from infancy to age 14 to be effective.
• Review dietary history with the family. A diet that includes large amounts of fish, mineral water, and tea provides about 5 mg/day of fluoride.

Breast-feeding patients
• Very little sodium fluoride appears in breast milk, and it increases only when daily intake exceeds 1.5 mg.

Pediatric patients
• Young children usually can't perform the rinse process necessary with oral solutions. Because prolonged ingestion or improper techniques may result in dental fluorosis and osseous changes, the dose must be carefully adjusted according to the amount of fluoride ion in drinking water.

Patient education
• Tell patient that sodium fluoride tablets and drops should be taken with meals, but not with dairy products.
• Advise patient that rinse and gel are most effective if used immediately after brushing or flossing and when taken just before going to bed.
• Tell patient to expectorate (and not swallow) excess liquid or gel.
• Warn patient not to eat, drink, or rinse mouth for 15 to 30 minutes after application. Tell patient to use a plastic container—not glass—to dilute drops or rinse, because the fluoride interacts with glass.
• Encourage patient to notify dentist if mottling of teeth occurs.
• Advise patient that if there is a change in water supply or if the patient moves to another area, then a dentist should be contacted because excessive fluoride causes mottled tooth enamel. If patient uses a private well, the water should be tested for fluoride.
• Warn parents to treat fluoride tablets as a drug and to keep them away from children.

sodium phosphates (sodium phosphate and sodium biphosphate)
Fleet Phospho-soda

Pharmacologic classification: acid salt
Therapeutic classification: saline laxative
Pregnancy risk category: C

Indications and dosages
➤ **Constipation.** *Adults and children age 12 and older:* 20 to 45 ml daily.
Children ages 10 to 11: 10 to 20 ml daily.
Children ages 5 to 9: 5 to 10 ml daily.

How supplied
Available without a prescription
Solution: 2.4 g monobasic sodium phosphate and 9 g dibasic sodium phosphate/5 ml

Pharmacodynamics
Laxative action: Sodium phosphate and sodium biphosphate exert an osmotic effect in the small intestine by drawing water into the intestinal lumen, producing distention that promotes peristalsis and bowel evacuation.

Pharmacokinetics
Absorption: The extent of phosphate and sodium absorption from oral phosphate laxatives is unknown. The extent of phosphate absorption from rectally administered phosphate enemas is unknown, but about 1% to 20% of the sodium and phosphate in such preparations is reportedly absorbed. With oral administration, action begins in 3 to 6 hours.
Distribution: Unknown.
Metabolism: Unknown.
Excretion: Unknown; probably in feces and urine.

Route	Onset	Peak	Duration
P.O.	Variable	Variable	Variable

Contraindications and precautions
Contraindicated in patients on sodium-restricted diets and patients with abdominal pain, nausea, vomiting, or other symptoms of appendicitis or acute surgical abdomen; intestinal obstruction or perforation; edema; heart failure; megacolon; or impaired renal function. Use cautiously in patients with large hemorrhoids or anal excoriations.

Interactions
Drug-drug. *Antacids:* May cause inactivation of both drugs. Don't use together.

Adverse reactions
GI: *abdominal cramping.*
Metabolic: fluid and electrolyte disturbances (hypernatremia, hyperphosphatemia) with daily use.
Other: laxative dependence with long-term or excessive use.

Overdose and treatment
No information available; probable clinical effects include abdominal pain and diarrhea.

Special considerations
● Dilute drug with water before giving orally (as directed by manufacturer). Follow drug administration with full glass of water.
● Drug isn't routinely used to treat constipation but is commonly used to evacuate the bowel.

Patient monitoring
● Monitor serum electrolyte levels; when drug is given as saline laxative, up to 10% of sodium content may be absorbed.

Breast-feeding patients
● It's not known if drug appears in human milk. Use cautiously in nursing women.

Patient education
● Teach patient how to mix drug.
● Instruct patient about dose schedule.
● Warn patient that frequent or prolonged use of drug may lead to laxative dependence.

● Teach patient about dietary sources of bulk, which include bran and other cereals, fresh fruit, and vegetables.
● Tell patient to drink 8 oz of cool water after taking Fleet Phospho-soda.
● Caution patient that rectal forms aren't intended for oral use.
● For children under age 5, tell parent to contact prescriber before use.

sodium polystyrene sulfonate
Kayexalate, SPS

Pharmacologic classification: cation-exchange resin
Therapeutic classification: potassium-removing resin
Pregnancy risk category: C

Indications and dosages
➤ *Hyperkalemia. Adults:* 15 g (4 teaspoonfuls of powder or 60 ml of available suspension) P.O. daily to q.i.d. in water or sorbitol. Or, give 30 to 50 g as needed as a retention enema. Dosage is individualized and depends on daily assessment of total body potassium.

How supplied
Available by prescription only
Oral powder: 1.25 g/5 ml suspension
Powder for oral or rectal administration: 454 g in 1-lb jar
Rectal suspension: 1.25 g/5 ml suspension

Pharmacodynamics
Potassium-removing action: Sodium polystyrene sulfonate is a cation-exchange resin that releases sodium in exchange for other cations in the GI tract. High levels of potassium ion are found in the large intestine and therefore are exchanged and eliminated.

Pharmacokinetics
Absorption: Not absorbed.
Distribution: None.
Metabolism: None.
Excretion: Excreted unchanged in feces.

Route	Onset	Peak	Duration
P.O.	2-12 hr	Unknown	Unknown
P.R.	Unknown	Unknown	Unknown

Contraindications and precautions
Contraindicated in patients hypersensitive to drug and in patients with hypokalemia. Use cautiously in patients with marked edema or severe heart failure or hypertension.

Interactions
Drug-drug. *Cardiac glycosides:* Toxic effects are exaggerated by hypokalemia, even when serum digoxin levels are in the normal range. Don't use together.

Reactions may be *common*, uncommon, *life-threatening*, or COMMON AND LIFE-THREATENING.

Magnesium- and calcium-containing antacids: Metabolic alkalosis in patients with renal impairment. Don't use together.

Adverse reactions
GI: *constipation,* fecal impaction (in elderly patients), anorexia, gastric irritation, nausea, vomiting, *diarrhea* (with sorbitol emulsions).
Metabolic: *hypokalemia,* hypocalcemia, sodium retention, altered serum magnesium level.

Overdose and treatment
Signs and symptoms of overdose reflect those of hypokalemia, such as irritability, confusion, arrhythmias, ECG changes, severe muscle weakness, and sometimes paralysis; they reflect those of digitalis toxicity in digitalized patients.

Drug may be discontinued or dose lowered when serum potassium level decreases to 4 to 5 mEq/L.

Special considerations
• For oral administration, mix resin only with water or sorbitol; never mix with orange juice because of its high potassium content.
• Chill oral suspension to increase palatability; don't heat because that inactivates resin.
• Use P.R. route when vomiting, P.O. restrictions, or upper GI tract problems are present.
• Fecal impaction can be prevented in geriatric patients by administering resin P.R. Cleaning enema should precede rectal administration.
• For rectal administration, mix polystyrene resin only with water and sorbitol for rectal use. Don't use other vehicles such as mineral oil for rectal administration to prevent impactions. Ion exchange requires aqueous medium. Sorbitol content prevents impaction. Prepare rectal dose at room temperature. Stir emulsion gently during administration.
• Constipation is more likely when drug is given with phosphate binders such as aluminum hydroxide. Monitor patient's bowel habits.

Patient monitoring
• Monitor serum potassium at least once daily. Watch for other signs of hypokalemia.
• Monitor patient for symptoms of other electrolyte deficiencies (magnesium, calcium) because drug is nonselective. Monitor serum calcium determination in patients receiving sodium polystyrene therapy for more than 3 days. Supplementary calcium may be needed.
• If hyperkalemia is severe, more drastic modalities should be added; for example, dextrose 50% with regular insulin I.V. push. Don't depend solely on polystyrene resin to lower serum potassium levels in severe hyperkalemia.

Pediatric patients
• Adjust dose in children by calculating 1 mEq of potassium bound for each 1 g of resin.

Geriatric patients
• Fecal impaction is more likely in elderly patients.

Patient education
• Instruct patient in the importance of following a prescribed low-potassium diet.
• Explain necessity of retaining enema to patient. Retention for 6 to 10 hours is ideal, but 30 to 60 minutes is acceptable.

somatropin
Genotropin, Humatrope, Norditropin, Nutropin, Nutropin AQ, Saizen, Serostim

Pharmacologic classification: anterior pituitary hormone
Therapeutic classification: purified growth hormone (GH)
Pregnancy risk category: C

Indications and dosages
➤ *Long-term treatment of growth failure in children with inadequate secretion of endogenous GH. Children:* 0.18 mg/kg S.C. or I.M. weekly, divided equally and given on 3 alternate days, six times weekly or daily using Humatrope. Or, 0.30 mg/kg S.C. weekly in daily divided doses using Nutropin. Or, 0.06 mg/kg I.M. or S.C. three times weekly using Saizen. Or, 0.024 to 0.034 mg/kg S.C., six to seven times weekly using Norditropin.
➤ *In children, growth failure from chronic renal insufficiency up to time of renal transplantation.* Nutropin and Nutropin AQ. *Children:* weekly dosage of up to 0.35 mg/kg S.C. divided into daily doses.
➤ *Long-term treatment of short stature related to Turner's syndrome. Children:* up to 0.375 mg/kg weekly (about 1.125 IU/kg weekly) S.C. divided into equal doses given three to seven times weekly.
➤ *Replacement of endogenous GH in adult patients with GH deficiency. Adults:* initially, not more than 0.006 mg/kg S.C. daily. May be increased to maximum of 0.025 mg/kg daily in patients younger than age 35 or 0.0125 mg/kg daily in patients older than age 35.
➤ *AIDS wasting or cachexia.* Serostim.
Adults and children who weigh more than 55 kg (121 lb): 6 mg S.C. h.s.
Adults and children who weigh 45 to 55 kg (99 to 121 lb): 5 mg S.C. h.s.
Adults and children who weigh 35 to 45 kg (77 to 99 lb): 4 mg S.C h.s.
Adults and children who weigh less than 35 kg: 0.1 mg/kg daily S.C. h.s.

How supplied
Available by prescription only
Genotropin injection: 1.5 mg (about 4 IU/ml),
5.8 mg (about 15 IU/ml)
Injection: 2-mg (about 6-IU [Humatrope]) vial,
5-mg (about 15-IU [Humatrope]) vial, 10-mg
(about 30-IU [Nutropin]) vial
Norditropin injection: 4 mg (about 12 IU/ml),
8 mg (about 24 IU/ml)
Nutropin AQ injection: 10 mg (about 30 IU/
vial)
Nutropin injection: 5 mg (about 15 IU/vial),
10 mg (about 30 IU/vial)
Saizen injection: 5 mg (about 15 IU/vial)
Serostim injection: 5 mg (about 15 IU/vial),
6 mg (about 18 IU/ml)

Pharmacodynamics
Growth-stimulating action: Somatropin is a
purified GH of recombinant DNA origin that stimulates skeletal, linear bone, muscle, and organ
growth.

Pharmacokinetics
Absorption: Absorbed from the injection site in
a similar fashion as somatrem (human growth
hormone).
Distribution: Localizes to highly perfused organs, notably the liver and kidney.
Metabolism: Metabolized in the liver.
Excretion: Returned to the systemic circulation
as amino acids.

Route	Onset	Peak	Duration
I.M., S.C.	Unknown	3-5 hr	12-48 hr

Contraindications and precautions
Contraindicated in patients with closed epiphyses or an active underlying intracranial lesion.
Humatrope shouldn't be reconstituted with the
supplied diluent for patients with known sensitivity to either m-Cresol or glycerin.
    Use cautiously in children with hypothyroidism
and in those whose GH deficiency results from
an intracranial lesion; these children should be
examined frequently for progression or recurrence of underlying disease.

Interactions
Drug-drug. *Glucocorticoid therapy:* May inhibit growth-promoting effect. Carefully adjust
glucocorticoid replacement dose in patients with
coexistent deficiency.

Adverse reactions
CNS: headache, weakness.
CV: mild, transient edema.
Hematologic: *leukemia.*
Metabolic: mild hyperglycemia; hypothyroidism;
increased inorganic phosphorus, alkaline phos-
phatase, and parathyroid hormone levels.
Musculoskeletal: carpal tunnel syndrome.
Other: injection site pain, localized muscle pain,
gynecomastia, antibody formation to GH.

Overdose and treatment
Long-term overdose may result in signs and symptoms of gigantism or acromegaly consistent with
the known effects of excess human GH.

Special considerations
⚠ **ALERT** Don't confuse somatropin with somatrem or sumatriptan.
● For Genotropin, reconstitute per manufacturer's directions provided with each device.
● To prepare solution, inject the supplied diluent into the vial containing the drug by aiming
the stream of the liquid against the glass wall of
the vial. Swirl the vial with a gentle rotary motion
until the contents are completely dissolved. Don't
shake the vial.
● After reconstitution, vial solution should be
clear. Don't use if it's cloudy or contains particles.
● Store reconstituted vial in refrigerator; refer to
product information for storage and stability information.
● If sensitivity to diluent occurs, vial may be reconstituted with sterile water for injection. When
drug is reconstituted in this manner, use only one
reconstituted dose per vial and refrigerate the solution if it isn't used immediately after reconstitution. Use reconstituted dose within 24 hours,
and discard unused portion.

Patient monitoring
● Monitor child's height regularly. Regular monitoring of blood and radiologic studies is also
necessary.
● Monitor patient's blood glucose levels regularly
because GH may induce a state of insulin resistance.
● Excessive glucocorticoid therapy inhibits the
growth-promoting effect of somatropin. Adjust
glucocorticoid replacement dose in patients with
a coexisting corticotropin deficiency to avoid an
inhibitory effect on growth.
● Frequently monitor patients with GH deficiency secondary to an intracranial lesion for progression or recurrence of the underlying disease
process.
● Carefully monitor patient for any malignant
transformation of skin lesions.
● Periodically monitor thyroid function tests for
hypothyroidism, which may require treatment
with a thyroid hormone.

Patient education
● Inform parents that children with endocrine
disorders including GH deficiency are more likely to develop slipped capital epiphyses. Tell them
to call if they notice their child limping.
● Stress to parents the importance of close follow-
up care.

Reactions may be *common*, uncommon, *life-threatening*, or COMMON AND LIFE-THREATENING.

sotalol
Betapace, Betapace AF

Pharmacologic classification: beta blocker
Therapeutic classification: antiarrhythmic
Pregnancy risk category: B

Indications and dosages
➤ *Documented, life-threatening ventricular arrhythmias.* **Betapace.** *Adults:* Initially, 80 mg P.O. b.i.d. Increase dose q 2 to 3 days as needed and tolerated. Most patients respond to daily dose of 160 to 320 mg given in divided doses b.i.d. A few patients with refractory arrhythmias have received as much as 640 mg daily given in divided doses b.i.d.

✦*Dosage adjustment.* For adults with renal failure and creatinine clearance above 60 ml/minute, no adjustment in dose interval is necessary. If creatinine clearance is 30 to 60 ml/minute, give q 24 hours; if 10 to 29 ml/minute, q 36 to 48 hours; if less than 10 ml/minute, individualized dosage.

➤ *Maintenance of normal sinus rhythm (delay in time to recurrence of atrial fibrillation or flutter) in patients with symptomatic atrial fibrillation or flutter who are currently in sinus rhythm.* **Betapace AF.** *Adults:* Initially, 80 mg P.O. once or twice daily depending on creatinine clearance. For patients with creatinine clearance above 60 ml/minute, give dose twice daily. For creatinine clearance of 40 to 60 ml/minute, give dose once daily. Don't give drug to patients with a creatinine clearance below 40 ml/minute.

If initial dose doesn't reduce the frequency of relapses of atrial fibrillation or flutter and is tolerated without excessive prolongation of QT interval (520 msec or above), the dose may be increased to 120 mg. If the 120-mg dose also doesn't reduce the frequency and is tolerated without excessive QT interval prolongation, an increase to 160 mg can be considered.

The baseline QT interval must be 450 msec or less to start a patient on Betapace AF. During start of therapy and adjustment of dosage, monitor QT interval 2 to 4 hours after each dose. If the QT interval is 500 msec or more, the dose must be reduced or the drug discontinued.

How supplied
Available by prescription only
Tablets: 80 mg, 120 mg, 160 mg, 240 mg (Betapace AF only)

Pharmacodynamics
Antiarrhythmic action: Sotalol is a nonselective beta blocker that depresses sinus heart rate, slows AV conduction, increases AV nodal refractoriness, prolongs the refractory period of atrial and ventricular muscle and AV accessory pathways in anterograde and retrograde directions, decreases cardiac output, and lowers systolic and diastolic blood pressure.

Pharmacokinetics
Absorption: Well absorbed after oral administration, with a bioavailability of 90% to 100%. After oral administration, steady state plasma levels are attained in 2 to 3 days (after five to six doses when given twice daily).
Distribution: Doesn't bind to plasma proteins and crosses the blood-brain barrier poorly.
Metabolism: Not metabolized.
Excretion: Excreted primarily in urine unchanged.

Route	Onset	Peak	Duration
P.O.	Unknown	2¼-4 hr	Unknown

Contraindications and precautions
Contraindicated in patients hypersensitive to drug, severe sinus node dysfunction, sinus bradycardia, second- and third-degree AV block in the absence of an artificial pacemaker, congenital or acquired long-QT syndrome, cardiogenic shock, uncontrolled heart failure, and bronchial asthma. Betapace AF is contraindicated in patients with creatinine clearance below 40 ml/minute.

Use cautiously in patients with impaired renal function or diabetes mellitus.

Interactions
Drug-drug. *Antacids:* Decreased effects of sotalol. Advise patient to take 2 hours apart.
Antiarrhythmics: Additive effects when administered with sotalol. Avoid use together.
Calcium channel blockers: Enhanced myocardial depression. Don't give with sotalol.
Catecholamine-depleting drugs, such as guanethidine and reserpine: Enhanced hypotensive effects of sotalol. Monitor patient closely.
Clonidine: Sotalol may enhance the rebound hypertensive effect after withdrawal of clonidine. Discontinue sotalol several days before withdrawing clonidine.
Insulin, oral antidiabetics: Increased blood glucose levels and possible masked symptoms of hypoglycemia. Adjust sotalol dosage if necessary.
Drug-food. *Any food:* Decreased absorption. Tell patient to take drug on an empty stomach.

Adverse reactions
CNS: asthenia, light-headedness, headache, dizziness, weakness, fatigue, sleep problems.
CV: *bradycardia, palpitations, chest pain, arrhythmias, heart failure, AV block, proarrhythmic events (ventricular tachycardia, PVCs, ventricular fibrillation),* edema, ECG abnormalities, hypotension.
GI: *nausea, vomiting,* diarrhea, dyspepsia.
Hepatic: elevated liver enzyme levels.
Metabolic: increased serum glucose level.
Respiratory: *dyspnea, bronchospasm.*

Overdose and treatment
The most common signs and symptoms of overdose are bradycardia, heart failure, hypotension, bronchospasm, and hypoglycemia.

If overdose occurs, discontinue sotalol. Because of the lack of protein-binding, hemodialysis is useful in reducing sotalol plasma levels. Observe patient carefully until QT intervals are normalized.

Atropine, another anticholinergic drug, a beta-adrenergic agonist, or transvenous cardiac pacing also may be used to treat bradycardia; transvenous cardiac pacing to treat second- or third-degree heart block; epinephrine to treat hypotension (depending on associated factors); aminophylline or an aerosol beta$_2$-receptor stimulant to treat bronchospasm; and DC cardioversion, transvenous cardiac pacing, epinephrine, or magnesium sulfate to treat torsades de pointes.

Special considerations
⚡ ALERT Don't substitute Betapace for Betapace AF.
• Because proarrhythmic events, such as sustained ventricular tachycardia or ventricular fibrillation, may occur at when therapy starts or dosage is adjusted, patient should be hospitalized. Facilities and personnel should be available for cardiac rhythm monitoring and ECG interpretation.
• Although patients receiving I.V. lidocaine have begun sotalol therapy without ill effect, other antiarrhythmics should be withdrawn before sotalol therapy begins. Sotalol therapy typically is delayed until two or three half-lives of the withdrawn drug have elapsed. After withdrawal of amiodarone, sotalol shouldn't be given until the QT interval normalizes.
• Patients with a history of symptomatic atrial fibrillation or flutter who are currently taking Betapace to maintain a normal sinus rhythm should be switched to Betapace AF because of significant differences in labeling between drugs.
• Anticoagulate patients who have atrial fibrillation according to standard practice.
• Adjust dosage slowly, allowing 3 days (or 5 to 6 doses if patient is receiving once-daily doses) between dose increments for adequate monitoring of QT intervals and for drug plasma levels to reach steady state.

Patient monitoring
• Monitor serum electrolyte levels regularly, especially if patient is receiving diuretics. Electrolyte imbalances, such as hypokalemia or hypomagnesemia, may enhance QT interval prolongation and increase risk of serious arrhythmias, such as torsades de pointes.

Pregnant patients
• Safety hasn't been established. Use only when potential benefits outweigh the risks to the fetus.

Breast-feeding patients
• Because drug may appear in breast milk, either breast-feeding or sotalol may be discontinued depending on importance of drug to woman's health.

Pediatric patients
• Safety and efficacy in children haven't been established.

Patient education
• Explain importance of taking sotalol as prescribed, even when feeling well.
• Caution patient not to stop drug suddenly.
• Tell patient not to take antacids within 2 hours of sotalol.
• Tell patient not to double the next dose if he misses one. Instead, tell him to take the next dose at the usual time.

sparfloxacin
Zagam

Pharmacologic classification: fluorinated quinolone
Therapeutic classification: broad-spectrum antibacterial
Pregnancy risk category: C

Indications and dosages
➤ *Acute bacterial exacerbation of chronic bronchitis caused by* **Staphylococcus aureus, Streptococcus pneumoniae, Chlamydia pneumoniae, Enterobacter cloacae, Klebsiella pneumoniae, Moraxella catarrhalis, Haemophilus influenzae,** *or* **H. parainfluenzae.** *Adults over age 18:* 400 mg P.O. on first day as a loading dose, then 200 mg daily for total of 10 days of therapy (total, 11 tablets).
➤ *Community-acquired pneumonia caused by* **C. pneumoniae, H. influenzae, H. parainfluenzae, M. catarrhalis, Mycoplasma pneumoniae,** *or* **S. pneumoniae.** *Adults over age 18:* 400 mg P.O. on first day as a loading dose, and then 200 mg daily for total of 10 days of therapy (total, 11 tablets).
✦ *Dosage adjustment.* If creatinine clearance is less than 50 ml/minute, give a loading dose of 400 mg P.O.; thereafter, give 200 mg P.O. q 48 hours for a total of 9 days of therapy (total, six tablets).

How supplied
Available by prescription only
Tablets: 200 mg

Pharmacodynamics
Antibactericidal action: Inhibits bacterial DNA gyrase and prevents DNA replication, transcription, repair, and deactivation in susceptible bacteria.

Pharmacokinetics

Absorption: Well absorbed following oral administration with an absolute bioavailability of 92%.

Distribution: Volume of distribution is about 3.9 L/kg, indicating distribution well into the tissues. Level of drug in respiratory tissues at 2 to 6 hours following dosing is about three to six times greater than plasma.

Metabolism: Metabolized by the liver, primarily by phase II glucuronidation. Its metabolism doesn't interfere with or use the cytochrome P-450 system.

Excretion: Excreted in both the urine (50%) and feces (50%). Terminal elimination half-life varies between 16 and 30 hours; mean, 20 hours.

Route	Onset	Peak	Duration
P.O.	Unknown	3-6 hr	Unknown

Contraindications and precautions

Contraindicated in patients with history of hypersensitivity or photosensitivity reactions to drugs and those who can't stay out of the sun. Don't use in patients with cardiac conditions that predispose them to arrhythmias. Contraindicated in patients taking drugs that prolong the QTc interval.

Use cautiously in patients with known or suspected CNS disorders, such as seizures, toxic psychoses, or tremors.

Interactions

Drug-drug. *Antacids containing aluminum or magnesium, iron salts, sucralfate, zinc:* May interfere with GI absorption of sparfloxacin. Don't give sparfloxacin within 2 hours before or 6 hours after an antacid.

Drugs that prolong the QTc interval, including amiodarone, bepridil, disopyramide, class Ia antiarrhythmics (procainamide, quinidine), class III drugs (sotalol); erythromycin, pentamidine, tricyclic antidepressants, and some antipsychotics including phenothiazines: May cause torsades de pointes. Don't administer together.

Drug-lifestyle. *Sun exposure:* May cause photosensitivity reactions. Advise patient to take precautions.

Adverse reactions

CNS: asthenia, dizziness, headache, insomnia, *seizures,* somnolence.

CV: *QT interval prolongation,* vasodilatation.

GI: dry mouth, taste perversion, abdominal pain, diarrhea, dyspepsia, flatulence, nausea, pseudomembranous colitis, vomiting.

GU: vaginal candidiasis.

Hematologic: elevated WBC count.

Hepatic: elevated liver enzyme levels.

Musculoskeletal: tendon rupture.

Skin: photosensitivity, pruritus, rash.

Other: *hypersensitivity reactions.*

Overdose and treatment

If overdose is suspected, have patient avoid sunlight exposure for 5 days. Monitor ECG for possible QTc interval prolongation. It isn't known if drug is dialyzable.

Special considerations

● Use cautiously in patients with a history of seizure disorder or other CNS diseases, such as cerebral arteriosclerosis.

● Acute hypersensitivity reactions may require treatment with epinephrine, oxygen, I.V. fluids, antihistamines, corticosteroids, pressor amines, and airway management.

● Drug may produce false-negative culture results for *Mycobacterium tuberculosis.*

Patient monitoring

● Monitor renal function.

● Obtain specimen for culture and sensitivity before starting therapy to determine whether bacterial resistance has occurred.

Breast-feeding patients

● Because drug appears in breast milk, discontinue either breast-feeding or drug.

Pediatric patients

● Safety and efficacy in children and adolescents under age 18 haven't been established.

Geriatric patients

● Pharmacokinetics of drug aren't altered in elderly patients with normal renal function. Monitor renal function carefully and adjust doses as recommended.

Patient education

● Inform patient that drug may be taken with food, milk, or products that contain caffeine.

● Tell patient to take drug as prescribed, even if symptoms disappear.

● Advise patient to take drug with plenty of fluids and to avoid antacids, sucralfate, and products containing iron or zinc for at least 4 hours after each dose.

● Warn patient to avoid hazardous tasks until adverse CNS effects of drug are known.

● Tell patient to discontinue drug and report pain or inflammation; tendon rupture can occur with drug. Tell patient to rest and refrain from exercise until a diagnosis is made.

● Tell patient to avoid exposure to sunlight, bright natural light and ultraviolet rays during and for 5 days after treatment is stopped.

spironolactone
Aldactone

Pharmacologic classification: potassium-sparing diuretic
Therapeutic classification: management of edema; antihypertensive; diagnosis of primary hyperaldosteronism; treatment of diuretic-induced hypokalemia
Pregnancy risk category: NR

Indications and dosages
➤ *Edema. Adults:* 25 to 200 mg P.O. daily in divided doses.
Children: Initially, 3.3 mg/kg or 60 mg/m² P.O. daily in divided doses.
➤ *Hypertension. Adults:* 50 to 100 mg P.O. daily in divided doses.
Children: 1 to 2 mg/kg P.O. b.i.d. has been used.
➤ *Diuretic-induced hypokalemia. Adults:* 25 to 100 mg P.O. daily when oral potassium supplements are considered inappropriate.
➤ *Detection of primary hyperaldosteronism. Adults:* 400 mg P.O. daily for 4 days (short test) or for 3 to 4 weeks (long test). If hypokalemia and hypertension are corrected, a presumptive diagnosis of primary hyperaldosteronism is made.
➤ *Hirsutism ◇. Adults:* 50 to 200 mg P.O. daily.
➤ *Premenstrual syndrome ◇. Adults:* 25 mg q.i.d. P.O. on day 14 of menstrual cycle.
➤ *Heart failure in patients receiving an ACE inhibitor and a loop diuretic with or without a cardiac glycoside ◇. Adults:* Initially, 12.5 to 25 mg P.O. daily.
➤ *To decrease risk of metrorrhagia ◇. Adults:* 50 mg b.i.d. P.O. on days 4 through 21 of menstrual cycle.
➤ *Acne vulgaris ◇. Adults:* 100 mg P.O. daily.

How supplied
Available by prescription only
Tablets: 25 mg
Tablets (film-coated): 25 mg, 50 mg, 100 mg

Pharmacodynamics
Diuretic and potassium-sparing actions: Spironolactone competitively inhibits aldosterone effects on the distal renal tubules, increasing sodium and water excretion and decreasing potassium excretion.

Spironolactone is used to treat edema associated with excessive aldosterone secretion, such as that associated with hepatic cirrhosis, nephrotic syndrome, and heart failure. It's also used to treat diuretic-induced hypokalemia.
Antihypertensive action: The mechanism of action is unknown; spironolactone may block the effect of aldosterone on arteriolar smooth muscle.
Diagnosis of primary hyperaldosteronism: Spironolactone inhibits the effects of aldosterone; therefore, correction of hypokalemia and hy-

pertension is presumptive evidence of primary hyperaldosteronism.

Pharmacokinetics
Absorption: About 90% is absorbed after oral administration.
Distribution: Drug and its major metabolite, canrenone, are more than 90% plasma protein-bound.
Metabolism: Rapidly and extensively metabolized to canrenone.
Excretion: Canrenone and other metabolites are excreted primarily in urine, and a small amount is excreted in feces via the biliary tract; half-life of canrenone is 13 to 24 hours. Half-life of parent compound is 1 to 2 hours.

Route	Onset	Peak	Duration
P.O.	1-2 days	2-3 days	2-3 days

Contraindications and precautions
Contraindicated in patients with anuria, acute or progressive renal insufficiency, or hyperkalemia or those receiving amiloride or triamterene. Use cautiously in patients with impaired renal function, hepatic disease, or fluid and electrolyte imbalances.

Interactions
Drug-drug. *ACE inhibitors, potassium supplements, potassium-containing drugs such as parenteral penicillin G:* Spironolactone increases the risk of hyperkalemia when administered with these drugs. Use together cautiously, especially in patients with renal impairment.
Anesthetics, norepinephrine: Reduced response to these drugs. Use together cautiously.
Antihypertensives: Spironolactone may potentiate hypotensive effects. May be used to therapeutic advantage.
Aspirin: May slightly decrease the response to spironolactone. Watch for diminished effect.
Cardiac glycosides: Increased serum digoxin levels and subsequent toxicity. Monitor drug levels of digoxin.
NSAIDs, such as ibuprofen or indomethacin: May impair renal function and thus affect potassium excretion. Avoid use together.
Potassium-sparing diuretics: Increased risk of hyperkalemia. Avoid use together.
Drug-herb. *Licorice:* Antiulcer and aldosterone-like effects of herb may be blocked. Discourge use together.
Drug-food. *Potassium-containing salt substitutes, potassium-rich foods (such as citrus fruit and tomatoes):* Increased risk of hyperkalemia. Advise caution.

Adverse reactions
CNS: headache, drowsiness, lethargy, confusion, ataxia.
GI: diarrhea, gastric bleeding, ulceration, cramping, gastritis, vomiting.

GU: inability to maintain erection, menstrual disturbances in women.
Hematologic: *agranulocytosis.*
Metabolic: *hyperkalemia,* dehydration, hyponatremia, transient elevation in BUN level, metabolic acidosis.
Skin: hirsutism, urticaria, maculopapular eruptions.
Other: gynecomastia, breast soreness in women, drug fever.

Overdose and treatment

Signs and symptoms of overdose are consistent with dehydration and electrolyte disturbance.

Treatment is supportive and symptomatic. In acute ingestion, empty stomach by emesis or lavage. In severe hyperkalemia (more than 6.5 mEq/L), reduce serum potassium levels with I.V. sodium bicarbonate or glucose with insulin. A cation exchange resin, sodium polystyrene sulfonate (Kayexalate), given orally or as a retention enema, may also reduce serum potassium levels.

Special considerations

Consider recommendations relevant to all potassium-sparing diuretics as well as the following.
● Give drug with meals to enhance absorption.
● Protect drug from light.
● Spironolactone is antiandrogenic and has been used to treat hirsutism in doses of 200 mg/day.
● Avoid unnecessary use of drug. Drug has been shown to induce tumors in laboratory animals.

Patient monitoring

● Diuretic effect may be delayed 2 to 3 days if drug is used alone; maximum antihypertensive effect may be delayed 2 to 3 weeks.
● Adverse reactions are related to dose levels and duration of therapy and usually disappear with withdrawal of drug; however, gynecomastia may persist.
● Watch for hyperchloremic metabolic acidosis.

Breast-feeding patients

● Safety during breast-feeding hasn't been established. Canrenone, a metabolite, appears in breast milk. Recommend an alternative feeding method during spironolactone therapy.

Pediatric patients

● When giving drug to children, crush tablets and mix in cherry syrup as an oral suspension.

Geriatric patients

● These patients are more susceptible to diuretic effects and may need lower doses to prevent excessive diuresis.

Patient education

● Instruct patient to report mental confusion or lethargy immediately.

● Explain that adverse reactions usually disappear after drug is discontinued; gynecomastia, however, may persist.
● Caution patient to avoid hazardous activities such as driving until response to drug is known.

stavudine (d4T)
Zerit

Pharmacologic classification: synthetic thymidine nucleoside analogue
Therapeutic classification: antiviral
Pregnancy risk category: C

Indications and dosages

➤ *Treatment of patients with HIV infection in combination with other antiretroviral agents. Adults who weigh 60 kg (132 lb) or more:* 40 mg P.O. q 12 hours.
Adults and children who weigh more than 30 kg (66 lb) but less than 60 kg: 30 mg P.O. q 12 hours.
Children who weigh less than 30 kg: 1 mg/kg q 12 hours.
✦ *Dosage adjustment.* For adults undergoing hemodialysis, give 20 mg q 24 hours if patient weighs 60 kg or more and 15 mg q 24 hours if patient weighs less than 60 kg. Data are inadequate for children with renal impairment, so a dose reduction or increase in time interval between doses should be considered. For adults with renal impairment, refer to the table below.

Creatinine clearance (ml/min)	Dosage for patients weighing ≥ 60 kg	Dosage for patients weighing < 60 kg
26-50	20 mg q 12 hours	15 mg q 12 hours
10-25	20 mg q 24 hours	15 mg q 24 hours

How supplied

Available by prescription only
Capsules: 15 mg, 20 mg, 30 mg, 40 mg
Oral solution: 1 mg/ml

Pharmacodynamics

Antiviral action: Stavudine is phosphorylated by cellular kinases to stavudine triphosphate, which retards HIV replication by inhibiting HIV reverse transcriptase and inhibiting viral DNA synthesis. The triphosphate also inhibits cellular DNA polymerase beta and gamma and reduces mitochondrial DNA synthesis.

Pharmacokinetics

Absorption: Rapidly absorbed with a mean absolute bioavailability of 86.4%.
Distribution: Mean volume of distribution is 58 L, suggesting distribution into extravascular space.

Drug is distributed equally between RBCs and plasma. It binds poorly to plasma proteins.
Metabolism: Not clearly defined.
Excretion: Renal elimination accounts for about 40% of overall clearance, regardless of administration route; there's active tubular secretion in addition to glomerular filtration.

Route	Onset	Peak	Duration
P.O.	Unknown	1 hr	Unknown

Contraindications and precautions
Contraindicated in patients hypersensitive to drug. Use cautiously in patients with impaired renal function or history of peripheral neuropathy and in pregnant women.

Interactions
Drug-drug. *Zidovudine:* May competitively inhibit intracellular phosphorylation of stavudine. Avoid use together.

Adverse reactions
CNS: *peripheral neuropathy, headache, malaise, insomnia, anxiety, depression, nervousness,* dizziness.
CV: chest pain.
EENT: conjunctivitis.
GI: *abdominal pain, diarrhea, nausea, vomiting, anorexia,* dyspepsia, constipation, weight loss.
Hematologic: *neutropenia, thrombocytopenia,* anemia.
Hepatic: elevated liver enzyme levels, *hepatotoxicity.*
Musculoskeletal: *myalgia, asthenia, back pain, arthralgia.*
Respiratory: *dyspnea.*
Skin: *rash, diaphoresis, pruritus,* maculopapular rash.
Other: *chills, fever,* lactic acidosis.

Overdose and treatment
Experience with adults who had received 12 to 24 times the recommended daily dose revealed no acute toxicity. Complications of chronic overdose include peripheral neuropathy and hepatic toxicity. It is removed by hemodialysis but it isn't known if drug is eliminated by peritoneal dialysis.

Special considerations
◪ **ALERT** Don't confuse this drug with other antivirals that may use initials for identification.
● Use cautiously in patients with renal impairment or history of peripheral neuropathy. Dosage adjustment may be necessary.
● Give drug with other antiretrovirals.
● Monitor patient for development of peripheral neuropathy, usually characterized by numbness, tingling, or pain in the feet or hands. If symptoms develop, interrupt drug therapy. They may resolve if therapy is withdrawn promptly, although they sometimes worsen temporarily af-

ter drug is stopped. If symptoms resolve completely, resume treatment using the following dosage: 20 mg twice daily if patient weighs 60 kg or more, 15 mg twice daily if patient weighs less than 60 kg. Manage clinically significant elevations of hepatic transaminase levels in same way.
● If neruopathy recurs after restarting drug, consider stopping drug permanently.
◪ **ALERT** Lactic acidosis and severe hepatomegaly with steatosis have been reported in patients taking stavudine and in patients receiving other nucleoside analogs.

Patient monitoring
● Monitor CBC and serum levels of creatinine, AST, ALT, and alkaline phosphatase.

Breast-feeding patients
● It isn't known if drug appears in breast milk. Because of the potential for adverse reactions in breast-fed infants, breast-feeding should be discontinued during therapy.

Patient education
● Inform patient that stavudine doesn't cure HIV infection and that the patient may continue to acquire illnesses related to AIDS or AIDS-related complex, including opportunistic infections.
● Inform patient that drug doesn't reduce risk of transmitting HIV to others through sexual contact or blood contamination.
● Instruct patient to report signs of peripheral neuropathy, such as tingling, burning, pain, or numbness in the hands and feet, because dose adjustments may be necessary.
● Advise patient not to use other medications, including OTC preparations, without contacting prescriber first.
● Explain that long-term effects of drug are currently unknown.

streptokinase
Streptase

Pharmacologic classification: plasminogen activator
Therapeutic classification: thrombolytic enzyme
Pregnancy risk category: C

Indications and dosages
➤ **Lysis of coronary artery thrombi after acute MI.** *Adults:* 1,500,000 IU by I.V. infusion over 60 minutes; intracoronary loading dose of 20,000 IU via coronary catheter, followed by a maintenance dosage of 2,000 IU/minute for 60 minutes as an infusion.
➤ **Venous thrombosis, pulmonary embolism, and arterial thrombosis and embolism.** *Adults:* Loading dose of 250,000 IU I.V. infusion over 30 minutes. *Sustaining dose:* 100,000 IU/hour I.V. infusion for 72 hours for

deep vein thrombosis, 100,000 IU/hour over 24 hours by I.V. infusion for pulmonary embolism, 100,000 IU/hour by I.V. infusion for 24 to 72 hours for arterial thrombosis or embolism.

➤ *Arteriovenous cannula occlusion. Adults:* 250,000 IU in 2 ml solution by I.V. infusion pump into each occluded limb of the cannula over 25 to 35 minutes. Clamp off cannula for 2 hours, then aspirate contents of cannula, flush with saline solution, and reconnect. The manufacturer doesn't recommend using drug to restore patency of occluded I.V. catheters.

How supplied
Available by prescription only
Injection: 250,000 IU, 750,000 IU, 1,500,000 IU in vials for reconstitution

Pharmacodynamics
Thrombolytic action: Streptokinase promotes thrombolysis by activating plasminogen in two steps. First, plasminogen and streptokinase form a complex, exposing plasminogen-activating site, and second, cleavage of peptide bond converts plasminogen to plasmin.

In treatment of acute MI, streptokinase prevents primary or secondary thrombus formation in microcirculation surrounding the necrotic area.

Pharmacokinetics
Absorption: Plasminogen activation begins promptly after infusion or instillation of streptokinase.
Distribution: Doesn't cross placenta, but antibodies do.
Metabolism: Insignificant.
Excretion: Removed from circulation by antibodies and reticuloendothelial system. Half-life is biphasic; initially it's 18 minutes (from antibody action) and then extends up to 83 minutes. Anticoagulant effect may persist for 12 to 24 hours after infusion is discontinued.

Route	Onset	Peak	Duration
I.V.	Immediate	20 min-2 hr	4 hr

Contraindications and precautions
Contraindicated in patients with ulcerative wounds, active internal bleeding, and recent CVA; recent trauma with possible internal injuries; visceral or intracranial malignant neoplasms; ulcerative colitis; diverticulitis; severe hypertension; acute or chronic hepatic or renal insufficiency; uncontrolled hypocoagulation; chronic pulmonary disease with cavitation; subacute bacterial endocarditis or rheumatic valvular disease; or recent cerebral embolism, thrombosis, or hemorrhage.

Also contraindicated within 10 days after intraarterial diagnostic procedure or any surgery, including liver or kidney biopsy, lumbar puncture, thoracentesis, paracentesis, or extensive or several cutdowns. I.M. injections and other invasive procedures are contraindicated during streptokinase therapy.

Use cautiously in patients with arterial embolism that originates from the left side of the heart.

Not recommended by manufacturer to restore patency of occluded I.V. catheters because of the risk of life-threatening reactions.

Interactions
Drug-drug. *Aminocaproic acid:* Inhibits streptokinase effects on plasminogen activation. Don't use together.
Anticoagulants: May cause hemorrhage. It may also be necessary to reverse effects of oral anticoagulants before beginning therapy. Monitor patient closely.
Aspirin, indomethacin, phenylbutazone, or other drugs that affect platelet activity: Increases risk of bleeding. Monitor patient closely.
Drug-herb. *Dong quai, feverfew, garlic, ginger, horse chestnut, red clover:* Increased risk of bleeding. Discourage use together.

Adverse reactions
CNS: polyradiculoneuropathy, headache.
CV: reperfusion arrhythmias, *hypotension,* vasculitis.
EENT: periorbital edema.
GI: nausea.
Hematologic: *bleeding.*
Musculoskeletal: musculoskeletal pain.
Respiratory: minor breathing difficulty, *bronchospasm, apnea.*
Skin: urticaria, pruritus, flushing.
Other: phlebitis at injection site, hypersensitivity reactions *(anaphylaxis),* delayed hypersensitivity reactions (interstitial nephritis, serum sickness-like reactions), *angioedema, fever.*

Overdose and treatment
Overdose may cause serious bleeding, which may result in bleeding gums, epistaxis, hematoma, spontaneous ecchymoses, oozing at catheter site, increased pulse, and pain from internal bleeding.

Discontinue drug, and restart therapy when bleeding stops.

Special considerations
Consider the recommendations relevant to all thrombolytic enzymes as well as the following.
● Reconstitute vial with 5 ml normal saline solution injection or 5% dextrose injection according to manufacturer product information; roll gently to mix. Don't shake. Use immediately; refrigerate remainder and discard after 8 hours. Store powder at room temperature.
● Rate of I.V. infusion depends on thrombin time and streptokinase resistance; higher loading dose may be necessary in patients with recent streptococcal infection or recent treatment with strep-

◇ Unlabeled clinical use

tokinase, to compensate for antibody drug neutralization.

• Don't discontinue therapy for minor allergic reactions that can be treated with antihistamines or corticosteroids; about one-third of patients experience a slight temperature elevation, and some have chills. Symptomatic treatment with acetaminophen (but not aspirin or other salicylates) is indicated if temperature reaches 104° F (40° C). Patients may be pretreated with corticosteroids, repeating doses during therapy, to minimize pyrogenic or allergic reactions.

• If minor bleeding can be controlled by local pressure, don't decrease dose so more plasminogen is available for conversion to plasmin.

• Antibodies to streptokinase can persist for 3 to 6 months or longer after the initial dose; if further thrombolytic therapy is needed, consider urokinase.

Patient monitoring
• Monitor pulse, color, and sensation of limbs every hour.

Pediatric patients
• Safety and efficacy in children haven't been established.

Geriatric patients
• Patients age 75 or older have a greater risk of cerebral hemorrhage because they're likely to have preexisting cerebrovascular disease.

Patient education
• Explain use and administration to patient and family.

---

streptomycin sulfate

Pharmacologic classification: aminoglycoside
Therapeutic classification: antibiotic
Pregnancy risk category: D

Indications and dosages
➤ **Tuberculosis.** *Adults:* 1 g or 15 mg/kg I.M. daily or 25 to 30 mg/kg (up to 1.5 g) two to three times weekly for at least 1 year.
Elderly patients: reduced daily doses based on age, renal function, and 8th cranial nerve function. Suggested dosage is 10 mg/kg (up to 750 mg) daily.
Children: 20 to 40 mg/kg (up to 1 gram) I.M. daily or 25 to 30 mg/kg (up to 1.5 g) two to three times weekly for at least 1year.
➤ **Enterococcal endocarditis.** *Adults:* 1 g I.M. q 12 hours for 2 weeks; then 500 mg I.M. q 12 hours for 4 weeks with penicillin.
➤ **Tularemia.** *Adults:* 1 to 2 g I.M. daily in divided doses for 7 to 14 days or until patient is afebrile for 5 to 7 days.
➤ **Plague.** *Adults:* 2 g (30 mg/kg) I.M. daily in 2 divided doses for at least 10 days.

Children: 30 mg/kg daily I.M. in two to three divided doses for 10 days.
➤ **Brucellosis.** *Adults:* 1g I.M. once or twice daily with doxycycline or tetracycline during the first week and once daily for at least one more week.
Children older than age 8: 20 mg/kg (up to 1 g) I.M. for 2 weeks in combination with tetracycline.
➤ **Penicillin-susceptible streptococcal endocarditis.** *Adults age 60 and younger:* 1 g I.M. twice daily for 1 week with a penicillin. Then 500 mg twice daily for 1 week.
Adults over age 60: 500 mg twice daily for 2 weeks with a penicillin.
✦ **Dosage adjustment.** Dose and frequency modified based on serum levels, which shouldn't peak above 20 to 25 mcg/ml. If serum levels aren't available, dosage may be based on creatinine clearance. After 1-g loading dose, patients with creatinine clearance of 50 to 80 ml/minute receive 7.5 mg/kg at 24 hour intervals. For those with clearance of 10 to 50 ml/minute, increase interval to q 24 to 72 hours. Those with clearance below 10 ml/minute may need interval of 72 to 96 hours.

If patient has renal failure and receives hemodialysis, some clinicians suggest supplemental doses of 50% to 75% of the loading dose at the end of each dialysis period. However, serum levels should be monitored and dosage adjusted to maintain a desired level.

How supplied
Available by prescription only
Injection: 400 mg/ml
Lyophilized cake/powder for injection: 200mg/ ml

Pharmacodynamics
Antibiotic action: Streptomycin is bactericidal; it binds directly to the 30S ribosomal subunit, inhibiting bacterial protein synthesis. Its spectrum of activity includes many aerobic gram-negative organisms and some aerobic gram-positive organisms. Streptomycin is generally less active against many gram-negative organisms than is tobramycin, gentamicin, amikacin, or netilmicin. Streptomycin is also active against *Mycobacterium* and *Brucella.*

Pharmacokinetics
Absorption: Absorbed poorly after oral administration and usually given by deep I.M. injection.
Distribution: Widely distributed after parenteral administration; intraocular penetration is poor. CSF penetration is low, even in patients with inflamed meninges. Streptomycin crosses the placenta, and is 36% protein-bound.
Metabolism: Not metabolized.
Excretion: Excreted primarily in urine by glomerular filtration; small amounts may be excreted in bile and breast milk. Elimination half-

---

life in adults is 2 to 3 hours. In severe renal damage, half-life may extend to 110 hours.

Route	Onset	Peak	Duration
I.M.	Unknown	1-2 hr	Unknown

Contraindications and precautions
Contraindicated in patients hypersensitive to drug or other aminoglycosides and in those with labyrinthine disease. Never administer I.V. Use cautiously in elderly patients and patients with impaired renal function or neuromuscular disorders.

Interactions
Drug-drug. *Amphotericin B, capreomycin, cephalosporins, cisplatin, methoxyflurane, polymyxin B, vancomycin, and other aminoglycosides:* Increased risk of nephrotoxicity, ototoxicity, and neurotoxicity. Avoid concurrent or sequential use.
Bumetanide, ethacrynic acid, furosemide, mannitol, urea: Increased risk of ototoxicity. Use together cautiously.
Dimenhydrinate, other antiemetic and antivertigo drugs: May mask streptomycin-induced ototoxicity. Use together cautiously.
General anesthetics or neuromuscular blockers, such as succinylcholine and tubocurarine: Streptomycin may potentiate neuromuscular blockade. Monitor patient closely.
Penicillin: Synergistic bactericidal effect against *Citrobacter, Enterobacter, Escherichia coli, Klebsiella, Proteus mirabilis, Pseudomonas aeruginosa,* and *Serratia;* however, drugs are physically and chemically incompatible and are inactivated when mixed or given together. Don't use together.

Adverse reactions
CNS: *neuromuscular blockade.*
EENT: *ototoxicity.*
GI: vomiting, nausea.
GU: some *nephrotoxicity* (not as often as other aminoglycosides).
Hematologic: eosinophilia, *leukopenia, thrombocytopenia.*
Respiratory: *apnea.*
Skin: *exfoliative dermatitis.*
Other: hypersensitivity reactions (rash, fever, urticaria, *angioedema*), *anaphylaxis.*

Overdose and treatment
Effects of overdose include ototoxicity, nephrotoxicity, and neuromuscular toxicity.
Remove drug by hemodialysis or peritoneal dialysis. Treatment with calcium salts or anticholinesterases reverses neuromuscular blockade.

Special considerations
● Protect hands when preparing drug because it irritates skin.

● In primary tuberculosis therapy, discontinue streptomycin when sputum culture is negative.
● Because streptomycin is dialyzable, patients undergoing hemodialysis may need dose adjustments.
● Streptomycin may cause false-positive reaction in copper sulfate test for urine glucose (Benedict's reagent or Clinitest).

Patient monitoring
● Check blood for peak streptomycin level 1 to 2 hours after I.M. injection; for trough levels, blood should be drawn just before next dose. Don't use heparinized tube because heparin is incompatible with aminoglycosides.

Pregnant patients
● Aminoglycosides have caused fetal harm.

Pediatric patients
● Use cautiously and at reduced doses in premature and full-term neonates because of renal immaturity.

Patient education
● Instruct patient to report adverse reactions promptly.
● Encourage adequate fluid intake.
● Emphasize the need for blood tests to monitor streptomycin levels and determine the effectiveness of therapy.

streptozocin
Zanosar

Pharmacologic classification: antibiotic antineoplastic nitrosourea (not specific to cell cycle phase)
Therapeutic classification: antineoplastic
Pregnancy risk category: D

Indications and dosages
Dosage and indications may vary. Check current literature for recommended protocol.
➤ *Metastatic islet cell carcinoma of the pancreas. Adults and children:* 500 mg/m² I.V. for 5 consecutive days q 6 weeks until maximum benefit or toxicity is observed. Or, 1,000 mg/m² at weekly intervals for first 2 weeks; may increase to a maximum single dose of 1,500 mg/m². On this schedule, the median time to onset of response is about 17 days and median time to maximum response is about 35 days.
✦ *Dosage adjustment.* In patients with impaired renal function, give 75% of dose if creatinine clearance is 10 to 50 ml/minute and 50% of dose if it's less than 10 ml/minute.

How supplied
Available by prescription only
Injection: 1-g vials

Pharmacodynamics

Antineoplastic action: Streptozocin exerts cytotoxic activity by selectively inhibiting DNA synthesis. It also causes cross-linking of DNA strands through an alkylation mechanism.

Pharmacokinetics

Absorption: Administered I.V.
Distribution: After an I.V. dose, drug and its metabolites distribute mainly into the liver, kidneys, intestines, and pancreas. Drug hasn't been shown to cross the blood-brain barrier; however, its metabolites achieve levels in the CSF equivalent to the level in the plasma.
Metabolism: Extensively metabolized in the liver and kidneys.
Excretion: Elimination of drug from the plasma is biphasic, with an initial half-life of 5 minutes and a terminal phase half-life of 35 to 40 minutes. Plasma half-life of metabolites is longer than parent drug. Drug and its metabolites are excreted primarily in urine and a small amount of dose may also be excreted in expired air.

Route	Onset	Peak	Duration
I.V.	Unknown	Unknown	Unknown

Contraindications and precautions

No known contraindications. Use cautiously in patients with renal and hepatic disease.

Interactions

Drug-drug. *Doxorubicin:* Prolonged elimination half-life of doxorubicin. Reduce doxorubicin dosage if necessary.
Other nephrotoxic drugs: May potentiate nephrotoxicity caused by streptozocin. Use cautiously.
Phenytoin: May decrease effects of streptozocin on the pancreas. Avoid concomitant use.

Adverse reactions

CNS: confusion, lethargy, depression.
GI: *nausea, vomiting,* diarrhea.
GU: *renal toxicity* (evidenced by azotemia, glycosuria, and renal tubular acidosis), mild proteinuria.
Hematologic: *anemia, leukopenia, thrombocytopenia.*
Hepatic: elevated liver enzyme levels, jaundice, *liver dysfunction, hepatotoxicity.*
Metabolic: hyperglycemia, hypoglycemia, diabetes mellitus.

Overdose and treatment

Signs and symptoms of overdose include myelosuppression, nausea, and vomiting. Treatment is usually supportive and includes transfusion of blood components and antiemetics.

Special considerations

● To reconstitute drug, use 9.5 ml of normal saline solution injection to yield 100 mg/ml.

● Use drug within 12 hours of reconstitution. Reconstituted solution is a golden color that changes to dark brown with decomposition.
● Product contains no preservatives and isn't intended as a multiple-dose vial.
● Drug may be given by rapid I.V. push.
● Drug may be further diluted in 10 to 200 ml of D$_5$W to infuse over 10 to 15 minutes. It also can be infused over 6 hours.
● Wear gloves to prevent contact with skin. If contact occurs, wash immediately with soap and water. Follow recommended procedures for safe handling and disposal of chemotherapy drugs.
● Extravasation may cause ulceration and tissue necrosis.
● Keep dextrose 50% at bedside because of risk of hypoglycemia from sudden release of insulin.
● Drug also has been used for colon cancer, pancreatic adenocarcinoma, and carcinoid tumors. These uses are unlabeled, and dosing schedules and protocols vary.
● Nausea and vomiting occur in almost all patients within 1 to 4 hours. Make sure patient receives an antiemetic.
● Mild proteinuria is one of the first signs of renal toxicity and may necessitate dose reduction.

Patient monitoring

● Test urine regularly for protein and glucose.
● Monitor CBC and liver function studies at least weekly.
● Renal toxicity resulting from therapy is dose-related and cumulative. Monitor renal function before and after each course of therapy.
● Obtain urinalysis, BUN levels, and creatinine clearance before therapy and at least weekly during drug administration. Continue weekly monitoring for 4 weeks after each course.

Breast-feeding patients

● It isn't known if drug appears in breast milk. However, because of the potential for serious adverse reactions, mutagenicity, and carcinogenicity in the infant, breast-feeding isn't recommended.

Patient education

● Encourage adequate fluid intake to increase urine output and reduce potential for renal toxicity.
● Remind diabetic patients that intensive monitoring of blood glucose levels is necessary.
● Tell patient to report symptoms of anemia, infection, or bleeding immediately.
● Warn patient that bruising may occur easily because of effect of drug on blood count.

Reactions may be *common*, uncommon, *life-threatening*, or COMMON AND LIFE-THREATENING.

succimer
Chemet

Pharmacologic classification: heavy metal
Therapeutic classification: chelating agent
Pregnancy risk category: C

Indications and dosages
➤ **Treatment of lead poisoning in children with blood lead levels greater than 45 mcg/dl.** *Children:* Initially, 10 mg/kg or 350 mg/m² P.O. q 8 hours for 5 days. Higher starting doses aren't recommended. Frequency of administration may be reduced to 10 mg/kg or 350 mg/m² q 12 hours for another 2 weeks. A course of treatment lasts 19 days, and repeated courses may be needed if indicated by weekly monitoring of blood lead levels. At least 2 weeks between courses is recommended unless blood lead levels mandate more prompt action.
✦ **Dosage adjustment.** Adjust dosage based on weight, as shown in the table.

PEDIATRIC DOSES

Weight		Dose	
(lb)	(kg)	(mg)	Capsules
18-35	8-15	100	1
36-55	16-23	200	2
56-75	24-34	300	3
76-100	35-44	400	4
> 100	> 45	500	5

How supplied
Available by prescription only
Capsules: 100 mg

Pharmacodynamics
Antidote action: Succimer forms water-soluble chelates and increases the urinary excretion of lead.

Pharmacokinetics
Absorption: Rapidly but variably absorbed after oral administration.
Distribution: Unknown.
Metabolism: Rapidly and extensively metabolized.
Excretion: Excreted 39% in feces as nonabsorbed drug; 9% in urine; 1% as carbon dioxide from the lungs. About 90% of absorbed drug is excreted in urine.

Route	Onset	Peak	Duration
P.O.	Unknown	1-2 hr	Unknown

Contraindications and precautions
Contraindicated in patients hypersensitive to drug. Use cautiously in patients with impaired renal function.

Interactions
Drug-drug. *Other chelating agents:* Interactions haven't been widely studied, but concurrent use isn't recommended.

Adverse reactions
CNS: *drowsiness, dizziness, sensory motor neuropathy, sleepiness, paresthesia, headache.*
CV: *arrhythmias.*
EENT: plugged ears, cloudy film in eyes, otitis media, watery eyes, sore throat, rhinorrhea, nasal congestion.
GI: *nausea, vomiting, diarrhea, loss of appetite, abdominal cramps, hemorrhoidal symptoms, metallic taste in mouth, loose stools.*
GU: decreased urination, difficult urination, proteinuria, candidiasis.
Hematologic: increased platelet count, intermittent eosinophilia.
Hepatic: *elevated serum AST, ALT, and alkaline phosphatase levels.*
Metabolic: *elevated cholesterol levels.*
Musculoskeletal: *leg, knee, back, stomach, rib, or flank pain.*
Respiratory: cough, head cold.
Skin: papular rash, herpetic rash, mucocutaneous eruptions, pruritus.
Other: *flulike symptoms.*

Overdose and treatment
No overdose has been reported. If necessary, induce vomiting with ipecac syrup or perform gastric lavage. Follow with activated charcoal slurry and appropriate supportive therapy.

Special considerations
● Identification and removal of lead sources in child's environment are critical to successful therapy. Chelation therapy isn't a substitute for preventing further exposure and shouldn't be used to permit continued exposure.
● Patients who have received ethylenediaminetetraacetic acid, with or without dimercaprol, may use succimer as subsequent therapy after an interval of 4 weeks. Use with other chelating agents isn't recommended.
● Consider the possibility of allergic or other mucocutaneous reactions each time drug is used, including during the initial course.
● False-positive results for ketones in urine using nitroprusside reagents (Ketostix) and false decreased levels of serum uric acid and CK have been reported.

Patient monitoring
● Monitor serum transaminase levels before and at least weekly during therapy. Patients with a history of hepatic disease should be monitored more closely.

• Elevated blood lead levels and resulting symptoms may return rapidly after drug is discontinued because of redistribution of lead from bone to soft tissues and blood. Monitor patients at least once weekly for rebound blood lead levels.
• Use the severity of lead intoxication as a guide for more frequent blood lead monitoring. This is measured by the initial blood lead level and the rate and degree of rebound of blood lead.

Pediatric patients
• For young children who can't swallow capsules, succimer capsule may be opened and sprinkled on a small amount of soft food, or medicated beads from the capsules may be poured onto a spoon for administration and followed with a fruit drink.

Patient education
• Instruct parents to maintain child's adequate fluid intake.
• Tell parents to report rash.
• Urge parents to identify and remove source of lead in environment.
• Tell parents to store capsules at room temperature, out of reach of children.

---

sucralfate
Carafate

Pharmacologic classification: pepsin inhibitor
Therapeutic classification: antiulcer agent
Pregnancy risk category: B

Indications and dosages
➤ *Short-term (up to 8 weeks) treatment of duodenal ulcer; aspirin-induced gastric erosion* ◊ . *Adults:* 1 g P.O. q.i.d. 1 hour before meals and h.s.
➤ *Maintenance therapy of duodenal ulcer. Adults:* 1 g P.O. b.i.d.

How supplied
Available by prescription only
Suspension: 1 g/10 ml
Tablets: 1 g

Pharmacodynamics
Antiulcer action: Sucralfate has a unique mechanism of action. It adheres to proteins at the ulcer site, forming a protective coating against gastric acid, pepsin, and bile salts. It also inhibits pepsin, exhibits a cytoprotective effect, and forms a viscous, adhesive barrier on the surface of the intact intestinal mucosa and the stomach.

Pharmacokinetics
Absorption: Only about 3% to 5% of a dose is absorbed. Drug activity isn't related to the amount absorbed.

Distribution: Acts locally, at the ulcer site. Absorbed drug is distributed to many body tissues, including the liver and kidneys.
Metabolism: None.
Excretion: About 90% of a dose is excreted in feces; absorbed drug is excreted unchanged in urine.

Route	Onset	Peak	Duration
P.O.	Unknown	Unknown	6 hr

Contraindications and precautions
No known contraindications. Use cautiously in patients with chronic renal failure.

Interactions
Drug-drug. *Antacids:* May decrease binding of drug to gastroduodenal mucosa, impairing effectiveness. Separate sucralfate and antacid doses by 30 minutes.
Anticoagulants: Increased risk of subtherapeutic PT. Separate adminstration time by 2 hours.
Cimetidine; digoxin; fat-soluble vitamins A, D, E, and K; ketoconazole; phenytoin; quinidine; quinolones; ranitidine; tetracycline; theophylline: Sucralfate decreases absorption of these drugs. Separate administration times by at least 2 hours.

Adverse reactions
CNS: dizziness, sleepiness, headache, vertigo.
GI: *constipation,* nausea, gastric discomfort, diarrhea, bezoar formation, vomiting, flatulence, dry mouth, indigestion.
Musculoskeletal: back pain.
Skin: rash, pruritus.
Other: hypersensitivity reaction.

Overdose and treatment
No information available.

Special considerations
• Drug is poorly water-soluble. For administration by nasogastric tube, prepare water-sorbitol suspension of sucralfate. Or, place tablet in 60-ml syringe; add 20 ml water. Let stand with tip up for about 5 minutes, occasionally shaking gently. The resultant suspension may be administered from the syringe. After administration, flush tube several times to ensure that the patient receives the entire dose.
• Patients who have trouble swallowing tablet may place it in 15 to 30 ml of water at room temperature, let it disintegrate, and then drink the resulting suspension. This is particularly useful for patients with esophagitis and painful swallowing.
• Some experts believe that 2 g given b.i.d. is as effective as the standard regimen.
• Drug treats ulcers as effectively as H_2-receptor antagonists.

Patient monitoring
• Monitor patient for constipation.
• Therapy exceeding 8 weeks isn't recommended.

Reactions may be *common,* uncommon, *life-threatening,* or COMMON AND LIFE-THREATENING.

Breast-feeding patients
• The risks to breast-feeding infants must be weighed against benefits.

Pediatric patients
• Safety and efficacy in children haven't been established.

Patient education
• Remind patient to take drug on an empty stomach and at least 1 hour before meals.
• Advise patient to continue taking drug as directed, even after pain begins to subside, to ensure adequate healing.
• Warn patient not to take drug for more than 8 weeks.

---

sufentanil citrate
Sufenta

Pharmacologic classification: opioid
Therapeutic classification: analgesic, adjunct to anesthesia, anesthetic
Controlled substance schedule: II
Pregnancy risk category: C

Indications and dosages
➤ *Adjunct to general anesthetic. Adults:* 1 to 8 mcg/kg I.V. with nitrous oxide and oxygen. Maintenance dosage, 10 to 50 mcg.
➤ *Primary anesthetic. Adults:* 8 to 30 mcg/kg I.V. with 100% oxygen and a muscle relaxant. Maintenance dosage, 25 to 50 mcg.
Children: 10 to 25 mcg/kg I.V. with 100% oxygen and a muscle relaxant. Maintenance dosage, up to 25 to 50 mcg.

How supplied
Available by prescription only
Injection: 50 mcg/ml

Pharmacodynamics
Analgesic action: Sufentanil has a high affinity for opiate receptors, exerting an agonistic effect to provide analgesia. It's also used as an adjunct to anesthesia or as a primary anesthetic because of its potent CNS depressant effects.

Pharmacokinetics
Absorption: Has a more rapid onset of action than morphine or fentanyl.
Distribution: Highly lipophilic and is rapidly and extensively distributed in animals. It's highly protein-bound (greater than 90%) and redistributed rapidly.
Metabolism: Appears to be metabolized mainly in the liver and small intestine. Relatively little accumulation occurs.
Excretion: Drug and its metabolites are excreted primarily in urine.

Route	Onset	Peak	Duration
I.V.	1-3 min	Unknown	Unknown

Contraindications and precautions
Contraindicated in patients hypersensitive to drug. Use cautiously in elderly or debilitated patients and in those with decreased respiratory reserve, head injuries, or renal, pulmonary, or hepatic disease.

Interactions
Drug-drug. *Anticholinergics:* Possible paralytic ileus. Monitor patient closely.
Beta blockers: If beta blockers have been used preoperatively, decrease dose of sufentanil.
Cimetidine: Increased respiratory and CNS depression. Reduce sufentanil dosage if necessary.
General anesthetics: Severe CV depression. Monitor patient closely.
Narcotic agonist-antagonist or a single dose of an antagonist: Acute withdrawal syndrome if physically dependent patient receives high doses of these drugs. Avoid use together.
Nitrous oxide: May produce CV depression when given with high doses of sufentanil. Monitor patient closely.
Other CNS depressants, such as antihistamines, barbiturates, benzodiazepines, general anesthetics, muscle relaxants, narcotic analgesics, phenothiazines, sedative-hypnotics, and tricyclic antidepressants: Additive CNS depression. Use together cautiously.
Pancuronium: May produce a dose-dependent elevation in heart rate during sufentanil and oxygen anesthesia. Use moderate doses of pancuronium or a less vagolytic neuromuscular blocking agent. Vagolytic effect of pancuronium may be reduced in patients given nitrous oxide with sufentanil.
Drug-lifestyle. *Alcohol use:* May cause additive effects. Discourage use together.

Adverse reactions
CNS: chills, somnolence.
CV: *hypotension, **bradycardia,*** hypertension, ***arrhythmias,*** tachycardia.
GI: nausea, vomiting.
Metabolic: increased plasma amylase, lipase, and serum prolactin levels.
Musculoskeletal: intraoperative muscle movement.
Respiratory: ***chest wall rigidity, apnea, bronchospasm.***
Skin: *pruritus,* erythema.

Overdose and treatment
There's no clinical experience with acute overdose of sufentanil, but signs and symptoms probably are similar to those caused by other opioids, with less CV toxicity. The most common signs and symptoms of acute opiate overdose are CNS depression, respiratory depression, and miosis (pinpoint pupils). Other acute toxic effects include hypotension, bradycardia, hypothermia, shock, apnea, cardiopulmonary arrest, circulatory collapse, pulmonary edema, and seizures.

To treat acute overdose, establish adequate respiratory exchange via a patent airway and ventilation, as needed; administer a narcotic antagonist (naloxone) to reverse respiratory depression. (Because the duration of action of sufentanil is longer than that of naloxone, repeated naloxone dosing is necessary.) Don't give naloxone unless the patient has clinically significant respiratory or CV depression. Monitor vital signs closely.

Provide symptomatic and supportive treatment (continued respiratory support, correction of fluid or electrolyte imbalance). Monitor laboratory parameters, vital signs, and neurologic status closely.

Special considerations
Consider the recommendations relevant to all opioids as well as the following.
• Sufentanil should be given only by persons specifically trained in the use of I.V. anesthetics.
• Sufentanil has a more rapid onset and shorter duration of action than fentanyl.

Patient monitoring
• When used at doses exceeding 8 mcg/kg, postoperative mechanical ventilation and observation are essential because of extended postoperative respiratory depression.
• Sufentanil may produce muscle rigidity involving all the skeletal muscles (risk and severity are dose-related). Choose a neuromuscular blocker appropriate for the patient's CV status.
• In patients weighing more than 20% above ideal body weight, determine dose based on ideal body weight.

Pediatric patients
• Safety and efficacy in children under age 2 have been documented in only a limited number of patients (who were undergoing CV surgery).

Geriatric patients
• Lower doses are usually indicated for elderly patients, who may be more sensitive to therapeutic and adverse effects of drug.

Patient education
• Assure patient and family of continuous monitoring.
• Answer questions and concerns about drug.

---

sulfadiazine

Pharmacologic classification: sulfonamide
Therapeutic classification: antibiotic
Pregnancy risk category: NR

Indications and dosages
➤ **Urinary tract infection.** *Adults:* Initially, 2 to 4 g P.O.; then 2 to 4 g daily in three to six divided doses.

Children age 2 months or older: Initially, 75 mg/kg or 2 g/m² P.O.; then 150 mg/kg daily P.O. in four to six divided doses. Maximum daily dose, 6 g.
➤ **Rheumatic fever prophylaxis, as an alternative to penicillin.** *Children who weigh more than 30 kg (66 lb):* 1 g P.O. daily.
Children who weigh less than 30 kg: 500 mg P.O. daily.
➤ **Adjunctive treatment in toxoplasmosis.** *Adults:* 1 to 1.5 g P.O. q.i.d. for 3 to 4 weeks; given with pyrimethamine.
Children: 100 to 200 mg/kg P.O. daily in divided doses q 6 hours for 3 to 4 weeks; given with pyrimethamine.
➤ **Prevention of toxoplasmosis relapse in patients with HIV infection.** *Adults and adolescents:* 0.5 to 1 g P.O. q 6 hours with pyrimethamine and lecovorin.
Infants and children: 85 to 120 mg/kg P.O. in two to four divided doses with pyrimethamine and leucovorin.
➤ **Nocardiasis.** *Adults:* 4 to 8 g P.O. daily in divided doses q 6 hours for 6 weeks.
➤ **Asymptomatic meningococcal carrier.** *Adults:* 1 g P.O. b.i.d. for 2 days.
Children ages 1 to 12: 500 mg P.O. b.i.d. for 2 days.
Children ages 2 months to 12 months: 500 mg P.O. daily for 2 days.

How supplied
Available by prescription only
Tablets: 500 mg

Pharmacodynamics
Antibacterial action: Sulfadiazine is bacteriostatic. It inhibits formation of tetrahydrofolic acid from para-aminobenzoic acid (PABA), preventing bacterial cell synthesis of folic acid. Drug is active against many gram-positive bacteria, *Chlamydia trachomatis,* many Enterobacteriaceae, and some strains of *Toxoplasma gondii* and *Plasmodium falciparum.*

Pharmacokinetics
Absorption: Absorbed from the GI tract after oral administration.
Distribution: Distributed widely into most body tissues and fluids, including synovial, pleural, amniotic, prostatic, peritoneal, and seminal fluids; CSF penetration, however, is poor. Drug crosses the placenta, and is 32% to 56% protein-bound.
Metabolism: Metabolized partially in the liver.
Excretion: Both unchanged drug and metabolites are excreted primarily in urine by glomerular filtration and, to a lesser extent, renal tubular secretion; some drug appears in breast milk. Urine solubility of unchanged drug increases as urine pH increases.

Route	Onset	Peak	Duration
P.O.	Unknown	4-6 hr	Unknown

Contraindications and precautions

Contraindicated in patients hypersensitive to sulfonamides, in those with porphyria, in infants under age 2 months (except in congenital toxoplasmosis), in pregnant women at term, and during breast-feeding.

Use cautiously in patients with impaired renal or hepatic function, bronchial asthma, multiple allergies, G6PD deficiency, or blood dyscrasia.

Interactions

Drug-drug. *Oral anticoagulants:* Inhibited hepatic metabolism of these drugs and enhanced anticoagulant effects. Monitor PT, INR, blood levels, and patient for bleeding.
Oral antidiabetics, including sulfonylureas: Enhanced hypoglycemic effects. Monitor blood glucose levels.
PABA: Antagonized sulfonamide effects. Don't use together.
Pyrimethamine and trimethoprim (folic acid antagonists with different mechanisms of action): Causes synergistic antibacterial effects and delays or prevents bacterial resistance. Don't use together.
Drug-lifestyle. *Sun exposure:* May cause photosensitivity reactions. Advise patient to take precautions.

Adverse reactions

CNS: headache, mental depression, *seizures,* hallucinations.
GI: *nausea, vomiting, diarrhea,* abdominal pain, anorexia, stomatitis.
GU: elevated serum creatinine level, *toxic nephrosis* with oliguria and anuria, crystalluria, hematuria.
Hematologic: *agranulocytosis, aplastic anemia, hemolytic anemia, thrombocytopenia,* megaloblastic anemia, *leukopenia.*
Hepatic: elevated liver enzyme levels, jaundice.
Skin: *erythema multiforme (Stevens-Johnson syndrome),* generalized skin eruption, *epidermal necrolysis, exfoliative dermatitis,* photosensitivity, urticaria, pruritus.
Other: hypersensitivity reactions (*serum sickness, drug fever, anaphylaxis*), local irritation, extravasation.

Overdose and treatment

Signs and symptoms of overdose include dizziness, drowsiness, headache, unconsciousness, anorexia, abdominal pain, nausea, and vomiting. More severe complications, including hemolytic anemia, agranulocytosis, dermatitis, acidosis, sensitivity reactions, and jaundice, may be fatal.

Treatment includes gastric lavage if ingestion has occurred within the preceding 4 hours followed by correction of acidosis, forced fluids, and urinary alkalinization to enhance solubility and excretion. Treatment of renal failure as well as transfusion of appropriate blood products (in severe hematologic toxicity) may be required.

Special considerations

Consider the recommendations relevant to all sulfonamides as well as the following.
⚡ ALERT Don't confuse sulfadiazine and sulfasalazine.
● Sulfadiazine is a less soluble sulfonamide; therefore, it's more likely to cause crystalluria. Avoid using drug with urine acidifiers and ensure adequate fluid intake. If adequate fluid intake can't be ensured, recommend sodium bicarbonate to reduce risk of crystalluria.
● Sulfadiazine should not be used for Group A B-hemolytic streptococcal infections.
● Sulfadiazine alters urine glucose tests using cupric sulfate (Benedict's reagent or Clinitest).

Patient monitoring

● Monitor renal and liver function test results.
● Monitor patient for signs of blood dyscrasia.
● Monitor urine cultures and CBCs, and conduct urinalyses before and during therapy.

Breast-feeding patients

● Drug appears in breast milk and shouldn't be used in breast-feeding women.

Pediatric patients

● Contraindicated in children under age 2 months.

Patient education

● Instruct patient to report adverse reactions promptly.
● Patient should drink a glass of water with each dose and extra water daily as tolerated to prevent crystalluria.

---

sulfamethoxazole

Gantanol

Pharmacologic classification: sulfonamide
Therapeutic classification: antibiotic
Pregnancy risk category: C

Indications and dosages

➤ *Urinary tract and systemic infections.*
Adults: Initially, 2 g P.O.; then 1 g P.O. b.i.d., up to t.i.d. for severe infections.
Children and infants over age 2 months: Initially, 50 to 60 mg/kg P.O.; then 25 to 30 mg/kg b.i.d. Maximum, 75 mg/kg daily.

How supplied

Available by prescription only
Tablets: 500 mg

Pharmacodynamics

Antibacterial action: Sulfamethoxazole is bacteriostatic. It acts by inhibiting formation of tetrahydrofolic acid from para-aminobenzoic acid (PABA), thus preventing bacterial cell synthesis of folic acid. Spectrum of action includes some gram-positive bacteria, *Chlamydia trachoma-*

---

tis, many Enterobacteriaceae, and some strains of *Toxoplasma* and *Plasmodium.*

Pharmacokinetics
Absorption: Absorbed from the GI tract after oral administration, but not as completely as sulfisoxazole.
Distribution: Distributed widely into most body tissues and fluids, including cerebrospinal, synovial, pleural, amniotic, prostatic, peritoneal, and seminal fluids. Sulfamethoxazole crosses the placenta, and is 50% to 70% protein-bound.
Metabolism: Metabolized partially in the liver.
Excretion: Both unchanged drug and metabolites are excreted primarily in urine by glomerular filtration and, to a lesser extent, renal tubular secretion; some drug appears in breast milk. Urinary solubility of unchanged drug increases as urine pH increases. Elimination half-life in patients with normal renal function is 7 to 12 hours.

Route	Onset	Peak	Duration
P.O.	Unknown	3-4 hr	Unknown

Contraindications and precautions
Contraindicated in patients hypersensitive to sulfonamides, patients with porphyria, infants under age 2 months (except in congenital toxoplasmosis), pregnant women at term, and breast-feeding women. Use cautiously in patients with renal or hepatic impairment, bronchial asthma, severe allergies, G6PD deficiency, or blood dyscrasia.

Interactions
Drug-drug. *Cyclosporine:* Decreased cyclosporine levels and increased risk of nephrotoxicity. Monitor patient.
Hydantoins: Possible increased hydantoin levels. Montior patient closely.
Methotrexate: Increased risk of methotrexate-induced bone marrow suppression. Monitor patient closely.
Oral anticoagulants: Enhanced anticoagulant effects. Monitor patient for bleeding.
Oral antidiabetics, including sulfonylureas: Enhanced hypoglycemic effects. Monitor blood glucose levels.
PABA: Antagonized sulfonamide effects. Don't use together.
Pyrimethamine and trimethoprim (folic acid antagonists with different mechanisms of action): Synergistic antibacterial effects and delayed or blocked bacterial resistance. Don't use together.
Drug-lifestyle. *Sun exposure:* May cause photosensitivity reactions. Advise patient to take precautions.

Adverse reactions
CNS: headache, mental depression, *seizures,* hallucinations, aseptic meningitis, apathy.
EENT: tinnitus.

GI: *nausea, vomiting, diarrbea,* abdominal pain, anorexia, stomatitis, ***pancreatitis,*** pseudomembranous colitis.
GU: *toxic nephrosis with oliguria and anuria,* crystalluria, hematuria, interstitial nephritis.
Hematologic: *agranulocytosis, bemolytic anemia, aplastic anemia,* megaloblastic anemia, *thrombocytopenia, leukopenia,* methemoglobinemia.
Hepatic: elevated liver enzyme levels, *jaundice.*
Skin: *erythema multiforme (Stevens-Johnson syndrome),* generalized skin eruption, *epidermal necrolysis, exfoliative dermatitis,* photosensitivity, urticaria, pruritus.
Other: hypersensitivity reactions *(serum sickness, drug fever, anaphylaxis).*

Overdose and treatment
Signs and symptoms of overdose include dizziness, drowsiness, headache, unconsciousness, anorexia, abdominal pain, nausea, and vomiting. More severe complications, including hemolytic anemia, agranulocytosis, dermatitis, acidosis, sensitivity reactions, and jaundice, may be fatal.

Treat by gastric lavage if ingestion has occurred within the preceding 4 hours, followed by correction of acidosis, forced fluids, and I.V. fluids if urine output is low and renal function is normal. Treatment of renal failure and transfusion of appropriate blood products (in severe hematologic toxicity) may be required. Follow hematologic parameters over the mext 10 days to 2 weeks after overdose. Methmoglobinuria can be reverse with 1 % methylene blue.

Special considerations
Consider the recommendations relevant to all sulfonamides as well as the following.
⚠ **ALERT** Don't confuse sulfamethoxazole with sulfamethizole. Don't confuse combination products (such as Azo Gantanol and Gantanol) with sulfamethoxazole alone.
• Sulfamethoxazole alters results of urine glucose tests using cupric sulfate (Benedict's reagent or Clinitest).

Patient monitoring
• Monitor urine cultures and CBCs, and conduct urinalyses before and during therapy.
• Monitor fluid intake and output.

Breast-feeding patients
• Sulfamethoxazole appears in breast milk and shouldn't be given to breast-feeding women.

Pediatric patients
• Sulfamethoxazole is contraindicated in children under age 2 months.

Patient education
• Instruct patient to take drug exactly as prescribed, even if he feels better.

Reactions may be *common,* uncommon, ***life-threatening***, or **common and life-threatening**.

• Tell patient to drink a glass of water with each dose, and extra water daily as tolerated to prevent crystalluria.

• Advise patient to use precautions and avoid sun exposure if possible.

sulfasalazine
Azulfidine, Azulfidine En-tabs

Pharmacologic classification: sulfonamide
Therapeutic classification: anti-inflammatory
Pregnancy risk category: B

How supplied
Available by prescription only
Suspension: 250 mg/5 ml
Tablets (with or without enteric coating): 500 mg

Indications and dosages
➤ *Mild to moderate ulcerative colitis, adjunctive therapy in severe ulcerative colitis. Adults:* Initially, 3 to 4 g P.O. daily in evenly divided doses. Maintenance dosage is 2 g P.O. daily in divided doses q 6 hours. May need to start with 1 to 2 g initially, with a gradual increase in dose to minimize adverse reactions.
Children over age 2: Initially, 40 to 60 mg/kg P.O. daily, divided into three to six doses; then 30 mg/kg daily in four doses. Maximum, 2 g daily. May need to start at lower dose if GI intolerance occurs.
➤ *Rheumatoid arthritis (enteric-coated tablets). Adults:* 2 g daily P.O. in 2 evenly divided doses. Start at lower dosage to minimize adverse GI effects.
➤ *Juvenile rheumatoid arthritis—polyarticular course. Children age 6 and older:* 30 to 50 mg/kg daily in 2 evenly divided doses. Maximum, 2 g daily. To reduce adverse GI effects, start with one-quarter to one-third of planned maintenance dose and increase weekly until reaching the maintenance dose at 1 month.

Pharmacodynamics
Antibacterial action: Exact mechanism of action of drug in ulcerative colitis is unknown; it's believed to be a prodrug metabolized by intestinal flora in the colon. One metabolite (5-aminosalicylic acid or mesalamine) is responsible for the anti-inflammatory effect; the other metabolite (sulfapyridine) may be responsible for antibacterial action and for some adverse effects.

Pharmacokinetics
Absorption: Absorbed poorly from the GI tract after oral administration; 70% to 90% is transported to the colon where intestinal flora metabolize drug to its active ingredients—sulfapyridine (antibacterial) and 5-aminosalicylic acid (anti-inflammatory)—which exert their effects locally. Sulfapyridine is absorbed from the colon, but only a small portion of 5-aminosalicylic acid is absorbed.
Distribution: Human data on sulfasalazine distribution are lacking; animal studies have identified drug and metabolites in serous fluid, liver, and intestinal walls. Parent drug and both metabolites cross the placenta.
Metabolism: Cleaved by intestinal flora in the colon.
Excretion: Systemically absorbed sulfasalazine is excreted chiefly in urine; some parent drug and metabolites appear in breast milk. Plasma half-life is about 6 to 8 hours.

Route	Onset	Peak	Duration
P.O.	Unknown	3-12 hr	Unknown

Contraindications and precautions
Contraindicated in patients hypersensitive to salicylates or sulfonamides or to other drugs containing sulfur, such as thiazides, furosemide, or oral sulfonylureas. Also contraindicated in pregnant women, breast-feeding women, infants and children under age 2, and patients with porphyria or severe renal or hepatic dysfunction. Sulfasalazine is also contraindicated in patients with intestinal or urinary tract obstructions because of the risk of local GI irritation and crystalluria.

Use cautiously in patients with mild to moderate renal or hepatic dysfunction, severe allergies, asthma, blood dyscrasia, or G6PD deficiency.

Interactions
Drug-drug. *Antacids:* Increased systemic absorption and hazard of toxicity. Monitor patient closely.
Antibiotics that alter intestinal flora: May interfere with conversion of sulfasalazine to sulfapyridine and 5-aminosalicylic acid, decreasing its effectiveness. Monitor patient closely.
Digoxin, folic acid: Sulfasalazine may reduce GI absorption of these drugs. Monitor patient closely.
Oral anticoagulants: Enhanced anticoagulant effects. Monitor patient for bleeding.
Oral antidiabetic agents including sulfonylureas: Enhanced hypoglycemic effects. Monitor blood glucose levels.
Urine acidifying agents, such as ammonium chloride and ascorbic acid: Increasing risk of crystalluria. Monitor patient closely.
Drug-lifestyle. *Sun exposure:* Photosensitivity may occur. Advise patient to take precautions.

Adverse reactions
CNS: headache, mental depression, *seizures,* hallucinations, tinnitus.
GI: *nausea, vomiting, diarrhea, abdominal pain, anorexia,* stomatitis.
GU: toxic nephrosis with oliguria and anuria, crystalluria, hematuria, oligospermia, infertility.
Hematologic: *agranulocytosis, aplastic anemia,* megaloblastic anemia, *thrombocytopenia, leukopenia, hemolytic anemia.*
Hepatic: jaundice, elevated liver enzyme levels.

Skin: *erythema multiforme (Stevens-Johnson syndrome)*, generalized skin eruption, *epidermal necrolysis, exfoliative dermatitis*, photosensitivity, urticaria, pruritus.
Other: *hypersensitivity reactions*, serum sickness, drug fever, *anaphylaxis*, bacterial and fungal superinfection.

Overdose and treatment
Signs and symptoms of overdose include dizziness, drowsiness, headache, unconsciousness, anorexia, abdominal pain, nausea, and vomiting. More severe complications, including hemolytic anemia, agranulocytosis, dermatitis, acidosis, sensitivity reactions, and jaundice, may be fatal.

Treat by gastric lavage, if ingestion has occurred within the preceding 4 hours, followed by correction of acidosis, forced fluids, and urinary alkalinization to enhance solubility and excretion. If kidney function is normal, force fluids. If anuria is present, restrict fluids and salt, and treat appropriately. Catheterization of the ureters may be indicated for complete renal blockage by crystals.

Special considerations
Consider the recommendations relevant to all sulfonamides as well as the following.
● Most adverse effects involve the GI tract; minimize reactions and facilitate absorption by spacing doses evenly and giving drug after food.
● Drug colors urine and it may color skin orange-yellow.
● Don't give antacids with enteric-coated sulfasalazine; they may alter absorption.
● Sulfasalazine alters results of urine glucose tests using cupric sulfate (Benedict's reagent or Clinitest).
● Drug should be discontinued if signs of toxicity or hypersensitivity occur; if hematologic abnormalities are accompanied by sore throat, pallor, fever, jaundice, purpura, or weakness; if crystalluria is accompanied by renal colic, hematuria, oliguria, proteinuria, urinary obstruction, urolithiasis, increased BUN levels, or anuria; if severe diarrhea indicates pseudomembranous colitis; or if severe nausea, vomiting, or diarrhea persists.

Patient monitoring
● Perform CBC, including differential white cell count and liver function tests before starting therapy and every second week during the first 3 months of therapy. During the second 3 months, perform the same tests once monthly and, thereafter, once every 3 months and as clinically indicated. Also perform urinalysis and an assessment of renal function periodically during treatment.
● Serum sulfapyridine levels may be useful because levels above 50 mcg/ml appear to be linked to an increased risk of adverse reactions.

Breast-feeding patients
● Drug appears in breast milk; use cautiously.

Pediatric patients
● Contraindicated in patients under age 2 months.

Patient education
● Tell patient that sulfasalazine normally turns urine orange-yellow. Warn that skin may also turn orange-yellow and that drug may permanently stain soft contact lenses yellow.
● Advise patient to take drug after meals to reduce GI distress and to facilitate passage into intestines.

sulfinpyrazone
Anturane

Pharmacologic classification: uricosuric
Therapeutic classification: renal tubular–blocking agent, platelet aggregation inhibitor
Pregnancy risk category: NR

Indications and dosages
➤ *Chronic gouty arthritis and intermittent gouty arthritis, or hyperuricemia related to gout.* Adults: initially, 200 to 400 mg P.O. daily in two divided doses, gradually increasing to maintenance dosage in 1 week. Maintenance dosage is 400 mg P.O. daily in two divided doses; may increase to 800 mg daily or decrease to 200 mg daily.
➤ *Prophylaxis of thromboembolic disorders, including angina, MI, transient (cerebral) ischemic attacks, and presence of prosthetic heart valves* ◇. Adults: 600 to 800 mg P.O. daily in divided doses to decrease platelet aggregation.

How supplied
Available by prescription only
Capsules: 200 mg
Tablets: 100 mg

Pharmacodynamics
Uricosuric action: Sulfinpyrazone competitively inhibits renal tubule reabsorption of uric acid. Sulfinpyrazone inhibits adenosine diphosphate and 5-HT, resulting in decreased platelet adhesiveness and increased platelet survival time.

Pharmacokinetics
Absorption: Absorbed completely after oral administration.
Distribution: 98% to 99% protein-bound.
Metabolism: Metabolized rapidly in the liver.
Excretion: Drug and its metabolites are eliminated in urine; about 50% is excreted unchanged.

Route	Onset	Peak	Duration
P.O.	Unknown	1-2 hr	4-6 hr

Contraindications and precautions
Contraindicated in patients hypersensitive to pyrazolone derivatives (including oxyphenbutazone and phenylbutazone) and in those with blood

dyscrasia, active peptic ulcer, or symptoms of GI inflammation or ulceration.

Use cautiously in patients with healed peptic ulcer and in pregnant patients.

Interactions
Drug-drug. *Cholestyramine:* Decreased sulfinpyrazone absorption. Give sulfinpyrazone 1 hour before or 4 to 6 hours after cholestyramine.
Diazoxide, diuretics, pyrazinamide: Increased serum uric acid. Increase sulfinpyrazone dosage.
Oral antidiabetics: Increased effects. Monitor blood glucose levels.
Penicillin, other beta-lactam antibiotics, nitrofurantoin, sulfonylureas: Reduced excretion of nitrofurantoin, decreasing the efficacy of sulfinpyrazone in urinary tract infections and increasing systemic toxicity; may cause hypoglycemia. Monitor patient closely.
Probenecid: Inhibited renal excretion of sulfinpyrazone. Use together cautiously.
Salicylates: Blocked uricosuric effects of sulfinpyrazone (high doses). Avoid use together.
Warfarin: Enhanced hypoprothrombinemic effect and risk of bleeding; increased bleeding in these patients also may result from the antiplatelet effect of sulfinpyrazone. Use together cautiously.
Drug-lifestyle. *Alcohol use:* May decrease effectiveness of drug. Advise patient to avoid alcohol.

Adverse reactions
GI: *nausea, dyspepsia,* epigastric pain, reactivation of peptic ulcerations.
GU: altered renal function test results, decreased urinary excretion of aminohippuric acid and phenolsulfonphthalein.
Hematologic: *blood dyscrasia* (such as anemia, *leukopenia, agranulocytosis, thrombocytopenia, aplastic anemia*).
Respiratory: *bronchoconstriction* in patients with aspirin-induced asthma.
Skin: rash.

Overdose and treatment
Signs and symptoms of overdose include nausea, vomiting, epigastric pain, ataxia, labored breathing, seizures, and coma.

Treat supportively; induce emesis or use gastric lavage as appropriate. Treat seizures with diazepam or phenytoin or both.

Special considerations
● Drug doesn't accumulate and tolerance to it doesn't develop; it's suitable for long-term use.
● Drug has no analgesic or anti-inflammatory actions.
● Give with food, milk, or prescribed antacids to lessen GI upset.
● Sulfinpyrazone is used investigationally to increase platelet survival time, to treat thromboembolic phenomena, and to prevent MI recurrence.

● Drug is not intended for relief of an acute gout attack.
● Drug may not be effective and should be avoided when creatinine clearance is less than 50 ml/minute.
● Maintain adequate hydration with high fluid intake to prevent formation of uric acid kidney stones.

Patient monitoring.
● Monitor renal function and CBC routinely.
● Monitor serum uric acid levels and adjust dose accordingly.

Breast-feeding patients
● Safety in breast-feeding women hasn't been established. An alternative feeding method is recommended during therapy.

Geriatric patients
● These patients are more likely to have glomerular filtration rates less than 50 ml/minute; sulfinpyrazone may be ineffective.

Patient education
● Explain that gouty attacks may increase during first 6 to 12 months of therapy and that patient shouldn't discontinue drug without medical approval.
● Encourage patient to comply with dose regimen and to keep scheduled follow-up visits.
● Tell patient to drink 8 to 10 glasses of fluid each day and to take drug with food to minimize GI upset; warn patient to avoid alcoholic beverages, which decrease the therapeutic effect of sulfinpyrazone.

sulfisoxazole, sulfisoxazole acetyl
Gantrisin

sulfisoxazole diolamine
Gantrisin (Ophthalmic Solution)

Pharmacologic classification: sulfonamide
Therapeutic classification: antibiotic
Pregnancy risk category: C

Indications and dosages
➤ *Urinary tract and systemic infections.*
Adults: Initially, 2 to 4 g P.O.; then 4 to 8 g P.O. daily in divided doses q 4 to 6 hours.
Children and infants over age 2 months: Initially, 75 mg/kg P.O.; then 150 mg/kg (or 4 g/m²) P.O. daily in divided doses q 4 to 6 hours. Maximum, 6 g in 24 hours.
➤ *Conjunctivitis, corneal ulcer, superficial ocular infections; adjunct in systemic treatment of trachoma. Adults:* Instill 1 to 2 drops in the lower conjuctival sac of affected eye daily q 1 to 4 hours.

How supplied
Available by prescription only
Liquid: 500 mg/5 ml (sulfisoxazole acetyl)
Ophthalmic solution: 4%
Tablets: 500 mg

Pharmacodynamics
Antibacterial action: Sulfisoxazole is bacteriostatic. It acts by inhibiting formation of tetrahydrofolic acid from para-aminobenzoic acid (PABA), preventing bacterial cell synthesis of folic acid. It acts synergistically with folic acid antagonists such as trimethoprim, which block folic acid synthesis at a later stage, thus delaying or preventing bacterial resistance. Sulfisoxazole is active against some gram-positive bacteria, *Chlamydia trachomatis*, many Enterobacteriaceae, and some strains of *Toxoplasma* and *Plasmodium*.

Pharmacokinetics
Absorption: Absorbed readily from the GI tract after oral administration.
Distribution: Distributed into extracellular compartments; CSF penetration is 8% to 57% of blood levels in uninflamed meninges. Sulfisoxazole crosses the placenta, and is 85% protein-bound.
Metabolism: Metabolized partially in the liver.
Excretion: Both unchanged drug and metabolites are excreted primarily in urine by glomerular filtration and, to a lesser extent, renal tubular secretion; some drug appears in breast milk. Urinary solubility of unchanged drug increases as urine pH increases. Plasma half-life in patients with normal renal function is about 4½ to 8 hours.

Route	Onset	Peak	Duration
P.O.	Unknown	1-4 hr	Unknown
Oph-thalmic	Unknown	Unknown	Unknown

Contraindications and precautions
Contraindicated in patients hypersensitive to sulfonamines, in infants under age 2 months (except in congenital toxoplasmosis [with oral form only]), in pregnant women at term, and in breast-feeding women.

Use oral form cautiously in patients with impaired renal or hepatic function, severe allergies, bronchial asthma, or G6PD deficiency. Use ophthalmic form cautiously in patients with severely dry eyes.

Interactions
Drug-drug. *Cyclosporine:* Decreased cyclosporine levels and increased risk of nephrotoxicity. Monitor patient closely.
Hydantoins: Increased hydantoin levels. Monitor patient closely.
Methotrexate: Increased risk of methotrexate-induced bone marrow suppression. Monitor patient closely.

Oral anticoagulants: Exaggerated anticoagulant effects. Monitor patient for bleeding.
Oral antidiabetics, including sulfonylureas: Enhanced hypoglycemic effects. Monitor blood glucose levels.
PABA: Antagonized effects of sulfonamides. Don't use together.
Pyrimethamine, trimethoprim (folic acid antagonists with different mechanisms of action): Results in synergistic antibacterial effects and delays or prevents bacterial resistance. Don't use together.
Urine acidifying agents, such as ammonium chloride and ascorbic acid: Increased risk of crystalluria. Monitor patient closely.
Drug-lifestyle. *Sun exposure:* Photosensitivity reaction may occur. Advise patient to take precautions.

Adverse reactions
CNS: headache; mental depression, hallucinations, *seizures* (with oral form).
CV: tachycardia, palpitations, syncope, cyanosis (with oral form).
EENT: *ocular irritation, itching, chemosis, periorbital edema* (with ophthalmic form).
GI: *nausea, vomiting, diarrhea,* abdominal pain, anorexia, stomatitis, pseudomembranous colitis (with oral form).
GU: *toxic nephrosis with oliguria and anuria, acute renal failure,* crystalluria, hematuria (with oral form).
Hematologic: *agranulocytosis, aplastic anemia, thrombocytopenia, hemolytic anemia,* megaloblastic anemia, *leukopenia* (with oral form).
Hepatic: elevated liver enzyme levels, jaundice (with oral administration), *hepatitis.*
Skin: *erythema multiforme, epidermal necrolysis, exfoliative dermatitis,* generalized skin eruption, photosensitivity, urticaria, pruritus (with oral form).
Other: hypersensitivity reactions (*serum sickness, drug fever, anaphylaxis*), **Stevens-Johnson syndrome,** overgrowth of nonsusceptible organisms (with ophthalmic form).

Overdose and treatment
Signs and symptoms of overdose include dizziness, drowsiness, headache, unconsciousness, anorexia, abdominal pain, nausea, and vomiting. More severe complications, including hemolytic anemia, agranulocytosis, dermatitis, acidosis, sensitivity reactions, and jaundice, may be fatal.

Treatment requires gastric lavage, if ingestion has occurred within the preceding 4 hours, followed by correction of acidosis, and forced fluids and urinary alkalinization to enhance solubility and excretion. Treatment of renal failure and transfusion of appropriate blood products (in severe hematologic toxicity) may be required.

Reactions may be *common,* uncommon, *life-threatening*, or COMMON AND LIFE-THREATENING.

Special considerations

Consider the recommendations relevant to all sulfonamides as well as the following.

⚠ ALERT Don't confuse sulfisoxazole with sulfasalazine. Also, don't confuse combination products (such as Azo Gantrisin and Gantrisin) with sulfamethoxazole alone.

• Sulfisoxazole-pyrimethamine is used to treat toxoplasmosis.

• Sulfisoxazole alters results of urine glucose tests using cupric sulfate (Benedict's reagent or Clinitest).

Patient monitoring

• Monitor urine cultures, CBCs, and PT, and conduct urinalyses before and during therapy.

• Monitor renal and liver function test results.

Breast-feeding patients

• Drug appears in breast milk and shouldn't be given to breast-feeding women.

Pediatric patients

• Contraindicated in children under age 2 months.

Patient education

• Tell patient to drink 8 oz (240 ml) of water with each oral dose and to take drug on an empty stomach.

• Tell patient to complete prescribed medication.

• Teach patient how to use ophthalmic preparations. Warn patient not to touch tip of dropper or tube to any surface.

• Warn patient that ophthalmic solution may cause blurred vision immediately after application. Tell patient to gently close eyes and keep closed for 1 to 2 minutes.

---

sulindac
Clinoril

Pharmacologic classification: NSAID
Therapeutic classification: nonnarcotic analgesic, antipyretic, anti-inflammatory
Pregnancy risk category: NR

Indications and dosages

➤ *Osteoarthritis, rheumatoid arthritis, ankylosing spondylitis. Adults:* 150 mg P.O. b.i.d. initially; may increase to 200 mg P.O. b.i.d.

➤ *Acute subacromial bursitis or supraspinatus tendinitis, acute gouty arthritis. Adults:* 200 mg P.O. b.i.d. for 7 to 14 days. Dose may be reduced as symptoms subside.

How supplied

Available by prescription only
Tablets: 150 mg, 200 mg

Pharmacodynamics

Analgesic, antipyretic, and anti-inflammatory actions: Mechanisms of action are unknown but are thought to inhibit prostaglandin synthesis

by sulindac's sulfide metabolite. Sulindac's sulfide metabolite inhibits cyclooxygenase-1 and cyclooxygenase-2.

Pharmacokinetics

Absorption: About 90% of an oral dose is absorbed.

Distribution: About 93% of sulindac and 98% of its sulfide metabolite are bound to human albumin.

Metabolism: Inactive and metabolized hepatically to the active sulfide metabolite.

Excretion: Excreted in urine. Half-life of parent drug is about 8 hours; half-life of active metabolite is about 16 hours.

Route	Onset	Peak	Duration
P.O.	Unknown	2-4 hr	Unknown

Contraindications and precautions

Contraindicated in patients hypersensitive to drug and in those for whom use of aspirin or NSAIDs leads to acute asthmatic attacks, urticaria, or rhinitis. Avoid use during pregnancy.

Use cautiously in patients with history of ulcer or GI bleeding, renal dysfunction, compromised cardiac function, hypertension, or conditions predisposing to fluid retention.

Interactions

Drug-drug. *Antacids:* Delayed and decreased sulindac absorption. Separate administration times.

Anticoagulants, thrombolytics: May be potentiated by platelet-inhibiting effect of sulindac. Monitor PT closely.

Aspirin, diflunisal: Decreased plasma levels of the active sulfide metabolite. Don't use together.

Cyclosporine: Increased nephrotoxic effects of cyclosporine. Use cautiously together, and monitor renal function closely.

Dimethyl sulfoxide: Possible decreased plasma levels of the active sulfide metabolite. Peripheral neuropathies have also been reported. Don't use together.

GI-irritating drugs, including antibiotics, corticosteroids, and NSAIDs: May potentiate the adverse GI effects of sulindac. Use together cautiously.

Highly protein-bound drugs, such as phenytoin, sulfonylureas, and warfarin: May cause displacement of either drug and adverse effects. Monitor therapy closely for both drugs.

Lithium carbonate: NSAIDs decrease renal clearance of this drug, thus increasing serum lithium levels and risks of adverse effects. Avoid use together.

Methotrexate: NSAIDs may inhibit renal elimination of methotrexate and increase risk of severe, sometimes fatal toxicity. Avoid use together.

Probenecid: Increased sulindac levels and decreased uricosuric effect of probenecid. Monitor patient for toxicity.

◇ Unlabeled clinical use

Drug-herb. *Dong quai, feverfew, garlic, ginger, horse chestnut, red clover:* Increased risk of bleeding. Discourage use together.

Adverse reactions
CNS: dizziness, headache, nervousness, psychosis.
CV: hypertension, *heart failure*, palpitations, edema.
EENT: tinnitus, transient visual disturbances.
GI: *epigastric distress, peptic ulceration, GI bleeding, pancreatitis*, occult blood loss, nausea, constipation, dyspepsia, flatulence, anorexia, vomiting, diarrhea.
GU: increased BUN and serum creatinine levels, interstitial nephritis, *nephrotic syndrome, renal failure.*
Hematologic: prolonged bleeding time, *aplastic anemia, thrombocytopenia, agranulocytosis, neutropenia*, hemolytic anemia.
Hepatic: elevated liver enzyme levels.
Metabolic: hyperkalemia.
Skin: *rash,* pruritus.
Other: drug fever, *anaphylaxis, hypersensitivity syndrome, angioedema.*

Overdose and treatment
Signs and symptoms of overdose include dizziness, drowsiness, mental confusion, disorientation, lethargy, paresthesias, numbness, vomiting, gastric irritation, nausea, abdominal pain, headache, stupor, coma, and hypotension.

To treat overdose, empty stomach immediately by inducing emesis with ipecac syrup or by gastric lavage. Administer activated charcoal via nasogastric tube. Provide symptomatic and supportive measures (respiratory support and correction of fluid and electrolyte imbalances). Dialysis is thought to be of minimal value because sulindac is highly protein-bound. Monitor laboratory parameters and vital signs closely.

Special considerations
• Sulindac may be the safest NSAID for patients with mild renal impairment. It may also be less likely to cause further renal toxicity.
• Impose safety measures to prevent injury, such as using raised side rails and supervised ambulation.
• Symptomatic improvement may take 7 days or longer.

Patient monitoring
• Assess cardiopulmonary status frequently. Monitor vital signs, especially heart rate and blood pressure, to detect abnormalities.
• Assess fluid balance status. Monitor intake and output and daily weight. Observe for presence and amount of edema.

Breast-feeding patients
• Safe use of sulindac during breast-feeding hasn't been established. Avoid use of drug in breast-feeding women.

Pediatric patients
• Safety of long-term drug use in children hasn't been established.

Geriatric patients
• Patients over age 60 are more sensitive to the adverse effects of sulindac. Use cautiously. Because of its effect on renal prostaglandins, drug may cause fluid retention and edema, which may be significant in elderly patients and those with heart failure.

Patient education
• Caution patient to avoid use of OTC medications unless medically approved.
• Teach patient how to recognize signs and symptoms of possible adverse reactions; instruct patient to report such adverse reactions.
• Instruct patient to check weight two or three times weekly and to report weight gain of 3 lb (1.4 kg) or more within 1 week, to prescriber.
• Advise patient to report edema and have blood pressure checked routinely.
• Instruct patient in safety measures; advise him to avoid hazardous activities that require alertness until CNS effects of drug are known.

sumatriptan succinate
Imitrex

Pharmacologic classification: selective 5-hydroxytryptamine (5HT₁)-receptor agonist
Therapeutic classification: antimigraine agent
Pregnancy risk category: C

Indications and dosages
➤ *Acute migraine attacks (with or without aura).* Adults: 6 mg S.C. Maximum recommended dose is two 6-mg injections in 24 hours, separated by at least 1 hour, or 25 to 100 mg P.O. initially. If response isn't achieved in 2 hours, may give second dose of 25 to 100 mg. Additional doses may be used in at least 2-hour intervals. Maximum daily dose, 200 mg.

For nasal spray, administer single dose of 5 mg, 10 mg, or 20 mg once in one nostril; may repeat once after 2 hours under prescriber's guidance for maximum daily dose of 40 mg. A 10-mg dose may be achieved by the administration of a single 5-mg dose in each nostril.

How supplied
Available by prescription only
Injection: 12 mg/ml (0.5 ml in 1-ml prefilled syringe), 6-mg single-dose vial (0.5 ml in 2 ml), and STAT dose system.
Nasal spray: 5 mg/0.1 ml, 20 mg/0.1 ml
Tablets: 25 mg, 50 mg

Pharmacodynamics
Antimigraine action: Sumatriptan selectively binds to a 5-HT₁ receptor subtype found in the basilar artery and vasculature of dura mater,

where it presumably exerts its antimigraine effect. In these tissues, sumatriptan activates the receptor to cause vasoconstriction, an action correlating with the relief of migraine.

Pharmacokinetics

Absorption: Bioavailability via S.C. injection is 97% of that obtained via I.V. injection. Bioavailability following oral or intranasal administration averages 15 or 17% respectively.
Distribution: Has a low protein-binding capacity (about 14% to 21%).
Metabolism: About 80% is metabolized in the liver, primarily to an inactive indoleacetic acid metabolite.
Excretion: Excreted primarily in urine, partly (20%) as unchanged drug and partly as the indoleacetic acid metabolite. Elimination half-life is about 2 hours.

Route	Onset	Peak	Duration
P.O.	½ hr	2-2½ hr	Unknown
S.C.	10-20 min	12 min	Unknown
Nasal	Unknown	Unknown	Unknown

Contraindications and precautions

Contraindicated in patients hypersensitive to drug, patients who have taken an MAO inhibitor within 14 days, and patients taking ergotamine. Also contraindicated in patients with uncontrolled hypertension; ischemic heart disease, such as angina pectoris, Prinzmetal's angina, history of MI, or documented silent ischemia; or hemiplegic or basilar migraine.

Use cautiously in patients who may be at risk for coronary artery disease (CAD) (such as postmenopausal women or men over age 40) or those with risk factors such as hypertension, hypercholesterolemia, obesity, diabetes, smoking, or family history. Use cautiously in women of childbearing age and during pregnancy.

Interactions

Drug-drug. *Ergot, ergot derivatives:* Prolonged vasospastic effects. These drugs shouldn't be used within 24 hours of sumatriptan.
MAO inhibitors: Increased sumatriptan effects. Avoid use within 2 weeks of discontinuing MAO inhibitor therapy.
Selective serotonin reuptake inhibitors (SSRIs): Risk of weakness, hyperreflexia, and incoordination. Monitor patient closely if concomitant therapy is clinically warranted.
Drug-herb. *Horehound:* May enhance serotonergic effects. Discourage use together.

Adverse reactions

CNS: *dizziness, vertigo,* drowsiness, headache, anxiety, malaise, fatigue.
CV: *atrial fibrillation, ventricular fibrillation, ventricular tachycardia, MI,* pressure or tightness in chest.
EENT: discomfort of throat, nasal cavity, sinus, mouth, jaw, or tongue; altered vision.

GI: abdominal discomfort, nausea, vomiting, dysphagia, unusual taste.
Musculoskeletal: myalgia, muscle cramps, neck pain.
Skin: flushing.
Other: *tingling; warm or hot sensation; burning sensation; heaviness, pressure or tightness;* anxious feeling; tight feeling in head; cold sensation; diaphoresis; *injection site reaction.*

Overdose and treatment

No specific information available. However, overdose would be expected to cause seizures, tremor, inactivity, erythema of the limbs, reduced respiratory rate, cyanosis, ataxia, mydriasis, injection site reactions, and paralysis.

Continue monitoring patient while signs and symptoms persist and for at least 10 hours thereafter. Effect of hemodialysis or peritoneal dialysis on serum sumatriptan levels is unknown.

Special considerations

● Don't use drug to manage hemiplegic or basilar migraine. Safety and effectiveness also haven't been established for cluster headache, which occurs in an older, predominantly male population.
● Don't give drug I.V. because coronary vasospasm may occur.
● Nasal spray is generally well tolerated; however, adverse reactions seen with the other forms of the drug can still occur.
● Clinical data on sumatriptan injection include rare reports of serious or life-threatening arrhythmias, such as atrial and ventricular fibrillation, ventricular tachycardia, and marked ischemic ST elevations. Data also include rare, but more frequent, reports of chest and arm discomfort thought to represent angina pectoris. Because such coronary events can occur, consider administering first dose in an outpatient setting to patients in whom unrecognized CAD is comparatively likely (postmenopausal women; men over age 40; and patients with risk factors for CAD, such as hypertension, hypercholesterolemia, obesity, diabetes, smoking, and strong family history of CAD).

Patient monitoring

● Patient response to nasal spray may be varied. The choice of dose should be made individually, weighing the possible benefit of the 20-mg dose with the potential for a greater risk of adverse events.

Pregnant patients

● Potential for harm to fetus. Use only when benefits outweigh risks to fetus. Tell pregnant women or those who intend to become pregnant during therapy to consult prescriber and discuss risks and benefits of drug use.

Breast-feeding patients

● Drug appears in breast milk. Use cautiously when administering to breast-feeding women.

Pediatric patients
● Safety and efficacy in children haven't been established.

Patient education
● Tell patient that drug may be given at any time during a migraine attack, but preferably as soon as symptoms begin. A second injection may be given if symptoms recur. Tell patient not to use more than two injections in 24 hours and to allow at least 1 hour between doses. Pain or redness at the injection site may occur but usually lasts less than 1 hour.
● Explain that drug is intended to relieve migraine, not to prevent or reduce the number of attacks.
● Tell patient not to use a second nasal spray dose if there was no response to the initial dose unless the prescriber is first contacted.
● Explain that drug is available in a spring-loaded injector system that facilitates self-administration. Review detailed information with patient. Be sure he understands how to load the injector, administer the injection, and dispose of the used syringes.
● Tell patient who feels persistent or severe chest pain to call the prescriber immediately. Tell patient who experiences pain or tightness in the throat, wheezing, heart throbbing, rash, lumps, hives, or swollen eyelids, face, or lips to stop using the drug and call at once.

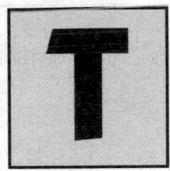

tacrine hydrochloride
Cognex

Pharmacologic classification: centrally acting reversible cholinesterase inhibitor
Therapeutic classification: psychotherapeutic agent (for Alzheimer's disease)
Pregnancy risk category: C

Indications and dosages
➤ **Mild to moderate dementia of the Alzheimer's type.** *Adults:* Initially, 40 mg daily (10 mg P.O. q.i.d.). Maintain therapy for at least 4 weeks. After 4 weeks of therapy, begin every-other-week monitoring of transaminase levels. If patient tolerates treatment and transaminase levels remain normal, increase to 80 mg daily (20 mg P.O. q.i.d.). Adjust to higher dosage at 4-week intervals to a total of 120 to 160 mg daily (30 to 40 mg P.O. q.i.d.).
✦ *Dosage adjustment.* In patients with an ALT level two to three times the upper limit of normal, monitor ALT level weekly. If ALT level is three to five times the upper normal limit, reduce dosage by 40 mg daily and monitor ALT level weekly. Resume usual pattern of dosage adjustment and every-other-week monitoring when ALT level returns to normal. If ALT level is above five times upper normal limit, stop treatment and monitor ALT level. Monitor patient for signs and symptoms related to hepatitis. Rechallenge when ALT level is normal, and monitor ALT level weekly.

How supplied
Available by prescription only
Capsules: 10 mg, 20 mg, 30 mg, 40 mg

Pharmacodynamics
Psychotherapeutic action: Tacrine presumably slows degradation of acetylcholine released by still-intact cholinergic neurons, thereby elevating acetylcholine levels in the cerebral cortex. If this theory is correct, the effects of tacrine may lessen as the disease process advances and fewer cholinergic neurons remain functionally intact. No evidence suggests that tacrine alters the course of the underlying dementia.

Pharmacokinetics
Absorption: Rapidly absorbed after oral administration. Absolute bioavailability of tacrine is about 17%. Food reduces tacrine bioavailability by about 30% to 40% if taken less than 1 hour before a meal.

Distribution: About 55% bound to plasma proteins.
Metabolism: Undergoes first-pass metabolism, which is dose dependent. It's extensively metabolized by the cytochrome P-450 system to multiple metabolites, not all of which have been identified.
Excretion: Elimination half-life is about 2 to 4 hours.

Route	Onset	Peak	Duration
P.O.	Unknown	½-3 hr	Unknown

Contraindications and precautions
Contraindicated in patients hypersensitive to drug or acridine derivatives and in patients with hypersensitivity reactions related to elevated ALT level. Also contraindicated in patients with tacrine-related jaundice that's been confirmed with an elevated total bilirubin level of more than 3 mg/dl.

Use cautiously in patients with sick sinus syndrome, bradycardia, renal disease, Parkinson's disease, asthma, prostatic hyperplasia, or other urinary outflow impairment. Also use cautiously in patients with a history of hepatic disease and in those at risk for peptic ulcer.

Interactions
Drug-drug. *Anticholinergics:* Decreased anticholinergic effectiveness. Monitor patient closely.
Cholinergics, cholinesterase inhibitors: Additive effects. Monitor patient for signs of toxicity.
Cimetidine: Increased tacrine level (by 54 %). Monitor patient.
Drugs that undergo extensive metabolism via cytochrome P-450: Possible drug interactions. Use together cautiously.
NSAIDs: May contribute to GI irritation and gastric bleeding. Monitor patient carefully.
Theophylline: Doubled theophylline elimination half-life and average plasma levels. Monitor plasma theophylline level.
Drug-food. *Any food:* Can delay drug absorption. Give drug 1 hour before meals.
Drug-lifestyle. *Smoking:* Significantly decreased drug levels. Advise patient to avoid smoking.

Adverse reactions
CNS: agitation, ataxia, insomnia, abnormal thinking, somnolence, depression, anxiety, *headache, dizziness,* fatigue, confusion, **seizures.**
CV: **bradycardia,** hypertension, palpitations, chest pain.
EENT: rhinitis.

GI: *nausea, vomiting, diarrhea,* dyspepsia, loose stools, changes in stool color, anorexia, abdominal pain, flatulence, constipation.
Hepatic: elevated liver enzyme levels.
Metabolic: hyperglycemia, weight loss.
Musculoskeletal: myalgia.
Respiratory: upper respiratory tract infection, cough.
Skin: rash, jaundice, facial flushing.
Other: increased sweating.

Overdose and treatment
Overdose with cholinesterase inhibitors can cause a cholinergic crisis by severe nausea, vomiting, salivation, sweating, bradycardia, hypotension, and seizures. Increasing muscle weakness may occur and can result in death if respiratory muscles are involved.

Provide supportive care. Tertiary anticholinergics, such as atropine, may be used as an antidote for tacrine overdose. I.V. atropine sulfate titrated to effect is recommended (initial dose of 1 to 2 mg I.V. in adults, with subsequent doses based on clinical response). In children, may give 0.05 mg/kg I.V. or I.M., repeated q 10 to 30 minutes until muscarinic signs and symptoms subside. It isn't known whether tacrine or its metabolites can be eliminated by dialysis.

Special considerations
● Tacrine as a cholinesterase inhibitor is likely to exaggerate succinylcholine-type muscle relaxation during anesthesia.
● Drug may have vagotonic effects on the heart rate, such as bradycardia. Use cautiously in patients with sick sinus syndrome.
● Dose escalation may be slowed if patient is intolerant to recommended titration schedule. Acceleration of titration schedule is never recommended.
● Cognitive function can worsen after abrupt discontinuation of tacrine or after a reduction in total daily dose of 80 mg or more.
● If drug is discontinued for 4 weeks or more, restart titration and monitoring schedule.
● The risk of transaminase elevations is higher among women. There are no other known predictors of risk of hepatocellular injury.

Patient monitoring
● Monitor serum ALT levels every other week from at least week 4 to week 16 following start of therapy, after which monitoring may be decreased to every 3 months if ALT level is less than or equal to two times the upper limit of normal. After each dose adjustment, resume monitoring schedule.
● Monitor patient for dose tolerance and cognitive changes.

Patient education
● Instruct caregiver to give drug between meals. If GI upset occurs, drug may be taken with food but plasma levels may be reduced.

● Inform caregiver that drug can alleviate symptoms but doesn't alter the underlying degenerative disease.
● Inform caregiver that effectiveness of therapy depends on drug administration at regular intervals.
● Caution caregiver that dose adjustment is an integral part of the safe use of drug. Abrupt discontinuation or a large reduction in daily dose (80 mg or more) may precipitate behavioral disturbances and a decline in cognitive function.
● Advise caregiver to promptly report significant adverse effects or changes in status.

tacrolimus (FK506)
Prograf

Pharmacologic classification: bacteria-derived macrolide
Therapeutic classification: immunosuppressant
Pregnancy risk category: C

Indications and dosages
➤ *Organ liver rejection prophylaxis.*
Adults: Initially, 0.05 to 0.1 mg/kg daily as a continuous I.V. infusion given no sooner than 6 hours after transplantation. Maintain I.V. route only until patient can tolerate oral administration (usually within 2 to 3 days); then give 0.15 to 0.3 mg/kg P.O. daily in two divided doses q 12 hours, beginning 8 to 12 hours after stopping infusion. May use oral dosing originally, if tolerated. Administer doses at lower end of range, if possible.
Children: 0.1 mg/kg I.V. daily or 0.3 mg/kg P.O. daily given no sooner than 6 hours after transplantation. Maintain I.V. route only until patient can tolerate oral administration (usually within 2 to 3 days); then give 0.3 mg/kg P.O. daily in two divided doses q 12 hours, beginning 8 to 12 hours after stopping infusion.

How supplied
Available by prescription only
Capsules: 1 mg, 5 mg
Injection: 5 mg/ml

Pharmacodynamics
Immunosuppressant action: Exact mechanism unknown. Inhibits T-lymphocyte activation. Evidence suggests that drug binds to an intracellular protein, FKBP-12. A complex of tacrolimus-FKBP-12, calcium, calmodulin, and calcineurin then forms, inhibiting the phosphatase activity of calcineurin. This effect may prevent the generation of nuclear factor of activated T cells, a nuclear component thought to initiate gene transcription for the formation of lymphocyte activation and, therefore, to cause immunosuppression.

Reactions may be *common*, uncommon, *life-threatening*, or COMMON AND LIFE-THREATENING.

Pharmacokinetics

Absorption: Absorption of oral drug from the GI tract varies. Absorption half-life in liver transplant patients is about 5½ hours. Levels in blood and plasma peak in 1½ to 3½ hours. Absolute bioavailability is 14% to 17%. Food reduces absorption and bioavailability.

Distribution: Bound to proteins, mainly albumin and α1-acid glycoprotein, and is highly bound to erythrocytes. Protein-binding is between 75% and 99%. Distribution of drug between whole blood and plasma depends on several factors, such as hematocrit, temperature of separation of plasma, drug level, and plasma protein level.

Metabolism: Extensively metabolized by mixed-function oxidase system, primarily cytochrome P-450.

Excretion: Less than 1% of dose is excreted unchanged in urine. Ten possible metabolites have been identified in human plasma. Two metabolites, a demethylated and a double demethylated tacrolimus, are shown to retain 10% and 7%, respectively, of inhibitory effect of tacrolimus on T-lymphocyte activation.

Route	Onset	Peak	Duration
P.O.	Unknown	1½-3½ hr	Unknown
I.V.	Rapid	1-2 hr	Unknown

Contraindications and precautions

Contraindicated in patients hypersensitive to drug. I.V. form is contraindicated in those hypersensitive to castor oil derivatives. Use cautiously in patients with impaired renal or hepatic function.

Interactions

Drug-drug. *Antifungals, bromocriptine, calcium channel blockers, cimetidine, clarithromycin, danazol, diltiazem, erythromycin, methylprednisolone, metoclopramide:* Possible interference with tacrolimus metabolism. Reduce tacrolimus dosage if needed.

Carbamazepine, phenobarbital, phenytoin, rifamycins: Decreased tacrolimus levels. Increase tacrolimus dosage.

Immunosuppressants (except adrenal corticosteroids): Increased susceptibility to infection. Avoid concomitant use.

Live-virus vaccines: Active infection. Avoid concomitant use.

Nephrotoxic drugs (aminoglycosides, amphotericin B, cisplatin, cyclosporine): Increased risk of nephrotoxicity. Avoid use of tacrolimus and cyclosporine; stop one at least 24 hours before starting other. With elevated tacrolimus or cyclosporine levels, further dosing with other drug is usually delayed.

Drug-food. *Any food:* Inhibited drug absorption. Give drug on empty stomach.

Grapefruit juice: Increased drug blood levels in liver transplant patients. Tell patient not to use together.

Adverse reactions

CNS: *headache, tremor, insomnia, paresthesia, asthenia.*
CV: *hypertension, peripheral edema.*
GI: *diarrhea, nausea, constipation, anorexia, vomiting, abdominal pain.*
GU: *abnormal renal function, increased creatinine or BUN levels, urinary tract infection, oliguria.*
Hematologic: *anemia, leukocytosis,* THROMBOCYTOPENIA.
Hepatic: *abnormal liver function test results.*
Metabolic: *hyperkalemia, hypokalemia, hyperglycemia, hypomagnesemia.*
Musculoskeletal: *back pain.*
Respiratory: *pleural effusion, atelectasis, dyspnea.*
Skin: *pruritus, rash.*
Other: *pain, fever, ascites, **anaphylaxis.***

Overdose and treatment

There's minimal experience with overdose. Patients who received inadvertent overdose developed no adverse reactions different from those reported at therapeutic doses.

Provide supportive care and systemic treatment. Because of its poor aqueous solubility and extensive erythrocyte and plasma protein–binding, tacrolimus probably isn't dialyzable to a significant extent.

Special considerations

● Give adult patients doses at lower end of dosing range. Adjust dosage based on assessment of rejection and tolerance. Lower doses may be sufficient as maintenance therapy. Tacrolimus should be used with adrenal corticosteroids in early posttransplant period.

● Because of risk of anaphylaxis, reserve injection for patients unable to take capsules.

● Drug is being investigated for use in kidney, bone marrow, cardiac, pancreas, pancreatic islet cell, and small bowel transplantation. It also may be used to treat autoimmune disease and severe recalcitrant psoriasis.

● Tacrolimus therapy is usually delayed 48 hours or longer in patients with postoperative oliguria.

● Because of risk of hyperkalemia (mild to severe hyperkalemia has been noted in 10% to 44% of liver transplant recipients given tacrolimus), monitor serum potassium levels and don't use potassium-sparing diuretics.

◾ **ALERT** Patients receiving drug are at increased risk for developing lymphomas and other malignancies, particularly of skin. Risk appears to be related to intensity and duration of immunosuppression rather than to use of any specific drug.

● A lymphoproliferative disorder (LPD) related to Epstein-Barr virus (EBV) has been reported in immunosuppressed organ transplant recipients. LPD risk appears greatest in young children who are at risk for primary EBV infection while immunosuppressed or who are switched to tacrolimus after long-term immunosuppressive therapy.

• Antihypertensive therapy may be needed to control blood pressure elevations linked to drug use. Likewise, therapy may be needed to control blood glucose elevations linked to drug use.

• Black renal transplant patients may need higher doses to maintain comparable whole blood trough drug levels.

• Dilute I.V. form with normal saline solution injection or D_5W injection to a level between 0.004 and 0.02 mg/ml before use.

• Store diluted infusion solution in glass or polyethylene container and discard after 24 hours. Don't store in polyvinyl chloride container because of decreased stability and potential for extraction of phthalates.

Patient monitoring

• Closely monitor patient with impaired renal function; dosage may need to be reduced. In patients with persistent elevations of serum creatinine level who are unresponsive to dosage adjustments, consider changing to another immunosuppressive therapy.

• Closely monitor patient experiencing posttransplant hepatic impairment because of increased risk of renal insufficiency related to high whole-blood levels of tacrolimus. Dosage adjustments may be needed.

• Continuously observe patient receiving drug I.V. for at least 30 minutes after start of infusion and frequently thereafter. Stop infusion if signs or symptoms of anaphylaxis occur. Have an aqueous solution of epinephrine 1:1,000 and a source of oxygen available at patient's bedside.

Breast-feeding patients

• Drug appears in breast milk. Avoid use in breast-feeding women.

Pediatric patients

• Children without renal or hepatic dysfunction have needed and tolerated higher doses than adults to achieve similar blood levels. Children should receive high end of recommended adult I.V. and oral dosing ranges (0.1 mg/kg I.V. daily and 0.3 mg/kg P.O. daily). Dosage adjustments may be needed.

Patient education

• Tell patient to take capsules on empty stomach because food impairs drug absorption.

• Inform patient of need for repeated laboratory tests during therapy to watch for adverse reactions and monitor drug effectiveness.

• Advise woman of childbearing age to call if she becomes pregnant or plans to become pregnant.

tamoxifen citrate
Nolvadex, Nolvadex-D*, Tamofen*

Pharmacologic classification: nonsteroidal antiestrogen
Therapeutic classification: antineoplastic
Pregnancy risk category: D

Indications and dosages
Dosages and indications may vary. Check current literature for recommended protocol.

➤ **Breast cancer.** *Adults:* 20 to 40 mg P.O. daily. Give amounts greater than 20 mg in divided doses (morning and evening).

➤ **Reduction of breast cancer risk in high-risk women.** *Adults:* 20 mg P.O. daily for 5 years.

➤ **Ductal carcinoma in situ.** *Adults:* 20 mg daily for 5 years.

➤ **Stimulation of ovulation** ◇. *Adults:* 5 to 40 mg P.O. b.i.d. for 4 days.

How supplied
Available by prescription only
Tablets: 10 mg, 20 mg
Tablets (enteric-coated): 20 mg*

Pharmacodynamics
Antineoplastic action: Exact mechanism of action is unclear. Tamoxifen may exert its cytotoxic action by blocking estrogen receptors within tumor cells that require estrogen to thrive. The estrogen receptor-tamoxifen complex may be translocated into the nucleus of the tumor cell, where it inhibits DNA synthesis.

Pharmacokinetics
Absorption: Appears to be well absorbed across the GI tract after oral administration. Steady state serum levels usually occur after 3 to 4 weeks.
Distribution: Distribution of drug and its metabolites into body tissues and fluids hasn't been fully established.
Metabolism: Metabolized extensively in the liver to several metabolites.
Excretion: Excreted primarily in feces, mostly as metabolites. Drug has a distribution phase half-life of 7 to 14 hours. Half-life of the terminal elimination phase is more than 7 days.

Route	Onset	Peak	Duration
P.O.	Unknown	5 hr	Unknown

Contraindications and precautions
Contraindicated in pregnant women and in patients hypersensitive to drug. Also contraindicated for risk reduction in high-risk women who also take coumarin-type anticoagulants or who have a history of deep vein thrombosis or pulmonary edema.

Use cautiously in patients who have leukopenia or thrombocytopenia.

Interactions
Drug-drug. *Antacids:* May affect absorption of enteric-coated tablets. Give drugs 2 hours apart.
Bromocriptine: Increased tamoxifen levels. Dosage adjustment may be needed. Monitor patient closely.
Coumadin: Significant increase in anticoagulation effect. Monitor PT and INR. Dosage adjustment may be needed.
Cytotoxic drugs: Increased risk of thromboembolic events. Avoid use together.

Adverse reactions
GI: *nausea, vomiting, diarrhea.*
GU: *vaginal discharge* and bleeding, *irregular menses, increased BUN and creatinine levels, amenorrhea.*
Hematologic: *leukopenia, thrombocytopenia.*
Hepatic: elevated liver enzyme levels.
Metabolic: hypercalcemia, increased serum triglycerides and cholesterol, increased thyroxine level, *weight changes.*
Musculoskeletal: temporary bone or tumor pain, brief exacerbation of pain from osseous metastases.
Skin: *skin changes.*
Other: *hot flashes, fluid retention.*

Overdose and treatment
Acute overdose hasn't been reported. No specific treatment is known. Treatment should include supportive measures. In advanced metastatic cancer, patients receiving loading doses above 400 mg/m^2 followed by 150 mg/m^2 b.i.d. have an increased risk of acute neurotoxicity (tremor, hyperreflexia, unsteady gait, and dizziness). Symptoms may arise within 3 to 5 days of starting therapy; they're expected to clear 2 to 5 days after stopping therapy. QT interval may be prolonged as well.

Special considerations
● Tamoxifen acts as an antiestrogen. Best results occur in patients with positive estrogen receptors.
● Adverse reactions are usually minor and well tolerated. They usually can be controlled by dose reduction.
● Clotting factor abnormalities may occur with prolonged tamoxifen therapy at usual doses.
● Variations on karyopyknotic index in vaginal smears and various degrees of estrogen effect on Papanicolaou smears have been seen in some postmenopausal patients. May increase serum thyroxine concentrations and may be explained by increases in thyroxine binding globulin.
● Initial adverse reactions (increased bone pain) may be a sign of good tumor response shortly after starting tamoxifen therapy.

Patient monitoring
● Monitor WBC count, platelet count, and periodic liver function tests.

● Monitor serum calcium levels; hypercalcemia may occur early in therapy in patients with bone metastases.

Pregnant patients
● Drug shouldn't be used during pregnancy or for at least 2 months before pregnancy because of risks to fetus.

Breast-feeding patients
● It isn't known whether drug appears in breast milk. However, because of the potential for serious adverse reactions and carcinogenicity in the infant, breast-feeding isn't recommended.

Pediatric patients
● Safety and efficacy haven't been established for use in children.

Geriatric patients
● The risk of serious adverse effects for women age 65 and older is the same as for women age 50 and older (the group identified in one study as being at highest risk for serious adverse effects).

Patient education
● Stress the importance of swallowing enteric-coated tablets without crushing or breaking them.
● Urge patient to continue taking drug despite nausea and vomiting.
● Tell patient to promptly report vomiting if it occurs shortly after dose ingestion.
● Reassure patient that acute exacerbation of bone pain during tamoxifen therapy usually indicates that drug will produce good response.
● Advise women to avoid becoming pregnant during drug therapy. Also recommend barrier or nonhormonal contraceptive measures for sexually active patients during treatment period.

tamsulosin hydrochloride
Flomax

Pharmacologic classification: alpha-adrenergic blocker
Therapeutic classification: BPH agent
Pregnancy risk category: B

Indications and dosages
➤ *BPH. Adult men:* 0.4 mg P.O. once daily, 30 minutes after same meal each day. For those who don't respond after 2 to 4 weeks, increase to 0.8 mg P.O. once daily. If either dosing regimen is interrupted for several days, restart therapy with 0.4 mg once daily.

How supplied
Available by prescription only
Capsules: 0.4 mg

Pharmacodynamics
Anti-BPH action: Drug selectively blocks alpha$_1$-receptors in the prostate, leading to relaxation

of smooth muscles in the bladder neck and prostate, improving urine flow, and reducing BPH symptoms.

Pharmacokinetics

Absorption: Completely absorbed following oral administration under fasting conditions.

Distribution: Studies suggest distribution into extracellular fluids and most tissues, including kidneys, prostate, gallbladder, heart, aorta, and brown fat, with minimal distribution into brain, spinal cord, and testes. Drug is extensively bound to plasma proteins but isn't thought to affect other highly bound drugs.

Metabolism: Metabolized by cytochrome P-450 in the liver, with less than 10% excreted unchanged; however, pharmacokinetic profile of metabolites hasn't been established. Metabolites undergo extensive conjugation to glucuronide or sulfate before renal excretion.

Excretion: Excreted primarily in urine (76%); about 21% excreted in feces. Elimination half-life is 5 to 7 hours, with apparent half-life from 9 to 15 hours secondary to rate-controlled absorption pharmacokinetics.

Route	Onset	Peak	Duration
P.O.	Unknown	4-7 hr	9-15 hr

Contraindications and precautions

Contraindicated in patients hypersensitive to drug or its components.

Interactions

Drug-drug. *Alpha-adrenergic blockers:* Presumed to interact with drug. Avoid use together.
Cimetidine: Decreased clearance of tamsulosin. Use together cautiously.

Adverse reactions

CNS: asthenia, *dizziness, headache,* insomnia, somnolence.
CV: chest pain, syncope.
EENT: amblyopia, pharyngitis, *rhinitis,* sinusitis.
GI: diarrhea, nausea.
GU: abnormal ejaculation.
Musculoskeletal: back pain.
Respiratory: increased cough.
Other: decreased libido, *infection,* tooth disorder, allergic reactions (rash, pruritus, urticaria, *angioedema*).

Overdose and treatment

Overdose can lead to hypotension. Treat by supporting CV system. Keep patient in supine position, and administer I.V. fluids if necessary. Give vasopressors, if needed, and monitor renal function, supporting as needed. Dialysis is unlikely to be beneficial.

Special considerations

⚠ **ALERT** Don't confuse Flomax and Volmax; they sound alike and look alike.

● Symptoms of BPH and carcinoma of the prostate are similar; rule out carcinoma before starting therapy with tamsulosin.
● If treatment is interrupted for several days, restart therapy at 1 capsule daily.

Patient monitoring
● Monitor patient for decreased blood pressure.

Breast-feeding patients
● Drug isn't indicated for use in women.

Pediatric patients
● Drug isn't indicated for use in children.

Geriatric patients
● Half-life may be prolonged because of diminishing intrinsic clearance that comes with aging.

Patient education
● Instruct patient not to crush, chew, or open capsules and to take drug at the same time each day 30 minutes after eating.
● Tell patient to get up slowly from chair or bed at start of therapy and to avoid situations in which injury could occur as a result of syncope.
● Instruct patient not to drive or perform hazardous tasks at start of therapy and for 12 hours following the initial dose or changes in dose until response can be monitored.

telmisartan
Micardis

Pharmacologic classification: angiotensin II receptor antagonist
Therapeutic classification: antihypertensive
Pregnancy risk category: C (D in second and third trimesters)

Indications and dosages
➤ **Hypertension (used alone or with other antihypertensives).** *Adults:* 40 mg P.O. once daily. Blood pressure response is dose-related over a range of 20 to 80 mg daily.

How supplied
Available by prescription only
Tablets: 40 mg, 80 mg

Pharmacodynamics
Antihypertensive action: Inhibits vasocontriction and aldosterone production by selectively blocking the binding of angiotensin II to its receptors.

Pharmacokinetics
Absorption: Absolute bioavailability is about 42% for a 40-mg dose. Peak plasma levels are reached in ½ to 1 hour following oral administration.
Distribution: More than 99.5% bound to plasma proteins.

Reactions may be *common*, uncommon, *life-threatening*, or COMMON AND LIFE-THREATENING.

Metabolism: Metabolized by glucuronide conjugation to an inactive metabolite.
Excretion: Half-life is about 24 hours. Most is excreted unchanged in the feces via biliary excretion.

Route	Onset	Peak	Duration
P.O.	Unknown	½-1 hr	24 hr

Contraindications and precautions
Contraindicated in pregnant women and in patients hypersensitive to drug or its components.

Use cautiously in patients with biliary obstruction disorders, renal stenosis, or renal or hepatic insufficiency and in those with an activated renin-angiotensin system, such as volume- or salt-depleted patients (such as those receiving high doses of diuretics).

Interactions
Drug-drug. *Digoxin:* Increased digoxin levels. Monitor digoxin levels closely.
Warfarin: Decreased warfarin levels. Monitor patient closely.
Drug-lifestyle. *Alcohol use:* Enhanced hypotensive effects. Discourage use together.

Adverse reactions
CNS: dizziness, pain, fatigue, headache.
CV: chest pain, hypertension, peripheral edema.
EENT: pharyngitis, sinusitis.
GI: abdominal pain, diarrhea, dyspepsia, nausea.
GU: urinary tract infection.
Hepatic: elevated liver enzyme levels.
Musculoskeletal: back pain, myalgia.
Respiratory: cough, upper respiratory tract infection.
Other: flulike symptoms.

Overdose and treatment
Limited data exist. Most likely, symptoms include hypotension, tachycardia, dizziness, and possibly bradycardia. Treatment should involve supportive care. Telmisartan isn't removed by hemodialysis.

Special considerations
• Blood pressure response in black patients is less than in white patients.
• Most of the antihypertensive effect is present within 2 weeks. Maximal blood pressure reduction usually is achieved after 4 weeks.
• Diuretic may be added if blood pressure isn't controlled by drug alone.
• Drug isn't removed by hemodialysis. Orthostatic hypotension may develop in patients undergoing dialysis.

Patient monitoring
• Monitor patient for hypotension following initiation of drug. Place patient in supine position if hypotension occurs and administer I.V. normal saline solution if necessary, as indicated.
• Closely monitor blood pressure.

Pregnant patients
• Use of drug is contraindicated during pregnancy because of potential risk of fetal and neonatal morbidity and death.

Breast-feeding patients
• It isn't known whether drug appears in breast milk. Assess risks and benefits before continuing drug in breast-feeding women.

Pediatric patients
• Safety and efficacy in children haven't been established.

Geriatric patients
• No significant difference has been reported compared to younger patients.

Patient education
• Inform patient that drug shouldn't be removed from blister-sealed packet until immediately before use.
• Inform women of childbearing age of the consequences of second- and third-trimester exposure to drug.
• Inform patient that transient hypotension may occur.

---

temazepam
Restoril

Pharmacologic classification: benzodiazepine
Therapeutic classification: sedative-hypnotic
Controlled substance schedule: IV
Pregnancy risk category: X

Indications and dosages
➤ *Insomnia.* *Adults:* 7.5 to 30 mg P.O. 30 minutes before bedtime.
Elderly patients: Initiate at 7.5 mg P.O. h.s. until individual response is determined.
✦ *Dosage adjustment.* In debilitated patients, 7.5 mg P.O. h.s. until individual response is determined.

How supplied
Available by prescription only
Capsules: 7.5 mg, 15 mg, 30 mg

Pharmacodynamics
Sedative-hypnotic action: Temazepam depresses the CNS at the limbic and subcortical levels of the brain. It produces a sedative-hypnotic effect by potentiating the effect of the neurotransmitter gamma-aminobutyric acid on its receptor in the ascending reticular activating system, which increases inhibition and blocks both cortical and limbic arousal.

Pharmacokinetics
Absorption: Well absorbed through the GI tract when administered orally.

Distribution: Widely distributed throughout the body. Drug is 96% protein-bound.
Metabolism: Metabolized in the liver primarily to inactive metabolites.
Excretion: Metabolites are excreted in urine as glucuronide conjugates. Half-life of drug is 4 to 20 hours.

Route	Onset	Peak	Duration
P.O.	½-1 hr	1¼-1½ hr	Unknown

Contraindications and precautions

Contraindicated in pregnant women and in patients hypersensitive to drug or other benzodiazepines.

Use cautiously in patients with impaired renal or hepatic function, chronic pulmonary insufficiency, severe or latent mental depression, suicidal tendencies, or a history of drug abuse.

Interactions

Drug-drug. *Antidepressants, antihistamines, barbiturates, general anesthetics, MAO inhibitors, narcotics, phenothiazines:* Enhanced CNS depressant effects. Use together cautiously.
Haloperidol: Increased haloperidol levels. Monitor patient closely.
Levodopa: Reduced levodopa therapeutic effect. Use together cautiously.
Drug-herb. *Catnip, kava, lady's slipper, lemon balm, passion flower, sassafras, skullcap, valerian:* Possible increased sedative effects. Discourage use together.
Drug-lifestyle. *Alcohol use:* Increased CNS depression. Discourage use together.
Smoking: Accelerated temazepam metabolism, which lowers effectiveness. Advise patient to avoid smoking.

Adverse reactions

CNS: *drowsiness, dizziness, lethargy,* disturbed coordination, daytime sedation, confusion, nightmares, vertigo, euphoria, weakness, headache, fatigue, nervousness, anxiety, depression, minor changes in EEG patterns.
EENT: blurred vision.
GI: diarrhea, nausea, dry mouth.
Hepatic: elevated liver enzyme levels.
Other: physical and psychological dependence.

Overdose and treatment

Signs and symptoms of overdose include somnolence, confusion, hypoactive or absent reflexes, dyspnea, labored breathing, hypotension, bradycardia, slurred speech, unsteady gait or impaired coordination, and, ultimately, coma.

Support blood pressure and respiration until drug effects subside; monitor vital signs. Mechanical ventilatory assistance via endotracheal tube may be required to maintain a patent airway and support adequate oxygenation. Flumazenil, a specific benzodiazepine antagonist, may be useful. Use I.V. fluids and vasopressors, such as dopamine and phenylephrine, to treat hypoten-

sion as needed. If patient is conscious, induce emesis. Use gastric lavage if ingestion was recent, but only if an endotracheal tube is present to prevent aspiration. After emesis or lavage, administer activated charcoal with a cathartic as a single dose. Don't use barbiturates if excitation occurs. Dialysis is of limited value.

Special considerations

● Prolonged use isn't recommended; however, drug has proved effective for up to 4 weeks of continuous use.
● After long-term use, avoid abrupt withdrawal and follow a gradual tapering dose schedule.
● Drug is useful for patients who have difficulty falling asleep or who awaken frequently in the night.

Patient monitoring

● Monitor hepatic function studies to prevent toxicity; lower doses are indicated in patients with hepatic dysfunction.

Pregnant patients

● Use is contraindicated during pregnancy because of potential risk of harm to fetus.

Breast-feeding patients

● Drug appears in breast milk. A breast-fed infant may become sedated, have feeding difficulties, or lose weight. Avoid use in breast-feeding women.

Pediatric patients

● Safe use in patients under age 18 hasn't been established.

Geriatric patients

● These patients are more susceptible to drug's CNS depressant effects. Use cautiously.

Patient education

● Instruct patient to seek medical approval before changing regimen.
● Inform patient of the risk for physical and psychological dependence with long-term use.
● Caution women about risks to fetus.
● Warn patient about risk of CNS depression with alcohol use and decreased therapeutic benefits related to heavy smoking.

temozolomide
Temodar

Pharmacologic classification: alkylating agent
Therapeutic classification: antineoplastic
Pregnancy risk category: D

Indications and dosages

➤ *Refractory anaplastic astrocytoma that has relapsed following chemotherapy regimen containing a nitrosourea and procarbazine. Adults:* Initial cycle—150 mg/m²

P.O. once daily for first 5 days of 28-day treatment cycle. Subsequent cycles—100 to 200 mg/m² P.O. once daily for first 5 days of subsequent 28-day treatment cycles. Timing and dosage of subsequent cycles must be adjusted according to absolute neutrophil count (ANC) and platelet count measured on cycle day 22 (expected nadir) and cycle day 29 (start of next cycle).

Dosage adjustments are based on the lowest of these ANC and platelet results. If ANC is less than 1,000/mm³ or platelet count is less than 50,000/mm³, hold therapy until ANC is greater than 1,500/mm³ and platelet count is greater than 100,000/mm³. Reduce dose by 50 mg/m² for subsequent cycle. Minimum dose is 100 mg/m².

If ANC is 1,000 to 1,500/mm³ or platelet count is 50,000 to 100,000/mm³, hold therapy until ANC is greater than 1,500/mm³ and platelet count is greater than 100,000/mm³. Maintain prior dose for subsequent cycle.

If ANC is greater than 1,500/mm³ and platelet count is greater than 100,000/mm³, increase dose to (or maintain at) 200 mg/m² for first 5 days of subsequent cycle.

How supplied
Available by prescription only
Capsules: 5 mg, 20 mg, 100 mg, 250 mg

Pharmacodynamics
Antineoplastic action: Temozolomide is a prodrug that's rapidly hydrolyzed to the active agent. It's thought to interfere with DNA replication in rapidly dividing tissues, primarily through alkylation (methylation) of guanine nucleotides in the DNA structure.

Pharmacokinetics
Absorption: Rapidly and completely absorbed from the GI tract following oral administration, with plasma levels peaking in 1 hour.
Distribution: 15% bound to plasma proteins.
Metabolism: Undergoes spontaneous hydrolysis to its active form and other metabolites. After 7 days, 38% of administered dose is recovered in urine and 0.8% in feces.
Excretion: Rapidly eliminated, with an elimination half-life of 1¾ hours.

Route	Onset	Peak	Duration
P.O.	Unknown	1 hr	Unknown

Contraindications and precautions
Contraindicated in patients hypersensitive to temozolomide or its components and in those allergic to dacarbazine, which is structurally similar to temozolomide. Also contraindicated in pregnant women. Use cautiously in patients with severe hepatic or renal impairment.

Interactions
Drug-drug. *Valproic acid:* Decreases oral clearance of temozolomide by about 5%. Use cautiously.

Drug-food. *Any food:* Reduces drug absorption; however, there are no dietary restrictions with drug administration. Give drug on an empty stomach to reduce nausea and vomiting.

Adverse reactions
CNS: *amnesia,* anxiety, *asthenia,* ataxia, confusion, *seizures, coordination abnormality,* depression, *dizziness,* dysphasia, *fatigue,* gait abnormality, *headache, hemiparesis, insomnia,* local seizures, paresis, *paresthesia, somnolence.*
EENT: abnormal vision, diplopia, pharyngitis, sinusitis.
GI: *abdominal pain, anorexia, constipation, diarrhea, nausea, vomiting.*
GU: increased urinary frequency, urinary incontinence, urinary tract infection.
Hematologic: anemia, *leukopenia, neutropenia, thrombocytopenia.*
Metabolic: weight increase.
Musculoskeletal: back pain, myalgia.
Respiratory: cough, upper respiratory tract infection.
Skin: pruritus, rash.
Other: breast pain, *fever,* hyperadrenocorticism, *peripheral edema, viral infection.*

Overdose and treatment
Neutropenia and thrombocytopenia have occurred after a single dose of 1,000 mg/m². Closely monitor patient's hematologic status and administer supportive therapies, as needed.

Special considerations
● Avoid skin contact with, or inhalation of, capsule contents if capsule is accidentally opened or damaged. Follow procedures for safe handling and disposal of antineoplastics.
● Store capsules at 59° to 86° F (15° to 30° C).

Patient monitoring
● Obtain a CBC on day 22 and then weekly until ANC is above 1,500/mm³ and platelet count is above 100,000/mm³.

Pregnant patients
● Drug shouldn't be used during pregnancy because of risk of harm to the fetus, unless potential benefit outweighs fetal risk.

Breast-feeding patients
● It's unknown whether temozolomide appears in breast milk; patient should discontinue breast-feeding while receiving drug.

Pediatric patients
● Safety and efficacy haven't been evaluated in children.

Geriatric patients
● Severe neutropenia and thrombocytopenia are more common following first treatment cycle in patients age 70 and older.

◇ Unlabeled clinical use

Patient education
• Emphasize importance of taking dose exactly as prescribed, to swallow capsules whole, and to take drug on an empty stomach or at bedtime.
• Stress importance of continuing drug despite nausea and vomiting.
• Tell patient to call immediately if vomiting (dose loss) occurs shortly after a dose is taken.
• Tell patient to promptly report sore throat, fever, unusual bruising or bleeding, rash, or seizures.
• Advise patient to avoid exposure to people with infections.
• Advise women of childbearing potential that drug may cause birth defects.

tenecteplase
TNKase

Pharmacologic classification: recombinant tissue plasminogen activator
Therapeutic classification: thrombolytic
Pregnancy risk category: C

Indications and dosages
➤**Reduction of mortality from acute MI.**
Adults who weigh less than 60 kg (132 lb):
30 mg (6 ml) by I.V. bolus over 5 seconds.
Adults who weigh 60 to 69 kg (132 to 152 lb):
35 mg (7 ml) by I.V. bolus over 5 seconds.
Adults who weigh 70 to 79 kg (154 to 174 lb):
40 mg (8 ml) by I.V. bolus over 5 seconds.
Adults who weigh 80 to 89 kg (176 to 196 lb):
45 mg (9 ml) by I.V. bolus over 5 seconds.
Adults who weigh 90 kg (198 lb) or more: 50 mg (10 ml) by I.V. bolus over 5 seconds.
Maximum dose is 50 mg.

How supplied
Available by prescription only
Injection: 50 mg

Pharmacodynamics
Thrombolytic action: A human tissue plasminogen activator that binds to fibrin and converts plasminogen to plasmin. The specificity to fibrin decreases systemic activation of plasminogen and the resulting breakdown of circulating fibrinogen.

Pharmacokinetics
Absorption: Administered I.V.
Distribution: Related to weight and is an approximation of plasma volume.
Metabolism: Primarily hepatic.
Excretion: Initial half-life is 20 to 24 minutes and terminal half-life is 90 to 130 minutes.

Route	Onset	Peak	Duration
I.V.	Immediate	Immediate	20-24 min

Contraindications and precautions
Contraindicated in patients with active internal bleeding; history of CVA; intracranial or intraspinal surgery or trauma within the previous 2 months; intracranial neoplasm, aneurysm, or arteriovenous malformation; severe uncontrolled hypertension; or known bleeding diathesis.

Use cautiously in patients who have had recent major surgery (such as coronary artery bypass graft), organ biopsy, obstetrical delivery, or previous puncture of noncompressible vessels. Also use cautiously in pregnant women, patients age 75 and older, and patients with recent trauma, recent GI or GU bleeding, high risk of left ventricular thrombus, acute pericarditis, hypertension (systolic 180 mm Hg or above, diastolic 110 mm Hg or above), severe hepatic dysfunction, hemostatic defects, subacute bacterial endocarditis, septic thrombophlebitis, diabetic hemorrhagic retinopathy, or cerebrovascular disease.

Interactions
Drug-drug: *Anticoagulants (heparin, vitamin K antagonists), drugs that alter platelet function (acetylsalicylic acid, dipyridamole, glycoprotein IIb/IIIa inhibitors):* Increased risk of bleeding when used before, during, or after therapy with tenecteplase. Use cautiously.

Adverse reactions
CNS: *intracranial hemorrhage.*
CV: *CVA.*
EENT: pharyngeal bleeding, epistaxis.
GI: GI bleeding.
GU: hematuria.
Hematologic: bleeding at puncture site.
Skin: *hematoma.*

Overdose and treatment
No data are available regarding overdose. Monitor patient for increased bleeding.

Special considerations
• Begin therapy as soon as possible after onset of MI symptoms.
• Avoid arterial and venous punctures during treatment.
• Avoid noncompressible arterial punctures and internal jugular and subclavian venous punctures.
• Use syringe prefilled with sterile water for injection and inject the entire contents into drug vial.
⚑ **ALERT** Gently swirl solution once mixed. Don't shake.
• Draw up the appropriate dose needed from the reconstituted vial with the syringe and discard any unused portion.
• Inspect product for particulates before administration.
• Administer the drug rapidly over 5 seconds.
• Give drug immediately once reconstituted, or refrigerate and use within 8 hours.
• Don't give drug in same I.V. line as dextrose. Flush dextrose-containing lines with normal saline solution before administration.
• Administer tenecteplase in a designated line.

Reactions may be *common*, uncommon, *life-threatening*, or COMMON AND LIFE-THREATENING.

● Give heparin with tenecteplase, but not in the same I.V. line.

Patient monitoring
● Monitor patient for bleeding. If serious bleeding occurs, discontinue heparin and antiplatelet drugs immediately.
● Monitor ECG for reperfusion arrhythmias.
● Cholesterol embolism is rarely related to thrombolytic use, but may be lethal. Signs and symptoms may include livedo reticularis "purple toe" syndrome, acute renal failure, gangrenous digits, hypertension, pancreatitis, MI, cerebral infarction, spinal cord infarction, retinal artery occlusion, bowel infarction, and rhabdomyolysis.

Breast-feeding patients
● It isn't known whether drug appears in breast milk. Give cautiously to breast-feeding women.

Pediatric patients
● Safety and efficacy haven't been established.

Geriatric patients
● Administer cautiously to patients age 75 and older. The drug benefit should be weighed against the risk of increased adverse effects.

Patient education
● Advise patient about proper dental care to avoid excessive gum bleeding.
● Advise patient to report any adverse effects or excess bleeding immediately.
● Explain use of drug to patient and family.

teniposide (VM-26)
Vumon

Pharmacologic classification: podophyllotoxin (specific to G_2 and late S phases of cell cycle)
Therapeutic classification: antineoplastic
Pregnancy risk category: D

Indications and dosages
Dosages and indications may vary. Check current literature for recommended protocol.
➤ *Acute lymphocytic leukemia. Children:* Optimum dose hasn't been established. One protocol reported by manufacturer is 165 mg/m² I.V. teniposide with cytarabine 300 mg/m² I.V. twice weekly for eight or nine doses.

How supplied
Available by prescription only
Injection: 50 mg/5 ml ampules

Pharmacodynamics
Antineoplastic action: Teniposide causes single- and double-stranded breaks in DNA and DNA protein cross-links, preventing cells from entering mitosis.

Pharmacokinetics
Absorption: Administered I.V.
Distribution: More than 99% bound to plasma proteins. Teniposide crosses the blood-brain barrier to a limited extent.
Metabolism: Metabolized extensively in the liver.
Excretion: About 4% to 12% of a dose is eliminated through the kidneys as unchanged drug or metabolites. Terminal half-life of drug is 5 hours.

Route	Onset	Peak	Duration
I.V.	Unknown	Unknown	Unknown

Contraindications and precautions
Contraindicated in patients hypersensitive to drug or to polyoxyethylated castor oil, an injection vehicle.

Interactions
Drug-drug. *Methotrexate:* May increase clearance and intracellular levels of methotrexate. Avoid use together.
Sodium salicylate, sulfamethizole, tolbutamide: May displace teniposide from protein-binding sites and increase toxicity. Don't administer together.

Adverse reactions
CV: hypotension from rapid infusion.
GI: *nausea, vomiting, mucositis, diarrhea.*
Hematologic: *leukopenia, neutropenia, thrombocytopenia, myelosuppression* (dose-limiting), bleeding, *anemia.*
Metabolic: elevated uric acid levels in blood and urine.
Skin: rash.
Other: *anaphylaxis, infection, hypersensitivity reactions* (chills, fever, urticaria, tachycardia, *bronchospasm*, dyspnea, hypotension, flushing), *phlebitis and extravasation* at injection site.

Overdose and treatment
Signs and symptoms of overdose include myelosuppression, nausea, and vomiting. Treatment is usually supportive and includes transfusion of blood components, antiemetics, and antibiotics for infections that may develop.

Special considerations
● Use glass or polyolefin bags or containers for infusion. Don't use polyvinyl chloride containers.
● Handle and prepare solution cautiously, and wear gloves.
● Dilute with D_5W or normal saline solution to give final teniposide levels of 0.1 mg/ml, 0.2 mg/ml, 0.4 mg/ml, or 1 mg/ml.
● Solutions that contain 0.1 mg/ml, 0.2 mg/ml, or 0.4 mg/ml are stable at room temperature for 24 hours. Solutions that contain 1 mg/ml should be given within 4 hours of preparation.

---

* Canada only   ◇ Unlabeled clinical use

• If teniposide solution contacts skin, immediately wash with soap and water. If it contacts mucous membranes, immediately flush with water.
• Don't administer drug through a membrane-type in-line filter because the diluent may dissolve the filter.
⚠ **ALERT** Keep diphenhydramine, hydrocortisone, epinephrine, and oral airway available in case of anaphylaxis.
• Administer I.V. infusion over 30 to 60 minutes to prevent hypotension. Avoid I.V. push because of increased risk of hypotension.
• Decrease dose in patients with renal or hepatic insufficiency and in patients with Down syndrome.

Patient monitoring
• Monitor patient for chemical phlebitis at injection site.
• Monitor blood pressure before infusion and at 30-minute intervals during infusion. If systolic blood pressure decreases below 90 mm Hg, stop infusion.
• Monitor CBC. Observe patient for signs of bone marrow depression.
• Monitor renal and hepatic function during therapy.

Pregnant patients
• Use of drug during pregnancy can harm fetus. Use during pregnancy only when expected benefits justify risk to fetus.

Breast-feeding patients
• It isn't known whether drug appears in breast milk. However, because of the risk of serious adverse reactions, mutagenicity, and carcinogenicity in the infant, breast-feeding isn't recommended.

Patient education
• Encourage adequate fluid intake to increase urine output and facilitate excretion of uric acid.
• Caution patient to avoid exposure to people with infections.
• Caution patient of potential for harm to fetus.
• Advise patient that hair should grow back after treatment ends.
• Tell patient to call promptly if a sore throat or fever develops or if unusual bruising or bleeding occurs.

---

terazosin hydrochloride
Hytrin

Pharmacologic classification: alpha₁-adrenergic blocker
Therapeutic classification: antihypertensive
Pregnancy risk category: C

Indications and dosages
➤ *Mild to moderate hypertension. Adults:* Initially, 1 mg P.O. h.s. Adjust dosage according to patient response. Recommended range is 1 to 5 mg daily or divided b.i.d.
If therapy stops for several days, resume using the initial dosing regimen of 1 mg P.O. h.s. Slowly increase dosage until desired blood pressure is attained. Doses of more than 20 mg don't appear to further affect blood pressure.
➤ *BPH. Adults:* Initially, 1 mg P.O. h.s. Dose may be increased based on patient response. Increase in a stepwise manner to 2 mg, 5 mg, and 10 mg. A daily dose of 10 mg may be required.

How supplied
Available by prescription only
Capsules: 1 mg, 2 mg, 5 mg, 10 mg
Tablets: 1 mg, 2 mg, 5 mg, 10 mg

Pharmacodynamics
Antihypertensive action: Terazosin reduces blood pressure by selectively inhibiting alpha₁ receptors in vascular smooth muscle, reducing peripheral vascular resistance. Because of its selectivity for alpha₁ receptors, heart rate increases minimally. Significant decreases in serum cholesterol, low-density lipoprotein, and very-low-density lipoprotein cholesterol fractions occur during therapy; the significance of these changes is unknown, as is the mechanism by which they occur.
Terazosin administration doesn't significantly alter potassium or glucose levels; it has been used successfully with diuretics, beta blockers, and other antihypertensive regimens.
Hypertrophic action: Alpha-blockade in non-vascular smooth muscle causes relaxation, notably in prostatic tissue, reducing urinary symptoms in men with BPH.

Pharmacokinetics
Absorption: Rapidly absorbed after oral administration. About 90% of oral dose is bioavailable; ingestion of food doesn't appear to alter bioavailability.
Distribution: About 90% to 94% is plasma protein-bound.
Metabolism: Metabolized in the liver. Pharmacokinetics of drug don't appear to be affected by hypertension, heart failure, or age.
Excretion: About 40% is excreted in urine, 60% in feces, mostly as metabolites. Up to 30% may be excreted unchanged. Elimination half-life is about 12 hours.

Route	Onset	Peak	Duration
P.O.	15 min	2-3 hr	24 hr

Contraindications and precautions
Contraindicated in patients hypersensitive to drug or other quinazoline derivatives.

Interactions
Drug-drug. *Alpha-adrenergic blockers:* Possible marked hypotension, especially with first dose

---

or first few days of therapy. Monitor patient's blood pressure.

Antihypertensives: Excessive hypotension. Use together cautiously.

Clonidine: Decreased antihypertensive effect of clonidine. Monitor patient closely.

Drug-herb. *Butcher's broom:* Possible reduction in terazosin effects. Discourage use together.

Adverse reactions

CNS: *asthenia, dizziness, headache,* nervousness, paresthesia, somnolence.

CV: *palpitations, peripheral edema,* orthostatic hypotension, tachycardia, syncope.

EENT: *nasal congestion,* sinusitis, blurred vision.

GI: *nausea.*

GU: impotence.

Musculoskeletal: back pain, muscle pain.

Respiratory: dyspnea.

Overdose and treatment

Signs and symptoms of overdose are exaggerated adverse reactions, particularly hypotension and shock.

Treatment is symptomatic and supportive. Dialysis may not be helpful because drug is highly protein-bound.

Special considerations

Consider the recommendations relevant to all alpha-adrenergic blockers as well as the following.

• Terazosin can cause marked hypotension, especially orthostatic hypotension, and syncope with the first dose or during the first few days of therapy. A similar response occurs if therapy is interrupted for more than a few doses.

• Terazosin therapy causes small but significant decreases in hematocrit, WBC count, and hemoglobin, total protein, and albumin levels; these decreases haven't been shown to worsen with time, suggesting the possibility of hemodilution.

Patient monitoring

• Monitor blood pressure closely.

Pregnant patients

• Safety during pregnancy hasn't been established.

Breast feeding patients

• It isn't known whether drug appears in breast milk. Avoid use in breast-feeding women.

Pediatric patients

• Safety and efficacy in patients under age 21 haven't been established.

Geriatric patients

• Patients over age 65 may be particularly susceptible to adverse reactions.

Patient education

• Instruct patient to take first dose at bedtime.

• Warn patient to avoid hazardous tasks that require alertness for 12 hours after the first dose and dose increases and when restarting dose after interruption of therapy.

• Caution patient to rise carefully and slowly from sitting and supine positions, and to report dizziness, light headedness, or palpitations. Dose adjustment may be necessary.

terbinafine hydrochloride
Lamisil, Lamisil AT, Lamisil DermGel

Pharmacologic classification: synthetic allylamine derivative
Therapeutic classification: antifungal
Pregnancy risk category: B

Indications and dosages

➤ *Interdigital tinea pedis, tinea cruris, or tinea corporis caused by* Epidermophyton floccosum, Trichophyton mentagrophytes, *or* Trichophyton rubrum. *Adults and children over age 12:* For interdigital tinea pedis, apply to cover the affected and immediately surrounding areas b.i.d. until signs and symptoms significantly improve (by day 7 for most patients). For tinea cruris or tinea corporis, apply to cover the affected and immediately surrounding areas once or twice daily until signs and symptoms significantly improve (by day 7 for most patients). Treatment should last at least 1 week and no longer than 4 weeks.

➤ *Onychomycosis of fingernails or toenails caused by dermatophytes (tinea unguium). Adults and children over age 12:* For fingernails, 250 mg P.O. daily for 6 weeks. For toenails, 250 mg P.O. daily for 12 weeks.

How supplied

Available by prescription only
Cream: 1%
Gel: 10 mg/g
Tablets: 250 mg
Available without a prescription
Cream: 1%

Pharmacodynamics

Antifungal action: Terbinafine exerts its antifungal effect by inhibiting squalene epoxidase, a key enzyme in sterol biosynthesis in fungi. This action results in a deficiency in ergosterol and a corresponding accumulation of squalene within the fungal cell and causes fungal cell death.

Pharmacokinetics

Topical form
Absorption: Systemic absorption of terbinafine is highly variable.
Distribution: No information available.
Metabolism: No information available.

Excretion: About 75% of cutaneously absorbed terbinafine is eliminated in urine, predominantly as metabolites.

Oral form

Absorption: More than 70% of drug is absorbed; food enhances absorption.

Distribution: Distributed to serum and skin. Plasma half-life is about 36 hours; half-life in tissue is 200 to 400 hours. More than 99% of drug is bound to plasma proteins.

Metabolism: First-pass metabolism is about 40%.

Excretion: About 70% of dose is eliminated in urine; clearance is decreased by 50% in patients with hepatic cirrhosis and impaired renal function.

Route	Onset	Peak	Duration
P.O.	Unknown	2 hr	Unknown
Topical	Unknown	Unknown	Unknown

Contraindications and precautions

Contraindicated in patients hypersensitive to drug. Oral form is also contraindicated in pregnant women and in patients with hepatic disease or impaired renal function (creatinine clearance of 50 ml/minute or less).

Interactions

None reported for topical form.

Drug-drug. *Cimetidine:* Decreased terbinafine clearance by 33%. Avoid use together.

Cyclosporine: Increased cyclosporine clearance. Monitor levels carefully.

I.V. caffeine: Decreased caffeine clearance. Monitor patient closely.

Rifampin: Increased terbinafine clearance by 100%. Monitor patient closely.

Adverse reactions

CNS: *headache.*

EENT: visual disturbances.

GI: taste disturbances, diarrhea, dyspepsia, abdominal pain, nausea, flatulence.

Hematologic: decreased absolute lymphocyte count, *neutropenia.*

Hepatic: elevated liver enzyme levels.

Skin: *Stevens-Johnson syndrome, toxic epidermal necrolysis,* irritation, burning, pruritus, dryness.

Overdose and treatment

Acute overdose with topical application is unlikely because of the limited absorption of topically applied drug and wouldn't be expected to lead to a life-threatening situation.

Special considerations

⚠ ALERT Don't confuse terbinafine and terbutaline.

● Before therapy starts, obtain nail specimens to confirm the diagnosis of onychomycosis.

● Diagnosis should be confirmed either by culture or by direct microscopic examination of scrapings from infected tissue mounted in a solution of potassium hydroxide.

● Don't use topical form for oral, ophthalmic, or intravaginal use.

● Tests of serum AST and ALT levels are advised for all patients before therapy starts.

Patient monitoring

● Many patients given shorter durations of therapy (1 to 2 weeks) continue to improve during the 2 to 4 weeks after drug therapy stops. Therefore, therapy shouldn't be considered a failure until patient has been observed for 2 to 4 weeks off therapy. If successful outcome isn't achieved during the post-treatment observation period, review the diagnosis.

● Monitor patient for irritation or sensitivity to drug. Discontinue therapy if irritation or sensitivity is present, and institute appropriate treatment measures.

⚠ ALERT The FDA has issued a health advisory regarding the use of terbinafine after reports of liver failure and death. The warning advises testing liver function before prescribing terbinafine tablets. When taking drug, patients should be instructed to report nausea, anorexia, fatigue, vomiting, upper abdominal pain, jaundice, dark urine, or pale stools. If any of these symptoms occurs, the drug should be stopped and liver function tests performed immediately.

Pregnant patients

● Not recommended for use during pregnancy.

Breast-feeding patients

● Drug appears in breast milk. A decision to discontinue either breast-feeding or drug must be made, taking into account the importance of drug to the woman.

● Women who are breast-feeding should avoid application of terbinafine cream to the breast.

Pediatric patients

● Safety and efficacy in children under age 12 haven't been established.

Patient education

● Advise patient to use drug as directed and to avoid contact with eyes, nose, mouth, or other mucous membranes.

● Stress importance of using drug for recommended treatment time.

⚠ ALERT If patient takes tablets, tell him to report persistent nausea, anorexia, fatigue, vomiting, right upper quadrant abdominal pain, jaundice, dark urine, or pale stools.

● Tell patient to notify prescriber if the area of application shows signs or symptoms of increased irritation or possible sensitization, such as redness, itching, burning, blistering, swelling, or oozing.

● Instruct patient not to use occlusive dressings unless directed.

Reactions may be *common*, uncommon, *life-threatening*, or COMMON AND LIFE-THREATENING.

terbutaline sulfate
Brethine, Bricanyl

Pharmacologic classification: adrenergic
(beta₂ agonist)
Therapeutic classification: bronchodilator,
premature labor inhibitor (tocolytic)
Pregnancy risk category: B

Indications and dosages
➤ *Relief of bronchospasm in patients
with reversible obstructive airway disease.* *Adults and adolescents age 15 or older:*
5 mg P.O. t.i.d. at 6-hour intervals. Reduce dosage
to 2.5 mg P.O. t.i.d. if adverse effects occur. Maximum dosage is 15 mg daily. Or, 0.25 mg S.C.
may be repeated in 15 to 30 minutes. Maximum
dosage is 0.5 mg q 4 hours.
Children ages 12 to 15: 2.5 mg P.O. t.i.d. Maximum dosage is 7.5 mg daily.
➤ *Premature labor◇. Adults:* Initially, 2.5 to
10 mcg/minute I.V. Increase dose gradually as
tolerated at 10- to 20-minute intervals until desired effects are achieved. Maximum dosages
range from 17.5 to 30 mcg/minute, although
dosages up to 80 mcg/minute have been used
cautiously. Continue infusion for at least 12 hours
after uterine contractions stop. Maintenance therapy is 2.5 to 10 mg P.O. q 4 to 6 hours.

How supplied
Available by prescription only
Injection: 1 mg/ml parenteral
Tablets: 2.5 mg, 5 mg

Pharmacodynamics
Bronchodilator action: Terbutaline acts directly on beta₂-adrenergic receptors to relax
bronchial smooth muscle, relieving bronchospasm and reducing airway resistance. Cardiac
and CNS stimulation may occur with high doses.
Tocolytic action: When used in premature labor, terbutaline relaxes uterine smooth muscle,
which inhibits uterine contractions.

Pharmacokinetics
Absorption: About 33% to 50% of an oral dose
is absorbed through the GI tract.
Distribution: Distributed widely throughout the
body.
Metabolism: Partially metabolized in the liver
to inactive compounds.
Excretion: After parenteral administration, 60%
of drug is excreted unchanged in urine, 3% in
feces through bile, and the remainder in urine
as metabolites. After oral administration, most
drug is excreted as metabolites.

Route	Onset	Peak	Duration
P.O.	½ hr	2-3 hr	4-8 hr
S.C.	15 min	½ hr	1½-4 hr

Contraindications and precautions
Contraindicated in patients hypersensitive to drug
or sympathomimetic amines. Use cautiously in
patients with CV disorders, hyperthyroidism, diabetes, or seizure disorders.

Interactions
Drug-drug. *Cardiac glycosides, cyclopropane,
halogenated inhaled anesthetics, levodopa:* Increased risk of arrhythmias. Monitor patient closely. Avoid use with levodopa.
CNS stimulants: Increased CNS stimulation. Avoid
use together.
MAO inhibitors: Potential for hypertensive crisis. Avoid use together.
Propranolol, other beta blockers: Blocked bronchodilation effects of terbutaline. Avoid use together.
Sympathomimetics: Possible additive adverse
CV effects. Don't use together.

Adverse reactions
CNS: *nervousness, tremor, drowsiness, dizzi-
ness, headache,* weakness.
CV: *palpitations,* tachycardia, **arrhythmias**,
flushing.
GI: *vomiting, nausea,* heartburn.
Metabolic: hypokalemia.
Respiratory: *paradoxical bronchospasm
with prolonged use,* dyspnea.
Skin: diaphoresis.

Overdose and treatment
Signs and symptoms of overdose include exaggeration of common adverse reactions, particularly arrhythmias, seizures, nausea, and vomiting.
  Treatment requires supportive measures. If
patient is conscious and ingestion was recent, induce emesis and follow with gastric lavage. If patient is comatose, after endotracheal tube is in
place with cuff inflated, perform gastric lavage;
then administer activated charcoal to reduce drug
absorption. Maintain adequate airway, provide
cardiac and respiratory support, and monitor vital signs closely.

Special considerations
Consider the recommendations relevant to all
adrenergics as well as the following.
⚠ ALERT Don't confused terbutaline with
terbinafine.
● Store injection solution away from light. Don't
use if discolored.
● CV effects are more likely with S.C. route and
when patient has arrhythmias.
● Most adverse reactions are transient; however,
tachycardia may persist for a relatively long time.
● Terbutaline may reduce the sensitivity of spirometry for diagnosis of bronchospasm.

Patient monitoring
● Carefully monitor patient for toxicity.
● When drug is used for tocolytic therapy, mon-
itor patient for CV effects, including tachycardia,

---

for 12 hours after discontinuation of drug. Monitor intake and output; fluid restriction may be necessary. Muscle tremor is common but may subside with continued use.
• Monitor neonate for hypoglycemia if the mother used terbutaline during pregnancy.

Pregnant patients
• Manufacturers state that drug shouldn't be used to treat preterm labor. Use drug during pregnancy only when expected benefits justify risk to fetus.

Breast-feeding patients
• Distributed into breast milk in minute amounts. Use drug cautiously in breast-feeding women.

Pediatric patients
• Drug isn't recommended for use in children under age 12.

Geriatric patients
• These patients are more sensitive to the effects of terbutaline; a lower dose may be required.

Patient education
• Instruct patient to use terbutaline only as directed. If drug produces no relief or if condition worsens, call prescriber promptly.
• Advise patient to take a missed dose within 1 hour. If missed dose is remembered more than 1 hour later, patient should skip the dose.
• Caution patient that many OTC cold and allergy remedies contain a sympathomimetic that may be harmful when combined with terbutaline.

---

terconazole
Terazol 3, Terazol 7

Pharmacologic classification: triazole derivative
Therapeutic classification: antifungal
Pregnancy risk category: C

Indications and dosages
➤ **Local treatment of vulvovaginal candidiasis.** *Adults:* For 0.4% strength—1 full applicator (5 g) intravaginally once daily h.s. for 7 consecutive days. For 0.8% strength—1 full applicator (5 g) intravaginally once daily h.s. for 3 consecutive days. Or, insert one suppository vaginally h.s. for 3 consecutive days.

How supplied
Available by prescription only
Vaginal cream: 0.4% in 45-g tube, 0.8% in 20-g tube with applicator
Vaginal suppositories: 80 mg

Pharmacodynamics
Antifungal action: Exact mechanism of action is unknown. Terconazole may disrupt fungal cell membrane permeability.

Pharmacokinetics
Absorption: Minimally absorbed, about 5% to 16%.
Distribution: Effect is mainly local.
Metabolism: Metabolized mainly by oxidative *N*- and *O*-dealkylation, dioxolane ring cleavage, and conjugation pathways.
Excretion: Following oral administration of terconazole, 32% to 56% of dose is excreted in urine and 47% to 52% is excreted in feces within 24 hours.

Route	Onset	Peak	Duration
Intra-vaginal	Unknown	Unknown	Unknown

Contraindications and precautions
Contraindicated in patients hypersensitive to terconazole or any inactive ingredient in drug.

Interactions
None reported.

Adverse reactions
CNS: *headache.*
GU: dysmenorrhea, genitalia pain, vulvovaginal burning.
Skin: irritation, *pruritus,* photosensitivity.
Other: fever, chills, body aches.

Overdose and treatment
None reported.

Special considerations
• Drug is only effective against vulvovaginitis caused by *Candida.* Confirm diagnosis by cultures or potassium hydroxide smears.
• Intractable candidiasis may be a sign of diabetes mellitus. Perform blood and urine glucose determinations to rule out undiagnosed diabetes mellitus.

Patient monitoring
• A persistent infection may be caused by reinfection. Evaluate patient for possible sources.

Pregnant patients
• There are no adequate and controlled studies regarding use of drug during first trimester. Drug was used during second and third trimesters in at least 100 women without adverse effects on the outcome of pregnancy.

Breast-feeding patients
• Safety isn't established. Breast-feeding isn't recommended during therapy with terconazole.

Patient education
• Instruct patient to insert cream high into the vagina.
• Tell patient to complete full course of therapy and to use it continuously, even during menstrual period. The therapeutic effect of terconazole isn't affected by menstruation.

Reactions may be *common,* uncommon, *life-threatening,* or COMMON AND LIFE-THREATENING.

● Inform patient to report burning or irritation.

testosterone
Histerone 100, Tesamone, Testandro, Testopel Pellets

testosterone cypionate
depAndro 100, depAndro 200, Depotest 100, Depotest 200, Depo-Testosterone, Duratest-100, Duratest-200, T-Cypionate, Virilon IM

testosterone enanthate
Andro L.A. 200, Andropository 200, Delatestryl, Durathate-200, Everone 200

testosterone propionate

Pharmacologic classification: androgen
Therapeutic classification: androgen replacement, antineoplastic
Controlled substance schedule: III
Pregnancy risk category: X

Indications and dosages
➤ *Male hypogonadism.* testosterone or testosterone propionate. *Adults:* 10 to 25 mg I.M. two or three times weekly.
testosterone cypionate or enanthate
Adults: 50 to 400 mg I.M. q 2 to 4 weeks.
➤ *Delayed puberty in males.* testosterone or testosterone propionate. *Children:* 25 to 50 mg I.M. two or three times weekly for up to 4 to 6 months.
testosterone cypionate or enanthate
Children: 50 to 200 mg I.M. q 2 to 4 weeks for up to 6 months.
➤ *Postpartum breast pain and engorgement.* testosterone or testosterone propionate. *Adults:* 25 to 50 mg I.M. daily for 3 to 4 days.
➤ *Inoperable breast cancer.* testosterone propionate. *Adults:* 50 to 100 mg I.M. three times weekly.
testosterone cypionate or enanthate
Adults: 200 to 400 mg I.M. q 2 to 4 weeks.
testosterone
Adults: 100 mg I.M. three times weekly.
➤ *Postpubertal cryptorchidism.* testosterone or testosterone propionate. *Adults:* 10 to 25 mg I.M. two or three times weekly.
➤ *Growth stimulation in Turner's syndrome.* testosterone propionate. *Adults:* 40 to 50 mg/m² I.M. once monthly for 6 months.

How supplied
Available by prescription only
testosterone
Injection (aqueous suspension): 25 mg/ml, 50 mg/ml, 100 mg/ml
Pellets for S.C. implantation: 75 mg

testosterone cypionate (in oil)
Injection: 100 mg/ml, 200 mg/ml
testosterone enanthate (in oil)
Injection: 100 mg/ml, 200 mg/ml
testosterone propionate (in oil)
Injection: 100 mg/ml

Pharmacodynamics
Androgenic action: Testosterone is the endogenous androgen that stimulates receptors in androgen-responsive organs and tissues to promote growth and development of male sexual organs and secondary sexual characteristics.
Antineoplastic action: Testosterone exerts inhibitory, antiestrogenic effects on hormone-responsive breast tumors and metastases.

Pharmacokinetics
Absorption: Testosterone and its esters must be administered parenterally because they're inactivated rapidly by the liver when given orally. The onset of action of cypionate and enanthate esters of testosterone is somewhat slower than that of testosterone itself.
Distribution: 98% to 99% plasma protein–bound, primarily to the testosterone-estradiol binding globulin.
Metabolism: Metabolized to several 17-keto-steroids by two main pathways in the liver. A large portion of these metabolites then form glucuronide and sulfate conjugates. Plasma half-life of testosterone ranges from 10 to 100 minutes. The cypionate and enanthate esters of testosterone have longer durations of action than testosterone. Cypionate half-life is about 8 days.
Excretion: Very little unchanged testosterone appears in urine or feces. About 90% of metabolized testosterone is excreted in urine in the form of sulfate and glucuronide conjugates.

Route	Onset	Peak	Duration
I.M.	Unknown	10-100 min	Unknown

Contraindications and precautions
Contraindicated in men with breast or prostate cancer; in patients with hypercalcemia or cardiac, hepatic, or renal decompensation; in pregnant women; and in breast-feeding women. Also contraindicated in patients hypersensitive to the drug and sensitive or allergic to mercury compounds (histerone).

Use cautiously in elderly patients and in women of childbearing age.

Interactions
Drug-drug. *Hepatotoxic medication:* Increased risk of hepatotoxicity. Monitor patient closely.
Insulin, oral antidiabetics: Decreased serum glucose levels; altered glucose levels in diabetic patients. Monitor patient closely. Dosage may require adjustment.
Oral anticoagulants: Prolonged PT and INR. Monitor patient closely.

Oxyphenbutazone: May increase serum oxyphenbutazone levels. Monitor patient closely.

Adverse reactions

CNS: headache, anxiety, depression, paresthesia, sleep apnea syndrome.
CV: edema.
GI: nausea.
Hematologic: prolonged PT and INR, polycythemia, suppression of clotting factors.
Hepatic: reversible jaundice, cholestatic hepatitis, abnormal liver enzyme levels.
Metabolic: hypercalcemia, hypernatremia, hyperkalemia, hyperphosphatemia, hypercholesterolemia, abnormal results of glucose tolerance tests, decreased thyroid function tests and serum 17-ketosteroid levels.
Skin: pain and induration at injection site, local edema, hypersensitivity reactions.
Other: hypoestrogenic effects in women (flushing; diaphoresis; vaginitis, including itching, drying, and burning; vaginal bleeding; menstrual irregularities), androgenic effects in women *(acne, edema, oily skin, weight gain, hirsutism, hoarseness,* clitoral enlargement, deepening voice, decreased or increased libido), excessive hormonal effects in men (prepubertal—premature epiphyseal closure, *acne,* priapism, *growth of body and facial hair,* phallic enlargement; postpubertal—testicular atrophy, oligospermia, decreased ejaculatory volume, impotence, gynecomastia, epididymitis), increased serum creatinine level.

Overdose and treatment

Not reported.

Special considerations

Consider the recommendations relevant to all androgens, as well as the following.
● When used to treat male hypogonadism, start therapy with full therapeutic doses and taper according to patient tolerance and response. Administering long-acting esters (enanthate or cypionate) at intervals greater than every 2 to 3 weeks may cause hormone levels to fall below those found in normal adults.
● Testosterone enanthate has been used for postmenopausal osteoporosis and to stimulate erythropoiesis.
● Androgens may decrease thyroxine-binding globulin concentrations, resulting in decreased total serum thyroxine (T_4) concentrations and increased resin uptake of triiodothyroxine (T_3) and T_4.

Patient monitoring

● Carefully observe women for signs of excessive virilization. If possible, stop therapy at first sign of virilization because some adverse effects, such as deepening of voice and clitoral enlargement, are irreversible. Patients with metastatic breast cancer should have regular determinations of serum calcium levels to avoid serious hypercalcemia.

Pregnant patients

● Drug isn't indicated for use during pregnancy.

Breast-feeding patients

● It's unknown whether drug appears in breast milk. An alternative feeding method is recommended because of potential for severe adverse effects of androgens on the infant.

Pediatric patients

● Use with extreme caution in children to avoid precocious puberty and premature closure of the epiphyses. Obtain X-ray examinations every 6 months to assess skeletal maturation.

Geriatric patients

● Observe elderly men for prostatic hyperplasia. Development of symptomatic prostatic hyperplasia or prostatic carcinoma mandates discontinuation of the drug.

Patient education

● Explain to women that virilization may occur, and advise them to report androgenic effects immediately. Stopping drug prevents further androgenic changes but probably won't reverse those already present.
● Tell women to report menstrual irregularities; drug may be discontinued pending determination of the cause.
● Inform men to report too frequent or persistent penile erections.
● Advise patient to report persistent GI distress, diarrhea, or the onset of jaundice.

testosterone transdermal system
Androderm, Testoderm, Testoderm TTS

Pharmacologic classification: androgen
Therapeutic classification: androgen replacement
Controlled substance schedule: III
Pregnancy risk category: X

Indications and dosages

➤ *Primary or hypogonadotropic hypogonadism.* Androderm. *Men age 18 and older:* Two systems (2.5 mg each) applied nightly for 24 hours, providing a total dose of 5 mg daily. Apply on dry area of skin on back, abdomen, upper arms, or thighs. Don't apply to scrotum.
Testoderm
Men age 18 and older: Apply one 6-mg patch to scrotal area daily for 22 to 24 hours. If scrotal area is too small for 6-mg patch, start therapy with 4-mg patch.

Testoderm TTS
Men age 18 and older: Apply one 5-mg patch on dry skin area on arm, back, or upper buttocks at the same time each day. Don't apply to scrotum. Wear the system for 24 hours a day.

How supplied
Available by prescription only
Transdermal system: 2.5 mg (Androderm), 4 mg (Testoderm), 5 mg (Testoderm TTS), 6 mg (Testoderm)

Pharmacodynamics
Androgenic action: Testosterone transdermal system releases testosterone, the endogenous androgen that stimulates receptors in androgen-responsive organs and tissues to promote growth and development of male sex organs and secondary sex characteristics.

Pharmacokinetics
Absorption: After placement of a testosterone transdermal system on scrotal skin. Daily application of two Androderm systems at bedtime results in a serum testosterone concentration profile that mimics the normal circadian variation observed in healthy young men.
Distribution: Circulating testosterone is chiefly bound in the serum to sex hormone binding globulin and albumin.
Metabolism: Metabolized to various 17-ketosteroids through two pathways; the major active metabolites are estradiol and dihydrotestosterone.
Excretion: Little unchanged testosterone appears in urine or feces.

Route	Onset	Peak	Duration
Trans-dermal	Unknown	2-4 hr	2 hr after removal

Contraindications and precautions
Contraindicated in patients hypersensitive to drug, in women, and in men with known or suspected breast or prostate cancer.
   Use cautiously in elderly men and patients with renal, cardiac, or hepatic disease.

Interactions
Drug-drug. *Hepatotoxic drugs:* Increased risk of hepatotoxicity. Monitor patient closely.
Insulin, oral antidiabetics: Decreased serum glucose levels; altered glucose levels in diabetic patients. Monitor patient closely. Dose may require adjustment.
Oral anticoagulants: Prolonged PT and INR. Monitor patient closely.
Oxyphenbutazone: May increase serum oxyphenbutazone levels. Monitor patient closely.

Adverse reactions
CNS: *CVA.*
GU: prostatitis, urinary tract infection.
Metabolic: altered thyroid function test results.
Skin: acne, *pruritus.*

Other: *gynecomastia;* breast tenderness, discomfort, and irritation.

Overdose and treatment
Testosterone levels of up to 11,400 ng/dl have been implicated in CVA. No other information is available.

Special considerations
● Testoderm form of testosterone transdermal system doesn't produce adequate serum testosterone level if applied to nongenital skin.
● Gynecomastia commonly develops and occasionally persists in patients receiving treatment for hypogonadism.
● Topical adverse reactions decrease over time.
● Store testosterone transdermal system at room temperature.
● Androgens may decrease thyroxine-binding globulin concentrations, resulting in decreased total serum thyroxine (T_4) concentrations and increased resin uptake of triidothyroxine (T_3) and T_4.
● If patient hasn't achieved desired results within 8 weeks, consider another form of testosterone replacement therapy.

Patient monitoring
● Check hemoglobin levels and hematocrit periodically (to detect polycythemia) in patients on long-term androgen therapy.
● Check liver function, prostatic acid phosphatase, prostatic specific antigen, cholesterol, and high-density lipoproteins periodically.
● After 3 to 4 weeks of daily system use in patients receiving Testoderm or Testoderm TTS, draw blood 2 to 4 hours after system application for determination of serum total testosterone. For patients receiving Androderm, monitor serum testosterone the morning following regular evening application. Because of variability in analytical values among diagnostic laboratories, this laboratory work and later analyses for assessing the effect of testosterone transdermal system should be performed at the same laboratory.

Pediatric patients
● Testosterone transdermal system hasn't been evaluated clinically in males under age 18.

Geriatric patients
● Androgens may increase the risk of prostatic hyperplasia and prostatic carcinoma in elderly men. Use testosterone transdermal system cautiously in this age-group.

Patient education
● Instruct patient regarding proper administration technique.
● Advise patient to report nausea, vomiting, skin color changes, ankle edema, and too-frequent or persistent penile erections.
● Inform patient that topical testosterone preparations used by men have caused virilization in

female partners. Changes in body hair distribution or significant increase in acne of the female partner should be reported.

● Advise patient to discontinue testosterone transdermal system if edema occurs.

---

tetanus immune globulin, human (TIG)
BayTet

Pharmacologic classification: immune serum
Therapeutic classification: tetanus prophylaxis
Pregnancy risk category: C

Indications and dosages
➤ *Tetanus prophylaxis. Adults and children age 7 and older:* 250 units I.M. For severe wounds or delay in starting prophylaxis, give 500 units I.M.
Children under age 7: 4 units/kg I.M.
➤ *Tetanus treatment. Adults and children:* Although optimal therapeutic doses haven't been established, single doses of 3,000 to 6,000 units I.M. have been used. Dosages should be adjusted based on severity of the infection. Don't give at same site as toxoid.

How supplied
Available by prescription only
Injection: 250 units/ml in 1-ml vial or syringe

Pharmacodynamics
Antitetanus action: TIG provides passive immunity to tetanus. Antibodies remain at effective levels for 3 weeks or longer. TIG protects the patient for the incubation period of most tetanus cases.

Pharmacokinetics
Absorption: Absorbed slowly.
Distribution: No information available.
Metabolism: No information available.
Excretion: Serum half-life is about 28 days.

Route	Onset	Peak	Duration
I.M.	Unknown	2-3 days	4 wk

Contraindications and precautions
Contraindicated in patients with thrombocytopenia or any coagulation disorder that contraindicates I.M. injection unless potential benefits outweigh risks. Contraindicated for use in patients hypersensitive to thimerosal or TIG. Not recommended for use in immunoglobulin A deficiency. Don't give I.V.

Interactions
None reported.

Adverse reactions
GU: *nephrotic syndrome.*

Other: slight fever, *hypersensitivity reactions, anaphylaxis, angioedema,* pain, stiffness, erythema at injection site.

Overdose and treatment
Not reported.

Special considerations
● Don't confuse drug with tetanus toxoid, which should be given at the same time (but at different sites) to produce active immunization.
● Have epinephrine solution 1:1,000 available to treat allergic reactions.
● TIG is used for prophylaxis in patients with dirty wounds if patient has had fewer than three previous tetanus toxoid injections or if the immunization history is unknown or uncertain.
● TIG hasn't been linked to an increase of AIDS cases. The immune globulin is devoid of HIV. Immune globulin recipients don't develop antibodies to HIV.
● Refrigerate TIG between 36° and 46° F (2° and 8° C). Don't freeze.

Patient monitoring
● Monitor patient for hypersensitivity reactions and site injection reactions.

Pregnant patients
● Tetanus increases risks of severe morbidity and mortality in both mother and fetus if untreated. No fetal risk from the use of immune globulin has been reported to date.

Breast-feeding patients
● It's unknown whether TIG appears in breast milk. Use cautiously in breast-feeding women.

Patient education
● Tell patient that current data indicate that TIG administration doesn't cause AIDS or hepatitis.
● Inform patient that he may experience some local pain, swelling, and tenderness at the injection site. Recommend acetaminophen to alleviate these minor effects.
● Instruct patient to report headache, skin changes, or difficulty breathing.

---

tetanus toxoid, adsorbed
tetanus toxoid

Pharmacologic classification: toxoid
Therapeutic classification: tetanus prophylaxis
Pregnancy risk category: C

Indications and dosages
➤ *Primary immunization.* adsorbed formulation. *Adults and children age 1 and older:* 0.5 ml I.M. 4 to 8 weeks apart for two doses; then a third dose 6 to 12 months after the second dose.

Children ages 2 months to 12 months: 0.5 ml I.M. 3 to 8 weeks apart for three doses, followed by a fourth dose of 0.5 ml 6 to 12 months after the third dose. Booster dosage is 0.5 ml I.M. q 5 to 10 years.

➤ *Primary immunization.* tetanus toxoid. *Adults and children:* 0.5 ml I.M. or S.C. 4 to 8 weeks apart for three doses; then a fourth dose 6 to 12 months after the third dose. Booster dosage is 0.5 ml I.M. or S.C. q 10 years.

How supplied
Available by prescription only
adsorbed toxoid
Injection: 5 to 10 Lf units of inactivated tetanus/ 0.5-ml dose, in 0.5-ml syringes and 5-ml vials
toxoid
Injection: 4 to 5 Lf units of inactivated tetanus/ 0.5-ml dose, in 0.5-ml syringes and 7.5-ml vials

Pharmacodynamics
Tetanus prophylaxis action: Tetanus toxoid promotes active immunity by inducing production of tetanus antitoxin.

Pharmacokinetics
Absorption: Absorbed slowly. Non-absorbed formulation provides quicker booster effect.
Distribution: No information available.
Metabolism: No information available.
Excretion: Unknown. Active immunity usually persists for 10 years. Adsorbed tetanus toxoid usually produces more persistent antitoxin titers than fluid tetanus toxoid.

Route	Onset	Peak	Duration
I.M., S.C.	2 doses	Unknown	> 10 yr

Contraindications and precautions
Contraindicated in immunosuppressed patients and in those with immunoglobulin abnormalities or severe hypersensitivity or neurologic reactions to the toxoid or its ingredients (such as thimerosal). Also contraindicated in patients with thrombocytopenia or any coagulation disorder that would contraindicate I.M. injection unless the potential benefits outweigh the risks. Defer vaccination in patients with acute illness; also defer vaccination during polio outbreaks, except in emergencies.

Use absorbed form cautiously in infants or children with cerebral damage, neurologic disorders, or history of febrile seizures.

Interactions
Drug-drug. *Chloramphenicol, corticosteroids, immunosuppressants:* May impair the immune response to tetanus toxoid. Avoid concomitant elective immunization.

Adverse reactions
CNS: headache, *seizures,* malaise.
CV: *tachycardia, hypotension.*

Skin: urticaria, pruritus, erythema, induration, nodule (at injection site).
Other: slight fever, chills, aches and pains, flushing, *anaphylaxis.*

Overdose and treatment
Not reported.

Special considerations
● Adsorbed toxoids induce higher antitoxin titers and more persistent antitoxin levels.
● Have epinephrine 1:1,000 solution available to treat allergic reactions.
● Don't confuse drug with tetanus immune globulin.
● Refrigerate at 36° to 46° F (2° to 8° C). Don't freeze.

Patient monitoring
● Monitor patient for hypersensitivity reactions, seizures, and injection site reactions.

Pregnant patients
● Although there's no evidence of teratogenicity, it's recommended that administration be deferred until second trimester.

Breast-feeding patients
● It isn't known whether tetanus toxoid appears in breast milk. Use cautiously in breast-feeding women.

Geriatric patients
● These patients develop lower antitoxin levels than younger patients after tetanus immunization. Therefore, skin test responsiveness may be delayed or reduced.

Patient education
● Inform patient of possible adverse reactions.
● Encourage patient to report distressing adverse reactions.
● Tell patient that immunization requires a series of injections. Stress the importance of keeping scheduled appointments for subsequent doses.

tetracycline hydrochloride
Achromycin, Novo-tetra*, Panmycin, Sumycin, Tetralan, Topicycline

Pharmacologic classification: tetracycline
Therapeutic classification: antibiotic
Pregnancy risk category: D (B for topical form)

Indications and dosages
➤ *Infections caused by sensitive organisms. Adults:* 1 to 2 g P.O., divided into two to four doses.
Children over age 8: 25 to 50 mg/kg P.O. daily, divided into two to four doses.
➤ *Uncomplicated urethral, endocervical, or rectal infection caused by* Chlamydia

trachomatis. *Adults:* 500 mg P.O. q.i.d. for at least 7 days.

➤**Brucellosis.** *Adults:* 500 mg P.O. q 6 hours for 3 weeks with streptomycin 1 g I.M. q 12 hours during week 1 and once daily during week 2.

➤**Gonorrhea in patients sensitive to penicillin.** *Adults:* Initially, 1.5 g P.O.; then 500 mg q 6 hours for 4 days.

➤**Syphilis in nonpregnant patients sensitive to penicillin.** *Adults:* 500 mg P.O. q.i.d. for 14 days.

Acne

Adults and adolescents: Initially, 500 to 1,000 mg P.O., divided into four doses; then 125 to 500 mg P.O. daily or every other day; apply topical ointment generously to affected areas b.i.d. until skin is thoroughly wet.

➤**Lyme disease**◊. *Adults:* 250 to 500 mg P.O. q.i.d. for 10 to 30 days.

➤**Acute transmitted epididymitis (children over age 8**◊**); pelvic inflammatory disease**◊**; infection with** Helicobacter pylori◊ **(all these indications use tetracycline as adjunctive therapy).** *Adults:* 500 mg P.O. q.i.d. for 10 to 14 days.

➤**Infection prophylaxis in minor skin abrasions and treatment of superficial infections caused by susceptible organisms.** *Adults and children:* Apply topical ointment to infected area one to five times daily.

How supplied

Available by prescription only
Capsules: 100 mg, 250 mg, 500 mg
Suspension: 125 mg/5 ml
Tablets: 250 mg, 500 mg
Available without a prescription
Topical ointment: 3%

Pharmacodynamics

Antibacterial action: Tetracycline is bacteriostatic; it binds reversibly to ribosomal subunits, inhibiting bacterial protein synthesis. Its spectrum of action includes many gram-negative and gram-positive organisms, *Mycoplasma, Rickettsia, Chlamydia,* and spirochetes.

Tetracycline is useful against brucellosis, glanders, mycoplasma pneumonia infections (some clinicians prefer erythromycin), leptospirosis, early stages of Lyme disease, rickettsial infections (such as Rocky Mountain spotted fever, Q fever, and typhus fever), and chlamydial infections. It's an alternative to penicillin for infection with *Neisseria gonorrhoeae,* but because of a high level of resistance in the United States, other antibiotics should be considered.

Pharmacokinetics

Absorption: 75% to 80% absorbed after oral administration. Food or milk products significantly reduce oral absorption.
Distribution: Widely distributed into body tissues and fluids, including synovial, pleural, prostatic, and seminal fluids, bronchial secretions,

saliva, and aqueous humor; CSF penetration is poor. Drug crosses the placenta and is 20% to 67% protein-bound.
Metabolism: Not metabolized.
Excretion: Excreted primarily unchanged in urine by glomerular filtration; plasma half-life is 6 to 12 hours in adults with normal renal function. Some drug appears in breast milk. Only minimal amounts of tetracycline are removed by hemodialysis or peritoneal dialysis.

Route	Onset	Peak	Duration
P.O.	Unknown	2-4 hr	Unknown
Topical	Unknown	Unknown	Unknown

Contraindications and precautions

Contraindicated in patients hypersensitive to tetracyclines. Use cautiously in patients with impaired renal or hepatic function. Use oral form cautiously in last half of pregnancy and in children under age 8.

Interactions

Drug-drug. *Antacids containing aluminum, calcium, magnesium; laxatives containing magnesium, oral iron, sodium bicarbonate:* Decreased absorption of tetracycline. Avoid use together.
Anticoagulants: Enhanced anticoagulation effects; monitor effects closely. Dosage adjustment may be needed.
Cimetidine: May decrease GI absorption of tetracycline. Avoid use together.
Digoxin: Because of increased bioavailability, dosage adjustment may be needed. Monitor patient closely.
Methoxyflurane: Increased risk of nephrotoxicity. Avoid use together.
Oral contraceptives: Decreased contraceptive effect. Advise patient to use another contraceptive method.
Penicillin: Inhibited cell growth from bacteriostatic action. Give penicillin 2 to 3 hours before tetracycline.
Drug-food. *Dairy products and food:* Decreased antibiotic absorption. Give antibiotic 1 hour before or 2 hours after ingesting dairy products or food.
Drug-lifestyle. *Sun exposure:* Enhanced photosensitivity reactions. Advise patient to take precautions.

Adverse reactions

Unless otherwise noted, the following adverse reactions refer to oral form of drug.
CNS: dizziness, headache, ***intracranial hypertension (pseudotumor cerebri).***
CV: ***cardiac arrest, arrhythmias,*** pericarditis.
EENT: sore throat, glossitis.
GI: anorexia, dysphagia, *epigastric distress, nausea,* vomiting, *diarrhea,* esophagitis, oral candidiasis, stomatitis, enterocolitis, inflammatory lesions in anogenital region.
GU: elevated BUN levels.

Reactions may be *common*, uncommon, *life-threatening*, or COMMON AND LIFE-THREATENING.

Hematologic: *neutropenia*, eosinophilia, *thrombocytopenia*.
Hepatic: elevated liver enzyme levels.
Respiratory: *respiratory arrest.*
Skin: *candidal superinfection, maculopapular and erythematous rashes, urticaria, photosensitivity, increased pigmentation*, temporary stinging or burning on application, slight yellowing of treated skin (especially in patients with light complexions), severe dermatitis (with topical administration).
Other: *anaphylactoid reactions, status asthmaticus, hypersensitivity reactions, permanent discoloration of teeth, enamel defects*, and *retardation of bone growth* when used in children under age 8.

Overdose and treatment

Signs and symptoms of overdose are usually limited to GI tract; give antacids or empty stomach by gastric lavage if ingestion was within 4 hours.

Special considerations

Consider the recommendations relevant to all tetracyclines as well as the following.
• Tetracycline causes false-negative results in urine tests using glucose oxidase reagent (Diastix, Chemstrip uG, or glucose enzymatic test strip) and false elevations in fluorometric tests for urinary catecholamines.
ALERT Check expiration date. Outdated or deteriorated tetracyclines have been linked to reversible nephrotoxicity (Fanconi's syndrome).
• During topical use, avoid contact with eyes, nose, and mouth.

Patient monitoring

• Monitor patient for hypersensitivity reactions.
• Monitor patient for resolution of symptoms.
• Discontinue drug if condition persists or worsens.

Pregnant patients

• Drug causes fetal harm and should be administered during pregnancy only when expected benefits justify risk to fetus.

Breast-feeding patients

• Because drug appears in breast milk, don't use in breast-feeding women.

Pediatric patients

• Don't use in children under age 8.

Patient education

• Inform patient using topical form that normal use of cosmetics may continue.
• Tell patient that stinging may occur with topical use but resolves quickly.
• Inform patient that tetracycline may stain clothing.
• Warn patient to avoid prolonged exposure to sunlight.

• Tell patient to report persistent nausea or vomiting and yellowing of skin or eyes.

tetrahydrozoline hydrochloride
Collyrium Fresh, Extra Eye Drops, Eyesine, Eye-Zine, Geneye, Mallazine Eye Drops, Murine Plus, Optigene 3, Tetra-Ide, Tetrasine, Tyzine, Tyzine Pediatric, Visine

Pharmacologic classification: sympathomimetic
Therapeutic classification: vasoconstrictor, decongestant
Pregnancy risk category: C

Indications and dosages

➤ *Nasal congestion. Adults and children over age 6:* Apply 2 to 4 drops in each nostril t.i.d. or q.i.d., p.r.n., or 3 to 4 sprays of 0.1% nasal solution in each nostril q.i.d., p.r.n.
Children age 2 to 6: Apply 2 or 3 drops of 0.05% solution in each nostril q 4 to 6 hours, p.r.n
➤ *Conjunctival congestion. Adults:* 1 or 2 drops of ophthalmic solution in each eye b.i.d. to q.i.d.

How supplied

Available by prescription only
Nasal solution: 0.05%, 0.1%
Available without a prescription
Ophthalmic solution: 0.05%

Pharmacodynamics

Decongestant action: In ocular use, vasoconstriction is produced by local adrenergic action on the blood vessels of the conjunctiva. After nasal application, drug acts on alpha-adrenergic receptors in nasal mucosa to produce constriction, decreasing blood flow and nasal congestion.

Pharmacokinetics

No information available.

Route	Onset	Peak	Duration
Oph-thalmic	Few min	Unknown	1-4 hr

Contraindications and precautions

Contraindicated in patients hypersensitive to drug or its components, in patients with angle-closure glaucoma or other serious eye diseases, and in patients taking an MAO inhibitor. Nasal solution is contraindicated in children under age 2; 0.1% solution is contraindicated in children under age 6.
   Use cautiously in patients with hyperthyroidism, hypertension, and diabetes mellitus. Use ophthalmic form cautiously in patients with cardiac disease.

Interactions
Drug-drug. *Beta blockers:* Systemic adverse re-actions may occur more rapidly. Monitor patient closely.
Guanethidine, MAO inhibitors, tricyclic anti-depressants: Increased adrenergic response and hypertensive crisis. Avoid use together.

Adverse reactions
CNS: headache, drowsiness, insomnia, dizziness, tremor (with ophthalmic form).
CV: *arrhythmias* (with ophthalmic form), tachy-cardia, palpitations.
EENT: transient eye stinging, pupillary dilation, increased intraocular pressure, keratitis, lacrima-tion, eye irritation (with ophthalmic form); tran-sient burning, stinging; sneezing, rebound nasal congestion with excessive or long-term use (with nasal form).

Overdose and treatment
Signs and symptoms of overdose include brady-cardia, decreased body temperature, shocklike hypotension, apnea, drowsiness, CNS depression, and coma.

   Because of rapid onset of sedation, emesis isn't recommended unless induced early. Acti-vated charcoal or gastric lavage may be used ini-tially. Monitor vital signs and ECG. Treat seizures with I.V. diazepam.

Special considerations
• Excessive use of either preparation may cause rebound effect.
• Drug shouldn't be used for more than 3 to 4 days.
• Use in glaucoma requires close medical su-pervision.

Patient monitoring
• Monitor cardiac status (ophthalmic solution).
• Monitor patient for resolution of symptoms.

Pregnant patients
• It isn't known whether drug causes fetal harm. Administer drug during pregnancy only when clearly indicated.

Breast-feeding patients
• It isn't known whether drug appears in breast milk. Use cautiously in breast-feeding women.

Pediatric patients
• The 0.1% nasal solution is contraindicated in children under age 6. All uses are contraindi-cated in children under age 2.

Geriatric patients
• Don't use in elderly patients to treat redness and inflammation, which may represent more se-rious eye conditions.
• These patients are more likely to experience adverse reactions to sympathomimetics.

Patient education
• Teach patient proper administration technique.
• Advise patient not to exceed recommended dose and to use drug only when needed.
• Tell patient to remove contact lenses before us-ing drug.

thalidomide
Thalomid

Pharmacologic classification: immunomodu-lator
Therapeutic classification: leprosy agent
Pregnancy risk category: X

Indications and dosages
➤ *Acute treatment of cutaneous effects of moderate to severe erythema nodosum leprosum (ENL).* *Adults:* 100 to 300 mg P.O. daily h.s. If patient weighs less than 110 lb (50 kg), start dosing at the lower end of range.
➤ *Maintenance therapy for prevention and suppression of the cutaneous effects of ENL recurrence.* *Adults:* Up to 400 mg P.O. daily h.s. or in divided doses at least 1 hour af-ter meals.
➤ *Recurrent aphthous stomatitis* ◊. *Adults:* 100 to 300 mg P.O. daily. Higher doses, up to 600 mg daily, may be necessary.
➤ *Graft versus host disease* ◊ . *Adults:* 800 to 1,600 mg P.O. daily. Drug shouldn't be used prophylactically.

How supplied
Available by prescription only
Capsules: 50 mg

Pharmacodynamics
An immunomodulatory agent whose mechanism of action in patients with ENL isn't fully under-stood.

Pharmacokinetics
Absorption: Slowly absorbed from GI tract.
Distribution: No information available.
Metabolism: Exact metabolic fate is unknown.
Excretion: Mean half-life is 5 to 7 hours. Route of elimination isn't fully understood.

Route	Onset	Peak	Duration
P.O.	Unknown	3-6 hr	Unknown

Contraindications and precautions
Contraindicated in patients hypersensitive to drug or its components; in pregnant women, and in those capable of becoming pregnant, except when alternative therapies are inappropriate and pa-tient meets all conditions listed in the System for Thalidomide Education and Prescribing Safety (S.T.E.P.S.) program.

Reactions may be *common*, uncommon, *life-threatening*, or COMMON AND LIFE-THREATENING.

Interactions
Drug-drug. *Barbiturates, chlorpromazine, reserpine:* May enhance sedative activity. Use together cautiously.
Drugs linked to peripheral neuropathy: Increased risk of peripheral neuropathy. Use together cautiously.
Drug-food. *Any food:* Decreased absorption of drug. Give drug at least 1 hour after meals at h.s.
Drug-lifestyle. *Alcohol use:* Increased sedation. Caution patient against using together.

Adverse reactions
CNS: *asthenia, drowsiness, somnolence, dizziness,* peripheral neuropathy, *headache,* agitation, insomnia, malaise, nervousness, *paresthesia,* tremor, vertigo.
CV: orthostatic hypotension, ***bradycardia,*** peripheral edema.
EENT: pharyngitis, sinusitis.
GI: dry mouth, oral candidiasis, abdominal pain, anorexia, constipation, *diarrhea,* flatulence, *nausea.*
GU: albuminuria, *hematuria,* impotence.
Hematologic: *neutropenia,* anemia, *lymphadenopathy,* LEUKOPENIA.
Hepatic: abnormal liver function test results, increased AST levels.
Musculoskeletal: back pain, neck pain, neck rigidity.
Skin: acne, fungal dermatitis, nail disorder, pruritus, *rash,* ***maculopapular rash,*** *sweating.*
Other: *teratogenicity, hypersensitivity reactions, increased HIV viral load,* facial edema, hyperlipidemia, lymphadenopathy, fever, chills, accidental injury, infection, pain.

Overdose and treatment
Three cases of overdose have been reported, none of which resulted in fatality. Overdose may cause prolonged sleep.

Special considerations
⚠ ALERT Thalidomide must be administered in compliance with all of the terms outlined in the S.T.E.P.S. program, prescribed only by doctors registered with the S.T.E.P.S. program, and dispensed by pharmacists registered with the S.T.E.P.S. program.
● All sexually mature patients, men or women, capable of reproduction must meet rigid S.T.E.P.S. program requirements, including ability to understand and carry out instructions, ability and willingness to comply with mandatory contraceptive measures (concurrent use of at least two highly effective means of contraception), and a written acknowledgment of understanding of all warnings concerning the hazards of fetal exposure to thalidomide and the risk of contraception failure.
● Sexually mature women who haven't undergone a hysterectomy or who haven't been postmenopausal for at least 24 consecutive months (who have had menses at some time in the preceding 24 consecutive months) are considered to be women of childbearing potential even with history of infertility.
● Pregnancy test is mandatory within 24 hours before thalidomide therapy for women of childbearing potential, then weekly during first month of therapy, then monthly for women with regular menstrual cycles. If menstrual cycles are irregular, pregnancy testing continues every 2 weeks during therapy. Retesting is performed if menstrual changes occur, including missed menses.
● Corticosteroids may be given with drug in patients with moderate to severe neuritis linked to severe ENL reaction. Corticosteroids can be tapered and discontinued when neuritis improves.
● A patient with a history of requiring prolonged treatment to prevent recurrence of cutaneous ENL or who experiences flare during tapering, should use minimum effective dose. Tapering should be attempted every 3 to 6 months, reducing dose 50 mg every 2 to 4 weeks.
● Report immediately suspected fetal exposure to FDA via MedWATCH at 1-800-332-1088 and report to manufacturer.

Patient monitoring
● Perform CBC and differential before starting therapy and periodically thereafter, as ordered. Patients with an absolute neutrophil count below 750/mm² while on treatment should be reevaluated.
● Monitor patient for signs and symptoms of neuropathy, such as numbness, tingling, or pain in hands or feet, at least once monthly during first 3 months of drug therapy, then periodically.

Pregnant patients
● Drug is highly dangerous to fetus in any amount. At least two highly reliable means of contraception must be used simultaneously and continuously from at least 1 month before thalidomide therapy until 1 month following completion of therapy.

Breast-feeding patients
● It isn't known whether drug appears in breast milk. Either the drug or nursing should be discontinued, depending on the importance of the drug to the woman.

Pediatric patients
● Safety and efficacy in children under age 12 haven't been established.

Geriatric patients
● Safety and efficacy don't differ significantly between elderly patients and younger patients.

Patient education
● Warn patient of dangers of fetal exposure to any amount of thalidomide and that blood and sperm donations are prohibited while taking thalidomide.

• Explain that at least two highly reliable means of contraception must be used simultaneously and continuously from at least 1 month before thalidomide therapy until 1 month after completion of therapy.

• Instruct patient to report signs or symptoms of pregnancy immediately without regard to probability or improbability of pregnancy.

• Inform women of childbearing potential about mandatory pregnancy testing schedule.

• Inform patient that drug must be discontinued immediately if pregnancy occurs.

• Explain to patient that it isn't known whether drug is present in ejaculate of men receiving drug, and that men receiving thalidomide must always use a latex condom when engaging in sexual activity with women of childbearing potential.

• Advise patient to read package insert carefully.

• Caution patient about potential for dizziness and orthostatic hypotension; instruct patient to change position slowly when rising.

• Inform patient that drug frequently causes drowsiness and somnolence. Advise patient to avoid hazardous activities and the use of alcohol or other medications that might cause drowsiness.

• Tell patient to take drug at bedtime with a glass of water, at least 1 hour after the evening meal.

• Tell patient that drug has caused hypersensitivity reactions and to report erythematous macular rash, fever, tachycardia, and hypotension or any other adverse reactions.

theophylline

Accurbron, Aerolate III, Aerolate Jr., Aerolate SR, Aquaphyllin, Asmalix, Bronkodyl, Elixophyllin, Lanophyllin, Quibron-T, Respbid, Slo-bid Gyrocaps, Slo-Phyllin, Sustaire, Theobid Duracaps, Theochron, Theoclear-80, Theoclear L.A., Theo-Dur, Theolair, Theo-Sav, Theo-24, Theospan-SR, Theostat 80, Theovent, Theo-X, T-Phyl, Uni-Dur, Uniphyl

Pharmacologic classification: xanthine derivative
Therapeutic classification: bronchodilator
Pregnancy risk category: C

Indications and dosages

➤ *Symptomatic relief of bronchospasm in patients not currently receiving theophylline who require rapid relief of acute symptoms. Loading dose:* 6 mg/kg anhydrous theophylline, then:
Adults (nonsmokers): 3 mg/kg P.O. q 6 hours for two doses; then 3 mg/kg q 8 hours.
Older adults with cor pulmonale: 2 mg/kg P.O. q 6 hours for two doses; then 2 mg/kg q 8 hours.
Adults with heart failure: 2 mg/kg P.O. q 8 hours for two doses; then 1 to 2 mg/kg q 12 hours.

Children and adolescents ages 9 to 16 and young adult smokers: 3 mg/kg P.O. q 4 hours for three doses; then 3 mg/kg q 6 hours.
Neonates and children ages 6 months to 9 years: 4 mg/kg P.O. q 4 hours for three doses; then 4 mg/kg q 6 hours.
Neonates and infants under age 6 months ◇: Dosage is highly individualized. Serum theophylline levels should be maintained at less than 10 mcg/ml in neonates and less than 20 mcg/ml in older infants. After loading dose of 1 mg/kg P.O. or I.V. for each 2 mcg/ml increase in theophylline level, infants ages 8 weeks to 6 months receive 1 to 3 mg/kg q 6 hours. Infants ages 4 to 8 weeks receive 1 to 2 mg/kg q 8 hours. Neonates up to age 4 weeks receive 1 to 2 mg/kg q 12 hours. And premature neonates (less than 40 weeks' gestational age) receive 1 mg/kg q 12 hours.

➤ *Parenteral theophylline for patients not currently receiving theophylline. Loading dose:* 4.7 mg/kg (equivalent to 6 mg/kg anhydrous aminophylline) I.V. slowly; then maintenance infusion.
Adults (nonsmokers): 0.55 mg/kg/hour (equivalent to 0.7 mg/kg/hour anhydrous aminophylline) for 12 hours, then 0.39 mg/kg/hour (equivalent to 0.5 mg/kg/hour anhydrous aminophylline).
Older adults with cor pulmonale: 0.47 mg/kg/hour (equivalent to 0.6 mg/kg/hour anhydrous aminophylline) for 12 hours; then 0.24 mg/kg/hour (equivalent to 0.3 mg/kg/hour anhydrous aminophylline).
Adults with heart failure or liver disease: 0.39 mg/kg/hour (equivalent to 0.5 mg/kg/hour anhydrous aminophylline) for 12 hours; then 0.08 to 0.16 mg/kg/hour (equivalent to 0.1 to 0.2 mg/kg/hour anhydrous aminophylline).
Children ages 9 to 16: 0.79 mg/kg/hour (equivalent to 1 mg/kg/hour anhydrous aminophylline) for 12 hours; then 0.63 mg/kg/hour (equivalent to 0.8 mg/kg/hour anhydrous aminophylline).
Infants and children ages 6 months to 9 years: 0.95 mg/kg/hour (equivalent to 1.2 mg/kg/hour anhydrous aminophylline) for 12 hours; then 0.79 mg/kg/hour (equivalent to 1 mg/kg/hour anhydrous aminophylline).
Switch to oral theophylline as soon as patient shows adequate improvement.

➤ *Symptomatic relief of bronchospasm in patients currently receiving theophylline. Adults and children:* Each 0.5 mg/kg I.V. or P.O. (loading dose) increases plasma levels by 1 mcg/ml. Ideally, dose is based on current theophylline level and lean body weight. In emergency situations, may use a 2.5 mg/kg P.O. dose of rapidly absorbed form if no obvious signs of theophylline toxicity are present.

➤ *Prophylaxis of bronchial asthma, bronchospasm of chronic bronchitis, and emphysema. Adults and children:* Using rapidly absorbed dose forms, initial dose is 16 mg/kg or 400 mg P.O. daily (whichever is less) divided q

6 to 8 hours; dose may be increased in approximate increments of 25% at 2- to 3-day intervals. Using extended-release dose forms, initial dose is 12 mg/kg or 400 mg P.O. daily (whichever is less) divided q 8 to 12 hours; dose may be increased, if tolerated, by 2 to 3 mg/kg daily at 3-day intervals. Regardless of dose form used, dose may be increased, if tolerated, up to the following maximum daily doses, without measurements of serum theophylline level.

Adults and adolescents ages 16 and older: 13 mg/kg P.O. or 900 mg P.O. daily in divided doses.

Adolescents age 12 to 16: 18 mg/kg P.O. daily in divided doses.

Children ages 9 to 12: 20 mg/kg P.O. daily in divided doses.

Children under age 9: 24 mg/kg P.O. daily in divided doses.

Note: Dose individualization is required. Use peak plasma and trough levels to estimate dose. Therapeutic range is 10 to 20 mcg/ml. All doses are based on theophylline anhydrous and lean body weight.

➤ **Cystic fibrosis**◇. *Infants:* 10 to 20 mg/kg I.V. daily.

➤ **Promotion of diuresis**◇; **treatment of Cheyne-Stokes respirations**◇; **paroxysmal nocturnal dyspnea**◇. *Adults:* 200 to 400 mg I.V. bolus (single dose).

How supplied
Available by prescription only
Capsules: 100 mg, 200 mg
Capsules (extended-release): 50 mg, 60 mg, 65 mg, 75 mg, 100 mg, 125 mg, 130 mg, 200 mg, 250 mg, 260 mg, 300 mg, 400 mg
D₅W injection: 200 mg in 50 ml or 100 ml; 400 mg in 100 ml, 250 ml, 500 ml, or 1,000 ml; 800 mg in 500 ml or 1,000 ml
Elixir: 50 mg/5 ml, 80 mg/15 ml
Syrup: 50 mg/5 ml, 80 mg/15 ml, 150 mg/15 ml
Tablets: 100 mg, 125 mg, 200 mg, 250 mg, 300 mg
Tablets (extended-release): 100 mg, 200 mg, 250 mg, 300 mg, 400 mg, 450 mg, 500 mg, 600 mg

Pharmacodynamics
Bronchodilator action: Drug may act by inhibiting phosphodiesterase, elevating cellular cyclic AMP levels, or antagonizing adenosine receptors in the bronchi, resulting in relaxation of the smooth muscle.

Drug also increases sensitivity of the medullary respiratory center to carbon dioxide, to reduce apneic episodes. It prevents muscle fatigue, especially that of the diaphragm. It also causes diuresis and cardiac and CNS stimulation.

Pharmacokinetics
Absorption: Well absorbed. Rate and onset of action depend on the dose form. Food may further alter absorption, especially of some extended-release preparations.

Distribution: Distributed throughout the extracellular fluids; equilibrium between fluid and tissues occurs within an hour of an I.V. loading dose. Therapeutic plasma levels are 10 to 20 mcg/ml, but many patients respond to lower levels.

Metabolism: Metabolized in the liver to inactive compounds. Half-life is 7 to 9 hours in adults, 4 to 5 hours in smokers, 20 to 30 hours in premature infants, and 3 to 5 hours in children.

Excretion: About 10% of dose is excreted in urine unchanged. The other metabolites include 1,3-dimethyluric acid, 1-methyluric acid, and 3-methylxanthine.

Route	Onset	Peak	Duration
P.O.			
Regular	15-60 min	1-2 hr	Unknown
Extended	15-60 min	4-7 hr	Unknown
I.V.	15 min	15-30 min	Unknown

Contraindications and precautions
Contraindicated in patients hypersensitive to xanthine compounds, such as caffeine and theobromine, and in those with active peptic ulcer and seizure disorders.

Use cautiously in elderly patients, neonates, infants, young children, and in patients with COPD, cardiac failure, cor pulmonale, renal or hepatic disease, peptic ulcer, hyperthyroidism, diabetes mellitus, glaucoma, severe hypoxemia, hypertension, compromised cardiac or circulatory function, angina, acute MI, or sulfite sensitivity.

Interactions
Drug-drug. *Activated charcoal, barbiturates, ketoconazole, phenytoin, rifampin:* Decreased theophylline levels. Monitor patient closely. Dosage adjustment may be needed if use together can't be avoided.

Allopurinol (high dose), calcium channel blockers, cimetidine, corticosteroids, erythromycin, interferon, mexiletine, oral contraceptives, propranolol, quinolones, troleandomycin: May increase theophylline levels. Monitor patient closely. Dosage adjustment may be needed if use together can't be avoided.

Beta blockers: Antagonistic pharmacologic effect. Avoid use together.

Carbamazepine, isoniazid, loop diuretics: May alter theophylline levels. Monitor patient closely. Dosage adjustment may be needed if use together can't be avoided.

Lithium: Increased lithium excretion. Lithium dosage may require adjustment. Monitor patient carefully.

Drug-herb. *Cacao tree:* Possible inhibition of theophylline metabolism. Discourage ingesting large amounts of cocoa when taking theophylline.

Caffeine, guarana: Additive CNS and CV effects. Discourage use together.

Ephedra: Increased risk of adverse reactions. Discourage concomitant use.

St. John's wort: Decreased theophylline levels and efficacy. Discourage concurrent use if possible. If not, monitor theophylline levels and adjust dosage as needed.
Drug-food. *Any food:* Accelerated absorption. Advise patient to take drug on an empty stomach.
Drug-lifestyle. *Smoking (cigarettes, marijuana):* Increased elimination of theophylline. Monitor theophylline response and serum levels. Dosage adjustment may be needed.

Adverse reactions
CNS: *restlessness, dizziness, insomnia,* headache, irritability, *seizures,* muscle twitching.
CV: *palpitations, sinus tachycardia, extrasystoles,* flushing, marked hypotension, *arrhythmias.*
GI: *nausea, vomiting,* diarrhea, epigastric pain.
Respiratory: tachypnea, *respiratory arrest.*

Overdose and treatment
Signs and symptoms of overdose include nausea, vomiting, insomnia, irritability, tachycardia, extrasystoles, tachypnea, or tonic-clonic seizures. The onset of toxicity may be sudden and severe, with arrhythmias and seizures as the first signs.
Induce emesis except in patients experiencing seizures, then use activated charcoal and cathartics. Treat arrhythmias with lidocaine and seizures with I.V. diazepam; support respiratory and CV systems.

Special considerations
● Theophylline has a low therapeutic index.
● Dosage is determined by monitoring response, tolerance, pulmonary function, and serum theophylline levels. Target range is 10 to 20 mcg/ml.
● Use cautiously in young children, infants, neonates, and the elderly.
● Depending on assay used, theophylline levels may be falsely elevated in the presence of furosemide, phenylbutazone, probenecid, theobromine, caffeine, tea, chocolate, cola beverages, and acetaminophen. Falsely elevates serum uric acid as measured by the Bittner or calorimetric method.

Patient monitoring
● Monitor vital signs and watch for signs and symptoms of toxicity.
● Obtain serum theophylline measurements in patients receiving long-term therapy. Ideal levels are between 10 and 20 mcg/ml, although some patients may respond adequately with lower serum levels. Check every 6 months. If levels are less than 10 mcg/ml, increase dose by about 25% each day. If levels are 20 to 25 mcg/ml, decrease dose by about 10% each day. If levels are 25 to 30 mcg/ml, skip next dose and decrease by 25% each day. If levels are more than 30 mcg/ml, skip next two doses and decrease by 50% each day. Repeat serum level determination.

Breast-feeding patients
● Drug appears in breast milk and may cause irritability, insomnia, or fretfulness in the breast-fed infant. A decision must be made to stop either breast-feeding or drug therapy.

Pediatric patients
● Use cautiously in neonates. Children usually require higher doses (on a mg/kg basis) than adults. Maximum recommended daily doses are 24 mg/kg in children under age 9; 20 mg/kg in children age 9 to 12; 18 mg/kg in adolescents ages 12 to 16; 13 mg/kg or 900 mg (whichever is less) in adolescents and adults age 16 or older.

Patient education
● Tell patient to take drug with food if GI upset occurs with liquid preparations or nonsustained-release forms.
● Instruct patient to continue to use the same brand of theophylline.
⚠ ALERT If patient smokes, tell him to notify prescriber if he quits because theophylline dose may need to be reduced to avoid toxicity.
● Advise patient to take drug at regular intervals as instructed, around-the-clock.
● If patient misses a dose, tell him to take it as soon as possible, but not to double the dose.
● Inform patient of adverse effects and possible signs of toxicity.

thiabendazole
Mintezol

Pharmacologic classification: benzimidazole
Therapeutic classification: anthelmintic
Pregnancy risk category: C

Indications and dosages
➤ *Systemic infections with pinworm, roundworm, threadworm, whipworm, visceral larva migrans, trichinosis. Adults and children who weigh 14 to 70 kg (30 to 154 lb):* 25 mg/kg P.O. q 12 hours for 2 successive days.
Adults and children who weigh more than 70 kg: 1.5 g P.O. q 12 hours for 2 successive days. Maximum dose is 3 g daily. For trichinosis, two doses daily for 2 to 4 successive days. For visceral larva migrans, two doses daily for 7 successive days.
➤ *Cutaneous infestations with larva migrans (creeping eruption). Adults and children:* 25 mg/kg P.O. b.i.d. for 2 to 5 days. Maximum dose is 3 g daily. If lesions persist after 2 days, repeat course.
➤ *Dracunculiasis◇; infections caused by* **Angiostrongylus costaricensis◇.** *Adults:* 25 to 37.5 mg/kg P.O. b.i.d. (25 mg t.i.d. for *A. costaricensis*) for 3 successive days.
➤ *Capillariasis◇. Adults:* 25 mg/kg P.O. q 12 hours for 30 days.

How supplied
Available by prescription only
Oral suspension: 500 mg/5 ml
Tablets (chewable): 500 mg

Pharmacodynamics
Anthelmintic action: Thiabendazole kills susceptible helminths by inhibiting fumarate reductase. It's the drug of choice for *Strongyloides stercoralis* (threadworm) infections and may be useful in disseminated strongyloidiasis. It's also preferred for oral and topical therapy of *Ancylostoma braziliense, Toxocara canis,* and *T. cati.* It has shown activity in certain other nematode infections, but other agents are preferred for the treatment of ascariasis, tricuriasis, uncinariasis, and enterobiasis.

Pharmacokinetics
Absorption: Absorbed readily; serum levels peak at 1 to 2 hours.
Distribution: No information available.
Metabolism: Metabolized almost completely by hydroxylation and conjugation.
Excretion: About 90% of dose is excreted in urine as metabolites within 48 hours; about 5% is excreted in feces.

Route	Onset	Peak	Duration
P.O.	Unknown	1-2 hr	Unknown

Contraindications and precautions
Contraindicated in patients hypersensitive to drug. Use cautiously in patients with renal or hepatic dysfunction, severe malnutrition, or anemia and in those who are vomiting.

Interactions
Drug-drug. *Theophylline:* Increased risk of theophylline toxicity. Monitor patient closely.

Adverse reactions
CNS: impaired mental alertness, impaired coordination, numbness, *seizures, drowsiness, fatigue, headache,* giddiness, dizziness.
CV: *hypotension.*
EENT: tinnitus, blurry or yellow vision, dry mouth and eyes, xanthopsia.
GI: *anorexia, nausea, vomiting,* diarrhea, epigastric distress, cholestasis.
GU: hematuria, enuresis, crystalluria, malodorous urine.
Hematologic: *leukopenia.*
Hepatic: *jaundice, parenchymal liver damage,* elevated AST levels.
Metabolic: hyperglycemia
Skin: *rash, pruritus, erythema multiforme, Stevens-Johnson syndrome.*
Other: lymphadenopathy, fever, flushing, chills, *angioedema, anaphylaxis.*

Overdose and treatment
Signs and symptoms of overdose may include visual disturbances and altered mental status.

Treatment includes induced emesis or gastric lavage if ingested within 4 hours, followed by supportive and symptomatic treatment.

Special considerations
● Drug may be given with milk, fruit juice, or food.
● Assess patient and review laboratory reports for signs of anemia, dehydration, or malnutrition before starting therapy.

Patient monitoring
● Monitor patient for adverse reactions, which usually occur 3 to 4 hours after drug is administered. Adverse effects are usually mild and related to dose and duration of therapy.

Pregnant patients
● Use drug during pregnancy only when potential benefit justifies risk to fetus.

Breast-feeding patients
● Safety in breast-feeding women hasn't been established.

Pediatric patients
● Drug shouldn't be used in children who weigh less than 13.6 kg (30 lb) for the treatment of strongloidiasis, ascariasis, hookworm infections, trichuriasis, and trichinosis unless benefits outweigh the risk.

Patient education
● Warn patient that drug causes drowsiness or dizziness and to avoid driving or other hazardous activities during therapy.
● Instruct patient to promptly report adverse reactions.

thiamine hydrochloride (vitamin B₁)
Thiamilate

Pharmacologic classification: water-soluble vitamin
Therapeutic classification: nutritional supplement
Pregnancy risk category: A (C if more than RDA)

Indications and dosages
The RDA of thiamine is as follows:
Neonates and infants up to age 6 months: 0.3 mg daily.
Infants ages 6 months to 1 year: 0.4 mg daily.
Children ages 1 to 3: 0.7 mg daily.
Children ages 4 to 6: 0.9 mg daily.
Children ages 7 to 10: 1 mg daily.
Males ages 11 to 14: 1.3 mg daily.
Men ages 15 to 50: 1.5 mg daily.
Men age 51 and older: 1.2 mg daily.
Women ages 11 to 50: 1.1 mg daily.
Women age 51 and older: 1 mg daily.

Pregnant women: 1.5 mg daily.
Breast-feeding women: 1.6 mg daily.
➤*Beriberi. Adults:* 10 to 20 mg I.M., depending on severity (can receive up to 100 mg I.M. or I.V. for severe cases), t.i.d. for 2 weeks, followed by dietary correction and multivitamin supplement containing 5 to 30 mg thiamine daily in single dose or three divided doses for 1 month.
Children: 10 to 25 mg, depending on severity, I.M. daily for several weeks with adequate dietary intake.

➤*Anemia secondary to thiamine deficiency; polyneuritis secondary to alcoholism, pregnancy, or pellagra. Adults and children:* P.O. dosage is based on RDA for age-group.
➤*Wernicke's encephalopathy. Adults:* Initially, 100 mg I.V., followed by 50 to 100 mg I.M. or I.V. daily.
➤*"Wet beriberi" with heart failure. Adults and children:* 10 to 30 mg I.V. for emergency treatment.

How supplied
Available by prescription only
Injection: 1-ml ampules (100 mg/ml), 1-ml vials (100 mg/ml), 1-ml syringes (100 mg/ml), 2-ml vials (100 mg/ml), 10-ml vials (100 mg/ml), 30-ml vials (100 mg/ml).
Available without a prescription
Tablets: 25 mg, 50 mg, 100 mg, 250 mg, 500 mg
Tablets (enteric-coated): 20 mg

Pharmacodynamics
Metabolic action: Exogenous thiamine is required for carbohydrate metabolism. Thiamine combines with ATP to form thiamine pyrophosphate, a coenzyme in carbohydrate metabolism and transketolation reactions. This coenzyme is also necessary in the hexose monophosphate shunt during pentose utilization. One sign of thiamine deficiency is an increase in pyruvic acid. The body's need for thiamine is greater when the carbohydrate content of the diet is high. Within 3 weeks of total absence of dietary thiamine, significant vitamin depletion can occur. Thiamine deficiency can cause beriberi.

Pharmacokinetics
Absorption: Absorbed readily after oral administration of small doses; after oral administration of a large dose, the total amount absorbed is limited to 4 to 8 mg. In patients with alcoholism, cirrhosis, or malabsorption, GI absorption of thiamine is decreased. When given with meals, GI drug absorption decreases, but total absorption remains the same. After I.M. administration, drug is absorbed rapidly and completely.
Distribution: Distributed widely into body tissues. When intake exceeds the minimal requirements, tissue stores become saturated. About 100 to 200 mcg of thiamine is distributed daily into the milk of breast-feeding women on a normal diet.

Metabolism: Metabolized in the liver.
Excretion: Excess thiamine is excreted in urine. After administration of large doses (more than 10 mg), both unchanged thiamine and metabolites are excreted in urine after tissue stores become saturated.

Route	Onset	Peak	Duration
P.O., I.V., I.M.	Unknown	Unknown	Unknown

Contraindications and precautions
Contraindicated in patients hypersensitive to thiamine products.

Interactions
Drug-drug. *Alkaline solutions, such as carbonates, citrates, and bicarbonates:* Thiamine is incompatible with these solutions. Avoid use together.
Neuromuscular blockers: Possible enhanced effects of these drugs.
Neutral or alkaline solutions: Thiamine is unstable in these solutions. Don't mix the drug in these solutions.
Sulfites: Solutions containing sulfites are incompatible with thiamine. Avoid use together.

Adverse reactions
CNS: restlessness.
CV: *angioedema, CV collapse,* cyanosis.
EENT: tightness of throat (allergic reaction).
GI: nausea, *hemorrhage.*
Respiratory: pulmonary edema.
Skin: feeling of warmth, pruritus, urticaria, diaphoresis.
Other: weakness, tenderness and induration following I.M. administration.

Overdose and treatment
Very large doses of thiamine administered parenterally may produce neuromuscular and ganglionic blockade and neurologic symptoms. Treatment is supportive.

Special considerations
• An intradermal skin test should be performed before I.V. thiamine administration if sensitivity is suspected.
• Keep epinephrine available when giving large parenteral doses.
• I.M. injection may be painful. Rotate injection sites.
• Total absence of dietary thiamine can produce a deficiency state in about 3 weeks.
• Accurate dietary history is important during vitamin replacement therapy.
• Store thiamine in light-resistant, nonmetallic container.
• Drug therapy may produce false-positive results in the phosphotungstate method for determination of uric acid and in urine spot tests with Ehrlich's reagent for urobilinogen.

Reactions may be *common,* uncommon, *life-threatening,* or COMMON AND LIFE-THREATENING.

- Large doses of thiamine interfere with the Schack and Waxler spectrophotometric determination of serum theophylline levels.

Patient monitoring
- Monitor patient for adverse reactions including injection site reactions.
- Monitor patient for symptom relief.

Breast-feeding patients
- Thiamine, in amounts that don't exceed the RDA, is safe to use in breast-feeding women. It appears in breast milk and fulfills a nutritional requirement of the infant.

Patient education
- Inform patient of potential adverse reactions.

---

thiopental sodium
Pentothal

Pharmacologic classification: barbiturate
Therapeutic classification: anesthetic
Controlled substance schedule: III
Pregnancy risk category: C

Indications and dosages
➤ **General anesthetic for short-term procedures.** *Adults and children:* 2 to 4 ml 2.5% solution (50 to 100 mg) administered I.V. for induction and repeated as a maintenance dosage; dose is individualized.
➤ **Convulsive states following anesthesia.** *Adults:* 50 to 125 mg (2 to 5 ml 2.5% solution) I.V.
➤ **Neurosurgical patients with increased ICP.** *Adults:* 1.5 to 3.5 mg/kg I.V. bolus. May give intermittently as long as patient is adequately ventilated.

How supplied
Available by prescription only
Injection: 250-mg (2.5%), 400-mg (2%), 500-mg (2.5%) syringes; 500-mg (2.5%), 1-g (2.5%), 2.5-g (2.5%), 5-g (2.5%), 1-g (2%), 2.5-g (2%), 5-g (2%) kits

Pharmacodynamics
Anesthetic action: Thiopental produces anesthesia by direct depression of the polysynaptic midbrain reticular activating system. Thiopental decreases presynaptic (by way of decreased neurotransmitter release) and postsynaptic excitation. These effects may be subsequent to increased gamma-aminobutyric acid (GABA) levels, enhancement of GABA effects, or a direct effect on GABA receptor sites.

Pharmacokinetics
Absorption: Depth of anesthesia may increase for up to 40 seconds. Consciousness returns in 20 to 30 minutes.

Distribution: Distributed throughout the body; highest initial level occurs in vascular areas of the brain, primarily gray matter; drug is 80% protein-bound. Redistribution of drug is primarily responsible for its short duration of action.
Metabolism: Metabolized extensively but slowly in the liver.
Excretion: Unchanged thiopental isn't excreted in significant amounts; duration of action depends on tissue redistribution.

Route	Onset	Peak	Duration
I.V.	Immediate	10-20 sec	Unknown

Contraindications and precautions
Contraindicated in patients with acute intermittent or variegate porphyria (not in other porphyrias); in patients hypersensitive to drug; and in patients in whom general anesthesia is contraindicated.

Use with extreme caution in patients with respiratory, cardiac, circulatory, renal, or hepatic dysfunction; severe anemia; shock; myxedema; and status asthmaticus because drug may worsen these conditions. Also use cautiously in breast-feeding women and in patients with hypotension, Addison's disease, myasthenia gravis, or increased intracranial pressure.

Interactions
Drug-drug. *Antihistamines, benzodiazepines, hypnotics, narcotics, phenothiazines, sedatives:* Increased CNS effect. Monitor patient closely.
Drug-lifestyle. *Alcohol use:* Increased CNS depressant effects. Discourage use together.

Adverse reactions
CNS: anxiety, restlessness, retrograde amnesia, prolonged somnolence, dose-dependent alteration in EEG patterns.
CV: thrombophlebitis, hypotension, tachycardia, peripheral vascular collapse, *myocardial depression, arrhythmias.*
GI: nausea and vomiting, abdominal pain, diarrhea, cramping.
Respiratory: cough, sneezing, *respiratory depression, apnea, laryngospasm, bronchospasm.*
Other: pain, swelling, ulceration, necrosis on extravasation (unlikely at levels less than 2.5%), gangrene after intra-arterial injection, *allergic reactions,* hiccups, shivering, local irritation.

Overdose and treatment
Effects of overdose include respiratory depression, respiratory arrest, hypotension, and shock.

Treat supportively, using mechanical ventilation if needed; give I.V. fluids or vasopressors (dopamine, phenylephrine) for hypotension. Monitor vital signs closely.

Special considerations
● Solutions of succinylcholine, tubocurarine, or atropine shouldn't be mixed with thiopental but can be given to the patient at the same time.
● A small test dose of 25 to 75 mg may be administered to assess tolerance or unusual sensitivity.
● Discontinue drug if peripheral vascular collapse, respiratory arrest, or hypersensitivity occurs.

Patient monitoring
● Monitor cardiac and respiratory status.

Pediatric patients
● Use cautiously in children.

Geriatric patients
● These patients may need lower dosages.

Patient education
● Reasure patient and family that patient will be monitored continuously throughout anesthesia.

thioridazine
Mellaril-S

thioridazine hydrochloride
Apo-Thioridazine*, Mellaril

Pharmacologic classification: phenothiazine (piperidine derivative)
Therapeutic classification: antipsychotic
Pregnancy risk category: C

Indications and dosages
➤ *Management of symptoms of psychotic disorders in patients intolerant of other antipsychotics.* Adults: Initially, 50 to 100 mg P.O. t.i.d., with gradual increments up to 800 mg daily in divided doses, if needed. Dosage varies.
➤ *Dysthymic disorder (neurotic depression), dementia in elderly patients, behavioral problems in children.* Adults: Initially, 25 mg P.O. t.i.d. Maintenance dosage is 20 to 200 mg daily.
Children over age 2: Usually, 0.5 to 3 mg/kg P.O. daily in divided doses. Give 10 mg b.i.d. or t.i.d. to children with moderate disorders and 25 mg b.i.d. or t.i.d. to hospitalized children.

How supplied
Available by prescription only
Oral concentrate: 30 mg/ml, 100 mg/ml (3% to 4.2% alcohol)
Suspension: 25 mg/5 ml, 100 mg/5 ml
Tablets: 10 mg, 15 mg, 25 mg, 50 mg, 100 mg, 150 mg, 200 mg

Pharmacodynamics
Antipsychotic action: Thioridazine is thought to exert antipsychotic effects by postsynaptic blockade of CNS dopamine receptors, inhibiting dopamine-mediated effects.

Thioridazine has many other central and peripheral effects: It produces both alpha and ganglionic blockade and counteracts histamine- and serotonin-mediated activity. Its most common adverse reactions are antimuscarinic and sedative; it causes fewer extrapyramidal effects than other antipsychotics.

Pharmacokinetics
Absorption: Absorption varies with administration route. Oral tablet absorption is erratic and variable, with onset ranging from ½ to 1 hour. Oral concentrates and suspensions are much more predictable.
Distribution: Distributed widely throughout the body, including breast milk. Steady state serum level is achieved within 4 to 7 days. Drug is 91% to 99% protein-bound.
Metabolism: Metabolized extensively by the liver and forms the active metabolite mesoridazine.
Excretion: Mostly excreted as metabolites in urine; some is excreted in feces by way of the biliary tract.

Route	Onset	Peak	Duration
P.O.	Unknown	2-4 hr	4-6 hr

Contraindications and precautions
Contraindicated in patients hypersensitive to drug or in those experiencing coma, CNS depression, or severe hypertensive or hypotensive cardiac disease. Mellaril is contraindicated in patients taking fluvoxamine, propranolol, pindolol, drugs that inhibit the cytochrome P-450 2D6 isozyme, and drugs that are known to prolong the QTc interval. Mellaril is also contraindicated in patients with reduced levels of the cytochrome P-450 2D6 isozyme and in patients with congenital long-QT syndrome or a history of cardiac arrhythmias.

Use cautiously in elderly or debilitated patients and in those with hepatic or CV disease, respiratory or seizure disorders, hypocalcemia, severe reactions to insulin or electroconvulsive therapy, and exposure to extreme cold or heat or to organophosphate insecticides.

Interactions
Drug-drug. *Aluminum- and magnesium-containing antacids and antidiarrheals, phenobarbital:* Decreased therapeutic effect. Avoid use together.
Analgesics, anesthetics (epidural, general, spinal), antiarrhythmics, anticholinergics (including atropine, disopyramide, quinidine), antidepressants, antihistamines, barbiturates, CNS depressants, MAO inhibitors, meperidine, narcotics, parenteral magnesium, phenothiazines, tranquilizers: Additive effect. Avoid use together.

Antiparkinsonians: Oversedation, paralytic ileus, visual changes, and severe constipation. Monitor patient closely.

Bromocriptine: Antagonized therapeutic effect on prolactin secretion. Monitor patient closely. Dosage adjustment may be needed.

Centrally acting antihypertensive drugs, clonidine, guanabenz, guanadrel, guanethidine, methyldopa, reserpine: Inhibited blood pressure response. Monitor patient; dosage adjustment may be needed.

Dopamine (high dose): Decreased vasoconstricting effects. Dosage may need adjustment; monitor patient closely.

Drugs that inhibit P-450 2D6 (fluoxetine, paroxetine): Increased thioridazine levels, increasing cardiotoxicity and life-threatening arrhythmias. Use together is contraindicated.

Drugs that prolong the QT interval: Increased risk of cardiotoxicity and life-threatening arrhythmias. Use together is contraindicated.

Levodopa: Decreased effectiveness and increased toxicity. Monitor patient carefully.

Lithium: Possible severe neurologic toxicity with an encephalitis-like syndrome. Avoid use together.

Metrizamide: Increased risk of seizures. Avoid use together.

Nitrates: Hypotension. Monitor patient closely.

Phenytoin: Increased toxicity. Avoid use together.

Procainamide: Increased risk of arrhythmias and conduction defects. Avoid use together.

Propranolol: Increased thioridazine plasma levels and toxicity. Avoid use together if possible. Monitor patient closely if drugs must be given together.

Propylthiouracil: Increased risk of agranulocytosis. Monitor patient closely.

Sympathomimetics, such as appetite suppressants, ephedrine (commonly found in nasal sprays), epinephrine, phenylephrine: Decreased stimulatory and pressor effects. Monitor patient closely.

Drug-herb. *Kava:* Possible increased risk or severity of dystonic reactions. Discourage use together.

Yohimbe: Phenothiazines may increase the risk of toxicity. Discourage use together.

Drug-food. *Caffeine:* Increased metabolism of drug. Discourage use together.

Drug-lifestyle. *Alcohol use:* Increased CNS depression. Discourage use together.

Sun exposure: Potentiation of photosensitivity reactions. Advise patient to avoid prolonged or unprotected sun exposure.

Heavy smoking: Increased metabolism of drug. Advise patient to avoid or limit smoking.

Adverse reactions

CNS: *neuroleptic malignant syndrome,* extrapyramidal reactions, *tardive dyskinesia, sedation,* EEG changes, dizziness.

CV: *orthostatic hypotension,* tachycardia, ECG changes, *arrythmias, torsades de pointes.*

EENT: *ocular changes, blurred vision,* retinitis pigmentosa.

GI: *dry mouth, constipation.*

GU: *urine retention,* dark urine, menstrual irregularities, inhibited ejaculation.

Hematologic: *transient leukopenia, agranulocytosis,* hyperprolactinemia.

Hepatic: cholestatic jaundice, elevated liver enzyme levels.

Metabolic: weight gain, increased appetite.

Skin: *mild photosensitivity,* allergic reactions.

Other: gynecomastia.

Overdose and treatment

CNS depression is characterized by deep, unarousable sleep and possible coma, hypotension or hypertension, extrapyramidal symptoms, abnormal involuntary muscle movements, agitation, seizures, arrhythmias, ECG changes, hypothermia or hyperthermia, and autonomic nervous system dysfunction.

Treatment is symptomatic and supportive and includes maintaining vital signs, airway, stable body temperature, and fluid and electrolyte balance. Patient should have ECG continuously monitored.

Don't induce vomiting; Drug inhibits cough reflex, and aspiration may occur. Use gastric lavage, then activated charcoal and sodium chloride cathartics; dialysis doesn't help. Regulate body temperature as needed. Treat hypotension with I.V. fluids: Don't give epinephrine. Treat seizures with parenteral diazepam or barbiturates; arrhythmias with parenteral phenytoin (1 mg/kg with rate adjusted to blood pressure); and extrapyramidal reactions with benztropine at 1 to 2 mg or parenteral diphenhydramine at 10 to 50 mg. Contact poison information center for specific instructions.

Special considerations

Consider the recommendations relevant to all phenothiazines as well as the following.

⚠ ALERT Serious dose-related cardiac events have been reported, including torsades de pointes and sudden death.

• Different liquid forms have different concentrations. Check dosage carefully.

• Doses of more than 300 mg daily are usually reserved for adults with severe psychosis. Don't exceed 800 mg daily because ophthalmic toxicity may result.

• Liquid forms may cause a rash if skin contact occurs.

• Drug can cause pink to brown discoloration of urine.

• Thioridazine is linked to a high risk of sedation, anticholinergic effects, orthostatic hypotension, photosensitivity reactions, and delayed or absent ejaculation. It has the lowest potential for extrapyramidal reactions of all phenothiazines.

• Oral forms may cause stomach upset. Administer with food or fluid.

• Concentrate must be diluted in 2 to 4 oz (60 to 120 ml) of liquid, preferably water, carbonated drinks, fruit juice, tomato juice, milk, or pudding.
• All liquid formulations must be protected from light.
• Thioridazine causes false-positive test results for urinary porphyrins, urobilinogen, amylase, and 5-hydroxyindoleacetic acid because of darkening of urine by metabolites. It also causes false-positive urine pregnancy results in tests using human chorionic gonadotropin as the indicator.

Patient monitoring
• Patient should have baseline ECG before starting therapy. If QT interval is greater than 450 milliseconds, don't give drug.
• Check baseline potassium and correct any imbalance before starting therapy.
• Check patient regularly (at least every 6 months)for abnormal body movements.

Breast-feeding patients
• Thioridazine may enter breast milk. Potential benefits to the woman should outweigh potential harm to infant.

Pediatric patients
• Drug isn't recommended for children under age 2.

Geriatric patients
• These patients tend to need lower doses, adjusted to individual response. Such patients also are more likely to develop adverse reactions, especially tardive dyskinesia and other extrapyramidal effects.

Patient education
• Explain risks of dystonic reactions and tardive dyskinesia, and tell patient to report abnormal body movements.
• Tell patient to avoid sun exposure and to wear sunscreen when going outdoors to prevent photosensitivity reactions. (Heat lamps and tanning beds also may cause burning of the skin or skin discoloration.)
• Warn patient not to spill the liquid on the skin; rash and irritation may result.
• Warn patient to avoid extremely hot or cold baths or exposure to temperature extremes, sunlamps, or tanning beds; drug may cause thermoregulatory changes.
• Advise patient to take drug exactly as prescribed and not to double missed doses.
• Explain that many drug interactions are possible. Patient should seek medical approval before taking any self-prescribed medication.
• Tell patient not to stop taking drug suddenly; most adverse reactions may be relieved by dose reduction. However, patient should report difficulty urinating, sore throat, dizziness, fainting, or visual changes.

• Patient may experience gastritis, nausea, vomiting, dizziness, tremor, feeling of warmth or cold, diaphoresis, tachycardia, headache, insomnia after abrupt withdrawal of long-term therapy.
• Warn patient to avoid hazardous activities that require alertness until the effect of drug is established. Reassure patient that excessive sedation usually subsides after several weeks.
• Tell patient not to drink alcohol or take other medications that may cause excessive sedation.
• Advise patient to maintain adequate hydration.
• Explain which fluids are appropriate for diluting the concentrate and the dropper technique of measuring dose.
• Tell patient to store drug safely away from children.

thiotepa
Thioplex

Pharmacologic classification: alkylating (not specific to cell cycle phase)
Therapeutic classification: antineoplastic
Pregnancy risk category: D

Indications and dosages
Dosages and indications may vary. Check current literature for recommended protocol.
➤ *Breast and ovarian cancer, Hodgkin's disease, lymphomas. Adults and adolescents age 12 and older:* 0.2 mg/kg I.V. daily for 4 to 5 days, repeated q 2 to 4 weeks. Or, 0.3 to 0.4 mg/kg I.V. q 1 to 4 weeks.
➤ *Bladder tumor. Adults and adolescents age 12 and older:* 60 mg in 30 to 60 ml of normal saline solution (thiotepa in distilled water) instilled in bladder once weekly for 4 weeks. Retain the solution for 2 hours. If the patient cannot retain it, give 30 ml.
➤ *Neoplastic effusions. Adults and adolescents age 12 and over:* 0.6 to 0.8 mg/kg intracavity or intratumor q 1 to 4 weeks.
➤ *Malignant meningeal neoplasm◇. Adults:* 1 to 10 mg/m² intrathecally, once to twice weekly.

How supplied
Available by prescription only
Injection: 15-mg vials

Pharmacodynamics
Antineoplastic action: Thiotepa exerts its cytotoxic activity as an alkylating agent, cross-linking strands of DNA and RNA and inhibiting protein synthesis, resulting in cell death.

Pharmacokinetics
Absorption: Incompletely absorbed across the GI tract; absorption from the bladder is variable, ranging from 10% to 100% of an instilled dose. Absorption is increased by certain pathologic conditions. I.M. and pleural membrane absorption of thiotepa is also variable.

Reactions may be *common*, uncommon, *life-threatening*, or COMMON AND LIFE-THREATENING.

Distribution: Distributed readily into CNS after I.V. administration.
Metabolism: Metabolized extensively in the liver.
Excretion: Drug and its metabolites are excreted in urine. Half-life is 2½ hours.

Route	Onset	Peak	Duration
I.V.	Unknown	Unknown	Unknown
Intra-vasical	15 min	1 hr	6 hr
Intra-peritoneal	Immediate	Immediate	Unknown

Contraindications and precautions

Contraindicated in patients hypersensitive to drug and in those with severe bone marrow, hepatic, or renal dysfunction. Use cautiously in patients with impaired renal or hepatic function or bone marrow suppression.

Interactions

Drug-drug. *Alkylating agents, irradiation therapy:* Toxicity. Avoid use together.
Anticoagulants, aspirin: Increased risk of bleeding. Avoid use together.
Myelosuppressive drugs: Additive myelosuppression. Monitor patient closely.
Neuromuscular blockers: Prolonged muscular paralysis. Monitor patient closely.
Succinylcholine: Prolonged respirations and apnea. Monitor patient closely. Avoid use together.

Adverse reactions

CNS: headache, dizziness, blurred vision, fatigue, weakness.
EENT: *laryngeal edema,* conjunctivitis.
GI: *nausea, vomiting,* abdominal pain, anorexia.
GU: amenorrhea, decreased spermatogenesis, dysuria, urine retention, hemorrhagic cystitis.
Hematologic: *leukopenia (begins within 5 to 10 days), thrombocytopenia, neutropenia,* anemia.
Metabolic: hyperuricemia, decreased plasma pseudocholinesterase levels.
Respiratory: asthma.
Skin: alopecia, hives, rash, dermatitis.
Other: fever, pain at injection site, *hypersensitivity, anaphylaxis.*

Overdose and treatment

Signs and symptoms of overdose are mainly extensions of adverse reactions, particularly leukopenia and thrombocytopenia, effects that may lead to infection or bleeding. Dosages within or slightly above the recommended therapeutic dosages have been linked to dose-related, life-threatening hematopoietic toxicity.

There's no known antidote for thiotepa overdose; whole blood or platelet transfusions have been beneficial. Thiotepa is removed by dialysis.

Special considerations

• Refrigerate dry powder; protect from light.

• Use only sterile water for injection to reconstitute. Refrigerated solution is stable for 8 hours.
• Drug can be given by all parenteral routes, including direct injection into the tumor.
• Drug may be mixed with procaine 2% or epinephrine 1:1,000, or both, for local use.
• Drug may be further diluted to larger volumes with normal saline solution, D_5W, or lactated Ringer's solution for I.V. infusion, intracavitary injection, or perfusion therapy.
• Filter solutions through a 0.22-micron filter before administration. Don't use solutions that are opaque or precipitate after filtration.
• To prevent hyperuricemia with resulting uric acid nephropathy, allopurinol may be given; keep patient well hydrated.
• Avoid all I.M. injections when platelet count is less than 100,000/mm³.
• Toxicity may be delayed and prolonged because drug binds to tissues and stays in body several hours.

Patient monitoring

• Stop drug or decrease dose if WBC count decreases to less than 4,000/mm³ or if platelet count decreases to less than 150,000/mm³.
• Monitor uric acid.
• Monitor CBC weekly for at least 3 weeks after last dose. Warn patient to report even mild infections.

Pregnant patients

• Drug shouldn't be used during pregnancy.

Breast-feeding patients

• It isn't known whether drug appears in breast milk. However, because of risk of serious adverse reactions, mutagenicity, and carcinogenicity in the infant, breast-feeding isn't recommended.

Pediatric patients

• Safety and efficacy haven't been established.

Patient education

• Encourage patient to maintain an adequate fluid intake to facilitate the excretion of uric acid.
• Instruct patient to avoid OTC products containing aspirin.
• Tell patient to avoid people with infections.
• Advise patient that hair should grow back.
• Tell patient to report sore throat, fever, or unusual bruising or bleeding.
• Instruct patient to use effective contraception measures; if patient becomes pregnant, she should notify prescriber immediately.

thiothixene
thiothixene hydrochloride
Navane

Pharmacologic classification: thioxanthene
Therapeutic classification: antipsychotic
Pregnancy risk category: C

Indications and dosages
➤*Acute agitation. Adults:* 4 mg I.M. b.i.d. to
q.i.d. Maximum dosage is 30 mg I.M. daily. Change
to P.O. form as soon as possible.
➤*Mild to moderate psychosis. Adults:* Initially, 2 mg P.O. t.i.d. May increase gradually to
15 mg daily. Maximum dosage is 60 mg daily.
➤*Severe psychosis. Adults:* Initially, 5 mg
P.O. b.i.d. May increase gradually to 20 to 30 mg
daily. Maximum recommended dosage is 60 mg
daily.

How supplied
Available by prescription only
Capsules: 1 mg, 2 mg, 5 mg, 10 mg, 20 mg
Injection: 2 mg/ml, 5 mg/ml, 10 mg/ml
Oral concentrate: 5 mg/ml (7% alcohol)

Pharmacodynamics
Antipsychotic action: Thiothixene is thought
to exert antipsychotic effects by postsynaptic
blockade of CNS dopamine receptors, thereby inhibiting dopamine-mediated effects.

Thiothixene has many other central and peripheral effects; it also acts as an alpha blocker.
Its most prominent adverse reactions are extrapyramidal.

Pharmacokinetics
Absorption: Rapidly absorbed.
Distribution: Widely distributed throughout the
body. Drug is 91% to 99% protein-bound.
Metabolism: Metabolized in the liver.
Excretion: Mostly excreted as parent drug in fe-
ces by way of the biliary tract.

Route	Onset	Peak	Duration
P.O., I.M.	10-30 min	1-6 hr	Unknown

Contraindications and precautions
Contraindicated in patients hypersensitive to drug
and in those experiencing circulatory collapse,
coma, CNS depression, or blood dyscrasia.

Use cautiously in geriatric or debilitated patients; in those with history of seizure disorders,
CV disease, heat exposure, glaucoma, or prostatic hyperplasia; and in those in a state of alcohol
withdrawal.

Interactions
Drug-drug. *CNS depressants:* Increased CNS
depression. Avoid use together.
Drug-herb. *Nutmeg:* May cause loss of symptom control. Discourage use together.

Drug-food. *Caffeine:* Increased metabolism of
drug. Advise patient to avoid caffeine.
Drug-lifestyle. *Alcohol use:* Increased CNS depression. Advise patient to avoid alcohol.
Heavy smoking: Increased metabolism of drug.
Advise patient to avoid or limit smoking.
Sun exposure: May potentiate photosensitivity
reactions. Advise patient to avoid prolonged or
unprotected sun exposure.

Adverse reactions
CNS: *neuroleptic malignant syndrome*,
extrapyramidal reactions, drowsiness, rest-
lessness, agitation, insomnia, *tardive dyskine-
sia,* sedation, pseudoparkinsonism, EEG changes,
dizziness.
CV: *hypotension,* tachycardia, ECG changes.
EENT: ocular changes, *blurred vision,* nasal con-
gestion.
GI: *dry mouth, constipation.*
GU: *urine retention,* menstrual irregularities,
inhibited ejaculation.
**Hematologic: *transient leukopenia, leuko-
cytosis, agranulocytosis.***
Hepatic: jaundice, elevated liver enzyme levels.
Metabolic: weight gain.
Skin: *mild photosensitivity,* allergic reactions,
pain at I.M. injection site, sterile abscess.
Other: gynecomastia.

Overdose and treatment
CNS depression is characterized by deep,
unarousable sleep and possible coma, hypotension or hypertension, extrapyramidal symptoms,
abnormal involuntary muscle movements, agitation, seizures, arrhythmias, ECG changes, hypothermia or hyperthermia, and autonomic nervous system dysfunction.

Treatment is symptomatic and supportive and
includes maintaining vital signs, airway, stable
body temperature, and fluid and electrolyte balance.

Don't induce vomiting: Drug inhibits cough
reflex, and aspiration may occur. Use gastric
lavage, then activated charcoal and sodium chloride cathartics; dialysis doesn't help. Regulate
body temperature as needed. Treat hypotension
with I.V. fluids: Don't give epinephrine. Seizures
may be treated with parenteral diazepam or barbiturates; arrhythmias with parenteral phenytoin
(1 mg/kg with rate titrated to blood pressure);
and extrapyramidal reactions with benztropine
at 1 to 2 mg or parenteral diphenhydramine at
10 to 50 mg.

Special considerations
• Drug is linked to a high risk of extrapyramidal
effects.
• Taper drug gradually. After abrupt withdrawal
of long-term therapy, patient may experience gastritis, nausea, vomiting, dizziness, tremor, feeling of warmth or cold, diaphoresis, tachycardia,
headache, and insomnia.

Reactions may be *common*, uncommon, *life-threatening*, or COMMON AND LIFE-THREATENING.

• Liquid and injectable formulations may cause a rash if skin contact occurs.

• Because stomach upset may occur, administer oral form with food or fluid.

• Dilute the concentrate in 2 to 4 oz (60 to 120 ml) of liquid, preferably water, carbonated drinks, fruit juice, tomato juice, milk, or pudding.

• Photosensitivity reactions may occur; advise patient to avoid exposure to sunlight or heat lamps.

• I.M. injection may cause skin necrosis.

• Solution for injection may be slightly discolored. Don't use if excessively discolored or if a precipitate is evident.

• Drug is stable after reconstitution for 48 hours at room temperature.

• Protect liquid formulation from light.

• Dosage adjustments may be necessary when changing from I.M. to P.O. or vice versa.

• Drug causes false-positive test results for urinary porphyrins, urobilinogen, amylase, and 5-hydroxyindoleacetic acid because of darkening of urine by metabolites; it also causes false-positive urine pregnancy results in tests using human chorionic gonadotropin as the indicator.

Patient monitoring

• Monitor blood pressure before and after parenteral administration.

• Check patient regularly for abnormal body movements (at least once every 6 months).

Pregnant patients

• Hyperreflexia has been reported in infants following in utero exposure. Use drug during pregnancy only when potential benefit justifies risk to fetus.

Pediatric patients

• Drug isn't recommended for children under age 12.

Geriatric patients

• Geriatric patients tend to require lower doses, adjusted to individual response. Adverse reactions are more likely to develop in such patients, especially tardive dyskinesia and other extrapyramidal effects.

Patient education

• Explain risks of dystonic reactions and tardive dyskinesia, and tell patient to report abnormal body movements.

• Tell patient to avoid sun exposure and to wear sunscreen when going outdoors to prevent photosensitivity reactions. Remind him that heat lamps and tanning beds also may cause burning of the skin or skin discoloration.

• Instruct patient not to spill the liquid on skin. Contact with skin may cause rash and irritation.

• Tell patient to take drug exactly as prescribed, not to double missed doses, and not to share drug with others.

• Explain that many drug interactions are possible. Patient should seek medical approval before taking any OTC or herbal medication.

• Tell patient not to stop taking drug suddenly; most adverse reactions may be relieved by reducing the dose. However, patient should report difficulty urinating, sore throat, dizziness, or fainting.

• Warn patient against hazardous activities that require alertness until effect of drug is established. Reassure patient that sedation usually subsides after several weeks.

• Tell patient not to drink alcohol or take other medications that may cause excessive sedation.

• Explain which fluids are appropriate for diluting the concentrate and the dropper technique of measuring dose.

• Tell patient to shake concentrate before administration.

• Instruct patient to store drug away from children.

thyroid, desiccated
Armour Thyroid

Pharmacologic classification: thyroid hormone
Therapeutic classification: thyroid
Pregnancy risk category: A

Indications and dosages

➤ *Adult hypothyroidism. Adults:* Initially, 30 mg P.O. daily, increased by 15 mg q 14 to 30 days depending on disease severity until desired response is achieved. Usual maintenance dosage is 60 to 180 mg P.O. daily as a single dose.

➤ *Congenital hypothyroidism. Children over age 12:* Dosage may approach adult dose (60 to 180 mg daily), depending on response.
Children ages 6 to 12: 60 to 90 mg P.O. daily.
Children ages 1 to 5: 45 to 60 mg P.O. daily.
Infants ages 6 to 12 months: 30 to 45 mg P.O. daily.
Neonates and infants up to age 6 months: 15 to 30 mg P.O. daily.

How supplied

Available by prescription only
Tablets: 15 mg, 30 mg, 60 mg, 90 mg, 120 mg, 180 mg, 240 mg, 300 mg

Pharmacodynamics

Thyrotropic action: Affects protein and carbohydrate metabolism, promotes gluconeogenesis, increases the utilization and mobilization of glycogen stores, stimulates protein synthesis, and regulates cell growth and differentiation. The major effect of thyroid is to increase the metabolic rate of tissue.

Pharmacokinetics

Absorption: Thyroid USP absorbed from GI tract.

Distribution: Not fully understood. Highly protein-bound.
Metabolism: Not fully understood.
Excretion: Not fully understood.

Route	Onset	Peak	Duration
P.O.	Unknown	Unknown	Unknown

Contraindications and precautions
Contraindicated in patients hypersensitive to drug and in those with acute MI uncomplicated by hypothyroidism, untreated thyrotoxicosis, or uncorrected adrenal insufficiency. Use cautiously in elderly patients and in patients with angina pectoris, hypertension, other CV disorders, renal insufficiency, or ischemia.

Interactions
Drug-drug. *Adrenocorticoids, corticotropin:* Changes in thyroid status. Dosage adjustments may be needed.
Anticoagulants: Altered anticoagulant effect. Reduced anticoagulant dosage may be needed.
Cholestyramine, colestipol: Decreased absorption. Monitor patient closely; adjust dosage.
Estrogens: Increased thyroid requirements. Adjust dosage.
Insulin, oral antidiabetics: May affect dosage requirements of these drugs. Monitor glucose levels; adjust dosage as needed.
I.V. phenytoin: May release free thyroid from thyroglobulin. Monitor patient closely; adjust dosage.
Somatrem: Accelerated epiphyseal maturation. Use together cautiously.
Sympathomimetics, tricyclic antidepressants: Increased effects of these drugs or of thyroid (desiccated); possible coronary insufficiency or cardiac arrhythmias. Monitor patient closely; adjust dosage.

Adverse reactions
CNS: *nervousness, insomnia,* tremor, headache.
CV: tachycardia, **arrhythmias, cardiac decompensation and collapse,** angina pectoris.
GI: diarrhea, vomiting.
GU: menstrual irregularities.
Metabolic: weight loss, heat intolerance.
Musculoskeletal: accelerated bone maturation in infants and children.
Skin: allergic skin reactions, diaphoresis.

Overdose and treatment
Evidence of overdose includes signs and symptoms of hyperthyroidism (weight loss, increased appetite, palpitations, nervousness, diarrhea, abdominal cramps, sweating, tachycardia, increased pulse rate and blood pressure, angina, arrhythmias, tremor, headache, insomnia, heat intolerance, fever, and menstrual irregularities).

Treatment of acute overdose requires reduction of GI absorption and efforts to counteract central and peripheral effects, primarily sympathetic activity. Use gastric lavage or induce eme-

sis (then activated charcoal, if less than 4 hours after ingestion). If patient is comatose or is having seizures, inflate cuff on endotracheal tube to prevent aspiration.

Treatment of overdose may include oxygen and artificial ventilation to support respiration along with measures to treat heart failure and control fever, hypoglycemia, and fluid loss.

Propranolol may be used to combat many of the effects of increased sympathetic activity. Thyroid USP therapy should be withdrawn gradually over 2 to 6 days, then resumed at a lower dose.

Special considerations
Consider the recommendations relevant to all thyroid hormones as well as the following.
● Levothyroxine is considered the drug of choice for thyroid hormone supplementation.
● Commercial preparations may have variable hormonal content and produce fluctuating liothyronine and levothyroxine levels. Because of this variability, the use of thyroid has decreased considerably.
● Enteric-coated tablets give unreliable absorption.
● Thyroid USP therapy alters ^{131}I thyroid uptake, protein-bound iodine levels, and liothyronine uptake.

Patient monitoring
● Monitor patient's pulse rate and blood pressure. Thyroid may cause CV adverse effects.
● Digoxin levels should be monitored closely as patient becomes euthyroid.
● In children, sleeping pulse rate and basal morning temperature are guides to treatment.

Breast-feeding patients
● Minimal amounts of drug appear in breast milk. Use cautiously in breast-feeding women.

Pediatric patients
● Partial hair loss may occur during the first few months of therapy. Reassure child and parents that this is temporary.

Geriatric patients
● Elderly patients are more sensitive to thyroid effects. In patients over age 60, initial dose should be 25% lower than usual recommended dose.

Patient education
● Urge patient to take dose at same time each day, preferably in morning to avoid insomnia.
● Advise patient to report headache, diarrhea, nervousness, excessive sweating, heat intolerance, chest pain, increased pulse rate, or palpitations.
● Tell patient not to store drug in warm, humid areas such as bathroom to prevent deterioration.
● Warn patient not to switch brands or dose.

Reactions may be *common,* uncommon, ***life-threatening,*** or COMMON AND LIFE-THREATENING.

thyrotropin (thyroid stimulating hormone, TSH)
Thytropar

Pharmacologic classification: anterior pituitary hormone
Therapeutic classification: thyrotropic hormone
Pregnancy risk category: C

Indications and dosages
➤ **Diagnosis of thyroid cancer remnant with** ^{131}I **after surgery.** *Adults and children:* 10 IU I.M. or S.C. for 3 to 7 days.
➤ **Differential diagnosis of primary and secondary hypothyroidism.** *Adults and children:* 10 IU I.M. or S.C. for 1 to 3 days.
➤ **In protein-bound iodine or** ^{131}I **uptake determinations for differential diagnosis of subclinical hypothyroidism or low thyroid reserve.** *Adults and children:* 10 IU I.M. or S.C.
➤ **Therapy for thyroid carcinoma (local or metastatic) with** ^{131}I. *Adults and children:* 10 IU I.M. or S.C. for 3 to 8 days.
➤ **To determine thyroid status of patient receiving thyroid.** *Adults and children:* 10 IU I.M. or S.C. for 1 to 3 days.

How supplied
Available by prescription only
Powder for injection: 10 IU/vial

Pharmacodynamics
Thyrotropic action: Increases uptake of iodine by the thyroid, and increases formation and release of thyroid hormone.

Pharmacokinetics
Absorption: Onset occurs within minutes after injection.
Distribution: Concentrated primarily in thyroid gland.
Metabolism: Not fully understood.
Excretion: Excreted rapidly in urine.

Route	Onset	Peak	Duration
I.M.	Rapid	Unknown	Unknown

Contraindications and precautions
Contraindicated in patients hypersensitive to drug and in those with coronary thrombosis or untreated Addison's disease. Use cautiously in patients with angina pectoris, heart failure, hypopituitarism, or adrenocortical suppression.

Interactions
None reported.

Adverse reactions
CNS: headache.
CV: *tachycardia*, hypotension.
GI: nausea, vomiting.

Other: thyroid hyperplasia (with large doses), hypersensitivity reactions (postinjection flare, urticaria, ANAPHYLAXIS), fever.

Overdose and treatment
Signs and symptoms of overdose include headache, irritability, nervousness, sweating, tachycardia, increased GI motility, and menstrual irregularities. Angina or heart failure may be aggravated. Shock may develop. Treatment includes administering propranolol (or another beta blocker) to treat adrenergic effects of hyperthyroidism. Adult dosage of propranolol is 1 mg over at least 1 minute, repeated every 2 to 5 minutes (maximum dose is 5 mg). Dosage in children is 0.01 to 0.1 mg/kg over 10 minutes (maximum dose is 1 mg). Monitor blood pressure and cardiac function.
Exchange transfusions may be useful in acute overdose. Diuresis and dialysis are ineffective.

Special considerations
Besides the recommendations relevant to all thyroid hormones, consider the following.
● Thyrotropin may cause thyroid hyperplasia.
● Three-day dose schedule may be used in longstanding pituitary myxedema or with prolonged use of thyroid medication.
● Thyrotropin therapy alters ^{131}I thyroid uptake.

Patient monitoring
● Monitor therapeutic effect.
● Monitor patient for symptoms of hypersensitivity.

Patient education
● Warn patient to report itching, redness, or swelling at injection site; rash; tightness of throat or wheezing; chest pain; irritability; nervousness; rapid heartbeat; shortness of breath; or unusual sweating.

tiagabine hydrochloride
Gabitril

Pharmacologic classification: gamma aminobutyric acid (GABA) enhancer
Therapeutic classification: anticonvulsant
Pregnancy risk category: C

Indications and dosages
➤ **Adjunctive therapy in the treatment of partial seizures.** *Adults:* Initially, 4 mg P.O. once daily. May increase total daily dose by 4 to 8 mg at weekly intervals until clinical response occurs or up to maximum of 56 mg daily. Give total daily dose in divided doses b.i.d. to q.i.d.
Adolescents ages 12 to 18: Initially, 4 mg P.O. once daily. May increase total daily dose by 4 at mg beginning of week 2 and thereafter by 4 to 8 mg at weekly intervals until clinical response

is seen or up to maximum of 32 mg daily. Give total daily dose in divided doses b.i.d. to q.i.d.
✦ *Dosage adjustment.* In patients with impaired liver function, initial and maintenance dosages may be reduced or dosing intervals increased.

How supplied
Available by prescription only
Tablets: 2 mg, 4 mg, 12 mg, 16 mg, 20 mg

Pharmacodynamics
Anticonvulsant action: Exact mechanism unknown. Tiagabine is thought to act by enhancing the activity of GABA, the major inhibitory neurotransmitter in the CNS. It binds to recognition sites related to the GABA uptake carrier and may thus permit more GABA to be available for binding to receptors on postsynaptic cells.

Pharmacokinetics
Absorption: Rapidly and nearly completely absorbed (more than 95%). Absolute bioavailability is about 90%.
Distribution: About 96% is bound to human plasma proteins, mainly to serum albumin and alpha-1 acid glycoprotein.
Metabolism: Likely to be metabolized by the cytochrome P-450 3A isoenzymes.
Excretion: About 2% is excreted unchanged, with 25% and 63% of dose excreted into urine and feces, respectively. Half-life is about 7 to 9 hours.

Route	Onset	Peak	Duration
P.O.	Rapid	45 min	7-9 hr

Contraindications and precautions
Contraindicated in patients hypersensitive to drug or its ingredients. Use cautiously in breast-feeding women.

Interactions
Drug-drug. *Carbamazepine, phenobarbital, phenytoin:* Increased tiagabine clearance. Monitor patient closely.
CNS depressants: Enhanced CNS effects. Use cautiously.
Valproate: Decreased valproate level. Monitor patient closely.
Drug-lifestyle. *Alcohol use:* Enhanced CNS effects. Advise patient to avoid alcohol.

Adverse reactions
CNS: *dizziness, asthenia, somnolence, nervousness,* tremor, difficulty with concentration and attention, insomnia, ataxia, confusion, speech disorder, difficulty with memory, paresthesia, depression, emotional lability, abnormal gait, hostility, language problems, agitation.
CV: vasodilation.
EENT: amblyopia, nystagmus, pharyngitis.
GI: abdominal pain, *nausea,* diarrhea, vomiting, increased appetite, mouth ulceration.

GU: urinary tract infection.
Musculoskeletal: myalgia, myasthenia.
Respiratory: increased cough.
Skin: rash, pruritus.
Other: flu syndrome.

Overdose and treatment
Common symptoms reported after an overdose include somnolence, impaired consciousness, impaired speech, agitation, confusion, speech difficulty, hostility, depression, weakness, and myoclonus. There's no specific antidote for tiagabine. If indicated, elimination of unabsorbed drug should be achieved by emesis or gastric lavage. Observe usual precautions to maintain the airway, and provide general supportive care.

Special considerations
• A therapeutic range for plasma drug levels hasn't been established.
⚠ ALERT Status epilepticus and sudden unexpected death in epilepsy have occurred in patients receiving tiagabine. Patients who aren't receiving at least one other enzyme-inducing antiepilepsy drug at the time of tiagabine initiation may require lower doses or a slower dose adjustment.
• Never withdraw drug suddenly because seizure frequency may increase. Withdraw tiagabine gradually unless safety concerns require a more rapid withdrawal.

Patient monitoring
• Because of the potential for pharmacokinetic interactions between tiagabine and drugs that induce or inhibit hepatic metabolizing enzymes, obtain plasma levels of tiagabine before and after changes are made in the therapeutic regimen.

Pregnant patients
• Drug shouldn't be used during pregnancy unless potential benefit justifies potential risk.

Breast-feeding patients
• Tiagabine and its metabolites appear in breast milk. Use in breast-feeding women only if the benefits clearly outweigh the risks.

Pediatric patients
• Drug hasn't been investigated in adequate and well-controlled trials in patients under age 12.

Geriatric patients
• Because few patients over age 65 were exposed to tiagabine hydrochloride during its clinical evaluation, safety or efficacy in this age-group isn't clear.

Patient education
• Advise patient to take drug only as prescribed and to take tiagabine with food.
• Warn patient that drug may cause dizziness, somnolence, and other symptoms and signs of CNS depression.

Reactions may be *common,* uncommon, ***life-threatening***, or COMMON AND LIFE-THREATENING.

• Advise patient to avoid driving and other potentially hazardous activities that require mental alertness until CNS effects of drug are known.

ticarcillin disodium
Ticar

Pharmacologic classification: extended-spectrum penicillin, alpha-carboxypenicillin
Therapeutic classification: antibiotic
Pregnancy risk category: B

Indications and dosages

➤ *Serious infections caused by susceptible organisms.* *Adults:* 200 to 300 mg/kg I.V. daily, divided into doses given q 4 or 6 hours.
Infants and children older than 1 month who weigh less than 40 kg (88 lb): 200 to 300 mg/kg I.V. daily, divided into doses given q 4 to 6 hours.
Neonates who weigh more than 2 kg (4.4 lb): 225 to 300 mg/kg daily, divided into doses given q 8 hours.
Neonates who weigh less than 2 kg: 150 to 225 mg/kg daily, divided into doses given q 8 to 12 hours. Give prescribed dose I.M. or via I.V. infusion over 10 to 20 minutes.
➤ *Urinary tract infection.* *Adults:* For complicated infection, give 150 to 200 mg/kg I.V. daily, divided into doses q 4 to 6 hours. For uncomplicated infection, give 1 g I.V. or I.M. q 6 hours.
Infants and children older than 1 month who weigh less than 40 kg: For complicated infection, give 150 to 200 mg/kg daily by I.V. infusion divided into doses given every 4 to 6 hours. For uncomplicated infection, give 50 to 100 mg/kg daily I.M. or direct I.V. divided into doses given every 6 to 8 hours.
✦ *Dosage adjustment.* For patient with renal impairment, give initial loading dose of 3 g I.V. Then if patient receives hemodialysis, give 2 g I.V. q 12 hours and 3 g I.V. after each treatment. If he receives peritoneal dialysis, give 3 g I.V. q 12 hours. If he doesn't receive dialysis, give subsequent doses based on the table.

Creatinine clearance (ml/min)	Dosage in adults
30-60	2 g I.V. q 4 hours
10-30	2 g I.V. q 8 hours
< 10	2 g I.V. q 12 hours or 1 g I.M. q 6 hours
< 10 with hepatic failure	2 g I.V. q 24 hours or 1 g I.M. q 12 hours

How supplied
Available by prescription only
Injection: 1 g, 3 g, 6 g
I.V. infusion: 3 g

Pharmacodynamics
Antibiotic action: Bactericidal. Adheres to bacterial penicillin-binding proteins, thus inhibiting bacterial cell-wall synthesis. Extended-spectrum penicillins are more resistant to inactivation by certain beta-lactamases, especially those produced by gram-negative organisms, but are still susceptible to inactivation by certain others.

Spectrum of activity includes many gram-negative aerobic and anaerobic bacilli, many gram-positive and gram-negative aerobic cocci, and some gram-positive aerobic and anaerobic bacilli. Drug may be effective against some strains of carbenicillin-resistant gram-negative bacilli.

In many cases, ticarcillin is more active (by weight) against *Pseudomonas aeruginosa* than is carbenicillin. Its primary use is in combination with an aminoglycoside to treat *P. aeruginosa* infections.

When ticarcillin is used alone, resistance develops rapidly. It's almost always used with other antibiotics (such as aminoglycosides).

Pharmacokinetics
Absorption: Plasma levels peak 30 to 75 minutes after I.M. dose. About 86% of dose is absorbed.
Distribution: Distributed widely. Minimal CSF penetration with uninflamed meninges. Crosses placenta. 45% to 65% protein-bound.
Metabolism: About 13% of dose is metabolized by hydrolysis to inactive compounds.
Excretion: 80% to 93% excreted in urine by renal tubular secretion and glomerular filtration; also excreted in bile and breast milk. Elimination half-life in adults is about 1 hour; in patients with severe renal impairment, half-life is extended to about 3 hours. Removed by hemodialysis but not by peritoneal dialysis.

Route	Onset	Peak	Duration
I.V.	Immediate	Immediate	Unknown
I.M.	Unknown	30-75 min	Unknown

Contraindications and precautions
Contraindicated in patients hypersensitive to drug or other penicillins. Use cautiously in patients with other drug allergies, especially to cephalosporins, and in those with impaired renal function, hemorrhagic conditions, hypokalemia, and sodium restrictions.

Interactions
Drug-drug. *Aminoglycoside antibiotics:* Synergistic bactericidal effects against *P. aeruginosa*, *Escherichia coli*, *Klebsiella*, *Citrobacter*, *Enterobacter*, *Serratia*, and *Proteus mirabilis*. However, drugs are physically and chemically incompatible and inactivated when mixed or given together. Don't administer concomitantly. Adjust dosage for therapeutic response.
Clavulanic acid: Synergistic bactericidal effect against certain beta-lactamase-producing bacteria. Adjust dosage for therapeutic response.

Methotrexate: Elevated serum levels of methotrexate. Adjust dosage.
Probenecid: Increased serum levels of ticarcillin. Adjust dosage.

Adverse reactions
CNS: *seizures,* neuromuscular excitability.
GI: nausea, diarrhea, vomiting, pseudomembranous colitis.
Hematologic: leukopenia, eosinophilia, *neutropenia, thrombocytopenia,* hemolytic anemia, positive Coombs' test, prolonged PT and INR.
Hepatic: elevated liver enzyme levels.
Metabolic: hypokalemia, hypernatremia.
Other: hypersensitivity reactions (rash, pruritus, urticaria, chills, fever, edema, *anaphylaxis*), overgrowth of nonsusceptible organisms, pain at injection site, vein irritation, phlebitis.

Overdose and treatment
Signs and symptoms of overdose include neuromuscular hypersensitivity or seizures resulting from CNS irritation by high drug levels. Drug can be removed by hemodialysis.

Special considerations
Besides the recommendations relevant to all penicillins, consider the following.
• Ticarcillin is almost always used with another antibiotic such as an aminoglycoside in life-threatening infections.
• Ticarcillin contains 5.2 mEq of sodium per gram of drug. Use cautiously in patients with sodium restriction.
• Because drug is dialyzable, patients undergoing hemodialysis may need dosage adjustments.
• Ticarcillin alters tests for urinary or serum proteins; it interferes with turbidimetric methods that use sulfosalicylic acid, trichloroacetic acid, acetic acid, or nitric acid. Ticarcillin doesn't interfere with tests using bromophenol blue (Albustix, Albutest, Multistix).
• Drug may falsely decrease serum aminoglycoside levels.

Patient monitoring
• Monitor serum electrolyte levels to prevent hypokalemia and hypernatremia.
• Monitor neurologic status. High levels of drug may cause seizures.
• Check CBC, differential, PT, and PTT. Drug may cause thrombocytopenia. Watch for signs of bleeding.

Breast-feeding patients
• Drug appears in breast milk; use cautiously in breast-feeding women.

Pediatric patients
• Ticarcillin reconstituted for I.M. use with bacteriostatic water for injection containing benzyl alcohol shouldn't be used in neonates because

of potential for toxicity. Children weighing more than 40 kg (88 lb) should receive adult dose.

Geriatric patients
• Half-life may be prolonged in elderly patients because of impaired renal function.

Patient education
• Warn patient about potential adverse reactions.
• Advise patient of need for monitoring.

---

ticarcillin disodium/ clavulanate potassium
Timentin

Pharmacologic classification: extended-spectrum penicillin, beta-lactamase inhibitor
Therapeutic classification: antibiotic
Pregnancy risk category: B

Indications and dosages
➤ *Infections of the lower respiratory tract, urinary tract, bones and joints, and skin and skin structure; intra-abdominal infections; septicemia when caused by susceptible organisms. Adults:* 3.1 g (contains 3 g ticarcillin and 0.1 g clavulanate potassium) diluted in 50 to 100 ml D₅W, saline solution, or lactated Ringer's injection and administered by I.V. infusion over 30 minutes q 4 to 6 hours.
Children ages 3 months to 16 years who weigh less than 60 kg (132 lb): For mild to moderate infections, 200 mg/kg daily (contains 3 g ticarcillin and 0.1 g clavulanate potassium) I.V. infusion given in divided doses q 6 hours. For severe infections, 300 mg/kg daily (contains 3 g ticarcillin and 0.1 g clavulanate potassium) I.V. given in divided doses q 4 hours.
➤ *Gynecologic infections. Adults who weigh 60 kg or more:* 200 mg/kg daily in divided doses q 6 hours. For more severe infections, 300 mg/kg daily in divided doses q 4 hours.
✦ *Dosage adjustment.* In patients with renal failure, loading dose is 3.1 g (3 g ticarcillin with 100 mg clavulanate).

Creatinine clearance (ml/min)	Dosage in adults
30-60	2 g I.V. q 4 hours
10-30	2 g I.V. q 8 hours
< 10	2 g I.V. q 12 hours
< 10 with hepatic failure	2 g I.V. q 24 hours

How supplied
Available by prescription only
Injection: 3 g ticarcillin and 100 mg clavulanic acid

Pharmacodynamics
Antibiotic action: Ticarcillin is bactericidal; it adheres to bacterial penicillin-binding proteins, inhibiting bacterial cell wall synthesis. Extended-spectrum penicillins are more resistant to inactivation by certain beta-lactamases, especially those produced by gram-negative organisms, but are still susceptible to inactivation by certain others.

Clavulanic acid has only weak antibacterial activity and doesn't affect the action of ticarcillin. However, clavulanic acid has a beta-lactam ring and is structurally similar to penicillin and cephalosporins; it binds irreversibly with certain beta-lactamases, preventing inactivation of ticarcillin and broadening its bactericidal spectrum.

Spectrum of activity of ticarcillin includes many gram-negative aerobic and anaerobic bacilli, many gram-positive and gram-negative aerobic cocci, and some gram-positive aerobic and anaerobic bacilli. The combination of ticarcillin and clavulanate potassium is also effective against many beta-lactamase-producing strains, including *Staphylococcus aureus, Haemophilus influenzae, Neisseria gonorrhoeae, Escherichia coli, Klebsiella, Providencia,* and *Bacteroides fragilis,* but not *Pseudomonas aeruginosa.*

Pharmacokinetics
Absorption: Administered I.V.
Distribution: Distributed widely. It penetrates minimally into CSF with uninflamed meninges; clavulanic acid penetrates into pleural fluid, lungs, and peritoneal fluid. Ticarcillin sodium achieves high levels in urine. Protein-binding is 45% to 65% for ticarcillin and 22% to 30% for clavulanic acid; both cross the placenta.
Metabolism: About 13% of a ticarcillin dose is metabolized by hydrolysis to inactive compounds; clavulanic acid is thought to undergo extensive metabolism, but its fate is as yet unknown.
Excretion: Ticarcillin is excreted primarily (83% to 90%) in urine by renal tubular secretion and glomerular filtration; it's also excreted in bile and in breast milk. Metabolites of clavulanate are excreted in urine by glomerular filtration and in breast milk. Elimination half-life of ticarcillin in adults is about 1 hour and that of clavulanate is about 1 hour; in severe renal impairment, half-life of ticarcillin is extended to about 8 hours and that of clavulanate to about 3 hours. Both drugs are removed by hemodialysis but only slightly by peritoneal dialysis.

Route	Onset	Peak	Duration
I.V.	Unknown	Immediate	Unknown

Contraindications and precautions
Contraindicated in patients hypersensitive to drug or other penicillins. Use cautiously in patients with other drug allergies, especially to cephalosporins, impaired renal function, hemorrhagic conditions, hypokalemia, or sodium restrictions.

Interactions
Drug-drug. *Aminoglycoside antibiotics:* Chemically incompatible. Don't mix in the same I.V. container.
Oral contraceptives: Decreased efficacy of contraceptive. Advise patient to use another contraceptive method.
Probenecid: Elevated serum ticarcillin level. Monitor patient carefully.

Adverse reactions
CNS: *seizures,* neuromuscular excitability, headache, giddiness.
GI: nausea, diarrhea, stomatitis, vomiting, epigastric pain, flatulence, pseudomembranous colitis, taste and smell disturbances.
Hematologic: *leukopenia, neutropenia,* eosinophilia, *thrombocytopenia,* hemolytic anemia, anemia, positive Coombs' test, prolonged PT and INR.
Hepatic: elevated liver enzyme levels.
Metabolic: hypokalemia, hypernatremia.
Other: hypersensitivity reactions (rash, pruritus, urticaria, chills, fever, edema, *anaphylaxis*), overgrowth of nonsusceptible organisms, pain at injection site, vein irritation, phlebitis.

Overdose and treatment
Overdose may cause neuromuscular hypersensitivity and seizures; ticarcillin and clavulanate potassium can be removed by hemodialysis.

Special considerations
Consider the recommendations relevant to all penicillins as well as the following.
● Ticarcillin disodium/clavulanate potassium is almost always used with another antibiotic such as an aminoglycoside in life-threatening situations.
● Administer aminoglycosides 1 hour before or after administration of ticarcillin disodium/clavulanate potassium.
● Ticarcillin contains 5.2 mEq of sodium per gram of drug. Use cautiously in patients with sodium restriction.
● Because ticarcillin disodium/clavulanate potassium is dializable, patients undergoing hemodialysis may need dosage adjustments.
● Ticarcillin disodium/clavulanate potassium alters tests for urinary or serum proteins; it interferes with turbidimetric methods that use sulfosalicylic acid, trichloroacetic acid, acetic acid, or nitric acid. Ticarcillin disodium/clavulanate potassium doesn't interfere with tests using bromophenol blue (Albustix, Albutest, MultiStix). It may falsely decrease serum aminoglycoside level.

Patient monitoring
● Monitor renal and hepatic function.
● Monitor serum electrolytes. Observe for signs of hypernatremia and hypokalemia.
● Monitor neurologic status. High blood levels may cause seizures.

◇ Unlabeled clinical use

Pregnant patients
● Use drug during pregnancy only when clearly needed.

Breast-feeding patients
● Ticarcillin and clavulanate potassium appear in breast milk; use cautiously in breast-feeding women.

Geriatric patients
● Half-life may be prolonged in geriatric patients because of impaired renal function.

Patient education
● Advise patient of adverse effects and advise limiting salt intake during drug therapy.

---

ticlopidine hydrochloride
Ticlid

Pharmacologic classification: platelet aggregation inhibitor
Therapeutic classification: antithrombotic
Pregnancy risk category: B

Indications and dosages
➤ **Reduction of risk of thrombotic CVA in patients with history of CVA, those who have experienced CVA precursors, or those who are intolerant to aspirin therapy.**
Adults: 250 mg P.O. b.i.d. with meals.

How supplied
Available by prescription only
Tablets (film-coated): 250 mg

Pharmacodynamics
Antithrombotic action: Ticlopidine blocks adenosine diphosphate–induced platelet-fibrinogen and platelet-platelet binding.

Pharmacokinetics
Absorption: Rapidly and extensively (more than 80%) absorbed after oral administration. Absorption is enhanced by food.
Distribution: 98% bound to serum proteins and lipoproteins.
Metabolism: Extensively metabolized by the liver. It's unknown whether parent drug or active metabolites are responsible for pharmacologic activity.
Excretion: About 60% is excreted in urine and 23% in feces; only trace amounts of intact drug are found in urine. After one dose, half-life is 12½ hours; with repeat dosing, half-life increases to 4 to 5 days.

Route	Onset	Peak	Duration
P.O.	Unknown	2 hr	Unknown

Contraindications and precautions
Contraindicated in patients hypersensitive to drug; in patients with hematopoietic disorders, such as neutropenia, thrombocytopenia, or disorders of hemostasis; in patients with active pathologic bleeding from peptic ulceration or active intracranial bleeding; and in patients with severe liver dysfunction.

Interactions
Drug-drug. *Antacids:* Decreased ticlopidine levels. Separate administration times by at least 2 hours.
Aspirin: Potentiated effects of aspirin on platelets. Avoid use together.
Cimetidine: Decreased ticlopidine clearance; increased toxicity risk. Don't use together.
Digoxin: Causes slightly decreased serum digoxin levels. Monitor serum digoxin levels.
Theophylline: Increased risk of theophylline toxicity. Monitor patient closely; adjust theophylline dose as needed.
Drug-herb. *Dong quai, feverfew, garlic, ginger, horse chestnut, red clover:* Increased risk of bleeding. Discourage use together.

Adverse reactions
CNS: dizziness, *intracerebral bleeding,* peripheral neuropathy.
CV: vasculitis.
EENT: epistaxis, conjunctival hemorrhage.
GI: *diarrhea, nausea, dyspepsia, abdominal pain,* anorexia, vomiting, flatulence, GI bleeding, light-colored stools.
GU: hematuria, **nephrotic syndrome,** dark-colored urine.
Hematologic: prolonged bleeding time, **neutropenia, pancytopenia, agranulocytosis, immune thrombocytopenia,** ecchymoses.
Hepatic: **hepatitis,** cholestatic jaundice, abnormal liver function test results.
Metabolic: *hyponatremia, increased serum cholesterol levels.*
Musculoskeletal: arthropathy, myositis.
Respiratory: *allergic pneumonitis.*
Skin: *rash,* pruritus, maculopapular rash, urticaria, **thrombocytopenic purpura.**
Other: *hypersensitivity reactions,* postoperative bleeding, systemic lupus erythematosus, **serum sickness.**

Overdose and treatment
Only one case of overdose has been reported. The patient, who ingested more than 6 g of drug, showed increased bleeding time and increased ALT levels. The patient recovered with supportive therapy.

Special considerations
● If drug is being substituted for a fibrinolytic or anticoagulant drug, stop previous drug before starting ticlopidine.
◗ **ALERT** Patients who receive ticlopidine may develop aplastic anemia. Development of the disorder seems to peak after about 4 to 8 weeks of

---

Reactions may be *common*, uncommon, **life-threatening**, or COMMON AND LIFE-THREATENING.

treatment; only a few of the reported cases developed after 3 months of treatment.
• If necessary, methylprednisolone 20 mg I.V. has been shown to normalize the bleeding time within 2 hours. Platelet transfusions also may be necessary.
• Drug has been used investigationally for many conditions, including intermittent claudication, chronic arterial occlusion, subarachnoid hemorrhage, primary glomerulonephritis, sickle cell disease, and uremic patients with AV shunts. When used preoperatively, it may decrease risk of graft occlusion in patients receiving coronary artery bypass grafts and reduce the severity of decreased platelet count in patients receiving extracorporeal hemoperfusion during open heart surgery.

Patient monitoring
• Perform baseline liver function tests and repeat whenever liver dysfunction is suspected. Monitor patient closely, especially during the first 4 months of treatment.
• Monitor CBC and WBC differential every 2 weeks for the first 3 months of therapy. Severe hematologic adverse events can occur with ticlopidine.
⚠ ALERT Monitor CBC—including neutrophil count, platelet count, and peripheral smear—every 2 weeks for the first 3 months of therapy. Patients with a simultaneous decrease in platelets and WBCs should be evaluated for aplastic anemia. Stop drug immediately if laboratory findings suggest aplastic anemia.

Pregnant patients
• Use drug during pregnancy only when clearly needed.

Breast-feeding patients
• It isn't known whether drug appears in breast milk. Breast-feeding isn't recommended.

Pediatric patients
• Safety and efficacy in children under age 18 haven't been established.

Patient education
• Tell patient to take drug with meals because food substantially increases bioavailability and improves GI tolerance.
• Emphasize that drug prolongs bleeding time. Tell patient to report unusual bleeding and to inform dentists and other health care providers that he's taking ticlopidine.
• Be sure patient understands the need to report for regular blood tests. Neutropenia can result in an increased risk of infection. Tell patient to immediately report signs and symptoms of infection, such as fever, chills, or sore throat.
• Warn patient to avoid aspirin and aspirin-containing products, which may prolong bleeding. Instruct him to call before taking OTC medications because many contain aspirin.

• Tell patient to report yellow skin or sclera, severe or persistent diarrhea, rash, subcutaneous bleeding, light-colored stools, or dark urine.

tiludronate disodium
Skelid

Pharmacologic classification: bisphosphonate analogue
Therapeutic classification: antihypercalcemic
Pregnancy risk category: C

Indications and dosages
➤ *Paget's disease. Adults:* 400 mg P.O. once daily taken with 6 to 8 oz (180 to 240 ml) of water for 3 months, given 2 hours before or after meals.

How supplied
Available by prescription only
Tablets: 200 mg

Pharmacodynamics
Antihypercalcemic action: Tiludronate is thought to suppress bone resorption by reducing osteoclastic activity through inhibition of the osteoclastic proton pump and through disruption of the cytoskeletal ring structure, possibly by inhibiting protein-tyrosine-phosphatase, leading to detachment of osteoclasts from the bone surface.

Pharmacokinetics
Absorption: Bioavailability of drug on an empty stomach is 8%. Food and beverages other than water can reduce bioavailability by up to 90%.
Distribution: Widely distributed in bone and soft tissue. Protein binding is about 90% (mainly albumin).
Metabolism: Probably not metabolized.
Excretion: Principally excreted in urine. Mean plasma half-life is 150 hours.

Route	Onset	Peak	Duration
P.O.	Unknown	2 hr	Unknown

Contraindications and precautions
Contraindicated in patients hypersensitive to any component of drug and in patients with creatinine clearance below 30 ml/minute. Use cautiously in patients with upper GI disease, such as dysphagia, esophagitis, esophageal ulcer, or gastric ulcer.

Interactions
Drug-drug. *Aluminum antacids, aspirin, calcium supplements, indomethacin, magnesium antacids:* Reduced bioavailability of tiludronate. Monitor patient closely and adjust dosage as needed.
Drug-food. *Any food:* Delayed drug absorption. Advise patient not to take drug within 2 hours of meals.

Beverages other than plain water: Reduced drug absorption. Tell patient to take drug with water only.

Adverse reactions
CNS: anxiety, dizziness, headache, insomnia, paresthesia, somnolence, vertigo.
CV: chest pain, hypertension.
EENT: cataracts, conjunctivitis, glaucoma, pharyngitis, sinusitis, rhinitis.
GI: anorexia, constipation, diarrhea, dry mouth, dyspepsia, flatulence, gastritis, nausea, vomiting.
Metabolic: vitamin D deficiency.
Musculoskeletal: involuntary muscle contractions, arthralgia, arthrosis, back pain.
Respiratory: bronchitis, cough, crackles.
Skin: pruritus.
Other: tooth disorder, edema, sweating, *whole body pain,* hyperparathyroidism.

Overdose and treatment
No specific information available. Use standard treatment for hypocalcemia or renal insufficiency, if they occur. Dialysis isn't beneficial.

Special considerations
• Use drug in patients with Paget's disease who have serum alkaline phosphatase level at least twice the upper limit of normal or who are symptomatic or at risk for future complications of disease.
• Administer drug for 3 months to assess response.
• Hypocalcemia and other disturbances of mineral metabolism such as vitamin D deficiency should be corrected before starting therapy.

Patient monitoring
• Monitor symptom control.
• Monitor patient for adverse reaction.

Breast-feeding patients
• It isn't known whether drug appears in breast milk. Use cautiously in breast-feeding women.

Pediatric patients
• Safety and efficacy in children haven't been established.

Geriatric patients
• Plasma levels may be increased in elderly patients. However, dose adjustment isn't necessary.

Patient education
• Instruct patient to take drug with 6 to 8 oz (180 to 240 ml) of water and not to take it within 2 hours of food or other beverages.
• Advise patient to maintain adequate vitamin D and calcium intake.
• Inform patient that calcium supplements, aspirin, and indomethacin shouldn't be taken within 2 hours before or after tiludronate.

• Tell patient that aluminum- and magnesium-containing antacids can be taken 2 hours after taking tiludronate.

timolol maleate
Blocadren, Timoptic, Timoptic-XE

Pharmacologic classification: beta blocker
Therapeutic classification: antihypertensive, adjunct in MI, antiglaucoma
Pregnancy risk category: C

Indications and dosages
➤ *Hypertension.* Adults: Initially, 10 mg P.O. b.i.d. Usual maintenance dosage is 20 to 40 mg daily. Maximum dosage is 60 mg daily. There should be an interval of at least 7 days between dose increases.
➤ *Reduction of risk of CV mortality and reinfarction after MI.* Adults: 10 mg P.O. b.i.d. started within 1 to 4 weeks after infarction.
➤ *Migraine headache.* Adults: 10 mg P.O. b.i.d.; then increase up to 20 mg. Or, 30-mg dose (10 mg P.O. in the morning and 20 mg P.O. in the evening).
➤ *Glaucoma.* Adults: 1 drop of 0.25% or 0.5% solution to the conjunctiva once or twice daily. Or, 1 drop of 0.25% or 0.5% gel to the conjunctiva once daily.
➤ *Angina ◊.* Adults: 15 to 45 mg P.O. daily given in three divided doses.

How supplied
Available by prescription only
Ophthalmic gel: 0.25%, 0.5%
Ophthalmic solution: 0.25%, 0.5%
Tablets: 5 mg, 10 mg, 20 mg

Pharmacodynamics
Antihypertensive action: Exact mechanism of antihypertensive effect of timolol is unknown. Timolol may reduce blood pressure by blocking adrenergic receptors (decreasing cardiac output), by decreasing sympathetic outflow from the CNS, and by suppressing renin release.
MI prophylactic action: Exact mechanism by which timolol decreases risk of mortality after MI is unknown. Timolol produces a negative chronotropic and inotropic activity. This decrease in heart rate and myocardial contractility results in reduced myocardial oxygen consumption.
Antiglaucoma action: Beta-blocking action of timolol decreases the production of aqueous humor, decreasing intraocular pressure.

Pharmacokinetics
Absorption: About 90% of an oral dose is absorbed from the GI tract.
Distribution: After oral administration, timolol is distributed throughout the body; depending on assay method, drug is 10% to 60% protein-bound.
Metabolism: About 80% of a given dose is metabolized in the liver to inactive metabolites.

Excretion: Drug and its metabolites are excreted primarily in urine; half-life is about 4 hours.

Route	Onset	Peak	Duration
P.O.	15-30 min	1-2 hr	6-12 hr
Oph-thalmic	30 min	1-2 hr	12-24 hr

Contraindications and precautions

Contraindicated in patients with bronchial asthma, severe COPD, sinus bradycardia and heart block greater than first degree, cardiogenic shock, heart failure, overt cardiac failure, or hypersensitivity to drug.

Use cautiously in patients with diabetes, hyperthyroidism, or respiratory disease (especially nonallergic bronchospasm or emphysema). Use oral form cautiously in patients with compensated heart failure and hepatic or renal disease. Use ophthalmic form cautiously in patients with cerebrovascular insufficiency.

Interactions

Drug-drug. *Antihypertensives, general anesthetics, fentanyl, NSAIDs:* Hypotension. Monitor patient closely.
Cardiac glycosides, diltiazem, verapamil: Excessive bradycardia and increased depressant effect on myocardium. Use together cautiously.
Indomethacin: Decreased antihypertensive effect. Monitor patient closely; dose may need adjustment.
Insulin, oral antidiabetics: Altered requirements for these drugs. Monitor glucose levels; dose may need adjustment.

Adverse reactions

CNS: fatigue, lethargy, dizziness; depression, hallucinations, confusion (with ophthalmic form).
CV: *arrhythmias, bradycardia,* hypotension, *heart failure,* peripheral vascular disease, *pulmonary edema* (with oral administration); *CVA, cardiac arrest, heart block,* palpitations (with ophthalmic form).
EENT: minor eye irritation, decreased corneal sensitivity with long-term use, conjunctivitis, blepharitis, keratitis, visual disturbances, diplopia, ptosis (with ophthalmic form).
GI: nausea, vomiting, diarrhea (with oral administration).
GU: increased BUN level.
Hematologic: decreased hemoglobin levels and hematocrit.
Metabolic: hyperkalemia, hyperuricemia, hyperglycemia.
Respiratory: dyspnea, *bronchospasm,* increased airway resistance (with oral administration); *asthmatic attacks in patients with history of asthma* (with ophthalmic form).
Skin: pruritus (with oral administration).

Overdose and treatment

Effects of overdose include severe hypotension, bradycardia, heart failure, and bronchospasm.

After acute ingestion, empty stomach by induced emesis or gastric lavage and give activated charcoal to reduce absorption. Subsequent treatment is usually symptomatic and supportive.

Special considerations

Consider the recommendations relevant to all beta blockers as well as the following.
● Dosage adjustment may be necessary for patient with renal or hepatic impairment.
● Although controversial, drug may need to be discontinued 48 hours before surgery in patients receiving ophthalmic timolol because systemic absorption occurs.
● Drug therapy may slightly increase BUN, serum potassium, uric acid, and blood glucose levels and may slightly decrease hemoglobin levels and hematocrit.

Patient monitoring

● Monitor patient for cardiac and respiratory symptoms.

Pregnant patients

● Use drug during pregnancy only when potential benefits justify possible risk to fetus.

Breast-feeding patients

● Timolol appears in breast milk. Because of the potential for serious adverse reactions in breast-fed infants, an alternative feeding method is recommended during therapy.

Pediatric patients

● Safety and efficacy in children haven't been established; use only if potential benefit outweighs risk.

Geriatric patients

● These patients may need lower oral maintenance dosages because of increased bioavailability or delayed metabolism; they also may experience enhanced adverse effects. Use cautiously because half-life may be prolonged in elderly patients.

Patient education

● For ophthalmic form of timolol, teach patient proper method of eye drop administration. Warn patient not to touch dropper to eye or surrounding tissue; lightly press lacrimal sac with finger after administration to decrease systemic absorption.
● Instruct patient to invert ophthalmic gel container once before each use.
● Instruct patient to administer other ophthalmic drugs at least 10 minutes before the ophthalmic gel.

tinzaparin sodium
Innohep

Pharmacologic classification: low molecular weight heparin
Therapeutic classification: anticoagulant
Pregnancy risk category: B

Indications and dosages
➤ *Symptomatic deep vein thrombosis with or without pulmonary embolism with warfarin sodium.* Adults: 175 anti-Xa IU/kg of body weight S.C. once daily for at least 6 days and until adequate anticoagulation occurs with warfarin sodium (INR of at least 2) for 2 consecutive days. Start warfarin sodium therapy when appropriate, usually within 1 to 3 days of tinzaparin initiation. Volume of dose to be given may be calculated as follows:
Patient weight in kg ? 0.00875 ml/kg = volume to be administered in ml.
✦ *Dosage adjustment.* Use cautiously in elderly patients and patients with renal insufficiency.

How supplied
Available by prescription only
Injection: 20,000 anti-Xa IU/ml, in 2-ml vials

Pharmacodynamics
Tinzaparin sodium is a low molecular weight heparin that inhibits reactions that lead to the clotting of blood, including the formation of fibrin clots. It also acts as a potent co-inhibitor of several activated coagulation factors, especially factors Xa and IIa (thrombin). The primary inhibitory activity is actviated by binding with the plasma protease inhibitor, antithrombin. Its binding with antithrombin causes an increased ability to inactivate coagulation enzymes factor Xa and thrombin. Tinzaparin sodium also induces release of tissue factor pathway inhibitor, which may contribute to the antithrombotic effect.

Pharmacokinetics
Absorption: Plasma levels peak in 4 to 5 hours.
Distribution: The volume of distribution of tinzaparin sodium is similar to that of blood volume, which suggests that distribution is limited to the central compartment.
Metabolism: Tinzaparin sodium is partially metabolized by desulphation and depolymerization, similar to that seen by other low molecular weight heparins.
Excretion: The primary route of elimination is renal. The elimination half-life is about 3 to 4 hours.

Route	Onset	Peak	Duration
S.C.	2-3 hr	4-5 hr	18-24 hr

Contraindications and precautions
Contraindicated in patients hypersensitive to tinzaparin sodium, heparin, sulfites, benzyl alcohol, or pork products. Also contraindicated in patients with active major bleeding or patients with or a known history of heparin-induced thrombocytopenia.

Use cautiously in patients with increased risk of hemorrhage, such as those with bacterial endocarditis, uncontrolled hypertension, diabetic retinopathy, congenital or acquired bleeding disorders such as hepatic failure and amyloidosis, GI ulceration, or hemorrhagic CVA. Also use cautiously in patients who have recently undergone brain, spinal, or ophthalmological surgery, or in patients being treated with platelet inhibitors. Use cautiously in the elderly and in patients with renal insufficiency.

Interactions
Drug-drug. *Oral anticoagulants, platelet inhibitors (such as dextran, dipyridamole, NSAIDs, salicylates, sulfinpyrazone), thrombolytics:* May increase risk of bleeding. Use together cautiously. If drugs must be given together, monitor patient.

Adverse reactions
CNS: headache, dizziness, insomnia, confusion, *cerebral or intracranial bleeding.*
CV: *arrhythmias,* chest pain, hypotension, hypertension, *MI, thromboembolism,* tachycardia, dependent edema, angina pectoris.
EENT: epistaxis, ocular hemorrhage.
GI: anorectal bleeding, constipation, flatulence, hematemesis, hemarthrosis, *GI hemorrhage,* melena, nausea, vomiting, dyspepsia, retroperitoneal or intra-abdominal bleeding.
GU: dysuria, hematuria, urinary tract infection, urine retention, vaginal hemorrhage.
Hematologic: granulocytopenia, *thrombocytopenia,* anemia, *agranulocytosis, pancytopenia, hemorrhage.*
Hepatic: elevated AST and ALT levels.
Musculoskeletal: back pain.
Respiratory: pneumonia, respiratory disorder, *pulmonary embolism,* dyspnea.
Skin: bullous eruption, cellulitis, *injection site hematoma,* pruritus, purpura, rash, skin necrosis, wound hematoma, bullous eruption.
Other: *hypersensitivity reaction, spinal or epidural hematoma,* fever, pain, infection, impaired healing, allergic reaction, congenital anomaly, fetal death, fetal distress.

Overdose and treatment
Overdose of tinzaparin sodium may lead to bleeding complications. The first signs of bleeding may be nosebleeds, hematuria, or tarry stools. Easy bruising or petechial hemorrhages may precede frank bleeding.

In the case of minor bleeding, discontinue tinzaparin sodium; apply pressure to the site and monitor patient for signs of more severe bleeding. In the case of serious bleeding or large overdoses, replace volume and hemostatic blood elements (e.g., red blood cells, fresh frozen plasma,

---

Reactions may be *common*, uncommon, *life-threatening*, or COMMON AND LIFE-THREATENING.

platelets) as required. If replacement is ineffective, protamine sulfate can be administered.

Special considerations
• Tinzaparin sodium isn't intended for intramuscular or intravenous administration, nor should it be mixed with other injections or infusions.
• Tinzaparin sodium shouldn't be interchanged (unit to unit) with heparin or other low molecular weight heparins.
• When administering tinzaparin sodium, the patient should be lying or sitting down. Administer by deep S.C. injection into the abdominal wall. Introduce the whole length of the needle into skin fold held between thumb and forefinger. Make sure to hold skin fold throughout injection. Rotate injection sites between the right and left anterolateral and posterolateral abdominal wall. To minimize bruising, don't rub the injection site after administration.
• Use an appropriate calibrated syringe to assure correct withdrawal of the volume of drug from tinzaparin sodium vials.
• Drug contains sodium metabisulfite, which may cause allergic reactions.
🔋 **ALERT** When neuraxial anesthesia (epidural/spinal anesthesia) or spinal puncture is employed, the patient is at risk for developing spinal hematoma, which can result in long-term or permanent paralysis. Monitor patient for signs and symptoms of neurological impairment. Consideration should be given to the risk versus benefit of neuraxial intervention in patients receiving anticoagulation therapy with low molecular weight heparins or heparinoids.
• If a patient becomes pregnant while taking tinzaparin sodium, she should be notified of the potential hazards to the fetus. Cases of "gasping syndrome" have occurred in premature infants when large amounts of benzyl alcohol have been administered.
• Store tinzaparin sodium at room temperature.

Patient monitoring
• Monitor platelet count during therapy. Discontinue drug if platelet count falls below 100,000/mm³.
• Periodically monitor CBC and stool tests for occult blood during treatment.
• Drug may affect PT and INR levels. Patients also receiving warfarin should have blood for PT and INR drawn just before the next scheduled dose of tinzaparin.

Breast-feeding patients
• It isn't known whether tinzaparin sodium appears in breast milk; use caution when giving tinzaparin sodium to breast-feeding women.

Pediatric patients
• Safety and efficacy in children haven't been established.

Geriatric patients
• Elderly patients and patients with renal insufficiency may show reduced elimination of tinzaparin sodium. Use drug cautiously in these patients.

Patient education
• Explain to patient importance of laboratory monitoring to ensure effectiveness of drugs while maintaining safety.
• Teach patient warning signs of bleeding and instruct him to report these signs immediately.
• Caution patient to take such safety measures as using a soft toothbrush and an electric razor to prevent cuts and bruises.
• Instruct patient that warfarin therapy will be started when appropriate, within 1 to 3 days of tinzaparin administration. Explain importance of warfarin therapy and monitoring to ensure safety and efficacy.

tioconazole
Monistat 1, Vagistat-1

Pharmacologic classification: imidazole derivative
Therapeutic classification: antifungal
Pregnancy risk category: C

Indications and dosages
➤ **Vulvovaginal candidiasis.** *Adults:* Insert 1 full applicator (about 4.6 g) intravaginally h.s. as a single dose.

How supplied
Available without a prescription
Vaginal ointment: 6.5%

Pharmacodynamics
Antifungal action: Tioconazole is a fungicidal imidazole that alters cell wall permeability.

Pharmacokinetics
Absorption: Small amounts are absorbed systemically when administered intravaginally.
Distribution: Generally persists in vaginal fluid for 24 to 72 hours.
Metabolism: No information available.
Excretion: The portion of drug absorbed is excreted in the urine as metabolites and 59% is excreted in the feces.

Route	Onset	Peak	Duration
Intra-vaginal	Unknown	2-24 hr	2-3 days

Contraindications and precautions
Contraindicated in patients hypersensitive to drug or other imidazole antifungals (miconazole, ketoconazole) and in breast-feeding women.

Interactions
None reported.

Adverse reactions
GU: *burning, pruritus,* vaginal discharge, vaginal pain, dysuria, dyspareunia, vulvar edema, irritation.

Overdose and treatment
Not reported.

Special considerations
● Because drug is useful only for candidal vulvovaginitis, the diagnosis should be confirmed by potassium hydroxide smears or cultures before treatment with tioconazole.

Patient monitoring
● Monitor patient for relief of symptoms.
● Monitor patient for adverse reactions.

Pregnant patients
● Limit course of treatment to 7 days during pregnancy.

Breast-feeding patients
● Instruct patient to temporarily stop breast-feeding during therapy.

Pediatric patients
● Safety and efficacy haven't been established.
● Tioconazole shouldn't be given to girls younger than 12 years old.

Patient education
● Review correct use of drug with patient.
● Tell patient to avoid sexual intercourse during therapy or advise partner to use a condom to prevent reinfection.
● Tell patient to promptly report irritation or symptoms of sensitivity.
● Emphasize need for patient to continue therapy for the full course, even if symptoms have improved, and during menstrual period.

tirofiban hydrochloride
Aggrastat

Pharmacologic classification: GP IIb/IIIa receptor antagonist
Therapeutic classification: Platelet aggregation inhibitor
Pregnancy risk category: B

Indications and dosages
➤ *Treatment of acute coronary syndrome, with heparin, including patients who are to be managed medically and those undergoing percutaneous transluminal coronary angioplasty (PTCA) or atherectomy.* Adults: I.V. loading dose of 0.4 mcg/kg/minute for 30 minutes followed by a continuous I.V. infusion of 0.1 mcg/kg/minute. Continue infusion through angiography and for 12 to 24 hours after angioplasty or atherectomy.

✦ *Dosage adjustment.* In patients with renal insufficiency (creatinine clearance of less than 30 ml/minute), use a loading dose of 0.2 mcg/kg/minute for 30 minutes, followed by a continuous infusion of 0.05 mcg/kg/minute. Continue infusion through angiography and for 12 to 24 hours after angioplasty or atherectomy.

How supplied
Available by prescription only
Injection: 50-ml vials (250 mcg/ml), 500-ml premixed vials (50 mcg/ml)

Pharmacodynamics
Platelet-inhibiting action: Drug is a reversible antagonist of fibrinogen binding to the GP IIb/IIIa receptor on platelets, producing a dose-dependent inhibition of platelet aggregation.

Pharmacokinetics
Absorption: Administered I.V.
Distribution: 65% protein bound. Volume of distribution ranges from 22 to 42 liters.
Metabolism: Metabolism is limited. Half-life is about 2 hours
Excretion: Renal clearance accounts for 39% to 69% of elimination; feces accounts for 25%.

Route	Onset	Peak	Duration
I.V.	Immediate	Immediate	4-8 hr after end of infusion

Contraindications and precautions
Contraindicated in patients hypersensitive to drug or its components; in patients receiving another parenteral GP IIb/IIIa inhibitor; in patients with active internal bleeding, a history of bleeding diathesis within the previous 30 days, or history of intracranial hemorrhage; in patients with intracranial neoplasm, arteriovenous malformation, or aneurysm; in patients with thrombocytopenia following exposure to drug; in patients who had a CVA within 30 days or a history of hemorrhagic CVA; in patients with symptoms or findings suggestive of aortic dissection; and in patients with severe hypertension (systolic blood pressure over 180 mm Hg or diastolic blood pressure over 110 mm Hg), acute pericarditis, or a major surgical procedure or severe physical trauma within previous month. Use cautiously in patients with platelet count below 150,000 mm^3 and patients with hemorrhagic retinopathy.

Interactions
Drug-drug. Anticoagulants such as *clopidogrel, dipyridamole, NSAIDs, thrombolytics, ticlopidine, warfarin:* Increased risk of bleeding. Monitor patient closely.
Levothyroxine, omeprazole: Increased renal clearance of tirofiban. Monitor patient carefully.
Drug-herb. *Dong quai, feverfew, garlic, ginger, horse chestnut, red clover:* Increased risk of bleeding. Discourage use together.

Adverse reactions

CNS: dizziness, fever, headache.
CV: *bradycardia, coronary artery dissection,* edema, vasovagal reaction.
GI: nausea, *occult bleeding.*
GU: pelvic pain.
Hematologic: *bleeding, thrombocytopenia,* decreased hemoglobin and hematocrit.
Musculoskeletal: leg pain.
Skin: sweating.
Other: bleeding at arterial access site.

Overdose and treatment

Overdose may be expected to produce bleeding. Treat overdose by assessing patient's clinical condition and by stopping or adjusting infusion. Drug is removed by dialysis.

Special considerations

• Don't infuse at levels greater than 50 mcg/ml.
• Minimize use of arterial and venous punctures, I.M. injections, urinary catheters, nasotracheal intubation, and nasogastric tubes. Avoid noncompressible I.V. access sites, such as subclavian or jugular veins.
⚠ ALERT Don't confuse Aggrastat (tirofiban) with Acova (agatroban).

Patient monitoring

• Drug is linked to increases in bleeding, particularly at the site of arterial access for femoral sheath placement. Before pulling the sheath, discontinue heparin for 3 to 4 hours and document activated clotting time of less than 180 seconds or aPTT of less than 45 seconds. Sheath hemostasis should be achieved at least 4 hours before hospital discharge.
• Monitor hemoglobin, hematocrit, and platelet counts before starting therapy, 6 hours following loading dose, and at least daily during therapy.

Pregnant patients

• Use drug during pregnancy only if expected benefit to mother justifies potential risk to fetus.

Breast-feeding patients

• It isn't known whether drug appears in breast milk. Depending on the importance of the drug to the woman, either breast-feeding or the drug should be discontinued.

Pediatric patients

• Safety and efficacy in patients under age 18 haven't been established.

Patient education

• Instruct patient to report chest discomfort or other adverse effects immediately.
• Inform patient that frequent blood sampling may be needed to evaluate therapy.

tobramycin

tobramycin ophthalmic

Tobrex

tobramycin sulfate

Nebcin, Nebcin Add-Vantage, Nebcin Pediatric

tobramycin solution for inhalation

TOBI

Pharmacologic classification: aminoglycoside
Therapeutic classification: antibiotic
Pregnancy risk category: D

Indications and dosages

➤ *Serious infections caused by sensitive* **Escherichia coli, Proteus, Klebsiella, Enterobacter, Serratia, Staphylococcus aureus, Pseudomonas, Citrobacter,** *or* **Providencia.**
Adults and children with normal renal function: 3 mg/kg I.M. or I.V. daily, divided q 8 hours. Up to 5 mg/kg I.M. or I.V. daily, divided q 6 to 8 hours for life-threatening infections.
Neonates under age 1 week: Up to 4 mg/kg I.M. or I.V. daily, divided q 12 hours. For I.V. use, dilute in 50 to 100 ml normal saline solution or D₅W for adults and in less volume for children. Infuse over 20 to 60 minutes.
✦ *Dosage adjustment.* In patients with impaired renal function, initial dosage is same as for those with normal renal function. Subsequent doses and frequency are determined by renal function study results and blood levels; keep peak serum levels between 4 and 10 mcg/ml and trough serum levels between 1 and 2 mcg/ml. Several methods have been used to calculate dosage in renal failure.

After a 1-mg/kg loading dose, adjust subsequent dosage by reducing doses administered at 8-hour intervals or by prolonging the interval between normal doses. Both of these methods are useful when serum levels of tobramycin can't be measured directly. They're based on either creatinine clearance (preferred) or serum creatinine because these values correlate with half-life of drug.

To calculate reduced dosage for 8-hour intervals, use available nomograms; or, if patient's steady state serum creatinine values are known, divide the normally recommended dose by patient's serum creatinine value. To determine frequency in hours for normal dosage (if creatinine clearance rate isn't available), divide the normal dose by patient's serum creatinine value. Dosage schedules derived from either method require careful clinical and laboratory observations of patient and should be adjusted as appropriate. These methods of calculation may be misleading in geriatric patients and in those with severe wasting; neither should be used when dialysis is performed.

Hemodialysis removes 50% to 75% of a dose in 6 hours. In anephric patients maintained by dialysis, 1.5 to 2 mg/kg after each dialysis usually maintains therapeutic, nontoxic serum levels. Patients receiving peritoneal dialysis twice a week should receive a 1.5 to 2 mg/kg loading dose followed by 1 mg/kg q 3 days. Those receiving dialysis q 2 days should receive a 1.5 mg/kg loading dose after first dialysis and 0.75 mg/kg after each subsequent dialysis.

➤*Intrathecally or intraventricularly, together with I.M. or I.V. administration*◇. *Adults:* 3 to 8 mg q 18 to 48 hours.

➤*Management of cystic fibrosis in patients with* Pseudomonas aeruginosa *infection. Adults and children over age 6:* 1 single-use ampule (300 mg) administered q 12 hours for 28 days, then off for 28 days, then on for 28 days as advised by prescriber. There's no dose adjustment for age or renal failure.

➤*Treatment of external ocular infection caused by susceptible gram-negative bacteria. Adults and children:* In mild to moderate infections, instill 1 or 2 drops into affected eye q 4 to 6 hours. In severe infections, instill 2 drops into affected eye hourly or apply a small amount of ointment into conjunctival sac t.i.d. or q.i.d.

How supplied
Available by prescription only
Injection: 40 mg/ml, 10 mg/ml (pediatric), 10 mg/ml (adult)
Nebulizer solution for inhalation: Single-use 5-ml (300-mg) ampule
Ophthalmic solution: 0.3%
Ophthalmic ointment: 0.3%

Pharmacodynamics
Antibiotic action: Tobramycin is bactericidal; it binds directly to the 30S ribosomal subunit, thereby inhibiting bacterial protein synthesis. Its spectrum of activity includes many aerobic gram-negative organisms, including most strains of *P. aeruginosa* and some aerobic gram-positive organisms. Tobramycin may act against some bacterial strains resistant to other aminoglycosides; many strains resistant to tobramycin are susceptible to amikacin, gentamicin, or netilmicin.

Pharmacokinetics
Absorption: Absorbed poorly after oral administration and usually is given parenterally. Inhaled drug remains concentrated in the airway, with serum level after 20 weeks of therapy being 1.05 mcg/ml 1 hour after dosing.
Distribution: Distributed widely after parenteral administration; intraocular penetration is poor. CSF penetration is low, even in patients with inflamed meninges. Protein binding is minimal; tobramycin crosses the placenta. Inhaled drug remains primarily concentrated in the airway.
Metabolism: Not metabolized.

Excretion: Excreted primarily in urine by glomerular filtration; small amounts may be excreted in bile and breast milk. Elimination half-life in adults is 2 to 3 hours. In severe renal damage, half-life may extend to 24 to 60 hours. With inhalation use, unabsorbed tobramycin is probably eliminated in the sputum.

Route	Onset	Peak	Duration
I.V.	Immediate	Immediate	8 hr
I.M.	Unknown	30-90 min	8 hr
Ophthalmic, inhalation	Unknown	Unknown	Unknown

Contraindications and precautions
Contraindicated in patients hypersensitive to drug or other aminoglycosides. Use injectable form cautiously in elderly patients and those with impaired renal function or neuromuscular disorders.

Interactions
Drug-drug. *Aminoglycosides, amphotericin B, capreomycin, cephalosporins, cisplatin, methoxyflurane, polymyxin B, vancomycin:* Increased risk of nephrotoxicity, ototoxicity, and neurotoxicity. Monitor patient carefully.
Antiemetics, antivertigo drugs, dimenhydrinate: May mask tobramycin-induced ototoxicity. Monitor patient closely.
Bumetanide, ethacrynic acid, furosemide, mannitol, urea: Increased risk of ototoxicity. Monitor patient closely.
General anesthetics, neuromuscular blockers, succinylcholine, tubocurarine: Potentiate neuromuscular blockade. Monitor patient closely.
Penicillins: Physically and chemically incompatible. Don't mix in same I.V. line.

Adverse reactions
CNS: headache, lethargy, confusion, *seizures*, disorientation (injectable form).
EENT: *ototoxicity* (injectable form); blurred vision (ophthalmic ointment); burning or stinging on instillation, lid itching or swelling, conjunctival erythema (ophthalmic administration).
GI: vomiting, nausea, diarrhea (injectable form).
GU: elevated BUN, nonprotein nitrogen, and serum creatinine levels; increased urinary excretion of casts; *nephrotoxicity* (injectable form).
Hematologic: anemia, eosinophilia, *leukopenia, thrombocytopenia, granulocytopenia* (injectable form).
Respiratory: *bronchospasm* (inhaled form).
Skin: rash, urticaria, pruritus (injectable form).
Other: fever, *hypersensitivity reactions*, overgrowth of nonsusceptible organisms (ophthalmic administration).

Overdose and treatment
Signs and symptoms of overdose include ototoxicity, nephrotoxicity, and neuromuscular toxici-

---

Reactions may be *common*, uncommon, *life-threatening*, or COMMON AND LIFE-THREATENING.

ty. Remove drug by hemodialysis or peritoneal dialysis. Treatment with calcium salts or anticholinesterases reverses neuromuscular blockade.

Special considerations

Consider the recommendations relevant to all aminoglycosides as well as the following.

⚑ ALERT Don't confuse tobramycin with Trobicin.

● For I.V. administration, the usual volume of diluent (normal saline solution injection or D_5W injection) for adult doses is 50 to 100 ml. For children, the volume should be proportionately less. Infusion should be over 20 to 60 minutes.

● Don't premix tobramycin with other drugs; administer separately at least 1 hour apart.

● Discontinue ophthalmic preparation if keratitis, erythema, lacrimation, edema, or lid itching occurs.

● Because tobramycin is dialyzable, patients undergoing hemodialysis may need dose adjustments.

● Inhalation form of tobramycin is an orphan drug used specifically for management of cystic fibrosis patients with *P. aeruginosa* infection.

Patient monitoring

● Monitor patient for symptoms of toxicity.

● Monitor peak and trough drug levels; peak shouldn't exceed 4 to 12 mcg/ml and trough shouldn't go below 2 mcg/ml.

Pregnant patients

● Use drug during pregnancy only when clearly indicated.

Breast-feeding patients

● A decision should be made to discontinue either medication or breast-feeding.

Patient education

● Advise patient that inhalation doses should be taken as close to 12 hours apart as possible and no less than 6 hours apart.

● Instruct patient on proper administration (inhalation).

---

tocainide hydrochloride
Tonocard

Pharmacologic classification: local anesthetic (amide type)
Therapeutic classification: ventricular antiarrhythmic
Pregnancy risk category: C

Indications and dosages

➤ *Suppression of symptomatic ventricular arrhythmias, including frequent PVCs.* Dosage must be individualized based on antiarrhythmic response and tolerance.

Adults: Initially, 400 mg P.O. q 8 hours. Usual dose is between 1,200 and 1,800 mg daily, divided into three doses. Drug may be given in a twice-daily regimen if patient is able to tolerate the t.i.d. regimen.

✦ *Dosage adjustment.* Patients with impaired renal or hepatic function may be adequately treated with less than 1,200 mg daily.

➤ *Myotonic dystrophy* ◊. *Adults:* 800 to 1,200 mg P.O. daily.

How supplied

Available by prescription only
Tablets: 400 mg, 600 mg

Pharmacodynamics

Antiarrhythmic action: Tocainide is structurally similar to lidocaine and possesses similar electrophysiologic and hemodynamic effects. A class IB antiarrhythmic, it suppresses automaticity and shortens the effective refractory period and action potential duration of His-Purkinje fibers and suppresses spontaneous ventricular depolarization during diastole. Conductive atrial tissue and AV conduction aren't affected significantly at therapeutic levels. Unlike quinidine and procainamide, tocainide doesn't significantly alter hemodynamics when administered in usual doses. Tocainide exerts its effects on the conduction system, causing inhibition of reentry mechanisms and cessation of ventricular arrhythmias; these effects may be more pronounced in ischemic tissue. Tocainide doesn't cause a significant negative inotropic effect. Its direct cardiac effects are less potent than those of lidocaine.

Pharmacokinetics

Absorption: Rapidly and completely absorbed from the GI tract; unlike lidocaine, it undergoes negligible first-pass effect in the liver. Bioavailability is nearly 100%.

Distribution: Distribution is only partially understood; however, it appears to be distributed widely and apparently crosses the blood-brain barrier and placenta in animals (it is, however, less lipophilic than lidocaine). Only about 10% to 20% is bound to plasma protein.

Metabolism: Apparently metabolized in the liver to inactive metabolites.

Excretion: Excreted in urine as unchanged drug and inactive metabolites. About 30% to 50% of an orally administered dose is excreted in urine as metabolites. Elimination half-life is about 11 to 23 hours, with an initial biphasic plasma level decline similar to that of lidocaine. Half-life may be prolonged in patients with renal or hepatic insufficiency. Urine alkalinization may substantially decrease the amount of unchanged drug excreted in urine.

Route	Onset	Peak	Duration
P.O.	Unknown	½-2 hr	8 hr

Contraindications and precautions

Contraindicated in patients hypersensitive to lidocaine or other amide-type local anesthetics and in those with second- or third-degree AV block in the absence of an artificial pacemaker.

Use cautiously in patients with heart failure, diminished cardiac reserve, bone marrow failure, cytopenia, or impaired renal or hepatic function.

Interactions

Drug-drug. *Allopurinol:* Increased allopurinol effects. Monitor patient carefully.

Antiarrhythmics: Additive, synergistic, or antagonistic effects. Monitor cardiac status closely.

Cimetidine, rifampin: Decreased elimination half-life and bioavailability of tocainide. Monitor patient carefully. Dosage adjustment may be needed.

Lidocaine: May cause CNS toxicity. Monitor patient closely.

Metoprolol: Decreased myocardial contractility and bradycardia. Monitor cardiac status.

Adverse reactions

CNS: *light-headedness, tremor,* paresthesia, *dizziness, vertigo,* drowsiness, fatigue, confusion, headache.

CV: hypotension, *new or worsened arrhythmias, heart failure, bradycardia,* palpitations.

EENT: blurred vision, tinnitus.

GI: *nausea, vomiting,* diarrhea, anorexia.

Hematologic: *blood dyscrasia.*

Hepatic: abnormal liver function test results, *hepatitis.*

Respiratory: *respiratory arrest,* pulmonary fibrosis, pneumonitis, *pulmonary edema.*

Skin: rash, diaphoresis.

Overdose and treatment

Effects of overdose include extensions of common adverse reactions, particularly those related to the CNS or GI tract.

Treatment generally involves symptomatic and supportive care. In acute overdose, induce emesis or perform gastric lavage. Respiratory depression necessitates immediate attention and maintenance of a patent airway with ventilatory assistance, if required. Seizures may be treated with small incremental doses of a benzodiazepine, such as diazepam or a short- or ultrashort-acting barbiturate, such as pentobarbital or thiopental.

Special considerations

● Drug is considered an oral lidocaine and may be used to ease transition from I.V. lidocaine to oral antiarrhythmic therapy.

● Use cautiously and with lower doses in patients with hepatic or renal impairment.

● A chest radiograph should be obtained if pulmonary symptoms exist.

● Adverse effects tend to be frequent and problematic.

Patient monitoring

● Monitor blood levels; therapeutic levels range from 4 to 10 mcg/ml.

● Monitor periodic blood counts for the first 3 months of therapy and frequently thereafter. Perform CBC promptly if signs of infection develop.

● Observe patient for tremors, a possible sign that maximum safe dose has been reached.

Pregnant patients

● Use drug during pregnancy only when potential benefits justify possible risks to fetus.

Breast-feeding patients

● Safety in breast-feeding women hasn't been established. An alternative feeding method is recommended.

Pediatric patients

● Safety and efficacy haven't been established.

Geriatric patients

● Use cautiously in elderly patients; increased serum drug levels and toxicity are more likely. Monitor patient carefully.

● Elderly patients are more likely to become dizzy and may need assistance walking.

Patient education

● Instruct patient to report unusual bleeding or bruising; signs or symptoms of infection, such as fever, sore throat, stomatitis, or chills; or pulmonary symptoms, such as cough, wheezing, or exertional dyspnea.

● Tell patient he may take tocainide with food to lessen GI upset.

● Tell patient that tocainide may cause drowsiness or dizziness, and he should be careful while performing tasks that require alertness.

tolazamide
Tolinase

Pharmacologic classification: sulfonylurea
Therapeutic classification: antidiabetic
Pregnancy risk category: C

Indications and dosages

➤*Adjunct to diet to lower blood glucose levels in patients with non-insulin-dependent diabetes mellitus (type 2).*
Adults: Initially, 100 mg P.O. daily with breakfast if fasting blood glucose level is below 200 mg/dl. Or, 250 mg P.O. daily if fasting blood glucose level is above 200 mg/dl. May adjust dose at weekly intervals in increments of 100 to 250 mg based on blood glucose response. Maximum dosage is 500 mg P.O. b.i.d. before meals.
Elderly patients: Initially, 100 mg P.O. daily.
✦ *Dosage adjustment.* Initially, malnourished or underweight patients may be given 100 mg P.O. daily.

Reactions may be *common,* uncommon, *life-threatening,* or COMMON AND LIFE-THREATENING.

How supplied

Available by prescription only
Tablets: 100 mg, 250 mg, 500 mg

Pharmacodynamics

Antidiabetic action: Tolazamide lowers blood glucose levels by stimulating insulin release from functioning beta cells of the pancreas. After prolonged administration, the hypoglycemic effects of drug appear to reflect extrapancreatic effects, possibly including reduction of basal hepatic glucose production and enhanced peripheral sensitivity to insulin.

Pharmacokinetics

Absorption: Absorbed well from the GI tract.
Distribution: Probably distributed into the extracellular fluid.
Metabolism: Metabolized probably by the liver to several mildly active metabolites.
Excretion: Excreted in urine primarily as metabolites, with small amounts excreted as unchanged drug. Half-life is 7 hours.

Route	Onset	Peak	Duration
P.O.	Unknown	3-4 hr	Unknown

Contraindications and precautions

Contraindicated in patients hypersensitive to drug or other sulfonylureas; in patients with type 1 diabetes (insulin-dependent) or diabetes that can be adequately controlled by diet; in patients with type 2 diabetes complicated by ketosis, acidosis, coma, or other acute complications such as major surgery, severe infection, or severe trauma; in patients with uremia; and in pregnant or breastfeeding women.

Use cautiously in geriatric, debilitated, or malnourished patients and in those with impaired renal or hepatic function or those with adrenal or pituitary insufficiency.

Interactions

Drug-drug. *Beta blockers, including ophthalmics:* Increased risk of hypoglycemia, masking its symptoms (increasing pulse rate and blood pressure) and prolonging it by blocking gluconeogenesis. Use together cautiously.
Calcium channel blockers, corticosteroids, estrogens, isoniazid, oral contraceptives, phenothiazines, phenytoin, sympathomimetics, thiazide diuretics, thyroid hormones, triamterene: Decreased hypoglycemic effect. Monitor blood glucose level and adjust dose accordingly.
Chloramphenicol, insulin, MAO inhibitors, NSAIDs, probenecid, salicylates, sulfonamides: Increased hypoglycemic effect. Monitor blood glucose level closely.
Oral anticoagulants: May increase hypoglycemic activity or enhance anticoagulant effect. Monitor blood glucose level and PT and INR.
Drug-herb. *Aloe, bitter melon, bilberry leaf, burdock, dandelion, fenugreek, garlic, ginseng:*

Possible improved blood glucose control, requiring a reduction in antidiabetic dosage. Advise patient to discuss the use of herbs before use.
Drug-lifestyle. *Alcohol use:* Disulfiram-like reaction (nausea, vomiting, abdominal cramps, headaches). Advise patient to avoid alcohol.

Adverse reactions

CNS: weakness, fatigue, dizziness, vertigo, malaise, headache.
GI: nausea, vomiting, epigastric distress, heartburn.
Hematologic: *leukopenia,* hemolytic anemia, ***thrombocytopenia, aplastic anemia, agranulocytosis,*** pancytopenia.
Metabolic: *hyponatremia, hypoglycemia.*
Skin: photosensitivity reactions.

Overdose and treatment

Signs and symptoms of overdose include low blood glucose levels, tingling of lips and tongue, hunger, nausea, decreased cerebral function (lethargy, yawning, confusion, agitation, nervousness), increased sympathetic activity (tachycardia, sweating, tremor), and ultimately seizures, stupor, and coma.

Mild hypoglycemia, without loss of consciousness or neurologic findings, responds to treatment with oral glucose and adjustments in drug doses and meal patterns. If patient loses consciousness or has neurologic findings, give rapid injection of $D_{50}W$ followed by continuous infusion of $D_{10}W$ at a rate to maintain blood glucose levels above 100 mg/dl. Monitor patient for 24 to 48 hours.

Special considerations

Consider the recommendations relevant to all sulfonylureas as well as the following.
● Over time, patients may become unresponsive (uncontrolled blood sugar) to therapy with this agent as well as other sulfonylureas; monitor patient appropriately.
● To avoid GI intolerance for those patients receiving doses of 500 mg or more daily and to improve control of hyperglycemia, divided doses are recommended; these are given before the morning and evening meals.
● Tablets may be crushed to ease administration.
● Use cautiously in women of childbearing age. Tolazamide isn't recommended for treatment of diabetes related to pregnancy.
● Oral antidiabetics have been linked to an increased risk of CV mortality compared with diet or diet and insulin therapy.
● To change from insulin to oral therapy with tolazamide, if insulin dose is less than 20 units daily, insulin may be stopped and oral therapy started at 100 mg P.O. daily in the morning. If insulin dose is 20 to 40 units daily, insulin may be stopped and oral therapy started at 250 mg P.O. daily in the morning. If insulin dose is more than 40 units daily, decrease insulin dose by 50% and start oral

therapy at 250 mg P.O. daily with breakfast. Increase doses as appropriate based on blood glucose response.

Patient monitoring
• When substituting tolazamide for chlorpropamide therapy, monitor patient closely for 1 to 2 weeks because of prolonged retention of chlorpropamide in the body, which may result in hypoglycemia.

Pregnant patients
• Use cautiously in pregnant women.

Breast-feeding patients
• Because of the risk of hypoglycemia in the breast-fed infant, a risk/benefit decision should be made to discontinue either the drug or breast-feeding.

Pediatric patients
• Tolazamide is ineffective in insulin-dependent (type 1, juvenile-onset) diabetes. Safety and efficacy in children haven't been established.

Geriatric patients
• These patients may be more sensitive to the effects of drug because of reduced metabolism and elimination. Hypoglycemia causes more neurologic symptoms in these patients. Geriatric patients usually require a lower initial dose.

Patient education
• Advise patient to take drug at the same time each day. If a dose is missed, it should be taken immediately, unless it's almost time to take the next dose; he shouldn't double the doses.
• Warn patient to avoid alcohol when taking tolazamide.
• Recommend that patient take the drug with food to minimize GI upset.

tolbutamide
Orinase

Pharmacologic classification: sulfonylurea
Therapeutic classification: antidiabetic
Pregnancy risk category: C

Indications and dosages
➤ *Adjunct to diet to lower blood glucose levels in patients with type 2 diabetes mellitus.* *Adults:* Initially, 1 to 2 g P.O. daily as single dose or divided b.i.d. or t.i.d. May adjust dosage to maximum of 3 g P.O. daily.

How supplied
Available by prescription only
Tablets: 500 mg

Pharmacodynamics
Antidiabetic action: Tolbutamide lowers blood glucose levels by stimulating insulin release from functioning beta cells of the pancreas. After prolonged administration, the hypoglycemic effects of the drug appear to reflect extrapancreatic effects, possibly including reduction of basal hepatic glucose production and enhanced peripheral sensitivity to insulin.

Pharmacokinetics
Absorption: Absorbed readily from the GI tract with peak levels occurring at 3 to 4 hours.
Distribution: Probably distributed into extracellular fluid. Drug is 95% bound to plasma proteins.
Metabolism: Metabolized in the liver to inactive metabolites.
Excretion: Drug and its metabolites are excreted in urine and feces. Half-life is 4½ to 6½ hours.

Route	Onset	Peak	Duration
P.O.	½-1 hr	3-5 hr	24 hr

Contraindications and precautions
Contraindicated in patients hypersensitive to drug or other sulfonylureas; pregnant women; breast-feeding women; patients with type 1 diabetes (insulin-dependent) or diabetes that can be adequately controlled by diet; patients with type 2 diabetes complicated by fever, ketosis, acidosis, coma, or other acute complications such as major surgery, severe infection, or severe trauma; and patients with severe renal insufficiency.

Use cautiously in elderly, debilitated, or malnourished patients and in those with impaired renal or hepatic function or porphyria.

Interactions
Drug-drug. *Anticoagulants:* Increased hypoglycemic activity, enhanced anticoagulant effect. Monitor blood glucose levels, PT, and INR. Dosage may need adjustment.
Beta blockers, including ophthalmics: Mask symptoms of hypoglycemia and may prolong hypoglycemia. Use together cautiously.
Calcium channel blockers, corticosteroids, estrogens, isoniazid, oral contraceptives, phenothiazines, phenytoin, sympathomimetics, thiazide diuretics, thyroid products, triamterene: Decreased hypoglycemic effect. Monitor blood glucose level; dosage may need adjustment.
Chloramphenicol, insulin, MAO inhibitors, NSAIDs, probenecid, salicylates, sulfonamides: Increased hypoglycemic effect. Monitor blood glucose levels closely.
Drug-herb. *Aloe, bitter melon, bilberry leaf, burdock, dandelion, fenugreek, garlic, ginseng:* Possible improved blood glucose control, requiring a reduction of antidiabetic dosage. Advise patient to discuss herbs before use.
Drug-lifestyle. *Alcohol use:* May produce a disulfiram-like reaction with nausea, vomiting, abdominal cramps, and headaches. Advise patient to avoid alcohol.

Adverse reactions

CNS: headache.

GI: taste alterations, nausea, heartburn, epigastric distress.

Hematologic: *leukopenia,* hemolytic anemia, *thrombocytopenia, aplastic anemia, agranulocytosis,* pancytopenia.

Hepatic: hepatic porphyria.

Metabolic: *hypoglycemia, dilutional hyponatremia.*

Skin: rash, pruritus, erythema, urticaria.

Other: SIADH, *hypersensitivity reactions, disulfiram-like reactions.*

Overdose and treatment

Signs and symptoms of overdose include low blood glucose levels, tingling of lips and tongue, hunger, nausea, decreased cerebral function (lethargy, yawning, confusion, agitation, nervousness), increased sympathetic activity (tachycardia, sweating, tremor), and ultimately, seizures, stupor, and coma.

Mild hypoglycemia, without loss of consciousness or neurologic findings, responds to treatment with oral glucose and dose adjustments. If patient loses consciousness or develops neurologic findings, the patient should receive rapid injection of $D_{50}W$, followed by a continuous infusion of $D_{10}W$ at a rate to maintain blood glucose levels greater than 100 mg/dl. Monitor patient for 24 to 48 hours.

Special considerations

Consider the recommendations relevant to all sulfonylureas as well as the following.

• To avoid GI intolerance for those patients on larger doses and to improve control of hyperglycemia, divided doses given before the morning and evening meals are recommended.

• Patients should avoid taking tolbutamide at bedtime because of the potential for nocturnal hypoglycemia.

• Tolbutamide may give a false-positive reading for albumin in urine if measured by the acidification-after-boiling test. There's no interference with the sulfosalicylic acid test. Tolbutamide decreases the uptake of radioactive iodine and may interfere with test results of radioactive iodine uptake.

• To change from insulin to oral therapy with tolbutamide, if insulin dose is less than 20 units daily, insulin may be stopped and oral therapy started at 1 to 2 g daily. If insulin dose is 20 to 40 units daily, insulin dose is reduced 30% to 50% and oral therapy started as above. If insulin dose is more than 40 units daily, insulin dose is decreased 20% and oral therapy started as above. Further reductions in insulin dose are based on patient's response to oral therapy.

Patient monitoring

• When substituting tolbutamide for chlorpropamide therapy, monitor patient closely for the first 2 weeks because of prolonged retention of chlorpropamide in the body, which may result in hypoglycemia.

Pregnant patients

• Use cautiously in women of childbearing age. Tolbutamide isn't recommended for treatment of diabetes related to pregnancy.

Breast-feeding patients

• Tolbutamide appears in breast milk. Because of the risk of hypoglycemia in the breast-fed infant, a decision should be made to discontinue either the drug or breast-feeding.

Pediatric patients

• Tolbutamide is ineffective in insulin-dependent and type 1, juvenile-onset diabetes. Safety and efficacy in children haven't been established.

Geriatric patients

• These patients may be more sensitive to the effects of drug because of reduced metabolism and elimination.

• Hypoglycemia causes more neurologic symptoms in these patients.

• Elderly patients usually require a lower initial dose.

Patient education

• Emphasize to patient the importance of following prescribed diet, exercise, and medical regimen.

• Instruct patient to take drug at the same time each day.

• Inform patient that, if a dose is missed, it should be taken immediately, unless it's almost time to take the next dose. Patient shouldn't double the doses.

• Advise patient to avoid products containing alcohol while taking tolbutamide because of prolonged hypoglycemic effect.

tolcapone
Tasmar

Pharmacologic classification: catechol-*O*-methyltransferase (COMT) inhibitor
Therapeutic classification: antiparkinsonian
Pregnancy risk category: C

Indications and dosages

➤ *Adjunct to levodopa and carbidopa for treatment of signs and symptoms of idiopathic Parkinson's disease. Adults:* Recommended initial dose is 100 mg (preferred) or 200 mg P.O. t.i.d. If starting treatment with 200 mg t.i.d. and dyskinesias occur, then a decrease in dose of levodopa may be necessary. Maximum dosage is 600 mg daily. Always give with levodopa-carbidopa. The first tolcapone dose of the day should always be taken with the first levodopa-carbidopa dose of the day.

✦ *Dosage adjustment.* Don't use doses over 100 mg t.i.d. in patients with severe hepatic or renal dysfunction.

How supplied
Available by prescription only
Tablets: 100 mg, 200 mg

Pharmacodynamics
Antiparkinsonian action: Exact mechanism of action isn't known. It's thought to reversibly inhibit erythrocyte COMT when given with levodopa/carbidopa, resulting in a decrease in the clearance of levodopa and a two-fold increase in the bioavailability of levodopa. The decrease in clearance of levodopa prolongs the elimination half-life of levodopa from 2 to 3½ hours.

Pharmacokinetics
Absorption: Rapidly absorbed and reaches peak plasma levels within 2 hours. Following oral administration, absolute bioavailability is 65%. Onset of effect occurs following administration of first dose. Absorption of tolcapone decreases when given within 1 hour before or 2 hours after food; however, drug can be administered without regard to meals.
Distribution: Highly bound to plasma proteins (greater than 99.9%), primarily to albumin. The steady state volume of distribution is small.
Metabolism: Completely metabolized before excretion. The main mechanism of metabolism is glucuronidation.
Excretion: Only 0.5% of dose is found unchanged in urine. Tolcapone is a low-extraction-ratio drug with a systemic clearance of 7 L/hour. Elimination half-life is 2 to 3 hours. Dialysis isn't expected to affect clearance because of the high protein binding.

Route	Onset	Peak	Duration
P.O.	Unknown	2 hr	Unknown

Contraindications and precautions
Contraindicated in patients hypersensitive to drug or its components; in patients with liver disease or two ALT or AST values exceeding the upper limit of normal; in patients withdrawn from therapy because of drug-induced hepatocellular injury; and in patients with a history of nontraumatic rhabdomyolysis or hyperpyrexia and confusion, possibly related to drug.

Use cautiously in patients with Parkinson's disease because syncope and orthostatic hypotension may worsen.

Interactions
Drug-drug. *Desipramine:* Increased risk of adverse effects. Use together cautiously.
MAO inhibitors: Hypertensive crisis may occur. Avoid use together.
Warfarin: Drug may increase the anticoagulant effect of warfarin. Monitor PTT.

Drug-food: When given 1 hour before or 2 hours after food, bioavailability is decreased by 10% to 20%.

Adverse reactions
CNS: *dyskinesia, sleep disorder, dystonia, excessive dreaming, somnolence, dizziness, confusion, headache, hallucinations,* hyperkinesia, fatigue, balance loss, depression, tremor, speech disorder, paresthesia.
CV: syncope, *orthostatic complaints,* chest pain, chest discomfort, palpitations, hypotension.
EENT: pharyngitis, tinnitus.
GI: *nausea, anorexia, diarrhea,* flatulence, *vomiting,* constipation, abdominal pain, dyspepsia, dry mouth.
GU: urinary tract infection, urine discoloration, hematuria, urinary incontinence, impotence.
Hepatic: *hepatotoxicity.*
Musculoskeletal: *muscle cramps,* myalgia, stiffness, arthritis, neck pain.
Respiratory: bronchitis, dyspnea, upper respiratory tract infection.
Skin: increased sweating, rash.
Other: falls.

Overdose and treatment
The highest dose used is 800 mg t.i.d.; nausea, vomiting, and dizziness were noted. Provide supportive care and hospitalize, if indicated.

Special considerations
• Because of the risk of potentially fatal, acute fulminant liver failure, use drug only in patients on levodopa/carbidopa who don't respond to or aren't suitable for other therapy.
• Diarrhea occurs commonly in patients taking tolcapone. It may occur 2 weeks after therapy begins or after 6 to 12 weeks. Although it usually resolves with discontinuation of drug, hospitalization may be required in rare cases.
• Dosage adjustments aren't needed in patients with mild to moderate renal dysfunction; use cautiously in patients with severe renal impairment.
• Withdraw drug in patients who fail to show clinical benefit within 3 weeks of treatment.

Patient monitoring
• Monitor liver enzyme levels at baseline, then every 2 weeks for the first year of therapy, and then every 8 weeks. Stop drug if hepatic transaminases exceed the upper limits of normal or if patient appears jaundiced.
• Monitor patient for clinical improvement, which should occur within 3 weeks.

Pregnant patients
• Use drug during pregnancy only when potential benefits justify risk to fetus.

Breast-feeding patients
• Because of the risk that drug may be appear in breast milk, use cautiously in breast-feeding women.

Reactions may be *common,* uncommon, *life-threatening,* or COMMON AND LIFE-THREATENING.

Pediatric patients
● There's no known use in children.

Patient education
● Advise patient to take drug exactly as prescribed.
● Warn patient about risk of orthostatic hypotension; tell him to use caution when rising from a seated or recumbent position.
● Caution patient to avoid hazardous activities until CNS effects of drug are known.
● Tell patient that nausea may occur and to report signs of liver injury immediately.
● Advise patient about risk of increased dyskinesia or dystonia.
● Inform patient that hallucinations may occur.
● Tell patient to report planned or suspected pregnancy during therapy.

tolmetin sodium
Tolectin, Tolectin DS

Pharmacologic classification: NSAID
Therapeutic classification: nonnarcotic analgesic, anti-inflammatory
Pregnancy risk category: C

Indications and dosages
➤ *Rheumatoid arthritis, osteoarthritis, juvenile rheumatoid arthritis.* Adults: Initially, 400 mg P.O. t.i.d. Maximum dosage is 1,800 mg daily. Usual dose ranges from 600 to 1,800 mg daily in three divided doses.
Children age 2 or older: Initially, 20 mg/kg P.O. daily in three or four divided doses. Usual dose ranges from 15 to 30 mg/kg daily in three or four divided doses.

How supplied
Available by prescription only
Capsules: 400 mg
Tablets: 200 mg, 600 mg

Pharmacodynamics
Analgesic and anti-inflammatory actions: Although the exact mechanism of action is unknown, inhibition of prostaglandin synthesis may be responsible for the anti-inflammatory effects of tolmetin. Drug also seems to possess analgesic and antipyretic activity.

Pharmacokinetics
Absorption: Absorbed rapidly from GI tract.
Distribution: Highly protein-bound.
Metabolism: Metabolized in the liver.
Excretion: Excreted in urine as an inactive metabolite or conjugates of tolmetin. Elimination is biphasic, consisting of a rapid phase with a half-life of 1 to 2 hours followed by a slower phase with a half-life of about 5 hours.

Route	Onset	Peak	Duration
P.O.	Unknown	½-1½ hr	24 hr

Contraindications and precautions
Contraindicated in patients hypersensitive to drug; in patients in whom acute asthmatic attacks, urticaria, or rhinitis is precipitated by aspirin or NSAIDs; and in breast-feeding women. Use cautiously in patients with renal or cardiac disease, GI bleeding, history of peptic ulcer, hypertension, and conditions predisposing to fluid retention.

Interactions
Drug-drug. *Anticoagulants, thrombolytics:* Increased risk of bleeding. Use together cautiously.
Aspirin: Decreased plasma levels of tolmetin. Monitor patient closely. Dosage adjustment may be required.
GI-irritating drugs, such as antibiotics, corticosteroids, and NSAIDs: Potentiate adverse GI effects. Use together cautiously.
Highly protein-bound drugs, such as phenytoin, salicylates, sulfonamides, sulfonylureas, and warfarin: Increased adverse effects. Monitor patient closely.
Methotrexate: Increased risk of methotrexate toxicity. Avoid use together. If given together, monitor patient closely.
Drug-herb. *Aloe, bitter melon, bilberry leaf, burdock, dandelion, fenugreek, garlic, ginseng:* Possible improved blood glucose control, requiring a reduction of antidiabetic dosage. Advise patient to discuss herbs before use.
Drug-food. *Any food:* Delayed and decreased absorption of tolmetin. Separate administration times.

Adverse reactions
CNS: headache, dizziness, drowsiness, asthenia, depression.
CV: chest pain, hypertension, edema.
EENT: tinnitus, visual disturbances.
GI: epigastric distress, peptic ulceration, occult blood loss, *nausea,* vomiting, abdominal pain, diarrhea, constipation, dyspepsia, flatulence, anorexia.
GU: urinary tract infection.
Hematologic: decreased hemoglobin and hematocrit.
Hepatic: abnormal liver function test results.
Metabolic: weight gain or loss, elevated BUN level.
Skin: irritation.
Other: *anaphylaxis.*

Overdose and treatment
Effects of overdose include dizziness, drowsiness, mental confusion, and lethargy.
To treat tolmetin overdose, empty stomach immediately by inducing emesis or by gastric lavage followed by administration of activated charcoal. Provide symptomatic and supportive measures (respiratory support and correction of fluid and electrolyte imbalances). Monitor laboratory parameters and vital signs closely. Alkalinization of urine by sodium bicarbonate ingestion may enhance renal excretion of tolmetin.

Special considerations
Consider the recommendations relevant to all NSAIDs as well as the following.
● Assess cardiopulmonary status closely.
● Therapeutic effect usually occurs within a few days to 1 week of therapy. Evaluate patient's response to drug as evidenced by relief of symptoms.
● Administer drug on empty stomach for maximum absorption. However, it may be administered with meals to lessen GI upset.
● Tolmetin falsely elevates results of urinary protein (pseudoproteinuria) in tests that rely on acid precipitation, such as those using sulfosalicylic acid.

Patient monitoring
● Monitor vital signs closely, especially heart rate and blood pressure.
● Assess renal function periodically during therapy; monitor fluid intake and output and daily weight.
● Monitor patient for edema.

Pregnant patients
● Use drug during pregnancy only when clearly needed.

Breast-feeding patients
● Because drug appears in breast milk, it may adversely affect neonates. Avoid use in breast-feeding women.

Pediatric patients
● Safety and efficacy in children under age 2 haven't been established.

Patient education
● Explain that therapeutic effects may occur in 1 week but could take 2 to 4 weeks.
● Advise patient to avoid use of OTC medications such as NSAIDs, unless medically approved.
● Instruct patient to follow prescribed regimen and recommended schedule of follow-up.
● Advise patient to report any signs of edema or other adverse reactions.

tolterodine tartrate
Detrol, Detrol LA

Pharmacologic classification: muscarinic receptor antagonist
Therapeutic classification: anticholinergic
Pregnancy risk category: C

Indications and dosages
➤ *Treatment of patients with overactive bladder with symptoms of urinary frequency, urgency, or urge incontinence.*
Adults: Initial dosage is 2 mg P.O. b.i.d. May lower to 1 mg b.i.d. based on response and tolerance. Or, using extended-release form, give 4 mg P.O. daily. Dose may be reduced to 2 mg P.O. daily of the extended-release formulation based on tolerance and response.
✦ *Dosage adjustment.* In patients who have significantly reduced hepatic function or who are currently taking a drug that inhibits the cytochrome P-450 3A4 isoenzyme system, recommended dose is 1 mg b.i.d. of regular form or 2 mg daily of extended-release form.

How supplied
Available by prescription only
Capsules (extended release): 2 mg, 4 mg
Tablets: 1 mg, 2 mg

Pharmacodynamics
Anticholinergic action: Tolterodine is a competitive muscarinic receptor antagonist. Both urinary bladder contraction and salivation are mediated by way of cholinergic muscarinic receptors.

Pharmacokinetics
Absorption: Well absorbed with about 77% bioavailability. Food increases bioavailability by 53%.
Distribution: Volume of distribution is about 113 L. Tolterodine is 96% protein-bound.
Metabolism: Metabolized by the liver primarily by oxidation by the cytochrome P-450 2D6 pathway; leads to formation of a pharmacologically active 5-hydroxymethyl metabolite.
Excretion: Excreted mostly via urine; the rest in feces. Less than 1% of a dose is recovered as unchanged drug, and 5% to 14% is recovered as the active metabolite. Half-life is 2 to 3½ hours.

Route	Onset	Peak	Duration
P.O.	Unknown	1-2 hr	Unknown

Contraindications and precautions
Contraindicated in patients with urine or gastric retention and uncontrolled narrow-angle glaucoma. Also contraindicated in patients hypersensitive to tolterodine or its ingredients.

Use cautiously in patients with significantly reduced hepatic or renal function.

Interactions
Drug-drug. *Antifungals, such as itraconazole, ketoconazole, and miconazole; cytochrome P-450 3A4 inhibitors, such as macrolide antibiotics (including clarithromycin and erythromycin):* Increased tolterodine levels. Doses should be reduced.
Drug-food. *Food:* Increases tolterodine absorption. May be used for this effect.

Adverse reactions
CNS: paresthesia, vertigo, dizziness, *headache,* nervousness, somnolence, fatigue.
CV: hypertension, chest pain.
EENT: abnormal vision (including accommodation), xerophthalmia, pharyngitis, rhinitis, sinusitis.
GI: *dry mouth,* abdominal pain, constipation, diarrhea, dyspepsia, flatulence, nausea, vomiting.

Reactions may be *common,* uncommon, *life-threatening,* or COMMON AND LIFE-THREATENING.

GU: dysuria, micturition frequency, urine retention, urinary tract infection.
Metabolic: weight gain.
Musculoskeletal: arthalgia, back pain.
Respiratory: bronchitis, cough, upper respiratory tract infection.
Skin: pruritus, rash, erythema, dry skin.
Other: flulike symptoms.

Overdose and treatment
Overdose can potentially result in severe central anticholinergic effects and should be treated accordingly. Perform ECG monitoring if an overdose occurs with close attention to QT interval.

Special considerations
• Food increases the absorption of tolterodine, but no dosage adjustment is needed.
• Dry mouth is the most frequently reported adverse effect.

Patient monitoring
• Monitor patient for urinary symptoms and adverse reactions.

Pregnant patients
• Use drug during pregnancy only when clearly needed.

Breast-feeding patients
• It isn't known whether drug appears in breast milk. Drug isn't recommended for use in breast-feeding women.

Pediatric patients
• Safety and efficacy in children haven't been established.

Geriatric patients
• No overall differences in safety have been observed between older and younger patients.

Patient education
• Inform patient that antimuscarinics such as tolterodine may produce blurred vision.
• Caution patient to avoid hazardous activities until effects of drug are known.
• Tell patient to swallow extended-release formulation whole.

topiramate
Topamax

Pharmacologic classification: sulfamate-substituted monosaccharide
Therapeutic classification: anticonvulsant
Pregnancy risk category: C

Indications and dosages
➤ *Adjunctive therapy of partial onset seizures or primary generalized tonic-clonic seizures.* *Adults:* Initially, 25 to 50 mg daily followed by adjustments of 25 to 50 mg

weekly. Adjust up to maximum daily dosage of 400 mg in two divided doses. Adjustment schedule is as follows.

Week	A.M. dose	P.M. dose
1	None	50 mg
2	50 mg	50 mg
3	50 mg	100 mg
4	100 mg	100 mg
5	100 mg	150 mg
6	150 mg	150 mg
7	150 mg	200 mg
8	200 mg	200 mg

Children ages 2 to 16: 5 to 9 mg/kg P.O. daily in two divided doses. Dosage adjustment should begin at 1 to 3 mg/kg daily for 1 week. Then increase at 1- to 2-week intervals by 1 to 3 mg/kg daily to achieve optimal clinical response. Dosage adjustment should be guided by clinical outcome.
✦ *Dosage adjustment.* In patients with moderate to severe renal impairment, reduce dose by 50%. A supplemental dose may be required during hemodialysis.

How supplied
Available by prescription only
Capsules: 15 mg, 25 mg
Tablets: 25 mg, 100 mg, 200 mg

Pharmacodynamics
Anticonvulsant action: Mechanism of action is unknown. Thought to block action potential, suggestive of a sodium channel-blocking action. Drug may potentiate activity of gamma-aminobutyric acid (GABA) and antagonize the ability of kainate to activate the kainate/AMPA subtype of excitatory amino acid (glutamate) receptor. Topiramate also has weak carbonic anhydrase inhibitor activity, which is unrelated to its anticonvulsant properties.

Pharmacokinetics
Absorption: Rapidly absorbed. Relative bioavailability of drug is about 80% compared with a solution and isn't affected by food.
Distribution: Plasma levels increase proportionately with dose; mean elimination half-life is 21 hours. Steady state is reached in 4 days in patients with normal renal function. Drug is 13% to 17% bound to plasma proteins.
Metabolism: Not extensively metabolized.
Excretion: About 70% of an administered dose is eliminated unchanged in urine. Mean plasma half-life is 21 hours.

Route	Onset	Peak	Duration
P.O.	Unknown	2 hr	Unknown

Contraindications and precautions
Contraindicated in patients hypersensitive to any component of the preparation.

Interactions
Drug-drug. *Carbamazepine, phenytoin:* Decreased topiramate levels. Monitor patient closely.
Carbonic anhydrase inhibitors, such as acetazolamide and dichlorphenamide: May increase the risk of renal stone formation. Avoid use together.
CNS depressants: Risk of topiramate-induced CNS depression and other adverse cognitive and neuropsychiatric events. Use together cautiously.
Oral contraceptives: Decreased contraceptive effect. Advise patient to use another method of contraception.
Phenobarbital, primidone, valproic acid: Increased phenytoin levels. Monitor patient closely.
Drug-lifestyle. *Alcohol use:* CNS depression and other adverse cognitive and neuropsychiatric events. Discourage alcohol use.

Adverse reactions
CNS: *fatigue;* malaise; abnormal coordination; agitation; apathy; asthenia; *ataxia; confusion;* depression; difficulty with concentration, attention, language, and memory; *dizziness;* emotional lability; euphoria; *generalized tonic-clonic seizures;* hallucination; hyperkinesia; hypertonia; hypoaesthesia; hypokinesia; insomnia; mood problems; *nervousness; nystagmus; paresthesia;* personality disorder; *psychomotor slowing;* psychosis; *somnolence; speech disorders;* stupor; *suicide attempts; tremor;* vertigo.
CV: edema, chest pain, palpitations.
EENT: *abnormal vision,* conjunctivitis, *diplopia,* eye pain, epistaxis, hearing or vestibular problems, pharyngitis, sinusitis, tinnitus.
GI: taste perversion, abdominal pain, anorexia, constipation, diarrhea, dry mouth, dyspepsia, flatulence, gastroenteritis, gingivitis, *nausea,* vomiting.
GU: amenorrhea, dysuria, dysmenorrhea, leukorrhea, hematuria, impotence, intermenstrual bleeding, menstrual disorder, menorrhagia, micturition frequency, renal calculus, urinary incontinence, urinary tract infection, vaginitis.
Hematologic: anemia, *leukopenia.*
Metabolic: weight changes.
Musculoskeletal: back pain, leg pain, myalgia.
Respiratory: bronchitis, cough, dyspnea, *upper respiratory tract infection.*
Skin: acne, alopecia, aggressive reaction, increased sweating, pruritus, rash.
Other: body odor, fever, flulike symptoms, hot flashes.

Overdose and treatment
In acute overdose after recent ingestion, institute gastric lavage or emesis. Activated charcoal isn't recommended. Institute supportive treatment. Hemodialysis is an effective means of removing drug.

Special considerations
● Because of their bitter taste, tablets shouldn't be broken.
● Capsules can be opened and contents sprinkled on soft food.
● If necessary, stop anticonvulsant drugs gradually to minimize the increased risk of seizures.
● Stop drug if patient has an ocular reaction: acute myopia or secondary angle-closure glaucoma.

Patient monitoring
● Monitor CBC.
● Monitor patient for seizures.

Breast-feeding patients
● It isn't known whether drug appears in breast milk. Use cautiously in breast-feeding women.

Pediatric patients
● Safety and efficacy in children under age 2 haven't been established.

Geriatric patients
● No age-related problems have been seen in elderly patients; however, age-related renal abnormalities should be considered.

Patient education
● Carefully review dosing schedule with patient to avoid under- or overmedication.
● Tell patient to maintain adequate fluid intake during therapy because of potential to form renal stones.
● Advise patient to avoid hazardous activities until effects of drug are known.
● Tell patient to report vision changes right away.

topotecan hydrochloride
Hycamtin

Pharmacologic classification: semisynthetic camptothecin derivative
Therapeutic classification: antineoplastic
Pregnancy risk category: D

Indications and dosages
➤ *Metastatic carcinoma of the ovary after failure of initial or subsequent chemotherapy.* Adults: 1.5 mg/m^2 daily as an I.V. infusion given over 30 minutes for 5 consecutive days, starting on day 1 of a 21-day cycle. Minimum of four cycles should be given.
✦ *Dosage adjustment.* In adults with renal impairment and creatinine clearance of 20 to 39 ml/minute, adjust dosage to 0.75 mg/m^2. In patients with mild renal impairment (creatinine clearance of 40 to 60 ml/minute), adjustment isn't required. There are insufficient data available for a dosage recommendation for patients with creatinine clearance of less than 20 ml/minute. In the event of severe neutropenia occurring during any course, reduce the dose by 0.25 mg/m^2 for subsequent courses. Or, give

granulocyte-colony stimulating factor (G CSF) starting from day 6 of subsequent courses (24 hours after completion of topotecan) before resorting to dosage reduction.

➤ *Treatment of small-cell lung cancer sensitive disease after failure of first-line chemotherapy.* Adults: 1.5 mg/m² I.V. infusion given over 30 minutes daily for 5 consecutive days, followed by a 16-day rest period for a 21-day treatment course. Minimum of four cycles should be given.

✦ *Dosage adjustment.* In patients with creatinine clearance of 20 to 39 ml/minute, dosage is decreased to 0.75 mg/m². If severe neutropenia occurs, dosage is decreased by 0.25 mg/m² for subsequent courses. Or, if severe neutropenia occurs, G-CSF may be given following the subsequent course (before resorting to dosage reduction) starting from day 6 of course (24 hours after completion of topotecan administration).

How supplied
Available by prescription only
Injection: 4-mg single-dose vial

Pharmacodynamics
Antineoplastic action: Topotecan relieves torsional strain in DNA by inducing reversible single-strand breaks. It binds to the topoisomerase I-DNA complex and prevents religation of these single-strand breaks. The cytotoxicity of topotecan is thought to be due to double-strand DNA damage produced during DNA synthesis when replication enzymes interact with the ternary complex formed by topotecan, topoisomerase I, and DNA.

Pharmacokinetics
Absorption: Administered I.V.
Distribution: About 35% is bound to plasma protein.
Metabolism: Undergoes a reversible pH-dependent hydrolysis of its lactone moiety; the lactone form is pharmacologically active.
Excretion: About 30% is excreted in the urine. Terminal half-life is 2 to 3 hours.

Route	Onset	Peak	Duration
I.V.	Unknown	Unknown	Unknown

Contraindications and precautions
Contraindicated in patients hypersensitive to drug or its components, in those with severe bone marrow depression, and in pregnant or breast-feeding women.

Interactions
Drug-drug. *Cisplatin:* Increased severity of myelosuppression. Use together with extreme caution.
G-CSF: Prolonged duration of neutropenia. Don't initiate G-CSF until day 6 of the course of therapy, 24 hours after completion of treatment with topotecan.

Adverse reactions
CNS: *fatigue, asthenia, headache,* paresthesia.
GI: *nausea, vomiting, diarrhea, constipation, abdominal pain, stomatitis, anorexia.*
Hematologic: *neutropenia, leukopenia, thrombocytopenia, anemia.*
Hepatic: transient elevations of liver enzyme levels.
Respiratory: *dyspnea.*
Skin: *alopecia.*
Other: *sepsis,* fever.

Overdose and treatment
The primary adverse effect linked to topotecan overdose is thought to be bone marrow suppression. Treatment should be supportive. There's no known antidote.

Special considerations
● Before first course, baseline neutrophil count should exceed 1,500 cells/mm³ and platelet count should exceed 100,000 cells/mm³.
● Protect unopened vials of drug from light. Reconstituted vials are stable at about 68° to 77° F (20° to 25° C) with ambient lighting conditions for 24 hours.
● Prepare drug under a vertical laminar flow hood wearing gloves and protective clothing. If drug solution contacts the skin, wash the skin immediately and thoroughly with soap and water. If mucous membranes are affected, flush areas thoroughly with water.
● Reconstitute each 4-mg vial with 4 ml sterile water for injection. Then dilute appropriate volume of reconstituted solution in either normal saline solution or D₅W before use.
● Bone marrow suppression (primarily neutropenia) is the dose-limiting toxicity of topotecan. The nadir occurs at about 11 days. If severe neutropenia occurs during therapy, reduce dose by 0.25 mg/m² for subsequent courses. Alternatively, administer G-CSF after the subsequent course (before dose is reduced) starting from day 6 (24 hours after completion of topotecan administration). Neutropenia isn't cumulative over time.
● Thrombocytopenia occurred with a median duration of 5 days and platelet nadir at a median of 15 days; anemia occurred with a median nadir at day 15. Blood or platelet (or both) transfusions may be necessary.
● Inadvertent extravasation with topotecan has been linked to only mild local reactions, such as erythema and bruising.

Patient monitoring
● Frequent monitoring of peripheral blood cell counts is necessary. Don't give patients subsequent courses of topotecan until neutrophil counts exceed 1,000 cells/mm³, platelet counts are more than 100,000 cells/mm³, and hemoglobin levels are 9 mg/dl (with transfusion if needed).

Pregnant patients
● Contraindicated during pregnancy.

Breast-feeding patients
● Because it isn't known whether drug appears in breast milk, avoid use of drug in breast-feeding women.

Pediatric patients
● Safety and efficacy in children haven't been established.

Patient education
● Instruct patient to promptly report sore throat, fever, chills, bruising, or unusual bleeding.
● Inform patient of need for frequent blood work to detect potential bone marrow suppression.

torsemide
Demadex

Pharmacologic classification: loop diuretic
Therapeutic classification: diuretic/anti-hypertensive
Pregnancy risk category: B

Indications and dosages
➤**Diuresis in patients with heart failure.** *Adults:* Initially, 10 to 20 mg P.O. or I.V. once daily. If response is inadequate, double the dose until response is obtained. Maximum dosage is 200 mg daily.
➤**Diuresis in patients with chronic renal failure.** *Adults:* Initially, 20 mg P.O. or I.V. once daily. If response is inadequate, double the dose until response is obtained. Maximum dosage is 200 mg daily.
➤**Diuresis in patients with hepatic cirrhosis.** *Adults:* Initially, 5 to 10 mg P.O. or I.V. once daily with an aldosterone antagonist or a potassium-sparing diuretic. If response is inadequate, double the dose until response is obtained. Maximum dosage is 40 mg daily.
➤**Hypertension.** *Adults:* Initially, 5 mg P.O. daily. Increase to 10 mg once daily in 4 to 6 weeks, if needed and tolerated. If response is still inadequate, add another antihypertensive.

How supplied
Available by prescription only
Solution: 2-ml ampule (10 mg/ml), 5-ml ampule (10 mg/ml)
Tablets: 5 mg, 10 mg, 20 mg, 100 mg

Pharmacodynamics
Diuretic and antihypertensive actions: Loop diuretics such as torsemide enhance excretion of sodium, chloride, and water by acting on the ascending portion of the loop of Henle. Torsemide doesn't significantly alter glomerular filtration rate, renal plasma flow, or acid-base balance.

Pharmacokinetics
Absorption: Absorbed with little first-pass metabolism; serum level reaches its peak within 1 hour after oral administration.

Distribution: Volume of distribution is 12 to 15 L in healthy patients and in those with mild to moderate renal failure or heart failure. In patients with hepatic cirrhosis, volume of distribution is about doubled. Drug is extensively (97% to 99%) bound to plasma protein.
Metabolism: Metabolized in the liver to an inactive major metabolite and to two lesser metabolites that have some diuretic activity; for practical purposes, metabolism terminates action of drug. Duration of action is 6 to 8 hours after oral or I.V. use.
Excretion: From 22% to 34% of dose is excreted unchanged in urine via active secretion of drug by the proximal tubules. The elimination half-life is about 3½ hours.

Route	Onset	Peak	Duration
P.O.	1 hr	1-2 hr	6-8 hr
I.V.	10 min	1 hr	6-8 hr

Contraindications and precautions
Contraindicated in patients hypersensitive to drug or other sulfonylurea derivatives and in patients with anuria. Use cautiously in patients with hepatic disease and associated cirrhosis and ascites.

Interactions
Drug-drug. *Aminoglycosides and other ototoxic drugs:* Auditory toxicity. Monitor patient carefully.
Cholestyramine: Decreased torsemide absorption. Separate administration by at least 3 hours.
Indomethacin, probenecid: Decreased diuretic effect. Avoid use together.
Lithium: Lithium toxicity. Monitor patient closely.
NSAIDs: Renal dysfunction. Use together cautiously.
Salicylates: Reduced salicylate excretion. Avoid use together.
Drug-herb. *Dandelion:* Possible interference with antidiuretic activity. Discourage concurrent use.
Licorice root: May contribute to the potassium depletion caused by thiazides. Discourage patient from using this herb.

Adverse reactions
CNS: asthenia, dizziness, headache, nervousness, insomnia, syncope.
CV: ECG abnormalities, chest pain, edema, *dehydration.*
EENT: rhinitis, sore throat.
GI: diarrhea, constipation, nausea, dyspepsia, *hemorrhage.*
GU: *excessive urination,* altered renal function test results.
Metabolic: electrolyte imbalance.
Musculoskeletal: arthralgia, myalgia.
Respiratory: *cough.*

Reactions may be *common,* uncommon, *life-threatening,* or COMMON AND LIFE-THREATENING.

Overdose and treatment
Although data specific to torsemide overdose are lacking, signs and symptoms would probably reflect excessive pharmacologic effect: dehydration, hypovolemia, hypotension, hyponatremia, hypokalemia, hypochloremic alkalosis, and hemoconcentration.

Treatment should consist of fluid and electrolyte replacement.

Special considerations
• Tinnitus and hearing loss (usually reversible) have been observed after rapid I.V. injection of other loop diuretics and have been noted after oral torsemide administration. Inject drug slowly over 2 minutes; single doses shouldn't exceed 200 mg.
• CV disease (especially in patients receiving cardiac glycosides) and diuretic-induced hypokalemia may be risk factors for the development of arrhythmias.
⚡ **ALERT** The risk of hypokalemia is greatest in patients with hepatic cirrhosis, brisk diuresis, inadequate oral intake of electrolytes, or concurrent therapy with corticosteroids or corticotropin. Perform periodic monitoring of serum potassium and other electrolytes.
• Excessive diuresis may cause dehydration, blood-volume reduction, and possibly thrombosis and embolism, especially in geriatric patients.

Patient monitoring
Monitor fluid intake and output, serum electrolyte levels, blood pressure, weight, and pulse rate during rapid diuresis and routinely with long-term use. If fluid and electrolyte imbalances occur, discontinue drug until the imbalances are corrected. Drug may then be restarted at a lower dose.

Breast-feeding patients
• It isn't known whether drug appears in breast milk. Use caution when administering drug to breast-feeding women.

Pediatric patients
• Safety and efficacy in children under age 18 haven't been established.

Geriatric patients
• Special dose adjustment usually isn't necessary. However, elderly patients are at greater risk for dehydration, blood-volume reduction, and possibly thrombosis and embolism with excessive diuresis.

Patient education
• Instruct patient to take torsemide in the morning to prevent nocturia and to change positions slowly to prevent dizziness.
• Instruct patient to report ringing in ears immediately because this may indicate toxicity.

tramadol hydrochloride
Ultram

Pharmacologic classification: synthetic derivative
Therapeutic classification: analgesic
Pregnancy risk category: C

Indications and dosages
➤ *Moderate to moderately severe pain.*
Adults: 50 to 100 mg P.O. q 4 to 6 hours, p.r.n. Maximum dosage is 400 mg daily.
✦ *Dosage adjustment.* In patients with creatinine clearance of less than 30 ml/minute, increase dosing interval to q 12 hours, to maximum of 200 mg daily. In patients with cirrhosis, recommended dosage is 50 mg q 12 hours.

How supplied
Available by prescription only
Tablets: 50 mg

Pharmacodynamics
Analgesic action: Mechanism of action is unknown. It's a centrally acting synthetic analgesic compound that isn't chemically related to opiates but is thought to bind to opioid receptors and inhibit reuptake of norepinephrine and serotonin.

Pharmacokinetics
Absorption: Almost completely absorbed. Mean absolute bioavailability of a 100-mg dose is about 75%.
Distribution: About 20% bound to plasma protein; it may cross the blood-brain barrier.
Metabolism: Extensively metabolized.
Excretion: About 30% of a dose is excreted unchanged in urine and 60% as metabolites. Half-life of drug is about 6 to 7 hours.

Route	Onset	Peak	Duration
P.O.	Unknown	2 hr	Unknown

Contraindications and precautions
Contraindicated in patients hypersensitive to drug; in patients experiencing acute intoxication with alcohol; and in those taking hypnotics, centrally acting analgesics, opioids, or psychotropic drugs.

Use cautiously in patients at risk for seizures or respiratory depression; in those with increased intracranial pressure or head injury, acute abdominal conditions, impaired renal or hepatic function; and in patients physically dependent on opioids.

Interactions
Drug-drug. *Carbamazepine:* Increases tramadol metabolism. Monitor patient closely. Dosage adjustment may be needed.
CNS depressants: Additive effects. Use together cautiously. Tramadol dose may need to be reduced.

MAO inhibitors, neuroleptic drugs: Increased risk of seizures. Monitor patient closely.
Drug-food. *Alcohol use:* Increased CNS depression. Advise patient to avoid alcohol.

Adverse reactions
CNS: *dizziness, vertigo, headache, somnolence, CNS stimulation, asthenia,* anxiety, confusion, coordination disturbance, euphoria, nervousness, sleep disorder, *seizures,* malaise.
CV: vasodilation.
EENT: visual disturbances.
GI: *nausea, constipation, vomiting,* dyspepsia, dry mouth, diarrhea, abdominal pain, anorexia, flatulence.
GU: urine retention, urinary frequency, increased creatinine clearance, proteinuria, menopausal symptoms.
Hematologic: decreased hemoglobin levels.
Hepatic: elevated liver enzyme levels.
Musculoskeletal: hypertonia.
Respiratory: *respiratory depression.*
Skin: *pruritus,* diaphoresis, rash.

Overdose and treatment
Cases of overdose have been reported. Serious potential consequences are respiratory depression and seizures. Because naloxone will reverse some, but not all, of the symptoms caused by tramadol overdose, supportive therapy is recommended. Hemodialysis removes only a small percentage of drug.

Special considerations
• Drug has been reported to reduce seizure threshold.
• Serious and rarely fatal anaphylactoid reactions have been reported (less than 1%).

Patient monitoring
• Monitor patient closely for seizures.
• Monitor patient's CV and respiratory status and stop dose if respirations decrease or rate is less than 12 breaths/minute or if patient exhibits signs of respiratory depression.
• Monitor patient for drug dependence. Because drug dependence similar to codeine or dextropropoxyphene can occur, the potential for abuse exists.

Pregnant patients
• Safe use during pregnancy hasn't been established.

Breast-feeding patients
• Use of drug in breast-feeding women isn't recommended.

Pediatric patients
• Safety and efficacy in children under age 16 haven't been established.

Geriatric patients
• Use cautiously in geriatric patients because serum levels are slightly elevated and the elimination half-life of drug is prolonged. Don't exceed daily dose of 300 mg in patients over age 75.

Patient education
• Instruct patient to take drug only as prescribed.
• Caution patient to avoid potentially hazardous activities that require mental alertness until adverse CNS effects of drug are known.

trandolapril
Mavik

Pharmacologic classification: angiotensin-converting enzyme (ACE) inhibitor
Therapeutic classification: antihypertensive
Pregnancy risk category: C (D in second and third trimesters)

Indications and dosages
➤ *Hypertension.* Adults: In patient not taking a diuretic, initially 1 mg for nonblack and 2 mg for black patient P.O. once daily. If control isn't adequate, dose can be increased at intervals of at least 1 week. Maintenance dosage ranges from 2 to 4 mg daily for most patients; there's little experience with doses of more than 8 mg. Patients receiving once-daily dosing at 4 mg may use b.i.d. dosing.
  For patient receiving a diuretic, initially 0.5 mg P.O. once daily. Subsequent dosage adjustment made based on blood pressure response.
➤ *Heart failure post-MI or left ventricular dysfunction post-MI. Adults:* Initially, 1 mg P.O. daily, adjusted to 4 mg P.O. daily. If patient can't tolerate 4 mg, continue at highest tolerated dose.
✦ *Dosage adjustment.* For hypertensive adults with creatinine clearance below 30 ml/minute, the usual initial dosage is 0.5 mg daily. In patients with hepatic cirrhosis, start at 0.5 mg daily.

How supplied
Available by prescription only
Tablets: 1 mg, 2 mg, 4 mg

Pharmacodynamics
Antihypertensive action: Although not fully understood, drug action is thought to result primarily from inhibition of circulating and tissue ACE activity, reducing angiotensin II formation, decreasing vasoconstriction, decreasing aldosterone secretion, and increasing plasma renin. Decreased aldosterone secretion leads to diuresis, natriuresis, and a small increase in serum potassium.

Pharmacokinetics
Absorption: Absolute bioavailability after oral administration of trandolapril is about 10% for

---

Reactions may be *common*, uncommon, *life-threatening*, or COMMON AND LIFE-THREATENING.

trandolapril and 70% for its metabolite, trandolaprilat.

Distribution: About 80% protein-bound.

Metabolism: Metabolized by the liver to the active metabolite, trandolaprilat, and at least seven other metabolites.

Excretion: About 66% excreted in feces; 33% in urine. Elimination half-lives of trandolapril and trandolaprilat are about 6 and 10 hours, respectively, but like all ACE inhibitors, trandolaprilat also has a prolonged terminal elimination phase.

Route	Onset	Peak	Duration
P.O.	Unknown	1-10 hr	24 hr

Contraindications and precautions
Contraindicated in patients hypersensitive to drug and in those with a history of angioedema related to previous treatment with an ACE inhibitor. Drug isn't recommended for use in pregnant women.

Use cautiously in patients with impaired renal function, heart failure, or renal artery stenosis.

Interactions
Drug-drug. *Diuretics:* Increased risk of excessive hypotension. Stop diuretic or lower dose of trandolapril.

Lithium: Lithium toxicity. Don't use together.

Potassium-sparing diuretics, potassium supplements: Increased risk of hyperkalemia. Monitor serum potassium closely.

Drug-herb. *Capsaicin:* Increased risk of cough. Discourage concomitant use.

Licorice: Possible sodium retention and increased blood pressure, interfering with therapeutic effects of ACE inhibitors. Discourage concomitant use.

Drug-food. *Salt substitutes that contain potassium:* Increased risk of hyperkalemia. Monitor serum potassium level closely.

Adverse reactions
CNS: dizziness, headache, fatigue, drowsiness, insomnia, paresthesia, vertigo, anxiety.

CV: chest pain, *AV first-degree block, bradycardia,* edema, flushing, hypotension, palpitations.

EENT: epistaxis, throat inflammation.

GI: diarrhea, dyspepsia, abdominal distention, abdominal pain or cramps, constipation, vomiting, *pancreatitis.*

GU: urinary frequency, increased creatinine clearance and BUN levels, impotence.

Hematologic: *neutropenia, leukopenia.*

Hepatic: elevated liver enzyme levels.

Metabolic: hyperkalemia, hyponatremia, hyperuricemia.

Respiratory: upper respiratory tract infection; dry, persistent, tickling, nonproductive cough; dyspnea.

Skin: rash, pruritus, pemphigus.

Other: decreased libido, *anaphylactoid reactions, angioedema.*

Overdose and treatment
It's thought that the effects of overdose are similar to those of other ACE inhibitors, with hypotension being the main adverse reaction. Because the hypotensive effect of trandolapril is achieved through vasodilation and effective hypovolemia, it's reasonable to treat trandolapril overdose by infusion of normal saline solution. In addition, renal function and serum potassium should be monitored. Trandolaprilat is removed by hemodialysis.

Special considerations
• Other ACE inhibitors have been linked to agranulocytosis and neutropenia.

• Angioedema of the tongue, glottis, or larynx may be fatal because of airway obstruction. Appropriate therapy, such as S.C. epinephrine 1:1,000 (0.3 to 0.5 ml) and equipment to ensure a patent airway, should be readily available.

• Obtain baseline CBC with differential counts before therapy, especially in patients who have collagen vascular disease with impaired renal function.

• If jaundice develops, discontinue drug. Although rare, ACE inhibitors have been linked to a syndrome of cholestatic jaundice, fulminant hepatic necrosis, and death.

Patient monitoring
• Assess patient's renal function before and periodically throughout therapy. Monitor serum potassium levels.

• Monitor patient for hypotension. Excessive hypotension can occur when drug is given with diuretics. If possible, discontinue diuretic therapy 2 to 3 days before starting trandolapril to decrease potential for excessive hypotensive response. If trandolapril doesn't adequately control blood pressure, diuretic therapy may be reinstituted with care.

Pregnant patients
• Drug is contraindicated for use during pregnancy.

Breast-feeding patients
• It isn't known whether drug appears in breast milk. Avoid use in breast-feeding women.

Pediatric patients
• Safety and efficacy in children haven't been established.

Patient education
• Advise patient to report signs of infection, easy bruising or bleeding; swelling of tongue, lips, face, eyes, mucous membranes, or limbs; difficulty swallowing or breathing; and hoarseness.

• Instruct patient to avoid products containing potassium, such as sodium substitutes.

• If syncope occurs, instruct patient to stop taking drug and notify prescriber immediately.

tranylcypromine sulfate
Parnate

Pharmacologic classification: MAO inhibitor
Therapeutic classification: antidepressant
Pregnancy risk category: C

Indications and dosages
➤ *Severe depression, panic disorder.*
Adults: 30 mg P.O. daily in divided doses. If there's no improvement after 2 weeks, increase daily dose by 10 mg q 1 to 3 weeks. Maximum dosage is 60 mg daily.

How supplied
Available by prescription only
Tablets: 10 mg

Pharmacodynamics
Antidepressant action: Endogenous depression is thought to result from low CNS levels of neurotransmitters, including norepinephrine and serotonin. Tranylcypromine inhibits effects of MAO, an enzyme that normally inactivates amine-containing substances, thus increasing their concentration and activity.

Pharmacokinetics
Absorption: Rapidly and completely absorbed from GI tract. Serum levels peak at 1 to 3 hours; onset of therapeutic activity may not occur for 3 to 4 weeks.
Distribution: Not fully understood. Dosage adjustments determined by therapeutic response and adverse reaction profile.
Metabolism: Metabolized in liver.
Excretion: Drug is excreted primarily in urine within 24 hours; some drug is excreted in feces via biliary tract. Half-life is 2½ hours. Enzyme inhibition prolonged and unrelated to half-life.

Route	Onset	Peak	Duration
P.O.	Unknown	1-3½ hr	≤ 10 days

Contraindications and precautions
Contraindicated in patients receiving MAO inhibitors, dibenzazepine derivatives, sympathomimetics (such as amphetamines), some CNS depressants (such as narcotics and alcohol), selective serotonin reuptake inhibitors, antihypertensives, diuretics, antihistamines, sedatives, anesthetics, bupropion hydrochloride, buspirone hydrochloride, dextromethorphan, or meperidine.

Also contraindicated in patients consuming foods with a high tyramine or tryptophan content or excessive quantities of caffeine; in those with a confirmed or suspected cerebrovascular defect, pheochromocytoma, history of liver disease, severe impairment of renal function, CV disease, hypertension, or history of headache; and in those undergoing elective surgery.

Use cautiously in patients with renal disease, diabetes, seizure disorders, Parkinson's disease, or hyperthyroidism; in those at risk for suicide; and in patients receiving antiparkinsonians or spinal anesthetics.

Interactions
Drug-drug. *Amphetamines, ephedrine, phenylephrine, phenylpropanolamine, other related drugs:* May result in serious CV toxicity. Don't use together.
Barbiturates, dextromethorphan, narcotics, other sedatives: Increased CNS depressant effects. Reduce dosage if concomitant use can't be avoided.
Cocaine, local anesthetics containing vasoconstrictors: May precipitate hypertension. Should be avoided.
Disulfiram: Possible tachycardia, flushing, or palpitations. Don't use together. If concomitant use can't be avoided, use cautiously.
General or spinal anesthetics normally metabolized by MAO inhibitors: Severe hypotension and excessive CNS depression. Tranylcypromine should be stopped for at least 1 week before using these drugs.
Local anesthetics (such as lidocaine, procaine): Decreased therapeutic effect; poor nerve block. Don't use together.
Meperidine: Circulatory collapse and death. Don't use together.
Tricyclic antidepressants: Enhanced adverse CNS effects. Wait at least 2 weeks before switching to these drugs.
Drug-herb. *Ginseng:* Possible adverse reactions, including headache, tremors, mania. Discourage concomitant use.
Drug-food. *Foods high in caffeine, tryptophan, tyramine:* Possible hypertensive crisis. Discourage use together.
Drug-lifestyle. *Alcohol use:* Potentiated CNS effects. Discourage use.

Adverse reactions
CNS: *dizziness,* headache, anxiety, agitation, paresthesia, drowsiness, weakness, numbness, tremor, jitters, confusion.
CV: *orthostatic hypotension, tachycardia,* paradoxical hypertension, palpitations, edema.
EENT: blurred vision, tinnitus.
GI: dry mouth, *anorexia,* nausea, diarrhea, constipation, abdominal pain.
GU: impotence, urine retention, elevated urinary catecholamine levels, impaired ejaculation.
Hematologic: anemia, *leukopenia, agranulocytosis, thrombocytopenia.*
Hepatic: elevated liver function test results, hepatitis.
Musculoskeletal: muscle spasm, myoclonic jerks.
Skin: rash.
Other: SIADH, chills.

Reactions may be *common*, uncommon, *life-threatening*, or COMMON AND LIFE-THREATENING.

Overdose and treatment

Signs and symptoms of overdose include exacerbations of adverse reactions or an exaggerated response to normal pharmacologic activity; such signs and symptoms become apparent slowly (24 to 48 hours) and may persist for up to 2 weeks. Agitation, flushing, tachycardia, hypotension, hypertension, palpitations, increased motor activity, twitching, increased deep tendon reflexes, seizures, hyperpyrexia, cardiorespiratory arrest, or coma may occur. Death has occurred with doses of 350 mg.

Treat symptomatically and supportively. Give 5 to 10 mg of phentolamine I.V. push for hypertensive crisis; treat seizures, agitation, or tremors with I.V. diazepam, tachycardia with beta blockers, and fever with cooling blankets. Monitor vital signs and fluid and electrolyte balance.

Special considerations

• Consider the inherent risk of suicide until significant improvement of depressive state occurs. Closely supervise high-risk patients during initial drug therapy. To reduce risk of suicidal overdose, prescribe smallest quantity of tablets consistent with good management.
• Tranylcypromine may have a more rapid onset of antidepressant effect compared with other MAO inhibitors (7 to 10 days versus 21 to 30 days). MAO activity also returns rapidly to pretreatment values.

Patient monitoring

• Watch closely for suicidal risk.
• Monitor patient for adverse effects.

Breast-feeding patients

• Safety in breast-feeding women hasn't been established.

Pediatric patients

• Drug isn't recommended for children under age 16.

Geriatric patients

• Drug isn't recommended for patients over age 60 because they have less compensatory reserve to cope with serious adverse effects of drug.

Patient education

• Warn patient to avoid taking alcohol, other CNS depressants, and self-prescribed drugs, such as cold, hay fever, or diet preparations, without medical approval.
• To minimize daytime sedation, tell patient to take drug at bedtime.
• Explain that many foods and beverages containing tyramine or tryptophan (such as wines, beer, cheeses, preserved fruits, meats, and vegetables) may interact with drug. A list of foods to avoid can be obtained from the hospital dietary department or pharmacy.

• Tell patient to avoid hazardous activities that require alertness until full effect of drug on CNS is known.
• Inform patient to lie down after taking drug and to avoid abrupt postural changes, especially when arising, to prevent dizziness induced by orthostatic blood pressure changes.
• Tell patient to take drug exactly as prescribed, not to double a missed dose, and not to stop taking drug abruptly. Patient should promptly report any adverse reactions. Dosage reduction can relieve most adverse reactions.
• Tell patient to inform dentist or other health care providers about the use of an MAO inhibitor.
• Inform patient to report severe headache, palpitations, tachycardia, sweating, tightness in throat and chest, dizziness, stiff neck, nausea, vomiting, or other unusual symptoms.
• Advise patient to store drug safely away from children.

trastuzumab
Herceptin

Pharmacologic classification: monoclonal antibody to human epidermal growth factor receptor 2 protein (HER2)
Therapeutic classification: antineoplastic
Pregnancy risk category: B

Indications and dosages

➤ *Single-agent treatment of metastatic breast cancer in patients whose tumors overexpress the HER2 protein and who have received one or more chemotherapy regimens for their metastatic disease, or with paclitaxel for metastatic breast cancer in patients whose tumors overexpress the HER2 protein and who haven't received chemotherapy for their metastatic disease.* Adults: Initial loading dose is 4 mg/kg I.V. over 90 minutes. If initial loading dose is well tolerated, maintenance dosage is 2 mg/kg I.V. weekly as a 30-minute I.V. infusion.

How supplied

Available by prescription only
Injection: lyophilized sterile powder containing 440 mg per vial

Pharmacodynamics

Antineoplastic action: Protein overexpression is observed in 25% to 30% of primary breast cancers. Drug is a recombinant DNA-derived monoclonal antibody that selectively binds to HER2, inhibiting the proliferation of human tumor cells that overexpress HER2.

Pharmacokinetics

Absorption: Administered I.V.
Distribution: Volume of distribution is about that of serum volume (44 ml/kg). Between weeks 16 and 32, serum levels reach steady state with

a mean trough of 79 mcg/ml and peak of 123 mcg/ml.

Metabolism: Not reported.

Excretion: Half-life and clearance are dose dependent. At the recommended dose, a mean half-life of 5¾ days (range 1 to 32 days) has been observed.

Route	Onset	Peak	Duration
I.V.	Unknown	Unknown	Unknown

Contraindications and precautions
Use cautiously in patients hypersensitive to drug or any of its components, in patients with cardiac dysfunction, and in the elderly.

Interactions
Drug-drug. *Anthracyclines:* Increased risk of cardiotoxicity. Avoid use together.
Paclitaxel: Increased trastuzumab levels. Monitor patient closely.

Adverse reactions
CNS: depression, *headache, dizziness, insomnia, asthenia,* neuropathy, paresthesia, peripheral neuritis.
CV: *heart failure, peripheral edema,* tachycardia, paroxysmal nocturnal dyspnea, cardiomyopathy, decreased ejection fraction.
EENT: *rhinitis, pharyngitis,* sinusitis.
GI: *anorexia, abdominal pain, diarrhea, nausea, vomiting.*
GU: urinary tract infection.
Hematologic: *leukopenia,* anemia.
Musculoskeletal: arthralgia, *back pain,* bone pain.
Respiratory: *dyspnea, increased cough.*
Skin: acne, herpes simplex, *rash.*
Other: *allergic reaction,* chills, edema, *fever, flu syndrome, infection, pain.*

Overdose and treatment
Not reported.

Special considerations
● Before beginning therapy, patients should undergo a thorough baseline cardiac assessment, including history and physical examination and other evaluation methods to identify those at risk of cardiotoxicity development.
● Drug should be used only in patients with metastatic breast cancer whose tumors have HER2 protein overexpression.
● A first-infusion symptom complex (chills or fever) was observed in about 40% of patients. Treat with acetaminophen, diphenhydramine, and meperidine (with or without reducing infusion rate). Other signs or symptoms may include nausea, vomiting, pain, rigors, headache, dizziness, dyspnea, hypotension, rash, and asthenia. These symptoms diminish with subsequent infusions.
● Stopping drug should be strongly considered in patients in whom a clinically significant decrease in left ventricular function develops.

Patient monitoring
● Monitor patient for dyspnea, increased cough, paroxysmal nocturnal dyspnea, peripheral edema, or S_3 gallop, especially if patient is receiving drug with anthracyclines and cyclophosphamide.
● Perform baseline cardiac evaluation including history, physical examination, and cardiac function tests.

Breast-feeding patients
● Because immunoglobulin G appears in milk and because the potential for harm to infant is unknown, advise women to discontinue breast-feeding during and for 6 months following therapy.

Pediatric patients
● Safety and efficacy in children haven't been established

Geriatric patients
● Risk of cardiac dysfunction may be increased in elderly patients.

Patient education
● Tell patient about risk of first-dose adverse effects.
● Instruct patient to notify prescriber immediately if signs or symptoms of cardiac dysfunction occur, such as shortness of breath, increased cough, or peripheral edema.

travoprost ophthalmic solution
Travatan

Pharmacologic classification: prostaglandin analogue
Therapeutic classification: antiglaucoma drug, ocular antihypertensive
Pregnancy risk category: C

Indications and dosages
➤ *Reduction of elevated intraocular pressure (IOP) in patients with open-angle glaucoma or ocular hypertension who are intolerant of other IOP-lowering drugs, or in patients who have had insufficient responses to other IOP-lowering drugs.*
Adults: One drop in conjunctival sac of affected eye once daily in evening.

How supplied
Available by prescription only
Ophthalmic solution: 0.004%

Pharmacodynamics
Exact mechanism of action unknown. Drug is thought to reduce IOP by increasing uveoscleral outflow.

Pharmacokinetics
Absorption: Absorbed through the cornea.

Reactions may be *common*, uncommon, ***life-threatening***, or COMMON AND LIFE-THREATENING.

Distribution: Plasma levels peak within 30 minutes following topical ocular administration.

Metabolism: Drug is an isopropyl ester prodrug, which is hydrolyzed by esterases in the cornea to its biologically active free acid. The active acid of drug reaching systemic circulation is primarily metabolized by the liver.

Excretion: Following ocular administration, travoprost free acid is rapidly eliminated from plasma within 1 hour.

Route	Onset	Peak	Duration
Oph-thelmic	Unknown	30 min	Unknown

Contraindications and precautions

Contraindicated in patients hypersensitive to travoprost, benzalkonium chloride, or other components. Not recommended for pregnant women or for women attempting to become pregnant.

Use cautiously in patients with renal or hepatic impairment, active intraocular inflammation (iritis, uveitis), or risk factors for macular edema. Also use cautiously in aphakic patients and pseudophakic patients with a torn posterior lens capsule.

Interactions

None reported.

Adverse reactions

CNS: anxiety, depression, headache.

CV: angina pectoris, *bradycardia,* chest pain, hypertension, hypotension.

EENT: *ocular hyperemia, decreased visual acuity, eye discomfort, foreign body sensation, eye pain, eye pruritus,* conjunctival hyperemia, abnormal vision, blepharitis, blurred vision, cataract, conjunctivitis, dry eye, eye disorder, iris discoloration, keratitis, lid margin crusting, photophobia, subconjunctival hemorrhage, tearing, sinusitis.

GI: dyspepsia, GI disorder.

GU: prostate disorder, urinary incontinence, urinary tract infection.

Metabolic: hypercholesterolemia.

Musculoskeletal: arthritis, back pain.

Respiratory: bronchitis.

Other: accidental injury, cold syndrome, infection, pain.

Overdose and treatment

Aside from ocular irritation and conjunctival hyperemia, ocular effects of drug at high doses are unknown. Treatment should be symptomatic if overdose occurs.

Special considerations

● Don't use in patients with angle closure glaucoma or inflammatory or neovascular glaucoma.

● Patient should remove contact lenses before administration of drug. Lenses may be reinserted 15 minutes after administration.

● If more than one ophthalmic drug is being used, the drugs should be administered at least 5 minutes apart.

● Store drug between 36° and 77° F (2° and 25° C).

Patient monitoring

● Temporary or permanent increased pigmentation of the iris and eyelid may occur, as well as increased pigmentation and growth of the eyelashes.

Pregnant patients

● If a pregnant woman or a woman attempting to become pregnant accidentally comes in contact with drug, thoroughly cleanse the exposed area with soap and water immediately.

Breast-feeding patients

● It's unknown whether drug appears in breast milk. Use cautiously in breast-feeding women.

Pediatric patients

● Safety and efficacy in children haven't been established.

Geriatric patients

● No overall differences in safety or effectiveness have been observed between elderly and other adult patients.

Patient education

● Teach patient how to instill drops, and advise him to wash hands before and after instilling solution. Warn him not to touch dropper or tip to eye or surrounding tissue.

● Tell patient receiving treatment in only one eye about the potential for increased brown pigmentation of the iris, eyelid skin darkening, and increased length, thickness, pigmentation, or number of lashes in the treated eye.

● Tell patient that, if eye trauma or infection occurs or if eye surgery is needed, he should seek medical advice before continuing to use the multidose container.

● Advise patient to immediately report conjunctivitis or lid reactions.

● Advise patient to apply light pressure on lacrimal sac for 1 minute after instillation to minimize systemic absorption of drug.

● Tell patient to remove contact lenses before administration of solution and that he can reinsert them 15 minutes after administration.

● Advise patient that, if more than one ophthalmic drug is being used, the drugs should be administered at least 5 minutes apart.

● Stress importance of compliance with recommended therapy.

● Tell patient to discard container within 6 weeks of removing it from the sealed pouch.

● If a pregnant woman or a woman attempting to become pregnant accidentally comes in contact with drug, tell her to thoroughly cleanse the exposed area with soap and water immediately.

trazodone hydrochloride
Desyrel

Pharmacologic classification: triazolopyridine derivative
Therapeutic classification: antidepressant
Pregnancy risk category: C

Indications and dosages
➤ *Depression. Adults:* Initial dosage is 150 mg daily in divided doses, which can be increased by 50 mg daily q 3 to 4 days. Average dosage ranges from 150 mg to 400 mg daily. Maximum dosage is 400 mg daily in outpatients; 600 mg daily in hospitalized patients.
➤ *Aggressive behavior* ◇. *Adults:* 50 mg P.O. b.i.d.
➤ *Panic disorder* ◇. *Adults:* 300 mg P.O. daily.

How supplied
Available by prescription only
Dividose tablets: 150 mg, 300 mg
Tablets (film-coated): 50 mg, 100 mg

Pharmacodynamics
Antidepressant action: Trazodone is thought to exert its antidepressant effects by inhibiting reuptake of norepinephrine and serotonin in CNS nerve terminals (presynaptic neurons), which enhances activity of these neurotransmitters in the synaptic cleft. Trazodone shares some properties with tricyclic antidepressants: It has antihistaminic, alpha-blocking, analgesic, and sedative effects as well as relaxant effects on skeletal muscle. Unlike tricyclic antidepressants, however, trazodone counteracts the pressor effects of norepinephrine, has limited effects on the CV system, and, in particular, has no direct quinidine-like effects on cardiac tissue; it also causes relatively fewer anticholinergic effects. Trazodone has been used in patients with alcohol dependence to decrease tremors and to alleviate anxiety and depression. Adverse reactions are somewhat dose-related; risk increases with higher dosages.

Pharmacokinetics
Absorption: Well absorbed from GI tract after oral administration. Taking drug with food delays absorption and increases amount absorbed by 20%.
Distribution: Widely distributed throughout the body. Drug isn't concentrated in any particular tissue, but small amounts may appear in breast milk. About 90% is protein-bound. Proposed therapeutic drug levels haven't been established. Steady state plasma levels are reached in 3 to 7

days, and onset of therapeutic activity occurs in 7 days.
Metabolism: Metabolized by the liver; more than 75% of metabolites are excreted within 3 days.
Excretion: Mostly excreted in urine; the rest is excreted in feces via the biliary tract.

Route	Onset	Peak	Duration
P.O.	Unknown	1-2 hr	Unknown

Contraindications and precautions
Contraindicated during initial recovery phase of MI or in patients hypersensitive to drug. Use cautiously in patients with cardiac disease and in those at risk for suicide.

Interactions
Drug-drug. *Antihypertensives, CNS depressants:* Additive effects of antihypertensives and CNS depressants. Monitor patient closely. Dosage adjustment may be needed.
Digoxin, phenytoin: Increased serum levels of digoxin and phenytoin. Monitor patient closely.
Drug-herb. *St. John's wort:* Increased risk of serotonin syndrome. Discourage concomitant use.
Drug-lifestyle. *Alcohol use:* Exacerbated CNS depression. Advise patient to avoid alcohol.

Adverse reactions
CNS: *drowsiness, dizziness,* nervousness, fatigue, confusion, tremor, weakness, hostility, anger, nightmares, vivid dreams, headache, insomnia, *generalized tonic-clonic seizures.*
CV: orthostatic hypotension, tachycardia, hypertension, prolonged conduction time on ECG, syncope.
EENT: blurred vision, tinnitus, nasal congestion.
GI: dry mouth, dysgeusia, constipation, nausea, vomiting, anorexia.
GU: urine retention; priapism, possibly leading to impotence; hematuria.
Hematologic: anemia, decreased WBC counts.
Hepatic: elevated liver function test results.
Metabolic: altered serum glucose levels.
Respiratory: shortness of breath.
Skin: rash, urticaria, diaphoresis.
Other: decreased libido.

Overdose and treatment
The most common signs and symptoms of drug overdose are drowsiness and vomiting; other signs and symptoms include orthostatic hypotension, tachycardia, seizures, respiratory arrest, ECG changes, priapism, headache, shortness of breath, dry mouth, and incontinence. Coma may occur.

Treatment is symptomatic and supportive and includes maintaining airway and stabilizing vital signs and fluid and electrolyte balance. Induce emesis if gag reflex is intact; follow with gastric lavage (begin with lavage if emesis isn't feasible) and activated charcoal to prevent further ab-

---

sorption. Forced diuresis may aid elimination. Dialysis usually isn't effective.

Special considerations
● Drug has fewer adverse cardiac and anticholinergic effects than tricyclic antidepressants.
● Consider the inherent risk of suicide until significant improvement of depressive state occurs.
● Tolerance to adverse effects (especially sedative effects) usually develops after 1 to 2 weeks of treatment.
● Drug may cause prolonged painful erections that may require surgical correction. An involuntary erection lasting more than 1 hour should be considered a medical emergency.
● Adverse effects are more common when doses exceed 300 mg daily.
● Don't withdraw drug abruptly.
● Discontinue drug at least 48 hours before surgical procedures.

Patient monitoring
● Closely monitor patients at high risk for suicide, especially during initial stage of drug therapy.
● Monitor blood pressure because hypotension may occur.

Pregnant patients
● Use drug during pregnancy only when potential benefits justify risk to fetus.

Breast-feeding patients
● Drug appears in breast milk; use cautiously in breast-feeding women.

Pediatric patients
● Drug isn't recommended for children under age 18.

Geriatric patients
● Elderly patients usually need lower initial doses because adverse reactions are more likely to develop. However, drug may be preferred in these patients because it has fewer adverse cardiac effects.

Patient education
● Tell patient that full effects of drug may not become apparent for up to 2 weeks.
● Tell patient to take drug exactly as prescribed.
● Instruct patient not to participate in activities that require mental alertness until full effects of drug are known.
● Tell patient to avoid alcoholic beverages and medicinal elixirs while taking drug.
● Advise patient to promptly report adverse reactions, including prolonged, painful erections; sexual dysfunction; dizziness; fainting; or rapid heartbeat.

tretinoin (systemic)
Vesanoid

Pharmacologic classification: retinoid
Therapeutic classification: antineoplastic
Pregnancy risk category: D

Indications and dosages
➤ *Induction of remission in patients with acute promyelocytic leukemia (APL), French-American-British classification M³ (including the M³ variant), characterized by the presence of the t(15,17) translocation or the presence of PML/RAR alpha gene, who are refractory to, or who have relapsed from, anthracycline chemotherapy or for whom anthracycline-based chemotherapy is contraindicated.* Adults and children age 1 and older: 45 mg/m² P.O. daily administered as two evenly divided doses until complete remission is documented. Discontinue therapy 30 days after achievement of complete remission or after 90 days of treatment, whichever occurs first.

How supplied
Available by prescription only
Capsules: 10 mg

Pharmacodynamics
Antineoplastic action: Exact mechanism of action of tretinoin is unknown. Tretinoin produces an initial maturation of primitive promyelocytes derived from the leukemic clone, followed by a repopulation of bone marrow and peripheral blood by normal, polyclonal hematopoietic cells.

Pharmacokinetics
Absorption: Well absorbed from the GI tract.
Distribution: About 95% is bound to plasma protein.
Metabolism: May induce its own metabolism.
Excretion: Excreted in urine and feces. Terminal elimination half-life is ½ to 2 hours.

Route	Onset	Peak	Duration
P.O.	Unknown	1-2 hr	Unknown

Contraindications and precautions
Contraindicated in patients hypersensitive to retinoids or parabens, which are used as preservatives in the gelatin capsule. Also contraindicated in pregnant or breast-feeding women.

Interactions
Drug-drug. *Ketoconazole:* Increased tretinoin plasma level. Use together cautiously.

Adverse reactions
CNS: *malaise,* dizziness, *paresthesia, headache, anxiety, insomnia, depression, confusion, cerebral hemorrhage,* intracranial hyper-

tension, agitation, hallucination, abnormal gait, agnosia, aphasia, asterixis, cerebellar edema, cerebellar disorders, *seizures, coma,* CNS depression, dysarthria, encephalopathy, facial paralysis, hemiplegia, hyporeflexia, hypotaxia, no light reflex neurologic reaction, spinal cord disorder, tremor, leg weakness, unconsciousness, dementia, forgetfulness, somnolence, slow speech.

CV: *chest discomfort, arrhythmias, heart failure,* hypotension, hypertension, peripheral edema, phlebitis, edema, *cardiac failure, cardiac arrest, MI,* enlarged heart, heart murmur, ischemia, *CVA,* myocarditis, pericarditis, secondary cardiomyopathy.

EENT: *ear fullness, visual disturbances, ocular disorders,* hearing loss, *mucositis.*

GI: *GI hemorrhage, nausea, vomiting, anorexia, abdominal pain, GI disorders, diarrhea, constipation, dyspepsia, abdominal distention,* hepatosplenomegaly, ulcer, unspecified liver disorder.

GU: *renal insufficiency, acute renal failure,* urinary frequency, dysuria, renal tubular necrosis, enlarged prostate.

Hematologic: leukocytosis, *hemorrhage, disseminated intravascular coagulation.*

Hepatic: elevated liver function study results, *hepatitis.*

Metabolic: acidosis, hypothermia, fluid imbalance, hypercholesterolemia, hypertriglyceridemia, *weight changes.*

Musculoskeletal: flank pain, *myalgia, bone pain,* bone inflammation.

Respiratory: *pneumonia, upper respiratory tract disorders, dyspnea, respiratory insufficiency, pleural effusion, crackles, expiratory wheezing,* lower respiratory tract disorders, pulmonary infiltrate, bronchial asthma, pulmonary or larynx edema, unspecified pulmonary disease, pulmonary hypertension.

Skin: *flushing, skin mucous membrane dryness, pruritus, decreased sweating, alopecia, skin changes.*

Other: *fever, infections, shivering, pain, injection site reactions, retinoic acid-APL syndrome, septicemia, multiorgan failure,* cellulitis, facial edema, pallor, lymph disorder, ascites.

Overdose and treatment

Not reported. Overdose with other retinoids has been linked to transient headache, facial flushing, cheilosis, abdominal pain, dizziness, and ataxia. These signs and symptoms have quickly resolved without apparent residual effects.

Special considerations

● Drug must be administered in a facility with laboratory and supportive services sufficient to monitor drug tolerance and protect and maintain patients compromised by drug toxicity.
● For women, a pregnancy test is required within 1 week before tretinoin therapy. When possi-

ble, therapy is delayed until a negative result is obtained.
● Patients with high WBC counts at diagnosis are at greater risk for rapid increases in WBC counts. Rapidly evolving leukocytosis is linked to a higher risk of life-threatening complications.
⚠ ALERT About 25% of patients given drug during clinical studies have experienced retinoic acid-APL syndrome, characterized by fever, dyspnea, weight gain, radiographic pulmonary infiltrates, and pleural or pericardial effusions. This syndrome has occasionally been accompanied by impaired myocardial contractility and episodic hypotension with or without leukocytosis. Some patients have died because of progressive hypoxemia and multiorgan failure. The syndrome generally occurs during the first month of therapy. Treatment with high-dose corticosteroids at the first signs of the syndrome may reduce morbidity and mortality risk.

Patient monitoring

● Monitor CBC and platelet counts regularly.
● Monitor patient, especially children, for symptoms of pseudotumor cerebri, such as papilledema, headache, nausea, vomiting, and visual disturbances.
● Monitor cholesterol and triglyceride levels and liver function studies.

Pregnant patients

● Drug use is contraindicated during pregnancy.

Breast-feeding patients

● It isn't known whether drug appears in breast milk. Because of the potential for serious adverse reactions in breast-fed infants, drug shouldn't be given to breast-feeding women.

Pediatric patients

● Safety and efficacy in children under age 1 haven't been established.

Patient education

● Instruct patient to report signs or symptoms of infection (fever, sore throat, fatigue) or bleeding (easy bruising, nosebleeds, bleeding gums, melena).
● Tell patient to record his temperature daily.

tretinoin (topical)
Avita, Renova, Retin-A, Retin-A Micro

Pharmacologic classification: vitamin A derivative
Therapeutic classification: antiacne
Pregnancy risk category: C

Indications and dosages
➤ *Acne vulgaris (especially grades I, II, and III). Adults and children:* Clean affected area and lightly apply solution once daily h.s. or as directed.

➤ *Treatment of photodamaged skin (wrinkles).* *Adults:* 0.05% solution or 0.025% to 0.1% cream applied daily for at least 4 months.
➤ *Mitigation of fine facial wrinkles, mottled hyperpigmentation and tactile roughness of facial skin in patients who use comprehensive skin care and sunlight avoidance programs.* Adults: 0.05% cream applied once daily, or apply a small, pearl-sized amount (¼ inch or 5 mm in diameter) of 0.02% cream to cover affected area lightly, once daily in the evening.

How supplied
Available by prescription only
Cream: 0.02%, 0.025%, 0.05%, 0.1%
Gel: 0.01%, 0.025%
Microsphere gel: 0.1%
Solution: 0.05%

Pharmacodynamics
Antiacne action: Mechanism of action of tretinoin hasn't been determined; however, it appears that tretinoin acts as a follicular epithelium irritant, preventing horny cells from sticking together and inhibiting the formation of additional comedones.

Pharmacokinetics
Absorption: Limited with topical use.
Distribution: None.
Metabolism: None.
Excretion: Minimal amount is excreted in the urine.

Route	Onset	Peak	Duration
Topical	Unknown	Unknown	Unknown

Contraindications and precautions
Contraindicated in patients hypersensitive to vitamin A or retinoic acid, and in pregnant women.
    Use cautiously in patients with eczema. Avoid contact of drug with eyes, mouth, angles of the nose, mucous membranes, or open wounds. Avoid use of topical preparations containing high levels of alcohol, menthol, spices, or lime because they may cause skin irritation. Avoid use of medicated cosmetics on treated skin. Use cautiously in patients that are on medications that increase photosensitivity (fluoroquinolones, thiazide diuretics, sulfonamides, phenothiazines).

Interactions
Drug-drug. *Topical drugs:* Risk of skin irritation. Avoid use together.
Drug-lifestyle. *Abrasive cleaners, medicated cosmetics, and skin preparations containing alcohol:* Increased risk of skin irritation. Tell patient to avoid use together.
Sun exposure: Potentiation of photosensitivity reactions. Advise patient to avoid prolonged or unprotected exposure to the sun.

Adverse reactions
Skin: peeling, erythema, blisters, crusting, hyperpigmentation, hypopigmentation, contact dermatitis.

Overdose and treatment
Not reported. Stop use and rinse area thoroughly. Oral ingestion of drug may lead to the same adverse effects as those linked to excessive oral intake of vitamin A.

Special considerations
● Discontinue drug if sensitization or extreme redness and blistering of skin occurs.
● Don't use drug in patients who can't or won't minimize sun exposure.
● Although tretinoin microsphere gel was developed to minimize dermal irritation, the skin of some patients may become excessively dry, red, swollen, blistered, or crusted.

Patient monitoring
● Therapeutic effect normally occurs in 2 to 3 weeks but may take 6 weeks or more. Relapses generally occur within 3 to 6 weeks of stopping medication.

Pregnant patients
● Drug use is contraindicated during pregnancy.

Breast-feeding patients
● It isn't known whether drug appears in breast milk. Because of the potential for serious adverse reactions in breast-fed infants, drug shouldn't be given to breast-feeding women.

Pediatric patients
● Safety and efficacy in children under age 1 haven't been established.

Patient education
● Advise patient on proper application technique. Stress importance of thorough removal of dirt and makeup before application and of hand washing after each use.
● Inform patient that application of medication may cause a temporary feeling of warmth and to promptly report discomfort.
● Advise patient that initial exacerbation of inflammatory lesions is common and that redness and scaling (usually occurring in 7 to 10 days) are normal skin responses that disappear when therapy is discontinued.
● Caution patient to minimize exposure to sunlight or ultraviolet light.
● Advise patient to keep medication away from eyes, mouth, angles of nose, and mucous membranes or open wounds.

triamcinolone (systemic)
Aristocort, Aristo-Pak, Kenacort

triamcinolone acetonide
Kenaject, Kenalog, Tac, Triam-A

triamcinolone diacetate
Amcort, Aristocort, Aristocort Forte, Aristocort Intralesional, Triam-Forte, Triamolone 40, Tristoject

triamcinolone hexacetonide
Aristospan Intra-articular, Aristospan Intralesional

Pharmacologic classification: glucocorticoid
Therapeutic classification: anti-inflammatory, immunosuppressant
Pregnancy risk category: C

Indications and dosages
➤ *Adrenal insufficiency.* triamcinolone.
Adults: 4 to 12 mg P.O. daily, in single or divided doses.
Children: 117 mcg/kg or 3.3 mg/m^2 P.O. daily, in single or divided doses.
➤ *Severe inflammation or immunosuppression.* triamcinolone. *Adults:* 8 to 16 mg P.O. daily, in single or divided doses.
Children: 416 mcg to 1.7 mg/kg or 12.5 to 50 mg/m^2 P.O. daily, in single or divided doses.
triamcinolone acetonide
Adults: Initially, 60 mg I.M. Additional doses of 20 to 100 mg may be given, p.r.n., at 6-week intervals. Alternatively, administer 2.5 to 15 mg intra-articularly, or up to 1 mg intralesionally, p.r.n.
Children ages 6 to 12: 0.03 to 0.2 mg/kg I.M. at 1- to 7-day intervals.
triamcinolone diacetate
Adults: 40 mg I.M. once weekly. Or, 2 to 40 mg intra-articularly, intrasynovially, or intralesionally q 1 to 8 weeks. Or, 4 to 48 mg P.O. divided into four doses.
Children: 0.117 to 1.66 mg/kg/day P.O. divided into four doses.
triamcinolone hexacetonide
Adults: 2 to 20 mg intra-articularly q 3 to 4 weeks, p.r.n. Or, up to 0.5 mg intralesionally per square inch of skin.
➤ *Systemic lupus erythematosus.* triamcinolone. *Adults:* 20 to 32 mg P.O. daily.
➤ *Acute rheumatic carditis.* triamcinolone. *Adults:* 20 to 60 mg P.O. daily.
➤ *Tuberculous meningitis.* triamcinolone. *Adults:* 32 to 48 mg P.O. daily.
➤ *Edematous states.* triamcinolone. *Adults:* 16 to 48 mg P.O. daily.
➤ *Collagen diseases.* triamcinolone. *Adults:* 30 to 48 mg P.O. daily.
➤ *Dermatologic disorders.* triamcinolone. *Adults:* 8 to 16 mg P.O. daily.

➤ *Allergic states.* triamcinolone. *Adults:* 8 to 12 mg P.O. daily.
➤ *Ophthalmic diseases.* triamcinolone. *Adults:* 12 to 40 mg P.O. daily.
➤ *Respiratory diseases.* triamcinolone. *Adults:* 16 to 48 mg P.O. daily.
➤ *Hematologic diseases.* triamcinolone. *Adults:* 16 to 60 mg P.O. daily.
➤ *Neoplastic diseases.* triamcinolone. *Adults:* 16 to 100 mg P.O. daily.

How supplied
Available by prescription only
triamcinolone
Syrup: 3 mg/ml, 4 mg/ml
Tablets: 4 mg, 8 mg
triamcinolone acetonide
Injection: 3 mg/ml, 10 mg/ml, 40 mg/ml suspension
triamcinolone diacetate
Injection: 25 mg/ml, 40 mg/ml suspension
triamcinolone hexacetonide
Injection: 5 mg/ml, 20 mg/ml suspension

Pharmacodynamics
Anti-inflammatory action: Triamcinolone stimulates the synthesis of enzymes needed to decrease the inflammatory response. It suppresses the immune system by reducing activity and volume of the lymphatic system, producing lymphocytopenia (primarily of T lymphocytes), decreasing immunoglobulin and complement levels, decreasing passage of immune complexes through basement membranes, and possibly depressing reactivity of tissue to antigen-antibody interactions.

Triamcinolone is an intermediate-acting glucocorticoid. The addition of a fluorine group in the molecule increases the anti-inflammatory activity, which is five times more potent than an equal weight of hydrocortisone. It has essentially no mineralocorticoid activity.

Triamcinolone may be administered orally. The diacetate and acetonide salts may be administered by I.M., intra-articular, intrasynovial, intralesional, sublesional, and soft-tissue injection. The diacetate suspension is slightly soluble, providing a prompt onset of action and a longer duration of effect (1 to 2 weeks). Triamcinolone acetonide is relatively insoluble and slowly absorbed. Its extended duration of action lasts for several weeks. Triamcinolone hexacetonide is relatively insoluble, is absorbed slowly, and has a prolonged action of 3 to 4 weeks. Don't administer any of the parenteral suspensions I.V.

Pharmacokinetics
Absorption: Absorbed readily after oral administration. After oral and I.V. administration, peak effects occur in about 1 to 2 hours. The suspensions for injection have variable onset and duration of action, depending on whether they're injected into an intra-articular space or a muscle, and on the blood supply to that muscle.

Reactions may be *common*, uncommon, *life-threatening*, or COMMON AND LIFE-THREATENING.

Distribution: Removed rapidly from the blood and distributed to muscle, liver, skin, intestines, and kidneys. Drug is extensively bound to plasma proteins (transcortin and albumin). Only the unbound portion is active. Adrenocorticoids are distributed into breast milk and through the placenta.

Metabolism: Metabolized in the liver to inactive glucuronide and sulfate metabolites.

Excretion: The inactive metabolites and small amounts of unmetabolized drug are excreted by the kidneys. Insignificant quantities of drug are also excreted in feces. Biologic half-life of triamcinolone is 18 to 36 hours.

Route	Onset	Peak	Duration
P.O., I.V., I.M., intra-lesional, intra-articular	Variable	Variable	Variable

Contraindications and precautions
Contraindicated in patients hypersensitive to any component of the formulation and in patients with systemic fungal infections.

Use cautiously in patients with GI ulcer, renal disease, hypertension, osteoporosis, diabetes mellitus, hypothyroidism, cirrhosis, diverticulitis, nonspecific ulcerative colitis, recent intestinal anastomosis, thromboembolic disorders, seizures, myasthenia gravis, heart failure, hepatitis, tuberculosis, ocular herpes simplex, emotional instability, or psychotic tendencies.

Interactions
Drug-drug. *Amphotericin B, diuretics:* Enhanced hypokalemia. Monitor patient closely.
Antacids, cholestyramine, colestipol: Decreased effect of triamcinolone. Dosage may need adjustment.
Barbiturates, phenytoin, rifampin: Decreased corticosteroid effects. Dosage may need adjustment.
Cardiac glycosides: Increased toxicity. Monitor patient closely.
Estrogens: Reduced metabolism of triamcinolone. Dosage may need adjustment.
Isoniazid, salicylates: Hyperglycemia. Dosage may need adjustment.
NSAIDs, ulcerogenic drugs: Increased risk of GI ulceration. Avoid use together.
Oral anticoagulants: Decreased anticoagulation. Monitor patient closely; dosage may need adjustment.

Adverse reactions
CNS: *euphoria, insomnia,* psychotic behavior, pseudotumor cerebri, vertigo, headache, paresthesia, *seizures.*
CV: *heart failure, thromboembolism,* hypertension, edema, *arrhythmias,* thrombophlebitis.
EENT: cataracts, glaucoma.

GI: *peptic ulceration,* GI irritation, increased appetite, *pancreatitis,* nausea, vomiting.
GU: menstrual irregularities, increased urine glucose and calcium levels.
Metabolic: hypokalemia, hyperglycemia, hypocalcemia, decreased T_3 and T_4 levels, hypercholesterolemia, carbohydrate intolerance.
Musculoskeletal: muscle weakness, osteoporosis.
Skin: delayed wound healing, acne, various skin eruptions.
Other: cushingoid state (moonface, buffalo hump, central obesity), hirsutism, susceptibility to infections; growth suppression in children; *acute adrenal insufficiency* with increased stress (infection, surgery, or trauma) or abrupt withdrawal after long-term therapy.

Overdose and treatment
Acute ingestion, even in massive doses, is rarely a clinical problem. Toxic signs and symptoms rarely occur if drug is used for less than 3 weeks, even at large doses. However, long-term use causes adverse physiologic effects, including suppression of the hypothalamic-pituitary-adrenal axis, cushingoid appearance, muscle weakness, and osteoporosis.

Special considerations
Recommendations for use of triamcinolone and for care and teaching of patients during therapy are the same as those for all systemic adrenocorticoids.

‼ **ALERT** Gradually taper dosage. After abrupt withdrawal, patient may experience rebound inflammation, fatigue, weakness, arthralgia, fever, dizziness, lethargy, depression, fainting, orthostatic hypotension, dyspnea, anorexia, and hypoglycemia. After prolonged use, sudden withdrawal may be fatal.
● Most adverse reactions to corticosteroids are dose- or duration-dependent.
● Triamcinolone suppresses reactions to skin tests; causes false-negative results in the nitroblue tetrazolium test for systemic bacterial infections; and decreases ^{131}I uptake and protein-bound iodine levels in thyroid function tests.

Patient monitoring
● Monitor patient for allergic reactions, adrenal insufficiency, and seizure activity.
● Monitor cardiac status.

Breast-feeding patients
● Use drug cautiously in breast-feeding women.

Pediatric patients
● Long-term use of drug in children and adolescents may delay growth and maturation.

Patient education
● Instruct patient to take drug exactly as prescribed and not to suddenly discontinue drug.

• Instruct patient to promptly report any adverse reactions or unusual symptoms.

---

triamcinolone acetonide (oral and nasal inhalant)
Azmacort, Nasacort, Nasacort AQ

Pharmacologic classification: glucocorticoid
Therapeutic classification: anti-inflammatory, antiasthmatic
Pregnancy risk category: C

Indications and dosages
➤ *Corticosteroid-dependent asthma.*
Adults: Two inhalations t.i.d. or q.i.d. Maximum dosage is 16 inhalations daily.
Children ages 6 to 12: One or two inhalations t.i.d. or q.i.d. Maximum dosage is 12 inhalations daily.
➤ *Rhinitis, allergic disorders, inflammatory conditions, nasal polyps.* *Adults:* Two sprays in each nostril daily; may increase to maximum of four sprays per nostril daily, if needed.
Children ages 6 to 12: One spray in each nostril once daily. Maximum dose is two sprays per nostril once daily.

How supplied
Available by prescription only
Nasal aerosol: 55 mcg/metered spray
Nasal spray: 120 actuations/bottle
Oral inhalation aerosol: 100 mcg/metered spray

Pharmacodynamics
Anti-inflammatory action: Glucocorticoids stimulate the synthesis of enzymes needed to decrease the inflammatory response. Triamcinolone acetonide is used as an oral inhalant to treat bronchial asthma in patients who require corticosteroids to control symptoms.

Pharmacokinetics
Absorption: Systemic absorption from the lungs is similar to oral administration.
Distribution: After oral inhalation, 10% to 25% is distributed to the lungs; the rest is swallowed or deposited within the mouth. After nasal use, only a small amount reaches systemic circulation.
Metabolism: Metabolized mainly by the liver. Some that reaches the lungs may be metabolized locally.
Excretion: The major portion of a dose is eliminated in feces. Biologic half-life of triamcinolone is 18 to 36 hours.

Route	Onset	Peak	Duration
Inhalation	Unknown	1-2 hr	Unknown

Contraindications and precautions
Oral form is contraindicated in patients hypersensitive to any component of the formulation and in those with status asthmaticus. Nasal form is contraindicated in patients with hypersensitivity or untreated localized infections.

Use oral form cautiously in patients with tuberculosis of the respiratory tract; untreated fungal, bacterial, or systemic viral infections; or ocular herpes simplex and in those receiving corticosteroids. Use both forms cautiously in breast-feeding women.

Interactions
None reported.

Adverse reactions
EENT: dry or irritated nose or throat, hoarseness.
GI: *oral candidiasis,* dry or irritated tongue or mouth.
Respiratory: cough, wheezing (oral form).
Other: facial edema (oral form).

Overdose and treatment
Not reported.

Special considerations
• Most adverse reactions to corticosteroids are dose- or duration-dependent.
• Recommendations for use of triamcinolone and for care and teaching of patients during therapy are the same as those for all inhalant adrenocorticoids.

Patient monitoring
• Monitor patient for symptom resolution.
• Monitor patient's respiratory status.

Breast-feeding patients
• Use drug cautiously in breast-feeding women.

Pediatric patients
• Safety and efficacy haven't been established for children under age 12 for nasal aerosol and under age 6 for oral aerosol.

Patient education
• Instruct patient to rinse mouth or gargle after inhaler use.
• Instruct patient to report lack of therapeutic effect or any adverse effects.

---

triamcinolone acetonide (topical)
Aristocort, Flutex, Kenalog, Kenalog in Orabase, Triacet, Triaderm*

Pharmacologic classification: topical adrenocorticoid
Therapeutic classification: anti-inflammatory
Pregnancy risk category: C

Indications and dosages
➤ *Inflammation of corticosteroid-responsive dermatoses.* *Adults and chil-*

---

dren: Apply cream, ointment, or lotion sparingly once to four times daily. Apply paste to oral lesions by pressing a small amount into lesion without rubbing until thin film develops. Apply b.i.d. or t.i.d. after meals and h.s. Spray aerosol for about 2 seconds from a distance of about 7.5 to 15 cm, three or four times daily.

How supplied
Available by prescription only
Cream, ointment: 0.025%, 0.1%, 0.5%
Lotion: 0.025%, 0.1%
Paste: 0.1%
Topical aerosol: 0.2 mg per 2-second spray

Pharmacodynamics
Anti-inflammatory action: Glucocorticoids stimulate the synthesis of enzymes needed to decrease the inflammatory response. Triamcinolone acetonide is a synthetic fluorinated corticosteroid. The 0.5% cream and ointment are recommended only for dermatoses refractory to treatment with lower levels.

Pharmacokinetics
Absorption: Absorption depends on potency of preparation, amount applied, and nature and condition of skin at application site. It ranges from about 1% in areas with a thick stratum corneum, such as the palms, soles, elbows, and knees, to as high as 36% in areas of the thinnest stratum corneum, such as the face, eyelids, and genitals. Absorption increases in areas of skin damage, inflammation, or occlusion. Some systemic absorption of steroids occurs, especially through the oral mucosa.
Distribution: Drug is distributed throughout the local skin layer. Drug absorbed into circulation is rapidly distributed into muscle, liver, skin, intestines, and kidneys.
Metabolism: Drug is metabolized primarily in the skin. The small amount that's absorbed into systemic circulation is metabolized primarily in the liver to inactive compounds.
Excretion: Inactive metabolites are excreted by the kidneys, primarily as glucuronides and sulfates, but also as unconjugated products. Small amounts of the metabolites are also excreted in feces.

Route	Onset	Peak	Duration
Topical	Unknown	Unknown	Unknown

Contraindications and precautions
Contraindicated in patients hypersensitive to drug.

Interactions
None reported.

Adverse reactions
Metabolic: *hyperglycemia, glycosuria.*
Skin: *burning, pruritus, irritation, dryness, erythema, folliculitis, hypertrichosis, hypopigmentation, acneiform eruptions, perioral*

dermatitis, allergic contact dermatitis, maceration, secondary infection, atrophy, striae, miliaria (with occlusive dressings).
Other: *hypothalamic-pituitary-adrenal axis suppression,* Cushing's syndrome.

Overdose and treatment
Not reported.

Special considerations
● Recommendations for use of triamcinolone acetonide and for care and teaching of patients during therapy are the same as those for all topical adrenocorticoids.

Patient monitoring
● Monitor patient for symptom resolution.
● Monitor patient's respiratory status.

Patient education
● Advise patient or family members of proper administration technique.
● If an occlusive dressing is ordered, advise patient not to leave it in place longer than 12 hours each day and not to use occlusive dressings on infected or exudative lesions.
● Tell patient to promptly report signs of systemic absorption, skin irritation or ulceration, hypersensitivity, infection, or no improvement.

---

triamterene
Dyrenium

Pharmacologic classification: potassium-sparing diuretic
Therapeutic classification: diuretic
Pregnancy risk category: B

Indications and dosages
➤ *Edema.* *Adults:* Initially, 100 mg P.O. b.i.d. after meals. Total daily dose shouldn't exceed 300 mg.

How supplied
Available by prescription only
Capsules: 50 mg, 100 mg

Pharmacodynamics
Diuretic action: Triamterene acts directly on the distal renal tubules to inhibit sodium reabsorption and potassium excretion, reducing potassium loss.

Triamterene is commonly used with other more effective diuretics to treat edema related to excessive aldosterone secretion, hepatic cirrhosis, nephrotic syndrome, and heart failure.

Pharmacokinetics
Absorption: Absorbed rapidly after oral administration, but the extent varies. Diuretic effect may be delayed 2 to 3 days if used alone; maximum antihypertensive effect may be delayed 2 to 3 weeks.

Distribution: About 67% protein-bound.
Metabolism: Metabolized by hydroxylation and sulfation.
Excretion: Excreted in urine; half-life of triamterene is 100 to 150 minutes.

Route	Onset	Peak	Duration
P.O.	2-4 hr	2-4 hr	7-9 hr

Contraindications and precautions

Contraindicated in patients receiving other potassium-sparing agents, such as spirolactone or amiloride hydrochloride; in those hypersensitive to drug; and in patients with anuria, severe or progressive renal disease or dysfunction, severe hepatic disease, or hyperkalemia.

Use cautiously in patients with impaired hepatic function or diabetes mellitus and in geriatric or debilitated patients.

Interactions

Drug-drug. *ACE inhibitors, such as captopril and enalapril; potassium-containing drugs, such as parenteral penicillin G; potassium-sparing diuretics; potassium supplements:* Increased risk of hyperkalemia. Monitor patient closely.
Antihypertensives: Enhanced hypoglycemia. Monitor patient closely. May be a therapeutic advantage.
Cimetidine: Increased bioavailability of triamterene. Monitor patient closely.
Lithium: Decreased lithium clearance. Avoid use together.
NSAIDs: Altered potassium excretion. Monitor patient closely.
Drug-herb. *Licorice root.* May contribute to potassium depletion caused by thiazides. Discourage use together.
Drug-food. *Potassium-containing salt substitutes, potassium-rich foods:* Increased risk of hyperkalemia. Discourage use together.
Drug-lifestyle. *Sun exposure:* Drug may cause photosensitivity reactions. Advise patient to avoid excessive sun exposure.

Adverse reactions

CNS: dizziness, weakness, fatigue, headache.
CV: hypotension.
GI: dry mouth, nausea, vomiting, diarrhea.
GU: transient elevation in BUN or creatinine levels, interstitial nephritis.
Hematologic: megaloblastic anemia related to low folic acid levels, *agranulocytosis, thrombocytopenia*.
Hepatic: jaundice, liver enzyme abnormalities.
Metabolic: *hyperkalemia*, acidosis, hypokalemia, azotemia.
Musculoskeletal: muscle cramps.
Skin: photosensitivity, rash.
Other: *anaphylaxis*.

Overdose and treatment

Signs include those indicative of dehydration and electrolyte disturbance. Treatment is supportive and symptomatic. For recent ingestion (less than 4 hours), empty stomach by induced emesis or gastric lavage. In severe hyperkalemia (more than 6.5 mEq/L), reduce serum potassium levels with I.V. sodium bicarbonate or glucose with insulin. A cation exchange resin, sodium polystyrene sulfonate (Kayexalate), given orally or as a retention enema, may also reduce serum potassium levels.

Special considerations

Consider the recommendations relevant to all potassium-sparing diuretics as well as the following:
● Drug is less potent than thiazides and loop diuretics and is useful as an adjunct to other diuretic therapy. Usually used with potassium-wasting diuretics. Full effect is delayed 2 to 3 days when used alone.
● To minimize excessive rebound potassium excretion, withdraw drug gradually.

Patient monitoring
● Monitor blood pressure, blood uric acid, CBC, blood glucose, BUN, and serum electrolyte levels.
● Watch for blood dyscrasia.

Pregnant patients
● Use drug during pregnancy only when potential benefits justify possible risk to fetus.

Breast-feeding patients
● Drug may appear in breast milk; safety during breast-feeding hasn't been established.

Pediatric patients
● Use cautiously; children are more susceptible to hyperkalemia.

Geriatric patients
● Elderly and debilitated patients need close observation because they're more susceptible to drug-induced diuresis and hyperkalemia. Reduced doses may be indicated.

Patient education
● To prevent serious hyperkalemia, warn patient to avoid excessive ingestion of potassium-rich foods, such as citrus fruits, tomatoes, bananas, dates, and apricots; potassium-containing salt substitutes; and potassium supplements.
● Advise patient to avoid direct sunlight, wear protective clothing, and use a sunblock to prevent photosensitivity reactions.
● Tell patient his urine may turn blue.
● Tell patient to promptly report weakness, sore throat, headache, fever, bruising, bleeding, mouth sores, nausea, vomiting, and dry mouth.

triazolam
Halcion

Pharmacologic classification: benzodiazepine
Therapeutic classification: sedative-hypnotic
Controlled substance schedule: IV
Pregnancy risk category: X

Indications and dosages
➤ *Insomnia. Adults:* 0.125 to 0.25 mg P.O. h.s.
(0.5 mg P.O. h.s. only in exceptional patients;
maximum dose is 0.5 mg).
Elderly patients: 0.125 mg P.O. h.s. May give up
to 0.25 mg.

How supplied
Available by prescription only
Tablets: 0.125 mg, 0.25 mg

Pharmacodynamics
Sedative-hypnotic action: Triazolam depresses the CNS at the limbic and subcortical levels of
the brain. It produces a sedative-hypnotic effect
by potentiating the effect of the neurotransmitter
gamma-aminobutyric acid on its receptor in the
ascending reticular activating system, which increases inhibition and blocks both cortical and
limbic arousal.

Pharmacokinetics
Absorption: Well-absorbed through the GI tract
after oral administration.
Distribution: Distributed widely throughout the
body. Drug is 90% protein-bound.
Metabolism: Metabolized in the liver primarily
to inactive metabolites.
Excretion: Metabolites are excreted in urine.
Half-life of triazolam ranges from about 1½ to
5½ hours.

Route	Onset	Peak	Duration
P.O.	15-20 min	1-2 hr	Unknown

Contraindications and precautions
Contraindicated in patients hypersensitive to benzodiazepines and in pregnant women. Also contraindicated in patients taking ketoconazole, itraconazole, nefazodone, or any other medications
that impair the oxidative metabolism of triazolam by cytochrome P-450 3A.
Use cautiously in patients with impaired renal or hepatic function, chronic pulmonary insufficiency, sleep apnea, mental depression, suicidal tendencies, or history of drug abuse.

Interactions
Drug-drug. *Antidepressants, antihistamines,
barbiturates, general anesthetics, MAO inhibitors, narcotics, phenothiazines:* Enhanced
CNS depressant effects. Avoid use together.
*Cimetidine, disulfiram, isoniazid, oral con-
traceptives:* Increased triazolam level. Monitor
patient carefully.

Erythromycin: Decreased triazolam clearance.
Monitor patient closely.
Haloperidol: Decreased haloperidol levels. Monitor patient closely.
Levodopa: Decreased levodopa effects. Avoid use
together.
Drug-herb. *Catnip, kava, lady's slipper, lemon
balm, passionflower, sassafras, skullcap, valerian:* Sedative effects may be enhanced. Discourage use together.
Drug-food. *Grapefruit juice:* Increased triazolam levels. Advise patient to use cautiously.
Monitor patient closely.
Drug-lifestyle. *Alcohol use:* Enhanced amnesia, excessive CNS depression. Advise patient to
avoid alcohol use.
Heavy smoking: Decreased triazolam effectiveness. Advise patient to avoid smoking.

Adverse reactions
CNS: *drowsiness, dizziness, headache,* rebound
insomnia, amnesia, light-headedness, lack of co-
ordination, mental confusion, depression, ner-
vousness, ataxia, minor changes in EEG patterns.
GI: nausea, vomiting.
Hepatic: elevated liver enzyme levels.
Other: physical or psychological dependence.

Overdose and treatment
Signs and symptoms of overdose include somnolence, confusion, hypoactive reflexes, dyspnea, labored breathing, hypotension, bradycardia, slurred speech, unsteady gait or impaired
coordination, and, ultimately, coma.
Support blood pressure and respiration until drug effects subside; monitor vital signs.
Flumazenil, a specific benzodiazepine antagonist,
may be useful. Mechanical ventilatory assistance
via endotracheal tube may be required to maintain a patent airway and support adequate oxygenation. Use I.V. fluids and vasopressors, such
as dopamine and phenylephrine, to treat hypotension as needed. If patient is conscious, induce emesis. Use gastric lavage if ingestion was
recent, but only if an endotracheal tube is present to prevent aspiration. After emesis or lavage,
administer activated charcoal with a cathartic as
a single dose. Don't use barbiturates if excitation
occurs. Dialysis is of limited value.

Special considerations
Consider the recommendations relevant to all
benzodiazepines as well as the following.
● Onset of sedation or hypnosis is rapid; patient
should be in bed when taking triazolam.

Patient monitoring
● Monitor liver and kidney function tests and perform blood counts regularly during long-term
therapy.

Breast-feeding patients
● Triazolam appears in breast milk. A breast-fed
infant may become sedated, have feeding diffi-

culties, or lose weight. Avoid use in breast-feeding women.

Pediatric patients
● Safety in children under age 18 hasn't been established.

Geriatric patients
● Geriatric patients are more susceptible to CNS depressant effects of drug and require supervision during start of therapy and after dosage increases.

Patient education
● Advise patient of the potential for physical and psychological dependence.
● Instruct patient not to take OTC drugs or to change medication regimen without medical approval.
● Advise patient that rebound insomnia may occur after stopping drug.
● Advise women to report suspected pregnancy immediately.
● Advise patient not to take triazolam when a full night's sleep and clearance of the drug from the body isn't possible before normal daily activities resume.

trifluoperazine hydrochloride
Apo-Trifluoperazine*, Solazine*, Stelazine, Terfluzine*

Pharmacologic classification: phenothiazine (piperazine derivative)
Therapeutic classification: antipsychotic, antiemetic
Pregnancy risk category: C

Indications and dosages
➤ *Anxiety states. Adults:* 1 to 2 mg P.O. b.i.d. Increase dosage, p.r.n., but don't exceed 6 mg daily.
➤ *Schizophrenia and other psychotic disorders. Adults:* For outpatients, 1 to 2 mg P.O. b.i.d., increased, p.r.n. For hospitalized patients, 2 to 5 mg P.O. b.i.d.; may increase gradually to 40 mg daily. For I.M. injection, 1 to 2 mg q 4 to 6 hours, p.r.n.
Children ages 6 to 12 (hospitalized or under close supervision): 1 mg P.O. daily or b.i.d. May increase dosage gradually to 15 mg daily. Or, give 1 mg I.M. once or twice daily.

How supplied
Available by prescription only
Injection: 2 mg/ml
Oral concentrate: 10 mg/ml
Tablets (regular and film-coated): 1 mg, 2 mg, 5 mg, 10 mg

Pharmacodynamics
Antipsychotic action: Trifluoperazine is thought to exert its antipsychotic effects by postsynaptic blockade of CNS dopamine receptors, inhibiting dopamine-mediated effects; antiemetic effects are attributed to dopamine receptor blockade in the medullary chemoreceptor trigger zone. Trifluoperazine has many other central and peripheral effects; it produces alpha and ganglionic blockade and counteracts histamine- and serotonin-mediated activity. Its most common adverse reactions are extrapyramidal; it has less sedative and autonomic activity than aliphatic and piperidine phenothiazines.

Pharmacokinetics
Absorption: Absorption varies with route of administration: Oral tablet absorption is erratic and variable, with onset of action ranging from ½ to 1 hour; oral concentrate absorption is much more predictable. I.M. drug is absorbed rapidly.
Distribution: Distributed widely throughout the body, including breast milk. Drug is 91% to 99% protein-bound; steady state serum levels are achieved within 4 to 7 days.
Metabolism: Metabolized extensively by the liver, but no active metabolites are formed.
Excretion: Mostly excreted in urine via the kidneys; some is excreted in feces by way of the biliary tract.

Route	Onset	Peak	Duration
P.O., I.M.	Unknown	2-4 hr	4-6 hr

Contraindications and precautions
Contraindicated in patients hypersensitive to phenothiazines or in patients with coma, CNS depression, bone marrow suppression, or liver damage.
  Use cautiously in elderly or debilitated patients; in those exposed to extreme heat; and in patients with CV disease, seizure disorders, glaucoma, or prostatic hyperplasia.

Interactions
Drug-drug. *Aluminum salts:* Increased GI absorption of trifluoperazine and decreased therapeutic effects. Administer 1 hour before or 2 hours after aluminum salts.
Barbiturates, lithium: Decreased phenothiazine effect. Monitor patient closely.
Beta blockers: Increased trifluoperazine levels and toxicity. Monitor patient closely.
Centrally acting antihypertensives, such as clonidine, guanabenz, guanadrel, guanethidine, methyldopa, and reserpine: Inhibition of blood pressure response. Monitor blood pressure.
CNS depressants: Enhanced CNS depression. Avoid use together.
Epinephrine: Further lowering of blood pressure. Monitor patient closely. Dosage adjustment may be necessary.
Lithium: Severe neurologic toxicity with an encephalitis-like syndrome, decreased therapeutic response to trifluoperazine. Avoid use together.

Reactions may be *common*, uncommon, *life-threatening*, or COMMON AND LIFE-THREATENING.

Propylthiouracil: Increased risk of agranulocytosis. Monitor patient closely.

Sympathomimetics: Decreased stimulatory and pressor effects. Monitor patient carefully.

Drug-food. *Caffeine:* Decreased therapeutic drug effects. Dosage adjustment may be necessary.

Drug-lifestyle. *Alcohol use:* Additive effects. Advise patient to avoid alcohol.

Smoking: Decreased therapeutic effects. Discourage use together.

Sun exposure: Increased photosensitivity reactions. Advise patient to avoid sun exposure.

Adverse reactions

CNS: *neuroleptic malignant syndrome, extrapyramidal reactions, tardive dyskinesia,* pseudoparkinsonism, dizziness, drowsiness, insomnia, fatigue, headache.

CV: *orthostatic hypotension,* tachycardia, ECG changes.

EENT: ocular changes, *blurred vision.*

GI: *dry mouth, constipation,* nausea.

GU: *urine retention,* menstrual irregularities.

Hematologic: transient leukopenia, *agranulocytosis.*

Hepatic: cholestatic jaundice, elevated liver function test results.

Metabolic: weight gain.

Skin: *photosensitivity,* allergic reactions, pain at I.M. injection site, sterile abscess, rash.

Other: gynecomastia, inhibited lactation.

Overdose and treatment

CNS depression is characterized by deep, unarousable sleep and possible coma, hypotension or hypertension, extrapyramidal symptoms, dystonia, abnormal involuntary muscle movements, agitation, seizures, arrhythmias, ECG changes, hypothermia or hyperthermia, and autonomic nervous system dysfunction.

Treatment is symptomatic and supportive and includes maintaining vital signs, airway, stable body temperature, and fluid and electrolyte balance.

Don't induce vomiting. Drug inhibits cough reflex, and aspiration may occur. Use gastric lavage, then activated charcoal and sodium chloride cathartics; dialysis is usually ineffective. Regulate body temperature as needed. Treat hypotension with I.V. fluids. Don't give epinephrine. Treat seizures with parenteral diazepam or barbiturates, arrhythmias with parenteral phenytoin (1 mg/kg with rate titrated to blood pressure), and extrapyramidal reactions with benztropine at 1 to 2 mg or parenteral diphenhydramine at 10 to 50 mg.

Special considerations

● Benzodiazepines are preferred for the treatment of anxiety. When trifluoperazine is given for anxiety, don't exceed 6 mg daily for longer than 12 weeks.

● Drug is linked to a high risk of extrapyramidal symptoms and photosensitivity reactions.

● Taper dose gradually. After abrupt withdrawal of long-term therapy, patient may experience gastritis, nausea, vomiting, dizziness, tremor, feeling of warmth or cold, diaphoresis, tachycardia, headache, insomnia, anorexia, muscle rigidity, altered mental status, and evidence of autonomic instability.

● Worsening anginal pain has been reported in patients receiving trifluoperazine; however, ECG reactions are less common with drug than with other phenothiazines.

● Liquid and injectable formulations may cause a rash after contact with skin.

● Drug may cause pink to brown discoloration of urine or blue-gray skin.

● Drug causes false-positive test results for urine porphyrins, urobilinogen, amylase, and 5-hydroxyindoleacetic acid levels from darkening of urine by metabolites; it also causes false-positive urine pregnancy results in tests using human chorionic gonadotropin as the indicator.

Patient monitoring

● Monitor blood pressure before and after parenteral administration

● Monitor patient regularly for abnormal body movements (at least once every 6 months).

Breast-feeding patients

● Drug may appear in breast milk. Potential benefits to the woman should outweigh the potential harm to the infant.

Pediatric patients

● Not recommended for children under age 6.

Geriatric patients

● Elderly patients tend to need lower doses, adjusted to effect. Adverse effects, especially tardive dyskinesia and other extrapyramidal effects and hypotension, are more likely to develop in such patients.

Patient education

● Explain risks of dystonic reactions, akathisia, and tardive dyskinesia, and tell patient to report abnormal body movements.

● Explain that many drug interactions are possible. Tell patient to seek medical approval before taking any other medication.

● Warn patient against hazardous activities that require alertness until the effect of drug is established.

● Tell patient to avoid sun exposure and to avoid exposure to temperature extremes because drug may cause thermoregulatory changes.

● Tell patient to take drug exactly as prescribed and to avoid alcohol and other medications that may cause excessive sedation.

trihexyphenidyl hydrochloride

Apo-Trihex*, Artane, Artane Sequels, Trihexy-2, Trihexy-5

Pharmacologic classification: anticholinergic
Therapeutic classification: antiparkinsonian
Pregnancy risk category: C

Indications and dosages

➤ *Idiopathic parkinsonism. Adults:* 1 mg P.O. on first day, 2 mg on second day, then increase 2 mg q 3 to 5 days until total of 6 to 10 mg is given daily. Usually given t.i.d. with meals and, if needed, q.i.d. (last dose should be before bedtime). Postencephalitic parkinsonism may require 12 to 15 mg total daily dose. Patients receiving levodopa may need 3 to 6 mg daily. Sustained-release capsules shouldn't be used as initial therapy, but after the patient has been stabilized on the conventional dose forms. Sustained-release capsules can be dosed on a mg-per-mg basis and administered as a single dose after breakfast or in two divided doses 12 hours apart.
➤ *Drug-induced parkinsonism. Adults:* 5 to 15 mg daily.

How supplied

Available by prescription only
Capsules (sustained-release): 5 mg
Elixir: 2 mg/5 ml
Tablets: 2 mg, 5 mg

Pharmacodynamics

Antiparkinsonian action: Trihexyphenidyl blocks central cholinergic receptors, helping to balance cholinergic activity in the basal ganglia. It may also prolong the effects of dopamine by blocking dopamine reuptake and storage at central receptor sites.

Pharmacokinetics

Absorption: Rapidly absorbed after oral administration.
Distribution: Crosses the blood-brain barrier; little else is known about its distribution.
Metabolism: Exact metabolic fate is unknown.
Excretion: Excreted in urine as unchanged drug and metabolites.

Route	Onset	Peak	Duration
P.O.	1 hr	Unknown	6-12 hr

Contraindications and precautions

Contraindicated in patients hypersensitive to drug. Use cautiously in patients with impaired renal, cardiac, or hepatic function, glaucoma, obstructive disease of the GI or GU tract, or prostatic hyperplasia.

Interactions

Drug-drug. *Amantadine:* Amplified anticholinergic adverse effects, including confusion and hallucinations. Reduce trihexyphenidyl dose before giving amantadine.
Antacids, antidiarrheals: May decrease absorption of trihexyphenidyl. Monitor patient closely. Dosage adjustment may be needed.
CNS depressants, including tranquilizers and sedative-hypnotics: Increased sedative effects. Avoid use together.
Haloperidol, phenothiazines: Decreased antipsychotic effectiveness. Dosage adjustment may be needed.
Levodopa: Synergistic anticholinergic effects, enhanced GI metabolism of levodopa. Monitor patient closely. Dosage adjustment may be needed
Phenothiazine: Increased risk of anticholinergic adverse effects. Adjust dosage as needed.
Drug-lifestyle. *Alcohol use:* Increased sedative effects. Advise patient to avoid alcohol.

Adverse reactions

CNS: nervousness, dizziness, headache, hallucinations, drowsiness, weakness.
CV: tachycardia, palpitations, hypotension, orthostatic hypotension.
EENT: blurred vision, mydriasis, increased intraocular pressure.
GI: *dry mouth, nausea,* constipation, vomiting.
GU: urinary hesitancy, urine retention.

Overdose and treatment

Signs and symptoms of overdose include central stimulation followed by depression, with such psychotic symptoms as disorientation, confusion, hallucinations, delusions, anxiety, agitation, and restlessness. Peripheral effects may include dilated, nonreactive pupils; blurred vision; flushed, dry, hot skin; dry mucous membranes; dysphagia; decreased or absent bowel sounds; urine retention; hyperthermia; headache; tachycardia; hypertension; and increased respiration.

Treatment is primarily symptomatic and supportive. Maintain patent airway. If the patient is alert, induce emesis (or use gastric lavage) and follow with sodium chloride cathartic and activated charcoal to prevent further drug absorption. In severe cases, physostigmine may be administered to block antimuscarinic effects of trihexyphenidyl. Give fluids, as needed, to treat shock; diazepam to control psychotic symptoms; and pilocarpine (instilled into the eyes) to relieve mydriasis. If urine retention occurs, catheterization may be necessary.

Special considerations

Consider the recommendations relevant to all anticholinergics as well as the following.
● Tolerance may develop to drug, necessitating higher doses.
● Use drug cautiously in hot weather due to the increased risk of heat prostration.

Patient monitoring

● Monitor patient for urinary hesitancy.

Reactions may be *common*, uncommon, *life-threatening*, or COMMON AND LIFE-THREATENING.

- Obtain gonioscopic evaluation and close intraocular pressure monitoring, especially in patients over age 40.

Breast-feeding patients
- Drug may appear in breast milk, possibly resulting in infant toxicity. It may also decrease milk production. Use cautiously in breast-feeding women.

Geriatric patients
- Use caution when administering drug to elderly patients. Lower doses are indicated.

Patient education
- Tell patient to avoid activities that require alertness until CNS effects of drug are known.
- Advise patient to report signs of urinary hesitation or urine retention.
- Tell patient to take drug with food if GI upset occurs.

trimethobenzamide hydrochloride
Tebamide, T-Gen, Ticon, Tigan, Trimazide

Pharmacologic classification: ethanolamine-related antihistamine
Therapeutic classification: antiemetic
Pregnancy risk category: C

Indications and dosages
➤ *Nausea and vomiting. Adults:* 250 mg P.O. t.i.d. or q.i.d. Or, 200 mg I.M. or P.R. t.i.d. or q.i.d.
Children who weigh 14 to 41 kg (30 to 90 lb): 100 to 200 mg P.O. or P.R. t.i.d. or q.i.d.
Children who weigh less than 14 kg: 100 mg P.R. t.i.d. or q.i.d.

How supplied
Available by prescription only
Capsules: 100 mg, 250 mg
Injection: 100 mg/ml
Suppositories: 100 mg, 200 mg

Pharmacodynamics
Antiemetic action: Trimethobenzamide is a weak antihistamine with limited antiemetic properties. Its exact mechanism of action is unknown. Drug effects may occur in the chemoreceptor trigger zone of the brain; however, drug apparently doesn't inhibit direct impulses to the vomiting center.

Pharmacokinetics
Absorption: About 60% of an oral dose is absorbed.
Distribution: Unknown.
Metabolism: About 50% to 70% of dose is metabolized, probably in the liver.

Excretion: Excreted in urine and feces.

Route	Onset	Peak	Duration
P.O.	10-20 min	Unknown	3-4 hr
I.M.	15-35 min	Unknown	2-3 hr
P.R.	Unknown	Unknown	Unknown

Contraindications and precautions
Contraindicated in patients hypersensitive to drug. Suppositories are contraindicated in patients hypersensitive to benzocaine hydrochloride or similar local anesthetic. Parenteral form is contraindicated in children, and suppositories are contraindicated in premature infants and neonates. Use cautiously in children and when used during acute febrile illness.

Interactions
Drug-drug. *CNS depressants, including antihypertensives, belladonna alkaloids, phenothiazines, and tricyclic antidepressants:* Increased trimethobenzamide toxicity. Avoid use together.
Drug-lifestyle. *Alcohol use:* Increased sedative effects. Discourage use together.

Adverse reactions
CNS: *drowsiness,* dizziness, headache, disorientation, depression, parkinsonian-like symptoms, *coma, seizures.*
CV: hypotension.
EENT: blurred vision.
GI: diarrhea.
Hepatic: jaundice.
Musculoskeletal: muscle cramps.
Other: *hypersensitivity reactions* (pain, stinging, burning, redness, swelling at I.M. injection site).

Overdose and treatment
Signs and symptoms of overdose may include severe neurologic reactions, such as opisthotonos, seizures, coma, and extrapyramidal reactions.
    Discontinue drug and provide supportive care.

Special considerations
- Drug may be less effective against severe vomiting than other agents.
- Drug has little or no value in treating motion sickness.

Patient monitoring
- Monitor patient for hypersensitivity reactions.
- Monitor patient for relief of symptoms.

Pregnant patients
- Safety during pregnancy hasn't been established.

Breast-feeding patients
- Safety in breast-feeding women hasn't been established.

Pediatric patients
- Use drug cautiously in children. Don't administer to children with viral illness because drug may contribute to development of Reye's syn-

drome. Don't use in newborn or premature infants.

Geriatric patients
• Use drug cautiously in elderly patients because they may be more susceptible to adverse CNS effects.

Patient education
• Warn patient to avoid hazardous activities that require alertness because drug may cause drowsiness, and to avoid consuming alcohol to prevent additive sedation.
• Instruct patient to report persistent vomiting.
• Instruct patient on proper administration and storage of suppositories.

trimethoprim
Primsol, Proloprim, Trimpex

Pharmacologic classification: synthetic folate antagonist
Therapeutic classification: antibiotic
Pregnancy risk category: C

Indications and dosages
➤ *Treatment of uncomplicated urinary tract infections. Adults:* 100 mg P.O. q 12 hours or 200 mg q 24 hours for 10 days.
➤ *Acute otitis media caused by susceptible strains of* Streptococcus pneumoniae *or* Haemophilus influenzae. Primsol. *Children age 6 months or older:* 10 mg/kg/day in divided doses q 12 hours for 10 days.
➤ *Prophylaxis of chronic and recurrent urinary tract infections◇. Adults:* 100 mg P.O. h.s. for 6 weeks to 6 months.
➤ *Traveler's diarrhea◇. Adults:* 200 mg P.O. b.i.d. for 3 to 5 days.
➤ *Pneumocystis carinii pneumonia◇. Adults:* 5 mg/kg P.O. t.i.d. with dapsone 100 mg daily for 21 days.
✦ *Dosage adjustment.* If creatinine clearance is 15 to 30 ml/minute, give 50 mg every 12 hours. If creatinine clearance is less than 15 ml/minute, manufacturer doesn't recommend use of this drug.

How supplied
Available by prescription only
Oral solution: 50 mg/5 ml
Tablets: 100 mg, 200 mg

Pharmacodynamics
Antibacterial action: By interfering with action of dihydrofolate reductase, drug inhibits bacterial synthesis of folic acid. Drug is effective against many gram-positive and gram-negative organisms, including most Enterobacteriaceae organisms (except *Pseudomonas*), *Proteus mirabilis, Klebsiella,* and *Escherichia coli.* Trimethoprim is usually bactericidal.

Pharmacokinetics
Absorption: Absorbed quickly and completely.
Distribution: Widely distributed. About 42% to 46% of dose is plasma protein-bound.
Metabolism: Less than 20% of dose is metabolized in the liver.
Excretion: Most of dose is excreted in urine via filtration and secretion. In patients with normal renal function, elimination half-life is 8 to 11 hours; in patients with impaired renal function, half-life is prolonged.

Route	Onset	Peak	Duration
P.O.	Unknown	1-4 hr	Unknown

Contraindications and precautions
Contraindicated in patients hypersensitive to drug and in those with megaloblastic anemia caused by folate deficiency. Use cautiously in patients with folate deficiency and impaired hepatic or renal function, especially those with creatinine clearance of 15 ml/minute or less.

Interactions
Drug-drug. *Phenytoin:* Increased serum phenytoin levels. Monitor patient closely.

Adverse reactions
GI: *epigastric distress, nausea, vomiting,* glossitis.
GU: increased BUN and serum creatinine levels.
Hematologic: *thrombocytopenia, leukopenia,* megaloblastic anemia, methemoglobinemia.
Hepatic: elevated liver enzyme levels.
Skin: *rash, pruritus,* exfoliative dermatitis.
Other: fever.

Overdose and treatment
Effects of acute overdose include nausea, vomiting, dizziness, headache, confusion, and bone marrow depression. Treatment includes gastric lavage and supportive measures. Urine may be acidified to enhance drug elimination.

Effects of chronic toxicity caused by prolonged high-dose therapy include bone marrow depression, leukopenia, thrombocytopenia, and megaloblastic anemia. Treatment includes drug discontinuation and administration of leucovorin, 3 to 6 mg I.M. daily for 3 days or 5 to 15 mg P.O. daily until normal hematopoiesis returns.

Special considerations
⚠ **ALERT** Trimethoprim is also used with sulfamethoxazole. Don't confuse the two products.
• Obtain urine specimen for culture and sensitivity tests before starting therapy.
• Drug is usually used with other antibiotics, especially sulfamethoxazole, because resistance develops rapidly when used alone.
• Advanced age, malnourishment, pregnancy, debilitation, renal impairment, and prolonged high-dose therapy increase risk of hematologic toxicity, as does use of drug with folate antagonist drugs such as phenytoin.

Reactions may be common, uncommon, ***life-threatening****, or* COMMON AND LIFE-THREATENING.

● Trimethoprim may falsely elevate creatinine values when the Jaffé reaction is used.

Patient monitoring
● If patient is receiving drug with phenytoin, monitor serum phenytoin levels.
● Sore throat, fever, pallor, and purpura may be early signs and symptoms of serious blood disorders. Monitor blood counts regularly.

Pregnant patients
● Use drug during pregnancy only when benefits justify risk to fetus.

Breast-feeding patients
● Drug appears in breast milk; alternative feeding method is recommended during trimethoprim therapy.

Pediatric patients
● Safety in children under age 2 months hasn't been established. Efficacy in children under age 12 hasn't been established. Drug isn't recommended for children under age 12.

Geriatric patients
● These patients may be more susceptible to hematologic toxicity.

Patient education
● Instruct patient to continue taking drug as directed, until course of therapy is completed.
● Advise patient to report signs or symptoms of blood disorders.

trimipramine maleate
Surmontil

Pharmacologic classification: tricyclic antidepressant
Therapeutic classification: antidepressant, antianxiety
Pregnancy risk category: C

Indications and dosages
➤ *Depression. Adults:* For outpatients, 75 mg P.O. daily in divided doses, increased to 200 mg daily. Maintenance dosage is 50 to 150 mg daily. For inpatients, 100 mg daily in divided doses, increased p.r.n. Maximum dosage is 300 mg daily. *Elderly patients and adolescents:* 50 to 100 mg P.O. daily.

How supplied
Available by prescription only
Capsules: 25 mg, 50 mg, 100 mg

Pharmacodynamics
Antidepressant action: Trimipramine is thought to exert its antidepressant effects by equally inhibiting reuptake of norepinephrine and serotonin in CNS nerve terminals (presynaptic neurons), which results in increased concentration

and enhanced activity of these neurotransmitters in the synaptic cleft. Trimipramine also has anxiolytic effects and inhibits gastric acid secretion.

Pharmacokinetics
Absorption: Absorbed rapidly from the GI tract after oral administration.
Distribution: Distributed widely throughout the body. Drug is 90% protein-bound; steady state occurs within 7 days.
Metabolism: Metabolized by the liver; a significant first-pass effect may explain variability of serum levels in different patients taking the same dose.
Excretion: Mostly excreted in urine; some is excreted in feces by way of the biliary tract.

Route	Onset	Peak	Duration
P.O.	Unknown	2 hr	Unknown

Contraindications and precautions
Contraindicated in patients hypersensitive to drug, in patients who have taken an MAO inhibitor within 14 days, and in patients who are in the acute recovery phase of MI.

Use cautiously in adolescents, elderly or debilitated patients, patients receiving thyroid medications, and patients with CV disease, increased intraocular pressure, hyperthyroidism, impaired hepatic function, or a history of seizures, urine retention, or angle-closure glaucoma.

Interactions
Drug-drug. *Antiarrhythmics (such as disopyramide, procainamide, and quinidine), pimozide, thyroid medication:* Increased risk of arrhythmias and conduction defects. Monitor patient closely.
Anticholinergics, including antihistamines, antiparkinsonians, atropine, meperidine, and phenothiazines: May cause oversedation, paralytic ileus, visual changes, and severe constipation. Monitor patient.
Barbiturates: Decreased trimipramine therapeutic efficacy. Dosage adjustment may be necessary.
Beta blockers, cimetidine, methylphenidate, oral contraceptives, propoxyphene: Increased trimipramine plasma levels and toxicity. Monitor patient closely.
Centrally acting antihypertensives, including clonidine, guanabenz, guanadrel, guanethidine, methyldopa, and reserpine: Decreased hypotensive effects. Monitor patient carefully.
CNS depressants, including analgesics, anesthetics, barbiturates, narcotics, and tranquilizers: May cause oversedation. Monitor patient.
Disulfiram, ethchlorvynol: May cause delirium and tachycardia. Monitor patient carefully.
Haloperidol, phenothiazines: Decreased trimipramine metabolism and decreased therapeutic efficacy. Dosage adjustment may be needed.
Metrizamide: Increased risk of seizures. Monitor patient closely.

Selective serotonin reuptake inhibitors, including fluoxetine, paroxetine, and sertraline: Increased pharmacologic and toxic effects of trimipramine. Monitor patient closely. Dosage adjustment may be needed.

Sympathomimetics, including ephedrine, epinephrine, and phenylephrine: Increased blood pressure. Monitor patient closely.

Warfarin: Increased PT and INR with bleeding. Monitor PT and INR. Dosage adjustment may be needed.

Drug-herb. *SAMe, St. John's wort, yohimbe:* Possible elevation of serotonin levels. Discourage concomitant use.

Drug-lifestyle. *Alcohol use:* Additive trimipramine effects. Advise patient to avoid alcohol. *Heavy smoking:* Decreased therapeutic efficacy. Advise patient to avoid smoking. *Sun exposure:* Increased risk of photosensitivity reactions. Advise patient to avoid sun exposure.

Adverse reactions
CNS: *drowsiness, dizziness,* paresthesia, ataxia, hallucinations, delusions, anxiety, agitation, insomnia, tremor, weakness, confusion, headache, EEG changes, **seizures,** extrapyramidal reactions.
CV: *orthostatic hypotension,* tachycardia, hypertension, **arrhythmias, heart block, MI, CVA,** prolonged conduction time on ECG.
EENT: *blurred vision,* tinnitus, mydriasis.
GI: *dry mouth, constipation,* nausea, vomiting, anorexia, paralytic ileus.
GU: *urine retention.*
Hematologic: decreased WBC counts, altered PT and INR.
Hepatic: elevated liver function test results.
Metabolic: altered serum glucose levels.
Skin: *diaphoresis,* rash, urticaria, photosensitivity.
Other: *hypersensitivity reaction.*
After abrupt withdrawal of long-term therapy: nausea, headache, malaise (doesn't indicate addiction).

Overdose and treatment
The first 12 hours after acute ingestion are a stimulatory phase characterized by excessive anticholinergic activity, including agitation, irritation, confusion, hallucinations, parkinsonian symptoms, seizure, urine retention, dry mucous membranes, pupillary dilation, constipation, and ileus. This is followed by CNS depressant effects, including hypothermia, decreased or absent reflexes, sedation, hypotension, cyanosis, and cardiac irregularities, including tachycardia, conduction disturbances, and quinidine-like effects on the ECG.

Severity of overdose is best indicated by prolongation of QRS interval beyond 100 milliseconds, which usually represents a serum level in excess of 1,000 ng/ml; serum levels are generally not helpful. Metabolic acidosis may follow hypotension, hypoventilation, and seizures.

Treatment is symptomatic and supportive and includes maintaining airway, stable body temperature, and fluid and electrolyte balance. Induce emesis with ipecac if patient is conscious; follow with gastric lavage and activated charcoal to prevent further absorption. Dialysis is of little use. Physostigmine given I.V. slowly has been used to reverse most CV and CNS effects of overdose. Treat seizures with parenteral diazepam or phenytoin; arrhythmias with parenteral phenytoin or lidocaine; and acidosis with sodium bicarbonate. Don't give barbiturates; these may enhance CNS and respiratory depressant effects.

Special considerations
Consider the recommendations relevant to all tricyclic antidepressants as well as the following.
• Consider the inherent risk of suicide until significant improvement of depressive state occurs.
• Tolerance generally develops to the sedative effects of drug.

Patient monitoring
• Watch for bleeding because drug may cause alterations in PT and INR.
• Closely monitor high-risk patients during initial drug therapy.

Geriatric patients
• Geriatric patients may be more vulnerable to adverse cardiac effects.

Patient education
• Explain that full effects of drug may not become apparent for up to 4 to 6 weeks after therapy begins.
• Tell patient to take drug exactly as prescribed.
• Warn patient that drug may cause drowsiness or dizziness and to avoid activities that require mental alertness until the full effects of drug are known.
• Warn patient not to drink alcoholic beverages or medicinal elixirs while taking drug.
• Suggest taking drug with food or milk if it causes stomach upset and to ease dry mouth with sugarless chewing gum, hard candy, or ice.
• Tell patient to report adverse reactions promptly, especially confusion, movement disorders, rapid heartbeat, dizziness, fainting, or difficulty urinating.

---

troleandomycin
Tao

Pharmacologic classification: macrolide antibiotic
Therapeutic classification: antibiotic
Pregnancy risk category: C

Indications and dosages
➤ *Pneumonia or respiratory tract infection caused by sensitive pneumococci or*

---

group A beta-hemolytic streptococci.
Adults: 250 to 500 mg P.O. q 6 hours.
Children: 125 to 250 mg P.O. q 6 hours.

How supplied
Available by prescription only
Capsules: 250 mg

Pharmacodynamics
Antibacterial action: Drug inhibits bacterial protein synthesis by binding to 50S ribosomal subunit. It produces bacteriostatic effects on susceptible bacteria, including gram-positive cocci and bacilli and a few gram-negative organisms, including *Haemophilus influenzae*, *Neisseria gonorrhoeae*, and *Neisseria meningitidis*.

Pharmacokinetics
Absorption: Absorbed rapidly but incompletely.
Distribution: Distributed widely to body fluids, except to CSF.
Metabolism: Metabolized in the liver.
Excretion: Excreted in bile, feces, and urine (10% to 25%).

Route	Onset	Peak	Duration
P.O.	Unknown	2 hr	12 hr

Contraindications and precautions
Contraindicated in patients hypersensitive to drug. Use cautiously in patients with hepatic dysfunction.

Interactions
Drug-drug. *Carbamazepine, methylprednisolone, theophylline:* Increased toxicity of drugs. Avoid use together.
Ergotamine: May precipitate severe ischemic reactions and peripheral vasospasms. Monitor patient closely.
Oral contraceptives: May cause marked cholestatic jaundice. Monitor patient closely.

Adverse reactions
GI: *abdominal cramps, discomfort,* vomiting, diarrhea.
Hematologic: eosinophilia, leukocytosis.
Hepatic: elevated liver enzyme levels, cholestatic jaundice.
Skin: urticaria, rash.
Other: *anaphylaxis.*

Overdose and treatment
None reported.

Special considerations
● Obtain culture and sensitivity tests before starting therapy.
⚡ **ALERT** Repeated courses of therapy or therapy exceeding 2 weeks may lead to allergic cholestatic hepatitis, as indicated by jaundice, right upper abdominal quadrant pain, fever, nausea, vomiting, eosinophilia, and leukocytosis.

● Discontinue drug if liver function test values increase or if signs or symptoms of cholestatic hepatitis occur.

Patient monitoring
● If patient is receiving drug with theophylline or carbamazepine, closely monitor serum theophylline or carbamazepine levels and assess patient frequently for signs and symptoms of theophylline or carbamazepine toxicity.
● Monitor total serum bilirubin and AST, ALT, and serum alkaline phosphatase levels.

Pregnant patients
● Safe use of troleandomycin during pregnancy hasn't been established.

Patient education
● Instruct patient to continue taking drug as prescribed, even if he's feeling better.
● Advise patient to take drug on an empty stomach for best absorption 1 hour before or 2 hours after meals, with full glass of water.
● Instruct patient to report abdominal pain or nausea immediately.

tromethamine
Tham

Pharmacologic classification: sodium-free organic amine
Therapeutic classification: systemic alkalinizer
Pregnancy risk category: C

Indications and dosages
➤ *Correction of metabolic acidosis (related to cardiac bypass surgery or cardiac arrest).* *Adults:* Dosage depends on base deficit. Calculate as follows: ml of 0.3 molar tromethamine solution needed = body weight (in kg) $\times$ base deficit (in mEq/L). Total dose should be administered over at least 1 hour and shouldn't exceed 500 mg/kg for an adult.

Usual dose of a 0.3 M solution (3.6 to 10.8 g tromethamine) may be administered into a large peripheral vein. If the chest is open, 55 to 165 ml of a 0.3 M solution (2 to 6 g tromethamine) has also been injected into ventricular cavity (not into cardiac muscle).

For systemic acidosis during cardiac bypass surgery, usual single dose of a 0.3 M solution is 9 ml/kg (324 mg/kg tromethamine) or about 500 ml (18 g tromethamine) for most adults.
➤ *To titrate excess acidity of stored blood used to prime the pump-oxygenator during cardiac bypass surgery.* *Adults:* Add 15 to 77 ml (500 mg to 2.5 g) of 0.3 M solution to each 500 ml of blood, depending on pH of blood.

How supplied
Available by prescription only
Injection: 18 g/500 ml

Pharmacodynamics

Systemic alkalinizing action: As a weak base, acts as a proton acceptor to prevent or correct acidosis; reduces hydrogen ion concentration. Also acts as a weak osmotic diuretic, increasing the flow of alkaline urine.

Pharmacokinetics

Absorption: Administered I.V.
Distribution: At pH of 7.4, about 25% of drug is un-ionized; this portion may enter cells to neutralize acidic ions of intracellular fluid.
Metabolism: None.
Excretion: Rapidly excreted renally as the bicarbonate salt.

Route	Onset	Peak	Duration
I.V.	Immediate	Immediate	Unknown

Contraindications and precautions

Contraindicated in patients with anuria, uremia, or chronic respiratory acidosis and during pregnancy (except in acute, life-threatening situations). Use cautiously in patients with renal disease or poor urine output.

Interactions

Drug-drug. *CNS and respiratory depressants:* Risk of respiratory depression. Avoid concomitant use.

Adverse reactions

Hepatic: hemorrhagic hepatic necrosis.
Metabolic: hypoglycemia, **hyperkalemia** (with decreased urine output).
Respiratory: *respiratory depression.*
Other: venospasm; I.V. thrombosis; inflammation, necrosis, and sloughing (if extravasation occurs).

Overdose and treatment

Signs and symptoms of overdose include respiratory or systemic alkalosis, arrhythmias secondary to hypokalemia, respiratory depression, and hypoglycemia.

Stop drug and correct pH; use decreased ventilation and systemic acidifiers, if necessary. Treat hypokalemia cautiously with potassium (serum potassium levels increase with correction of alkalosis) and hypoglycemia with I.V. glucose as needed.

Special considerations

• Administer drug by slow I.V. into the largest antecubital vein or via a large needle, indwelling catheter, or pump-oxygenator. If extravasation occurs, aspirate as much fluid as possible. Infiltrating area with 1% procaine hydrochloride to which hyaluronidase has been added may lessen extravasation and venospasm. Local injection of phentolamine can be used to reverse venospasm.

Patient monitoring

• Monitor vital signs, blood pH levels, carbon dioxide tension, and bicarbonate, glucose, and electrolyte levels before, during, and after infusion.
• Check infusion site frequently to avoid extravasation of solution and prevent tissue damage.

Pediatric patients

• Use drug cautiously; severe hepatic necrosis has occurred in infants and neonates after receiving a 1.2 M solution through umbilical vein. Hypoglycemia may occur when given to premature or full-term neonates.

Geriatric patients

• Patients with severe renal dysfunction or chronic respiratory acidosis are at increased risk when receiving tromethamine; use drug cautiously.

Patient education

• Explain drug to patient and family.
• Tell patient to report adverse reactions.

---

trovafloxacin mesylate
Trovan Tablets

alatrofloxacin mesylate
Trovan I.V.

Pharmacologic classification: fluoroquinolone derivative
Therapeutic classification: antibiotic
Pregnancy risk category: C

Indications and dosages

The following dosages are administered once every 24 hours.
➤ *Gynecologic and pelvic infections, complicated intra-abdominal and postsurgical infections. Adults:* 300 mg I.V. daily followed by 200 mg P.O. daily for 7 to 14 days.
➤ *Nosocomial pneumonia. Adults:* 300 mg I.V. daily followed by 200 mg P.O. daily for 10 to 14 days.
➤ *Community-acquired pneumonia. Adults:* 200 mg P.O. or I.V. daily followed by 200 mg P.O. daily for 7 to 14 days.
➤ *Complicated skin and skin structure infections, including diabetic foot infections. Adults:* 200 mg P.O. or I.V. daily followed by 200 mg P.O. daily for 10 to 14 days.
✦ *Dosage adjustment.* Dosage adjustments are unnecessary when switching from I.V. to oral forms. An adjustment in dose isn't needed in patients with renal impairment; however, in patients with mild to moderate hepatic disease (cirrhosis), the following dose reductions are recommended: Reduce 300 mg I.V. to 200 mg I.V., reduce 200 mg I.V. or P.O. to 100 mg I.V. or P.O.; no reduction needed for 100 mg P.O.

Reactions may be *common*, uncommon, *life-threatening*, or COMMON AND LIFE-THREATENING.

How supplied
Available by prescription only
Tablets: 100 mg, 200 mg
Injection: 5 mg/ml, in 40 ml (200 mg) and 60 ml (300 mg) vials

Pharmacodynamics
Antibiotic action: Trovafloxacin is related to the fluoroquinolones with in vitro activity against a wide range of gram-positive and gram-negative aerobic and anaerobic microorganisms. The bactericidal action of trovafloxacin results from inhibition of DNA gyrase and topoisomerase IV, two enzymes involved in bacterial replication.

Pharmacokinetics
Absorption: Well absorbed after oral administration with an absolute bioavailability of about 88%. Steady state levels are obtained by the third day of oral or I.V. administration.
Distribution: Widely and rapidly distributed throughout the body, resulting in significantly higher tissue levels than in plasma or serum. Mean plasma protein bound fraction is about 76%. Trovafloxacin is found in measurable levels in breast milk.
Metabolism: Primarily metabolized by conjugation, although there's minimal oxidative metabolism by cytochrome P-450. About 13% of a dose appears in urine as the glucuronide ester and 9% as the *N*-acetyl metabolite.
Excretion: Primary route of elimination is fecal. About 50% of an oral dose is excreted as unchanged drug (43% in feces and 6% in urine).

Route	Onset	Peak	Duration
P.O., I.V.	Unknown	1 hr	Unknown

Contraindications and precautions
Contraindicated in patients hypersensitive to trovafloxacin, alatrovafloxacin, or other quinolone antimicrobials. Use cautiously in patients with history of seizures, psychosis, or increased intracranial pressure.

Interactions
Drug-drug. *Aluminum-, iron-, and magnesium-containing preparations, such as antacids and vitamin-minerals, and divalent and trivalent cations such as didanosine:* Reduces oral bioavailability of drug. Separate administration times by at least 2 hours.
I.V. morphine, sucralfate: Reduced trovafloxacin plasma levels. Give I.V. morphine at least 2 hours after oral trovafloxacin in fasting state and at least 4 hours after oral trovafloxacin is taken with food.
Warfarin: Enhanced anticoagulation effect. Monitor PT and INR.
Drug-lifestyle. *Sun exposure:* Photosensitivity reaction. Advise patient to avoid sun exposure.

Adverse reactions
CNS: *dizziness,* light-headedness, headache, *seizures.*

GI: diarrhea, nausea, vomiting, abdominal pain, pseudomembranous colitis.
GU: vaginitis.
Hematologic: *bone marrow aplasia (anemia, thrombocytopenia, leukopenia).*
Hepatic: elevated hepatic transaminases, *hepatitis,* jaundice, *liver failure.*
Musculoskeletal: arthralgia, arthropathy, myalgia.
Skin: pruritus, rash, injection site reaction (I.V.), photosensitivity.

Overdose and treatment
Trovafloxacin has a low risk of acute toxicity. Signs of overdose include decreased activity and respiration, ataxia, ptosis, tremors, and seizures.
     Treat by emptying the stomach and providing symptomatic and supportive treatment. Drug isn't efficiently removed by hemodialysis.

Special considerations
ALERT Only available by the manufacturer to inpatient health-care facilities due to the potential of fatal liver toxicity.
● Reserve for use in patients with serious, life-threatening or limb-threatening infections.
● Oral form is more cost-effective and carries less risk; both forms have similar clinical efficacy and pharmacokinetics. Patients started with I.V. therapy may be switched to oral therapy when clinically indicated and at the discretion of the prescriber.
● Alatrofloxacin mesylate is supplied in single-use vials which must be further diluted with a compatible solution, such as D_5W or half-normal saline solution, before administration. Don't dilute drug with normal saline solution or lactated Ringer's solution. Follow package insert for specific instructions regarding preparation of desired dose.
● After dilution, administer I.V. drug as a 60-minute infusion.
● Changes in laboratory values during trovafloxacin therapy didn't produce clinical abnormalities, and levels generally returned to normal 1 to 2 months after discontinuation of therapy.
● Duration of therapy shouldn't exceed 2 weeks.

Patient monitoring
● Monitor liver function tests in patients who develop signs and symptoms of hepatitis. Consider discontinuing the drug in those who show abnormal liver function tests.
● Monitor patient for neurologic complications.

Breast-feeding patients
● Drug appears in breast milk in measurable levels. Because of unknown effects in infants, the risks of therapy and breast-feeding should be evaluated.

Pediatric patients
● Safety and efficacy in children under age 18 haven't been established.

Geriatric patients
● At recommended doses, drug is as well tolerated and efficient in patients age 65 and older as in younger patients.

Patient education
● Inform patient that drug may be taken without regard to meals; however, tell him to take vitamins, minerals, and antacids at least 2 hours before or after a trovafloxacin dose.
● Warn patient to avoid excessive sunlight or artificial ultraviolet light.
● Instruct patient to discontinue treatment, refrain from exercise, and seek medical advice if pain, inflammation, or rupture of a tendon occurs.
● Advise patient to promptly report symptoms of allergic reaction or diarrhea.
● Advise patient to promptly report signs of liver dysfunction (nausea, vomiting, abdominal pain, jaundice, dark urine, anorexia, pale stools, or fatigue) and stop the medication.

tuberculosis skin test antigens

tuberculin purified protein derivative (PPD)
Aplisol, Tubersol

tuberculin cutaneous multiple-puncture device
Aplitest (PPD), Mono-Vacc Test (Old Tuberculin), Tine Test (Old Tuberculin), Tine Test PPD

Pharmacologic classification: Mycobacterium tuberculosis and *Mycobacterium bovis* antigen
Therapeutic classification: diagnostic skin test antigen
Pregnancy risk category: C

Indications and dosages
➤ *Diagnosis of tuberculosis; evaluation of immunocompetence in patients with cancer or malnutrition. Adults and children:* I.D. injection of 5 tuberculin units/0.1 ml.

A single-use, multiple-puncture device is used for determining tuberculin sensitivity. All multiple-puncture tests are equivalent to or more potent than 5 tuberculin units of PPD. However, doses in multi-puncture devices cannot precisely be controlled. These devices shouldn't be used for periodic checks of individuals who are likely to be exposed to TB. Apply unit firmly and without any twisting to the upper one-third of the forearm for about 3 seconds; this ensures stabilizing the dried tuberculin B in the tissue lymph. Exert enough pressure to ensure that all four tines have entered the skin of the test area and a circular depression is visible.

How supplied
Available by prescription only
tuberculin PPD
Injection (I.D.): 1 tuberculin unit/0.1 ml, 5 tuberculin units/0.1 ml, 250 tuberculin units/0.1 ml
tuberculin cutaneous multiple-puncture device
Test: 25, 100, and 250 devices/pack

Pharmacodynamics
Diagnosis of tuberculosis: Administration to a patient who is natural infected with *M. tuberculosis* usually results in sensitivity to tuberculin and a delayed hypersensitivity reaction (after administration of old tuberculin or PPD). The cell-mediated immune reaction to tuberculin in tuberculin-sensitive individuals, which results mainly from cellular infiltrates of the dermis of the skin, usually causes local edema.
Evaluation of immunocompetence in patients with cancer or malnutrition: PPD is given I.D. with three or more antigens to detect anergy, the absence of an immune response to the test. The reaction may not be evident. Injection into a site subject to excessive exposure to sunlight may cause a false-negative reaction.

Pharmacokinetics
Absorption: Local.
Distribution: Local.
Metabolism: None reported.
Excretion: None reported.

Route	Onset	Peak	Duration
I.D.	5-6 hr	48-72 hr	Unknown

Contraindications and precautions
Severe reactions to tuberculin PPD are rare and usually result from extreme sensitivity to the tuberculin. Inadvertent S.C. administration of PPD may result in a febrile reaction in highly sensitized patients. Old tubercular lesions aren't activated by administration of PPD. Don't use PPD solution containing 250 TU/0.1 ml for initial testing due to skin necrosis at the site of injection.

Interactions
Drug-drug. *Aminocaproic acid, systemic corticosteroids:* False-negative reactions may occur. Don't use together.
Live- or inactivated-virus vaccines: Suppressed reaction. PPD antigen is used 4 to 6 weeks after immunization.
Topical alcohol: May inactivate the PPD antigen and invalidate the test. Avoid use together.

Adverse reactions
Other: Local pain, pruritus, vesiculation, ulceration, or necrosis, hypersensitivity, *anaphylaxis,* Arthus reaction (type III hypersensitivity reaction).

Overdose and treatment
Not reported.

Reactions may be *common,* uncommon, *life-threatening,* or COMMON AND LIFE-THREATENING.

Special considerations

• Pregnancy may caused a falsely insignificant re-action (old tuberculin multiple-puncture test). Avoid testing during pregnancy if possible.
• A positive reaction is induration greater than 2 mm. (Consider further diagnostic procedures.) A negative reaction is induration less than 2 mm.
• A tuberculin PPD injection must be given I.D. or by skin puncture; an S.C. injection invalidates the test.
• Reaction to a multiple-puncture device may be supressed in patients with malnutrition, im-munosuppression, or miliary tuberculosis.

Patient monitoring

• Read a PPD test in 48 to 72 hours. An indura-tion of 10 mm or greater is a significant reaction in patients who aren't suspected to have tuber-culosis and who haven't been exposed to active tuberculosis, indicating present or past infection. An induration of 5 mm or more is significant in patients with AIDS or in those suspected to have tuberculosis or who have recently been exposed to active tuberculosis. An induration of 5 to 9 mm is inconclusive in patients not suspected of having been exposed to or having tuberculosis infection; therefore, test should be repeated if there's more than 10 mm of erythema without induration. The amount of induration at the site, not the erythe-ma, determines the significance of the reaction.
• Read a multiple-puncture test at 48 to 72 hours.

Pregnant patients

• Use during pregnancy only when clearly need-ed and with the understanding that result can be falsely insignificant reaction (old tuberculin multiple-puncture test).

Breast-feeding patients

• There appears to be no risk to breast-feeding infants.

Geriatric patients

• Geriatric patients not having a cell-mediated immune reaction to the test may be anergic or they may test negative.

Patient education

• Advise patient that test must be read in 48 to 72 hours.
• Instruct patient to promptly report any unex-pected adverse effects.

---

tubocurarine chloride

Pharmacologic classification: nondepolariz-ing neuromuscular blocker
Therapeutic classification: skeletal muscle relaxant
Pregnancy risk category: C

Indications and dosages

➤ *Adjunct to general anesthesia to in-duce skeletal muscle relaxation, facili-*
tate intubation, and reduce fractures and
dislocations. Dose depends on anesthetic used, individual needs, and response. Doses listed are representative and must be adjusted. Dose may be calculated on the basis of 0.165 mg/kg.
Adults: Initially, 6 to 9 mg I.V. or I.M., followed by 3 to 4.5 mg in 3 to 5 minutes if needed. Ad-ditional doses of 3 mg may be given, if needed, during prolonged anesthesia.
➤ *To assist with mechanical ventilation.*
Adults: Initially, 0.0165 mg/kg I.V. or I.M. (aver-age 1 mg), then adjust subsequent doses to pa-tient's response.
➤ *To weaken muscle contractions in*
pharmacologically or electrically induced
seizures. Adults: Initially, 0.165 mg/kg I.V. or I.M. slowly. As a precaution, 3 mg less than the calculated dose should be administered initially.
➤ *Diagnosis of myasthenia gravis. Adults:*
Single I.V. or I.M. dose of 0.004 to 0.033 mg/kg.

How supplied

Available by prescription only
Injection: 3 mg/ml parenteral

Pharmacodynamics

Skeletal muscle relaxant action: Tubocu-rarine prevents acetylcholine from binding to re-ceptors on motor end-plate, blocking depolar-ization. Tubocurarine has histamine-releasing and ganglionic-blocking properties, and is usu-ally antagonized by anticholinesterase agents.

Pharmacokinetics

Absorption: I.V. direct. I.M., none reported.
Distribution: After I.V. injection, drug is dis-tributed in extracellular fluid and rapidly reach-es its site of action. After tissue compartment is saturated, drug may persist in tissues for up to 24 hours; 40% to 45% is bound to plasma pro-teins, mainly globulins.
Metabolism: Undergoes *N*-demethylation in the liver.
Excretion: About 33% to 75% of a dose is ex-creted unchanged in urine in 24 hours; up to 11% is excreted in bile.

Route	Onset	Peak	Duration
I.V.	1 min	2-5 min	25-90 min (first dose, longer for subsequent doses)
I.M.	10-25 min	Unknown	Unknown

Contraindications and precautions

Contraindicated in patients hypersensitive to drug and in those for whom histamine release is a haz-ard (asthmatic patients).
    Use cautiously in geriatric or debilitated pa-tients; in those with impaired hepatic or pul-monary function, hypothermia, respiratory de-pression, myasthenia gravis, myasthenic syndrome of lung cancer or bronchiogenic carcinoma, de-

hydration, thyroid disorders, collagen diseases, porphyria, electrolyte disturbances, fractures, or muscle spasms; in women undergoing cesarean section; and in patients with poor renal perfusion or renal impairment.

Interactions
Drug-drug. *Aminoglycoside antibiotics, beta blockers, calcium salts, clindamycin, depolarizing neuromuscular blockers, furosemide, general anesthetics, lincomycin, local anesthetics, other nondepolarizing neuromuscular blockers, other potassium-depleting drugs, parenteral magnesium salts, polymyxin antibiotics, quinidine, quinine, thiazide diuretics:* Enhanced or prolonged tubocurarine-induced neuromuscular blockade. Use cautiously. Monitor patient closely.
Opioid analgesics, quinidine, quinine: Increased respiratory depression. Monitor patient closely. Use cautiously.

Adverse reactions
CV: hypotension, *arrhythmias, cardiac arrest, bradycardia.*
Musculoskeletal: profound and prolonged muscle relaxation, idiosyncrasy, residual muscle weakness.
Respiratory: *respiratory depression or apnea, bronchospasm.*
Other: *hypersensitivity reactions,* increased salivation.

Overdose and treatment
Signs and symptoms of overdose include apnea or prolonged muscle paralysis, which can be treated with controlled ventilation.

Use a peripheral nerve stimulator to monitor effects and to determine nature and degree of blockade. Anticholinesterase agents may antagonize tubocurarine. Atropine given before or with the antagonist counteracts its muscarinic effects.

Special considerations
● The margin of safety between therapeutic dose and dose causing respiratory paralysis is small.
● Drug doesn't affect consciousness or relieve pain.
● Don't mix with barbiturates or other alkaline solutions in same syringe.
● I.V. administration requires direct medical supervision. Give drug I.V. slowly over 60 to 90 seconds or I.M. by deep injection in deltoid muscle. Tubocurarine is usually administered by I.V. injection, but if patient's veins are inaccessible, drug may be given I.M. in same dose as given I.V.
● Renal dysfunction prolongs drug action.

Patient monitoring
● Assess baseline tests of renal function and serum electrolyte levels before drug administration. Electrolyte imbalance, particularly of potassium and magnesium, can potentiate effects of drug.

● Monitor respirations closely for early symptoms of paralysis.
● A nerve stimulator may be used to evaluate recovery from neuromuscular blockade.
● Monitor blood pressure, vital signs, and airway until patient recovers from drug effects. Ganglionic blockade (hypotension), histamine liberation (increased salivation, bronchospasm), and neuromuscular blockade (respiratory depression) are known effects of tubocurarine.
● After neuromuscular blockade dissipates, watch for residual muscle weakness.

Breast-feeding patients
● It isn't known whether drug appears in breast milk. Use cautiously in breast-feeding women.

Pediatric patients
● Administer cautiously to children because the preservative, benzyl alcohol, has been linked to toxicity.

Geriatric patients
● Administer cautiously to geriatric patients.

Patient education
● Explain all events and procedures to patient because he can still hear.

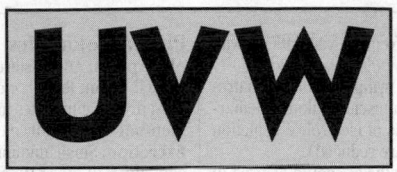

urea (carbamide)
Ureaphil

Pharmacologic classification: carbonic acid salt
Therapeutic classification: osmotic diuretic
Pregnancy risk category: C

Indications and dosages
➤ **Reduction of intracranial or intraocular pressure.** *Adults:* 1 to 1.5 g/kg as a 30% solution given by slow I.V. infusion over 1 to 2½ hours.
Children over age 2: 0.5 to 1.5 g/kg by slow I.V. infusion.
Children up to age 2: As little as 0.1 g/kg by slow I.V. infusion may be given. Maximum, 4 ml/minute.

   Maximum adult dose is 120 g daily. To prepare 135 ml of 30% solution, mix contents of a 40-g vial of urea with 105 ml of D_5W or $D_{10}W$ with 10% invert sugar in water. Each milliliter of 30% solution provides 300 mg of urea.
➤ **SIADH** ◊. *Adults:* 80 g as a 30% solution I.V. over 6 hours.
➤ **Diuresis** ◊. *Adults and children over age 2:* 500 mg to 1.5 g/kg as a 30% solution given by slow I.V. infusion over 30 minutes to 2 hours.
Children up to age 2: 100 mg to 1.5 g/kg as a 30% solution given by slow I.V. infusion over 30 minutes to 2 hours.

How supplied
Available by prescription only
Injectable: 40-g vial

Pharmacodynamics
Diuretic action: Elevates plasma osmolality, enhancing the flow of water into extracellular fluid such as blood, and reducing intracranial and intraocular pressure.

Pharmacokinetics
Absorption: I.V. urea produces diuresis and maximal reduction of intraocular and intracranial pressure within 1 to 2 hours; even though administered I.V., it's hydrolyzed and absorbed from GI tract.
Distribution: Distributed into intracellular and extracellular fluid, including lymph, bile, and CSF.
Metabolism: Hydrolyzed in GI tract by bacterial urease.

Excretion: Excreted by kidneys.

Route	Onset	Peak	Duration
I.V.	30-45 min	1-2 hr	3-10 hr

Contraindications and precautions
Contraindicated in patients with severely impaired renal function, marked dehydration, frank hepatic failure, active intracranial bleeding, or sickle-cell disease with CNS involvement. Use cautiously in pregnant women, breast-feeding women, and patients with cardiac disease or impaired renal or hepatic function.

Interactions
Drug-drug. *Lithium:* Enhanced renal excretion of lithium; lowered serum lithium levels. Monitor lithium levels closely.

Adverse reactions
CNS: *headache,* syncope, disorientation.
GI: *nausea, vomiting.*
Metabolic: altered electrolyte balance.
Other: irritation or necrotic sloughing with extravasation.

Overdose and treatment
Signs and symptoms of overdose include unusually elevated BUN levels, polyuria, cellular dehydration, hypotension, and CV collapse. Stop infusion and institute supportive measures.

Special considerations
● Avoid rapid I.V. infusion, which may cause hemolysis or increased capillary bleeding. Also avoid extravasation, which may cause reactions ranging from mild irritation to necrosis.
● Use only freshly reconstituted urea for I.V. infusion; solution turns to ammonia when left standing. Use within minutes of reconstitution.
● Don't administer through same infusion line as blood.
● Don't infuse into leg veins; this may cause phlebitis or thrombosis, especially in elderly patients.
● Maintain adequate hydration.
● If satisfactory diuresis doesn't occur in 6 to 12 hours, stop urea and reevaluate renal function.
● Urea has been used orally on an investigational basis for migraine prophylaxis, acute sickle-cell crisis prevention, and correction of SIADH.

Patient monitoring
● Monitor fluid and electrolyte balance.

- Monitor BUN levels frequently in patients with renal disease.
- Watch for signs and symptoms of hyponatremia or hypokalemia (muscle weakness, lethargy) as early indications of electrolyte depletion (before serum levels are reduced).
- Indwelling urinary catheter should be used in comatose patients to ensure bladder emptying. Use of an hourly urometer collection bag facilitates accurate measurement of urine output.

Breast-feeding patients
- It isn't known if drug appears in breast milk. Safety in breast-feeding women hasn't been established.

Geriatric patients
- Elderly or debilitated patients will need close observation and may need lower doses. Excessive diuresis promotes rapid dehydration and hypovolemia, hypokalemia, and hyponatremia.

Patient education
- Advise patient of need to monitor fluid balance, electrolyte balance, and BUN level.
- Advise patient to report muscle weakness and lethargy.

urokinase
Abbokinase, Abbokinase Open-Cath

Pharmacologic classification: thrombolytic enzyme
Therapeutic classification: thrombolytic enzyme
Pregnancy risk category: B

Indications and dosages
➤ *Lysis of acute massive pulmonary emboli and of pulmonary emboli accompanied by unstable hemodynamics.* Adults: For I.V. infusion only by constant infusion pump; priming dose: 4,400 IU/kg over 10 minutes, followed by 4,400 IU/kg hourly for 12 hours.
➤ *Coronary artery thrombosis.* Adults: 6,000 IU/minute of urokinase intra-arterial via a coronary artery catheter until artery is maximally opened, usually within 15 to 30 minutes; however, drug has been administered for up to 2 hours. Average total dose, 500,000 IU.
➤ *Venous catheter occlusion.* Adults: Instill 5,000 IU into occluded line.

How supplied
Available by prescription only
Injection: 5,000 IU/ml unit-dose vial; 250,000-IU/vial

Pharmacodynamics
Thrombolytic action: Urokinase promotes thrombolysis by directly activating conversion of plasminogen to plasmin.

Pharmacokinetics
Absorption: Administered I.V.
Distribution: Rapidly cleared from circulation; most drug accumulates in the kidneys and liver.
Metabolism: Rapidly metabolized by the liver.
Excretion: Small amount is eliminated in urine and bile. Half-life is 10 to 20 minutes; longer in patients with hepatic dysfunction.

Route	Onset	Peak	Duration
I.V.	Immediate	20 min-4 hr	4 hr

Contraindications and precautions
Contraindicated in patients with active internal bleeding, history of CVA, aneurysm, arteriovenous malformation, known bleeding diathesis, recent trauma with possible internal injuries, visceral or intracranial malignancy, ulcerative colitis, diverticulitis, severe hypertension, hemostatic defects including those resulting from severe hepatic or renal insufficiency, uncontrolled hypocoagulation, chronic pulmonary disease with cavitation, subacute bacterial endocarditis or rheumatic valvular disease, and recent cerebral embolism, thrombosis, or hemorrhage.

Also contraindicated during pregnancy and first 10 days postpartum, within 10 days after intra-arterial diagnostic procedure or surgery (including liver or kidney biopsy, lumbar puncture, thoracentesis, paracentesis, or extensive or multiple cutdowns), or within 2 months after intracranial or intraspinal surgery.

I.M. injections and other invasive procedures are contraindicated during urokinase therapy.

Interactions
Drug-drug. *Aminocaproic acid:* Inhibits urokinase-induced activation of plasminogen. Avoid use together.
Anticoagulants, including heparin and oral anticoagulants: Hemorrhage. Heparin must be stopped and its effects allowed to diminish. It may also be necessary to reverse effects of oral anticoagulants before beginning therapy.
Aspirin, indomethacin, phenylbutazone, other drugs that affect platelet activity: Increased risk of bleeding. Avoid use together.

Adverse reactions
CV: *reperfusion arrhythmias,* tachycardia, transient hypotension or hypertension.
Hematologic: *bleeding;* increased thrombin time, aPTT, PT, and INR; decreased hematocrit.
Respiratory: *bronchospasm,* minor breathing difficulties.
Other: phlebitis at injection site, fever, rash, *anaphylaxis,* chills, nausea, vomiting.

Overdose and treatment
Signs and symptoms of overdose reflect potentially serious bleeding: bleeding gums, epistaxis, hematoma, spontaneous ecchymoses, oozing at catheter site, increased pulse, and pain from in-

---

ternal bleeding. Discontinue drug and restart when bleeding stops.

Special considerations
Consider the recommendations relevant to all thrombolytic enzymes as well as the following.
• Don't use bacteriostatic water to reconstitute.
• Product contains no preservatives; discard unused portion.
• Drug may affect platelet function.

Patient monitoring
• Patient should be monitored for signs of hemorrhage.

Pregnant patients
• There are no adequate or controlled studies using urokinase in pregnant women. The drug shouldn't be used during pregnancy unless clearly needed.

Breast-feeding patients
• It isn't known if drug appears in breast milk; use it cautiously in breast-feeding women.

Pediatric patients
• Safety and efficacy in children haven't been established.

Geriatric patients
• Patients age 75 or older have a greater risk of cerebral hemorrhage because they're more apt to have cerebrovascular disease.

Patient education
• Explain use and administration of urokinase to patient and family.
• Instruct patient to report adverse reactions promptly.

---

valacyclovir hydrochloride
Valtrex

Pharmacologic classification: synthetic purine nucleoside
Therapeutic classification: antiviral
Pregnancy risk category: B

Indications and dosages
➤ *Herpes zoster in immunocompetent patients.* Adults: 1 g P.O. t.i.d. daily for 7 days.
➤ *Initial episode of genital herpes.* Adults: 1 g P.O. b.i.d. for 10 days.
➤ *Recurrent genital herpes in immunocompetent patients.* Adults: 500 mg P.O. b.i.d. for 3 days.
➤ *Long-term suppressive therapy of recurrent genital herpes.* Adults: 1 g P.O. once daily.
✦ *Dosage adjustment.* For patients with renal impairment, see the table at the top of the next column.

Creatinine clearance (ml/min)	Herpes zoster	Genital herpes
30-49	1 g q 12 hours	500 mg q 12 hours
10-29	1 g q 24 hours	500 mg q 24 hours
< 10	500 mg q 24 hours	500 mg q 24 hours

How supplied
Available by prescription only
Caplets: 500 mg, 1000 mg

Pharmacodynamics
Antiviral action: Rapidly becomes converted to acyclovir. Acyclovir becomes incorporated into viral DNA and inhibits viral DNA polymerase, thus inhibiting viral multiplication.

Pharmacokinetics
Absorption: Rapidly absorbed from GI tract; absolute bioavailability about 54.5%.
Distribution: Protein-binding ranges from 13.5% to 17.9%.
Metabolism: Rapidly and nearly completely converted to acyclovir and L-valine by first-pass intestinal or hepatic metabolism.
Excretion: Excreted in urine and feces. Half-life is about 2½ to 3⅓ hours.

Route	Onset	Peak	Duration
P.O.	30 min	Unknown	Unknown

Contraindications and precautions
Contraindicated in immunocompromised patients and patients hypersensitive to or intolerant of valacyclovir, acyclovir, or their components. Use cautiously in patients with impaired renal function and in those receiving other nephrotoxic drugs.

Interactions
Drug-drug. *Cimetidine, probenecid:* Reduced rate of renal clearance of acyclovir; increased acyclovir blood levels. Monitor patient for possible toxicity.

Adverse reactions
CNS: *headache,* dizziness, asthenia.
GI: *nausea,* vomiting, diarrhea, constipation, abdominal pain, anorexia.

Overdose and treatment
No report of overdose. However, precipitation of acyclovir in renal tubules may occur when the solubility (2.5 mg/ml) is exceeded in the intratubular fluid.

If acute renal failure and anuria occur, hemodialysis may be helpful until renal function is restored.

Special considerations

• Preferably, start therapy within 24 hours after onset of signs or symptoms of an episode; treatment is most effective when started within 48 hours of zoster rash onset.
• The manufacturer maintains a registry of women exposed to drug during pregnancy. Follow-up studies to date haven't shown an increased risk of birth defects.
• Thrombotic thrombocytopenic purpura and hemolytic uremic syndrome have occurred, resulting in death in some patients with advanced HIV infection, and also in bone marrow transplant and renal transplant recipients participating in clinical trials of valacyclovir.
◼ **ALERT** Don't confuse valacyclovir with valganciclovir.

Patient monitoring
• Monitor therapeutic effect.

Breast-feeding patients
• It isn't known if drug appears in breast milk. Use in breast-feeding women isn't recommended.

Pediatric patients
• Safety and effectiveness in children haven't been established.

Geriatric patients
• Dosage adjustment may be needed in elderly patients based on underlying renal status.

Patient education
• Inform patient that drug may be taken without regard to meals.
• Advise patient to call immediately at the first sign of an episode.
• Tell patient to avoid contact with lesions and to avoid intercourse when lesions or symptoms are present.

---

valganciclovir hydrochloride
Valcyte

Pharmacologic classification: synthetic nucleoside
Therapeutic classification: antiviral
Pregnancy risk category: C

Indications and dosages
➤ *Active cytomegalovirus (CMV) retinitis in patients with AIDS. Adults:* 900 mg (two 450-mg tablets) P.O. b.i.d. with food for 21 days. Maintenance, 900 mg (two 450-mg tablets) P.O. once daily with food.
➤ *Inactive CMV retinitis. Adults:* 900 mg (two 450-mg tablets) P.O. once daily with food.
✦ *Dosage adjustment.* For patients with impaired renal function, see the table at the top of the next column.

Creatinine clearance (ml/min)	Induction dosage	Maintenance dosage
40-59	450 mg P.O. b.i.d.	450 mg P.O. daily
25-39	450 mg P.O. daily	450 mg P.O. every 2 days
10-24	450 mg P.O. every 2 days	450 mg P.O. twice weekly

How supplied
Tablets: 450 mg

Pharmacodynamics
Drug is a prodrug that is converted to ganciclovir, which inhibits replication of viral DNA synthesis of CMV.

Pharmacokinetics:
Absorption: Well absorbed from GI tract. Has higher absorption when taken with food.
Distribution: Minimal binding to plasma proteins.
Metabolism: Metabolized in intestinal wall and liver to ganciclovir.
Excretion: Eliminated renally.

Route	Onset	Peak	Duration
P.O.	Unknown	1-3 hr	Unknown

Contraindications and precautions
Contraindicated in patients hypersensitive to valganciclovir or ganciclovir. Don't use in patients receiving hemodialysis. Use cautiously in patients with cytopenias and in those who have received immunosuppressants or radiation.

Interactions
Drug-drug. *Didanosine:* Possible increased absorption of didanosine. Monitor patient closely for didanosine toxicity.
Immunosuppressants, zidovudine: Possible enhanced neutropenia, anemia, thrombocytopenia, and bone marrow depression. Monitor CBC.
Mycophenolate mofetil: Possible increased levels of both drugs in renally impaired patients. Use together carefully.
Probenecid: Decreased renal clearance of ganciclovir. Monitor patient for ganciclovir toxicity.
Drug-food. *Any food:* Increased absorption of drug. Give drug with food.

Adverse reactions
CNS: *headache, insomnia,* peripheral neuropathy, paresthesia, ***seizures,*** psychosis, hallucinations, confusion, agitation.
EENT: *retinal detachment.*
GI: *diarrhea, nausea, vomiting, abdominal pain.*
GU: *decreased creatinine clearance.*

Reactions may be *common*, uncommon, *life-threatening*, or COMMON AND LIFE-THREATENING.

Hematologic: NEUTROPENIA, *anemia*, ***thrombocytopenia, pancytopenia, bone marrow depression, aplastic anemia.***
Other: catheter-related infection, ***sepsis***, local or systemic infections, *pyrexia*, ***hypersensitivity reactions.***

Overdose and treatment
Overdose may cause severe, fatal bone marrow depression, and renal toxicity.

To treat, maintain adequate hydration, and consider hematopoietic growth factors. Dialysis may be useful in reducing serum levels.

Special considerations
⚠ ALERT Adhere to dosing guidelines for valganciclovir because ganciclovir and valganciclovir aren't interchangeable, and overdose may occur.
• Cytopenia may occur at any time during treatment and increase with continued dosing. Cell counts usually recover 3 to 7 days after stopping drug.
⚠ ALERT Don't confuse valganciclovir with valacyclovir.
• No drug interaction studies have been conducted with valganciclovir; however, because drug is converted to ganciclovir, it can be assumed that drug interactions would be similar.
• Drug may cause temporary or permanent inhibition of spermatogenesis.
• Women of childbearing potential must use contraception during treatment. Men should use barrier contraception during and for 90 days after treatment.
⚠ ALERT Clinical toxicities include severe leukopenia, neutropenia, anemia, pancytopenia, bone marrow depression, aplastic anemia, and thrombocytopenia. Don't use drug if patient's absolute neutrophil count is less than 500 cells/mm³, platelets are less than 25,000/mm³, or hemoglobin is less than 8 g/dl.

Patient monitoring
• Monitor CBC, platelet counts, and serum creatinine levels or creatinine clearance values frequently during treatment.

Breast-feeding patients
• It isn't known if drug appears in breast milk. Because of the possibility of serious adverse reactions in infants who are breast-fed, don't use in breast-feeding women.

Pediatric patients
• Safety and effectiveness in children haven't been established.

Geriatric patients
• Carefully monitor renal function before and during treatment. Use cautiously, keeping in mind the increased frequency of decreased hepatic, renal, or cardiac function; concomitant disease; or other drug therapy.

valproic acid
Depakene, Epival*

divalproex sodium
Depakote, Depakote Sprinkle, Depakote ER

valproate sodium
Depacon

Pharmacologic classification: carboxylic acid derivative
Therapeutic classification: anticonvulsant
Pregnancy risk category: D

Indications and dosages
Note: Doses of divalproex sodium (Depakote) and valproate sodium are expressed as valproic acid.

➤ *Complex partial seizures. Adults and children age 10 and older:* Initially, 10-15 mg/kg daily as monotherapy or adjunctive therapy when being added to a current therapeutic regimen. Increase by 5 to 10 mg/kg weekly until seizures are controlled or adverse effects preclude further increases. Maximum, 60 mg/kg daily.
➤ *Simple and complex absence seizures. Adults and children:* Initially, 15 mg/kg daily, may increase by 5 to 10 mg/kg daily at weekly intervals until seizures are controlled or adverse effects prevent further increases in dosage. Maximum, 60 mg/kg daily. If daily dose is greater than 250 mg, give drug in two or more divided doses.
➤ *Mania. Adults:* 750 mg P.O. in divided doses (divalproex sodium). Maximum, 60 mg/kg daily.
➤ *Migraine prophylaxis. Adults:* 250 mg P.O. b.i.d. Some patients may benefit from doses up to 1 g daily. Or 500 mg (extended-release tablets) once daily for 1 week; dosage may be increased to 1 g/day.
➤ *Status epilepticus refractory to I.V. diazepam◇. Adults:* 400 to 600 mg P.R. q 6 hours.

How supplied
Available by prescription only
valproic acid
Capsules: 250 mg
Syrup: 250 mg/5 ml
divalproex sodium
Capsules (sprinkle): 125 mg
Tablets (delayed-release): 125 mg, 250 mg, 500 mg
Tablets (extended release): 500 mg
valproate sodium
Injection: 5 ml single-dose vials

Pharmacodynamics
Anticonvulsant action: Mechanism unknown; effects may be from increased brain levels of gamma-aminobutyric acid (GABA), an inhibitory transmitter. Also may decrease GABA's enzymatic catabolism. Onset of therapeutic effects

may require a week or more. May be used with other anticonvulsants.

Pharmacokinetics
Absorption: Valproate sodium and divalproex sodium quickly convert to valproic acid after administration of oral dose; plasma levels peak in 1 to 5 hours, 15 minutes to 2 hours with syrup, and immediately with I.V.; same bioavailability for all dose forms.
Distribution: Distributed rapidly throughout body; 80% to 95% protein-bound.
Metabolism: Metabolized by liver.
Excretion: Excreted in urine; some drug excreted in feces and exhaled air. Breast milk levels are 1% to 10% of serum levels.

Route	Onset	Peak	Duration
P.O.	Unknown	15 min-4 hr	Unknown
I.V.	Unknown	1 hr	Unknown

Contraindications and precautions
Contraindicated in patients hypersensitive to drug. Use cautiously in patients with history of hepatic dysfunction. Don't give valproate sodium injection to patients with hepatic disease or significant hepatic dysfunction.

Interactions
Drug-drug. *Antidepressants, MAO inhibitors, oral anticoagulants:* Potentiated effects of these drugs. Monitor patient closely.
Carbamazepine: Decreased carbamazepine levels and increased metabolite levels. Monitor patient.
Clonazepam: Increased risk of absence seizures. Avoid concomitant use.
Diazepam: Valproate displaces diazepam from albumin binding sites and inhibits its metabolism. Monitor patient.
Ethosuximide: Valproate inhibits ethosuximide metabolism. Monitor plasma levels of both drugs.
Felbamate, lamotrigine, salicylates: Increased valproate levels. Monitor valproate levels.
Phenobarbital, phenytoin, primidone: Increased serum levels of these drugs; excessive somnolence. Monitor patient carefully.
Rifampin: Increased oral clearance of valproate. Adjust valproate dosage if necessary.
Drug-lifestyle. *Alcohol use:* Decreased valproic acid effectiveness; increased adverse CNS effects. Discourage use.

Adverse reactions
Because drug usually is used with other anticonvulsants, adverse reactions may not be caused by valproic acid alone.
CNS: *sedation,* emotional upset, depression, psychosis, aggressiveness, hyperactivity, behavioral deterioration, tremor, ataxia, headache, dizziness, incoordination.
EENT: nystagmus, diplopia.
GI: *nausea, vomiting, indigestion,* diarrhea, abdominal cramps, constipation, increased appetite and weight gain, anorexia, *pancreatitis.*

Hematologic: *thrombocytopenia,* increased bleeding time, petechiae, bruising, eosinophilia, *hemorrhage, leukopenia, bone marrow suppression.*
Hepatic: elevated liver enzyme levels, *toxic hepatitis.*
Musculoskeletal: muscle weakness.
Skin: rash, alopecia, pruritus, photosensitivity, *erythema multiforme.*

Overdose and treatment
Signs and symptoms of overdose include somnolence and coma.

Treat supportively. Maintain adequate urine output, and monitor vital signs and fluid and electrolyte balance carefully. Naloxone reverses CNS and respiratory depression but also may reverse anticonvulsant effects of valproic acid. Hemodialysis and hemoperfusion have been used.

Special considerations
● Administer drug with food to minimize GI irritation.
● Administer I.V. as 60-minute infusion at no more than 20 mg/minute.
● Use of valproate sodium injection for periods of more than 14 days hasn't been studied. Patients should be switched to oral products as soon as clinically feasible. When switching from I.V. to oral therapy or from oral to I.V. therapy, the total daily dose should be equivalent and given with the same frequency.
● Don't withdraw drug abruptly.
● Valproic acid may cause false-positive test results for urinary ketones.
● Divalproex sodium extended-release tablets and divalproex sodium delayed-release tablets are not bioequivalent.
● Valproic acid reportedly alters thyroid function test results. Clinical significance is unknown.
● A ketone metabolite in the urine of patients taking valproic acid may produce a false-positive result for urine ketones.

Patient monitoring
● Monitor plasma level and make dosage adjustments as needed; therapeutic range of drug is 50 to 100 mcg/ml.
● Watch for tremors; they may indicate need for dosage reduction.
● Evaluate liver function, platelet count, and PT at baseline and monthly intervals—especially during first 6 months of therapy.

Breast-feeding patients
● Drug appears in breast milk at 1% to 10% of serum levels. An alternative to breast-feeding is recommended during therapy.

Pediatric patients
● Not recommended for use in children under age 2; this age-group is at highest risk for adverse effects.

- Hyperexcitability and aggressiveness have occurred in a few children.
- Divalproex sodium extended-release tablets aren't recommended for children.

Geriatric patients
- Drug is eliminated more slowly in elderly patients; lower dosages are recommended.

Patient education
- Tell patient to swallow tablets or capsules whole to avoid local mucosal irritation. If necessary, tell patient to take with food but not carbonated beverages because tablet may dissolve before swallowing, causing irritation and unpleasant taste.
- Warn patient to avoid alcohol while taking drug; it may decrease drug effectiveness and increase adverse CNS effects.
- Advise patient to avoid tasks that require mental alertness until CNS sedative effects are known. Drowsiness and dizziness may occur. Bedtime administration of drug may minimize CNS depression.
- Teach patient signs and symptoms of hypersensitivity and adverse effects and the need to report them
- Advise patient not to stop drug suddenly, not to alter dosage without approval, and to call before changing brand or using generic drug because therapeutic effect may change.
- Encourage patient taking anticonvulsants to wear a medical identification bracelet or necklace that lists drug and seizure disorder.

valrubicin
Valstar

Pharmacologic classification: anthracycline
Therapeutic classification: antineoplastic
Pregnancy risk category: C

Indications and dosages
➤ *Intravesical therapy carcinoma in situ (CIS) of the urinary bladder refractory to bacillus calmette-guerin vaccine and in patients for whom immediate cystectomy would risk unacceptable morbidity or mortality.* Adults: 800 mg intravesically once weekly for six weeks.

How supplied
Available by prescription only
Solution for intravesical instillation: 200 mg/5 ml

Pharmacodynamics
Antineoplastic action: Anthracycline exerts cytotoxic activity by penetrating cells and inhibiting the incorporation of nucleosides into nucleic acids. It also causes extensive chromosomal damage and arrests the cell cycle in G_2. And it interferes with the normal breaking-resealing action of DNA topoisomerase II, thereby inhibiting DNA synthesis.

Pharmacokinetics
Absorption: Only small quantities absorbed into plasma after intravesical administration.
Distribution: Penetrates into bladder wall after intravesical administration. Systemic exposure dependent on condition of bladder wall.
Metabolism: Metabolites found in blood.
Excretion: After retention, almost completely excreted by voiding the instillate.

Route	Onset	Peak	Duration
Intra-vesical	Unknown	Unknown	Unknown

Contraindications and precautions
Contraindicated in patients hypersensitive to drug, other anthracyclines, or Cremophor EL (polyoxyethyleneglycol triricinoleate). Also contraindicated in patients with urinary tract infections, small bladder capacity (unable to tolerate a 75 ml instillation), or perforated bladder. Also contraindicated in those with compromised integrity of the bladder mucosa.

Use cautiously in patients with severe irritable bladder symptoms.

Interactions
None reported.

Adverse reactions
CNS: asthenia, headache, malaise, dizziness.
CV: vasodilation, chest pain, peripheral edema.
GI: diarrhea, flatulence, nausea, vomiting, abdominal pain.
GU: urine retention, urinary tract infection, urinary frequency, dysuria, urinary urgency, bladder spasm, hematuria, bladder pain, urinary incontinence, pelvic pain, urethral pain, nocturia, cystitis, local burning symptoms.
Hematologic: anemia.
Metabolic: hyperglycemia.
Musculoskeletal: myalgia, back pain.
Respiratory: pneumonia.
Skin: rash.
Other: fever.

Overdose and treatment
There is no known antidote for overdose. Anticipated complications linked to intravesical overdose would be consistent with irritable bladder symptoms.

Special considerations
⚠ **ALERT** Drug should be administered intravesically only by those experienced in the use of intravesical antineoplastics. Don't give I.V. or I.M.
- In patients with severe irritable bladder symptoms, bladder spasm and spontaneous discharge of the intravesical instillate may occur. Clamping the urinary catheter isn't advised.

• For patients undergoing transurethral resection of the bladder, evaluate bladder status before intravesical instillation of drug to avoid dangerous systemic exposure.

• In case of bladder perforation, delay administration until bladder integrity has been restored.

• If there isn't a complete response of CIS to valrubicin treatment after 3 months or if CIS recurs, cystectomy must be reconsidered because delaying cystectomy could lead to metastatic bladder cancer.

• Myelosuppression is possible if drug is inadvertently given systemically or if significant systemic exposure occurs after intravesical administration, such as in patients with bladder rupture or perforation.

• Use gloves during dose preparation and administration. Prepare and store solution in glass, polypropylene, or polyolefin containers and tubing. It's recommended that polyethylene-lined administration sets be used. Don't use polyvinyl chloride I.V. bags and tubing.

⚠ **ALERT** Don't confuse Valstar with valsartan.

• Store unopened vials under refrigeration at 36° to 46° F (2° to 8° C). Diluted drug is stable for 12 hours at temperatures up to 77° F (25° C).

Patient monitoring

• Monitor patient closely for disease recurrence or progression by cystoscopy, biopsy, and urine cytology every 3 months.

• If drug is administered when bladder rupture or perforation is suspected, CBC should be monitored weekly for 3 weeks. Myelosuppression begins during the first week, with the nadir by the second week, and recovery by the third week.

Breast-feeding patients

• It isn't known if drug appears in breast milk. Because drug is highly lipophilic and exposure of infants to drug could cause serious health risks, women should stop breast-feeding before therapy begins.

Pediatric patients

• Safety and effectiveness in children haven't been established.

Patient education

• Advise patient that drug induces complete response in only about 1 in 5 patients with refractory CIS. If CIS fails to respond completely after 3 months or if it recurs, discuss risks of cystectomy versus risks of metastatic bladder cancer with patient.

• Advise patient to retain drug for 2 hours before voiding, if possible. Instruct patient to void at the end of 2 hours.

• Instruct patient to maintain adequate hydration after treatment.

• Advise patient that major adverse reactions are related to irritable bladder symptoms that may occur during instillation and retention of drug and for a limited period after voiding. For the first 24 hours after administration, red-tinged urine is typical. Tell patient to report prolonged irritable bladder symptoms or prolonged passage of red-colored urine immediately.

• Advise a woman of childbearing age to avoid becoming pregnant during treatment. Men who take the drug should avoid fathering a child.

valsartan
Diovan

Pharmacologic classification: angiotensin II receptor antagonist
Therapeutic classification: antihypertensive
Pregnancy risk category: C (first trimester) D (second and third trimesters)

Indications and dosages

➤ *Hypertension, alone or with other antihypertensives. Adults:* Initially, 80 mg P.O. once daily as monotherapy in patients who aren't volume-depleted. Blood pressure reduction should occur in 2 to 4 weeks. If additional antihypertensive effect is needed, dosage may be increased to 160 or 320 mg daily or diuretic may be added. (Addition of diuretic has greater effect than dose increases beyond 80 mg.) Usual dosage range is 80 to 320 mg daily.

How supplied

Available by prescription only
Capsules: 80 mg, 160 mg

Pharmacodynamics

Antihypertensive action: Blocks binding of angiotensin II to receptor sites in vascular smooth muscle and adrenal gland, which inhibits the pressor effects of the renin-angiotensin system.

Pharmacokinetics

Absorption: Absolute bioavailability about 25%. Plasma level peaks 2 to 4 hours after dosing.
Distribution: Isn't distributed extensively into tissues; 95% bound to serum proteins, mainly to serum albumin.
Metabolism: Only about 20% is metabolized. Enzyme responsible for metabolism not yet identified; doesn't appear to be a cytochrome P-450 enzyme.
Excretion: 83% of dose excreted through feces; about 13% in urine. Average elimination half-life is about 6 hours.

Route	Onset	Peak	Duration
P.O.	2 hr	2-4 hr	24 hr

Contraindications and precautions

Contraindicated in patients hypersensitive to drug. Use cautiously in patients with renal or hepatic disease.

Interactions
Drug-drug. *Diuretics:* Increased risk of excessive hypotension. Use together cautiously. Monitor patient closely.

Adverse reactions
CNS: fatigue, dizziness, headache, insomnia.
CV: edema.
EENT: pharyngitis, rhinitis, sinusitis.
GI: abdominal pain, diarrhea, nausea, dyspepsia.
Hematologic: *neutropenia.*
Metabolic: hyperkalemia.
Musculoskeletal: arthralgia.
Respiratory: cough, upper respiratory tract infection.
Other: viral infection.

Overdose and treatment
The most likely effects of overdose are hypotension and tachycardia; bradycardia could occur from parasympathetic (vagal) stimulation. Treat supportively.

Special considerations
● Excessive hypotension can occur when drug is given with high doses of diuretics. Correct volume and salt depletions before therapy.
● Don't use in pregnant women because fetal and neonatal morbidity and death may occur.
⚠ ALERT Don't confuse valsartan with Valstar.

Patient monitoring
● Monitor fluid and electrolyte balance.
● Monitor cardiac status.

Breast-feeding patients
● It isn't known if drug appears in breast milk; use cautiously in breast-feeding women.

Pediatric patients
● Safety and effectiveness in children haven't been established.

Geriatric patients
● Although no overall difference in efficacy or safety has been observed, greater sensitivity of some older patients to drug can't be ruled out.

Patient education
● Advise woman to avoid pregnancy during therapy and to call immediately if pregnancy is suspected.
● Advise patient to report dizziness.

---

vancomycin hydrochloride
Vancocin, Vancoled

Pharmacologic classification: glycopeptide
Therapeutic classification: antibiotic
Pregnancy risk category: C

Indications and dosages
➤ *Severe staphylococcal infections when other antibiotics are ineffective or con-*
traindicated. Adults: 500 mg I.V. q 6 hours. Or, 1 g q 12 hours.
Children: 40 mg/kg I.V. daily divided q 6 hours.
Neonates: Initially, 15 mg/kg. Then, 10 mg/kg I.V. q 12 hours for first week after birth. Then, q 8 hours up to age 1 month.
➤ *Antibiotic-related pseudomembranous and staphylococcal enterocolitis. Adults:* 125 to 500 mg P.O. q 6 hours for 7 to 10 days.
Children: 40 mg/kg P.O. daily divided q 6 to 8 hours for 7 to 10 days. Don't exceed 2 g daily in children.
➤ *Endocarditis prophylaxis for dental, GI, biliary, and GU instrumentation procedures; surgical prophylaxis in patients allergic to penicillin. Adults:* 1 g I.V., given slowly over 1 to 2 hours with the infusion complete within 30 minutes of the start of the procedure.
Children: 20 mg/kg I.V. given slowly over 1 to 2 hours with the infusion complete within 30 minutes of the start of the procedure.
✦ *Dosage adjustment.* In renal failure, adjust dosage based on degree of renal impairment, severity of infection, and susceptibility of causative organism. Base dosage on serum levels of drug.

Recommended initial dose is 15 mg/kg. Subsequent doses should be adjusted, p.r.n. Some clinicians use the following schedule.

Creatinine clearance (mg/dl)	Adult dosage
< 1.5	1 g q 12 hours
1.5-5	1 g q 3 to 6 days
> 5	1 g q 10 to 14 days

How supplied
Available by prescription only
Powder for injection: 500-mg, 1-g, 5-g vials; 10-g pharmacy bulk package
Powder for oral solution: 1-g, 10-g bottles
Pulvules: 125 mg, 250 mg

Pharmacodynamics
Antibacterial action: Bactericidal. Hinders cell-wall synthesis and blocks glycopeptide polymerization. Spectrum of activity includes many gram-positive organisms, including those resistant to other antibiotics. Useful for *Staphylococcus epidermidis* and methicillin-resistant *S. aureus.* Also useful for penicillin-resistant *S. pneumococcus.*

Pharmacokinetics
Absorption: Minimal systemic absorption with oral use. However, drug may accumulate in patients with colitis or renal failure.
Distribution: Distributed widely in body fluids, including pericardial, pleural, ascitic, synovial, and placental fluid. Achieves therapeutic levels in CSF in patients with inflamed meninges. Therapeutic levels are 18 to 26 mcg/ml for 2-hour,

postinfusion peaks and 5 to 10 mcg/ml for pre-infusion troughs; values may vary depending on laboratory and sampling time.
Metabolism: No information available.
Excretion: When administered parenterally, excreted renally, mainly by filtration. When administered orally, excreted in feces. In patients with normal renal function, plasma half-life is 4 to 6 hours; in those with creatinine clearance of 10 to 60 ml/minute, plasma half-life is about 32 hours; if creatinine clearance is below 10 ml/minute, plasma half-life is 146 hours.

Route	Onset	Peak	Duration
P.O.	Unknown	Unknown	Unknown
I.V.	Immediate	Immediate	Unknown

Contraindications and precautions
Contraindicated in patients hypersensitive to drug. Use cautiously in patients over age 60; patients with impaired renal or hepatic function, hearing loss, or allergies to other antibiotics; and patients receiving other neurotoxic, nephrotoxic, or ototoxic drugs.

Interactions
Drug-drug. *Aminoglycosides, amphotericin B, capreomycin, cisplatin, colistin, methoxyflurane, polymyxin B:* Additive effect of these drugs. Monitor patient closely; adjust dosages as needed.
Nondepolarizing muscle relaxants: Enhanced neuromuscular blockade. Use together cautiously.

Adverse reactions
CV: hypotension.
EENT: tinnitus, ototoxicity.
GI: nausea.
GU: increased BUN and serum creatinine levels, ***nephrotoxicity.***
Hematologic: ***neutropenia,*** eosinophilia.
Respiratory: wheezing, dyspnea.
Skin: "red-neck" syndrome with rapid I.V. infusion (maculopapular rash on face, neck, trunk, and limbs).
Other: chills, fever, ***anaphylaxis,*** superinfection, pain or thrombophlebitis at injection site.

Overdose and treatment
Little information is available on acute toxicity.
   Treatment includes providing supportive care and maintaining glomerular filtration rate. Hemodialysis and hemoperfusion have been used.

Special considerations
• Administer intermittent I.V. infusion over at least 60 minutes.
• Oral form isn't for systemic infections and can't be interchanged with I.V. form.
• If patient has auditory dysfunction or needs prolonged therapy, auditory function tests may be indicated before and during therapy.
• Obtain culture and sensitivity tests before starting therapy (unless drug is being used for prophylaxis).

• I.M. administration is contraindicated because drug is highly irritating.
• Hemodialysis and peritoneal dialysis remove only minimal drug amounts. Patients receiving these treatments need usual dose only once every 5 to 7 days; however, some dialysis centers are using high flux hemodialysis, which can remove up to 50% of vancomycin, creating a need for supplemental doses. Dose should be based on serum level of drug.

Patient monitoring
• Monitor blood counts and BUN, serum creatinine, and drug levels.
• If patient develops maculopapular rash on face, neck, trunk, and arms, slow infusion rate.

Breast-feeding patients
• Drug appears in breast milk. Use cautiously in breast-feeding women.

Geriatric patients
• Elderly patients may be more susceptible to ototoxic effects. Monitor serum drug levels closely and adjust dosage as needed.

Patient education
• Advise patient receiving drug orally to continue taking as directed for full course of therapy, even when feeling better.
• Advise patient not to take antidiarrheals with drug unless prescribed.
• Instruct patient to promptly report onset of ringing in ears.

varicella virus vaccine, live
Varivax

Pharmacologic classification: vaccine
Therapeutic classification: viral vaccine
Pregnancy risk category: C

Indications and dosages
➤ *Prevention of varicella-zoster (chickenpox) infections. Adults and children age 13 and older:* Administer 0.5 ml S.C.; then give a second dose of 0.5 ml 4 to 8 weeks later.
Children ages 1 to 12: 0.5 ml S.C. as a single dose.

How supplied
Available by prescription only
Injection: Single-dose vial containing 1,350 plaque-forming units of Oka/Merck varicella virus

Pharmacodynamics
Antiviral vaccine action: Prevents chickenpox by inducing production of antibodies to varicella-zoster virus.

Pharmacokinetics
Absorption: Antibodies usually noted 4 to 6 weeks after S.C. injection. Varicella antibodies

have been detected 99.5% of the time 4 years postvaccination.
Distribution: No information available.
Metabolism: No information available.
Excretion: No information available.

Route	Onset	Peak	Duration
S.C.	7-10 days	28 days	> 10 yr

Contraindications and precautions
Contraindicated in patients hypersensitive to drug, in pregnant women, in patients with history of anaphylactoid reaction to neomycin, and in patients with blood dyscrasias, leukemia, lymphomas, neoplasms affecting bone marrow or the lymphatic system, primary and acquired immunosuppressive states, active untreated tuberculosis, or any febrile respiratory illness or other active febrile infection.

Interactions
Drug-drug. *Blood products, immune globulin:* May inactivate vaccine. Defer vaccination for at least 5 months after blood or plasma transfusions or administration of immune globulin or varicella-zoster immune globulin.
Immunosuppressants: Increased risk of severe reactions to live-virus vaccines. Postpone routine vaccination.
Salicylates. Risk of developing Reye's syndrome. Avoid salicylates for 6 weeks after vaccination.

Adverse reactions
Other: *fever, injection site reactions (swelling, redness, pain, rash),* varicella-like rash.

Overdose and treatment
No information available.

Special considerations
● Have epinephrine readily available.
● Administer vaccine immediately after reconstitution. Discard if not used within 30 minutes.
● Vaccine contains a live attenuated virus. Children who develop a rash may be capable of transmitting virus.
● Vaccine has been safely and effectively used with measles, mumps, and rubella vaccine.
● Vaccine appears to be less effective in adults than in children.
● Studies are underway to determine how often herpes zoster occurs after a latent period.
● Pregnancy should be avoided for 3 months after receiving vaccine.

Patient monitoring
● Monitor patient for rash; patient may be capable of transmitting virus.

Breast-feeding patients
● It isn't known if vaccine virus appears in breast milk; use cautiously in breast-feeding women.

Pediatric patients
● A safety study protocol program is available for children and adolescents (ages 12 to 17) with acute lymphocytic leukemia. Clinicians can enroll patients in this program by contacting Omnicare at (484) 679-2680.
● Safety and efficacy in children under age 1 haven't been established.

Patient education
● Inform patient or parents about adverse reactions associated with vaccine.
● Caution woman of childbearing age to call if pregnancy is suspected before receiving vaccine.

varicella-zoster immune globulin (VZIG)

Pharmacologic classification: immune serum
Therapeutic classification: varicella-zoster prophylaxis
Pregnancy risk category: C

Indications and dosages
➤ *Passive immunization of susceptible patients, primarily immunocompromised patients after exposure to varicella (chickenpox or herpes zoster). Adults and children:* 125 units per 10 kg of body weight I.M., to maximum of 625 units. Higher doses may be needed in immunocompromised adults.

How supplied
Available by prescription only
Injection: 10% to 18% solution of the globulin fraction of human plasma containing 125 units of varicella-zoster virus antibody in 2.5 ml or less

Pharmacodynamics
Postexposure prophylaxis: Provides passive immunity to varicella-zoster virus.

Pharmacokinetics
Absorption: After I.M. absorption, persistence of antibodies is unknown, but protection should last at least 3 weeks. Protection is sufficient to prevent or lessen severity of varicella infections.
Distribution: No information available.
Metabolism: No information available.
Excretion: No information available.

Route	Onset	Peak	Duration
I.M.	Unknown	Unknown	1 mo

Contraindications and precautions
Contraindicated in patients with thrombocytopenia, coagulation disorders, immunoglobulin A deficiency, or history of severe reaction to human immune serum globulin or thimerosal.

Interactions
Drug-drug. *Corticosteroids, immunosuppressants:* May interfere with immune response

to this immune globulin. Whenever possible, avoid using these drugs during postexposure immunization period.
Live-virus vaccines (such as those for measles, mumps, rubella): Drug may interfere with immune response. Don't administer live-virus vaccines within 2 weeks before or 3 months after VZIG. If you must administer VZIG with a live-virus vaccine, confirm seroconversion with follow-up serologic testing.

Adverse reactions
CNS: malaise, headache.
CV: chest tightness.
GI: GI distress.
GU: *nephrotic syndrome.*
Musculoskeletal: myalgia.
Respiratory: respiratory distress.
Skin: rash.
Other: *anaphylaxis,* discomfort at injection site, *angioedema, angioneurotic edema,* fever.

Overdose and treatment
No information available.

Special considerations
● Have epinephrine solution 1:1,000 available to treat allergic reactions.
● For maximum benefit, administer VZIG within 96 hours of presumed exposure.
● Although usually used only in children under age 15, VZIG may be administered to adults, if needed.
● VZIG is recommended primarily for immunodeficient patients under age 15 and certain infants exposed in utero, although use in other patients (especially immunocompromised patients of any age, normal adults, pregnant women, and premature and full-term infants) should be considered on a case-by-case basis. Not routinely recommended for use in immunocompetent pregnant women because chickenpox is much less severe than in immunosuppressed patients. Moreover, vaccine won't protect fetus. VZIG isn't for use in immunodeficient patients with history of varicella, unless immunosuppression is caused by bone marrow transplantation.
● Administer only by deep I.M. injection, never I.V. Use gluteal muscle in infants and small children and deltoid or anterolateral thigh in adults and larger children. For patients over 10 kg (22 lb), give no more than 2.5 ml at a single injection site.

Patient monitoring
● Monitor patient for immediate postadministration reactions, including anaphylaxis.

Breast-feeding patients
● It isn't known if VZIG appears in breast milk. Use cautiously in breast-feeding women.

Patient education
● Advise patient that the chance of contracting AIDS or hepatitis from VZIG is very small.
● Inform patient that some pain, swelling, and tenderness may occur at injection site. Acetaminophen may be taken to alleviate these minor effects.
● Encourage patient to immediately report severe reactions.

---

vasopressin
Pitressin Synthetic

Pharmacologic classification: posterior pituitary hormone
Therapeutic classification: antidiuretic hormone, peristaltic stimulant, hemostatic
Pregnancy risk category: C

Indications and dosages
➤ *Nonnephrogenic, nonpsychogenic diabetes insipidus. Adults:* 5 to 10 units I.M. or S.C. b.i.d. to q.i.d., p.r.n.
Children: 2.5 to 10 units I.M. or S.C. b.i.d. to q.i.d., p.r.n.
➤ *Postoperative abdominal distention. Adults:* 5 units I.M. initially; then q 3 to 4 hours, increasing dose to 10 units, if needed. Reduce dosage for children proportionately.
➤ *To expel gas before abdominal X-ray. Adults:* Inject 5 to 15 units S.C. at 2 hours; then again at 30 minutes before X-ray. Enema before first dose may also help to eliminate gas.
➤ *Upper GI tract hemorrhage. Adults:* 0.2 to 0.4 units/minute I.V. or 0.1 to 0.5 units/minute intra-arterially.

How supplied
Available by prescription only
Injection: 0.5-ml and 1-ml ampules, 20 units/ml; 0.5-ml, 1-ml vials, 20 units/ml

Pharmacodynamics
Antidiuretic action: Used as an antidiuretic to control or prevent signs and complications of neurogenic diabetes insipidus. Acting primarily at the renal tubular level, drug increases cAMP, which increases water permeability at the renal tubule and collecting duct, resulting in increased urine osmolality and decreased urine flow rate.
Peristaltic stimulant action: Used to treat postoperative abdominal distention and to facilitate abdominal radiographic procedures, vasopressin induces peristalsis by directly stimulating contraction of smooth muscle in the GI tract.
Hemostatic action: In patients with GI hemorrhage, vasopressin, administered I.V. or intra-arterially into the superior mesenteric artery, controls bleeding of esophageal varices by directly stimulating vasoconstriction of capillaries and small arterioles.

Pharmacokinetics
Absorption: Destroyed by trypsin in GI tract; must be given intranasally or parenterally.
Distribution: Distributed throughout extracellular fluid, with no evidence of protein-binding.
Metabolism: Most of dose destroyed rapidly in liver and kidneys.
Excretion: About 5% of S.C. dose excreted unchanged in urine after 4 hours. Duration of action after I.M. or S.C. administration is 2 to 8 hours. Half-life, 10 to 20 minutes.

Route	Onset	Peak	Duration
I.M., S.C., intranasal	2-8 hr	Unknown	Unknown

Contraindications and precautions
Contraindicated in patients hypersensitive to vasopressin or its components and in patients with anaphylactoid reactions to them. Also contraindicated in patients with chronic nephritis accompanied by nitrogen retention. Use cautiously in children, pregnant patients, elderly patients, preoperative or postoperative patients who are polyuric, and patients with seizure disorders, migraine headache, asthma, CV or renal disease, heart failure, goiter with cardiac complications, arteriosclerosis, or fluid overload.

Interactions
Drug-drug. *Carbamazepine, chlorpropamide, clofibrate, fludricortisone, phenformin urea, tricyclic antidepressants:* May potentiate antidiuretic effect. Monitor therapeutic effect.
Demeclocycline, epinephrine, heparin, lithium, norepinephrine: Decreased antidiuretic effect. Monitor therapeutic effect.
Drug-lifestyle. *Alcohol use:* Reduced antidiuretic activity. Discourage use.

Adverse reactions
CNS: tremor, headache, vertigo.
CV: angina in patients with vascular disease, vasoconstriction, **arrhythmias, cardiac arrest,** myocardial ischemia, circumoral pallor, decreased cardiac output.
GI: abdominal cramps, nausea, vomiting, flatulence.
Skin: cutaneous gangrene, diaphoresis.
Other: *water intoxication* (drowsiness, listlessness, headache, confusion, weight gain, *seizures, coma*), hypersensitivity reactions (urticaria, **angioedema, bronchospasm, anaphylaxis**).

Overdose and treatment
Signs and symptoms of overdose include drowsiness, listlessness, headache, confusion, anuria, and weight gain (water intoxication).
Treatment requires water restriction and temporary withdrawal of vasopressin until polyuria occurs. Severe water intoxication may require osmotic diuresis with mannitol, hypertonic dextrose, or urea, either alone or with furosemide.

Special considerations
Consider the recommendations relevant to all posterior pituitary hormones as well as the following.
• Never inject during first stage of labor; this may cause ruptured uterus.
• Use extreme caution to avoid extravasation because of risk of necrosis and gangrene.

Patient monitoring
• Establish baseline vital signs and intake and output ratio at start of therapy.
• Monitor patient's blood pressure twice daily. Watch for excessively elevated blood pressure or lack of response to drug, which may be indicated by hypotension.
• Monitor fluid intake and output and daily weight.
• Observe patient for signs of early water intoxication —drowsiness, listlessness, headache, confusion, and weight gain—to prevent seizures, coma, and death.
• Monitor abdominal distention and GI function; a rectal tube will facilitate gas expulsion after vasopressin injection.

Breast-feeding patients
• It isn't known if drug appears in breast milk. Use cautiously in breast-feeding women.

Pediatric patients
• Children show increased sensitivity to drug's effects. Use cautiously.

Geriatric patients
• Elderly patients show increased sensitivity to drug's effects. Use cautiously.

Patient education
• Advise patient to rotate injection sites.
• Tell patient to drink one or two glasses of water with each dose of vasopressin to reduce adverse reactions such as unusual paleness, nausea, abdominal cramps, and vomiting.
• Tell patient to call immediately if he develops chest pain, confusion, fever, hives, rash, headache, problems with urination, seizures, weight gain, unusual drowsiness, wheezing, trouble with breathing, or swelling of face, hands, feet, or mouth.

vecuronium bromide
Norcuron

Pharmacologic classification: nondepolarizing neuromuscular blocker
Therapeutic classification: skeletal muscle relaxant
Pregnancy risk category: C

Indications and dosages
➤*Adjunct to anesthesia, to facilitate intubation, and to provide skeletal muscle relaxation during surgery or me-*

chanical ventilation. Dosages are representative and must be adjusted based on anesthetic used and individual needs and response. *Adults and children age 10 and over:* Initially, 0.08 to 0.1 mg/kg I.V. bolus. Higher initial doses (up to 0.28 mg/kg) may be used for rapid onset. Maintenance doses of 0.01 to 0.015 mg/kg within 25 to 40 minutes of initial dose should be administered during prolonged surgical procedures. Maintenance doses may be given q 12 to 15 minutes in patients receiving balanced anesthetic.

Or, after the initial dosing of 0.08 to 0.1 mg/kg, a continuous infusion of 1 mcg/kg/minute may be started 20 to 40 minutes later.

How supplied
Available by prescription only
Injection: 10 mg (with or without diluent), 20 mg (without diluent)

Pharmacodynamics
Skeletal muscle relaxant action: Prevents acetylcholine from binding to receptors on motor end plate, thus blocking depolarization. Exhibits minimal CV effects and doesn't appear to alter heart rate or rhythm, systolic or diastolic blood pressure, cardiac output, systemic vascular resistance, or mean arterial pressure. Has little or no histamine-releasing effect.

Pharmacokinetics
Absorption: Administered I.V.
Distribution: After I.V. administration, distributed in extracellular fluid and rapidly reaches site of action. 60% to 90% plasma protein–bound. Volume of distribution decreased in children under age 1; may be decreased in elderly patients.
Metabolism: Undergoes rapid and extensive hepatic metabolism.
Excretion: Drug and metabolites appear to be primarily excreted in feces by biliary elimination; also excreted in urine.

Route	Onset	Peak	Duration
I.V.	1 min	3-5 min	15-25 min

Contraindications and precautions
Contraindicated in patients hypersensitive to vecuronium and bromides. Use cautiously in elderly patients and in patients with altered circulation caused by CV disease and edematous states, hepatic disease, severe obesity, bronchogenic carcinoma, electrolyte disturbances, or neuromuscular diseases.

Interactions
Drug-drug. *Aminoglycosides, clindamycin, depolarizing neuromuscular blockers, furosemide, general anesthetics, lincomycin, nondepolarizing neuromuscular blockers, parenteral magnesium salts, polymyxin antibiotics, potassium-depleting drugs, quinidine, quinine, thiazide diuretics:* Increased vecuronium-induced neuromuscular blockade. Don't use together. When concomitant use can't be avoided, use together cautiously. Decrease dosage by 15%, especially with enflurane and isoflurane.
Anticholinesterases: Antagonized effects of vecuronium. Monitor patient closely. Adjust dosage as needed.
Narcotic (opioid) analgesics: Increased central respiratory depression. Monitor respiratory status closely.

Adverse reactions
Musculoskeletal: skeletal muscle weakness.
Respiratory: *prolonged, dose-related respiratory insufficiency or apnea.*

Overdose and treatment
Signs and symptoms of overdose include prolonged duration of neuromuscular blockade, skeletal muscle weakness, decreased respiratory reserve, low tidal volume, and apnea.

Treatment is supportive and symptomatic. Keep airway clear and maintain adequate ventilation.

Special considerations
● Keep emergency respiratory support equipment immediately available.
● Administration of vecuronium must be accompanied by adequate anesthesia. Drug doesn't relieve pain or affect consciousness.
● Administer by rapid I.V. injection or I.V. infusion. Don't give I.M.
● Diluent supplied by manufacturer contains benzyl alcohol, which isn't intended for use in newborns.
● Don't mix in same syringe or give through same needle as barbiturates or other alkaline solutions.
● Protect solution from light.
● Use peripheral nerve stimulator to determine and monitor degree of blockade. Give anticholinesterase (edrophonium, neostigmine, or pyridostigmine) to reverse neuromuscular blockade and atropine or glycopyrrolate to overcome muscarinic effects.

Patient monitoring
● Assess baseline serum electrolyte levels, acid-base balance, and renal and hepatic function before administration.
● Peripheral nerve stimulator may be used to identify residual paralysis during recovery and is especially useful during administration to high-risk patients.
● After procedure, monitor vital signs at least every 15 minutes until patient is stable, and then every 30 minutes for next 2 hours. Monitor airway and pattern of respirations until patient has recovered from drug effects.
● Evaluate recovery from neuromuscular blockade by checking strength of patient's hand grip and his ability to breathe naturally, take deep

breaths and cough, keep eyes open, and lift head keeping mouth closed.

Breast-feeding patients
• It isn't known if drug appears in breast milk. Use cautiously in breast-feeding women.

Pediatric patients
• Safety and efficacy haven't been established in infants under age 7 weeks.
• Infants ages 7 weeks to 1 year are more sensitive to neuromuscular blocking effects; less frequent administration may be needed.
• Higher doses may be needed in children ages 1 to 9.

Geriatric patients
• Administer cautiously to elderly patients.

Patient education
• Advise patient that drug won't relieve pain or affect consciousness.
• Inform patient that postprocedure monitoring will involve patient demonstrating hand grip, breathing, and coughing.

venlafaxine hydrochloride
Effexor, Effexor XR

Pharmacologic classification: neuronal serotonin, norepinephrine, and dopamine reuptake inhibitor
Therapeutic classification: antidepressant
Pregnancy risk category: C

Indications and dosages
➤ *Depression. Adults:* Initially, 75 mg P.O. daily, in two or three divided doses with food. Increase dosage as tolerated and needed in increments of 75 mg daily at intervals of no less than 4 days. For moderately depressed outpatients, usual maximum dose is 225 mg daily. In certain severely depressed patients, dosage may be as high as 375 mg daily divided into three doses. For extended-release capsules, 75 mg P.O. daily, in a single dose. For some patients, it may be desirable to start at 37.5 mg P.O. daily for 4 to 7 days before increasing to 75 mg daily. Dosage may be increased at increments of 75 mg daily q 4 days to a maximum of 225 mg daily.
➤ *Generalized anxiety disorder. Adults:* Initally, 75 mg daily (extended-release) in a single dose. Increase dosage as needed in 75-mg daily increments at intervals of at least 4 days. Maximum, 225 mg daily.
✦ *Dosage adjustment.* Reduce dosage by 50% in patients with impaired hepatic function. In patients with moderate renal impairment (glomerular filtration rate of 10 to 70 ml/minute), total daily dose should be reduced by 25% to 50%. In hemodialysis patients, reduce dosage by 50% and withhold drug until after dialysis treatment.

➤ *Prevention of major depressive disorder relapse. Adults:* 75 to 225 mg/day P.O. of Effexor, or 75 to 150 mg daily P.O. of Effexor XR.

How supplied
Available by prescription only
Capsules (extended-release): 37.5 mg, 75 mg, 150 mg
Tablets: 25 mg, 37.5 mg, 50 mg, 75 mg, 100 mg

Pharmacodynamics
Antidepressant action: Thought to potentiate neurotransmitter activity in the CNS. Venlafaxine and its active metabolite, O-desmethylvenlafaxine (ODV) are potent inhibitors of neuronal serotonin and norepinephrine reuptake and weak inhibitors of dopamine reuptake.

Pharmacokinetics
Absorption: About 92% of drug absorbed after oral administration.
Distribution: 25% to 29% protein-bound in plasma.
Metabolism: Extensively metabolized in liver, with ODV the only major active metabolite.
Excretion: About 87% of dose recovered in urine within 48 hours (5% as unchanged venlafaxine, 29% as unconjugated ODV, 26% as conjugated ODV, 27% as minor inactive metabolites). Elimination half-life is about 5 hours for venlafaxine and 11 hours for ODV.

Route	Onset	Peak	Duration
P.O.	Unknown	Unknown	Unknown

Contraindications and precautions
Contraindicated in patients hypersensitive to drug and within 14 days of MAO inhibitor therapy. Use cautiously in patients with impaired renal or hepatic function, diseases or conditions that could affect hemodynamic responses or metabolism, or history of seizures or mania.

Interactions
Drug-drug. *Cimetidine, CNS-active drugs:* Pronounced increase in venlafaxine level in elderly patients and those with hepatic dysfunction or hypertension. Use cautiously together.
MAO inhibitors: May precipitate a syndrome similar to neuroleptic malignant syndrome when used with venlafaxine. Don't start venlafaxine within 14 days of stopping an MAO inhibitor; don't start MAO inhibitor within 7 days of stopping venlafaxine.
Drug-herb. *Yohimbé:* Possible additive stimulation. Use together cautiously.

Adverse reactions
CNS: *headache, somnolence, dizziness, nervousness, insomnia,* anxiety, tremor, abnormal dreams, paresthesia, agitation, *asthenia.*
CV: hypertension, vasodilation.
EENT: blurred vision.

GI: *nausea, constipation,* vomiting, *dry mouth, anorexia,* diarrhea, dyspepsia, flatulence.
GU: *abnormal ejaculation,* impotence, urinary frequency, impaired urination.
Metabolic: weight loss.
Skin: *diaphoresis,* rash.
Other: yawning, chills, infection, decreased libido (extended release).

Overdose and treatment
Signs and symptoms of overdose may range from none (most commonly) to somnolence, generalized seizures, and prolongation of QT interval.

Treatment should consist of general measures used in managing any antidepressant overdose (ensuring an adequate airway, providing oxygenation and ventilation, monitoring cardiac rhythm and vital signs). General supportive and symptomatic measures also are recommended. Use of activated charcoal, induction of emesis, or gastric lavage should be considered. No specific antidote is known for venlafaxine overdose.

Special considerations
• When ending therapy after more than 1 week, taper dose. If patient has received drug for at least 6 weeks, gradually taper over 2 weeks.
• Stop drug in patient who develops seizures.

Patient monitoring
• Because drug may cause sustained increases in blood pressure, monitor blood pressure regularly. For patients who have sustained increase in blood pressure, consider either dosage reduction or discontinuation of drug.
• Monitor patients with major affective disorders; drug may activate mania or hypomania.

Breast-feeding patients
• Drug appears in breast milk. Because of the potential for serious adverse effects in the breastfed infant, a decision should be made to discontinue drug or breast-feeding.

Pediatric patients
• Safety and effectiveness in children under age 18 haven't been established.

Patient education
• Caution patient to avoid hazardous activities until drug's effects are known.
• Advise woman to report suspected, planned, or known pregnancy during therapy.
• Instruct patient to call before taking other drugs, including OTC medications, because of potential interactions.
• Tell patient to avoid alcohol during therapy.
• Instruct patient to report rash, hives, or a related allergic reaction.

verapamil hydrochloride
Calan, Calan SR, Covera-HS, Isoptin, Isoptin SR, Verelan, Verelan PM

Pharmacologic classification: calcium channel blocker
Therapeutic classification: antianginal, antihypertensive, antiarrhythmic
Pregnancy risk category: C

Indications and dosages
➤ *Management of Prinzmetal's or variant angina or unstable or chronic stable angina pectoris. Adults:* Initial dose, 80 to 120 mg P.O. t.i.d. Dosage may be increased at weekly intervals. Some patients may need up to 480 mg daily.
➤ *Supraventricular tachyarrhythmias. Adults:* 0.075 to 0.15 mg/kg (5 to 10 mg) I.V. push over 2 minutes. If no response occurs, give a second dose of 10 mg (0.15 mg/kg) 15 to 30 minutes after the initial dose. Give over at least 3 minutes in geriatric patients.
Children ages 1 to 15: 0.1 to 0.3 mg/kg (2 to 5 mg) as I.V. bolus over 2 minutes. Dose shouldn't exceed 5 mg. Dose may be repeated in 30 minutes if no response occurs (shouldn't exceed 10 mg).
Children under age 1: 0.1 to 0.2 mg/kg (0.75 to 2 mg) as I.V. bolus over 2 minutes. Dose may be repeated in 30 minutes if no response occurs.
➤ *Control of ventricular rate in digitalized patients with chronic atrial flutter or fibrillation. Adults:* 240 to 320 mg P.O. daily in three to four divided doses.
➤ *Prophylaxis of repetitive paroxysmal supraventricular tachycardia. Adults:* 240 to 480 mg daily given in three to four divided doses.
➤ *Hypertension. Adults:* Usual starting dose is 80 mg P.O. t.i.d. Daily dose may be increased to 360 to 480 mg. Initial dose of extended release tablets or capsules is 120 to 240 mg daily in the morning. Initial dose of Covera-HS is 180 mg h.s. and Verelan PM 200 mg h.s. Start therapy with sustained-release capsules at 180 mg (240 mg for Verelan) daily in the morning. Adjust dosage based on effectiveness 24 hours after dosing. Increase by 120 mg daily until a maximum dose of 480 mg daily is given. Sustained-release capsules should be given only once daily. Antihypertensive effects are usually seen within the first week of therapy. Most patients respond to 240 mg daily.

How supplied
Available by prescription only
Capsules (extended release): 120 mg, 180 mg, 240 mg
Capsules (sustained-release): 100 mg, 120 mg, 180 mg, 200 mg, 240 mg, 300 mg, 360 mg
Injection: 2.5 mg/ml

Reactions may be *common,* uncommon, **life-threatening**, or COMMON AND LIFE-THREATENING.

Tablets: 40 mg, 80 mg, 120 mg
Tablets (extended release): 120 mg, 180 mg, 240 mg
Tablets (sustained-release): 120 mg, 180 mg, 240 mg

Pharmacodynamics

Antianginal action: Manages unstable and chronic stable angina by reducing afterload, both at rest and with exercise, thereby decreasing oxygen consumption. Also decreases myocardial oxygen demand and cardiac work by exerting a negative inotropic effect, reducing heart rate, relieving coronary artery spasm (via coronary artery vasodilation), and dilating peripheral vessels. The net result of these effects is relief of angina-related ischemia and pain. In patients with Prinzmetal's variant angina, verapamil inhibits coronary artery spasm, resulting in increased myocardial oxygen delivery.

Antihypertensive action: Reduces blood pressure mainly by dilating peripheral vessels. Drug's negative inotropic effect blocks reflex mechanisms that lead to increased blood pressure.

Antiarrhythmic action: Drug's combined effects on the SA and AV nodes help manage arrhythmias. Its primary effect is on the AV node; slowed conduction reduces the ventricular rate in atrial tachyarrhythmias and blocks reentry paths in paroxysmal supraventricular arrhythmias.

Pharmacokinetics

Absorption: Absorbed rapidly and completely from GI tract after oral administration; however, only about 20% to 35% reaches systemic circulation because of first-pass effect. When administered orally, peak plasma concentrations are reached within 1 to 2 hours with conventional tablets; within 4 to 11 hours with sustained-release preparations. When administered I.V., effects occur within minutes after injection and usually last about 30 to 60 minutes (may last up to 6 hours). Therapeutic serum levels are 80 to 300 ng/ml.

Distribution: Steady state distribution volume in healthy adults ranges from about 4.5 to 7 L/kg; may increase to 12 L/kg in patients with hepatic cirrhosis. About 90% of circulating drug is bound to plasma proteins.

Metabolism: Metabolized in liver.

Excretion: Excreted in urine as unchanged drug and active metabolites. Elimination half-life normally 6 to 12 hours; increases to as much as 16 hours in patients with hepatic cirrhosis. In infants, elimination half-life may be 5 to 7 hours.

Route	Onset	Peak	Duration
P.O.			
Regular	½ hr	1-2 hr	8-10 hr
Extended	½ hr	5-9 hr	24 hr
I.V.	Immediate	1-5 min	1-6 hr

Contraindications and precautions

Contraindicated in patients hypersensitive to drug and in those with severe left ventricular dysfunction, cardiogenic shock, second- or third-degree AV block or sick sinus syndrome except in presence of functioning pacemaker, atrial flutter or fibrillation and accessory bypass tract syndrome, severe heart failure (unless secondary to verapamil therapy), and severe hypotension. In addition, I.V. verapamil is contraindicated in patients receiving I.V. beta blockers and in those with ventricular tachycardia.

Use cautiously in elderly patients and patients with impaired renal or hepatic function or increased intracranial pressure.

Interactions

Drug-drug. *Antihypertensives, drugs that attenuate alpha-adrenergic response (such as methyldopa, prazosin), quinidine (to treat hypertrophic cardiomyopathy):* Hypotension. Monitor blood pressure closely. Adjust dosage of either drug as needed.

Beta blockers: Additive effects leading to heart failure, conduction disturbances, arrhythmias, and hypotension, especially with high beta-blocker doses, drugs administered I.V., or moderately severe to severe heart failure, severe cardiomyopathy, or recent MI. Monitor cardiac status closely.

Carbamazepine: Increased serum carbamazepine levels and subsequent toxicity. Use together cautiously; watch for signs of toxicity.

Cyclosporine: Increased serum cyclosporine levels. Monitor therapeutic effect; adjust cyclosporine dosage as needed.

Dantrolene: Possible hyperkalemia and myocardial depression. Consider using a dihydropyridine calcium blocker.

Digoxin: May increase serum digoxin levels by 50% to 75% during first week of therapy. Adjust digoxin dosage; monitor cardiac status closely.

Disopyramide: Combined negative inotropic effects. Monitor patient closely.

Etomidate: Anesthetic effect of etomidate may be increased, with prolonged respiratory depression and apnea. Use cautiously.

Flecainide: May add to negative inotropic effect and prolong AV conduction. Monitor cardiac status.

Hydantoins: Serum verapamil levels may be decreased. Use cautiously.

Inhaled anesthetics: Excessive CV depression. Avoid concomitant use.

Lithium: May increase lithium effects. Adjust lithium dosage as needed.

Neuromuscular blockers: Drug may potentiate their action. Adjust dosage of neuromuscular blockers as needed; monitor patient closely.

Phenobarbital: May increase verapamil clearance. Monitor cardiac status.

Rifampin: May substantially reduce verapamil's oral bioavailability. Monitor therapeutic effect; adjust dosage of verapamil as needed.

◇ Unlabeled clinical use

Sulfinpyrazone: Clearance of verapamil may be increased. Montior patient closely.
Theophylline: Increased plasma theophylline levels. Monitor patient closely; adjust theophylline dosage as needed.
Vitamin D: Therapeutic effect of verapamil may be reduced. Monitor patient closely.
Drug-herb. *Black catechu:* May cause additive effects. Discourage use together.
Yerba maté: May decrease clearance of yerba maté methylxanthines and cause toxicity. Tell patient to use together cautiously.
Drug-food. *Any food:* Increased absorption. Patient should take drug with food.
Drug-lifestyle. *Alcohol use:* Prolonged intoxication effect. Discourage use.

Adverse reactions

CNS: dizziness, headache, asthenia.
CV: *transient hypotension,* **heart failure, pulmonary edema, bradycardia, AV block, ventricular asystole, ventricular fibrillation,** peripheral edema.
GI: *constipation,* nausea.
Hepatic: elevated liver enzyme levels.
Respiratory: pulmonary edema.
Skin: rash.

Overdose and treatment

Effects of overdose are primarily extensions of adverse reactions. Heart block, asystole, and hypotension are the most serious reactions and require immediate attention.

Treatment may include administering I.V. isoproterenol, norepinephrine, epinephrine, atropine, or calcium gluconate in usual doses. Ensure adequate hydration.

In patients with hypertrophic cardiomyopathy, alpha-adrenergic drugs, such as methoxamine, phenylephrine, and metaraminol, should be used to maintain blood pressure. (Avoid isoproterenol and norepinephrine.) Inotropic drugs, such as dobutamine and dopamine, may be used if needed.

If severe conduction disturbances, such as heart block and asystole, occur with hypotension that doesn't respond to drug therapy, start cardiac pacing immediately, with CPR measures as indicated.

In patients with Wolff-Parkinson-White or Lown-Ganong-Levine syndrome and a rapid ventricular rate caused by hemodynamically significant antegrade conduction, synchronized cardioversion may be used. Lidocaine and procainamide may be used as adjuncts.

Special considerations

● If verapamil is started in patient receiving carbamazepine, a 40% to 50% reduction in carbamazepine dosage may be necessary. Monitor patient closely for signs of toxicity.
● If verapamil is added to therapy of patient receiving digoxin, reduce digoxin dosage by half and monitor subsequent serum drug levels.

● Reduce verapamil dosage in patients with renal or hepatic impairment, those with severely compromised cardiac function, and those receiving beta blockers.
● Stop disopyramide 48 hours before starting verapamil, and don't resume until 24 hours after verapamil has been stopped.
● Generic sustained-release verapamil tablets may be substituted only for Isoptin SR and Calan SR, not Verelan capsules. The capsule form should be given only once daily. When using sustained-release tablets, doses over 240 mg should be given b.i.d.

Patient monitoring

● During long-term therapy with verapamil and digoxin, monitor ECG periodically to observe for AV block and bradycardia.
● Obtain periodic liver function tests.
● If patient is receiving verapamil I.V., monitor ECG and blood pressure continuously.

Breast-feeding patients

● Drug appears in breast milk. To avoid possible adverse effects in infants, mother shouldn't breast-feed during therapy.

Pediatric patients

● Currently, only the I.V. form is indicated for use in children to treat supraventricular tachyarrhythmias.

Geriatric patients

● Elderly patients may need lower doses.
● Give I.V. doses over at least 3 minutes to minimize risk of adverse effects.

Patient education

● Instruct patient to report signs of heart failure, such as swelling of hands and feet or shortness of breath.
● Urge patient who is receiving nitrate therapy while verapamil dosage is being adjusted to comply with prescribed therapy.

vidarabine (adenine arabinoside)
Vira-A

Pharmacologic classification: purine nucleoside
Therapeutic classification: antiviral
Pregnancy risk category: C

Indications and dosages

➤ *Acute keratoconjunctivitis and recurrent epithelial keratitis caused by herpes simplex virus types 1 and 2.* *Adults and children:* Administer ½ inch (1.3 cm) of ointment into lower conjunctival sac five times daily at 3-hour intervals.

How supplied
Available by prescription only
Ophthalmic ointment: 3% in 3.5-g tube (equivalent to 2.8% vidarabine)

Pharmacodynamics
Antiviral action: Exact mechanism unknown. Adenine analogue; presumably involves inhibition of DNA polymerase and viral replication by incorporation into viral DNA.

Pharmacokinetics
Absorption: No systemic absorption occurs with ophthalmic use.
Distribution: Only trace amounts of drug detected in aqueous humor if cornea is intact.
Metabolism: Metabolized into active metabolite arabinosyl-hypoxanthine.
Excretion: No information available.

Route	Onset	Peak	Duration
Oph-thalmic	Unknown	Unknown	Unknown

Contraindications and precautions
Contraindicated in patients hypersensitive to drug and in those with sterile trophic ulcers. Use cautiously in patients receiving corticosteroids.

Interactions
None reported.

Adverse reactions
EENT: temporary burning, itching, mild irritation, pain, lacrimation, foreign body sensation, conjunctival injection, punctal occlusion, sensitivity, superficial punctate keratitis, photophobia.
Other: hypersensitivity reactions.

Overdose and treatment
No information available

Special considerations
● Drug is effective only if patient has at least minimal immunocompetence.
● Definitive diagnosis of herpes simplex conjunctivitis should be made before administration of ophthalmic form.

Patient monitoring
● Monitor therapeutic effect. If there are no signs of improvement after 7 days or if reepithelialization hasn't occurred in 21 days, consider other forms of therapy. Patients with severe cases may need longer treatment. Continue drug for 5 to 7 days, b.i.d., to prevent recurrence.
● Monitor patient for adverse effects.

Patient education
● Warn patient receiving ophthalmic ointment not to exceed recommended frequency or duration of therapy. Instruct him to wash hands before and after applying ointment, and warn him against allowing tip of tube to touch eye or surrounding area.
● Advise patient to wear sunglasses if photosensitivity occurs.
● Instruct patient to store ophthalmic ointment in tightly sealed, light-resistant container.

vinblastine sulfate (VLB)
Velban, Velbe*

Pharmacologic classification: vinca alkaloid (specific to M phase of cell cycle)
Therapeutic classification: antineoplastic
Pregnancy risk category: D

Indications and dosages
Dosage and indications may vary. Check current literature for recommended protocol.
➤ **Breast or testicular cancer, Hodgkin's and malignant lymphomas, choriocarcinoma, lymphosarcoma, neuroblastoma, lung cancer, mycosis fungoides, histiocytosis, Kaposi's sarcoma.** *Adults:* 0.1 mg/kg or 3.7 mg/m^2 I.V. weekly or q 2 weeks. May be increased in weekly increments of 50 mcg/kg or 1.8 to 1.9 mg/m^2 to maximum dose of 0.5 mg/kg or 18.5 mg/m^2 I.V. weekly, based on response. Dose shouldn't be repeated if WBC count falls below 4,000/mm^3.
Children: 2.5 mg/m^2 I.V. as a single dose every week, increased weekly in increments of 1.25 mg/m^2 to maximum of 12.5 mg/m^2.

How supplied
Available by prescription only
Injection: 10-mg vials (lyophilized powder), 1 mg/ml in 10-ml and 25-ml vials

Pharmacodynamics
Antineoplastic action: Exerts cytotoxic activity by arresting the cell cycle in the metaphase portion of cell division, resulting in a blockade of mitosis. Drug also inhibits DNA-dependent RNA synthesis and interferes with amino acid metabolism, inhibiting purine synthesis.

Pharmacokinetics
Absorption: Administered I.V.
Distribution: Distributed widely into body tissues. Drug crosses blood-brain barrier but doesn't achieve therapeutic levels in CSF.
Metabolism: Metabolized partially in liver to an active metabolite.
Excretion: Excreted primarily in bile as unchanged drug. Smaller portion excreted in urine. Triphasic plasma elimination; half-lives of 3.7 minutes, 1.6 hours, and 24.8 hours for alpha, beta, and terminal phases, respectively.

Route	Onset	Peak	Duration
I.V.	Unknown	Unknown	Unknown

Contraindications and precautions

Contraindicated in patients with severe leukopenia, granulocytopenia (unless result of disease being treated), or bacterial infection. Use cautiously in patients with hepatic dysfunction.

Interactions

Drug-drug. *Erythromycin:* May cause vinblastine toxicity. Watch closely for toxicity.
Mitomycin: Acute shortness of breath and severe bronchospasm. Use cautiously together.
Phenytoin: May reduce plasma phenytoin levels. Increase phenytoin dosage, as needed.

Adverse reactions

CNS: depression, *paresthesia, peripheral neuropathy and neuritis, numbness, loss of deep tendon reflexes, muscle pain and weakness, seizures, CVA,* headache.
CV: hypertension, *MI.*
EENT: pharyngitis.
GI: *nausea, vomiting,* ulcer, bleeding, *constipation, ileus, anorexia,* diarrhea, abdominal pain, *stomatitis.*
Hematologic: *anemia, leukopenia* (nadir occurs days 4 to 10 and lasts another 7 to 14 days), *thrombocytopenia.*
Metabolic: hyperuricemia, *weight loss.*
Respiratory: *acute bronchospasm,* shortness of breath.
Skin: vesiculation, reversible alopecia.
Other: *irritation, phlebitis,* cellulitis, necrosis with extravasation.

Overdose and treatment

Signs and symptoms of overdose include stomatitis, ileus, mental depression, paresthesia, loss of deep reflexes, permanent CNS damage, and myelosuppression.

Treatment is usually supportive and includes transfusion of blood components and appropriate symptomatic therapy.

Special considerations

• Give an antiemetic before drug to reduce nausea.
• Drug may be given by I.V. push injection over 1 minute into the tubing of a freely flowing I.V. infusion.
• Dilution into larger volume isn't recommended for infusion into peripheral veins. This method increases risk of extravasation. Drug may be administered as an I.V. infusion through a central venous catheter.
• Don't administer more often than every 7 days to allow review of effect on leukocytes before next dose. Leukopenia may develop.
• Reduced dosages may be needed in patients with liver disease.
• Prevent uric acid nephropathy with generous oral fluid intake and administration of allopurinol.
ALERT Don't confuse vinblastine with vincristine, vindesine, or vinorelbin.

• Drug is less neurotoxic than vincristine.

Patient monitoring

• Watch for life-threatening acute bronchospasm reaction. This reaction is most likely to occur in patients also receiving mitomycin.

Breast-feeding patients

• It isn't known if drug appears in breast milk. However, because of risk of serious adverse reactions, mutagenicity, and carcinogenicity in infants, breast-feeding isn't recommended.

Geriatric patients

• Patients with cachexia or skin ulceration (which is more common in elderly patients) may be more susceptible to leukopenic effect of drug.

Patient education

• Encourage adequate fluid intake to increase urine output and facilitate excretion of uric acid.
• Reassure patient that therapeutic response isn't immediate. Adequate trial is 12 weeks.
• Advise patient to avoid exposure to people with infections and to report signs of infection or unusual bleeding immediately.
• Reassure patient that hair should grow back after treatment has ended.

vincristine sulfate
Oncovin, Vincasar PFS

Pharmacologic classification: vinca alkaloid (specific to M phase of cell cycle)
Therapeutic classification: antineoplastic
Pregnancy risk category: D

Indications and dosages

Dosage and indications may vary. Check current literature for recommended protocol.
➤ *Acute lymphoblastic and other leukemias; Hodgkin's disease; lymphosarcoma; reticulum cell, osteogenic, and other sarcomas; neuroblastoma; rhabdomyosarcoma; Wilms' tumor; lung cancer; breast cancer*◇. *Adults:* 1.4 mg/m² I.V. weekly. Maximum single dose (adults and children) is 2 mg.
Children: 2 mg/m² I.V. weekly.
Children who weigh less than 10 kg (22 lb) or have a body surface area less than 1 m²: 0.05 mg/kg once weekly.
✦ *Dosage adjustment.* Reduce dosage by 50% in patients with direct serum bilirubin level exceeding 3 ml/dl or other evidence of significant hepatic impairment.

How supplied

Available by prescription only
Injection: 1 mg/1 ml, 2 mg/2 ml, 5 mg/5 ml in multiple-dose vials; 1 mg/1 ml, 2 mg/2 ml, 5 mg/ml in preservative-free vials

---

Pharmacodynamics

Antineoplastic action: Exerts cytotoxic activity by arresting the cell cycle in the metaphase portion of cell division, resulting in a blockade of mitosis. Also inhibits DNA-dependent RNA synthesis and interferes with amino acid metabolites, inhibiting purine synthesis.

Pharmacokinetics

Absorption: Administered I.V.
Distribution: Rapidly and widely distributed into body tissues; bound to erythrocytes and platelets. Drug crosses blood-brain barrier but doesn't achieve therapeutic levels in CSF.
Metabolism: Extensively metabolized in liver.
Excretion: Drug and metabolites primarily excreted into bile. Smaller portion eliminated through kidneys. Triphasic plasma elimination; half-lives of about 4 minutes, 2¼ hours, and 85 hours for distribution, second, and terminal phases, respectively.

Route	Onset	Peak	Duration
I.V.	Unknown	Unknown	Unknown

Contraindications and precautions

Contraindicated in patients hypersensitive to drug and in those who have the demyelinating form of Charcot-Marie-Tooth syndrome. Don't give to patients who are receiving radiation therapy through ports that include the liver. Use cautiously in patients with hepatic dysfunction, neuromuscular disease, or infection.

Interactions

Drug-drug. *Asparaginase:* Decreased hepatic clearance of vincristine. Adjust vincristine dosage.
Calcium channel blockers: Enhanced vincristine accumulation in cells. Monitor patient closely; adjust vincristine dosage.
Digoxin: Decreased digoxin levels. Monitor serum digoxin levels.
Methotrexate: Increased therapeutic effect of methotrexate. May require a lower dosage of methotrexate.
Mitomycin: Possible increased frequency of bronchospasm and acute pulmonary reactions. Avoid concomitant use.
Neurotoxic drugs: Increased neurotoxicity; additive effect. Monitor patient closely; adjust vincristine dosage as needed.
Phenytoin: May decrease plasma phenytoin levels. Monitor phenytoin levels.

Adverse reactions

CNS: *peripheral neuropathy,* sensory loss, *loss of deep tendon reflexes, paresthesia, wristdrop and footdrop,* **seizures, coma,** headache, ataxia, cranial nerve palsies, *jaw pain,* hoarseness, vocal cord paralysis, *muscle weakness and cramps.* Some neurotoxicities may be permanent.
CV: hypotension, hypertension.

EENT: diplopia, optic and extraocular neuropathy, ptosis, photophobia, transient cortical blindness, optical atrophy.
GI: diarrhea, *constipation, cramps,* ileus that mimics surgical abdomen, paralytic ileus, *nausea, vomiting,* anorexia, dysphagia, *intestinal necrosis, stomatitis.*
GU: urine retention, dysuria, acute uric acid neuropathy, polyuria.
Hematologic: anemia, *leukopenia, thrombocytopenia.*
Metabolic: *hyperuricemia,* hyponatremia, weight loss.
Respiratory: *acute bronchospasm,* dyspnea.
Skin: *reversible alopecia.*
Other: fever, severe local reaction with extravasation, *phlebitis,* SIADH, cellulitis at injection site.

Overdose and treatment

Signs and symptoms of overdose include alopecia, myelosuppression, paresthesia, neuritic pain, motor difficulties, loss of deep tendon reflexes, nausea, vomiting, and ileus.

Treatment is usually supportive and includes transfusion of blood components, antiemetics, enemas for ileus, phenobarbital for seizures, and other appropriate symptomatic therapy. Administration of calcium leucovorin at a dosage of 15 mg I.V. every 3 hours for 24 hours, and then every 6 hours for 48 hours may help protect cells from the toxic effects of vincristine.

Special considerations

● Drug may be administered by I.V. push injection over 1 minute into the tubing of a freely flowing I.V. infusion.
● Dilution into larger volumes isn't recommended for infusion into peripheral veins; this method increases risk of extravasation. Drug may be administered as an I.V. infusion through a central venous catheter.
● Necrosis may result from extravasation. Manufacturer recommends treatment with moderate heat to the area and prompt administration of intradermal hyaluronidase. See package insert for additional recommendations.
● Because of potential for neurotoxicity, don't give drug more than once weekly. Children are more resistant to neurotoxicity than adults. Neurotoxicity is dose-related and usually reversible; reduce dosage if symptoms of neurotoxicity develop.
● Prevent uric acid nephropathy with generous oral fluid intake and administration of allopurinol. Alkalinization of urine may be required if serum uric acid level is increased.
● Reduced dosage may be needed in patients with obstructive jaundice or liver disease.
◼ ALERT Don't confuse vincristine with vinblastine or vindesine.
● Drug may cause SIADH secretion. Treatment requires fluid restriction and a loop diuretic.

• Management of patients mistakenly receiving intrathecal vincristine is a medical emergency. Prognosis is generally poor.

Patient monitoring

• After administering drug, monitor patient for life-threatening bronchospasm. It's most likely to occur in patients also receiving mitomycin.
• Watch for neurotoxicity by checking for depression of Achilles tendon reflex, numbness, tingling, footdrop or wristdrop, difficulty in walking, ataxia, and slapping gait. Also check ability to walk on heels.
• Monitor patient's bowel function. Patient should have stool softener, laxative, or water before dosing. Constipation may be an early indication of neurotoxicity.

Breast-feeding patients

• It isn't known if drug appears in breast milk. However, because of risk of serious adverse reactions, mutagenicity, and carcinogenicity in infant, breast-feeding isn't recommended.

Geriatric patients

• Elderly patients who are weak or bedridden may be more susceptible to neurotoxic effects. Use cautiously.

Patient education

• Encourage adequate fluid intake to increase urine output and facilitate excretion of uric acid.
• Tell patient to call regarding use of laxatives if constipation or stomach pain occurs.
• Assure patient that hair should grow back after therapy ends.

vinorelbine tartrate
Navelbine

Pharmacologic classification: semisynthetic vinca alkaloid
Therapeutic classification: antineoplastic
Pregnancy risk category: D

Indications and dosages

➤ *Alone or as adjunct therapy with cisplatin for first-line treatment of ambulatory patients with nonresectable advanced non-small-cell lung cancer (NSCLC); alone or with cisplatin in stage IV of NSCLC; with cisplatin in stage III of NSCLC. Adults:* 30 mg/m² I.V. weekly. In combination treatment, same dosage used with 120 mg/m² of cisplatin, given on days 1 and 29, and then q 6 weeks.
✦ *Dosage adjustment.* Adjust dosage based on hematologic toxicity or hepatic insufficiency, whichever results in a lower dose. Reduce dose by 50% if patient's granulocyte count falls below 1,500 cells/mm³ but exceeds 1,000 cells/mm³. If three consecutive doses are skipped because of granulocytopenia, stop further drug therapy.

How supplied

Available by prescription only
Injection: 10 mg/ml in 1-ml and 5-ml single-use vials

Pharmacodynamics

Antineoplastic action: Exerts antineoplastic effect by disrupting microtubule assembly, which disrupts spindle formation and prevents mitosis.

Pharmacokinetics

Absorption: Administered I.V.
Distribution: Drug-binding to plasma constituents ranges from 79.6% to 91.2%. It demonstrates high binding to platelets and lymphocytes.
Metabolism: Undergoes substantial hepatic metabolism.
Excretion: About 18% of drug excreted in urine; 46% excreted in feces. Terminal phase half-life averages 28 to 44 hours.

Route	Onset	Peak	Duration
I.V.	Unknown	Unknown	Unknown

Contraindications and precautions

Contraindicated in patients with pretreatment granulocyte counts below 1,000 cells/m³. Use with extreme caution in patients whose bone marrow may have been compromised by previous exposure to radiation or chemotherapy or whose bone marrow is still recovering from previous chemotherapy. Also use cautiously in patients with impaired hepatic function.

Interactions

Drug-drug. *Cisplatin:* Increased risk of bone marrow suppression. When concomitant use can't be avoided, use cautiously. Monitor patient's hematologic status.
Mitomycin: Pulmonary reactions. Monitor patient's respiratory status.

Adverse reactions

CNS: *fatigue, peripheral neuropathy, asthenia.*
CV: chest pain.
GI: *nausea, vomiting, anorexia, diarrhea, constipation, stomatitis.*
Hematologic: **bone marrow suppression (agranulocytosis, LEUKOPENIA, thrombocytopenia,** anemia*).*
Hepatic: *abnormal liver function test results, bilirubinemia.*
Musculoskeletal: jaw pain, myalgia, arthralgia.
Respiratory: dyspnea.
Skin: *alopecia,* rash, *injection pain or reaction.*
Other: SIADH.

Overdose and treatment

The primary anticipated complications of overdose are bone marrow suppression and peripheral neurotoxicity.

Reactions may be *common*, uncommon, *life-threatening*, or COMMON AND LIFE-THREATENING.

Treatment includes general supportive measures and appropriate blood transfusions and antibiotics as needed. There's no known antidote.

Special considerations
● Dilute drug before administration. Administer I.V. over 6 to 10 minutes into side port of a free-flowing I.V. closest to I.V. bag; then flush with at least 75 to 125 ml of D_5W or normal saline solution.

⚠ ALERT Don't confuse vinorelbine with vinblastine.

● Drug can cause considerable irritation if extravasation occurs.
● Use gloves. Avoid inhalation of vapors and contact with skin or mucous membranes, especially eyes. If contact occurs, wash with water for at least 15 minutes.

Patient monitoring
● Check patient's granulocyte count before starting therapy. It should be 1,000 or more cells/mm³ for drug to be administered.
● Monitor patient for hypersensitivity reactions.
● Monitor patient's peripheral blood count and bone marrow to guide effects of therapy.

Breast-feeding patients
● It isn't known if drug appears in breast milk. Because of risk of adverse effects in breast-fed infant, don't use drug in breast-feeding women.

Pediatric patients
● Safety and effectiveness in children haven't been established.

Patient education
● Tell patient not to take other drugs, including OTC preparations, unless instructed.
● Instruct patient to report signs and symptoms of infection (fever, chills, malaise) because drug has immunosuppressive activity.
● Tell woman to avoid becoming pregnant during therapy.

vitamin A (retinol)
Aquasol A, Del-Vi-A, Palmitate-A 5000

Pharmacologic classification: fat-soluble vitamin
Therapeutic classification: vitamin
Pregnancy risk category: C (doses larger than 800 mcg retinol equivalents), A (doses smaller than 800 mcg retinol equivalents), X (Aquasol)

Indications and dosages
➤ *Severe vitamin A deficiency with xerophthalmia.* *Adults and children over age 8:* 500,000 IU P.O. daily for 3 days. Then 50,000 IU P.O. daily for 14 days. Then maintenance dose of 10,000 to 20,000 IU P.O. daily for 2 months. Then adequate dietary nutrition and RDA vitamin A supplements.

➤ *Severe vitamin A deficiency.* *Adults and children over age 8:* 100,000 IU P.O. or I.M. daily for 3 days. Then 50,000 IU P.O. or I.M. daily for 14 days. Then maintenance dose of 10,000 to 20,000 IU P.O. daily for 2 months. Then adequate dietary nutrition and RDA vitamin A supplements.
Children ages 1 to 8: 17,500 to 35,000 IU I.M. daily for 10 days.
Infants under age 1: 7,500 to 15,000 IU I.M. daily for 10 days.
➤ *RDA for vitamin A.* See following table.

	Vitamin A RDA (RE)	Vitamin A and beta carotene RDA
Infants		
Birth to 12 months	375	1,875 IU
Children		
Age 1 to 3	400	2,000 IU
Age 4 to 6	500	2,500 IU
Age 7 to 10	700	3,500 IU
Men		
Age 11 and over	1,000	5,000 IU
Women		
Age 11 and over	800	4,000 IU
Pregnant	800	4,000 IU
Breast-feeding	1,300 (1st 6 months)	6,500 IU
	1,200 (2nd 6 months)	6,000 IU

RE = retinol equivalents
IU = combination of retinol and beta-carotene

How supplied
Available by prescription only
Capsules: 25,000 IU
Injection: 2-ml vials (50,000 IU/ml with 0.5% chlorobutanol, polysorbate 80, butylated hydroxyanisole, and butylated hydroxytoluene)
Available without a prescription
Capsules: 10,000 IU, 15,000 IU
Tablets: 5,000 IU

Pharmacodynamics
Metabolic action: One IU of vitamin A is equivalent to 0.3 mcg of retinol or 0.6 mcg of beta-carotene. Betacarotene, or provitamin A, yields retinol after absorption from the intestinal tract. Retinol's use with opsin, the red pigment in the retina, helps form rhodopsin, which is needed for visual adaptation to darkness. Vitamin A pre-

vents growth retardation and preserves the integrity of the epithelial cells. Vitamin A deficiency is characterized by nyctalopia (night blindness), keratomalacia (necrosis of the cornea), keratinization and drying of the skin, low resistance to infection, growth retardation, bone thickening, diminished cortical steroid production, and fetal malformations.

Pharmacokinetics

Absorption: In normal doses, absorbed readily and completely if fat absorption is normal. Larger doses, or regular doses in patients with fat malabsorption, low protein intake, or hepatic or pancreatic disease may be absorbed incompletely. Because vitamin A is fat-soluble, absorption needs bile salts, pancreatic lipase, and dietary fat.
Distribution: Stored (primarily as palmitate) in Kupffer's cells of liver. Normal adult liver stores are sufficient to provide vitamin A requirements for 2 years. Lesser amounts of retinyl palmitate are stored in kidneys, lungs, adrenal glands, retinas, and intraperitoneal fat. Vitamin A circulates bound to a specific alpha$_1$ protein, retinol-binding protein (RBP). Blood level assays may not reflect liver storage of vitamin A because serum levels depend partly on circulating RBP. Liver storage should be adequate before therapy ends. Distributed into breast milk; doesn't readily cross placenta.
Metabolism: Metabolized in liver.
Excretion: Retinol (fat-soluble) is conjugated with glucuronic acid and then further metabolized to retinal and retinoic acid. Retinoic acid is excreted in feces via biliary elimination. Retinal, retinoic acid, and other water-soluble metabolites excreted in urine and feces. Normally, no unchanged retinol excreted in urine, except in patients with pneumonia or chronic nephritis.

Route	Onset	Peak	Duration
P.O.	Unknown	3-5 hr	Unknown
I.M.	Unknown	Unknown	Unknown

Contraindications and precautions

Oral form contraindicated in patients with malabsorption syndrome; if malabsorption is from inadequate bile secretion, oral route may be used with concurrent administration of bile salts (dehydrocholic acid). Also contraindicated in those with hypervitaminosis A and hypersensitivity to any ingredient in product. I.V. route contraindicated except for special water-miscible forms intended for infusion with large parenteral volumes. I.V. push of vitamin A of any type also contraindicated (anaphylaxis or anaphylactoid reactions and death have resulted). Use cautiously in pregnant women.

Interactions

Drug-drug. *Cholestyramine, mineral oil (prolonged use), neomycin:* Decreased absorption of vitamin A. Avoid concomitant use of mineral oil or neomycin. Daily vitamin A supplements

have been recommended during long-term cholestyramine therapy.
Oral contraceptives: Significantly increased vitamin plasma levels. Adjust vitamin dosage.
Retinoids (such as etretinate, isotretinoin): Potential for additive adverse effects. Avoid concomitant use.
Warfarin: Large doses of vitamin A may interfere with hypoprothrombinemic effect of warfarin. Avoid concomitant use.

Adverse reactions

Adverse reactions usually occur only with toxicity.
CNS: irritability, headache, ***increased intracranial pressure,*** fatigue, lethargy, malaise.
EENT: papilledema, exophthalmos.
GI: anorexia, epigastric pain, vomiting, polydipsia.
GU: hypomenorrhea, polyuria.
Hepatic: jaundice, hepatomegaly, ***cirrhosis,*** elevated liver enzyme levels.
Musculoskeletal: slow growth, decalcification, hypercalcemia, periostitis, premature closure of epiphyses, migratory arthralgia, cortical thickening over the radius and tibia.
Skin: alopecia; dry, cracked, scaly skin; pruritus; lip fissures; erythema; inflamed tongue, lips, and gums; massive desquamation; increased pigmentation; night sweats.
Other: splenomegaly, ***anaphylaxis.***

Overdose and treatment

In cases of acute toxicity, a few hours after administration of a dose of 25,000 units/kg, irritability, drowsiness, vertigo, delirium, coma, vomiting and diarrhea may occur. Increased intracranial pressure develops within 8 to 12 hours; cutaneous desquamation follows in a few days. Toxicity can follow a single dose of 25,000 IU/kg, which in infants would represent about 75,000 IU and in adults over 2 million IU.

Chronic toxicity results from administration of 4,000 IU/kg for 6 to 15 months. In infants (ages 3 to 6 months) this would represent about 18,500 IU/day for 1 to 3 months; in adults, 1 million IU/day for 3 days, 50,000 IU/day for more than 18 months, or 500,000 IU/day for 2 months.

To treat toxicity, stop vitamin A if hypercalcemia persists; administer I.V. saline solution, prednisone, and calcitonin, if indicated. Perform liver function tests to detect possible liver damage.

Special considerations

● In any dietary deficiency, multiple vitamin deficiency should be suspected.
● Give vitamin A with bile salts to patients with malabsorption caused by inadequate bile secretion.
⚠ ALERT Vitamin A given by I.V. push is contraindicated; it can cause anaphylaxis and death.
● Use special water-miscible form of vitamin A when adding to large parenteral volumes.
● Vitamin A therapy may falsely increase serum cholesterol level readings by interfering with the

Zlatkis-Zak reaction. Vitamin A has also been reported to falsely elevate bilirubin levels.

Patient monitoring
● Monitor therapeutic effect.
● Monitor patient for adverse effects.
● Patients receiving more than 25,000 units of vitamin A should be closely supervised.

Pregnant patients
● Safety of amounts exceeding 5,000 IU/day (oral) or 6,000 IU/day (parenteral) during pregnancy is unknown.

Breast-feeding patients
● Vitamin A appears in breast milk. The RDA of vitamin A for breast-feeding women in the United States is 1,300 and 1,200 retinol equivalents for the first 6 months and second 6 months, respectively. Unless the maternal diet is grossly inadequate, infants can usually obtain sufficient vitamin A from breast-feeding. The effect of large maternal doses of vitamin A on breast-fed infants is unknown.

Pediatric patients
● Liquid preparations may be mixed with fruit juice or cereal.

Geriatric patients
● Liquid preparations are available to administer by nasogastric tube.

Patient education
● Explain that patient must avoid prolonged use of mineral oil while taking drug because mineral oil reduces vitamin A absorption in the intestine.
● Tell patient not to exceed recommended dosage.
● Instruct patient to report promptly symptoms of overdose (nausea, vomiting, anorexia, malaise, drying or cracking of skin or lips, irritability, headache, or loss of hair) and to stop drug immediately if they occur.
● Advise patient to consume adequate protein, vitamin E, and zinc, which, along with bile, are necessary for vitamin A absorption.
● Tell patient to store vitamin A in a tight, light-resistant container.

vitamin E (alpha tocopherol)
Aquavit-E, d'ALPHA E 1000

Pharmacologic classification: fat-soluble vitamin
Therapeutic classification: vitamin
Pregnancy risk category: A (C if greater than RDA)

Indications and dosages
➤ *Vitamin E deficiency in premature infants and in patients with impaired fat absorption (including patients with cys-*
tic fibrosis), biliary atresia. Adults: 60 to 75 IU P.O. daily, depending on severity. Maximum dose is 300 IU daily.
Children: 1 unit/kg P.O. daily.
Premature neonates: 5 units P.O. daily.
Full-term neonates: 5 units P.O. per liter of formula.
➤ *RDA for vitamin E.* (α-TE is alpha tocopherol equivalent equal to 1 mg d-α-tocopherol or 1.49 IU). *Infants up to age 6 months:* 3 α-TE or 4 IU.
Children ages 6 months to 1 year: 4 α-TE or 6 IU.
Children ages 1 to 3: 6 α-TE or 9 IU.
Children ages 4 to 10: 7 α-TE or 10 IU.
Men over age 11: 10 α-TE or 15 IU.
Women over age 11: 8 α-TE or 12 IU.
Pregnant women: 10 α-TE or 15 IU.
Breast-feeding women: First 6 months, 12 α-TE or 18 IU, over 6 months, 11 α-TE or 16 IU.

How supplied
Available without a prescription, as appropriate
Capsules: 100 IU, 200 IU, 400 IU, 1,000 IU
Drops: 15 IU/0.03 ml
Oral solution: 50 IU/ml
Tablets: 100 IU, 200 IU, 400 IU, 500 IU, 800 IU, 1,000 IU

Pharmacodynamics
Nutritional action: As a dietary supplement, exact biochemical mechanism unclear, although it's believed to act as an antioxidant. Vitamin E protects cell membranes, vitamin A, vitamin C (ascorbic acid), and polyunsaturated fatty acids from oxidation. It also may act as a cofactor in enzyme systems, and some evidence exists that it decreases platelet aggregation.

Pharmacokinetics
Absorption: GI absorption depends on presence of bile. Only 20% to 60% of vitamin obtained from dietary sources is absorbed. As dose increases, the fraction of vitamin E absorbed decreases.
Distribution: Distributed to all tissues; stored in adipose tissue.
Metabolism: Metabolized in liver by glucuronidation.
Excretion: Vitamin E excreted primarily in bile. Some enterohepatic circulation may occur. Small amounts of metabolites excreted in urine.

Route	Onset	Peak	Duration
P.O.	Unknown	Unknown	Unknown

Contraindications and precautions
No known contraindications. Use cautiously in patients with liver or gallbladder disease.

Interactions
Drug-drug. *Cholestyramine, colestipol, mineral oil, sucralfate:* Increased vitamin E re-

quirements. Give drugs at well-spaced intervals; monitor result.

Iron: Vitamin E may may impair hematologic response to iron therapy in children with iron deficiency anemia. Monitor patient closely.

Oral anticoagulants: Risk of hemorrhage after large doses of vitamin E. Avoid concomitant use.

Orlistat: May decrease GI absorption of vitamin E. Separate doses by at least 2 hours.

Vitamin K: Possible anti–vitamin K effects. Monitor therapeutic effect; adjust dosage as needed.

Adverse reactions

None reported with recommended doses. Hypervitaminosis E symptoms include fatigue, weakness, nausea, headache, blurred vision, flatulence, intestinal cramps and diarrhea.

Overdose and treatment

Signs and symptoms of overdose include a possible increase in blood pressure. Treatment is generally supportive.

Special considerations

• Give with bile salts if patient has malabsorption caused by lack of bile.

• Vitamin E has been used for investigational purposes to prevent retrolental fibroplasia and bronchopulmonary dysplasia in neonates and periventricular hemorrhage in premature infants, and to decrease the severity of hemolytic anemia in infants.

Patient monitoring

• Monitor therapeutic effect.

• Monitor patient for hypervitaminosis E.

Patient education

• Inform patient about dietary sources of vitamin E.

• Instruct patient to swallow capsules whole and not to crush or chew them.

• Tell patient to store vitamin E in a tight, light-resistant container.

vitamin K derivatives

phytonadione

AquaMEPHYTON, Mephyton

Pharmacologic classification: vitamin K
Therapeutic classification: blood coagulation modifier
Pregnancy risk category: C

Indications and dosages

➤ *Hypoprothrombinemia secondary to vitamin K malabsorption or drug therapy, or when oral administration is desired and bile secretion is inadequate.* *Adults:* 5 to 10 mg P.O. daily, or adjusted to patient's needs.

➤ *Hypoprothrombinemia secondary to vitamin K malabsorption, drug therapy, or excess vitamin A.* *Adults:* 2 to 25 mg P.O. or parenterally, repeated and increased up to 50 mg, if needed.

Children: 5 to 10 mg P.O. or parenterally.

Infants: 2 mg P.O. or parenterally.

➤ *Hypoprothrombinemia secondary to effect of oral anticoagulants.* *Adults:* 2.5 to 10 mg P.O., S.C., or I.M., based on PT and INR, repeated, if needed, 12 to 48 hours after oral dose or 6 to 8 hours after parenteral dose. In emergency, give 10 to 50 mg slow I.V., rate not to exceed 1 mg/minute, repeated q 4 hours, p.r.n.

➤ *Prevention of hemorrhagic disease in neonates.* *Neonates:* 0.5 to 1 mg S.C. or I.M. immediately (within 1 hour) after birth, repeated in 2 to 3 weeks, if needed, especially if mother received oral anticoagulants or long-term anticonvulsant therapy during pregnancy.

➤ *Prevention of hypoprothrombinemia related to vitamin K deficiency in long-term parenteral nutrition.* *Adults:* 5 to 10 mg I.M. weekly.

Children: 2 to 5 mg I.M. weekly.

➤ *RDA for vitamin K.* *Infants up to age 6 months:* 5 mcg.

Children ages 6 months to 1 year: 10 mcg.

Children ages 1 to 3: 15 mcg.

Children ages 4 to 6: 20 mcg.

Children ages 7 to 10: 30 mcg.

Boys ages 11 to 14: 45 mcg.

Boys ages 15 to 18: 65 mcg.

Men ages 19 to 24: 70 mcg.

Men over age 24: 80 mcg.

Girls ages 11 to 14: 45 mcg.

Girls ages 15 to 18: 55 mcg.

Women ages 19 to 24: 60 mcg.

Women over age 24: 65 mcg.

Pregnant or breast-feeding women: 65 mcg.

How supplied

Available by prescription only
Injection (aqueous colloidal solution): 2 mg/ml
Injection (aqueous dispersion): 10 mg/ml
Tablets: 5 mg

Pharmacodynamics

Coagulation modifying action: Vitamin K is a lipid-soluble vitamin that promotes hepatic formation of active prothrombin and several other coagulation factors (specifically factors II, VII, IX, and X).

Phytonadione (vitamin K_1) is a synthetic form of vitamin K and is also lipid-soluble. Vitamin K doesn't counteract the action of heparin.

Pharmacokinetics

Absorption: Phytonadione needs the presence of bile salts for GI tract absorption. Once absorbed, vitamin K enters blood directly. Onset of action after I.V. injection more rapid, but of shorter duration, than after S.C. or I.M. injection.

Distribution: Concentrated in liver for a short time. Action of parenteral phytonadione begins in 1 to 2 hours; hemorrhage usually controlled within 3 to 6 hours, and normal prothrombin levels in 12 to 14 hours. Oral phytonadione begins to act within 6 to 10 hours.

Metabolism: Metabolized rapidly by liver; little tissue accumulation occurs.

Excretion: Limited data; high levels in feces; however, intestinal bacteria can synthesize vitamin K.

Route	Onset	Peak	Duration
P.O.	6-12 hr	Unknown	Unknown
I.V., I.M., S.C.	1-2 hr	Unknown	Unknown

Contraindications and precautions
Contraindicated in patients hypersensitive to drug.

Interactions
Drug-drug. *Broad-spectrum antibiotics (especially cefoperazone, cefotetan):* May interfere with actions of vitamin K, producing hypoprothrombinemia. Avoid concomitant use; adjust dosage as needed.

Mineral oil: Inhibited absorption of oral vitamin K. Give drugs at well-spaced intervals; monitor result.

Oral anticoagulants: Antagonized effects of oral anticoagulants. Avoid concomitant use.

Orlistat: Decreased GI absorption of fat-soluble vitamins such as vitamin K. Separate doses by at least 2 hours.

Adverse reactions
CNS: headache, dizziness, convulsive movements.
CV: transient hypotension after I.V. administration, rapid and weak pulse, *arrhythmias.*
GI: nausea, vomiting.
Hematologic: *fatal kernicterus, severe hemolytic anemia in neonates.*
Hepatic: hyperbilirubinemia.
Respiratory: *bronchospasm,* dyspnea.
Skin: diaphoresis, flushing, erythema, urticaria, pruritus, allergic rash.
Other: cramplike pain, *anaphylaxis and anaphylactoid reactions* (usually after too-rapid I.V. administration), pain, swelling, hematoma at injection site.

Overdose and treatment
Excessive doses of vitamin K may cause hepatic dysfunction in adults; in neonates and premature infants, large doses may cause hemolytic anemia, kernicterus, and death. Treatment of overdose is supportive.

Special considerations
● When I.V. administration is unavoidable, inject drug very slowly, not exceeding 1 mg/minute.
● If severity of condition warrants I.V. infusion, mix with preservative-free normal saline solution, D₅W, or dextrose 5% in normal saline solution.
● Stop drug if allergic or severe CNS reactions appear.
● Excessive use of vitamin K may temporarily defeat oral anticoagulant therapy; higher doses of oral anticoagulant or interim use of heparin may be needed.
● Phytonadione for hemorrhagic disease in infants causes fewer adverse reactions than do other vitamin K analogues; phytonadione is the vitamin K analogue of choice to treat oral anticoagulant overdose.
● Patients receiving phytonadione who have bile deficiency need concurrent use of bile salts to ensure adequate absorption.
● Phytonadione can falsely elevate urine steroid levels.

Patient monitoring
● During I.V. administration, watch for flushing, weakness, tachycardia, and hypotension; shock may follow. Deaths have occurred.
● Monitor PT and INR to determine effectiveness.
● Monitor patient response, and watch for adverse effects; failure to respond to vitamin K may indicate coagulation defects or irreversible hepatic damage.

Breast-feeding patients
● It isn't known if vitamin K appears in breast milk. Use cautiously in breast-feeding women.

Pediatric patients
● Don't exceed recommended dosage. Hemolysis, jaundice, and hyperbilirubinemia in newborns, particularly premature infants, may be related to vitamin K administration.

Patient education
● For patient receiving oral form, explain rationale for drug therapy and stress importance of complying with medical regimen and keeping follow-up appointments.
● Tell patient to take a missed dose as soon as possible (but not if it's almost time for next dose) and to report missed doses.

warfarin sodium
Coumadin

Pharmacologic classification: coumarin derivative
Therapeutic classification: anticoagulant
Pregnancy risk category: X

Indications and dosages
➤ *Pulmonary emboli, deep vein thrombosis, MI, rheumatic heart disease with heart valve damage, atrial arrhythmias.*
Adults: Initially, 2 to 5 mg P.O. or I.V.; then daily. PT and INR are used to establish optimal dose. Usual maintenance dosage, 2 to 10 mg P.O. daily.

How supplied

Available by prescription only
Injection: 5 mg/vial
Tablets: 1 mg, 2 mg, 2.5 mg, 3 mg, 4 mg, 5 mg, 6 mg, 7.5 mg, 10 mg

Pharmacodynamics

Anticoagulant action: Warfarin inhibits vitamin K–dependent activation of clotting factors II, VII, IX, and X, which are formed in the liver; it has no direct effect on established thrombi and can't reverse ischemic tissue damage. However, warfarin may prevent additional clot formation, extension of formed clots, and secondary complications of thrombosis.

Pharmacokinetics

Absorption: Rapidly and completely absorbed from GI tract.
Distribution: Highly bound to plasma protein, especially albumin; it crosses placenta but doesn't appear to accumulate in breast milk.
Metabolism: Warfarin is hydroxylated by liver into inactive metabolites.
Excretion: Metabolites are reabsorbed from bile and excreted in urine. Half-life of parent drug is 1 to 3 days, but is highly variable. Because therapeutic effect is relatively more dependent on clotting factor depletion (factor X has half-life of 40 hours).

Route	Onset	Peak	Duration
P.O.	½-3 days	Unknown	2-5 days
I.V.	Unknown	Unknown	Unknown

Contraindications and precautions

Contraindicated in pregnant women and in patients with bleeding or hemorrhagic tendencies, GI ulcerations, severe hepatic or renal disease, severe uncontrolled hypertension, subacute bacterial endocarditis, aneurysm, ascorbic acid deficiency, and a history of warfarin-induced necrosis, threatened abortion, eclampsia, preeclampsia, regional or lumbar block anesthesia, polycythemia vera, and vitamin K deficiency. Also contraindicated in patients in whom diagnostic tests or therapeutic procedures may cause uncontrolled bleeding; unsupervised patients with senility, alcoholism, psychosis, or lack of cooperation; and patients who had recent eye, brain, or spinal cord surgery.

Use cautiously in breast-feeding patients and in patients with diverticulitis, colitis, hypertension, hepatic or renal disease, drainage tubes in any orifice, infectious disease or disturbance of intestinal flora, trauma, surgery resulting in large exposed surface, indwelling catheters, known or suspected deficiency in protein C or S, heart failure, severe diabetes, vasculitis, polycythemia vera, concurrent use of NSAIDs, or risk of hemorrhage.

Interactions

Drug-drug. *Acetaminophen:* May increase bleeding with use of acetaminophen longer than 2 weeks and doses above 2 g daily. Monitor patient closely.

Allopurinol, amiodarone, anabolic steroids, azithromycin, capecitabine, celecoxib, cephalosporins, chloramphenicol, cimetidine, ciprofloxacin, clofibrate, co-trimoxazole, danazol, diazoxide, diflunisal, disulfiram, erythromycin, fenofibrate, fenoprofen calcium, fluoroquinolones, fluoxetine, flutamide, fluvoxamine, glucagon, heparin, ibuprofen, influenza virus vaccine, isoniazid, itraconazole, ketoprofen, lovastatin, meclofenamate, metronidazole, methimazole, miconazole, neomycin (oral), norfloxacin, ofloxacin, omeprazole, pentoxifylline, propafenone, propoxyphene, propylthiouracil, quinidine,quinine, rofecoxib, salicylates, sertraline, simvastatin, streptokinase, sulfinpyrazone, sulfonamides, sulindac, tamoxifen, tetracyclines, thiazides, thyroid drugs, tramadol, tricyclic antidepressants, urokinase, vitamin E, zafirlukast, zileuton: Increased PT. Monitor patient closely for bleeding. Reduce warfarin dosage as necessary.

Aminoglutethimide, atorvastatin, carbamazepine, corticosteroids, ethchlorvynol, glutethimide, griseofulvin, mercaptopurine, methaqualone, nafcillin, oral contraceptives, rifampin, spironolactone, trazodone, sucralfate, vitamin K: Decreased anticoagulant effect. Avoid use together.

Anticonvulsants: Increased serum levels of phenytoin and phenobarbital. Monitor patient closely.

Barbiturates: May inhibit anticoagulant effect for several weeks after barbiturate withdrawal, and fatal hemorrhage can occur after cessation of barbiturate effect. Monitor patient closely. If barbiturates are withdrawn, reduce anticoagulant dose.

Chloral hydrate: May increase or decrease anticoagulant effect. Avoid use together.

Ethacrynic acid, indomethacin, mefenamic acid, phenylbutazone, sulfinpyrazone: Increased anticoagulant effect and increased risk of severe GI irritation (may be ulcerogenic). Avoid use together.

Cholestyramine: Decreased anticoagulant effect. Administer 6 hours after warfarin.

Drug-herb. *Angelica root, anise, arnica flower, asafetida, bromelain, celery, chamomile, clove, Dan-shen, devil's claw, dong quai, fenugreek, feverfew, garlic, ginger, ginkgo biloba, horse chestnut, licorice, meadowsweet, motherwort, onion, papain, parsley, passion flower, quassia, reishi mushroom, rue, sweet clover, turmeric:* Increased risk of bleeding. Discourage concurrent use.

Angelica sinensis: May significantly prolong PT. Discourage concurrent use.

Ginseng, St. John's wort, ubiquinone: Anticoagulant effect may be decreased. Discourage concurrent use.

Green tea: Decreased anticoagulant effect from vitamin K content of green tea. Tell patient to min-

---

Reactions may be *common,* uncommon, **_life-threatening,_** or COMMON AND LIFE-THREATENING.

imize variable consumption of green tea and other foods or nutritional supplements containing vitamin K.

Drug-food. *Foods or enteral products that contain vitamin K:* May impair warfarin effects. Advise patient to maintain a consistent daily intake of leafy green vegetables.

Drug-lifestyle. *Alcohol use:* Possible enhanced anticoagulation. Advise patient to avoid alcohol.

Adverse reactions

GI: anorexia, nausea, vomiting, cramps, *diarrhea*, mouth ulcerations, sore mouth.

GU: hematuria.

Hematologic: prolonged PT, INR, and partial thromboplastin time; *hemorrhage* (with excessive dosage).

Hepatic: hepatitis, elevated liver function test results, jaundice.

Skin: dermatitis, urticaria, necrosis, *gangrene*, alopecia, *rash*.

Other: *fever,* enhanced uric acid excretion.

Overdose and treatment

Signs and symptoms of overdose vary with severity and may include internal or external bleeding or skin necrosis of fat-rich areas, but most common sign is hematuria. Excessive prolongation of PT and INR or minor bleeding mandates withdrawal of therapy; withholding one or two doses may be adequate in some cases.

Treatment to control bleeding may include oral or I.V. phytonadione (vitamin K_1) and, in severe hemorrhage, fresh frozen plasma or whole blood. Use of phytonadione may interfere with subsequent oral anticoagulant therapy.

Special considerations

● Store drug in light-resistant containers at 59° to 86° F (15° to 30° C).

● After reconstitution, warfarin injection is stable for 4 hours at controlled room temperature.

● I.V. warfarin provides an alternative for patients who can't tolerate or receive oral medication.

● PT and INR are used to determine optimal dose.

ALERT Use of a large loading dose may increase the risk of hemorrhage or other complications and does not offer faster protection against thrombi formation.

● Warfarin causes false-negative serum theophylline levels.

Patient monitoring

● Monitor PT and INR closely.

● Monitor patient for signs of bleeding.

Pregnant patients

● Drug use is contraindicated during pregnancy.

Breast-feeding patients

● Although drug doesn't appear to accumulate in breast milk, use cautiously in breast-feeding women.

Pediatric patients

● Infants, especially neonates, may be more susceptible to anticoagulants because of vitamin K deficiency. Safety and efficacy haven't been established in children under age 18.

Geriatric patients

● These patients are more susceptible to effects of anticoagulants and have an increased risk of hemorrhage. This may be caused by altered hemostatic mechanisms or age-related deterioration of hepatic and renal functions.

Patient education

● Tell patient to promptly report any unusual bruising or bleeding.

● Warn patient to avoid taking OTC products containing aspirin, other salicylates, or drugs that may interact with the anticoagulant, causing an increase or decrease in action of drug, and to seek medical approval before stopping or starting medication.

● Advise patient not to substantially alter daily intake of foods that contain vitamin K, such as asparagus, broccoli, cabbage, lettuce, turnip greens, spinach, watercress, fish, pork, beef liver, green tea, or tomatoes. Widely varying daily intake may alter anticoagulant effect of warfarin.

● Instruct patient to inform all health care providers (including dentists) about use of warfarin.

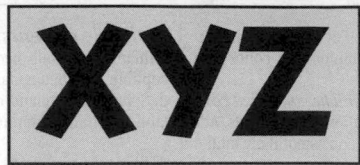

xylometazoline hydrochloride
Otrivin, Otrivin Pediatric Nasal Drops

Pharmacologic classification: sympathomimetic
Therapeutic classification: decongestant, vasoconstrictor
Pregnancy risk category: C

Indications and dosages
➤**Nasal congestion.** *Adults and children over age 12:* 2 or 3 drops or sprays of 0.1% solution to nasal mucosa q 8 to 10 hours, not to exceed three times in 24 hours.
Infants and children ages 6 months to 12 years: 2 or 3 drops of 0.05% solution to nasal mucosa q 8 to 10 hours, not to exceed three times in 24 hours.
Infants under age 6 months: 1 drop of 0.05% solution in each nostril q 6 hours, p.r.n., under medical direction.

How supplied
Available without a prescription
Nasal drops: 0.05%, 0.1% (pediatric use)
Nasal spray: 0.1%

Pharmacodynamics
Decongestant action: Acts on alpha-adrenergic receptors in nasal mucosa to produce constriction, decreasing blood flow and nasal congestion.

Pharmacokinetics
None reported.

Route	Onset	Peak	Duration
Nasal	5-10 min	Unknown	5-6 hr

Contraindications and precautions
Contraindicated in patients hypersensitive to drug and patients with acute angle-closure glaucoma. Use cautiously in patients with hyperthyroidism, cardiac disease, hypertension, diabetes mellitus, and advanced arteriosclerosis.

Interactions
Drug-drug. *Tricyclic antidepressants, xylometazoline:* May potentiate the pressor effects of tricyclic antidepressants if significant systemic absorption occurs. Monitor patient closely.

Adverse reactions
EENT: transient burning or stinging, dryness or ulceration of nasal mucosa, sneezing, rebound nasal congestion, irritation (with excessive or long-term use).

Overdose and treatment
Signs and symptoms of overdose include somnolence, sedation, sweating, CNS depression with hypertension, bradycardia, decreased cardiac output, rebound hypotension, CV collapse, depressed respirations, coma.

Because of rapid onset of sedation, emesis isn't recommended in therapy unless given early. Activated charcoal or gastric lavage may be used initially. Monitor vital signs and ECG. Treat seizures with I.V. diazepam.

Special considerations
● Systemic absorption is less likely and drug is more effective if 3 to 5 minutes elapse between sprays and nose is cleared before next spray.

Patient monitoring
● Watch carefully for adverse effects in patients with CV disease, diabetes mellitus, or hyperthyroidism.

Pediatric patients
● Keep in mind that children may be prone to greater systemic absorption and increased adverse effects.

Geriatric patients
● Use cautiously in elderly patients with cardiac disease, diabetes mellitus, or poorly controlled hypertension.

Patient education
● Inform patient that drug should be used only for short-term relief of symptoms (3 to 5 days maximum).
● Instruct patient on correct method of administration.
● Caution patient not to exceed recommended dose to avoid rebound congestion.
● Instruct patient to promptly report insomnia, dizziness, weakness, tremor, or irregular heartbeat.

Reactions may be *common*, uncommon, *life-threatening*, or COMMON AND LIFE-THREATENING.

yellow fever vaccine
YF-Vax

Pharmacologic classification: vaccine
Therapeutic classification: viral vaccine
Pregnancy risk category: C

Indications and dosages
➤ *Primary vaccination. Adults and children over age 6 months:* 0.5 ml deep S.C. Booster dose is 0.5 ml S.C. q 10 years.

How supplied
Available by prescription only
Injection: Live, attenuated 17D yellow fever virus in 1-dose, 5-dose, 20-dose, and 100-dose vials, with diluent; supplied only to designated yellow fever vaccination centers authorized to issue yellow fever vaccination certificates

Pharmacodynamics
Yellow fever prophylaxis: Promotes active immunity to yellow fever.

Pharmacokinetics
Absorption: Immunity usually develops within 7 to 10 days; lasts for 10 years or longer.
Distribution: No information available.
Metabolism: No information available.
Excretion: No information available.

Route	Onset	Peak	Duration
S.C.	7-10 days	28 days	> 10 yr

Contraindications and precautions
Contraindicated in patients hypersensitive to chicken or eggs, in those with cancer or gamma globulin deficiency, in immunosuppressed patients, and in those receiving corticosteroid or radiation therapy. Also contraindicated in pregnant women and in infants under age 4 months, except in high-risk areas. Information regarding these areas can be obtained from the Centers for Disease Control and Prevention, Division of Vector-Borne Infectious Diseases, at (970) 221-6400.

Interactions
Drug-drug. *Blood, plasma transfusion.* May impair vaccine effectiveness. Defer vaccination for 2 months.
Cholera vaccines: Administration within 3 weeks of each other may reduce antibody responses to both vaccines. Give more than 3 weeks apart.
Corticosteroids, immunosuppressants: May impair immune response to vaccine. Avoid concomitant use.

Adverse reactions
CNS: *malaise,* headache.
Musculoskeletal: myalgia.
Other: *anaphylaxis, fever,* mild swelling, pain (at injection site).

Overdose and treatment
No information available.

Special considerations
● Keep epinephrine solution 1:1,000 available to treat allergic reactions.
● Don't give yellow fever vaccine less than 1 month before or after immunization with other live-virus vaccines except for live, attenuated measles virus vaccine; bacillus Calmette-Guérin vaccine and hepatitis B vaccine may also be given concurrently.
● Whenever possible, administer cholera and yellow fever vaccines at least 3 weeks apart; however, if time constraints require it, they may be given simultaneously.
● Reconstitute vaccine only with diluent provided. Follow package directions carefully for reconstitution. Swirl and agitate reconstituted vial but don't shake vigorously to avoid foaming of suspension. Use vaccine within 60 minutes of preparation.
● Unreconstituted vials must be stored between −22° and 41° F (−30° and 5° C). Don't use unless shipping case contains some dry ice upon arrival.
● Discard unused reconstituted vaccine.

Patient monitoring
● Watch for postadministration anaphylaxis.

Pregnant patients
● Because of theoretical risk of maternal-fetal transmission of infection through vaccination, don't give yellow fever vaccine to pregnant women unless they are at high risk for exposure in an epidemic focus. There are no data to show teratogenicity or ill effects in fetus after maternal immunization.

Breast-feeding patients
● It isn't known if vaccine appears in breast milk. Use cautiously in breast-feeding women.

Pediatric patients
● Never give vaccine to children under age 4 months.
● Vaccination of children ages 4 to 9 months may be needed in high-risk areas or when travel to high-risk areas can't be postponed and a high level of protection against mosquito exposure isn't feasible.

Patient education
● Advise patient to expect some pain or swelling at injection site and fever or general malaise after injection. Recommend acetaminophen to alleviate fever.
● Advise patient to report adverse reactions.
● Inform patient about need for revaccination in 10 years to maintain his traveler's vaccination certificate.

zafirlukast
Accolate

Pharmacologic classification: leukotriene
receptor antagonist
Therapeutic classification: antasthmatic
Pregnancy risk category: B

Indications and dosages
➤ *Prophylaxis and long-term treatment
of asthma. Adults and children age 12 and
older:* 20 mg P.O. b.i.d. taken 1 hour before or
2 hours after meals.
Children ages 7 to 11: 10 mg P.O. b.i.d. taken 1
hour before or 2 hours after meals.
➤ *Prophylaxis for seasonal allergic rhinitis ◇. Adults:* 20 to 40 mg P.O. single dose before environmental exposure to allergen.

How supplied
Available by prescription only
Tablets: 10 mg, 20 mg

Pharmacodynamics
Antasthmatic action: Selectively competes for
leukotriene receptor (LTD_4 and LTE_4) sites, blocking inflammatory action.

Pharmacokinetics
Absorption: Rapidly absorbed after oral administration. Plasma levels peak 3 hours after
dosing.
Distribution: Over 99% of drug is protein-bound
to plasma proteins, predominantly albumin.
Metabolism: Extensively metabolized through
cytochrome P-450 2C9 (CYP 2C9) system. Drug
also inhibits the CYP 3A4 and CYP 2C9 isoenzymes.
Excretion: Primarily excreted in feces. Mean
terminal half-life is about 10 hours.

Route	Onset	Peak	Duration
P.O.	Rapid	3 hr	Unknown

Contraindications and precautions
Contraindicated in patients hypersensitive to drug
or its components. Use cautiously in elderly patients and in patients with hepatic impairment.

Interactions
Drug-drug. *Aspirin, erythromycin, theophylline:* Increased plasma zafirlukast levels. If concomitant use can't be avoided, monitor plasma
levels and adjust dosage.
Warfarin: Increased PT and INR. Monitor PT and
INR; adjust anticoagulant dosage.

Adverse reactions
CNS: asthenia, dizziness, *headache.*
GI: abdominal pain, diarrhea, dyspepsia, nau-
sea, vomiting.
Hepatic: elevated liver enzyme levels.

Musculoskeletal: back pain, myalgia.
Other: accidental injury, fever, infection, pain.

Overdose and treatment
There is no experience with zafirlukast overdose.
Treat patient symptomatically and provide supportive measures, as needed. If indicated, remove
unabsorbed drug from GI tract.

Special considerations
● Drug isn't indicated for reversal of bronchospasm in acute asthma attacks.
● Drug is known to inhibit CYP 3A4 and CYP 2C9
in vitro; it's reasonable to use appropriate clinical monitoring when drugs metabolized by this
isoenzyme system are administered together.
🄴 **ALERT** Zafirlukast should be discontinued if
patient has evidence of hepatic dysfunction, such
as right upper quadrant abdominal pain, nausea,
fatigue, lethargy, pruritus, jaundice, flu-like symptoms, anorexia, or enlarged liver.

Patient monitoring
● Liver function tests should be measured immediately if patient shows signs of hepatic dysfunction, with special consideration given to the
ALT level. If hepatic dysfunction is confirmed with
these tests, zafirlukast therapy should not be resumed.
● Monitor therapeutic effect.
● Monitor patient for adverse effects.

Breast-feeding patients
● Drug appears in breast milk. Don't use in breast-
feeding women.

Pediatric patients
● The effective dose in children ages 5 and 6
hasn't been established. Safety and efficacy in
children under age 5 hasn't been established.

Geriatric patients
● Drug clearance is reduced in elderly patients;
use drug cautiously. Elderly patients have an increased frequency of infections.

Patient education
● Tell patient that drug is used for long-term treatment of asthma and to keep taking drug even if
his symptoms disappear.
● Advise patient to continue taking other antasthmatics as prescribed.
● Instruct patient not to take drug with food. Drug
should be taken 1 hour before or 2 hours after
meals.

Reactions may be *common*, uncommon, *life-threatening*, or COMMON AND LIFE-THREATENING.

zalcitabine (dideoxycytidine, ddC)
Hivid

Pharmacologic classification: nucleoside analogue
Therapeutic classification: antiviral
Pregnancy risk category: C

Indications and dosages
➤ *Patients with advanced HIV infection (CD4+ count below 300 cells/mm³) who have significant clinical or immunologic deterioration.* Adults and children age 13 and older: 0.75 mg P.O. q 8 hours. Can be taken with zidovudine (200 mg P.O. q 8 hours).
✦ *Dosage adjustment.* Adjustment may be necessary in patients with impaired renal function and creatinine clearance of 40 ml/minute or below, as shown.

Creatinine clearance (ml/min)	Adult dosage
10-40	0.75 mg P.O. q 12 hours
<10	0.75 mg P.O. q 24 hours

How supplied
Available by prescription only
Tablets (film-coated): 0.375 mg, 0.75 mg

Pharmacodynamics
Antiviral action: Active against HIV. Within cells, drug is converted by cellular enzymes into its active metabolite, dideoxycytidine 5'-triphosphate. Inhibits replication of HIV by blocking viral DNA synthesis. Also inhibits reverse transcriptase by acting as an alternative for the enzyme's substrate, deoxycytidine triphosphate.

Pharmacokinetics
Absorption: Mean absolute bioavailability above 80%; food decreases rate and extent of absorption.
Distribution: Steady state volume of distribution is 0.534 to 0.127 L/kg. Drug enters CNS.
Metabolism: Doesn't appear to undergo significant hepatic metabolism; phosphorylation to the active form occurs within cells.
Excretion: Primarily excreted by kidneys; about 70% of dose appears in urine within 24 hours. Mean elimination half-life is 2 hours.

Route	Onset	Peak	Duration
P.O.	Unknown	1-2 hr	Unknown

Contraindications and precautions
Contraindicated in patients hypersensitive to drug or its components. Use cautiously in patients with peripheral neuropathy, impaired renal function, hepatic failure, or history of pancreatitis, heart failure, or cardiomyopathy.

Interactions
Drug-drug. *Antacids that contain magnesium or aluminum:* Decreased zalcitabine absorption. Avoid giving simultaneously.
Cimetidine, probenecid: Decreased zalcitabine elimination. Monitor patient closely; adjust dosage as needed.
Drugs that cause peripheral neuropathy (such as chloramphenicol, cisplatin, dapsone, didanosine, disulfiram, ethionamide, glutethimide, gold salts, hydralazine, iodoquinol, isoniazid, metronidazole, nitrofurantoin, phenytoin, ribavirin, vincristine): Increased risk of peripheral neuropathy. Monitor patient closely; adjust dosage as needed.
Drugs that may impair renal function (aminoglycosides, amphotericin, foscarnet): Increased risk of zalcitabine-induced adverse effects. Limit concomitant use; monitor patient closely.
Pentamidine: Risk of pancreatitis. Avoid concomitant use.

Adverse reactions
CNS: *peripheral neuropathy, headache, fatigue,* dizziness, confusion, *seizures,* impaired concentration, amnesia, insomnia, mental depression, tremor, hypertonia, anxiety.
EENT: pharyngitis, ocular pain, abnormal vision, ototoxicity, nasal discharge.
GI: nausea, vomiting, diarrhea, abdominal pain, anorexia, constipation, stomatitis, esophageal ulcer, glossitis, *pancreatitis.*
Hematologic: anemia, *leukopenia, neutropenia, thrombocytopenia,* eosinophilia.
Respiratory: cough.
Skin: rash, prutitis, urticaria.

Overdose and treatment
There's little experience with acute overdose and it's unknown if drug is dialyzable. Treat overdose symptomatically.

Special considerations
● If drug is stopped because of toxicity, resume recommended dosage for zidovudine alone, which is 100 mg every 4 hours.
● If symptoms indicating peripheral neuropathy occur, stop drug if they're bilateral and persist beyond 72 hours. If these symptoms persist or worsen beyond 1 week, permanently stop drug. However, if all findings relevant to peripheral neuropathy have resolved to minor symptoms, drug may be reintroduced at 0.375 mg P.O. every 8 hours.
● When drug alone is only treatment, peripheral neuropathy has occurred in 17% to 31% of patients. The peripheral neuropathy seen with zalcitabine therapy is a sensorimotor neuropathy, initially characterized by numbness and burning in the limbs. If drug isn't withdrawn, symptoms can progress to sharp, shooting pain or severe,

continuous burning pain requiring narcotic analgesics; pain may or may not be reversible.
• Women of childbearing age should use an effective contraceptive while taking drug.
• Patients who had long-term exposure to doses about six times higher than the current recommended dosage experienced peripheral neuropathy within 10 weeks; patients exposed to twice the recommended dosage experienced peripheral neuropathy within 12 weeks.

Patient monitoring

• Watch for toxic effects. They may cause abnormalities in several laboratory tests, including CBC, leukocyte count, reticulocyte count, granulocyte count, hemoglobin level, platelet count, and AST, ALT, and alkaline phosphatase levels.
• Monitor patient for peripheral neuropathy.

Breast-feeding patients

• It isn't known if drug appears in breast milk. Because of risk of transmitting virus, HIV-positive women shouldn't breast-feed.

Pediatric patients

• Safety and efficacy in children under age 13 haven't been established.
• An oral solution is available from the manufacturer through a compassionate use program.

Patient education

• Explain that drug doesn't cure HIV infection and that HIV can still be transmitted. Opportunistic infections may continue to occur despite use of drug.
• Tell patient that drug may cause peripheral neuropathy and life-threatening pancreatitis. Review signs and symptoms of these reactions, and instruct patient to report them immediately.

zaleplon
Sonata

Pharmacologic classification: pyrazolopyrimidine
Therapeutic classification: hypnotic
Controlled substance schedule: IV
Pregnancy risk category: C

Indications and dosages

➤ **Insomnia.** *Adults:* 5 to 20 mg P.O. daily, immediately before h.s.
Elderly patients: 5 to 10 mg P.O. daily, immediately before h.s.; doses over 10 mg aren't recommended.
✦ **Dosage adjustment.** For debilitated patients, initially 5 mg P.O. daily, immediately before h.s.; doses over 10 mg aren't recommended. For patients with mild to moderate hepatic impairment or those receiving cimetidine concurrently, 5 mg by P.O. daily immediately before bedtime.

How supplied

Available by prescription only
Capsules: 5 mg, 10 mg

Pharmacodynamics

Hypnotic action: Hypnotic with a chemical structure unrelated to benzodiazepines; interacts with the gamma-aminobutyric acid benzodiazepine receptor complex in the CNS. Modulation of this complex is hypothesized to be responsible for sedative, anxiolytic, muscle relaxant, and anticonvulsant effects of benzodiazepines.

Pharmacokinetics

Absorption: Rapidly and almost completely absorbed; levels peak within 1 hour. Dosing after a high-fat or heavy meal delays peak levels by about 2 hours.
Distribution: Distributed substantially into extravascular tissues. Plasma protein–binding about 60%.
Metabolism: Extensively metabolized, primarily by aldehyde oxidase and, to a lesser extent, CYP 3A4 to inactive metabolites. Less than 1% of dose excreted unchanged in urine.
Excretion: Rapidly excreted, with a mean half-life of about 1 hour.

Route	Onset	Peak	Duration
P.O.	1 hr	1 hr	3-4 hr

Contraindications and precautions

Contraindicated in patients with severe hepatic impairment. Use cautiously in elderly and debilitated patients, those with compromised respiratory function, and those with evidence of depression.

Interactions

Drug-drug. *Carbamazepine, phenobarbital, phenytoin, rifampin, and other drugs that affect CYP 344 enzyme:* Reduced bioavailability and peak levels of zaleplon by about 80%. Consider alternative hypnotic.
Cimetidine: Increased zaleplon bioavailability and peak levels by 85%. For patient taking cimetidine, give initial zaleplon dose of 5 mg.
CNS depressants (imipramine, thioridazine): Possible additive CNS effects. Use cautiously together.
Drug-food. *Heavy meals, high-fat foods:* Prolong absorption, delaying peak zaleplon levels by about 2 hours; sleep onset may be delayed. Tell patient to separate administration from meals.
Drug-lifestyle. *Alcohol use:* Concurrent use may increase CNS effects. Discourage use.

Adverse reactions

CNS: *headache,* amnesia, dizziness, somnolence, depression, hypertonia, nervousness, depersonalization, hallucinations, vertigo, difficulty concentrating, anxiety, paresthesia, hypesthesia, tremor, asthenia, migraine, malaise.
CV: chest pain, peripheral edema.

Reactions may be *common,* uncommon, **life-threatening**, or COMMON AND LIFE-THREATENING.

EENT: abnormal vision, conjunctivitis, eye pain, ear pain, hyperacusis, epistaxis, parosmia.
GI: constipation, dry mouth, anorexia, dyspepsia, nausea, abdominal pain, colitis.
GU: dysmenorrhea.
Musculoskeletal: arthritis, myalgia, back pain.
Respiratory: bronchitis.
Skin: pruritus, rash, photosensitivity reaction.
Other: fever.

Overdose and treatment
Overdose signs and symptoms usually include exaggerated CNS depressant effects of drug, ranging from drowsiness to coma. Use immediate gastric lavage when appropriate and general supportive measures for symptomatic management.

Special considerations
• Because drug works rapidly, it should only be ingested immediately before bedtime or after patient has gone to bed and has experienced difficulty falling asleep.
• Don't administer drug with or after a high-fat or heavy meal.
• Zaleplon may be used up to 5 weeks. Reevaluate patient if hypnotics are to be taken for more than 2 to 3 weeks.
• Start treatment only after careful evaluation of patient because sleep disturbances may be a symptom of an underlying physical or psychiatric disorder.
• Adverse reactions are usually dose related. Use the lowest effective dose.
• Potential for drug abuse and dependence exists. Don't give drug in quantities exceeding 1-month supply.

Patient monitoring
• Closely monitor therapeutic effect.
• Monitor patients for signs of adverse effects, especially patients with compromised respiratory function due to preexisting illness, and elderly or debilitated patients.

Breast-feeding patients
• A small amount of drug appears in breast milk. Avoid use in breast-feeding women.

Pediatric patients
• Safety and effectiveness in children haven't been established.

Geriatric patients
• Elderly patients appear to be more sensitive to the effects of hypnotics. Monitor these patients closely for impaired motor or cognitive performance.

Patient education
• Advise patient that drug works rapidly and should only be taken immediately before bedtime or after patient has gone to bed and has had difficulty falling asleep.

• Advise patient to take drug only if he will be able to sleep for at least 4 undisturbed hours.
• Caution patient that drowsiness, dizziness, light-headedness, and difficulty with coordination most often occur within 1 hour after taking drug.
• Advise patient to avoid performing activities that require mental alertness until CNS effects of drug are known.
• Advise patient to avoid alcohol while taking drug and to call before taking any prescription or OTC drugs.
• Tell patient not to take drug after a high-fat or heavy meal.
• Advise patient to report any continued sleep problems despite use of drug.
• Notify patient that dependence can occur and that drug is recommended for short-term use only.
• Warn patient not to abruptly stop drug because withdrawal symptoms (including unpleasant feelings, stomach and muscle cramps, vomiting, sweating, shakiness, and seizures) may occur.
• Notify patient that insomnia may recur for a few nights after stopping drug, but should resolve on its own.
• Advise patient that drug may cause changes in behavior and thinking, including outgoing or aggressive behavior, loss of personal identity, confusion, strange behavior, agitation, hallucinations, worsening of depression, or suicidal thoughts. Tell patient to call immediately if any of these symptoms occur.

zanamivir
Relenza

Pharmacologic classification: neuraminidase inhibitor
Therapeutic classification: antiviral
Pregnancy risk category: C

Indications and dosages
➤ *Uncomplicated acute illness caused by influenza virus in patients who have been symptomatic for no more than 2 days.* *Adults and adolescents age 7 and older:* Two oral inhalations (one 5-mg blister per inhalation for a total dose of 10 mg) twice daily using the Diskhaler inhalation device for 5 days. Two doses should be taken on the first day of treatment provided there are at least 2 hours between doses. Subsequent doses should be about 12 hours apart (in the morning and evening) at about the same time each day.

How supplied
Available by prescription only
Powder for inhalation: 5 mg per blister pack

Pharmacodynamics
Antiviral action: Most likely inhibits neuraminidase on the surface of the influenza virus, potentially altering virus particle aggregation and release. With the inhibition of neuraminidase, the

virus can't escape from its host cell to attack others, thereby inhibiting the process of viral proliferation.

Pharmacokinetics

Absorption: About 4% to 17% of orally inhaled drug systemically absorbed; serum levels peak 1 to 2 hours after a 10-mg dose.
Distribution: Less than 10% plasma protein–binding.
Metabolism: Not metabolized; excreted by kidneys as unchanged drug.
Excretion: Excreted unchanged in urine within 24 hours. Unabsorbed drug excreted in feces; serum half-life ranges from 2½ to 5 hours.

Route	Onset	Peak	Duration
Inhalation	Unknown	1-2 hr	Unknown

Contraindications and precautions

Contraindicated in patients hypersensitive to drug or its components. Drug isn't recommended for patients with severe or decompensated COPD, asthma, or other underlying respiratory disease.

Interactions

None reported.

Adverse reactions

CNS: headache, dizziness.
EENT: nasal signs and symptoms; sinusitis; ear, nose, and throat infections.
GI: diarrhea, nausea, vomiting.
Respiratory: bronchitis, cough.

Overdose and treatment

None reported.

Special considerations

● Patient with underlying respiratory disease should have a fast-acting bronchodilator available in case of wheezing while taking zanamivir. Patients scheduled to use an inhaled bronchodilator for asthma should use their bronchodilator before taking zanamivir.
🛨 **ALERT** Drug may cause serious respiratory adverse reactions in patients with or without known underlying respiratory disease.
● Safety and efficacy of drug haven't been established in patients who begin treatment after 48 hours of symptom onset.
● Safety and efficacy of drug haven't been established for influenza prophylaxis. Use of zanamivir shouldn't affect the evaluation of patients for their annual influenza vaccination.
● Lymphopenia, neutropenia, and a rise in liver enzyme and CK levels have been reported during therapy.

Patient monitoring

● Monitor patient for bronchospasm and decline in lung function. Stop drug, as needed, in such situations.
● Monitor therapeutic effect.

Breast-feeding patients

● It's unknown if drug appears in breast milk. Because many drugs do, use cautiously in breast-feeding women.

Pediatric patients

● Safety and effectiveness in children under age 7 haven't been established.

Patient education

● Tell patient to carefully read instructions regarding proper use. Tell him to keep Diskhaler level when loading and inhaling, always check inside mouthpiece to make sure it's free of foreign objects, exhale fully before putting mouthpiece in mouth, close lips around mouthpiece, breathe in steadily and deeply, and hold breath for a few seconds after inhaling to prolong drug's presence in lungs.
● Advise patient with underlying respiratory disease who is scheduled to use an inhaled bronchodilator to do so before taking zanamivir. Tell patient to have a fast-acting bronchodilator available in case of wheezing while taking zanamivir.
● Inform patient that it's important to finish entire 5-day course of treatment even if feeling better.
● Advise patient that drug hasn't been shown to reduce risk of transmitting influenza virus to others.

zidovudine (AZT)
Retrovir

Pharmacologic classification: thymidine analogue
Therapeutic classification: antiviral
Pregnancy risk category: C

Indications and dosages

➤ **Symptomatic HIV, AIDS, or advanced AIDS-related complex.** *Adults and children over age 12:* 100 mg P.O. q 4 hours (600 mg daily dose). Or give by I.V. infusion 1 to 2 mg/kg (at constant rate over 1 hour) q 4 hours for total of 6 mg/kg daily.
Children ages 3 months to 12 years: 180 mg/m² q 6 hours (720 mg/m² daily). Don't exceed 200 mg q 6 hours.
➤ **Asymptomatic HIV infection (CD4⁺ count below 500 cells/mm³).** *Adults and children over age 12:* 100 mg P.O. q 4 hours while awake (for total of five doses or 500 mg daily). Or give 1 mg/kg I.V. over 1 hour q 4 hours while awake (5 mg/kg daily).
Children ages 3 months to 12 years: 180 mg/m² q 6 hours (720 mg/m² P.O. daily) in divided doses q 6 hours. Don't exceed 200 mg q 6 hours.
➤ **Maternal-fetal transmission of HIV.** *Adults:* For maternal dosing, give 100 mg P.O. q 4 hours while awake (for total of five doses daily). Start at 14 to 34 weeks of pregnancy and continue until labor starts. During labor and delivery, give 2 mg/kg I.V. over 1 hour; then a

continuous infusion of 1 mg/kg/hour until clamping of umbilical cord. For infant dosing, give 2 mg/kg P.O. q 6 hours starting 12 hours after birth and continuing until 6 weeks old. Or, give 1.5 mg/kg via I.V. infusion over 30 minutes q 6 hours.

✦ *Dosage adjustment.* Because drug is partially removed by dialysis, dosage adjustment may be needed in affected patients. Dosage adjustment also may be warranted in patients with decreased liver function.

How supplied
Available by prescription only
Capsules: 100 mg
Injection: 10 mg/ml
Syrup: 50 mg/5 ml
Tablets: 300 mg

Pharmacodynamics
Antiviral action: Converted intracellularly to an active triphosphate compound that inhibits reverse transcriptase (an enzyme essential for retroviral DNA synthesis), thereby inhibiting viral replication. When used in vitro, drug inhibits certain other viruses and bacteria; however, this has undetermined clinical significance.

Pharmacokinetics
Absorption: Absorbed rapidly from GI tract. Average systemic bioavailability 65% of dose (drug undergoes first-pass metabolism).
Distribution: Preliminary data reveal good CSF penetration. About 36% of dose is bound to plasma protein.
Metabolism: Metabolized rapidly to inactive compound.
Excretion: Parent drug and metabolite excreted by glomerular filtration and tubular secretion in kidneys. Urine recovery of parent drug and metabolite is 14% and 74%, respectively. Elimination half-lives of these compounds, 1 hour.

Route	Onset	Peak	Duration
P.O., I.V.	Unknown	½-1½ hr	Unknown

Contraindications and precautions
Contraindicated in patients hypersensitive to drug. Use cautiously in patients in advanced stages of HIV and in those with severe bone marrow suppression, renal insufficiency, or hepatomegaly, hepatitis, or other risk factors for hepatic disease.

Interactions
Drug-drug. *Acetaminophen:* May inhibit glucuronidation of zidovudine. Monitor patient closely.
Acyclovir: Severe drowsiness and lethargy. Use cautiously together.
Drugs that are nephrotoxic or affect bone marrow function or formation of bone marrow elements (such as amphotericin B, dapsone, doxorubicin, flucytosine, ganciclovir, interferon, *pentamidine, vinblastine, vincristine):* May increase risk of toxicity of these drugs. Use cautiously together.
Fluconazole: Concomitant use interferes with the metabolism and clearance of zidovudine. Monitor patient closely.
Nucleoside analogs affecting DNA replication: May antagonize the activity of zidovudine against HIV. Avoid concomitant use.
Probenecid: Impaired zidovudine elimination. Monitor patient closely; adjust dosage as needed.

Adverse reactions
CNS: headache, *seizures,* paresthesia, malaise, asthenia, insomnia, dizziness, somnolence.
GI: taste perversion, nausea, anorexia, abdominal pain, vomiting, constipation, diarrhea, dyspepsia.
Hematologic: *severe bone marrow suppression (resulting in anemia), agranulocytosis, thrombocytopenia.*
Musculoskeletal: myalgia.
Skin: *rash,* diaphoresis.
Other: *fever.*

Overdose and treatment
No information available.

Special considerations
● Zidovudine injection should not be given by rapid or bolus I.V. injection and should not be given I.M.
● Neither optimum duration of treatment nor dosage for optimum effectiveness and minimum toxicity is known.
● I.V. dosage equivalent to 100 mg P.O. every 4 hours is about 1 mg/kg I.V. every 4 hours.
● Store undiluted injection, capsules, and syrup at 77° F (25° C); protect from light. Dilute I.V. form to less than 4 mg/ml with D₅W before administering. Don't mix with solutions containing protein. To minimize potential for microbial contamination, administer within 8 hours of mixing if left at room temperature or within 24 hours if refrigerated (36° to 46° F [2° to 8° C]).
● Drug doesn't cure HIV infection or AIDS but may reduce morbidity resulting from opportunistic infections and thus prolong patient's life.

Patient monitoring
● Monitor CBC and platelet count at least every 2 weeks. Significant anemia (hemoglobin level less than 7.5 g/dl or reduction of over 25% of baseline) or significant neutropenia (granulocyte count below 750 cells/mm³ or reduction of more than 50% from baseline) may need interruption of drug until evidence of bone marrow recovery occurs. In patients with less severe anemia or neutropenia, a dosage reduction may be adequate.
● Watch for signs and symptoms of opportunistic infection (including pneumonia, meningitis, and sepsis).

Breast-feeding patients
● Drug appears in breast milk. To avoid transmitting HIV to infant, HIV-positive women shouldn't breast-feed.

Patient education
● Because drug frequently causes a low RBC count, advise patient that he may need blood transfusions or epoetin alfa therapy during treatment.
● Teach proper drug administration; explain importance of maintaining an adequate blood level.
● Warn patient not to take other drugs for AIDS without medical approval.
● Advise patient that drug doesn't reduce the ability to transmit HIV.
● Advise patient to protect capules and syrup from light.

zileuton
Zyflo Filmtab

Pharmacologic classification: 5-lipoxygenase inhibitor
Therapeutic classification: antasthmatic
Pregnancy risk category: C

Indications and dosages
➤ **Prophylaxis and long-term treatment of asthma.** *Adults and children age 12 and older:* 600 mg P.O. q.i.d.

How supplied
Available by prescription only
Tablets: 600 mg

Pharmacodynamics
Antasthmatic action: Inhibits enzyme responsible for formation of leukotrienes, thus reducing inflammatory response.

Pharmacokinetics
Absorption: Rapidly absorbed with oral administration; mean time to peak levels is 1.7 hours.
Distribution: Apparent volume of distribution is 1.2 L/kg. 93% bound to plasma proteins, primarily albumin.
Metabolism: Oxidatively metabolized by cytochrome P-450 system. Several
active and inactive metabolites identified.
Excretion: Elimination predominantly via metabolism with a mean terminal half-life of 2½ hours.

Route	Onset	Peak	Duration
P.O.	Rapid	2 hr	Unknown

Contraindications and precautions
Contraindicated in patients hypersensitive to drug or its components and in those with active hepatic disease or transaminase elevations at least
three times upper limit of normal. Use cautiously in patients with hepatic impairment or history of heavy alcohol use.

Interactions
Drug-drug. *Beta blockers, propranolol:* Increased beta blocker effect. Monitor patient; reduce beta blocker dosage.
Drugs metabolized by P-450 isoenzymes 1A2, 2C9 & 3A4 (cyclosporine, dihydropyridine calcium channel blockers, estradiol, ethinyl, prednisone): No formal interaction studies have been conducted. Administer cautiously.
Theophylline: Decreased theophylline clearance (on average, serum theophylline levels double). Reduce theophylline dosage; monitor serum levels.
Warfarin: Increased PT and INR. Monitor PT and INR; adjust anticoagulant dosage.

Adverse reactions
CNS: malaise, asthenia, dizziness, headache, insomnia, nervousness, somnolence.
CV: chest pain.
EENT: conjunctivitis.
GI: abdominal pain, constipation, dyspepsia, flatulence, nausea.
GU: urinary tract infection, vaginitis.
Hematologic: *leukopenia.*
Hepatic: elevated liver enzyme levels.
Musculoskeletal: arthralgia, hypertonia, myalgia, neck pain and rigidity.
Skin: pruritus.
Other: accidental injury, fever, lymphadenopathy, pain.

Overdose and treatment
Data on acute overdose are limited. Treat patient symptomatically and provide supportive measures. If indicated, eliminate unabsorbed drug by emesis or gastric lavage. Drug isn't removed by dialysis.

Special considerations
● Drug may be taken with meals and at bedtime.
● Drug isn't indicated for use in the reversal of bronchospasm in acute asthma attacks.

Patient monitoring
● Obtain liver enzyme levels at baseline, once a month for the first 3 months, every 2 to 3 months for the remainder of the first year, and periodically thereafter.
● Monitor patient for adverse effects.

Breast-feeding patients
● It isn't known if drug appears in breast milk. Use cautiously in breast-feeding women.

Pediatric patients
● Safety and effectiveness in children under age 12 haven't been studied.

Reactions may be *common*, uncommon, *life-threatening*, or COMMON AND LIFE-THREATENING.

Patient education
• Advise patient that drug is used for long-term treatment of asthma and that he should continue taking drug even if his symptoms disappear.
• Caution patient that drug isn't a bronchodilator and shouldn't be used to treat an acute asthma attack.
• Advise patient to continue taking other antasthmatics.
• Instruct patient to call if short-acting bronchodilator isn't effective in relieving symptoms.
• Advise patient to call immediately if signs and symptoms of hepatic dysfunction develop (right upper quadrant pain, nausea, fatigue, pruritus, jaundice, malaise).
• Advise patient to avoid alcohol and to call before taking OTC or new prescription drugs.

zinc
Orazinc, Verazinc, Zinc 15, Zinc-220, Zincate, Zinca-Pak

zinc sulfate (ophthalmic)
Eye-Sed

Pharmacologic classification: trace element; miscellaneous anti-infective
Therapeutic classification: nutritional supplement; topical anti-infective
Pregnancy risk category: C

Indications and dosages
➤ *RDA of zinc. Infants up to age 1:* 5 mg P.O.
Children ages 1 to 10: 10 mg P.O.
Men age 11 and older: 15 mg P.O.
Women age 11 and older: 12 mg P.O.
Pregnant women: 15 mg P.O.
Breast-feeding women (first 6 months): 19 mg P.O.
Breast-feeding women (second 6 months): 16 mg P.O.
➤ *Metabolically stable zinc deficiency.*
Adults: 2.5 to 4 mg daily I.V. Add 2 mg daily for acute catabolic states.
➤ *Stable zinc deficiency with fluid loss from the small bowel. Adults:* Add 12.2 mg/L of total parenteral nutrition solution or 17.1 mg/kg of stool or ileostomy output.
➤ *Zinc deficiency. Children under age 5:* 100 mcg/kg daily I.V.
Premature infants: 300 mcg/kg daily I.V.
➤ *Dietary supplementation. Adults:* 25 to 50 mg P.O. daily.
➤ *Minor eye irritation. Adults:* 1 to 2 drops ophthalmic solution into eye b.i.d. to q.i.d. Patients should report irritation that persists for more than 3 days.

How supplied
Available by prescription only
Capsules: 220 mg (50 mg zinc)

Injection: 10 ml (1 mg/ml), 30 ml (1 mg/ml with 0.9% benzyl alcohol), 5 ml (5 mg/ml); 10 ml (5 mg/ml)
Available without a prescription, as appropriate
Capsules: 220 mg (50 mg zinc)
Solution: 1 ml (0.25%)
Tablets: 66 mg (15 mg zinc), 110 mg (25 mg zinc), 200 mg (47 mg zinc)

Pharmacodynamics
Metabolic action: Zinc serves as a cofactor for more than 70 different enzymes. It facilitates wound healing, normal growth rates, and normal skin hydration and helps maintain the senses of taste and smell.

Adequate zinc provides normal growth and tissue repair. In patients receiving total parenteral nutrition with low plasma levels of zinc, dermatitis has been followed by alopecia. Zinc is an integral part of many enzymes important to carbohydrate and protein mobilization of retinal-binding protein.

Zinc sulfate ophthalmic solution exhibits astringent and weak antiseptic activity, which may result from precipitation of protein by the zinc ion and by clearing mucus from the outer surface of the eye. Drug has no decongestant action and produces mild vasodilation.

Pharmacokinetics
Absorption: Zinc sulfate is absorbed poorly from the GI tract; only 20% to 30% of dietary zinc is absorbed. After administration, zinc resides in muscle, bone, skin, kidneys, liver, pancreas, retina, prostate, and particularly RBCs and WBCs. Binds to plasma albumin, alpha-2 macroglobulin, and some plasma amino acids, including histidine, cysteine, threonine, glycine, and asparagine.
Distribution: Major zinc stores in skeletal muscle, skin, bone, and pancreas.
Metabolism: Zinc is a cofactor in many enzymatic reactions; is needed for synthesis and mobilization of retinal binding protein.
Excretion: After parenteral administration, 90% excreted in stool, urine, and sweat. After oral use, major route of excretion is secretion into duodenum and jejunum. Small amounts excreted in urine (0.3 to 0.5 mg daily) and sweat (1.5 mg daily).

Route	Onset	Peak	Duration
P.O.	Unknown	Unknown	Unknown
I.V.	Immediate	Immediate	Unknown
Ophthalmic	Unknown	Unknown	Unknown

Contraindications and precautions
Parenteral use of zinc sulfate is contraindicated in patients with renal failure or biliary obstruction (and requires caution in all patients); monitor zinc plasma levels frequently. Don't exceed prescribed dosages. In patients with renal dysfunction or GI malfunction, trace metal supple-

ments may need to be reduced, adjusted, or omitted. Hypersensitivity may result. Routine use of zinc supplementation during pregnancy isn't recommended.

Administering copper in the absence of zinc or administering zinc in the absence of copper may result in decreased serum levels of either element. When only one trace element is needed, it should be added separately and serum levels monitored closely. To avoid overdose, administer multiple trace elements only when clearly needed. In patients with extreme vomiting or diarrhea, large amounts of trace element replacement may be needed. Excessive intake in healthy persons may be deleterious.

Interactions
Drug-drug. *Certain proteins, methylcellulose suspensions:* Precipitation of these drugs. Avoid concomitant use.
Fluoroquinolones, tetracyclines: Impaired antibiotic absorption. Avoid concomitant use.
Sodium borate: Precipitation of zinc borate when using ocular preparation. Glycerin may prevent interaction.
Drug-herb. *Acacia:* Zinc ophthalmic solution may precipitate acacia. Discourage concurrent use.
Drug-food. *Dairy products:* Possible reduction in zinc absorption. Discourage concurrent use.

Adverse reactions
CNS: restlessness.
GI: distress and irritation, nausea, vomiting with high doses, gastric ulceration, diarrhea.
Skin: rash.
Other: dehydration.

Overdose and treatment
Signs and symptoms of severe toxicity include hypotension, pulmonary edema, diarrhea, vomiting, jaundice, and oliguria. If toxicity occurs, stop drug and provide support measures.

Special considerations
● Results may not appear for 6 to 8 weeks in zinc-depleted patients.
● Zinc decreases absorption of tetracyclines and fluoroquinolones.
● Calcium supplements may confer a protective effect against zinc toxicity.
● Because of potential for infusion phlebitis and tissue irritation, an undiluted direct injection must not be administered into a peripheral vein.
● Don't exceed prescribed dosage of oral zinc; if oral zinc is administered in single 2-g doses, emesis will occur.
● If ophthalmic use causes increasing irritation, stop drug.

Patient monitoring
● Monitor patient for severe vomiting and dehydration, which may indicate overdose.

Patient education
● Advise patient not to take zinc with dairy products, which can reduce zinc absorption.
● Teach patient how to instill ophthalmic solution and to prevent contamination. Tell him to avoid contacting lip of container with other surface and to tightly close container after use.
● Warn patient about self-medication with zinc sulfate ophthalmic solution, which shouldn't continue longer than 3 days. Patient should report increased irritation or redness.
● Advise patient that GI upset may occur after oral administration but may decrease if zinc is taken with food. Tell him to avoid foods high in calcium, phosphorus, or phytate during therapy.

ziprasidone
Geodon

Pharmacologic classification: atypical antipsychotic
Therapeutic classification: psychotropic
Pregnancy risk category: C

Indications and dosages
➤ *Symptoms of schizophrenia. Adults:* Initially, 20 mg b.i.d. with food. Dosages are highly individualized. Dosage adjustments, if necessary, should occur no sooner than every 2 days, but to allow for lowest possible doses, the interval should be several weeks for symptom response. Effective dosage range is usually 20 to 80 mg b.i.d. Maximum recommended dosage is 100 mg b.i.d.

How supplied
Capsules: 20 mg, 40 mg, 60 mg, 80 mg

Pharmacodynamics
Unknown, although drug probably works through dopamine and serotonin antagonism. These two neurotransmitters usually are targeted for treatment of positive and negative symptoms of schizophrenia. Blocking them allows improvement of symptoms with minimal adverse extrapyramidal effects.

Pharmacokinetics
Absorption: Serum levels peak in about 6 to 8 hours. Absorption doubles when drug is taken with food, and administration with food is recommended.
Distribution: Highly protein-bound.
Metabolism: Hepatic, with no active metabolites. Less than one-third of drug is metabolized through the cytochrome P-450 system. CYP3A4 (major) and CYP1A2 (minor) are the pathways involving the cytochrome P-450 system.
Excretion: Half-life is about 7 hours.

Route	Onset	Peak	Duration
P.O.	1-3 days	6-8 hr	12 hr

Adverse reactions
CNS: *somnolence,* akathesia, dizziness, extrapyramidal symptoms, dystonia, hypertonia, asthenia.
CV: tachycardia, orthostatic hypotension.
EENT: rhinitis, abnormal vision.
GI: *nausea,* constipation, dyspepsia, diarrhea, dry mouth, anorexia.
Musculoskeletal: myalgia.
Respiratory: cough.
Skin: rash.

Interactions
Drug-drug. *Carbamazepine:* May decrease ziprasidone levels. Higher ziprasidone dosage may be needed.
Drugs that decrease serum potassium or magnesium levels, such as diuretics: May increase risk of arrhythmias. Monitor serum potassium and magnesium levels if giving together.
Drugs that increase dopamine levels, such as levodopa and dopamine agonists: Possible antagonistic effect on ziprasidone. Use cautiously together.
Drugs that prolong QT interval, including dofetilide, moxifloxacin, pimozide, quinidine, sotalol, sparfloxacin, thioridazine: May increase risk of arrhythmias. Don't give together.
Ketoconazole: May increase ziprasidone levels. Lower ziprasidone dosage may be needed.

Overdose and treatment
Signs and symptoms of overdose include sedation, slurred speech, and hypotension. They may also include obtundation, seizures, extrapyramidal reactions, dystonia, and arrhythmias.

There's no antidote for ziprasidone, and dialysis isn't effective. Consider giving activated charcoal, a laxative, or both. If the patient is unconscious, an I.V. line should be established. Otherwise, symptomatic monitoring and treatment is recommended, particularly ECG monitoring for arrhythmias.

Contraindications and precautions
Contraindicated in patients hypersensitive to drug and patients who take other drugs known to prolong the QT interval. Also contraindicated in patients with a history of QT prolongation, congenital QT syndrome, recent MI, or uncompensated heart failure. Use cautiously in patients with a history of bradycardia, hypokalemia, or hypomagnesemia and in patients with acute diarrhea.

Special considerations
• Patients who take antipsychotics are at risk for developing neuroleptic malignant syndrome, tardive dyskinesia, or both.
• Dosage shouldn't be adjusted more than every 2 days. Longer intervals may be necessary since symptom response may not be seen for up to 4 to 6 weeks.
• Ziprasidone has been linked to prolongation of the QT interval. Other antipsychotics should

be considered instead of ziprasidone in patients with a history of QT interval prolongation, acute MI, congenital QT syndrome, and other conditions that place the patient at risk for life-threatening arrhythmias.
• Patients who develop symptoms of arrhythmias should have further CV monitoring.
• Patients who develop symptoms of neuroleptic malignant syndrome should receive immediate treatment because this condition can be life-threatening.
• Dosage adjustment should occur at appropriate intervals. Symptom response may not occur in some patients for 4 to 6 weeks.
• Ziprasidone should be taken with food, which increases drug effect.
• Ziprasidone should be discontinued in patients who have a QT interval greater than 500 msec.

Patient monitoring
• Electrolyte disturbances, such as hypokalemia or hypomagnesemia, increase the risk of arrhythmia. Monitor potassium and magnesium levels before starting therapy, and correct imbalances.
• Monitor patient for prolonged QT interval during therapy.
• Monitor patient for tardive dyskinesia.
• Patients who experience dizziness, palpitations, or syncope should have further evaluation and monitoring.

Breast-feeding patients
• Patients who are breast-feeding shouldn't take ziprasidone.

Patient education
• Tell patient to take drug with food.
• Tell patient to immediately report dizziness, fainting, irregular heart beat, or relevant cardiac problems.
• Advise patient to report any recent episodes of diarrhea.
• Advise patient to report abnormal movements.
• Tell patient to report sudden fever, muscle rigidity, or change in mental status.

zolmitriptan
Zomig, Zomig-ZMT

Pharmacologic classification: selective 5-hydroxytryptamine (5-HT) receptor agonist
Therapeutic classification: antimigraine
Pregnancy risk category: C

Indications and dosages
➤ *Acute migraine headaches with or without aura.* **Tablets.** *Adults:* Initially, 2.5 mg or less P.O. A dose lower than 2.5 mg can be achieved by breaking a 2.5 mg tablet in half. If headache returns after first dose, a second dose may be given after 2 hours. Maximum dose is 10 mg in 24-hour period.

Orally disintegrating tablets
Adults: Initially, 2.5 mg P.O. Don't break tablets in half. If headache returns after initial dose, a second dose may be given after 2 hours. Maximum dose is 10 mg in 24-hour period.

✦ *Dosage adjustment.* In patients with liver disease, use doses under 2.5 mg. Don't use orally disintegrating tablets because they shouldn't be broken in half.

How supplied
Available by prescription only
Orally disintegrating tablets: 2.5 mg
Tablets: 2.5 mg, 5 mg

Pharmacodynamics
Antimigraine action: Binds with high affinity to 5-HT_{1D} and 5-HT_{1B} receptors, aborting migraine headaches by causing constriction of cranial blood vessels and inhibition of proinflammatory neuropeptide release.

Pharmacokinetics
Absorption: Well absorbed after oral administration; plasma level peaks in 2 hours. Mean absolute bioavailability about 40%.
Distribution: Apparent volume of distribution is 7 L/kg. Plasma protein–binding is 25%.
Metabolism: Converted to an active N-desmethyl metabolite. Time to maximum concentration for the metabolite is 2 to 3 hours. Mean elimination half-life of zolmitriptan and active N-desmethyl metabolite is 3 hours.
Excretion: Mean total clearance is 31.5 ml/minute/kg; one-sixth is renal clearance. The renal clearance is greater than the glomerular filtration rate, suggesting renal tubular secretion. About 65% of dose excreted in urine, 30% in feces.

Route	Onset	Peak	Duration
P.O.			
Regular	Unknown	2 hr	3 hr
Disintegrating	Unknown	2 hr	Unknown

Contraindications and precautions
Contraindicated in patients hypersensitive to drug or its components and in those with uncontrolled hypertension, ischemic heart disease (angina pectoris, history of MI or documented silent ischemia), or other significant heart disease (including Wolff-Parkinson-White syndrome).

Avoid use within 2 weeks of stopping an MAO inhibitor or within 24 hours of other 5-HT_1 agonists or ergot-containing drugs. Also avoid use in patients with hemiplegic or basilar migraine.

Use cautiously in patients with liver disease and in pregnant or breast-feeding women.

Interactions
Drug-drug. *Cimetidine:* Doubled half-life of zolmitriptan. Monitor patient closely.

Drugs containing ergot: Additive vasospastic reactions. Avoid concomitant use.
Fluoxetine, fluvoxamine, paroxetine, sertraline: Possible weakness, hyperreflexia, and incoordination. Use cautiously together.
MAO inhibitors: Increased plasma levels of zolmitriptan. Monitor zolmitriptan levels; adjust dosage as needed. Avoid use of drug within 2 weeks of stopping MAO inhibitor therapy.
Oral contraceptives: Increased mean plasma levels of zolmitriptan. Adjust dosage as needed.

Adverse reactions
CNS: somnolence, vertigo, *dizziness,* hyperesthesias, paresthesia, asthenia.
CV: palpitations, *pain or heaviness in chest, pain, tightness, or pressure in the neck, throat, or jaw.*
GI: dry mouth, dyspepsia, dysphagia, nausea.
Musculoskeletal: myalgia.
Skin: sweating.
Other: warm or cold sensations.

Overdose and treatment
There's no specific antidote for overdose. If severe intoxication occurs, intensive care procedures are recommended, including establishing and maintaining a patent airway, ensuring adequate oxygenation and ventilation, and monitoring and supporting CV system. The effect of hemodialysis or peritoneal dialysis on drug plasma levels is unknown.

Special considerations
● Drug isn't intended for prophylactic therapy of migraine headaches or for use in hemiplegic or basilar migraines.
● Safety of drug hasn't been established for cluster headaches.
● Serious cardiac events, including some that have been fatal, have occurred rarely after use of 5-HT_1 agonists. Events reported have included coronary artery vasospasm, transient myocardial ischemia, MI, ventricular tachycardia, and ventricular fibrillation.

Patient monitoring
● Monitor blood pressure in patients with liver disease.
● Monitor therapeutic effect.

Breast-feeding patients
● It's unknown if drug appears in breast milk. Use cautiously in breast-feeding women.

Pediatric patients
● Safety and effectiveness in children haven't been established.

Patient education
● Advise patient that drug is intended to relieve migraine symptoms, not prevent them.
● Advise patient to take drug only as prescribed and not to take a second dose unless instructed.

Reactions may be *common*, uncommon, *life-threatening*, or COMMON AND LIFE-THREATENING.

If a second dose is indicated, he should take it 2 hours after first dose.

● Advise patient to immediately report pain or tightness in chest or throat, heart throbbing, rash, skin lumps, or swelling of face, lips, or eyelids.
● Caution woman to avoid pregnancy during therapy.
● Advise patient that drug shouldn't be taken with other migraine drugs.
● Instruct patient to not release the orally disintegrating tablets from their blister pack until just before use and then to open the pack and dissolve on tongue.
● Advise patient not to break the orally disintegrating tablets in half.

zolpidem tartrate
Ambien

Pharmacologic classification: imidazopyridine
Therapeutic classification: hypnotic
Controlled substance schedule: IV
Pregnancy risk category: B

Indications and dosages
➤ *Short-term management of insomnia.*
Adults: 10 mg P.O. immediately before h.s.
✦ *Dosage adjustment.* In elderly or debilitated patients or patients with hepatic insufficiency, 5 mg P.O. immediately before h.s. Maximum daily dose is 10 mg.

How supplied
Available by prescription only
Tablets: 5 mg, 10 mg

Pharmacodynamics
Hypnotic action: Hypnotic with a chemical structure unrelated to benzodiazepines, barbiturates, or other drugs with known hypnotic properties; however, it interacts with a gamma-aminobutyric acid-benzodiazepine or omega-receptor complex and shares some of the pharmacologic properties of the benzodiazepines. It exhibits no muscle relaxant or anticonvulsant properties.

Pharmacokinetics
Absorption: Absorbed rapidly from GI tract; mean peak concentration time of 1.6 hours. Food delays absorption.
Distribution: Protein-binding is about 92.5%.
Metabolism: Converted to inactive metabolites in liver.
Excretion: Primarily eliminated in urine; elimination half-life about 2.5 hours.

Route	Onset	Peak	Duration
P.O.	Rapid	½-2 hr	Unknown

Contraindications and precautions
No known contraindications. Use cautiously in patients with conditions that could affect metabolism or hemodynamic response and in those with decreased respiratory drive, depression, or history of alcohol or drug abuse.

Interactions
Drug-drug. *CNS depressants:* Enhanced CNS depression of zolpidem. Avoid concomitant use.
Drug-lifestyle. *Alcohol use:* Excessive CNS depression. Tell patient to use together cautiously.

Adverse reactions
CNS: daytime drowsiness, light-headedness, abnormal dreams, amnesia, dizziness, *headache*, hangover, sleep disorder, lethargy, depression.
CV: palpitations, chest pain.
EENT: sinusitis, pharyngitis.
GI: dry mouth, nausea, vomiting, diarrhea, dyspepsia, constipation, abdominal pain.
Musculoskeletal: back pain, myalgia, arthralgia.
Skin: rash.
Other: flulike symptoms, *hypersensitivity reactions.*

Overdose and treatment
Effects of overdose may range from somnolence to light coma. CV and respiratory compromise also may occur. Provide general symptomatic and supportive measures, along with immediate gastric lavage when appropriate. Give I.V. fluids as needed. Flumazenil may be useful. Monitor and treat hypotension and CNS depression. Withhold sedatives after zolpidem overdose even if excitation occurs.

Special considerations
● Limit drug therapy to 7 to 10 days; reevaluate patient if drug is to be taken for over 2 weeks.
● Because sleep disturbance may be a sign or symptom of a physical or psychiatric disorder, initiate symptomatic treatment of insomnia only after careful evaluation of patient.
● Zolpidem has CNS depressant effects similar to other sedative-hypnotic drugs. Because of its rapid onset of action, drug should be taken immediately before patient goes to bed.
● Dosage adjustments may be needed when drug is given with other CNS depressants because of potentially additive effects.
● Prevent hoarding or intentional overdosing by hospitalized patients who are depressed, suicidal, or known to abuse drug.

Patient monitoring
● Closely monitor patient with history of addiction to or abuse of drugs or alcohol because of risk of habituation and dependence.
● Monitor patient for hypersensitivity reactions.

Breast-feeding patients
● Because drug appears in breast milk, its use in breast-feeding women isn't recommended.

Pediatric patients
● Safety and effectiveness in children under age 18 haven't been established.

Geriatric patients
● Impaired motor or cognitive performance after repeated exposure or unusual sensitivity to sedative-hypnotics may occur in elderly patients. Recommended dose is 5 mg rather than 10 mg.

Patient education
● Tell patient not to take drug with or immediately after a meal.
● Stress importance of taking drug only as prescribed; inform patient of potential drug dependency associated with hypnotics taken for long periods.
● Inform patient that tolerance may occur if drug is taken for more than a few weeks.
● Warn patient against use of alcohol or other sleep preparations during therapy to avoid serious adverse effects.
● Caution patient to avoid activities that require alertness, such as driving, until adverse CNS effects of drug are known.
● Tell patient not to increase dose and to call if he feels drug is no longer effective.

zonisamide
Zonegran

Pharmacologic classification: sulfonamide
Therapeutic classification: antiseizure drug
Pregnancy risk category: C

Indication and dosages
➤**Adjunct therapy for partial seizures in adults with epilepsy.** *Adults over age 16:* Initially, 100 mg P.O. as a single daily dose for 2 weeks. After 2 weeks, may increase to 200 mg daily for at least 2 weeks. May be increased to 300 mg and 400 mg P.O. daily, with the dose stable for at least 2 weeks to achieve steady state at each level. Doses can be given once or twice daily except for the daily dose of 100 mg at start of therapy. Can be taken with or without food.
✦ **Dosage adjustment.** Use cautiously in patients with hepatic and renal disease; they may need slower adjustment and more frequent monitoring. If glomerular filtration rate is less than 50 ml/minute, don't give drug.

How supplied
Available by prescription only
Capsules: 100 mg

Pharmacodynamics
Unknown, but drug is thought to produce antiseizure effects through action at the sodium and calcium channels, thereby stabilizing neuronal membranes and suppressing neuronal hypersynchronization. Other models suggest that synaptically driven electrical activity is suppressed with-

out potentiation of synaptic activity by gamma-aminobutyric acid. Drug also may facilitate dopaminergic and serotonergic neurotransmission.

Pharmacokinetics
Absorption: Plasma levels peak in 2 to 6 hours. Food delays but doesn't alter bioavailability.
Distribution: Extensively binds to erythrocytes. Drug is about 40% bound to plasma proteins. Protein-binding is unaffected in the presence of therapeutic levels of phenytoin, phenobarbital, or carbamazepine.
Metabolism: Metabolized by cytochrome P-450 3A4. Clearance increases in patients who are receiving enzyme-inducing drugs.
Excretion: Excreted mainly in urine as parent drug and as glucuronide of a metabolite. Half-life of zonisamide in plasma is about 63 hours.

Route	Onset	Peak	Duration
P.O.	Unknown	Unknown	Unknown

Contraindications and precautions
Contraindicated in patients hypersensitive to sulfonamides or zonisamide. Use cautiously in patients with renal and hepatic dysfunction. If glomerular filtration rate is less than 50 ml/minute, don't give drug.

Interactions
Drug-drug: *Drugs that induce or inhibit CYP3A4:* May alter zonisamide levels. Monitor patient.

Adverse reactions
CNS: *headache, dizziness,* ataxia, asthenia, nystagmus, paresthesia, confusion, difficulty with concentration or memory, mental slowing, agitation, irritability, depression, insomnia, anxiety, nervousness, schizophrenic or schizophreniform behavior, *somnolence,* fatigue, tiredness, speech abnormalities, difficulty with verbal expression, tremor, *seizures,* abnormal gait, hyperethesia, lack of coordination.
EENT: diplopia, rhinitis, pharyngitis, amblyopia, tinnitis.
GI: taste perversion, *anorexia,* nausea, diarrhea, dyspepsia, constipation, dry mouth, abdominal pain, vomiting.
Hematologic: ecchymoses.
Metabolic: weight loss.
Respiratory: increased cough.
Skin: rash, pruritis.
Other: flu syndrome, accidental injury.

Overdose and treatment
Overdose probably would cause CNS signs and symptoms, although information is limited. No antidote is available. After a suspected overdose, induce emesis or perform gastric lavage with precautions to protect the airway. Provide supportive care and frequent monitoring of vital signs. Dialysis may not be effective. Contact a poison

---

Reactions may be *common*, uncommon, *life-threatening*, or COMMON AND LIFE-THREATENING.

control center for information on managing zonisamide overdose.

Special considerations
● Consider discontinuing zonisamide in patients who develop an unexplained rash.

Patient monitoring
● Monitor patient for symptoms of hypersensitivty.
● Monitor body temperatures, especially in the summer, since decreased sweating and increased body temperature has occurred (especially in patients age 17 and younger) causing heatstroke and dehydration.
● Abrupt withdrawal of zonisamide may increase frequency of seizures or status epilepticus; reduce dose or discontinue drug gradually.
● Increase fluid intake and urine output to help prevent kidney stones, especially in patients with predisposing factors.
● Monitor renal function periodically. If patient develops acute renal failure or a clinically significant sustained increase in creatinine or BUN levels, the drug should be discontinued.

Breast-feeding patients
● It isn't known if drug appears in breast milk. A decision should be made to discontinue breast-feeding or drug, taking into account the importance of the drug to the mother. This drug should be used in nursing mothers only if benefits outweigh the risk.

Pediatric patients
● Safety and efficacy in children under age 16 haven't been established.

Geriatric patients
● Use cautiously, and start at lower end of dosage range.

Patient education
● Tell patient to take drug with or without food. Caution against biting or breaking the capsule.
● Urge patient to contact prescriber immediately if any of the following occurs: rash, fever, sore throat, mouth sores, easy bruising easily, sudden back pain, abdominal pain, pain when urinating, bloody or dark urine, decreased sweating, increased body temperature, depression, or speech or language problems.
● Caution patient to avoid hazardous activities until drug effects are known because drug can cause drowsiness.
● Warn patient not to stop taking drug without prescriber's approval.
● Urge patient to drink 6 to 8 glasses of water daily to help reduce the risk of kidney stones.
● Tell women to report planned, suspected, or known pregnancy during therapy. Also, tell them to report an intention to breast-feed.
● Urge women of childbearing potential to use contraception while taking this drug.

Prescribing authority by state for advanced practice nurses

As of 2001, nurse practitioners held prescribing authority in all 50 states and Washington, DC, as indicated on the map below.

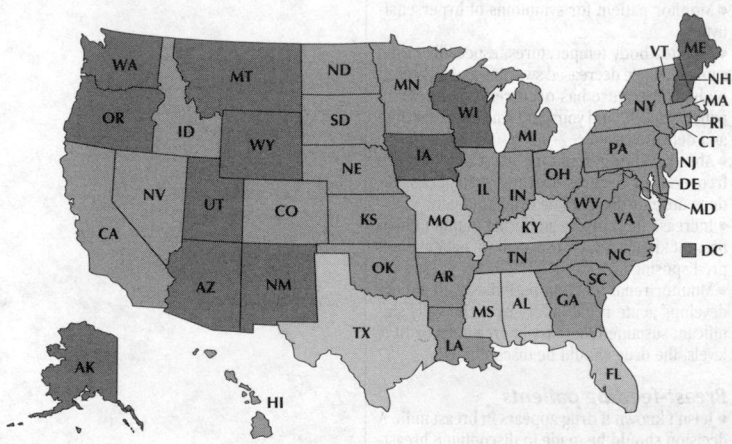

■ States where nurse practitioners† can prescribe (including controlled substances) independent of any required physician involvement in prescriptive authority: **AK, AZ, DC, IA, ME, MT, NH, NM, OR, UT‡, WA, WI, WY**

■ States where nurse practitioners† can prescribe (including controlled substances) with some degree of physician involvement or delegation of prescription writing: **AR, CA, CO, CT, DE, GA§, HI, ID, IL, IN, KS, LA, MA, MD, MI, MN, NC, ND, NE, NJ, NV, NY, OH, OK, PA, RI, SC‡, SD, TN, VA, VT, WV**

■ States where nurse practitioners† can prescribe (excluding controlled substances) with some degree of physician involvement or delegation of prescription writing: **AL, FL, KY, MO, MS, TX**

---

† The information may apply to other advanced practice nurses (clinical nurse specialists, nurse midwives, and nurse anesthetists).

‡ Schedule IV and V controlled substances only.

§ Nurse practitioners do not have written prescribing or dispensing authority; the process falls under delegated medical authority.

Adapted with permission from "Fourteenth Annual Legislative Update," *Nurse Practitioner* 27(1):15, January 2002.

Selected nonnarcotic analgesic combination products

Many common analgesics are combinations of two or more generic drugs. This table reviews common nonnarcotic analgesics.

Trade names	Generic drugs	Indications and adult dosages
Alka-Seltzer Plus Cold & Sinus Caplets, Allerest No-Drowsiness Tablets, Coldrine, Ornex No Drowsiness Caplets, Sinus-Relief Tablets, Sinutab Without Drowsiness	• acetaminophen 325 mg • pseudoephedrine hydrochloride 30 mg	For common cold, nasal congestion, sinus congestion, sinus pain. Give 2 tablets q 6 hours. Maximum, 8 tablets in 24 hours.
Amaphen, Anoquan, Butace, Endolor, Fsgic, Femcet, Fioricet, Fiorpap, Isocet, Medigesic, Repan, Triad	• acetaminophen 325 mg • caffeine 40 mg • butalbital 50 mg	For headache, mild to moderate pain, migraine. Give 1–2 tablets or capsules q 4 hours. Maximum, 6 tablets or capsules in 24 hours.
Anacin, Gensan, P-A-C Analgesic Tablets	• aspirin 400 mg • caffeine 32 mg	For headache, mild pain, myalgia. Give 2 tablets q 6 hours. Maximum, 8 tablets in 24 hours.
Ascriptin, Magnaprin	• aspirin 325 mg • magnesium hydroxide 50 mg • aluminum hydroxide 50 mg • calcium carbonate 50 mg	For fever, mild to moderate pain. Give 1–2 tablets q 4 hours.
Ascriptin A/D, Magnaprin Arthritis Strength Caplets	• aspirin 325 mg • magnesium hydroxide 75 mg • aluminum hydroxide 75 mg • calcium carbonate 75 mg	For mild to moderate pain. Give 1–2 tablets q 4 hours.
Aspirin-free Anacin PM, Excedrine PM, Extra Strength Tylenol PM, Sominex Pain Relief	• acetaminophen 500 mg • diphenhydramine 25 mg	For allergic rhinitis, headache, insomnia from pain or pruritus. Give 1 tablet at bedtime.
Axocet, Bucet, Butex Forte, Phrenilin Forte, Tencon	• acetaminophen 650 mg • butalbital 50 mg	For headache, mild to moderate pain. Give 1 tablet or capsule q 4 hours. Maximum, 4 tablets or capsules in 24 hours.
Bayer Select Head Cold Caplets, Dristan Cold Caplets, Maximum Strength Sudafed, Sinus Excedrin Extra Strength	• acetaminophen 500 mg • pseudoephedrine hydrochloride 30 mg	For common cold, nasal and sinus congestion, sinus pain. Give 2 tablets q 6 hours. Maximum, 8 tablets in 24 hours.
Bufferin AF Nite Time, Excedrin P.M. Caplets	• acetaminophen 500 mg • diphenhydramine citrate 3 mg	For insomnia from pain or pruritus. Give 1 tablet at bedtime.
Cama Arthritis Pain Reliever	• aspirin 500 mg • magnesium oxide 150 mg • aluminum hydroxide 125 mg	For mild to moderate pain. Give 1–2 tablets q 4 hours. Maximum, 8 tablets in 24 hours. *(continued)*

* Available in Canada only

Trade names	Generic drugs	Indications and adult dosages
Comtrex Allergy-Sinus, Sine-Off Medicine Caplets, Sinutab Maximum Strength	• acetaminophen 500 mg • pseudoephedrine hydrochloride 30 mg • chlorpheniramine maleate 2 mg	For allergic rhinitis, common cold, flu symptoms. Give 2 tablets q 4 hours. Maximum, 8 tablets in 24 hours.
Esgic-Plus	• acetaminophen 500 mg • caffeine 40 mg • butalbital 50 mg	For headache, migraine, mild to moderate pain. Give 1–2 tablets or capsules q 4 hours. Maximum, 6 tablets or capsules in 24 hours.
Excedrin Extra Strength, Excedrin Migraine	• aspirin 250 mg • acetaminophen 250 mg • caffeine 65 mg	For headache, migraine. Give 2 tablets q 4 hours. Maximum, 8 tablets in 24 hours.
Fiorinal, Fiortal, Lanorinal	• aspirin 325 mg • caffeine 40 mg • butalbital 50 mg	For headache, mild to moderate pain. Give 1–2 tablets or capsules q 4 hours. Maximum, 6 tablets or capsules in 24 hours.
Marten Tab, Phrenilin	• acetaminophen 325 mg • butalbital 50 mg	For headache, mild to moderate pain. Give 1–2 tablets q 4 hours. Maximum, 6 tablets in 24 hours.
Midrin	• isometheptene mucate 65 mg • dichloralphenazone 100 mg • acetaminophen 325 mg	For migraine, tension headache. For migraine, give 2 capsules initially; then 1 capsule q 1 hour to a maximum of 5 capsules in 12 hours. For tension headache, give 1–2 capsules q 4 hours to a maximum of 8 capsules in 24 hours.
Sinutab Regular*	• acetaminophen 325 mg • chlorpheniramine 2 mg • pseudoephedrine hydrochloride 30 mg	For allergic rhinitis, common cold, flu symptoms. Give 2 tablets q 6 hours. Maximum, 8 tablets in 24 hours.
Tecnal*	• aspirin 330 mg • caffeine 40 mg • butalbital 5 mg	For headache, mild to moderate pain. Give 1–2 tablets or capsules q 4 hours. Maximum, 6 tablets or capsules in 24 hours.
Vanquish	• aspirin 227 mg • acetaminophen 194 mg • caffeine 33 mg • aluminum hydroxide 25 mg • magnesium hydroxide 50 mg	For minor aches and pains. Give 2 caplets q 4 hours. Maximum, 12 caplets in 24 hours.

* Available in Canada only

Selected narcotic analgesic combination products

Many common analgesics are combinations of two or more generic drugs. This table reviews common narcotic analgesics.

Trade names and controlled substance schedule (CSS)	Generic drugs	Indications and adult dosages
Aceta with Codeine *CSS III*	• acetminophen 30 mg • codeine phosphate 30 mg	For fever, mild to moderate pain. Give 1–2 tablets q 4 hours. Maximum, 12 tablets in 24 hours.
Alor 5/500 Tablets, Damason-P, Lortab ASA *CSS III*	• aspirin 500 mg • hydrodocone bitartrate 5 mg	For moderate to moderately severe pain. Give 1–2 tablets q 4 hours. Maximum, 8 tablets in 24 hours.
Anexsia 7.5/650, Lorcet Plus *CSS III*	• acetaminophen 650 mg • hydrocodone bitartrate 7.5 mg	For arthralgia, bone pain, dental pain, headache, migraine, moderate pain. Give 1–2 tablets q 4 hours. Maximum, 6 tablets in 24 hours.
Capital with Codeine, Tylenol with Codeine Elixir *CSS V*	• acetaminophen 120 mg • codeine phosphate 12 mg/5 ml	For mild to moderate pain. Give 15 ml q 4 hours.
Darvocet-N 50 *CSS IV*	• acetaminophen 325 mg • propoxyphene napsylate 50 mg	For mild to moderate pain. Give 1–2 tablets q 4 hours. Maximum, 12 tablets in 24 hours.
Darvocet-N 100, Propacet 100 *CSS IV*	• acetaminophen 650 mg • propoxyphene napsykate 100 mg	For mild to moderate pain. Give 1 tablet q 4 hours. Maximum, 6 tablets in 24 hours.
Empirin with Codeine No. 3 *CSS III*	• aspirin 325 mg • codeine phosphate 30 mg	For fever, mild to moderate pain. Give 1–2 tablets q 4 hours. Maximum, 12 tablets in 24 hours.
Empirin with Codeine No. 4 *CSS III*	• aspirin 325 mg • codeine phosphate 60 mg	For fever, mild to moderate pain. Give 1 tablet q 4 hours. Maximum, 6 tablets in 24 hours.
Fioricet with Codeine *CSS III*	• acetaminophen 325 mg • butalbital 50 mg • caffeine 40 mg • codeine phosphate 30 mg	For headache, mild to moderate pain. Give 1–2 capsules q 4 hours. Maximum, 6 capsules in 24 hours.
Fiorinal with Codeine *CSS III*	• aspirin 325 mg • butalbital 50 mg • caffeine 40 mg • codeine phosphate 30 mg	For headache, mild to moderate pain. Give 1–2 tablets or capsules q 4 hours. Maximum, 6 tablets or capsules in 24 hours.
Lorcet 10/650 *CSS III*	• acetaminophen 650 mg • hydrocodone bitartrate 10 mg	For moderate to moderately severe pain. Give 1 tablet q 4 hours. Maximum, 6 tablets in 24 hours.
Lortab 2.5/500 *CSS III*	• acetaminophen 500 mg • hydrocodone bitartrate 2.5 mg	For moderate to moderately severe pain. Give 1–2 tablets q 4 hours. Maximum, 8 tablets in 24 hours.
Lortab 5/500 *CSS III*	• acetaminophen 500 mg • hydrocodone bitartrate 5 mg	For moderate to moderately severe pain. Give 1–2 tablets q 4 hours. Maximum, 8 tablets in 24 hours.

(continued)

Trade names and controlled substance schedule (CSS)	Generic drugs	Indications and adult dosages
Lortab 7.5/500 *CSS III*	• acetaminophen 500 mg • hydrocodone bitartrate 7.5 mg	For moderate to moderately severe pain. Give 1 tablet q 4 hours. Maximum, 8 tablets in 24 hours.
Lortab 10/500 *CSS III*	• acetaminophen 500 mg • hydrocodone bitartrate 10 mg	For moderate to moderately severe pain. Give 1 tablet q 4-6 hours. Maximum, 6 tablets in 24 hours.
Percocet 2.5/325 *CSS II*	• acetaminophen 325 mg • oxycodone hydrochloride 2.5 mg	For moderate to moderately severe pain. Give 1–2 tablets q 4-6 hours. Maximum, 12 tablets in 24 hours.
Percocet *CSS II*	• acetaminophen 325 mg • oxycodone hydrochloride 5 mg	For moderate to moderately severe pain. Give 1–2 tablets q 4 hours. Maximum, 12 tablets in 24 hours.
Percocet 7.5/500 *CSS II*	• acetaminophen 500 mg • oxycodone hydrochloride 7.5 mg	For moderate to moderately severe pain. Give 1–2 tablets q 4-6 hours. Maximum, 8 tablets in 24 hours.
Percocet 10/650 *CSS II*	• acetaminophen 650 mg • oxycodone hydrochloride 10 mg	For moderate to moderately severe pain. Give 1–2 tablets q 4-6 hours. Maximum, 6 tablets in 24 hours.
Percodan-Demi *CSS II*	• aspirin 325 mg • oxycodone hydrochloride 2.25 mg • oxycodone terephthalate 0.19 mg	For moderate to moderately severe pain. Give 1–2 tablets q 6 hours. Maximum, 8 tablets in 24 hours.
Percodan, Roxiprin *CSS II*	• aspirin 325 mg • oxycodone hydrochloride 4.5 mg • oxycodone terephthalate 0.38 mg	For moderate to moderately severe pain. Give 1 tablet q 6 hours. Maximum, 4 tablets in 24 hours.
Phenaphen/Codeine No. 3 *CSS III*	• acetaminophen 325 mg • codeine phosphate 30 mg	For fever, mild to moderate pain. Give 1–2 tablets q 4 hours. Maximum, 12 tablets in 24 hours.
Phenaphen/Codeine No. 4 *CSS III*	• acetaminophen 325 mg • codeine phosphate 60 mg	For fever, mild to moderate pain. Give 1 tablet q 4 hours. Maximum, 6 tablets in 24 hours.
Propoxyphene Napsylate/ Acetaminophen *CSS IV*	• acetaminophen 650 mg • propoxyphene napsylate 100 mg	For mild to moderate pain. Give 1 tablet q 4 hours. Maximum, 6 tablets in 24 hours.
Roxicet *CSS II*	• acetaminophen 325 mg • oxycodone hydrochloride 5 mg	For moderate to moderately severe pain. Give 1–2 tablets q 4 hours. Maximum, 12 tablets in 24 hours.
Roxicet 5/500, Roxilox *CSS II*	• acetaminophen 500 mg • oxycodone hydrochloride 5 mg	For moderate to moderately severe pain. Give 1–2 tablets q 4-6 hours. Maximum, 8 tablets in 24 hours.
Roxicet Oral Solution *CSS II*	• acetaminophen 325 mg • oxycodone hydrochloride 5 mg/5 ml	For moderate to moderately severe pain. Give 5–10 ml q 4-6 hours. Maximum, 60 ml in 24 hours.
Talacen *CSS IV*	• acetaminophen 650 mg • pentazocine hydrochloride 25 mg	For mild to moderate pain. Give 1 tablet q 4 hours. Maximum, 6 tablets in 24 hours.

Trade names and controlled substance schedule (CSS)	Generic drugs	Indications and adult dosages
Talwin Compound *CSS IV*	• aspirin 325 mg • pentazocine hydro-chloride 12.5 mg	For moderate pain. Give 2 tablets q 6 hours. Maximum, 8 tablets in 24 hours.
ylenol with Codeine No. 2 *CSS III*	• acetaminophen 300 mg • codeine phosphate 15 mg	For fever, mild to moderate pain. Give 1–2 tablets q 4 hours. Maximum, 12 tablets in 24 hours.
Tylenol with Codeine No. 3 *CSS III*	• acetaminophen 300 mg • codeine phosphate 30 mg	For fever, mild to moderate pain. Give 1–2 tablets q 4 hours. Maximum, 12 tablets in 24 hours.
Tylenol with Codeine No. 4 *CSS III*	• acetaminophen 300 mg • codeine phosphate 60 mg	For fever, mild to moderate pain. Give 1 tablet q 4 hours. Maximum, 6 tablets in 24 hours.
Tylox *CSS II*	• acetaminophen 500 mg • oxycodone hydro-chloride 5 mg	For moderate to moderately severe pain. Give 1–2 tablets q 4 hours. Maximum, 12 tablets in 24 hours.
Vicodin *CSS III*	• acetaminophen 500 mg • hydrocodone bitartrate 5 mg	For moderate to moderately severe pain. Give 1–2 tablets q 4 hours. Maximum, 8 tablets in 24 hours.
Vicodin ES *CSS III*	• acetaminophen 750 mg • hydrocodone bitartrate 7.5 mg	For moderate to moderately severe pain. Give 1 tablet q 4–6 hours. Maximum, 5 tablets in 24 hours.
Wygesic *CSS IV*	• acetaminophen 650 mg • propoxyphene nap-sylate 65 mg	For mild to moderate pain. Give 1 tablet q 4 hours. Maximum, 6 tablets in 24 hours.
Zydone *CSS III*	• acetaminophen 400 mg • hydrocodone bitartrate 10 mg	For moderate to moderately severe pain. Give 1 tablet q 4–6 hours. Maximum, 6 tablets in 24 hours

Guidelines for use of selected antimicrobials

This table provides guidelines for the first-line (denoted by the numeral 1) and second-line (numeral 2) management of selected organisms and should be used as a general reference only. Use patient condition, sensitivities, institutional policies, and recent research when initiating new therapy.

	Aminoglycosides				Cephalosporins								
	Amikacin	Gentamicin	Netilmicin	Tobramycin	Cefazolin	Cefepime	Cefixime	Cefotaxime	Cefoxitin	Ceftazidime	Ceftizoxime	Ceftriaxone	Cefuroxime
Acinetobacter	1	2	2	2									
Bacillus anthracis													
Bacteroides fragilis									2				
Borrelia burgdorferi (skin)												2	2
Campylobacter jejuni													
Chlamydia pneumoniae													
Chlamydia psittaci													
Chlamydia trachomatis													
Citrobacter freundii		1		1									
Clostridium difficile													
Clostridium perfringens					2			2	2		2	2	
Enterobacter sp.	1	1	1	1		2							
Enterococcus faecalis													
Enterococcus faecium													
Escherichia coli	2	2	2	2	1		1	1	1	1	1	1	1
Haemophilus influenzae†								1			1	1	
Haemophilus influenzae‡							2						2
Klebsiella pneumoniae (UTI)					1		1	1	1		1	1	1
Klebsiella pneumoniae (pneumonia)	2	2	2	2			1	1	1	1	1	1	1
Legionella pneumophila													
Listeria monocytogenes		1		1									
Moraxella catarrhalis						2	2	2	2	2	2	2	2
Mycoplasma pneumoniae													
Neisseria gonorrhoeae							1					1	
Nocardia asteroides													
Pneumocystis carinii													
Proteus mirabilis						2	2	2	2	2	2	2	2
Proteus vulgaris							1	1		1	1	1	
Pseudomonas aeruginosa	2	2	2	1		2				1			
Serratia marcescens	2	2	2	2				1			2	2	1
Shigella sp.													
Staphylococcus aureus					1								
Staphylococcus saprophyticus													
Streptococcus pneumoniae								2				2	
Streptococcus pyogenes (group A)					1	1	1	1	1		1	1	1
Streptococcus (anaerobic sp.)													
Streptococcus (viridans group)		1										2	
Vibrio cholerae													

† life-threatening   ‡ non-life-threatening

	Miscellaneous													Penicillins						
	Azithromycin	Aztreonam	Chloramphenicol	Clarithromycin	Clindamycin	Eyrthromycin	Imipenem/Cilastatin	Meropenem	Metronidazole	Pentamidine	Rifampin	Trimethoprim/Sulfamethoxazole	Vancomycin	Amoxicillin	Ampicillin	Mezlocillin	Nafcillin	Penicillin G	Piperacillin	Ticarcillin
							1	1				2								
				2		2													1	
						2	2	2	1											
	2			2		2								1				2		
	2			2	2	1														
	2			2		2														
			2																	
	1					2														
		2					1	1												
									1			2								
					2														1	
							1	1												
												2		1	1			1		
			2										1							
		2					2	2				2								
		2					2	2												
	2			2								1								
		2										2								
		2					2	2				2								
	1			2	2						2									
												2					1	1		
	2			2								1								
	2			2	1															
												1								
									2			1								
			2									1								
												1								
			2				2	2									1		1	1
		2										1								
												1					2			
					2						2	2		1			1			
					2															
														1	1	1		1		
	2			2	2	2								1				1		
					2													1		
	2			2	2	2												1		
												2								

(continued)

	Combination with β-lactamase inhibitors				Tetracyclines		Fluoroquinolones			
	Amoxicillin/Clavulanic acid	Ampicillin/Sulbactam	Pipericillin/Tazobactam	Ticarcillin/Clavulanic acid	Doxycyline	Minocycline	Ciprofloxacin	Levofloxacin	Norfloxacin	Ofloxacin
Acinetobacter		2					2			2
Bacillus anthracis					1					
Bacteroides fragilis	2	2	2	2						
Borrelia burgdorferi (skin)					1					
Campylobacter jejuni							2			2
Chlamydia pneumoniae					1			2		
Chlamydia psittaci					1					
Chlamydia trachomatis					1					2
Citrobacter freundii							1			
Clostridium difficile										
Clostridium perfringens										
Enterobacter sp.							1			
Enterococcus faecalis										
Enterococcus faecium					2					
Escherichia coli			2				2	2	2	2
Haemophilus influenzae†		1	2	1			1	1		1
Haemophilus influenzae‡	1	1					2	2		2
Klebsiella pneumoniae (UTI)	2			2			1	2	2	2
Klebsiella pneumoniae (pneumonia)	2	2	2	2			2	2		2
Legionella pneumophila					2		1	1		1
Listeria monocytogenes										
Moraxella catarrhalis	1	1					2	2		2
Mycoplasma pneumoniae					1			2		
Neisseria gonorrhoeae							2			2
Nocardia asteroides						2				
Pneumocystis carinii										
Proteus mirabilis										
Proteus vulgaris	2						1	1	1	1
Pseudomonas aeruginosa							2			
Serratia marcescens							2	2		2
Shigella sp.					2		1		1	1
Staphylococcus aureus	2	2	2	2			2	2		2
Staphylococcus saprophyticus							2		1	2
Streptococcus pneumoniae					1			1		
Streptococcus pyogenes (group A)										
Streptococcus (anaerobic sp.)										
Streptococcus (viridans group)										
Vibrio cholerae					1		1			1

† life-threatening   ‡ non-life-threatening

Dialyzable drugs

The amount of a drug removed by dialysis differs among patients and depends on several factors, including the patient's condition, the drug's properties, length of dialysis and dialysate used, rate of blood flow or dwell time, and purpose of dialysis. This table indicates the effect of hemodialysis on selected drugs.

Drug	Level reduced by hemodialysis	Drug	Level reduced by hemodialysis
acetaminophen	Yes (may not influence toxicity)	chlorambucil	No
		chlordiazepoxide	No
acyclovir	Yes	chloroquine	No
allopurinol	Yes	chlorpheniramine	No
alprazolam	No	chlorpromazine	No
amikacin	Yes	chlorthalidone	No
amiodarone	No	cimetidine	Yes
amitriptyline	No	ciprofloxacin	Yes (only by 20%)
amoxicillin	Yes	cisplatin	No
amoxicillin/clavulanate potassium	Yes	clindamycin	No
		clofibrate	No
amphotericin B	No	clonazepam	No
ampicillin	Yes	clonidine	No
ampicillin/clavulanate potassium	Yes	clorazepate	No
		cloxacillin	No
aspirin	Yes	codeine	No
atenolol	Yes	colchicine	No
azathioprine	Yes	cortisone	No
aztreonam	Yes	co-trimoxazole	Yes
captopril	Yes	cyclophosphamide	Yes
carbamazepine	No	diazepam	No
carbenicillin	Yes	diclofenac	No
carmustine	No	dicloxacillin	No
cefaclor	Yes	digoxin	No
cefadroxil	Yes	diltiazem	No
cefamandole	Yes	diphenhydramine	No
cefazolin	Yes	dipyridamole	No
cefepime	Yes	disopyramide	Yes
cefonicid	Yes (only by 20%)	doxazosin	No
cefoperazone	Yes	doxepin	No
cefotaxime	Yes	doxorubicin	No
cefotetan	Yes (only by 20%)	doxycycline	No
cefoxitin	Yes	enalapril	Yes
ceftazidime	Yes	erythromycin	Yes (only by 20%)
ceftizoxime	Yes	ethambutol	Yes (only by 20%)
ceftriaxone	No	ethchlorvynol	Yes
cefuroxime	Yes	ethosuximide	Yes
cephalexin	Yes	famotidine	No
cephalothin	Yes	fenoprofen	No
cephapirin	Yes	flecainide	No
chloral hydrate	Yes		

Drug	Level reduced by hemodialysis	Drug	Level reduced by hemodialysis
fluconazole	Yes	methotrexate	Yes
flucytosine	Yes	methyldopa	Yes
fluorouracil	Yes	methylprednisolone	No
fluoxetine	No	metoclopramide	No
flurazepam	No	metolazone	No
fosinopril	No	metoprolol	No
furosemide	No	metronidazole	Yes
gabapentin	Yes	mexiletine	Yes
ganciclovir	Yes	mezlocillin	Yes
gemfibrozil	No	miconazole	No
gentamicin	Yes	midazolam	No
glipizide	No	minocycline	No
glutethimide	Yes	minoxidil	Yes
glyburide	No	misoprostol	No
guanfacine	No	morphine	No
haloperidol	No	nabumetone	No
heparin	No	nadolol	Yes
hydralazine	No	nafcillin	No
hydrochlorothiazide	No	naproxen	No
hydroxyzine	No	nelfinavir	No
ibuprofen	No	netilmicin	Yes
imipenem/cilastatin	Yes	nifedipine	No
imipramine	No	nimodipine	No
indapamide	No	nitrofurantoin	Yes
indomethacin	No	nitroglycerin	No
insulin	No	nitroprusside	Yes
irbesartan	No	nizatidine	No
iron dextran	No	norfloxacin	No
isoniazid	Yes	nortriptyline	No
isosorbide	No	ofloxacin	Yes
isradipine	No	olanzapine	No
kanamycin	Yes	omeprazole	No
ketoconazole	No	oxazepam	No
ketoprofen	Yes	paroxetine	No
labetalol	No	penicillin G	Yes
levofloxacin	No	pentamidine	No
lidocaine	No	pentazocine	Yes
lithium	Yes	phenobarbital	Yes
lomustine	No	phenylbutazone	No
loracarbef	Yes	phenytoin	No
loratidine	No	piperacillin	Yes
lorazepam	No	piroxicam	No
mechlorethamine	No	prazosin	No
meperidine	No	prednisone	No
methadone	No	primidone	Yes
methicillin	No	procainamide	Yes

Drug	Level reduced by hemodialysis
promethazine	No
propoxyphene	No
propranolol	No
protriptyline	No
quinidine	Yes
ramipril	No
ranitidine	Yes
rifampin	No
rofecoxib	No
sertraline	No
sotalol	Yes
stavudine	Yes
streptomycin	Yes
sucralfate	No
sulbactam	Yes
sulfamethoxazole	Yes
sulindac	No
temazepam	No
theophylline	Yes
ticarcillin	Yes
timolol	No
tobramycin	Yes
tocainide	Yes
tolbutamide	No
topiramate	Yes
trazodone	No
triazolam	No
trimethoprim	Yes
valacyclovir	Yes
valproic acid	No
valsartan	No
vancomycin	No
verapamil	No
warfarin	No

Topical drugs

This table shows commonly used topical drugs and their indications, dosages, and actions. It also provides special considerations for topical administration.

	Drug	Indications and dosages
Antibacterials and antifungals	**alcohol, ethyl and isopropyl**	*To disinfect skin, instruments, and ampules:* Disinfect, p.r.n. Isopropyl alcohol is superior to ethyl alcohol as an anti-infective (70%). *Antipyresis:* Apply 25% solution. *Anhidrosis:* Apply 50% solution p.r.n.
	hydrogen peroxide (Peroxyl)	*Cleaning wounds:* Use 1.5% to 3% solution, p.r.n. *Mouthwash for necrotizing ulcerative gingivitis:* Gargle with 3% solution, p.r.n. *Cleaning minor wounds or irritations of the mouth or gums:* Use 1.5% gel, p.r.n. *Cleaning douche:* Use 2% solution q.i.d., p.r.n.
Antiseptics and germicidals	**benzalkonium chloride** (Benza, Mycocide NS, Ony-Clear, Zephiran Chloride)	*Preoperative disinfection of unbroken skin:* Apply 1:750 tincture or spray. *Disinfection of mucous membranes and denuded skin:* Apply 1:10,000 to 1:5,000 aqueous solution. *Irrigation of vagina:* Instill 1:5,000 to 1:2,000 aqueous solution. *Irrigation of deep infected wounds:* Instill 1:20,000 to 1:3,000 aqueous solution. *Irrigation of urinary bladder and urethra:* 1:20,000 to 1:5,000 aqueous solution.
	hexachlorophene (pHisoHex, Septisol)	*Surgical scrub, bacteriostatic skin cleanser:* Use 0.23% to 3% concentrations, p.r.n.
	iodine	*Preoperative disinfection of skin (small wounds and abraded areas):* Apply p.r.n.
	povidone-iodine (Acu-dyne, Aerodine, Betadine, Betagen, Biodine, Etodine, Iodex, Operand, Polydine)	*Preoperative skin preparation and scrub; germicide for surface wounds; postoperative application to incisions; prophylactic application to urinary meatus of catheterized patients; miscellaneous disinfection; scaling and itching from dandruff (shampoo):* Apply p.r.n., or use as scrub, p.r.n.
Keratolytics	**podophyllum resin** (Podocon, Podofin)	*Venereal warts:* Apply podophyllum resin preparation to the lesion, cover with waxed paper, and bandage. The first application should remain on skin for 30 to 40 minutes; subsequent applications may last 1 to 4 hours, depending on lesion and patient's condition. Wash lesion to remove medication. Repeat at weekly intervals, if indicated. *Multiple superficial epitheliomatosis and keratosis:* Apply daily with applicator and allow to dry. Remove necrotic tissue before each application.
	salicylic acid (Calicylic, Compound W, DuoFilm, Freezone, Gordofilm, Hydrisalic, Keralyt, Occlusal, Off-Ezy, Sal-Acid, Wart-Off)	*Scaling dermatoses, hyperkeratosis, calluses, warts:* Apply to affected area and cover with occlusive dressing at night.
Protectants	**benzoin tincture compound**	*Demulcent and protectant (cutaneous ulcers, bedsores, cracked nipples, fissures of lips and anus):* Apply locally once daily or b.i.d.
	zinc oxide with calamine and gelatin (Dome-Paste)	*Protectant (lesions or injuries of lower legs or arms):* Wrap the wet bandage in place and retain for about 1 week. Dome-Paste, in 3" to 4" bandages, can be applied directly to arm or leg.
Wet dressings, soaks	**aluminum acetate, aluminum sulfate** (Bluboro Powder, Boropak Powder, Burow's Solution, Domeboro Powder)	*Mild skin irritation from exposure to soaps, chemicals, diaper rash, acne, eczema:* Apply p.r.n. *Skin inflammation, contact dermatoses:* Mix powder or tablet with 1 pint of lukewarm water. Apply to loose dressing q 15 to 30 minutes for 4 to 8 hours.

Action	Special considerations
Antibacterial effect through reduction of surface tension of bacterial cell walls, inhibiting bacterial growth. Also antipyretic and astringent effects.	• Avoid contact with eyes and mucous membranes. • Contraindicated in patients taking disulfiram if used over large surface area. • Do not apply to open wounds.
Antibacterial effect through oxidation.	• Do not instill into closed body cavities or abscesses because released gas cannot escape. • Store in a tightly capped, dark container in a cool, dry place. • Do not confuse with peroxide (6% to 20%) used for bleaching hair.
Cationic surface action producing bacteriostatic or bactericidal effect, depending on the concentration used.	• Do not use with occlusive dressings or packs. • Inactivated by anionic compounds such as soap. • Rinse area thoroughly after each application. • Skin inflammation and irritation may require lower concentration or discontinuation.
Bacteriostatic effect against staphylococci and other gram-positive bacteria, probably due to inhibition of bacterial membrane-bound enzymes.	• Do not use on broken skin, skin lesions, burns, wounds, or under occlusive dressings. Do not use around eyes or mucous membranes. • Discontinue promptly if CNS irritability occurs. • Rinse thoroughly after use. • Do not use in infants; use cautiously in children.
Germicidal effect against bacteria, fungi, protozoa, yeast, and viruses, probably from protein disruption.	• Do not cover after application to avoid irritation. • Avoid contact with eyes and mucous membranes. • Toxic if ingested; sodium thiosulfate is an antidote.
Germicidal effect against bacteria, fungi, and viruses; has same action as iodine without its irritating effects.	• Contraindicated in patients with known sensitivity to iodine. • Do not use around eyes; do not use full-strength solution on mucous membranes. May stain skin and mucous membranes. • Avoid using solution that contains a detergent when treating open wounds.
Caustic and erosive action from disruption of epithelial cell division.	• Should not be used in pregnant patients. • May be toxic if applied to large surface area or applied too frequently. • Wash hands thoroughly after applying. • Protect surrounding area with petrolatum. • Wash off thoroughly with soap and water after prescribed time. • May cause abnormal pigmentation. • To be applied by only a health care provider. • Don't use on inflamed or irritated warts. Avoid contact with healthy tissue and eyes.
Causes desquamation of cornified epithelium by increasing hydration.	• Don't use on birthmarks, moles, or areas of hair follicle involvement. • Avoid contact with eyes, face, genitals, mucous membranes, and normal skin. Don't use in aspirin sensitive patients. • Hydrate skin for at least 5 minutes before application. • Apply emollient to surrounding skin for protection. • Wash off thoroughly after overnight use.
Protects skin from external environment by coating action.	• Clean and dry area before applying. • Useful in protection of skin from adhesive.
Protects skin by forming occlusive barrier.	• Watch for signs of infection. • Warn patient not to shower or bathe with gel on. • Remove by soaking in warm water. Remove all of previous application before reapplying. • Apply with nap of hair to avoid folliculitis. • Do not use with constrictive bandage.
Reduces friction and provides soothing relief through astringent action.	• Avoid use around eyes and mucous membranes. • Do not use with occlusive dressings. • Discontinue if irritation occurs.

Selected local and topical anesthetics

Drug, indications, dosage	Adverse reactions
Local	

bupivacaine hydrochloride
(Marcaine, Sensorcaine)
Dosages given are for the drug without epinephrine and for adults. Volume listed below refers to the total volume of anesthetic given, sometimes in incremental doses of 2 to 6 ml.
Epidural block—
0.25% solution: 10 to 20 ml (25 to 50 mg)
0.5% solution: 10 to 20 ml (50 to 100 mg)
0.75% solution: 10 to 20 ml (75 to 150 mg), single-dose only
Caudal block—
0.25% solution: 15 to 30 ml (37.5 to 75 mg)
0.5% solution: 15 to 30 ml (75 to 150 mg)
Spinal block—
0.75% solution (in dextrose 8.25%): 0.8 to 1.6 ml (6 to 12 mg)
Peripheral nerve block—
0.25% solution: 5 ml (12.5 mg)
0.5% solution: 5 ml (25 mg)

CNS: anxiety, nervousness, *seizures* followed by drowsiness.
CV: *arrhythmias, bradycardia, cardiac arrest,* hypotension, myocardial depression.
EENT: blurred vision, tinnitus.
GI: nausea, vomiting.
Respiratory: *respiratory arrest.*
Skin: dermatologic reactions, *status asthmaticus.*
Other: *anaphylactoid reactions, anaphylaxis,* edema.

---

chloroprocaine hydrochloride
(Nesacaine, Nesacaine-MPF)
Dosages given are for the drug without epinephrine and for adults. Volume listed below refers to the total volume of anesthetic given, sometimes in incremental doses of 2 to 6 ml.
Infiltration and nerve block—
1% solution: 3 to 20 ml (30 to 200 mg)
2% solution: 2 to 40 ml (40 to 800 mg)
Caudal and epidural block—
2% to 3% solution: 15 to 25 ml (300 to 750 mg)
  May be repeated with smaller doses q 40 to 50 minutes. Dose and interval may be increased when combined with epinephrine. Maximum adult dose is 800 mg; when combined with epinephrine, maximum dose is 1 g.

CNS: anxiety, nervousness, *seizures* followed by drowsiness.
CV: *arrhythmias, bradycardia, cardiac arrest,* hypotension, myocardial depression.
EENT: blurred vision, tinnitus.
GI: nausea, vomiting.
Respiratory: *respiratory arrest, status asthmaticus.*
Skin: dermatologic reactions.
Other: *anaphylactoid reactions, anaphylaxis,* edema.

---

etidocaine hydrochloride
(Duranest, Duranest MPF)
Dosages given are for the drug without epinephrine and for adults.
  Dose limit is 4 mg/kg or 300 mg per injection. When combined with epinephrine, dose limit is 5.5 mg/kg or 400 mg per injection. May be repeated q 2 to 3 hours.
Peripheral nerve block—
1% solution: 5 to 40 ml (50 to 400 mg)
Central neural block (lower limbs, cesarean section, lumbar, epidural)—
1% solution: 10 to 30 ml (100 to 300 mg)
Transvaginal block—
1% solution: 5 to 20 ml (50 to 200 mg)
Caudal block—
1% solution: 10 to 30 ml (100 to 300 mg)

CNS: anxiety, apprehension, nervousness, *seizures* followed by drowsiness.
CV: *arrhythmias, bradycardia, cardiac arrest,* hypotension, myocardial depression.
EENT: blurred vision, tinnitus.
GI: nausea, vomiting.
Respiratory: *respiratory arrest, status asthmaticus.*
Skin: dermatologic reactions.
Other: *anaphylactoid reactions, anaphylaxis,* edema.

Reactions may be *common,* uncommon, *life-threatening,* or COMMON AND LIFE-THREATENING.

Interactions	Nursing considerations

Beta blockers: enhanced sympatho-mimetic effects when used with bupi-vacaine and epinephrine. Use with caution.
Butyrophenones, phenothiazines: may reduce or reverse pressor effect of ep-inephrine. Monitor patient.
Chloroprocaine: may lessen bupiva-caine's action. Don't use together.
CNS depressants: may cause additive CNS effects. Reduce dosage of CNS depressants.
Cyclic antidepressants, MAO in-hibitors: severe, sustained hyperten-sion when used with bupivacaine and epinephrine. Use with extreme cau-tion.
Enflurane, halothane, isoflurane, relat-ed drugs: arrhythmias when used with bupivacaine and epinephrine. Use with extreme caution.

- Contraindicated in children under 12 years, for spinal or topical anesthesia or paracervical block, and in patients with known history of hypersensitivity reactions to local anesthetics of the amide type.
- Some solutions contain sulfites and should be avoided in patients with sulfite hypersensitivity.
- Should not be used for I.V. regional anesthesia (Bier block, Bier's local anesthesia).
- Don't use 0.75% solution for obstetric surgery; lower concentrations are effective and less hazardous.
- Use cautiously in debilitated, elderly, or acutely ill pa-tients and in patients with severe hepatic disease or drug allergies.
- Use solutions with epinephrine cautiously in patients with CV disorders and in body areas with limited blood supply (ears, nose, fingers, toes).
- Keep resuscitation equipment and drugs available.
- Don't use solution with preservatives for caudal or epidural block.
- Discard partially used vials without preservatives.
- Check solution for particles.
- Protect solutions containing epinephrine from light.

Bupivacaine: chloroprocaine may lessen bupivacaine's action. Monitor for effect.
CNS depressants: may cause additive CNS effects. Reduce dosage of CNS depressants.
Sulfonamides: chloroprocaine inhibits the action of sulfonamides. Don't use in conditions in which a sulfonamide drug is required.

- Contraindicated in patients with hypersensitivity to pro-caine, tetracaine, or other PABA derivatives and for spinal or topical anesthesia. Epidural and caudal blocks are contraindicated in patients with CNS disease.
- Use cautiously in debilitated, elderly, or acutely ill pa-tients; in children; and in patients with drug allergies, paracervical block, or CV disease.
- Keep resuscitation equipment and drugs available.
- Don't use solution with preservatives for caudal or epidural block.
- Don't use discolored solution.
- Check solution for particles.
- Discard partially used vials without preservatives.

Cyclic antidepressants, MAO in-hibitors, phenothiazines: severe, sus-tained hypertension or hypotension with etidocaine and epinephrine. Use with extreme caution.
Enflurane, halothane, isoflurane, relat-ed drugs: arrhythmias when used with etidocaine and epinephrine. Use with extreme caution.
CNS depressants: may cause additive CNS effects. Reduce dosage of CNS depressants.

- Contraindicated in patients with inflammation or infec-tion in puncture region, septicemia, severe hyperten-sion, spinal deformities, or neurologic disorders; in chil-dren under 14 years; and for spinal anesthesia.
- Contraindicated in patients with known history of hy-persensitivity to local anesthetics of the amide type.
- Some solutions contain sulfites and should be avoided in patients with sulfite hypersensitivity.
- Use cautiously in debilitated, elderly, or acutely ill pa-tients; in patients with severe shock, heart block, gener-al drug allergies, or hepatic and renal disease; and as epidural block in obstetric patients.
- Use solutions with epinephrine cautiously in patients with CV disease and in body areas with limited blood supply (ears, nose, fingers, toes).
- Don't use solution with preservatives for caudal or epidural block; check solution for particles.
- Keep resuscitation equipment and drugs available.

(continued)

Drug, indications, dosage	Adverse reactions
Local	

lidocaine hydrochloride
[lignocaine hydrochloride]
(Dilocaine, Lidoject-1, Lidoject-2, Nervocaine, Octocaine, Xylocaine)
Dosages given are for drug without epinephrine and for adults. Volume listed below refers to total volume of anesthetic given, sometimes in incremental doses of 2 to 6 ml.
For anesthesia other than spinal—
Maximum single dose is 4.5 mg/kg or 300 mg. With epinephrine, maximum dose is 7 mg/kg or 500 mg.
Caudal (obstetric) or epidural (thoracic) block—
1% solution: 20 to 30 ml (200 to 300 mg)
Epidural (lumbar anesthesia) block—
1% solution: 25 to 30 ml (250 to 300 mg)
1.5% solution: 15 to 20 ml (225 to 300 mg)
2% solution: 10 to 15 ml (200 to 300 mg)
Spinal surgical anesthesia—
5% (with 7.5% dextrose): 1.5 to 2 ml (75 to 100 mg)
Caudal (surgery) block—
1.5% solution: 15 to 20 ml (225 to 300 mg)

CNS: anxiety, nervousness, *seizures* followed by drowsiness.
CV: *arrhythmias, bradycardia, cardiac arrest,* myocardial depression, hypotension.
EENT: blurred vision, tinnitus.
GI: nausea, vomiting.
Respiratory: *respiratory arrest, status asthmaticus.*
Skin: dermatologic reactions.
Other: *anaphylactoid reactions, anaphylaxis,* edema.

procaine hydrochloride
(Novocain)
Spinal anesthesia—
Adults: initial dose should not exceed 1 g. Before using, dilute 10% solution with normal saline solution injection, sterile distilled water, or CSF. For hyperbaric technique, use dextrose solution.
Perineum: 0.5 ml of 10% solution (50 mg) and 0.5 ml diluent injected at the L4 interspace
Perineum and lower extremities: 1 ml of 10% solution (100 mg) and 1 ml diluent injected at the L3 or L4 interspace
Up to costal margin: 2 ml of 10% solution (200 mg) and 1 ml diluent injected at the L2, L3, or L4 interspace
Peripheral nerve block—
1% solution: 100 ml (1 g)
2% solution: 50 ml (1 g)
Infiltration
350 to 600 mg in 0.25% to 0.5% solution. Maximum initial dose is 1 g.

CNS: anxiety, nervousness, *seizures* followed by drowsiness.
CV: *arrhythmias, bradycardia, cardiac arrest,* hypotension, myocardial depression.
EENT: blurred vision, tinnitus.
GI: nausea, vomiting.
Respiratory: *respiratory arrest, status asthmaticus.*
Skin: dermatologic reactions.
Other: *anaphylactoid reactions, anaphylaxis,* edema.

ropivacaine hydrochloride
(Naropin)
Avoid rapid injection of large volume of local anesthetic and use incremental doses. Use smallest dose and concentration required to produce desired result.
Lumbar epidural block in surgery—
0.5% solution: 15 to 30 ml (75 to 150 mg)
0.75% solution: 15 to 25 ml (119 to 188 mg)
1.0% solution: 15 to 30 ml (150 to 200 mg)
Lumbar epidural block for cesarean section—
0.5% solution: 20 to 30 ml (100 to 150 mg)
Thoracic epidural administration to establish block for postoperative pain relief—
0.5% solution: 5 to 15 ml (25 to 75 mg)
Major nerve block (brachial plexus)—
0.5 % solution: 35 to 50 ml (175 to 250 mg)
Field block (minor nerve blocks and infiltration)—
0.5% solution: 1 to 10 ml (5 to 200 mg)
Lumbar epidural block in labor—
Initially, 0.2% solution: 10 to 20 ml (20 to 40 mg); then 6 to 14 ml/hour (12 to 28 mg/hour) as continuous infusion or 10 to 15 ml/hour (20 to 30 mg/hour) as incremental "top-up" injections

CNS: anxiety, dizziness, headache, hypoesthesia, pain, paresthesia.
CV: *bradycardia,* chest pain, hypotension, hypertension, tachycardia.
GI: nausea, vomiting.
GU: oliguria, urine retention.
Hematologic: anemia.
Skin: pruritus.
Other: back pain, fever, chills, postoperative complications, rigors.
Neonatal—vomiting, jaundice, tachypnea, respiratory distress.
Fetal— bradycardia, fever, tachycardia, distress.

Reactions may be *common,* uncommon, *life-threatening,* or COMMON AND LIFE-THREATENING.

Interactions	Nursing considerations
Beta blockers: enhanced sympathomimetic effects. Don't use with lidocaine and epinephrine. *Butyrophenones, phenothiazines:* may reduce or reverse the pressor effect of epinephrine. Monitor patient. *CNS depressants:* may cause additive CNS effects. Reduce dosage of CNS depressants. *Cyclic antidepressants, MAO inhibitors:* severe, sustained hypertension when used with lidocaine and epinephrine. Use with extreme caution. *Enflurane, halothane, isoflurane, related drugs:* arrhythmias when used with lidocaine and epinephrine. Use with extreme caution.	• Contraindicated in patients with inflammation or infection in puncture region, septicemia, severe hypertension, spinal deformities, and neurologic disorders. • Also contraindicated in patients with known history of hypersensitivity to local anesthetics of the amide type. • Use cautiously in debilitated, elderly, or acutely ill patients; in patients with severe shock, heart block, or general drug allergies; in obstetric patients; and for paracervical block. • Dose and interval are increased with epinephrine. • Use solutions with epinephrine cautiously in patients with CV disorders and in body areas with limited blood supply (ears, nose, fingers, toes). • Don't use solution with preservatives for spinal, epidural, or caudal block. • Keep resuscitation equipment and drugs available. • Discard partially used vials without preservatives. • Check solution for particles. • Some solutions contain sulfites; they shouldn't be given to patients hypersensitivie to sulfites.
CNS depressants: may cause additive CNS effects. Reduce dosage of CNS depressants. *Echothiophate iodide:* reduced hydrolysis of procaine. Use together cautiously. *Succinylcholine:* prolonged neuromuscular blockade. Use cautiously together. *Sulfonamides:* procaine inhibits the action of sulfonamides. Don't use in conditions in which a sulfonamide drug is required.	• Contraindicated in patients with traumatized urethras and in those with hypersensitivity to chloroprocaine, tetracaine, or other PABA derivatives. • Also contraindicated in obstetric patients with cephalopelvic disproportion, placenta previa, abruptio placentae, floating fetal head, and intrauterine manipulation. • Use cautiously in hyperexcitable patients; in those with CNS disease, infection at puncture site, shock, profound anemia, cachexia, sepsis, hypertension, hypotension, GI hemorrhage, bowel perforation or strangulation, peritonitis, cardiac decompensation, massive pleural effusion, or increased intra-abdominal pressure; and in obstetric patients. • Keep resuscitation equipment and drugs available. • Use preservative-free solution for epidural block. • Discard partially used vials without preservatives.
Amide-type anesthetics: additive effects if given with ropivacaine. Use with caution. *CNS depressants:* may cause additive CNS effects. Reduce dosage of CNS depressants. *Fluvoxamine, imipramine, theophylline, verapamil:* may interact with ropivacaine. Use with caution.	• Contraindicated in patients with known hypersensitivity to drug or local anesthetics of amide type. • Use cautiously (especially when giving repeat doses) in debilitated, elderly, acutely ill, or breast-feeding patients and in patients with hypotension, hypovolemia, impaired CV function, heart block, or hepatic disease. • Don't inject drug rapidly. • Aspiration for blood should be done before all doses to avoid intravascular or subarachnoid injection. • Drug should only be used by personnel familiar with use of drug. Have emergency equipment and personnel available. • Don't use in emergency situations. • Drug should not be used for the production of obstetric paracervical block anesthesia, retrobulbar block, or spinal anesthesia (subarachnoid block). • Should not be used for I.V. regional anesthesia (Bier block). • Use an adequate test dose (3 to 5 ml of short-acting local anesthetic solution containing epinephrine) before induction of complete block.

(continued)

Drug, indications, dosage	Adverse reactions

Local

ropivacaine hydrochloride *(continued)*
Lumbar epidural block in postoperative pain management—
0.2% solution: 6 to 10 ml/hour (12 to 20 mg/hour) as continuous infusion
Thoracic epidural block in postoperative pain management—
0.2% solution: 4 to 8 ml/hour (8 to 16 mg/hour) as continuous infusion
Infiltration (minor nerve block) in postoperative pain management—
0.2% solution: 1 to 100 ml (2 to 200 mg)
0.5% solution: 1 to 40 ml (5 to 200 mg)

---

tetracaine hydrochloride
(Pontocaine)
Dosage for adults varies according to extent of block.
Low spinal (saddle) block in vaginal delivery—
2 to 5 mg as hyperbaric solution (in 10% dextrose)
Perineum and lower extremities: 5 to 10 mg
Up to costal margin: 15 to 20 mg

CNS: anxiety, nervousness, *seizures* followed by drowsiness. **CV:** *arrhythmias, bradycardia, cardiac arrest,* hypotension, myocardial depression. **EENT:** blurred vision, tinnitus. **GI:** nausea, vomiting. **Respiratory:** *respiratory arrest, status asthmaticus.* **Skin:** dermatologic reactions. **Other:** *anaphylactoid reactions, anaphylaxis,* edema.

Topical

proparacaine hydrochloride
(AK-Taine, Alcaine, Ophthaine, Ophthetic)
Anesthesia for tonometry, gonioscopy—
Adults and children: 1 or 2 drops of 0.5% solution instilled in eye just before procedure.
Anesthesia for cataract extraction, glaucoma surgery—
Adults and children: 1 or 2 drops of 0.5% solution instilled in eye q 5 to 10 minutes for five to seven doses.
Removal of foreign bodies or sutures—
Adults and children: 1 or 2 drops 2 to 3 minutes before procedure or q 5 to 10 minutes for one to three doses.

EENT: conjunctival redness, transient eye pain. **Other:** hypersensitivity reactions.

---

tetracaine
(Pontocaine Solution)
tetracaine hydrochloride
(Pontocaine)
Anesthesia for tonometry, gonioscopy; removal of corneal foreign bodies, suture removal from cornea; other diagnostic and minor surgical procedures—
Adults and children: 1 to 2 drops of 0.5% in eye just before procedure.

EENT: transient stinging in eye 30 seconds after initial instillation, epithelial damage in excessive or long-term use. **Other:** sensitization with repeated use (allergic skin rash, urticaria).

Reactions may be *common,* uncommon, *life-threatening,* or COMMON AND LIFE-THREATENING.

Interactions	Nursing considerations

| | • Restlessness, anxiety, incoherent speech, light-headedness, numbness and tingling of mouth and lips, metallic taste, tinnitus, dizziness, blurred vision, tremors, twitching, depression, or drowsiness may be early warning signs or symptoms of CNS toxicity.
• Don't use in ophthalmic surgery. |

CNS depressants: may cause additive CNS effects. Reduce dosage of CNS depressants. *Sulfonamides:* tetracaine inhibits the action of sulfonamides. Don't use in conditions in which a sulfonamide drug is required.	• Safety and efficacy in children haven't been established. • Contraindicated in patients with infection at injection site, CNS disease, or hypersensitivity to procaine or related agents. • Saddle block is contraindicated in patients with cephalopelvic disproportion, placenta previa, abruptio placentae, intrauterine manipulation, and floating fetal head. • Use cautiously in patients with shock, profound anemia, cachexia, hypertension, hypotension, peritonitis, cardiac decompensation, massive pleural effusion, increased intracranial pressure, and infection. Beware of possible sulfite sensitivity. • Keep resuscitation equipment and drugs available. • When CSF is added to powdered drug or solution during spinal anesthesia, solution may be cloudy. Don't use discolored or crystallized solutions. • Protect from light; store in refrigerator.

None significant.	• Contraindicated in patients with hypersensitivity to ester-type local anesthetics, PABA or its derivatives, or to other ingredients in these preparations. • Use cautiously in patients with cardiac disease and hyperthyroidism. • Not for long-term use; may delay wound healing. • Warn patients not to rub or touch eye while cornea is anesthetized. • Warn patients with corneal abrasion that pain is relieved only temporarily. • Check solution for particles. • Don't use discolored solution. • Store in tightly closed container. Refrigerate opened containers.

Cholinesterase inhibitors: prolonged ocular anesthesia and increased risk of toxicity. Use with caution. *Sulfonamides:* interference with sulfonamide antibacterial activity. Wait 30 minutes after anesthesia before instilling sulfonamide.	• Contraindicated in patients with hypersensitivity to drug or similar drugs (such as ester-type local anesthetics), PABA or its derivatives, or other ingredients in these preparations. • Drug doesn't dilate pupils, paralyze accommodation, or increase intraocular pressure. • Don't use discolored, cloudy, or crystallized solution. Keep container tightly closed and refrigerated. • Warn patient not to touch eye while cornea is anesthetized. • Avoid long-term use.

Therapeutic drug monitoring guidelines

Drug	Laboratory test monitored	Therapeutic ranges of test
aminoglycoside antibiotics (amikacin, gentamicin, tobramycin)	Serum amikacin peak trough	20 to 25 mcg/ml 5 to 10 mcg/ml
	Serum gentamicin/ tobramycin	
	peak	4 to 8 mcg/ml
	trough	1 to 2 mcg/ml
	Serum creatinine	0.6 to 1.3 mg/dl
amphotericin B	Serum creatinine	0.6 to 1.3 mg/dl
	BUN	5 to 20 mg/dl
	Serum electrolytes (especially potassium and magnesium)	Potassium: 3.5 to 5 mEq/L Magnesium: 1.5 to 2.5 mEq/L Sodium: 135 to 145 mEq/L Chloride: 98 to 106 mEq/L
	Liver function tests	*
	CBC with differential and platelets	*****
antibiotics	WBC with differential	*****
	Cultures and sensitivities	
biguanides (metformin)	Serum creatinine	0.6 to 1.3 mg/dl
	Fasting serum glucose	70 to 110 mg/dl
	Glycosolated hemoglobin	5.5% to 8.5% of total hemoglobin
	CBC	*****
clozapine	WBC with differential	*****
digoxin	Serum digoxin	0.8 to 2 ng/ml
	Serum electrolytes (especially potassium, magnesium, and calcium)	Potassium: 3.5 to 5 mEq/L Magnesium: 1.7 to 2.1 mEq/L Sodium: 135 to 145 mEq/L Chloride: 98 to 106 mEq/L Calcium: 8.6 to 10 mg/dl
	Serum creatinine	0.6 to 1.3 mg/dl
diuretics	Serum electrolytes	Potassium: 3.5 to 5 mEq/L Magnesium: 1.7 to 2.1 mEq/L Sodium: 135 to 145 mEq/L Chloride: 98 to 106 mEq/L Calcium: 8.6 to 10 mg/dl
	Serum creatinine	0.6 to 1.3 mg/dl
	BUN	5 to 20 mg/dl
	Uric acid	2 to 7 mg/dl
	Fasting serum glucose	70 to 110 mg/dl
erythropoietin	Hematocrit	Women: 36% to 48% Men: 42% to 52%
ethosuximide	Serum ethosuximide	40 to 100 mcg/ml

Note: ***** For those areas marked with asterisks, the following values can be used:

Hemoglobin: Women: 12 to 16 g/dl
  Men: 14 to 18 g/dl
Hematocrit: Women: 37% to 48%
  Men: 42% to 52%
RBCs: 4 to 5.5 x 10^6/mm^3
WBCs: 5 to 10 x 10^3/mm^3

Differential: Neutrophils: 45% to 74%
  Bands: 0% to 8%
  Lymphocytes: 16% to 45%
  Monocytes: 4% to 10%
  Eosinophils: 0% to 7%
  Basophils: 0% to 2%

Monitoring guidelines

Wait until the administration of the third dose to check drug levels. Obtain blood for peak level 30 minutes after I.V. infusion or 60 minutes after I.M. administration. For trough levels, draw blood just before next dose. Dosage may need to be adjusted accordingly. Recheck after three doses. Monitor serum creatinine and BUN levels and urine output for signs of decreasing renal function.

Monitor serum creatinine, BUN, and serum electrolyte levels at least weekly during therapy. Also, regularly monitor blood counts and liver function tests during therapy.

Specimen cultures and sensitivities will determine the cause of the infection and the best treatment. Monitor WBC with differential weekly during therapy.

Check renal function and hematologic parameters before initiating therapy and at least annually thereafter. If the patient has impaired renal function, don't use metformin because it may cause lactic acidosis. Monitor response to therapy by periodically evaluating fasting glucose and glycosolated hemoglobin levels. A patient's home monitoring of blood glucose levels helps monitor compliance and response.

Obtain WBC with differential before initiating therapy, weekly during therapy, and 4 weeks after discontinuing the drug.

Check serum digoxin levels at least 12 hours, but preferably 24 hours, after the last dose is administered. To monitor maintenance therapy, check drug levels at least 1 to 2 weeks after therapy is initiated or changed. Make any adjustments in therapy based on entire clinical picture, not solely on drug levels. Also, check electrolyte levels and renal function periodically during therapy.

To monitor fluid and electrolyte balance, perform baseline and periodic determinations of serum electrolyte, serum calcium, BUN, uric acid, and serum glucose levels.

After therapy is initiated or changed, monitor the hematocrit twice weekly for 2 to 6 weeks until stabilized in the target range and a maintenance dose determined. Monitor hematocrit regularly thereafter.

Check drug level 8 to 10 days after therapy is initiated or changed.

(continued)

---

* For those areas marked with one asterisk, the following values can be used:

ALT: 7 to 56 U/L
AST: 5 to 40 U/L
Alkaline phosphatase: 17 to 142 U/L
LD: 60 to 220 U/L
GGT: < 40 U/L
Total bilirubin: 0.2 to 1 mg/dl

Drug	Laboratory test monitored	Therapeutic ranges of test
gemfibrozil	Serum lipids	Total cholesterol: < 200 mg/dl LDL: < 130 mg/dl HDL: Women: 40 to 75 mg/dl Men: 37 to 70 mg/dl Triglycerides: 10 to 160 mg/dl
heparin	Activated partial thrombo-plastin time (aPTT)	1.5 to 2 times control
HMG-CoA reduc-tase inhibitors (fluvastatin, lova-statin, pravastatin, simvastatin)	Serum lipids Liver function tests	Total cholesterol: < 200 mg/dl LDL: < 130 mg/dl HDL: Women: 40 to 75 mg/dl Men: 37 to 70 mg/dl Triglycerides: 10 to 160 mg/dl *
insulin	Fasting serum glucose Glycosylated hemoglobin	70 to 110 mg/dl 5.5% to 8.5% of total hemoglobin
lithium	Serum lithium Serum creatinine CBC Serum electrolytes (espe-cially potassium and sodium) Fasting serum glucose Thyroid function tests	0.5 to 1.4 mEq/L 0.6 to 1.3 mg/dl ***** Potassium: 3.5 to 5 mEq/L Magnesium: 1.7 to 2.1 mEq/L Sodium: 135 to 145 mEq/L Chloride: 98 to 106 mEq/L 70 to 110 mg/dl TSH: 0.2 to 5.4 microU/ml T_3: 80 to 200 ng/dl T_4: 5.4 to 11.5 mcg/dl
methotrexate	Serum methotrexate CBC with differential Platelet count Liver function tests Serum creatinine	Normal elimination: < 10 micromol 24 hours postdose < 1 micromol 48 hours postdose < 0.2 micromol 72 hours postdose ***** 150 to 450 × 10^3/mm³ * 0.6 to 1.3 mg/dl
phenytoin	Serum phenytoin CBC	10 to 20 mcg/ml *****
potassium chloride	Serum potassium	3.5 to 5 mEq/L
procainamide	Serum procainamide Serum N-acetylpro-cainamide CBC	4 to 8 mcg/ml (procainamide) 5 to 30 mcg/ml (combined procainamide and NAPA) *****
quinidine	Serum quinidine CBC Liver function tests Serum creatinine Serum electrolytes (espe-cially potassium)	2 to 6 mcg/ml ***** * 0.6 to 1.3 mg/dl Potassium: 3.5 to 5 mEq/L Magnesium: 1.7 to 2.1 mEq/L Sodium: 135 to 145 mEq/L Chloride: 98 to 106 mEq/L

Note: ***** For those areas marked with asterisks, the following values can be used:

Hemoglobin: Women: 12 to 16 g/dl
   Men: 14 to 18 g/dl
Hematocrit: Women: 37% to 48%
   Men: 42% to 52%
RBCs: 4 to 5.5 x 10⁶/mm³
WBCs: 5 to 10 x 10³/mm³

Differential: Neutrophils: 45% to 74%
   Bands: 0% to 8%
   Lymphocytes: 16% to 45%
   Monocytes: 4% to 10%
   Eosinophils: 0% to 7%
   Basophils: 0% to 2%

Monitoring guidelines

Therapy is usually withdrawn after 3 months if response is inadequate. Patient must be fasting to measure triglyceride levels.

When drug is given by continuous I.V. infusion, check aPTT every 4 hours in the early stages of therapy. When drug is given by deep S.C. injection, check aPTT 4 to 6 hours after injection.

Perform liver function tests at baseline, 6 to 12 weeks after therapy is initiated or changed, and periodically thereafter. If adequate response isn't achieved within 6 weeks, consider changing the therapy.

Monitor response to therapy by evaluating serum glucose and glycosolated hemoglobin levels. Glycosylated hemoglobin level is a good measure of long-term control. A patient's home monitoring of blood glucose levels helps measure compliance and response.

Checking blood lithium levels is crucial to the safe use of the drug. Obtain serum lithium levels immediately before next dose. Monitor levels twice weekly until stable. Once at steady state, levels should be checked weekly; when the patient is on the appropriate maintenance dose, levels should be checked every 2 to 3 months. Monitor serum creatinine, serum electrolyte, and fasting serum glucose levels; CBC; and thyroid function tests before therapy is inititated and periodically during therapy.

Monitor methotrexate levels according to dosing protocol. Monitor CBC with differential, platelet count, and liver and renal function tests more frequently when therapy is initiated or changed and when methotrexate levels may be elevated, such as when the patient is dehydrated.

Monitor serum phenytoin levels immediately before next dose and 2 to 4 weeks after therapy is initiated or changed. Obtain a CBC at baseline and monthly early in therapy. Watch for toxic effects at therapeutic levels. Adjust the measured level for hypoalbuminemia or renal impairment, which can increase free drug levels.

Check level weekly after oral replacement therapy is initiated until stable and every 3 to 6 months thereafter.

Measure procainamide levels 6 to 12 hours after a continuous infusion is started or immediately before the next oral dose. Combined (procainamide and NAPA) levels can be used as an index of toxicity when renal impairment exists. Obtain CBC periodically during longer-term therapy.

Obtain levels immediately before next oral dose and 30 to 35 hours after therapy is initiated or changed. Periodically obtain blood counts, liver and kidney function tests, and serum electrolyte levels.

(continued)

* For those areas marked with one asterisk, the following values can be used:

ALT: 7 to 56 U/L
AST: 5 to 40 U/L
Alkaline phosphatase: 17 to 142 U/L
LD: 60 to 220 U/L
GGT: < 40 U/L
Total bilirubin: 0.2 to 1 mg/dl

Drug	Laboratory test monitored	Therapeutic ranges of test
sulfonylureas	Fasting serum glucose Glycosylated hemoglobin	70 to 110 mg/dl 5.5% to 8.5% of total hemoglobin
theophylline	Serum theophylline	10 to 20 mcg/ml
thyroid hormone	Thyroid function tests	TSH: 0.2 to 5.4 microU/ml T_3: 80 to 200 ng/dl T_4: 5.4 to 11.5 mcg/dl
vancomycin	Serum vancomycin Serum creatinine	20 to 35 mcg/ml (peak) 5 to 10 mcg/ml (trough) 0.6 to 1.3 mg/dl
warfarin	INR	For an acute MI, atrial fibrillation, treatment of pulmonary embolism, prevention of systemic embolism, tissue heart valves, valvular heart disease, or prophylaxis or treatment of venous thrombosis: 2 to 3 For mechanical prosthetic valves or recurrent systemic embolism: 2.5 to 3.5

Note: ***** For those areas marked with asterisks, the following values can be used:

Hemoglobin: Women: 12 to 16 g/dl
    Men: 14 to 18 g/dl
Hematocrit: Women: 37% to 48%
    Men: 42% to 52%
RBCs: 4 to 5.5 x 10⁶/mm³
WBCs: 5 to 10 x 10³/mm³

Differential: Neutrophils: 45% to 74%
    Bands: 0% to 8%
    Lymphocytes: 16% to 45%
    Monocytes: 4% to 10%
    Eosinophils: 0% to 7%
    Basophils: 0% to 2%

Monitoring guidelines

Monitor response to therapy by periodically evaluating fasting glucose and glycosolated hemoglobin levels. A patient's home monitoring of blood glucose levels helps measure compliance and response.

Obtain serum theophylline levels immediately before next dose of sustained-release oral product and at least 2 days after therapy is initiated or changed.

Monitor thyroid function tests every 2 to 3 weeks until appropriate maintenance dose is determined.

Serum vancomycin levels may be checked with the third dose administered, at the earliest. Draw peak levels ½ hour after the I.V. infusion is completed. Draw trough levels immediately before the next dose is administered. Renal function can be used to adjust dosing and intervals.

Check INR daily, beginning 3 days after therapy is initiated. Continue checking it until therapeutic goal is achieved, and monitor it periodically thereafter. Also, check levels 7 days after any change in warfarin dose or concomitant, potentially interacting therapy.

* For those areas marked with one asterisk, the following values can be used:

ALT: 7 to 56 U/L
AST: 5 to 40 U/L
Alkaline phosphatase: 17 to 142 U/L
LD: 60 to 220 U/L
GGT: < 40 U/L
Total bilirubin: 0.2 to 1 mg/dl

Therapeutic management guidelines: Asthma (adults and children over age 5)

Asthma management involves a steplike approach to treatment. The two approaches to controlling asthma are either:

1. Start therapy at level indicated for severity of patient's asthma and "step up" if control isn't achieved.

2. Start therapy at higher level than patient's step of severity and, once control is gained, "step down."

Therapy may move from step 1 to step 2, 3, or 4 if asthma is uncontrolled or it may move from step 2 directly to step 4. Or therapy may start at step 4, 3, or 2 and move down step by step as control is achieved, or therapy can bypass a step, going from step 4 to step 2. The clinician must assess each patient's needs and circumstances to determine the best therapy.

This diagram illustrates the steplike approach to therapy and the best possible therapeutic goals and outcomes of asthma management. Treatment should be reviewed every 1 to 6 months if the patient's symptoms are being well controlled.

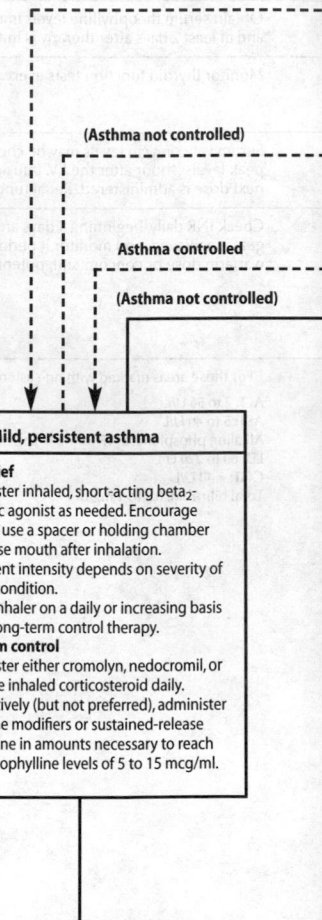

(Asthma not controlled)

Asthma controlled

(Asthma not controlled)

Asthma controlled

(Asthma not controlled)

Step 2: Mild, persistent asthma

Quick relief
- Administer inhaled, short-acting beta₂-adrenergic agonist as needed. Encourage patient to use a spacer or holding chamber and to rinse mouth after inhalation.
- Treatment intensity depends on severity of patient's condition.
- Use of inhaler on a daily or increasing basis requires long-term control therapy.

Long-term control
- Administer either cromolyn, nedocromil, or a low-dose inhaled corticosteroid daily.
- Alternatively (but not preferred), administer leukotriene modifiers or sustained-release theophylline in amounts necessary to reach serum theophylline levels of 5 to 15 mcg/ml.

Step 1: Mild, intermittent asthma

Quick relief
- Administer inhaled, short-acting beta₂-adrenergic agonist as needed. Encourage patient to use a spacer or holding chamber and to rinse mouth after inhalation.
- Treatment intensity depends on severity of patient's condition.
- Use of inhaler more than twice weekly may require long-term control therapy.

Long-term control
- No daily medications used.

Asthma controlled

Asthma controlled

Based on National Institutes of Health (NIH) National Heart, Lung, and Blood Institute recommendations for asthma management. (Guidelines for the Diagnosis and Management of Asthma. NIH pub. 97-4051. Washington, D.C.: U.S. Government Printing Office, April, 1997.)

Asthma controlled

Step 4: Severe, persistent asthma

Quick relief
- Administer inhaled, short-acting beta$_2$-adrenergic agonist as needed. Encourage patient to use a spacer or holding chamber and to rinse mouth after inhalation.
- Treatment intensity depends on severity of patient's condition.
- Use of inhaler on a daily or increasing basis requires long-term control therapy.

Long-term control
- Administer daily doses of a high-dose inhaled corticosteroid and a long-acting inhaled beta$_2$-adrenergic agonist (or sustained-release theophylline or a long-acting beta$_2$-adrenergic agonist in tablet form).
- If needed, use oral corticosteroids 2 mg/kg daily. Maximum, 60 mg daily. Make repeated attempts to reduce oral corticosteroids.

Asthma controlled

(Asthma not controlled)

Step 3: Moderate, persistent asthma

Quick relief
- Administer inhaled, short-acting beta$_2$-adrenergic agonist as needed. Encourage patient to use a spacer or holding chamber and to rinse mouth after inhalation.
- Treatment intensity depends on severity of patient's condition.
- Use of inhaler on a daily or increasing basis requires long-term control therapy.

Long-term control
- Administer daily doses of either a medium-dose inhaled corticosteroid alone or a low-to-medium–dose inhaled corticosteroid and a long-acting inhaled beta$_2$-adrenergic agonist. Combination therapy is preferred for managing nighttime symptoms.
- If needed, administer medium-to-high–dose inhaled corticosteroid and either a long-acting, inhaled beta$_2$-adrenergic agonist, sustained-release theophylline, or a long-acting beta$_2$-adrenergic agonist in tablet form.

Asthma controlled

Asthma controlled

Therapeutic goals
- Prevention of chronic and bothersome symptoms, such as coughing or shortness of breath in the early morning, at night, or following exertion.
- Maintenance of normal or nearly normal pulmonary function.
- Maintenance of normal activity, including exercise and other physical activity.
- Prevention of recurrent episodes of asthma and minimal need for treatment in an emergency department or hospital.
- Provide optimal treatment with minimal or no adverse effects.
- Fulfillment of the patient's and family's expectations of care.
- Peak expiratory flow at 80% of personal best or higher.

Therapeutic management guidelines: Cancer pain

Managing a patient with cancer-related pain involves regular assessment, a step-up approach to analgesic use, and the empowerment of patients or their caregivers to control pain therapy. Pain control options should be individualized according to the specific needs of each patient, family, and setting. Analgesics should be administered on time using a logical, coordinated effort on the part of the entire health care team.

Schedule administration of analgesics at regular intervals. Add "break-through" doses (10% to 20% of the total daily dose every 2 hours) as needed. Use oral route for analgesics whenever possible. Rectal or transdermal routes may be used during periods of nausea or vomiting.

The patient should be assessed for pain at regular intervals, after each new report of pain, and after each administration of an analgesic or adjuvant drug, such as hydroxyzine or dexamethasone. Some anticonvulsants (such as gabapentin) are being evaluated for their effects on peripheral nerve pain, which affects many patients with cancer pain. Adjuvant drugs enhance the analgesic effects of opioids, treat conditions that may exacerbate pain, or provide independent analgesia for specific types of pain. These agents may be used at any point in pain therapy.

This diagram illustrates the steps in the management of an adult patient with cancer-related pain.

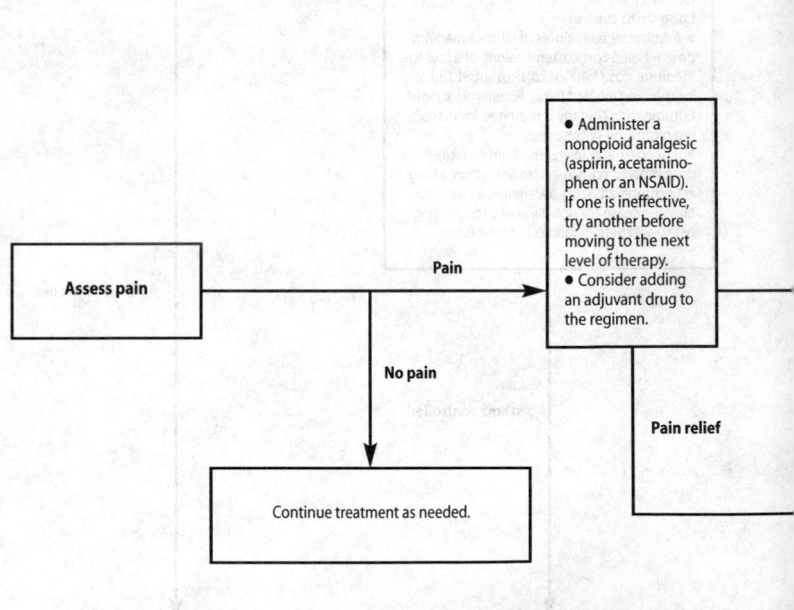

Based on guidelines from the Agency for Health Care Policy and Research (AHCPR). (AHCPR. Management of Cancer Pain: Adults. No. 94-0593. Rockville, MD: U.S. Department of Health and Human Services Public Health Service Agency for Health Care Policy and Research, 1994.)

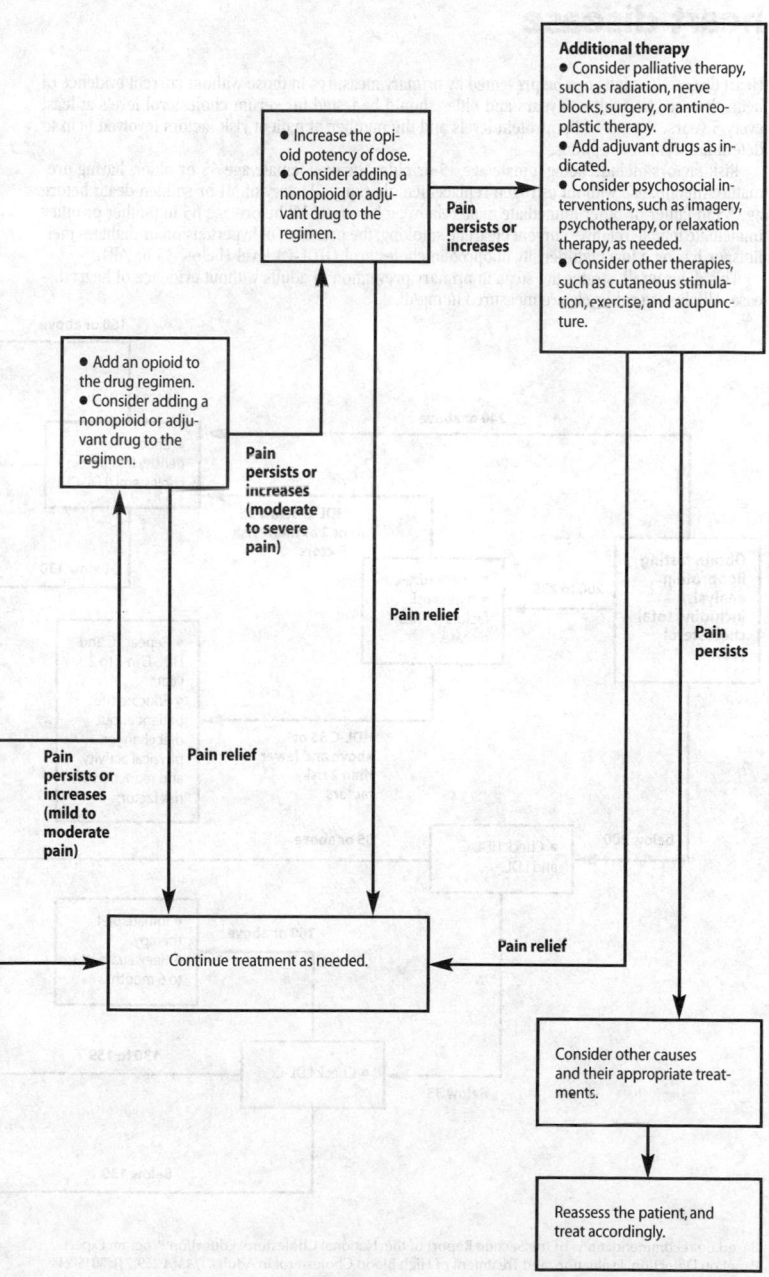

Additional therapy
- Consider palliative therapy, such as radiation, nerve blocks, surgery, or antineoplastic therapy.
- Add adjuvant drugs as indicated.
- Consider psychosocial interventions, such as imagery, psychotherapy, or relaxation therapy, as needed.
- Consider other therapies, such as cutaneous stimulation, exercise, and acupuncture.

- Increase the opioid potency of dose.
- Consider adding a nonopioid or adjuvant drug to the regimen.

Pain persists or increases

- Add an opioid to the drug regimen.
- Consider adding a nonopioid or adjuvant drug to the regimen.

Pain persists or increases (moderate to severe pain)

Pain relief

Pain persists

Pain persists or increases (mild to moderate pain)

Pain relief

Pain relief

Continue treatment as needed.

Pain relief

Consider other causes and their appropriate treatments.

Reassess the patient, and treat accordingly.

Therapeutic management guidelines: Dyslipidemia without evidence of heart disease

Heart disease in adults can be prevented by primary measures in those without current evidence of heart disease. All adults 20 years and older should be tested for serum cholesterol levels at least every 5 years. Results of lipoprotein levels and the number of patient risk factors involved help to determine treatment options.

Risk factors include being a male age 45 or older; being a female age 55 or older; having premature menopause without estrogen replacement therapy; a history of MI or sudden death before age 55 in father or other immediate male relative; a history of MI before age 65 in mother or other immediate female relative; current cigarette smoking; the presence of hypertension or diabetes mellitus; or having a low high-density lipoprotein cholesterol (HDL-C) level (below 35 mg/dl).

This diagram illustrates the steps in primary prevention in adults without evidence of heart disease. All cholesterol levels are measured in mg/dl.

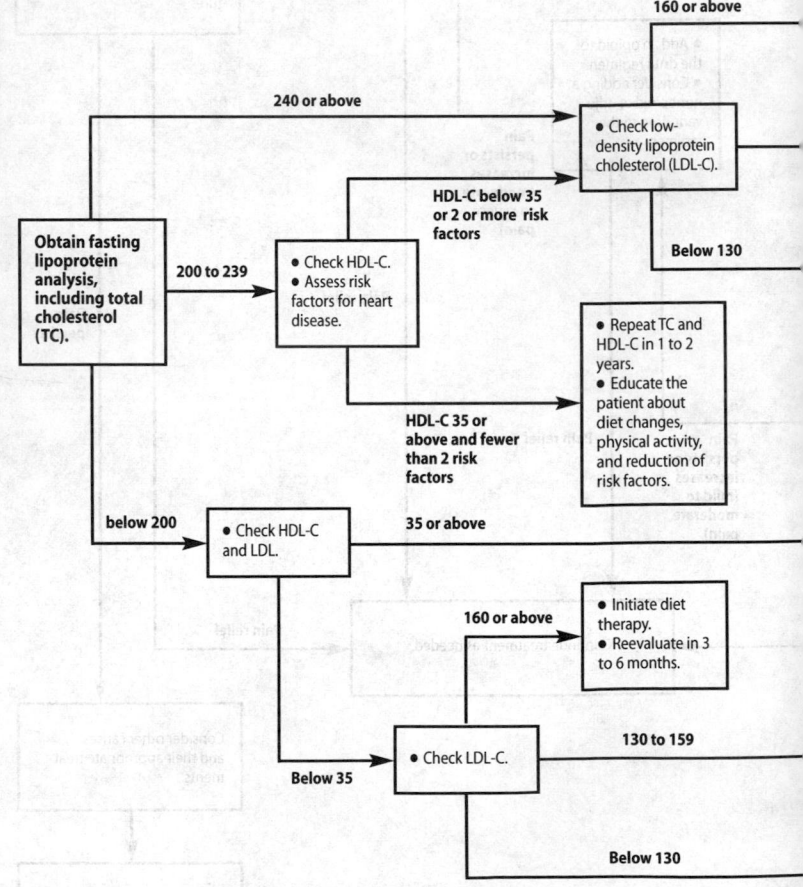

Based on recommendations of the Second Report of the National Cholesterol Education Program Expert Panel on Detection, Evaluation, and Treatment of High Blood Cholesterol in Adults. (*JAMA* 269[23]: 3015-23, 1993.)

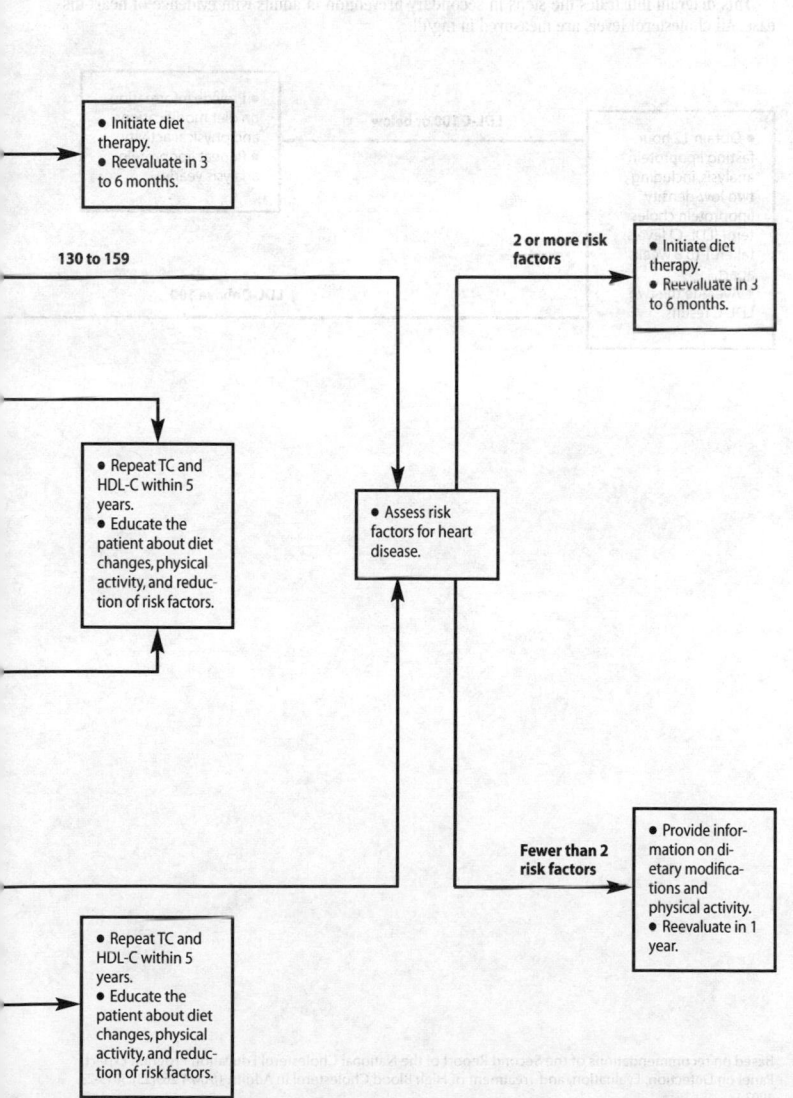

- Initiate diet therapy.
- Reevaluate in 3 to 6 months.

130 to 159

2 or more risk factors

- Initiate diet therapy.
- Reevaluate in 3 to 6 months.

- Repeat TC and HDL-C within 5 years.
- Educate the patient about diet changes, physical activity, and reduction of risk factors.

- Assess risk factors for heart disease.

Fewer than 2 risk factors

- Provide information on dietary modifications and physical activity.
- Reevaluate in 1 year.

- Repeat TC and HDL-C within 5 years.
- Educate the patient about diet changes, physical activity, and reduction of risk factors.

Therapeutic management guidelines: Dyslipidemia with evidence of heart disease

Secondary prevention of heart disease in adults—used for those with current evidence of heart disease—involves ongoing assessment of the patient's lipoprotein levels; instruction in diet, activity, and risk factors; and appropriate diet and pharmacologic treatment. Lowering of cholesterol levels through diet and drug therapies is associated with a reduction not only in recurrent heart disease but also in total mortality rates.

This diagram illustrates the steps in secondary prevention in adults with evidence of heart disease. All cholesterol levels are measured in mg/dl.

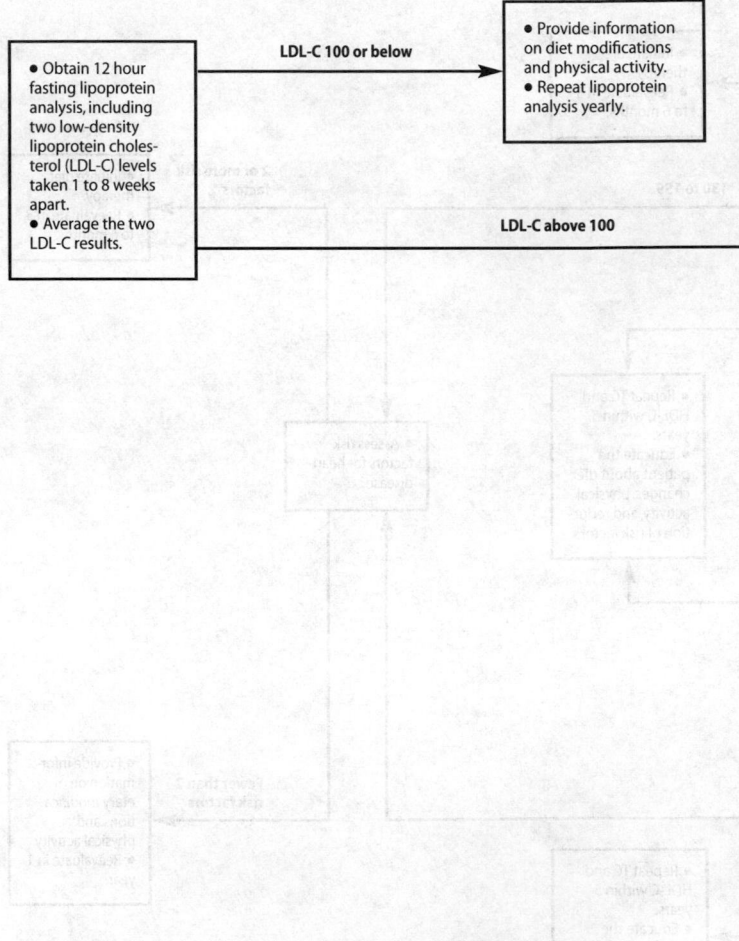

Based on recommendations of the Second Report of the National Cholesterol Education Program Expert Panel on Detection, Evaluation, and Treatment of High Blood Cholesterol in Adults. (*JAMA* 269[23]:3015-23, 1993.)

• Conduct complete health assessment.
• Evaluate patient for secondary causes of high LDL-C.
• Check for presence of familial disorders.
• Consider influence of modifiable risk factors for heart disease.
• Begin treatment, including diet, physical activity, smoking cessation, and weight loss, as needed. Consider drug therapy.

Initiate diet therapy if:
• LDL-C is 160 or above and patient has fewer than 2 risk factors without evidence of heart disease.
• LDL-C is 130 or above and patient has 2 or more risk factors without evidence of heart disease.
• LDL-C is above 100 and patient has evidence of heart disease.

Initiate drug therapy if:
• LDL-C is 190 or above and patient has fewer than 2 risk factors without evidence of heart disease.
• LDL-C is 160 or above and patient has 2 or more risk factors without evidence of heart disease.
• LDL-C is 130 or above and patient has evidence of heart disease.

Therapeutic management guidelines: Hypertension

Hypertension in adults is generally categorized according to a person's risk of developing hypertension-related diseases. Optimal blood pressure (below 120 mm Hg systolic and 80 mm Hg diastolic) is associated with the lowest cardiovascular risk. Other categories include normal (below 130 mm Hg systolic and 85 mm Hg diastolic), high-normal (130 to 139 mm Hg systolic or 85 to 89 mm Hg diastolic), or hypertension.

Hypertension is further classified as stage 1 (140 to 159 mm Hg systolic or 90 to 99 mm Hg diastolic), stage 2 (160 to 179 mm Hg systolic or 100 to 109 mm Hg diastolic), or stage 3 (180 mm Hg or above systolic or 110 mm Hg or above diastolic). This diagram illustrates recommended treatment options for hypertension.

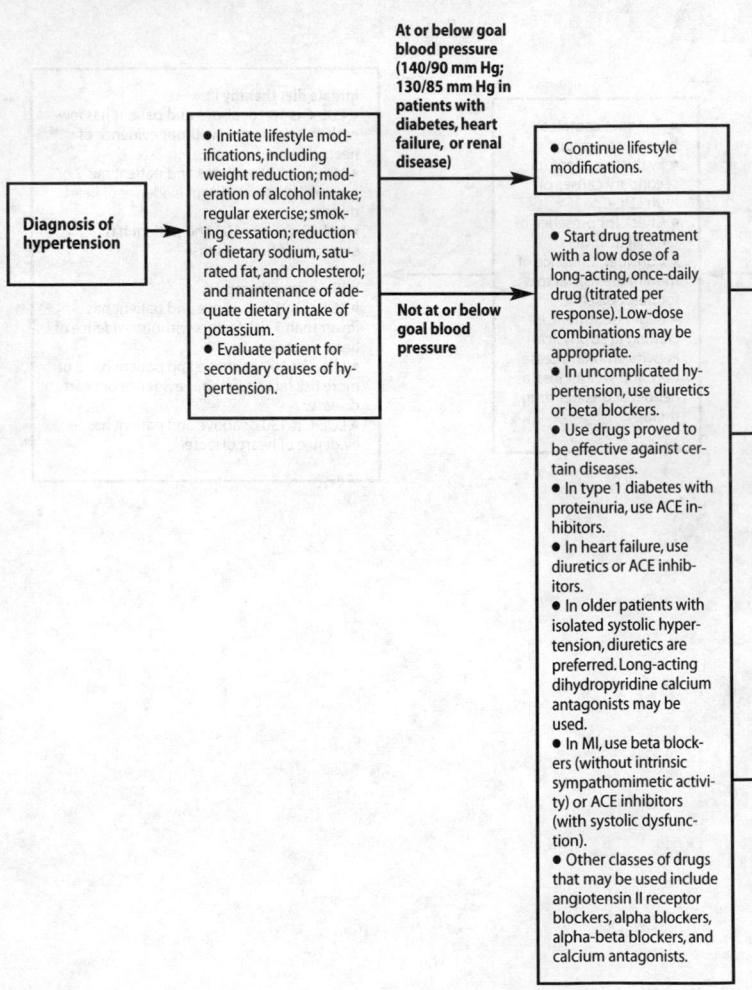

Diagnosis of hypertension

- Initiate lifestyle modifications, including weight reduction; moderation of alcohol intake; regular exercise; smoking cessation; reduction of dietary sodium, saturated fat, and cholesterol; and maintenance of adequate dietary intake of potassium.
- Evaluate patient for secondary causes of hypertension.

At or below goal blood pressure (140/90 mm Hg; 130/85 mm Hg in patients with diabetes, heart failure, or renal disease)

- Continue lifestyle modifications.

Not at or below goal blood pressure

- Start drug treatment with a low dose of a long-acting, once-daily drug (titrated per response). Low-dose combinations may be appropriate.
- In uncomplicated hypertension, use diuretics or beta blockers.
- Use drugs proved to be effective against certain diseases.
- In type 1 diabetes with proteinuria, use ACE inhibitors.
- In heart failure, use diuretics or ACE inhibitors.
- In older patients with isolated systolic hypertension, diuretics are preferred. Long-acting dihydropyridine calcium antagonists may be used.
- In MI, use beta blockers (without intrinsic sympathomimetic activity) or ACE inhibitors (with systolic dysfunction).
- Other classes of drugs that may be used include angiotensin II receptor blockers, alpha blockers, alpha-beta blockers, and calcium antagonists.

Based on recommendations of the Sixth Report of the Joint National Committee on Prevention, Detection, Evaluation, and Treatment of High Blood Pressure. (*Arch Intern Med* 157[21]:2413-46, 1997.)

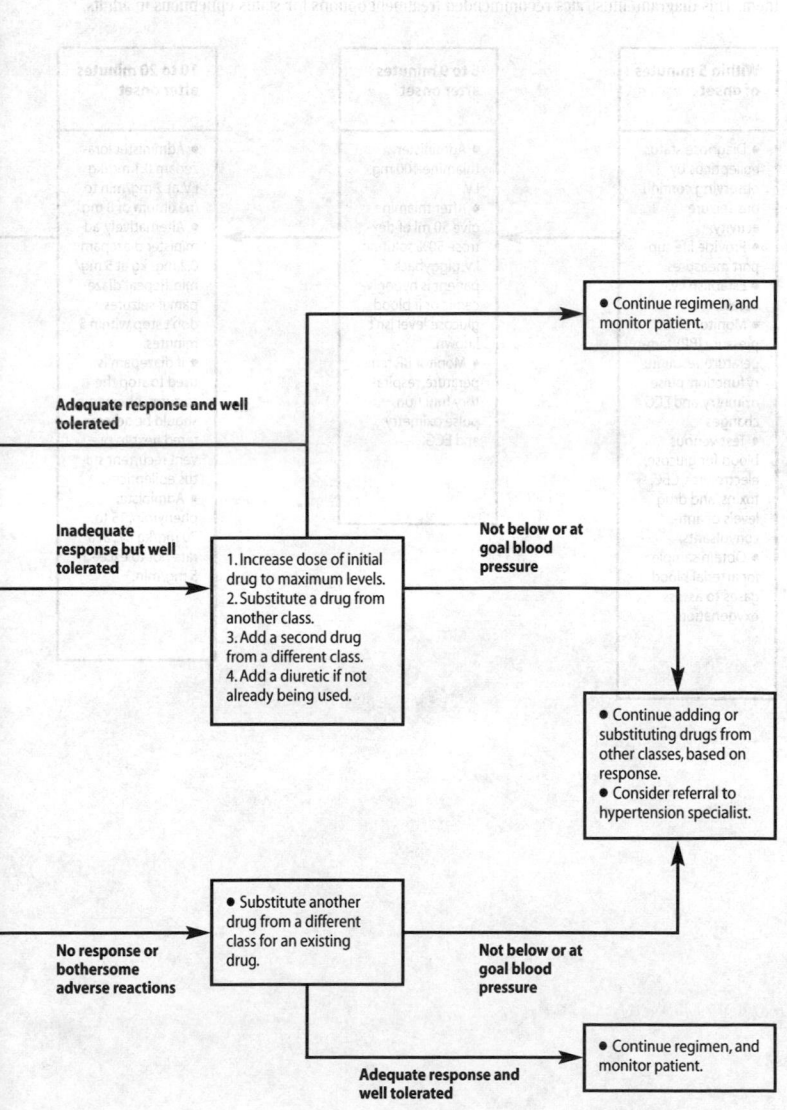

Therapeutic management guidelines: Status epilepticus

Status epilepticus is defined as a period of continuous seizure activity lasting longer than 30 minutes or as the occurrence of two or more successive seizures without return of consciousness between them. This diagram illustrates recommended treatment options for status epilepticus in adults.

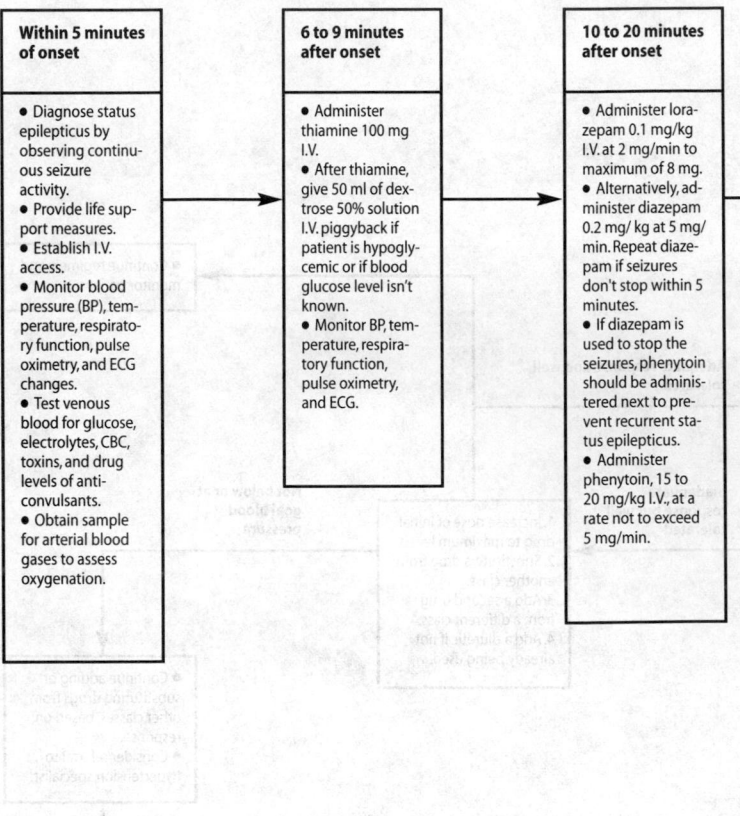

Within 5 minutes of onset

- Diagnose status epilepticus by observing continuous seizure activity.
- Provide life support measures.
- Establish I.V. access.
- Monitor blood pressure (BP), temperature, respiratory function, pulse oximetry, and ECG changes.
- Test venous blood for glucose, electrolytes, CBC, toxins, and drug levels of anticonvulsants.
- Obtain sample for arterial blood gases to assess oxygenation.

6 to 9 minutes after onset

- Administer thiamine 100 mg I.V.
- After thiamine, give 50 ml of dextrose 50% solution I.V. piggyback if patient is hypoglycemic or if blood glucose level isn't known.
- Monitor BP, temperature, respiratory function, pulse oximetry, and ECG.

10 to 20 minutes after onset

- Administer lorazepam 0.1 mg/kg I.V. at 2 mg/min to maximum of 8 mg.
- Alternatively, administer diazepam 0.2 mg/kg at 5 mg/min. Repeat diazepam if seizures don't stop within 5 minutes.
- If diazepam is used to stop the seizures, phenytoin should be administered next to prevent recurrent status epilepticus.
- Administer phenytoin, 15 to 20 mg/kg I.V., at a rate not to exceed 5 mg/min.

Based on recommendations of the Epilepsy Foundation of America's Working Group on Status Epilepticus. ("Treatment of Convulsive Status Epilepticus," *JAMA* 270[7]: 854-59, 1993. Copyrighted 1993, American Medical Association.)

21 to 60 minutes after onset

- Administer phenytoin 15 to 20 mg/kg I.V. at a rate not to exceed 50 mg/min by I.V. bolus or I.V. piggyback in normal saline solution. Final concentration should not exceed 5 mg/ml. Flush catheter with saline before and after administration.
- Or, administer fosphenytoin 15 to 20 mg PE (phenytoin sodium equivalent)/kg I.V. at a rate not to exceed 150 mg PE/min by I.V. bolus or I.V. piggyback in normal saline solution or dextrose 5% in water.
- Monitor for changes in ECG, BP, and respiratory function. If changes occur, decrease infusion rate.

More than 60 minutes after onset

- If status epilepticus doesn't stop with phenytoin 20 mg/kg, administer additional doses of phenytoin 5 mg/kg I.V. to maximum cumulative dose of 30 mg/kg.
- If status epilepticus persists, administer phenobarbital to a total of 20 mg/kg I.V. at 60 mg/min. Monitor BP and respiratory function.

Status epilepticus persists

- Obtain neurologic consultation.
- Consider initiating barbiturate-induced coma using phenobarbital or pentobarbital I.V.
- Monitor vital signs continuously.
- Provide ventilatory assistance and vasopressors as needed.

Herbal medicines

Herb names	Reported uses	Special considerations	Patient education
ALOE Aloe Gel, Aloe Latex, Aloe Vera, Cape	Aloe latex is used orally as a cathartic. It's used to treat constipation; to provide evacuation relief for patient with anal fissures, hemorrhoids, or recent anorectal surgery; and to prepare a patient for diagnostic testing of the GI tract. Aloe gel is used to treat minor burns and skin irritation and to aid in wound healing. It may also be effective as an antibacterial.	• Find out why patient is using the herb. • Aloe's laxative effects are apparent within 10 hours of taking it. • Monitor patient for signs of dehydration. Geriatric patients are particularly at risk. • Monitor electrolyte levels, especially potassium, after long-term use. • If patient is using aloe topically, monitor wound for healing.	• Advise patient to consult with his health care provider before using an herbal preparation because a treatment with proven efficacy may be available. • Tell patient to remind pharmacist of any herbal or dietary supplement that he's taking, when filling a new prescription. • Caution patient that if he delays seeking medical diagnosis and treatment, his condition could worsen. • If patient is taking digoxin or another drug to control his heart rate, a diuretic, or a corticosteroid, warn him not to take aloe without consulting his health care provider. • Advise patient to reduce dose if cramping occurs after a single dose and not to take aloe for longer than 1 to 2 weeks at a time without consulting his health care provider. • Advise patient to notify his health care provider immediately if he experiences feelings of dehydration, weakness, or confusion, especially if he has been using aloe for a prolonged period.
ANGELICA Nature's Answer Angelica Root Liquid	Angelica seed is used as a diuretic and diaphoretic. It's also used to treat conditions of the kidneys and the urinary, GI, and respiratory tracts as well as rheumatic and neuralgic symptoms.	• Find out why patient is using the herb. • Monitor patient for persistent diarrhea, which may be a sign of something more serious. • Monitor patient for dermatologic reactions. • Photodermatosis is possible after contact with the plant juice or plant extract.	• Advise patient to consult with his health care provider before using an herbal preparation because a treatment with proven efficacy may be available. • Tell patient to remind pharmacist of any herbal or dietary supplement that he's taking, when filling a new prescription. • Caution patient not to delay seeking medical treatment for symptoms that may be related to a serious medical condition. • Advise patient not to take angelica if pregnant or if taking a gastric acid blocker or anticoagulant. • Advise patient to notify his health care provider if he develops a rash.
BITTER MELON BitterMelon, Bitter Melon Juice, Bitter Melon Power, Bitter Melon Tincture	Used to treat diabetes symptoms. May help treat GI disorders.	• Find out why patient is using the herb. • The juice of bitter melon has a bitter taste. • Bitter melon should be taken only in small doses, for no longer than 4 weeks. • The hypoglycemic effects of bitter melon are dose related, so dosage	• Advise patient to consult with his health care provider before using an herbal preparation because a treatment with proven efficacy may be available. • Tell patient to remind pharmacist of any herbal or dietary supplement that he's taking, when filling a new prescription.

Herb names	Reported uses	Special considerations	Patient education

BITTER MELON
(continued)

should be adjusted gradually.
• **ALERT:** Bitter melon seeds contain vicine, which may cause an acute condition characterized by headache, fever, abdominal pain, and coma.

CAPSICUM
Topical capsaicin products: Capsin (0.025% or 0.075% lotion), CapzasIn-P (0.025% cream), Dolorac (0.025% cream in emollient base), No Pain-HP (0.075% roll-on), Pain Doctor (0.025% cream with methylsalicylate and menthol), Pain-X(0.05% gel), R-Gel (0.025% gel), Zostrix (0.025% cream in emollient base), Zostrix0HP (0.075% cream in emollient base)
Oral capsaicin products: Cayenne Pepper Capsules and Alcoholic Extract

The FDA has approved topical capsaicin for temporary relief of pain from rheumatoid arthritis, osteoarthritis, postherpetic neuralgia (shingles), and diabetic neuropathy. It's being tested for treatment of psoriasis, intractable pruritus, vitiligo, phantom limb pain, mastectomy pain, Guillain-Barré syndrome, neurogenic bladder, vulvar vestibulitis, apocrine chromhidrosis and reflex sympathetic dystrophy. It's also used in personal defense sprays.

Oral capsaicin is used for various GI complaints, including dyspepsia, flatulence, ulcers, and stomach cramps. It's used to treat hypertension and improve circulation. It's also used in some weight-loss and metabolic-enhancement products.

• Find out why patient is using the herb.
• Alcoholic extract may be unsuitable for children, alcoholic patients, patients with liver disease, and those taking disulfiram or metronidazole.
• Topical product shouldn't be used on broken or irritated skin or covered with a tight bandage.
• Adverse skin reactions to topically applied capsaicin are treated by washing the area thoroughly with soap and water. Soaking the area in vegetable oil after washing provides a slower onset but longer duration of relief than cold water. Vinegar water irrigation is moderately successful. Rubbing alcohol may also help.
• EMLA, an emulsion of lidocaine and prilocaine, provides pain relief in about 1 hour to skin that has been severely irritated by capsaicin.
• **ALERT:** Capsicum shouldn't be taken orally for longer than 2 days and then shouldn't be used again for 2 weeks.

• Advise patient to consult with his health care provider before using an herbal preparation because a treatment with proven efficacy may be available.
• Tell patient to remind pharmacist of any herbal or dietary supplement that he's taking, when filling a new prescription.
• If patient is pregnant or breast-feeding or is planning pregnancy, advise her not to use this herb.
• If patient is applying capsicum topically, inform him that it may take 1 to 2 weeks for him to experience maximum pain control.
• If patient is using capsicum topically, instruct him to wash his hands before and immediately after applying it and to avoid contact with eyes. Advise contact lens wearer to wash his hands and to use gloves or an applicator if handling his lenses after applying capsicum.
• If patient is using capsicum topically, advise him not to use topical capsicum on broken or irritated skin and instruct him not to tightly bandage any area to which he has applied it.
• Inform patient not to delay treatment for an illness that doesn't resolve after taking capsicum. If he's applying it topically, advise him to promptly contact his health care provider if his condition worsens or if symptoms persist for 2 to 4 weeks.
• Tell patient to store capsicum in a tightly sealed container, away from light.

CHAMOMILE
Azulon, Chamomile Flowers, Chamomile Tea, Kid Chamomile, Standardized Chamomile Extract, Wild Chamomile

Used orally to treat diarrhea, anxiety, restlessness, stomatitis, hemorrhagic cystitis, flatulence and motion sickness.
Used topically to stimulate skin metabolism, reduce inflammation, encourage

• Find out why patient is using the herb.
• **ALERT:** People sensitive to ragweed and chrysanthemums or other Compositae family members (arnica, yarrow, feverfew, tansy, artemisia) may be more susceptible to contact allergies and anaphylaxis. Patients with hay fever or bronchial asthma caused by pollens are

• Advise patient to consult with his health care provider before using an herbal preparation because a treatment with proven efficacy may be available.
• Tell patient to remind pharmacist of any herbal or dietary supplement that he's taking, when filling a new prescription.
• If patient is pregnant or is planning pregnancy, advise her not to use chamomile.

(continued)

Herb names	Reported uses	Special considerations	Patient education
CHAMOMILE *(continued)*	the healing of wounds, and treat cutaneous burns. Also used for its antibacterial and antiviral effects. Teas are mainly used for sedation or relaxation.	more susceptible to anaphylactic reactions.	• If patient is taking an anticoagulant, advise him not to use chamomile because of possible enhanced anticoagulant effects. • Advise patient that chamomile may enhance an allergic reaction or make existing symptoms worse in susceptible patients. • Instruct parent not to give chamomile to any child before checking with a knowledgeable practitioner.
CRANBERRY Cran-Actin, Cranberry-Plus, Emergen-C Cranberry, Ultra Cranberry	Used to prevent urinary tract infections, particularly in women prone to recurrent infection. Also used to prevent kidney stones and to treat asthma, fever, and active urinary tract infection (UTI).	• Find out why patient is using the herb. • Tinctures may contain up to 45% alcohol. • Contrary to early investigations focusing on cranberry's ability to acidify the urine, its ability to prevent bacteria from adhering to the bladder wall seems to be more important in preventing UTIs. • Only the unsweetened, unprocessed form of cranberry juice is effective in preventing bacteria from adhering to the bladder wall. • Cranberry is safe for use in pregnant and breast-feeding patients. • When consumed regularly, cranberry may be effective in reducing the frequency of bacteriuria with pyuria in women with recurrent UTIs.	• Advise patient to consult with his health care provider before using an herbal preparation because a treatment with proven efficacy may be available. • Tell patient to remind pharmacist of any herbal or dietary supplement that he's taking, when filling a new prescription. • Advise patient that an appropriate antibiotic is usually needed to treat an active UTI. • If patient is using cranberry to prevent a UTI, advise him to notify his health care provider if signs or symptoms of a UTI appear. • If patient has diabetes, inform him that cranberry juice contains sugar but that sugar-free cranberry supplements and juices are available.
ECHINACEA Coneflower Extract, EchinaCare Liquid, Echinacea, Echinacea Angustifolia Herb, Echinacea Extract, Echinacea Fresh Freeze Dried, Echinacea Glycerite, Echinacea Herbal Comfort, Echinacea Red Root Supreme, Echinacea Root Complex, Echinacea Root Extract, Echinacea Xtra, Echina Fresh, Echinagel,	Used to stimulate the immune system and treat acute and chronic upper respiratory tract infections and urinary tract infections. Used also to heal wounds, including abscesses, burns, eczema, and skin ulcers. Used as an adjunct to a conventional antineoplastic and to provide prophylaxis against upper respiratory tract infections and the common cold.	• Find out why patient is using the herb. • Daily dose depends on the preparation and potency but shouldn't exceed 8 weeks. Consult specific manufacturer's instructions for parenteral administration, if applicable. • Echinacea is considered supportive treatment for infection; it shouldn't be used in place of antibiotic therapy. • Some active components may be water-insoluble. • Echinacea is usally taken at the first sign of illness and continued for up to 14 days. Regular prophylactic use isn't recommended. • Herbalists recommend using liquid preparations because it's believed that echinacea functions in	• Advise patient to consult with his health care provider before using an herbal preparation because a treatment with proven efficacy may be available. • Tell patient to remind pharmacist of any herbal or dietary supplement that he's taking, when filling a new prescription. • Advise patient not to delay seeking appropriate medical evaluation for a prolonged illness. • Advise patient that prolonged use may result in overstimulation of the immune system and possible immune suppression. Echinacea shouldn't be used longer than 14 days for supportive treatment of infection. • The herb should be stored away from direct light. • Warn patients to keep all herbal products away from children and pets.

Herb names	Reported uses	Special considerations	Patient education
ECHINACEA (continued) EchinaGuard Liquid, EchinaGuard Pro, Echinex, Enhanced Echinacea, Standardized Echinacea Extract		the mouth and should have direct contact with the lymph tissues at the back of the throat. • Some tinctures contain between 15% and 90% alcohol, which may be unsuitable for children and adolescents, alcoholics, and patients with hepatic disease.	
EPHEDRA Available as combination products, including Chromemate, Escalation, Excel, Herbal Ecstasy, Herbal Fen-Phen, Herbalife, Metabolife, Power Trim, Up Your Gas	Used to treat respiratory tract diseases with mild bronchospasm. Allopathic practitioners have used it since the 1930s to treat asthma, but the herb has become less popular as more specific beta agonists have become available. Also used as a CV stimulant. Pseudoephedrine remains a common ingredient in many OTC cough and cold preparations. Ephedrine is used to treat various other conditions, including chills, coughs, colds, flu, fever, headaches, edema, and nasal congestion; it's also used as an appetite suppressant. The alkaloid-free North American species is used to treat venereal disease.	• Find out why patient is using the herb. • Compounds containing ephedra have been linked to several deaths and more than 800 adverse effects, many of which appear to be dose related. • Monitor patient's pulse and blood pressure. • Ephedra shouldn't be used for more than 7 consecutive days because of the risk of anaphylaxis and dependence. • Patients with eating disorders may abuse this herb. • **ALERT:** Pills containing ephedra have been combined with other stimulants like caffeine and sold as "natural" stimulants in weight loss products. Deaths from overstimulation have been reported. • **ALERT:** Dosages high enough to produce psychoactive or hallucinogenic effects are toxic to the heart and shouldn't be used. • Signs and symptoms of toxic reaction include diaphoresis, dilated pupils, muscle spasms, fever, and cardiac and respiratory failure. • If overdose occurs, perform gastric lavage and administer activated charcoal. Treat spasms with diazepam, replace electrolytes with I.V. fluids, and prevent acidosis with sodium bicarbonate infusions.	• Advise patient to consult with his health care provider before using an herbal preparation because a treatment with proven efficacy may be available. • Tell patient to remind pharmacist of any herbal or dietary supplement that he's taking, when filling a new prescription. • Advise patient not to use this herb in place of getting the proper medical evaluation for a prolonged illness. • Advise patient with thyroid disease, hypertension, CV disease, or diabetes to avoid using ephedra. • Recommend standard pharmaceutical formulations of ephedrine or pseudoephedrine for those with a valid need for these compounds because preparations may differ in ephedrine alkaloid content by 130%. • Advise patient not to use ephedra-containing products for longer than 7 consecutive days. • Advise patient not to use ephedra at dosages that are purported to produce psychoactive or hallucinogenic effects because such dosages are toxic to the heart. • Advise patient to watch for adverse reactions, particularly chest pain, shortness of breath, palpitations, dizziness, and fainting. • Instruct patient to store ephedra away from direct light. • Warn patients to keep all herbal products away from children and pets.
FEVERFEW Feverfew, Feverfew Extract, Feverfew Extract Complex,	Used most commonly to prevent or treat migraine headaches and to treat rheumatoid arthritis. Used to	• Find out why patient is using the herb. • If patient is taking an anticoagulant, monitor appropriate coagulation values, such as INR, PTT,	• Advise patient to consult with his health care provider before using an herbal preparation because a treatment with proven efficacy may be available. *(continued)*

Herb names	Reported uses	Special considerations	Patient education
FEVERFEW (continued) Feverfew Leaf, Feverfew Leaf and Flower, Feverfew LF and FL-GBE, Feverfew Power, Fresh Freeze-Dried Feverfew, Migracare Feverfew Extract, Migracin, MigraSpray, MygraFew, Partenelle, Tanacet	treat asthma, psoriasis, menstrual cramps, digestion problems, and intestinal parasites; to debride wounds; and to promote menstrual flow. Also used as a mouthwash after tooth extraction, a tranquilizer, and abortifacient, and an external antiseptic and insecticide.	and PT. Also, observe patient for abnormal bleeding. • Rash or contact dermatitis may indicate sensitivity to feverfew. Patient should discontinue use immediately. • Abruptly stopping the herb may cause "postfeverfew syndrome," involving tension headaches, insomnia, joint stiffness and pain, and lethargy.	• Tell patient to remind pharmacist of any herbal or dietary supplement that he's taking, when filling a new prescription. • If patient is pregnant, planning to become pregnant, or breastfeeding, advise her not to use feverfew. • Educate patient about the potential risk of abnormal bleeding when combining herb with an anticoagulant, such as warfarin or heparin, or an antiplatelet, such as aspirin or another NSAID. • Caution patient that a rash or abnormal skin alteration may indicate an allergy to feverfew. Instruct patient to stop taking the herb if a rash appears.
FLAX Dakota Flax Gold, Fax Seed Oil, Flax Seed Whole	Used internally to treat diarrhea, constipation, diverticulitis, irritable bowel, colons damaged by laxative abuse, gastritis, enteritis, and bladder inflammation. Used externally to remove foreign objects from the eye. Also used as a poultice for skin inflammation.	• Find out why patient is using the herb. • When flax is used internally, it should be taken with more than 5 oz of liquid per tablespoon of flaxseed. • Cyanogenic glycosides may release cyanide; however, the body only metabolizes these to a certain extent. At therapeutic doses, flax doesn't elevate cyanide ion level. • Even though flax may decrease a patient's cholesterol level or increase bleeding time, it isn't necessary to monitor cholesterol level or platelet aggregation.	• Advise patient to consult with his health care provider before using an herbal preparation because a treatment with proven efficacy may be available. • Tell patient to remind pharmacist of any herbal or dietary supplement that he's taking, when filling a new prescription. • Warn patient not to treat chronic constipation or other GI disturbances or ophthalmic injury with flax before seeking appropriate medical evaluation because doing so my delay diagnosis of a potentially serious medical condition. • If patient is pregnant, plans to become pregnant, or is breastfeeding, advise her not to use flax. • Instruct patient to drink plenty of water when taking flaxseed. • Instruct patient not to take any drug for at least 2 hours after taking flax.
GARLIC Garlicin, Garlic Powermax, Garlinase 4,000, GarliPure, Garlique, Garlitrin 4,000, Kwai, Kyolic Liquid, Wellness Garlicell	Used most commonly to decrease total cholesterol and triglyceride levels and increase HDL cholesterol level. Also used to help prevent atherosclerosis because of its effect on blood pressure and platelet aggregation. Used to decrease the risk of cancer, especially cancer of the GI tract. Used to decrease the risk of stroke and heart attack and to treat	• Find out why patient is using the herb. • Garlic isn't recommended for patients with diabetes, insomnia, pemphigus, organ transplants, and rheumatoid arthritis, and in postsurgical patients. • Consuming excessive amounts of raw garlic increases the risk of adverse reactions. • Monitor patient for signs and symptoms of bleeding. • Garlic may lower blood glucose level. If patient is taking an antihyperglycemic, watch for signs and symptoms of hypo-	• Advise patient to consult with his health care provider before using an herbal preparation because a treatment with proven efficacy may be available. • Tell patient to remind pharmacist of any herbal or dietary supplement that he's taking, when filling a new prescription. • .Advise patient not to delay seeking appropriate medical evaluation because doing so may delay diagnosis of a potentially serious medical condition. • Advise patient to consume garlic in moderation, to minimize the risk of adverse reactions. • Discourage heavy use of garlic before surgery. • If patient is using garlic to lower his serum cholesterol levels, ad-

Herb names	Reported uses	Special considerations	Patient education
GARLIC (continued)	coughs, colds, fevers, and sore throats. Used orally and topically to fight infection through its antibacterial and antifungal effects.	glycemia and monitor his serum glucose level. • **ALERT:** Garlic oil shouldn't be used to treat inner ear infection in children.	vise him to notify his health care provider and to have his serum cholesterol levels monitored. • Advise patient that using garlic with anticoagulants may increase the risk of bleeding. • If patient is using garlic as a topical antiseptic, avoid prolonged exposure to the skin because burns can occur.
GINGER Alcohol-Free Ginger Root, Caffeine Free Ginger Root, Ginger Aid Tea, Ginger Kid, Ginger-Max, Ginger Powder, Ginger Root, Quanterra Stomach Comfort, Travellers, Travel Sickness, Zintona	Used most commonly as an antiemetic in those with motion sickness, morning sickness, and generalized nausea. Used to treat colic, flatulence, and indigestion. Used to treat hypercholesterolemia, burns, ulcers, depression, impotence, and liver toxicity. Used as an antiinflammatory for those with arthritis and as an antispasmodic. Also used for its antitumorigenic activity in patients with cancer.	• Find out why patient is using the herb. • Adverse reactions are uncommon. • Monitor patient for signs and symptoms of bleeding. If patient is taking an anticoagulant, monitor PTT, PT, and INR carefully. • Use in pregnant patients is questionable, although small amounts used in cooking are safe. It's unknown if ginger appears in breast milk. • Ginger may interfere with the intended therapeutic effect of conventional drugs. • If overdose occurs, monitor patient for arrhythmias and CNS depression.	• Advise patient to consult with his health care provider before using an herbal preparation because a treatment with proven efficacy may be available. • Tell patient to remind pharmacist of any herbal or dietary supplement that he's taking, when filling a new prescription. • If patient is pregnant, advise her to consult with a knowledgeable practitioner before using ginger medicinally. • Educate patients to look for signs and symptoms of bleeding, such as nosebleeds or excessive bruising. • Tell patient to remind pharmacist of any herbal or dietary supplement that he's taking, when filling a new prescription. • Warn patient to keep all herbal products away from children and pets.
GINKGO Bioginkgo, Gincosan, Ginkgo Go!, Ginkgo Liquid Extract Herb, Ginkgo Nut, Ginkgo Power, Ginkgo Capsules, Ginkgo, Quanterra Mental Sharpness	Primarily used to manage cerebral insufficiency, dementia, and circulatory disorders such as intermittent claudication. Also used to treat headaches, asthma, colitis, impotence, depression, altitude sickness, tinnitus, cochlear deafness, vertigo, premenstrual syndrome, macular degeneration, diabetic retinopathy, and allergies. Used as an adjunctive treatment for pancreatic cancer and schizophrenia. Also used in addition to physical therapy for Fontaine stage IIb peripheral arterial disease to decrease pain during ambulation with a minimum	• Find out why the patient is using the herb. • Ginkgo extracts are considered standardized if they contain 24% ginkgo flavonoid glycosides and 6% terpene lactones. • Treatment should continue for at least 6 to 8 weeks, but therapy beyond 3 months isn't recommended. • **ALERT:** Seizures have been reported in children after ingestion of more than 50 seeds. • Patients must be monitored for possible adverse reaction such as GI problems, headaches, dizziness, allergic reactions, and serious bleeding. • Toxicity may cause atonia and adynamia.	• Advise patient to consult with his health care provider before using an herbal preparation because a treatment with proven efficacy may be available. • Tell patient to remind pharmacist of any herbal or dietary supplement that he's taking, when filling a new prescription. • If patient is taking the herb for motion sickness, advise him to begin taking it 1 to 2 days before taking the trip and to continue taking it for the duration of his trip. • Inform patient that the therapeutic and toxic components of ginkgo can vary significantly from product to product. Advise him to obtain his ginkgo from a reliable source. • Warn patient to keep all herbal products away from children and pets. • Advise patient to discontinue use at least 2 weeks before surgery.

(continued)

Herb names	Reported uses	Special considerations	Patient education
GINKGO (continued)	of 6 weeks of treatment. In Germany, standardized ginkgo extract must contain 22% to 27% ginkgo flavonoids and 5% to 7% terpenoids.		
GINSENG, ASIAN American Ginseng, American Ginseng Root, Centrum Ginseng, Chikusetsu Ginseng, Chinese Red Panax Ginseng, Concentrate, Ginseng Manchurian, Ginseng Natural, Ginseng Power Max 004X G-Sana, Ginseng Up, Gin Zip, Herbal Sure Chinese Red Ginseng, Herbal Sure Korean Ginseng, Himalayan Ginseng, Korean Ginseng, Korean Ginseng Root, Forean White Ginseng, Lynae Ginse-Cool, Manchurian Ginseng, Natural Ginseng, Power Herb Korean Ginseng, Premium Blend Korean Ginseng Extract, Sanchi Ginseng, The Ginseng Solution, Time Release Korean Ginseng Power, Zhuzishen	Used to manage fatigue and lack of concentration and to treat atherosclerosis, bleeding disorders, colitis, diabetes, depression, and cancer. Also used to help recover health and strength after sickness or weakness.	• Find out why patient is using the herb. • The German Commission E doesn't recommend using ginseng for longer than 3 months. • Ginseng is believed by some to strengthen the body and increase resistance to disease. • **ALERT:** Reports have circulated of a severe reaction known as the ginseng abuse syndrome in patients taking large doses—more than 3 g per day for up to 2 years. Patients experiencing this syndrome report a feeling of increased motor and cognitive activity combined with significant diarrhea, nervousness, insomnia, hypertension, edema, and skin eruptions.	• Advise patient to consult with his health care provider before using an herbal preparation because a treatment with proven efficacy may be available. • Tell patient to remind pharmacist of any herbal or dietary supplement that he's taking, when filling a new prescription. • Inform patient that the therapeutic and toxic components of ginseng can vary significantly from product to product. Advise him to obtain his ginseng from a reliable source.
GREEN TEA Chinese Green Tea Bags, Green Tea (*various manufacturers*), Green	Used to prevent cancer, hyperlipidemia, atherosclerosis, dental caries, and headaches, and to treat wounds,	• Find out why patient is using the herb. • Dosage varies with the form of the herb. • Look for products standardized to 80%	• Advise patient to consult with his health care provider before using an herbal preparation because a treatment with proven efficacy may be available. • Tell patient to remind pharmacist of any herbal or dietary

Herb names	Reported uses	Special considerations	Patient education
GREEN TEA (continued) Tea Extract, Green Tea Power, Green Tea Power Caffeine Free, Standardized Green Tea Extract	skin disorders, stomach disorders, and infectious diarrhea. Also used as a CNS stimulant, a mild diuretic, and antibacterial and, topically, as an astringent.	polyphenol and 55% epigallocatechin gallate. • Daily consumption should be limited to fewer than 5 cups, or the equivalent of 300 mg of caffeine, per day to avoid the adverse effects of caffeine. • Prolonged high caffeine intake may cause restlessness, irritability, insomnia, palpitations, vertigo, headache, and adverse GI effects. Monitor patient's intake. • The adverse GI effects of chlorogenic acid and tannin can be avoided if milk is added to the tea mixture. • The tannin content in tea increases the longer it's left to brew; this increases the antidiarrheal properties of the tea. • In children, administering green tea with iron supplements or multivitamins with iron prevents the absorption of iron. • The first signs of a toxic reaction are vomiting and abdominal spasm.	supplement that he's taking, when filling a new prescription. • Instruct patient not to consume more than 5 cups a day, or 300 mg of caffeine, to avoid or minimize adverse effects. • Advise patient that heavy consumption may be associated with esophageal cancer secondary to the tannin content in the mixture. • Tell patient that the first signs of toxic reaction are vomiting and abdominal spasm.
HAWTHORNE Hawthorne Berry, Hawthorne Extract, Hawthorne Formula, Hawthorne Power	Used to regulate blood pressure and heart rate and to treat atherosclerosis. Used as a cardiotonic and as a sedative for sleep. Used in mild cardiac insufficiency, heart conditions not requiring digoxin, mild stable forms of angina pectoris, and mild forms of bradycardia and palpitations.	• Find out why patient is using the herb. • High doses may cause hypotension and sedation. Monitor patient for CNS adverse effects, and monitor blood pressure. • Hawthorne may interfere with digoxin's effects and serum monitoring. • If patient has heart failure, he should only use hawthorne under close medical supervision and in combination with other standard treatments, only as directed. • Observe patient closely for adverse reactions, especially adverse CNS reactions.	• Advise patient not to delay seeking appropriate medical evaluation because doing so may delay diagnosis of a potentially serious medical condition. • Advise patient to consult with his health care provider before using an herbal preparation because a treatment with proven efficacy may be available. • Tell patient to remind pharmacist of any herbal or dietary supplement that he's taking, when filling a new prescription. • Advise patient to avoid use because of toxic adverse effects and narrow therapeutic index. • Warn patient to keep all herbal products away from children and pets.
HORSE CHESTNUT Horse Chestnut (some products that contain varying amounts of horse chestnut include: Arthro-Therapy, Cell-	Used to treat chronic venous insufficiency, varicose veins, leg pain, tiredness, tension, and leg swelling and edema. Extract is used as a conjunctive treatment for lymph-	• Find out why patient is using the herb. • The nuts, seeds, twigs, sprouts, and leaves of horse chestnut are poisonous. Standardized formulations remove most of the toxins and standardize the amount of aescin.	• Advise patient to consult with his health care provider before using an herbal preparation because a treatment with proven efficacy may be available. • Tell patient to remind pharmacist of any herbal or dietary supplement that he's taking, when filling a new prescription.

(continued)

Herb names	Reported uses	Special considerations	Patient education
HORSE CHESTNUT *(continued)* U-Var Cream, Varicare, Varicosin, and VenoCare Ultra-Joint Response), Venastat	edema, hemorrhoids, and enlarged prostate. Horse chestnut has been used as an analgesic, anticoagulant, antipyretic, astringent, expectorant, and tonic. It has also been used to treat skin ulcers, phlebitis, leg cramps, cough, and diarrhea.	• **ALERT:** High doses and nonstandardized forms can be lethal. • Signs and symptoms of toxicity include loss of coordination, salivation, hemolysis, headache, dilated pupils, muscle twitching, seizures, vomiting, diarrhea, depression, paralysis, respiratory and cardiac failure, and death. • Monitor patient for signs of toxicity and discontinue horse chestnut immediately if any occur. • Monitor blood glucose level in patients taking antidiabetics for hypoglycemia.	• Inform patient that the FDA classifies horse chestnut as an unsafe herb and that deaths have occurred. • Advise patient to use only a standardized extract containing 16% to 21% aescin, at recommended doses, and to discontinue use if he experiences sign of toxic reaction. • Tell patient that this is only symptomatic treatment of chronic venous insufficiency and not a cure. • Advise patient not to confuse horse chestnut with sweet chestnut, used as a food. • Advise patient to keep the herb away from children. Consumption of amounts of leaves, twigs, and seeds equaling 1% of a child's weight may be lethal.
KAVA Contained in a variety of products including, but not limited to, the following: Alcohol-Free Fava-Kava, Kavacin, Kava Kava Plus, Kava Kava Root, Fava Tone, St. John's Plus Kava Kava, and Standardized Kava Extract.	Used to treat nervous anxiety, stress, and restlessness. It's used orally to produce sedation, to promote wound healing, and to treat headaches, seizure disorders, the common cold, respiratory tract infection, tuberculosis, and rheumatism. It's also used to treat urogenital infections, including chronic cystitis, veneral disease, uterine inflammation, menstrual problems, and vaginal prolapse. Some herbal practitioners consider kava an aphrodisiac. Kava juice is used to treat skin diseases, including leprosy. It's also used as a poultice for intestinal problems, otitis, and abscesses.	• Find out why patient is using the herb. • Patient shouldn't use kava with conventional sedative-hypnotics, anxiolytics, MAO inhibitors, other psychopharmacologic drugs, levodopa, or antiplatelet drugs without first consulting a health care provider. • Adverse effects of kava are mild at suggested dosages. They may occur at start of therapy but are transient. • Oral use is probably safe for 3 months or less; use for longer than 3 months may be habit forming. • Kava can cause drowsiness and may impair motor reflexes. • Patients should avoid taking herb with alcohol because of increased risk of CNS depression and liver damage. • Periodic monitoring of liver function tests and CBC may be needed. • Heavy kava users are more likely to complain of poor health: 20% are underweight with reduced levels of albumin, total protein, bilirubin, urea, platelets, and lymphocytes; increased HDL cholesterol and RBCs; hematuria; puffy faces; scaly rashes; and some evidence of pulmonary hypertension. These symptoms resolve several weeks after the herb is	• Advise patient to consult with his health care provider before using an herbal preparation because a treatment with proven efficacy may be available. • Tell patient to remind pharmacist of any herbal and dietary supplements that he's taking, when filling a new prescription. • Encourage patients to seek medical diagnosis before taking kava. • Advise patient that usual doses can affect motor function; caution him against performing hazardous activities. • Tell patient oral use is probably safe for 3 months or less, but use for longer than 3 months may be habit forming. • Warn patient to avoid taking herb with alcohol because of increased risk of CNS depression and liver damage.

Herb names	Reported uses	Special considerations	Patient education
KAVA (continued)		stopped. Toxic doses can cause progressive ataxia, muscle weakness, and ascending paralysis, all of which resolve when herb is stopped. Extreme use (more than 300 g per week) may increase gammaglutamyltransferase levels.	
MELATONIN Circadian (controlled-release, not available in U.S.), Mela-T, Melatonex	Used for treating insomnia, jet lag, shift-work disorder, blind entrainment (a condition in which blind people develop insomnia or daytime sleepiness because they feel no circadian rhythm), immune system enhancement, tinnitus, depression, and benzodiazepine withdrawal in geriatric patients with insomnia. Also, used as a cancer therapy adjuvant, anti-aging product, contraceptive, and a prophylactic therapy for cluster headaches. Topically, it's used for skin protection against ultraviolet light.	• Find out why patient is using herb. • Monitor patient for excessive daytime drowsiness. • May increase human growth hormone levels.	• Advise patient to consult with his health care provider before using an herbal preparation or supplement because a treatment with proven efficacy may be available. • Tell patient to remind pharmacist of any herbal and dietary supplements that he's taking, when filling a new prescription. • Warn patient to avoid hazardous activities until full extent of CNS depressant effect is known. • If patient wishes to conceive, tell her that melatonin may have a contraceptive effect. However, herb shouldn't be used as birth control. • Although no chemical interactions have been reported in clinical studies, tell patient that melatonin may interfere with therapeutic effects of conventional drugs. • Warn patient about possible additive effects if taken with alcohol. • Advise patient to use only the synthetic form (not the animal-derived product) because of concerns about contamination and viral transmission. • Advise patient not to use melatonin for prolonged periods because safety data aren't available.
MILK THISTLE Liver Formula with Milk Thistle, Milk Thistle Extract, Milk Thistle Phytosome, Milk Thistle Plus, Milk Thistle Power, Milk Thistle Super Complex, Silybin Phytosome, Silymarin Milk Thistle, Simply Milk Thistle, Thisilyn	Used for dyspesia, liver damage from chemicals, *Amanita* mushroom poisoning, supportive therapy for inflammatory liver disease and cirrhosis, loss of appetite, and gallbladder and spleen disorders. It's also used as a liver protectant.	• Find out why patient is using herb. • Mild allergic reactions may occur, especially in people allergic to members of the Astertaceae family, including ragweed, chrysanthemums, marigolds, and daisies. • Don't confuse milk thistle seeds or fruit with other parts of the plant or with blessed thistle (*Cnictus benedictus*). • Silymarin has poor water solubility; therefore, efficacy when prepared as a tea is questionable.	• Advise patient to consult with his health care provider before using an herbal preparation because a treatment with proven efficacy may be available. • Tell patient to remind pharmacist of any herbal and dietary supplements that he's taking, when filling a new prescription. • Although no chemical interactions have been reported in clinical studies, advise patient that herb may interfere with therapeutic effect of conventional drugs. • Warn patient not to take this herb while pregnant or breast-feeding. • Tell patient to stay alert for possible allergic reactions, espe- *(continued)*

Herb names	Reported uses	Special considerations	Patient education
MILK THISTLE (continued)			cially if allergic to ragweed, chrysanthemums, marigolds, or daisies. • Warn patient not to take herb for liver inflammation or cirrhosis before seeking appropriate medical evaluation because doing so may delay diagnosis of a potentially serious medical condition. • Warn patient to keep all herbal products away from children and pets.
NETTLE Freeze-Dried Nettle Capsules, Fresh Nettle Leaf, Nettle Blend, Nettle Leaf, Nettle Leaf Tea, Nettle Organic Tea, Netttle Root, Nettle Seed	Used to treat allergic rhinitis, osteoarthritis, rheumatoid arthritis, kidney stones, asthma, and BPH. Also used as a diuretic, an expectorant, a general health tonic, a blood builder and purifier, a pain reliever and anti-inflammatory, and a lung tonic for ex-smokers. Also used for eczema, hives, bursitis, tendinitis, laryngitis, sciatica, and premenstrual syndrome. Nettle is being investigated for treatment of hay fever and irrigation of the urinary tract.	• Find out why patient is using the herb. • Nettle is reported to be an abortifacient and may affect the menstrual cycle. • Allergic adverse effects from internal use are rare.	• Advise patient to consult with his health care provider before using an herbal preparation because a treatment with proven efficacy may be available. • Tell patient to remind pharmacist of any herbal and dietary supplements that he's taking, when filling a new prescription. • Recommend caution if patient takes an antihypertensive or antidiabetic. • Warn patient that external adverse effects result from skin contact and include burning and stinging that may persist for 12 hours or longer. • Inform patient that capsules and extracts should be stored at room temperature, away from heat and direct light. • Instruct women taking herb to notify health care provider about planned, suspected, or known pregnancy. • Advise patient not to breastfeed while taking this herb.
PASSION FLOWER Passion Flower, Alcohol Free Passion Flower Liquid	Used as a sedative, a hypnotic, an analgesic, and an antispasmodic for treating muscle spasms caused by indigestion, menstrual cramping, pain, or migraines. Also used for neuralgia, generalized seizures, hysteria, nervous agitation, and insomnia. Crushed leaves and flowers are used topically for cuts and bruises.	• Find out why patient is using the herb. • Monitor patient for possible adverse CNS effects. • No adverse effects have been observed with recommended doses. • A disulfiram-like reaction may produce nausea, vomiting, flushing, headache, hypotension, tachycardia, ventricular arrhythmias, and shock leading to death. • Patients with liver disease or alcoholism shouldn't use herbal products that contain alcohol.	• Advise patient to consult with his health care provider before using an herbal preparation because a treatment with proven efficacy may be available. • Tell patient to remind pharmacist of any herbal and dietary supplements that he's taking, when filling a new prescription. • Because sedation is possible, caution patient to avoid hazardous activities. • Warn patient not to take herb for chronic pain or insomnia before seeking medical attention because doing so may delay diagnosis of a potentially serious medical condition. • Caution pregnant patients to avoid this herb.
SAW PALMETTO Centrum Saw Palmetto, Herbal Sure Saw Palmetto,	Used to treat symptoms of BPH and coughs and congestion from colds, bronchitis, or asthma. Also	• Find out why patient is using the herb. • Herb should be used cautiously for conditions other than BPH because data about its effective-	• Advise patient to consult with his health care provider before using an herbal preparation because a treatment with proven efficacy may be available.

Herb names	Reported uses	Special considerations	Patient education
SAW PALMETTO (continued) Permixon, PlusStrogen, Premium Blend Saw Palmetto, Pro-active Saw Palmetto, Propalmex, Quanterra Prostate, Saw Palmetto Power, Standardized Saw Palmetto ExtractCap, Super Saw Palmetto	used as a mild diuretic, urinary antiseptic, and astringent.	ness in other conditions is lacking. • Obtain a baseline prostate-specific antigen (PSA) test before patient starts taking herb because it may cause a false-negative PSA result. • Saw palmetto may not alter prostate size. • Laboratory values didn't change significantly in clinical trials using dosages of 160 mg to 320 mg daily.	• Tell patient to remind pharmacist of any herbal and dietary supplements that he's taking, when filling a new prescription. • Warn patient not to take herb for bladder or prostate problems before seeking medical attention because doing so could delay diagnosis of a potentially serious medical condition. • Tell patient to take herb with food to minimize GI effects. • Caution patient to promptly notify health care provider about new or worsened adverse effects. • Warn women to avoid herb if planning pregnancy, if pregnant, or if breast-feeding.
ST. JOHN'S WORT Alterra, Hypercalm, Kira, Quanterra Emotional Balance, St. John's Wort Extracts, Tension Tamer, various combination products	Used orally for mild to moderate depression, anxiety, psychovegetative disorders, sciatica, and viral infections, including herpes simplex virus types 1 and 2, hepatitis C, influenza virus, murine cytomegalovirus, and poliovirus. St. John's wort has also been used to treat bronchitis, asthma, gallbladder disease, nocturnal enuresis, gout, and rheumatism, although it hasn't proven effective in these cases.	• Find out why patient is using the herb. • St. John's wort has been effective in treating mild to moderate depression. • Recommended duration of therapy for depression is 4 to 6 weeks; if no improvement occurs, a different therapy should be considered. • Monitor patient for response to herbal therapy, as evidenced by improved mood and lessened depression. • By using standardized extracts, patient can better control the dosage. Clinical studies have used formulations of standardized 0.3% hypericin as well as hyperforin-stabilized version of the extract. • St. John's wort interacts with many other products; they must be considered before patient takes it with other prescription or OTC products. • Serotonin syndrome may cause dizziness, nausea, vomiting, headache, epigastric pain, anxiety, confusion, restlessness, and irritability. • Because St. John's wort decreases the effect of certain prescription drugs, watch for signs of drug toxicity if patient stops using the herb. Drug dosage may need to be reduced. • St. John's wort has mutagenic effects on sperm cells and oocytes and ad-	• Advise patient to consult with his health care provider before using an herbal preparation because a treatment with proven efficacy may be available. • Tell patient to remind pharmacist of any herbal and dietary supplements that he's taking, when filling a new prescription. • Instruct patient to consult a health care provider for a thorough medical evaluation before using St. John's wort. • Encourage patient to discuss depression and to seek regular psychiatric help, as indicated. • If patient takes St. John's wort for mild to moderate depression, explain that several weeks may pass before effects occur. Tell patient that a new therapy may be needed if no improvement occurs in 4 to 6 weeks. • Inform patient that St. John's wort interacts with many other prescription and OTC products and may reduce their effectiveness. • Tell patient that St. John's wort may cause increased sensitivity to direct sunlight. Recommend protective clothing, sunscreen, and limited sun exposure. • Inform patient that a sufficient wash-out period is needed after stopping an antidepressant before switching to St. John's wort. • Tell patient to report adverse effects to a health care provider. • Warn patient to keep all herbal products away from children and pets.

(continued)

Herb names	Reported uses	Special considerations	Patient education
ST. JOHN'S WORT *(continued)*		verse effects on reproductive cells; therefore, it shouldn't be used by pregnant patients or those planning pregnancy (including men). • Topically, the volatile plant oil is an irritant. Monitor affected site for adverse effects and improvement. • Monitor patient for sedative effects and GI complaints.	
TEA TREE OIL Tea Tree Oil, Tea Tree Oil Lotion, Tea Tree Soap	Used topically for contusions, inflammation, myalgia, burns, hemorrhoids, and vitiligo. In traditional Chinese medicine, tea tree oil has been used as a gargle for tonsillitis and as a lotion for dermatoses.	• Find out why patient is using the herb. • Because of systemic toxicity, tea tree oil shouldn't be used internally. • Essential oil should be used externally only after being diluted, especially by people with sensitive skin. • Tea tree oil may cause burns or itching in tender areas and shouldn't be used around nose, eyes, and mouth. • Diluted essential oil, even as low as 0.25% or 0.5%, is active against microbes. • Vaginal douches using concentrations as strong as 40% require extreme caution and supervision by a health care provider. • Pure (100%) essential tea tree oil is rarely used and only with close supervision by a health care provider. • Other related *Melaleuca* species are also known as tea trees, such as *M. cajeputi, M. dissitifolia,* and *M. linariiflora,* but tea tree oil can be obtained only from *M. alternifolia.*	• Advise patient to consult with his health care provider before using an herbal preparation because a treatment with proven efficacy may be available. • Tell patient to remind pharmacist of any herbal and dietary supplements that he's taking, when filling a new prescription. • Tell patient to use very dilute tea tree oil (0.25% to 0.5%) as topical anti-infective. • Explain that a few drops are sufficient in mouthwash, shampoo, or sitz bath. • Caution patient not to apply oil to wounds or to skin that's dry or cracked. • If patient will be using the douche form of this product, stress the need for medical supervision. • Warn patient to keep all herbal products away from children and pets.

Index

A

abacavir sulfate, 81-82
Abbokinase, 1254
Abbokinase Open-Cath, 1254
abciximab, 82-83
Abdominal distention, post-operative
neostigmine for, 906
vasopressin for, 1264
Abdominal trauma during pregnancy, Rh$_o$(D) immune globulin for, 1086
Abdominal X-ray, vasopressin for, 1264
Abelcet, 141
Abortion
carboprost tromethamine for, 260
dinoprostone for, 444
mifepristone for, 853
oxytocin for, 957
Rh$_o$(D) immune globulin for, 1085-1086
Abreva, 459
acarbose, 83-85
Accolate, 1284
Accupril, 1067
Accurbron, 1184
Accutane, 711
acebutolol, 85-86
Acel-Imune, 450
Aceon, 987
Acephen, 86
acetaminophen, 86-88
Acetaminophen toxicity, acetylcysteine for, 90
Aceta with Codeine, 1301t
acetazolamide, 88-89
acetazolamide sodium, 88-89
acetylcholine chloride, 89-90
acetylcysteine, 90-91
Achromycin, 1179
Acid indigestion. See Stomach acid, neutralizing.
Aciphex, 1074
Aclovate, 99
Acne
azelaic acid cream for, 180
clindamycin for, 340
erythromycin for, 514
isotretinoin for, 711
minocycline for, 858
spironolactone for, 1138

Acne (continued)
tetracycline for, 1180
tretinoin for, 1232
Acne rosacea, metronidazole for, 846
Acova, 160
Acquired immunodeficiency syndrome. See also HIV infection.
filgrastim for, 562
somatropin for, 1133
zidovudine for, 1288
Acromegaly
bromocriptine for, 224
octreotide for, 934
ACT, 1130
ACTH, 360-362
Acthar, 360
ActHIB, 642
Acticin, 988
Acticort 100, 657
Actidose-Aqua, 92
Actimmune, 696
actinomycin D, 386-387
Actiq, 555
Activase, 109
activated charcoal, 92-93
Activella, 524
Actos, 1009
Acu-dyne, 1310t
Acular, 720
Acute coronary syndrome, tirofiban for, 1208
Acute leukemia myelodysplastic syndrome, filgrastim for, 562
Acute renal failure, mannitol for, 788
Acute rheumatic carditis, triamcinolone for, 1234
acycloguanosine, 93-95
acyclovir, 93-95
acyclovir sodium, 93-95
Adalat, 914
Adalat CC, 914
adenine arabinoside, 1270-1271
Adenocard, 95
adenosine, 95-96
Adipex-P, 996
Adrenalin Chloride, 500
Adrenal insufficiency
cortisone for, 362
dexamethasone for, 407
fludrocortisone for, 572
hydrocortisone for, 655
triamcinolone for, 1234

Adrenergics, direct- and indirect-acting, 1-3
Adrenocortical function, testing
corticotropin for, 360
cosyntropin for, 364
Adrenocorticoids
nasal, 3-6
oral inhalation, 3-6
systemic, 6-9
topical, 9-11
adrenocorticotropic hormone, 360-362
Adriamycin PFS, 476
Adriamycin RDF, 476
Adrucil, 577
Adsorbocarpine, 1004
Advair Diskus 100/50, 590
Advair Diskus 250/50, 590
Advair Diskus 500/50, 590
Advil, 668
Adynamic ileus, postoperative, dexpanthenol for, 411
AeroBid, 574
AeroBid-M, 574
Aerodine, 1310t
Aerolate Jr., 1184
Aerolate SR, 1184
Aerolate III, 1184
Aeroseb-HC, 657
Afrin, 955
Agammaglobulinemia, immune globulin for, 676-677
Agenerase, 148
Aggrastat, 1208
Aggressive behavior, trazodone for, 1230
Agitation
lorazepam for, 773
thiothixene for, 1194
Agranulocytosis
co-trimoxazole for, 365
filgrastim for, 562
Agrylin, 150
A-hydroCort, 655
AIDS-related complex, zidovudine for, 1288
Airet, 97
Akarpine Isopto Carpine, 1004
AKBeta, 740
AK-Con, 895
AK-Dex, 406, 407
AK-Dilate, 998
Akineton, 213
AK-Nefrin, 998

---

t refers to a table; i refers to an illustration.

---

t refers to a table; i refers to an illustration.

---

t refers to a table; i refers to an illustration.

---

t refers to a table; i refers to an illustration.

mivacurium chloride, 867-868
M-M-R II, 789
Moban, 871
Mobic, 800
Mobidin, 785
modafinil, 868-870
Modane, 215
Modane Soft, 460
Modecate, 582
Modicon 21, 527
Modicon 28, 527
Moditen Enanthate, 582
moexipril hydrochloride, 870-871
molindone hydrochloride, 871-873
Mol-Iron, 560
Monistat 1, 1207
Monistat 3, 850
Monistat 7, 850
Monistat-Derm, 850
Monoclate-P, 153
Monodox, 480
Monoket, 709
Mononine, 545
Monopril, 602
Mono-Vacc Test, 1250
montelukast sodium, 873-874
Monurol, 602
moricizine hydrochloride, 874-875
morphine hydrochloride, 875-877
morphine sulfate, 875-877
Morphitec, 875
M.O.S., 875
Motion sickness
  cyclizine for, 371
  dimenhydrinate for, 442
  diphenhydramine for, 446
  meclizine for, 796
  promethazine for, 1047
  scopolamine for, 1114
Motrin, 668
Motrin IB, 668
Mountain sickness, aceta-zolamide for, 88
Mouth irritation, carbamide peroxide for, 258
moxifloxacin hydrochlo-ride, 877-879
M-oxy, 953
M-R-Vax II, 790
MS Contin, 875
MSIR, 875
MS/L, 875
MS/S, 875
MSTA, 879
MTC, 864-865

Mucocutaneous lymph node syndrome, as-pirin for, 166-167
Muco-Fen-LA, 636
Mucomyst, 90
Mucosil, 90
Multipax, 664
Multiple endocrine adeno-mas. *See* Hypersecre-tory conditions.
Multiple myeloma
  carmustine for, 263
  cyclophosphamide for, 374
  melphalan for, 802
  pamidronate for, 961
Multiple sclerosis
  baclofen for, 189
  corticotropin for, 361
  glatiramer for, 619
  interferon beta-1a for, 694
  interferon beta-1b for, 695
  methylprednisolone for, 834
  mitoxantrone for, 866
mumps skin test antigen, 879-880
Mumpsvax, 880
mumps virus vaccine, live, 880-881
mupirocin, 881-882
mupirocin calcium, 881-882
Murine Ear, 258
Murine Plus, 1181
muromonab-CD3, 882-883
Muscarinic effects, block-ing, atropine for, 175
Muscle contractions, weak-ening, tubocurarine for, 1251
Muscle fasciculations, drug-induced, dantrolene for, 391
Muscle pain, postoperative, dantrolene for, 391
Muscle spasm
  diazepam for, 420
Musculoskeletal conditions
  carisoprodol for, 261
  chlorzoxazone for, 319
  cyclobenzaprine for, 372
  methocarbamol for, 826
  naproxen for, 896
  orphenadrine for, 943
Muse, 107
Mutamycin, 864
Myambutol, 535
Myasthenia gravis
  edrophonium for, 489
  ephedrine for, 498
  neostigmine for diagnos-ing, 906

Myasthenia gravis
  (continued)
  pyridostigmine for, 1061
  tubocurarine for diagnos-ing, 1251
Mycelex, 352
Mycelex-7, 352
Mycelex-G, 352
Mycelex OTC, 352
Mycifradin, 904
Myciguent, 904
Mycobacterial infections
  ciprofloxacin for, 329
  clofazimine for, 342
  minocycline for, 858
Mycobutin, 1089
Mycocide NS, 1310t
mycophenolate mofetil, 883-884
Mycoplasmal infections, amoxicillin trihydrate for, 135
Mycosis fungoides
  cladribine for, 336
  cyclophosphamide for, 374
  fludarabine for, 571
  methotrexate for, 827
  vinblastine for, 1271
Mycostatin, 932
Mydfrin, 998
Mydriasis
  cyclopentolate for proce-dures requiring, 373
  phenylephrine for, 998
Mydriatic effects, counter-acting, pilocarpine for, 1004
Myelodysplasia, filgrastim for, 562
Myelodysplastic syndrome, sargramostim for, 1113
Myelofibrosis, busulfan for, 236
Mykrox, 841
Myleran, 236
Mylicon, 1123
Mylotarg, 616
Myocardial infarction
  alteplase for, 109
  aspirin for, 166
  atenolol for, 169
  cholestyramine for, 321
  clopidogrel for, 349
  enoxaparin for, 496
  eptifibatide for, 508-509
  heparin sodium for, 645
  lisinopril for, 761
  magnesium sulfate for, 786
  metoprolol for, 842
  morphine for, 875

---

t refers to a table; i refers to an illustration.

t refers to a table; i refers to an illustration.

t refers to a table; i refers to an illustration.

---

t refers to a table; i refers to an illustration.

---

t refers to a table; i refers to an illustration.